Handbook
on
Injectable
Drugs

11

11th edition

Lawrence A. Trissel

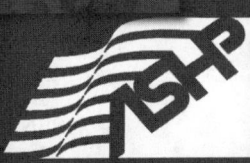

LAWRENCE A. TRISSEL, F.A.S.H.P., the author of the *Handbook on Injectable Drugs*, is Director, Clinical Pharmaceutics Research Program, Division of Pharmacy, The University of Texas, M. D. Anderson Cancer Center, Houston, Texas.

Any correspondence regarding this publication should be sent to the publisher, American Society of Health-System Pharmacists®, 7272 Wisconsin Avenue, Bethesda, MD 20814, attn: Special Publishing.

The information presented herein reflects the opinions of the author and reviewers. It should not be interpreted as an official policy of ASHP or as an endorsement of any product.

Drug information and its applications are constantly evolving because of ongoing research and clinical experience and are often subject to professional judgment and interpretation by the practitioner and to the uniqueness of a clinical situation. The author, reviewers, and ASHP have made every effort to ensure the accuracy and completeness of the information presented in this book. However, the reader is advised that the publisher, author, contributors, editors, and reviewers cannot be responsible for the continued currency of the information, for any errors or omissions, and/or for any consequences arising from the use of the information in the clinical setting.

The reader is cautioned that ASHP makes no representation, guarantee, or warranty, express or implied, that the use of the information contained in this book will prevent problems with insurers and will bear no responsibility or liability for the results or consequences of its use.

Produced by the Special Publishing Department of the American Society of Health-System Pharmacists
Managing Editor/Development Editor: Cynthia Reilly
Assistant Development Editor: Con Ann Ling
Production Manager: Bruce Hawkins
Technical Editor: Bill Fogle

Cover Design: David A. Wade

ISBN: 1-58528-016-X

To Cyndi with love and joy,
To P.D. with fond memories,
and, as always,
To Pam for all you do

Now go, write it before them in a table,
and note it in a book, that it may be
for the time to come...
Isaiah 30:8

CONTENTS

ACKNOWLEDGMENTS

I would like to gratefully acknowledge the contributions of the following individuals, who served as reviewers for the eleventh edition of the *Handbook:*

MICHAEL A. ALLWOOD, Ph.D., F.R.Pharm.S.G.B., Head of Pharmacy Academic Practice Unit, School of Health and Community Studies, University of Derby, Kingsway House, Kingsway, Derby, United Kingdom

DANIEL P. HAAS, M.S., Director of Pharmacy for Pharmacy Systems, Inc., Memorial Hospital of Union County, Marysville, Ohio; and Clinical Instructor, The Ohio State University College of Pharmacy, Columbus, Ohio

KAREN NAQUIN HALE, M.P.H., Senior Research Specialist, The Ohio State University Medical Center, and Clinical Assistant Professor, The Ohio State University College of Pharmacy, Columbus, Ohio

N. PAULINE THOMAS PARKS, M.S., Consultant Pharmacist, Houston, Texas

JUDITH A. SMITH, Pharm.D., Clinical Pharmacology Section, Division of Pharmacy, The University of Texas, M. D. Anderson Cancer Center, Houston, Texas

PREFACE

The *Handbook on Injectable Drugs*, 11th edition, is the most recent contribution in this continuing series. With its publication, all previous editions are considered out of date.

For proper use of this reference work, the reader must review the *How to Use the Handbook* section that immediately follows this preface. This section will acquaint the user of the *Handbook* with its organization, content, structure, summarization strategy, interpretation of the information presented, and limitations of the published literature on which the *Handbook* is based. Without a good working knowledge of these points, the *Handbook* may not be used to its best advantage or even interpreted correctly.

The 11th edition of the *Handbook on Injectable Drugs* brings together a wealth of information on 297 parenteral drugs commercially available in the United States, plus 25 additional parenteral drugs available only in other countries. The information in the 11th edition is accumulated from over 2230 references, including 174 new to this edition. As for each previous edition, the monographs have been completely updated. In addition to the updated monographs, 13 additional monographs on parenteral drugs available commercially in the United States that are new to this edition are presented. These include the following drugs:

Adenosine
Allopurinol sodium
Amphotericin B cholesteryl sulfate complex
Busulfan
Cisatracurium besylate
Docetaxel
Doxorubicin HCl liposome injection
Fosphenytoin sodium
Gemcitabine HCl
Mepivacaine HCl
Remifentanil HCl
Topotecan
Torsemide

In addition, the section on drugs available outside the United States has been completely updated and expanded. Five new drug monographs are presented in this section, including:

Clarithromycin
Omeprazole
Propafenone HCl
Tramadol
Tropisetron HCl

My initial conceptualization of the project that led to the *Handbook on Injectable Drugs* did not foresee in any way the vast growth of this work nor its enduring nature. Beginning in 1977 with a small amount of information from only 297 references, the *Handbook* has grown to incorporate the information from nearly eight times that many references based principally on laboratory research but also including observations from practice. Initially, it was physically small; it was truly a "handbook." Now, over 20 years later, the work has grown into a major reference source. Throughout this 23-year series of *Handbook* editions,

the intent of this work has remained unchanged: to organize and summarize in a concise, standardized format the results of the primary research in parenteral drug stability and compatibility to facilitate its use in clinical practice settings for the benefit of our patients.

Recently, the safety of medications and medical care has been getting a lot of attention from both health care professionals and from the public, quite justifiably. While the profession of pharmacy has always been active in improving the medication use process and in improving pharmaceutical care, a more broadly based interest is certainly welcome and may be pivotal in creating effective improvements to the overall system.

One aspect of the safe use of parenteral drugs remains the assurance of the drug's pharmaceutical integrity, including stability and compatibility. Although few pharmacists would question this premise, the profession seems to be moving away from involvement with this issue, at least in the United States. De-emphasizing pharmaceutics, compounding, and other drug product related course work in schools of pharmacy, an apparent decrease in the publishing of parenteral drug stability and compatibility information in pharmacy journals, and the potential for a lack of new drug stability and compatibility researchers are a few examples that are emblematic of the changes. The ramifications to patient care and a safe medication use process that a dwindling commitment to the assurance of drug stability and compatibility represent should be considered. This is a responsibility that the profession of pharmacy should not ignore.

Note of Appreciation

I want to express my gratitude to the panel of reviewers for the 11th edition of the *Handbook on Injectable Drugs:* Dr. Michael Allwood, Mr. Daniel Haas, Ms. Karen Hale, Ms. N. Pauline Thomas Parks, and Dr. Judith Smith. Working through a challenging review process, they have made a great contribution toward making the *Handbook* a better reference. The commitment and effort that each individual had to put forth in performing the review is certainly appreciated. Thank you.

Thanks also go to Ms. Cynthia Reilly and Mr. Bruce Hawkins of ASHP, who tackled the difficult editorial aspects of this 11th edition. I certainly recognize that this is a complicated manuscript and a difficult revision process at best. Your efforts and perseverance in bringing the 11th edition of the *Handbook on Injectable Drugs* into existence are greatly appreciated.

Special thanks go to those users of the *Handbook* who continue to make valuable suggestions for its improvement, call my attention to new articles and relevant information, and point out errors. I appreciate your interest and help. If any reader has input for improvement of the *Handbook*, please feel free to contact me through the publisher, the American Society of Health-System Pharmacists.

Finally, but most important, my deepest gratitude continues to go to my wife, Pam, whose forbearance in the face of this enormous time commitment is greatly appreciated. Her support makes it possible for me to undertake the demanding challenge the *Handbook* represents.

LAT
June 2000

HOW TO USE THE HANDBOOK

What Is the Handbook?

The *Handbook on Injectable Drugs* is a collection of summaries of information from the published literature on the pharmaceutics of parenteral medications as applied to the clinical setting. The *Handbook* is constructed from information derived from over 2230 original research reports with the information presented in the standardized structure described below. The purpose of the *Handbook* is to facilitate the use of this clinical pharmaceutics research by knowledgeable health care professionals for the benefit of patients. The summary information from published research is supplemented with information from the labeling of each product and from other references.

The information base summarized in the *Handbook on Injectable Drugs* is large and highly complex, requiring thoughtful consideration for proper use. The *Handbook* is not, nor should it be considered, elementary in nature or a primer. A single quick glance in a table is not adequate for proper interpretation of this highly complex information base. Proper interpretation includes the obvious need to consider and evaluate all relevant research information and results. Additionally, information on the formulation components, product attributes (especially pH), and the known stability behaviors of each parenteral drug, as well as the clinical situation of the patient, must be included in a thoughtful, reasoned evaluation of clinical pharmaceutics questions.

Who Should Use the Handbook?

The *Handbook on Injectable Drugs* is designed for use as a professional reference and guide to the literature on the clinical pharmaceutics of parenteral medications. The intended audience consists of knowledgeable health care professionals, particularly pharmacists, well versed in the formulation and clinical use of parenteral medications and who have the highly specialized knowledge base, training, and skills set necessary to interpret and apply the information. Practitioners who are not well versed in the formulation, essential properties, and clinical application of parenteral drugs should seek the assistance of more knowledgeable and experienced health care professionals to ensure patient safety.

Users of the *Handbook* must recognize that no reference work, including this one, can substitute for adequate decision-making by health care professionals. Proper clinical decisions must be made considering all aspects of the patient's condition and needs, with particular attention to the special demands imposed by parenteral medications. The *Handbook* cannot make decisions for its users. However, in knowledgeable hands, it is a valuable tool for the proper use of parenteral medications.

Organization of the Handbook

The *Handbook on Injectable Drugs* has been organized as a collection of monographs on each of 297 commercially available drugs. In addition, information on 25 drugs available outside the United States has been included. The monographs on the commercial drugs are arranged alphabetically by nonproprietary name. The names of the drugs follow the style of *USAN and the USP Dictionary of Drug Names*. Also included are some of the trade names and manufacturers of the drug products; this listing is not necessarily comprehensive and should not be considered an endorsement of any product or manufacturer.

All of the information included in the *Handbook* is referenced so that those who wish to study the original sources may find them. In addition, the *American Hospital Formulary Service* Classification System numbers have been included to facilitate the location of therapeutic information on the drugs.

The monographs have been divided into the subheadings described below:

Products—lists many of the sizes, strengths, volumes, and forms in which the drug is supplied, along with other components of the formulation. Instructions for reconstitution (when applicable) are included in this section.

The products cited do not necessarily constitute a comprehensive list of all available products. Rather, some common representative products are described. Furthermore, dosage forms, sizes, and container configurations of parenteral products may undergo significant changes during the lifespan of this edition of the *Handbook*.

Following the product descriptions, the pH of the drug products, the osmotic value(s) of the drug and/or dilutions (when available), and other miscellaneous product information such as the sodium content and definition of units are presented.

Practitioners have not always recognized the value and importance of incorporating product formulation information into the thought process that leads to their decision on handling drug compatibility and stability questions. However, consideration of the product information and formulation components as well as the properties and attributes of the products, especially pH, is essential to proper interpretation of the information presented in the *Handbook*.

Administration—includes route(s) by which the drug can be given, rates of administration (when applicable), and other related administration details.

The administration information is a condensation derived primarily from the product's official labeling and the *American Hospital Formulary Service*. For complete information, including dosage information sufficient for prescribing, the reader should refer to the official labeling and therapeutically comprehensive references such as the *American Hospital Formulary Service*.

Stability—describes the drug's stability and storage requirements. The storage condition terminology of *The United States Pharmacopeia*, 24th ed., is used in the *Handbook on Injectable Drugs*.

The United States Pharmacopeia defines controlled room temperature as "A temperature maintained thermostatically that encompasses the usual and customary working environment of 20 ° to 25 °; that results in a mean kinetic temperature calculated to be not more than 25 °; and that allows for excursions between 15 ° and 30 ° that are experienced in pharmacies, hospitals, and warehouses."[1] (All temperatures are Celsius.)

Protection from excessive heat is often required; excessive heat is defined as any temperature above 40 °C. Similarly, protection from freezing may be required for products that are subject to loss of strength or potency, or destructive alteration of their characteristics in addition to the risk of container breakage.[1]

Some products may require storage at a cool temperature, which is defined as any temperature between 8 and 15 °C, or a cold temperature, which is defined as any temperature not exceeding 8 °C. A refrigerator is defined as a cold place in which the temperature is maintained thermostati-

Table 1.
Solution Compatibility

				Monograph drug name		
Solution	Mfr	Mfr	Conc/L	Remarks	Ref	C/I
(1)	(2)	(3)	(4)	(5)	(6)	(7)

1. Solution in which the test was conducted.
2. Manufacturer of the solution.
3. Manufacturer of the drug about which the monograph is written.
4. Concentration of the drug about which the monograph is written.
5. Description of the results of the test.
6. Reference to the original source of the information.
7. Designation of the compatibility (C) or incompatibility (I) of the test result according to conventional guidelines.

Table 2.
Additive Compatibility

			Monograph drug name					
Drug	Mfr	Conc/L	Mfr	Conc/L	Test Soln	Remarks	Ref	C/I
(1)	(2)	(3)	(4)	(5)	(6)	(7)	(8)	(9)

1. Test drug.
2. Manufacturer of the test drug.
3. Concentration of the test drug.
4. Manufacturer of the drug about which the monograph is written.
5. Concentration of the drug about which the monograph is written.
6. Infusion solution in which the test was conducted.
7. Description of the results of the test.
8. Reference to the original source of the information.
9. Designation of the compatibility (C) or incompatibility (I) of the test result according to conventional guidelines.

Table 3.
Drugs in Syringe Compatibility

			Monograph drug name				
Drug (in syringe)	Mfr	Amt	Mfr	Amt	Remarks	Ref	C/I
(1)	(2)	(3)	(4)	(5)	(6)	(7)	(8)

1. Test drug.
2. Manufacturer of the test drug.
3. Actual amount of the test drug.
4. Manufacturer of the drug about which the monograph is written.
5. Actual amount of the drug about which the monograph is written.
6. Description of the results of the test.
7. Reference to the original source of the information.
8. Designation of the compatibility (C) or incompatibility (I) of the test result according to conventional guidelines.

Table 4.
Y-Site Injection Compatibility (1:1 Mixture)

			Monograph drug name				
Drug	Mfr	Conc	Mfr	Conc	Remarks	Ref	C/I
(1)	(2)	(3)	(4)	(5)	(6)	(7)	(8)

1. Test drug.
2. Manufacturer of the test drug.
3. Concentration of the test drug prior to mixing at the Y-site.
4. Manufacturer of the drug about which the monograph is written.
5. Concentration of the drug about which the monograph is written prior to mixing at the Y-site.
6. Description of the results of the test.
7. Reference to the original source of the information.
8. Designation of the compatibility (C) or incompatibility (I) of the test result according to conventional guidelines.

cally between 2 and 8 °C. Freezer storage refers to a place in which the temperature is maintained thermostatically between –25 and –10 °C.[1]

In addition to storage requirements, aspects of drug stability related to pH, freezing, and exposure to light are presented in this section. Also presented is information on repackaging of the drugs or their dilutions in container/closure systems other than the original package (e.g., prefilling into syringes or in ambulatory pumps). Sorption and filtration characteristics of the drugs are provided as well when this information is available. The information is derived principally from the primary published research literature and is supplemented by the product labeling and the *AHFS Drug Information*.

Compatibility Information—tabulates the results of published reports from primary research on the compatibility of the subject drug with infusion solutions and the other drugs. The various citations are listed alphabetically by solution or drug name; the information is completely cross-referenced among the monographs.

Four types of tables are utilized to present the available information, depending on the kind of test being reported. The first type is for information on the compatibility of a drug in various infusion solutions and is depicted in Table 1. The second type of table presents information on two or more drugs in intravenous solutions and is shown in Table 2. The third type of table is used for tests of two or more drugs in syringes and is shown in Table 3. The fourth table format is used for reports of simulated or actual injection into Y-sites of administration sets and is shown in Table 4.

Many published articles, especially older ones, do not include all of the information necessary to complete the tables. However, the tables have been completed as fully as possible from the original articles.

Additional Compatibility Information—provides additional information and discussions of compatibility presented largely in narrative form. In addition to primary published research, the information in this section is derived from reliable secondary sources. Examples of such sources include the product labeling and the *AHFS Drug Information*. For information from secondary sources, the research on which the information is based is not available for review. However, the sources are sufficiently reliable that inclusion in the *Handbook* is warranted.

Other Information—contains any relevant auxiliary information concerning the drug which does not fall into the previous categories.

The Listing of Concentration

The concentrations of all admixtures in intravenous solutions in the tables have been indicated in terms of concentration per liter to facilitate comparison of the various studies. In some cases, this may result in amounts of the drug that are greater or lesser than those normally administered (as when the recommended dose is tested in 100 ml of vehicle), but the listings do accurately reflect the actual concentrations tested, expressed in standardized terms.

For studies involving syringes, the amounts actually used are indicated. The volumes are also listed if indicated in the original article.

For studies of actual or simulated Y-site injection of drugs, the concentrations are cited in terms of concentration per milliliter of each drug solution prior to mixing at the Y-site. Most published research reports have presented the drug concentrations in this manner, and the *Handbook* follows this convention. For those few published reports that presented the drug concentrations after mixing at the Y-site, the concentrations have been recalculated to be consistent with the more common presentation style to maintain the consistency of presentation in the *Handbook*. Note that the Y-Site Injection Compatibility table is designed with the assumption of a 1:1 mixture of the subject drug and infusion solution or admixture. For citations reporting other than a 1:1 mixture, the actual amounts tested are specifically noted.

Designating Compatibility or Incompatibility

Each summary of a published research report appearing in the Compatibility Information tables bears a compatibility indicator (*C*, *I*, or *?*). A report receives a designation of *C* when the study results indicate that compatibility of the test samples existed under the test conditions. If the study determined an incompatibility existed under the test conditions, then an *I* designation is assigned for the *Handbook* entry for that study result. Specific standardized guidelines are used to assign these compatibility designations. The citation is designated as a report of compatibility when results of the original article indicated one or more of the following criteria were met:

1. Physical or visual compatibility of the combination was reported (no visible or electronically detected indication of particulate formation, haze, precipitation, color change, or gas evolution).
2. Stability of the components for at least 24 hours in an admixture under the specified conditions was reported (decomposition of 10% or less).
3. Stability of the components for the entire test period, although in some cases it was less than 24 hours, was reported (time periods less than 24 hours have been noted).

The citation is designated as a report of incompatibility when the results of the original article indicated either or both of the following criteria were met:

1. A physical or visual incompatibility was reported (visible or electronically detected particulate formation, haze, precipitation, color change, or gas evolution).
2. Greater than 10% decomposition of one or more components in 24 hours or less under the specified conditions was reported (time periods of less than 24 hours have been noted in the table).

Reports of test results that do not clearly fit into the compatibility or incompatibility definitions cannot be designated as either. These are indicated with a question mark.

Although these criteria have become the conventional definitions of compatibility and incompatibility, the reader should recognize that the criteria may need to be tempered with professional judgment. Inflexible adherence to the compatibility designations should be avoided. Instead, they should be used as aids in the exercising of professional judgment.

Therapeutic incompatibilities or other drug interactions are not within the scope of the *Handbook* and have not been included.

Interpreting Compatibility Information in the Handbook

As mentioned above, the body of information summarized in the *Handbook* is large and complicated. With the possible exception of a report of immediate gross precipitation, it usually takes some degree of thoughtful consideration and judgment to properly evaluate and appropriately act on the research results that are summarized in this book.

Nowhere is the need for judgment more obvious than when apparently contradictory information appears in two or more published reports. The body of literature in drug–drug and drug–vehicle compatibility is replete with apparently contradictory results. Except for study results that have been documented later to be incorrect, the conflicting information has been included in the *Handbook* to provide practitioners with all of the information for their consideration. The conflicting information will be readily apparent to the reader because of the content of the Remarks section as well as the *C*, *I*, and *?* designations following each citation.

Many or most of the apparently conflicting citations may be the result of differing conditions or materials used in the studies. A variety of factors that can influence the compatibility and stability of drugs must be considered in evaluating such conflicting results, and absolute statements are often difficult or impossible to make. Differences in concentrations, buffering systems, preservatives, vehicles, temperatures, and order of mixing may all play a role. By reviewing a variety of reports, the user of the *Handbook* is better able to exercise professional judgment with regard to compatibility and stability.

The reader must guard against misinterpretation of research results, which may lead to extensions of compatibility and stability that are inappropriate. As an example, a finding of precipitate formation two hours after two drugs are mixed does not imply nor should it be interpreted to mean that the combination is compatible until that time point, when a sudden precipitation occurs. Rather, it should be interpreted to mean that precipitation occurred at some point between mixing and the first observation point at two hours. Such a result would lead to a designation of incompatibility in the *Handbook*.

Precipitation reports can be particularly troublesome for practitioners to deal with because of the variability of the time frames in which they may occur. Apart from combinations that repeatedly result in immediate precipitation, the formation of a precipitate can be unpredictable to some degree. Numerous examples of variable precipitation time frames can be found in the literature, including paclitaxel, etoposide, and sulfamethoxazole-trimethoprim in infusion solutions and calcium and phosphates precipitation in parenteral nutrition mixtures. Differing drug concentrations can also play a role in creating variability in results. A good example of this occurs with co-administered vancomycin HCl and beta-lactam antibiotics. Users of the information in the *Handbook* must always be aware that a marginally incompatible combination might exhibit precipitation earlier or later than that reported in the literature. It has been suggested that in many such cases, the precipitation is ultimately going to occur, it is just the timing that is in question. This is of particular importance for precipitate formation because of the potential for serious adverse clinical consequences, including death, which have occurred. Certainly, users of the *Handbook* information should always keep in mind and anticipate the possibility of precipitation and its clinical ramifications.

In addition, many research reports cite test solutions or concentrations that may not be appropriate for clinical use. An example would be a report of a drug's stability in unsterile water. Although the *Handbook* summary will accurately reflect the test solutions and conditions that existed in a study, it is certainly inappropriate to misinterpret a stability report like this as being an authorization to use the product clinically. In such cases, the researchers may have used the clinically inappropriate diluent to evaluate the drug's stability for extrapolation to a more suitable vehicle that is similar, or they may not have recognized that the diluent is clinically unsuitable. In either event, it is incumbent on the practitioner in the clinical setting to use professional judgment to apply the information in an appropriate manner and recognize what is not acceptable clinically.

Further, it should be noted that many of the citations designated incompatible are not absolute. While a particular admixture may incur more than 10% decomposition within 24 hours, the combination may be useful for a shorter time period. The concept of "utility time" or the time to 10% decomposition may be useful in these cases. Unfortunately, such information is often not available. Included in the Remarks columns of the tables are the amount of decomposition, the time period involved, and the temperature at which the study was conducted when this information is available.

Users of the *Handbook* information should always keep in mind that the information in the *Handbook* must be used as a tool and a guide to the research that has been conducted and published. It is not a replace-ment for thoughtfully considered professional judgment. It falls to the practitioner to interpret the information in light of the clinical situation, including the patient's needs and status. What is certain is that relying solely on the *C* or *I* designation without the application of professional judgment is inappropriate.

Limitations of the Literature

In addition to conflicting information, many of the published articles have provided only partial evaluations, not looking at all aspects of a drug's stability and compatibility. This is not surprising considering the complexity, difficulty, and costs of conducting such research. There are, in fact, some articles that do provide evaluations of both physical stability/compatibility and chemical stability. But others are devoted only to physical issues, while others examine only chemical stability. Although a finding of precipitation, haze, or other physical effect may constitute an incompatibility (unless transient), the lack of such changes does not rule out chemical deterioration. In some cases, drugs initially designated as compatible because of a lack of visual change were later shown to undergo chemical decomposition. Similarly, the determination of chemical stability does not rule out the presence of unacceptable levels of particulates and/or turbidity in the combination. In a classic case, the drugs leucovorin calcium and fluorouracil were determined to be chemically stable for extended periods by stability-indicating HPLC assays in several studies, but years later, repeated episodes of filter clogging led to the discovery of unacceptable quantities of particulates in combinations of these drugs. The reader must always bear in mind these possibilities when only partial information is available.

And, finally, contemporary practitioners have come to expect that the analytical methods used in reports on the chemical stability of drugs will be validated stability-indicating methods. However, many early studies used methods that were not demonstrated to be stability indicating.

Literature Search for Updating the Handbook

To gather the bulk of the published compatibility and stability information for updating the *Handbook*, a literature search is performed using the *International Pharmaceutical Abstracts* database. By using key terms (e.g., stability), a listing of candidate articles for inclusion in the *Handbook* is generated. From this list, truly relevant articles are selected. As a supplement to this automated literature searching, a manual search of the references of the articles is also conducted, and any articles not included previously are obtained. Although this labor-intensive approach yields a very high percentage of the relevant articles published in the world's literature, it is not 100% inclusive. Occasionally, users of the *Handbook* come across articles that were overlooked. The author encourages anyone who finds an article that has been missed to bring it to his attention.

Reference

1. *The United States Pharmacopeia*, 24th ed, United States Pharmacopeial Convention: Rockville, MD; 2000.

Solution Abbreviations

AA	Amino acids (percentage specified)
D	Dextrose solution (percentage unspecified)
D5LR	Dextrose 5% in Ringer's injection, lactated
D5R	Dextrose 5% in Ringer's injection
D–S	Dextrose–saline combinations
D2.5½S	Dextrose 2.5% in sodium chloride 0.45%
D2.5S	Dextrose 2.5% in sodium chloride 0.9%
D5¼S	Dextrose 5% in sodium chloride 0.225%
D5½S	Dextrose 5% in sodium chloride 0.45%

D5S	Dextrose 5% in sodium chloride 0.9%
D10S	Dextrose 10% in sodium chloride 0.9%
D5W	Dextrose 5% in water
D10W	Dextrose 10% in water
DXN–S	Dextran 6% in sodium chloride 0.9%
IDCM	Ionosol DCM
IG	Ionosol G
IM	Isolyte M
IP	Isolyte P
IS	Invert sugar
LR	Ringer's injection, lactated
NM	Normosol M
NR	Normosol R
NS	Sodium chloride 0.9%
PH	Protein hydrolysate
R	Ringer's injections
S	Saline solution (percentage unspecified)
½S	Sodium chloride 0.45%
SL	Sodium lactate $\frac{1}{6}$ M
TPN	Total parenteral nutrition solution
W	Sterile water for injection

Manufacturer and Compendium Abbreviations

AB	Abbott
ACC	American Critical Care
AD	Adria
AGT	Aguettant
AH	Allen & Hanburys
AHP	Ascot Hospital Pharmaceuticals
ALZ	Alza
AMG	Amgen
AMR	American Regent
ANT	Antigen
AP	Asta-Pharma
APC	Apothecon
AQ	American Quinine
AR	Armour
ARC	American Red Cross
AS	Arnar-Stone
ASC	Ascot
AST	Astra
AT	Alpha Therapeutic
AW	Asta Werke
AY	Ayerst
BA	Baxter
BAY	Bayer
BC	Bencard
BE	Beecham
BED	Bedford
BEL	R. Bellon
BFM	Bieffe Medital
BI	Boehringer Ingelheim
BK	Berk
BKN	Baker Norton
BM	Boehringer Mannheim
BMS	Bristol-Myers Squibb
BN	Breon
BP	British Pharmacopoeia[a]
BPC	British Pharmaceutical Codex[a]
BR	Bristol
BRN	Braun
BRT	Britanna
BT	Boots
BTK	Biotika
BV	Ben Venue
BW	Burroughs Wellcome
BX	Berlex
BY	Bayer
CA	Calmic
CE	Carlo Erba
CER	Cerenex
CET	Cetus
CH	Lab. Choay Societe Anonyme
CHI	Chiron
CL	Ciba
CL	Clintec
CN	Connaught
CNF	Centrafarm
CO	Cole
CP	Continental Pharma
CPP	CP Pharmaceuticals
CR	Critikon
CU	Cutter
CY	Cyanamid
DAK	Dakota
DB	David Bull Laboratories
DCC	Dupont Critical Care
DI	Dista
DIA	Diamant
DM	Dome
DME	Dupont Merck Pharma
DMX	Dumex
DU	DuPont
DW	Delta West
EA	Eaton
EN	Endo
ES	Elkins-Sinn
EV	Evans
EX	Essex
FA	Farmitalia
FAU	Faulding
FC	Frosst & Cie
FI	Fisons
FRE	Fresenius
FUJ	Fujisawa
GEM	Geneva-Marsam
GEN	Genentech
GG	Geigy
GIL	Gilead
GL	Glaxo
GNS	Gensia
GRI	Grifols
GRP	Gruppo
GRU	Grunenthal
GW	Glaxo Wellcome
HC	Hillcross
HO	Hoechst-Roussel
HR	Horner
HY	Hyland
ICI	ICI Pharmaceuticals
IMM	Immunex
IMS	IMS Ltd.

IN	Intra
IV	Ives
IVX	Ivex
IX	Invenex
JC	Janssen-Cilag
JN	Janssen
KA	Kabi
KN	Knoll
KP	Kabi Pharmacia
KV	Kabi-Vitrum
KY	Kyowa
LA	Lagap
LE	Lederle
LEM	Lemmon
LEO	Leo Laboratories
LI	Lilly
LY	Lyphomed
LZ	Labaz Laboratories
MA	Mallinckrodt
MAR	Marsam
MB	May & Baker
ME	Merck
MG	McGaw
MI	Miles
MJ	Mead Johnson
MN	McNeil
MMD	Marion Merrell Dow
MRD	Merrill-Dow
MRN	Merrill-National
MSD	Merck Sharp & Dohme
MUN	Mundi Pharma
MY	Maney
NA	National
NAP	NAPP Pharmaceuticals
NCI	National Cancer Institute
NE	Norwich-Eaton
NF	National Formulary[a]
NO	Nordic
NOV	Novo
OHM	Ohmeda
OM	Omega
OMJ	OMJ Pharmaceuticals
ON	Orion
OR	Organon
ORT	Ortho
PD	Parke-Davis
PE	Pentagone
PF	Pfizer
PFM	Pfrimmer
PH	Pharmacia
PHT	Pharma-Tek
PHU	Pharmacia & Upjohn
PHX	Phoenix
PO	Poulenc
PR	Pasadena Research
PRK	Parkfields
PX	Pharmax
QLM	Qualimed Labs
QU	Quad
RB	Robins
RC	Roche

RI	Riker
RKC	Reckitt-Colman
ROR	Rorer
RP	Rhone-Poulenc
RPR	Rhone-Poulenc Rorer
RR	Roerig
RS	Roussel
RU	Rugby
SA	Sankyo
SC	Schering
SCN	Schein
SCS	SCS Pharmaceuticals
SE	Searle
SEQ	Sequus
SKB	SmithKline Beecham
SKF	Smith Kline & French
SM	Smith
SN	Smith + Nephew
SO	SoloPak
SQ	Squibb
ST	Sterilab
STR	Sterling
STS	Steris
STU	Stuart
SV	Savage
SW	Sanofi Winthrop
SX	Sabex
SY	Syntex
SZ	Sandoz
TAK	Takeda
TE	Teva
TL	Tillotts
TO	Torigian
TR	Travenol
UP	Upjohn
USB	US Bioscience
USP	United States Pharmacopeiea[a]
USV	USV Pharmaceuticals
VI	Vitarine
VT	Vitrum
WAS	Wasserman
WB	Winthrop-Breon
WC	Warner-Chilcott
WED	Weddel
WEL	Wellcome
WI	Winthrop
WL	Warner Lambert
WY	Wyeth
YAM	Yamanouchi
ZEN	Zeneca

---

[a]*While reference to a compendium does not indicate the specific manufacturer of a product, it does help to indicate the formulation that was used in the test.*

DRUG STABILITY AND COMPATIBILITY ISSUES IN DRUG DELIVERY

Lawrence A. Trissel

Drug stability and compatibility are critical elements in the accurate and appropriate delivery of drug therapy to patients. Both the therapeutic adequacy of the treatment and the safety of the therapy can be adversely affected by drug instability or incompatibility.

The term *instability* is usually applied to chemical reactions that are incessant, irreversible, and result in distinctly different chemical entities (degradation products) that can be both therapeutically inactive and possibly exhibit greater toxicity. Examples include hydrolysis and oxidative reactions.[1]

Incompatibility generally refers to physicochemical phenomena such as concentration-dependent precipitation and acid-base reactions with the products of reaction manifested as a change in physical state or protonation-deprotonation equilibria.[1] When the incompatibilities result in visible change(s) such as precipitation, turbidity or haziness, changes in color or viscosity, effervescence, or the formation of immiscible liquid layers, the term *physical incompatibility* or, more accurately, *visual incompatibility is* used.

Expiration time, shelf life, or *utility time* restrictions result from drug instability or incompatibility as well as from other factors such as the maintenance of sterility. Typically, these terms indicate the period for which a minimum of 90% of the drug remains intact and available for delivery.[2] Most often, an expiration date is applied to the intact formulation from the manufacturer, while a much shorter utility time is determined for the drug when constituted and diluted for administration. The term shelf life has been applied to both of these situations.[2]

Types of Common Incompatibilities

Common incompatibilities are often classified as "chemical" and "physical," even though all incompatibilities have a chemical basis. Physical incompatibilities may be related to solubility changes or container interactions rather than molecular changes to the drug entity itself.

Physical Incompatibilities—A drug can be maintained in aqueous solution as long as its concentration is less than its saturation solubility. A drug may not necessarily precipitate from a supersaturated solution immediately, but precipitation can begin at any time. Erratic and unpredictable precipitation times often result. Trimethoprim–sulfamethoxazole, etoposide, and teniposide exhibit variable precipitation times.[3–7] Drugs that are poorly water-soluble are often formulated using water-miscible cosolvents such as ethanol, propylene glycol, and polyethylene glycol. Drug products that use a cosolvent formulation approach include digoxin, phenytoin, trimethoprim–sulfamethoxazole, etoposide, and teniposide.[6,7]

A classic example of a cosolvent formulation resulting in precipitation problems is diazepam injection. Diazepam is formulated at a 5-mg/mL concentration in a vehicle composed of propylene glycol, 40%; ethanol, 10%; benzyl alcohol, 1.5%; and water for injection. Numerous reports have focused on the problems with precipitation of this drug.[8–14] Dilution of the dosage form results in precipitation in some concentrations, but sufficient dilution to a point below diazepam's saturation solubility results in a physically stable admixture. Morris[11] reported that a visible precipitate is produced in dilutions of 1:1 to 1:10. Haziness was reported at 1:15, and delayed precipitate formation after 6 to 8 hours was seen in some solutions at 1:20; however, dilutions of 1:40 to 1:100 remained clear for 24 hours. Maloney[14] noted similar diazepam behavior, and similar findings were reported for trimethoprim–sulfamethoxazole by Lesko et al.[3] and Jarosinski et al.,[5] for digoxin,[15] and for etoposide, teniposide, and taxol by Trissel et al.[7]

For drugs that are weak acids or bases, solubility is a direct function of solution pH. Along with the drug's dissociation constant(s), pH controls the portion of drug in its ionized form and the solubility of the un-ionized form. A drug that is a weak acid may be formulated at a pH sufficient to yield the desired solubility. Examples include sodium salts of barbiturates, phenytoin, methotrexate, mercaptopurine, thioguanine, and bromodeoxyuridine. All these drugs are formulated at high pH values to achieve adequate solubility.[6–7] If the solution pH of these drugs is lowered, the drug's solubility at the final pH may be exceeded, resulting in possible precipitation. Numerous examples of barbiturate precipitation from admixture with acidic drugs have been cited in the literature.[6] A similar rationale for possible precipitation exists for the salts of weak bases in alkaline media.[2]

Precipitation may also occur due to the formation of salts that are relatively insoluble. A well-known example of this phenomenon results from the mixture of a calcium salt with phosphates, typically in parenteral nutrition solutions. Dozens of articles have dealt with various aspects of calcium phosphate precipitation from parenteral solutions.[6] Graphic depictions of solubility curves for specific admixtures have been created,[16–19] but the phenomenon is very complex, being dependent on a multiplicity of factors (Table 1). Although exact predictions are not possible, enhanced precipitate formation would be expected from high concentrations of calcium and phosphate, increases in solution pH, decreases in amino acid concentrations, increases in temperature, addition of calcium before phosphate, lengthy time delays or slow infusion rates, and use of the chloride salt of calcium.[20]

Originally published in *The Cancer Bulletin.* 1990;42:393–398. Copyright 1990. Medical Arts Publishing Foundation, Houston, Texas.

Table 1. Factors That Play a Role In Calcium and Phosphate Precipitation

Concentration of calcium
Salt form of calcium
Concentration of phosphate
Concentration of amino acids
Amino acids composition
Concentration of dextrose
Temperature of solution
pH of solution
Presence of other additives
Order of mixing

Large organic anions and cations may also form precipitates or insoluble complexes. A group of well-documented examples is the interaction between heparin, an anionic polysulfonated mucopolysaccharide, and aminoglycoside antibiotics, which are large cationic drugs. Precipitation has been demonstrated for heparin with amikacin,[21-23] gentamicin,[23-27] netilmicin,[22,23] and tobramycin.[22,23] It has been postulated that these are heparin salts of the cationic drug that are relatively insoluble in water.[2] In these cases, precipitation may or may not occur, depending on whether the solubility product of the salt is exceeded. Consequently, precipitation may occur at high drug concentrations but may not occur if sufficiently diluted. Even in dilute solution, a transient precipitation may occur due to a locally high drug concentration; the precipitate dissipates as the effects of full dilution are realized.

Sorption Phenomena—Sorption phenomena are also classified as physical incompatibilities. In cases of sorption, the intact drug is lost from the solution to be administered by adsorption to the surface or absorption into the matrix of the container material, administration set, or filter. As a result of the pioneering work by Moorhatch and Chiou[28] and follow-up studies by other researchers, numerous drugs exhibiting sorption have been identified, including nitroglycerin, diazepam, warfarin, vitamin A, dactinomycin, and insulin.[6]

Adsorption to surfaces commonly results from interactions of functional groups within the drug molecule to binding sites on the surfaces. Glass surfaces can be treated to block the polar silanol binding sites, but this process of silanization does not prevent binding to nonpolar hydrophobic sites.[2] Adsorption also readily occurs to plastic surfaces of bags, administration sets, and filters. The adsorption phenomenon becomes important to drug delivery for agents administered in small quantities or low concentration because a clinically relevant amount of the agent may be removed from solution. Drugs administered in larger quantities lose a smaller percentage of the total dose. This difference occurs because of the saturation of binding sites on the container surface. At higher drug concentrations, binding site saturation can occur with only an insignificantly small drug loss from a therapeutic standpoint. Of course, the small amounts of drug present in biologic samples often result in a major portion of drug being lost to adsorption, even for a drug not exhibiting such losses at therapeutic concentrations. Examples include doxorubicin hydrochloride and mitoxantrone dihydrochloride.[29]

Absorption into the matrix of plastic containers and administration sets, especially those made of polyvinyl chloride (PVC), is a source of drug loss from solution for lipid-soluble drugs. The PVC is made pliable and flexible by incorporating substantial amounts of phthalate plasticizers. Lipid-soluble drugs diffuse from the solution into the plasticizer in the plastic matrix.[30] Plastics that contain little or no phthalate plasticizers, such as polyethylene and polypropylene, do not readily absorb lipid-soluble drugs into the polymer core. This difference in absorption potential serves as the basis for specialized administration sets such as those for nitroglycerin and fat emulsion.

The opposite effect, leaching of phthalate plasticizers into the solution, may also occur. The presence of surface-active agents or large amounts of organic cosolvents in the formulation may enhance leaching of the plasticizer.[31]

Other Physical Incompatibilities—Physical incompatibilities also include salting out, complexation, color changes, and gas evolution.

The *salting out* of a drug refers to the decreased solubility of nonelectrolytes and weakly hydrated organic ions in the presence of strong electrolytes such as sodium, potassium, and calcium chlorides.[1] A nonionized organic drug molecule, such as diazepam or chlorpromazine hydrochloride, may precipitate from solution, depending on the drug and salt concentration, temperature, and solution pH.[1]

Complexation is another possible physical phenomenon. Tetracyclines are well documented to form insoluble chelates with Al^{+3}, Ca^{+2}, Fe^+, and Mg^{+2} under the necessary conditions of concentration and pH.[1] Amphotericin B and erythromycin gluceptate apparently form poorly soluble complexes with antibacterial preservatives such as those in bacteriostatic water for injection.[6]

Color changes are common visual incompatibilities that are in reality chemical interactions resulting in molecular changes in the drug entities. The color formation or changes of sympathomimetic amines, anthracyclines, amsacrine, and tetracycline with alkaline drugs such as aminophylline and ganciclovir are the result of chemical degradation to colored decomposition products.[6]

Similarly, *gas evolution* results from a chemical reaction, often between carbonates or bicarbonates and acidic drugs. It is not just sodium bicarbonate injection that poses the potential of gas evolution. Some cephalosporins such as cephalothin sodium, cephradine, cefamandole nafate, and ceftazidime contain sodium carbonate or bicarbonate in the formulations.[6] Indeed, carbon dioxide is generated during the normal constitution of cefamandole and ceftazidime and has resulted in explosive-like reactions in syringes.[32-34]

Chemical Degradation Pathways

Although color changes and gas evolution result from chemical reactions, most chemical incompatibilities, those interactions resulting in molecular changes or rearrangements to different chemical entities, are not visibly observable. Drugs may undergo a variety of chemical degradation pathways.

Hydrolysis is a common mode of chemical decomposition causing the bulk of drug instabilities. Hydrolysis generally involves attack by water on labile bonds in dissolved drug molecules with resulting molecular changes. Functional groups that are labile to hydrolysis include carboxylic acid and phosphate esters, amides, lactams, and imines. In esters, a rupture of a covalent linkage between a carbon atom and an oxygen atom occurs. For carboxylic acid ester hydrolysis, the functional group RCOOR′ yields an alcohol (R′OH) and a carboxylic acid (RCOOH) or its conjugate base (RCOO⁻).[1] Amide hydrolysis products are carboxylic acids and amines. Ester hydrolysis is catalyzed by hydrogen or hydroxyl ions.[35] Phosphate esters, such as hydrocortisone sodium phosphate, may readily hydrolyze at acidic pH; imines such as diazepam and oximes like pralidoxime are both acid-labile and subject to base-catalyzed hydrolysis as well.[2]

Oxidation and *reduction* reactions involve exchange of electrons and valence changes in the drug molecules. Oxidation is electron loss that causes a positive increase in valence. Most drugs are present in reduced form, so the atmospheric oxygen creates stability problems.[1] Pharmaceuticals susceptible to oxidation include steroids, tricyclic compounds, and phenolic drugs such as epinephrine.[2] *Autoxidation* is a spontaneous reaction under ambient conditions of a substrate with atmospheric oxygen.[1] Phenolic compounds such as the sympathomimetic amines readily undergo oxidation in neutral or alkaline pH. The reaction occurs much more slowly at pH below 4.[2] Even small amounts of oxidized epinephrine result in highly discolored solutions due to the formation of adrenochrome, the primary oxidation product.[2] To control this process in pharmaceuticals, oxygen may be excluded from the dosage forms, pH may be adjusted, chelating agents like ethylenediaminetetraacetic acid (EDTA) may be incorporated, and antioxidants such as sodium bisulfite and metabisulfite or ascorbic acid may be added to the formulation.

Reduction reactions involve electron gain with a reduction in valence and the addition of halogens or hydrogen to C=C bonds.[1] Although much rarer than oxidation reactions in drugs, beta-lactam antibiotics such as the penicillins can produce reducing aldehydes upon hydrolysis. The displacement of aluminum from needles by cisplatin is another example, resulting in the precipitation of platinum metal.[36,37]

Photolysis or *photodegradation* is the catalysis by light of degradation reactions such as oxidation or hydrolysis. A variety of decomposition mechanisms may occur from the absorption of radiation energy, but the net effect is that sufficient energy becomes concentrated at a chemical bond that decomposes or rearranges into a new chemical entity.[2] A number of drugs undergo photolytic degradation including amphotericin B, furosemide, dacarbazine, doxorubicin hydrochloride, sodium nitroprusside, and vitamin A.[6] The energy imparted to the degradation reaction per photon of light increases as the wavelength increases. Consequently, ultraviolet light is more deleterious than visible light; daylight is more deleterious than fluorescent light. These

photodegradation reactions also depend on the intensity as well as the wavelength of light. The more intense a light source and/or the closer the photolabile drugs are to these light sources, the greater the rate and degree of photodegradation.[1] To effectively deliver drugs that are highly subject to photolytic degradation, such as sodium nitroprusside, exclusion of light from the container and possibly the tubing by wrapping with foil is necessary.[38–42]

Racemization and *epimerization* can occur to drugs that are optically active due to a chiral carbon center in the molecule. If one isomer is more pharmacologically active than another, this process results in the loss of therapeutic activity. This occurs with epinephrine, in which the *l*-isomer is about 15 times more active than the *d*-isomer. If a drug has only one chiral center, the process of racemization leads to a 50:50 mixture of the two isomers. If more than one chiral center exists in a molecule, one isomer may be favored over another, resulting in equilibrium at something other than a 50:50 mixture. This process is called epimerization.[1]

Factors Influencing Chemical Degradation Rates

The most important factors that influence the rate of drug decomposition in drug delivery systems are solution pH and temperature. Drug concentration, light exposure, and solution ionic strength are also important factors.

Effects of Solution pH—Just as solution pH is an important factor influencing solubility phenomena of some drugs, it can have a similarly profound impact on drug delivery to patients. The degradation of many drugs is catalyzed by extremes of pH, the reactions being affected by the presence of hydrogen or hydroxide ions. Drug reaction rates are generally less at intermediate pH values than at high or low ranges.[35] A pH-rate profile is a graphic or tabular representation of a drug's stability at various pH values. The pH profile of a drug will often determine the pH at which the product is formulated. This usually corresponds to the pH of maximum stability but can be a pH to enhance solubility. Many times a buffer system will be incorporated to ensure the maintenance of the proper pH. Most drugs are sufficiently stable in the pH range of 4 to 8 to be administered over convenient time periods; however, drugs formulated at more extreme pH values can lead to increasingly rapid decomposition of other drugs if admixed in the same solution. The pH of each component of a potential drug admixture should be evaluated for unacceptable differences before mixing for administration to the patient. Possible drug–drug or drug–vehicle incompatibilities can be avoided if potentially unacceptable pH shifts are anticipated.

Effects of Temperature—Temperature is another primary variable affecting the rate of degradation reactions. Each 10 °C elevation in temperature may increase reaction rates two- to fivefold.[1] Even though this estimated effect may be fairly accurate for some drugs, the rule cannot be applied indiscriminately. Some degradation reactions are not affected by a 10 °C temperature change while other reactions undergo extremely rapid changes.[35] In some cases, reduced temperature may actually increase the reaction rate. Savello and Shangraw[43] determined the stability of

Table 2. Percentage Degradation in 4 Hours of 1% Ampicillin Sodium at Several Temperatures*

Temperature	Diluent	
(°C)	5% Dextrose	0.9% Sodium Chloride
−20	13.6	1.2
0	6.2	0.4
5	10.1	1.0
27	21.3	1.8

Adapted from Savello and Shangraw.[43]

ampicillin sodium at various temperatures (Table 2). As the temperature decreases from 27 °C to 5 °C and down to 0 °C, the rate of decomposition declines. However, as the temperature falls further, the decomposition rate in dilute solutions increases. At −20 °C, small pockets of concentrated ampicillin sodium solution are trapped in an ice matrix, resulting in increased decomposition due to self-catalyzed hydrolysis. The impact of the dextrose catalysis is also evident.

For most drugs, an Arrhenius plot of the reaction rate constant vs. the reciprocal absolute temperature yields a linear relationship from which a shelf life at a given temperature can be estimated.[1,2] However, expiration periods or utility times based on Arrhenius predictions may be erroneous and invalid in a variety of situations. If higher temperatures evaporate solvents and concentrate the drugs or produce variable moisture contents, reaction rates may be affected. Similarly, at high temperatures, reduced humidity and oxygen may occur and affect the predictability of degradation.[35] The mechanism of degradation may be altered. Peptides degrade by hydrolysis and oxidation at low temperatures and by denaturation at higher temperatures.[2] Reactions catalyzed by enzymes may be temperature dependent until the enzyme begins to denature, reducing its ability to catalyze a reaction.[44]

Consequently, the effects of temperature on drug degradation can be complicated. Prediction of long-term degradation rates based on elevated temperature data alone is problematic.

Effects of Other Factors—Increases in drug concentration will usually increase the degradation rate exponentially. Autocatalysis and pH–buffer effects, such as for ampicillin, yield these decomposition rate increases.[1] Savello and Shangraw[43] described ampicillin decomposition at various concentrations and reported increasing decomposition with increasing concentration (Table 3). Some drugs appear to undergo lower rates of decomposition at higher concentrations. Examples that have been noted include the autoxidation of catecholamines[45] and the reduced hydrolysis of nafcillin in the presence of aminophylline.[46] Presumably, the greater buffer concentration at higher nafcillin concentrations protects the drug to some extent from aminophylline's high pH and slows the hydrolysis.[1] Obviously, concentration dependency has assumed greater importance with the proliferation of ambulatory infusion therapy, which utilizes much greater drug concentrations.

Exposure to light can greatly influence the degradation rate of drugs that undergo extensive photodegradation. In the case of sodium nitroprusside, light exposure is the single most important determinant of solution stability.[38–42]

Changes in the ionic strength of a drug product may increase, decrease, or have no effect on degradation rate.[35] A positively charged drug undergoing hydrogen ion catalysis will show an increased rate of degradation with increased sodium chloride concentrations; however, a decreased rate will occur if the positively charged drug is undergoing hydroxyl ion catalysis. If the drug is neutral, changes in the ionic strength will not affect the rate of degradation.[35]

Impact of Drug Delivery Systems on Drug Stability

When the multiplicity of factors that can affect drug stability and compatibility is considered, it is obvious that drug delivery technology will play a role. It can affect both the nature and extent of drug degradation mechanisms. Conversely, consideration of a drug's stability and compatibility may influence the choice of delivery technology.

Over the years, parenteral drugs have often been administered via large-volume parenteral solutions. One or several drugs would be added to a standard infusion solution. The worst case can be found with parenteral nutrition solutions combining dozens of components. The number of potential permutations of components of parenteral nutrition solutions has been estimated to be in the millions[47] without even considering differences in concentration. Obviously, the potential for drug stability and compatibility problems is great because of the long duration of contact time and exposure to ambient conditions of temperature and light.

Another common approach is the administration of drugs via syringes, whether for intravenous, intramuscular, or subcutaneous injection. In general, this approach entails a much more concentrated drug solution than that used for infusions. If more than one concentrated drug is combined in a syringe, the potential for an adverse compatibility interaction is greatly enhanced. Until recent years, syringe delivery of drug combinations meant keeping the drugs' contact time short, generally no more than a few minutes. With the proliferation of syringe pumps, highly concentrated drugs are given over extended periods, often continuously for

Table 3. Percentage Degradation of Ampicillin Sodium at Various Concentrations in Water for Injection at 5 °C after 8 Hours*

Concentration (%)	Degradation (%)
1	0.8
5	3.6
10	5.8
15	10.4
20	12.3
25	13.3

Adapted from Savello and Shangraw.[43]

many days, increasing the contact times unless Y-site administration is utilized.

The use of Y-site or piggyback drug delivery has helped prevent or avoid drug stability and compatibility problems. Often, Y-site delivery permits administration of drugs that cannot be given in combination in the same solution. The contact time of multiple solutions being administered via Y-site is short, often in the range of 15 minutes and hardly ever more than 60 minutes.[48] Relatively few drug combinations are so chemically unstable that Y-site administration of the combination is precluded.[6] If the drug combination is physically compatible, often it can be administered by Y-site injection.

Temperature can be an important factor in drug stability and delivery in the clinical setting. Drugs may be stored frozen at −20 °C or under refrigeration. Warming to room temperature (approximately 22 °C to 25 °C) occurs during preparation for administration. Some drugs are administered at ambient temperature, as with normal continuous or intermittent infusion using fixed gravity or pump systems. Portable pumps may be carried near the body so that the drug solution is warmed to approximately 30 °C to 32 °C. With implantable pumps, drug solutions are at about 37 °C. Because generalizations are not applicable, each drug entity's stability at a variety of temperatures should be assessed to ensure adequate drug therapy by whatever delivery device is selected.

Conclusion

Drug stability and compatibility issues are important considerations in assuring the adequacy of drug delivery to the patient. The nature and extent of a drug's stability and compatibility characteristics are the result of the interrelationship of a complex set of factors, some inherent in the drug molecule itself and others in the drug's environment. The goal is to use the knowledge of drug stability and compatibility that has accumulated over decades in conjunction with the advances in drug delivery technology to assure the safe and efficacious administration of drug therapy.

References

1. Newton DW. Physicochemical determinants of incompatibility and instability of drugs for injection and infusion. *Am J Hosp Pharm.* 1978;35:1213–1222.
2. Stella VJ. Chemical and physical bases determining the instability and incompatibility of formulated injectable drugs. *J Parenter Sci Technol.* 1986;40:142–163.
3. Lesko LJ, Marion A, Ericson J, et al. Stability of trimethoprim-sulfamethoxazole injection in two infusion fluids. *Am J Hosp Pharm.* 1981;38:1004–1006.
4. Deans KW, Lang JR, Smith DE. Stability of trimethoprim-sulfamethoxazole injection in five infusion fluids. *Am J Hosp Pharm.* 1982;39:1681–1684.
5. Jarosinski PF, Kennedy PF, Gallelli JF. Stability of concentrated trimethoprim-sulfamethaxazole admixtures. *Am J Hosp Pharm.* 1989;46:732–737.
6. Trissel LA. *Handbook on Injectable Drugs.* 5th ed. Bethesda, Md: American Society of Hospital Pharmacists; 1988.
7. Trissel LA, Davignon IP, Kleinman LM, et al. *NCI Investigational Drugs—Pharmaceutical Data 1988.* Bethesda, Md: National Cancer Institute; 1988.
8. Jusko WJ, Gretch M, Gassett R. Precipitation of diazepam from intravenous preparations. *JAMA.* 1973;225:176. Letter.
9. Dam M, Christiansen J. Diazepam: intravenous infusion in the treatment of status epilepticus. *Acta Neurol Scand.* 1976;54:278–280.
10. Kortilla K, Sothman A, Andersson P. Polyethylene glycol as a solvent for diazepam: bioavailability and clinical effects after intramuscular administration, comparison of oral, intramuscular, and rectal administration and precipitation from intravenous solutions. *Acta Pharmacol Toxicol.* 1976;39:104–117.
11. Morris ME. Compatibility and stability of diazepam injection following dilution from intravenous fluids. *Am J Hosp Pharm.* 1978;35:669–672.
12. Newton DW, Driscoll DF, Goudreau JL, et al. Solubility characteristics of diazepam in aqueous admixture solutions: theory and practice. *Am J Hosp Pharm.* 1981;38:179–182.
13. Mason NA, Cline S, Hyneck ML, et al. Factors affecting diazepam infusion: solubility, administration-set composition, and flow rate. *Am J Hosp Pharm.* 1981;38:1449–1454.
14. Maloney TJ. Dilution of diazepam injection prior to intravenous administration. *Aust J Hosp Pharm.* 1983;13:79.
15. McEvoy G, ed. *American Hospital Formulary Service 89.* Bethesda, Md: American Society of Hospital Pharmacists, 1989.
16. Schuetz DH, King JC. Compatibility and stability of electrolytes, vitamins and antibiotics in combination with 8% amino acids solution. *Am J Hosp Pharm.* 1978;35:33–44.
17. Henry RS, Jurgens RW, Sturgeon R, et al. Compatibility of calcium chloride and calcium gluconate with sodium phosphate in a mixed TPN solution. *Am J Hosp Pharm.* 1980;37:673–674.
18. Eggert LD, Ruska WJ, MacKay MW, et al. Calcium and phosphorus compatibility in parenteral nutrition solutions for neonates. *Am J Hosp Pharm.* 1982;39:49–53.
19. Fitzgerald KA, MacKay MW. Calcium and phosphate solubility in neonatal parenteral nutrient solutions containing TrophAmine. *Am J Hosp Pharm.* 1986;43:88–93.
20. Niemiec PW, Vanderveen TW. Compatibility considerations in parenteral nutrient solutions. *Am J Hosp Pharm.* 1984;41:893-911.
21. Nunning BC, Granatek AP. Physical compatibility and chemical stability of amikacin sulfate in combination with non-antibiotic drugs in large-volume parenteral solutions, part IV. *Curr Ther Res Clin Exp.* 1976;20:417–491.
22. Hutchison SM. Heparin and aminoglycosides instability. *Drug Intell Clin Pharm.* 1986;20:886. Letter.
23. Schutz VH, Schroder F. Heparin-natrium kompatibal bei gleichzeitiger applikation anderer pharmaka. *Krankenhauspharmazie.* 1985;6:7–11.

24. Riley BB. Incompatibilities in intravenous solutions. *J Hosp Pharm.* 1970;28:228–240.

25. Jacobs J, Kletter D, Superstine E, et al. Intravenous infusions of heparin and penicillins. *J Clin Pathol.* 1973;26:742–746.

26. Koup JR, Gerbracht L. Reduction in heparin activity by gentamicin. *Drug Intell Clin Pharm.* 1975;9:568. Letter.

27. Neil JM. A rational approach to intravenous additives. *Proc Guild.* 1979;7:3–33.

28. Moorhatch P, Chiou WL. Interactions between drugs and plastic intravenous fluid bags: I. Sorption studies in 17 drugs. *Am J Hosp Pharm.* 1974;31:72–78.

29. Bosanquet AG. Stability of solutions of antineoplastic agents during preparation and storage for in vitro assays: general considerations, the nitrosoureas and alkylating agents. *Cancer Chemother Pharmacol.* 1985;16:83–95.

30. Illium L, Bundgaard H. Sorption of drugs by plastic infusion bags. *Int J Pharmaceutics.* 1982;10:339–351.

31. Moorhatch P, Chiou WL. Interactions between drugs and plastic fluid bags: II. Leaching of chemicals from bags containing various solvent media. *Am J Hosp Pharm.* 1974;31:149–152.

32. Palmer MA, Fraterrigo CC. Production of carbon dioxide gas after reconstitution of cefamandole nafate. *Am J Hosp Pharm.* 1979;36:596–597.

33. Klink PR, McKeecham CW. Production of carbon dioxide gas after reconstitution of cefamandole nafate. *Am J Hosp Pharm.* 1979;36:597. Letter.

34. Palmer MA, Fraterrigo CC. Clarification of "explosive-like" reaction occurring when reconstituted cefamandole nafate was stored in syringes. *Am J Hosp Pharm.* 1979;36:1025. Letter.

35. Lachman L, DeLuca P, Akers MJ. Kinetic principles and stability testing. In: Lachman L, Lieberman HA, Kanig JL, eds. *Theory and Practice of Industrial Pharmacy.* 3rd ed. Philadelphia, Pa: Lea & Febiger; 1986:760–803.

36. Bohart RD, Ogawa G. An observation on the stability of *cis*-dichlorodiammineplatinum (II): a caution regarding its administration. *Cancer Treat Rep.* 1979;63:2117–2118.

37. Prestayko AW, Cadiz M, Crooke ST. Incompatibility of aluminum-containing iv administration equipment with *cis*-dichlorodiammineplatinum (II) administration. *Cancer Treat Rep.* 1979;63:2118–2119.

38. Frank MJ, Johnson JB, Rubin SH. Spectrophotometric determination of sodium nitroprusside and its photodegradation products. *J Pharm Sci.* 1976;65:44–48.

39. Vesey CJ, Batistona GA. Determination and stability of sodium nitroprusside in aqueous solutions (determination and stability of SNP). *J Clin Pharm.* 1977;2:105–117.

40. Mahoney C, Brown JE. Starget WW, et al. In vitro stability of sodium nitroprusside solutions for intravenous administration. *J Pharm Sci.* 1984;73:838–839.

41. Sewell GJ, Forbes DR, Munton TI. Stability of sodium nitroprusside infusion during the administration by motorized syringe-pump. *J Clin Hosp Pharm.* 1985;10:351–360.

42. Baaske DM, Smith MD, Karnatz N, et al. High-performance liquid chromatographic determination of sodium nitroprusside. *J Chromatogr.* 1981;212:339–346.

43. Savello DR, Shangraw RF. Stability of sodium, ampicillin solutions in the frozen and liquid states. *Am J Hosp Pharm.* 1971;28:754–759.

44. Moore JW, Pearson RG. *Kinetics and Mechanisms: A Study of Homogeneous Chemical Reactions.* 3rd ed. New York, NY: John Wiley & Sons Inc; 1981:31–36, 83–191.

45. Newton DW, Fung EYY, Williams DA. Stability of five catecholamines and terbutaline sulfate in 5% dextrose injection in the absence and presence of aminophylline. *Am J Hosp Pharm.* 1981;38:1314–1319.

46. Parker EA, Levin HJ. Unipen injection. *Am J Hosp Pharm.* 1975;32:943–944.

47. Kramer W, Inglott A, Cluxton R. Some physical and chemical incompatibilities of drugs for i.v. administration. *Drug Intell Clin Pharm.* 1971;5:211–228.

48. Leissing NC, Story KO, Zaske D. Inline fluid dynamics in piggy-back and manifold drug delivery systems. *Am J Hosp Pharm.* 1989;46:89–97.

COMMERCIAL DRUG
MONOGRAPHS

ACETAZOLAMIDE SODIUM
AHFS 52:10

Bedford

Products— Acetazolamide as the sodium salt is available in 500-mg vials with sodium hydroxide and, if necessary, hydrochloric acid to adjust the pH. Reconstitute the solution with at least 5 ml of sterile water for injection to yield a solution containing not more than 100 mg/ml (4).

pH— Approximately 9.2 to 9.6 (1-7/98; 4).

Osmolality— The osmolality of acetazolamide sodium 500 mg was calculated for the following dilutions (1054):

Diluent	Osmolality (mOsm/kg)	
	50 ml	100 ml
Dextrose 5% in water	321	291
Sodium chloride	348	317

Sodium Content— 2.049 mEq/500 mg (calculated) (846).

Administration— Administration by direct intravenous injection is preferred. Intramuscular injection is painful due to the alkaline pH and is not recommended (1-7/98; 4).

Stability— The manufacturer states that the reconstituted solution is stable for three days if refrigerated or for 12 hours at room temperature (1-7/98). Other information indicates that the reconstituted solution is stable for one week under refrigeration. However, because the product contains no preservatives, use of the solution within 24 hours after reconstitution is recommended (4).

pH Effects— The stability of acetazolamide sodium in aqueous solution appears to decrease as the pH increases above 9. At pH 8.8, a 0.25-mg/ml solution retained 96% of the initial amount after three days at 25 °C; at pH 10.8 and 12.7, the remaining drug was 88 and 83%, respectively, after four days (1230). Acetazolamide exhibits maximum stability at pH 4 (1424).

Freezing Solutions— Acetazolamide sodium (Lederle) 375 mg/L in dextrose 5% in water and sodium chloride 0.9% in PVC bags lost less than 3% after 44 days at −10 °C (1085).

Sorption— Acetazolamide sodium (Lederle) 19 mg/L in sodium chloride 0.9% (Travenol) in PVC bags did not exhibit significant sorption to the plastic during one week of storage at room temperature (15 to 20 °C) (536).

Acetazolamide sodium (Lederle) 19 mg/L in sodium chloride 0.9% did not exhibit any loss due to sorption during a seven-hour simulated infusion through an infusion set (Travenol) consisting of a cellulose propionate burette chamber and 170 cm of PVC tubing (606).

The drug was also tested as a simulated infusion over at least one hour by a syringe pump system. A glass syringe on a syringe pump was fitted with 20 cm of polyethylene tubing or 50 cm of Silastic tubing. No loss of drug due to sorption was observed with either tubing (606).

A 25-ml aliquot of acetazolamide sodium (Lederle) 19 mg/L in sodium chloride 0.9% was stored in all-plastic syringes composed of polypropylene barrels and polyethylene plungers for 24 hours at room temperature in the dark. No loss due to sorption occurred (606).

Compatibility Information

Solution Compatibility

Acetazolamide sodium

Solution	Mfr	Mfr	Conc/L		Remarks	Ref	C/I
Dextran 6% in dextrose 5%	AB	LE	375	mg	Physically compatible	3	C
Dextran 6% in sodium chloride 0.9%	AB	LE	375	mg	Physically compatible	3	C
Dextrose–Ringer's injection combinations	AB	LE	375	mg	Physically compatible	3	C
Dextrose–Ringer's injection, lactated, combinations	AB	LE	375	mg	Physically compatible	3	C
Dextrose–saline combinations	AB	LE	375	mg	Physically compatible	3	C
Dextrose 2½% in water	AB	LE	375	mg	Physically compatible	3	C
Dextrose 5% in water	AB	LE	375	mg	Physically compatible	3	C
	TR[a]	LE	375	mg	Physically compatible with 7% acetazolamide loss in 5 days at 25 °C and 5% loss in 44 days at 5 °C	1085	C
Dextrose 10% in water	AB	LE	375	mg	Physically compatible	3	C
Fructose 10% in sodium chloride 0.9%	AB	LE	375	mg	Physically compatible	3	C
Fructose 10% in water	AB	LE	375	mg	Physically compatible	3	C
Invert sugar 5 and 10% in sodium chloride 0.9%	AB	LE	375	mg	Physically compatible	3	C
Invert sugar 5 and 10% in water	AB	LE	375	mg	Physically compatible	3	C

Solution Compatibility (Cont.)

Acetazolamide sodium

Solution	Mfr	Mfr	Conc/L	Remarks	Ref	C/I
Ionosol products	AB	LE	375 mg	Physically compatible	3	C
Ringer's injection	AB	LE	375 mg	Physically compatible	3	C
Ringer's injection, lactated	AB	LE	375 mg	Physically compatible	3	C
Sodium chloride 0.45%	AB	LE	375 mg	Physically compatible	3	C
Sodium chloride 0.9%	AB	LE	375 mg	Physically compatible	3	C
	TR[a]	LE	375 mg	Physically compatible with 7% acetazolamide loss in 5 days at 25 °C and 5% loss in 44 days at 5 °C	1085	C
Sodium lactate ⅙ M	AB	LE	375 mg	Physically compatible	3	C

[a]Tested in PVC containers.

Additive Compatibility

Acetazolamide sodium

Drug	Mfr	Conc/L	Mfr	Conc/L	Test Soln	Remarks	Ref	C/I
Cimetidine HCl	SKF	3 g	LE	5 g	D5W	Physically compatible and cimetidine chemically stable for 24 hr at room temperature. Acetazolamide not tested	551	C
Ranitidine HCl	GL	50 mg and 2 g		5 g	D5W	Physically compatible and ranitidine chemically stable by HPLC for 24 hr at 25 °C. Acetazolamide not tested	1515	C

Y-Site Injection Compatibility (1:1 Mixture)

Acetazolamide sodium

Drug	Mfr	Conc	Mfr	Conc	Remarks	Ref	C/I
Diltiazem HCl	MMD	5 mg/ml	LE	100 mg/ml	Precipitate forms	1807	I
	MMD	1 mg/ml[b]	LE	100 mg/ml	Visually compatible	1807	C
TPN #203 and #204[a]			LE	100 mg/ml	White precipitate forms immediately	1974	I

[a]Refer to Appendix I for the composition of parenteral nutrition solutions. TPN indicates a 2-in-1 admixture.
[b]Tested in sodium chloride 0.9%.

Additional Compatibility Information

Acetazolamide sodium is stated to be physically incompatible with multivitamins (Astra) (1-4/98).

ACYCLOVIR SODIUM
AHFS 8:18

Zovirax   **Glaxo Wellcome**

Products— Acyclovir sodium (Glaxo Wellcome) is available in vials containing 500 mg or 1 g of acyclovir as the sodium salt. Reconstitute the 500-mg vial with 10 ml and the 1-g vial with 20 ml of sterile water for injection; shake well to ensure complete dissolution. The final acyclovir concentration is 50 mg/ml. Do not use bacteriostatic water for injection containing parabens or benzyl alcohol (2).

pH— The reconstituted solution has a pH of 10.5 to 11.6 (4).

Osmolality— Acyclovir sodium (Glaxo Wellcome) 50 mg/ml in sterile water for injection has an osmolality of 348 mOsm/kg (2043).

The osmolality of acyclovir sodium 500 mg was calculated for the following dilutions (1054):

	Osmolality (mOsm/kg)	
Diluent	50 ml	100 ml
Dextrose 5% in water	316	289
Sodium chloride 0.9%	342	316

The osmolality of acyclovir sodium 7 mg/ml was determined to be 278 mOsm/kg in dextrose 5% in water and 299 mOsm/kg in sodium chloride 0.9% (1375).

Sodium Content— Acyclovir sodium (Glaxo Wellcome) contains 4.2 mEq of sodium per gram of drug (4).

Administration— Acyclovir sodium is administered by slow intravenous infusion at concentrations of 7 mg/ml or less over a period of one hour. Rapid intravenous administration over less than one hour and administration by other routes must be avoided (2; 4).

Stability— The reconstituted solution should be used within 12 hours. Refrigeration of the reconstituted solution may cause a precipitate, but this precipitate will dissolve at room temperature, apparently without affecting potency. After dilution for administration, the dose may be stored at room temperature; it should be used within 24 hours (2; 4). However, storage of acyclovir admixtures at room temperature does not guarantee that no precipitate will form. Precipitation has also been observed in acyclovir sodium infusions in PVC containers after a few days' storage at room temperature (2190).

Short-term refrigerated storage of acyclovir sodium admixtures with concentrations exceeding 1 mg/ml may result in formation of a precipitate that redissolves upon warming to room temperature. However, such solutions should be used immediately after warming to room temperature because of the subsequent appearance of persistent microprecipitates (2098).

Physical instability is the principal limitation to long-term storage of acyclovir sodium admixtures. Persistent subvisual microprecipitate formation as well as frank persistent precipitation may occur in variable time periods. Such precipitation has been reported to occur after as little as seven days and in varying time periods throughout a 35-day observation period; the appearance of a precipitate is not precisely predictable (2098).

The formation of large amounts of subvisual particulates has been attributed to an interaction of the highly alkaline acyclovir sodium solution with PVC containers. Some increase in the number of particulates was observed in as little as one day, with substantial increases in seven days. When packaged in ethylene vinyl acetate (EVA) containers, no significant increase in subvisual particulates occurs, even after 28 days of storage (2190).

Elastomeric Reservoir Pumps— Acyclovir sodium (Burroughs Wellcome) 5 mg/ml in both dextrose 5% in water and sodium chloride 0.9% was evaluated for binding potential to natural rubber elastomeric reservoirs (Baxter). No loss was found after storage for two weeks at 35 °C with gentle agitation (2014).

Compatibility Information

Solution Compatibility

Acyclovir sodium

Solution	Mfr	Mfr	Conc/L	Remarks	Ref	C/I
Dextrose 5% in water	TR[a]	BW	5 g	Visually compatible with no loss by HPLC in 37 days at 25 and 5 °C	1343	C
	BA[a]	BW	1 g	Physically compatible with no loss by HPLC after 35 days at 23 °C and after 35 days at 4 °C followed by 2 days at 23 °C protected from light	2098	C
	BA[a]	BW	7 g	Physically compatible with 3% or less loss by HPLC after 28 days at 23 °C protected from light. Subvisual microprecipitate forms by 35 days	2098	C
	BA[a]	BW	7 g	Precipitate forms on refrigeration that redissolves on warming. No loss by HPLC after 35 days at 4 °C protected from light, but subvisual precipitate forms after 2 more days at 23 °C	2098	C

Solution Compatibility (Cont.)

Acyclovir sodium

Solution	Mfr	Mfr	Conc/L	Remarks	Ref	C/I
	BA[a]	BW	10 g	Physically compatible with no loss by HPLC after 21 days at 23 °C protected from light. Subvisual microprecipitate forms in 28 days, and visible precipitate forms in 35 days	2098	**C**
	BA[a]	BW	10 g	Precipitate forms on refrigeration that redissolves on warming. No loss by HPLC after 35 days at 4 °C protected from light, but subvisual precipitate forms after 2 more days at 23 °C	2098	**C**
Sodium chloride 0.9%	TR[a]	BW	5 g	No acyclovir loss by HPLC in 37 days at 25 and 5 °C. Storage at 5 °C resulted in white precipitate that dissolved on warming to 25 °C	1343	**C**
	BA[a]	BW	1, 7, 10 g	Physically compatible with no loss by HPLC after 7 days at 23 °C protected from light. Visible precipitate formed within 14 days	2098	**C**
	BA[a]	BW	1, 7, 10 g	Physically compatible with no loss by HPLC after 35 days at 4 °C followed by 2 days at 23 °C protected from light	2098	**C**
	BA[a]	WEL	2.5 and 5 g	No loss of acyclovir by HPLC in 28 days at 25 °C, but subvisual particulates increased significantly after 7 days due to interaction with PVC containers	2190	**C**
	BA[b]	WEL	2.5 and 5 g	No loss of acyclovir by HPLC and little or no change in subvisual particulates in 28 days at 25 °C in EVA containers	2190	**C**

[a]Tested in PVC containers.
[b]Tested in ethylene vinyl acetate (EVA) containers.

Additive Compatibility

Acyclovir sodium

Drug	Mfr	Conc/L	Mfr	Conc/L	Test Soln	Remarks	Ref	C/I
Dobutamine HCl	LI	1 g	BW	5 g	D5W	Discoloration developed in 25 min and cloudiness and brown color developed in 2 hr due to dobutamine oxidation. No acyclovir loss found	1343	**I**
Dopamine HCl	SO	1.6 g	BW	5 g	D5W	Yellow color developed in 1.5 hr due to dopamine oxidation. No acyclovir loss found	1343	**I**
Fluconazole	PF	1 g	BW	5 g	D5W	Visually compatible with no fluconazole loss by HPLC in 72 hr at 25 °C under fluorescent light. Acyclovir not tested	1677	**C**
Meropenem	ZEN	1 g	BW	5 g	NS	Visually compatible for 4 hr at room temperature	1994	**C**
	ZEN	20 g	BW	5 g	NS	Immediate precipitation	1994	**I**

Y-Site Injection Compatibility (1:1 Mixture)

Acyclovir sodium

Drug	Mfr	Conc	Mfr	Conc	Remarks	Ref	C/I
Allopurinol sodium	BW	3 mg/ml[b]	BW	7 mg/ml[b]	Physically compatible with no change in measured turbidity or increase in particle content in 4 hr at 22 °C	1686	C
Amifostine	USB	10 mg/ml[a]	BW	7 mg/ml[a]	Subvisual needles form in 1 hr. Visible particles form in 4 hr	1845	I
Amikacin sulfate	BR	5 mg/ml[a]	BW	5 mg/ml[a]	Physically compatible for 4 hr at 25 °C	1157	C
Amphotericin B cholesteryl sulfate complex	SEQ	0.83 mg/ml[a]	GW	7 mg/ml[a]	Physically compatible with little or no change in measured turbidity or increase in particle content in 4 hr at 23 °C under fluorescent light	2117	C
Ampicillin sodium	WY	20 mg/ml[b]	BW	5 mg/ml[a]	Physically compatible for 4 hr at 25 °C	1157	C
Amsacrine	NCI	1 mg/ml[a]	BW	7 mg/ml[a]	Immediate dark orange turbidity, becoming brownish orange in 1 hr	1381	I
Aztreonam	SQ	40 mg/ml[a]	BW	7 mg/ml[a]	White crystalline needles form immediately and become dense flocculent precipitate in 4 hr	1758	I
Cefamandole nafate	LI	20 mg/ml[a]	BW	5 mg/ml[a]	Physically compatible for 4 hr at 25 °C	1157	C
Cefazolin sodium	SKF	20 mg/ml[a]	BW	5 mg/ml[a]	Physically compatible for 4 hr at 25 °C	1157	C
Cefepime HCl	BR	20 mg/ml[a]	BW	7 mg/ml[a]	Tiny crystals form in 4 hr	1689	I
Cefoperazone sodium	RR	20 mg/ml[a]	BW	5 mg/ml[a]	Physically compatible for 4 hr at 25 °C	1157	C
Cefotaxime sodium	HO	20 mg/ml[a]	BW	5 mg/ml[a]	Physically compatible for 4 hr at 25 °C	1157	C
Cefoxitin sodium	MSD	20 mg/ml[a]	BW	5 mg/ml[a]	Physically compatible for 4 hr at 25 °C	1157	C
Ceftazidime[g]	SKF	20 mg/ml[a]	BW	5 mg/ml[a]	Physically compatible for 4 hr at 25 °C	1157	C
Ceftizoxime sodium	SKF	20 mg/ml[a]	BW	5 mg/ml[a]	Physically compatible for 4 hr at 25 °C	1157	C
Ceftriaxone sodium	RC	20 mg/ml[a]	BW	5 mg/ml[a]	Physically compatible for 4 hr at 25 °C	1157	C
Cefuroxime sodium	GL	15 mg/ml[a]	BW	5 mg/ml[a]	Physically compatible for 4 hr at 25 °C	1157	C
Chloramphenicol sodium succinate	ES	20 mg/ml[a]	BW	5 mg/ml[a]	Physically compatible for 4 hr at 25 °C	1157	C
Cimetidine HCl	SKF	6 mg/ml[a]	BW	5 mg/ml[a]	Physically compatible for 4 hr at 25 °C	1157	C
Cisatracurium besylate	GW	0.1 and 2 mg/ml[a]	BW	7 mg/ml[a]	Physically compatible with no change in measured turbidity or increase in particle content in 4 hr at 23 °C	2074	C
	GW	5 mg/ml[a]	BW	7 mg/ml[a]	White cloudiness forms immediately	2074	I
Clindamycin phosphate	UP	12 mg/ml[a]	BW	5 mg/ml[a]	Physically compatible for 4 hr at 25 °C	1157	C
Dexamethasone sodium phosphate	ES	0.2 mg/ml[a]	BW	5 mg/ml[a]	Physically compatible for 4 hr at 25 °C	1157	C
Diltiazem HCl	MMD	5 mg/ml	BW	5[a] and 7[b] mg/ml	Cloudiness and precipitate form	1807	I
	MMD	1 mg/ml[b]	BW	5[a] and 7[b] mg/ml	Visually compatible	1807	C
Dimenhydrinate	SE	1 mg/ml[a]	BW	5 mg/ml[a]	Physically compatible for 4 hr at 25 °C	1157	C
Diphenhydramine HCl	ES	1 mg/ml[a]	BW	5 mg/ml[a]	Physically compatible for 4 hr at 25 °C	1157	C
Dobutamine HCl	LI	1 mg/ml[a]	BW	5 mg/ml[a]	Solution turns cloudy and brown in 1 hr at 25 °C under fluorescent light	1157	I

Y-Site Injection Compatibility (1:1 Mixture) (Cont.)

Acyclovir sodium

Drug	Mfr	Conc	Mfr	Conc	Remarks	Ref	C/I
Docetaxel	RPR	0.9 mg/ml[a]	GW	7 mg/ml[a]	Physically compatible with no change in measured turbidity or increase in particle content in 4 hr at 23 °C	2224	C
Dopamine HCl	AB	1.6 mg/ml[a]	BW	5 mg/ml[a]	Solution turns dark brown in 2 hr at 25 °C under fluorescent light	1157	I
Doxorubicin HCl liposome injection	SEQ	0.4 mg/ml[a]	GW	7 mg/ml[a]	Physically compatible with little or no change in measured turbidity and no increase in particle content in 4 hr at 23 °C	2087	C
Doxycycline hyclate	PF	1 mg/ml[a]	BW	5 mg/ml[a]	Physically compatible for 4 hr at 25 °C	1157	C
Erythromycin lactobionate	AB	4 mg/ml[a]	BW	5 mg/ml[a]	Physically compatible for 4 hr at 25 °C	1157	C
Etoposide phosphate	BR	5 mg/ml[a]	GW	7 mg/ml[a]	Physically compatible with no change in measured turbidity or increase in particle content in 4 hr at 23 °C	2218	C
Famotidine	ME	2 mg/ml[b]	BW	7 mg/ml[a]	Visually compatible for 4 hr at 22 °C	1936	C
Filgrastim	AMG	30 μg/ml[a]	BW	7 mg/ml[a]	Physically compatible with no change in measured turbidity or increase in particle content in 4 hr at 22 °C	1687	C
Fluconazole	RR	2 mg/ml	BW	10 mg/ml	Physically compatible for 24 hr at 25 °C	1407	C
Fludarabine phosphate	BX	1 mg/ml[a]	BW	7 mg/ml[a]	Darker color visible with high intensity light within 4 hr	1439	I
Foscarnet sodium	AST	24 mg/ml	BW	10 mg/ml	Immediate precipitation	1335	I
	AST	24 mg/ml	BW	7 mg/ml[c]	Acyclovir crystals form immediately	1393	I
Gemcitabine HCl	LI	10 mg/ml[b]	GW	7 mg/ml[b]	Gross precipitation occurs immediately	2226	I
Gentamicin sulfate	TR	1.6 mg/ml[a]	BW	5 mg/ml[a]	Physically compatible for 4 hr at 25 °C	1157	C
Granisetron HCl	SKB	0.05 mg/ml[a]	BW	7 mg/ml[a]	Physically compatible with no change in measured turbidity or increase in particle content in 4 hr at 23 °C	2000	C
Heparin sodium	ES	50 units/ml[a]	BW	5 mg/ml[a]	Physically compatible for 4 hr at 25 °C	1157	C
Hydrocortisone sodium succinate	LY	1 mg/ml[a]	BW	5 mg/ml[a]	Physically compatible for 4 hr at 25 °C	1157	C
Hydromorphone HCl	WB	0.04 mg/ml[a]	BW	5 mg/ml[a]	Physically compatible for 4 hr at 25 °C	1157	C
Idarubicin HCl	AD	1 mg/ml[b]	BW	5 mg/ml[b]	Haze forms and color changes immediately. Precipitate forms in 12 min	1525	I
Imipenem–cilastatin sodium	MSD	5 mg/ml[b]	BW	5 mg/ml[a]	Physically compatible for 4 hr at 25 °C	1157	C
Lorazepam	WY	0.04 mg/ml[a]	BW	5 mg/ml[a]	Physically compatible for 4 hr at 25 °C	1157	C
Magnesium sulfate	LY	20 mg/ml[a]	BW	5 mg/ml[a]	Physically compatible for 4 hr at 25 °C	1157	C
Melphalan HCl	BW	0.1 mg/ml[b]	BW	7 mg/ml[b]	Physically compatible with no change in measured turbidity or increase in particle content in 3 hr at 22 °C	1557	C
Meperidine HCl	WB	1 mg/ml[a]	BW	5 mg/ml[a]	Physically compatible for 4 hr at 25 °C	1157	C
	AB	10 mg/ml	BW	5 mg/ml[a]	White crystalline precipitate forms within 1 hr at 25 °C under fluorescent light	1397	I
	WY	100 mg/ml	BW	5 mg/ml[c]	Visually compatible for 24 hr at room temperature in test tubes. No precipitate found on filter from Y-site delivery	2063	C

Y-Site Injection Compatibility (1:1 Mixture) (Cont.)

Acyclovir sodium

Drug	Mfr	Conc	Mfr	Conc	Remarks	Ref	C/I
Meropenem	ZEN	1 mg/ml[b]	BW	5 mg/ml[d]	Visually compatible for 4 hr at room temperature	1994	C
	ZEN	50 mg/ml[b]	BW	5 mg/ml[d]	Precipitate forms	2068	I
Methylprednisolone sodium succinate	LY	0.8 mg/ml[a]	BW	5 mg/ml[a]	Physically compatible for 4 hr at 25 °C	1157	C
Metoclopramide HCl	ES	0.2 mg/ml[a]	BW	5 mg/ml[a]	Physically compatible for 4 hr at 25 °C	1157	C
Metronidazole	SE	5 mg/ml	BW	5 mg/ml[a]	Physically compatible for 4 hr at 25 °C	1157	C
Morphine sulfate	WB	0.08 mg/ml[a]	BW	5 mg/ml[a]	Physically compatible for 4 hr at 25 °C	1157	C
	AB	1 mg/ml	BW	5 mg/ml[a]	White crystalline precipitate forms within 2 hr at 25 °C under fluorescent light	1397	I
Multivitamins	LY	0.01 ml/ml[a]	BW	5 mg/ml[a]	Physically compatible for 4 hr at 25 °C	1157	C
Nafcillin sodium	WY	20 mg/ml[a]	BW	5 mg/ml[a]	Physically compatible for 4 hr at 25 °C	1157	C
Ondansetron HCl	GL	1 mg/ml[b]	BW	7 mg/ml[a]	Immediate precipitation	1365	I
Oxacillin sodium	BE	20 mg/ml[a]	BW	5 mg/ml[a]	Physically compatible for 4 hr at 25 °C	1157	C
Paclitaxel	NCI	1.2 mg/ml[a]	BW	7 mg/ml[a]	Physically compatible with no change in measured turbidity in 4 hr at 22 °C	1556	C
Penicillin G potassium	PF	40,000 units/ml[a]	BW	5 mg/ml[a]	Physically compatible for 4 hr at 25 °C	1157	C
Pentobarbital sodium	WY	2 mg/ml[a]	BW	5 mg/ml[a]	Physically compatible for 4 hr at 25 °C	1157	C
Perphenazine	SC	0.1 mg/ml[a]	BW	5 mg/ml[a]	Physically compatible for 4 hr at 25 °C	1157	C
Piperacillin sodium	LE	60 mg/ml[a]	BW	5 mg/ml[a]	Physically compatible for 4 hr at 25 °C	1157	C
Piperacillin sodium–tazobactam sodium	LE	40 + 5 mg/ml[a]	BW	7 mg/ml[a]	Particles form in 1 hr	1688	I
Potassium chloride	IX	0.04 mEq/ml[a]	BW	5 mg/ml[a]	Physically compatible for 4 hr at 25 °C	1157	C
Propofol	ZEN	10 mg/ml	BW	7 mg/ml[a]	Physically compatible for 1 hr at 23 °C with no increase in particle content	2066	C
Ranitidine HCl	GL	1 mg/ml[a]	BW	5 mg/ml[a]	Physically compatible for 4 hr at 25 °C	1157	C
Remifentanil HCl	GW	0.025 and 0.25 mg/ml[b]	BW	7 mg/ml[a]	Physically compatible with no change in measured turbidity or increase in particle content in 4 hr at 23 °C	2075	C
Sargramostim	IMM	10 μg/ml[b]	BW	7 mg/ml[b]	Few small white particles form in 4 hr	1436	I
Sodium bicarbonate	IX	0.5 mEq/ml[a]	BW	5 mg/ml[a]	Physically compatible for 4 hr at 25 °C	1157	C
Tacrolimus	FUJ	1 mg/ml[b]	BW	10 mg/ml[a]	Visually compatible for 24 hr at 25 °C	1630	C
Teniposide	BR	0.1 mg/ml[a]	BW	7 mg/ml[a]	Physically compatible with no subvisual haze or particle formation in 4 hr at 23 °C	1725	C
Theophylline	TR	1.6 mg/ml[a]	BW	5 mg/ml[a]	Physically compatible for 4 hr at 25 °C	1157	C
Thiotepa	IMM[e]	1 mg/ml[a]	BW	7 mg/ml[a]	Physically compatible with no change in measured turbidity or increase in particle content in 4 hr at 23 °C	1861	C
Ticarcillin disodium	TR	30 mg/ml[a]	BW	5 mg/ml[a]	Physically compatible for 4 hr at 25 °C	1157	C
TNA #218 to #226[f]			GW	7 mg/ml[a]	White precipitate forms immediately	2215	I
Tobramycin sulfate	DI	1.6 mg/ml[a]	BW	5 mg/ml[a]	Physically compatible for 4 hr at 25 °C	1157	C
TPN #203 and #204[f]			BW	7 mg/ml	White precipitate forms immediately	1974	I

Y-Site Injection Compatibility (1:1 Mixture) (Cont.)

Acyclovir sodium

Drug	Mfr	Conc	Mfr	Conc	Remarks	Ref	C/I
TPN #212 to #215[f]			BW	7 mg/ml[a]	Crystalline needles form immediately, becoming a gross precipitate in 1 hr	2109	**I**
Trimethoprim–sulfamethoxazole	RC	0.8 + 4 mg/ml[a]	BW	5 mg/ml[a]	Physically compatible for 4 hr at 25 °C	1157	**C**
Vancomycin HCl	LI	5 mg/ml[a]	BW	5 mg/ml[a]	Physically compatible for 4 hr at 25 °C	1157	**C**
Vinorelbine tartrate	BW	1 mg/ml[b]	BW	7 mg/ml[b]	Heavy white precipitate forms immediately	1558	**I**
Zidovudine	BW	4 mg/ml[a]	BW	7 mg/ml[a]	Physically compatible for 4 hr at 25 °C under fluorescent light by visual and microscopic examination	1193	**C**

[a]*Tested in dextrose 5% in water.*
[b]*Tested in sodium chloride 0.9%.*
[c]*Tested in both dextrose 5% water and sodium chloride 0.9%.*
[d]*Tested in sterile water for injection.*
[e]*Lyophilized formulation tested.*
[f]*Refer to Appendix I for the composition of parenteral nutrition solutions. TNA indicates a 3-in-1 admixture, and TPN indicates a 2-in-1 admixture.*
[g]*Sodium carbonate–containing formulation tested.*

Additional Compatibility Information

Recommended infusion solutions are dextrose 5% in water, sodium chloride 0.9%, dextrose 5%–sodium chloride combinations, and Ringer's injection, lactated (857). Biologic or colloidal fluids are not recommended (2).

If acyclovir sodium is diluted in solutions with dextrose concentrations greater than 10%, a yellow discoloration may appear. This discoloration does not affect the drug's potency (4).

ADENOSINE
AHFS 24:04

Adenocard IV   **Fujisawa**
Adenoscan   **Fujisawa**

Products— Adenosine is available under the name Adenocard IV as a 3-mg/ml solution in 2-ml vials and 2- and 4-ml disposable syringes for intravenous bolus injection. Adenosine is also available under the name Adenoscan as a 3-mg/ml solution in 20- and 30-ml vials for intravenous infusion only. Each of these products also contains sodium chloride 9 mg/ml (2).

pH— Adenocard IV: from 5.5 to 7.5. Adenoscan: from 4.5 to 7.5 (2).

Administration— Adenosine injections are administered intravenously. Adenocard IV is given as a rapid bolus injection by the peripheral intravenous route directly into a vein or into an intravenous line close to the patient and is followed by a sodium chloride 0.9% flush. Adenoscan is given by continuous peripheral intravenous infusion only (2).

Stability— Intact containers of adenosine injections should be stored at controlled room temperatures of 15 to 30 °C. They should not be refrigerated, because of possible crystal formation. If crystallization occurs, let the solution warm to room temperature to dissolve the crystals. The solution must be clear prior to administration (2).

Adenosine 6 μg/ml in sodium chloride 0.9% was packaged in 5-ml glass ampuls. Based on HPLC analysis of high-temperature-accelerated decomposition, it was projected that the drug solution would be stable for at least five years at 4 and 25 °C (2115).

Syringes— Undiluted adenosine (Fujisawa) 3 mg/ml was packaged as 25 ml in 60-ml polypropylene syringes (Becton-Dickinson) and sealed with polyolefin tip caps (Sherwood Medical). The syringes were stored at 25, 5, and −15 °C. The solutions remained visually clear, and HPLC analysis showed no loss of adenosine in 7 days at 25 °C, 14 days at 5 °C, and 28 days at −15 °C. The drug's stability in glass vials was essentially identical under the same conditions (2114).

Adenosine (Fujisawa) diluted to 0.75 mg/ml with several infusion solutions was packaged as 25 ml in 60-ml polypropylene syringes (Becton-Dickinson) and sealed with polyolefin tip caps (Sherwood Medical). The syringes were stored at 25, 5, and −15 °C. The solutions remained visually clear, and HPLC analysis showed no loss of adenosine in 14 days for dextrose 5% in lactated Ringer's and lactated Ringer's injection and 16 days for dextrose 5% in water and sodium chloride 0.9% (2114).

Sorption— No loss due to sorption was found for adenosine (Fujisawa) undiluted at 3 mg/ml in polypropylene syringes and diluted to 0.75 mg/ml with infusion solutions in polypropylene syringes and PVC bags (2114).

Compatibility Information

Solution Compatibility

Adenosine

Solution	Mfr	Mfr	Conc/L	Remarks	Ref	C/I
Dextrose 5% in Ringer's injection, lactated	BA[a]	FUJ	750 mg	Visually compatible with no loss by HPLC in 14 days at 25, 5, and −15 °C	2114	C
Dextrose 5% in water	BA[a]	FUJ	750 mg	Visually compatible with no loss by HPLC in 16 days at 25, 5, and −15 °C	2114	C
Ringer's injection, lactated	BA[a]	FUJ	750 mg	Visually compatible with no loss by HPLC in 14 days at 25, 5, and −15 °C	2114	C
Sodium chloride 0.9%	BA[a]	FUJ	750 mg	Visually compatible with no loss by HPLC in 16 days at 25, 5, and −15 °C	2114	C

[a]*Tested in PVC containers.*

NORMAL HUMAN SERUM ALBUMIN
AHFS 16:00

Products— Normal human serum albumin (Immuno-US) is available in 20-, 50-, and 100-ml vials as a 25% aqueous solution. Each 100 ml of solution contains 25 g of serum albumin. Normal human serum albumin is also available as a 5% aqueous solution in 50-, 250-, 500-, and 1000-ml sizes. The products also contain sodium carbonate, sodium bicarbonate, sodium hydroxide, and/or acetic acid to adjust the pH (1-7/98; 4). The products are heat-treated for inactivation of hepatitis viruses. Sodium caprylate 0.08 mmol/g and sodium *N*-acetyltryptophanate 0.08 mmol/g of albumin are added to the products as stabilizers to prevent denaturation during the heat treatment (1-7/98).

pH— From 6.4 to 7.4 (1-7/98; 4).

Sodium Content— From 130 to 160 mEq/L (1-7/98; 4).

Administration— Normal human serum albumin is administered intravenously either undiluted or diluted in an intravenous infusion solution (1-7/98; 4).

Stability— Normal human serum albumin has been variously described as clear amber to deep orange-brown and as a transparent or slightly opalescent pale straw to dark brown solution. The solution should not be used if it is turbid or contains a deposit. Since it contains no preservative, the manufacturer recommends use within four hours after opening the vial (1-7/98; 4). The expiration date is five years after issue from the manufacturer if the labeling recommends storage between 2 and 10 °C, or not more than three years after issue from the manufacturer if the labeling recommends storage at temperatures not greater than 37 °C.

Freezing the albumin solutions may damage the container and result in contamination (4).

Compatibility Information

Solution Compatibility

Normal human serum albumin

Solution	Mfr	Mfr	Conc/L	Remarks	Ref	C/I
Dextran 6% in dextrose 5%	AB		5 g	Physically compatible	3	C
Dextran 6% in sodium chloride 0.9%	AB		5 g	Physically compatible	3	C
Dextrose–Ringer's injection combinations	AB		5 g	Physically compatible	3	C
Dextrose–Ringer's injection, lactated, combinations	AB		5 g	Physically compatible	3	C
Dextrose–saline combinations	AB		5 g	Physically compatible	3	C
Dextrose 2½% in water	AB		5 g	Physically compatible	3	C

Solution Compatibility (Cont.)

Normal human serum albumin

Solution	Mfr	Mfr	Conc/L	Remarks	Ref	C/I
Dextrose 5% in water	AB		5 g	Physically compatible	3	C
Dextrose 10% in water	AB		5 g	Physically compatible	3	C
Fructose 10% in sodium chloride 0.9%	AB		5 g	Physically compatible	3	C
Fructose 10% in water	AB		5 g	Physically compatible	3	C
Invert sugar 5 and 10% in sodium chloride 0.9%	AB		5 g	Physically compatible	3	C
Invert sugar 5 and 10% in water	AB		5 g	Physically compatible	3	C
Ionosol products (except as noted below)	AB		5 g	Physically compatible	3	C
Ionosol D-CM	AB		5 g	Haze or precipitate forms within 24 hr	3	I
Ringer's injection	AB		5 g	Physically compatible	3	C
Ringer's injection, lactated	AB		5 g	Physically compatible	3	C
Sodium chloride 0.45%	AB		5 g	Physically compatible	3	C
Sodium chloride 0.9%	AB		5 g	Physically compatible	3	C
Sodium lactate ⅙ M	AB		5 g	Physically compatible	3	C

Additive Compatibility

Normal human serum albumin

Drug	Mfr	Conc/L	Mfr	Conc/L	Test Soln	Remarks	Ref	C/I
Verapamil HCl	KN	80 mg	ARC	25 g	D5W, NS	Cloudiness develops within 8 hr	764	I

Y-Site Injection Compatibility (1:1 Mixture)

Normal human serum albumin

Drug	Mfr	Conc	Mfr	Conc	Remarks	Ref	C/I
Diltiazem HCl	MMD	5 mg/ml	AR, AT	5 and 25%	Visually compatible	1807	C
Lorazepam	WY	0.33 mg/ml[b]		200 mg/ml	Visually compatible for 24 hr at 22 °C	1855	C
Midazolam HCl	RC	5 mg/ml		200 mg/ml	White precipitate forms immediately	1855	I
Vancomycin HCl		20 mg/ml[a]		0.1 and 1%[b]	Heavy turbidity forms immediately and precipitate develops subsequently	1701	I
Verapamil HCl	LY	0.2 mg/ml[a]	HY	250 mg/ml[a]	Slight haze in 1 hr	1316	I
	LY	0.2 mg/ml[b]	HY	250 mg/ml[b]	Slight haze in 3 hr	1316	I

[a]*Tested in dextrose 5% in water.*
[b]*Tested in sodium chloride 0.9%.*

Additional Compatibility Information

Vehicles— Dextrose 5% in water, dextrose 10% in water, and sodium chloride 0.9% have been recommended as infusion vehicles. Normal human serum albumin has been stated to be compatible with whole blood, plasma, and sodium lactate solutions as well as dextrose and sodium chloride injections (4).

CAUTION—Substantial reduction in tonicity, creating the potential for fatal hemolysis and acute renal failure, may result from the use of sterile water as a diluent. The hemolysis and acute renal failure that result from the use of a sufficient volume of sterile water as a diluent may be life-threatening (4; 1942; 2072; 2073).

Parenteral Nutrition Solutions— The addition of albumin to parenteral nutrition solutions appears to result in visually compatible admixtures for 24 hours. However, occlusion of filters has occurred if the albumin concentration exceeded 25 g/L (854) and, occasionally, even at concentrations of 19.4 and 10.8 g/L (1634). Snyder studied the filtration of albumin 25%, from several suppliers, through

0.22-μm filters using a syringe pump. Four products were filtered over 20 minutes, but the Armour product activated the occlusion alarm after only 3.2 minutes. Use of albumin from suppliers other than Armour in parenteral nutrition solutions resulted in no additional occlusions or flow problems (1634). However, Feldman and Bergman noted that although all U.S. manufacturers of albumin and other plasma proteins use the same cold-alcohol fractionation process, batch-to-batch variations in polymer content occur within all manufacturers' products. Furthermore, parenteral nutrition solution composition, additives, filter composition, and kind of pump may affect flow rates as much as differences in batches or manufacturers (1635).

Albumin has also been found to increase the potential of parenteral nutrition solutions to support the growth of fungi and bacteria. Administration of albumin separately was recommended (573).

ALDESLEUKIN
(INTERLEUKIN-2; IL-2)
AHFS 10:00

Proleukin   **Chiron**

Products— Aldesleukin (Chiron) is available in single-use vials containing 22 million I.U. (1.3 mg of protein). When reconstituted with 1.2 ml of sterile water for injection, each milliliter contains aldesleukin 18 million I.U. (1.1 mg) along with mannitol 50 mg, sodium dodecyl sulfate 0.18 mg, monobasic sodium phosphate 0.17 mg, and dibasic sodium phosphate 0.89 mg. During reconstitution, the sterile water for injection should be directed at the vial's sides. Swirl the contents gently to cause dissolution and avoid excess foaming. Do not shake the vial (2).

pH— The reconstituted product has a pH of 7.2 to 7.8 (2).

Administration— Aldesleukin is administered intravenously; the reconstituted solution should be diluted in 50 ml of dextrose 5% in water and infused over 15 minutes. Inline filters should not be used (2; 4). The drug should be diluted within the concentration range of 30 to 70 μg/ml for administration. Concentrations of aldesleukin below 30 μg/ml and above 70 μg/ml have shown increased variability in drug delivery. Dilution and drug delivery outside this concentration range should be avoided (2).

Only dextrose 5% in water is recommended for intravenous infusion of aldesleukin. Reconstitution or dilution with sodium chloride 0.9% or bacteriostatic water for injection increases aggregation (2; 4).

If aldesleukin concentrations less than 30 μg/ml are necessary for short-term intravenous infusion of 15 minutes, the manufacturer recommends diluting the dose in dextrose 5% in water that contains human serum albumin 0.1% (1890).

Stability— Aldesleukin is a white to off-white powder; it becomes a colorless to slightly yellow liquid when reconstituted (2).

Intact vials should be stored under refrigeration (2). However, aldesleukin in intact vials is stable for at least two months at controlled room temperature (1890). The reconstituted solution, as well as dilutions in infusion solutions for intravenous administration, should also be stored under refrigeration and protected from freezing. Intravenous infusions should be brought to room temperature before administration (2).

The manufacturer indicates that reconstituted and diluted aldesleukin is stable for 48 hours when stored at room temperature or under refrigeration. Refrigeration is recommended because the product contains no antibacterial preservative (2).

The manufacturer also states that reconstitution and dilution procedures other than those recommended may alter aldesleukin delivery and/or pharmacology and should not be used (2).

Syringes— Aldesleukin (Cetus), reconstituted according to label directions, was evaluated for stability when stored in 1-ml plastic syringes (Becton-Dickinson). One- and 0.5-ml aliquots were drawn into these syringes and refrigerated for five days. The product was physically stable and retained activity by biological analysis (cell proliferation assay) throughout the study period (1821).

Reconstituted aldesleukin diluted to a concentration of 220 μg/ml with dextrose 5% in water was repackaged aseptically as 1 ml drawn into tuberculin syringes and stored under refrigeration at 2 to 8 °C. The drug was found to be stable for the 14-day study period (1890).

Ambulatory Infusion Pumps— For continuous intravenous infusion of aldesleukin in concentrations of 70 μg/ml or less via an ambulatory pump at the accompanying higher temperature of near 32 °C, the dose should be diluted in dextrose 5% in water to which human serum albumin at a concentration of 0.1% has been added to maintain aldesleukin stability (1890). The albumin helps keep aldesleukin in its microaggregate state and helps decrease sorption to surfaces, especially at concentrations below 10 μg/ml (4). In the absence of albumin, visually observed precipitation and loss of aldesleukin activity has been found (1890). At concentrations greater than 70 and less than 100 μg/ml at 32 °C, aldesleukin is unstable whether human serum albumin is present or not. In an ambulatory pump at 32 °C at a concentration above 100 μg/ml, it is not necessary to add albumin to maintain aldesleukin stability (1890).

Aldesleukin (Cetus) 5 to 500 μg/ml in dextrose 5% in water was evaluated for stability in PVC containers during simulated administration from pumps (CADD-1, Pharmacia Deltec). At 100 to 500 μg/ml, aldesleukin was stable by biological analysis (cell proliferation assay) for six days at 32 °C and remained visually clear throughout the study period. At concentrations of 5 and 40 μg/ml, however, human serum albumin 0.1% was necessary to maintain physical stability. The aldesleukin solutions with albumin remained clear and retained activity for six days at 32 °C. Without albumin, precipitation occurred within a few hours (1821).

Sorption— Aldesleukin in low concentrations, particularly less than 10 μg/ml, undergoes sorption to surfaces such as plastic bags, tubing, and administration devices. Addition of 0.1% human albumin to the solution decreases the extent of sorption (4).

Filtration— Inline filters should not be used for aldesleukin (2; 4).

Compatibility Information

Y-Site Injection Compatibility (1:1 Mixture)

IL-2

Drug	Mfr	Conc	Mfr	Conc	Remarks	Ref	C/I
Amikacin sulfate	BR	250 mg/ml	RC[c]	4800 I.U./ml[b]	Visually compatible and IL-2 activity by bioassay retained. Amikacin not tested	1552	C
Amphotericin B	SQ	1.6 mg/ml[a]	CHI	33,800 I.U./ml[a]	Visually compatible for 2 hr. Bioassay not possible	1857	C
Calcium gluconate	LY	100 mg/ml	CHI	33,800 I.U./ml[a]	Visually compatible with little or no loss of aldesleukin activity by bioassay	1857	C
Diphenhydramine HCl	SCN	50 mg/ml	CHI	33,800 I.U./ml[a]	Visually compatible for 2 hr. Bioassay not possible	1857	C
Dopamine HCl	ES	1.6 mg/ml[a]	CHI	33,800 I.U./ml[a]	Visually compatible with little or no loss of aldesleukin activity by bioassay	1857	C
Fat emulsion, intravenous	KA	20%	RC[c]	4800 I.U./ml[b]	Visually compatible and IL-2 activity by bioassay retained. Fat emulsion not tested	1552	C
Fluconazole	RR	2 mg/ml[a]	CHI	33,800 I.U./ml[a]	Visually compatible with little or no loss of aldesleukin activity by bioassay	1857	C
Foscarnet sodium	AST	24 mg/ml	CHI	33,800 I.U./ml[a]	Visually compatible with little or no loss of aldesleukin activity by bioassay	1857	C
Ganciclovir sodium	SY	10 mg/ml[a]	CHI	33,800 I.U./ml[a]	Aldesleukin bioactivity inhibited	1857	I
Gentamicin sulfate	ES	40 mg/ml	RC[c]	4800 I.U./ml[b]	Visually compatible and IL-2 activity by bioassay retained. Gentamicin not tested	1552	C
Heparin sodium	BA	100 units/ml	CHI	33,800 I.U./ml[a]	Visually compatible with little or no loss of aldesleukin activity by bioassay	1857	C
Lorazepam	WY	2 mg/ml	CHI	33,800 I.U./ml[a]	Globules form immediately	1857	I
Magnesium sulfate	LY	20 mg/ml[a]	CHI	33,800 I.U./ml[a]	Visually compatible with little or no loss of aldesleukin activity by bioassay	1857	C
Metoclopramide HCl	DU	5 mg/ml	CHI	33,800 I.U./ml[a]	Visually compatible with little or no loss of aldesleukin activity by bioassay	1857	C
Morphine sulfate	SCN	1 mg/ml	RC[c]	4800 I.U./ml[b]	Visually compatible and IL-2 activity by bioassay retained. Morphine not tested	1552	C
Ondansetron HCl	GL	0.7 mg/ml[a]	CHI	33,800 I.U./ml[a]	Visually compatible with little or no loss of aldesleukin activity by bioassay	1857	C
Pentamidine isethionate	FUJ	6 mg/ml[a]	CHI	33,800 I.U./ml[a]	Aldesleukin bioactivity inhibited	1857	I
Piperacillin sodium	LE	200 mg/ml	RC[c]	4800 I.U./ml[b]	Visually compatible and IL-2 activity by bioassay retained. Piperacillin not tested	1552	C
Potassium chloride	AB	0.2 mEq/ml	CHI	33,800 I.U./ml[a]	Visually compatible with little or no loss of aldesleukin activity by bioassay	1857	C
Prochlorperazine edisylate	SKB	5 mg/ml	CHI	33,800 I.U./ml[a]	Aldesleukin bioactivity inhibited	1857	I
Promethazine HCl	ES	25 mg/ml	CHI	33,800 I.U./ml[a]	Aldesleukin bioactivity inhibited	1857	I
Ranitidine HCl	AB	1 mg/ml[d]	CHI	33,800 I.U./ml[a]	Visually compatible with little or no loss of aldesleukin activity by bioassay	1857	C

Y-Site Injection Compatibility (1:1 Mixture) (Cont.)

IL-2

Drug	Mfr	Conc	Mfr	Conc	Remarks	Ref	C/I
Thiethylperazine malate	SZ	0.4 mg/ml[a]	CHI	33,800 I.U./ml[a]	Visually compatible with little or no loss of aldesleukin activity by bioassay	1857	C
Ticarcillin disodium	BE	200 mg/ml	RC[c]	4800 I.U./ml[b]	Visually compatible and IL-2 activity by bioassay retained. Ticarcillin not tested	1552	C
Tobramycin sulfate	LI	40 mg/ml	RC[c]	4800 I.U./ml[b]	Visually compatible and IL-2 activity by bioassay retained. Tobramycin not tested	1552	C
TPN #145[e]			RC[c]	4800 I.U./ml[b]	Visually compatible and IL-2 activity by bioassay retained	1552	C
Trimethoprim-sulfamethoxazole	BW	1.6 + 8 mg/ml[a]	CHI	33,800 I.U./ml[a]	Visually compatible with little or no loss of aldesleukin activity by bioassay	1857	C

[a]*Tested in dextrose 5% in water.*
[b]*Tested in sodium chloride 0.9%.*
[c]*The Roche product is a different form of IL-2 than the Chiron product.*
[d]*Tested in sodium chloride 0.45%.*
[e]*Refer to Appendix I for the composition of parenteral nutrition solutions. TPN indicates a 2-in-1 admixture.*

Additional Compatibility Information

Additives— The manufacturer recommends that aldesleukin not be co-administered with other drugs in the same container (2).

Container Compatibility— Both glass and PVC containers have been used to infuse aldesleukin with comparable clinical results. However, drug delivery may be more consistent with PVC containers (2).

Units— The biological potency of aldesleukin is determined by the lymphocyte proliferation bioassay and is expressed in International Units (I.U.). Aldesleukin 18 million I.U. equals 1.1 mg of protein (2). During the development of aldesleukin, various unit systems were employed. However, the International Unit is now the standard measure of its activity.

ALFENTANIL HCL
AHFS 28:08.08

Alfenta   **Taylor**

Products— Alfentanil HCl (Taylor) is available at a concentration equivalent to alfentanil base 500 μg/ml with sodium chloride for isotonicity in 2-, 5-, 10-, and 20-ml ampuls (1-3/98).

pH— From 4 to 6 (1-3/98).

Administration— Alfentanil HCl is administered by intravenous injection or infusion. For infusion, dilution to 25 to 80 μg/ml in a compatible solution has been utilized (1-3/98).

Stability— Alfentanil HCl injection is stable at controlled room temperature when protected from light (1-3/98).

Syringes— Alfentanil HCl (Janssen) 0.5 mg/ml in 5% dextrose injection was packaged in 20-ml polypropylene syringes (Becton-Dickinson) and stored at 20 °C exposed to light and at 8 °C for 16 weeks. The solutions were visually clear and colorless throughout the study. HPLC analysis found no loss of alfentanil HCl and no peaks for leached substances from the plastic syringes (2191).

Alfentanil HCl (Janssen) 0.167 mg/ml in sodium chloride 0.9% packaged in polypropylene syringes (Sherwood) was physically stable and exhibited little or no loss by stability-indicating HPLC analysis in 24 hours stored at 4 and 23 °C (2199).

Compatibility Information

Solution Compatibility

Alfentanil HCl

Solution	Mfr	Mfr	Conc/L	Remarks	Ref	C/I
Dextrose 5% in water	[a]	JN	500 mg	Visually compatible and no loss by HPLC in 16 weeks at 20 °C exposed to light and at 4 °C	2191	**C**

[a]*Packaged in 20-ml polypropylene syringes.*

Drugs in Syringe Compatibility

Alfentanil HCl

Drug (in syringe)	Mfr	Amt	Mfr	Amt	Remarks	Ref	C/I
Atracurium besylate	BW	10 mg/ml		0.5 mg/ml	Physically compatible and atracurium chemically stable for 24 hr at 5 and 30 °C	1694	**C**
Midazolam HCl	RC	0.2 mg/ml[a]	JN	0.5 mg/ml[a]	Visually compatible with 8% midazolam and 2% alfentanil loss in 3 weeks at 20 °C exposed to light. No alfentanil loss and 7% midazolam loss in 4 weeks at 6 °C in the dark	2133	**C**
Ondansetron HCl	GW	1.33 mg/ml[a]	JN	0.167 mg/ml[a]	Physically compatible with no measured increase in particulates and little or no loss of either drug by HPLC in 24 hr at 4 or 23 °C	2199	**C**

[a]*Diluted with sodium chloride 0.9%.*

Y-Site Injection Compatibility (1:1 Mixture)

Alfentanil HCl

Drug	Mfr	Conc	Mfr	Conc	Remarks	Ref	C/I
Amphotericin B cholesteryl sulfate complex	SEQ	0.83 mg/ml[a]	JN	0.5 mg/ml	Gross precipitate forms	2117	**I**
Cisatracurium besylate	GW	0.1, 2, 5 mg/ml[a]	JN	0.125 mg/ml[a]	Physically compatible with no change in measured turbidity or increase in particle content in 4 hr at 23 °C	2074	**C**
Etomidate	AB	2 mg/ml	JN	0.5 mg/ml	Visually compatible for 7 days at 25 °C	1801	**C**
Propofol	ZEN	10 mg/ml	JN	0.5 mg/ml	Physically compatible for 1 hr at 23 °C with no increase in particle content	2066	**C**
Remifentanil HCl	GW	0.025 and 0.25 mg/ml[b]	JN	0.125 mg/ml[a]	Physically compatible with no change in measured turbidity or increase in particle content in 4 hr at 23 °C	2075	**C**
Thiopental sodium	AB	25 mg/ml	JN	0.5 mg/ml	White pellets form within 24 hr at 25 °C	1801	**I**

[a]*Tested in dextrose 5% in water.*
[b]*Tested in sodium chloride 0.9%.*

Additional Compatibility Information

Solutions— The manufacturer states that alfentanil HCl is physically and chemically stable in dextrose 5% in sodium chloride 0.9%, dextrose 5% in Ringer's injection, lactated, dextrose 5% in water, and sodium chloride 0.9%. The recommended concentration range is 25 to 80 µg/ml (1-3/98).

ALLOPURINOL SODIUM
AHFS 92:00

Aloprim   **Nabi**

Products—— Allopurinol sodium (Nabi) is available in single-use vials containing the equivalent of 500 mg of allopurinol in lyophilized form. Reconstitute with 25 ml of sterile water for injection to yield an almost colorless concentrated solution that is clear to slightly opalescent (1-6/99).

pH— 11.1 to 11.8 (1-6/99).

Administration—— The reconstituted solution must be diluted for use in sodium chloride 0.9% or dextrose 5% in water to a final concentration of no greater than 6 mg/ml. Sodium bicarbonate–containing solutions should not be used for this dilution. The diluted infusion is given as a single infusion daily or in equally divided infusions at 6-, 8-, or 12-hour intervals. The rate of infusion depends on the volume to be infused (1-6/99).

Stability—— Allopurinol sodium is supplied as a white lyophilized powder. The intact vials should be stored at controlled room temperature. Administration should begin within 10 hours of reconstitution. The reconstituted solution and diluted infusion solution should not be refrigerated (1-6/99).

Compatibility Information

Y-Site Injection Compatibility (1:1 Mixture)

Allopurinol sodium

Drug	Mfr	Conc	Mfr	Conc	Remarks	Ref	C/I
Acyclovir sodium	BW	7 mg/ml[b]	BW	3 mg/ml[b]	Physically compatible with no change in measured turbidity or increase in particle content in 4 hr at 22 °C	1686	C
Amikacin sulfate	BR	5 mg/ml[b]	BW	3 mg/ml[b]	Crystals and flakes form within 1 hr	1686	I
Aminophylline	AB	2.5 mg/ml[b]	BW	3 mg/ml[b]	Physically compatible with no change in measured turbidity or increase in particle content in 4 hr at 22 °C	1686	C
Amphotericin B	SQ	0.6 mg/ml[a,b]	BW	3 mg/ml[b]	Natural haze of amphotericin B lost immediately	1686	I
Aztreonam	SQ	40 mg/ml[b]	BW	3 mg/ml[b]	Physically compatible with no change in measured turbidity or increase in particle content in 4 hr at 22 °C	1686	C
Bleomycin sulfate	BR	1 unit/ml[b]	BW	3 mg/ml[b]	Physically compatible with no change in measured turbidity or increase in particle content in 4 hr at 22 °C	1686	C
Bumetanide	RC	0.04 mg/ml[b]	BW	3 mg/ml[b]	Physically compatible with no change in measured turbidity or increase in particle content in 4 hr at 22 °C	1686	C
Buprenorphine HCl	RKC	0.04 mg/ml[b]	BW	3 mg/ml[b]	Physically compatible with no change in measured turbidity or increase in particle content in 4 hr at 22 °C	1686	C
Butorphanol tartrate	BR	0.04 mg/ml[b]	BW	3 mg/ml[b]	Physically compatible with no change in measured turbidity or increase in particle content in 4 hr at 22 °C	1686	C
Calcium gluconate	AMR	40 mg/ml[b]	BW	3 mg/ml[b]	Physically compatible with no change in measured turbidity or increase in particle content in 4 hr at 22 °C	1686	C
Carboplatin	BR	5 mg/ml[b]	BW	3 mg/ml[b]	Physically compatible with no change in measured turbidity or increase in particle content in 4 hr at 22 °C	1686	C
Carmustine	BR	1.5 mg/ml[b]	BW	3 mg/ml[b]	Gas evolves immediately	1686	I
Cefazolin sodium	GEM	20 mg/ml[b]	BW	3 mg/ml[b]	Physically compatible with no change in measured turbidity or increase in particle content in 4 hr at 22 °C	1686	C

Y-Site Injection Compatibility (1:1 Mixture) (Cont.)

Allopurinol sodium

Drug	Mfr	Conc	Mfr	Conc	Remarks	Ref	C/I
Cefoperazone sodium	RR	40 mg/ml[b]	BW	3 mg/ml[b]	Physically compatible with no change in measured turbidity or increase in particle content in 4 hr at 22 °C	1686	**C**
Cefotaxime sodium	HO	20 mg/ml[b]	BW	3 mg/ml[b]	Tiny particles form immediately	1686	**I**
Cefotetan sodium	STU	20 mg/ml[b]	BW	3 mg/ml[b]	Physically compatible with no change in measured turbidity or increase in particle content in 4 hr at 22 °C	1686	**C**
Ceftazidime	LI[c]	40 mg/ml[b]	BW	3 mg/ml[b]	Physically compatible with no change in measured turbidity or increase in particle content in 4 hr at 22 °C	1686	**C**
Ceftizoxime sodium	FUJ	20 mg/ml[b]	BW	3 mg/ml[b]	Physically compatible with no change in measured turbidity or increase in particle content in 4 hr at 22 °C	1686	**C**
Ceftriaxone sodium	RC	20 mg/ml[b]	BW	3 mg/ml[b]	Physically compatible with no change in measured turbidity or increase in particle content in 4 hr at 22 °C	1686	**C**
Cefuroxime sodium	GL	20 mg/ml[b]	BW	3 mg/ml[b]	Physically compatible with no change in measured turbidity or increase in particle content in 4 hr at 22 °C	1686	**C**
Chlorpromazine HCl	RU	2 mg/ml[b]	BW	3 mg/ml[b]	Heavy white turbidity and precipitate form immediately	1686	**I**
Cimetidine HCl	SKB	12 mg/ml[b]	BW	3 mg/ml[b]	Tiny crystals form in 1 hr and become large crystals in 4 hr	1686	**I**
Cisplatin	BR	1 mg/ml	BW	3 mg/ml[b]	Physically compatible with no change in measured turbidity or increase in particle content in 4 hr at 22 °C	1686	**C**
Clindamycin phosphate	AB	10 mg/ml[b]	BW	3 mg/ml[b]	Tiny particles form immediately and become more numerous over 4 hr	1686	**I**
Cyclophosphamide	MJ	10 mg/ml[b]	BW	3 mg/ml[b]	Physically compatible with no change in measured turbidity or increase in particle content in 4 hr at 22 °C	1686	**C**
Cytarabine	SCN	50 mg/ml	BW	3 mg/ml[b]	Tiny particles form within 4 hr	1686	**I**
Dacarbazine	MI	4 mg/ml[b]	BW	3 mg/ml[b]	Small particles form within 1 hr and become large pink pellets in 24 hr	1686	**I**
Dactinomycin	MSD	0.01 mg/ml[b]	BW	3 mg/ml[b]	Physically compatible with no change in measured turbidity or increase in particle content in 4 hr at 22 °C	1686	**C**
Daunorubicin HCl	WY	1 mg/ml[b]	BW	3 mg/ml[b]	Reddish-purple color and haze form immediately. Reddish-brown particles form within 1 hr	1686	**I**
Dexamethasone sodium phosphate	LY	1 mg/ml[b]	BW	3 mg/ml[b]	Physically compatible with no change in measured turbidity or increase in particle content in 4 hr at 22 °C	1686	**C**
Diphenhydramine HCl	PD	2 mg/ml[b]	BW	3 mg/ml[b]	Heavy white turbidity and precipitate form immediately	1686	**I**
Doxorubicin HCl	CET	2 mg/ml	BW	3 mg/ml[b]	Dark red color and haze form immediately. Reddish-brown particles form within 1 hr	1686	**I**

Y-Site Injection Compatibility (1:1 Mixture) (Cont.)

Allopurinol sodium

Drug	Mfr	Conc	Mfr	Conc	Remarks	Ref	C/I
Doxorubicin HCl liposome injection	SEQ	0.4 mg/ml[a]	BW	3 mg/ml	Physically compatible with little or no change in measured turbidity and no increase in particle content in 4 hr at 23 °C	2087	**C**
Doxycycline hyclate	ES	1 mg/ml[b]	BW	3 mg/ml[b]	Small brown particles form immediately. Hazy brown solution with precipitate develops in 4 hr	1686	**I**
Droperidol	JN	0.4 mg/ml[b]	BW	3 mg/ml[b]	Heavy turbidity with particles forms immediately	1686	**I**
Enalaprilat	MSD	0.1 mg/ml[b]	BW	3 mg/ml[b]	Physically compatible with no change in measured turbidity or increase in particle content in 4 hr at 22 °C	1686	**C**
Etoposide	BR	0.4 mg/ml[b]	BW	3 mg/ml[b]	Physically compatible with no change in measured turbidity or increase in particle content in 4 hr at 22 °C	1686	**C**
Famotidine	MSD	2 mg/ml[b]	BW	3 mg/ml[b]	Physically compatible with no change in measured turbidity or increase in particle content in 4 hr at 22 °C	1686	**C**
Floxuridine	RC	3 mg/ml[b]	BW	3 mg/ml[b]	Tiny particles form in 1 to 4 hr	1686	**I**
Fluconazole	RR	2 mg/ml	BW	3 mg/ml[b]	Physically compatible with no change in measured turbidity or increase in particle content in 4 hr at 22 °C	1686	**C**
Fludarabine phosphate	BX	1 mg/ml[b]	BW	3 mg/ml[b]	Physically compatible with no change in measured turbidity or increase in particle content in 4 hr at 22 °C	1686	**C**
Fluorouracil	RC	16 mg/ml[b]	BW	3 mg/ml[b]	Physically compatible with no change in measured turbidity or increase in particle content in 4 hr at 22 °C	1686	**C**
Furosemide	ES	3 mg/ml[b]	BW	3 mg/ml[b]	Physically compatible with no change in measured turbidity or increase in particle content in 4 hr at 22 °C	1686	**C**
Ganciclovir sodium	SY	20 mg/ml[b]	BW	3 mg/ml[b]	Physically compatible with no change in measured turbidity or increase in particle content in 4 hr at 22 °C	1686	**C**
Gentamicin sulfate	ES	5 mg/ml[b]	BW	3 mg/ml[b]	Hazy solution with crystals forms in 1 hr	1686	**I**
Haloperidol lactate	MN	0.2 mg/ml[b]	BW	3 mg/ml[b]	Heavy turbidity forms immediately. Crystals form within 1 hr	1686	**I**
Heparin sodium	ES	100 units/ml[b]	BW	3 mg/ml[b]	Physically compatible with no change in measured turbidity or increase in particle content in 4 hr at 22 °C	1686	**C**
Hydrocortisone sodium phosphate	MSD	1 mg/ml[b]	BW	3 mg/ml[b]	Physically compatible with no change in measured turbidity or increase in particle content in 4 hr at 22 °C	1686	**C**
Hydrocortisone sodium succinate	UP	1 mg/ml[b]	BW	3 mg/ml[b]	Physically compatible with no change in measured turbidity or increase in particle content in 4 hr at 22 °C	1686	**C**
Hydromorphone HCl	KN	0.5 mg/ml[b]	BW	3 mg/ml[b]	Physically compatible with no change in measured turbidity or increase in particle content in 4 hr at 22 °C	1686	**C**

Y-Site Injection Compatibility (1:1 Mixture) (Cont.)

Allopurinol sodium

Drug	Mfr	Conc	Mfr	Conc	Remarks	Ref	C/I
Hydroxyzine HCl	ES	4 mg/ml[b]	BW	3 mg/ml[b]	Heavy white turbidity and precipitate form immediately	1686	I
Idarubicin HCl	AD	0.5 mg/ml[b]	BW	3 mg/ml[b]	Reddish-purple color forms immediately. Particles form within 1 hr. Complete color loss in 24 hr	1686	I
Ifosfamide	MJ	25 mg/ml[b]	BW	3 mg/ml[b]	Physically compatible with no change in measured turbidity or increase in particle content in 4 hr at 22 °C	1686	C
Imipenem–cilastatin sodium	MSD	10 mg/ml[b]	BW	3 mg/ml[b]	Haze and particles form in 1 hr	1686	I
Lorazepam	WY	0.1 mg/ml[b]	BW	3 mg/ml[b]	Physically compatible with no change in measured turbidity or increase in particle content in 4 hr at 22 °C	1686	C
Mannitol	BA	15%	BW	3 mg/ml[b]	Physically compatible with no change in measured turbidity or increase in particle content in 4 hr at 22 °C	1686	C
Mechlorethamine HCl	MSD	1 mg/ml	BW	3 mg/ml[b]	Haze and small particles form immediately and become numerous large particles in 4 hr	1686	I
Meperidine HCl	WY	4 mg/ml[b]	BW	3 mg/ml[b]	Tiny particles form immediately and increase in number over 4 hr	1686	I
Mesna	MJ	10 mg/ml[b]	BW	3 mg/ml[b]	Physically compatible with no change in measured turbidity or increase in particle content in 4 hr at 22 °C	1686	C
Methotrexate sodium	LE	15 mg/ml[b]	BW	3 mg/ml[b]	Physically compatible with no change in measured turbidity or increase in particle content in 4 hr at 22 °C	1686	C
Methylprednisolone sodium succinate	AB	5 mg/ml[b]	BW	3 mg/ml[b]	Haze forms in 1 hr with white precipitate in 24 hr	1686	I
Metoclopramide HCl	DU	5 mg/ml	BW	3 mg/ml[b]	Heavy white precipitate forms immediately	1686	I
Metronidazole	BA	5 mg/ml	BW	3 mg/ml[b]	Physically compatible with no change in measured turbidity or increase in particle content in 4 hr at 22 °C	1686	C
Minocycline HCl	LE	0.2 mg/ml[b]	BW	3 mg/ml[b]	Greenish-yellow color forms in 4 hr	1686	I
Mitoxantrone HCl	LE	0.5 mg/ml[b]	BW	3 mg/ml[b]	Physically compatible with no change in measured turbidity or increase in particle content in 4 hr at 22 °C	1686	C
Morphine sulfate	WI	1 mg/ml[b]	BW	3 mg/ml[b]	Physically compatible with no change in measured turbidity or increase in particle content in 4 hr at 22 °C	1686	C
Nalbuphine HCl	DU	10 mg/ml	BW	3 mg/ml[b]	Tiny particles form in 1 hr, becoming numerous crystals in 4 hr	1686	I
Netilmicin sulfate	SC	5 mg/ml[b]	BW	3 mg/ml[b]	Haze increases and flakes form in 1 hr	1686	I
Ondansetron HCl	GL	1 mg/ml[b]	BW	3 mg/ml[b]	Heavy turbidity forms immediately, becoming white flocculent precipitate	1686	I
Piperacillin sodium	LE	40 mg/ml[b]	BW	3 mg/ml[b]	Physically compatible with no change in measured turbidity or increase in particle content in 4 hr at 22 °C	1686	C

Y-Site Injection Compatibility (1:1 Mixture) (Cont.)

		Allopurinol sodium					
Drug	*Mfr*	*Conc*	*Mfr*	*Conc*	*Remarks*	*Ref*	*C/I*
Plicamycin	MI	0.01 mg/ml[b]	BW	3 mg/ml[b]	Physically compatible with no change in measured turbidity or increase in particle content in 4 hr at 22 °C	1686	**C**
Potassium chloride	AB	0.1 mEq/ml[b]	BW	3 mg/ml[b]	Physically compatible with no change in measured turbidity or increase in particle content in 4 hr at 22 °C	1686	**C**
Prochlorperazine edisylate	SKB	0.5 mg/ml[b]	BW	3 mg/ml[b]	Heavy turbidity forms immediately	1686	**I**
Promethazine HCl	WY	2 mg/ml[b]	BW	3 mg/ml[b]	Heavy turbidity forms immediately, developing white particles in 4 hr	1686	**I**
Ranitidine HCl	GL	2 mg/ml[b]	BW	3 mg/ml[b]	Physically compatible with no change in measured turbidity or increase in particle content in 4 hr at 22 °C	1686	**C**
Sodium bicarbonate	AB	1 mEq/ml	BW	3 mg/ml[b]	Small and large crystals form in 1 hr	1686	**I**
Streptozocin	UP	40 mg/ml[b]	BW	3 mg/ml[b]	Haze and small particles form in 1 hr and increase in 4 hr	1686	**I**
Thiotepa	LE[d]	1 mg/ml[b]	BW	3 mg/ml[b]	Physically compatible with no change in measured turbidity or increase in particle content in 4 hr at 22 °C	1686	**C**
Ticarcillin disodium	BE	30 mg/ml[b]	BW	3 mg/ml[b]	Physically compatible with no change in measured turbidity or increase in particle content in 4 hr at 22 °C	1686	**C**
Ticarcillin disodium–clavulanate potassium	SKB	31 mg/ml[b]	BW	3 mg/ml[b]	Physically compatible with no change in measured turbidity or increase in particle content in 4 hr at 22 °C	1686	**C**
Tobramycin sulfate	LI	5 mg/ml[b]	BW	3 mg/ml[b]	Haze and crystals form in 1 hr	1686	**I**
Trimethoprim–sulfamethoxazole	ES	0.8 + 4 mg/ml[b]	BW	3 mg/ml[b]	Physically compatible with no change in measured turbidity or increase in particle content in 4 hr at 22 °C	1686	**C**
Vancomycin HCl	LY	10 mg/ml[b]	BW	3 mg/ml[b]	Physically compatible with no change in measured turbidity or increase in particle content in 4 hr at 22 °C	1686	**C**
Vinblastine sulfate	LI	0.12 mg/ml[b]	BW	3 mg/ml[b]	Physically compatible with no change in measured turbidity or increase in particle content in 4 hr at 22 °C	1686	**C**
Vincristine sulfate	LI	0.05 mg/ml[b]	BW	3 mg/ml[b]	Physically compatible with no change in measured turbidity or increase in particle content in 4 hr at 22 °C	1686	**C**
Vinorelbine tartrate	BW	1 mg/ml[b]	BW	3 mg/ml[b]	Heavy gelatinous white precipitate forms immediately	1686	**I**
Zidovudine	BW	4 mg/ml[b]	BW	3 mg/ml[b]	Physically compatible with no change in measured turbidity or increase in particle content in 4 hr at 22 °C	1686	**C**

[a]*Tested in dextrose 5% in water.*
[b]*Tested in sodium chloride 0.9%.*
[c]*Sodium carbonate–containing formulation tested.*
[d]*Powder fill formulation tested.*

ALTEPLASE
AHFS 20:40

Activase   **Genentech**

Products— Alteplase (Genentech) is available as a sterile lyophilized powder in 50- and 100-mg vials. The products contain (2):

Alteplase	50 mg	100 mg
L-Arginine	1.7 g	3.5 g
Phosphoric acid	0.5 g	1 g
Polysorbate 80	≤4 mg	≤11 mg

The pH may have been adjusted with phosphoric acid and/or sodium hydroxide. Intact 50-mg vials contain a vacuum, but the 100-mg vials do not (2).

The alteplase vials are accompanied by 50- and 100-ml vials of sterile water for injection for the 50- and 100-mg sizes, respectively. Alteplase should be reconstituted with sterile water for injection only; do not use solutions containing preservatives. Use of the accompanying diluent results in a 1-mg/ml concentration. The manufacturer recommends use of a large bore needle to direct the stream into the lyophilized cake of the 50-mg vials. For the 100-mg vials, the special transfer device should be used. The vials should be swirled gently—not shaken—to dissolve the drug. Although slight foaming may occur, the bubbles will dissipate after standing for several minutes (2).

pH— Approximately 7.3 (2).

Specific Activity— Alteplase is a purified glycoprotein with a specific activity of 580,000 I.U./mg. The 50-mg vial contains 29 million I.U., and the 100-mg vial contains 58 million I.U. (2).

Osmolality— The product has an osmolality of 215 mOsm/kg (2).

Administration— Alteplase is administered by intravenous infusion, directly after reconstitution to a 1-mg/ml concentration or diluted with an equal volume of sodium chloride 0.9% or dextrose 5% in water to a 0.5-mg/ml concentration (2; 4). Dilution to a lower concentration may result in precipitation (4; 1425).

Stability— Alteplase, an off-white lyophilized powder, becomes a colorless to pale yellow solution on reconstitution. Intact vials should be refrigerated or stored at room temperature with protection from extended exposure to light. The 50-mg vials should not be used unless a vacuum is present (2).

Because alteplase has no bacteriostat, the manufacturer recommends reconstitution immediately before use. However, the solution may be administered within eight hours when stored at room temperature or under refrigeration (2). Equal-volume dilutions (0.5 mg/ml) in dextrose 5% in water or sodium chloride 0.9% in either glass bottles or PVC containers are also stable for up to eight hours at room temperature. No other solutions should be used for dilution (2). Exposure to light does not affect the potency of either reconstituted solutions of alteplase or dilutions in compatible infusion solutions (2; 4).

pH Effects— Alteplase in solution is stable at pH 5 to 7.5 (4).

Syringes— A 50-mg vial of alteplase (Genentech), reconstituted with sterile water for injection to a concentration of 1 mg/ml, was diluted with balanced saline solution to a final concentration of 250 μg/ml. Then 0.3-ml (75 μg) portions of the diluted solution were drawn into 1-ml tuberculin syringes and frozen at −70 °C. Alteplase activity was retained for at least one year (2157).

Sodium chloride 0.9% has also been suggested as a suitable diluent for alteplase solution for frozen storage (1822).

However, others have objected to frozen storage of diluted alteplase solution. It was noted that the alteplase formulation has been designed for optimal stability, and dilution to a concentration lower than 500 μg/ml might adversely affect the drug's solubility by diluting the formulation's solubilizing components. Furthermore, it was noted that the calcium or magnesium salts contained in some diluents might interact with the phosphates present in the alteplase formulation to form a precipitate. Indeed, precipitated protein has been found in diluted alteplase after room temperature storage for 24 hours. Frozen storage at −20 °C with subsequent thawing has resulted in changed patterns of light scattering as well. It was recommended that dilution with balanced saline solution and storage of dilutions for any length of time at room temperature or frozen should be avoided (2158).

Use of a diluent containing polysorbate 80, L-arginine, and phosphoric acid to reconstitute and dilute alteplase to 50 μg/ml is reported to permit frozen storage. Although the report did not specify the exact concentrations of the diluent components, it may have duplicated the alteplase vehicle after reconstitution. Use of this diluent for dilution prevented precipitation of the protein upon frozen storage at −20 °C. In addition, the activity in ophthalmic use was found to be unchanged after storage for six months in the frozen state (2159).

Precipitation— Dilution of alteplase (Genentech) to 0.16 and 0.09 mg/ml in dextrose 5% in water (McGaw) resulted in precipitation immediately and in four hours, respectively, due to dilution of the arginine solubilizer. In sodium chloride 0.9%, dilution to 0.2 mg/ml did not result in precipitation (1425).

Compatibility Information

Solution Compatibility

Alteplase

Solution	Mfr	Mfr	Conc/L	Remarks	Ref	C/I
Dextrose 5% in water	MG	GEN	160 mg	Immediate precipitation	1425	I
	MG	GEN	90 mg	Precipitate forms in 4 hr	1425	I

Additive Compatibility

		Alteplase						
Drug	*Mfr*	*Conc/L*	*Mfr*	*Conc/L*	*Test Soln*	*Remarks*	*Ref*	*C/I*
Dobutamine HCl	LI	5 g	GEN	0.5 g	D5W, NS	Yellow discoloration and precipitate form	1856	**I**
Dopamine HCl	ACC	5 g	GEN	0.5 g	D5W, NS	About 30% alteplase clot-lysis activity loss in 24 hr at 25 °C	1856	**I**
Heparin sodium	ES	40,000 units	GEN	0.5 g	NS	Heparin interacts with alteplase. Opalescence forms within 5 min with peak intensity at 4 hr at 25 °C. Alteplase clot-lysis activity reduced slightly	1856	**I**
Lidocaine HCl	AST	4 g	GEN	0.5 g	D5W	Visually compatible with no alteplase clot-lysis activity loss in 24 hr at 25 °C	1856	**C**
	AST	4 g	GEN	0.5 g	NS	Visually compatible with 7% alteplase clot-lysis activity loss in 24 hr at 25 °C	1856	**C**
Morphine sulfate	WY	1 g	GEN	0.5 g	D5W, NS	Visually compatible with 5 to 8% alteplase clot-lysis activity loss in 24 hr at 25 °C	1856	**C**
Nitroglycerin	ACC	400 mg	GEN	0.5 g	D5W, NS	Visually compatible with 2% or less alteplase clot-lysis activity loss in 24 hr at 25 °C	1856	**C**

Y-Site Injection Compatibility (1:1 Mixture)

		Alteplase					
Drug	*Mfr*	*Conc*	*Mfr*	*Conc*	*Remarks*	*Ref*	*C/I*
Dobutamine HCl	LI	2 mg/ml[a]	GEN	1 mg/ml	Haze noted in 20 min by spectrophotometric examination and in 2 hr by visual examination	1340	**I**
Dopamine HCl	DU	8 mg/ml[a]	GEN	1 mg/ml	Haze noted in 4 hr by visual examination	1340	**I**
Heparin sodium	ES	100 units/ml[a]	GEN	1 mg/ml	Haze noted in 24 hr by visual examination. Erratic spectrophotometer readings	1340	**I**
Lidocaine HCl	AB	8 mg/ml[a]	GEN	1 mg/ml	Physically compatible for 12 days by spectrophotometric and visual examination	1340	**C**
Metoprolol tartrate	CI	1 mg/ml	GEN	1 mg/ml	Visually compatible with no alteplase clot-lysis activity loss in 24 hr at 25 °C	1856	**C**
Nitroglycerin	DU	0.2 mg/ml[a]	GEN	1 mg/ml	Haze noted in 24 hr by visual examination. Erratic spectrophotometer readings	1340	**I**
Propranolol HCl	AY	1 mg/ml	GEN	1 mg/ml	Visually compatible with 2% or less alteplase clot-lysis activity loss in 24 hr at 25 °C	1856	**C**

[a]*Tested in dextrose 5% in water.*

Additional Compatibility Information

Preservatives— Alteplase is stated to be incompatible with bacteriostatic water for injection because preservatives can interact with the alteplase molecule (4).

Miscellaneous— Lidocaine HCl, metoprolol tartrate, and propranolol HCl are physically compatible with alteplase when administered by Y-site injection into the running alteplase solution (4).

AMIFOSTINE
AHFS 92:00

Ethyol   **Alza/U.S. Bioscience**

Products— Amifostine (Alza/US Bioscience) is available in vials containing, in lyophilized form, 500 mg of amifostine on the anhydrous basis. The vial contents are reconstituted with 9.7 ml of sodium chloride 0.9% to yield a solution containing amifostine 50 mg/ml (2).

pH— Approximately 7 (234).

Administration— In adults, amifostine is administered once daily as a 15-minute intravenous infusion. The infusion is started 30 minutes before chemotherapy. Patients should be well hydrated prior to intravenous infusion of amifostine and should maintain a supine position during the infusion. Only limited experience in administration to children or elderly patients is available (2; 4).

Stability— The intact vials may be stored at controlled room temperatures of 20 to 25 °C. The manufacturer states that the reconstituted solution is chemically stable for 24 hours under refrigeration but only five hours at 25 °C. The product should not be used if cloudiness or a precipitate is observed (2).

Admixed in PVC bags of sodium chloride 0.9%, amifostine concentrations between 5 and 40 mg/ml are also stable for 24 hours under refrigeration and five hours at 25 °C. The manufacturer does not recommend the use of infusion solutions other than sodium chloride 0.9% (2; 4).

Compatibility Information

Y-Site Injection Compatibility (1:1 Mixture)

				Amifostine			
Drug	*Mfr*	*Conc*	*Mfr*	*Conc*	*Remarks*	*Ref*	*C/I*
Acyclovir sodium	BW	7 mg/ml[a]	USB	10 mg/ml[a]	Subvisual needles form in 1 hr. Visible particles form in 4 hr	1845	I
Amikacin sulfate	DU	5 mg/ml[a]	USB	10 mg/ml[a]	Physically compatible with no change in measured turbidity or increase in particle content in 4 hr at 23 °C	1845	C
Aminophylline	AMR	2.5 mg/ml[a]	USB	10 mg/ml[a]	Physically compatible with no change in measured turbidity or increase in particle content in 4 hr at 23 °C	1845	C
Amphotericin B	AD	0.6 mg/ml[a]	USB	10 mg/ml[a]	Turbidity forms immediately	1845	I
Ampicillin sodium	WY	20 mg/ml[b]	USB	10 mg/ml[a]	Physically compatible with no change in measured turbidity or increase in particle content in 4 hr at 23 °C	1845	C
Ampicillin sodium–sulbactam sodium	RR	20 + 10 mg/ml[b]	USB	10 mg/ml[a]	Physically compatible with no change in measured turbidity or increase in particle content in 4 hr at 23 °C	1845	C
Aztreonam	SQ	40 mg/ml[a]	USB	10 mg/ml[a]	Physically compatible with no change in measured turbidity or increase in particle content in 4 hr at 23 °C	1845	C
Bleomycin sulfate	MJ	1 unit/ml[b]	USB	10 mg/ml[a]	Physically compatible with no change in measured turbidity or increase in particle content in 4 hr at 23 °C	1845	C
Bumetanide	RC	0.04 mg/ml[a]	USB	10 mg/ml[a]	Physically compatible with no change in measured turbidity or increase in particle content in 4 hr at 23 °C	1845	C
Buprenorphine HCl	RKC	0.04 mg/ml[a]	USB	10 mg/ml[a]	Physically compatible with no change in measured turbidity or increase in particle content in 4 hr at 23 °C	1845	C
Butorphanol tartrate	BR	0.04 mg/ml[a]	USB	10 mg/ml[a]	Physically compatible with no change in measured turbidity or increase in particle content in 4 hr at 23 °C	1845	C
Calcium gluconate	AMR	40 mg/ml[a]	USB	10 mg/ml[a]	Physically compatible with no change in measured turbidity or increase in particle content in 4 hr at 23 °C	1845	C

Y-Site Injection Compatibility (1:1 Mixture) (Cont.)

		Amifostine					
Drug	*Mfr*	*Conc*	*Mfr*	*Conc*	*Remarks*	*Ref*	*C/I*
Carboplatin	BR	5 mg/ml[a]	USB	10 mg/ml[a]	Physically compatible with no change in measured turbidity or increase in particle content in 4 hr at 23 °C	1845	**C**
Carmustine	BR	1.5 mg/ml[a]	USB	10 mg/ml[a]	Physically compatible with no change in measured turbidity or increase in particle content in 4 hr at 23 °C	1845	**C**
Cefazolin sodium	MAR	20 mg/ml[a]	USB	10 mg/ml[a]	Physically compatible with no change in measured turbidity or increase in particle content in 4 hr at 23 °C	1845	**C**
Cefoperazone sodium	RR	40 mg/ml[a]	USB	10 mg/ml[a]	Haze forms immediately, becoming cloudy with microprecipitation in 4 hr	1845	**I**
Cefotaxime sodium	HO	20 mg/ml[a]	USB	10 mg/ml[a]	Physically compatible with no change in measured turbidity or increase in particle content in 4 hr at 23 °C	1845	**C**
Cefotetan disodium	STU	20 mg/ml[a]	USB	10 mg/ml[a]	Physically compatible with no change in measured turbidity or increase in particle content in 4 hr at 23 °C	1845	**C**
Cefoxitin sodium	MSD	20 mg/ml[a]	USB	10 mg/ml[a]	Physically compatible with no change in measured turbidity or increase in particle content in 4 hr at 23 °C	1845	**C**
Ceftazidime	LI[c]	40 mg/ml[a]	USB	10 mg/ml[a]	Physically compatible with no change in measured turbidity or increase in particle content in 4 hr at 23 °C	1845	**C**
Ceftizoxime sodium	FUJ	20 mg/ml[a]	USB	10 mg/ml[a]	Physically compatible with no change in measured turbidity or increase in particle content in 4 hr at 23 °C	1845	**C**
Ceftriaxone sodium	RC	20 mg/ml[a]	USB	10 mg/ml[a]	Physically compatible with no change in measured turbidity or increase in particle content in 4 hr at 23 °C	1845	**C**
Cefuroxime sodium	GL	30 mg/ml[a]	USB	10 mg/ml[a]	Physically compatible with no change in measured turbidity or increase in particle content in 4 hr at 23 °C	1845	**C**
Chlorpromazine HCl	SCN	2 mg/ml[a]	USB	10 mg/ml[a]	Subvisual haze forms immediately	1845	**I**
Cimetidine HCl	SKB	12 mg/ml[a]	USB	10 mg/ml[a]	Physically compatible with no change in measured turbidity or increase in particle content in 4 hr at 23 °C	1845	**C**
Ciprofloxacin	MI	1 mg/ml[a]	USB	10 mg/ml[a]	Physically compatible with no change in measured turbidity or increase in particle content in 4 hr at 23 °C	1845	**C**
Cisplatin	BR	1 mg/ml	USB	10 mg/ml[a]	Subvisual haze forms in 4 hr	1845	**I**
Clindamycin phosphate	AST	10 mg/ml[a]	USB	10 mg/ml[a]	Physically compatible with no change in measured turbidity or increase in particle content in 4 hr at 23 °C	1845	**C**
Cyclophosphamide	MJ	10 mg/ml[a]	USB	10 mg/ml[a]	Physically compatible with no change in measured turbidity or increase in particle content in 4 hr at 23 °C	1845	**C**
Cytarabine	CET	50 mg/ml	USB	10 mg/ml[a]	Physically compatible with no change in measured turbidity or increase in particle content in 4 hr at 23 °C	1845	**C**

Y-Site Injection Compatibility (1:1 Mixture) (Cont.)

Drug	Mfr	Conc	Mfr	Conc	Remarks	Ref	C/I
				Amifostine			
Dacarbazine	MI	4 mg/ml[a]	USB	10 mg/ml[a]	Physically compatible with no change in measured turbidity or increase in particle content in 4 hr at 23 °C	1845	C
Dactinomycin	ME	0.01 mg/ml[a]	USB	10 mg/ml[a]	Physically compatible with no change in measured turbidity or increase in particle content in 4 hr at 23 °C	1845	C
Daunorubicin HCl	WY	1 mg/ml[a]	USB	10 mg/ml[a]	Physically compatible with no change in measured turbidity or increase in particle content in 4 hr at 23 °C	1845	C
Dexamethasone sodium phosphate	AMR	1 mg/ml[a]	USB	10 mg/ml[a]	Physically compatible with no change in measured turbidity or increase in particle content in 4 hr at 23 °C	1845	C
Diphenhydramine HCl	PD	2 mg/ml[a]	USB	10 mg/ml[a]	Physically compatible with no change in measured turbidity or increase in particle content in 4 hr at 23 °C	1845	C
Dobutamine HCl	LI	4 mg/ml[a]	USB	10 mg/ml[a]	Physically compatible with no change in measured turbidity or increase in particle content in 4 hr at 23 °C	1845	C
Docetaxel	RPR	0.9 mg/ml[a]	ALZ	10 mg/ml[b]	Physically compatible with no change in measured turbidity or increase in particle content in 4 hr at 23 °C	2224	C
Dopamine HCl	AST	3.2 mg/ml[a]	USB	10 mg/ml[a]	Physically compatible with no change in measured turbidity or increase in particle content in 4 hr at 23 °C	1845	C
Doxorubicin HCl	CET	2 mg/ml	USB	10 mg/ml[a]	Physically compatible with no change in measured turbidity or increase in particle content in 4 hr at 23 °C	1845	C
Doxycycline hyclate	LY	1 mg/ml[a]	USB	10 mg/ml[a]	Physically compatible with no change in measured turbidity or increase in particle content in 4 hr at 23 °C	1845	C
Droperidol	JN	0.4 mg/ml[a]	USB	10 mg/ml[a]	Physically compatible with no change in measured turbidity or increase in particle content in 4 hr at 23 °C	1845	C
Enalaprilat	MSD	0.1 mg/ml[a]	USB	10 mg/ml[a]	Physically compatible with no change in measured turbidity or increase in particle content in 4 hr at 23 °C	1845	C
Etoposide	BR	0.4 mg/ml[a]	USB	10 mg/ml[a]	Physically compatible with no change in measured turbidity or increase in particle content in 4 hr at 23 °C	1845	C
Famotidine	ME	2 mg/ml[a]	USB	10 mg/ml[a]	Physically compatible with no change in measured turbidity or increase in particle content in 4 hr at 23 °C	1845	C
Floxuridine	RC	3 mg/ml[a]	USB	10 mg/ml[a]	Physically compatible with no change in measured turbidity or increase in particle content in 4 hr at 23 °C	1845	C
Fluconazole	RR	2 mg/ml	USB	10 mg/ml[a]	Physically compatible with no change in measured turbidity or increase in particle content in 4 hr at 23 °C	1845	C

Y-Site Injection Compatibility (1:1 Mixture) (Cont.)

		Amifostine					
Drug	Mfr	Conc	Mfr	Conc	Remarks	Ref	C/I
Fludarabine phosphate	BX	1 mg/ml[a]	USB	10 mg/ml[a]	Physically compatible with no change in measured turbidity or increase in particle content in 4 hr at 23 °C	1845	C
Fluorouracil	AD	16 mg/ml[a]	USB	10 mg/ml[a]	Physically compatible with no change in measured turbidity or increase in particle content in 4 hr at 23 °C	1845	C
Furosemide	AB	3 mg/ml[a]	USB	10 mg/ml[a]	Physically compatible with no change in measured turbidity or increase in particle content in 4 hr at 23 °C	1845	C
Ganciclovir sodium	SY	20 mg/ml[a]	USB	10 mg/ml[a]	Subvisual needles form immediately, becoming a dense flocculent precipitate in 1 hr	1845	I
Gemcitabine HCl	LI	10 mg/ml[b]	USB	10 mg/ml[b]	Physically compatible with no change in measured turbidity or increase in particle content in 4 hr at 23 °C	2226	C
Gentamicin sulfate	ES	5 mg/ml[a]	USB	10 mg/ml[a]	Physically compatible with no change in measured turbidity or increase in particle content in 4 hr at 23 °C	1845	C
Granisetron HCl	SKB	0.05 mg/ml[a]	USB	10 mg/ml[a]	Physically compatible with no change in measured turbidity or increase in particle content in 4 hr at 23 °C	2000	C
Haloperidol lactate	MN	0.2 mg/ml[a]	USB	10 mg/ml[a]	Physically compatible with no change in measured turbidity or increase in particle content in 4 hr at 23 °C	1845	C
Heparin sodium	ES	100 units/ml[a]	USB	10 mg/ml[a]	Physically compatible with no change in measured turbidity or increase in particle content in 4 hr at 23 °C	1845	C
Hydrocortisone sodium phosphate	MSD	1 mg/ml[a]	USB	10 mg/ml[a]	Physically compatible with no change in measured turbidity or increase in particle content in 4 hr at 23 °C	1845	C
Hydrocortisone sodium succinate	UP	1 mg/ml[a]	USB	10 mg/ml[a]	Physically compatible with no change in measured turbidity or increase in particle content in 4 hr at 23 °C	1845	C
Hydromorphone HCl	AST	0.5 mg/ml[a]	USB	10 mg/ml[a]	Physically compatible with no change in measured turbidity or increase in particle content in 4 hr at 23 °C	1845	C
Hydroxyzine HCl	WI	4 mg/ml[a]	USB	10 mg/ml[a]	Subvisual haze forms immediately	1845	I
Idarubicin HCl	AD	0.5 mg/ml[a]	USB	10 mg/ml[a]	Increase in turbidity no greater than dilution with D5W alone. No change in particle content in 4 hr at 23 °C	1845	C
Ifosfamide	MJ	25 mg/ml[a]	USB	10 mg/ml[a]	Physically compatible with no change in measured turbidity or increase in particle content in 4 hr at 23 °C	1845	C
Imipenem–cilastatin sodium	MSD	10 mg/ml[a]	USB	10 mg/ml[a]	Physically compatible with no change in measured turbidity or increase in particle content in 4 hr at 23 °C	1845	C
Leucovorin calcium	LE	2 mg/ml[a]	USB	10 mg/ml[a]	Physically compatible with no change in measured turbidity or increase in particle content in 4 hr at 23 °C	1845	C

Y-Site Injection Compatibility (1:1 Mixture) (Cont.)

			Amifostine				
Drug	*Mfr*	*Conc*	*Mfr*	*Conc*	*Remarks*	*Ref*	*C/I*
Lorazepam	WY	0.1 mg/ml[a]	USB	10 mg/ml[a]	Physically compatible with no change in measured turbidity or increase in particle content in 4 hr at 23 °C	1845	**C**
Magnesium sulfate	AST	100 mg/ml[a]	USB	10 mg/ml[a]	Physically compatible with no change in measured turbidity or increase in particle content in 4 hr at 23 °C	1845	**C**
Mannitol	BA	15%	USB	10 mg/ml[a]	Physically compatible with no change in measured turbidity or increase in particle content in 4 hr at 23 °C	1845	**C**
Mechlorethamine HCl	MSD	1 mg/ml	USB	10 mg/ml[a]	Physically compatible with no change in measured turbidity or increase in particle content in 4 hr at 23 °C	1845	**C**
Meperidine HCl	WY	4 mg/ml[a]	USB	10 mg/ml[a]	Physically compatible with no change in measured turbidity or increase in particle content in 4 hr at 23 °C	1845	**C**
Mesna	MJ	10 mg/ml[a]	USB	10 mg/ml[a]	Physically compatible with no change in measured turbidity or increase in particle content in 4 hr at 23 °C	1845	**C**
Methotrexate sodium	LE	15 mg/ml[a]	USB	10 mg/ml[a]	Physically compatible with no change in measured turbidity or increase in particle content in 4 hr at 23 °C	1845	**C**
Methylprednisolone sodium succinate	AB	5 mg/ml[a]	USB	10 mg/ml[a]	Physically compatible with no change in measured turbidity or increase in particle content in 4 hr at 23 °C	1845	**C**
Metoclopramide HCl	ES	5 mg/ml	USB	10 mg/ml[a]	Physically compatible with no change in measured turbidity or increase in particle content in 4 hr at 23 °C	1845	**C**
Metronidazole	BA	5 mg/ml	USB	10 mg/ml[a]	Physically compatible with no change in measured turbidity or increase in particle content in 4 hr at 23 °C	1845	**C**
Minocycline HCl	LE	0.2 mg/ml[a]	USB	10 mg/ml[a]	Bright yellow discoloration forms immediately	1845	**I**
Mitomycin	BR	0.5 mg/ml	USB	10 mg/ml[a]	Physically compatible with no change in measured turbidity or increase in particle content in 4 hr at 23 °C	1845	**C**
Mitoxantrone HCl	LE	0.5 mg/ml[a]	USB	10 mg/ml[a]	Physically compatible with no change in measured turbidity or increase in particle content in 4 hr at 23 °C	1845	**C**
Morphine sulfate	AST	1 mg/ml[a]	USB	10 mg/ml[a]	Physically compatible with no change in measured turbidity or increase in particle content in 4 hr at 23 °C	1845	**C**
Nalbuphine HCl	AST	10 mg/ml	USB	10 mg/ml[a]	Physically compatible with no change in measured turbidity or increase in particle content in 4 hr at 23 °C	1845	**C**
Netilmicin sulfate	SC	5 mg/ml[a]	USB	10 mg/ml[a]	Physically compatible with no change in measured turbidity or increase in particle content in 4 hr at 23 °C	1845	**C**

Y-Site Injection Compatibility (1:1 Mixture) (Cont.)

Amifostine

Drug	Mfr	Conc	Mfr	Conc	Remarks	Ref	C/I
Ondansetron HCl	GL	1 mg/ml[a]	USB	10 mg/ml[a]	Physically compatible with no change in measured turbidity or increase in particle content in 4 hr at 23 °C	1845	**C**
Piperacillin sodium	LE	40 mg/ml[a]	USB	10 mg/ml[a]	Physically compatible with no change in measured turbidity or increase in particle content in 4 hr at 23 °C	1845	**C**
Plicamycin	MI	0.01 mg/ml[a]	USB	10 mg/ml[a]	Physically compatible with no change in measured turbidity or increase in particle content in 4 hr at 23 °C	1845	**C**
Potassium chloride	AB	0.1 mEq/ml[a]	USB	10 mg/ml[a]	Physically compatible with no change in measured turbidity or increase in particle content in 4 hr at 23 °C	1845	**C**
Prochlorperazine edisylate	SN	0.5 mg/ml[a]	USB	10 mg/ml[a]	Immediate increase in subvisual haze	1845	**I**
Promethazine HCl	ES	2 mg/ml[a]	USB	10 mg/ml[a]	Physically compatible with no change in measured turbidity or increase in particle content in 4 hr at 23 °C	1845	**C**
Ranitidine HCl	GL	2 mg/ml[a]	USB	10 mg/ml[a]	Physically compatible with no change in measured turbidity or increase in particle content in 4 hr at 23 °C	1845	**C**
Sodium bicarbonate	AST	1 mEq/ml	USB	10 mg/ml[a]	Physically compatible with no change in measured turbidity or increase in particle content in 4 hr at 23 °C	1845	**C**
Streptozocin	UP	40 mg/ml[a]	USB	10 mg/ml[a]	Physically compatible with no change in measured turbidity or increase in particle content in 4 hr at 23 °C	1845	**C**
Teniposide	BR	0.1 mg/ml[a]	USB	10 mg/ml[a]	Physically compatible with no change in measured turbidity or increase in particle content in 4 hr at 23 °C	1845	**C**
Thiotepa	LE	1 mg/ml[a]	USB	10 mg/ml[a]	Physically compatible with no change in measured turbidity or increase in particle content in 4 hr at 23 °C	1845	**C**
Ticarcillin disodium	BE	30 mg/ml[a]	USB	10 mg/ml[a]	Physically compatible with no change in measured turbidity or increase in particle content in 4 hr at 23 °C	1845	**C**
Ticarcillin disodium–clavulanate potassium	SKB	31 mg/ml[a]	USB	10 mg/ml[a]	Physically compatible with no increase in measured turbidity or increase in particle content in 4 hr at 23 °C	1845	**C**
Tobramycin sulfate	LI	5 mg/ml[a]	USB	10 mg/ml[a]	Physically compatible with no change in measured turbidity or increase in particle content in 4 hr at 23 °C	1845	**C**
Trimethoprim–sulfamethoxazole	ES	0.8 + 4 mg/ml[a]	USB	10 mg/ml[a]	Physically compatible with no change in measured turbidity or increase in particle content in 4 hr at 23 °C	1845	**C**
Trimetrexate glucuronate	USB	2 mg/ml[a]	USB	10 mg/ml[a]	Physically compatible with no change in measured turbidity or increase in particle content in 4 hr at 23 °C	1845	**C**
Vancomycin HCl	AB	10 mg/ml[a]	USB	10 mg/ml[a]	Physically compatible with no change in measured turbidity or increase in particle content in 4 hr at 23 °C	1845	**C**

Y-Site Injection Compatibility (1:1 Mixture) (Cont.)

Amifostine

Drug	Mfr	Conc	Mfr	Conc	Remarks	Ref	C/I
Vinblastine sulfate	LI	0.12 mg/ml[a]	USB	10 mg/ml[a]	Physically compatible with no change in measured turbidity or increase in particle content in 4 hr at 23 °C	1845	C
Vincristine sulfate	LI	0.05 mg/ml[a]	USB	10 mg/ml[a]	Physically compatible with no change in measured turbidity or increase in particle content in 4 hr at 23 °C	1845	C
Zidovudine	BW	4 mg/ml[a]	USB	10 mg/ml[a]	Physically compatible with no change in measured turbidity or increase in particle content in 4 hr at 23 °C	1845	C

[a]*Tested in dextrose 5% in water.*
[b]*Tested in sodium chloride 0.9%.*
[c]*Sodium carbonate–containing formulation tested.*

AMIKACIN SULFATE
AHFS 8:12.02

Products— Amikacin sulfate is available in concentrations of 50 mg/ml in 2-ml vials and 250 mg/ml in 2- and 4-ml vials and 2-ml disposable syringes. The two strengths have the following compositions (2; 29; 154):

	50 mg/ml	250 mg/ml
Amikacin sulfate		
Sodium bisulfite	0.13%	0.66%
Sodium citrate	0.5%	2.5%
Sulfuric acid	to adjust pH	to adjust pH

pH— 4.5 (291). The range is 3.5 to 5.5 (4).

Osmolality— Amikacin sulfate (Apothecon) 250 mg/ml has an osmolality of 913 mOsm/kg; the 50-mg/ml concentration has an osmolality of 186 mOsm/kg (2043).

The osmolality of amikacin sulfate 500 mg was calculated for the following dilutions (1054):

	Osmolality (mOsm/kg)	
Diluent	50 ml	100 ml
Dextrose 5% in water	353	319
Sodium chloride 0.9%	383	349

Sodium Content— The sodium content of amikacin sulfate 50 mg/ml is 0.064 mEq/ml; for the 250-mg/ml concentration, the sodium content is 0.319 mEq/ml (291).

Administration— Amikacin sulfate may be administered by intramuscular injection and intravenous infusion; for intravenous infusion 500 mg may be diluted in 100 to 200 ml of compatible infusion solution and administered to adults over 30 to 60 minutes. The diluent volume should be sufficient for drug infusion over one to two hours in infants and over 30 to 60 minutes in older children (2; 4).

Stability— Amikacin sulfate is supplied as a colorless to pale yellow or light straw-colored solution which is stable for at least two years at controlled room temperature (4). It was reported that aqueous solutions of amikacin sulfate in concentrations of 37.5 to 250 mg/ml retained greater than 90% potency for up to 36 months at 25 °C, 12 months at 37 °C, and three months at 56 °C (291). Aqueous solutions of amikacin sulfate are subject to color darkening because of air oxidation. However, this change in color has no effect on potency (291).

Autoclaving commercially available vials of amikacin sulfate of 50- and 250-mg/ml concentrations at 15 pounds pressure at 120 °C for 60 minutes resulted in no decrease in potency (291).

Amikacin sulfate (Bristol) in concentrations of 250 mg/L and 5 g/L was found to be stable under the following conditions in almost all of the solutions listed under Compatibility Information (except as noted below) (292):

1. Stored for 60 days at 4 °C and then stored for 24 hours at 25 °C.
2. Frozen at −15 °C for 30 days, thawed, and then stored for 24 hours at 25 °C.
3. Frozen at −15 °C for 30 days, thawed, and then stored for 24 hours at 4 °C followed by 24 hours at 25 °C.

Exceptions to storage condition 1 were noted for amikacin sulfate 250 mg/L in Normosol R in dextrose 5% in water and in Surbex T with dextrose 5% in water. Greater than 10% potency loss of amikacin sulfate was noted within 24 hours of room temperature storage in these solutions. The stability of the 5-g/L concentration was satisfactory under these conditions. If storage of the 250-mg/L concentration at 4 °C was limited to 30 days, the amikacin sulfate potency was retained for 24 hours at 25 °C (292).

Amikacin sulfate (Bristol) 750 mg diluted with 1 ml of sodium chloride 0.9% to a final volume of 4 ml was stable, showing about a 2% loss when stored in polypropylene syringes (Becton-Dickinson) for 48 hours at 25 °C under fluorescent light (1159).

Freezing Solutions— Amikacin sulfate (Bristol) 1 g/50 ml of dextrose 5% in water in PVC bags frozen at −20 °C for 30 days and then thawed by exposure to ambient temperature or microwave radiation had no evidence of precipitation or color change and showed 6% or less loss of potency as determined microbiologically. Subsequent storage of the admixture at room temperature for 24 hours also yielded a physically compatible solution which exhibited little or no additional loss of activity (555).

Compatibility Information

Solution Compatibility

Amikacin sulfate

Solution	Mfr	Mfr	Conc/L	Remarks	Ref	C/I
Dextran 75 6% in sodium chloride 0.9%	BA	BR	250 mg and 5 g	Physically compatible and potency retained for 24 hr at 25 °C	292	C
Dextrose 5% in Ringer's injection	BA	BR	250 mg and 5 g	Physically compatible and potency retained for 24 hr at 25 °C	292	C
Dextrose 5% in Ringer's injection, lactated	BA	BR	250 mg and 5 g	Physically compatible and potency retained for 24 hr at 25 °C	292	C
Dextrose 2½% in sodium chloride 0.45%	BA	BR	250 mg and 5 g	Physically compatible and potency retained for 24 hr at 25 °C	292	C
Dextrose 2½% in sodium chloride 0.9%	BA	BR	250 mg and 5 g	Physically compatible and potency retained for 24 hr at 25 °C	292	C
Dextrose 5% in sodium chloride 0.2%	BA	BR	250 mg and 5 g	Physically compatible and potency retained for 24 hr at 25 °C	292	C
Dextrose 5% in sodium chloride 0.33%	BA	BR	250 mg and 5 g	Physically compatible and potency retained for 24 hr at 25 °C	292	C
Dextrose 5% in sodium chloride 0.45%	BA	BR	250 mg and 5 g	Physically compatible and potency retained for 24 hr at 25 °C	292	C
Dextrose 5% in sodium chloride 0.9%	BA	BR	250 mg and 5 g	Physically compatible and potency retained for 24 hr at 25 °C	292	C
Dextrose 10% in sodium chloride 0.9%	BA	BR	250 mg and 5 g	Physically compatible and potency retained for 24 hr at 25 °C	292	C
Dextrose 5% in water	BA	BR	250 mg and 5 g	Physically compatible and potency retained for 24 hr at 25 °C	292	C
	TR[a]	BR	5 g	Physically compatible and potency retained for 24 hr at room temperature	518	C
	TR[a]	BR	20 g	Physically compatible and approximately 2 to 4% loss of potency in 24 hours at room temperature	555	C
	MG[b]	BR	4 g	Activity retained for 48 hr at 25 °C under fluorescent light	981	C
	AB[a]	BR	5 g	Visually compatible and potency by immunoassay retained for 48 hr at 25 °C under fluorescent light and 4 °C in the dark	1541	C
Dextrose 10% in water	BA	BR	250 mg and 5 g	Physically compatible and potency retained for 24 hr at 25 °C	292	C
	SO	BR	250 mg/ 21 ml[c]	Visually compatible with no amikacin loss by TDx in 30 days at 5 °C	1731	C
	SO	BR	500 mg/ 22 ml[c]	Visually compatible with no amikacin loss by TDx in 30 days at 5 °C	1731	C
Dextrose 20% in water	BA	BR	250 mg and 5 g	Physically compatible and potency retained for 24 hr at 25 °C	292	C
Invert sugar 10% in sodium chloride 0.9%	BA	BR	250 mg and 5 g	Physically compatible and potency retained for 24 hr at 25 °C	292	C

Solution Compatibility (Cont.)

Amikacin sulfate

Solution	Mfr	Mfr	Conc/L	Remarks	Ref	C/I
Invert sugar 10% in water	BA	BR	250 mg and 5 g	Physically compatible and potency retained for 24 hr at 25 °C	292	C
Ionosol DCM	AB	BR	250 mg and 5 g	Physically compatible and potency retained for 24 hr at 25 °C	292	C
Mannitol 20% in water	BA	BR	250 mg and 5 g	Physically compatible and potency retained for 24 hr at 25 °C	292	C
Normosol M in dextrose 5% in water	AB	BR	250 mg and 5 g	Physically compatible and potency retained for 24 hr at 25 °C	292	C
Normosol R	AB	BR	250 mg and 5 g	Physically compatible and potency retained for 24 hr at 25 °C	292	C
Normosol R in dextrose 5% in water	AB	BR	250 mg and 5 g	Physically compatible and potency retained for 24 hr at 25 °C	292	C
Sodium chloride 0.25%	BA	BR	250 mg and 5 g	Physically compatible and potency retained for 24 hr at 25 °C	292	C
Sodium chloride 0.45%	BA	BR	250 mg and 5 g	Physically compatible and potency retained for 24 hr at 25 °C	292	C
Sodium chloride 0.9%	BA	BR	250 mg and 5 g	Physically compatible and potency retained for 24 hr at 25 °C	292	C
	TR[a]	BR	5 g	Physically compatible and potency retained for 24 hr at room temperature	518	C
	MG[b]	BR	4 g	Activity retained for 48 hr at 25 °C under fluorescent light	981	C
	AB[a]	BR	5 g	Visually compatible and potency by immunoassay retained for 48 hr at 25 °C under fluorescent light and 4 °C in the dark	1541	C
Sodium chloride 5%	BA	BR	250 mg and 5 g	Physically compatible and potency retained for 24 hr at 25 °C	292	C
Sodium lactate 1/6 M	BA	BR	250 mg and 5 g	Physically compatible and potency retained for 24 hr at 25 °C	292	C
TPN #107[d]			150 mg	Physically compatible and amikacin activity retained for 24 hr at 21 °C by microbiological assay	1326	C

[a]*Tested in PVC containers.*
[b]*Tested in glass containers.*
[c]*Tested as a concentrate in glass vials.*
[d]*Refer to Appendix I for the composition of parenteral nutrition solutions. TPN indicates a 2-in-1 admixture.*

Additive Compatibility

Amikacin sulfate

Drug	Mfr	Conc/L	Mfr	Conc/L	Test Soln	Remarks	Ref	C/I
Aminophylline	SE	5 g	BR	5 g	LR, NS, R, SL	Physically compatible and amikacin potency retained for 24 hr at 25 °C. Aminophylline not analyzed	294	C
	SE	5 g	BR	5 g	D5LR, D5R, D5S, D5W, D10W, IS10	Greater than 10% amikacin decomposition after 8 hr but within 24 hr at 25 °C. Aminophylline not analyzed	294	I

Additive Compatibility (Cont.)

Amikacin sulfate

Drug	Mfr	Conc/L	Mfr	Conc/L	Test Soln	Remarks	Ref	C/I
Amobarbital sodium	LI	100 mg	BR	5 g	a	Physically compatible and potency of both retained for 24 hr at 25 °C	294	**C**
Amphotericin B	SQ	100 mg	BR	5 g	a	Immediate precipitate	293	**I**
Ampicillin sodium	BR	30 g	BR	5 g	a	Greater than 10% ampicillin decomposition in 4 hr at 25 °C	293	**I**
Ascorbic acid injection[b]	CO	5 g	BR	5 g	a	Physically compatible and potency of both retained for 24 hr at 25 °C	294	**C**
Bleomycin sulfate	BR	20 and 30 units	BR	1.25 g	NS	Physically compatible and bleomycin activity retained for 1 week at 4 °C. Amikacin not tested	763	**C**
Calcium chloride	UP	1 g	BR	5 g	a	Physically compatible and potency of both retained for 24 hr at 25 °C	294	**C**
Calcium gluconate	UP	500 mg	BR	5 g	a	Physically compatible and potency of both retained for 24 hr at 25 °C	294	**C**
Cefazolin sodium	LI	20 g	BR	5 g	a	Potency of both retained for at least 8 hr at 25 °C. Turbidity observed at 24 hr	293	**I**
Cefepime HCl	BR	4 g	BR	6 g	D5W, NS	Visually compatible with 6% cefepime loss by HPLC in 24 hr at room temperature and 4% loss in 7 days at 5 °C. No amikacin loss by bioassay	1681	**C**
Cefoxitin sodium	MSD	5 g	BR	5 g	D5S	9% cefoxitin decomposition at 25 °C and none at 5 °C over 48 hr. No amikacin decomposition at 25 °C and 1% at 5 °C over 48 hr	308	**C**
Chloramphenicol sodium succinate	PD	10 g	BR	5 g	a	Physically compatible and potency of both retained for 24 hr at 25 °C	293	**C**
Chlorothiazide sodium	MSD	10 mg	BR	5 g	a	Precipitate forms within 4 hr at 25 °C	294	**I**
Chlorpheniramine maleate	SC	40 mg	BR	5 g	a	Physically compatible and potency of both retained for 24 hr at 25 °C	294	**C**
Cimetidine HCl	SKF	1.5 g	BR	2.5 g	D5W	Physically compatible and cimetidine chemically stable for 24 hr at room temperature. Amikacin not tested	551	**C**
Ciprofloxacin	MI	1.6 g	BR	4.1 g	D5W, NS	Visually compatible and ciprofloxacin potency by HPLC and amikacin potency by immunoassay retained for 48 hr at 25 °C under fluorescent light	1541	**C**
Clindamycin phosphate	UP	6 g	BR	5 g	a	Physically compatible and amikacin potency retained for 24 hr at 25 °C. Clindamycin not analyzed	293	**C**
	UP	9 g	AB	4 g	D5W, NS[c]	Physically compatible and potency of both drugs retained for 48 hr at room temperature with exposure to light and for 1 week frozen	174	**C**
	UP	9 g	AB	4 g	D5W, NS[c]	Potency of both drugs retained for 48 hr at 25 °C under fluorescent light	981	**C**
Colistimethate sodium	WC	500 mg	BR	5 g	a	Physically compatible and amikacin potency retained for 24 hr at 25 °C. Colistimethate not analyzed	293	**C**

Additive Compatibility (Cont.)

Amikacin sulfate

Drug	Mfr	Conc/L	Mfr	Conc/L	Test Soln	Remarks	Ref	C/I
Dexamethasone sodium phosphate	MSD	40 mg	BR	5 g	[a]	Physically compatible and potency of both retained for 24 hr at 25 °C	294	C
	MSD	40 mg	BR	5 g	D2.5S	16% dexamethasone decomposition in 4 hr at 25 °C	294	I
Dimenhydrinate	SE	100 mg	BR	5 g	[a]	Physically compatible and potency of both retained for 24 hr at 25 °C	294	C
Diphenhydramine HCl	PD	100 mg	BR	5 g	[a]	Physically compatible and potency of both retained for 24 hr at 25 °C	294	C
Epinephrine HCl	PD	2.5 mg	BR	5 g	[a]	Physically compatible and potency of both retained for 24 hr at 25 °C	294	C
Ergonovine maleate	LI	0.2 mg	BR	5 g	[a]	Physically compatible and amikacin potency retained for 24 hr at 25 °C. Ergonovine not analyzed	294	C
Fluconazole	PF	1 g	BR	2.5 g	D5W	Visually compatible with no fluconazole loss by HPLC in 72 hr at 25 °C under fluorescent light. Amikacin not tested	1677	C
Furosemide	HO	160 mg	BR	2 g	D5W, NS	Transient cloudiness during admixture. Then physically compatible for 24 hr at 21 °C	876	C
Heparin sodium	AB	30,000 units	BR	5 g	[a]	Immediate precipitation	294	I
Hyaluronidase	SE	150 units	BR	5 g	[a]	Physically compatible and amikacin potency retained for 24 hr at 25 °C. Hyaluronidase not analyzed	294	C
Hydrocortisone sodium phosphate	MSD	250 mg	BR	5 g	[a]	Physically compatible and potency of both retained for 24 hr at 25 °C	294	C
Hydrocortisone sodium succinate	UP	200 mg	BR	5 g	[a]	Physically compatible and potency of both retained for 24 hr at 25 °C	294	C
Lincomycin HCl	UP	10 g	BR	5 g	[a]	Physically compatible and potency of both retained for 24 hr at 25 °C	293	C
Metaraminol bitartrate	BR	200 mg	BR	5 g	[a]	Physically compatible and potency of both retained for 24 hr at 25 °C	294	C
Metronidazole	RP	5 g[d]	BR	5 g		Physically compatible with little or no pH change for at least 12 hr at 23 °C	807	C
Metronidazole HCl with sodium bicarbonate	SE AB	5 g 50 mEq	BR	2.25 g	D5W, NS	Physically compatible for 48 hr	765	C
Norepinephrine bitartrate	WI	8 mg	BR	5 g	[a]	Physically compatible and potency of both retained for 24 hr at 25 °C	294	C
Oxacillin sodium	BR	2 g	BR	5 g	D5LR, D5R, D5S, D5W, D10W, IS10, LR, NS, R	Physically compatible and potency of both retained for 24 hr at 25 °C	293	C
	BR	2 g	BR	5 g	NR, SL	Oxacillin potency retained through 8 hr at 25 °C. Greater than 10% decomposition in 24 hr	293	I

Additive Compatibility (Cont.)

Amikacin sulfate

Drug	Mfr	Conc/L	Mfr	Conc/L	Test Soln	Remarks	Ref	C/I
Penicillin G potassium	LI	20 million units	BR	5 g	D5LR, D5R, D5S, D5W, D10W, LR, NS, R, SL	Physically compatible and potency of both retained for 24 hr at 25 °C	293	C
	LI	20 million units	BR	5 g	IG–D5W, IS10	Potency of penicillin retained through 8 hr at 25 °C. Greater than 10% decomposition in 24 hr	293	I
Pentobarbital sodium	AB	100 mg	BR	5 g	a	Physically compatible and potency of both retained for 24 hr at 25 °C	294	C
Phenobarbital sodium	LI	300 mg	BR	5 g	a	Physically compatible and potency of both retained for 24 hr at 25 °C	294	C
Phenytoin sodium	PD	250 mg	BR	5 g	a	Immediate precipitation	294	I
Phytonadione	MSD	200 mg	BR	5 g	a	Physically compatible and amikacin potency retained for 24 hr at 25 °C. Phytonadione not analyzed	294	C
Polymyxin B sulfate	BW	200 mg	BR	5 g	a	Physically compatible and amikacin potency retained for 24 hr at 25 °C. Polymyxin not analyzed	293	C
Potassium chloride	LI	3 g	BR	5 g	a	Physically compatible and potency of both retained for 24 hr at 25 °C	294	C
	LI	3 g	BR	5 g	DXN–S	14% amikacin decomposition in 4 hr at 25 °C	294	I
Prochlorperazine edisylate	SKF	20 mg	BR	5 g	a	Physically compatible and potency of both retained for 24 hr at 25 °C	294	C
Promethazine HCl	WY	100 mg	BR	5 g	a	Physically compatible and potency of both retained for 24 hr at 25 °C	294	C
Ranitidine HCl	GL	100 mg	BR	1 g	D5W	Physically compatible for 24 hr at ambient temperature under fluorescent light	1151	C
	GL	50 mg and 2 g		2.5 g	D5W	Physically compatible and ranitidine chemically stable by HPLC for 24 hr at 25 °C. Amikacin not tested	1515	C
Sodium bicarbonate	BR	15 g	BR	5 g	a	Physically compatible and potency of both retained for 24 hr at 25 °C	294	C
Succinylcholine chloride	SQ	2 g	BR	5 g	a	Physically compatible and potency of both retained for 24 hr at 25 °C	294	C
Thiopental sodium	AB	4 g	BR	5 g	a	Immediate precipitation	294	I
Vancomycin HCl	LI	2 g	BR	5 g	a	Physically compatible and amikacin potency retained for 24 hr at 25 °C. Vancomycin not analyzed	293	C
Verapamil HCl	KN	80 mg	BR	2 g	D5W, NS	Physically compatible for 24 hr	764	C
Vitamin B complex with C	AB	5 ml	BR	5 g	a	Red precipitate forms within 24 hr	294	I

[a]*Tested in the following solutions: D5R, D5LR, D5¼S, D5½S, D5S, D5W, D10W, IS10, NS, LR, R, and SL.*
[b]*Present as calcium ascorbate.*
[c]*Tested in glass containers.*
[d]*Minibags (100 ml) containing metronidazole 500 mg with disodium phosphate 150 mg, citric acid 44 mg, and sodium chloride 740 mg. This product differs from the Searle product.*

Drugs in Syringe Compatibility

		Amikacin sulfate					
Drug (in syringe)	Mfr	Amt	Mfr	Amt	Remarks	Ref	C/I
Clindamycin phosphate	UP	900 mg/ 6 ml	BR	750 mg/ 4 ml[a]	Physically compatible with little or no loss of either drug in 48 hr at 25 °C in polypropylene syringes	1159	**C**
Doxapram HCl	RB	400 mg/ 20 ml		100 mg/ 2 ml	Physically compatible with no doxapram loss in 24 hr	1177	**C**
Heparin sodium		2500 units/ 1 ml		100 mg	Turbidity or precipitate forms within 5 min	1053	**I**

[a]Diluted to 4 ml with 1 ml of sodium chloride 0.9%.

Y-Site Injection Compatibility (1:1 Mixture)

		Amikacin sulfate					
Drug	Mfr	Conc	Mfr	Conc	Remarks	Ref	C/I
Acyclovir sodium	BW	5 mg/ml[a]	BR	5 mg/ml[a]	Physically compatible for 4 hr at 25 °C	1157	**C**
Allopurinol sodium	BW	3 mg/ml[b]	BR	5 mg/ml[b]	Crystals and flakes form within 1 hr	1686	**I**
Amifostine	USB	10 mg/ml[a]	DU	5 mg/ml[a]	Physically compatible with no change in measured turbidity or increase in particle content in 4 hr at 23 °C	1845	**C**
Amiodarone HCl	LZ	4 mg/ml[c]	BR	5 mg/ml[c]	Physically compatible for 4 hr at room temperature	1444	**C**
Amphotericin B cholesteryl sulfate complex	SEQ	0.83 mg/ml[a]	AB	5 mg/ml[a]	Gross precipitate forms	2117	**I**
Amsacrine	NCI	1 mg/ml[a]	BR	5 mg/ml[a]	Physically compatible for 4 hr at room temperature under fluorescent light	1381	**C**
Aztreonam	SQ	40 mg/ml[a]	BMS	5 mg/ml[a]	Physically compatible with no subvisual haze or particle formation in 4 hr at 23 °C	1758	**C**
Cefpirome sulfate	HO	50 mg/ml[d]	APC	0.5 mg/ml[d]	Visually and microscopically compatible with less than 6% cefpirome loss and less than 10% amikacin loss by HPLC in 8 hr at 23 °C	2044	**C**
Cisatracurium besylate	GW	0.1, 2, 5 mg/ml[a]	AB	5 mg/ml[a]	Physically compatible with no change in measured turbidity or increase in particle content in 4 hr at 23 °C	2074	**C**
Cyclophosphamide	MJ	20 mg/ml[a]	BR	5 mg/ml[a]	Physically compatible for 4 hr at 25 °C	1194	**C**
Dexamethasone sodium phosphate	AMR	4 mg/ml	SQ	50 mg/ml[e]	Visually compatible for 24 hr at room temperature in test tubes. No precipitate found on filter from Y-site delivery	2063	**C**
Diltiazem HCl	MMD	5 mg/ml	BR	5[b] and 250 mg/ml	Visually compatible	1807	**C**
Docetaxel	RPR	0.9 mg/ml[a]	AB	5 mg/ml[a]	Physically compatible with no change in measured turbidity or increase in particle content in 4 hr at 23 °C	2224	**C**
Enalaprilat	MSD	0.05 mg/ml[b]	BR	2 mg/ml[a]	Physically compatible for 24 hr at room temperature under fluorescent light	1355	**C**
Esmolol HCl	DCC	10 mg/ml[a]	BR	5 mg/ml[a]	Physically compatible for 24 hr at 22 °C	1169	**C**

Y-Site Injection Compatibility (1:1 Mixture) (Cont.)

Amikacin sulfate

Drug	Mfr	Conc	Mfr	Conc	Remarks	Ref	C/I
Etoposide phosphate	BR	5 mg/ml[a]	APC	5 mg/ml[a]	Physically compatible with no change in measured turbidity or increase in particle content in 4 hr at 23 °C	2218	C
Filgrastim	AMG	30 μg/ml[a]	ES	5 mg/ml[a]	Physically compatible with no change in measured turbidity or increase in particle content in 4 hr at 22 °C	1687	C
	AMG	10[f] and 40[a] μg/ml	BMS	5 mg/ml[a]	Visually compatible with little or no loss of filgrastim activity by bioassay and amikacin by immunoassay in 4 hr at 25 °C	2060	C
Fluconazole	RR	2 mg/ml	BR	20 mg/ml	Physically compatible for 24 hr at 25 °C	1407	C
Fludarabine phosphate	BX	1 mg/ml[a]	BR	5 mg/ml[a]	Physically compatible for 4 hr at room temperature under fluorescent light	1439	C
Foscarnet sodium	AST	24 mg/ml	BR	20 mg/ml	Physically compatible for 24 hr at room temperature under fluorescent light	1335	C
Furosemide	HO	10 mg/ml	BR	2 mg/ml[c]	Physically compatible for 24 hr at 21 °C	876	C
Gemcitabine HCl	LI	10 mg/ml[b]	APC	5 mg/ml[b]	Physically compatible with no change in measured turbidity or increase in particle content in 4 hr at 23 °C	2226	C
Granisetron HCl	SKB	0.05 mg/ml[a]	AB	5 mg/ml[a]	Physically compatible with no change in measured turbidity or increase in particle content in 4 hr at 23 °C	2000	C
Hetastarch	DCC	6%	BR	5 mg/ml[a]	Small crystals formed immediately after mixing and persisted for 4 hr	1313	I
Idarubicin HCl	AD	1 mg/ml[b]	BR	5 mg/ml[a]	Physically compatible for 24 hr at 25 °C	1525	C
IL-2	RC	4800 I.U./ml[b]	BR	250 mg/ml	Visually compatible and IL-2 activity by bioassay retained. Amikacin not tested	1552	C
Labetalol HCl	SC	1 mg/ml[a]	BR	5 mg/ml[a]	Physically compatible for 24 hr at 18 °C	1171	C
Lorazepam	WY	0.33 mg/ml[b]	BMS	5 mg/ml	Visually compatible for 24 hr at 22 °C	1855	C
Magnesium sulfate	IX	16.7, 33.3, 66.7, 100 mg/ml[a]	BR	5 mg/ml[a]	Physically compatible for at least 4 hr at 32 °C	813	C
Melphalan HCl	BW	0.1 mg/ml[b]	BR	5 mg/ml[b]	Physically compatible with no change in measured turbidity or increase in particle content in 3 hr at 22 °C	1557	C
Midazolam HCl	RC	5 mg/ml	BMS	5 mg/ml	Visually compatible for 24 hr at 22 °C	1855	C
Morphine sulfate	WI	1 mg/ml[a]	BR	5 mg/ml[a]	Physically compatible for at least 4 hr at 25 °C under fluorescent light	987	C
Ondansetron HCl	GL	1 mg/ml[b]	BR	5 mg/ml[a]	Physically compatible for 4 hr at 22 °C	1365	C
Paclitaxel	NCI	1.2 mg/ml[a]	BR	5 mg/ml[a]	Physically compatible with no change in measured turbidity in 4 hr at 22 °C	1556	C
Perphenazine	SC	0.02 mg/ml[a]	BR	5 mg/ml[a]	Physically compatible for 4 hr at 25 °C	1155	C
Propofol	ZEN	10 mg/ml	DU	5 mg/ml[a]	White precipitate and yellow color form immediately	2066	I
Remifentanil HCl	GW	0.025 and 0.25 mg/ml[b]	AB	5 mg/ml[a]	Physically compatible with no change in measured turbidity or increase in particle content in 4 hr at 23 °C	2075	C

Y-Site Injection Compatibility (1:1 Mixture) (Cont.)

Amikacin sulfate

Drug	Mfr	Conc	Mfr	Conc	Remarks	Ref	C/I
Sargramostim	IMM	10 µg/ml[b]	BR	5 mg/ml[b]	Physically compatible for 4 hr at 22 °C	1436	C
Teniposide	BR	0.1 mg/ml[a]	BR	5 mg/ml[a]	Physically compatible with no subvisual haze or particle formation in 4 hr at 23 °C	1725	C
Thiotepa	IMM[g]	1 mg/ml[a]	DU	5 mg/ml[a]	Physically compatible with no change in measured turbidity or increase in particle content in 4 hr at 23 °C	1861	C
TNA #97 to #104[h]			BR	250 mg/ml	Broken fat emulsion with oil floating in admixtures	1324	I
TNA #218 to #226[h]			AB	5 mg/ml[a]	Visually compatible with no precipitate or emulsion damage apparent in 4 hr at 23 °C	2215	C
TPN #54[h]				250 mg/ml	Physically compatible and amikacin activity retained over 6 hr at 22 °C by microbiological assay	1045	C
TPN #61[h]		[i]	BR	37.5 mg/0.15 ml[j]	Physically compatible	1012	C
		[k]	BR	225 mg/0.9 ml[j]	Physically compatible	1012	C
TPN #91[h]		[l]		15 mg[m]	Physically compatible	1170	C
TPN #203 and #204[h]			APC	5 mg/ml	Visually compatible for 2 hr at 23 °C	1974	C
TPN #212 to #215[h]			AB	5 mg/ml[a]	Physically compatible with no change in measured turbidity or increase in particle content in 4 hr at 23 °C	2109	C
Vinorelbine tartrate	BW	1 mg/ml[b]	BR	5 mg/ml[b]	Physically compatible with no change in measured turbidity or increase in particle content in 4 hr at 22 °C	1558	C
Warfarin sodium	DU	0.1[c] and 2 mg/ml[n]	AB	5 mg/ml[c]	Physically compatible with no change in measured turbidity or increase in particle content in 24 hr at 23 °C	2011	C
Zidovudine	BW	4 mg/ml[a]	BR	4 mg/ml[a]	Physically compatible for 4 hr at 25 °C under fluorescent light by visual and microscopic examination	1193	C

[a]Tested in dextrose 5% in water.
[b]Tested in sodium chloride 0.9%.
[c]Tested in both dextrose 5% in water and sodium chloride 0.9%.
[d]Tested in dextrose 5% in water, Ringer's injection, lactated, sodium chloride 0.45%, and sodium chloride 0.9%.
[e]Tested in sodium chloride 0.45%.
[f]Tested in dextrose 5% in water with human albumin 2 mg/ml.
[g]Lyophilized formulation tested.
[h]Refer to Appendix I for the composition of parenteral nutrition solutions. TNA indicates a 3-in-1 admixture, and TPN indicates a 2-in-1 admixture.
[i]Run at 21 ml/hr.
[j]Given over 30 minutes by syringe pump.
[k]Run at 94 ml/hr.
[l]Run at 10 ml/hr.
[m]Given over one hour by syringe pump.
[n]Tested in sterile water for injection.

Additional Compatibility Information

The manufacturer recommends that other drugs not be physically combined with amikacin sulfate but be administered separately (2).

Vehicles— Amikacin sulfate 250 mg/L and 5 g/L is stable for 24 hours at room temperature in the following infusion solutions (2):

Dextrose 5% in sodium chloride 0.2%
Dextrose 5% in sodium chloride 0.45%
Dextrose 5% in water
Normosol M in dextrose 5%
Normosol R in dextrose 5%
Plasma-Lyte 56 in dextrose 5%
Plasma-Lyte 148 in dextrose 5%
Ringer's injection, lactated
Sodium chloride 0.9%

β-Lactam Antibiotics— In common with other aminoglycoside antibiotics, amikacin activity may be impaired by β-lactam antibiotics. This inactivation is dependent on concentration, temperature, and time of exposure. However, amikacin appears to be less affected by the β-lactam antibiotics than other aminoglycosides such as gentamicin and tobramycin.

Incubation of amikacin 10 mg/L in sodium chloride 0.9% with 500 mg/L of carbenicillin or ticarcillin at 37 °C for 24 hours resulted in about a 25% reduction in amikacin activity. When serum was substituted for the sodium chloride solution, only 10% or less reduction in activity was reported. However, when the drugs were buffered to pH 7.4 in aqueous solution, about a 30 to 40% loss of activity was noted. Ticarcillin appeared to affect the amikacin less than did carbenicillin (574).

In another study, amikacin 10 and 20 μg/ml dissolved in human serum and incubated with carbenicillin and ticarcillin 100 to 600 μg/ml at 37 °C demonstrated greater rates of amikacin decomposition at the higher concentration of the penicillins. In 24 hours, little or no loss of amikacin activity occurred at 100 μg/ml, but about a 20% loss occurred at 600 μg/ml of carbenicillin. Approximately a 4% loss at 100 μg/ml to a 40% loss at 600 μg/ml occurred in 72 hours with carbenicillin. Ticarcillin affected amikacin less under these conditions. Little or no loss of amikacin activity occurred at the lower concentrations, but about a 10% loss occurred at 600 μg/ml in 72 hours (575).

Both of these studies indicated that amikacin was more stable in the presence of carbenicillin and ticarcillin than other aminoglycosides (574; 575). This relatively greater stability was also demonstrated in vivo in nephrectomized dogs (576).

Flournoy noted the relative degree of inactivation of tobramycin, gentamicin, netilmicin, and amikacin 10 mg/L in serum when combined with carbenicillin 125 to 1000 mg/L over temperatures ranging from −20 to 42 °C. Tobramycin was more susceptible to inactivation than the others. Amikacin was the least susceptible, and gentamicin and netilmicin were similar in intermediate susceptibility to inactivation (617).

Although piperacillin sodium and aminoglycosides act synergistically and have been used successfully clinically when recommended doses of each drug were administered, mixing piperacillin sodium directly in a syringe or infusion bottle with an aminogly-coside can result in substantial inactivation of the aminoglycoside (740).

The inactivation of amikacin 10 μg/ml in sterile distilled water by several β-lactam antibiotics stored at 37 °C was reported by Jorgensen and Crawford. Ticarcillin 500 μg/ml caused a 16% amikacin loss in six hours, but no significant loss occurred at 100 μg/ml. Cephalothin and moxalactam 100 μg/ml caused a 16% amikacin loss, and a 500-μg/ml concentration of either drug caused a 30% loss. Amikacin was not inactivated by 500- or 100-μg/ml concentrations of penicillin G, carbenicillin, and cefotaxime. No loss of β-lactam antibiotic activity was detected in any combination (973).

Cefotaxime sodium (Hoechst-Roussel) should not be mixed with aminoglycosides in the same solution, but they may be administered to the same patient separately (2; 792). Cefotetan disodium is stated to be physically incompatible with aminoglycosides (4).

Hale et al. evaluated piperacillin and carbenicillin, at concentrations of 62.5 to 1000 μg/ml in human serum in combination with amikacin, gentamicin, or tobramycin 10 μg/ml at 37 °C for up to 24 hours, by bioassay and radioimmunoassay. Penicillin concentrations of 62.5 and 125 μg/ml had relatively little effect on the aminoglycoside concentration, even after 24 hours. However, increasing the penicillin concentration to 250 or 500 μg/ml greatly increased decomposition. After 24 hours with carbenicillin 500 μg/ml, the amounts of aminoglycosides remaining were amikacin, 82%; gentamicin, 43%; and tobramycin, 27%. After 24 hours with piperacillin 500 μg/ml, the remaining concentrations were 95, 45, and 52%, respectively. Even greater inactivation occurred at 1000 μg/ml of the penicillins, including the essentially complete loss of tobramycin in 24 hours. The authors concluded that amikacin is much more resistant to inactivation than the other aminoglycosides tested and that carbenicillin appears to be somewhat more aggressive in its inactivation than piperacillin (816).

Pickering and Rutherford evaluated several aminoglycosides combined with a number of penicillins. Gentamicin sulfate, netilmicin sulfate, and tobramycin sulfate 5 and 10 μg/ml and amikacin 10 and 20 μg/ml were combined in human serum with 125, 250, and 500 μg/ml of azlocillin, carbenicillin disodium, amdinocillin, mezlocillin, and piperacillin individually. Tobramycin and gentamicin sustained greater losses than netilmicin and amikacin at each of the penicillin concentrations. Significant decomposition of all aminoglycosides occurred in 24 hours at 37 °C at a penicillin concentration of 500 μg/ml. Tobramycin and gentamicin had losses of 40 to 60%, while 15 to 30% losses occurred for netilmicin. Amikacin sustained the least inactivation with losses of about 10 to 20%. At penicillin concentrations of 125 to 250 μg/ml, smaller losses of aminoglycosides were observed (68).

To determine if spurious aminoglycoside levels could result from a delay in assaying blood samples, Tindula et al. evaluated the inactivation of amikacin 35 μg/ml and gentamicin and tobramycin 10 μg/ml in human serum by 400-μg/ml concentrations of several penicillins and cephalosporins. Samples were stored for 24 hours at room temperature and frozen at −20 °C. For the room temperature samples, cefazolin and cefamandole caused relatively little inactivation. Nafcillin, cephapirin, and cefoxitin caused moderate inactivation, 20% or less. Penicillin, ampicillin, carbenicillin, and ticarcillin generally caused 25% or more inactivation of gentamicin and tobramycin. Amikacin was somewhat less affected. Freezing samples at −20 °C retarded the reaction sufficiently to prevent significant inactivation of amikacin and gentamicin by any of the drugs.

Freezing the tobramycin samples was satisfactory for most of the drugs except penicillin, ampicillin, and carbenicillin, which still exhibited a 15 to 20% loss in 24 hours (824).

The inactivation of gentamicin, tobramycin, and amikacin, each 5 μg/ml, by seven β-lactam antibiotics, 250 and 500 μg/ml, in serum at 25 °C over 24 hours was studied using bioassay, enzyme-mediated immunoassay technique (EMIT), fluorescence polarization immunoassay (TDx), and radioimmunoassay. No inactivation of any aminoglycoside by the cephalosporins moxalactam, cefotaxime, and cefazolin occurred within the study period. Results with the penicillins varied, depending on the assay technique used. The bioassay was the most sensitive to loss, TDx and radioimmunoassay were intermediate, and EMIT was the least sensitive. Azlocillin, carbenicillin, mezlocillin, and piperacillin all caused variable but extensive inactivation (up to 70%) of gentamicin and tobramycin in 24 hours. Amikacin, however, had only minor losses compared to the other aminoglycosides (654).

The comparative inactivation of five aminoglycosides by seven β-lactam antibiotics in human serum at 37 °C was reported by Riff and Thomason. Amikacin, followed by netilmicin, had the lowest degree of inactivation; tobramycin sustained the most pronounced losses. Gentamicin and kanamycin were intermediate in the extent of losses. The six penicillins that were tested all produced aminoglycoside inactivation; the greatest extent of inactivation was caused by carbenicillin followed by ticarcillin, penicillin G, oxacillin, methicillin, and ampicillin, in approximate descending order. Cephalothin produced minimal inactivation (5 to 10% in 24 hours). The rate of inactivation could be reduced by storage at 4 °C and further reduced by storage at −20 °C. The authors suggested processing blood samples rapidly to avoid inaccurate serum determinations. Storage of specimens at low temperature until analysis may be helpful (1052).

Roberts et al. studied the stability of azlocillin sodium 500 mg/L combined with the aminoglycosides amikacin sulfate 20 mg/L, gentamicin sulfate 8 mg/L, and netilmicin sulfate 7.5 mg/L in peritoneal dialysis solution (Dianeal 1.36%) stored at 37 °C. No azlocillin sodium loss occurred by HPLC during the eight-hour study period. However, the aminoglycosides tested by EMIT showed 10% losses in about six hours for gentamicin sulfate and netilmicin sulfate and in about 30 minutes for amikacin sulfate (1179).

The clinical significance of these interactions appears to be primarily confined to patients with renal failure (218; 334; 361; 364; 616; 816; 847). Literature reports of greatly reduced aminoglycoside levels in such patients have appeared frequently (363; 365–367; 614; 615; 962). In addition, the interaction may be clinically important if assays for aminoglycoside levels in serum are sufficiently delayed (576; 618; 814; 824; 847; 1052).

Most authors believe that in vitro mixing of penicillins, such as ticarcillin disodium, with aminoglycoside antibiotics should be avoided but that clinical use of the drugs in combination can be of great value. It is generally recommended that the drugs be given separately in such combined therapy (157; 218; 222; 224; 361; 364; 368–370).

Heparin— A white precipitate may result from the administration of amikacin sulfate through a heparinized intravenous cannula (976). Flushing heparin locks with sterile water for injection or sodium chloride 0.9% before and after administering drugs incompatible with heparin has been recommended (4).

Peritoneal Dialysis Solutions— Amikacin base (Bristol) 10 and 50 mg/L in peritoneal dialysis concentrate with 50% dextrose (McGaw) retained about 70% of initial activity in seven hours and about 40 to 50% in 24 hours at room temperature as determined by microbiological assay (1044).

Amikacin sulfate (Bristol) 25 μg/ml combined separately with the cephalosporins cefazolin sodium (Lilly), cefamandole nafate (Lilly), and cefoxitin sodium (MSD) at a concentration of 125 μg/ml in peritoneal dialysis solution (Dianeal 1.5%) exhibited enhanced rates of lethality to *Staphylococcus aureus, Escherichia coli,* and *Pseudomonas aeruginosa* compared to any of the drugs alone (1623).

Other Information

Heating Plasma— Heating plasma samples to 56 °C for one hour to inactivate potential human immunodeficiency virus (HIV) content resulted in no amikacin loss as determined by TDx (1615).

AMINO ACID INJECTION
AHFS 40:20

Products— Amino acid injections are supplied in a variety of concentrations and sizes, both alone and in kits with dextrose 50% injection. The approximate concentrations of amino acids and electrolytes in various representative solutions are listed in Table 1.

Administration— Parenteral nutrition solutions composed of amino acids and high-concentration dextrose, which are strongly hypertonic, may be safely administered only through an indwelling intravenous catheter with the tip in the superior vena cava; they are used for severely depleted patients or those requiring long-term therapy. For moderately depleted patients, parenteral nutrition solutions with dextrose concentrations of 5 to 10%, which are substantially less hypertonic, may be administered peripherally (4; 154).

Stability— Solution containers should be visually inspected for cloudiness, haze, discoloration, precipitates, and bottle cracks and checked for the presence of vacuum before mixing and prior to administration. Only clear solutions should be administered. It is also recommended that the containers be protected from light until ready for use and from extremes of temperature such as freezing or over 40 °C. Because of the risk of microbiological contamination, manufacturers recommend storing mixed parenteral nutrition solutions for as little time as possible after preparation. Administration of a single bottle should not exceed 24 hours.

A study of the original FreAmine showed that the mixed solution was stable at 4 °C for 12 weeks. Increased temperature enhanced degradation. Decomposition due to the Maillard reaction is visible as a color change from the clear, light, pale yellow of the freshly prepared solution to yellow to red to dark brown. It was noted that the possibility of microbiological contamination limits the desirable storage time. It was recommended that solutions be stored under refrigeration and used as soon as possible after mixing (186).

The previous study did not report on the stability of tryptophan because of variable and nonreproducible results (186). In another study, it was shown that the tryptophan content of the original FreAmine was reduced approximately 20% by the presence of the sodium bisulfite 0.1% antioxidant (187).

An evaluation of amino acid 4.25% injection with dextrose 25% (prepared from FreAmine II 8.5%), without additional additives, stored at 4 °C for two weeks showed little or no change in the concentrations of amino acids, including tryptophan, as well as pH. Particle counts were also normal over the period. When stored at 25 °C, approximately 6% tryptophan loss occurred, but no other changes were observed (581).

In contrast, parenteral nutrition solutions composed of amino acids solution with ethanol and vitamins (Aminofusin, Pfrimmer) along with dextrose and a variety of electrolytes exhibited a darkening of color on storage at 37, 25, and 5 °C for 60 days. The rate of color change was less at the lowest temperature. A loss of ascorbic acid in the mixture was also demonstrated and was shown to be associated with the color changes. The rate of ascorbic acid decomposition was dependent on air space in the container and storage temperature. In addition, fine white crystals of calcium phosphate precipitated on day 12 at 25 and 37 °C and on day 25 at 5 °C (580).

A photoreaction of the L-tryptophan in Nephramine essential amino acid injection was reported. The L-tryptophan in combination with bisulfite stabilizer, oxygen, and light yielded an indigo blue color. Although no toxicity was associated with the L-tryptophan degradation and blue color formation, it was recommended that Nephramine remain in its original carton until ready to be mixed with dextrose and that Nephramine mixtures be covered with amber, UV-light-resistant bags to retard the formation of the blue color. It was further noted that a slightly blue solution need not be changed for a colorless one, nor is it necessary to change a slightly blue filter for a white one (579). However, it has been emphasized that the clinical importance of this reaction is largely undetermined and may not be entirely benign (1055).

The effects of photoirradiation on a FreAmine II–dextrose 10% parenteral nutrition solution containing 1 ml/500 ml of multivitamins (USV) were evaluated. During simulated continuous adminis-tration to an infant at 0.156 ml/min, the amino acids did not change when the bottle, infusion tubing, and collection bottle were shielded with foil. Only 20 cm of tubing in the incubator was exposed to light. However, if the flow was stopped, a marked reduction in methionine (40%), tryptophan (44%), and histidine (22%) occurred in the solution exposed to light for 24 hours. In a similar solution without vitamins, only the tryptophan concentration decreased. The difference was attributed to the presence of riboflavin, a photosensitizer. The authors recommended administering the multivitamin separately and shielding from light (833).

The stability of amino acids in a parenteral nutrition solution composed of amino acids 3.5%, dextrose 25%, and electrolytes in PVC bags was assessed at 4 and 25 °C over 30 days. No significant decreases of the amino acids occurred in the refrigerated samples. However, the sample stored at room temperature showed significant losses of methionine (10.2%) and arginine (8.2%) in 30 days (1057).

The long-term stability of the components of a parenteral nutrition solution composed of amino acids, dextrose, electrolytes, and trace metals in PVC bags was determined over a six-month period of storage at 4 °C. None of the amino acids decomposed more than 10% during the first two months. However, at six months, all of the amino acids except tyrosine, lysine, and histidine had degraded by more than 10%; some losses exceeded 25%. The dextrose, electrolytes, and trace elements remained constant for the six-month period. Water loss through the PVC bag was only 0.2%. Visually the color remained unchanged (1058).

The long-term stability of the components of six parenteral nutrition solutions containing variable amounts of amino acids, dextrose, electrolytes, trace elements, and vitamins, stored in PVC bags at 4 and 25 °C, was evaluated. No significant changes to the amino acids, dextrose, electrolytes, or trace elements were noted during 28 days (1063).

Freezing Solutions— The acceptability of frozen storage of some parenteral nutrition solutions has been determined. Parenteral nutrition solutions composed of equal parts of Travasol 8.5% with electrolytes and dextrose 70% injection (final concentrations of amino acids and dextrose were 4.25 and 35%, respectively), in PVC containers were stored frozen at −20 °C for 60 days. Both overnight room temperature thawing and 30-minute microwave thawing were utilized. The results indicated that, with either thawing technique, the amino acids, electrolytes, and dextrose were unchanged after 60 days of frozen storage and subsequent thawing (578).

Table 1. Concentration of Amino Acids and Electrolytes in Selected Solutions

	Aminess 5.2%	Aminosyn 3.5%	Aminosyn 5%	Aminosyn 8.5%	Aminosyn II 7%	Aminosyn II 8.5%	Aminosyn II 10%	Aminosyn-HBC 7%	Aminosyn-PF 7%	Aminosyn-RF 5.2%	BranchAmin 4%
Protein equivalent (g/100 ml)	5.2	3.5	5	8.5	7	8.5	10	7	7	5.2	4
Total nitrogen (g/100 ml)	0.66	0.55	0.79	1.34	1.07	1.30	1.53	1.12	1.07	0.787	0.443
Osmolarity (mOsm/L)	416	357	500	850	612	742	873	665	586	475	316
pH	6.4	5.3	5.3	5.3	5–6.5	5–6.5	5–6.5	5.2	5.4	5.2	6.0
Essential Amino Acids (mg/100 ml)											
L-Isoleucine	525	252	360	620	462	561	660	789	534	462	1380
L-Leucine	825	329	470	810	700	850	1000	1576	831	726	1380
L-Lysine	600	252	360	624	735	893	1050	265	475	535	
L-Methionine	825	140	200	340	120	146	172	206	125	726	
L-Phenylalanine	825	154	220	380	209	253	298	228	300	726	
L-Threonine	375	182	260	460	280	340	400	272	360	330	
L-Trytophan	188	56	80	150	140	170	200	88	125	165	
L-Valine	600	280	400	680	350	425	500	789	452	528	1240
Nonessential Amino Acids (mg/100 ml)											
L-Alanine		448	640	1100	695	844	993	660	490		
L-Arginine		343	490	850	713	865	1018	507	861	600	
L-Histidine	412	105	150	260	210	255	300	154	220	429	
L-Proline		300	430	750	505	614	722	448	570		
L-Serine		147	210	370	371	450	530	221	347		
L-Tyrosine		31	44	44					33	44	
N-Acetyl-L-tyrosine					189	230	270				
Glycine (aminoacetic acid)		448	640	1100	350	425	500	660	270		
L-Cysteine HCl • H_2O											
Glutamic acid					517	627	738		576		
Aspartic acid					490	595	700		370		
Taurine									50		
Electrolytes (mEq/L)					a	a	a	a			
Sodium		7			31.3	33.3	45.3	7	3.4		
Potassium			5.4	5.4						5.4	
Magnesium											
Phosphorus											
Chloride				35							
Acetate	50	46	86	90	50.3	61.1	71.8	72	32.5	105	
Calcium											

[a]Also available with added electrolytes.

FreAmine III 3% with electrolytes	FreAmine III 8.5%	FreAmine III 10%	FreAmine HBC 6.9%	HepatAmine 8%	NephrAmine 5.4%	Novamine 15%	ProcalAmine 3% with glycerin 3%	RenAmin 6.5%	Travasol 3.5% with electrolytes	Travasol 5.5%	Travasol 8.5%	Travasol 10%	TrophAmine 6%	TrophAmine 10%
3	8.5	10	6.13	7.6	4	15	2.9	6.5	3.5	5.5	8.5	10	6	10
0.46	1.3	1.53	0.97	1.2	0.64	2.3	0.46	1	0.59	0.925	1.43	1.65	0.93	1.5
405	810	950	620	785	435	1300	735	600	450	569	880	998	525	875
6.8	6.5	6.5	6.5	6.5	6.5	5.6	6.8	6.0	6.0	6.0	6.0	6.0	5.5	5.5
210	590	690	760	900	560	749	210	500	168	263	406	600	490	820
270	770	910	1370	1100	880	1040	270	600	217	340	526	730	840	1400
220	620	730	410	610	640	1180	220	450	203	318	492	580	490	820
160	450	530	250	100	880	749	160	500	203	318	492	400	200	340
170	480	560	320	100	880	1040	170	490	217	340	526	560	290	480
120	340	400	200	450	400	749	120	380	147	230	356	420	250	420
46	130	150	90	66	200	250	46	160	63	99	152	180	120	200
200	560	660	880	840	640	960	200	820	161	252	390	580	470	780
210	600	710	400	770		2170	210	560	728	1140	1760	2070	320	540
290	810	950	580	600		1470	290	630	364	570	880	1150	730	1200
85	240	280	160	240	250	894	85	420	154	241	372	480	290	480
340	950	1120	630	800		894	340	350	147	230	356	680	410	680
180	500	590	330	500		592	180	300				500	230	380
						39		40	14	22	34	40	140	240
420	1190	1400	330	900		1040	420	300	728	1140	1760	1030	220	360
<20	<20	<24	<20	<20	<20		<20						<14	<16
						749							300	500
						434							190	320
													15	25
	a									a	a			
35	10	10	10	10	5		35		25				5	5
24.5							24		15					
5							5		5					
3.5	10	10		10			3.5		7.5					
mM	mM	mM	mM	mM			mM		mM					
41	<3	<3	<3	<3	<3		41	31	25	22	34	40	<3	<3
44	72	89	57	62	44	151	47	60	54	43	67	88	56	97
							3							

Compatibility Information

Solution Compatibility

				Amino acid injection		
Solution	*Mfr*	*Mfr*	*Conc/L*	*Remarks*	*Ref*	*C/I*
Fat emulsion 10%, intravenous	VT	MG	AA 8.5%	Mixed in equal parts. Physically compatible for 48 hr at 4 °C and room temperature	32	**C**
	CU	MG AB TR	8.5% 7% 8.5%	Mixed in equal parts. Physically compatible for 72 hr at room temperature	656	**C**
	VT		AA 10%	Mixed in equal parts. Changes observed in 20 min. Globule coalescence and creaming in 8 hr at 25 and 8 °C	825	**I**

Additive Compatibility

				Amino acid injection			
Drug	*Mfr*	*Conc/L*	*Mfr*	*Test Soln*	*Remarks*	*Ref*	*C/I*
Amikacin sulfate		150 mg		TPN #107[a]	Physically compatible and amikacin activity retained for 24 hr at 21 °C by microbiological assay	1326	**C**
Aminophylline	SE	500 mg	MG	AA 4.25%, D 25%	No increase in particulate matter in 24 hr at 4 °C	349	**C**
	SE	250 mg, 500 mg, 1 g, 1.5 g		TPN #25 to #27[a]	Physically compatible and aminophylline chemically stable for at least 24 hr at 25 °C	755	**C**
	SE	1 g		TPN #25 to #27[a]	Physically compatible and aminophylline chemically stable for at least 24 hr at 4 °C	755	**C**
	SE	1 g		TPN #28 to #30[a]	Physically compatible and aminophylline chemically stable for at least 24 hr at 25 °C	755	**C**
		29.3 mg		[b]	No significant change in aminophylline content over 24 hr at 24 to 26 °C	852	**C**
		284 and 638 mg		TNA #180[a]	Little or no theophylline loss by EMIT and no substantial increase in fat particle size in 24 hr at room temperature	1617	**C**
Amphotericin B	SQ	100 mg	MG	AA 4.25%, D 25%	Turbidity and fine yellow particles form	349	**I**
Ampicillin sodium	BR	1 g	MG	TPN #21[a]	Antibiotic potency retained for 24 hr at 4 °C	87	**C**
	BR	1 g	MG	TPN #21[a]	10% ampicillin decomposition in 6 hr and 25% decomposition in 24 hr at 25 °C	87	**I**
	BR	1 g	MG	AA 4.25%, D 25%	Increase in microscopic particles noted over 24 hr at 5 °C	349	**I**
	BR	1 g		TPN #1[a]	Physically compatible for 12 hr. Precipitate noted in 24 hr at 22 °C	313	**I**
	BR	1 g		TPN #2, #3, #5 to #9[a]	Physically incompatible with precipitate in 1 to 4 hr at 22 °C	313	**I**
	BR	1 g		TPN #4[a]	Physically compatible for 24 hr at 22 °C	313	**C**
	BR	20 mg		TPN #1[a]	Antibiotic potency retained for at least 12 hr at 22 °C	313	**C**
	BR	500 mg and 1 g		TPN #10[a]	Physically compatible for 24 hr and antibiotic potency retained for at least 12 hr at 22 °C	313	**C**

Additive Compatibility (Cont.)

Amino acid injection

Drug	Mfr	Conc/L	Mfr	Test Soln	Remarks	Ref	C/I
	AST	1.5 g		TPN #52[a]	69% ampicillin loss in 24 hr at 29 °C by microbiological assay	440	I
	AST	1.5 g		TPN #53[a]	22% ampicillin loss in 24 hr at 29 °C by microbiological assay	440	I
		1 and 3 g		TPN #107[a]	Physically compatible and ampicillin activity retained for 24 hr at 21 °C by microbiological assay	1326	C
Azlocillin sodium		2 g		TPN #107[a]	26% azlocillin loss in 24 hr at 21 °C by microbiological assay	1326	I
Aztreonam		2 g		TPN #107[a]	Physically compatible and aztreonam activity retained for 24 hr at 21 °C by microbiological assay	1326	C
Calcium gluconate	PR	100 mEq	CU	AA 4%, D 25%	Physically compatible for 24 hr at 22 °C	313	C
Cefamandole nafate	LI	2 g	AB	AA 3.5%	Physically compatible with 6% cefamandole loss in 48 hr at 25 °C and no loss in 10 days at 5 °C	788	C
	LI	2 g	AB	AA 7%	Physically compatible with 7% cefamandole loss in 48 hr at 25 °C and 2% loss in 10 days at 5 °C	788	C
	LI	2 g	MG	AA 8.5%	Physically compatible with 8% cefamandole loss in 48 hr at 25 °C and 4% loss in 10 days at 5 °C	788	C
	LI	2 g	TR	AA 8.5%	Physically compatible with 6% cefamandole loss in 48 hr at 25 °C and 2% loss in 10 days at 5 °C	788	C
	LI	2 g	TR	AA 8.5%, electrolytes	Physically compatible with 7% cefamandole loss in 48 hr at 25 °C and 1% loss in 10 days at 5 °C	788	C
		1.5 g		TPN #107[a]	Physically compatible and cefamandole activity retained for 24 hr at 21 °C by microbiological assay	1326	C
Cefazolin sodium	LI	1 g	MG	AA 4.25%, D 25%	No increase in particulate matter in 24 hr at 4 °C	349	C
	SKF	10 g	TR	TPN #22[a]	Physically compatible with no loss of activity by microbiological assay in 24 hr at 22 °C in the dark	837	C
		1 g		TPN #107[a]	Physically compatible with 9% cefazolin loss in 24 hr at 21 °C by microbiological assay	1326	C
Cefepime HCl	BR	1 and 4 g	AB	AA 4.25%, D 25%, electrolytes	5 to 6% cefepime loss by HPLC in 8 hr at room temperature and 3 days at 5 °C	1682	C
Cefoperazone sodium		1 g		TPN #107[a]	50% cefoperazone loss in 24 hr at 21 °C by microbiological assay	1326	I
Cefotaxime sodium		1 g		TPN #107[a]	Physically compatible and cefotaxime activity retained for 24 hr at 21 °C by microbiological assay	1326	C
Cefoxitin sodium		1 g		TPN #107[a]	Physically compatible and cefoxitin activity retained for 24 hr at 21 °C by microbiological assay	1326	C

Additive Compatibility (Cont.)

Amino acid injection

Drug	Mfr	Conc/L	Mfr	Test Soln	Remarks	Ref	C/I
Ceftazidime		1 g		TPN #107[a]	Physically compatible and ceftazidime activity retained for 24 hr at 21 °C by microbiological assay	1326	**C**
	GL[k]	6 g	AB	AA 5%, D 25%	No substantial amino acid degradation in 48 hr at 22 °C and 10 days at 4 °C. Ceftazidime stability the determining factor	1535	**C**
	GL[k]	1 g		TPN #141 to #143[a]	Visually compatible with 8% ceftazidime loss in 6 hr and 10% loss in 24 hr at 22 °C by HPLC. 8% ceftazidime loss in 3 days at 4 °C	1535	**C**
	GL[k]	6 g		TPN #141 to #143[a]	Visually compatible with 6% ceftazidime loss in 12 hr and 11 to 13% loss in 24 hr at 22 °C by HPLC. 7 to 9% ceftazidime loss in 3 days at 4 °C	1535	**C**
Ceftriaxone sodium		1 g		TPN #107[a]	Physically compatible and ceftriaxone activity retained for 24 hr at 21 °C by microbiological assay	1326	**C**
Cefuroxime sodium		1 g		TPN #107[a]	Physically compatible and cefuroxime activity retained for 24 hr at 21 °C by microbiological assay	1326	**C**
Cimetidine HCl	SKF	1.2 and 5 g	AB	AA 3.5%, electrolytes	Physically compatible and chemically stable for 1 week at room temperature	549	**C**
	SKF	1.2 and 5 g	TR	AA 5.5%	Physically compatible and chemically stable for 1 week at room temperature protected from light	550	**C**
	SKF	1.2 and 5 g	TR	AA 5.5%, electrolytes	Physically compatible and chemically stable for 1 week at room temperature protected from light	550	**C**
	SKF	1.2 and 5 g	TR	AA 8.5%	Physically compatible and chemically stable for 1 week at room temperature protected from light	550	**C**
	SKF	1.2 and 5 g	TR	AA 8.5%, electrolytes	Physically compatible and chemically stable for 1 week at room temperature protected from light	550	**C**
	SKF	300 mg	TR	TPN #34, #35, #37[a]	Physically compatible and cimetidine chemically stable for 24 hr at room temperature and 4 °C	781	**C**
	SKF	300 mg	TR	TPN #36[a]	Physically compatible and cimetidine chemically stable for 24 hr at 4 °C. Room temperature sample gave spurious result	781	**C**
	SKF	400, 800, 1200 mg		TNA #72[a]	Physically compatible and no cimetidine loss in 24 hr at 25 °C. Fat emulsion particle size increased in 48 hr	998	**C**
	SKF	1 g		TPN #75[a]	Physically compatible and cimetidine chemically stable for 48 hr at room temperature	140	**C**
		600 mg		TPN #93[a]	Physically compatible and cimetidine chemically stable for 48 hr at room temperature	1320	**C**
		600 mg		TPN #94[a]	Physically compatible and cimetidine and copper chemically stable for 48 hr at room temperature	1320	**C**

Additive Compatibility (Cont.)

Amino acid injection

Drug	Mfr	Conc/L	Mfr	Test Soln	Remarks	Ref	C/I
	SKF	400 and 900 mg		TNA #179[a]	Visually compatible with less than 3% cimetidine loss by HPLC in 72 hr at room temperature protected from light	1622	**C**
	SKF	450 mg		TNA #197 to #200[a]	Physically compatible with 7% or less cimetidine loss by HPLC in 48 hr at 22 °C exposed to light	1921	**C**
	SKF	450 mg		TPN #196[a]	Physically compatible and no cimetidine loss by HPLC in 48 hr at 22 °C exposed to light	1921	**C**
Clindamycin phosphate	UP	250 mg	MG	TPN #21[a]	Antibiotic potency retained for 24 hr at 4 and 25 °C	87	**C**
	UP	600 mg	MG	AA 4.25%, D 25%[a]	No increase in particulate matter in 24 hr at 4 °C	349	**C**
	UP	3 g	TR	TPN #22[a]	Physically compatible with no loss of activity by microbiological assay in 24 hr at 22 °C in the dark	837	**C**
		400 mg[c]		TPN #107[a]	Physically compatible and clindamycin activity retained for 24 hr at 21 °C by microbiological assay	1326	**C**
Cyanocobalamin	SQ	0.5 and 1 mg	CU	TPN #16 to #20[a]	Physically compatible for 24 hr at 22 °C. UV spectra of amino acids unaltered	313	**C**
	SQ	1 mg	CU	TPN #11 to #15[a]	Physically compatible for 24 hr at 22 °C. TLC changes of amino acids in similar solutions attributed to M.V.I. or vitamin B complex with C	313	**C**
Cyclophosphamide	MJ	500 mg	MG	AA 4.25%, D 25%[a]	No increase in particulate matter in 24 hr at 4 °C	349	**C**
Cyclosporine	SZ	150 mg	MG	AA 5%, D 25%[a]	Visually compatible with no cyclosporine loss by HPLC in 72 hr at 21 °C	1616	**C**
Cytarabine	UP	100 mg	MG	AA 4.25%, D 25%[a]	No increase in particulate matter in 24 hr at 4 °C	349	**C**
	UP	50 mg		TPN #57[a]	Physically compatible with no cytarabine loss in 48 hr at 25 or 8 °C	996	**C**
Dopamine HCl	AS	400 mg	MG	AA 4.25%, D 25%[a]	No increase in particulate matter in 24 hr at 4 °C	349	**C**
Epoetin alfa	ORT	100 units		[d]	98% of the epoetin alfa by bioassay delivered[e] over 24 hr	1878	**C**
Famotidine	MSD	20 and 40 mg		TPN #109 and #110[a]	Physically compatible with little or no famotidine loss and little change in amino acids in 48 hr at 21 °C and in 7 days at 4 °C	1331	**C**
	MSD	20 and 50 mg		TNA #111 and #112[a]	Physically compatible with little or no famotidine loss and no change in fat particle size in 48 hr at 4 and 21 °C	1332	**C**
	MSD	20 mg		TPN #113[a]	Physically compatible with little or no famotidine loss in 35 days at 4 °C protected from light	1334	**C**
	MSD	20 and 40 mg		TNA #114[a]	Physically compatible with little or no famotidine loss and no change in fat particle size in 72 hr at 21 °C under fluorescent light	1333	**C**

Additive Compatibility (Cont.)

Amino acid injection

Drug	Mfr	Conc/L	Mfr	Test Soln	Remarks	Ref	C/I
	MSD	20 mg		[f]	0 to 5% loss in 48 hr at 25 °C in light or dark and at 5 °C	1344	C
	MSD	16.7 and 33.3 mg		TPN #115 and #116[a]	No famotidine loss in 7 days at 23 and 4 °C	1352	C
	MSD	20 mg		TNA #182[a]	Visually compatible with no famotidine loss by HPLC in 24 hr at 24 °C under fluorescent light	1576	C
	MSD	20 mg		TNA #197 to #200[a]	Physically compatible with no famotidine loss by HPLC in 48 hr at 22 °C exposed to light	1921	C
	MSD	20 mg		TPN #196[a]	Physically compatible with no famotidine loss by HPLC in 48 hr at 22 °C exposed to light	1921	C
Fluorouracil	RC	500 mg	MG	AA 4.25%, D 25%	No increase in particulate matter in 24 hr at 4 °C	349	C
	RC	1 and 4 g		TPN #23[a]	Physically compatible for 42 hr at room temperature in ambient light. HPLC results erratic	562	?
	RC	1 g		TPN #23[a]	Physically compatible and fluorouracil chemically stable for 48 hr at room temperature in ambient light	826	C
Folic acid	LE	2.5 and 5 mg	CU	TPN #11 to #15[a]	Physically compatible for 24 hr at 22 °C. UV spectra of amino acids unaltered	313	C
	LE	5 mg		TPN #43 to #47[a]	Physically compatible for 24 hr at 22 °C. TLC changes of amino acids in similar solutions attributed to M.V.I. or vitamin B complex with C	313	C
		1 mg		TPN #74[a]	Folic acid stable over 8 hr at room temperature exposed to fluorescent light or sunlight	842	C
	USP	0.2 and 10 mg	MG	AA 4.25%, D 25%	Physically compatible and stable for at least 7 days at 4 °C or room temperature protected from light	895	C
	USP	0.4 mg		TPN #69[a]	Physically compatible and folic acid stable for at least 7 days at 4 and 25 °C protected from light	895	C
	LE	0.25 to 1 mg		TPN #70[a]	Folic acid stable for at least 48 hr at 6 and 21 °C in light or dark conditions	896	C
Fosphenytoin sodium	PD	1, 8, 20 mg PE/ml[j]	BA	AA 10%[h]	Visually compatible with little or no loss of fosphenytoin by HPLC in 7 days at 25 °C under fluorescent light	2083	C
Furosemide	HO	40 mg	MG	AA 4.25%, D 25%	No increase in particulate matter in 24 hr at 4 °C	349	C
Ganciclovir sodium	SY	3 and 5 g		TPN #183 to #185[a]	Precipitate forms	1744	I
	SY	2 g		TPN #183[a]	Precipitate forms	1744	I
Gentamicin sulfate	SC	80 mg	CU	AA 4%, D 25%	Physically compatible for 24 hr and antibiotic potency retained for at least 12 hr at 22 °C	313	C
	SC	80 mg	MG	AA 4.25%, D 25%	No increase in particulate matter in 24 hr at 4 °C	349	C
	SC	80 mg		TPN #1, #4, #5, #7[a]	Physically compatible for 24 hr at 22 °C	313	C

Additive Compatibility (Cont.)

Amino acid injection

Drug	Mfr	Conc/L	Mfr	Test Soln	Remarks	Ref	C/I
	SC	80 mg		TPN #2, #3, #6, #8, #9[a]	Physically incompatible with a precipitate in 8 to 24 hr at 22 °C	313	I
	SC	80 mg		TPN #1[a]	Antibiotic potency retained for at least 12 hr at 22 °C	313	C
	SC	80 mg		TPN #10[a]	Physically compatible for 24 hr and antibiotic potency retained for at least 12 hr at 22 °C	313	C
	SC	800 mg	TR	TPN #22[a]	Physically compatible with no loss of activity by microbiological assay in 24 hr at 22 °C in the dark	837	C
	SC	50 mg		TPN #52 and #53[a]	Physically compatible with no loss of gentamicin in 24 hr at 29 °C by microbiological assay	440	C
		75 mg		TPN #107[a]	Physically compatible and gentamicin activity retained for 24 hr at 21 °C by microbiological assay	1326	C
Heparin sodium	RI	20,000 units	MG	AA 4.25%, D 25%	No increase in particulate matter in 24 hr at 4 °C	349	C
		35,000 units		TPN #48 to #51[a]	Heparin activity retained for 24 hr at 25 °C but fell significantly after 24 hr	900	C
	LY	3000 to 20,000 units		TPN #200[a]	Heparin activity retained for 28 days at 4 °C	2025	C
Hydrochloric acid		40, 60, 100 mEq	MG	TPN #24[a]	Physically compatible and changes in amino acid concentrations considered negligible over 24 hr at 25 °C. Hydrochloric acid available from solution	582	C
Imipenem–cilastatin sodium		500 mg		TPN #107[a]	57% imipenem loss in 24 hr at 21 °C by microbiological assay	1326	I
Insulin, regular	LI	100 units	MG	AA 4.25%, D 25%	No increase in particulate matter in 24 hr at 4 °C	349	C
Iron dextran	FI	100 mg	TR	TPN #31 to #33[a]	Physically compatible with minimal changes to iron dextran and amino acids for 18 hr at room temperature	692	C
	FI	50 mg		TNA #122[a]	Lipid oiling out in 18 to 19 hr with formation of yellow-brown layer on admixture surface	1383	I
	FI	2 mg		TNA #159 to #166[a]	Physically compatible with no change by visual and microscopic examination and no change in particle size distribution in 48 hr at 4 and 25 °C	1648	C
	SCN	10 mg		TPN #207 and #208[a]	Rust-colored precipitate forms in 12 hr at 19 °C protected from sunlight	2103	I
	SCN	10 mg		TPN #209[a]	Rust-colored precipitate forms in some samples in 18 to 24 hr at 19 °C protected from sunlight	2103	I
	SCN	10 mg		TPN #210[a]	Visually compatible for 48 hr at 19 °C protected from sunlight. Trace iron precipitation found by filtration and analysis after 48 hr	2103	?
	SCN	10 mg		TPN #211[a]	Visually compatible for 48 hr at 19 °C protected from sunlight. No iron precipitation found by filtration and analysis after 48 hr	2103	C

Additive Compatibility (Cont.)

Amino acid injection

Drug	Mfr	Conc/L	Mfr	Test Soln	Remarks	Ref	C/I
Isoproterenol HCl	WI	2 mg	MG	AA 4.25%, D 25%	No increase in particulate matter in 24 hr at 4 °C	349	C
Kanamycin sulfate	BR	250 mg	MG	TPN #21[a]	Antibiotic potency retained for 24 hr at 4 °C	87	C
	BR	250 mg	MG	TPN #21[a]	13% kanamycin decomposition in 24 hr at 25 °C	87	I
	BR	500 mg	MG	AA 4.25%, D 25%	No increase in particulate matter in 24 hr at 4 °C	349	C
	BR	500 mg		TPN #2, #4, #5, #7, #8[a]	Physically compatible for 24 hr at 22 °C	313	C
	BR	500 mg		TPN #1, #3, #6, #9[a]	Physically incompatible with a precipitate in 8 to 12 hr at 22 °C	313	I
	BR	400 mg		TPN #1[a]	Antibiotic potency retained for at least 12 hr at 22 °C	313	C
	BR	500 mg		TPN #10[a]	Physically compatible for 24 hr and antibiotic potency retained for at least 12 hr at 22 °C	313	C
Lidocaine HCl	AST	1 g	MG	AA 4.25%, D 25%	No increase in particulate matter in 24 hr at 4 °C	349	C
Meperidine HCl	WI	100 mg		TPN #71[a,g]	Physically compatible with no meperidine loss in 36 hr at 22 °C	1000	C
Metaraminol bitartrate	MSD	100 mg	MG	AA 4.25%, D 25%	No increase in particulate matter in 24 hr at 4 °C	349	C
Methotrexate sodium	LE	50 mg	MG	AA 4.25%, D 25%	No increase in particulate matter in 24 hr at 4 °C	349	C
Methyldopate HCl	MSD	500 mg	MG	AA 4.25%, D 25%	No increase in particulate matter in 24 hr at 4 °C	349	C
Methylprednisolone sodium succinate	UP	250 mg	MG	AA 4.25%, D 25%	No increase in particulate matter in 24 hr at 4 °C	349	C
Metoclopramide HCl	RB	5 and 20 mg	TR	AA 2.75%, D 25%, electrolytes	Metoclopramide chemically stable for 72 hr at room temperature	854	C
	RB	5 mg		TPN #89[a]	Physically compatible with no metoclopramide loss in 24 hr and 10% loss in 48 hr at 25 °C	1167	C
	RB	20 mg		TPN #89[a]	Physically compatible with no metoclopramide loss in 72 hr at 25 °C	1167	C
	RB	5 mg		TPN #90[a]	Physically compatible with no metoclopramide loss in 72 hr at 25 °C	1167	C
	RB	20 mg		TPN #90[a]	Physically compatible with 3% metoclopramide loss in 72 hr at 25 °C	1167	C
Metronidazole HCl with sodium bicarbonate	SE AB	5 g 50 mEq	AB	AA 10%	Initial yellow color becomes dark yellow in 24 hr	765	I
Midazolam HCl	RC	600 mg to 1 g		TPN #174 to #176[a]	Immediate precipitation	1624	I
	RC	100 and 500 mg		TPN #174 to #176[a]	Visually compatible with little or no midazolam loss and less than 10% loss of any amino acid by HPLC in 5 hr at 22 °C under fluorescent light	1624	C
Morphine sulfate	LI	100 mg		TPN #71[a,g]	Physically compatible with no morphine loss in 36 hr at 22 °C	1000	C

Additive Compatibility (Cont.)

Amino acid injection

Drug	Mfr	Conc/L	Mfr	Test Soln	Remarks	Ref	C/I
Multivitamins	USV	1 vial	TR	AA 10%	40% loss of thiamine HCl in 22 hr at 30 °C due to sulfite content	843	**I**
	USV	1 vial	TR	AA 4.25%, D 25%	No loss of thiamine HCl in 22 hr at 30 °C	843	**C**
(Berocca PN)	RC	4 ml	MG	AA 8.5%	97% loss of thiamine in 24 hr at 23 °C due to bisulfite content of solution. 63% loss in 24 hr at 7 °C	774	**I**
	RC	4 ml	TR	AA 5.5%	About 70% loss of thiamine in 24 hr at 23 °C due to bisulfite content of solution. 33% loss in 24 hr at 7 °C	774	**I**
(Multivitamin additive)	AB		MG	AA 8.5%	96% loss of thiamine in 24 hr at 23 °C due to bisulfite content of solution	774	**I**
(M.V.I.-12)	USV		MG	AA 8.5%	92% loss of thiamine in 24 hr at 23 °C due to bisulfite content of solution	774	**I**
(M.V.I. Pediatric)	ROR	5 ml		AA 2%, D 12.5%, electrolytes	7% phytonadione loss in 4 hr and 27% loss in 24 hr by HPLC under ambient temperature and light	1815	**I**
Nafcillin sodium		1 and 2 g		TPN #107[a]	Physically compatible and nafcillin activity retained for 24 hr at 21 °C by microbiological assay	1326	**C**
Netilmicin sulfate	SC	3 g	MG	AA 8.5%	Physically compatible and chemically stable for 7 days at 25 and 4 °C	558	**C**
		75 mg		TPN #107[a]	Physically compatible and netilmicin activity retained for 24 hr at 21 °C by microbiological assay	1326	**C**
Nizatidine	LI	0.75 and 1.5 g	TR[g]	AA 8.5%	Visually compatible and nizatidine potency by HPLC retained for 7 days at 4 and 25 °C. Amino acids not tested	1533	**C**
	LI	3 g	TR[g]	AA 8.5%	Visually compatible with 8% nizatidine loss in 3 days and 13% loss in 7 days at 25 °C by HPLC. 5% nizatidine loss in 7 days at 4 °C. Amino acids not tested	1533	**C**
	LI	150 mg		TPN #134 and TNA #135 to #138[a]	Physically compatible with no increase in fat particle size and 2 to 7% nizatidine loss by HPLC in 48 hr at 22 °C under fluorescent light	1534; 1921	**C**
Norepinephrine bitartrate	WI	4 mg	MG	AA 4.25%, D 25%	No increase in particulate matter in 24 hr at 4 °C	349	**C**
Octreotide acetate	SZ	1.5 mg		TPN #119 and #120[a,h]	Little octreotide loss over 48 hr at room temperature in ambient room light	1373	**C**
	SZ	450 µg		TNA #139[a,i]	Physically compatible with no change in lipid particle size in 48 hr at 22 °C under fluorescent light and 7 days at 4 °C. Octreotide activity highly variable by radioimmunoassay	1540	**?**
Ondansetron HCl	GL	0.03 and 0.3 g		TNA #190[a]	Physically compatible with little or no ondansetron loss by HPLC in 48 hr at 24 °C under fluorescent light	1766	**C**
Oxacillin sodium	BR	500 mg	MG	AA 4.25%, D 25%	No increase in particulate matter in 24 hr at 4 °C	349	**C**

Additive Compatibility (Cont.)

Amino acid injection

Drug	Mfr	Conc/L	Mfr	Test Soln	Remarks	Ref	C/I
Penicillin G potassium	SQ	5 million units	MG	TPN #21[a]	Antibiotic potency retained for 24 hr at 4 and 25 °C	87	C
	LI	1 million units	MG	AA 4.25%, D 25%	No increase in particulate matter in 24 hr at 4 °C	349	C
	AY	25 million units	TR	TPN #22[a]	Physically compatible with no loss of activity by microbiological assay in 24 hr at 22 °C in the dark	837	C
		2 g		TPN #107[a]	Physically compatible and penicillin G activity retained for 24 hr at 21 °C by microbiological assay	1326	C
Penicillin G sodium		2 g		TPN #107[a]	Physically compatible and penicillin G activity by microbiological assay retained for 24 hr at 21 °C	1326	C
Phytonadione	MSD	5 and 10 mg	CU	TPN #16 to #20[a]	Physically compatible for 24 hr at 22 °C. UV spectra of amino acids unaltered	313	C
	MSD	5 and 10 mg	CU	TPN #11 to #15[a]	Physically compatible for 24 hr at 22 °C. TLC changes of amino acids in similar solutions attributed to M.V.I. or vitamin B complex with C	313	C
	MSD	10 mg	MG	AA 4.25%, D 25%	No increase in particulate matter in 24 hr at 4 °C	349	C
Piperacillin sodium		2 g		TPN #107[a]	43% piperacillin loss in 24 hr at 21 °C by microbiological assay	1326	I
Polymyxin B sulfate	NOV	40 mg		TPN #52 and #53[a]	Physically compatible with no polymyxin loss in 24 hr at 29 °C by microbiological assay	440	C
Potassium phosphate	MG	100 mEq	CU	AA 4%, D 25%	Physically compatible for 24 hr at 22 °C	313	C
Ranitidine HCl	GL	83, 167, 250 mg		TPN #58[a]	10% ranitidine loss in 48 hr at 23 °C	997	C
	GL	50 and 100 mg		TPN #59 and #60[a,h]	No color change and 7 to 9% ranitidine loss in 24 hr at 24 °C under fluorescent light. Amino acids not substantially affected. Darkened color and 10 to 12% ranitidine loss in 48 hr	1010	C
	GL	50 and 100 mg		TNA #92[a,i]	7 to 10% ranitidine loss in 12 hr and 20 to 28% loss in 24 hr at 23 °C under fluorescent light	1183	I
	GL	50 and 100 mg		TPN #117[a]	Physically compatible and no more than 5% ranitidine loss in 48 hr under refrigeration and at 25 °C	1360	C
	GL	50 and 100 mg		TNA #118[a]	Physically compatible with no effect on emulsion stability and about 6 to 10% ranitidine loss in 36 hr under refrigeration and at 25 °C with or without light protection	1360	C
	GL	50 mg and 2 g	TR	AA 8.5%	Physically compatible and ranitidine chemically stable by HPLC for 24 hr at 25 °C	1515	C
	GL	75 mg		TNA #197 to #200[a]	Physically compatible with 7% or less ranitidine loss by HPLC in 24 hr at 22 °C exposed to light. About 15% loss in 48 hr	1921	C

Additive Compatibility (Cont.)

Amino acid injection

Drug	Mfr	Conc/L	Mfr	Test Soln	Remarks	Ref	C/I
	GL	75 mg		TPN #201[a]	Physically compatible with 7% or less ranitidine loss by HPLC in 24 hr at 22 °C exposed to light. About 12% loss in 48 hr	1921	**C**
Sodium bicarbonate		50 and 150 mEq		TPN #62 to #65 and TNA #66 to #68[a]	Physically compatible with 10% or less carbon dioxide loss and unchanged pH in 7 days at 25 °C protected from light	1011	**C**
Tacrolimus	FUJ	100 mg		TPN #201[a,g]	Visually compatible with no loss by HPLC in 24 hr at 24 °C	1922	**C**
Ticarcillin disodium	BE	10 mg		TPN #86 to #88[a]	10% ticarcillin loss in 24 hr at room temperature exposed to light	1160	**C**
	BE	20 mg		TPN #86 to #88[a]	12 to 15% ticarcillin loss in 4 hr at room temperature exposed to light	1160	**I**
		2 g		TPN #107[a]	50% ticarcillin loss in 24 hr at 21 °C by microbiological assay	1326	**I**
Tobramycin sulfate	LI	80 mg	MG	AA 4.25%, D 25%	No increase in particulate matter in 24 hr at 4 °C	349	**C**
Vancomycin HCl		400 mg		TPN #95 and #96[a]	Physically compatible and vancomycin content retained for 8 days at room temperature and under refrigeration, with and without heparin, by TDx	1321	**C**
		1 and 6 g		TPN #105 and #106[a]	Physically compatible with little or no vancomycin loss in 4 hr at 22 °C by HPLC	1325	**C**
		200 mg		TPN #107[a]	Physically compatible and vancomycin activity retained for 24 hr at 21 °C by microbiological assay	1326	**C**
	LI	500 mg and 1 g		TPN #202[a,h]	Visually compatible and vancomycin activity by bioassay and immunoassay retained for 35 days at 4 °C and an additional 24 hr at 22 °C	1933	**C**

[a]*Refer to Appendix I for the composition of parenteral nutrition solutions. TNA indicates a 3-in-1 admixture, and TPN indicates a 2-in-1 admixture.*
[b]*Tested in a pediatric parenteral nutrition solution containing 150 ml of dextrose 5% in water and 30 ml of Vamin glucose with electrolytes and vitamins.*
[c]*Expressed as clindamycin base.*
[d]*TPN composed of amino acids (TrophAmine) 0.5 or 2.25% with dextrose 12.5%, vitamins, trace elements, magnesium sulfate, calcium gluconate, sodium chloride, potassium acetate, and heparin sodium.*
[e]*Delivered from a syringe through microbore tubing, T-connector, and a Teflon neonatal 24-gauge intravenous catheter.*
[f]*Tested in Vamin 14, Vamin 18, Vamin glucose, and Vamin N.*
[g]*Tested in glass bottles.*
[h]*Tested in PVC containers.*
[i]*Tested in ethylene vinyl acetate containers.*
[j]*Concentration expressed in milligrams of phenytoin sodium equivalents (PE) per milliliter.*
[k]*Sodium carbonate–containing formulation tested.*

Y-Site Injection Compatibility (1:1 Mixture)

Amino acid injection

Drug	Mfr	Conc	Mfr	Conc	Remarks	Ref	C/I
Acetazolamide sodium	LE	100 mg/ml		TPN #203 and #204[g]	White precipitate forms immediately	1974	**I**
Acyclovir sodium	BW	7 mg/ml		TPN #203 and #204[g]	White precipitate forms immediately	1974	**I**
	BW	7 mg/ml[a]		TPN #212 to #215[g]	Crystalline needles form immediately, becoming a gross precipitate in 1 hr	2109	**I**

Y-Site Injection Compatibility (1:1 Mixture) (Cont.)

			Amino acid injection				
Drug	*Mfr*	*Conc*	*Mfr*	*Conc*	*Remarks*	*Ref*	*C/I*
	GW	7 mg/ml[a]		TNA #218 to #226[g]	White precipitate forms immediately	2215	I
Amikacin sulfate		250 mg/ml		TPN #54[g]	Physically compatible and amikacin activity retained over 6 hr at 22 °C by microbiological assay	1045	C
	BR	37.5 mg/0.15 ml[j]		TPN #61[c,g]	Physically compatible	1012	C
	BR	225 mg/0.9 ml[j]		TPN #61[d,g]	Physically compatible	1012	C
	BR	15 mg[e]		TPN #91[f,g]	Physically compatible	1170	C
	BR	250 mg/ml		TNA #97 to #104[g]	Broken fat emulsion with oil floating in admixtures	1324	I
	APC	5 mg/ml		TPN #203 and #204[g]	Visually compatible for 2 hr at 23 °C	1974	C
	AB	5 mg/ml[a]		TPN #212 to #215[g]	Physically compatible with no change in measured turbidity or increase in particle content in 4 hr at 23 °C	2109	C
	AB	5 mg/ml[a]		TNA #218 to #226[g]	Visually compatible with no precipitate or emulsion damage apparent in 4 hr at 23 °C	2215	C
Aminophylline	DB	1 mg/ml[b]		TPN #189[g]	Visually compatible for 24 hr at 22 °C	1767	C
	AMR	5 mg/ml		TPN #203 and #204[g]	White precipitate forms immediately	1974	I
	AB	2.5 mg/ml[a]		TPN #212 to #215[g]	Physically compatible with no change in measured turbidity or increase in particle content in 4 hr at 23 °C	2109	C
	AB	2.5 mg/ml[a]		TNA #218 to #226[g]	Visually compatible with no precipitate or emulsion damage apparent in 4 hr at 23 °C	2215	C
Amoxicillin sodium		50 mg/ml[b]		TPN #189[g]	Visually compatible for 24 hr at 22 °C	1767	C
Amphotericin B	PH	0.6 mg/ml[a]		TPN #212 to #215[g]	Gross flocculent precipitate forms immediately	2109	I
	PH	0.6 mg/ml[a]		TNA #218 to #226[g]	Yellow precipitate forms immediately	2215	I
Ampicillin sodium	BR	2 g/50 ml[b]		TNA #73[g,h]	Physically compatible for 4 hr at 25 °C by visual observation	1008	C
	WY	250 mg/1.3 ml[i]		TPN #61[c,g]	Heavy precipitate of calcium phosphate due to increased pH	1012	I
	WY	1.5 g/7.5 ml[i]		TPN #61[d,g]	Heavy precipitate of calcium phosphate due to increased pH	1012	I
				TPN #54[g]	Precipitate forms in 30 min at 22 °C	1045	I
	APC	100 and 250 mg/ml		TPN #203 and #204[g]	White precipitate forms immediately	1974	I
	SKB	20 mg/ml[b]		TPN #212 to #215[g]	Physically compatible with no change in measured turbidity or increase in particle content in 4 hr at 23 °C	2109	C
	SKB	20 mg/ml[b]		TNA #218 to #226[g]	Visually compatible with no precipitate or emulsion damage apparent in 4 hr at 23 °C	2215	C
Ampicillin sodium–sulbactam sodium	RR	20 + 10 mg/ml[b]		TPN #212 to #215[g]	Physically compatible with no change in measured turbidity or increase in particle content in 4 hr at 23 °C	2109	C

Y-Site Injection Compatibility (1:1 Mixture) (Cont.)

Amino acid injection

Drug	Mfr	Conc	Mfr	Conc	Remarks	Ref	C/I
	PF	20 + 10 mg/ml[b]		TNA #218 to #226[g]	Visually compatible with no precipitate or emulsion damage apparent in 4 hr at 23 °C	2215	**C**
Ascorbic acid injection	DB	20 mg/ml[b]		TPN #189[g]	Visually compatible for 24 hr at 22 °C	1767	**C**
Atracurium besylate	WEL	10 mg/ml		TPN #189[g]	Visually compatible for 24 hr at 22 °C	1767	**C**
Azlocillin sodium		133 and 200 mg/ml		TPN #54[g]	Physically compatible and azlocillin activity retained over 6 hr at 22 °C by microbiological assay	1045	**C**
	MI	250 mg/2.5 ml[i]		TPN #61[c,g]	Physically compatible	1012	**C**
	MI	1.5 mg/15 ml[i]		TPN #61[d,g]	Physically compatible	1012	**C**
Aztreonam	SQ	40 mg/ml[a]		TPN #212 to #215[g]	Physically compatible with no change in measured turbidity or increase in particle content in 4 hr at 23 °C	2109	**C**
	SQ	40 mg/ml[a]		TNA #218 to #226[g]	Visually compatible with no precipitate or emulsion damage apparent in 4 hr at 23 °C	2215	**C**
Bumetanide	RC	0.04 mg/ml[a]		TPN #212 to #215[g]	Physically compatible with no change in measured turbidity or increase in particle content in 4 hr at 23 °C	2109	**C**
	RC, BV	0.04 mg/ml[a]		TNA #218 to #226[g]	Visually compatible with no precipitate or emulsion damage apparent in 4 hr at 23 °C	2215	**C**
Buprenorphine HCl	RKC	0.04 mg/ml[a]		TPN #212 to #215[g]	Physically compatible with no change in measured turbidity or increase in particle content in 4 hr at 23 °C	2109	**C**
	RKC	0.04 mg/ml[a]		TNA #218 to #226[g]	Visually compatible with no precipitate or emulsion damage apparent in 4 hr at 23 °C	2215	**C**
Butorphanol tartrate	APC	0.04 mg/ml[a]		TPN #212 to #215[g]	Physically compatible with no change in measured turbidity or increase in particle content in 4 hr at 23 °C	2109	**C**
	APC	0.04 mg/ml[a]		TNA #218 to #226[g]	Visually compatible with no precipitate or emulsion damage apparent in 4 hr at 23 °C	2215	**C**
Calcium gluconate	DB	10 mg/ml[b]		TPN #189[g]	Visually compatible for 24 hr at 22 °C	1767	**C**
	AB	40 mg/ml[a]		TPN #212 to #215[g]	Physically compatible with no change in measured turbidity or increase in particle content in 4 hr at 23 °C	2109	**C**
	AB	40 mg/ml[a]		TNA #218 to #226[g]	Visually compatible with no precipitate or emulsion damage apparent in 4 hr at 23 °C	2215	**C**
Carboplatin	BMS	5 mg/ml[a]		TPN #212 to #215[g]	Physically compatible with no change in measured turbidity or increase in particle content in 4 hr at 23 °C	2109	**C**
	BMS	5 mg/ml[a]		TNA #218 to #226[g]	Visually compatible with no precipitate or emulsion damage apparent in 4 hr at 23 °C	2215	**C**

Y-Site Injection Compatibility (1:1 Mixture) (Cont.)

				Amino acid injection			
Drug	*Mfr*	*Conc*	*Mfr*	*Conc*	*Remarks*	*Ref*	*C/I*
Cefamandole nafate		250 mg/ml		TPN #54[g]	Physically compatible and cefamandole activity retained over 6 hr at 22 °C by microbiological assay	1045	C
	LI	2 g/50 ml[a]		TNA #73[g,h]	Physically compatible for 4 hr at 25 °C by visual observation	1008	C
	LI	200 mg/ 0.7 ml[i]		TPN #61[c,g]	Physically compatible	1012	C
	LI	1.2 g/4.2 ml[i]		TPN #61[d,g]	Physically compatible	1012	C
Cefazolin sodium	SKF	1 g/50 ml[a]		TNA #73[g,h]	Physically compatible by visual observation for 4 hr at 25 °C	1008	C
	SKF	200 mg/ 0.9 ml[i]		TPN #61[c,g]	Physically compatible	1012	C
	SKF	1.2 g/5.3 ml[i]		TPN #61[d,g]	Physically compatible	1012	C
	SKB	20 mg/ml[a]		TPN #212 and #213[g]	Physically compatible with no change in measured turbidity or increase in particle content in 4 hr at 23 °C	2109	C
	SKB	20 mg/ml[a]		TPN #214 and #215[g]	Small amount of subvisual precipitate forms immediately	2109	I
	SKB	20 mg/ml[a]		TNA #218 to #226[g]	Visually compatible with no precipitate or emulsion damage apparent in 4 hr at 23 °C	2215	C
Cefoperazone sodium	RR	250 mg/ 1 ml[i]		TPN #61[c,g]	Physically compatible	1012	C
	RR	1.5 g/6 ml[i]		TPN #61[d,g]	Physically compatible	1012	C
	RR	40 mg/ml[a]		TPN #212 to #215[g]	Physically compatible with no change in measured turbidity or increase in particle content in 4 hr at 23 °C	2109	C
	PF	40 mg/ml[a]		TNA #218 to #226[g]	Visually compatible with no precipitate or emulsion damage apparent in 4 hr at 23 °C	2215	C
Cefotaxime sodium	HO	200 mg/ 0.7 ml[i]		TPN #61[c,g]	Physically compatible	1012	C
	HO	1.2 g/4 ml[i]		TPN #61[d,g]	Physically compatible	1012	C
	RS	200 mg/ml[k]		TPN #189[g]	Visually compatible for 24 hr at 22 °C	1767	C
	HO	60 mg/ml		TPN #203 and #204[g]	Visually compatible for 2 hr at 23 °C	1974	C
	HO	20 mg/ml[a]		TPN #212 to #215[g]	Physically compatible with no change in measured turbidity or increase in particle content in 4 hr at 23 °C	2109	C
	HO	20 mg/ml[a]		TNA #218 to #226[g]	Visually compatible with no precipitate or emulsion damage apparent in 4 hr at 23 °C	2215	C
Cefotetan sodium	STU	20 mg/ml[a]		TPN #212 to #215[g]	Physically compatible with no change in measured turbidity or increase in particle content in 4 hr at 23 °C	2109	C
	ZEN	20 mg/ml[a]		TNA #218 to #226[g]	Visually compatible with no precipitate or emulsion damage apparent in 4 hr at 23 °C	2215	C
Cefoxitin sodium	MSD	1 g/50 ml[a]		TNA #73[g,h]	Physically compatible for 4 hr at 25 °C by visual observation	1008	C
	MSD	200 mg/ 2.1 ml[i]		TPN #61[c,g]	Physically compatible	1012	C

Y-Site Injection Compatibility (1:1 Mixture) (Cont.)

				Amino acid injection			
Drug	*Mfr*	*Conc*	*Mfr*	*Conc*	*Remarks*	*Ref*	*C/I*
	MSD	1.2 g/ 12.6 ml[i]		TPN #61[d,g]	Physically compatible	1012	C
	MSD	200 mg/ml[k]		TPN #189[g]	Visually compatible for 24 hr at 22 °C	1767	C
	ME	20 mg/ml[a]		TPN #212 to #215[d]	Physically compatible with no change in measured turbidity or increase in particle content in 4 hr at 23 °C	2109	C
	ME	20 mg/ml[a]		TNA #218 to #226[g]	Visually compatible with no precipitate or emulsion damage apparent in 4 hr at 23 °C	2215	C
Ceftazidime	GL[v]	40 mg/ml[l]		TPN #141 to #143[g]	Visually compatible with 4% or less ceftazidime loss in 2 hr at 22 °C in 1:1 and 1:3 ratios	1535	C
	GL[v]	200 mg/ml[k]		TPN #189[g]	Visually compatible for 24 hr at 22 °C	1767	C
	LI[v]	60 mg/ml		TPN #203 and #204[g]	Visually compatible for 2 hr at 23 °C	1974	C
	SKB[v]	40 mg/ml[a]		TPN #212 to #215[g]	Physically compatible with no change in measured turbidity or increase in particle content in 4 hr at 23 °C	2109	C
	SKB[v]	40 mg/ml[a]		TNA #218 to #226[g]	Visually compatible with no precipitate or emulsion damage apparent in 4 hr at 23 °C	2215	C
	GL[w]	40 mg/ml[a]		TNA #218 to #226[g]	Visually compatible with no precipitate or emulsion damage apparent in 4 hr at 23 °C	2215	C
Ceftizoxime sodium	FUJ	20 mg/ml[a]		TPN #212 to #215[g]	Physically compatible with no change in measured turbidity or increase in particle content in 4 hr at 23 °C	2109	C
	FUJ	20 mg/ml[a]		TNA #218 to #226[g]	Visually compatible with no precipitate or emulsion damage apparent in 4 hr at 23 °C	2215	C
Ceftriaxone sodium	RC	100 mg/ml[k]		TPN #189[g]	Visually compatible for 24 hr at 22 °C	1767	C
	RC	20 mg/ml[a]		TPN #212 to #215[g]	Physically compatible with no change in measured turbidity or increase in particle content in 4 hr at 23 °C	2109	C
	RC	20 mg/ml[a]		TNA #218 to #226[g]	Visually compatible with no precipitate or emulsion damage apparent in 4 hr at 23 °C	2215	C
Cefuroxime sodium	LI	30 mg/ml[a]		TPN #212 to #215[g]	Physically compatible with no change in measured turbidity or increase in particle content in 4 hr at 23 °C	2109	C
	GL	30 mg/ml[a]		TNA #218 to #226[g]	Visually compatible with no precipitate or emulsion damage apparent in 4 hr at 23 °C	2215	C
Chloramphenicol sodium succinate	PD	125 mg/ 1.25 ml[i]		TPN #61[c,g]	Physically compatible	1012	C
	PD	750 mg/ 7.5 ml[i]		TPN #61[d,g]	Physically compatible	1012	C
Chlorothiazide sodium	ME	28 mg/ml		TPN #203 and #204[g]	White precipitate forms immediately	1974	I
Chlorpromazine HCl	SCN	2 mg/ml[a]		TPN #212 to #215[g]	Physically compatible with no change in measured turbidity or increase in particle content in 4 hr at 23 °C	2109	C

Y-Site Injection Compatibility (1:1 Mixture) (Cont.)

			Amino acid injection				
Drug	*Mfr*	*Conc*	*Mfr*	*Conc*	*Remarks*	*Ref*	*C/I*
	SCN	2 mg/ml[a]		TNA #218 to #226[g]	Visually compatible with no precipitate or emulsion damage apparent in 4 hr at 23 °C	2215	**C**
Cimetidine HCl	SKB	10 mg/ml[b]		TPN #189[g]	Visually compatible for 24 hr at 22 °C	1767	**C**
	SKB	12 mg/ml[a]		TPN #212 to #215[g]	Physically compatible with no change in measured turbidity or increase in particle content in 4 hr at 23 °C	2109	**C**
	SKB	12 mg/ml[a]		TNA #218 to #226[g]	Visually compatible with no precipitate or emulsion damage apparent in 4 hr at 23 °C	2215	**C**
Ciprofloxacin	MI	2 mg/ml[a]	AB	AA 5%, D 25%	Visually compatible for 2 hr at 25 °C under fluorescent light	1628	**C**
	MI	1 mg/ml[a]		TPN #212 to #215[g]	Amber discoloration forms in 1 to 4 hr	2109	**I**
	BAY	1 mg/ml[a]		TNA #218 to #226[g]	Visually compatible with no precipitate or emulsion damage apparent in 4 hr at 23 °C	2215	**C**
Cisplatin	BMS	1 mg/ml		TPN #212 to #215[g]	Amber discoloration forms in 1 to 4 hr	2109	**I**
	BMS	1 mg/ml		TNA #218 to #226[g]	Visually compatible with no precipitate or emulsion damage apparent in 4 hr at 23 °C	2215	**C**
Clindamycin phosphate	UP	600 mg/ 50 ml[a]		TNA #73[g,h]	Physically compatible for 4 hr at 25 °C by visual observation	1008	**C**
	UP	50 mg/ 0.33 ml[m]		TPN #61[c,g]	Physically compatible	1012	**C**
	UP	300 mg/ 2 ml[m]		TPN #61[d,g]	Physically compatible	1012	**C**
	AB	10 mg/ml[a]		TPN #212 to #215[g]	Physically compatible with no change in measured turbidity or increase in particle content in 4 hr at 23 °C	2109	**C**
	AST	10 mg/ml[a]		TNA #218 to #226[g]	Visually compatible with no precipitate or emulsion damage apparent in 4 hr at 23 °C	2215	**C**
Clonazepam	RC	1 mg/ml[k]		TPN #189[g]	Visually compatible for 24 hr at 22 °C	1767	**C**
Cyclophosphamide	MJ	10 mg/ml[a]		TPN #212 to #215[g]	Physically compatible with no change in measured turbidity or increase in particle content in 4 hr at 23 °C	2109	**C**
	MJ	10 mg/ml[a]		TNA #218 to #226[g]	Visually compatible with no precipitate or emulsion damage apparent in 4 hr at 23 °C	2215	**C**
Cyclosporine	SZ	5 mg/ml[a]		TPN #212 and #213[g]	Physically compatible with no change in measured turbidity or increase in particle content in 4 hr at 23 °C	2109	**C**
	SZ	5 mg/ml[a]		TPN #214 and #215[g]	Small amount of subvisual precipitate forms in 4 hr	2109	**I**
	SZ	5 mg/ml[a]		TNA #220 and #223[g]	Small amount of precipitate forms immediately	2215	**I**
	SZ	5 mg/ml[a]		TNA #218, #219, #221, #222, #224 to #226[g]	Visually compatible with no precipitate or emulsion damage apparent in 4 hr at 23 °C	2215	**C**

Y-Site Injection Compatibility (1:1 Mixture) (Cont.)

			Amino acid injection				
Drug	*Mfr*	*Conc*	*Mfr*	*Conc*	*Remarks*	*Ref*	*C/I*
Cytarabine	CHI	50 mg/ml		TPN #212 to #215[g]	Substantial loss of natural subvisual turbidity occurs immediately	2109	**I**
	BED	50 mg/ml		TNA #218 to #226[g]	Visually compatible with no precipitate or emulsion damage apparent in 4 hr at 23 °C	2215	**C**
Dexamethasone sodium phosphate	AMR	4 mg/ml		TPN #203 and #204[g]	Visually compatible for 2 hr at 23 °C	1974	**C**
	AMR	1 mg/ml[a]		TPN #212 to #215[g]	Physically compatible with no change in measured turbidity or increase in particle content in 4 hr at 23 °C	2109	**C**
	FUJ, ES	1 mg/ml[a]		TNA #218 to #226[g]	Visually compatible with no precipitate or emulsion damage apparent in 4 hr at 23 °C	2215	**C**
Diazepam	DB	5 mg/ml		TPN #189[g]	Visually compatible for 24 hr at 22 °C	1767	**C**
Digoxin	BW	0.625 mg/ 50 ml[l]		TNA #73[g]	Physically compatible for 4 hr by visual observation	1009	**C**
	BW	0.25 mg/ml		TPN #212 to #215[g]	Physically compatible with no change in measured turbidity or increase in particle content in 4 hr at 23 °C	2109	**C**
	ES, WY	0.25 mg/ml		TNA #218 to #226[g]	Visually compatible with no precipitate or emulsion damage apparent in 4 hr at 23 °C	2215	**C**
Diphenhydramine HCl	SCN	2 mg/ml[a]		TPN #212 to #215[g]	Physically compatible with no change in measured turbidity or increase in particle content in 4 hr at 23 °C	2109	**C**
	SCN	50 mg/ml		TPN #212 to #215[g]	Physically compatible with no change in measured turbidity or increase in particle content in 4 hr at 23 °C	2109	**C**
	SCN, PD	2[a] and 50 mg/ml		TNA #218 to #226[g]	Visually compatible with no precipitate or emulsion damage apparent in 4 hr at 23 °C	2215	**C**
Dobutamine HCl	LI	1 mg/ml[n]		TPN #91[f,g]	Physically compatible	1170	**C**
	LI	50 mg/ml[b]		TPN #189[g]	Visually compatible for 24 hr at 22 °C	1767	**C**
	LI	5 mg/ml		TPN #203 and #204[g]	Visually compatible for 4 hr at 23 °C	1974	**C**
	LI	4 mg/ml[a]		TPN #212 to #215[g]	Physically compatible with no change in measured turbidity or increase in particle content in 4 hr at 23 °C	2109	**C**
	AST	4 mg/ml[a]		TNA #218 to #226[g]	Visually compatible with no precipitate or emulsion damage apparent in 4 hr at 23 °C	2215	**C**
Dopamine HCl	AB	80 mg/ 50 ml[l]		TNA #73[g]	Physically compatible for 4 hr by visual observation	1009	**C**
	DB	1.6 mg/ml[b]		TPN #189[g]	Visually compatible for 24 hr at 22 °C	1767	**C**
	AMR	3.2 mg/ml		TPN #203 and #204[g]	Visually compatible for 4 hr at 23 °C	1974	**C**
	AB	3.2 mg/ml[a]		TPN #212 to #215[g]	Physically compatible with no change in measured turbidity or increase in particle content in 4 hr at 23 °C	2109	**C**
	AB	3.2 mg/ml[a]		TNA #222 and #223[g]	Precipitate forms immediately	2215	**I**

Y-Site Injection Compatibility (1:1 Mixture) (Cont.)

Drug	Mfr	Conc	Mfr	Conc	Remarks	Ref	C/I
				Amino acid injection			
	AB	3.2 mg/ml[a]		TNA #218 to #221 and #224 to #226[g]	Visually compatible with no precipitate or emulsion damage apparent in 4 hr at 23 °C	2215	**C**
Doxorubicin HCl	PH	2 mg/ml		TPN #212 to #215[g]	Substantial loss of natural subvisual turbidity occurs immediately	2109	**I**
	PH, GEN	2 mg/ml		TNA #218 to #226[g]	Damage to emulsion integrity occurs immediately with free oil formation possible	2215	**I**
Doxycycline hyclate	PF	10 mg/1 ml[j]		TPN #61[c,g]	Physically compatible	1012	**C**
	PF	60 mg/6 ml[j]		TPN #61[d,g]	Physically compatible	1012	**C**
	LY	1 mg/ml[a]		TPN #212 to #215[g]	Physically compatible with no change in measured turbidity or increase in particle content in 4 hr at 23 °C	2109	**C**
	FUJ	1 mg/ml[a]		TNA #218 to #226[g]	Damage to emulsion integrity occurs immediately with free oil formation possible	2215	**I**
Droperidol	AB	0.4 mg/ml[a]		TPN #212 to #215[g]	Physically compatible with no change in measured turbidity or increase in particle content in 4 hr at 23 °C	2109	**C**
	AB	0.4 mg/ml[a]		TNA #218 to #226[g]	Damage to emulsion integrity occurs in 1 to 4 hr with free oil formation possible	2215	**I**
Enalaprilat	MSD	0.1 mg/ml[a]		TPN #212 to #215[g]	Physically compatible with no change in measured turbidity or increase in particle content in 4 hr at 23 °C	2109	**C**
	ME	0.1 mg/ml[a]		TNA #218 to #226[g]	Visually compatible with no precipitate or emulsion damage apparent in 4 hr at 23 °C	2215	**C**
Epinephrine HCl	AST	0.2 mg/ml[b]		TPN #189[g]	Visually compatible for 24 hr at 22 °C	1767	**C**
Erythromycin lactobionate	AB	1 g/50 ml[b]		TNA #73[g,h]	Physically compatible for 4 hr at 25 °C by visual observation	1008	**C**
	AB	50 mg/1 ml[j]		TPN #61[c,g]	Physically compatible	1012	**C**
	AB	300 mg/ 6 ml[j]		TPN #61[d,g]	Physically compatible	1012	**C**
	DB	10 mg/ml[b]		TPN #189[g]	Visually compatible for 24 hr at 22 °C	1767	**C**
Famotidine HCl	ME	2 mg/ml[a]		TPN #212 to #215[g]	Physically compatible with no change in measured turbidity or increase in particle content in 4 hr at 23 °C	2109	**C**
	ME	2 mg/ml[a]		TNA #218 to #226[g]	Visually compatible with no precipitate or emulsion damage apparent in 4 hr at 23 °C	2215	**C**
Fentanyl citrate	ES	0.05 mg/ml		TPN #203 and #204[g]	Visually compatible for 4 hr at 23 °C	1974	**C**
	ES	0.01 mg/ml[k]		TPN #216[g]	Mixed 1 ml of fentanyl with 9 ml of TPN. Visually compatible for 24 hr	2104	**C**
	AB	0.05 mg/ml		TPN #212 to #215[g]	Physically compatible with no change in measured turbidity or increase in particle content in 4 hr at 23 °C	2109	**C**
	JN	0.0125 mg/ ml[a]		TPN #212 to #215[g]	Physically compatible with no change in measured turbidity or increase in particle content in 4 hr at 23 °C	2109	**C**

Y-Site Injection Compatibility (1:1 Mixture) (Cont.)

Drug	Mfr	Conc	Mfr	Conc	Remarks	Ref	C/I
	AB	0.0125[a] and 0.05 mg/ml		TNA #218 to #226[g]	Visually compatible with no precipitate or emulsion damage apparent in 4 hr at 23 °C	2215	C
Flucloxacillin sodium	BE	50 mg/ml[b]		TPN #189[g]	Visually compatible for 24 hr at 22 °C	1767	C
Fluconazole	PF	0.5 and 1.75 mg/ml[o]		TPN #146[g,o]	Visually compatible with no fluconazole loss by HPLC in 2 hr at 24 °C under fluorescent light. Amino acid concentrations by HPLC greater than 93%	1554	C
	PF	0.5 and 1.75 mg/ml[o]		TPN #147 and #148[g,o]	Visually compatible with no fluconazole loss by HPLC in 2 hr at 24 °C under fluorescent light. Amino acids not analyzed	1554	C
	RR	2 mg/ml		TPN #212 to #215[g]	Physically compatible with no change in measured turbidity or increase in particle content in 4 hr at 23 °C	2109	C
	PF	2 mg/ml		TNA #218 to #226[g]	Visually compatible with no precipitate or emulsion damage apparent in 4 hr at 23 °C	2215	C
Fluorouracil	PH	16 mg/ml[a]		TPN #212 and #213[g]	Slight subvisual haze, crystals, and amber discoloration form in 1 to 4 hr	2109	I
	PH	16 mg/ml[a]		TPN #214 and #215[g]	Turbidity forms immediately	2109	I
	PH	16 mg/ml[a]		TNA #220 and #223[g]	Small amount of white precipitate forms immediately	2215	I
	PH	16 mg/ml[a]		TNA #218, #219, #221, #222, #224 to #226[g]	Visually compatible with no precipitate or emulsion damage apparent in 4 hr at 23 °C	2215	C
Folic acid	AB	15 mg/ml		TPN #189[g]	Visually compatible for 24 hr at 22 °C	1767	C
Foscarnet sodium	AST	24 mg/ml		TPN #121[g]	Physically compatible for 24 hr at 25 °C under fluorescent light by visual and microscopic examination	1393	C
Furosemide	ES	165 mg/50 ml[l]		TNA #73[g]	Physically compatible for 4 hr by visual observation	1009	C
		10 mg/ml[b]		TPN #189[g]	Visually compatible for 24 hr at 22 °C	1767	C
	AMR	10 mg/ml		TPN #203 and #204[g]	Visually compatible for 2 hr at 23 °C	1974	C
	AB	3 mg/ml[a]		TPN #212 to #215[g]	Small amount of subvisual precipitate forms immediately	2109	I
	AB	3 mg/ml[a]		TNA #218 to #226[g]	Visually compatible with no precipitate or emulsion damage apparent in 4 hr at 23 °C	2215	C
Ganciclovir sodium	SY	1 and 5 mg/ml[a]		TPN #144[g]	Visually compatible for 2 hr at 20 °C under fluorescent light	1522	C
	SY	10 mg/ml[a]		TPN #144[g]	Heavy precipitate forms within 30 min	1522	I
	SY	3 and 5 mg/ml		TPN #183 to #185[g]	Precipitate forms	1744	I
	SY	2 mg/ml		TPN #183[g]	Precipitate forms	1744	I
	SY	1 mg/ml[p]		TPN #183[g]	Visually compatible with no ganciclovir loss by HPLC in 3 hr at 24 °C under fluorescent light. Less than 10% amino acids loss by HPLC in 2 hr	1744	C

Y-Site Injection Compatibility (1:1 Mixture) (Cont.)

				Amino acid injection			
Drug	*Mfr*	*Conc*	*Mfr*	*Conc*	*Remarks*	*Ref*	*C/I*
	SY	2 mg/ml[q]		TPN #184 and #185[g]	Visually compatible with no ganciclovir loss by HPLC in 3 hr at 24 °C under fluorescent light. Less than 10% amino acids loss by HPLC in 3 hr	1744	**C**
	SY	20 mg/ml[a]		TPN #212 to #215[g]	Gross white precipitate forms immediately	2109	**I**
	RC	20 mg/ml[a]		TNA #218 to #226[g]	Large amount of white precipitate forms immediately	2215	**I**
Gentamicin sulfate	SC	80 mg/ 50 ml[a]		TNA #73[g,h]	Physically compatible for 4 hr at 25 °C by visual observation	1008	**C**
	IX	12.5 mg/ 1.25 ml[j]		TPN #61[c,g]	Physically compatible	1012	**C**
	IX	75 mg/ 1.9 ml[j]		TPN #61[d,g]	Physically compatible	1012	**C**
		13 and 20 mg/ml		TPN #54[g]	Physically compatible and gentamicin activity retained over 6 hr at 22 °C by microbiological assay	1045	**C**
	IX	5 mg[e]		TPN #91[f,g]	Physically compatible	1170	**C**
	ES	40 mg/ml		TNA #97 to #104[g]	Physically compatible and gentamicin content retained for 6 hr at 21 °C by TDx	1324	**C**
	DB	1 mg/ml[b]		TPN #189[g]	Visually compatible for 24 hr at 22 °C	1767	**C**
	ES	10 mg/ml		TPN #203 and #204[g]	Visually compatible for 2 hr at 23 °C	1974	**C**
	AB	5 mg/ml[a]		TPN #212 to #215[g]	Physically compatible with no change in measured turbidity or increase in particle content in 4 hr at 23 °C	2109	**C**
	AB, FUJ	5 mg/ml[a]		TNA #218 to #226[g]	Visually compatible with no precipitate or emulsion damage apparent in 4 hr at 23 °C	2215	**C**
Granisetron HCl	SKB	0.05 mg/ml[a]		TPN #212 to #215[g]	Physically compatible with no change in measured turbidity or increase in particle content in 4 hr at 23 °C	2109	**C**
	SKB	0.05 mg/ml[a]		TNA #218 to #226[g]	Visually compatible with no precipitate or emulsion damage apparent in 4 hr at 23 °C	2215	**C**
Haloperidol lactate	SE	10 mg/ml		TPN #189[g]	Visually compatible for 24 hr at 22 °C	1767	**C**
	MN	0.2 mg/ml[a]		TPN #212 to #215[g]	Physically compatible with no change in measured turbidity or increase in particle content in 4 hr at 23 °C	2109	**C**
	MN	0.2 mg/ml[a]		TNA #218 to #226[g]	Damage to emulsion integrity occurs immediately with free oil formation possible	2215	**I**
Heparin sodium	DB	500 units/ml[b]		TPN #189[g]	Visually compatible for 24 hr at 22 °C	1767	**C**
	AB	100 units/ml		TPN #212 to #215[g]	Physically compatible with no change in measured turbidity or increase in particle content in 4 hr at 23 °C	2109	**C**
	AB	100 units/ml		TNA #218 to #226[g]	Damage to emulsion integrity occurs immediately with free oil formation possible	2215	**I**
Hydrocortisone sodium phosphate	ME	1 mg/ml[a]		TPN #212 to #215[g]	Physically compatible with no change in measured turbidity or increase in particle content in 4 hr at 23 °C	2109	**C**

Y-Site Injection Compatibility (1:1 Mixture) (Cont.)

			Amino acid injection				
Drug	*Mfr*	*Conc*	*Mfr*	*Conc*	*Remarks*	*Ref*	*C/I*
	ME	1 mg/ml[a]		TNA #218 to #226[g]	Visually compatible with no precipitate or emulsion damage apparent in 4 hr at 23 °C	2215	**C**
Hydrocortisone sodium succinate	UP	50 mg/ml[b]		TPN #189[g]	Visually compatible for 24 hr at 22 °C	1767	**C**
	AB	1 mg/ml[a]		TPN #212 to #215[g]	Physically compatible with no change in measured turbidity or increase in particle content in 4 hr at 23 °C	2109	**C**
	AB	1 mg/ml[a]		TNA #218 to #226[g]	Visually compatible with no precipitate or emulsion damage apparent in 4 hr at 23 °C	2215	**C**
Hydromorphone HCl	ES	0.5 mg/ml[a]		TPN #212 to #215[g]	Physically compatible with no change in measured turbidity or increase in particle content in 4 hr at 23 °C	2109	**C**
	ES	0.5 mg/ml[a]		TNA #219, #222, #224 to #226[g]	Damage to emulsion integrity occurs immediately with free oil formation possible	2215	**I**
	ES	0.5 mg/ml[a]		TNA #218, #220, #221, #223[g]	Visually compatible with no precipitate or emulsion damage apparent in 4 hr at 23 °C	2215	**C**
Hydroxyzine HCl	ES	2 mg/ml[a]		TPN #212 to #215[g]	Physically compatible with no change in measured turbidity or increase in particle content in 4 hr at 23 °C	2109	**C**
	ES	2 mg/ml[a]		TNA #218 to #226[g]	Visually compatible with no precipitate or emulsion damage apparent in 4 hr at 23 °C	2215	**C**
Idarubicin HCl	AD	1 mg/ml[b]		TPN #140[g]	Visually compatible for 24 hr at 25 °C under fluorescent light	1525	**C**
Ifosfamide	MJ	25 mg/ml[a]		TPN #212 to #215[g]	Physically compatible with no change in measured turbidity or increase in particle content in 4 hr at 23 °C	2109	**C**
	MJ	25 mg/ml[a]		TNA #218 to #226[g]	Visually compatible with no precipitate or emulsion damage apparent in 4 hr at 23 °C	2215	**C**
IL-2	RC	4800 I.U./ml[b]		TPN #145[g]	Visually compatible and IL-2 activity by bioassay retained	1552	**C**
Imipenem–cilastatin sodium	ME	10 mg/ml[b]		TPN #212 to #215[g]	Physically compatible with no change in measured turbidity or increase in particle content in 4 hr at 23 °C	2109	**C**
	ME	10 mg/ml[b]		TNA #218 to #226[g]	Visually compatible with no precipitate or emulsion damage apparent in 4 hr at 23 °C	2215	**C**
Indomethacin sodium trihydrate	MSD	1 mg/ml[b]	MG[r]	AA 1 and 2%, D 10%	Haze forms in 2 hr and white precipitate forms in 4 hr	1527	**I**
	MSD	1 mg/ml[b]	MG[r]	AA 1 and 2%, W	Haze forms in 30 min and white precipitate forms in 1 hr	1527	**I**
Insulin, regular	NOV	2 units/ml[s]		TPN #189[g]	Visually compatible for 24 hr at 22 °C	1767	**C**
	NOV	1 unit/ml[a]		TPN #212 to #215[g]	Physically compatible with no change in measured turbidity or increase in particle content in 4 hr at 23 °C	2109	**C**

Y-Site Injection Compatibility (1:1 Mixture) (Cont.)

Drug	Mfr	Conc	Mfr	Conc	Remarks	Ref	C/I
	NOV	1 unit/ml[a]		TNA #218 to #226[g]	Visually compatible with no precipitate or emulsion damage apparent in 4 hr at 23 °C	2215	**C**
Isoproterenol HCl	BR	0.2 mg/ 50 ml[l]		TNA #73[g]	Physically compatible for 4 hr by visual observation	1009	**C**
Kanamycin sulfate	BR	500 mg/ 50 ml[a]		TNA #73[g]	Physically compatible for 4 hr at 25 °C by visual observation	1008	**C**
Leucovorin calcium	IMM	2 mg/ml[a]		TPN #212 to #215[g]	Physically compatible with no change in measured turbidity or increase in particle content in 4 hr at 23 °C	2109	**C**
	IMM	2 mg/ml[a]		TNA #218 to #226[g]	Visually compatible with no precipitate or emulsion damage apparent in 4 hr at 23 °C	2215	**C**
Levorphanol tartrate	RC	0.5 mg/ml[a]		TPN #212 to #215[g]	Physically compatible with no change in measured turbidity or increase in particle content in 4 hr at 23 °C	2109	**C**
	RC	0.5 mg/ml[a]		TNA #218 to #226[g]	Damage to emulsion integrity occurs immediately with free oil formation possible	2215	**I**
Lidocaine HCl	ES	200 mg/ 50 ml[l]		TNA #73[g]	Physically compatible for 4 hr by visual observation	1009	**C**
Lorazepam	WY	0.1 mg/ml[a]		TPN #212 to #215[g]	Physically compatible with no change in measured turbidity or increase in particle content in 4 hr at 23 °C	2109	**C**
	WY	0.1 mg/ml[a]		TNA #218 to #226[g]	Damage to emulsion integrity occurs in 1 hr	2215	**I**
Magnesium sulfate	AB	100 mg/ml[a]		TPN #212 to #215[g]	Physically compatible with no change in measured turbidity or increase in particle content in 4 hr at 23 °C	2109	**C**
	AB	100 mg/ml[a]		TNA #218 to #226[g]	Visually compatible with no precipitate or emulsion damage apparent in 4 hr at 23 °C	2215	**C**
Mannitol	BA	15%		TPN #212 to #215[g]	Physically compatible with no change in measured turbidity or increase in particle content in 4 hr at 23 °C	2109	**C**
	BA	15%		TNA #218 to #226[g]	Visually compatible with no precipitate or emulsion damage apparent in 4 hr at 23 °C	2215	**C**
Meperidine HCl	AB	10 mg/ml		TPN #131 and #132[g]	Physically compatible for 4 hr at 25 °C under fluorescent light	1397	**C**
	DB	50 mg/ml		TPN #189[g]	Visually compatible for 24 hr at 22 °C	1767	**C**
	AST	4 mg/ml[a]		TPN #212 to #215[g]	Physically compatible with no change in measured turbidity or increase in particle content in 4 hr at 23 °C	2109	**C**
	AST	4 mg/ml[a]		TNA #218 to #226[g]	Visually compatible with no precipitate or emulsion damage apparent in 4 hr at 23 °C	2215	**C**
Meropenem	ZEN	20 mg/ml[a]		TNA #218 to #226[g]	Visually compatible with no precipitate or emulsion damage apparent in 4 hr at 23 °C	2215	**C**

Y-Site Injection Compatibility (1:1 Mixture) (Cont.)

Amino acid injection

Drug	Mfr	Conc	Mfr	Conc	Remarks	Ref	C/I
Mesna	MJ	10 mg/ml[a]		TPN #212 to #215[g]	Physically compatible with no change in measured turbidity or increase in particle content in 4 hr at 23 °C	2109	C
	MJ	10 mg/ml[a]		TNA #218 to #226[g]	Visually compatible with no precipitate or emulsion damage apparent in 4 hr at 23 °C	2215	C
Methotrexate sodium	LE	15 mg/ml[a]		TPN #212 to #215[g]	Substantial loss of natural subvisual turbidity with a hazy subvisual precipitate in 0 to 1 hr	2109	I
	IMM	15 mg/ml[a]		TNA #218 to #226[g]	Visually compatible with no precipitate or emulsion damage apparent in 4 hr at 23 °C	2215	C
Methyldopate HCl	MSD	250 mg/ 50 ml[a]		TNA #73[g]	Cracked the lipid emulsion	1009	I
	MSD	250 mg/ 50 ml[b]		TNA #73[g]	Physically compatible for 4 hr by visual observation	1009	C
Methylprednisolone sodium succinate	AB	5 mg/ml[a]		TPN #212 to #215[g]	Physically compatible with no change in measured turbidity or increase in particle content in 4 hr at 23 °C	2109	C
	AB	5 mg/ml[a]		TNA #218 to #226[g]	Visually compatible with no precipitate or emulsion damage apparent in 4 hr at 23 °C	2215	C
Metoclopramide HCl	AB	5 mg/ml		TPN #212 to #215[g]	Substantial loss of natural subvisual turbidity occurs immediately	2109	I
	AB	5 mg/ml		TNA #218 to #226[g]	Visually compatible with no precipitate or emulsion damage apparent in 4 hr at 23 °C	2215	C
Metronidazole	DB	5 mg/ml		TPN #189[g]	Visually compatible for 24 hr at 22 °C	1767	C
	AB	5 mg/ml		TPN #203 and #204[g]	Visually compatible for 2 hr at 23 °C	1974	C
	SCS	5 mg/ml		TPN #212 to #215[g]	Physically compatible with no change in measured turbidity or increase in particle content in 4 hr at 23 °C	2109	C
	AB	5 mg/ml		TNA #218 to #226[g]	Visually compatible with no precipitate or emulsion damage apparent in 4 hr at 23 °C	2215	C
Midazolam HCl	RC	5 mg/ml		TPN #189[g]	White haze and light white precipitate form immediately. Crystals form in 24 hr	1767	I
	RC	2 mg/ml[a]		TPN #212 to #215[g]	White cloudiness forms rapidly	2109	I
	RC	2 mg/ml[a]		TNA #218 to #226[g]	Damage to emulsion integrity occurs immediately with free oil formation possible	2215	I
Milrinone lactate	SW	0.4 mg/ml[a]		TPN #217[g]	Visually compatible with no loss of milrinone by HPLC in 4 hr at 23 °C	2214	C
Minocycline HCl	LE	0.2 mg/ml[a]		TPN #212 to #215[g]	Bright yellow discoloration forms immediately	2109	I
	LE	0.2 mg/ml[a]		TNA #218 to #226[g]	Damage to emulsion integrity occurs immediately with free oil formation possible	2215	I

Y-Site Injection Compatibility (1:1 Mixture) (Cont.)

			Amino acid injection				
Drug	*Mfr*	*Conc*	*Mfr*	*Conc*	*Remarks*	*Ref*	*C/I*
Mitoxantrone HCl	IMM	0.5 mg/ml[a]		TPN #212 to #215[g]	Substantial loss of natural subvisual turbidity occurs immediately	2109	I
	IMM	0.5 mg/ml[a]		TNA #218 to #226[g]	Visually compatible with no precipitate or emulsion damage apparent in 4 hr at 23 °C	2215	C
Morphine sulfate	AB	1 mg/ml		TPN #131 and #132[g]	Physically compatible for 4 hr at 25 °C under fluorescent light	1397	C
	DB	30 mg/ml		TPN #189[g]	Visually compatible for 24 hr at 22 °C	1767	C
	ES	1 mg/ml		TPN #203 and #204[g]	Visually compatible for 2 hr at 23 °C	1974	C
	AST	1 mg/ml[a]		TPN #212 to #215[g]	Physically compatible with no change in measured turbidity or increase in particle content in 4 hr at 23 °C	2109	C
	ES	1 mg/ml[a]		TNA #218 to #226[g]	Visually compatible with no precipitate or emulsion damage apparent in 4 hr at 23 °C	2215	C
	ES	15 mg/ml		TNA #218 to #226[g]	Damage to emulsion integrity occurs immediately with free oil formation possible	2215	I
Multivitamins (M.V.I.-12)	RR			TPN #189[g]	Visually compatible for 24 hr at 22 °C	1767	C
Nafcillin sodium	WY	250 mg/ 1 ml[i]		TPN #61[c,g]	Physically compatible	1012	C
	WY	1.5 g/6 ml[i]		TPN #61[d,g]	Physically compatible	1012	C
		250 mg/ml		TPN #54[g]	Physically compatible and nafcillin activity retained over 6 hr at 22 °C by microbiological assay	1045	C
	BE	20 mg/ml[a]		TPN #212 to #215[g]	Physically compatible with no change in measured turbidity or increase in particle content in 4 hr at 23 °C	2109	C
	BE, APC	20 mg/ml[a]		TNA #218 to #226[g]	Visually compatible with no precipitate or emulsion damage apparent in 4 hr at 23 °C	2215	C
Nalbuphine HCl	AB	10 mg/ml		TPN #212 to #215[g]	Physically compatible with no change in measured turbidity or increase in particle content in 4 hr at 23 °C	2109	C
	AB, AST	10 mg/ml		TNA #218 to #226[g]	Damage to emulsion integrity occurs immediately with free oil formation possible	2215	I
Netilmicin sulfate	SC	12.5 mg/ 0.13 ml[j]		TPN #61[c,g]	Physically compatible	1012	C
	SC	75 mg/ 0.75 ml[j]		TPN #61[d,g]	Physically compatible	1012	C
	SC	5 mg/ml[a]		TPN #212 to #215[g]	Physically compatible with no change in measured turbidity or increase in particle content in 4 hr at 23 °C	2109	C
	SC	5 mg/ml[a]		TNA #218 to #226[g]	Visually compatible with no precipitate or emulsion damage apparent in 4 hr at 23 °C	2215	C
Nitroglycerin	DU	0.4 mg/ml[a]		TPN #212 to #215[g]	Physically compatible with no change in measured turbidity or increase in particle content in 4 hr at 23 °C	2109	C

Y-Site Injection Compatibility (1:1 Mixture) (Cont.)

			Amino acid injection				
Drug	*Mfr*	*Conc*	*Mfr*	*Conc*	*Remarks*	*Ref*	*C/I*
	DU	0.4 mg/ml[a]		TNA #218 to #226[g]	Visually compatible with no precipitate or emulsion damage apparent in 4 hr at 23 °C	2215	**C**
Norepinephrine bitartrate	BN	0.4 mg/ 50 ml[i]		TNA #73[g]	Physically compatible for 4 hr by visual observation	1009	**C**
	AB	0.016 mg/ ml[a]		TPN #212 to #215[g]	Physically compatible with no change in measured turbidity or increase in particle content in 4 hr at 23 °C	2109	**C**
Octreotide acetate	SZ	0.01 mg/ml[a]		TPN #212 to #215[g]	Physically compatible with no change in measured turbidity or increase in particle content in 4 hr at 23 °C	2109	**C**
	SZ	0.01 mg/ml[a]		TNA #218 to #226[g]	Visually compatible with no precipitate or emulsion damage apparent in 4 hr at 23 °C	2215	**C**
Ofloxacin	ORT	4 mg/ml[a]		TPN #212 to #215[g]	Physically compatible with no change in measured turbidity or increase in particle content in 4 hr at 23 °C	2109	**C**
	ORT	4 mg/ml[a]		TNA #218 to #226[g]	Visually compatible with no precipitate or emulsion damage apparent in 4 hr at 23 °C	2215	**C**
Ondansetron HCl	GL	1 mg/ml[a]		TPN #212 to #215[g]	Physically compatible with no change in measured turbidity or increase in particle content in 4 hr at 23 °C	2109	**C**
	CER	1 mg/ml[a]		TNA #218 to #226[g]	Damage to emulsion integrity occurs immediately with free oil formation possible	2215	**I**
Oxacillin sodium	BE	1 g/50 ml[a]		TNA #73[g,h]	Physically compatible for 4 hr at 25 °C by visual observation	1008	**C**
	BE	250 mg/ 1.5 ml[i]		TPN #61[c,g]	Physically compatible	1012	**C**
	BE	1.5 g/9 ml[i]		TPN #61[d,g]	Physically compatible	1012	**C**
		100 and 150 mg/ml		TPN #54[g]	Physically compatible and 88 to 94% oxacillin activity retained over 6 hr at 22 °C by microbiological assay	1012	**C**
Paclitaxel	MJ	1.2 mg/ml[a]		TPN #212 to #215[g]	Physically compatible with no change in measured turbidity or increase in particle content in 4 hr at 23 °C	2109	**C**
	MJ	1.2 mg/ml[a]		TNA #218 to #226[g]	Visually compatible with no precipitate or emulsion damage apparent in 4 hr at 23 °C	2215	**C**
Penicillin G	PF	200,000 units/2 ml[i]		TPN #61[c,g]	Physically compatible	1012	**C**
	PF	1.2 million units/12 ml[i]		TPN #61[d,g]	Physically compatible	1012	**C**
		320,000 and 500,000 units/ml		TPN #54[g]	Physically compatible and 88% penicillin activity retained over 6 hr at 22 °C by microbiological assay	1045	**C**
		300 mg/ml[b]		TPN #189[g]	Visually compatible for 24 hr at 22 °C	1767	**C**
Penicillin G potassium	SQ	2 million units/50 ml[a]		TNA #73[g,h]	Physically compatible for 4 hr at 25 °C by visual observation	1008	**C**
	MAR	500,000 units/ml		TPN #203 and #204[g]	Visually compatible for 2 hr at 23 °C	1974	**C**

Y-Site Injection Compatibility (1:1 Mixture) (Cont.)

Amino acid injection

Drug	Mfr	Conc	Mfr	Conc	Remarks	Ref	C/I
Pentobarbital sodium	AB	5 mg/ml[a]		TPN #212 to #215[g]	Physically compatible with no change in measured turbidity or increase in particle content in 4 hr at 23 °C	2109	**C**
	AB	5 mg/ml[a]		TNA #218 to #226[g]	Damage to emulsion integrity occurs immediately with free oil formation possible	2215	**I**
Phenobarbital sodium	WY	5 mg/ml[a]		TPN #212 to #215[g]	Physically compatible with no change in measured turbidity or increase in particle content in 4 hr at 23 °C	2109	**C**
	WY	5 mg/ml[a]		TNA #218 to #226[g]	Damage to emulsion integrity occurs immediately with free oil formation possible	2215	**I**
Phenytoin sodium	PD	50 mg/ml		TPN #189[g]	Heavy white precipitate forms immediately	1767	**I**
Piperacillin sodium	LE	250 mg/ 1.25 ml[i]		TPN #61[c,g]	Physically compatible	1012	**C**
	LE	1.5 g/7.5 ml[i]		TPN #61[d,g]	Physically compatible	1012	**C**
		133 and 200 mg/ml		TPN #54[g]	Physically compatible and 90 to 100% piperacillin activity retained over 6 hr at 22 °C by microbiological assay	1045	**C**
	LE	40 mg/ml[a]		TPN #212 to #215[g]	Physically compatible with no change in measured turbidity or increase in particle content in 4 hr at 23 °C	2109	**C**
	LE	40 mg/ml[a]		TNA #218 to #226[g]	Visually compatible with no precipitate or emulsion damage apparent in 4 hr at 23 °C	2215	**C**
Piperacillin sodium–tazobactam sodium	CY	40 + 5 mg/ ml[a]		TPN #212 to #215[g]	Physically compatible with no change in measured turbidity or increase in particle content in 4 hr at 23 °C	2109	**C**
	LE	40 + 5 mg/ ml[a]		TNA #218 to #226[g]	Visually compatible with no precipitate or emulsion damage apparent in 4 hr at 23 °C	2215	**C**
Potassium chloride	AST	30 mg/ml[b]		TPN #189[g]	Visually compatible for 24 hr at 22 °C	1767	**C**
	AB	0.1 mEq/ml[a]		TPN #212 to #215[g]	Physically compatible with no change in measured turbidity or increase in particle content in 4 hr at 23 °C	2109	**C**
	AB	0.1 mEq/ml[a]		TNA #218 to #226[g]	Visually compatible with no precipitate or emulsion damage apparent in 4 hr at 23 °C	2215	**C**
Potassium phosphates	AB	3 mmol/ml		TPN #212 to #215[g]	Increased turbidity forms immediately	2109	**I**
	AB	3 mmol/ml		TNA #218 to #226[g]	Damage to emulsion integrity occurs immediately with free oil formation possible	2215	**I**
Prochlorperazine edisylate	SCN	0.5 mg/ml[a]		TPN #212 to #215[g]	Physically compatible with no change in measured turbidity or increase in particle content in 4 hr at 23 °C	2109	**C**
	SCN, SO	0.5 mg/ml[a]		TNA #218 to #226[g]	Visually compatible with no precipitate or emulsion damage apparent in 4 hr at 23 °C	2215	**C**

Y-Site Injection Compatibility (1:1 Mixture) (Cont.)

			Amino acid injection				
Drug	*Mfr*	*Conc*	*Mfr*	*Conc*	*Remarks*	*Ref*	*C/I*
Promethazine HCl	SCN	2 mg/ml[a]		TPN #212 and #214[g]	Physically compatible with no change in measured turbidity or increase in particle content in 4 hr at 23 °C	2109	**C**
	SCN	2 mg/ml[a]		TPN #213 and #215[g]	Amber discoloration forms in 4 hr	2109	**I**
	SCN	2 mg/ml[a]		TNA #218 to #226[g]	Visually compatible with no precipitate or emulsion damage apparent in 4 hr at 23 °C	2215	**C**
Propofol	STU	2 and 3 g		TPN #186 to #188[g]	Physically compatible with no change in particle size distribution and 6% or less propofol loss by HPLC in 5 hr at 22 °C	1805	**C**
	STU	500 mg		TPN #186[g]	Physically compatible with no change in particle size distribution but 28% propofol loss by HPLC in 5 hr at 22 °C	1805	**I**
	STU	500 mg		TPN #187 and #188[g]	Physically compatible with no change in particle size distribution and 6% or less propofol loss by HPLC in 5 hr at 22 °C	1805	**C**
Ranitidine HCl	GL	2.5 mg/ml[b]		TPN #189[g]	Visually compatible for 24 hr at 22 °C	1767	**C**
	GL	25 mg/ml		TPN #203 and #204[g]	Visually compatible for 2 hr at 23 °C	1974	**C**
	GL	2 mg/ml[a]		TPN #212 to #215[g]	Physically compatible with no change in measured turbidity or increase in particle content in 4 hr at 23 °C	2109	**C**
	GL	2 mg/ml[a]		TNA #218 to #226[g]	Visually compatible with no precipitate or emulsion damage apparent in 4 hr at 23 °C	2215	**C**
Salbutamol	AH	0.5 mg/ml[b]		TPN #189[g]	Visually compatible for 24 hr at 22 °C	1767	**C**
Sargramostim	IMM	10 μg/ml[b]		TPN #133[g]	Physically compatible for 4 hr at 22 °C under fluorescent light	1436	**C**
	IMM	6[t] and 15 μg/ml[b]		TPN #181[g]	Visually compatible for 2 hr	1618	**C**
Sodium bicarbonate	AB	1 mEq/ml		TPN #212 and #214[g]	Small amount of hazy subvisual precipitate forms in 1 hr and settles	2109	**I**
	AB	1 mEq/ml		TPN #213 and #215[g]	Physically compatible with no change in measured turbidity or increase in particle content in 4 hr at 23 °C	2109	**C**
	AB	1 mEq/ml		TNA #218 to #226[g]	Visually compatible with no precipitate or emulsion damage apparent in 4 hr at 23 °C	2215	**C**
Sodium nitroprusside	AB	0.4 mg/ml[a]		TPN #212 to #215[g]	Physically compatible with no change in measured turbidity or increase in particle content in 4 hr at 23 °C protected from light	2109	**C**
	AB	0.4 mg/ml[a]		TNA #218 to #226[g]	Visually compatible with no precipitate or emulsion damage apparent in 4 hr at 23 °C protected from light	2215	**C**
Sodium phosphates	AB	3 mmol/ml		TPN #212 to #215[g]	Increased turbidity forms immediately	2109	**I**
	AB	3 mmol/ml		TNA #218 to #226[g]	Damage to emulsion integrity occurs immediately with free oil formation possible	2215	**I**

Y-Site Injection Compatibility (1:1 Mixture) (Cont.)

				Amino acid injection			
Drug	*Mfr*	*Conc*	*Mfr*	*Conc*	*Remarks*	*Ref*	*C/I*
Tacrolimus	FUJ	1 mg/ml[a]		TPN #212 to #215[g]	Physically compatible with no change in measured turbidity or increase in particle content in 4 hr at 23 °C	2109	C
	FUJ	1 mg/ml[a]		TNA #218 to #226[g]	Visually compatible with no precipitate or emulsion damage apparent in 4 hr at 23 °C	2215	C
Thiotepa	IMM[u]	1 mg/ml[a]		TPN #193[g]	Physically compatible with no change in measured turbidity or increase in particle content in 4 hr at 23 °C	1861	C
Ticarcillin disodium	BE	3 g/50 ml[a]		TNA #73[g,h]	Physically compatible for 4 hr at 25 °C by visual observation	1008	C
	BE	250 mg/ 1 ml[i]		TPN #61[c,g]	Physically compatible	1012	C
	BE	1.5 g/6 ml[i]		TPN #61[d,g]	Physically compatible	1012	C
		267 and 400 mg/ml		TPN #54[g]	Physically compatible and 89 to 94% ticarcillin activity retained over 6 hr at 22 °C by microbiological assay	1045	C
	SKB	30 mg/ml[a]		TPN #212 to #215[g]	Physically compatible with no change in measured turbidity or increase in particle content in 4 hr at 23 °C	2109	C
	SKB	30 mg/ml[a]		TNA #218 to #226[g]	Visually compatible with no precipitate or emulsion damage apparent in 4 hr at 23 °C	2215	C
Ticarcillin disodium–clavulanate potassium	BE	30 mg/ml[b]		TPN #189[g]	Visually compatible for 24 hr at 22 °C	1767	C
	SKB	31 mg/ml[a]		TPN #212 to #215[g]	Physically compatible with no change in measured turbidity or increase in particle content in 4 hr at 23 °C	2109	C
	SKB	31 mg/ml[a]		TNA #218 to #226[g]	Visually compatible with no precipitate or emulsion damage apparent in 4 hr at 23 °C	2215	C
Tobramycin sulfate	LI	80 mg/ 50 ml[a]		TNA #73[g,h]	Physically compatible for 4 hr at 25 °C by visual observation	1008	C
	DI	12.5 mg/ 1.25 ml[j]		TPN #61[c,g]	Physically compatible	1012	C
	DI	75 mg/ 1.9 ml[j]		TPN #61[d,g]	Physically compatible	1012	C
		20 mg/ml		TPN #54[g]	Physically compatible and tobramycin activity retained over 6 hr at 22 °C by microbiological assay	1045	C
	LI	5 mg[e]		TPN #91[f,g]	Physically compatible	1170	C
	LI	40 mg/ml		TNA #97 to #104[g]	Physically compatible and tobramycin content retained for 6 hr at 21 °C by TDx	1324	C
	LI	10 mg/ml		TPN #203 and #204[g]	Visually compatible for 2 hr at 23 °C	1974	C
	AB	5 mg/ml[a]		TPN #212 to #215[g]	Physically compatible with no change in measured turbidity or increase in particle content in 4 hr at 23 °C	2109	C
	AB	5 mg/ml[a]		TNA #218 to #226[g]	Visually compatible with no precipitate or emulsion damage apparent in 4 hr at 23 °C	2215	C
Trace elements	DB			TPN #189[g]	Blue discoloration forms immediately	1767	I

Y-Site Injection Compatibility (1:1 Mixture) (Cont.)

Amino acid injection

Drug	Mfr	Conc	Mfr	Conc	Remarks	Ref	C/I
Trimethoprim–sulfamethoxazole	ES	0.8 + 4 mg/ml[a]		TPN #212 to #215[g]	Physically compatible with no change in measured turbidity or increase in particle content in 4 hr at 23 °C	2109	C
	ES	0.8 + 4 mg/ml[a]		TNA #218 to #226[g]	Visually compatible with no precipitate or emulsion damage apparent in 4 hr at 23 °C	2215	C
Urokinase	AB	2500 I.U./ml[b]		TPN #55 and #56[g]	No loss of urokinase activity when assayed immediately after mixing	1046	C
Vancomycin HCl	LI	50 mg/1 ml[j]		TPN #61[c,g]	Physically compatible	1012	C
	LI	300 mg/6 ml[j]		TPN #61[d,g]	Physically compatible	1012	C
	LI	30 mg[e]		TPN #91[f,g]	Physically compatible	1170	C
	DB	10 mg/ml[b]		TPN #189[g]	Visually compatible for 24 hr at 22 °C	1767	C
	LI	5 mg/ml		TPN #203 and #204[g]	Visually compatible for 2 hr at 23 °C	1974	C
	AB	10 mg/ml[a]		TPN #212 to #215[g]	Physically compatible with no change in measured turbidity or increase in particle content in 4 hr at 23 °C	2109	C
	AB	10 mg/ml[a]		TNA #218 to #226[g]	Visually compatible with no precipitate or emulsion damage apparent in 4 hr at 23 °C	2215	C
Vecuronium bromide	OR	2 mg/ml[k]		TPN #189[g]	Visually compatible for 24 hr at 22 °C	1767	C
Zidovudine	BW	4 mg/ml		TPN #203 and #204[g]	Visually compatible for 2 hr at 23 °C	1974	C
	BW	4 mg/ml[a]		TPN #212 to #215[g]	Physically compatible with no change in measured turbidity or increase in particle content in 4 hr at 23 °C	2109	C
	GW	4 mg/ml[a]		TNA #218 to #226[g]	Visually compatible with no precipitate or emulsion damage apparent in 4 hr at 23 °C	2215	C

[a]*Tested in dextrose 5% in water.*
[b]*Tested in sodium chloride 0.9%.*
[c]*Run at 21 ml/hr.*
[d]*Run at 94 ml/hr.*
[e]*Given over one hour by syringe pump.*
[f]*Run at 10 ml/hr.*
[g]*Refer to Appendix I for the composition of parenteral nutrition solutions. TNA indicates a 3-in-1 admixture, and TPN indicates a 2-in-1 admixture.*
[h]*A 32.5-ml sample of parenteral nutrition solution and 50 ml of antibiotic in a minibottle.*
[i]*Given over five minutes by syringe pump.*
[j]*Given over 30 minutes by syringe pump.*
[k]*Tested in sterile water for injection.*
[l]*Tested in both dextrose 5% in water and sodium chloride 0.9%.*
[m]*Given over 10 minutes by syringe pump.*
[n]*Tested in dextrose 5% in water infused at 1.2 ml/hr.*
[o]*Varying volumes to simulate varying administration rates.*
[p]*Ganciclovir sodium concentration after mixing was 0.83 mg/ml.*
[q]*Ganciclovir sodium concentration after mixing was 1.4 mg/ml.*
[r]*TrophAmine.*
[s]*Tested in Haemaccel (Behring).*
[t]*With human albumin 0.1%.*
[u]*Lyophilized formulation tested.*
[v]*Sodium carbonate–containing formulation.*
[w]L-*Arginine–containing formulation.*

Additional Compatibility Information

Compatibility of Some Parenteral Nutrition Solutions— Parenteral nutrition solutions #38 through #47 (Appendix I) have been tested and found to be physically compatible for 24 hours at 22 °C. However, those solutions containing multivitamin infusion concentrate or vitamin B complex with C exhibited changes in the UV spectra of both amino acids–dextrose and the vitamins. Additionally, TLC changes were observed in similar solutions in 12 hours (313).

Calcium and Phosphate— UNRECOGNIZED CALCIUM PHOSPHATE PRECIPITATION IN A 3-IN-1 PARENTERAL NUTRITION MIXTURE RESULTED IN PATIENT DEATH.

The potential for the formation of a calcium phosphate precipitate in parenteral nutrition solutions is well studied and documented (1771; 1777), but the information is complex and difficult to apply to the clinical situation (1770; 1772; 1777). The incorporation of fat emulsion in 3-in-1 parenteral nutrition solutions obscures any precipitate that may be present, which has led to substantial debate about the dangers associated with 3-in-1 parenteral nutrition mixtures and when or if the danger to the patient is warranted therapeutically (1770-1772; 2031-2036). Because such precipitation may be life threatening to patients (2037), the Food and Drug Administration issued a Safety Alert containing the following recommendations (1769):

"1. The amounts of phosphorus and of calcium added to the admixture are critical. The solubility of the added calcium should be calculated from the volume at the time the calcium is added. It should not be based upon the final volume.

Some amino acid injections for TPN admixtures contain phosphate ions (as a phosphoric acid buffer). These phosphate ions and the volume at the time the phosphate is added should be considered when calculating the concentration of phosphate additives. Also, when adding calcium and phosphate to an admixture, the phosphate should be added first.

The line should be flushed between the addition of any potentially incompatible components.

2. A lipid emulsion in a three-in-one admixture obscures the presence of a precipitate. Therefore, if a lipid emulsion is needed, either (1) use a two-in-one admixture with the lipid infused separately, or (2) if a three-in-one admixture is medically necessary, then add the calcium before the lipid emulsion and according to the recommendations in number 1 above.

If the amount of calcium or phosphate which must be added is likely to cause a precipitate, some or all of the calcium should be administered separately. Such separate infusions must be properly diluted and slowly infused to avoid serious adverse events related to the calcium.

3. When using an automated compounding device, the above steps should be considered when programming the device. In addition, automated compounders should be maintained and operated according to the manufacturer's recommendations.

Any printout should be checked against the programmed admixture and weight of components.

4. During the mixing process, pharmacists who mix parenteral nutrition admixtures should periodically agitate the admix-

ture and check for precipitates. Medical or home care personnel who start and monitor these infusions should carefully inspect for the presence of precipitates both before and during infusion. Patients and care givers should be trained to visually inspect for signs of precipitation. They also should be advised to stop the infusion and seek medical assistance if precipitates are noted.

5. A filter should be used when infusing either central or peripheral parenteral nutrition admixtures. At this time, data have not been submitted to document which size filter is most effective in trapping precipitates.

Standards of practice vary, but the following is suggested: a 1.2-μm air-eliminating filter for lipid-containing admixtures and a 0.22-μm air-eliminating filter for non-lipid-containing admixtures.

6. Parenteral nutrition admixtures should be administered within the following time frames: if stored at room temperature, the infusion should be started within 24 hours after mixing; if stored at refrigerated temperatures, the infusion should be started within 24 hours of rewarming. Because warming parenteral nutrition admixtures may contribute to the formation of precipitates, once administration begins, care should be taken to avoid excessive warming of the admixture.

Persons administering home care parenteral nutrition admixtures may need to deviate from these time frames. Pharmacists who initially prepare these admixtures should check a reserve sample for precipitates over the duration and under the conditions of storage.

7. If symptoms of acute respiratory distress, pulmonary emboli, or interstitial pneumonitis develop, the infusion should be stopped immediately and thoroughly checked for precipitates. Appropriate medical interventions should be instituted. Home care personnel and patients should immediately seek medical assistance."

Calcium Phosphate Precipitation Fatalities— Hill et al. reported fatal cases of paroxysmal respiratory failure in two previously healthy women receiving peripheral vein parenteral nutrition. The patients experienced sudden cardiopulmonary arrest consistent with pulmonary emboli. The authors used in vitro simulations and an animal model to conclude that unrecognized calcium phosphate precipitation in a 3-in-1 total nutrition admixture caused the fatalities. The precipitation resulted during compounding by introducing calcium and phosphate near to one another in the compounding sequence and prior to complete fluid addition. This resulted in a temporarily high concentration of the drugs and precipitation of calcium phosphate. Observation of the precipitate was obscured by the incorporation of 20% fat emulsion, intravenous into the nutrition mixture. No filter was used during infusion of the fatal nutrition admixtures (2037).

Calcium and Phosphate Conditional Compatibility— Calcium salts are conditionally compatible with potassium phosphate in parenteral nutrition solutions. The incompatibility is dependent on a solubility and concentration phenomenon and is not entirely predictable. Precipitation may occur during compounding or at some time after compounding is completed.

NOTE: Some amino acids solutions inherently contain calcium and phosphate, which must be considered in any projection of compatibility. See Table 1.

It also was noted that the order of mixing of calcium gluconate and potassium phosphate may affect compatibility at elevated concentrations. Addition of potassium phosphate should precede that of calcium gluconate (313).

A study by Henry et al. (608) determined the maximum concentrations of calcium (as chloride and gluconate) and phosphate that can be maintained without precipitation in a parenteral nutrition solution consisting of FreAmine II 4.25 and dextrose 25% for 24 hours at 30 °C. Their results are depicted in Figure 1.

Henry et al. noted that the amino acids in parenteral nutrition solutions form soluble complexes with calcium and phosphate, reducing the available free calcium and phosphate that can form insoluble precipitates. The concentration of calcium available for precipitation is greater with the chloride salt compared to the gluconate salt, at least in part because of differences in dissociation characteristics. This can be seen in Figure 1 by the greater concentration of calcium gluconate that can be mixed with sodium phosphate (608).

In addition to the concentrations of phosphate and calcium and the salt form of the calcium, Henry et al. noted that the concentration of amino acids and the time and temperature of storage altered the formation of calcium phosphate in parenteral nutrition solutions. As the temperature was increased, the incidence of precipitate formation also increased. This finding was attributed, at least in part, to a greater degree of dissociation of the calcium and phosphate complexes and the decreased solubility of calcium phosphate. Therefore, a solution possibly may be stored at 4 °C with no precipitation, but on warming to room temperature a precipitate will form over time (608).

Eggert et al. (609) evaluated the compatibility of calcium and phosphate in several parenteral nutrition formulas for newborn infants. Calcium gluconate 10% (Cutter) and potassium phosphate (Abbott) were used to achieve concentrations of 2.5 to 100 mEq/L of calcium and 2.5 to 100 mmol/L of phosphorus added. The parenteral nutrition solutions evaluated were as shown in Table 2. The results were reported as graphic depictions.

Eggert et al. noted the pH dependence of the phosphate–calcium precipitation. Dibasic calcium phosphate is very insoluble, while monobasic calcium phosphate is relatively soluble. At low pH, the soluble monobasic form predominates; but as the pH increases, more dibasic phosphate becomes available to bind with calcium and precipitate. Therefore, the lower the pH of the parenteral nutrition solution, the more calcium and phosphate can be solubilized. Once again, the effects of temperature were observed. As the temperature

Table 2. Parenteral Nutrition Solutions Used by Eggert et al. (609)

Component	Solution Number			
	#1	#2	#3	#4
FreAmine III	4%	2%	1%	1%
Dextrose	25%	20%	10%	10%
pH	6.3	6.4	6.6	7.0[a]

[a]Adjusted with sodium hydroxide.

is increased, more calcium ion becomes available and more dibasic calcium phosphate is formed. Therefore, temperature increases will increase the amount of precipitate (609).

Fitzgerald and MacKay reported similar calcium and phosphate solubility curves for neonatal parenteral nutrition solutions using TrophAmine (McGaw) 2, 1.5, and 0.8% as the sources of amino acids. The solutions also contained dextrose 10%, with cysteine and pH adjustment being used in some admixtures. Calcium and phosphate solubility followed the patterns reported by Eggert et al. (609). A slightly greater concentration of phosphate could be used in some mixtures, but this finding was not consistent (1024).

Using a similar study design, Fitzgerald and MacKay also studied six neonatal parenteral nutrition solutions based on Aminosyn-PF (Abbott) 2, 1.5, and 0.8%, with and without added cysteine HCl and dextrose 10%. Calcium concentrations ranged from 2.5 to 50 mEq/L, and phosphate concentrations ranged from 2.5 to 50 mmol/L. Solutions sat for 18 hours at 25 °C and then were warmed to 37 °C in a water bath to simulate the clinical situation of warming prior to infusion into a child. Solubility curves were markedly different than those for TrophAmine in the previous study (1024). Solubilities were reported to decrease by 15 mEq/L for calcium and 15 mmol/L for phosphate. The solutions remained clear during room temperature storage, but crystals often formed on warming to 37 °C (1211).

However, these data were questioned by Mikrut, who noted the similarities between the Aminosyn-PF and TrophAmine products and found little difference in calcium and phosphate solubilities in a preliminary report (1212). In the full report (1213), parenteral nutrition solutions containing Aminosyn-PF or TrophAmine 1 or 2.5% with dextrose 10 or 25%, respectively, plus electrolytes and trace metals, with or without cysteine HCl, were evaluated under the same conditions used by Fitzgerald and MacKay. Calcium concentrations ranged from 2.5 to 50 mEq/L, and phosphate concentrations ranged from 5 to 50 mmol/L. In contrast to the results of Fitzgerald and MacKay, the solubility curves were very similar for the Aminosyn-PF and TrophAmine parenteral nutrition solutions but very different from those of the previous Aminosyn-PF study (1211). The authors again showed that the solubility of calcium and phosphate is greater in solutions containing higher concentrations of amino acids and dextrose (1213).

Dunham et al. also reported calcium and phosphate solubility curves for TrophAmine 1 and 2% with dextrose 10% and electrolytes, vitamins, heparin, and trace elements. Calcium concentrations ranged from 10 to 60 mEq/L, and phosphorus concentrations ranged from 10 to 40 mmol/L. Calcium and phosphate solubilities were assessed by analysis of the calcium concentrations and followed patterns similar to those reported by Henry et al. (608) and Eggert et al. (609). The higher percentage of amino acids (TrophAmine 2%) permitted a slightly greater solubility of calcium and phosphate, especially in the 10 to 50-mEq/L and 10 to 35-mmol/L ranges, respectively (1614).

Knight et al. reported the maximal product of the amount of calcium (as gluconate) times phosphate (as potassium) that can be

Figure 1. Maximum solubilities of calcium chloride (○) and calcium gluconate (△) with sodium phosphate in an amino acid 4.25% – dextrose 25% solution at 30 °C

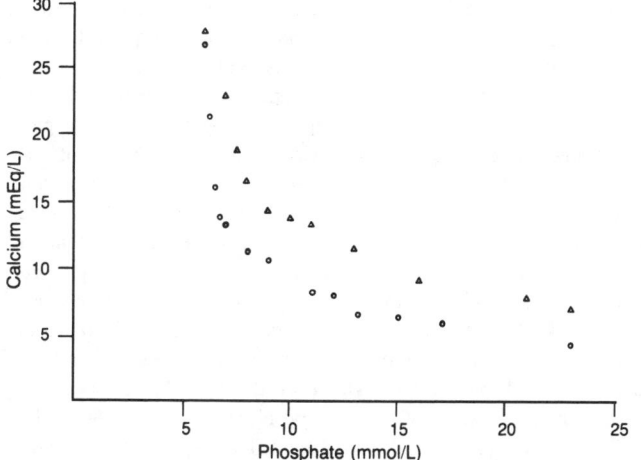

added to a parenteral nutrition solution, composed of amino acids 1% (Travenol) and dextrose 10%, for preterm infants. Turbidity was observed on initial mixing when the solubility product was around 115 to 130 mmol^2 or greater. After storage at 7 °C for 20 hours, visible precipitates formed at solubility products of 130 mmol^2 or greater. If the solution was administered through a barium-impregnated silicone rubber catheter, crystalline precipitates obstructed the catheters in 12 hours at a solubility product of 100 mmol^2 and in 10 days at 79 mmol^2, much lower than the in vitro results (1041).

Poole et al. determined the solubility characteristics of calcium and phosphate in pediatric parenteral nutrition solutions composed of Aminosyn 0.5, 2, and 4% with dextrose 10 to 25%. Also present were electrolytes and vitamins. Sodium phosphate was added sequentially in phosphorus concentrations from 10 to 30 mmol/L. Calcium gluconate was added last in amounts ranging from 1 to 10 g/L. The solutions were stored at 25 °C for 30 hours and examined visually and microscopically for precipitation. The authors found that higher concentrations of Aminosyn increased the solubility of calcium and phosphate. Precipitation occurred at lower calcium and phosphate concentrations in the 0.5% solution compared to the 2 and 4% solutions. For example, at a phosphorus concentration of 30 mmol/L, precipitation occurred at calcium gluconate concentrations of about 1, 2, and 4 g/L in the 0.5, 2, and 4% Aminosyn mixtures, respectively. Similarly, at a calcium gluconate concentration of 8 g/L and above, precipitation occurred at phosphorus concentrations of about 13, 17, and 22 mmol/L in the 0.5, 2, and 4% solutions, respectively. The dextrose concentration did not appear to affect the calcium and phosphate solubility significantly (1042).

Alexander and Arena evaluated the compatibility of calcium gluconate (American Quinine) and potassium phosphate (Lyphomed) in a parenteral nutrition solution, composed of dextrose 12.5% and amino acid injection (FreAmine III, McGaw) 1.33% and having a pH of 6.6, for premature infants. Potassium phosphate was added in varying amounts to samples of this solution. The samples were then titrated with calcium gluconate 10%. From the resulting data, an equation was derived to predict when precipitation would occur:

$$Y = -0.455X + 2.951$$

where Y is the Log_{10} of the calcium gluconate concentration (as mg/100 ml) and X is the phosphate concentration (as mmol/100 ml). The equation can be solved to determine the maximum concentration of calcium gluconate for a given phosphate concentration or vice versa. If either additive is sufficiently dilute, then the other can be added in high concentrations without precipitation occurring, obviating the need for the equation. These lower limits were set at 60 mg/100 ml for calcium gluconate and 0.6 mmol/100 ml for phosphate (1004).

While the authors noted that this equation technically applies to the specific solution being tested and that other variables such as temperature can affect precipitation, in practice they found it applicable to a variety of parenteral nutrition solutions, having similar components and pH values, for premature infants. The equation is *not* applicable to parenteral nutrition solutions with amino acid and dextrose concentrations, other components, or pH values that are much different (1004).

Venkaraman et al. evaluated the solubility of calcium and phosphorus in neonatal parenteral nutrition solutions composed of amino acids (Abbott) 1.25 and 2.5% with dextrose 5 and 10%, respectively. Also present were multivitamins and trace elements. The solutions contained calcium (as gluconate) in amounts ranging from 25 to

Table 3. Maximum Calcium and Phosphorus Concentrations Physically Compatible for 48 Hours at 4 °C (1210)

Calcium (mg/100 ml)	Phosphorus (mg/100 ml)	
	Amino Acids 1.25% + Dextrose 5%[a]	Amino Acids 2.5% + Dextrose 10%[a]
200[b]	50	75
150	50	100
100	75	100
50	100	125
25	150[b]	150[b]

[a]*Plus multivitamins and trace elements.*
[b]*Maximum concentration tested.*

200 mg/100 ml. The phosphorus (as potassium phosphate) concentrations evaluated ranged from 25 to 150 mg/100 ml. If calcium gluconate was added first, cloudiness occurred immediately. If potassium phosphate was added first, substantial quantities could be added with no precipitate formation in 48 hours at 4 °C (Table 3). However, if stored at 22 °C, the solutions were stable for only 24 hours, and all contained precipitates after 48 hours (1210).

Kirkpatrick et al. reported the physical compatibility of calcium gluconate 10 to 40 mEq/L and potassium phosphates 10 to 40 mmol/L in three neonatal parenteral nutrition solutions (TPN #123 to #125 in Appendix I), alone and with retrograde administration of aminophylline 7.5 mg diluted with 1.5 ml of sterile water for injection. Contact of the alkaline aminophylline solution with the parenteral nutrition solutions resulted in the precipitation of calcium phosphate at much lower concentrations than were compatible in the parenteral nutrition solutions alone (1404).

MacKay et al. reported additional calcium and phosphate solubility curves for specialty parenteral nutrition solutions based on NephrAmine and also HepatAmine at concentrations of 0.8, 1.5, and 2% as the sources of amino acids. The solutions also contained dextrose 10%, with cysteine and pH adjustment to simulate addition of fat emulsion used in some admixtures. Calcium and phosphate solubility followed the hyperbolic patterns reported by Eggert et al. (609). Temperature, time, and pH affected calcium and phosphate solubility, with pH having the greatest effect (2038).

Shatsky et al. reported the maximum sodium phosphate concentrations for given amounts of calcium gluconate that could be admixed in parenteral nutrition solutions containing TrophAmine in varying quantities (with cysteine HCl 40 mg/g of amino acid) and dextrose 10%. The solutions also contained magnesium sulfate 4 mEq/L, potassium acetate 24 mEq/L, sodium chloride 32 mEq/L, pediatric multivitamins, and trace elements. The presence of cysteine HCl reduces the solution pH and increases the amount of calcium and phosphate that can be incorporated before precipitation occurs. The results of this study cannot be safely extrapolated to TPN solutions with compositions other than the ones tested. The admixtures were compounded with the sodium phosphate added last after thorough mixing of all other components. The authors noted that this is not the preferred order of mixing (usually phosphate is added first and thoroughly mixed before adding calcium last); however, they believed this reversed order of mixing would provide a margin of error in cases in which the proper order is not followed. After compounding, the solutions were stored for 24 hours at 40 °C. The maximum calcium and phosphate amounts that could be mixed in the various solutions were reported tabularly and are shown in Table 4 (2039). However, these results are not entirely consistent with the study of Hoie and Narducci (2196). See below.

The temperature dependence of the calcium–phosphate precipita-

Table 4. Maximum Amount of Phosphate (as Sodium) (mmol/L) Not Resulting in Precipitation According to the Study of Shatsky et al. (2039). See CAUTION Below.[a]

Calcium (as gluconate)	Amino Acid (as TrophAmine) plus Cysteine HCl 40 mg/g Amino Acid				
	0%	0.4%	1%	2%	3%
9.8 mEq/L	0	27	42	60	66
14.7 mEq/L	0	15	18	30	36
19.6 mEq/L	0	6	15	27	30
29.4 mEq/L	0	3	6	21	24

[a]*CAUTION: The results cannot be safely extrapolated to solutions with formulas other than the ones tested. See text.*

tion has resulted in the occlusion of a subclavian catheter by a solution apparently free of precipitation. The parenteral nutrition solution consisted of FreAmine III 500 ml, dextrose 70% 500 ml, sodium chloride 50 mEq, sodium phosphate 40 mmol, potassium acetate 10 mEq, potassium phosphate 40 mmol, calcium gluconate 10 mEq, magnesium sulfate 10 mEq, and Shil's trace metals solution 1 ml. Although there was no evidence of precipitation in the bottle, tubing and pump cassette, and filter (all at approximately 26 °C) during administration, the occluded catheter and Vicra Loop Lock (next to the patient's body at 37 °C) had numerous crystals identified as calcium phosphate. In vitro, this parenteral nutrition solution had a precipitate in 12 hours at 37 °C but was clear for 24 hours at 26 °C (610).

Similarly, a parenteral nutrition solution that was clear and free of particulates after two weeks under refrigeration developed a precipitate in four to six hours when stored at room temperature. When the solution was warmed in a 37 °C water bath, precipitation occurred in one hour. Administration of the solution before the precipitate was noticed led to interstitial pneumonitis due to deposition of calcium phosphate crystals (1427).

Koorenhof and Timmer reported the maximum allowable concentrations of calcium and phosphate in a 3-in-1 parenteral nutrition mixture for children (TNA #192 in Appendix I). Added calcium was varied from 1.5 to 150 mmol/L, and added phosphate was varied from 21 to 300 mmol/L. These mixtures were stable for 48 hours at 22 and 37 °C as long as the pH was not greater than 5.7, the calcium concentration was below 16 mmol/L, the phosphate concentration was below 52 mmol/L, and the product of the calcium and phosphate concentrations was below 250 mmol²/L² (1773).

Fausel et al. evaluated calcium phosphate precipitation phenomena in a series of parenteral nutrition admixtures composed of dextrose 22%, amino acids (FreAmine III) 2.7%, and fat emulsion (Abbott) 0, 1, and 3.2%. Incorporation of calcium gluconate 19 to 24 mEq/L and phosphate (as sodium) 22 to 28 mmol/L resulted in visible precipitation in the fat-free admixtures. New precipitate continued to form over 14 days, even after repeated filtrations of the solutions through 0.2-μm filters. The presence of the amino acids increased calcium and phosphate solubility, compared with simple aqueous solutions. However, the incorporation of the fat emulsion did not result in a statistically significant increase in calcium and phosphate solubility. The authors noted that the kinetics of calcium phosphate precipitate formation do not appear to be entirely predictable; both transient and permanent precipitation can occur either during the compounding process or at some time afterward. Because calcium phosphate precipitation can be very dangerous clinically, the use of inline filters was recommended. The authors suggested that the filters should have a porosity appropriate to the parenteral

nutrition admixture—1.2 μm for fat-containing and 0.2 or 0.45 μm for fat-free nutrition mixtures (2061).

Hoie and Narducci used laser particle analysis to evaluate the formation of calcium phosphate precipitation in pediatric TPN solutions containing TrophAmine in concentrations ranging from 0.5 to 3% and also containing L-cysteine HCl 1 g/L. The solutions also contained in each liter sodium chloride 20 mEq, sodium acetate 20 mEq, magnesium sulfate 3 mEq, trace elements 3 ml, and heparin sodium 500 units. The presence of L-cysteine HCl reduces the solution pH and increases the amount of calcium and phosphate that can be incorporated before precipitation occurs. The results of this study cannot be safely extrapolated to TPN solutions with compositions other than the ones tested. The maximum amount of phosphate that was incorporated without the appearance of a measurable increase in particulates in 24 hours at 37 °C for each of the amino acids concentrations is shown in Table 5 (2196). These results are not entirely consistent with those of Shatsky et al. See above. The use of more sensitive electronic particle measurement for the formation of subvisual particulates in this study may contribute to the differences in the results.

The presence of magnesium in solutions may also influence the reaction between calcium and phosphate, including the nature and extent of precipitation (158; 159).

The interaction of calcium and phosphate in parenteral nutrition solutions is a complex phenomenon. Various factors play a role in the solubility or precipitation of a given combination, including (608; 609; 1042; 1063; 1427; 2038; 2039; 2061):

1. Concentration of calcium
2. Salt form of calcium
3. Concentration of phosphate
4. Concentration of amino acids
5. Amino acids composition
6. Concentration of dextrose
7. Temperature of solution
8. pH of solution
9. Presence of other additives
10. Order of mixing

Enhanced precipitate formation would be expected from such factors as high concentrations of calcium and phosphate, increases in

Table 5. Maximum Amount of Phosphate (as Potassium) (mmol/L) Not Resulting in Precipitation According to the Study of Hoie and Narducci (2196). See CAUTION Below.[a]

Calcium (as Gluconate) (mEq/L)	Amino Acid (as TrophAmine) plus Cysteine HCl 1 g/L					
	0.5%	1%	1.5%	2%	2.5%	3%
10	22	28	38	38	38	43
14	18	18	18	38	38	43
19	18	18	18	33	33	38
24	12	18	18	22	28	28
28	12	18	18	18	18	18
33	12	12	12	12	12	12
37	12	12	12	12	12	12
41	9	9	9	12	12	12
45	0	9	9	12	12	12
49	0	9	9	9	12	12
53	0	9	9	9	9	9

[a]*CAUTION: The results cannot be safely extrapolated to solutions with formulas other than the ones tested. See text.*

solution pH, decreased amino acid concentrations, increases in temperature, addition of calcium prior to the phosphate, lengthy standing times or slow infusion rates, and use of calcium as the chloride salt (854).

Even if precipitation does not occur in the bottle, it has been reported that crystallization of calcium phosphate may occur in a Silastic infusion pump chamber or tubing if the rate of administration is slow, as for premature infants. Water vapor may be transmitted outward and be replaced by air rapidly enough to produce supersaturation (202). Several other cases of catheter occlusion also have been reported (610; 1427–1429).

The UV spectrum of an equal parts mixture of amino acids 8%–dextrose 50% solution was not altered in 24 hours at 22 °C by the addition of calcium gluconate 20 mEq and potassium phosphate 25 mEq (313).

Multicomponent (3-in-1; TNA) Admixtures— Because of the potential benefits in terms of simplicity, efficiency, time, and cost, the concept of mixing amino acids, carbohydrates, electrolytes, fat emulsion, and other nutritional components together in the same container has been explored. Within limits, the feasibility of preparing such 3-in-1 parenteral nutrition admixtures has been demonstrated.

However, these 3-in-1 mixtures are very complex and inherently unstable. Emulsion stability is dependent on both zeta potential and van der Waals forces, influenced by the presence of dextrose (2029). The ultimate stability of each unique mixture depends on numerous complicated factors, making definitive stability predictions impossible. Injury and death have resulted from administration of unrecognized precipitation in 3-in-1 parenteral nutrition admixtures (1769; 1782; 1783). See the section on Calcium and Phosphate. In addition, the use of 3-in-1 admixtures is associated with a higher rate of catheter occlusion and reduced catheter life compared with giving the fat emulsion separately from the parenteral nutrition solution (2194).

Combining an amino acids–glucose parenteral nutrition solution containing various electrolytes with fat emulsion 20%, intravenous (Intralipid, Vitrum), resulted in a mixture which, although apparently stable for a limited time, ultimately exhibited a creaming phenomenon. Within 12 hours, a distinct 2-cm layer separated on the upper surface. Microscopic examination revealed aggregates believed to be clumps of fat droplets. Fewer and smaller aggregates were noted in the lower layer (560; 561).

Black and Popovich reported that amino acids had no adverse effect on the emulsion stability of Intralipid 10%. In addition, the amino acids appeared to prevent the adverse impact of dextrose and to slow the flocculation and coalescence resulting from mono- and divalent cations. However, significant coalescence did result after a longer time. Therefore, it was recommended that such cations not be mixed with fat emulsion, intravenous (656).

The compatibility and stability of parenteral nutrition solutions consisting of amino acids, dextrose, fat emulsion, and various additives, all in a single admixture, were evaluated by Cutter Laboratories. The study entailed combining, in glass bottles, various amino acid products with Intralipid 10 or 20% and dextrose 70 or 10% along with electrolytes, vitamins, and trace minerals. These parenteral nutrition solutions were stored at 5 °C for three days followed by 25 °C for two days. The compatibility and stability of the emulsion were evaluated initially and again after storage. Additive compatibility and stability were not evaluated. Cutter Laboratories concluded that most of the admixtures were compatible and stable over the test period with minimal chemical and physical

changes (Table 6). The exceptions were admixtures prepared with Aminosyn 7%. In the Aminosyn 7%-containing admixtures, the emulsion broke within 24 hours at room temperature and had oil globules floating on the surface. Refrigeration prevented the breaking of the emulsion, as did exclusion of the electrolytes. Presumably, the lower pH of Aminosyn 7% compared to the other amino acid products tested was associated with the disruption of the emulsion.

Although dextrose 70 and 10% were the only concentrations evaluated, Cutter Laboratories indicated that intermediate dextrose concentrations may be used as long as the amino acids–dextrose–Intralipid ratio is 1:1:1 or 1:1:½. Other ratios also have been recommended (703; 1068).

The disruptive effects of divalent ions are not as severe in these parenteral nutrition admixtures as they are in Intralipid alone. However, they do represent complex and somewhat unpredictable interactions. Consequently, Cutter Laboratories recommends using only combinations that have been evaluated. Concentrations of additive components may be at or below the maximum amounts indicated in Table 6.

Although some admixtures were stable over longer periods, Cutter Laboratories recommends use of these combined multicomponent admixtures within 24 hours (791).

Travenol states that 1:1:1 mixtures of amino acids 5.5, 8.5, or 10% (Travenol), fat emulsion 10 to 20% (Travenol), and dextrose 10 to 70% are physically stable but recommends administration within 24 hours. M.V.I.-12 3.3 ml/L and electrolytes may also be added to the admixtures up to the maximum amounts listed below (850):

Calcium	8.3 mEq/L
Magnesium	3.3 mEq/L
Sodium	23.3 mEq/L
Potassium	20.0 mEq/L
Chloride	23.3 mEq/L
Phosphate	20 mEq/L
Zinc	3.33 mg/L
Copper	1.33 mg/L
Manganese	0.33 mg/L
Chromium	13.33 μg/L

Knutsen et al. reported that a mixture of soybean oil emulsion 10% with amino acids 8.5%, concentrated dextrose, multivitamins, and electrolytes had good physical stability. Visual and microscopic examination of samples stored at 4 °C for one week showed the emulsion to be uniform with no flocculence (891).

Burnham et al. evaluated the stability of mixtures of 1 L of Intralipid 20%, 1.5 L of Vamin glucose (amino acids with dextrose 10%), and 0.5 L of dextrose 10% with various electrolytes and vitamins. Initial emulsion particle size was around 1 μm. The mixture containing only monovalent cations was stable for at least nine days at 4 °C, with little change in particle size. The mixtures containing the divalent cations, such as calcium and magnesium, demonstrated much greater particle size increases, with mean diameters of around 3.3 to 3.5 μm after nine days at 4 °C. After 48 hours of storage, however, these increases were more modest, around 1.5 to 1.85 μm. After storage at 4 °C for 48 hours followed by 24 hours at room temperature, few particles exceeded 5 μm. It was found that the effect of particle aggregation caused by electrolytes demonstrates a critical concentration before the effect begins. For calcium and magnesium chlorides, the critical concentrations were 2.4 and 2.6 mmol/L, respectively. Sodium and potassium chloride had critical concentrations of 110 and 150 mmol/L, respectively. The rate of

Table 6. Intralipid-Containing Parenteral Nutrition Admixtures Found to be Compatible and Stable (791)

Component	Amount (ml)				
	FreAmine II 8.5%	FreAmine III 8.5%	Travasol 8.5% without Electrolytes	Travasol 10% without Electrolytes	Veinamine 8%
Amino acids	500	500	500	500	500
Dextrose 70 or 10%	500	500	500	500	500
Intralipid 20 or 10%	500 or 250	500 or 250	500 or 250	500 or 250	500 or 250
	Maximum Total Concentration				
Calcium	10 mEq	10 mEq	10 mEq	10 mEq	10 mEq
Magnesium	13 mEq	13 mEq	13 mEq	13 mEq	13 mEq
Sodium	134 mEq	134 mEq	129 mEq	129 mEq	149 mEq
Potassium	105 mEq	105 mEq	105 mEq	105 mEq	120 mEq
Chloride	244 mEq	245 mEq	261 mEq	264 mEq	279 mEq
Sulfate	13 mEq	13 mEq	13 mEq	13 mEq	13 mEq
Phosphorus	12.5 mmol	12.5 mmol	7.5 mmol	7.5 mmol	7.5 mmol
Acetate	21 mEq	37 mEq	26 mEq	44 mEq	25 mEq
Zinc	4 mg	4 mg	4 mg	4 mg	4 mg
Copper	1.5 mg	1.5 mg	1.5 mg	1.5 mg	1.5 mg
Manganese	0.8 mg	0.8 mg	0.8 mg	0.8 mg	0.8 mg
Chromium	15 μg	15 μg	15 μg	15 μg	15 μg
Multivitamin infusion concentrate (USV)	5 ml	5 ml	5 ml	5 ml	5 ml

particle aggregation increased linearly with increasing electrolyte concentration. Heparin 667 units/L had no effect on emulsion stability. The quantity of emulsion in the mixture had a relatively small influence on stability, but higher concentrations exhibited a somewhat greater coalescence (892).

Davis and Galloway noted that instability of the emulsion systems is manifested by (1) flocculation of oil droplets to form aggregates, producing a cream-like layer on top; or (2) coalescence of oil droplets, leading to an increase in the average droplet size and eventually a separation of free oil. The lowering of pH and the adding of electrolytes can adversely affect the mechanical and electrical properties at the oil–water interface, eventually leading to flocculation and coalescence. Amino acids act as buffering agents and provide a protective effect on emulsion stability. Adding electrolytes, especially the divalent ions Mg^{++} and Ca^{++} in excess of 2.5 mmol/L, to simple fat emulsions will cause flocculation. But in mixed parenteral nutrition solutions, the stability of the emulsion will be enhanced, depending on the quantity and nature of the amino acids present. The authors recommended a careful examination of emulsion mixtures for signs of instability prior to administration (849).

Lawrence et al. reported good stability for an amino acid 4% (Travenol), dextrose 14%, and fat emulsion 4% (Pharmacia) parenteral nutrition solution. The solution also contained electrolytes, vitamins, and heparin sodium 4000 units/L. The aqueous solution was prepared first, with the fat emulsion added subsequently. This procedure allowed visual inspection of the aqueous phase and reduced the risk of emulsion breakdown by the divalent cations. Sample mixtures were stored at 18 to 25 and 3 to 8 °C for up to five days. They were evaluated visually and with a Coulter counter for particle size measurements. Both room temperature and refrigerated mixtures were stable for 48 hours. A marked increase in particle size was noted in the room temperature sample after 72 hours, but re-

frigeration delayed the changes. The authors' experience with over 1400 mixtures for administration to patients resulted in one emulsion creaming and another cracking, but the authors had no explanation for the failure of these particular emulsions (848).

Turner reported on six parenteral nutrition solutions having various concentrations of amino acids, dextrose, soybean oil emulsion (Kabi-Vitrum), electrolytes, and multivitamins. All of the admixtures were stable for one week under refrigeration followed by 24 hours at room temperature, with no visible changes, changes in pH, or significant changes in particle size (1013). However, other researchers questioned this interpretation of the results (1014; 1015).

Iliano et al. reported that the addition of trace elements to a 3-in-1 parenteral nutrition solution with electrolytes had no adverse effect on the particle size of the fat emulsion after eight days of storage at 4 °C (1017).

Harrie et al. reported on the stability of 3-in-1 parenteral nutrition solutions prepared with 500 ml of Intralipid 20% compared to Soyacal 20%, along with 500 or 1000 ml of FreAmine III 8.5% and 500 ml of dextrose 70%. Also present were relatively large amounts of electrolytes and other additives. All mixtures were similarly stable for 28 days at 4 °C followed by five days at 21 to 25 °C, with little change in the emulsion. A slight white cream layer appeared after five days at 4 °C but was easily redispersed with gentle agitation. The appearance of this cream layer did not statistically affect particle size distribution. The authors concluded that the emulsion mixture remained suitable for clinical use throughout the study period. The stability of other components was not evaluated (1019).

Sayeed et al. reported on the stability of 3-in-1 parenteral nutrition admixtures prepared with Liposyn II 10 and 20%, Aminosyn pH 6, and dextrose along with electrolytes, trace metals, and vitamins. Thirty-one different combinations were evaluated. Samples were stored at: (1) 25 °C for one day, (2) 5 °C for two days followed by

30 °C for one day, and (3) 5 °C for nine days followed by 25 °C for one day. In all cases, there was no visual evidence of creaming, free oil droplets, and other signs of emulsion instability. Furthermore, little or no change in the particle size or zeta potential (electrostatic surface charge of lipid particles) was found, indicating emulsion stability. The dextrose and amino acids remained stable over the 10-day storage period. The greatest change of an amino acid occurred with tryptophan, which lost 6% in 10 days. Vitamin stability was not tested (1025).

Hardy et al. reported on the stability of four parenteral nutrition admixtures, ranging from 1 L each of amino acids 5.5% (Travenol), dextrose 10%, and fat emulsion 10% (Travenol) up to a "worst case" of 1 L each of amino acids 10% with electrolytes (Travenol), dextrose 70%, and fat emulsion 10% (Travenol). The admixtures were stored at 48 hours at 5 to 9 °C followed by 24 hours at room temperature. There were no visible signs of creaming, flocculation, and free oil. The mean emulsion particle size remained within acceptable limits for all admixtures, and there were no significant changes in glucose, soybean oil, and amino acid concentrations. The authors noted that two factors were predominant in determining the stability of such admixtures: electrolyte concentrations and pH (1065).

Hardy and Klim reported that several parenteral nutrition solutions containing amino acids (Travenol), glucose, and lipid, with and without electrolytes and trace elements, produced no visible flocculation or any significant change in mean emulsion particle size during 24 hours at room temperature (1066).

Jeppsson and Sjoberg reported on the compatibility of 10 parenteral nutrition admixtures, evaluated over 96 hours while stored at 20 to 25 °C in both glass bottles and ethylene vinyl acetate bags. A slight creaming occurred in all admixtures, but the cream layer was easily redispersed with gentle shaking. No fat globules were visually apparent. The mean drop size was larger in the cream layer, but no globules were larger than 5 μm. Analyses of the concentrations of amino acids, dextrose, and electrolytes showed no changes over the study period. The authors concluded that such parenteral nutrition admixtures could be safely prepared as long as the component concentrations are within the following ranges (1067):

Vamin glucose or Vamin N (amino acids 7%)	1000 to 2000 ml
Dextrose 10 to 30%	100 to 550 ml
Intralipid 10 or 20%	500 to 1000 ml

Electrolyte (mmol/L)	
Sodium	20 to 70
Potassium	20 to 55
Calcium	2.3 to 2.9
Magnesium	1.1 to 3.1
Phosphorus	0 to 9.2
Chloride	27 to 71
Zinc	0.005 to 0.03

Parry et al. reported on the stability of eight parenteral nutrition admixtures with various ratios of amino acids, carbohydrates, and fat. FreAmine III 8.5%, dextrose 70%, and Soyacal 10 and 20% (mixed in ratios of 2:1:1, 1:1:1, 1:1:½, and 1:1:¼ , where 1 = 500 ml) were evaluated. Additive concentrations were high to stress the admixtures and represent maximum doses likely to be encountered clinically:

Sodium acetate	150 mEq
Sodium chloride	210 mEq
Potassium acetate	45 mEq
Potassium chloride	90 mEq
Potassium phosphate	15 mM
Calcium gluconate	20 mEq
Magnesium sulfate	36 mEq
Trace elements	present
Folic acid	5 mg
M.V.I.-12	10 ml

The admixtures were stored at 4 °C for 14 days followed by four days at 22 to 25 °C. After 24 hours, all admixtures developed a thin white cream layer, which readily redispersed on gentle agitation. No free oil droplets were observed. The mean particle diameter remained near the original size of the Soyacal throughout the study. Few particles were larger than 3 μm. Osmolality and pH also remained relatively unchanged (1068).

Bettner and Stennett had somewhat less success than others in preparing stable 3-in-1 parenteral nutrition admixtures with Aminosyn and Liposyn. Standard admixtures were prepared using Aminosyn 7% 1000 ml, dextrose 50% 1000 ml, and Liposyn 10% 500 ml. Concentrated admixtures were prepared using Aminosyn 10% 500 ml, dextrose 70% 500 ml, and Liposyn 20% 500 ml. Vitamins and trace elements were added to the admixtures along with the following electrolytes:

Electrolyte	Standard Admixture	Concentrated Admixture
Sodium	125 mEq	75 mEq
Potassium	95 mEq	74 mEq
Magnesium	25 mEq	25 mEq
Calcium	28 mEq	28 mEq
Phosphate	37 mM	36 mM
Chloride	83 mEq	50 mEq

Samples of each admixture were: (1) stored at 4 °C, (2) adjusted to pH 6.6 with sodium bicarbonate and stored at 4 °C, or (3) adjusted to pH 6.6 and stored at room temperature. The compatibility was evaluated for three weeks.

Visible signs of emulsion deterioration were evident by 96 hours in the standard admixture and by 48 hours in the concentrated admixture. Clear rings formed at the meniscus, becoming thicker, yellow, and oily over time. Free-floating oil was obvious in three weeks in the standard admixture and one week in the concentrated admixture. The samples adjusted to pH 6.6 developed visible deterioration later than the others. The authors indicated that pH may play a greater role than temperature in emulsion stability. However, precipitation (probably calcium phosphate and possibly carbonate) occurred in 36 hours in the pH 6.6 concentrated admixture but not the unadjusted (pH 5.5) samples. Mean particle counts increased for all samples over time but were greatest in the concentrated admixtures. The authors concluded that the concentrated admixtures were unsatisfactory for clinical use because of the early increase in particles and precipitation. Furthermore, they recommended that the standard admixtures be prepared immediately prior to use (1069).

Raupp et al. reported flocculation of fat emulsion (Kabi-Vitrum) during Y-site administration into a line used to infuse a parenteral nutrition solution containing both calcium gluconate and heparin sodium. Subsequent evaluation indicated that the combination of calcium gluconate (0.46 and 1.8 mmol/125 ml) and heparin sodium

(25 and 100 units/125 ml) in amino acids plus dextrose induced flocculation of the fat emulsion within two to four minutes at concentrations that resulted in no visually apparent flocculation in 30 minutes with either agent alone (1214).

This result was confirmed by Johnson et al. Calcium chloride quantities of 1 to 20 mmol normally result in slow flocculation of fat emulsion 20% over several hours. When heparin sodium 5 units/ml was added, the flocculation rate was accelerated greatly and a cream layer was observed visually in a few minutes. This effect was not observed when sodium ion was substituted for the divalent calcium (1406).

Barat et al. studied the physical stability of 10 parenteral nutrition admixtures with different amino acid sources. The admixtures contained 500 ml each of dextrose 70%, fat emulsion 20% (Alpha Therapeutic), and amino acids in various concentrations from each manufacturer. Also present were standard electrolytes, trace elements, and vitamins. The admixtures were stored for 14 days at 4 °C, followed by four days at 22 to 25 °C. Slight creaming was evident in all admixtures but redispersed easily with agitation. Emulsion particles were uniform in size, showing no tendency to aggregate. No cracked emulsions occurred (1217).

Cripps (1218) and Davis and Galloway (1219) described the stability of parenteral nutrition solutions containing amino acids, dextrose, and fat emulsion along with electrolytes, trace elements, and vitamins. Cripps reported that the admixtures were stable for 24 hours at room temperature and for eight days at 4 °C. The visual appearance and particle size of the fat emulsion showed little change over the observation periods (1218). Davis and Galloway reported variable stability periods, depending on electrolyte concentrations. Stability ranged from four to 25 days at room temperature (1219).

Ang et al. studied the physical stability and clinical safety of a 3-in-1 parenteral nutrition admixture composed of amino acids (Cutter), dextrose, and fat emulsion (Cutter) plus electrolytes and vitamins. The admixture was physically stable for up to six weeks at 4 °C. Furthermore, continuous infusion to 25 adult patients did not result in any adverse reaction or abnormal laboratory parameter (1220).

du Plesis et al. studied the effects of dilution, dextrose concentration, amino acids, and electrolytes on the physical stability of 3-in-1 parenteral nutrition admixtures prepared with Intralipid 10% or Travamulsion 10%. Travamulsion was affected by dilution up to 1:14, exhibiting an increase in mean particle size, while Intralipid remained virtually unchanged for 24 hours at 25 °C and for 72 hours at 4 °C. At dextrose concentrations above 15%, fat droplets larger than 5 μm formed during storage at either 4 °C or room temperature for 24 hours. The presence of amino acids increased the stability of the fat emulsions in the presence of dextrose. Fat droplets larger than 5 μm formed at a total electrolyte concentration above approximately 240 mmol/L (monovalent cation equivalent) for Travamulsion 10% and 156 mmol/L for Intralipid 10% in 24 hours at room temperature, although creaming or breaking of the emulsion was not observed visually (1221).

Sayeed et al. evaluated the stability of 43 parenteral nutrition admixtures composed of various ratios of amino acid products, dextrose 10 to 70%, and four lipid emulsions 10 and 20% with electrolytes, trace elements, and vitamins. One group of admixtures included Travasol 5.5, 8.5, and 10%, FreAmine III 8.5 and 10%, Novamine 8.5 and 11.4%, Nephramine 5.4%, and RenAmine 6.5% with Liposyn II 10 and 20%. In another group, Aminosyn II 7, 8.5, and 10% was combined with Intralipid, Travamulsion, and Soyacal 10 and 20%. A third group was comprised of Aminosyn II 7, 8.5,

and 10% with electrolytes combined with the latter three lipid emulsions. The admixtures were stored for 24 hours at 25 °C and for nine days at 5 °C followed by 24 hours at 25 °C. A few admixtures containing FreAmine III and Novamine with Liposyn II developed faint yellow streaks after 10 days of storage. The streaks readily dispersed with gentle shaking, as did the creaming present in most admixtures. Other properties such as pH, zeta-potential, and osmolality underwent little change in all of the admixtures. Particle size increased fourfold in one admixture (Novamine 8.5%, dextrose 50%, and Liposyn II in a 1:1:1 ratio), which the authors noted signaled the onset of particle coalescence. Nevertheless, the authors concluded that all of the admixtures were stable for the storage conditions and time periods tested (1222).

Sayeed et al. also evaluated the stability of 24 parenteral nutrition admixtures composed of various ratios of Aminosyn II 7, 8.5, or 10%, dextrose, and Liposyn II 10 and 20% with electrolytes, trace elements, and vitamins. Four admixtures were stored for 24 hours at 25 °C, six admixtures were stored for two days at 5 °C followed by one day at 30 °C, and 14 admixtures were stored for nine days at 5 °C followed by one day at 25 °C. No visible instability was evident. Creaming was present in most admixtures but disappeared with gentle shaking. Other properties such as pH, zeta potential, particle size, and potency of the amino acids and dextrose showed little or no change during storage (1223).

Tripp reported the emulsion stability of five parenteral nutrition formulas (TNA #126 through #130 in Appendix I) containing Liposyn II in concentrations ranging from 1.2 to 7.1%. The parenteral nutrition solutions were prepared using simultaneous pumping of the components into empty containers (as with the Nutrimix compounder) and sequential pumping of the components (as with Automix compounders). The solutions were stored for two days at 5 °C followed by 24 hours at 25 °C. Similar results were obtained for both methods of preparation using visual assessment and oil globule size distribution (1426).

Tripp et al. evaluated the stability of 24 parenteral nutrition admixtures containing various concentrations of Aminosyn II, dextrose, and Liposyn II with a variety of electrolytes, trace elements, and multivitamins in dual-chamber, flexible, Nutrimix containers. No instability was visible in the admixtures stored at 25 °C for 24 hours or in those stored for nine days at 5 °C followed by 24 hours at 25 °C. Creaming was observed, but neither particle coalescence nor free oil was noted. The pH, particle size distribution, and amino acid and dextrose concentrations remained acceptable during the observation period (1432).

Thomas studied two parenteral nutrition solutions composed of amino acids, dextrose 50%, fat emulsion (Intralipid) 20%, electrolytes, and vitamins. Their lipid particle sizes stayed within the manufacturer's range specifications when the solutions were stored at 23 or 4 °C and when frozen at −20 °C for 72 hours (1488).

Bullock et al. evaluated the physical stability of 10 parenteral nutrition formulas (TNA #149 through #158 in Appendix I) containing TrophAmine and Intralipid 20%, Liposyn II 20%, and Nutrilipid 20% in varying concentrations with low and high electrolyte concentrations. All test formulas were prepared with an automatic compounder and protected from light. TNA #149 through #156 were stored for 48 hours at 4 °C followed by 24 hours at 21 °C; TNA #157 and #158 were stored for 24 hours at 4 °C followed by 24 hours at 21 °C. Although some minor creaming occurred in all formulas, it was completely reversible with agitation. No other changes were visible, and particle size analysis indicated little variation during the study period. The addition of cysteine HCl 1 g/25 g of amino acids, alone or with L-carnitine 16 mg/g fat, to TNA #157 and #158 did not adversely affect the physical stability of 3-in-1 admixtures within the study period (1620).

Washington and Sizer evaluated the physical stability of five 3-in-1 parenteral nutrition solutions (TNA #167 through #171 in Appendix I) by visual observation, pH and osmolality determinations, and particle size distribution analysis. All five solutions were physically stable for 90 days at 4 °C. However, some irreversible flocculation occurred in all combinations after 180 days (1651).

Tu et al. studied the stability of several parenteral nutrition formulas (TNA #159 through #166), with and without iron dextran 2 mg/L. All formulas were physically compatible both visually and microscopically for 48 hours at 4 and 25 °C, and particle size distribution remained unchanged. The order of mixing and deliberate agitation had no effect on physical compatibility (1648).

Driscoll et al. evaluated the influence of six factors on the stability of fat emulsion in 45 different 3-in-1 parenteral nutrition mixtures. The factors evaluated were amino acid concentration (2.5 to 7%); dextrose concentration (5 to 20%); fat emulsion, intravenous, concentration (2 to 5%); monovalent cations (0 to 150 mEq/L); divalent cations (4 to 20 mEq/L); and trivalent cations from iron dextran (0 to 10 mg elemental iron/L). Although many formulations were unstable, visual examination could identify the instability in only 65% of these samples. Electronic particle size evaluation was required to identify the other unstable mixtures. Furthermore, only the concentration of trivalent ferric ions significantly and consistently affected emulsion stability during the 30-hour test. Of the parenteral nutrition mixtures containing iron dextran, 16% exhibited emulsion cracking. The authors suggested that iron dextran not be incorporated into 3-in-1 mixtures (1814).

The drop size of 3-in-1 parenteral nutrition solutions in drip chambers is variable, being altered by the constituents of the mixture. In one study, multivitamins (Multibionta, E. Merck) caused the greatest reductions in drop size, up to 37%. This change may affect the rate of delivery if the flow is estimated from drops per minute (1016). Similarly, flow rates delivered by infusion controllers dependent on predictable drop size may be inaccurate. Flow rates up to 29% less than expected have been reported. Therefore, variable pressure volumetric pumps, which are independent of drop size, should be used rather than infusion controllers (1215).

When multicomponent, 3-in-1, parenteral nutrition admixtures are used, the following points should be considered (490; 703; 892; 893; 1025; 1064; 1070; 1951; 2029; 2030):

1. The order of mixing is important. The amino acid solution should be added to either the fat emulsion or the dextrose before final mixing. This practice ensures the protective effect of the amino acids to emulsion disruption by changes in pH and the presence of electrolytes.

2. Electrolytes should not be added directly to the fat emulsions. Instead, they should be added to the amino acids or dextrose before the final mixing.

3. Such 3-in-1 admixtures containing electrolytes (especially divalent cations) are unstable and will eventually aggregate. The mixed systems should be carefully examined visually before use to ensure that a uniform emulsion still exists.

4. The admixtures should be stored under refrigeration if not used immediately.

5. The ultimate stability of the admixtures will be the result of a complex interaction of pH, component concentrations,

electrolyte concentrations, and, probably, storage temperature.

Furthermore, the use of a 1.2-μm filter to remove large lipid particles, electrolyte precipitates, and *Candida albicans* contaminants has been recommended (1657; 1769; 2061), although others recommend a 5-μm filter to minimize the frequency of occlusion alarms (1951).

Vitamins— Howard et al. reported on a patient receiving 3000 I.U. of retinol daily in a parenteral nutrition solution; nevertheless, this patient experienced two episodes of night blindness. The pharmacy prepared the parenteral nutrition solution in 1-L PVC bags in weekly batches and stored them at 4 °C in the dark until use. A subsequent in vitro study showed losses of vitamin A of 23 and 77% in three- and 14-day periods, respectively, under these conditions. About 30% of the lost vitamin A could be extracted from the PVC bag (1038).

Shenai et al. reported on losses of vitamin A from multivitamins (USV) in a neonatal parenteral nutrition solution. The solution was prepared in colorless glass bottles and run through an administration set with a burette (Travenol). The total loss of vitamin A was 75% in 24 hours, with about 16% as decomposition in the glass bottle. The decomposition was not noticeable during the first 12 hours, but then vitamin A levels fell rather precipitously to about one-third of the initial amount. The balance of the loss, averaging about 59%, occurred during transit through the administration set. Removal of the inline filter and treatment of the set with albumin had no effect on vitamin A delivery. The authors recommended a three- to four-fold increase in the amount of vitamin A to compensate for the losses (1039).

Kishi et al. reported on a parenteral nutrition solution in glass bottles exposed to sunlight. Vitamin A decomposed rapidly, losing more than 50% in three hours. The decomposition could be slowed by covering the bottle with a light-resistant vinyl bag, resulting in about a 25% loss in three hours (1040).

Kishi et al. also reported that vitamin E was stable in the parenteral nutrition solution in glass bottles exposed to sunlight, with no loss occurring during six hours of exposure (1040).

McKenna and Bieri reported that 40% retinol losses occurred in two hours and 60% in five hours from parenteral nutrition solutions pumped at 10 ml/hr through standard infusion sets at room temperature. The retinol concentration in the bottle remained constant while the retinol in the effluent decreased. Antioxidants had no effect. Much of the vitamin A was recoverable from hexane washings of the tubing (1050).

No loss of vitamin A to PVC delivery systems of *enteral* feeding solutions, after six hours of storage without protection from light and with exposure to ambient temperature, was reported by Bryant and Neufeld. The authors attributed this result to the presence of other (undefined) substances in the enteral feeding mixtures (1051).

Gillis et al. evaluated the delivery of vitamins A, D, and E from a parenteral nutrition solution composed of amino acids 3% solution (Pharmacia) in dextrose 10% with electrolytes, trace elements, vitamin K, folate, and vitamin B_{12}. To this solution was added 6 ml of multivitamin infusion (USV). The solution was prepared in PVC bags (Travenol), and administration was simulated through a fluid chamber (Buretrol) and infusion tubing with a 0.5-μm filter at 10 ml/hr. During the first 60 to 90 minutes, minimal delivery of the vitamins occurred. This was followed by a rise and plateau in the delivered vitamins, which were attributed to an increasing saturation of adsorptive binding sites in the tubing. Total amounts delivered over 24 hours were 31% for vitamin A, 68% for vitamin D, and 64% for vitamin E. Sorption of the vitamins was found in the PVC bag, fluid chamber, and tubing. Decomposition was not a factor (836).

Allwood found that vitamin A was rapidly and significantly decomposed when exposed to daylight. The extent and rate of loss were dependent on the degree of exposure to daylight which, in turn, depended on various factors such as the direction of the radiation, time of day, and climatic conditions. Delivery of less than 10% of the expected amount was reported (1047). In controlled light experiments, the decomposition initially progressed exponentially. Subsequently, the rate of decomposition slowed. This result was attributed to a protective effect of the degradation products on the remaining vitamin A. The presence of amino acids provided greater protection. Compared to degradation rates in dextrose 5% in water, decomposition was reduced by up to 50% in some amino acid mixtures (1048).

In a parenteral nutrition solution composed of amino acids, dextrose, electrolytes, trace elements, and multivitamins in PVC bags stored at 4 and 25 °C, vitamin A rapidly deteriorated to 10% of the initial concentration in eight hours at 25 °C while exposed to light. The decomposition was slowed by light protection and refrigeration, with a loss of about 25% in four days. Folic acid concentration dropped 40% initially on admixture and then remained relatively constant for 28 days of storage. About 35% of the ascorbic acid was lost in 39 hours at 25 °C with exposure to light. The loss was reduced to a negligible amount in four days by refrigeration and light protection. Thiamine content dropped by about 50% initially but then remained unchanged over 120 hours of storage (1063).

Riggle et al. noted a 50% loss of vitamin A from a bottle of parenteral nutrition solution prepared with multivitamin infusion (USV) after 5.5 hours of infusion. The amount delivered through an Ivex-2 filter set was only 6.3% of the added amount. Similar quantities were found after 20 hours of infusion. A reduced light exposure and use of ^{3}H-labeled vitamin A confirmed binding to the infusion bottles and tubing (704).

Subsequently, Riggle and Brandt incubated solutions containing multivitamins (USV) spiked with ^{3}H-labeled retinol in intravenous tubing protected from light and agitated to simulate flow for five hours. About half of the vitamin A was lost in 30 minutes, and 88 to 96% was lost in five hours. Spectrophotometric assays correlated closely with the radioisotope assays. Hexane rinses and radioactivity determinations on the tubing accounted for the decrease in radioactivity (1049).

In another experiment, neonatal parenteral nutrition solutions containing multivitamins prepared in bags were delivered at 10 ml/hr through Buretrol sets (Travenol). The bags and sets were protected from light. Spectrophotometric and radioisotope assays showed that about 26% of the vitamin A was lost before the flow was started. At 10 ml/hr, about 67% was lost from the effluent. More rapid flow reduced the extent of loss. Analysis of clinical samples of parenteral nutrition solutions showed losses of 21 to 57% after 20 hours. Because losses after five hours were of the same magnitude, the authors concluded that the loss occurs fairly rapidly and is not due to gradual decomposition (1049).

The quantity of retinol delivered from an M.V.I.-containing 2-in-1 parenteral nutrition solution and when M.V.I. was added to Intralipid 10% was evaluated during simulated administration through a PVC administration set. The parenteral nutrition solution was composed of amino acids 2.8%, dextrose 10%, and standard electrolytes; M.V.I. was added to yield a nominal retinol concentration of 455

μg/150 ml. Retinol losses were about 80% of the admixed amount after being delivered through the PVC set. When M.V.I. was added to Intralipid 10% in a retinol concentration of 455 μg/20 ml, retinol losses were reduced to about 10% of the admixed amount. As in the study by Bluhm et al. (1607), the fat emulsion provides retinol protection from sorption to the PVC administration set (2027).

Substantially higher amounts of retinol were found to be delivered using polyolefin administration set tubing when compared with PVC tubing during simulated neonatal intensive care administration. Retinol was added to a 2-in-1 parenteral nutrition solution (TPN #206) in concentrations of 25 and 50 I.U./ml and run at 4 and 10 ml/hr through three meter lengths of polyolefin (MiniMed) and PVC (Baxter) intravenous extension set tubing protected from light and passed through a 37 °C water bath. Using HPLC analysis, delivered quantities of retinol varied from 19 to 74% through the PVC tubing and 47 to 87% through the polyolefin tubing. The authors noted that the loss of retinol to the PVC tubing appeared to be saturable. Even so, the use of polyolefin tubing increases the amount of retinol delivered during simulated neonatal administration (2028).

Billion-Rey et al. reported substantial loss by HPLC analysis of retinol all-*trans* palmitate and phytonadione from both TPN and TNA admixtures due to exposure to sunlight. In three hours of exposure to sunlight, essentially total loss of retinol and 50% loss of phytonadione had occurred. The presence or absence of lipids did not affect stability. In contrast, tocopherol concentrations remained essentially unchanged by exposure to sunlight through 12 hours. The container material used to store the nutrition admixtures affected the concentration of the vitamins as well. Losses were greatest (10 to 25%) in PVC containers and were slightly better in EVA and glass containers (2049).

McGee et al. evaluated the stability of vitamin E (alphatocopherol acetate from M.V.I.-1000 or Soluzyme) and selenium (from Selepen) in amino acids (Abbott) and dextrose in PVC bags. Exposure to fluorescent light and room temperature (23 °C) for 24 hours and simulated infusion at 50 ml/hr for eight hours through a Medlon TPN administration set with a 0.22-μm filter did not affect the concentrations of vitamin E and selenium (1224).

Dahl et al. reported the stability of numerous vitamins in parenteral nutrition solutions composed of amino acids (Kabi-Vitrum), dextrose 30%, and fat emulsion 20% (Kabi-Vitrum) in a 2:1:1 ratio with electrolytes, trace elements, and both fat- and water-soluble vitamins. The admixtures were stored in darkness at 2 to 8 °C for 96 hours with no significant loss of retinyl palmitate, alphatocopherol, thiamine mononitrate, sodium riboflavin-5'-phosphate, pyridoxine HCl, nicotinamide, folic acid, biotin, sodium pantothenate, and cyanocobalamin. Sodium ascorbate and its biologically active degradation product, dehydroascorbic acid, totaled 59 and 42% of the nominal starting concentration at 24 and 96 hours, respectively. However, the actual initial concentration was only 66% of the nominal concentration (1225).

When the admixture was subjected to simulated infusion over 24 hours at 20 °C, either exposed to room light or light protected, or stored for six days in the dark under refrigeration and then subjected to the same simulated infusion, once again the retinyl palmitate, alpha-tocopherol, and sodium riboflavin-5'-phosphate did not undergo significant loss. However, sodium ascorbate and its degradation product, dehydroascorbic acid, had initial combined concentrations of 51 to 65% of the nominal initial concentration, with further declines during infusion. Light protection did not significantly alter the loss of total ascorbic acid (1225).

Smith et al. reported the stability of several vitamins from

M.V.I.-12 (Armour) admixed in parenteral nutrition solutions composed of different amino acid products, with or without Intralipid 10%, when stored in glass bottles and PVC bags at 25 and 5 °C for 48 hours. Riboflavin, folic acid, and vitamin E were stable in all samples. No vitamin A was lost in any formula in glass bottles, but samples in PVC containers lost as much as 35 and 60% at 5 and 25 °C, respectively, in 48 hours. Thiamine HCl was stable in the parenteral nutrition solutions prepared with amino acid products without sulfites. However, amino acid products containing sulfites (Travasol and FreAmine III) had a 25% thiamine loss in 12 hours and a 50% loss in 24 hours when the solutions were stored at 25 °C; no loss occurred when the solutions were stored at 5 °C. Ascorbic acid was lost from all samples stored at 25 °C, with the greatest losses occurring in solutions stored in plastic bags. No losses occurred in any sample stored at 5 °C (1431).

Samples from 24 1-L and four 2-L parenteral nutrition solutions, containing one vial each of multivitamin concentrate (USV), were evaluated for thiamine HCl content at 48 to 72 hours after mixing. The parenteral nutrition solutions contained amino acids 2.75 to 5%, dextrose 15 to 25%, and electrolytes. Thiamine HCl was stable in all of the solutions tested in spite of an approximate 0.05% sulfite content (843).

In another experiment, multivitamin concentrate (USV) was added to 500-ml glass bottles of amino acids 10% (Travenol) containing 0.1% sulfite and also to 1000-ml PVC bags containing amino acids 4.25%–dextrose 25% (Travenol) with about 0.05% sulfite. After 22 hours of storage at 30 °C, a 40% loss of thiamine HCl occurred in the amino acid 10% solution, but no loss occurred in the PVC bags of parenteral nutrition solution. The authors concluded that the thiamine HCl content is retained in usual clinical parenteral nutrition solutions, probably because of the dilution of the sulfite and buffering of pH. However, direct addition to solutions with a high sulfite content (0.1%) may result in significant decomposition (843).

The stability of five B vitamins was studied over an eight-hour period in representative parenteral nutrition solutions exposed to fluorescent light, indirect sunlight, and direct sunlight. One 5-ml vial of multivitamin concentrate (Lyphomed) and 1 mg of folic acid (Lederle) were added to a liter of parenteral nutrition solution composed of amino acids 4.25%–dextrose 25% (Travenol) with standard electrolytes and trace elements. All five B vitamins tested were stable for eight hours at room temperature when exposed to fluorescent light. In addition, folic acid and niacinamide were stable over eight hours in direct or indirect sunlight. Exposure to indirect sunlight appeared to have little or no effect on thiamine HCl and pyridoxine HCl in eight hours, but 47% of riboflavin-5-phosphate was lost in that period. Direct sunlight caused a 26% loss of thiamine HCl and an 86% loss of pyridoxine HCl in eight hours. Four-hour exposures of riboflavin-5-phosphate to direct sunlight resulted in a 98% loss (842).

The effects of photoirradiation on a FreAmine II–dextrose 10% parenteral nutrition solution containing 1 ml/500 ml of multivitamins (USV) were evaluated. During simulated continuous administration to an infant at 0.156 ml/min, no changes to the amino acids occurred when the bottle, infusion tubing, and collection bottle were shielded with foil. Only 20 cm of tubing in the incubator was exposed to light. However, if the flow was stopped, a marked reduction in methionine (40%), tryptophan (44%), and histidine (22%) occurred in the solution exposed to light for 24 hours. In a similar solution without vitamins, only the tryptophan concentration decreased. The difference was attributed to the presence of riboflavin,

a photosensitizer. The authors recommended administering the multivitamins separately and shielding from light (833).

In further work, the authors simulated more closely conditions occurring during phototherapy in neonatal intensive care units. Riboflavin 1 mg/100 ml was added to a solution of amino acids 2% (Abbott) with dextrose 10%. Infusion was simulated from glass bottles through PVC tubing with a Buretrol at a rate of 4 ml/hr. In addition to the fluorescent room lights, eight daylight bulbs delivered phototherapy. After a simulated 24-hour infusion, riboflavin decreased to about 50% of its initial level. Also, a 7% reduction in total amino acids was noted, including individual losses of glycine (10%), leucine (14%), methionine (24%), proline (10%), serine (9%), tryptophan (35%), and tyrosine (16%). Although the authors did not believe that these losses of amino acids were nutritionally important, they were concerned about the possibility of toxicity from photo-oxidation products. In the same solution without riboflavin, the individual amino acids decreased only slightly (974).

Allwood reported on the extent and rapidity of ascorbic acid decomposition in parenteral nutrition solutions composed of amino acids, dextrose, electrolytes, multivitamins, and trace elements in 3-L PVC bags stored at 3 to 7 °C. About 30 to 40% was lost in 24 hours. The degradation then slowed as the oxygen supply was reduced to the diffusion through the bag. About a 55 to 65% loss occurred after seven days of storage. The oxidation was catalyzed by metal ions, especially copper. In the absence of copper from the trace elements additive, less than 10% degradation of ascorbic acid occurred in 24 hours. The author estimated that 150 to 200 mg is degraded in two to four hours at ambient temperature in the presence of copper but that only 20 to 30 mg is broken down in 24 hours without copper. To minimize ascorbic acid loss, copper must be excluded. Alternatively, inclusion of excess ascorbic acid was suggested (1056).

Extensive decomposition of ascorbic acid and folic acid was reported in a parenteral nutrition solution composed of amino acids 3.3%, dextrose 12.5%, electrolytes, trace elements, and M.V.I.-12 (USV) in PVC bags. Half-lives were 1.1, 2.9, and 8.9 hours for ascorbic acid and 2.7, 5.4, and 24 hours for folic acid stored at 24 °C in daylight, 24 °C protected from light, and 4 °C protected from light, respectively. The decomposition was much greater than for solutions not containing catalyzing metal ions. Also, it was greater than for the vitamins singly because of interactions with the other vitamins present (1059).

The stability of ascorbic acid in parenteral nutrition solutions, with and without fat emulsion, was studied using HPLC analysis. Both with and without fat emulsion, the total vitamin C content (ascorbic acid plus dehydroascorbic acid) remained above 90% for 12 hours when the solutions were exposed to fluorescent light and for 24 hours when they were protected from light. When stored in a cool dark place, the solutions were stable for seven days (1227).

The influence of several factors on the rate of ascorbic acid oxidation in parenteral nutrition solutions was evaluted. Ascorbic acid is regarded as the least stable component in TPN admixtures. The type of amino acid used in the TPN was important. Some, such as FreAmine III and Vamin 14, contain antioxidant compounds (e.g., sodium metabisulfite or cysteine). Ascorbic acid stability was better in such solutions compared with those amino acid solutions having no antioxidant present. Furthermore, the pH of the solution may play a small role, with greater degradation as the pH rises from about 5 to about 7. Adding air to a compounded TPN container can also accelerate ascorbic acid decomposition. The most important factor was the type of plastic container used for the TPN. Ethylene vinyl acetate (EVA) containers (Mixieva, Miramed) allow more oxygen permeation, which results in substantial losses of ascorbic acid in relatively short time periods. In multilayer TPN bags (Ultrastab, Miramed) designed to reduce gas permeability, the rate of ascorbic acid degradation was greatly reduced. HPLC analysis of TPNs without antioxidants packaged in EVA bags found that an almost total loss of ascorbic acid activity occurred in one or two days at 5 °C. In contrast, in TPNs containing FreAmine III or Vamin 14 packaged in the multilayer bags, most of the ascorbic acid content was retained for 28 days at 5 °C. The authors concluded that TPNs made with antioxidant-containing amino acids and packaged in multilayer bags that reduce gas permeability can safely be given extended expiration dates and still retain most of the ascorbic acid activity (2163).

Because of these interactions, recommendations to separate the administration of vitamins and trace elements have been made (1056; 1060; 1061). Other researchers have termed such recommendations premature based on differing reports (895; 896) and the apparent absence of epidemic vitamin deficiency in parenteral nutrition patients (1062).

Shenkin et al. evaluated the vitamin and trace element status of 22 postoperative surgical patients. Twelve patients were given parenteral nutrition with the fat emulsion containing vitamins separate from amino acids and other water-soluble nutrients; 10 patients received all nutrients in one large bag. No clinically significant differences were noted after administration periods of seven to 38 days (1226).

Phytonadione stability in a total parenteral nutrition solution containing amino acids 2%, dextrose 12.5%, "standard" electrolytes, and multivitamins (M.V.I. Pediatric) was evaluated by HPLC over 24 hours while exposed to light. Vitamin loss, about 7% in four hours and 27% in 24 hours, was attributed partly to the light sensitivity of phytonadione (1815).

Trace Elements— The stability of a 3-in-1 parenteral nutrition mixture (TNA #191 in Appendix I) was compared with trace elements added as gluconate salts or chloride salts. TNA #191 with copper 0.24 mg/L, iron 0.5 mg/L, and zinc 2 mg/L in either salt form was physically stable for seven days at 4 and 25 °C (1787).

Trace elements additives, especially those containing copper ions, have the potential to be incompatible in TPN solutions, resulting in precipitation. In a TPN admixture containing 5% Synthamin 17, 25% dextrose, 1 g of ascorbic acid injection, 14 mmol of calcium chloride, and trace elements solution (David Bull), storage at 20 to 25 °C and 2 to 8 °C, protected from light, resulted in the formation of a discolored solution in three to seven days and an off-white to yellow precipitate in eight to 12 days, respectively. Electron microscopy revealed the presence of numerous bipyramidal, eight-sided crystals in sizes from 3 to 30 μm. The authors proposed that the crystals were calcium oxalate. They suggested that the ascorbic acid decomposed to oxalic acid; the oxalic acid then interacted with calcium ions to form calcium oxalate. The authors did not verify their supposition. They noted that the crystals were conformationally different from calcium phosphate crystals and that no phosphate had been added to the admixture. In addition, mixing ascorbic acid injection 500 mg/5 ml with trace elements solution 5 ml results in the formation of a transparent gel that becomes an opaque flocculent precipitate after five minutes. The authors recommended adding trace elements well away from injections that can act as ligands and with thorough mixing after each addition. Introduction of air and prolonged storage should be avoided. Incorporating trace elements and ascorbic acid on alternate days was also suggested (2197).

Iron— Mayhew and Quick evaluated the effect of amino acid concentration on precipitation of iron from iron dextran (INFeD, Schein) 10 mg/L in neonatal parenteral nutrition mixtures (TPN #207 to #211) formulated with TrophAmine (McGaw). Rust-colored precipitate formed in the neonatal formulations having amino acids concentrations of 1.5% or less. The precipitate formed more rapidly and in greater amount at lower amino acid concentrations. Parenteral nutrition admixtures with amino acids concentrations of 2 and 2.5% wre visually compatible for 48 hr at 19 °C, but trace precipitation was found upon filtration and analysis of the 2% admixture. Extrapolation of the information to other iron dextran products may not be appropriate because of possible product differences (2103).

Bicarbonate— Due to acidity, the addition of bicarbonate ion may result in the loss of some of this ion as carbon dioxide. Also, adding bicarbonate ions to a solution containing calcium or magnesium may result in the precipitation of insoluble carbonates (189).

While mixing potentially incompatible ions in separate bottles has been advocated by some (193; 200), it has been discouraged by others if the incompatibilities do not actually occur because potential fluctuations of ions in serum may result (192; 201).

Insulin— Regular insulin (Lilly) in concentrations of 10 to 50 units/L was tested in parenteral nutrition solutions #38 through #47 (Appendix I). The solutions were physically compatible for 24 hours at 22 °C in all but TPN #46 at 40 and 50 units/L of insulin. In these cases, a white crystalline precipitate was noted on the surface of the solution at 24 hours. At lower concentrations of insulin in TPN #46, no precipitate was observed (313).

It has also been stated that crystalline insulin is not inactivated by amino acids, but a physical separation may occur if not mixed thoroughly. An occasional shaking was recommended to prevent a bolus of insulin from being administered (189).

Cimetidine— Cimetidine HCl (SKF) 13 to 19 mg/kg/24 hr was administered to patients by continuous infusion in parenteral nutrition solutions composed of essential amino acids, dextrose 50% in water with varying amounts of vitamins, electrolytes, trace elements, and albumin. The admixtures were prepared within 24 hours prior to use. No physical incompatibilities were noted, and cimetidine blood levels were in the range achieved by long-term oral treatment (570).

When compounding parenteral nutrition mixtures, cimetidine should be admixed in a sequence that separates it from the copper sulfate present in trace elements injections to avoid formation of a green-colored copper-cimetidine complex (1951).

Ranitidine HCl— The stability of ranitidine HCl has been evaluated in a number of TPN solutions with variable results. See Solutions table above. The major mechanism of ranitidine HCl decomposition is oxidation. A number of factors have been found to contribute to ranitidine HCl instability in TPN solutions, including the presence or absence of antioxidants (such as sodium metabisulfite) in the amino acids, the addition of trace elements (which can catalyze ranitidine oxidation), solution pH, and type of plastic container used. In a study of rantidine HCl stability in several TPN solutions stored at 5 °C, the drug was most stable in FreAmine III–based (contains sodium metabisulfite) admixtures with additives when packaged in multilayer gas impermeable plastic containers (Ultrastab) with about 8% loss by HPLC in 28 days. In contrast, in ethylene vinyl acetate (EVA) bags, which are permeable to oxygen, losses of approximately 50% occurred in this time period. If Vamin 14 with no antioxidant present was used as the amino acid source, and the solution was packaged in EVA bags, ranitidine HCl losses of approximately 65% occurred in 28 days. Similarly, the addition of air to the bags during compounding increases the extent of rantidine HCl oxidation substantially (2195).

Gentamicin— Kern et al. evaluated the serum concentrations of gentamicin following intermittent 15 to 30-minute administration in piggyback infusions of 50 ml of dextrose 5% in water or 50 ml of TPN #177 (see Appendix I). Gentamicin serum concentrations were equivalent using both administration methods (1573).

Miscellaneous— It has been stated that antibiotics, steroids, and pressor agents should not be added to parenteral nutrition solutions. They may be administered through a Y-tube or into another vein (193; 195; 206).

Other information indicates that heparin sodium and hydrocortisone sodium succinate are physically and chemically compatible with amino acid injection (189). Additionally, the frequency of phlebitis was reported to have dropped from 50 to 25% upon addition of heparin (500 units/L) and hydrocortisone (5 mg/L) to amino acid–glucose nutrition solutions for peripheral administration (592).

Amino acids injection should not be administered simultaneously with blood through the same infusion set because of possible pseudoagglutination (341).

Other Information

Plasticizer Extraction— Mazur et al. reported that a parenteral nutrition solution containing an amino acid solution, dextrose, and electrolytes in a PVC bag did not leach measurable quantities of diethylhexylphthalate (DEHP) plasticizer during 21 days of storage at 4 and 25 °C. However, addition of fat emulsion 10 or 20% to the formula caused detectable leaching of DEHP from the PVC containers stored for 48 hours. Higher DEHP levels were found in the 25 °C samples than in the 4 °C samples. The authors recommended limiting the use of lipid-containing parenteral nutrition solutions to 24 to 36 hours. Use of non-PVC containers is another option (1430).

Titratable Acidity— The acidity of parenteral nutrition solutions can be a factor in the development of metabolic acidosis by a patient (577; 851). Titratable acidity is a measure of the hydrogen ion content that must be neutralized to raise the pH to a given endpoint and is often expressed as milliequivalents of titrant per liter of reactant. In a study (577) of five amino acid injections and mixtures, the titratable acidities were determined for pH 7.4 by titrating with 0.1220 N sodium hydroxide and 7.54% (0.898 M) sodium bicarbonate. The following results were observed:

	Titratable Acidity	
	NaOH (mEq/L)	NaHCO$_3$ (mEq/L)
Aminosyn 7%	37	314
FreAmine II 8.5%	16.8	176
Travasol 8.5%	34.7	354
Travasol 8.5% with electrolytes	45.2	420
Veinamine 8%	13.4	135

Corresponding (although somewhat lower) values were also obtained for 1:1 mixtures with dextrose 50%. It was concluded that use of sodium bicarbonate to adjust to pH 7.4 was not usually feasible given the large volumes of fluid and increased sodium ion required. However, smaller amounts could be used for smaller pH adjustments (577).

AMINOCAPROIC ACID
AHFS 20:12.16

Amicar   Immunex

Products— Aminocaproic acid (Immunex) is available as a 250-mg/ml concentration in 20-ml vials containing 5 g of drug. Also present are benzyl alcohol 0.9% and hydrochloric acid (2; 4) and/or sodium hydroxide for pH adjustment (4).

pH— The pH is adjusted to approximately 6.8 (2) with a range of 6 to 7.6 (4).

Administration— Aminocaproic acid is administered by continuous intravenous infusion after dilution in a suitable infusion solution. Rapid intravenous injection of the undiluted drug should be avoided (2; 4).

Intravenous solutions recommended for administering aminocaproic acid are sodium chloride 0.9%, dextrose 5% in water, and Ringer's injection (2; 4).

Compatibility Information

Solution Compatibility

Aminocaproic acid

Solution	Mfr	Mfr	Conc/L	Remarks	Ref	C/I
Dextrose 5% in water	BA[a]	IMM	10 and 100 g	Physically compatible with little or no loss by HPLC in 7 days at 4 and 23 °C. Yellow discoloration forms after 24 hr at 23 °C but is not associated with drug loss	2096	C

Solution Compatibility (Cont.)

Aminocaproic acid

Solution	Mfr	Mfr	Conc/L	Remarks	Ref	C/I
Sodium chloride 0.9%	BA[a]	IMM	10 and 100 g	Physically compatible with little or no loss by HPLC in 7 days at 4 and 23 °C	2096	C

[a]*Tested in PVC containers.*

Additive Compatibility

Aminocaproic acid

Drug	Mfr	Conc/L	Mfr	Conc/L	Test Soln	Remarks	Ref	C/I
Netilmicin sulfate	SC	3 g	LE	10 g	D5S	Physically compatible and netilmicin chemically stable for 7 days at 25 and 4 °C. Aminocaproic acid not tested	558	C

AMINOPHYLLINE
AHFS 86:16

Abbott

Products— Aminophylline is available as a 25-mg/ml solution in 10-ml (250 mg) and 20-ml (500 mg) ampuls and vials for intravenous injection. Aminophylline is a 2:1 complex of theophylline and ethylenediamine. It contains excess ethylenediamine to ensure stability (6) and is approximately 79 to 80% theophylline by weight. Aminophylline 25 mg is equivalent to 19.7 mg of theophylline (1-1/97).

pH— From 8.6 to 9 (4).

Osmotic Values— The calculated osmolarity of the injection is 170 mOsm/L (1-1/97). The osmolality was determined to be 114 mOsm/kg by freezing-point depression (1071).

The osmolality of aminophylline 250 mg was calculated for the following dilutions (1054):

Diluent	Osmolality (mOsm/kg)	
	50 ml	100 ml
Dextrose 5% in water	300	291
Sodium chloride 0.9%	327	318

Administration— Aminophylline may be administered by intravenous infusion or slow direct intravenous injection. Slow administration at a rate not exceeding 17 (1-1/97) to 20 mg/min (4) has been recommended.

Stability— The containers should be stored at controlled room temperature and protected from freezing and light (1-1/97). Although Searle indicated that refrigeration would not adversely affect its aminophylline, Elkins-Sinn recommended against refrigerated storage for its product because of possible reduction in solubility with crystallization (593). Containers of aminophylline should be inspected for particulate matter and discoloration prior to use. Do not use if crystals are present (1-1/97; 4).

The intact ampuls are stated to be stable indefinitely at room temperature (6). Stability is reported to be maintained at pH 3.5 to 8.6 for at least 48 hours at 25 °C (6), providing aminophylline concentrations do not exceed 40 mg/ml (4). Others have indicated that theophylline crystals may deposit below pH 8 (41).

Although some aminophylline products are labeled for storage with protection from light (1-1/97), one study of aminophylline (Squibb) 50 mg/ml found no change in theophylline potency after eight weeks of storage with exposure to fluorescent light (1231).

Aminophylline (Abbott) 5 mg/ml in bacteriostatic water for injection containing benzyl alcohol 0.9% in plastic syringes (Becton-Dickinson) exhibited 2 and 3% losses by HPLC at 4 and 22 °C, respectively, after 91 days of storage (1586).

Sorption— Aminophylline 9 mg/L in sodium chloride 0.9% (Travenol) in PVC bags did not exhibit significant sorption to the plastic during one week of storage at room temperature (15 to 20 °C) (536).

Aminophylline (David Bull Laboratories) 9 mg/L in sodium chloride 0.9% did not exhibit any loss due to sorption during a seven-hour simulated infusion through an infusion set (Travenol) consisting of a cellulose propionate burette chamber and 170 cm of PVC tubing (606).

The drug was also tested as a simulated infusion over at least one hour by a syringe pump system. A glass syringe on a syringe pump was fitted with 20 cm of polyethylene tubing or 50 cm of Silastic tubing. No loss of drug due to sorption was observed with either tubing (606).

A 25-ml aliquot of aminophylline (David Bull Laboratories) 9 mg/L in sodium chloride 0.9% was stored in all-plastic syringes composed of polypropylene barrels and polyethylene plungers for 24 hours at room temperature in the dark. No loss due to sorption occurred (606).

In another study, aminophylline, BP, 10 mg/2 ml diluted in dextrose 5% in water or sodium chloride 0.9% was stored for 18 hours at room temperature in the following plastic syringes: Brunswick (Sherwood Medical), Plastipak (Becton-Dickinson), Steriseal (Needle Industries), and Sabre (Gillette U.K.). The first three syringes have polypropylene barrels; the Sabre has a combination polypropylene–polystyrene barrel. No significant loss of aminophylline occurred due to sorption (784).

Filtration— Aminophylline (American Quinine) 500 mg/L in dextrose 5% in water in PVC bags was passed through an Ivex-2 inline filter assembly at a rate of 2 ml/min. No decrease in the delivered aminophylline concentration or any change in the physicochemical properties occurred over the eight-hour study period (556).

Compatibility Information

Solution Compatibility

Aminophylline

Solution	Mfr	Mfr	Conc/L	Remarks	Ref	C/I
Alcohol 5%, dextrose 5% in water	BA	SE	10 g	Physically compatible for 24 hr	315	C
Amino acids 4.25%, dextrose 25%	MG	SE	500 mg	No increase in particulate matter in 24 hr at 5 °C	349	C
Dextran 6% in dextrose 5%	AB		500 mg	Physically compatible	3	C
Dextran 6% in sodium chloride 0.9%	AB		500 mg	Physically compatible	3	C
Dextrose–Ringer's injection combinations	AB		500 mg	Physically compatible	3	C
Dextrose–Ringer's injection, lactated, combinations	AB		500 mg	Physically compatible	3	C
Dextrose 5% in Ringer's injection, lactated	BA	SE	10 mg	Physically compatible for 24 hr	315	C
Dextrose–saline combinations	AB		500 mg	Physically compatible	3	C
Dextrose 4% in sodium chloride 0.18%	TR[a]		1 g	Yellow discoloration in 2 hr but theophylline content by HPLC retained for at least 24 hr	1571	C
Dextrose 5% in sodium chloride 0.2%	MG	AQ	750 mg	Physically compatible with no aminophylline decomposition in 48 hr at 25 °C. Yellow tinge at 48 hr due to slight dextrose decomposition	556	C
Dextrose 5% in sodium chloride 0.9%			250 mg	Physically compatible	74	C
	BA	SE	10 g	Physically compatible for 24 hr	315	C
	TR[a]	AQ	750 mg	Physically compatible with no aminophylline decomposition in 48 hr at 25 °C. Yellow tinge at 48 hr due to slight dextrose decomposition	556	C
Dextrose 2½% in water	AB		500 mg	Physically compatible	3	C
Dextrose 5% in water			500 mg to 2 g	Potency retained for 24 hr at room temperature	56	C
			250 mg	Physically compatible	74	C
	AB		500 mg	Physically compatible	3	C
	AB	SE	450 mg	Potency retained for at least 24 hr at room temperature	6	C
	BA	SE	10 g	Physically compatible for 24 hr	315	C
	AB	ES	5 and 10 g	Physically compatible with little or no decomposition in 96 hr under refrigeration	537	C
	TR[a]	AQ	750 mg	Physically compatible with no aminophylline decomposition in 48 hr at 25 °C and 7 days at 5 °C. Yellow tinge in the 25 °C admixture at 48 hr due to slight dextrose decomposition	556	C
	TR[a]	AQ	250 and 500 mg	Physically compatible with no aminophylline decomposition in 48 hr at 25 °C. Yellow tinge in the admixture at 48 hr due to slight dextrose decomposition	556	C
			250 mg	Aminophylline chemically stable for at least 24 hr at 24 to 26 °C	852	C
	TR[a]	IX	500 mg	Physically compatible with little or no loss in 48 hr at room temperature	1186	C
	AB	SE	1 g	Physically compatible with no loss in 24 hr at 24 °C under fluorescent light	1198	C
	TR[a]	LY	1 g	Physically compatible with no loss in 24 hr at room temperature under fluorescent light	1358	C
	TR[a]		1 g	Yellow discoloration in 2 hr but theophylline content by HPLC retained for at least 24 hr	1571	C

Solution Compatibility (Cont.)

Aminophylline

Solution	Mfr	Mfr	Conc/L	Remarks	Ref	C/I
	TR[a]	ES	0.5 and 2 g	Visually compatible with little or no aminophylline loss by HPLC in 48 hr at room temperature	1802	**C**
Dextrose 10% in water	AB		500 mg	Physically compatible	3	**C**
	BA	SE	10 g	Physically compatible for 24 hr	315	**C**
			250 mg	Aminophylline chemically stable for at least 24 hr at 24 to 26 °C. Yellow discoloration at 2 hr and increased with time	852	**C**
Dextrose 20% in water	BA	SE	10 g	Physically compatible for 24 hr	315	**C**
			250 mg	Aminophylline chemically stable for at least 24 hr at 24 to 26 °C. Yellow discoloration at 2 hr and increased with time	852	**C**
Fat emulsion 10%, intravenous	VT	ES	1 g	Physically compatible for 48 hr at 4 °C and room temperature	32	**C**
	VT	DB	500 mg	Microscopic globule coalescence in 24 hr at 25 and 8 °C	825	**I**
Fructose 10% in sodium chloride 0.9%	AB		500 mg	Color change	3	**I**
Fructose 10% in water	BA	SE	10 g	Physically compatible for 24 hr	315	**C**
	AB		500 mg	Color change	3	**I**
Invert sugar 5% in sodium chloride 0.9%	AB		500 mg	Physically compatible	3	**C**
Invert sugar 5% in water	AB		500 mg	Physically compatible	3	**C**
Invert sugar 10% in Electrolyte #1	BA	SE	10 g	Physically compatible for 24 hr	315	**C**
Invert sugar 10% in Electrolyte #2	BA	SE	10 g	Physically compatible for 24 hr	315	**C**
Invert sugar 10% in sodium chloride 0.9%	AB		500 mg	Color change	3	**I**
Invert sugar 10% in water	AB		500 mg	Color change	3	**I**
Ionosol products	AB		500 mg	Physically compatible	3	**C**
Polysal M with dextrose 5%	BA	SE	10 g	Physically compatible for 24 hr	315	**C**
Ringer's injection	AB		500 mg	Physically compatible	3	**C**
Ringer's injection, lactated			250 mg	Physically compatible	74	**C**
	AB		500 mg	Physically compatible	3	**C**
	BA	SE	10 g	Physically compatible for 24 hr	315	**C**
Sodium chloride 0.45%	AB		500 mg	Physically compatible	3	**C**
Sodium chloride 0.9%	AB		500 mg	Physically compatible	3	**C**
			250 mg	Physically compatible	74	**C**
	TR	SE		Potency retained for 24 hr	45	**C**
	BA	SE		Potency retained for 24 hr	45	**C**
	BA	SE	10 g	Physically compatible for 24 hr	315	**C**
	TR[a]	AQ	750 mg	Physically compatible with no decomposition in 48 hr at 25 °C	556	**C**
	TR[a]		1 g	Theophylline content by HPLC retained for at least 24 hr	1571	**C**
	TR[a]	ES	0.5 and 2 g	Visually compatible with little or no aminophylline loss by HPLC in 48 hr at room temperature	1802	**C**
Sodium lactate ⅙ M	AB		500 mg	Physically compatible	3	**C**
	BA	SE	10 g	Physically compatible for 24 hr	315	**C**

Solution Compatibility (Cont.)

Aminophylline

Solution	Mfr	Mfr	Conc/L	Remarks	Ref	C/I
TNA #180[b]			234 and 638 mg	Little or no theophylline loss by EMIT and no substantial increase in fat particle size in 24 hr at room temperature	1617	C
TPN #25 to #27[b]		SE	250 mg, 500 mg, 1 g, 1.5 g	Physically compatible and aminophylline chemically stable for at least 24 hr at 25 °C	755	C
		SE	1 g	Physically compatible and aminophylline chemically stable for at least 24 hr at 4 °C	755	C
TPN #28 to #30[b]		SE	1 g	Physically compatible and aminophylline chemically stable for at least 24 hr at 25 °C	755	C
TPN[c]			29.3 mg	No significant change in aminophylline content over 24 hr at 24 to 26 °C	852	C

[a]Tested in PVC containers.
[b]Refer to Appendix I for the composition of parenteral nutrition solutions. TNA indicates a 3-in-1 admixture, and TPN indicates a 2-in-1 admixture.
[c]Tested in a pediatric parenteral nutrition solution containing 150 ml of dextrose 5% in water and 30 ml of Vamin glucose with electrolytes and vitamins.

Additive Compatibility

Aminophylline

Drug	Mfr	Conc/L	Mfr	Conc/L	Test Soln	Remarks	Ref	C/I
Amikacin sulfate	BR	5 g	SE	5 g	LR, NS, R, SL	Physically compatible and amikacin potency retained for 24 hr at 25 °C. Aminophylline not analyzed	294	C
	BR	5 g	SE	5 g	D5LR, D5R, D5S, D5W, D10W, IS10	Greater than 10% amikacin decomposition after 8 hr but within 24 hr at 25 °C. Aminophylline not analyzed	294	I
Amobarbital sodium	LI	500 mg	SE	500 mg		Physically compatible	6	C
Ascorbic acid injection	AB	500 mg	SE	500 mg		Physically compatible	6	C
						Physically incompatible	9	I
	UP	500 mg	SE	1 g	D5W	Physically incompatible	15	I
Atracurium besylate	BW	500 mg		1 g	D5W	Atracurium chemically unstable due to high pH	1694	I
Bleomycin sulfate	BR	20 and 30 units	ES	250 mg	NS	50% loss of bleomycin activity in 1 week at 4 °C	763	I
Bretylium tosylate	ACC	1 g	ES	1 g	D5W, NS	Physically compatible for 48 hr at 25 °C	756	C
Calcium gluconate		1 g		250 mg	D5W	Physically compatible	74	C
Cefepime HCl	BR	4 g	LY	1 g	NS	37% cefepime loss by HPLC in 18 hr at room temperature and 32% loss in 3 days at 5 °C. No aminophylline loss	1681	I
Ceftazidime	GL[a]	2 g	ES	1 g	D5W, NS	20 to 23% ceftazidime loss by HPLC in 6 hr at room temperature	1937	I
	GL[a]	6 g	ES	1 g	D5W, NS	8 to 10% ceftazidime loss and 13% theophylline loss by HPLC in 6 hr at room temperature	1937	I
	GL[a]	2 g	ES	2 g	D5W, NS	35 to 40% ceftazidime loss by HPLC in 6 hr at room temperature	1937	I

Additive Compatibility (Cont.)

Aminophylline

Drug	Mfr	Conc/L	Mfr	Conc/L	Test Soln	Remarks	Ref	C/I
	GL[a]	6 g	ES	2 g	D5W, NS	22% ceftazidime loss by HPLC in 6 hr at room temperature	1937	I
Ceftriaxone sodium	RC	20 g	AMR	1 g	D5W, NS[b]	Yellow color forms immediately. 3 to 6% ceftriaxone loss and 8 to 12% aminophylline loss by HPLC in 24 hr	1727	I
	RC	20 g	AMR	4 g	D5W, NS[b]	Yellow color forms immediately. 15 to 20% ceftriaxone loss and 7 to 9% aminophylline loss by HPLC in 24 hr	1727	I
	RC	40 g	AMR	1 g	D5W, NS[b]	Yellow color forms immediately. 15 to 18% ceftriaxone loss and 1 to 3% aminophylline loss by HPLC in 24 hr	1727	I
Chloramphenicol sodium succinate	PD	500 mg		250 mg	D5W	Physically compatible	74	C
	PD	10 g	SE	1 g	D5W	Physically compatible	15	C
Chlorpromazine HCl	BP	200 mg	BP	1 g	D5W, NS	Immediate precipitation	26	I
Cibenzoline succinate		2 g	IX	10 g	D5W, NS	Physically compatible for 24 hr at 25 °C by visual and microscopic examination	1182	C
Cimetidine HCl	SKF	1.2 g	IX	500 mg	D5W[c]	Physically compatible with about 3 to 5% cimetidine loss and little or no aminophylline loss in 48 hr at room temperature	1186	C
Ciprofloxacin	MI	1.6 g	LY	2 g	D5W, NS	Ciprofloxacin precipitate forms in 4 hr at 4 and 25 °C	1541	I
Clindamycin phosphate	UP	600 mg	SE	600 mg		Physically incompatible	101	I
Corticotropin		500 units		250 mg	D5W	Physically compatible	74	C
	AR, NA	40 units	SE	500 mg		Precipitate forms within 1 hr	6	I
Dexamethasone sodium phosphate		30 mg		625 mg	D5W	Physically compatible and chemically stable for 24 hr at 4 and 30 °C	521	C
Dimenhydrinate	SE	50 mg		250 mg	D5W	Physically compatible	74	C
	SE	500 mg	SE	1 g	D5W	Physically incompatible	15	I
Diphenhydramine HCl	PD	50 mg	SE	500 mg		Physically compatible	6	C
Dobutamine HCl	LI	1 g	SE	1 g	D5W, NS	Cloudy in 6 hr at 25 °C	789	I
	LI	1 g	ES	2.5 g	D5W, NS	White precipitate forms within 12 hr at 21 °C	812	I
Dopamine HCl	ACC	800 mg	SE	500 mg	D5W	Physically compatible. At 25 °C, 10% dopamine decomposition in 111 hr	527	C
Doxorubicin HCl	AD					Solution color darkens from red to blue-purple	524	I
Epinephrine HCl	PD	4 mg	SE	500 mg	D5W	At 25 °C, 10% epinephrine decomposition in 1.2 hr in light and 3 hr in dark	527	I
		4 mg		500 mg	D5W	Pink to brown discoloration of solution in 8 to 24 hr at room temperature	845	I
Erythromycin lactobionate	AB	1 g	SE	500 mg		Physically compatible. Erythromycin potency retained for 24 hr at 25 °C	20	C
Esmolol HCl	DU	6 g	LY	1 g	D5W	Physically compatible with no loss of either drug in 24 hr at room temperature under fluorescent light	1358	C

Additive Compatibility (Cont.)

Aminophylline

Drug	Mfr	Conc/L	Mfr	Conc/L	Test Soln	Remarks	Ref	C/I
Floxacillin sodium	BE	20 g	ANT	1 g	NS	Physically compatible for 72 hr at 15 and 30 °C	1479	C
Flumazenil	RC	20 mg	AMR	2 g	D5W[c]	Visually compatible with no flumazenil loss by HPLC in 24 hr at 23 °C under fluorescent light. Aminophylline not tested	1710	C
Furosemide	HO	1 g	ANT	1 g	NS	Physically compatible for 72 hr at 15 and 30 °C	1479	C
Heparin sodium		12,000 units		250 mg	D5W	Physically compatible	74	C
	UP	4000 units	SE	1 g	D5W	Physically compatible	15	C
Hydralazine HCl	BP	80 mg	BP	1 g	D5W	Yellow color produced	26	I
Hydrocortisone sodium succinate	UP	100 mg		250 mg	D5W	Physically compatible	74	C
	UP	500 mg	SE	1 g	D5W	Physically compatible	15	C
	UP	100 mg	SE	500 mg		Physically compatible	6	C
		250 mg		625 mg	D5W	Physically compatible and aminophylline chemically stable for 24 hr at 4 and 30 °C. Total hydrocortisone content changed little but substantial ester hydrolysis noted	521	C
Hydrocortisone sodium succinate with cephalothin sodium	UP LI	100 mg 1 g	SE	1 g	D5S	pH outside stability range for cephalothin. Precipitate seen in 12 hr	41	I
Hydroxyzine HCl	RR	250 mg	SE	1 g	D5W	Physically incompatible	15	I
Insulin, regular[d]	LI	20 units	SE	1 g	D5W	pH outside stability range for insulin	41	I
Isoproterenol HCl	BN	2 mg	SE	500 mg	D5W	At 25 °C, 10% isoproterenol decomposition in 2.2 to 2.5 hr in light and dark	527	I
Levorphanol bitartrate	RC					Physically incompatible	9	I
Lidocaine HCl	AST	2 g	SE	500 mg		Physically compatible	24	C
	AST	2 g	AQ	1 g	D5W, LR, NS	Physically compatible for 24 hr at 25 °C	775	C
Meperidine HCl	WI					Physically incompatible	9	I
Mephentermine sulfate		750 mg		625 mg	D5W	Physically compatible and chemically stable for 24 hr at 3 and 30 °C	520	C
Meropenem	ZEN	1 and 20 g	AMR	1 g	NS	Visually compatible for 4 hr at room temperature	1994	C
Methyldopate HCl	MSD	1 g	SE	500 mg	D, D–S, S	Physically compatible	23	C
	MSD	1 g	SE	500 mg	D5W	Physically compatible. At 25 °C, 10% methyldopate decomposition in 90 hr	527	C
Methylprednisolone sodium succinate	UP	40 to 250 mg		500 mg	D5W, NS	Clear solution for 24 hr	329	C
	UP	80 mg		1 g	D5W	Clear solution for 24 hr	329	C
	UP	125 mg	SE	500 mg		Precipitate forms after 6 hr but within 24 hr	6	I
	UP	250 mg to 1 g		1 g	D5W	Precipitate forms	329	I
	UP	10 to 20 g		~400 mg	D5S, D5W, LR	Yellow color forms	329	I

Additive Compatibility (Cont.)

Aminophylline

Drug	Mfr	Conc/L	Mfr	Conc/L	Test Soln	Remarks	Ref	C/I
	UP	500 mg and 2 g	SE	1 g	D5W	Physically compatible with no loss of aminophylline or methylprednisolone alcohol in 3 hr at room temperature. 7 to 10% ester hydrolysis termed not clinically important	1022	C
	UP	500 mg and 2 g	SE	1 g	NS	Physically compatible with no loss of aminophylline or methylprednisolone alcohol in 3 hr at room temperature. 12 to 18% ester hydrolysis termed not clinically important	1022	C
Metronidazole HCl with sodium bicarbonate	SE AB	5 g 50 mEq	SE	2 g	D5W, NS	Physically compatible for 48 hr	765	C
Morphine sulfate						Physically incompatible	9	I
Nafcillin sodium	WY	30 g	SE	500 mg	D5W	Nafcillin potency retained for 24 hr at 25 °C	27	C
	WY	2 g	SE	500 mg	D5W	14% nafcillin decomposition in 24 hr at 25 °C	27	I
Nitroglycerin	ACC	400 mg	IX	1 g	D5W[e]	Physically compatible with 4% nitroglycerin loss in 24 hr and 6% loss in 48 hr at 23 °C. Aminophylline not tested	929	C
	ACC	400 mg	IX	1 g	NS[e]	Physically compatible with no nitroglycerin loss in 24 hr and 5% loss in 48 hr at 23 °C. Aminophylline not tested	929	C
Norepinephrine bitartrate	WI	8 mg	SE	500 mg	D5W	At 25 °C, 10% norepinephrine decomposition in 3.6 hr	527	I
Papaverine HCl with trimecaine HCl		120 mg 600 mg		480 mg	D5W	Papaverine precipitation within 3 hr due to alkaline pH	835	I
Penicillin G potassium	SQ	1 million units	SE	500 mg	D5W	44% penicillin decomposition in 24 hr at 25 °C	47	I
	[f]	900,000 units	SE	500 mg	D5W	22% penicillin decomposition in 6 hr at 25 °C	48	I
Pentazocine lactate	WI	300 mg	SE	1 g	D5W	Physically incompatible	15	I
Pentobarbital sodium	AB	500 mg		500 mg		Physically compatible	3	C
	AB	1 g	SE	1 g	D5W	Physically compatible	15	C
	AB	500 mg	SE	500 mg		Physically compatible	6	C
Phenobarbital sodium	WI	200 mg	SE	1 g	D5W	Physically compatible	15	C
	AB	100 mg	SE	500 mg		Physically compatible	6	C
Potassium chloride	AB	3 g		250 mg	D5W	Physically compatible	74	C
	AB	40 mEq	SE	500 mg		Physically compatible	6	C
Procaine HCl	AB	1 g	SE	500 mg		Physically compatible	6	C
						Physically incompatible	9	I
	WI	1 g	SE	1 g	D5W	Physically incompatible	15	I
Prochlorperazine edisylate	SKF	100 mg	SE	1 g	D5W	Physically incompatible	15	I
Prochlorperazine mesylate	BP	100 mg	BP	1 g	D5W, NS	Immediate precipitate	26	I
Promazine HCl	BP	200 mg	BP	1 g	D5W, NS	Immediate precipitate	26	I
	WY	1 g	SE	1 g	D5W	Physically incompatible	15	I

Additive Compatibility (Cont.)

Aminophylline

Drug	Mfr	Conc/L	Mfr	Conc/L	Test Soln	Remarks	Ref	C/I
Promethazine HCl	BP	100 mg	BP	1 g	D5W, NS	Immediate precipitate	26	I
	WY	250 mg	SE	1 g	D5W	Physically incompatible	15	I
Ranitidine HCl	GL	50 mg and 2 g	ES	500 mg and 2 g	D5W, NS[c]	Physically compatible with 4% or less ranitidine loss in 24 hr at room temperature under fluorescent light. Aminophylline not tested	1361	C
	GL	50 mg and 2 g	ES	0.5 and 2 g	D5W, NS[c]	Visually compatible with little or no loss of either drug by HPLC in 48 hr at room temperature	1802	C
Sodium bicarbonate	AB	80 mEq	SE	1 g	D5W	Physically compatible	15	C
	AB	40 mEq	SE	500 mg		Physically compatible	6	C
	AB	2.4 mEq[g]	SE	500 mg	D5W	Physically compatible for 24 hr	772	C
Terbutaline sulfate	CI	4 mg	SE	500 mg	D5W	Physically compatible. At 25 °C, 10% terbutaline decomposition in 44 hr exposed to light	527	C
Vancomycin HCl	LI	1 g		250 mg	D5W	Physically compatible	74	C
	LI	5 g	SE	1 g	D5W	Physically incompatible	15	I
Verapamil HCl	KN	80 mg	SE	1 g	D5W, NS	Transient precipitate clears rapidly. Solution physically compatible for 48 hr	739	C
	KN	400 mg	SE	1 g	D5W	Visible turbidity forms immediately. Filtration removes all verapamil	1198	I
	KN	100 mg	SE	1 g	D5W	Visually clear, but precipitate found by microscopic examination. Filtration removes all verapamil	1198	I
Vitamin B complex with C	RC	2 ml	SE	1 g	D5S	High pH destroys vitamin activity	41	I
Zinc (salt unspecified)		50 mg		2.5 g	D5W, NS	Precipitate forms within a few minutes	1898	I
		40 mg		2 g	D5W, NS	Precipitate forms within a few minutes	1898	I
		20 mg		1 g	D5W, NS	Precipitate forms within 24 hr at room temperature less than 25 °C	1898	I
		20 mg		1 g	AA10, D25[h]	Visually compatible for 24 hr at room temperature less than 25 °C	1898	C

[a]*Sodium carbonate–containing formulation tested.*
[b]*Tested in polyolefin containers.*
[c]*Tested in PVC containers.*
[d]*Test performed prior to the availability of neutral regular insulin.*
[e]*Tested in glass containers.*
[f]*A buffered preparation was specified.*
[g]*One vial of Neut added to a liter of admixture.*
[h]*Also contained ascorbic acid 500 mg/L and vitamin B complex with C 2 ml/L.*

Drugs in Syringe Compatibility

Aminophylline

Drug (in syringe)	Mfr	Amt	Mfr	Amt	Remarks	Ref	C/I
Doxapram HCl	RB	400 mg/ 20 ml		250 mg/ 10 ml	Immediate turbidity and precipitation	1177	I
Heparin sodium		2500 units/ 1 ml		0.24 g/ 10 ml	Physically compatible for at least 5 min	1053	C
Metoclopramide HCl	RB	10 mg/ 2 ml	ES	80 mg/ 3.2 ml	Physically compatible for 24 hr at room temperature	924	C

Drugs in Syringe Compatibility (Cont.)

Aminophylline

Drug (in syringe)	Mfr	Amt	Mfr	Amt	Remarks	Ref	C/I
	RB	10 mg/ 2 ml	ES	500 mg/ 20 ml	Physically compatible for 24 hr at room temperature	924	C
	RB	10 mg/ 2 ml	ES	80 mg/ 3.2 ml	Physically compatible for 24 hr at 25 °C	1167	C
	RB	10 mg/ 2 ml	ES	500 mg/ 20 ml	Physically compatible for 24 hr at 25 °C	1167	C
	RB	160 mg/ 32 ml	ES	500 mg/ 20 ml	Physically compatible for 24 hr at 25 °C	1167	C
Pentobarbital sodium	AB	500 mg/ 10 ml		500 mg/ 2 ml	Physically compatible	55	C
Thiopental sodium	AB	75 mg/ 3 ml	SE	500 mg/ 2 ml	Physically compatible for at least 30 min	21	C
	AB	75 mg/ 3 ml		500 mg/ 2 ml	Physically compatible	55	C

Y-Site Injection Compatibility (1:1 Mixture)

Aminophylline

Drug	Mfr	Conc	Mfr	Conc	Remarks	Ref	C/I
Allopurinol sodium	BW	3 mg/ml[b]	AB	2.5 mg/ml[b]	Physically compatible with no change in measured turbidity or increase in particle content in 4 hr at 22 °C	1686	C
Amifostine	USB	10 mg/ml[a]	AMR	2.5 mg/ml[a]	Physically compatible with no change in measured turbidity or increase in particle content in 4 hr at 23 °C	1845	C
Amiodarone HCl	LZ	4 mg/ml[c]	ES	5 mg/ml[c]	Haze within 15 min and white precipitate within 6 hr at 21 °C	1032	I
Amphotericin B cholesteryl sulfate complex	SEQ	0.83 mg/ml[a]	AB	2.5 mg/ml[a]	Physically compatible with little or no change in measured turbidity or increase in particle content in 4 hr at 23 °C under fluorescent light	2117	C
Amrinone lactate	WB	3 mg/ml[b]	LY	2 mg/ml[a]	Physically compatible for at least 4 hr at 25 °C under fluorescent light	992	C
Aztreonam	SQ	40 mg/ml[a]	AMR	2.5 mg/ml[a]	Physically compatible with no subvisual haze or particle formation in 4 hr at 23 °C	1758	C
Ceftazidime	GL[d]	40 mg/ml[a]	ES	2 mg/ml[a]	Visually compatible with 4% ceftazidime loss and 9% theophylline loss by HPLC in 2 hr at room temperature	1937	C
	GL[d]	40 mg/ml[b]	ES	2 mg/ml[a]	Visually compatible with 5% ceftazidime loss and 4% theophylline loss by HPLC in 2 hr at room temperature	1937	C
	GL[e]	40 mg/ml	ES	2 mg/ml[a]	Visually compatible with no ceftazidime or theophylline loss by HPLC in 2 hr at room temperature	1937	C
	GL[f]	40 mg/ml[a]	ES	2 mg/ml[a]	Visually compatible with 5% ceftazidime loss and 7% theophylline loss by HPLC in 2 hr at room temperature	1937	C
	GL[f]	40 mg/ml[b]	ES	2 mg/ml[a]	Visually compatible with 2% ceftazidime loss and no theophylline loss by HPLC in 2 hr at room temperature	1937	C

Y-Site Injection Compatibility (1:1 Mixture) (Cont.)

Aminophylline

Drug	Mfr	Conc	Mfr	Conc	Remarks	Ref	C/I
Cimetidine HCl	SKF	6 mg/ml[c]	ES	4 mg/ml[c]	Physically compatible for 3 hr	1316	C
Ciprofloxacin	MI	2 mg/ml[c]	AB	2 mg/ml[c]	Fine white crystals form in 20 min in D5W and 2 min in NS	1655	I
Cisatracurium besylate	GW	0.1 and 2 mg/ml[a]	AB	2.5 mg/ml[a]	Physically compatible with no change in measured turbidity or increase in particle content in 4 hr at 23 °C	2074	C
	GW	5 mg/ml[a]	AB	2.5 mg/ml[a]	Gray subvisual haze forms in 1 hr	2074	I
Cladribine	ORT	0.015[b] and 0.5[g] mg/ml	AMR	2.5 mg/ml[b]	Physically compatible with no change in measured turbidity or increase in particle content in 4 hr at 23 °C	1969	C
Clarithromycin	AB	4 mg/ml[a]	EV	2 mg/ml[a]	Needle-like crystals form in 2 hr at 30 °C and 4 hr at 17 °C	2174	I
Diltiazem HCl	MMD	5 mg/ml	AMR	25 mg/ml[b]	Cloudiness forms	1807	I
	MMD	1 mg/ml[b]	AMR	25 mg/ml[b]	Visually compatible	1807	C
	MMD	5 mg/ml	AMR	2 mg/ml[c]	Visually compatible	1807	C
Dobutamine HCl	LI	4 mg/ml[c]	ES	4 mg/ml[c]	Slight haze or precipitate and color change in 1 hr	1316	I
Docetaxel	RPR	0.9 mg/ml[a]	AB	2.5 mg/ml[a]	Physically compatible with no change in measured turbidity or increase in particle content in 4 hr at 23 °C	2224	C
Doxorubicin HCl liposome injection	SEQ	0.4 mg/ml[a]	AB	2.5 mg/ml[a]	Physically compatible with little or no change in measured turbidity and no increase in particle content in 4 hr at 23 °C	2087	C
Enalaprilat	MSD	0.05 mg/ml[b]	ES	1 mg/ml[a]	Physically compatible for 24 hr at room temperature under fluorescent light	1355	C
Esmolol HCl	DCC	10 mg/ml[a]	ES	1 mg/ml[a]	Physically compatible for 24 hr at 22 °C	1169	C
Etoposide phosphate	BR	5 mg/ml[a]	AB	2.5 mg/ml[a]	Physically compatible with no change in measured turbidity or increase in particle content in 4 hr at 23 °C	2218	C
Famotidine	MSD	0.2 mg/ml[a]	LY	2.5 mg/ml[b]	Physically compatible for 14 hr	1196	C
	ME	2 mg/ml[d]		2.5 mg/ml[a]	Visually compatible for 4 hr at 22 °C	1936	C
Filgrastim	AMG	30 μg/ml[a]	AB	2.5 mg/ml[a]	Physically compatible with no change in measured turbidity or increase in particle content in 4 hr at 22 °C	1687	C
Fluconazole	RR	2 mg/ml	ES	25 mg/ml	Physically compatible for 24 hr at 25 °C	1407	C
	PF	0.5 and 1.5 mg/ml[c]	AMR	0.8 and 1.5 mg/ml[c]	Visually compatible with no loss of either drug by HPLC in 3 hr at 24 °C	1626	C
Fludarabine phosphate	BX	1 mg/ml[a]	ES	2.5 mg/ml[a]	Physically compatible for 4 hr at room temperature under fluorescent light	1439	C
Foscarnet sodium	AST	24 mg/ml	LY	25 mg/ml	Physically compatible for 24 hr at room temperature under fluorescent light	1335	C
Gemcitabine HCl	LI	10 mg/ml[b]	AB	2.5 mg/ml[b]	Physically compatible with no change in measured turbidity or increase in particle content in 4 hr at 23 °C	2226	C
Granisetron HCl	SKB	0.05 mg/ml[a]	AB	2.5 mg/ml[a]	Physically compatible with no change in measured turbidity or increase in particle content in 4 hr at 23 °C	2000	C

Y-Site Injection Compatibility (1:1 Mixture) (Cont.)

Aminophylline

Drug	Mfr	Conc	Mfr	Conc	Remarks	Ref	C/I
Heparin sodium with hydrocortisone sodium succinate	RI UP	1000 units + 100 mg/L[h]	SE	25 mg/ml	Physically compatible for at least 4 hr at room temperature by visual and microscopic examination	322	**C**
Hydralazine HCl	SO SO	1 mg/ml[a] 1 mg/ml[b]	ES ES	4 mg/ml[a] 4 mg/ml[b]	Gross color change in 1 hr Moderate color change in 1 hr and slight haze in 3 hr	1316 1316	**I** **I**
Labetalol HCl	SC	1 mg/ml[a]	ES	1 mg/ml[a]	Physically compatible for 24 hr at 18 °C	1171	**C**
Melphalan HCl	BW	0.1 mg/ml[b]	AB	2.5 mg/ml[b]	Physically compatible with no change in measured turbidity or increase in particle content in 3 hr at 22 °C	1557	**C**
Meropenem	ZEN	1 and 50 mg/ml[b]	AMR	25 mg/ml	Visually compatible for 4 hr at room temperature	1994	**C**
Morphine sulfate	WY	0.2 mg/ml[c]	ES	4 mg/ml[c]	Physically compatible for 3 hr	1316	**C**
Netilmicin sulfate	SC	5 mg/ml[i]	ES	800 µg/ml	Physically compatible and no netilmicin loss in 2 hr at 24 °C	1021	**C**
Ondansetron HCl	GL	1 mg/ml[b]	AMR	2.5 mg/ml[a]	Immediate turbidity and precipitation	1365	**I**
Paclitaxel	NCI	1.2 mg/ml[a]	AB	2.5 mg/ml[a]	Physically compatible with no change in measured turbidity in 4 hr at 22 °C	1556	**C**
Pancuronium bromide	ES	0.05 mg/ml[a]	AB	1 mg/ml[a]	Physically compatible for 24 hr at 28 °C	1337	**C**
Piperacillin sodium–tazobactam sodium	LE	40 + 5 mg/ml[a]	AB	2.5 mg/ml[a]	Physically compatible with no change in measured turbidity or increase in particle content in 4 hr at 22 °C	1688	**C**
Potassium chloride		40 mEq/L	SE	25 mg/ml	Physically compatible for at least 4 hr at room temperature by visual and microscopic examination	322	**C**
Propofol	ZEN	10 mg/ml	AMR	2.5 mg/ml[a]	Physically compatible for 1 hr at 23 °C with no increase in particle content	2066	**C**
Ranitidine HCl	GL	0.5 mg/ml[e]	LY	4 mg/ml[a]	Physically compatible for 24 hr	1323	**C**
Remifentanil HCl	GW	0.025 and 0.25 mg/ml[b]	AB	2.5 mg/ml[a]	Physically compatible with no change in measured turbidity or increase in particle content in 4 hr at 23 °C	2075	**C**
Sargramostim	IMM	10 µg/ml[b]	ES	2.5 mg/ml[b]	Physically compatible for 4 hr at 22 °C	1436	**C/I**
Tacrolimus	FUJ	1 mg/ml[b]	ES	2 mg/ml[a]	Visually compatible for 24 hr at 25 °C	1630	**C**
Teniposide	BR	0.1 mg/ml[a]	AB	2.5 mg/ml[a]	Physically compatible with no subvisual haze or particle formation in 4 hr at 23 °C	1725	**C**
Thiotepa	IMM[j]	1 mg/ml[b]	AMR	2.5 mg/ml[b]	Physically compatible with no change in measured turbidity or increase in particle content in 4 hr at 23 °C	1861	**C**
TNA #218 to #226[k]			AB	2.5 mg/ml[a]	Visually compatible with no precipitate or emulsion damage apparent in 4 hr at 23 °C	2215	**C**
Tolazoline HCl		0.1 mg/ml[a]	AB	5[a] and 25 mg/ml	Physically compatible for 24 hr at 22 °C	1363	**C**
TPN #189[k]			DB	1 mg/ml[b]	Visually compatible for 24 hr at 22 °C	1767	**C**
TPN #203 and #204[k]			AMR	5 mg/ml	White precipitate forms immediately	1974	**I**

Y-Site Injection Compatibility (1:1 Mixture) (Cont.)

Aminophylline

Drug	Mfr	Conc	Mfr	Conc	Remarks	Ref	C/I
TPN #212 to #215[k]			AB	2.5 mg/ml[a]	Physically compatible with no change in measured turbidity or increase in particle content in 4 hr at 23 °C	2109	C
Vecuronium bromide	OR	0.1 mg/ml[a]	AB	1 mg/ml[a]	Physically compatible for 24 hr at 28 °C	1337	C
Vinorelbine tartrate	BW	1 mg/ml[b]	AB	2.5 mg/ml[b]	Initial light haze becomes visible in room light along with large particles in 1 hr	1558	I
Vitamin B complex with C	RC	2 ml/L	SE	25 mg/ml	Physically compatible for at least 4 hr at room temperature by visual and microscopic examination	322	C
Warfarin sodium	DME	2 mg/ml[l]	ES	4 mg/ml[a]	Haze forms in 4 hr	2078	I

[a]*Tested in dextrose 5% in water.*
[b]*Tested in sodium chloride 0.9%.*
[c]*Tested in both dextrose 5% in water and sodium chloride 0.9%.*
[d]*Sodium carbonate–containing formulation tested.*
[e]*Tested in premixed infusion solution.*
[f]*Arginine formulation tested.*
[g]*Tested in bacteriostatic sodium chloride 0.9% preserved with benzyl alcohol 0.9%.*
[h]*Tested in dextrose 5% in water, sodium chloride 0.9%, and Ringer's injection, lactated.*
[i]*Tested in dextrose 5% in sodium chloride 0.2%.*
[j]*Lyophilized formulation tested.*
[k]*Refer to Appendix I for the composition of parenteral nutrition solutions. TNA indicates a 3-in-1 admixture, and TPN indicates a 2-in-1 admixture.*
[l]*Tested in sterile water for injection.*

Additional Compatibility Information

Acidic Additives— Reports in the literature of aminophylline precipitating in acidic media do not apply to the dilute solutions found in intravenous infusions. Aminophylline should not be mixed in a syringe with other components of an admixture but should be added separately (6).

Alkali-Labile Drugs— Because of the alkalinity of aminophylline-containing solutions, drugs known to be alkali labile should be avoided in admixtures, including epinephrine HCl, norepinephrine bitartrate, isoproterenol HCl, and penicillin G potassium (6). Cefotaxime sodium should not be mixed in alkaline solutions such as those containing aminophylline (792).

Calcium and Phosphate— Kirkpatrick et al. reported the physical compatibility of calcium gluconate 10 to 40 mEq/L and potassium phosphates 10 to 40 mM/L in three neonatal parenteral nutrition solutions (TPN #123 to #125 in Appendix I), alone and with retrograde administration of aminophylline 7.5 mg diluted with 1.5 ml of sterile water for injection. Contact of the alkaline aminophylline solution with the parenteral nutrition solutions resulted in the precipitation of calcium phosphate at much lower concentrations than were compatible in the parenteral nutrition solutions alone (1404).

Methylprednisolone— Studies of the compatibility of methylprednisolone sodium succinate (Upjohn) with aminophylline added to an auxiliary medication infusion unit have been performed. Primary admixtures were prepared by adding aminophylline 500 mg/L to dextrose 5% in water, dextrose 5% in sodium chloride 0.9%, and Ringer's injection, lactated. Up to 100 ml of the primary admixture was added along with methylprednisolone sodium succinate (Up-

john) to the auxiliary medication infusion unit with the following results (329):

Methylprednisolone Sodium Succinate	Aminophylline 500 mg/L Primary Solution	Results
500 mg	D5S, D5W qs 100 ml	Clear solution for 24 hr
500 mg	LR qs 100 ml	Clear solution for 24 hr
500 mg	Added to 100 ml LR	Clear solution for 1 hr
1000 mg	D5W qs 100 ml	Yellow solution, clear for 24 hr
1000 mg	D5S qs 100 ml	Yellow solution, clear for 6 hr
1000 mg	Added to 100 ml D5S	Yellow solution, clear for 24 hr
1000 mg	LR qs 100 ml or added to 100 ml LR	Yellow solution, clear for 4 hr
2000 mg	D5S, D5W, LR qs 100 ml	Yellow solution, clear for 24 hr

Dextrose-Containing Solutions— The addition of aminophylline 750 mg/L to the dextrose-containing solutions dextrose 5% in water and dextrose 5% in sodium chloride 0.9% resulted in a yellow discoloration. The yellow color developed after 48, 24, and 6 hours of storage at 25, 35, and 55 °C, respectively. When stored in the refrigerator, these solutions remained colorless for seven days. The color intensity was increased by elevated temperatures and longer exposures. Additional peaks appeared on HPLC chromatograms as the yellow color intensified. Because the aminophylline concentration remained constant in all admixtures and the yellow color did not form in solutions lacking dextrose, it was believed that the discoloration resulted from the decomposition of dextrose. However, the dextrose decomposition products were well within compendial limits. Therefore, the authors concluded that these solutions were compatible admixtures (556). Adams et al. reached the same conclusion in independent testing (1571).

Storage of aminophylline 12.5 mg/50 ml of water for injection and dextrose 5, 10, and 20% in polypropylene syringes (Plastipak, Becton-Dickinson) and glass flasks for 24 hours at 24 to 26 °C resulted in no loss of aminophylline. However, a yellow discoloration of the solution began in two hours and intensified with time in the dextrose 10 and 20% mixtures (852).

Concentrated Solutions— The following incompatibility determinations were performed with concentrated solutions. The drugs in dry form were reconstituted according to manufacturers' recommendations. Particulate matter was noted within two hours after adding 1 ml of aminophylline to 5 ml of sterile distilled water along with 1 ml of each of the following drugs (28):

    Dimenhydrinate (Searle)
    Hydroxyzine HCl (Pfizer)
    Phenytoin sodium (Parke-Davis)
    Prochlorperazine edisylate (SKF)
    Promazine HCl (Wyeth)
    Promethazine HCl (Wyeth)
    Vancomycin HCl (Lilly)

AMIODARONE HCL
AHFS 24:04

Cordarone Intravenous   **Wyeth-Ayerst**

Products— Amiodarone HCl (Wyeth-Ayerst) is available in 3-ml ampuls. Each milliliter of the pale yellow solution contains (2):

Amiodarone HCl	50 mg
Polysorbate (Tween) 80	100 mg
Benzyl alcohol	20.2 mg
Water for injection	qs 1 ml

pH— The pH is reported to be 4.08 (1053).

Administration— Amiodarone HCl is a concentrate that is administered by intravenous infusion after dilution in a compatible diluent. Intravenous infusion is performed using a volumetric pump and a dedicated central venous catheter with an inline filter when possible; concentrations greater than 2 mg/ml require a central venous catheter (2; 4). The injection contains polysorbate 80, a surface active agent that alters drop size. The drop size reduction may lead to substantial underdosage if a drop counter infusion set is used. Consequently, the drug must be delivered with a volumetric infusion pump (2; 1445).

Stability— Amiodarone HCl should be stored at room temperature and protected from light and excessive heat. Light protection is not necessary during administration. It is recommended that amiodarone HCl be added only to dextrose 5% in water (2). Information on the drug's compatibility in sodium chloride 0.9% has been conflicting. Amiodarone HCl 0.6 mg/ml in sodium chloride 0.9% precipitated in 24 hours at room temperature (1443). In another study, a 1.8-mg/ml concentration in sodium chloride 0.9% was physically and chemically compatible for 24 hours at 24 °C. This difference could have been due to higher polysorbate 80 concentrations in the latter admixtures (1031). Amiodarone HCl 0.6 mg/ml in dextrose 5% in water is stable for five days at room temperature (1443). Solutions containing less than 0.6 mg/ml of amiodarone HCl in dextrose 5% in water are unstable and should not be used (1442).

Amiodarone HCl (Wyeth-Ayerst) 2 mg/ml in dextrose 5% in water and also in sodium chloride 0.9% in amber glass containers was stored at 40 °C, being representative of the highest temperature to which drug solutions may be exposed. The solutions turned cloudy after 18 days of storage. HPLC analysis showed that 6 to 10% loss had occurred in sodium chloride 0.9% and dextrose 5% in water, respectively, in 18 days, with losses increasing to 11 to 14% in 24 days (2110).

Sorption— At concentrations of 1 to 6 mg/ml in dextrose 5% in water in polyolefin or glass containers, amiodarone HCl is physically compatible, with no loss in 24 hours. In PVC containers, however, the amiodarone HCl loss due to sorption occurs; acceptable potency (less than 10% loss) exists for two hours. Consequently, the manufacturer recommends that all infusions longer than two hours be made from glass or polyolefin containers only (2). Amiodarone HCl (Labaz) 0.6 mg/ml in dextrose 5% in water did not exhibit any loss due to sorption in rigid PVC containers (PVC Container Corp.) or glass bottles (Travenol). However, losses were observed in flexible PVC bags (Travenol). The losses totaled approximately 25% in 24 hours at room temperature (1443).

Similarly, amiodarone HCl is lost due to sorption to PVC infusion sets (2; 1443). However, the manufacturer states that these losses are accounted for by the recommended dosage schedule. Consequently, PVC sets should be used with this drug, but the recommended infusion regimen must be followed (2).

Precipitation— Amiodarone HCl may precipitate when diluted. Studies found little or no precipitation when the formulation was diluted to very small or very large concentrations. In the middle range, however, at concentrations between 45 mg/ml (90% amiodarone HCl formulation) and about 0.0025 mg/ml in phosphate buffer (pH 7.4), the drug concentration exceeds the solubility of amiodarone HCl in the mixture. Precipitation may occur immediately or on standing. Such precipitation may occur when the drug enters the bloodstream, contributing to the phlebitis associated with amiodarone HCl (1818; 1819).

Filtration— Amiodarone HCl (Labaz) 0.6 mg/ml in dextrose 5% in water and sodium chloride 0.9% was filtered through a 0.22-μm cellulose ester membrane filter (Ivex-HP, Millipore) over six hours. No significant drug loss due to binding to the filter was noted (1034). The use of an inline filter during administration is recommended (2; 4).

Compatibility Information

Solution Compatibility

Amiodarone HCl

Solution	Mfr	Mfr	Conc/L	Remarks	Ref	C/I
Dextrose 5% in water	MG[a]	LZ	1.8 g	Physically compatible with little or no amiodarone loss in 24 hr at 24 °C under fluorescent light	1031	C
	TR[b]	LZ	0.6 g	Approximately 25% drug loss in 24 hr at room temperature	1443	I
	TR[c]	LZ	0.6 g	Physically compatible with little or no drug loss in 5 days at room temperature	1443	C
	BA[d]	WY	2 g	Visually compatible with no loss at 5 °C and 3% loss at 25 °C in 32 days	2110	C
Sodium chloride 0.9%	MG[a]	LZ	1.8 g	Physically compatible with little or no amiodarone loss in 24 hr at 24 °C under fluorescent light	1031	C
	TR[c]	LZ	0.6 g	Physically incompatible in 24 hr at room temperature	1443	I
	BA[d]	WY	2 g	Visually compatible with no loss at 5 °C and 3% loss at 25 °C in 32 days	2110	C

[a]Tested in polyolefin containers.
[b]Tested in PVC containers.
[c]Tested in glass containers.
[d]Tested in amber glass containers.

Additive Compatibility

Amiodarone HCl

Drug	Mfr	Conc/L	Mfr	Conc/L	Test Soln	Remarks	Ref	C/I
Dobutamine HCl	LI	1 g	LZ	2.5 g	D5W, NS	Physically compatible for 24 hr at 21 °C	812	C
Floxacillin sodium	BE	20 g	LZ	4 g	D5W	Immediate precipitation	1479	I
Furosemide	ES	200 mg	LZ	1.8 g	D5W, NS[a]	Physically compatible with 8% or less amiodarone loss in 24 hr at 24 °C under fluorescent light	1031	C
	HO	1 g	LZ	4 g	D5W	Haze forms in 5 hr and precipitate forms in 24 to 72 hr at 30 °C. No change at 15 °C	1479	I
Lidocaine HCl	AB	4 g	LZ	1.8 g	D5W, NS[a]	Physically compatible with 9% or less amiodarone loss in 24 hr at 24 °C under fluorescent light	1031	C
Potassium chloride	AB	40 mEq	LZ	1.8 g	D5W, NS[a]	Physically compatible with no amiodarone loss in 24 hr at 24 °C under fluorescent light	1031	C
Procainamide HCl	SQ	4 g	LZ	1.8 g	D5W, NS[a]	Physically compatible with 5% or less amiodarone loss in 24 hr at 24 °C under fluorescent light	1031	C
Propafenone HCl	KN	0.625 g	LZ	1.25 g[d]	D5W	Visually compatible with no propafenone loss by HPLC in 24 hr at 22 °C exposed to fluorescent light. Amiodarone not tested	412	C

Additive Compatibility (Cont.)

Amiodarone HCl

Drug	Mfr	Conc/L	Mfr	Conc/L	Test Soln	Remarks	Ref	C/I
Quinidine gluconate	LI	1 g	LZ	1.8 g	D5W[b]	Precipitation causes milky appearance. 13% amiodarone loss in 6 hr and 23% loss in 24 hr at 24 °C under fluorescent light	1031	I
	LI	1 g	LZ	1.8 g	D5W[c]	Precipitation causes milky appearance. No amiodarone loss in 24 hr at 24 °C under fluorescent light	1031	I
	LI	1 g	LZ	1.8 g	NS[b]	Physically compatible with 4% amiodarone loss in 6 hr and 13% loss in 24 hr at 24 °C under fluorescent light	1031	I
	LI	1 g	LZ	1.8 g	NS[c]	Physically compatible with no amiodarone loss in 24 hr at 24 °C under fluorescent light	1031	C
Verapamil HCl	KN	50 mg	LZ	1.8 g	D5W, NS[a]	Physically compatible with 8% or less amiodarone loss in 24 hr at 24 °C under fluorescent light	1031	C

[a]Tested in both polyolefin and PVC containers.
[b]Tested in PVC containers.
[c]Tested in polyolefin containers.
[d]Approximate concentration.

Drugs in Syringe Compatibility

Amiodarone HCl

Drug (in syringe)	Mfr	Amt	Mfr	Amt	Remarks	Ref	C/I
Heparin sodium		2500 units/ 1 ml	LZ	150 mg/ 3 ml	Turbidity or precipitate forms within 5 min	1053	I

Y-Site Injection Compatibility (1:1 Mixture)

Amiodarone HCl

Drug	Mfr	Conc	Mfr	Conc	Remarks	Ref	C/I
Amikacin sulfate	BR	5 mg/ml[c]	LZ	4 mg/ml[c]	Physically compatible for 4 hr at room temperature	1444	C
Aminophylline	ES	5 mg/ml[c]	LZ	4 mg/ml[c]	Haze forms within 15 min and white precipitate forms within 6 hr at 21 °C	1032	I
Bretylium tosylate	ACC	8 mg/ml[c]	LZ	4 mg/ml[c]	Physically compatible for 24 hr at 21 °C	1032	C
Cefamandole nafate	LI	20 and 40 mg/ml[c]	LZ	4 mg/ml[c]	Precipitate forms	1444	I
Cefazolin sodium	LI	20 mg/ml[a]	LZ	4 mg/ml[a]	Precipitate forms	1444	I
	LI	20 mg/ml[b]	LZ	4 mg/ml[b]	Physically compatible for 4 hr at room temperature	1444	C
Clarithromycin	AB	4 mg/ml[a]	SW	3 mg/ml[a]	Visually compatible for 72 hr at both 30 and 17 °C	2174	C
Clindamycin phosphate	UP	6 mg/ml[c]	LZ	4 mg/ml[c]	Physically compatible for 4 hr at room temperature	1444	C
Dobutamine HCl	LI	2 mg/ml[c]	LZ	4 mg/ml[c]	Physically compatible for 24 hr at 21 °C	1032	C
Dopamine HCl	ES	1.6 mg/ml[c]	LZ	4 mg/ml[c]	Physically compatible for 24 hr at 21 °C	1032	C

Y-Site Injection Compatibility (1:1 Mixture) (Cont.)

Amiodarone HCl

Drug	Mfr	Conc	Mfr	Conc	Remarks	Ref	C/I
Doxycycline hyclate	ACC	0.25 mg/ml[c]	LZ	4 mg/ml[c]	Physically compatible for 4 hr at room temperature	1444	**C**
Erythromycin lactobionate	AB	2 mg/ml[c]	LZ	4 mg/ml[c]	Physically compatible for 4 hr at room temperature	1444	**C**
Esmolol HCl	DU	40 mg/ml[a]	WY	4.8 mg/ml[a]	Visually compatible for 24 hr at 23 °C	1877	**C**
Gentamicin sulfate	LY	0.8 mg/ml[c]	LZ	4 mg/ml[c]	Physically compatible for 4 hr at room temperature	1444	**C**
Heparin sodium		50 units/ml/min[b]	LZ	150 mg/3 ml[d]	Yellow solution with opalescence	1053	**I**
Insulin, regular	LI	1 unit/ml[a]	WY	4.8 mg/ml[a]	Visually compatible for 24 hr at 23 °C	1877	**C**
Isoproterenol HCl	ES	0.004 mg/ml[c]	LZ	4 mg/ml[c]	Physically compatible for 24 hr at 21 °C	1032	**C**
Labetalol HCl	GL	5 mg/ml	WY	4.8 mg/ml[a]	Visually compatible for 24 hr at 23 °C	1877	**C**
Lidocaine HCl	AST	8 mg/ml[c]	LZ	4 mg/ml[c]	Physically compatible for 24 hr at 21 °C	1032	**C**
Metaraminol bitartrate	MSD	0.2 mg/ml[c]	LZ	4 mg/ml[c]	Physically compatible for 24 hr at 21 °C	1032	**C**
Metronidazole HCl	LY	5 mg/ml[c]	LZ	4 mg/ml[c]	Physically compatible for 4 hr at room temperature	1444	**C**
Midazolam HCl	RC	1 mg/ml[a]	WY	4.8 mg/ml[a]	Visually compatible for 24 hr at 23 °C	1877	**C**
Morphine sulfate	SX	1 mg/ml[a]	WY	4.8 mg/ml[a]	Visually compatible for 24 hr at 23 °C	1877	**C**
Nitroglycerin	AB	0.24 mg/ml[c]	LZ	4 mg/ml[c]	Physically compatible for 24 hr at 21 °C	1032	**C**
Norepinephrine bitartrate	BN	0.064 mg/ml[c]	LZ	4 mg/ml[c]	Physically compatible for 24 hr at 21 °C	1032	**C**
Penicillin G potassium	PF	100,000 units/ml[c]	LZ	4 mg/ml[c]	Physically compatible for 4 hr at room temperature	1444	**C**
Phentolamine mesylate	CI	0.04 mg/ml[c]	LZ	4 mg/ml[c]	Physically compatible for 24 hr at 21 °C	1032	**C**
Phenylephrine HCl	WI	0.04 mg/ml[c]	LZ	4 mg/ml[c]	Physically compatible for 24 hr at 21 °C	1032	**C**
Potassium chloride	AB	0.04 mg/ml[c]	LZ	4 mg/ml[c]	Physically compatible for 24 hr at 21 °C	1032	**C**
Procainamide HCl	AHP	8 mg/ml[c]	LZ	4 mg/ml[c]	Physically compatible for 24 hr at 21 °C	1032	**C**
Sodium bicarbonate	AB	1 mEq/ml	WY	3 mg/ml[a]	Precipitate forms immediately	1851	**I**
Tobramycin sulfate	LI	0.8 mg/ml[c]	LZ	4 mg/ml[c]	Physically compatible for 4 hr at room temperature	1444	**C**
Vancomycin HCl	LI	5 mg/ml[c]	LZ	4 mg/ml[c]	Physically compatible for 4 hr at room temperature	1444	**C**

[a]*Tested in dextrose 5% in water.*
[b]*Tested in sodium chloride 0.9%.*
[c]*Tested in both dextrose 5% in water and sodium chloride 0.9%.*
[d]*Given over three minutes via a Y-site into a running infusion solution of heparin sodium in sodium chloride 0.9%.*

Additional Compatibility Information

Miscellaneous— The manufacturer states that a precipitate forms when amiodarone HCl 4 mg/ml in dextrose 5% in water is admixed with aminophylline, cefamandole nafate, or cefazolin sodium and at 3 mg/ml with sodium bicarbonate (2).

Evacuated Containers— Amiodarone HCl (Wyeth-Ayerst) 1.2 mg/ml in 250 ml of dextrose 5% in water has been reported to develop cloudiness upon standing when prepared in glass evacuated bottles (Abbott). The precipitation was attributed to the acetate buffers present in the small amount of residual fluid left in evacuated bottles from steam sterilization (1982).

AMITRIPTYLINE HCL
AHFS 28:16.04

Elavil   **Zeneca**

Products— Amitriptyline HCl (Zeneca) is available as a colorless solution in 10-ml vials. Each milliliter of solution contains (2):

Amitriptyline HCl	10 mg
Dextrose	44 mg
Methylparaben	1.5 mg
Propylparaben	0.2 mg
Water for injection	qs 1 ml

pH— From 4 to 6 (4).

Administration— Amitriptyline HCl is administered intramuscularly (2; 4).

Stability— Amitriptyline HCl injection should be protected from light and stored at 15 to 30 °C (4). Freezing and temperatures over 30 °C should be avoided (4). Exposure to light results in the formation of ketone and, in three to four days, a precipitate. In solutions protected from light, these effects were not observed (476).

Decomposition of amitriptyline HCl was observed when solutions in water or phosphate buffer (pH 6.8) were autoclaved at 115 °C for 30 minutes in the presence of excess oxygen (477).

Sorption— Amitriptyline HCl (Roche) (concentration unspecified) in dextrose 5% in water in PVC containers was delivered over four hours through PVC administration sets. Little or no loss due to sorption was found by UV spectroscopy (2045).

Compatibility Information

Sodium metabisulfite greatly increases the rate of decomposition of amitriptyline HCl. The presence of ferric or cupric ions also enhances decomposition (478).

AMMONIUM CHLORIDE
AHFS 40:04

Abbott

Products— Ammonium chloride additive solution (Abbott) is available in 20-ml vials containing 5.35 g of ammonium chloride, which provides 100 mEq (5 mEq/ml) of NH_4^+ and Cl^- ions. The solution also contains 2 mg/ml of disodium edetate as a stabilizer and hydrochloric acid to adjust the pH. The additive solution is intended to be used only after further dilution in a larger volume of sodium chloride 0.9% injection (4).

One gram of ammonium chloride contains 18.7 mEq each of ammonium and chloride ions (4).

pH— From 4 to 6 (17).

Osmolarity— 10 mOsm/ml (calculated) (4).

Administration— Ammonium chloride injection is generally administered by slow intravenous infusion after dilution of one or two vials (100 to 200 mEq) in 500 to 1000 ml of sodium chloride 0.9% injection. The infusion rate in adults of the diluted solution should not exceed 5 ml/min (4).

Stability— Store at controlled room temperature and protect from freezing. Highly concentrated solutions of ammonium chloride may crystallize when exposed to low temperatures. If such crystallization does occur, warming to room temperature in a water bath is recommended (4).

Compatibility Information

Solution Compatibility

Ammonium chloride

Solution	Mfr	Mfr	Conc/L	Remarks	Ref	C/I
Dextran 6% in dextrose 5%	AB	AB	400 mEq	Physically compatible	3	C
Dextran 6% in sodium chloride 0.9%	AB	AB	400 mEq	Physically compatible	3	C
Dextrose–Ringer's injection combinations	AB	AB	400 mEq	Physically compatible	3	C
Dextrose–Ringer's injection, lactated, combinations	AB	AB	400 mEq	Physically compatible	3	C
Dextrose–saline combinations	AB	AB	400 mEq	Physically compatible	3	C
Dextrose 2½% in water	AB	AB	400 mEq	Physically compatible	3	C
Dextrose 5% in water	AB	AB	400 mEq	Physically compatible	3	C
Dextrose 10% in water	AB	AB	400 mEq	Physically compatible	3	C
Fructose 10% in sodium chloride 0.9%	AB	AB	400 mEq	Physically compatible	3	C

Solution Compatibility (Cont.)

Ammonium chloride

Solution	Mfr	Mfr	Conc/L	Remarks	Ref	C/I
Fructose 10% in water	AB	AB	400 mEq Physically compatible		3	**C**
Invert sugar 5 and 10% in sodium chloride 0.9%	AB	AB	400 mEq Physically compatible		3	**C**
Invert sugar 5 and 10% in water	AB	AB	400 mEq Physically compatible		3	**C**
Ionosol products	AB	AB	400 mEq Physically compatible		3	**C**
Ringer's injection	AB	AB	400 mEq Physically compatible		3	**C**
Ringer's injection, lactated	AB	AB	400 mEq Physically compatible		3	**C**
Sodium chloride 0.45%	AB	AB	400 mEq Physically compatible		3	**C**
Sodium chloride 0.9%	AB	AB	400 mEq Physically compatible		3	**C**
Sodium lactate ⅙ M	AB	AB	400 mEq Physically compatible		3	**C**

Additive Compatibility

Ammonium chloride

Drug	Mfr	Conc/L	Mfr	Conc/L	Test Soln	Remarks	Ref	C/I
Dimenhydrinate	SE					Physically incompatible	9	**I**
	SE	500 mg	AB	20 g	D5W	Physically compatible	15	**C**
Levorphanol bitartrate	RC					Physically incompatible	9	**I**

Y-Site Injection Compatibility (1:1 Mixture)

Ammonium chloride

Drug	Mfr	Conc	Mfr	Conc	Remarks	Ref	C/I
Warfarin sodium	DU	0.1 mg/ml[a]	AB	5 mEq/ml	Subvisual haze forms immediately	2011	**I**
	DU	0.1 mg/ml[b]	AB	5 mEq/ml	Physically compatible with no change in measured turbidity or increase in particle content in 24 hr at 23 °C	2011	**C**
	DU	2 mg/ml[c]	AB	5 mEq/ml	Heavy white turbidity forms immediately and becomes flocculent precipitate in 24 hr at 23 °C	2011	**I**

[a]*Tested in dextrose 5% in water.*
[b]*Tested in sodium chloride 0.9%.*
[c]*Tested in sterile water for injection.*

Additional Compatibility Information

It has been stated that potassium chloride 20 and 40 mEq/L can be added to ammonium chloride injection (128).

Ammonium chloride is stated to be incompatible with alkalies and their carbonates (4).

AMOBARBITAL SODIUM
(AMYLOBARBITONE SODIUM)
AHFS 28:24.04

Amytal Sodium   **Ranbaxy**

Products— Amobarbital sodium (Ranbaxy) is available in vials containing 500 mg. Reconstitute the vials with sterile water for injection. The following table shows the amount of diluent to use to achieve various concentrations (1-3/13/98; 4; 108):

Vial Size	Concentration (mg/ml)				
	10	25	50	100	200
500 mg	50 ml	20 ml	10 ml	5 ml	2.5 ml

Ordinarily, a 100-mg/ml concentration is used. After the addition of the sterile water for injection, rotate the vial but do not shake it. Several minutes are usually necessary to dissolve the drug, but any solution that has not become completely clear within five minutes should not be used (1-3/13/98; 4).

pH— A 5% solution of amobarbital sodium in sterile water for injection has a pH of 9.6 to 10.4 (4).

Administration— Amobarbital sodium may be administered by deep intramuscular or slow intravenous injection. No more than 5 ml of solution (regardless of concentration) should be injected intramuscularly at any one site. Subcutaneous and superficial intramuscular injections can be painful and result in tissue damage. The intravenous injection rate should not exceed 50 (1-3/13/98; 4) to 100 mg/min in adults or 60 mg/m^2/min for children (4).

Stability— Amobarbital sodium hydrolyzes in solution or when exposed to air. The contents of the vial should be injected within 30 minutes after reconstitution (1-3/13/98; 4).

Amobarbital sodium should not be added to acidic solutions because the drug may precipitate if the resulting pH is 9.2 or less (4). No solution containing a precipitate should be used (1-3/13/98; 4).

Compatibility Information

Solution Compatibility

Amobarbital sodium

Solution	Mfr	Mfr	Conc/L	Remarks	Ref	C/I
Alcohol 5%, dextrose 5%	BA	LI	10 g	Physically compatible for 24 hr	315	C
Dextrose 5% in Ringer's injection, lactated	BA	LI	10 g	Physically compatible for 24 hr	315	C
Dextrose 5% in sodium chloride 0.9%	BA	LI	10 g	Physically compatible for 24 hr	315	C
Dextrose 5% in water	BA	LI	10 g	Physically compatible for 24 hr	315	C
Dextrose 10% in water	BA	LI	10 g	Physically compatible for 24 hr	315	C
Dextrose 20% in water	BA	LI	10 g	Physically compatible for 24 hr	315	C
Fructose 10% in water	BA	LI	10 g	Physically compatible for 24 hr	315	C
Invert sugar 10% in Electrolyte #1	BA	LI	5 and 10 g	Precipitate forms within 24 hr	315	I
Invert sugar 10% in Electrolyte #2	BA	LI	5 and 10 g	Precipitate forms within 24 hr	315	I
Polysal M with dextrose 5%	CU	LI	10 g	Physically compatible for 24 hr	315	C
Ringer's injection, lactated	BA	LI	10 g	Physically compatible for 24 hr	315	C
Sodium chloride 0.9%	BA	LI	10 g	Physically compatible for 24 hr	315	C
Sodium lactate ⅙ M	BA	LI	10 g	Physically compatible for 24 hr	315	C

Additive Compatibility

Amobarbital sodium

Drug	Mfr	Conc/L	Mfr	Conc/L	Test Soln	Remarks	Ref	C/I
Amikacin sulfate	BR	5 g	LI	100 mg	D5LR, D5R, D5S, D5W, D10W, IS10, LR, NS, R, SL	Physically compatible. Potency of both retained for 24 hr at 25 °C	294	C

Additive Compatibility (Cont.)

Amobarbital sodium

Drug	Mfr	Conc/L	Mfr	Conc/L	Test Soln	Remarks	Ref	C/I
Aminophylline	SE	500 mg	LI	500 mg		Physically compatible	6	C
Dimenhydrinate	SE					Physically incompatible	9	I
	SE	500 mg	LI	1 g	D5W	Physically compatible	15	C
Diphenhydramine HCl	PD					Physically incompatible	9	I
	PD	80 mg	LI	1 g	D5W	Physically incompatible	15	I
Hydrocortisone sodium succinate						Physically incompatible	9	I
	UP	500 mg	LI	1 g	D5W	Physically compatible	15	C
Hydroxyzine HCl	PF					Physically incompatible	9	I
	RR	250 mg	LI	1 g	D5W	Physically incompatible	15	I
Insulin, regular[a]						Physically incompatible	9	I
Levorphanol bitartrate	RC					Physically incompatible	9	I
Meperidine HCl	WI					Physically incompatible	9	I
Morphine sulfate						Physically incompatible	9	I
Norepinephrine bitartrate	WI					Physically incompatible	9	I
	WI	2 mg	LI	1 g	D5W	Physically incompatible	15	I
Pentazocine lactate	WI	300 mg	LI	1 g	D5W	Physically incompatible	15	I
Procaine HCl						Physically incompatible	9	I
	WI	1 g	LI	1 g	D5W	Physically incompatible	15	I
Sodium bicarbonate	AB	2.4 mEq[b]	LI	500 mg	D5W	Physically compatible for 24 hr	772	C
Streptomycin sulfate						Physically incompatible	9	I
Vancomycin HCl	LI					Physically incompatible	9	I
	LI	5 g	LI	1 g	D5W	Physically incompatible	15	I

[a]*Test performed prior to availability of neutral regular insulin.*
[b]*One vial of Neut added to a liter of admixture.*

Additional Compatibility Information

Additives— Drugs stated to be incompatible with barbiturate salts include pentazocine lactate (4), clindamycin phosphate (106), cefazolin sodium (278), cimetidine HCl (360), pancuronium bromide (4), and droperidol (4).

Acidic Solutions— Drugs such as amobarbital sodium exhibit poor solubility in an acidic medium and may precipitate (22). Metaraminol bitartrate is acidic and may cause precipitation, depending on the concentrations of the additives (7). Also, the acidic methyldopate HCl imparts some buffer capacity to admixtures and may pose solubility problems with barbiturate salts (23).

When barbiturates are mixed with succinylcholine chloride, either the free barbiturate will precipitate or the succinylcholine chloride will be hydrolyzed, depending on the final pH of the admixture (21). Atracurium besylate may also be inactivated by alkaline solutions, such as barbiturates, and precipitation of a free acid of the admixed drug may occur, depending on the resultant pH of the admixture (4).

Alkali-Labile Drugs— Amobarbital sodium may raise the pH of admixture solutions to the alkaline range and, therefore, should not be mixed with alkali-labile drugs such as penicillin G (47). Significant decomposition of isoproterenol HCl and norepinephrine bitartrate may also occur. If either of these two drugs is mixed with amobarbital sodium, the admixture should be used immediately after preparation (59; 77).

AMPHOTERICIN B
AHFS 8:12.04 and 84:04.08

Fungizone Intravenous   **Apothecon**

Products— Amphotericin B (Apothecon) is available in vials containing 50 mg of drug with sodium desoxycholate 41 mg and sodium phosphates 20.2 mg (1-10/98). Reconstitute with 10 ml of sterile water for injection without preservatives and shake until a clear colloidal dispersion is obtained. The resultant concentration is 5 mg/ml of amphotericin B. Use only sterile water for injection without preservatives for reconstitution because other diluents, such as sodium chloride 0.9% or solutions containing a bacteriostatic agent such as benzyl alcohol, may result in the precipitation of the antibiotic. For infusion, amphotericin B must be further diluted with dextrose 5% in water with a pH above 4.2 (1-10/98; 4).

pH— The pH of amphotericin B (Squibb) 100 mg/L in dextrose 5% in water has been reported as 5.7 (149).

Osmolality— The osmolality of amphotericin B (Squibb) 0.1 mg/ml in dextrose 5% in water was determined to be 256 mOsm/kg (1375).

Administration— Amphotericin B is administered by slow intravenous infusion over approximately two to six hours. The recommended concentration of the infusion is 0.1 mg/ml (1-10/98; 4). The drug has also been given intra-articularly, intrathecally, intrapleurally, and by irrigation (4).

Stability— Store intact vials at 2 to 8 °C and protect from light (1-10/98; 4). Although refrigeration is recommended, intact vials of amphotericin B (Squibb) are reported to be stable at room temperature for two weeks (853) to one month (60). The manufacturer indicates that a 5 to 10% potency loss occurs in one month at room temperature (1433).

Amphotericin B reconstituted with sterile water for injection without preservatives and stored in the dark is stable for 24 hours at room temperature and for one week under refrigeration at 2 to 8 °C (1-10/98; 4; 108). One report indicates that aqueous solutions may be stable for over a week at both 5 and 28 °C (352).

Although the manufacturer recommends light protection for aqueous solutions of amphotericin B (1-10/98), several reports indicate that for short-term exposure of eight to 24 hours, little difference in potency is observed between light-protected and light-exposed solutions (150; 335; 353). Longer exposure periods may result in unacceptable potency loss, however (150).

The pH range for optimum clarity and stability is 6 to 7 (148). At a pH of less than approximately 6, the colloidal dispersion may become turbid (40; 148). Colloidal particles tend to coagulate rapidly at a pH of less than 5 (4).

Filtration— Various studies have assessed the effects of filtration on the amphotericin B colloidal dispersion with differing results. Huber and Riffkin reported that the use of a 0.22-μm membrane filter was unacceptable with colloidal solutions adjusted to pH 4.7, 5.6, and 6.5. The concentration of amphotericin B in the filtrate decreased substantially after several hours. A 0.45-μm filter was satisfactory for infusions with a pH of 6.5, but the results at pH 5.6 were inconclusive. At pH 5.6 and 6.5, 1- and 5-μm filters both proved satisfactory in that they did not reduce the concentration of amphotericin B. For the turbid mixtures resulting at pH 4.7, however, all filters sharply reduced the concentration (148). A report by Rebagay et al. tended to support this finding for the 0.22-μm filter. At pH 5.7, fine particles of amphotericin B formed and were retained by the 0.22-μm filter (149). Gotz and Simon, using a method similar to that of Huber and Riffkin, found no appreciable reduction in concentration with the 0.45-μm filter; but with a 0.22-μm filter, after one hour the concentration of amphotericin B delivered was about 30% of the initial concentration (152). Tipple et al. reported that when amphotericin B 50 mg/500 ml in dextrose 5% in water was filtered through a 0.22-μm circular cellulose ester membrane (Swinnex) or a 0.22-μm cylindrical cellulose ester filter (Ivex-2), the flow rate decreased dramatically after passage of as little as 30 ml. Flow ceased altogether after 100 to 200 ml. The last sample filtered contained no drug. With a 0.45-μm circular cellulose ester membrane (Swinnex), no loss of activity was determined after filtration of 200 ml. However, the flow rate had decreased (598). On the other hand, Piecoro et al. found no significant difference in the amount or potency of amphotericin B in dextrose 5% in water with phosphate buffer after filtration with 0.22-, 0.45-, and 5-μm filters (151).

For amphotericin B infusions, only filters with a pore size not less than 1 μm should be used for filtration (1-10/98; 4; 148). This would allow a margin for error that would compensate for possible variations in particle size (148). Also, limiting the use of filtration to situations where it is believed to be necessary has been recommended (598; 599).

Elastomeric Reservoir Pumps— Amphotericin B (Lyphomed) 0.25 mg/ml in dextrose 5% in water was evaluated for binding potential to natural rubber elastomeric reservoirs (Baxter). No loss was found after storage for two weeks at 35 °C with gentle agitation (2014).

Compatibility Information

Solution Compatibility

Amphotericin B

Solution	Mfr	Mfr	Conc/L	Remarks	Ref	C/I
Amino acids 4.25%, dextrose 25%	MG	SQ	100 mg	Turbidity and fine yellow particles form	349	I
Dextrose 5% in Ringer's injection, lactated	MG[a]	SQ	100 mg	Precipitate forms in 30 min. Drug concentration of 43 to 53% of initial amount in 30 min	539	I
Dextrose 5% in sodium chloride 0.2%	BA	SQ	50 mg	Bioactivity not significantly affected over 24 hr at 25 °C with or without exposure to light	353	C

Solution Compatibility (Cont.)

Amphotericin B

Solution	Mfr	Mfr	Conc/L	Remarks	Ref	C/I
Dextrose 5% in sodium chloride 0.9%	MG[a]	SQ	100 mg	Precipitate forms within 2 hr. Drug concentration of 30 to 60% of initial amount in 2 hr	539	**I**
Dextrose 5% in water		SQ	70 and 140 mg	Bioactivity not significantly affected over 24 hr at 25 °C with or without light exposure	335	**C**
	MG[a]	SQ	100 mg	Physically compatible and drug concentration unchanged after 48 hr	539	**C**
		SQ	50 and 100 mg	No loss of bioactivity in normal light at 25 °C for 24 hr	540	**C**
	MG[b]	SQ	0.9, 1.2, 1.4 g	Physically compatible with little or no loss in 36 hr at 6 and 25 °C	1434	**C**
	MG[b]	SQ	470, 660, 750 mg	Visually compatible with no amphotericin B loss by HPLC in 24 hr at 25 °C	1537	**C**
	BA[c]	SQ	100 mg	Visually compatible with no amphotericin B loss by HPLC in 24 hr at 15 to 25 °C	1544	**C**
	BA[c]	SQ	100 and 250 mg	Visually compatible with 4% amphotericin B loss in 35 days at 4 °C in the dark	1546	**C**
	BA[c]	SQ	0.2, 0.5, 1 g	Visually compatible with little or no amphotericin B loss by HPLC in 5 days at 4 and 25 °C. Normal turbidity observed at 1 g/L	1728	**C**
	AB[a]	BMS	50 mg	Visually compatible with no loss by HPLC protected from light and 5% loss exposed to fluorescent light in 24 hr at 24 °C	2093	**C**
	AB[a]	BMS	500 mg	Visually compatible with no loss by HPLC protected from or exposed to fluorescent light in 24 hr at 24 °C	2093	**C**
Dextrose 10% in water	BA[c]	SQ	100 mg	Visually compatible with no amphotericin B loss by HPLC in 24 hr at 15 to 25 °C	1544	**C**
Dextrose 15% in water	BA[c]	SQ	100 mg	Visually compatible with no amphotericin B loss by HPLC in 24 hr at 15 to 25 °C	1544	**C**
Dextrose 20% in water	BA[c]	SQ	100 mg	Visually compatible with no amphotericin B loss by HPLC in 24 hr at 15 to 25 °C	1544	**C**
Fat emulsion 10 and 20%, intravenous	CL	APC, PHT	0.6 g	Precipitate forms immediately but is concealed by opaque emulsion	1808	**I**
Fat emulsion 20%, intravenous			90 mg	Yellow precipitate forms in 2 hr. HPLC found cumulative delivery of only 56% of the total dose	1872	**I**
	CL	APC	10, 50, 100, and 500 mg, 1 and 5 g	Emulsion separation occurred rapidly with visible creaming within 4 hr at 27 and 8 °C	1987	**I**
	KA	SQ	500 mg, 1 and 2 g	Precipitated amphotericin noted on bottom of containers within 4 hr	1988	**I**
	CL[d]	BMS	50 mg	Fat emulsion separates into two phases within 8 hr. No amphotericin B loss by HPLC protected from light and 4% loss exposed to fluorescent light in 24 hr at 24 °C	2093	**I**
	CL[d]	BMS	500 mg	Fat emulsion separates into two phases within 8 hr. No loss by HPLC protected from or exposed to fluorescent light in 24 hr at 24 °C	2093	**I**

Solution Compatibility (Cont.)

Amphotericin B

Solution	Mfr	Mfr	Conc/L	Remarks	Ref	C/I
Ringer's injection, lactated	MG[a]	SQ	100 mg	Precipitate forms within 2 hr. Drug concentration of 72% of initial amount in 2 hr	539	I
Sodium chloride 0.9%	AB	SQ	100 mg	Physically incompatible	15	I
	MG[a]	SQ	100 mg	Precipitate forms within 2 hr. Drug concentration of 43% of initial amount in 2 hr	539	I

[a]Tested in both glass and polyolefin containers.
[b]Tested in polyolefin containers.
[c]Tested in PVC containers.
[d]Tested in glass bottles.

Additive Compatibility

Amphotericin B

Drug	Mfr	Conc/L	Mfr	Conc/L	Test Soln	Remarks	Ref	C/I
Amikacin sulfate	BR	5 g	SQ	100 mg	D5LR, D5R, D5S, D5W, D10W, IS10, LR, NS, R, SL	Immediate precipitate	293	I
Calcium chloride	BP	4 g		200 mg	D5W	Haze develops over 3 hr	26	I
Calcium gluconate	BP	4 g		200 mg	D5W	Haze develops over 3 hr	26	I
Chlorpromazine HCl	BP	200 mg		200 mg	D5W	Immediate precipitate	26	I
Cimetidine HCl	SKF	600 mg	SQ	100 mg	D5W	Immediate haze formation. Precipitate observed at 24 hr at room temperature	551	I
Diphenhydramine HCl	PD	80 mg	SQ	100 mg	D5W	Physically incompatible	15	I
Dopamine HCl	AS	800 mg	SQ	200 mg	D5W	Immediate precipitate	78	I
Edetate calcium disodium	RI	4 g		200 mg	D5W	Haze develops over 3 hr	26	I
Fluconazole	PF	1 g	LY	50 mg	D5W	Visually compatible with no fluconazole loss by HPLC in 72 hr at 25 °C under fluorescent light. Amphotericin B not tested	1677	C
Gentamicin sulfate		320 mg		200 mg	D5W	Haze develops over 3 hr	26	I
Heparin sodium	UP	4000 units	SQ	100 mg	D5W	Physically compatible	15	C
	AB	4000 units	SQ	100 mg	D	Physically compatible	21	C
		2000 units	SQ	70 and 140 mg	D5W	Bioactivity not significantly affected over 24 hr at 25 °C with or without light exposure	335	C
Heparin sodium with hydrocortisone sodium phosphate	AB MSD	1500 units 50 and 100 mg	SQ	50 and 100 mg	D5W	Physically compatible and amphotericin B bioactivity retained in normal light at 25 °C for 24 hr. Hydrocortisone and heparin activity not tested	540	C
Hydrocortisone sodium phosphate	MSD	50 and 100 mg	SQ	50 and 100 mg	D5W	Physically compatible and amphotericin B bioactivity retained in normal light at 25 °C for 24 hr. Hydrocortisone not tested	540	C

Additive Compatibility (Cont.)

Amphotericin B

Drug	Mfr	Conc/L	Mfr	Conc/L	Test Soln	Remarks	Ref	C/I
Hydrocortisone sodium succinate	UP	500 mg	SQ	100 mg	D5W	Physically compatible	15	C
		50 mg	SQ	70 and 140 mg	D5W	Bioactivity not significantly affected over 24 hr at 25 °C with or without light exposure	335	C
Kanamycin sulfate	BPC	4 g		200 mg	D5W	Haze develops over 3 hr	26	I
Magnesium sulfate	IMS	2 and 4 g	SQ	40 and 80 mg	D5W	Physically incompatible in 3 hr at 24 °C with decreased clarity and development of supernatant. Total loss of amphotericin B in supernatant by HPLC	1578	I
Meropenem	ZEN	1 and 20 g	SQ	200 mg	NS	Precipitate forms	2068	I
Metaraminol bitartrate	BP	200 mg		200 mg	D5W	Haze develops over 3 hr	26	I
Methyldopate HCl		1 g		200 mg	D5W	Haze develops over 3 hr	26	I
Penicillin G potassium	SQ	20 million units	SQ	100 mg	D5W	Physically incompatible	15	I
	SQ	5 million units	SQ	50 mg		Precipitate forms within 1 hr	47	I
	BP	10 million units		200 mg	D5W	Haze develops over 3 hr	26	I
Penicillin G sodium	UP	20 million units	SQ	100 mg	D5W	Physically incompatible	15	I
	BP	10 million units		200 mg	D5W	Haze develops over 3 hr	26	I
Polymyxin B sulfate	BP	20 mg		200 mg	D5W	Haze develops over 3 hr	26	I
Potassium chloride	AB	100 mEq	SQ	100 mg	D5W	Physically incompatible	15	I
	BP	4 g		200 mg	D5W	Haze develops over 3 hr	26	I
Prochlorperazine mesylate	BP	100 mg		200 mg	D5W	Haze develops over 3 hr	26	I
Ranitidine HCl	GL	100 mg	SQ	200 mg	D5W	Color change and particle formation	1151	I
Sodium bicarbonate	AB	2.4 mEq[a]	SQ	50 mg	D5W	Physically compatible for 24 hr	772	C
Streptomycin sulfate	BP	4 g		200 mg	D5W	Haze develops over 3 hr	26	I
Verapamil HCl	KN	80 mg	SQ	100 mg	D5W	Physically incompatible after 8 hr	764	I
	KN	80 mg	SQ	100 mg	NS	Immediate physical incompatibility	764	I

[a]One vial of Neut added to a liter of admixture.

Drugs in Syringe Compatibility

Amphotericin B

Drug (in syringe)	Mfr	Amt	Mfr	Amt	Remarks	Ref	C/I
Heparin sodium		2500 units/ 1 ml		50 mg	Physically compatible for at least 5 min	1053	C

Y-Site Injection Compatibility (1:1 Mixture)

Amphotericin B

Drug	Mfr	Conc	Mfr	Conc	Remarks	Ref	C/I
Aldesleukin	CHI	33,800 I.U./ml[a]	SQ	1.6 mg/ml[a]	Visually compatible for 2 hr. Bioassay not possible	1857	C
Allopurinol sodium	BW	3 mg/ml[a]	SQ	0.6 mg/ml[a]	Natural haze of amphotericin B lost immediately	1686	I
Amifostine	AD	0.6 mg/ml[a]	AMR	2.5 mg/ml[a]	Turbidity forms immediately	1845	I
Amsacrine	NCI	1 mg/ml[a]	SQ	0.6 mg/ml[a]	Immediate light yellow turbidity, becoming yellow flocculent precipitate in 15 min	1381	I
Aztreonam	SQ	40 mg/ml[a]	PHT	0.6 mg/ml[a]	Yellow turbidity forms immediately and becomes flocculent precipitate in 4 hr	1758	I
Cefepime HCl	BR	20 mg/ml[a]	SQ	0.6 mg/ml[a]	Heavy yellow flocculent precipitate forms immediately	1689	I
Cefpirome sulfate	HO	50 mg/ml[c]	SQ	0.1 mg/ml[c]	Little or no cefpirome loss but up to 45% amphotericin B loss by HPLC in 4 hr at 23 °C	2044	I
Cisatracurium besylate	GW	0.1 mg/ml[a]	PH	0.6 mg/ml[a]	Physically compatible with no change in measured turbidity or increase in particle content in 4 hr at 23 °C	2074	C
	GW	2 mg/ml[a]	PH	0.6 mg/ml[a]	Cloudiness forms immediately; gel-like precipitate forms in 1 hr	2074	I
	GW	5 mg/ml[a]	PH	0.6 mg/ml[a]	Turbidity forms immediately	2074	I
Diltiazem HCl	MMD	5 mg/ml	SQ	0.1 mg/ml[a]	Visually compatible	1807	C
Docetaxel	RPR	0.9 mg/ml[a]	PH	0.6 mg/ml[a]	Visible turbidity forms immediately	2224	I
Doxorubicin HCl liposome injection	SEQ	0.4 mg/ml[a]	APC	0.6 mg/ml[a]	Fivefold increase in measured particulates in 4 hr	2087	I
Enalaprilat	MSD	1.25 mg/ml	SQ	0.1 mg/ml[a]	Layered haze develops in 4 hr at 21 °C	1409	I
Etoposide phosphate	BR	5 mg/ml[a]	GEN	0.6 mg/ml[a]	Yellow-orange flocculent precipitate forms immediately	2218	I
Filgrastim	AMG	30 μg/ml[a]	SQ	0.6 mg/ml[a]	Yellow turbidity forms immediately and becomes flocculent precipitate	1687	I
Fluconazole	RR	2 mg/ml	SQ	5 mg/ml	Cloudiness and yellow precipitation	1407	I
Fludarabine phosphate	BX	1 mg/ml[a]	SQ	0.6 mg/ml[a]	Small amount of precipitate forms within 4 hr at room temperature	1439	I
Foscarnet sodium	AST	24 mg/ml	SQ	5 mg/ml	Delayed formation of cloudy yellow precipitate	1335	I
	AST	24 mg/ml	SQ	0.6 mg/ml[a]	Dense haze develops immediately	1397	I
Gemcitabine HCl	LI	10 mg/ml[b]	PH	0.6 mg/ml[a]	Gross precipitation occurs immediately	2226	I
Granisetron HCl	SKB	0.05 mg/ml[a]	PH	0.6 mg/ml[a]	Large increase in measured turbidity occurs immediately	2000	I
Melphalan HCl	BW	0.1 mg/ml[b]	SQ	0.6 mg/ml[a]	Immediate two- to fourfold increase in measured turbidity due to sodium chloride	1557	I
	BW	0.1 mg/ml[a]	SQ	0.6 mg/ml[a]	Physically compatible but rapid melphalan loss in D5W precludes use	1557	I
Meropenem	ZEN	1 and 50 mg/ml[b]	SQ	5 mg/ml	Precipitate forms	2068	I

Y-Site Injection Compatibility (1:1 Mixture) (Cont.)

Amphotericin B

Drug	Mfr	Conc	Mfr	Conc	Remarks	Ref	C/I
Ondansetron HCl	GL	1 mg/ml[a]	SQ	0.6 mg/ml[a]	Immediate pale yellow turbidity and precipitation	1365	**I**
Paclitaxel	NCI	1.2 mg/ml[a]	SQ	0.6 mg/ml[a]	Immediate increase in measured turbidity followed by separation into layers in 24 hr at 22 °C	1556	**I**
Piperacillin sodium–tazobactam sodium	LE	40 + 5 mg/ml[a]	SQ	0.6 mg/ml[a]	Heavy yellow flocculent precipitate forms immediately	1688	**I**
Propofol	ZEN	10 mg/ml	APC	0.6 mg/ml[a]	Gel-like precipitate forms immediately	2066	**I**
Remifentanil HCl	GW	0.025 mg/ml[a]	PHT	0.6 mg/ml[a]	Physically compatible with no change in measured turbidity or increase in particle content in 4 hr at 23 °C	2075	**C**
	GW	0.25 mg/ml[a]	PHT	0.6 mg/ml[a]	Yellow precipitate forms immediately	2075	**I**
Sargramostim	IMM	10 μg/ml[a]	SQ	0.6 mg/ml[a]	Physically compatible for 4 hr at 22 °C	1436	**C**
	IMM	10 μg/ml[b]	SQ	0.6 mg/ml[b]	Moderately heavy yellow precipitate forms immediately	1436	**I**
Tacrolimus	FUJ	1 mg/ml[d]	LY	5 mg/ml[a]	Visually compatible for 24 hr at 25 °C	1630	**C**
Teniposide	BR	0.1 mg/ml[a]	SQ	0.6 mg/ml[a]	Physically compatible with no subvisual haze or particle formation in 4 hr at 23 °C	1725	**C**
Thiotepa	IMM[e]	1 mg/ml[a]	APC	0.6 mg/ml[a]	Physically compatible with no change in measured turbidity or increase in particle content in 4 hr at 23 °C	1861	**C**
TNA #218 to #226[g]			PH	0.6 mg/ml[a]	Yellow precipitate forms immediately	2215	**I**
TPN #212 to #215[g]			PH	0.6 mg/ml[a]	Gross flocculent precipitate forms immediately	2109	**I**
Vinorelbine tartrate	BW	1 mg/ml[b]	SQ	0.6 mg/ml[f]	Heavy yellow precipitate forms immediately	1558	**I**
Zidovudine	BW	4 mg/ml[a]	SQ	600 μg/ml[a]	Physically compatible for 4 hr at 25 °C under fluorescent light by visual and microscopic examination	1193	**C**

[a]*Tested in dextrose 5% in water.*
[b]*Tested in sodium chloride 0.9%.*
[c]*Tested in dextrose 5% in water, Ringer's injection, lactated, sodium chloride 0.45%, and sodium chloride 0.9%.*
[d]*Tested in sterile water.*
[e]*Lyophilized formulation tested.*
[f]*Tested in both dextrose 5% in water and sodium chloride 0.9%.*
[g]*Refer to Appendix I for the composition of parenteral nutrition solutions. TNA indicates a 3-in-1 admixture, and TPN indicates a 2-in-1 admixture.*

Additional Compatibility Information

Additives— When 17.5 mg of amphotericin B was added to 125 ml of a 20% mannitol solution and this was further diluted to 1000 ml with dextrose 5% in water for administration by infusion, serum amphotericin B levels were satisfactory during therapy (84; 357).

Amphotericin B in infusions appears to be compatible with limited amounts of heparin sodium (4; 356), hydrocortisone sodium succinate, and methylprednisolone sodium succinate (4). However, amphotericin B is stated to be incompatible with antihistamines and vitamins (40). Local anesthetics such as procaine HCl and lidocaine

HCl cause precipitation of amphotericin B (107). It also is stated to be incompatible with ranitidine HCl (1515).

Fat Emulsion— In an effort to reduce toxicity, amphotericin B has been admixed in Intralipid instead of the more usual dextrose 5% in water (1809–1811; 2178). However, amphotericin B 0.75 mg/kg/day administered using this approach in 250 ml of Intralipid 20% has been associated with acute pulmonary toxicities, including sudden onset of coughing, tachypnea, cyanosis, and deterioration of oxygen saturation following administration. The temporal relationship between the drug administration and respiratory symptoms suggested a causal relationship. Furthermore, no reduction in renal toxicity or other side effects was observed. It was concluded amphotericin B should not be administered in Intralipid (2177).

At a concentration of 0.6 mg/ml in Intralipid 10 or 20%, amphotericin B precipitates immediately or almost immediately. The precipitate is not visible to the unaided eye because of the emulsion's dense opacity. Particle size evaluation found thousands of particles larger than 10 μm per milliliter. In dextrose 5% in water, very few particles were larger than 10 μm. Centrifuging the Intralipid admixtures resulted in rapid visualization of the precipitate as a mass at the bottom of the test tubes (1808).

However, amphotericin B precipitation is observed in fat emulsion within two to four hours without centrifuging. In concentrations ranging from 90 mg to 2 g/L in Intralipid 20%, amphotericin B precipitate is easily seen as yellow particulate matter on the bottom of the lipid emulsion containers (1872; 1988). Damage to the emulsion integrity with creaming has also been reported (1987).

In other reports, the appearance of problems was observed in as little as 15 minutes, and actual amphotericin B precipitate formed within 20 minutes of mixing. Analysis of the precipitate confirmed its identity as amphotericin B. The authors hypothesized that amphotericin B precipitates as a consequence of the excipient deoxycholic acid, which is an anion, attracting oppositely charged choline groups from the egg yolk components of the fat emulsion. As a consequence, deoxycholic acid and phosphatidylcholine form a precipitate and insufficient surfactant remains to keep the amphotericin B dispersed (2204; 2205).

Evacuated Containers— Amphotericin B (Squibb) was reported to be physically incompatible with Abbott evacuated containers. These containers have a small residual amount of fluid composed of acetic acid and sodium acetate buffer. Preparation of amphotericin B in these containers resulted in a precipitate. Similarly, Travenol evacuated containers have a small residual amount of sodium chloride 0.9% solution, which also causes amphotericin B precipitation. McGaw uses only sterile water in its evacuated containers, and they should be satisfactory for preparing amphotericin B admixtures (1232).

Heparin Lock Flush Solution— Amphotericin B (Squibb) 0.1 mg/ml in dextrose 5% in water was combined in equal volumes with heparin lock flush solution (SoloPak) containing heparin sodium 100 units/ml in sodium chloride 0.9%, sodium chloride 0.9%, and sterile water for injection as a control. The heparin lock flush solution and sodium chloride 0.9% behaved identically. At room tem-

perature, the mixtures were clear at 15 minutes, turbid in 30 minutes, and markedly precipitated in four hours. At 37 °C, the process was accelerated, with marked precipitation in 45 minutes. The control solutions remained clear throughout. The authors recommended flushing sodium chloride-containing solutions from venous access devices with dextrose 5% in water before and after amphotericin B administration (1435).

Other Amphotericin B Formulations— Although various lipid complex and liposomal products of amphotericin B exist, they are sufficiently different from conventional amphotericin B formulations that extrapolating compatibility data to the other forms would be inappropriate.

Other Information

Dilution for Infusion— Reconstituted amphotericin B may be added to dextrose 5% in water with a pH above 4.2. Buffers present in the formulation raise the pH of the admixture. If the dextrose 5% in water has a pH less than 4.2, additional buffer must be added (1-10/98; 4). One or 2 ml of a buffer solution with the following composition should be added:

Dibasic sodium phosphate (anhydrous)	1.59 g
Monobasic sodium phosphate (anhydrous)	0.96 g
Water for injection	qs 100 ml

The buffer solution should be sterilized either by filtration or by autoclaving for 30 minutes at 121 °C at 15 pounds pressure (1-10/98). Failure to sterilize this buffer solution coupled with prolonged storage at room temperature has resulted in severe infection (328).

Turbidity may appear in solutions in which the final pH is less than approximately 6 (40; 148). Amphotericin B in dextrose 5% in water retained clarity for three days at pH 5.94 when stored at 5 °C. At pH 5.22, however, turbidity appeared within one day (40). An infusion containing a precipitate or foreign matter should not be used (4).

AMPHOTERICIN B CHOLESTERYL SULFATE COMPLEX
AHFS 8:12.04

Amphotec   **Alza**

Products— Amphotericin B cholesteryl sulfate complex (Alza) is available as a lyophilized powder in 50- and 100-mg vials. The product consists of a 1:1 molar ratio complex of amphotericin B and cholesteryl sulfate along with other components (2). The complete formulations are described in Table 1.

Amphotericin B cholesteryl sulfate complex should be reconstituted with sterile water for injection to form a colloidal dispersion of microscopic, disc-shaped particles. Add 10 ml to the 50-mg vial

Table 1. Amphotericin B Cholesteryl Sulfate Complex Products (2)

Component	50-mg vial	100-mg vial
Amphotericin B	50 mg	100 mg
Sodium cholesteryl sulfate	26.4 mg	52.8 mg
Tromethamine	5.64 mg	11.28 mg
Disodium edetate dihydrate	0.372 mg	0.744 mg
Lactose monohydrate	950 mg	1.9 g
Hydrochloric acid	to adjust pH	to adjust pH

and 20 ml to the 100-mg vial. Shake gently and rotate the vial until all of the solid material has dissolved. Reconstitution as directed yields opalescent or clear colloidal dispersions containing amphotericin B 5 mg/ml (2).

Amphotericin B cholesteryl sulfate complex must not be reconstituted with sodium chloride or dextrose solutions or mixed with solutions containing sodium chloride or other electrolytes. Furthermore, solutions containing a bacteriostatic agent such as benzyl alcohol should be avoided. Use of any solution other than those recommended may cause precipitate formation (2).

Administration— Amphotericin B cholesteryl sulfate complex is administered intravenously only after dilution in dextrose 5% in water to a concentration of 0.16 to 0.83 mg/ml. A test dose of 10 ml of the final admixed solution containing 1.6 to 8.3 mg of drug given over 15 to 30 minutes immediately preceding each new course of treatment is recommended. The patient should be observed for the next 30 minutes. Intravenous infusion of the diluted solution is performed at a rate of 1 mg/kg/hr. The infusion time may be shortened to a minimum of two hours for patients who exhibit no evidence of intolerance or reactions. The infusion time may need to be extended for patients who experience reactions or cannot tolerate the fluid volume (2).

The functional properties of a drug incorporated into a lipid complex like this one may differ substantially from the functional properties of the original formulation and alternative formulations, including other lipid complexes or liposome formulations (2). CAUTION: Care should be taken to ensure that the correct drug product, dose, and administration procedure are used and that no confusion with other products occurs.

Stability— Intact vials of amphotericin B cholesteryl sulfate complex should be stored at 15 to 30 °C. After reconstitution, the colloidal dispersion should be stored at 2 to 8 °C, protected from freezing, and used within 24 hours. Partially used vials should be discarded (2).

The reconstituted colloidal dispersion diluted to a concentration of 0.16 to 0.83 mg/ml in dextrose 5% in water should be stored at 2 to 8 °C and used within 24 hours (2).

Filtration— Amphotericin B cholesteryl sulfate complex is a colloidal dispersion; filtration, including inline filtration, should not be performed (2).

Compatibility Information

Solution Compatibility

Amphotericin B cholesteryl sulfate complex

Solution	Mfr	Mfr	Conc/L	Remarks	Ref	C/I
Dextrose 5% in water	BA	SEQ	415 mg	Physically compatible with little or no change in measured turbidity or increase in particle content in 4 hr at 23 °C under fluorescent light	2117	C
Sodium chloride 0.9%	BA	SEQ	415 mg	Microprecipitation or aggregation occurred immediately	2117	I

Y-Site Injection Compatibility (1:1 Mixture)

Amphotericin B cholesteryl sulfate complex

Drug	Mfr	Conc	Mfr	Conc	Remarks	Ref	C/I
Acyclovir sodium	GW	7 mg/ml[a]	SEQ	0.83 mg/ml[a]	Physically compatible with little or no change in measured turbidity or increase in particle content in 4 hr at 23 °C under fluorescent light	2117	C
Alfentanil HCl	JN	0.5 mg/ml	SEQ	0.83 mg/ml[a]	Gross precipitate forms	2117	I
Amikacin sulfate	AB	5 mg/ml[a]	SEQ	0.83 mg/ml[a]	Gross precipitate forms	2117	I
Aminophylline	AB	2.5 mg/ml[a]	SEQ	0.83 mg/ml[a]	Physically compatible with little or no change in measured turbidity or increase in particle content in 4 hr at 23 °C under fluorescent light	2117	C
Ampicillin sodium	SKB	20 mg/ml[b]	SEQ	0.83 mg/ml[a]	Gross precipitate forms	2117	I
Ampicillin sodium–sulbactam sodium	RR	20 + 10 mg/ml[b]	SEQ	0.83 mg/ml[a]	Gross precipitate forms	2117	I
Atenolol	ZEN	0.5 mg/ml	SEQ	0.83 mg/ml[a]	Gross precipitate forms	2117	I
Aztreonam	SQ	40 mg/ml[a]	SEQ	0.83 mg/ml[a]	Gross precipitate forms	2117	I
Bretylium tosylate	AST	50 mg/ml	SEQ	0.83 mg/ml[a]	Gross precipitate forms	2117	I
Buprenorphine HCl	RKC	0.04 mg/ml[a]	SEQ	0.83 mg/ml[a]	Microprecipitate forms in 4 hr at 23 °C under fluorescent light	2117	I

Y-Site Injection Compatibility (1:1 Mixture) (Cont.)

Amphotericin B cholesteryl sulfate complex

Drug	Mfr	Conc	Mfr	Conc	Remarks	Ref	C/I
Butorphanol tartrate	APC	0.04 mg/ml[a]	SEQ	0.83 mg/ml[a]	Decreased natural turbidity occurs immediately	2117	I
Calcium chloride	AST	40 mg/ml[a]	SEQ	0.83 mg/ml[a]	Gross precipitate forms	2117	I
Calcium gluconate	AB	40 mg/ml[a]	SEQ	0.83 mg/ml[a]	Gross precipitate forms	2117	I
Carboplatin	BR	5 mg/ml[a]	SEQ	0.83 mg/ml[a]	Increased turbidity forms immediately	2117	I
Cefazolin sodium	SKB	20 mg/ml[a]	SEQ	0.83 mg/ml[a]	Increased turbidity forms immediately	2117	I
Cefepime HCl	BMS	20 mg/ml[a]	SEQ	0.83 mg/ml[a]	Gross precipitate forms	2117	I
Cefoperazone sodium	RR	40 mg/ml[a]	SEQ	0.83 mg/ml[a]	Gross precipitate forms	2117	I
Cefoxitin sodium	ME	20 mg/ml[a]	SEQ	0.83 mg/ml[a]	Physically compatible with little or no change in measured turbidity or increase in particle content in 4 hr at 23 °C under fluorescent light	2117	C
Ceftazidime	SKB[c]	40 mg/ml[a]	SEQ	0.83 mg/ml[a]	Increased turbidity forms in 4 hr at 23 °C under fluorescent light	2117	I
	GW[d]	40 mg/ml[a]	SEQ	0.83 mg/ml[a]	Gross precipitate forms	2117	I
Ceftizoxime sodium	FUJ	20 mg/ml[a]	SEQ	0.83 mg/ml[a]	Physically compatible with little or no change in measured turbidity or increase in particle content in 4 hr at 23 °C under fluorescent light	2117	C
Ceftriaxone sodium	RC	20 mg/ml[a]	SEQ	0.83 mg/ml[a]	Decreased natural turbidity occurs immediately	2117	I
Chlorpromazine HCl	ES	2 mg/ml[a]	SEQ	0.83 mg/ml[a]	Gross precipitate forms	2117	I
Cimetidine HCl	AMR	12 mg/ml[a]	SEQ	0.83 mg/ml[a]	Gross precipitate forms	2117	I
Cisatracurium besylate	GW	2 mg/ml[a]	SEQ	0.83 mg/ml[a]	Gross precipitate forms	2117	I
Cisplatin	BR	1 mg/ml	SEQ	0.83 mg/ml[a]	Gross precipitate forms	2117	I
Clindamycin phosphate	UP	10 mg/ml[a]	SEQ	0.83 mg/ml[a]	Physically compatible with little or no change in measured turbidity or increase in particle content in 4 hr at 23 °C under fluorescent light	2117	C
Cyclophosphamide	MJ	10 mg/ml[a]	SEQ	0.83 mg/ml[a]	Increased turbidity forms immediately	2117	I
Cyclosporine	SZ	5 mg/ml[a]	SEQ	0.83 mg/ml[a]	Decreased natural turbidity occurs immediately	2117	I
Cytarabine	BED	50 mg/ml	SEQ	0.83 mg/ml[a]	Gross precipitate forms	2117	I
Dexamethasone sodium phosphate	ES	2 mg/ml[a]	SEQ	0.83 mg/ml[a]	Physically compatible with little or no change in measured turbidity or increase in particle content in 4 hr at 23 °C under fluorescent light	2117	C
Diazepam	SW	5 mg/ml	SEQ	0.83 mg/ml[a]	Gross precipitate forms	2117	I
Digoxin	WY	0.25 mg/ml	SEQ	0.83 mg/ml[a]	Microprecipitate forms in 4 hr at 23 °C under fluorescent light	2117	I
Diphenhydramine HCl	SCN	2 mg/ml[a]	SEQ	0.83 mg/ml[a]	Microprecipitate and increased turbidity form immediately	2117	I
Dobutamine HCl	AST	4 mg/ml[a]	SEQ	0.83 mg/ml[a]	Gross precipitate forms	2117	I
Dopamine HCl	AB	3.2 mg/ml[a]	SEQ	0.83 mg/ml[a]	Gross precipitate forms	2117	I
Doxorubicin HCl	CHI	2 mg/ml	SEQ	0.83 mg/ml[a]	Gross precipitate forms	2117	I

Y-Site Injection Compatibility (1:1 Mixture) (Cont.)

Amphotericin B cholesteryl sulfate complex

Drug	Mfr	Conc	Mfr	Conc	Remarks	Ref	C/I
Doxorubicin HCl liposome injection	SEQ	2 mg/ml	SEQ	0.83 mg/ml[a]	Gross precipitate forms	2117	I
Droperidol	AST	2.5 mg/ml	SEQ	0.83 mg/ml[a]	Gross precipitate forms	2117	I
Enalaprilat	ME	0.1 mg/ml[a]	SEQ	0.83 mg/ml[a]	Decreased natural turbidity occurs immediately	2117	I
Esmolol HCl	OHM	10 mg/ml[a]	SEQ	0.83 mg/ml[a]	Microprecipitate forms in 4 hr at 23 °C under fluorescent light	2117	I
Famotidine	ME	2 mg/ml[a]	SEQ	0.83 mg/ml[a]	Microprecipitate and increased turbidity form immediately	2117	I
Fentanyl citrate	AB	0.05 mg/ml	SEQ	0.83 mg/ml[a]	Physically compatible with little or no change in measured turbidity or increase in particle content in 4 hr at 23 °C under fluorescent light	2117	C
Fluconazole	RR	2 mg/ml	SEQ	0.83 mg/ml[a]	Gross precipitate forms	2117	I
Fluorouracil	PH	16 mg/ml[a]	SEQ	0.83 mg/ml[a]	Microprecipitate forms immediately	2117	I
Furosemide	AMR	3 mg/ml[a]	SEQ	0.83 mg/ml[a]	Physically compatible with little or no change in measured turbidity or increase in particle content in 4 hr at 23 °C under fluorescent light	2117	C
Ganciclovir sodium	RC	20 mg/ml[a]	SEQ	0.83 mg/ml[a]	Physically compatible with little or no change in measured turbidity or increase in particle content in 4 hr at 23 °C under fluorescent light	2117	C
Gentamicin sulfate	FUJ	5 mg/ml[a]	SEQ	0.83 mg/ml[a]	Gross precipitate forms	2117	I
Granisetron HCl	SKB	0.05 mg/ml[a]	SEQ	0.83 mg/ml[a]	Physically compatible with little or no change in measured turbidity or increase in particle content in 4 hr at 23 °C under fluorescent light	2117	C
Haloperidol lactate	MN	0.2 mg/ml[a]	SEQ	0.83 mg/ml[a]	Gross precipitate forms	2117	I
Heparin sodium	WY	1000 units/ml[a]	SEQ	0.83 mg/ml[a]	Gross precipitate forms	2117	I
Hydrocortisone sodium succinate	AB	1 mg/ml[a]	SEQ	0.83 mg/ml[a]	Physically compatible with little or no change in measured turbidity or increase in particle content in 4 hr at 23 °C under fluorescent light	2117	C
Hydromorphone HCl	ES	0.5 mg/ml[a]	SEQ	0.83 mg/ml[a]	Decreased natural turbidity occurs immediately	2117	I
Hydroxyzine HCl	ES	2 mg/ml[a]	SEQ	0.83 mg/ml[a]	Gross precipitate forms	2117	I
Ifosfamide	MJ	25 mg/ml[a]	SEQ	0.83 mg/ml[a]	Physically compatible with little or no change in measured turbidity or increase in particle content in 4 hr at 23 °C under fluorescent light	2117	C
Imipenem–cilastatin sodium	ME	10 mg/ml[b]	SEQ	0.83 mg/ml[a]	Gross precipitate forms	2117	I
Labetalol HCl	AH	5 mg/ml	SEQ	0.83 mg/ml[a]	Gross precipitate forms	2117	I
Leucovorin calcium	IMM	2 mg/ml[a]	SEQ	0.83 mg/ml[a]	Gross precipitate forms	2117	I
Lidocaine HCl	AST	10 mg/ml	SEQ	0.83 mg/ml[a]	Gross precipitate forms	2117	I

Y-Site Injection Compatibility (1:1 Mixture) (Cont.)

Amphotericin B cholesteryl sulfate complex

Drug	Mfr	Conc	Mfr	Conc	Remarks	Ref	C/I
Lorazepam	WY	0.1 mg/ml[a]	SEQ	0.83 mg/ml[a]	Physically compatible with little or no change in measured turbidity or increase in particle content in 4 hr at 23 °C under fluorescent light	2117	C
Magnesium sulfate	AST	100 mg/ml[a]	SEQ	0.83 mg/ml[a]	Gross precipitate forms	2117	I
Mannitol	BA	15%	SEQ	0.83 mg/ml[a]	Physically compatible with little or no change in measured turbidity or increase in particle content in 4 hr at 23 °C under fluorescent light	2117	C
Meperidine HCl	AST	4 mg/ml[a]	SEQ	0.83 mg/ml[a]	Increased turbidity forms immediately	2117	I
Mesna	MJ	10 mg/ml[a]	SEQ	0.83 mg/ml[a]	Microprecipitate forms immediately	2117	I
Methotrexate sodium	IMM	15 mg/ml[a]	SEQ	0.83 mg/ml[a]	Physically compatible with little or no change in measured turbidity or increase in particle content in 4 hr at 23 °C under fluorescent light	2117	C
Methylprednisolone sodium succinate	PHU	5 mg/ml[a]	SEQ	0.83 mg/ml[a]	Physically compatible with little or no change in measured turbidity or increase in particle content in 4 hr at 23 °C under fluorescent light	2117	C
Metoclopramide HCl	FAU	5 mg/ml	SEQ	0.83 mg/ml[a]	Gross precipitate forms	2117	I
Metoprolol tartrate	GEN	1 mg/ml	SEQ	0.83 mg/ml[a]	Gross precipitate forms	2117	I
Metronidazole	AB	5 mg/ml	SEQ	0.83 mg/ml[a]	Gross precipitate forms	2117	I
Midazolam HCl	RC	2 mg/ml[a]	SEQ	0.83 mg/ml[a]	Gross precipitate forms	2117	I
Mitoxantrone HCl	IMM	0.5 mg/ml[a]	SEQ	0.83 mg/ml[a]	Gross precipitate forms	2117	I
Morphine sulfate	ES	1 mg/ml[a]	SEQ	0.83 mg/ml[a]	Increased turbidity forms immediately	2117	I
Nalbuphine HCl	AST	10 mg/ml	SEQ	0.83 mg/ml[a]	Gross precipitate forms	2117	I
Naloxone HCl	AST	0.4 mg/ml	SEQ	0.83 mg/ml[a]	Gross precipitate forms	2117	I
Netilmicin sulfate	SC	5 mg/ml[a]	SEQ	0.83 mg/ml[a]	Gross precipitate forms	2117	I
Nitroglycerin	AMR	0.4 mg/ml[a]	SEQ	0.83 mg/ml[a]	Physically compatible with little or no change in measured turbidity or increase in particle content in 4 hr at 23 °C under fluorescent light	2117	C
Ofloxacin	ORT	4 mg/ml[a]	SEQ	0.83 mg/ml[a]	Gross precipitate forms	2117	I
Ondansetron HCl	CER	1 mg/ml[a]	SEQ	0.83 mg/ml[a]	Gross precipitate forms	2117	I
Paclitaxel	MJ	0.6 mg/ml[a]	SEQ	0.83 mg/ml[a]	Decreased natural turbidity occurs immediately	2117	I
Pentobarbital sodium	AB	5 mg/ml[a]	SEQ	0.83 mg/ml[a]	Decreased natural turbidity occurs immediately	2117	I
Phenobarbital sodium	WY	5 mg/ml[a]	SEQ	0.83 mg/ml[a]	Increased turbidity forms immediately	2117	I
Phenytoin sodium	ES	50 mg/ml[a]	SEQ	0.83 mg/ml[a]	Gross precipitate forms	2117	I
Piperacillin sodium	LE	40 mg/ml[a]	SEQ	0.83 mg/ml[a]	Microprecipitate forms in 4 hr at 23 °C under fluorescent light	2117	I
Piperacillin sodium–tazobactam sodium	CY	40 + 5 mg/ml[a]	SEQ	0.83 mg/ml[a]	Microprecipitate forms immediately	2117	I
Potassium chloride	AB	0.1 mEq/ml[a]	SEQ	0.83 mg/ml[a]	Gross precipitate forms	2117	I

Y-Site Injection Compatibility (1:1 Mixture) (Cont.)

Amphotericin B cholesteryl sulfate complex

Drug	Mfr	Conc	Mfr	Conc	Remarks	Ref	C/I
Prochlorperazine edisylate	SKB	0.5 mg/ml[a]	SEQ	0.83 mg/ml[a]	Gross precipitate forms	2117	I
Promethazine HCl	ES	2 mg/ml[a]	SEQ	0.83 mg/ml[a]	Gross precipitate forms	2117	I
Propranolol HCl	WY	1 mg/ml	SEQ	0.83 mg/ml[a]	Gross precipitate forms	2117	I
Ranitidine HCl	GL	2 mg/ml[a]	SEQ	0.83 mg/ml[a]	Microprecipitate and increased turbidity form immediately	2117	I
Remifentanil HCl	GW	0.5 mg/ml[a]	SEQ	0.83 mg/ml[a]	Gross precipitate forms	2117	I
Sodium bicarbonate	AB	1 mEq/ml	SEQ	0.83 mg/ml[a]	Gross precipitate forms	2117	I
Sufentanil citrate	JN	0.05 mg/ml	SEQ	0.83 mg/ml[a]	Physically compatible with little or no change in measured turbidity or increase in particle content in 4 hr at 23 °C under fluorescent light	2117	C
Ticarcillin disodium	SKB	30 mg/ml[a]	SEQ	0.83 mg/ml[a]	Microprecipitate forms immediately	2117	I
Ticarcillin disodium–clavulanate potassium	SKB	31 mg/ml[a]	SEQ	0.83 mg/ml[a]	Gross precipitate forms	2117	I
Tobramycin sulfate	AB	5 mg/ml[a]	SEQ	0.83 mg/ml[a]	Gross precipitate forms	2117	I
Trimethoprim–sulfamethoxazole	ES	0.8 + 4 mg/ml[a]	SEQ	0.83 mg/ml[a]	Physically compatible with little or no change in measured turbidity or increase in particle content in 4 hr at 23 °C under fluorescent light	2117	C
Vancomycin HCl	AB	10 mg/ml[a]	SEQ	0.83 mg/ml[a]	Gross precipitate forms	2117	I
Vecuronium bromide	MAR	1 mg/ml[a]	SEQ	0.83 mg/ml[a]	Gross precipitate forms	2117	I
Verapamil HCl	AMR	2.5 mg/ml	SEQ	0.83 mg/ml[a]	Gross precipitate forms	2117	I
Vinblastine sulfate	FAU	0.12 mg/ml[a]	SEQ	0.83 mg/ml[a]	Physically compatible with little or no change in measured turbidity or increase in particle content in 4 hr at 23 °C under fluorescent light	2117	C
Vincristine sulfate	FAU	0.05 mg/ml[a]	SEQ	0.83 mg/ml[a]	Physically compatible with little or no change in measured turbidity or increase in particle content in 4 hr at 23 °C under fluorescent light	2117	C
Vinorelbine tartrate	BW	1 mg/ml[a]	SEQ	0.83 mg/ml[a]	Gross precipitate forms	2117	I
Zidovudine	BW	4 mg/ml[a]	SEQ	0.83 mg/ml[a]	Physically compatible with little or no change in measured turbidity or increase in particle content in 4 hr at 23 °C under fluorescent light	2117	C

[a]*Tested in dextrose 5% in water.*
[b]*Tested in sodium chloride 0.9%.*
[c]*Sodium carbonate–containing formulation tested.*
[d]*L-Arginine–containing formulation tested.*

Additional Compatibility Information

Solutions— Amphotericin B cholesteryl sulfate complex should be reconstituted with sterile water for injection. (See Products section above.) Sodium chloride and dextrose solutions as well as solutions containing a preservative such as benzyl alcohol must not be used, because of the potential for precipitation. The reconstituted drug should be diluted in dextrose 5% in water to a concentration of 0.16 to 0.83 mg/ml for administration. Sodium chloride or other electrolyte solutions must not be used for this dilution to avoid possible precipitate formation (2).

Other Drugs— The manufacturer also recommends not mixing amphotericin B cholesteryl sulfate complex with other drug products and separating administration from other drugs given through existing intravenous lines by using a sufficient flush of the line with dextrose 5% in water to avoid contact with the other drugs (2). Flushes both before and after administering amphotericin B cholesteryl sulfate complex would be required to avoid inadvertent mixing with other drugs in line. Given the high number of incompatibilities that have been documented with amphotericin B cholesteryl sulfate complex (2117), care should be taken to avoid inadvertent contact with incompatible drugs in administration lines.

Other Amphotericin B Products— Although other lipid complex and liposomal amphotericin B products exist, they are sufficiently different from amphotericin B cholesteryl sulfate complex that extrapolating compatibility data to other forms would be inappropriate.

AMPICILLIN SODIUM
AHFS 8:12.16

Apothecon

Products— Ampicillin sodium is available in vials containing the equivalent of ampicillin 125 mg, 250 mg, 500 mg, 1 g, or 2 g. For intramuscular injection, reconstitute the vials with sterile water for injection or bacteriostatic water for injection in the following amounts (4; 154):

Vial Size	Volume of Diluent	Withdrawable Volume	Concentration
125 mg	1.2 ml	1 ml	125 mg/ml
250 mg	1.0 ml	1 ml	250 mg/ml
500 mg	1.8 ml	2 ml	250 mg/ml
1 g	3.5 ml	4 ml	250 mg/ml
2 g	6.8 ml	8 ml	250 mg/ml

For intravenous injection, reconstitute the 125-, 250-, and 500-mg vials with 5 ml of sterile water for injection or bacteriostatic water for injection. For the 1- or 2-g vials, 10 ml of sterile water for injection or bacteriostatic water for injection is recommended (1-6/17/94).

pH— Reconstituted solutions of ampicillin sodium have a pH of 8 to 10 (4). The pH values of various ampicillin sodium solutions are shown below (213):

Percent Ampicillin Sodium	Diluent	Initial pH
2	Sterile water	8.80
5	Sterile water	8.92
10	Sterile water	9.15
2	Sodium chloride 0.9%	8.7
5	Sodium chloride 0.9%	8.9
10	Sodium chloride 0.9%	9.2
2	Dextrose 5% in water	8.9
5	Dextrose 5% in water	9.3
10	Dextrose 5% in water	9.3

Osmolality— Reconstituted with sterile water for injection, ampicillin sodium (Wyeth) 100 mg/ml has an osmolality of 602 mOsm/kg (50). At 125 mg/ml, Wyeth's product was 702 mOsm/kg and Bristol's product was 675 mOsm/kg (1071).

In another study, the osmolality of ampicillin sodium (Bristol) diluted in sodium chloride 0.9% was determined to be 493 mOsm/kg at 50 mg/ml and 664 mOsm/kg at 100 mg/ml (1375).

The osmolality of ampicillin sodium 1 and 2 g was calculated for the following dilutions (1054):

Diluent	Osmolality (mOsm/kg)	
	50 ml	100 ml
1 g		
Dextrose 5% in water	341	302
Sodium chloride 0.9%	368	328
2 g		
Dextrose 5% in water	418	346
Sodium chloride 0.9%	444	372

Robinson et al. recommended the following maximum ampicillin sodium concentrations to achieve osmolalities suitable for peripheral infusion in fluid-restricted patients (1180):

Diluent	Maximum Concentration (mg/ml)	Osmolality (mOsm/kg)
Dextrose 5% in water	62	583
Sodium chloride 0.9%	56	576
Sterile water for injection	112	588

Sodium Content— Ampicillin sodium contains approximately 2.9 to 3.1 mEq of sodium per gram of drug (4).

Administration— Ampicillin sodium is administered by intramuscular or direct intravenous injection or intravenous infusion. Direct intravenous injection should be made slowly over 10 to 15 minutes (4; 154).

Stability— The stability of ampicillin sodium in solution under various conditions has been the subject of much work and numerous articles. Several characteristics of the stability of ampicillin sodium have emerged from these studies:

1. The stability is concentration dependent and decreases as the concentration increases.
2. Sodium chloride 0.9% appears to be a suitable diluent for the intravenous infusion of ampicillin sodium.
3. The stability is greatly decreased in dextrose solutions.
4. Storage temperature and the pH of solution affect the stability.

Concentration Effects— The effect of concentration on ampicillin sodium stability has been attributed to a self-catalyzing effect (210). As the concentration increases, so does the rate of decomposition (170; 210). Savello and Shangraw reported that, even though the initial pH values of various concentrations were 9.2 to 9.3, the higher concentrations of the drug maintained their pH longer because of their greater buffer capacity. This fact, along with greater probability of collision, helps explain the higher degradation rates at higher concentrations (210). (See Table 1.)

This concentration dependence of the stability of ampicillin sodium has been related to the polymerization of penicillins in concentrated solutions (601; 602). Dimerization is the predominant form of degradation with high ampicillin concentrations. The extent of this effect declines as the concentration drops but still remains significant in a 2% solution. At lower concentrations, hydrolysis becomes the determining factor (603).

In a 50% concentration, ampicillin sodium formed dimer, trimer, tetramer, and pentamer during 24 hours of storage at 24 °C in the dark. The polymer formed through a chain process by linkage of the amino group on the side chain to another molecule with a cleaved β-lactam ring (1400).

In a 20% ampicillin sodium aqueous solution adjusted to pH 8.5 and stored at 22 °C, 90% of all decomposition products formed within 72 hours were di- and polymers. In a 5% solution, 70% of the decomposition products were di- and polymers. However, a 1% solution formed α-aminobenzylpenicilloic acid as the predominant decomposition product and a dimer concentration of 1 to 2%. The rate of dimerization was almost independent of pH in the range of 7 to 10 but increased strongly with increases in the initial ampicillin sodium concentration (858).

However, one study showed that if the pH of the solution was held constant at 8 or 9.15, there was little dependence of the rate of

Table 1. Percent Degradation of Ampicillin Sodium Solutions after Reconstitution with Water for Injection at 5 °C after Eight Hours (210)

Percent Concentration	Percent Degradation
1	0.8
5	3.6
10	5.8
15	10.4
20	12.3
25	13.3

Table 2. Percent Degradation of 1% Ampicillin Sodium in Sodium Chloride 0.9% According to Temperature and Time (210)

Temperature (°C)	4 hr	8 hr	24 hr
−20	1.2	1.8	3.6
0	0.4	0.8	0.9
5	1.0	2.2	3.3
27	1.8	2.6	8.3

Table 3. Percent Degradation of 1% Ampicillin Sodium in Dextrose 5% in Water According to Temperature and Time (210)

Temperature (°C)	4 hr	8 hr	24 hr
−20	13.6	22.3	45.6
0	6.2	11.6	26.3
5	10.1	15.2	29.7
27	21.3	31.1	46.5

decomposition on concentration in the concentration range of 2 to 10% (213).

Infusion Diluents— Infusion diluents also affect the stability of ampicillin sodium. Although one report stated that there was no loss of ampicillin potency in a solution of ampicillin sodium 5 g/L in sodium chloride 0.9% in 14 days at 25 °C (144), the use of more accurate test methods has determined that this is not the case. For example, see the results of Savello and Shangraw in Table 2.

The work of Hiranaka et al. tends to support this result. In the concentration range of 5 to 40 g/L in sodium chloride 0.9%, approximately 1 to 6% loss of potency of ampicillin sodium was reported at 5 °C in 24 hours, and 6 to 15% was found at 25 °C in 24 hours (212).

Warren et al. reported similar results for ampicillin sodium 20 g/L in sodium chloride 0.9%. They noted approximately 3 to 4% decomposition at 5 °C and 12 to 18% at 25 °C in 24 hours (208).

Stjernstrom et al. found that ampicillin sodium 2 to 15 g/L in sodium chloride 0.9% exhibited 10% decomposition in time periods varying from over 48 hours in the more dilute solution to 33 hours in the more concentrated solutions when stored at 25 °C (604).

Dextrose is thought to exhibit an immense catalytic effect on the hydrolysis of ampicillin sodium (210), decreasing the stability about one-half when compared to sterile water or sodium chloride 0.9% (213). This has been well documented and has been regarded as an incompatibility (210; 213). (See Table 3.) This accelerated decomposition associated with dextrose extends to fructose as well, although it is not as extensive. It occurs in the alkaline pH range. Below pH 6 or 7, the decomposition rate with both dextrose and fructose appears to coincide with simple aqueous solutions (604).

Once again, other reports support these data. Hiranaka et al. found a 35 to 44% loss of ampicillin sodium in 24 hours at 25 °C in the

Table 4. Percent Degradation of 1% Ampicillin Sodium at 5 °C According to Dextrose Concentration and Time (210)

Percent Dextrose	3 hr	7 hr
5	7.4	13.9
10	10.3	19.4
20	14.2	27.8

Table 5. Percent Degradation of Ampicillin Sodium in the Reconstituted Vial (250 mg/ml) According to Temperature and Time (210)

Temperature (°C)	4 hr	8 hr	24 hr	48 hr
−20	2.2	2.8	5.0	8.4
−12	4.2	5.7	10.9	
0	5.8	10.4	21.9	
5	7.1	13.3	26.6	
27	11.2[a]			

[a]*Determined after two hours.*

Table 6. Percent Degradation of 1% Ampicillin Sodium in Water According to Temperature and Time (210)

Temperature (°C)	4 hr	8 hr	24 hr
−20	1.3	1.9	5.2
5	0.4	0.8	2.0

concentration range of 5 to 40 g/L in dextrose 5% in water. At 5 °C, the loss was reported to be 19 to 28% (212).

Warren et al., testing a concentration of 20 g/L in dextrose 5% in water, reported approximately 40% decomposition in 24 hours at 25 °C and up to 11% decomposition at 5 °C in 24 hours (208).

Stjernstrom et al. found that ampicillin sodium 2 to 15 g/L in dextrose 5% in water exhibited 10% decomposition at three and a half hours in the more dilute solutions and at two hours in the more concentrated solution when stored at 25 °C (604).

Savello and Shangraw further showed that increasing the concentration of dextrose decreased the stability of ampicillin sodium. (See Table 4.)

Stjernstrom et al. found that increasing the dextrose concentration from 5 to 10% increased the rate of ampicillin decomposition by a factor of about two (604).

Temperature Effects— The storage temperature of ampicillin sodium solutions may also affect stability. It has been stated that freezing ampicillin sodium solutions at −20 °C increases the rate of decomposition over that at 5 °C. For this reason, it has been recommended that ampicillin sodium solutions not be stored in the frozen state (123; 213).

However, Lynn noted a 20% loss of potency in six hours when 500 mg of ampicillin sodium reconstituted with 1.5 ml of water was stored at 5 °C. When stored at −20 °C, a 10% loss in 20 hours was noted (99). Further, Savello and Shangraw reported the results in Table 5 for the temperature dependence of the stability of vials of ampicillin sodium reconstituted with sterile distilled water.

Salvello and Shangraw found apparent increased ampicillin decomposition at −20 °C over that at 5 °C in two of the 1% solutions they tested (Tables 3 and 6). Warren et al. also noted this effect in their study of ampicillin sodium 2%, finding about 4 to 6% greater loss at −20 °C than at 5 °C in 24 hours in both dextrose 5% in water and sodium chloride 0.9% (208).

An explanation of this phenomenon was proposed by Pincock and Kiovsky. Below the freezing point but above the eutectic tempera-

ture, there exists a liquid and solid phase in equilibrium. If it is assumed that −20 °C is above the eutectic temperature, then liquid regions of a saturated solution of ampicillin sodium exist, which result in increased decomposition (214). Solutions of ampicillin sodium stored at −78 °C showed no decomposition within 24 hours (210).

In a study of long-term storage, Dinel et al. tested ampicillin sodium (Ayerst) 1 g/50 ml in dextrose 5% in water and also sodium chloride 0.9% in PVC containers frozen at −20 °C for 30 days. In sodium chloride 0.9%, they reported approximately 10% decomposition in one day and approximately 70% decomposition in 30 days. In dextrose 5% in water, even greater decomposition occurred. They reported about 50% decomposition in one day and virtually total decomposition in 30 days (299).

Holmes et al. tested ampicillin sodium (Wyeth) 1 g/50 ml of dextrose 5% in water in PVC bags frozen at −20 °C for 30 days and then thawed by exposure to ambient temperature or microwave radiation. The admixtures showed essentially total loss of ampicillin activity determined microbiologically (554). At −30 °C, only 18% of the ampicillin remained in 30 days. A storage temperature of −70 °C was required to retain at least 90% of the original activity for 30 days (555).

The same concentration in sodium chloride 0.9% showed a 29% loss of ampicillin activity at −20 °C but only about a 4% loss at −30 and −70 °C after 30 days. Subsequent thawing of the −30 and −70 °C samples by exposure to microwave radiation and storage at room temperature for eight hours resulted in additional losses of activity, with the final concentration totaling about 90% of the initial amount. The authors concluded that ampicillin sodium in sodium chloride 0.9% could be stored for 30 days at −30 °C, which was presumably below the eutectic point for this admixture. However, −30 °C was believed to be above the eutectic point for the dextrose 5% in water admixture because decomposition continued to occur (555).

Ampicillin sodium (Wyeth) 1 g/50 ml of sodium chloride 0.9% exhibited a 13% loss (by HPLC) in four days at −7 °C but only a 10% loss in the same time period at 4 °C (1035).

Even within acceptable limits for room temperature, significant differences in the rate of ampicillin decomposition can occur. In one solution at 20 °C, a 10% ampicillin loss resulted in 44 hours. This same solution at 30 °C exhibited a 10% loss in 12 hours. Over the range of 20 to 35 °C, each 5 °C rise approximately doubled the rate of decomposition (604).

pH Effects— The pH of the solution also plays a role in its stability. Hydrolysis has been shown to be catalyzed by hydroxide ion. An increase of 1 pH unit in an ampicillin sodium solution has been shown to increase the rate of decomposition 10-fold (213).

The optimum pH for ampicillin sodium stability has been variously reported as 5.8 (1072), 5.85 at 35 °C (215), approximately 5.2 at 25 °C (604), and 7.5 at room temperature (209). The pH of ampicillin sodium solutions, however, is in the alkaline range, with higher pH values having been reported at higher concentrations (213). (See the pH section above.)

Ampicillin sodium (Bristol) 10 g/L was tested for stability at pH 3.4 to 9.2 in various buffer additives. A 7.6% potency loss was reported in 12 hours at room temperature at pH 7.5. Significantly higher degradation rates occurred as the pH varied from 7.5, with about 70% degradation occurring in 12 hours at room temperature at pH 3.4 and 9.2 (209).

In another evaluation, rate constants for ampicillin degradation at various pH values were calculated for an aqueous solution at 25 °C.

Table 7. Suggested Storage Conditions for Ampicillin Sodium Solutions (210)

Solution	Temperature (°C)	Maximum Storage
Constituted vial	−20	48 hr
	5	4 hr
	27	1 hr
Ampicillin sodium 1% in sodium chloride 0.9%	5	5 days
	27	24 hr
Ampicillin sodium 1% in dextrose 5% in water	5	4 hr
	27	2 hr

Table 8. Recommended Maximum Concentrations and Usage Times in Intravenous Solutions (154)

Solution	Concentration	Temperature (°C)	Stability Period
Dextrose 5% in sodium chloride 0.45%	up to 2 mg/ml	25	4 hr
	up to 10 mg/ml	4	4 hr
Dextrose 5% in water	up to 20 mg/ml	25	2 hr
	up to 20 mg/ml	4	4 hr
Invert sugar 10% in water	up to 2 mg/ml	25	4 hr
	up to 20 mg/ml	4	3 hr
Ringer's injection, lactated	up to 30 mg/ml	25	8 hr
	up to 30 mg/ml	4	24 hr
Sodium chloride 0.9%	up to 30 mg/ml	25	8 hr
	up to 20 mg/ml	4	72 hr
	30 mg/ml	4	48 hr
Sodium lactate ⅙ M	up to 30 mg/ml	25	8 hr
	up to 30 mg/ml	4	8 hr
Sterile water for injection	up to 30 mg/ml	25	8 hr
	up to 20 mg/ml	4	72 hr
	30 mg/ml	4	48 hr

The pH providing maximum stability was 5.2. When tested in dextrose 10% in water, a minimum rate of decomposition was observed at approximately pH 5 to 5.5. The amount of ampicillin degradation was 10% or less in 24 hours at 25 °C within a pH range of about 2.75 to 6.75. At pH 8, the time to 10% decomposition was only about two hours (604).

The stability of ampicillin sodium (Beecham) 250 mg/50 ml and 1 g/100 ml in sodium chloride 0.9% in PVC bags was compared to the stability of the same solutions buffered with potassium acid phosphate 13.6% injection. The 50- and 100-ml containers were buffered with 1 and 2 ml, respectively, lowering the pH by nearly two pH units. Larger quantities of buffer caused precipitation. When stored at 5 °C, the 250-mg/50-ml solution had a shelf life (t_{90}) of 12 days while the 1-g/100-ml solution had a shelf life of six days. This finding compares favorably to the shelf life of one to two days for the unbuffered solutions (1820).

Storage and Usage Times— Savello and Shangraw offered the recommendations in Table 7 regarding storage conditions for ampicillin sodium solutions.

For ampicillin sodium (Apothecon), the manufacturer recommends using only freshly prepared solutions within one hour of reconstitution. In intravenous solutions, the maximum concentrations and stability periods in Table 8 have been recommended to ensure that not more than 10% ampicillin decomposition will result at the temperature specified.

Portable Pumps— Stiles et al. evaluated the stability of ampicillin

sodium (Wyeth) 60 mg/ml in sterile water for injection and sodium chloride 0.9% in 100-ml portable pump reservoirs (Pharmacia Deltec) during simulated administration for 24 hours. The drug solutions were tested by HPLC analysis when administered immediately after preparation and after storage for 24 hours at 5 °C before 24-hour administration. During simulated administration, some reservoirs were kept at 30 °C; others were placed in insulated pouches with frozen (−20 °C) gel packs to keep them chilled below the ambient temperature. All ampicillin sodium solutions, whether freshly prepared or after storage, exhibited little or no potency loss. However, solutions not chilled in the insulated pouches during administration exhibited about a 10% loss in six hours and a 20 to 27% loss in 24 hours. To complete the infusions with adequate drug stability, chilling of the drug reservoirs was necessary; the insulated pouches enhanced stability substantially during the study period (1779).

Elastomeric Reservoir Pumps— Ampicillin sodium (Apothecon) 20 mg/ml in sodium chloride 0.9% 100 ml was packaged in latex elastomeric reservoirs (Secure Medical). About 4% loss by HPLC analysis occurred in eight hours at 25 °C and 7% loss in three days at 5 °C (1970).

Syringes— Ampicillin sodium (Berk) 125 mg/ml in sterile water for injection was packaged as 0.25 ml in 1-ml syringes (Injekt, Braun) and sealed with blind hubs. When the syringes were stored at about 6 °C, approximately 36% of the antibiotic activity against *Micrococcus luteus* was lost in two days (1697).

Sorption— Ampicillin (as the trihydrate) 1.4 g/L in sodium chloride 0.9% (Travenol) in PVC bags did not exhibit significant sorption to the plastic during one week of storage at room temperature (15 to 20 °C) (536).

Ampicillin sodium (Beecham) 1.4 g/L in sodium chloride 0.9% did not exhibit any loss due to sorption during a seven-hour simulated infusion through an infusion set (Travenol) consisting of a cellulose propionate burette chamber and 170 cm of PVC tubing (606).

The drug was also tested as a simulated infusion over at least one hour by a syringe pump system. A glass syringe on a syringe pump was fitted with 20 cm of polyethylene tubing or 50 cm of Silastic tubing. No loss of drug due to sorption was observed with either tubing (606).

A 25-ml aliquot of ampicillin sodium (Beecham) 1.4 g/L in sodium chloride 0.9% was stored in all-plastic syringes composed of polypropylene barrels and polyethylene plungers for 24 hours at room temperature in the dark. No loss due to sorption occurred (606).

Picard et al. reported little or no loss due to sorption of ampicillin sodium (Bristol) 250 mg/100 ml in dextrose 5% in water and sodium chloride 0.9% in trilayer solution bags (Bieffe Medital) composed of polyethylene, polyamide, and polypropylene. The admixtures were evaluated by HPLC analysis up to two hours after preparation. Similarly, no loss was found during one-hour simulated infusion (1918).

Filtration— Filtration of ampicillin sodium (Wyeth) is stated to result in no adsorption, yielding solutions that maintain their potency (829).

Ampicillin sodium (Bristol) 1.97 mg/ml in sodium chloride 0.9% was filtered through a 0.22-μm cellulose ester membrane filter (Ivex-HP, Millipore) over five hours. No significant drug loss due to binding to the filter was noted (1034).

Compatibility Information

Solution Compatibility

Ampicillin sodium

Solution	Mfr	Mfr	Conc/L	Remarks	Ref	C/I
Amino acids 4.25%, dextrose 25%	MG	BR	1 g	Increase in microscopic particles noted in 24 hr at 5 °C	349	I
Dextran 40 10% in sodium chloride 0.9%	PH	AY	8 g	25% ampicillin decomposition in 24 hr at room temperature	99	I
	PH	BY	2 g	10% ampicillin decomposition in 2.8 hr at 25 °C	604	I
	PH	BY	5 g	10% ampicillin decomposition in 2.5 hr at 25 °C	604	I
	PH	BY	15 g	10% ampicillin decomposition in 2.3 hr at 25 °C	604	I
Dextran 40 10% in dextrose 5% in water	PH	AY	8 g	50% ampicillin decomposition in 24 hr at room temperature	99	I
	PH	BY	2 g	10% ampicillin decomposition in 3.5 hr at 25 °C	604	I
	PH	BY	5 g	10% ampicillin decomposition in 2.3 hr at 25 °C	604	I
	PH	BY	15 g	10% ampicillin decomposition in 1.5 hr at 25 °C	604	I
			4 g	46% ampicillin decomposition in 24 hr at 20 °C	834	I
Dextran 70 6% in sodium chloride 0.9%	PH	BY	2 g	10% ampicillin decomposition in 6.5 hr at 25 °C	604	I
	PH	BY	5 g	10% ampicillin decomposition in 4.3 hr at 25 °C	604	I
	PH	BY	15 g	10% ampicillin decomposition in 3.3 hr at 25 °C	604	I
Dextran 70 6% in dextrose 5% in water	PH	BY	2 g	10% ampicillin decomposition in 3.5 hr at 25 °C	604	I
	PH	BY	5 g	10% ampicillin decomposition in 2.5 hr at 25 °C	604	I
	PH	BY	15 g	10% ampicillin decomposition in 1.8 hr at 25 °C	604	I
			4 g	10% ampicillin decomposition in 6 hr and 40% decomposition in 24 hr at 20 °C	834	I
Dextrose 5% in sodium chloride 0.9%	MG	BR	1 g	19% ampicillin decomposition in 4 hr at 4 °C and 17% decomposition in 2 hr at 25 °C	105	I
Dextrose 5% in water		BE	1 g	24% ampicillin decomposition in 8 hr at 25 °C	211	I
		AY	2 and 4 g	10% ampicillin decomposition in 4 hr at room temperature	99	I
	MG	BR	1 g	11% ampicillin decomposition in 24 hr at 4 °C and 21% decomposition in 24 hr at 25 °C	105	I
	AB	AY	2 g	10% ampicillin decomposition in 24 hr at 5 °C and 20% decomposition in 24 hr at 25 °C	88	I
		BR	20 g	As much as 19% ampicillin decomposition in 4 hr at 25 °C. Approximately 40% decomposition in 24 hr at 25 °C	208	I
		BR	10 g	Approximately 46% ampicillin decomposition in 24 hr at −20 °C. Approximately 30% ampicillin decomposition in 24 hr at 5 °C. Approximately 47% ampicillin decomposition in 24 hr at 27 °C	210	I
	BA[a], TR	AY	20 g	40% decomposition in 24 hr at 22 °C and 30% decomposition in 24 hr at 5 °C	298	I

Solution Compatibility (Cont.)

Ampicillin sodium

Solution	Mfr	Mfr	Conc/L	Remarks	Ref	C/I
			2 g	5% decomposition in 2 hr and 38% decomposition in 24 hr at 20 to 25 °C	307	I
			4 g	10% decomposition in 2 hr and 45% decomposition in 24 hr at 20 to 25 °C	307	I
			10 g	12% decomposition in 2 hr and 50% decomposition in 24 hr at 20 to 25 °C	307	I
	TR[b]	WY	20 g	Ampicillin activity loss of 35% in 8 hr and 52% in 24 hr at room temperature	554	I
	PH	BY	2 g	10% ampicillin decomposition in 3.5 hr at 25 °C	604	I
	PH	BY	5 g	10% ampicillin decomposition in 2.5 hr at 25 °C	604	I
	PH	BY	15 g	10% ampicillin decomposition in 2 hr at 25 °C	604	I
			4 g	10% loss in 4 hr and 28% loss in 24 hr at room temperature	768	I
			5 g	7% loss in 2 hr and 15% loss in 4 hr at 29 °C. 8% loss in 8 hr at 4 °C	773	I
	TR[b]	WY	10 and 20 g	Approximately 60% ampicillin loss in 48 hr at 25 °C and in 7 days at 4 °C	1001	I
	TR[b]	WY	20 g	50% ampicillin loss at 24 °C and 28% at 4 °C in 1 day	1035	I
	[b]	BR	20 g	No drug loss by HPLC during 2 hr storage and 1-hr simulated infusion	1774	C
Dextrose 10% in water	MG	BR	1 g	17% ampicillin decomposition in 6 hr at 4 °C and 18% decomposition in 4 hr at 25 °C	105	I
Fat emulsion 10%, intravenous			20 g	15% ampicillin decomposition in 24 hr at 23 °C. Potency was retained through 6 hr	37	I
	VT	BE	2 g	Microscopic globule coalescence in 24 hr at 25 and 8 °C	825	I
Fructose 5.25%		BE	20 g	21% ampicillin decomposition in 6 hr at 25 °C	89	I
Hetastarch 6%			4 g	18% ampicillin decomposition in 6 hr and 35% decomposition in 24 hr at 20 °C	834	I
Invert sugar 7.5% with electrolytes		AST	1.5 g	52% ampicillin loss in 24 hr at 29 °C by microbiological assay	440	I
Invert sugar 10% in water		BY	2 g	10% ampicillin decomposition in 4 hr at 25 °C	604	I
		BY	5 g	10% ampicillin decomposition in 2.8 hr at 25 °C	604	I
		BY	15 g	10% ampicillin decomposition in 1.5 hr at 25 °C	604	I
Isolyte M with dextrose 5%	MG	BR	1 g	Potency retained for 24 hr at 4 and 25 °C	105	C
Isolyte P with dextrose 5%	MG	BR	1 g	Potency retained for 24 hr at 4 and 25 °C	105	C
Ringer's injection		AY	2 and 4 g	Less than 10% decomposition in 24 hr at room temperature	99	C
		BY	2 g	10% ampicillin decomposition in 40 hr at 25 °C	604	C
		BY	5 g	10% ampicillin decomposition in 25 hr at 25 °C	604	C
		BY	15 g	10% ampicillin decomposition in 20 hr at 25 °C	604	I
			5 g	9% loss in 8 hr and 18% loss in 24 hr at 29 °C. 3% loss in 24 hr at 4 °C	773	I
Ringer's injection, lactated		BE	1 g	17% ampicillin decomposition in 4 hr at 25 °C	211	I
		BR	1 g	14% ampicillin decomposition in 12 hr at 25 °C	87	I

Solution Compatibility (Cont.)

Ampicillin sodium

Solution	Mfr	Mfr	Conc/L	Remarks	Ref	C/I
	MG	BR	1 g	17% ampicillin decomposition in 6 hr at 4 °C and 25% decomposition in 6 hr at 25 °C	105	I
			5 g	20% loss in 2 hr at 29 °C and 11% loss in 4 hr at 4 °C	773	I
Sodium bicarbonate 1.4%		AY	2 and 4 g	10% ampicillin decomposition in 6 hr at room temperature	99	I
		BY	2 g	10% ampicillin decomposition in 17 hr at 25 °C	604	I
		BY	5 g	10% ampicillin decomposition in 14 hr at 25 °C	604	I
		BY	15 g	10% ampicillin decomposition in 10 hr at 25 °C	604	I
Sodium chloride 0.9%		BY	2 g	10% ampicillin decomposition in over 48 hr at 25 °C	604	C
		BY	5 g	10% ampicillin decomposition in 38 hr at 25 °C	604	C
		BY	15 g	10% ampicillin decomposition in 33 hr at 25 °C	604	C
		BE	10 g	Less than 10% decomposition in 24 hr at 25 °C	113	C
		BR	6 g	Approximately 9% decomposition in 24 hr at room temperature. Approximately 1% decomposition in 24 hr under refrigeration	127	C
	MG	BR	1 g	Potency retained for 24 hr at 4 and 25 °C	105	C
		AY	2 to 30 g	10% decomposition in 24 hr at room temperature	99	C
		BR	20 g	Approximately 4% decomposition in 24 hr at 5 °C. Approximately 12 to 16% decomposition in 24 hr at 25 °C	208	C
		BR	10 g	Approximately 4% decomposition in 24 hr at −20 °C. Approximately 3% decomposition in 24 hr at 5 °C. Approximately 8% decomposition in 24 hr at 27 °C	210	C
		BR	5, 10, 15, 20 g	Approximately 6 to 12% decomposition in 24 hr at 25 °C	212	C
		BR	5, 10, 15, 20, 30, 40 g	Approximately 1 to 6% decomposition in 24 hr at 5 °C	212	C
	BA[a], TR	AY	20 g	Potency retained for 24 hr at 5 and 22 °C	298	C
			2, 4, 10 g	Approximately 10% decomposition in 24 hr at 20 to 25 °C	307	C
	TR[b]	WY	10 and 20 g	10% ampicillin loss in 24 hr at 25 °C and in 48 hr at 4 °C	1001	C
		BE	1 g	12% ampicillin decomposition in 8 hr at 25 °C and 28% decomposition in 24 hr at 25 °C	211	I
		BR	30 and 40 g	Approximately 15% ampicillin decomposition in 24 hr at 25 °C	212	I
			4 g	10% loss in 8 hr and 19% loss in 24 hr at room temperature	768	I
			5 g	10% loss in 8 hr at 29 °C and 3% loss in 24 hr at 4 °C	773	I
	TR[b]	WY	20 g	15% ampicillin loss in 1 day and 30% in 4 days at 24 °C. 6% loss in 1 day and 10% in 4 days at 4 °C.	1035	I
	[b]	BR	20 g	No drug loss by HPLC during 2 hr storage and 1-hr simulated infusion	1774	C
	AB[c]	WY	60 g	Stable by HPLC for 24 hr at 5 °C. 10% ampicillin loss in 6 hr and 20% loss in 24 hr during administration at 30 °C via portable pump	1779	C
	BA[b]	BE	10 g	Visually compatible with 10% ampicillin loss by HPLC in 2 days at 5 °C	1820	C

Solution Compatibility (Cont.)

				Ampicillin sodium			
Solution	Mfr	Mfr	Conc/L	Remarks	Ref	C/I
	BA[b]	BE	5 g	Visually compatible with 10% ampicillin loss by HPLC in 1 day at 5 °C	1820	**C**
	AB[d]	APC	20 g	2 to 4% loss by HPLC in 8 hr at 25 °C and 7% loss in 3 days at 5 °C	1970	**C**
Sodium lactate ⅙ M		BR	1 g	37% ampicillin decomposition in 4 hr at 25 °C	211	**I**
		AY	up to 30 g	10% ampicillin decomposition in 6 hr at room temperature	99	**I**
TPN #1[e]		BR	1 g	Physically compatible for 12 hr. Precipitate noted in 24 hr at 22 °C	313	**I**
		BR	20 mg	Antibiotic potency retained for at least 12 hr at 22 °C	313	**C**
TPN #2, #3, #5 to #9[e]		BR	1 g	Physically incompatible with a precipitate noted in 1 to 4 hr at 22 °C	313	**I**
TPN #4[e]		BR	1 g	Physically compatible for 24 hr at 22 °C	313	**C**
TPN #10[e]		BR	500 mg and 1 g	Physically compatible for 24 hr, and antibiotic potency retained for at least 12 hr at 22 °C	313	**C**
TPN #21[e]		BR	1 g	Antibiotic potency retained for 24 hr at 4 °C	87	**C**
		BR	1 g	12 to 25% ampicillin decomposition in 24 hr at 25 °C	87	**I**
TPN #52[e]		AST	1.5 g	69% ampicillin loss in 24 hr at 29 °C by microbiological assay	440	**I**
TPN #53[e]		AST	1.5 g	22% ampicillin loss in 24 hr at 29 °C by microbiological assay	440	**I**
TPN #107[e]			1 and 3 g	Physically compatible and ampicillin activity retained for 24 hr at 21 °C by microbiological assay	1326	**C**

[a]Tested in both PVC and glass containers.
[b]Tested in PVC containers.
[c]Tested in portable pump reservoirs (Pharmacia Deltec).
[d]Tested in glass containers and latex elastomeric reservoirs (Secure Medical).
[e]Refer to Appendix I for the composition of parenteral nutrition solutions. TPN indicates a 2-in-1 admixture.

Additive Compatibility

				Ampicillin sodium				
Drug	Mfr	Conc/L	Mfr	Conc/L	Test Soln	Remarks	Ref	C/I
Amikacin sulfate	BR	5 g	BR	30 g	D5LR, D5R, D5S, D5W, D10W, IS10, LR, NS, R, SL	Greater than 10% ampicillin decomposition within 4 hr at 25 °C	293	**I**
Aztreonam	SQ	10 g	WY	20 g	D5W[a]	10% ampicillin loss in 2 hr and 10% aztreonam loss in 3 hr at 25 °C. 10% ampicillin loss in 24 hr and 10% aztreonam loss in 8 hr at 4 °C	1001	**I**
	SQ	10 g	WY	5 g	D5W[a]	10% ampicillin loss in 3 hr and 10% aztreonam loss in 7 hr at 25 °C. 10% loss of both drugs in 48 hr at 4 °C	1001	**I**

Additive Compatibility (Cont.)

Drug		Ampicillin sodium						
	Mfr	Conc/L	Mfr	Conc/L	Test Soln	Remarks	Ref	C/I
	SQ	20 g	WY	20 g	D5W[a]	10% ampicillin loss in 4 hr and 10% aztreonam loss in 5 hr at 25 °C. 10% loss of both drugs in 24 hr at 4 °C	1001	**I**
	SQ	20 g	WY	5 g	D5W[a]	10% ampicillin loss in 5 hr and 10% aztreonam loss in 8 hr at 25 °C. 10% ampicillin loss in 48 hr and 10% aztreonam loss in 72 hr at 4 °C	1001	**I**
	SQ	10 g	WY	20 g	NS[a]	10% ampicillin loss in 24 hr and 2% aztreonam loss in 48 hr at 25 °C. 10% ampicillin loss in 2 days and 9% aztreonam loss in 7 days at 4 °C	1001	**C**
	SQ	10 g	WY	5 g	NS[a]	10% ampicillin loss and no aztreonam loss in 48 hr at 25 °C. 10% ampicillin loss in 3 days and 8% aztreonam loss in 7 days at 4 °C	1001	**C**
	SQ	20 g	WY	20 g	NS[a]	10% ampicillin loss in 24 hr and 5% aztreonam loss in 48 hr at 25 °C. 10% ampicillin loss in 2 days and 7% loss in 7 days at 4 °C	1001	**C**
	SQ	20 g	WY	5 g	NS[a]	10% ampicillin loss and no aztreonam loss in 48 hr at 25 °C. 10% ampicillin loss and 5% aztreonam loss in 7 days at 4 °C	1001	**C**
Cefepime HCl	BR	40 g	BR	1 g	D5W	4% ampicillin loss by HPLC in 8 hr at room temperature and 5 °C. 7% cefepime loss by HPLC in 8 hr at room temperature and no loss in 8 hr at 5 °C	1682	**?**
	BR	40 g	BR	1 g	NS	No ampicillin loss by HPLC in 24 hr at room temperature and 9% loss in 48 hr at 5 °C. 5% cefepime loss by HPLC in 24 hr at room temperature and 2% loss in 72 hr at 5 °C	1682	**C**
	BR	40 g	BR	10 g	D5W	6% ampicillin loss by HPLC in 2 hr at room temperature and 2% loss in 8 hr at 5 °C. 7% cefepime loss by HPLC in 2 hr at room temperature and 8 hr at 5 °C	1682	**I**
	BR	40 g	BR	10 g	NS	6% ampicillin loss by HPLC in 8 hr at room temperature and 9% loss in 48 hr at 5 °C. 8% cefepime loss by HPLC in 8 hr at room temperature and 10% loss in 48 hr at 5 °C	1682	**I**
	BR	4 g	BR	40 g	D5W	10% ampicillin loss by HPLC in 1 hr at room temperature and 9% loss in 2 hr at 5 °C. 25% cefepime loss by HPLC in 8 hr at room temperature and 9% loss in 2 hr at 5 °C	1682	**I**
	BR	4 g	BR	40 g	NS	5% ampicillin loss by HPLC in 8 hr at room temperature and 4% loss in 8 hr at 5 °C. 4% cefepime loss by HPLC in 8 hr at room temperature and 6% loss in 8 hr at 5 °C	1682	**?**
Cefotiam HCl	TAK	20 g	GRU	20 g	W	Visually compatible with 4% or less loss of each drug by HPLC in 2 hr	1738	**C**

Additive Compatibility (Cont.)

Ampicillin sodium

Drug	Mfr	Conc/L	Mfr	Conc/L	Test Soln	Remarks	Ref	C/I
Chlorpromazine HCl	BP	200 mg	BP	2 g	D5W, NS	Immediate precipitate	26	I
Cimetidine HCl	SKF	1.2 and 5 g	SKF	1 g	D5W, NS	Physically compatible and cimetidine stable for 24 hr at room temperature. Ampicillin instability is determining factor	551	?
Clindamycin phosphate	UP	24 g	WY	10 and 20 g	NS	Physically compatible	1035	C
	UP	3 g	WY	3.7 g	NS	Physically compatible with 4% ampicillin loss in 1 day at 24 °C	1035	C
Dopamine HCl	AS	800 mg	BR	4 g	D5W	36% ampicillin decomposition in 6 hr at 23 to 25 °C. Apparent dopamine decomposition in 6 hr also; color change and second spot on TLC	78	I
Erythromycin lactobionate	AB	3 g	WY	3.7 g	NS	Physically compatible with 6% ampicillin loss in 1 day at 24 °C	1035	C
Floxacillin sodium	BE	20 g	BE	20 g	NS	Physically compatible for 72 hr at 15 and 30 °C	1479	C
Furosemide	HO	1 g	BE	20 g	NS	Physically compatible for 72 hr at 15 and 30 °C	1479	C
Gentamicin sulfate	RS	160 mg	BE	8 g	D5¼S, D5W, NS	50% gentamicin decomposition in 2 hr at room temperature	157	I
		100 mg		1 g	TPN #107[b]	42% gentamicin loss and 25% ampicillin loss in 24 hr at 21 °C by microbiological assay	1326	I
Heparin sodium		32,000 units		2 g	NS	Physically compatible and heparin activity retained for 24 hr	57	C
		12,000 units	BR	1 g	D5W, D10W, IM, IP, LR, NS	Ampicillin potency retained for 24 hr at 4 °C	87	C
	OR	20,000 units	BE	10 g	NS	Potency of both retained for 24 hr at 25 °C	113	C
		12,000 units	BR	1 g	D5S	15% ampicillin decomposition in 24 hr at 4 °C	87	I
		12,000 units	BR	1 g	D5W, D10W, LR	20 to 25% ampicillin decomposition in 24 hr at 25 °C	87	I
Hydralazine HCl	BP	80 mg	BP	2 g	D5W	Yellow color produced	26	I
Hydrocortisone sodium succinate		200 and 400 mg	BR	1 g	LR	Ampicillin potency retained for 24 hr at 25 °C	87	C
		50 and 100 mg	BR	1 g	LR	14% ampicillin decomposition in 12 hr at 25 °C	87	I
		200 mg	BE	20 g	D–S	32% ampicillin decomposition in 6 hr at 25 °C	89	I
		200 mg	BE	20 g	D5W	23% ampicillin decomposition in 6 hr at 25 °C	89	I
		200 mg	BE	20 g	NS	18% ampicillin decomposition in 6 hr at 25 °C	89	I
		1.8 g	BR	1 g	D5S, D10W, IM, IP, LR	11 to 28% ampicillin decomposition in 24 hr at 25 °C	87	I

Additive Compatibility (Cont.)

Ampicillin sodium

Drug	Mfr	Conc/L	Mfr	Conc/L	Test Soln	Remarks	Ref	C/I
		1.8 g	BR	1 g	D5S, D5W, D10W, IM, IP, LR, NS	Ampicillin potency retained for 24 hr at 4 °C	87	**C**
Metronidazole	RP	5 g[c]	AY	20 g		Physically compatible for at least 24 hr at 23 °C, but solution had a significant change in pH	807	**?**
	SE	5 g	BR	20 g		9% ampicillin loss in 22 hr at 25 °C and in 12 days at 5 °C. No metronidazole loss	993	**C**
Metronidazole HCl with sodium bicarbonate	SE AB	5 g 50 mEq	BR	2 g	D5W, NS	Physically compatible for 48 hr. Ampicillin instability may be determining factor	765	**?**
Prochlorperazine mesylate	BP	100 mg	BP	2 g	D5W, NS	Immediate precipitate	26	**I**
Ranitidine HCl	GL	100 mg		2 g	D5W	Physically compatible for 24 hr at ambient temperature under fluorescent light. Ampicillin instability is determining factor	1151	**?**
	GL	50 mg and 2 g		1 g	NS	Physically compatible and ranitidine chemically stable by HPLC for 24 hr at 25 °C. Ampicillin not tested	1515	**C**
Sodium bicarbonate	AB	2.4 mEq[d]	BR	500 mg	D5W	Physically compatible for 24 hr. Ampicillin instability is determining factor	772	**?**
Verapamil HCl	KN SE	80 mg [e]	BR WY	4 g 40 g	D5W, NS D5W, NS	Physically compatible for 24 hr Cloudy solution clears with agitation	764 1166	**C** **?**

[a]Tested in PVC containers.
[b]Refer to Appendix I for the composition of parenteral nutrition solutions. TPN indicates a 2-in-1 admixture.
[c]Minibags (100 ml) containing metronidazole 500 mg with disodium phosphate 150 mg, citric acid 44 mg, and sodium chloride 740 mg. This product differs from the Searle product.
[d]One vial of Neut added to a liter of admixture.
[e]Final concentration unspecified.

Drugs in Syringe Compatibility

Ampicillin sodium

Drug (in syringe)	Mfr	Amt	Mfr	Amt	Remarks	Ref	C/I
Chloramphenicol sodium succinate	PD	250 and 400 mg/ml in 1.5 to 2 ml	AY	500 mg	No precipitate or color change within 1 hr at room temperature	99	**C**
	PD	250 mg/1 ml	AY	500 mg	Physically compatible for 1 hr at room temperature	300	**C**
	PD	400 mg/1 ml	AY	500 mg	Physically compatible for 1 hr at room temperature	300	**C**
Colistimethate sodium	PX	40 mg/2 ml	AY	500 mg	No precipitate or color change within 1 hr at room temperature	99	**C**
	PX	500 mg/2 ml	AY	500 mg	Physically compatible for 1 hr at room temperature	300	**C**
Diatrizoate meglumine 52%, diatrizoate sodium 8%	MA	5 ml	BR	30 mg/1 ml	Physically compatible for at least 2 hr	1438	**C**

Drugs in Syringe Compatibility (Cont.)

Ampicillin sodium

Drug (in syringe)	Mfr	Amt	Mfr	Amt	Remarks	Ref	C/I
Diatrizoate sodium 60%	WI	5 ml	BR	30 mg/ 1 ml	Physically compatible for at least 2 hr	1438	C
Erythromycin lactobionate	AB	300 mg/ 6 ml	AY	500 mg	Precipitate forms in 1 hr at room temperature	300	I
Gentamicin sulfate		80 mg/ 2 ml	AY	500 mg	Physically incompatible within 1 hr at room temperature	99	I
Heparin sodium		2500 units/ 1 ml		2 g	Physically compatible for at least 5 min	1053	C
Hydromorphone HCl	KN	2, 10, 40 mg/ 1 ml	AY	250 mg/ 1 ml	Visually compatible but 10% loss of ampicillin by HPLC in 5 hr at room temperature	2082	I
Iohexol	WI	64.7%, 5 ml	BR	30 mg/ 1 ml	Physically compatible for at least 2 hr	1438	C
Iopamidol	SQ	61%, 5 ml	BR	30 mg/ 1 ml	Physically compatible for at least 2 hr	1438	C
Iothalamate meglumine 60%	MA	5 ml	BR	30 mg/ 1 ml	Physically compatible for at least 2 hr	1438	C
Ioxaglate meglumine 39.3%, ioxaglate sodium 19.6%	MA	5 ml	BR	30 mg/ 1 ml	Physically compatible for at least 2 hr	1438	C
Kanamycin sulfate		1 g/4 ml	AY	500 mg	Physically incompatible within 1 hr at room temperature	99	I
		1 g/2 ml	AY	500 mg	Precipitate forms in 1 hr at room temperature	300	I
Lidocaine HCl		0.5 and 2.5% in 2.5 ml	BE	500 mg	Physically compatible	89	C
		0.5 and 2.5% in 1.5 ml	BE	250 mg	Occasional turbidity	89	I
Lincomycin HCl	UP	600 mg/ 2 ml	AY	500 mg	Physically incompatible within 1 hr at room temperature	99	I
	UP	600 mg/ 2 ml	AY	500 mg	Precipitate forms in 1 hr at room temperature	300	I
Metoclopramide HCl	RB	10 mg/ 2 ml	BR	250 mg/ 2.5 ml	Incompatible. If mixed, use immediately	1167	I
	RB	10 mg/ 2 ml	BR	1 g/ 10 ml	Incompatible. If mixed, use immediately	1167	I
	RB	160 mg/ 32 ml	BR	1 g/ 10 ml	Incompatible. If mixed, use immediately	1167	I
Polymyxin B sulfate	BW	25 mg/ 1.5 ml	AY	500 mg	Physically compatible for 1 hr at room temperature	300	C
	BW	25 mg/ 1.5 ml	AY	250 mg	Precipitate forms in 1 hr at room temperature	300	I
Procaine HCl			BE		Physically compatible	89	C
Streptomycin sulfate		1 g/2 ml	AY	500 mg	No precipitate or color change within 1 hr at room temperature	99	C

Drugs in Syringe Compatibility (Cont.)

Ampicillin sodium

Drug (in syringe)	Mfr	Amt	Mfr	Amt	Remarks	Ref	C/I
	BP	1 g/2 ml	AY	500 mg	Physically compatible for 1 hr at room temperature	300	C
	BP	1 g/ 1.5 ml	AY	500 mg	Syrupy solution forms	300	I
Streptomycin sulfate stabilized	BP	0.75 g/ 1.5 ml	AY	500 mg	Precipitate forms in 1 hr at room temperature	300	I

Y-Site Injection Compatibility (1:1 Mixture)

Ampicillin sodium

Drug	Mfr	Conc	Mfr	Conc	Remarks	Ref	C/I
Acyclovir sodium	BW	5 mg/ml[a]	WY	20 mg/ml[b]	Physically compatible for 4 hr at 25 °C	1157	C
Amifostine	USB	10 mg/ml[a]	WY	20 mg/ml[b]	Physically compatible with no change in measured turbidity or increase in particle content in 4 hr at 23 °C	1845	C
Amphotericin B cholesteryl sulfate complex	SEQ	0.83 mg/ml[a]	SKB	20 mg/ml[b]	Gross precipitate forms	2117	I
Aztreonam	SQ	40 mg/ml[a]	WY	20 mg/ml[b]	Physically compatible with no subvisual haze or particle formation in 4 hr at 23 °C	1758	C
Calcium gluconate	AST	4 mg/ml[b]	WY	40 mg/ml[b]	Physically compatible for 3 hr	1316	C
	AST	4 mg/ml[a]	WY	40 mg/ml[a]	Slight color change in 1 hr	1316	I
Cisatracurium besylate	GW	0.1 and 2 mg/ml[a]	SKB	20 mg/ml[b]	Physically compatible with no change in measured turbidity or increase in particle content in 4 hr at 23 °C	2074	C
	GW	5 mg/ml[a]	SKB	20 mg/ml[b]	Gray subvisual haze forms in 1 hr	2074	I
Clarithromycin	AB	4 mg/ml[a]	BE	40 mg/ml[a]	Visually compatible for 72 hr at both 30 and 17 °C	2174	C
Cyclophosphamide	MJ	20 mg/ml[a]	BR	20 mg/ml[b]	Physically compatible for 4 hr at 25 °C	1194	C
Diltiazem HCl	MMD	5 mg/ml	WY	100 mg/ml[b]	Cloudiness forms	1807	I
	MMD	1 mg/ml[b]	WY	100 mg/ml[b]	Visually compatible	1807	C
	MMD	5 mg/ml	WY	10 and 20 mg/ml[b]	Visually compatible	1807	C
Docetaxel	RPR	0.9 mg/ml[a]	SKB	20 mg/ml[b]	Physically compatible with no change in measured turbidity or increase in particle content in 4 hr at 23 °C	2224	C
Doxorubicin HCl liposome injection	SEQ	0.4 mg/ml[a]	SKB	20 mg/ml[b]	Physically compatible with little or no change in measured turbidity and no increase in particle content in 4 hr at 23 °C	2087	C
Enalaprilat	MSD	0.05 mg/ml[b]	BR	10 mg/ml[b]	Physically compatible for 24 hr at room temperature under fluorescent light	1355	C
Epinephrine HCl	ES	0.032 mg/ ml[c]	WY	40 mg/ml[c]	Slight color change in 3 hr	1316	I
Esmolol HCl	DCC	10 mg/ml[a]	WY	20 mg/ml[b]	Physically compatible for 24 hr at 22 °C	1169	C
Etoposide phosphate	BR	5 mg/ml[a]	APC	20 mg/ml[b]	Physically compatible with no change in measured turbidity or increase in particle content in 4 hr at 23 °C	2218	C

Y-Site Injection Compatibility (1:1 Mixture) (Cont.)

Ampicillin sodium

Drug	Mfr	Conc	Mfr	Conc	Remarks	Ref	C/I
Famotidine	MSD	0.2 mg/ml[a]	ES	20 mg/ml[b]	Physically compatible for 14 hr	1196	**C**
	ME	2 mg/ml[b]		20 mg/ml[b]	Visually compatible for 4 hr at 22 °C	1936	**C**
Filgrastim	AMG	30 μg/ml[a]	WY	20 mg/ml[a]	Physically compatible with no change in measured turbidity or increase in particle content in 4 hr at 22 °C	1687	**C**
Fluconazole	RR	2 mg/ml	WY	20 mg/ml	Cloudiness	1407	**I**
Fludarabine phosphate	BX	1 mg/ml[a]	BR	20 mg/ml[b]	Physically compatible for 4 hr at room temperature under fluorescent light	1439	**C**
Foscarnet sodium	AST	24 mg/ml	WY	20 mg/ml	Physically compatible for 24 hr at room temperature under fluorescent light	1335	**C**
Gemcitabine HCl	LI	10 mg/ml[b]	SKB	20 mg/ml[b]	Physically compatible with no change in measured turbidity or increase in particle content in 4 hr at 23 °C	2226	**C**
Granisetron HCl	SKB	0.05 mg/ml[a]	MAR	20 mg/ml[b]	Physically compatible with no change in measured turbidity or increase in particle content in 4 hr at 23 °C	2000	**C**
Heparin sodium	TR	50 units/ml	WY	20 mg/ml[b]	Visually compatible for 6 hr at 25 °C	1793	**C**
Heparin sodium with hydrocortisone sodium succinate	RI UP	1000 units + 100 mg/L[d]	BR	25, 50, 100, 135 mg/ml	Physically compatible for at least 4 hr at room temperature by visual and microscopic examination	322	**C**
Hetastarch	DCC	6%	BR	20 mg/ml[a]	Physically compatible for 4 hr at room temperature by visual examination	1313	**C**
	DCC	6%	BR	20 mg/ml[a]	One or two particles in one of five vials. Fine white strands appeared immediately during Y-site infusion	1315	**I**
Hydralazine HCl	SO	1 mg/ml[b]	WY	40 mg/ml[b]	Moderate color change in 3 hr	1316	**I**
	SO	1 mg/ml[a]	WY	40 mg/ml[a]	Moderate color change in 1 hr	1316	**I**
Hydromorphone HCl	WY	0.2 mg/ml[a]	BR	20 mg/ml[b]	Physically compatible for at least 4 hr at 25 °C under fluorescent light	987	**C**
	KN	2, 10, 40 mg/ml	AY	20[a] and 250 mg/ml	Visually compatible and hydromorphone potency by HPLC retained for 24 hr. 10% ampicillin loss by HPLC in 5 hr with or without hydromorphone	1532	**I**
Insulin, regular	LI	0.2 unit/ml[b]	WY	20 mg/ml[b]	Physically compatible for 2 hr at 25 °C	1395	**C**
Labetalol HCl	SC	1 mg/ml[a]	WY	10 mg/ml[b]	Physically compatible for 24 hr at 18 °C	1171	**C**
Magnesium sulfate	IX	16.7, 33.3, 66.7, 100 mg/ml[a]	WY	20 mg/ml[b]	Physically compatible for at least 4 hr at 32 °C	813	**C**
Melphalan HCl	BW	0.1 mg/ml[b]	WY	20 mg/ml[b]	Physically compatible with no change in measured turbidity or increase in particle content in 3 hr at 22 °C	1557	**C**
Meperidine HCl	WY	10 mg/ml[a]	BR	20 mg/ml[b]	Physically compatible for at least 4 hr at 25 °C under fluorescent light	987	**C**
Midazolam HCl	RC	1 mg/ml[a]	WY	20 mg/ml[b]	Haze forms immediately	1847	**I**
Morphine sulfate	WI	1 mg/ml[a]	BR	20 mg/ml[b]	Physically compatible for at least 4 hr at 25 °C under fluorescent light	987	**C**
Multivitamins	USV	5 ml/L[a]	AY	1 g/50 ml[c]	Physically compatible for 24 hr at room temperature	323	**C**

Y-Site Injection Compatibility (1:1 Mixture) (Cont.)

Ampicillin sodium

Drug	Mfr	Conc	Mfr	Conc	Remarks	Ref	C/I
Ofloxacin	HO	2.2 mg/ml	HO	21.3 mg/ml	Visually compatible with no loss of either drug by HPLC in 2 hr at room temperature	1734	C
Ondansetron HCl	GL	1 mg/ml[b]	BR	20 mg/ml[b]	Immediate turbidity and precipitation	1365	I
Perphenazine	SC	0.02 mg/ml[a]	BR	20 mg/ml[b]	Physically compatible for 4 hr at 25 °C	1155	C
Phytonadione	MSD	0.4 mg/ml[c]	WY	40 mg/ml[b]	Physically compatible for 3 hr	1316	C
Potassium chloride		40 mEq/L[d]	BR	25, 50, 100, 135 mg/ml	Physically compatible for at least 4 hr at room temperature by visual and microscopic examination	322	C
Propofol	ZEN	10 mg/ml	WY	20 mg/ml[b]	Physically compatible for 1 hr at 23 °C with no increase in particle content	2066	C
Remifentanil HCl	GW	0.025 and 0.25 mg/ml[b]	SKB	20 mg/ml[b]	Physically compatible with no change in measured turbidity or increase in particle content in 4 hr at 23 °C	2075	C
Sargramostim	IMM	10 μg/ml[b]	BR	20 mg/ml[b]	Few small particles form in 4 hr	1436	I
Tacrolimus	FUJ	1 mg/ml[b]	WY	20 mg/ml[a]	Visually compatible for 24 hr at 25 °C	1630	C
Teniposide	BR	0.1 mg/ml[a]	WY	20 mg/ml[b]	Physically compatible with no subvisual haze or particle formation in 4 hr at 23 °C	1725	C
Theophylline	TR	4 mg/ml	WY	20 mg/ml[b]	Visually compatible for 6 hr at 25 °C	1793	C
Thiotepa	IMM[e]	1 mg/ml[a]	WY	20 mg/ml[b]	Physically compatible with no change in measured turbidity or increase in particle content in 4 hr at 23 °C	1861	C
TNA #73[f]		32.5 ml[g]	BR	2 g/50 ml[b]	Physically compatible for 4 hr at 25 °C by visual observation	1008	C
TNA #218 to #226[f]			SKB	20 mg/ml[b]	Visually compatible with no precipitate or emulsion damage apparent in 4 hr at 23 °C	2215	C
Tolazoline HCl		0.1 mg/ml[a]	WY	30 mg/ml[b]	Physically compatible for 24 hr at 22 °C	1363	C
TPN #54[f]					Precipitate forms within 30 min at 22 °C	1045	I
TPN #61[f]		[h]	WY	250 mg/ 1.3 ml[i]	Heavy precipitate of calcium phosphate due to increased pH	1012	I
		[j]	WY	1.5 g/7.5 ml[i]	Heavy precipitate of calcium phosphate due to increased pH	1012	I
TPN #203 and #204[f]			APC	100 and 250 mg/ml	White precipitate forms immediately	1974	I
TPN #212 to #215[f]			SKB	20 mg/ml[b]	Physically compatible with no change in measured turbidity or increase in particle content in 4 hr at 23 °C	2109	C
Vancomycin HCl	AB	20 mg/ml[a]	SKB	250 mg/ml[k]	Transient precipitate forms followed by clear solution	2189	?
	AB	20 mg/ml[a]	SKB	1, 10, and 50 mg/ml[b]	Physically compatible with no change in measured turbidity or increase in particle content in 4 hr at 23 °C	2189	C
	AB	2 mg/ml[a]	SKB	1[b], 10[b], 50[b], and 250[k] mg/ ml	Physically compatible with no change in measured turbidity or increase in particle content in 4 hr at 23 °C	2189	C

Y-Site Injection Compatibility (1:1 Mixture) (Cont.)

Ampicillin sodium

Drug	Mfr	Conc	Mfr	Conc	Remarks	Ref	C/I
Verapamil HCl	SE	2.5 mg/ml	WY	40 mg/ml[c]	White milky precipitate forms immediately and persists. 91% of verapamil precipitated	1166	I
Vinorelbine tartrate	BW	1 mg/ml[b]	WY	20 mg/ml[b]	Tiny particles form immediately, becoming large white particles in cloudy solution in 1 hr	1558	I
Vitamin B complex with C	RC	2 ml/L[d]	BR	25, 50, 100, 135 mg/ml	Physically compatible for at least 4 hr at room temperature by visual and microscopic examination	332	C
	RC	4 and 20 ml/L[a]		1 g/50 ml[c]	Physically compatible for 24 hr at room temperature	323	C

[a]*Tested in dextrose 5% in water.*
[b]*Tested in sodium chloride 0.9%.*
[c]*Tested in both dextrose 5% in water and sodium chloride 0.9%.*
[d]*Tested in dextrose 5% in water, sodium chloride 0.9%, and Ringer's injection, lactated.*
[e]*Lyophilized formulation tested.*
[f]*Refer to Appendix I for the composition of parenteral nutrition solutions. TNA indicates a 3-in-1 admixture, and TPN indicates a 2-in-1 admixture.*
[g]*A 32.5-ml sample of parenteral nutrition solution mixed with 50 ml of antibiotic solution.*
[h]*Run at 21 ml/hr.*
[i]*Given over five minutes by syringe pump.*
[j]*Run at 94 ml/hr.*
[k]*Tested in sterile water for injection.*

Additional Compatibility Information

Ampicillin sodium is stated to be physically compatible for 24 hours at room temperature with lincomycin HCl in infusion solutions (154).

Clindamycin phosphate has been stated to be physically incompatible with ampicillin sodium (4).

Aminoglycosides— Noone and Pattison evaluated the inactivation of gentamicin by a variety of penicillins and cephalosporins, including ampicillin sodium. They noted a 50% loss of gentamicin in two hours at room temperature when gentamicin sulfate (Roussel) 160 mg/L was combined with ampicillin sodium (Beecham) 8 g/L in several intravenous solutions (157).

Rank et al. evaluated the inactivation of tobramycin 6 μg/ml in human serum with the sodium salts of cloxacillin and piperacillin 150 and 300 μg/ml, ampicillin 100 and 200 μg/ml, and penicillin G 75 and 150 I.U./ml at 25 and 37 °C for up to 12 hours. Piperacillin induced the greatest inactivation among the penicillins, with up to a 15% loss in 12 hours at 37 °C, in the 300-μg/ml concentration. Cloxacillin and ampicillin had an intermediate effect, causing about a 5% loss in 12 hours at 37 °C in the highest concentrations. Penicillin G did not yield significant tobramycin inactivation (817).

The inactivation of tobramycin sulfate 8 μg/ml in human serum by ampicillin, carbenicillin disodium, and penicillin G potassium, each at 200 μg/ml, was studied at 0, 23, and 37 °C by O'Bey et al. For the tobramycin–ampicillin mixture, essentially no differences were observed at the various temperatures. The t_{90} values were 19, 16.5, and 20 hours at 0, 23, and 37 °C, respectively. Carbenicillin displayed a temperature-dependent inactivation of tobramycin. At 0 °C, the t_{90} was 36 hours; but at 23 and 37 °C, the t_{90} values were 10 and 12 hours, respectively. With penicillin G potassium, the t_{90}

values for tobramycin inactivation at 0, 23, and 37 °C were 48, 44, and 16 hours, respectively. Inaccurate pharmacokinetic dosing of tobramycin may occur if serum samples are not properly handled (832).

To determine if spurious aminoglycoside levels could result from a delay in assaying blood samples, Tindula et al. evaluated the inactivation of amikacin 35 μg/ml and gentamicin and tobramycin 10 μg/ml in human serum by 400-μg/ml concentrations of several penicillins and cephalosporins. Samples were stored for 24 hours at room temperature and frozen at −20 °C. For the room temperature samples, cefazolin and cefamandole caused relatively little inactivation. Nafcillin, cephapirin, and cefoxitin caused moderate inactivation, 20% or less. Penicillin, ampicillin, carbenicillin, and ticarcillin generally caused 25% or more inactivation of gentamicin and tobramycin. Amikacin was somewhat less affected. Freezing samples at −20 °C prevented significant inactivation of amikacin and gentamicin by any of the drugs. Freezing the tobramycin samples was satisfactory for most of the drugs except penicillin, ampicillin, and carbenicillin, which still exhibited a 15 to 20% loss in 24 hours (824).

The comparative inactivation of five aminoglycosides by seven β-lactam antibiotics in human serum at 37 °C was reported by Riff and Thomason. Amikacin, followed by netilmicin, had the lowest degree of inactivation; tobramycin sustained the most pronounced losses. Gentamicin and kanamycin were intermediate in the extent of losses. The six penicillins that were tested all produced aminoglycoside inactivation; the greatest extent of inactivation was caused by carbenicillin followed by ticarcillin, penicillin G, oxacillin, methicillin, and ampicillin, in approximate descending order. Cephalothin produced minimal inactivation (5 to 10% in 24 hours). The rate of inactivation could be reduced by storage at 4 °C and further reduced by storage at −20 °C. The authors suggested processing blood samples rapidly to avoid inaccurate serum determinations.

Storage of specimens at low temperatures until analysis may be helpful (1052).

Townsend reported the apparent inactivation of gentamicin sulfate by ampicillin sodium in blood samples held for 12 hours prior to assay (1382).

Vancomycin—— The compatibility or incompatibility of vancomycin HCl mixed with or administered simultaneously with ampicillin sodium may be concentration dependent (2189). See Y-Site Compatibility above. Vancomycin HCl has a low pH and is variably compatible with drugs having neutral to mildly alkaline pH, including cephalosporins and penicillins. The compatibility may depend on a number of factors, including concentration of each drug, dilution vehicle, actual pH of solutions, and completeness of mixing during administration. Combinations that are compatible when well mixed may result in precipitation if only partially mixed, presumably due to regionally different concentrations and pH values. If attempting to administer vancomycin HCl with ampicillin sodium, take care to ensure that the specific combination and the concentrations are compatible under the exact administration conditions to be used. An inline filter should be used as a final safety measure (2189).

Peritoneal Dialysis Solutions—— The stability of ampicillin sodium (Bristol) 50 mg/L in peritoneal dialysis solutions (Dianeal 137 and PD2) with heparin sodium 500 units/L was evaluated at 25 °C by microbiological assay. Approximately 93 ± 10% activity remained after 24 hours (1228).

AMPICILLIN SODIUM–SULBACTAM SODIUM
AHFS 8:12.16

Unasyn   **Pfizer**

Products—— Ampicillin sodium–sulbactam sodium (Pfizer) is available in vials and piggyback bottles containing 1.5 g (ampicillin 1 g plus sulbactam 0.5 g) or 3 g (ampicillin 2 g plus sulbactam 1 g) as the sodium salts (2).

For intramuscular injection, reconstitute vials with sterile water for injection or lidocaine HCl 0.5 or 2% in the following amounts (2):

Vial Size	Volume of Diluent	Withdrawable Volume	Concentration
1.5 g	3.2 ml	4 ml[a]	375 mg/ml[b]
3.0 g	6.4 ml	8 ml[a]	375 mg/ml[b]

[a]*Sufficient excess is present to permit withdrawal of the volume noted.*
[b]*Ampicillin 250 mg plus sulbactam 125 mg per milliliter.*

For intravenous use, reconstitute piggyback bottles directly with a compatible diluent to the desired concentration between 3 and 45 mg/ml (ampicillin 2 to 30 mg plus sulbactam 1 to 15 mg per milliliter). Standard vials of 1.5 and 3 g may be reconstituted with 3.2 and 6.4 ml of sterile water for injection, respectively, to yield 375-mg/ml solutions (ampicillin 250 mg plus sulbactam 125 mg per milliliter). The reconstituted solution should be diluted immediately in a compatible infusion solution to yield the desired concentration between 3 and 45 mg/ml (2).

Allow reconstituted solutions to stand so that any foaming may dissipate before inspecting them visually to ensure complete dissolution (2).

pH—— From 8 to 10 (2).

Osmolality—— Ampicillin sodium–sulbactam sodium 375 mg/ml in sterile water for injection has an osmolality exceeding 2000 mOsm/kg (1689).

Sodium Content—— Each 1.5 g (ampicillin 1 g plus sulbactam 0.5 g as the sodium salts) contains 5 mEq (115 mg) of sodium (2).

Administration—— Ampicillin sodium–sulbactam sodium may be administered by deep intramuscular injection or intravenous injection or infusion. By direct intravenous injection, the drug should be given slowly over at least 10 to 15 minutes. By infusion, it may be diluted in 50 to 100 ml of compatible diluent and infused over 15 to 30 minutes (2; 4).

Stability—— Intact vials of the white to off-white powder should be stored at or below 30 °C. Aqueous solutions are pale yellow to yellow. Dilute solutions are pale yellow to colorless. The manufacturer recommends that intramuscular solutions be used within one hour after preparation. The administration of diluted solutions for intravenous infusion should be completed within eight hours of preparation to ensure that the potency is maintained throughout the infusion (2; 4).

Compatibility Information

Solution Compatibility

Ampicillin sodium–sulbactam sodium

Solution	Mfr	Mfr	Conc/L	Remarks	Ref	C/I
Sodium chloride 0.9%	[a]	PF	20 + 10 g	Visually compatible with 10% ampicillin loss by HPLC in 32 hr at 24 °C and 68 hr at 5 °C	1691	C

[a]*Tested in PVC containers.*

Additive Compatibility

Ampicillin sodium–sulbactam sodium

Drug	Mfr	Conc/L	Mfr	Conc/L	Test Soln	Remarks	Ref	C/I
Aztreonam	SQ	10 g	PF	20 + 10 g	NS[a]	Visually compatible with 10% ampicillin loss by HPLC in 30 hr at 24 °C and 94 hr at 5 °C. Ampicillin loss is determining factor	1691	**C**

[a]*Tested in PVC containers.*

Y-Site Injection Compatibility (1:1 Mixture)

Ampicillin sodium–sulbactam sodium

Drug	Mfr	Conc	Mfr	Conc	Remarks	Ref	C/I
Amifostine	USB	10 mg/ml[a]	WY	20 + 10 mg/ml[b]	Physically compatible with no change in measured turbidity or increase in particle content in 4 hr at 23 °C	1845	**C**
Amphotericin B cholesteryl sulfate complex	SEQ	0.83 mg/ml[a]	RR	20 + 10 mg/ml[b]	Gross precipitate forms	2117	**I**
Aztreonam	SQ	40 mg/ml[a]	RR	20 + 10 mg/ml[b]	Physically compatible with no subvisual haze or particle formation in 4 hr at 23 °C	1758	**C**
Cefepime HCl	BR	20 mg/ml[a]	RR	20 + 10 mg/ml[a]	Physically compatible with no change in measured turbidity or increase in particle content in 4 hr at 22 °C	1689	**C**
Ciprofloxacin		400 mg[c]		3 + 1.5 g[c]	Administered sequentially through a Y-site into running D5S. White crystals formed immediately	1887	**I**
Cisatracurium besylate	GW	0.1 and 2 mg/ml[a]	RR	20 + 10 mg/ml[b]	Physically compatible with no change in measured turbidity or increase in particle content in 4 hr at 23 °C	2074	**C**
	GW	5 mg/ml[a]	RR	20 + 10 mg/ml[b]	Subvisual haze develops in 15 min	2074	**I**
Diltiazem HCl	MMD	5 mg/ml	RR	45 + 22.5 mg/ml[b]	Cloudiness forms	1807	**I**
	MMD	1 mg/ml[b]	RR	45 + 22.5 mg/ml[b]	Visually compatible	1807	**C**
	MMD	5 mg/ml	RR	15 + 7.5 mg/ml[b]	Visually compatible	1807	**C**
	MMD	5 mg/ml	RR	2 + 1 mg/ml[b]	Visually compatible	1807	**C**
Docetaxel	RPR	0.9 mg/ml[a]	RR	20 + 10 mg/ml[b]	Physically compatible with no change in measured turbidity or increase in particle content in 4 hr at 23 °C	2224	**C**
Enalaprilat	MSD	0.05 mg/ml[b]	PF	10 + 5 mg/ml[b]	Physically compatible for 24 hr at room temperature under fluorescent light	1355	**C**
Etoposide phosphate	BR	5 mg/ml[a]	RR	20 + 10 mg/ml[b]	Physically compatible with no change in measured turbidity or increase in particle content in 4 hr at 23 °C	2218	**C**
Famotidine	MSD	0.2 mg/ml[a]	RR	20 + 10 mg/ml[b]	Physically compatible for 14 hr	1196	**C**

Y-Site Injection Compatibility (1:1 Mixture) (Cont.)

Ampicillin sodium–sulbactam sodium

Drug	Mfr	Conc	Mfr	Conc	Remarks	Ref	C/I
Filgrastim	AMG	30 μg/ml[a]	RR	20 + 10 mg/ml[a]	Physically compatible with no change in measured turbidity or increase in particle content in 4 hr at 22 °C	1687	C
Fluconazole	RR	2 mg/ml	RR	40 + 20 mg/ml	Physically compatible for 24 hr at 25 °C	1407	C
Fludarabine phosphate	BX	1 mg/ml[a]	RR	20 + 10 mg/ml[b]	Physically compatible for 4 hr at room temperature under fluorescent light	1439	C
Gemcitabine HCl	LI	10 mg/ml[b]	RR	20 + 10 mg/ml[b]	Physically compatible with no change in measured turbidity or increase in particle content in 4 hr at 23 °C	2226	C
Granisetron HCl	SKB	0.05 mg/ml[a]	RR	20 + 10 mg/ml[b]	Physically compatible with no change in measured turbidity or increase in particle content in 4 hr at 23 °C	2000	C
Heparin sodium	TR	50 units/ml	PF	20 + 10 mg/ml[b]	Visually compatible for 6 hr at 25 °C	1793	C
Idarubicin HCl	AD	1 mg/ml[b]	RR	20 + 10 mg/ml[b]	Haze forms and color changes immediately. Precipitate forms within 20 min	1525	I
Insulin, regular	LI	0.2 unit/ml[b]	RR	20 + 10 mg/ml[b]	Physically compatible for 2 hr at 25 °C	1395	C
Meperidine HCl	WY	10 mg/ml[b]	RR	20 + 10 mg/ml[b]	Physically compatible for 1 hr at 25 °C	1338	C
Morphine sulfate	ES	1 mg/ml[b]	RR	20 + 10 mg/ml[b]	Physically compatible for 1 hr at 25 °C	1338	C
Ondansetron HCl	GL	1 mg/ml[b]	RR	20 + 10 mg/ml[b]	Immediate turbidity and precipitation	1365	I
Paclitaxel	NCI	1.2 mg/ml[a]	RR	20 + 10 mg/ml[b]	Physically compatible with no change in measured turbidity in 4 hr at 22 °C	1556	C
Remifentanil HCl	GW	0.025 and 0.25 mg/ml[b]	RR	20 + 10 mg/ml[b]	Physically compatible with no change in measured turbidity or increase in particle content in 4 hr at 23 °C	2075	C
Sargramostim	IMM	10 μg/ml[b]	RR	20 + 10 mg/ml[b]	Few small particles in 4 hr in one of two samples	1436	I
Tacrolimus	FUJ	1 mg/ml[b]	RR	33.3 + 16.7 mg/ml[a]	Visually compatible for 24 hr at 25 °C	1630	C
Teniposide	BR	0.1 mg/ml[a]	RR	20 + 10 mg/ml[b]	Physically compatible with no subvisual haze or particle formation in 4 hr at 23 °C	1725	C
Theophylline	TR	4 mg/ml	PF	20 + 10 mg/ml[b]	Visually compatible for 6 hr at 25 °C	1793	C
Thiotepa	IMM[d]	1 mg/ml[a]	RR	20 + 10 mg/ml[b]	Physically compatible with no change in measured turbidity or increase in particle content in 4 hr at 23 °C	1861	C
TNA #218 to #226[e]			PF	20 + 10 mg/ml[b]	Visually compatible with no precipitate or emulsion damage apparent in 4 hr at 23 °C	2215	C
TPN #212 to #215[e]			RR	20 + 10 mg/ml[b]	Physically compatible with no change in measured turbidity or increase in particle content in 4 hr at 23 °C	2109	C

Y-Site Injection Compatibility (1:1 Mixture) (Cont.)

Ampicillin sodium–sulbactam sodium

Drug	Mfr	Conc	Mfr	Conc	Remarks	Ref	C/I
Vancomycin HCl	AB	20 mg/ml[a]	PF	250 + 125 mg/ml[f]	Transient precipitate forms followed by clear solution	2189	?
	AB	20 mg/ml[a]	PF	1 + 0.5, 10 + 5, and 50 + 25 mg/ml[b]	Physically compatible with no change in measured turbidity or increase in particle content in 4 hr at 23 °C	2189	C
	AB	2 mg/ml[a]	PF	1 + 0.5[b], 10 + 5[b], 50 + 25[b], and 250 + 125[f] mg/ml	Physically compatible with no change in measured turbidity or increase in particle content in 4 hr at 23 °C	2189	C

[a]*Tested in dextrose 5% in water.*
[b]*Tested in sodium chloride 0.9%.*
[c]*Concentration and volume not specified.*
[d]*Lyophilized formulation tested.*
[e]*Refer to Appendix I for the composition of parenteral nutrition solutions. TNA indicates a 3-in-1 admixture, and TPN indicates a 2-in-1 admixture.*
[f]*Tested in sterile water for injection.*

Additional Compatibility Information

The compatibility information on ampicillin sodium should be considered. See previous monograph.

Solutions— The manufacturer recommends the following use periods for ampicillin sodium–sulbactam sodium diluted in the infusion solutions noted (2):

Infusion Solution	Maximum Concentration (mg/ml) (Ampicillin/ Sulbactam)	Storage Temperature (°C)	Use Period (hr)
Dextrose 5% in sodium chloride 0.45%	3 (2/1)	25	4
	15 (10/5)	4	4
Dextrose 5% in water	30 (20/10)	25	2
	30 (20/10)	4	4
	3 (2/1)	25	4
Invert sugar 10%	3 (2/1)	25	4
	30 (20/10)	4	3
Ringer's injection, lactated	45 (30/15)	25	8
	45 (30/15)	4	24
Sodium chloride 0.9%	45 (30/15)	25	8
	45 (30/15)	4	48
	30 (20/10)	4	72
Sodium lactate ⅙ M	45 (30/15)	25	8
	45 (30/15)	4	8
Sterile water for injection	45 (30/15)	25	8
	45 (30/15)	4	48
	30 (20/10)	4	72

Aminoglycosides— The manufacturer indicates that ampicillin sodium–sulbactam sodium should be reconstituted and administered separately from aminoglycosides because of possible in vitro inactivation (2).

Vancomycin— The compatibility or incompatibility of vancomycin HCl mixed with or administered simultaneously with ampicillin sodium–sulbactam sodium may be concentration dependent (2189). See Y-Site Compatibility above. Vancomycin HCl has a low pH and is variably compatible with drugs having neutral to mildly alkaline pH, including cephalosporins and penicillins. The compatibility may depend on a number of factors, including concentration of each drug, dilution vehicle, actual pH of solutions, and completeness of mixing during administration. Combinations that are compatible when well mixed may result in precipitation if only partially mixed, presumably because of regionally different concentrations and pH values. If attempting to administer vancomycin HCl with ampicillin sodium–sulbactam sodium, take care to ensure that the specific combination and the concentrations are compatible under the exact administration conditions to be used. An inline filter should be used as a final safety measure (2189).

AMRINONE LACTATE
AHFS 24:04

Inocor   **Sanofi Winthrop**

Products— Amrinone lactate (Sanofi Winthrop) is available as an aqueous solution in 20-ml ampuls. Each milliliter of solution contains 5 mg of amrinone base (as the lactate), 0.25 mg of sodium metabisulfite, and lactic acid or sodium hydroxide to adjust the pH. The total lactic acid concentration may range from 5 to 7.5 mg/ml (4; 154).

pH— From 3.2 to 4 (4).

Osmolality— 101 mOsm/kg (4).

Administration— Amrinone lactate may be administered by slow direct intravenous injection or continuous intravenous infusion. Direct intravenous injection should be performed slowly over two or three minutes directly into a vein or the tubing of a running infusion solution (4).

Stability— Amrinone lactate injection is a clear, yellow solution; it may be stored at room temperature and should be protected from light. The injection is stable for two years following manufacture (4).

pH Effects— The solubilities of amrinone at pH 4.1, 6, and 8 are 25, 0.9, and 0.7 mg/ml, respectively (4).

Compatibility Information

Solution Compatibility

Amrinone lactate

Solution	Mfr	Mfr	Conc/L	Remarks	Ref	C/I
Dextrose 5% in water		WI	1.25 g	Physically compatible with 5 to 6% loss in 4 hr at 22 °C	1419	I[a]
		WI	2.5 g	Physically compatible with 8% loss in 4 hr at 22 °C	1419	I[a]
Sodium chloride 0.45%		WI	1.25 and 2.5 g	Physically compatible with no loss in 4 hr at 22 °C	1419	C

[a]*Unacceptable losses occur in 24 hours.*

Additive Compatibility

Amrinone lactate

Drug	Mfr	Conc/L	Mfr	Conc/L	Test Soln	Remarks	Ref	C/I
Propafenone HCl	KN	0.5 g	SW	1 and 2.5 g[a]	NS	Visually compatible with little or no propafenone loss by HPLC in 24 hr at 22 °C exposed to fluorescent light. Amrinone not tested	412	C

[a]*Approximate concentration.*

Drugs in Syringe Compatibility

Amrinone lactate

Drug (in syringe)	Mfr	Amt	Mfr	Amt	Remarks	Ref	C/I
Propranolol HCl	LY	1 mg/ 1 ml	WI	5 mg/ 1 ml	Physically compatible with little or no loss of either drug in 4 hr at 22 °C	1419	C
Verapamil HCl	LY	10 mg/ 4 ml	WI	5 mg/ 1 ml	Physically compatible with little or no loss of either drug in 4 hr at 22 °C	1419	C

Y-Site Injection Compatibility (1:1 Mixture)

Amrinone lactate

Drug	Mfr	Conc	Mfr	Conc	Remarks	Ref	C/I
Aminophylline	LY	2 mg/ml[a]	WB	3 mg/ml[b]	Physically compatible for at least 4 hr at 25 °C under fluorescent light	992	C

Y-Site Injection Compatibility (1:1 Mixture) (Cont.)

Amrinone lactate

Drug	Mfr	Conc	Mfr	Conc	Remarks	Ref	C/I
Atropine sulfate	AB	0.1 mg/ml[a]	WB	3 mg/ml[b]	Physically compatible for at least 4 hr at 25 °C under fluorescent light	992	C
Bretylium tosylate	ACC	10 mg/ml[a]	WB	3 mg/ml[b]	Physically compatible for at least 4 hr at 25 °C under fluorescent light	992	C
Calcium chloride	AB	100 mg/ml	WB	3 mg/ml[b]	Physically compatible for at least 4 hr at 25 °C under fluorescent light	992	C
Cimetidine HCl	SKF	15 mg/ml[a]	WB	3 mg/ml[b]	Physically compatible for at least 4 hr at 25 °C under fluorescent light	992	C
Cisatracurium besylate	GW	0.1, 2, 5 mg/ml[a]	SW	2.5 mg/ml[b]	Physically compatible with no change in measured turbidity or increase in particle content in 4 hr at 23 °C	2074	C
Digoxin	ES	0.25 mg/ml	WI	2.5 mg/ml[c]	Physically compatible with little or no loss of either drug in 4 hr at 22 °C	1419	C
Dobutamine HCl	LI	4 mg/ml[a]	WB	3 mg/ml[b]	Physically compatible for at least 4 hr at 25 °C under fluorescent light	992	C
Dopamine HCl	ACC	1.6 mg/ml[a]	WB	3 mg/ml[b]	Physically compatible for at least 4 hr at 25 °C under fluorescent light	992	C
Epinephrine HCl	AB	0.1 mg/ml[a]	WB	3 mg/ml[b]	Physically compatible for at least 4 hr at 25 °C under fluorescent light	992	C
Famotidine	MSD	0.2 mg/ml[a]	WI	2 mg/ml[a]	Physically compatible for 4 hr at 25 °C	1188	C
Hydrocortisone sodium succinate	ES	1 mg/ml[a]	WB	3 mg/ml[b]	Physically compatible for at least 4 hr at 25 °C under fluorescent light	992	C
Isoproterenol HCl	BR	0.004 mg/ml[a]	WB	3 mg/ml[b]	Physically compatible for at least 4 hr at 25 °C under fluorescent light	992	C
Lidocaine HCl	ES	8 mg/ml[a]	WB	3 mg/ml[b]	Physically compatible for at least 4 hr at 25 °C under fluorescent light	992	C
Metaraminol bitartrate	MSD	0.2 mg/ml[a]	WB	3 mg/ml[b]	Physically compatible for at least 4 hr at 25 °C under fluorescent light	992	C
Methylprednisolone sodium succinate	ES	1 mg/ml[a]	WB	3 mg/ml[b]	Physically compatible for at least 4 hr at 25 °C under fluorescent light	992	C
Nitroglycerin		0.8 mg/ml[a]	WB	3 mg/ml[b]	Physically compatible for at least 4 hr at 25 °C under fluorescent light	992	C
Nitroprusside sodium	AB	0.2 mg/ml[a]	WB	3 mg/ml[b]	Physically compatible for at least 4 hr at 25 °C under fluorescent light	992	C
Norepinephrine bitartrate	BR	0.004 mg/ml[a]	WB	3 mg/ml[b]	Physically compatible for at least 4 hr at 25 °C under fluorescent light	992	C
Phenylephrine HCl	WI	0.02 mg/ml[a]	WB	3 mg/ml[b]	Physically compatible for at least 4 hr at 25 °C under fluorescent light	992	C
Potassium chloride	IX	0.04 mEq/ml[a]	WB	3 mg/ml[b]	Physically compatible for at least 4 hr at 25 °C under fluorescent light	992	C
	LY	80 mEq/L[c]	WI	5 mg/ml	Physically compatible with little or no loss of either drug in 4 hr at 22 °C	1419	C
	LY	80 mEq/L[c]	WI	2.5 mg/ml[c]	Physically compatible with little or no loss of either drug in 4 hr at 22 °C	1419	C
Procainamide HCl	SQ	4 mg/ml[a]	WB	3 mg/ml[b]	Physically compatible for at least 4 hr at 25 °C under fluorescent light	992	C

Y-Site Injection Compatibility (1:1 Mixture) (Cont.)

Amrinone lactate

Drug	Mfr	Conc	Mfr	Conc	Remarks	Ref	C/I
	LY	20 mg/ml[c]	WI	2.5 mg/ml[c]	Physically compatible with little or no loss of either drug in 4 hr at 22 °C	1419	C
	LY	20 mg/ml[a]	WI	2.5 mg/ml[a]	18% procainamide loss and 10% amrinone loss in 4 hr at 22 °C due to dextrose diluent	1419	I
	LY	4 mg/ml[c]	WI	5 mg/ml	Physically compatible with little or no loss of either drug in 4 hr at 22 °C	1419	C
	LY	4 mg/ml[a]	WI	5 mg/ml	20% procainamide loss and 8% amrinone loss in 4 hr at 22 °C due to dextrose diluent	1419	I
	LY	4 mg/ml[c]	WI	2.5 mg/ml[c]	Physically compatible with little or no loss of either drug in 4 hr at 22 °C	1419	C
	LY	4 mg/ml[a]	WI	2.5 mg/ml[a]	17% procainamide loss in 4 hr at 22 °C due to dextrose diluent	1419	I
Propofol	ZEN	10 mg/ml	WI	1 mg/ml[a]	Physically compatible for 1 hr at 23 °C with no increase in particle content	2066	C
Propranolol HCl	LY	1 mg/ml	WI	2.5 mg/ml[c]	Physically compatible with little or no loss of either drug in 4 hr at 22 °C	1419	C
Remifentanil HCl	GW	0.025 and 0.25 mg/ml[b]	SW	2.5 mg/ml[a]	Physically compatible with no change in measured turbidity or increase in particle content in 4 hr at 23 °C	2075	C
Sodium bicarbonate	AB	1 mEq/ml	WB	3 mg/ml[b]	Immediate color change from yellow to colorless	992	I
	AST	75 mg/ml	WI	5 mg/ml	Immediate precipitation	1419	I
	AST	75 mg/ml	WI	2.5 mg/ml[c]	Precipitate forms within 10 min	1419	I
Verapamil HCl	SE	0.1 mg/ml[a]	WB	3 mg/ml[b]	Physically compatible for at least 4 hr at 25 °C under fluorescent light	992	C
	LY	2.5 mg/ml	WI	2.5 mg/ml[c]	Physically compatible with little or no loss of either drug in 4 hr at 22 °C	1419	C

[a]*Tested in dextrose 5% in water.*
[b]*Tested in sodium chloride 0.9%.*
[c]*Tested in sodium chloride 0.45%.*

Additional Compatibility Information

For intravenous infusions, dilution of amrinone lactate in sodium chloride 0.45 or 0.9% to a concentration of 1 to 3 mg/ml is recommended. These solutions are stable for 24 hours at room temperature or under refrigeration in normal lighting conditions (4).

Amrinone lactate undergoes a slow chemical interaction with dextrose (4). At a concentration of 2.5 mg/ml in dextrose 5% in water, an 11 to 13% loss of potency occurs in 24 hours at room temperature. Therefore, the manufacturer states that the drug should not be diluted with dextrose-containing solutions prior to administration. However, amrinone lactate may be injected into running dextrose infusions through a Y-site or directly into the tubing (4).

Furosemide— A precipitate forms immediately when furosemide is injected into the tubing of a running amrinone lactate infusion (4).

ASCORBIC ACID INJECTION
AHFS 88:12

Cenolate   **Abbott**

Products— Ascorbic acid injection (Abbott) is provided as a sodium ascorbate solution equivalent to 500 mg/ml of ascorbic acid in 1- and 2-ml ampuls. The pH may be adjusted with sodium bicarbonate and ascorbic acid. Sodium hydrosulfite 0.5% is present as an antioxidant (1-10/95).

Pressure may build up during storage of ampuls of ascorbic acid injection. At room temperature, the pressure may become excessive. When opening ascorbic acid injection, the ampuls should be wrapped in a protective covering (1-10/95).

pH— From 5.5 to 7 (4; 17).

Osmolality— Ascorbic acid injection 500 mg/ml has an osmolality exceeding 2000 mOsm/kg (1689).

Administration— Intramuscular injection of ascorbic acid injection is preferred, but it may also be given subcutaneously or intravenously (1-10/95; 4). Intravenously, it should be added to a large volume of a compatible diluent and infused slowly (1-10/95).

Stability— Ascorbic acid gradually darkens on exposure to light. A slight color developed during storage does not impair the therapeutic activity (4). However, Abbott recommends protecting the intact ampuls from light by keeping them in the carton until ready for use (1-10/95).

The stability of ascorbic acid from a multiple vitamin product in dextrose 5% in water and sodium chloride 0.9%, in both PVC and ClearFlex containers, was evaluated. HPLC analysis showed that ascorbic acid was stable at 23 °C when protected from light, exhibiting less than a 10% loss. When exposed to light, however, ascorbic acid had losses of approximately 50 to 65% (1509).

To avoid excessive pressure inside the ampuls, they should be stored in the refrigerator and not allowed to stand at room temperature before use (1-10/95).

Although refrigeration is recommended, Lilly has stated that its ascorbic acid injection had a maximum room temperature stability of 96 hours (853). Intact ampuls of commercial ascorbic acid injection (Vitarine) have been reported to be stable for four years at room temperatures not exceeding 25 °C (60).

Ascorbic acid in solution is rapidly oxidized in air and alkaline media (4).

Ascorbic acid injection (Abbott) develops a grayish-brown color if left exposed to a stainless steel 5-μm filter needle (Monoject) for as little as one hour (1645).

Sorption— Pure ascorbic acid (Merck) did not display significant sorption to a PVC plastic test strip in 24 hours (12).

Compatibility Information

Solution Compatibility

Ascorbic acid injection

Solution	Mfr	Mfr	Conc/L	Remarks	Ref	C/I
Dextran 6% in dextrose 5%	AB	AB	1 g	Physically compatible	3	**C**
Dextran 6% in sodium chloride 0.9%	AB	AB	1 g	Physically compatible	3	**C**
Dextrose–Ringer's injection combinations	AB	AB	1 g	Physically compatible	3	**C**
Dextrose–Ringer's injection, lactated, combinations	AB	AB	1 g	Physically compatible	3	**C**
Dextrose–saline combinations	AB	AB	1 g	Physically compatible	3	**C**
Dextrose 5% in sodium chloride 0.45%		BTK	1.25 g	5% loss by UV spectroscopy in 24 hr at room temperature	1775	**C**
Dextrose 2½% in water	AB	AB	1 g	Physically compatible	3	**C**
Dextrose 5% in water	AB	AB	1 g	Physically compatible	3	**C**
		BTK	1.25 g	5% loss by UV spectroscopy in 24 hr at room temperature	1775	**C**
Dextrose 10% in water	AB	AB	1 g	Physically compatible	3	**C**
		BTK	1.25 g	4% loss by UV spectroscopy in 24 hr at room temperature	1775	**C**
Fat emulsion 10%, intravenous	VT	VI	1 g	Physically compatible for 48 hr at 4 °C and room temperature	32	**C**
	VT	DB	500 mg	Microscopic globule coalescence in 24 hr at 25 and 8 °C	825	**I**
	KA	KAª	7.2 g	Physically compatible for 24 hr at 26 °C with little loss by HPLC of most vitamins; up to 52% ascorbate loss	2050	**C**
Fructose 10% in sodium chloride 0.9%	AB	AB	1 g	Physically compatible	3	**C**
Fructose 10% in water	AB	AB	1 g	Physically compatible	3	**C**

Solution Compatibility (Cont.)

Ascorbic acid injection

Solution	Mfr	Mfr	Conc/L	Remarks	Ref	C/I
Invert sugar 5 and 10% in sodium chloride 0.9%	AB	AB	1 g	Physically compatible	3	C
Invert sugar 5 and 10% in water	AB	AB	1 g	Physically compatible	3	C
Ionosol products	AB	AB	1 g	Physically compatible	3	C
Ringer's injection	AB	AB	1 g	Physically compatible	3	C
		BTK	1.25 g	6% loss by UV spectroscopy in 24 hr at room temperature	1775	C
Ringer's injection, lactated	AB	AB	1 g	Physically compatible	3	C
		BTK	1.25 g	6% loss by UV spectroscopy in 24 hr at room temperature	1775	C
Sodium chloride 0.45%	AB	AB	1 g	Physically compatible	3	C
Sodium chloride 0.9%	AB	AB	1 g	Physically compatible	3	C
		BTK	1.25 g	4% loss by UV spectroscopy in 24 hr at room temperature	1775	C
Sodium lactate ⅙ M	AB	AB	1 g	Physically compatible	3	C

[a]*From multivitamins.*

Additive Compatibility

Ascorbic acid injection

Drug	Mfr	Conc/L	Mfr	Conc/L	Test Soln	Remarks	Ref	C/I
Amikacin sulfate	BR	5 g	CO[a]	5 g	D5LR, D5R, D5S, D5W, D10W, IS10, LR, NS, R, SL	Physically compatible. Potency of both retained for 24 hr at 25 °C	294	C
Aminophylline	SE	500 mg	AB	500 mg		Physically compatible	6	C
						Physically incompatible	9	I
	SE	1 g	UP	500 mg	D5W	Physically incompatible	15	I
Bleomycin sulfate	BR	20 and 30 units	PD	2.5 and 5 g	NS	Loss of all bleomycin activity in 1 week at 4 °C	763	I
Calcium chloride	UP	1 g	UP	500 mg	D5W	Physically compatible	15	C
Calcium gluconate	UP	1 g	UP	500 mg	D5W	Physically compatible	15	C
Chloramphenicol sodium succinate	PD	1 g	AB	1 g		Physically compatible	3; 6	C
Chlorpromazine HCl	SKF	250 mg	UP	500 mg	D5W	Physically compatible	15	C
Colistimethate sodium	WC	500 mg	UP	500 mg	D5W	Physically compatible	15	C
Cyanocobalamin	AB	1000 μg	AB	1 g		Physically compatible	3	C
Diphenhydramine HCl	PD	80 mg	UP	500 mg	D5W	Physically compatible	15	C
Erythromycin lactobionate	AB	1 g	AB	1 g		Physically compatible	3	C
	AB	5 g	UP	500 mg	D5W	Physically incompatible	15	I
Heparin sodium	UP	4000 units	UP	500 mg	D5W	Physically compatible	15	C
Kanamycin sulfate	BR	4 g	UP	500 mg	D5W	Physically compatible	15	C

Additive Compatibility (Cont.)

Ascorbic acid injection

Drug	Mfr	Conc/L	Mfr	Conc/L	Test Soln	Remarks	Ref	C/I
Methyldopa HCl	MSD	1 g	AB	1 g	D, D–S, S	Physically compatible	23	C
Nafcillin sodium	WY	5 g	UP	500 mg	D5W	Physically incompatible	15	I
Penicillin G potassium		1 million units	AB	1 g		Physically compatible	3	C
	SQ	10 million units	PD	500 mg	D5W	99% penicillin potency retained for at least 8 hr	166	C
Polymyxin B sulfate	BW	200 mg	UP	500 mg	D5W	Physically compatible	15	C
Procaine HCl	WI	1 g	UP	500 mg	D5W	Physically compatible	15	C
Prochlorperazine edisylate	SKF	100 mg	UP	500 mg	D5W	Physically compatible	15	C
Promethazine HCl	WY	250 mg	UP	500 mg	D5W	Physically compatible	15	C
Sodium bicarbonate	AB	80 mEq	UP	500 mg	D5W	Physically incompatible	15	I
Theophylline		2 g		1.9 g	D5W	Yellow discoloration with 8% ascorbic acid loss in 6 hr and 15% in 24 hr. No loss of theophylline	1909	I
Verapamil HCl	KN	80 mg	LI	1 g	D5W, NS	Physically compatible for 24 hr	764	C

[a]*As calcium ascorbate.*

Drugs in Syringe Compatibility

Ascorbic acid injection

Drug (in syringe)	Mfr	Amt	Mfr	Amt	Remarks	Ref	C/I
Cefazolin sodium	LI	1 g/3 ml	LI	1 ml	Precipitate forms within 3 min at 32 °C	766	I
Doxapram HCl	RB	400 mg/ 20 ml		500 mg/ 2 ml	Immediate turbidity changing to precipitation in 24 hr	1177	I
Metoclopramide HCl	RB	10 mg/ 2 ml	AB	250 mg/ 0.5 ml	Physically compatible for 48 hr at room temperature	924	C
	RB	10 mg/ 2 ml	AB	250 mg/ 0.5 ml	Physically compatible for 48 hr at 25 °C	1167	C
	RB	160 mg/ 32 ml	AB	250 mg/ 0.5 ml	Physically compatible for 48 hr at 25 °C	1167	C

Y-Site Injection Compatibility (1:1 Mixture)

Ascorbic acid injection

Drug	Mfr	Conc	Mfr	Conc	Remarks	Ref	C/I
Etomidate	AB	2 mg/ml	AB	500 mg/ml	Yellow discoloration and fine precipitate form in 24 hr	1801	I
Propofol	STU	2 mg/ml	AB	500 mg/ml	Yellow discoloration forms within 7 days at 25 °C. No visible change in 24 hr	1801	?
Thiopental sodium	AB	25 mg/ml	AB	500 mg/ml	Yellow discoloration and fine precipitate form in 24 hr	1801	I
TPN #189[c]			DB	20 mg/ml[b]	Visually compatible for 24 hr at 22 °C	1767	C

Y-Site Injection Compatibility (1:1 Mixture) (Cont.)

Ascorbic acid injection

Drug	Mfr	Conc	Mfr	Conc	Remarks	Ref	C/I
Warfarin sodium	DU	0.1[a,b] and 2[d] mg/ml	SCN	0.5 mg/ml[a,b]	Physically compatible with no change in measured turbidity or increase in particle content in 24 hr at 23 °C	2011	C

[a]*Tested in dextrose 5% in water.*
[b]*Tested in sodium chloride 0.9%.*
[c]*Refer to Appendix I for the composition of parenteral nutrition solutions. TPN indicates a 2-in-1 admixture.*
[d]*Tested in sterile water for injection.*

Additional Compatibility Information

Additives— Ascorbic acid with cyanocobalamin is stated to be compatible for 24 hours at room temperature protected from light without loss of activity (52).

Ascorbic acid has been stated to be incompatible with estrogens, conjugated (204), bleomycin sulfate which is inactivated in vitro (4), and chlorothiazide sodium since the final pH may be below 7.4, resulting in precipitation (7). However, it was not specified whether these reports refer to pure ascorbic acid or ascorbic acid injection.

In vitro testing of ascorbic acid at a concentration of 0.1% with kanamycin sulfate 0.025% in sterile distilled water showed a significant reduction in antibiotic activity in one hour at 25 °C (314).

Acid-Labile Drugs— Literature reports of incompatibilities between various acid-labile drugs such as penicillin G potassium (47; 165) and erythromycin lactobionate (20) with pure ascorbic acid do not pertain to ascorbic acid injection, USP. The official product has a pH of 5.5 to 7 (4; 17) and exists as a mixture of sodium ascorbate and ascorbic acid, with the sodium salt predominating. Pure ascorbic acid is quite acidic. A solution of ascorbic acid 500 mg in 2 ml of diluent had a pH of 2. The incompatibilities between pure ascorbic acid and penicillin G potassium have been attributed to the pH rather than being a characteristic of the ascorbate ion (166).

Chloramphenicol and Hydrocortisone— Ascorbic acid injection (Upjohn) in dextrose 5% in water has been reported to be conditionally compatible with both chloramphenicol sodium succinate (Parke-Davis) and hydrocortisone sodium succinate (Upjohn). The incompatibility that may occur is concentration dependent. Therefore, if attempting to combine either chloramphenicol sodium succinate or hydrocortisone sodium succinate with ascorbic acid injection, mix the solution thoroughly and observe it closely for any sign of incompatibility (15).

Parenteral Nutrition Solutions— Shine and Farwell reported a 35% ascorbic acid loss from a parenteral nutrition solution, composed of amino acids, dextrose, electrolytes, trace elements, and multivitamins, in 39 hours at 25 °C with exposure to light. The loss was reduced to a negligible amount in four days by refrigeration and light protection (1063).

Allwood reported on the extent and rapidity of ascorbic acid decomposition in parenteral nutrition solutions composed of amino acids, dextrose, electrolytes, multivitamins, and trace elements in 3-L PVC bags stored at 3 to 7 °C. About 30 to 40% was lost in 24 hours. The degradation then slowed as the oxygen supply was reduced to the diffusion through the bag. About a 55 to 65% loss occurred after seven days of storage. The oxidation was catalyzed by metal ions, especially copper. In the absence of copper from the trace elements additive, less than 10% degradation of ascorbic acid occurred in 24 hours. The author estimated that 150 to 200 mg is degraded in two to four hours at ambient temperature in the presence of copper but that only 20 to 30 mg is broken down in 24 hours without copper. To minimize ascorbic acid loss, copper must be excluded. Alternatively, inclusion of excess ascorbic acid was suggested (1056).

Extensive decomposition of ascorbic acid and folic acid was reported in a parenteral nutrition solution composed of amino acids 3.3%, dextrose 12.5%, electrolytes, trace elements, and M.V.I.-12 (USV) in PVC bags. Half-lives were 1.1, 2.9, and 8.9 hours for ascorbic acid and 2.7, 5.4, and 24 hours for folic acid stored at 24 °C in daylight, 24 °C protected from light, and 4 °C protected from light, respectively. The decomposition was much greater than for solutions not containing catalyzing metal ions. Also, it was greater than for the vitamins singly because of interactions with the other vitamins present (1059).

Dahl et al. reported the stability of numerous vitamins in parenteral nutrition solutions composed of amino acids (Kabi-Vitrum), dextrose 30%, and fat emulsion 20% (Kabi-Vitrum) in a 2:1:1 ratio with electrolytes, trace elements, and both fat- and water-soluble vitamins. The admixtures were stored in darkness at 2 to 8 °C for 96 hours with no significant loss of retinyl palmitate, alpha-tocopherol, thiamine mononitrate, sodium riboflavin-5'-phosphate, pyridoxine HCl, nicotinamide, folic acid, biotin, sodium pantothenate, and cyanocobalamin. Sodium ascorbate and its biologically active degradation product, dehydroascorbic acid, totaled 59 and 42% of the nominal starting concentration at 24 and 96 hours, respectively. However, the actual initial concentration was only 66% of the nominal concentration (1225).

When the admixture was subjected to simulated infusion over 24 hours at 20 °C, either exposed to room light or light protected, or stored for six days in the dark under refrigeration and then subjected to the same simulated infusion, once again the retinyl palmitate, alpha-tocopherol, and sodium riboflavin-5'-phosphate did not undergo significant loss. However, sodium ascorbate and its degradation product, dehydroascorbic acid, had initial combined concentrations of 51 to 65% of the nominal initial concentration, with further declines during infusion. Light protection did not significantly alter the loss of total ascorbic acid (1225).

The stability of ascorbic acid in parenteral nutrition solutions, with and without fat emulsion, was studied using HPLC analysis. Both with and without fat emulsion, the total vitamin C content (ascorbic acid plus dehydroascorbic acid) remained above 90% for 12 hours when the solutions were exposed to fluorescent light and for 24 hours when they were protected from light. When stored in a cool dark place, the solutions were stable for seven days (1227).

Smith et al. reported the stability of several vitamins from M.V.I.-12 (Armour) admixed in parenteral nutrition solutions composed of different amino acid products, with or without Intralipid 10%, when stored in glass bottles and PVC bags at 25 and 5 °C for 48 hours. Ascorbic acid was lost from all samples stored at 25 °C, with the greatest losses occurring in solutions stored in plastic bags. No losses occurred in any sample stored at 5 °C (1431).

Because of these interactions, recommendations to separate the administration of vitamins and trace elements have been made (1056; 1060; 1061). Other researchers have termed such recommendations premature based on differing reports (895; 896) and the apparent absence of epidemic vitamin deficiency in parenteral nutrition patients (1062).

The influence of several factors on the rate of ascorbic acid oxidation in parenteral nutrition solutions was evaluated. Ascorbic acid is regarded as the least stable component in TPN admixtures. The type of amino acid used in the TPN was important. Some, such as FreAmine III and Vamin 14, contain antioxidant compounds (e.g., sodium metabisulfite or cysteine). Ascorbic acid stability was better in such solutions compared with those amino acid solutions having no antioxidant present. Furthermore, the pH of the solution may play a small role, with greater degradation as the pH rises from about 5 to about 7. Adding air to a compounded TPN container can also accelerate ascorbic acid decomposition. The most important factor was the type of plastic container used for the TPN. Ethylene vinyl acetate (EVA) containers (Mixieva, Miramed) allow more oxygen permeation, which results in substantial losses of ascorbic acid in relatively short time periods. In multilayer TPN bags (Ultrastab, Miramed) designed to reduce gas permeability, the rate of ascorbic acid degradation was greatly reduced. HPLC analysis of TPNs without antioxidants packaged in EVA bags found that an almost total loss of ascorbic acid activity occurred in one or two days at 5 °C. In contrast, in TPNs containing FreAmine III or Vamin 14 and packaged in the multilayer bags, most of the ascorbic acid content was retained for 28 days at 5 °C. The authors concluded that TPNs made with antioxidant-containing amino acids and packaged in multilayer bags that reduce gas permeability can safely be given extended expiration dates and still retain most of the ascorbic acid activity (2163).

ASPARAGINASE
AHFS 10:00

Elspar　　　　　　　　　　　　　　　　　　**Merck**

Products— Asparaginase (Merck) is available in vials containing 10,000 I.U. of asparaginase and 80 mg of mannitol in lyophilized form (2).

For intravenous administration, reconstitute with 5 ml of sterile water for injection or sodium chloride 0.9% to yield a solution containing 2000 I.U./ml. For intramuscular injection, reconstitute with 2 ml of sodium chloride 0.9% (2).

To prepare a skin test solution for intradermal administration, 0.1 ml of the 2000-I.U./ml reconstituted solution (200 I.U.) is added to 9.9 ml of diluent to yield a 20-I.U./ml solution (2).

Units— The International Unit (I.U.) of asparaginase is defined as the quantity of enzyme that will release 1 μmol of ammonia per minute from asparagine under the assay conditions (4). The specific activity of asparaginase (MSD) is at least 225 I.U./mg of protein (2).

pH— Approximately 7.4. The enzyme is active over a pH range of 6.5 to 8 (4).

Osmolality— Asparaginase 2000 I.U./ml in sterile water for injection has an osmolality of 169 mOsm/kg (1689).

Administration— Asparaginase is administered intravenously, over not less than 30 minutes, through the sidearm of a running intravenous infusion of sodium chloride 0.9% or dextrose 5% in water. It may also be administered intramuscularly using a volume no greater than 2 ml; larger volumes require two injection sites (2; 4).

Stability— It is recommended that intact vials of asparaginase be stored under refrigeration (2). However, Merck Sharp & Dohme has indicated that asparaginase is stable for at least 48 hours at room temperature (853).

The manufacturer indicates that the reconstituted solution should be stored under refrigeration and can be used within eight hours as long as the solution is clear. If the solution becomes turbid, it should be discarded (2).

Ordinary shaking during reconstitution does not result in inactivation (4). However, one source indicates that vigorous shaking may result in some loss of potency (284). Vigorous shaking also can cause foaming, making it difficult to withdraw the entire vial contents (4).

Reconstituted solutions of asparaginase may occasionally develop small numbers of gelatinous fibers on standing. Filtration through a 5-μm filter will remove the fibers with no loss of potency, but filtration through a 0.2-μm filter may result in some potency loss (2).

Compatibility Information

Y-Site Injection Compatibility (1:1 Mixture)

					Asparaginase		
Drug	Mfr	Conc	Mfr	Conc	Remarks	Ref	C/I
Methotrexate sodium		30 mg/ml	BEL	120 I.U./ml[a]	Visually compatible for 4 hr at room temperature	1788	C

Y-Site Injection Compatibility (1:1 Mixture) (Cont.)

Asparaginase

Drug	Mfr	Conc	Mfr	Conc	Remarks	Ref	C/I
Sodium bicarbonate		1.4%	BEL	120 I.U./ml[a]	Visually compatible for 4 hr at room temperature	1788	C

[a]*Tested in dextrose 5% in water.*

Additional Compatibility Information

Solutions— Dextrose 5% in water and sodium chloride 0.9% have been recommended as diluents for asparaginase. The manufacturer indicates that such solutions may be used for up to eight hours as long as they remain clear (2).

ATENOLOL
AHFS 24:04

Tenormin I.V.   **Zeneca**

Products— Atenolol (Zeneca) is available in 10-ml ampuls. Each milliliter of solution contains atenolol 0.5 mg with sodium chloride for isotonicity and citric acid and sodium hydroxide to adjust the pH (2).

pH— From 5.5 to 6.5 (2).

Tonicity— The injection is isotonic (2).

Administration— Atenolol is administered undiluted by slow intravenous injection at 1 mg/min or is diluted with dextrose 5% in water or sodium chloride 0.9% (2; 4).

Stability— Intact ampuls should be stored at room temperature and protected from light. According to the manufacturer, admixtures in dextrose- and sodium chloride-containing infusion solutions are stable for 48 hours (2).

Compatibility Information

Y-Site Injection Compatibility (1:1 Mixture)

Atenolol

Drug	Mfr	Conc	Mfr	Conc	Remarks	Ref	C/I
Amphotericin B cholesteryl sulfate complex	SEQ	0.83 mg/ml[a]	ZEN	0.5 mg/ml	Gross precipitate forms	2117	I
Meperidine HCl	AB	10 mg/ml	ICI	0.5 mg/ml	Physically compatible for 4 hr at 25 °C	1397	C
Meropenem	ZEN	1 and 50 mg/ml[b]	ICI	0.5 mg/ml	Visually compatible for 4 hr at room temperature	1994	C
Morphine sulfate	AB	1 mg/ml	ICI	0.5 mg/ml	Physically compatible for 4 hr at 25 °C	1397	C

[a]*Tested in dextrose 5% in water.*
[b]*Tested in sodium chloride 0.9%.*

Additional Compatibility Information

Solutions— The manufacturer recommends the use of dextrose injections, sodium chloride injections, and combinations of the two for dilution of atenolol. Admixtures in these solutions are stable for 48 hours (2).

ATRACURIUM BESYLATE
AHFS 12:20

Tracrium   **Glaxo Wellcome**

Products— Atracurium besylate (Glaxo Wellcome) is available as a 10-mg/ml aqueous solution in 5-ml single-use vials and 10-ml multiple-dose vials with benzyl alcohol 0.9% as a preservative. The pH is adjusted with benzenesulfonic acid (2).

pH— Adjusted to 3.25 to 3.65 (2).

Osmolality— Atracurium besylate 10 mg/ml has an osmolality of 22 mOsm/kg (1689).

Administration— Atracurium besylate is administered by rapid intravenous injection or by intravenous infusion in concentrations of 0.2 and 0.5 mg/ml. It must not be given by intramuscular injection. Do not administer in the same syringe or through the same needle as an alkaline solution (2; 4).

Stability— Atracurium besylate injection is a clear, colorless solution; it should be stored under refrigeration and protected from freezing. Nevertheless, the drug undergoes slow decomposition of about 6% per year (2; 4). The estimated t_{90} at 5 °C is approximately 18 months (859). At 25 °C, the rate of decomposition increases to about 5% per month (2; 4). Glaxo Wellcome has indicated that intact vials of atracurium besylate may be used for 14 days when stored at room temperature (2; 1181).

Atracurium besylate is unstable in the presence of both acids and bases (4). Maximum stability in aqueous solution was observed at about pH 2.5. At 37 °C, aqueous solutions with pH values of 7.1 and 7.6 yielded t_{50} values of 75 and 30 minutes, respectively (859).

Repackaging in Syringes— Atracurium besylate (Burroughs Wellcome) 10 mg/ml was repackaged as 10 ml of solution in 12-ml plastic syringes (Monoject) and stored at 5, 25, and 40 °C. The samples remained visually clear throughout the study. HPLC analysis found no loss in the refrigerated samples and about 4% loss in the room temperature samples after 42 days of storage. The samples stored at elevated temperature lost about 15% in 21 days, indicating that exposure of atracurium to extreme temperature conditions should be avoided. (2141).

The stability of atracurium (salt form unspecified) 10 mg/ml repackaged in polypropylene syringes was evaluated by spectrophotometric and potentiometric methods. Little or no change in concentration was found after four weeks of storage at room temperature when not exposed to direct light (2164).

Compatibility Information

Solution Compatibility

Atracurium besylate

Solution	Mfr	Mfr	Conc/L	Remarks	Ref	C/I
Dextrose 5% in sodium chloride 0.9%		BW	200 and 500 mg	Physically compatible and chemically stable for 24 hr at 5 and 30 °C	1692	C
Dextrose 5% in water		BW	200 and 500 mg	Physically compatible and chemically stable for 24 hr at 5 and 30 °C	1692	C
		BW	1 and 5 g	Chemically stable for 48 hr	1693	C
	BA[a]	BW	0.5 g	About 50% loss by HPLC in 14 days stored at 5 and 25 °C	2141	I
Ringer's injection, lactated		BW	200 and 500 mg	Increased rate of atracurium degradation limits utility time to 8 hr at 25 °C	1692	I
Sodium chloride 0.9%		BW	200 and 500 mg	Physically compatible and chemically stable for 24 hr at 5 and 30 °C	1692	C
		BW	1 and 5 g	Chemically stable for 24 hr	1693	C
	BA[a]	BW	0.5 g	About 60% loss by HPLC in 14 days stored at 5 and 25 °C	2141	I

[a]*Tested in glass containers.*

Additive Compatibility

Atracurium besylate

Drug	Mfr	Conc/L	Mfr	Conc/L	Test Soln	Remarks	Ref	C/I
Aminophylline		1 g	BW	500 mg	D5W	Atracurium chemically unstable due to high pH	1694	I
Bretylium tosylate		4 g	BW	500 mg	D5W	Physically compatible and atracurium chemically stable for 24 hr at 5 and 30 °C	1694	C

Additive Compatibility (Cont.)

Atracurium besylate

Drug	Mfr	Conc/L	Mfr	Conc/L	Test Soln	Remarks	Ref	C/I
Cefazolin sodium		10 g	BW	500 mg	D5W	Atracurium chemically unstable and particles form	1694	I
Cimetidine HCl		5 g	BW	500 mg	D5W	Physically compatible and atracurium chemically stable for 24 hr at 5 and 30 °C	1694	C
Dobutamine HCl		1 g	BW	500 mg	D5W	Physically compatible and atracurium chemically stable for 24 hr at 5 and 30 °C	1694	C
Dopamine HCl		1.6 g	BW	500 mg	D5W	Physically compatible and atracurium chemically stable for 24 hr at 5 and 30 °C	1694	C
Esmolol HCl		10 g	BW	500 mg	D5W	Physically compatible and atracurium chemically stable for 24 hr at 5 and 30 °C	1694	C
Gentamicin sulfate		2 g	BW	500 mg	D5W	Physically compatible and atracurium chemically stable for 24 hr at 5 and 30 °C	1694	C
Heparin sodium		40,000 units	BW	500 mg	D5W	Particles form at 5 and 30 °C	1694	I
Isoproterenol HCl		4 mg	BW	500 mg	D5W	Physically compatible and atracurium chemically stable for 24 hr at 5 and 30 °C	1694	C
Lidocaine HCl		2 g	BW	500 mg	D5W	Physically compatible and atracurium chemically stable for 24 hr at 5 and 30 °C	1694	C
Morphine sulfate		1 g	BW	500 mg	D5W	Physically compatible and atracurium chemically stable for 24 hr at 5 and 30 °C	1694	C
Potassium chloride		80 mEq	BW	500 mg	D5W	Physically compatible and atracurium chemically stable for 24 hr at 5 and 30 °C	1694	C
Procainamide HCl		4 g	BW	500 mg	D5W	Physically compatible and atracurium chemically stable for 24 hr at 5 and 30 °C	1694	C
Quinidine gluconate		8.3 g	BW	500 mg	D5W	Particles form and atracurium chemically unstable at 5 and 30 °C	1694	I
Ranitidine HCl		500 mg	BW	500 mg	D5W	Atracurium chemically unstable due to high pH	1694	I
Sodium nitroprusside		2 g	BW	500 mg	D5W	Physically incompatible. Haze, particles, and yellow color form	1694	I
Vancomycin HCl		5 g	BW	500 mg	D5W	Physically compatible and atracurium chemically stable for 24 hr at 5 and 30 °C	1694	C

Drugs in Syringe Compatibility

Atracurium besylate

Drug (in syringe)	Mfr	Amt	Mfr	Amt	Remarks	Ref	C/I
Alfentanil HCl		0.5 mg/ml	BW	10 mg/ml	Physically compatible and atracurium chemically stable for 24 hr at 5 and 30 °C	1694	**C**
Fentanyl citrate		50 μg/ml	BW	10 mg/ml	Physically compatible and atracurium chemically stable for 24 hr at 5 and 30 °C	1694	**C**
Midazolam HCl		5 mg/ml	BW	10 mg/ml	Physically compatible and atracurium chemically stable for 24 hr at 5 and 30 °C	1694	**C**
Sufentanil citrate		50 μg/ml	BW	10 mg/ml	Physically compatible and atracurium chemically stable for 24 hr at 5 and 30 °C	1694	**C**

Y-Site Injection Compatibility (1:1 Mixture)

Atracurium besylate

Drug	Mfr	Conc	Mfr	Conc	Remarks	Ref	C/I
Cefazolin sodium	LY	10 mg/ml[a]	BW	0.5 mg/ml[a]	Physically compatible for 24 hr at 28 °C	1337	**C**
Cefuroxime sodium	GL	7.5 mg/ml[a]	BW	0.5 mg/ml[a]	Physically compatible for 24 hr at 28 °C	1337	**C**
Cimetidine HCl	SKF	6 mg/ml[a]	BW	0.5 mg/ml[a]	Physically compatible for 24 hr at 28 °C	1337	**C**
Clarithromycin	AB	4 mg/ml[a]	GW	1 mg/ml[a]	Visually compatible for 72 hr at both 30 and 17 °C	2174	**C**
Diazepam	ES	5 mg/ml[a]	BW	0.5 mg/ml[a]	Cloudy solution forms immediately	1337	**I**
Dobutamine HCl	LI	1 mg/ml[a]	BW	0.5 mg/ml[a]	Physically compatible for 24 hr at 28 °C	1337	**C**
Dopamine HCl	SO	1.6 mg/ml[a]	BW	0.5 mg/ml[a]	Physically compatible for 24 hr at 28 °C	1337	**C**
Epinephrine HCl	AB	4 μg/ml[a]	BW	0.5 mg/ml[a]	Physically compatible for 24 hr at 28 °C	1337	**C**
Esmolol HCl	DCC	10 mg/ml[a]	BW	0.5 mg/ml[a]	Physically compatible for 24 hr at 28 °C	1337	**C**
Etomidate	AB	2 mg/ml	BW	10 mg/ml	Visually compatible for up to 7 days at 25 °C	1801	**C**
Fentanyl citrate	ES	10 μg/ml[a]	BW	0.5 mg/ml[a]	Physically compatible for 24 hr at 28 °C	1337	**C**
Gentamicin sulfate	ES	2 mg/ml[a]	BW	0.5 mg/ml[a]	Physically compatible for 24 hr at 28 °C	1337	**C**
Heparin sodium	SO	40 units/ml[a]	BW	0.5 mg/ml[a]	Physically compatible for 24 hr at 28 °C	1337	**C**
Hydrocortisone sodium succinate	AB	1 mg/ml[a]	BW	0.5 mg/ml[a]	Physically compatible for 24 hr at 28 °C	1337	**C**
Isoproterenol HCl	ES	4 μg/ml[a]	BW	0.5 mg/ml[a]	Physically compatible for 24 hr at 28 °C	1337	**C**
Lorazepam	WY	0.5 mg/ml[a]	BW	0.5 mg/ml[a]	Physically compatible for 24 hr at 28 °C	1337	**C**
Midazolam HCl	RC	0.05 mg/ml[a]	BW	0.5 mg/ml[a]	Physically compatible for 24 hr at 28 °C	1337	**C**
	RC	0.1 mg/ml[a]	GW	1 and 5 mg/ml[a]	Visually compatible with no loss of either drug by HPLC in 3 hr at 25 °C under fluorescent light	2112	**C**
	RC	0.5 mg/ml[a]	GW	5 mg/ml[a]	Visually compatible with no loss of either drug by HPLC in 3 hr at 25 °C under fluorescent light	2112	**C**
	RC	0.5 mg/ml[a]	GW	1 mg/ml[a]	Visually compatible with no loss of midazolam and 4% loss of atracurium by HPLC in 3 hr at 25 °C under fluorescent light	2112	**C**
Milrinone lactate	SW	0.4 mg/ml[a]	BW	1 mg/ml[a]	Visually compatible with little or no loss of either drug by HPLC in 4 hr at 23 °C	2214	**C**

Y-Site Injection Compatibility (1:1 Mixture) (Cont.)

Atracurium besylate

Drug	Mfr	Conc	Mfr	Conc	Remarks	Ref	C/I
Morphine sulfate	WY	1 mg/ml[a]	BW	0.5 mg/ml[a]	Physically compatible for 24 hr at 28 °C	1337	**C**
Nitroglycerin	SO	0.4 mg/ml[a]	BW	0.5 mg/ml[a]	Physically compatible for 24 hr at 28 °C	1337	**C**
Propofol	STU	2 mg/ml	BW	10 mg/ml	Oil droplets form within 24 hr followed by phase separation at 25 °C	1801	**I**
	ZEN	10 mg/ml	BW	10 mg/ml	Emulsion broke and oiled out	2066	**I**
Ranitidine HCl	GL	0.5 mg/ml[a]	BW	0.5 mg/ml[a]	Physically compatible for 24 hr at 28 °C	1337	**C**
Sodium nitroprusside	ES	0.2 mg/ml[a]	BW	0.5 mg/ml[a]	Physically compatible for 24 hr at 28 °C	1337	**C**
Thiopental sodium	AB	25 mg/ml	BW	10 mg/ml	White cloudiness forms immediately but clears within 24 hr at 25 °C	1801	**I**
TPN #189[b]			WEL	10 mg/ml	Visually compatible for 24 hr at 22 °C	1767	**C**
Trimethoprim–sulfamethoxazole	ES	0.64 + 3.2 mg/ml[a]	BW	0.5 mg/ml[a]	Physically compatible for 24 hr at 28 °C	1337	**C**
Vancomycin HCl	ES	5 mg/ml[a]	BW	0.5 mg/ml[a]	Physically compatible for 24 hr at 28 °C	1337	**C**

[a]*Tested in dextrose 5% in water.*
[b]*Refer to Appendix I for the composition of parenteral nutrition solutions. TPN indicates a 2-in-1 admixture.*

Additional Compatibility Information

Vehicles— Atracurium besylate 0.2 and 0.5 mg/ml is physically and chemically compatible for 24 hours at 5 and 25 °C in dextrose 5% in water, sodium chloride 0.9%, and dextrose 5% in sodium chloride 0.9%. In Ringer's injection, lactated, at 0.5 mg/ml, it is stable for eight hours at 25 °C, although use of this solution is not generally recommended because of an increased rate of drug degradation (4).

Alkaline Solutions— Atracurium besylate, which has an acid pH, should not be mixed with alkaline solutions such as barbiturates. Atracurium besylate may be inactivated and precipitation of a free acid of the admixed drug may occur, depending on the resultant pH (2; 4).

ATROPINE SULFATE
AHFS 12:08.08

Fujisawa
Abbott

Products— Atropine sulfate injection (Fujisawa) is available in a concentration of 0.4 mg/ml in 1-ml and 20-ml multiple-dose vials. It is also available in concentrations of 0.5 and 1 mg/ml in 1-ml multiple-dose vials. Each formulation also contains in each milliliter methylparaben 0.1% and sulfuric acid to adjust the pH (if needed) in water for injection (1-7/95).

Atropine sulfate (Abbott) is available in a concentration of 0.1 mg/ml in 5- and 10-ml prefilled syringes. Each milliliter of the formulation also contains sodium chloride 9 mg and sulfuric acid and/or sodium hydroxide to adjust the pH (1-11/93).

pH— From 3 to 6.5 (4).

Administration— Atropine sulfate injection may be administered by subcutaneous, intramuscular, or direct (usually rapid) intravenous injection (4).

Stability— Atropine sulfate injection should be stored below 40 °C, preferably at room temperature. Freezing should be avoided (4). Minimum hydrolysis occurs at pH 3.5 (1072).

Atropine sulfate (Wyeth) 1 mg/ml was found to retain potency for three months at room temperature when 0.5 or 1 ml of solution was packaged in Tubex (13).

Syringes— The stability of atropine (salt form unspecified) 1 mg/ml repackaged in polypropylene syringes was evaluated by spectrophotometric and potentiometric methods. Little or no change in concentration was found after four weeks of storage at room temperature not exposed to direct light (2164).

Compatibility Information

Additive Compatibility

Atropine sulfate

Drug	Mfr	Conc/L	Mfr	Conc/L	Test Soln	Remarks	Ref	C/I
Dobutamine HCl	LI	167 mg	AB	16.7 mg	NS	Physically compatible for 24 hr	552	C
	LI	1 g	ES	50 mg	D5W, NS	Physically compatible for 24 hr at 21 °C	812	C
Floxacillin sodium	BE	20 g	ANT	60 mg	W	Haze forms in 24 hr and precipitate forms in 48 hr at 30 °C. No change at 15 °C	1479	I
Furosemide	HO	1 g	ANT	60 mg	W	Physically compatible for 72 hr at 15 and 30 °C	1479	C
Meropenem	ZEN	1 and 20 g	ES	40 mg	NS	Visually compatible for 4 hr at room temperature	1994	C
Netilmicin sulfate	SC	3 g	BW	40 mg	D5S	Physically compatible and netilmicin chemically stable for 7 days at 4 and 25 °C. Atropine not tested	558	C
Sodium bicarbonate	AB	2.4 mEq[a]		0.4 mg	D5W	Physically compatible for 24 hr	772	C
Verapamil HCl	KN	80 mg	IX	0.8 mg	D5W, NS	Physically compatible for 24 hr	764	C

[a]One vial of Neut added to a liter of admixture.

Drugs in Syringe Compatibility

Atropine sulfate

Drug (in syringe)	Mfr	Amt	Mfr	Amt	Remarks	Ref	C/I
Butorphanol tartrate	BR	4 mg/ 2 ml	ST	0.4 mg/ 1 ml	Physically compatible both macroscopically and microscopically for 30 min at room temperature	566	C
Chlorpromazine HCl	SKF	50 mg/ 2 ml		0.6 mg/ 1.5 ml	Physically compatible for at least 15 min	14	C
	PO	50 mg/ 2 ml	ST	0.4 mg/ 1 ml	Physically compatible for at least 15 min	326	C
Cimetidine HCl	SKF	300 mg/ 2 ml	LI	0.6 mg/ 1.5 ml	Physically compatible and chemically stable for 90 min at room temperature	542	C
	SKF	300 mg/ 2 ml	LI	0.4 mg/ 1 ml	Physically compatible and chemically stable for 90 min at room temperature	542	C
Cimetidine HCl with pentobarbital sodium	SKF AB	300 mg/ 2 ml 100 mg/ 2 ml	LI	0.6 mg/ 1.5 ml	Immediate precipitation	542	I
Dimenhydrinate	HR	50 mg/ 1 ml	ST	0.4 mg/ 1 ml	Physically compatible for at least 15 min	326	C
Diphenhydramine HCl	PD	50 mg/ 1 ml	ST	0.4 mg/ 1 ml	Physically compatible for at least 15 min	326	C
Droperidol	MN	2.5 mg/ 1 ml	ST	0.4 mg/ 1 ml	Physically compatible for at least 15 min	326	C
Fentanyl citrate	MN	100 μg/ 1 ml		0.6 mg/ 1.5 ml	Physically compatible for at least 15 min	14	C
	MN	0.05 mg/ 1 ml	ST	0.4 mg/ 1 ml	Physically compatible for at least 15 min	326	C
Glycopyrrolate	RB	0.2 mg/ 1 ml	ES	0.4 mg/ 1 ml	Physically compatible and pH in stability range for glycopyrrolate for 48 hr at 25 °C	331	C

Drugs in Syringe Compatibility (Cont.)

Atropine sulfate

Drug (in syringe)	Mfr	Amt	Mfr	Amt	Remarks	Ref	C/I
	RB	0.2 mg/ 1 ml	ES	0.8 mg/ 2 ml	Physically compatible and pH in stability range for glycopyrrolate for 48 hr at 25 °C	331	**C**
	RB	0.4 mg/ 2 ml	ES	0.4 mg/ 1 ml	Physically compatible and pH in stability range for glycopyrrolate for 48 hr at 25 °C	331	**C**
Heparin sodium		2500 units/ 1 ml		0.5 mg/ 1 ml	Physically compatible for at least 5 min	1053	**C**
Hydromorphone HCl	KN	4 mg/ 2 ml	ES	0.4 mg/ 0.5 ml	Physically compatible for 30 min	517	**C**
Hydroxyzine HCl	PF	100 mg/ 4 ml		0.6 mg/ 1.5 ml	Physically compatible for at least 15 min	14	**C**
	NF	50 mg/ 1 ml	USP	0.4 mg/ 0.4 ml	Hydroxyzine potency retained for at least 10 days at 3 and 25 °C	49	**C**
	PF	50 mg/ 1 ml	ST	0.4 mg/ 1 ml	Physically compatible for at least 15 min	326	**C**
	PF	100 mg/ 2 ml		0.4 mg/ 1 ml	Physically compatible	771	**C**
	PF	50 mg/ 1 ml		0.4 mg/ 1 ml	Physically compatible	771	**C**
Hydroxyzine HCl with meperidine HCl[a]	PF WI	50 mg 50 mg	ES	0.4 mg/ 2.5 ml	No alteration of UV spectra in 10 days at 3 and 25 °C	301	**C**
Meperidine HCl	WY	100 mg/ 1 ml		0.6 mg/ 1.5 ml	Physically compatible for at least 15 min	14	**C**
	WI	50 mg/ 1 ml	ST	0.4 mg/ 1 ml	Physically compatible for at least 15 min	326	**C**
Meperidine HCl with hydroxyzine HCl[a]	WI PF	50 mg 50 mg	ES	0.4 mg/ 2.5 ml	No alteration of UV spectra in 10 days at 3 and 25 °C	301	**C**
Meperidine HCl with promethazine HCl	WY WY	100 mg/ 1 ml 50 mg/ 2 ml		0.6 mg/ 1.5 ml	Physically compatible	14	**C**
Meperidine HCl with promethazine HCl	WI WY	50 mg/ 1 ml 25 mg/ 1 ml	LI	0.4 mg/ 1 ml	No loss of any drug in 24 hr at 25 °C. Slight haze at 24 hr but not at 6 hr	991	**C**
Metoclopramide HCl	NO	10 mg/ 2 ml	GL	0.4 mg/ 1 ml	Physically compatible both macroscopically and microscopically for 15 min at room temperature	565	**C**
Midazolam HCl	RC	5 mg/ 1 ml	IX	0.4 mg/ 1 ml	Physically compatible for 4 hr at 25 °C	1145	**C**
Milrinone lactate	WI	5.25 mg/ 5.25 ml	IX	2 mg/ 2 ml	Physically compatible with no loss of either drug in 20 min at 23 °C	1410	**C**
Morphine sulfate	WY	15 mg/ 1 ml		0.6 mg/ 1.5 ml	Physically compatible for at least 15 min	14	**C**
	ST	15 mg/ 1 ml	ST	0.4 mg/ 1 ml	Physically compatible for at least 15 min	326	**C**
Nalbuphine HCl	EN	10 mg/ 1 ml	WY	0.2 mg	Physically compatible for 36 hr at 27 °C	762	**C**
	EN	5 mg/ 0.5 ml	WY	0.2 mg	Physically compatible for 36 hr at 27 °C	762	**C**

Drugs in Syringe Compatibility (Cont.)

Atropine sulfate

Drug (in syringe)	Mfr	Amt	Mfr	Amt	Remarks	Ref	C/I
	EN	10 mg/ 1 ml	WY	0.5 mg	Physically compatible for 36 hr at 27 °C	762	C
	EN	5 mg/ 0.5 ml	WY	0.5 mg	Physically compatible for 36 hr at 27 °C	762	C
	DU	10 mg/ 1 ml		0.4 mg	Physically compatible for 48 hr	128	C
	DU	20 mg/ 1 ml		0.4 mg	Physically compatible for 48 hr	128	C
	DU	10 mg/ 1 ml		1 mg	Physically compatible for 48 hr	128	C
	DU	20 mg/ 1 ml		1 mg	Physically compatible for 48 hr	128	C
Ondansetron HCl	GW	1.33 mg/ ml[b]	GNS	0.133 mg/ ml[b]	Physically compatible with no measured increase in particulates and less than 6% ondansetron loss and less than 7% atropine loss by HPLC in 24 hr at 4 or 23 °C	2199	C
Pentazocine lactate	WI	30 mg/ 1 ml		0.6 mg/ 1.5 ml	Physically compatible for at least 15 min	14	C
	WI	30 mg/ 1 ml	ST	0.4 mg/ 1 ml	Physically compatible for at least 15 min	326	C
Pentobarbital sodium	WY	100 mg/ 2 ml		0.6 mg/ 1.5 ml	Physically compatible for at least 15 min	14	C
	AB	50 mg/ 1 ml	ST	0.4 mg/ 1 ml	Physically compatible for at least 15 min	326	C
	AB	100 mg/ 2 ml	LI	0.6 mg/ 1.5 ml	Precipitate forms within 24 hr at room temperature	542	I
Pentobarbital sodium with cimetidine HCl	AB SKF	100 mg/ 2 ml 300 mg/ 2 ml	LI	0.6 mg/ 1.5 ml	Immediate precipitation	542	I
Perphenazine	SC	5 mg/ 1 ml	ST	0.4 mg/ 1 ml	Physically compatible both macroscopically and microscopically for 30 min at room temperature	566	C
Prochlorperazine edisylate	SKF			0.6 mg/ 1.5 ml	Physically compatible for at least 15 min	14	C
	PO	5 mg/ 1 ml	ST	0.4 mg/ 1 ml	Physically compatible for at least 15 min	326	C
Promazine HCl	WY	50 mg/ 1 ml	ST	0.4 mg/ 1 ml	Physically compatible for at least 15 min	326	C
Promethazine HCl	WY	50 mg/ 2 ml		0.6 mg/ 1.5 ml	Physically compatible for at least 15 min	14	C
	PO	50 mg/ 2 ml	ST	0.4 mg/ 1 ml	Physically compatible for at least 15 min	326	C
Promethazine HCl with meperidine HCl	WY WY	50 mg/ 2 ml 100 mg/ 1 ml		0.6 mg/ 1.5 ml	Physically compatible	14	C
Promethazine HCl with meperidine HCl	WY WI	25 mg/ 1 ml 50 mg/ 1 ml	LI	0.4 mg/ 1 ml	No loss of any drug in 24 hr at 25 °C. Slight haze at 24 hr but not at 6 hr	991	C

Drugs in Syringe Compatibility (Cont.)

Atropine sulfate

Drug (in syringe)	Mfr	Amt	Mfr	Amt	Remarks	Ref	C/I
Propiomazine HCl	WY	20 mg/ 1 ml	WY	0.5 mg/ 0.5 ml	Potency retained for 1 month under refrigeration in Tubex	13	**C**
	WY	40 mg/ 2 ml	WY	0.5 mg/ 0.5 ml	Potency retained for 1 month under refrigeration in Tubex	13	**C**
Ranitidine HCl	GL	50 mg/ 2 ml	GL	0.4 mg/ 1 ml	Physically compatible for 1 hr at 25 °C by macroscopic and microscopic inspection	978	**C**
Scopolamine HBr	ST	0.4 mg/ 1 ml	ST	0.4 mg/ 1 ml	Physically compatible for at least 15 min	326	**C**
Sufentanil citrate	JN	50 μg/ml	LY	0.4 mg/ ml	Physically compatible with no subvisual haze or particle formation in 24 hr at 23 °C	1711	**C**

[a]Tested in both glass and plastic syringes.
[b]Tested in sodium chloride 0.9%.

Y-Site Injection Compatibility (1:1 Mixture)

Atropine sulfate

Drug	Mfr	Conc	Mfr	Conc	Remarks	Ref	C/I
Amrinone lactate	WB	3 mg/ml[b]	AB	0.1 mg/ml	Physically compatible for at least 4 hr at 25 °C under fluorescent light	992	**C**
Etomidate	AB	2 mg/ml	GNS	0.4 mg/ml	Visually compatible for up to 7 days at 25 °C	1801	**C**
Famotidine	MSD	0.2 mg/ml[a]	AST	0.1 mg/ml[a]	Physically compatible for at least 4 hr at 25 °C under fluorescent light	1188	**C**
Heparin sodium	UP	1000 units/L[c]	BW	0.5 mg/ml	Physically compatible for at least 4 hr at room temperature by visual and microscopic examination	534	**C**
Hydrocortisone sodium succinate	UP	10 mg/L[c]	BW	0.5 mg/ml	Physically compatible for at least 4 hr at room temperature by visual and microscopic examination	534	**C**
Meropenem	ZEN	1 and 50 mg/ml[b]	ES	0.4 mg/ml[d]	Visually compatible for 4 hr at room temperature	1994	**C**
Nafcillin sodium	WY	33 mg/ml[b]		0.4 mg/ml	No precipitation	547	**C**
Potassium chloride	AB	40 mEq/L[c]	BW	0.5 mg/ml	Physically compatible for at least 4 hr at room temperature by visual and microscopic examination	534	**C**
Propofol	STU	2 mg/ml	GNS	0.4 mg/ml	Oil droplets form within 7 days at 25 °C. No visible change in 24 hr	1801	**?**
	ZEN	10 mg/ml	AST	0.1 mg/ml[a]	Physically compatible for 1 hr at 23 °C with no increase in particle content	2066	**C**
Sufentanil citrate	JN	12.5 μg/ml[a]	LY	0.4 mg/ml[a]	Physically compatible with no subvisual haze or particle formation in 24 hr at 23 °C	1711	**C**
Thiopental sodium	AB	25 mg/ml	GNS	0.4 mg/ml	White particles form immediately and yellow discoloration forms within 24 hr at 25 °C	1801	**I**

Y-Site Injection Compatibility (1:1 Mixture) (Cont.)

Atropine sulfate

Drug	Mfr	Conc	Mfr	Conc	Remarks	Ref	C/I
Vitamin B complex with C	RC	2 ml/L[c]	BW	0.5 mg/ml	Physically compatible for at least 4 hr at room temperature by visual and microscopic examination	534	C

[a]*Tested in dextrose 5% in water.*
[b]*Tested in sodium chloride 0.9%.*
[c]*Tested in dextrose 5% in water, dextrose 5% in Ringer's injection, dextrose 5% in Ringer's injection, lactated, Ringer's injection, lactated, and sodium chloride 0.9%.*
[d]*Tested in sterile water for injection.*

Additional Compatibility Information

Additives— Atropine sulfate has been reported to be compatible with butorphanol tartrate (481) and buprenorphine HCl (4). Atropine sulfate is stated to be incompatible with sodium bicarbonate, norepinephrine bitartrate, and metaraminol bitartrate (4).

A haze or precipitate forms in 15 minutes when atropine sulfate is mixed with methohexital sodium (4).

AZATHIOPRINE SODIUM
AHFS 92:00

Imuran   **Glaxo Wellcome**

Products— Azathioprine sodium (Glaxo Wellcome) is available in 20-ml vials containing the equivalent of 100 mg of azathioprine with sodium hydroxide to adjust the pH. Reconstitute by adding 10 ml of sterile water for injection and swirling until a clear solution results (2).

pH— Approximately 9.6 (2).

Administration— Azathioprine sodium is administered intravenously by direct injection or intermittent or continuous infusion (8). Infusions are usually administered over 30 to 60 minutes but have been given over five minutes to eight hours (2; 4).

Stability— Azathioprine, a pale yellow powder, should be stored at controlled room temperature and protected from light. It is stated to be stable in neutral or acid solutions but is hydrolyzed to mercaptopurine in alkaline solutions (2; 4), especially on warming (2).

Maximum stability occurs at pH 5.5 to 6.5 (1633). Hydrolysis to mercaptopurine also occurs in the presence of sulfhydryl compounds such as cysteine (2; 4).

Use of azathioprine sodium within 24 hours after reconstitution is recommended because the product contains no preservatives (2; 4). Chemically, azathioprine sodium 10 mg/ml in aqueous solution is stable for about two weeks at room temperature (4). After this time, hydrolysis of azathioprine to mercaptopurine increases.

Storage of the reconstituted solution in the original vial and in plastic syringes (Jelco) at 20 to 25 °C under fluorescent light resulted in no decomposition or precipitation in 16 days. At 4 °C in the dark, a visible precipitate formed after four days (605).

Azathioprine sodium (Burroughs Wellcome) 100 mg/50 ml diluted in dextrose 5% in water, sodium chloride 0.9%, or sodium chloride 0.45% in PVC bags (Travenol) was stored at 20 to 25 °C under fluorescent light and at 4 °C in the dark. No decomposition occurred in the solutions over 16 days of storage. However, a precipitate formed in the dextrose 5% in water admixtures by the 16th day. No precipitate was observed after eight days of storage (605).

Compatibility Information

Solution Compatibility

Azathioprine sodium

Solution	Mfr	Mfr	Conc/L	Remarks	Ref	C/I
Dextrose 5% in water	TR[a]	BW	2 g	Physically compatible and chemically stable for 8 days at 23 and 4 °C. Precipitate forms in 16 days	605	C
Sodium chloride 0.45%	TR[a]	BW	2 g	Physically compatible and chemically stable for 16 days at 23 and 4 °C	605	C

Solution Compatibility (Cont.)

Azathioprine sodium

Solution	Mfr	Mfr	Conc/L	Remarks	Ref	C/I
Sodium chloride 0.9%	TR[a]	BW	2 g	Physically compatible and chemically stable for 16 days at 23 and 4 °C	605	C

[a]Tested in PVC containers.

Additional Compatibility Information

Preservatives— Azathioprine sodium is stated to be incompatible with methyl and propyl parabens and phenol (108).

Other Information

Inactivation— In the event of spills or leaks, the manufacturer recommends the use of sodium hypochlorite 5% (household bleach) and sodium hydroxide (concentration unspecified) to inactivate azathioprine (1200).

AZTREONAM
AHFS 8:12.07

Azactam   **Bristol-Myers Squibb**

Products— Aztreonam (Bristol-Myers Squibb) is available in vials and 100-ml infusion bottles containing 500 mg, 1 g, or 2 g of drug. Approximately 780 mg of arginine per gram of drug is also present (2).

For intramuscular injection, reconstitute each gram of drug in vials with at least 3 ml of one of the following diluents (2):

Sterile water for injection
Bacteriostatic water for injection
   (benzyl alcohol or parabens)
Sodium chloride 0.9%
Bacteriostatic sodium chloride 0.9%
   (benzyl alcohol)

For intravenous bolus injection, use the vials. Reconstitute with 6 to 10 ml of sterile water for injection (2).

For intravenous infusion, use the 100-ml bottle. Reconstitute each gram of drug with at least 50 ml of any compatible infusion solution to yield a solution containing not more than 2% (w/v) of aztreonam. Alternatively, reconstitute a vial of aztreonam with at least 3 ml of sterile water for injection per gram and further dilute with a compatible infusion solution (2).

On adding the diluent to the vial or bottle, shake the contents immediately and vigorously (2).

pH— Aqueous solutions of aztreonam have pH values of 4.5 to 7.5 (2).

Sodium Content— Aztreonam is sodium free (2).

Administration— Aztreonam may be administered by intravenous injection or infusion or by deep intramuscular injection into a large muscle mass. By intravenous injection, the dose should be given slowly, over three to five minutes, directly into a vein or the tubing of a compatible infusion solution. Intermittent infusion at concentrations not exceeding 1 g/50 ml should be completed within 20 to 60 minutes (2; 4).

Stability— The intact vials should be stored at controlled room temperature and protected from temperatures above 40 °C. Exposure to strong light may cause yellowing of the powder (2; 4).

Aztreonam solutions range from colorless to light straw to yellow. They may develop a slight pink tint on standing without potency being affected (2).

Aztreonam solutions at concentrations of 2% (w/v) or less should be used within 48 hours if stored at room temperature or seven days if refrigerated. Solutions with concentrations exceeding 2% (w/v) should be used immediately after preparation unless sterile water for injection or sodium chloride 0.9% is used. In these two excepted solutions, aztreonam at concentrations exceeding 2% (w/v) may be used up to 48 hours at room temperature or seven days under refrigeration (2).

Aztreonam (Squibb) 2 g in sodium chloride 0.9% (volume unspecified), stored in polypropylene syringes (3M) at 25 °C under fluorescent light, exhibited a 5% loss in 48 hours (1164).

Freezing Solutions— Aztreonam in any compatible infusion solution is stable for up to three months when frozen at −20 °C. Frozen solutions should be thawed at room temperature or by overnight refrigeration and should not be refrozen. Thawed solutions should be used within 24 hours at room temperature or 72 hours under refrigeration (4).

The commercially available frozen injection should be thawed at room temperature or under refrigeration and should not be refrozen. The manufacturer indicates that thawed solutions are stable for 48 hours at room temperature or 14 days under refrigeration (4).

Aztreonam (Squibb) 20 mg/ml in sodium chloride 0.9% exhibited no loss by HPLC after 120 days when stored at −20 °C. Storage of the solution at 4 °C resulted in a 10% loss in a time period greater than 120 days and has the advantage of not requiring thawing (1600).

pH Effects— In aqueous solutions, aztreonam undergoes hydrolysis of the β-lactam ring. Specific base catalysis occurs at pH greater than 6. At pH 2 to 5, isomerization of the side chain predominates. The lowest rates of decomposition occur at pH 5 to 7, with maximum stability occurring at pH 6 (1072).

Compatibility Information

Solution Compatibility

Aztreonam

Solution	Mfr	Mfr	Conc/L	Remarks	Ref	C/I
Dextrose 5% in water	TR[a]	SQ	10 g	Physically compatible with 6% aztreonam loss in 48 hr at 25 °C and 3% in 7 days at 4 °C	1001	C
	TR[a]	SQ	20 g	Physically compatible with 2% aztreonam loss in 48 hr at 25 °C and 3% in 7 days at 4 °C	1001	C
	MG[b]	SQ	20 g	Physically compatible with no aztreonam loss in 48 hr at 25 °C under fluorescent light	1026	C
Sodium chloride 0.9%	TR[a]	SQ	10 and 20 g	Physically compatible with little or no aztreonam loss in 48 hr at 25 °C and 7 days at 4 °C	1001	C
	MG[b]	SQ	20 g	Physically compatible with no aztreonam loss in 48 hr at 25 °C under fluorescent light	1026	C
	BA	SQ	20 g	10% loss by HPLC in 37 days at 25 °C and more than 120 days at 4 °C. No loss in 120 days at −20 °C	1600	C
	[a]	SQ	10 g	Visually compatible with no aztreonam loss by HPLC in 96 hr at 5 and 24 °C	1739	C
TPN #107[c]			2 g	Physically compatible and aztreonam activity retained for 24 hr at 21 °C by microbiological assay	1326	C

[a]Tested in PVC containers.
[b]Tested in glass containers.
[c]Refer to Appendix I for the composition of parenteral nutrition solutions. TPN indicates a 2-in-1 admixture.

Additive Compatibility

Aztreonam

Drug	Mfr	Conc/L	Mfr	Conc/L	Test Soln	Remarks	Ref	C/I
Ampicillin sodium	WY	20 g	SQ	10 g	D5W[a]	10% ampicillin loss in 2 hr and 10% aztreonam loss in 3 hr at 25 °C. 10% ampicillin loss in 24 hr and 10% aztreonam loss in 8 hr at 4 °C	1001	I
	WY	5 g	SQ	10 g	D5W[a]	10% ampicillin loss in 3 hr and 10% aztreonam loss in 7 hr at 25 °C. 10% loss of both drugs in 48 hr at 4 °C	1001	I
	WY	20 g	SQ	20 g	D5W[a]	10% ampicillin loss in 4 hr and 10% aztreonam loss in 8 hr at 25 °C. 10% ampicillin loss in 48 hr and 10% aztreonam loss in 72 hr at 4 °C	1001	I
	WY	5 g	SQ	20 g	D5W[a]	10% ampicillin loss in 5 hr and 10% aztreonam loss in 48 hr at 25 °C. 10% ampicillin loss in 48 hr and 10% aztreonam loss in 72 hr at 4 °C	1001	I
	WY	20 g	SQ	10 g	NS[a]	10% ampicillin loss in 24 hr and 2% aztreonam loss in 48 hr at 25 °C. 10% ampicillin loss in 2 days and 9% aztreonam loss in 7 days at 4 °C	1001	C
	WY	5 g	SQ	10 g	NS[a]	10% ampicillin loss and no aztreonam loss in 48 hr at 25 °C. 10% ampicillin loss in 3 days and 8% aztreonam loss in 7 days at 4 °C	1001	C

Additive Compatibility (Cont.)

	Aztreonam							
Drug	*Mfr*	*Conc/L*	*Mfr*	*Conc/L*	*Test Soln*	*Remarks*	*Ref*	*C/I*
	WY	20 g	SQ	20 g	NS[a]	10% ampicillin loss in 24 hr and 5% aztreonam loss in 48 hr at 25 °C. 10% ampicillin loss in 2 days and 7% aztreonam loss in 7 days at 4 °C	1001	**C**
	WY	20 g	SQ	5 g	NS[a]	10% ampicillin loss and no aztreonam loss in 48 hr at 25 °C. 10% ampicillin loss and 5% aztreonam loss in 7 days at 4 °C	1001	**C**
Ampicillin sodium–sulbactam sodium	PF	20 + 10 g	SQ	10 g	NS[a]	Visually compatible with 10% ampicillin loss by HPLC in 30 hr at 24 °C and 94 hr at 5 °C. Ampicillin loss is determining factor	1691	**C**
Cefazolin sodium	LI	5 and 20 g	SQ	10 and 20 g	D5W, NS[a]	Physically compatible and little or no loss of either drug in 48 hr at 25 °C and 7 days at 4 °C protected from light	1002	**C**
Cefoxitin sodium	MSD	10 and 20 g	SQ	10 and 20 g	NS[a]	3 to 5% aztreonam loss and no cefoxitin loss in 7 days at 4 °C	1023	**C**
	MSD	10 and 20 g	SQ	10 and 20 g	D5W[a]	3 to 6% cefoxitin loss and no aztreonam loss in 7 days at 4 °C	1023	**C**
	MSD	10 and 20 g	SQ	10 and 20 g	D5W, NS[a]	Both drugs stable for 12 hr at 25 °C. Yellow color accompanied 6 to 12% aztreonam loss and 9 to 15% cefoxitin loss in 48 hr at 25 °C	1023	**I**
Ciprofloxacin	MI	1 g	SQ	20 g	D5W, NS	Physically compatible for 24 hr at 22 °C under fluorescent light	1189	**C**
Clindamycin phosphate	UP	3 and 6 g	SQ	10 and 20 g	D5W, NS[a]	Physically compatible and little or no loss of either drug in 48 hr at 25 °C and 7 days at 4 °C	1002	**C**
	UP	9 g	SQ	20 g	D5W[b]	Physically compatible with 3% clindamycin loss and 5% aztreonam loss in 48 hr at 25 °C under fluorescent light	1026	**C**
	UP	9 g	SQ	20 g	NS[b]	Physically compatible with 2% clindamycin loss and no aztreonam loss in 48 hr at 25 °C under fluorescent light	1026	**C**
Gentamicin sulfate	SC	200 and 800 mg	SQ	10 and 20 g	D5W, NS[a]	Little or no aztreonam loss in 48 hr at 25 °C and 7 days at 4 °C. Gentamicin potency retained for 12 hr at 25 °C and 24 hr at 4 °C with up to 10% loss in 48 hr at 25 °C and 7 days at 4 °C	1023	**C**
Metronidazole	MG	5 g	SQ	10 and 20 g		Pink color develops in 12 hr, becoming cherry red in 48 hr at 25 °C. Pink color develops in 3 days at 4 °C. No loss of either drug detected	1023	**I**
Nafcillin sodium	BR	20 g	SQ	20 g	D5W, NS[a]	Cloudiness with fine precipitation forms gradually. 6 to 7% aztreonam loss and 10 to 11% nafcillin loss in 24 hr at room temperature	1028	**I**
Tobramycin sulfate	LI	200 and 800 mg	SQ	10 and 20 g	D5W, NS[a]	Little or no loss of either drug in 48 hr at 25 °C and 7 days at 4 °C	1023	**C**

Additive Compatibility (Cont.)

Drug	Mfr	Conc/L	Mfr	Conc/L	Test Soln	Remarks	Ref	C/I
Vancomycin HCl	AB	10 g	SQ	40 g	D5W, NS	Microcrystalline precipitate forms immediately. Gross turbidity and precipitate form over 24 hours	1848	I
	AB	1 g	SQ	4 g	D5W	Physically compatible with little or no loss of either drug in 31 days at 4 °C. About 8 to 10% aztreonam loss in 14 days at 23 °C and 7 days at 32 °C	1848	C
	AB	1 g	SQ	4 g	NS	Physically compatible with little or no loss of either drug in 31 days at 4 °C. About 5 to 8% aztreonam loss in 31 days at 23 °C and 7 days at 32 °C	1848	C

[a]Tested in PVC containers.
[b]Tested in glass containers.

Drugs in Syringe Compatibility

Drug (in syringe)	Mfr	Amt	Mfr	Amt	Remarks	Ref	C/I
Clindamycin phosphate	UP	600 mg/4 ml	SQ	2 g	Physically compatible with 2% clindamycin loss and 8% aztreonam loss in 48 hr at 25 °C under fluorescent light in polypropylene syringes	1164	C

Y-Site Injection Compatibility (1:1 Mixture)

Drug	Mfr	Conc	Mfr	Conc	Remarks	Ref	C/I
Acyclovir sodium	BW	7 mg/ml[a]	SQ	40 mg/ml[a]	White crystalline needles form immediately and become dense flocculent precipitate in 4 hr	1758	I
Allopurinol sodium	BW	3 mg/ml[b]	SQ	40 mg/ml[b]	Physically compatible with no change in measured turbidity or increase in particle content in 4 hr at 22 °C	1686	C
Amifostine	USB	10 mg/ml[a]	WY	20 mg/ml[a]	Physically compatible with no change in measured turbidity or increase in particle content in 4 hr at 23 °C	1845	C
Amikacin sulfate	BMS	5 mg/ml[a]	SQ	40 mg/ml[a]	Physically compatible with no subvisual haze or particle formation in 4 hr at 23 °C	1758	C
Aminophylline	AMR	2.5 mg/ml[a]	SQ	40 mg/ml[a]	Physically compatible with no subvisual haze or particle formation in 4 hr at 23 °C	1758	C
Amphotericin B	PHT	0.6 mg/ml[a]	SQ	40 mg/ml[a]	Yellow turbidity forms immediately and becomes flocculent precipitate in 4 hr	1758	I
Amphotericin B cholesteryl sulfate complex	SEQ	0.83 mg/ml[a]	SQ	40 mg/ml[a]	Gross precipitate forms	2117	I
Ampicillin sodium	WY	20 mg/ml[b]	SQ	40 mg/ml[a]	Physically compatible with no subvisual haze or particle formation in 4 hr at 23 °C	1758	C

Y-Site Injection Compatibility (1:1 Mixture) (Cont.)

		Aztreonam					
Drug	*Mfr*	*Conc*	*Mfr*	*Conc*	*Remarks*	*Ref*	*C/I*
Ampicillin sodium–sulbactam sodium	RR	20 + 10 mg/ml[b]	SQ	40 mg/ml[a]	Physically compatible with no subvisual haze or particle formation in 4 hr at 23 °C	1758	**C**
Amsacrine	NCI	1 mg/ml[a]	SQ	40 mg/ml[a]	Immediate light yellow-orange turbidity, developing into flocculent precipitate in 4 hr	1381	**I**
Bleomycin sulfate	MJ	1 unit/ml[b]	SQ	40 mg/ml[a]	Physically compatible with no subvisual haze or particle formation in 4 hr at 23 °C	1758	**C**
Bumetanide	RC	0.04 mg/ml[a]	SQ	40 mg/ml[a]	Physically compatible with no subvisual haze or particle formation in 4 hr at 23 °C	1758	**C**
Buprenorphine HCl	RKC	0.04 mg/ml[a]	SQ	40 mg/ml[a]	Physically compatible with no subvisual haze or particle formation in 4 hr at 23 °C	1758	**C**
Butorphanol tartrate	BMS	0.04 mg/ml[a]	SQ	40 mg/ml[a]	Physically compatible with no subvisual haze or particle formation in 4 hr at 23 °C	1758	**C**
Calcium gluconate	AMR	40 mg/ml[a]	SQ	40 mg/ml[a]	Physically compatible with no subvisual haze or particle formation in 4 hr at 23 °C	1758	**C**
Carboplatin	BMS	5 mg/ml[a]	SQ	40 mg/ml[a]	Physically compatible with no subvisual haze or particle formation in 4 hr at 23 °C	1758	**C**
Carmustine	BMS	1.5 mg/ml[a]	SQ	40 mg/ml[a]	Physically compatible with no subvisual haze or particle formation in 4 hr at 23 °C	1758	**C**
Cefazolin sodium	MAR	20 mg/ml[a]	SQ	40 mg/ml[a]	Physically compatible with no subvisual haze or particle formation in 4 hr at 23 °C	1758	**C**
Cefepime HCl	BR	20 mg/ml[a]	SQ	40 mg/ml[a]	Physically compatible with no change in measured turbidity or increase in particle content in 4 hr at 22 °C	1689	**C**
Cefoperazone sodium	RR	40 mg/ml[a]	SQ	40 mg/ml[a]	Physically compatible with no subvisual haze or particle formation in 4 hr at 23 °C	1758	**C**
Cefotaxime sodium	HO	20 mg/ml[a]	SQ	40 mg/ml[a]	Physically compatible with no subvisual haze or particle formation in 4 hr at 23 °C	1758	**C**
Cefotetan disodium	STU	20 mg/ml[a]	SQ	40 mg/ml[a]	Physically compatible with no subvisual haze or particle formation in 4 hr at 23 °C	1758	**C**
Cefoxitin sodium	MSD	20 mg/ml[a]	SQ	40 mg/ml[a]	Physically compatible with no subvisual haze or particle formation in 4 hr at 23 °C	1758	**C**
Ceftazidime	LI[f]	40 mg/ml[a]	SQ	40 mg/ml[a]	Physically compatible with no subvisual haze or particle formation in 4 hr at 23 °C	1758	**C**

Y-Site Injection Compatibility (1:1 Mixture) (Cont.)

					Aztreonam		
Drug	*Mfr*	*Conc*	*Mfr*	*Conc*	*Remarks*	*Ref*	*C/I*
Ceftizoxime sodium	FUJ	20 mg/ml[a]	SQ	40 mg/ml[a]	Physically compatible with no subvisual haze or particle formation in 4 hr at 23 °C	1758	**C**
Ceftriaxone sodium	RC	20 mg/ml[a]	SQ	40 mg/ml[a]	Physically compatible with no subvisual haze or particle formation in 4 hr at 23 °C	1758	**C**
Cefuroxime sodium	LI	30 mg/ml[a]	SQ	40 mg/ml[a]	Physically compatible with no subvisual haze or particle formation in 4 hr at 23 °C	1758	**C**
Chlorpromazine HCl	SCN	2 mg/ml[a]	SQ	40 mg/ml[a]	Dense white turbidity forms immediately	1758	**I**
Cimetidine HCl	SKB	12 mg/ml[a]	SQ	40 mg/ml[a]	Physically compatible with no subvisual haze or particle formation in 4 hr at 23 °C	1758	**C**
Ciprofloxacin	MI	1 mg/ml[a]	SQ	20 mg/ml[c]	Physically compatible for 24 hr at 22 °C	1189	**C**
	MI	1 mg/ml[a]	SQ	40 mg/ml[a]	Physically compatible with no subvisual haze or particle formation in 4 hr at 23 °C	1758	**C**
Cisatracurium besylate	GW	0.1, 2, 5 mg/ml[a]	SQ	40 mg/ml[a]	Physically compatible with no change in measured turbidity or increase in particle content in 4 hr at 23 °C	2074	**C**
Cisplatin	BMS	1 mg/ml	SQ	40 mg/ml[a]	Physically compatible with no subvisual haze or particle formation in 4 hr at 23 °C	1758	**C**
Clindamycin phosphate	AST	10 mg/ml[a]	SQ	40 mg/ml[a]	Physically compatible with no subvisual haze or particle formation in 4 hr at 23 °C	1758	**C**
Cyclophosphamide	MJ	10 mg/ml[a]	SQ	40 mg/ml[a]	Physically compatible with no subvisual haze or particle formation in 4 hr at 23 °C	1758	**C**
Cytarabine	CET	50 mg/ml	SQ	40 mg/ml[a]	Physically compatible with no subvisual haze or particle formation in 4 hr at 23 °C	1758	**C**
Dacarbazine	MI	4 mg/ml[a]	SQ	40 mg/ml[a]	Physically compatible with no subvisual haze or particle formation in 4 hr at 23 °C	1758	**C**
Dactinomycin	ME	0.01 mg/ml[a]	SQ	40 mg/ml[a]	Physically compatible with no subvisual haze or particle formation in 4 hr at 23 °C	1758	**C**
Daunorubicin HCl	WY	1 mg/ml[a]	SQ	40 mg/ml[a]	Haze forms immediately	1758	**I**
Dexamethasone sodium phosphate	AMR	1 mg/ml[a]	SQ	40 mg/ml[a]	Physically compatible with no subvisual haze or particle formation in 4 hr at 23 °C	1758	**C**
Diltiazem HCl	MMD	5 mg/ml	SQ	20 and 333 mg/ml[b]	Visually compatible	1807	**C**
	MMD	1 mg/ml[b]	SQ	333 mg/ml[b]	Visually compatible	1807	**C**
Diphenhydramine HCl	PD	2 mg/ml[a]	SQ	40 mg/ml[a]	Physically compatible with no subvisual haze or particle formation in 4 hr at 23 °C	1758	**C**

Y-Site Injection Compatibility (1:1 Mixture) (Cont.)

			Aztreonam				
Drug	*Mfr*	*Conc*	*Mfr*	*Conc*	*Remarks*	*Ref*	*C/I*
Dobutamine HCl	LI	4 mg/ml[a]	SQ	40 mg/ml[a]	Physically compatible with no subvisual haze or particle formation in 4 hr at 23 °C	1758	C
Docetaxel	RPR	0.9 mg/ml[a]	BMS	40 mg/ml[a]	Physically compatible with no change in measured turbidity or increase in particle content in 4 hr at 23 °C	2224	C
Dopamine HCl	AST	3.2 mg/ml[a]	SQ	40 mg/ml[a]	Physically compatible with no subvisual haze or particle formation in 4 hr at 23 °C	1758	C
Doxorubicin HCl	CET	2 mg/ml	SQ	40 mg/ml[a]	Physically compatible with no subvisual haze or particle formation in 4 hr at 23 °C	1758	C
Doxorubicin HCl liposome injection	SEQ	0.4 mg/ml[a]	SQ	40 mg/ml[a]	Physically compatible with little or no change in measured turbidity and no increase in particle content in 4 hr at 23 °C	2087	C
Doxycycline hyclate	ES	1 mg/ml[a]	SQ	40 mg/ml[a]	Physically compatible with no subvisual haze or particle formation in 4 hr at 23 °C	1758	C
Droperidol	JN	0.4 mg/ml[a]	SQ	40 mg/ml[a]	Physically compatible with no subvisual haze or particle formation in 4 hr at 23 °C	1758	C
Enalaprilat	MSD	0.05 mg/ml[b]	SQ	10 mg/ml[a]	Physically compatible for 24 hr at room temperature under fluorescent light	1355	C
	MSD	0.1 mg/ml[a]	SQ	40 mg/ml[a]	Physically compatible with no subvisual haze or particle formation in 4 hr at 23 °C	1758	C
Etoposide	BMS	0.4 mg/ml[a]	SQ	40 mg/ml[a]	Physically compatible with no subvisual haze or particle formation in 4 hr at 23 °C	1758	C
Etoposide phosphate	BR	5 mg/ml[a]	SQ	40 mg/ml[a]	Physically compatible with no change in measured turbidity or increase in particle content in 4 hr at 23 °C	2218	C
Famotidine	ME	2 mg/ml[a]	SQ	40 mg/ml[a]	Physically compatible with no subvisual haze or particle formation in 4 hr at 23 °C	1758	C
Filgrastim	AMG	30 μg/ml[a]	SQ	40 mg/ml[a]	Physically compatible with no change in measured turbidity or increase in particle content in 4 hr at 22 °C	1687	C
	AMG	30 μg/ml[a]	SQ	40 mg/ml[a]	Physically compatible with no subvisual haze or particle formation in 4 hr at 23 °C	1758	C
Floxuridine	RC	3 mg/ml[a]	SQ	40 mg/ml[a]	Physically compatible with no subvisual haze or particle formation in 4 hr at 23 °C	1758	C
Fluconazole	RR	2 mg/ml	SQ	40 mg/ml	Visually compatible for 24 hr at 25 °C	1407	C
	RR	2 mg/ml	SQ	40 mg/ml[a]	Physically compatible with no subvisual haze or particle formation in 4 hr at 23 °C	1758	C

Y-Site Injection Compatibility (1:1 Mixture) (Cont.)

		Aztreonam					
Drug	Mfr	Conc	Mfr	Conc	Remarks	Ref	C/I
Fludarabine phosphate	BX	1 mg/ml[a]	SQ	40 mg/ml[a]	Physically compatible for 4 hr at room temperature under fluorescent light	1439	**C**
	BX	1 mg/ml[a]	SQ	40 mg/ml[a]	Physically compatible with no subvisual haze or particle formation in 4 hr at 23 °C	1758	**C**
Fluorouracil	AD	16 mg/ml[a]	SQ	40 mg/ml[a]	Physically compatible with no subvisual haze or particle formation in 4 hr at 23 °C	1758	**C**
Foscarnet sodium	AST	24 mg/ml	SQ	40 mg/ml	Physically compatible for 24 hr at room temperature under fluorescent light	1335	**C**
	AST	24 mg/ml	SQ	40 mg/ml[c]	Physically compatible for 24 hr at 25 °C under fluorescent light by visual and microscopic examination	1393	**C**
Furosemide	AB	3 mg/ml[a]	SQ	40 mg/ml[a]	Physically compatible with no subvisual haze or particle formation in 4 hr at 23 °C	1758	**C**
Ganciclovir sodium	SY	20 mg/ml[a]	SQ	40 mg/ml[a]	White crystalline needles form immediately and become dense flocculent precipitate in 1 hr	1758	**I**
Gemcitabine HCl	LI	10 mg/ml[b]	SQ	40 mg/ml[b]	Physically compatible with no change in measured turbidity or increase in particle content in 4 hr at 23 °C	2226	**C**
Gentamicin sulfate	ES	5 mg/ml[a]	SQ	40 mg/ml[a]	Physically compatible with no subvisual haze or particle formation in 4 hr at 23 °C	1758	**C**
Granisetron HCl	SKB	0.05 mg/ml[a]	SQ	40 mg/ml[a]	Physically compatible with no change in measured turbidity or increase in particle content in 4 hr at 23 °C	2000	**C**
Haloperidol lactate	MN	0.2 mg/ml[a]	SQ	40 mg/ml[a]	Physically compatible with no subvisual haze or particle formation in 4 hr at 23 °C	1758	**C**
Heparin sodium	ES	100 units/ml[a]	SQ	40 mg/ml[a]	Physically compatible with no subvisual haze or particle formation in 4 hr at 23 °C	1758	**C**
	TR	50 units/ml	BV	20 mg/ml[a]	Visually compatible for 6 hr at 25 °C	1793	**C**
Hydrocortisone sodium phosphate	MSD	1 mg/ml[a]	SQ	40 mg/ml[a]	Physically compatible with no subvisual haze or particle formation in 4 hr at 23 °C	1758	**C**
Hydrocortisone sodium succinate	UP	1 mg/ml[a]	SQ	40 mg/ml[a]	Physically compatible with no subvisual haze or particle formation in 4 hr at 23 °C	1758	**C**
Hydromorphone HCl	KN	0.5 mg/ml[a]	SQ	40 mg/ml[a]	Physically compatible with no subvisual haze or particle formation in 4 hr at 23 °C	1758	**C**
Hydroxyzine HCl	WI	4 mg/ml[a]	SQ	40 mg/ml[a]	Physically compatible with no subvisual haze or particle formation in 4 hr at 23 °C	1758	**C**

Y-Site Injection Compatibility (1:1 Mixture) (Cont.)

Drug		Aztreonam					
	Mfr	Conc	Mfr	Conc	Remarks	Ref	C/I
Idarubicin HCl	AD	0.5 mg/ml[a]	SQ	40 mg/ml[a]	Increase in measured turbidity no greater than dilution of idarubicin with NS. No increase in particle content in 4 hr at 23 °C	1758	C
Ifosfamide	MJ	25 mg/ml[a]	SQ	40 mg/ml[a]	Physically compatible with no subvisual haze or particle formation in 4 hr at 23 °C	1758	C
Imipenem–cilastatin sodium	MSD	10 mg/ml[a]	SQ	40 mg/ml[a]	Physically compatible with no subvisual haze or particle formation in 4 hr at 23 °C	1758	C
Insulin, regular	LI	0.2 unit/ml[b]	SQ	20 mg/ml	Physically compatible for 2 hr at 25 °C	1395	C
Leucovorin calcium	LE	2 mg/ml[a]	SQ	40 mg/ml[a]	Physically compatible with no subvisual haze or particle formation in 4 hr at 23 °C	1758	C
Lorazepam	WY	0.1 mg/ml[a]	SQ	40 mg/ml[a]	Haze forms within 1 hr	1758	I
Magnesium sulfate	AST	100 mg/ml[a]	SQ	40 mg/ml[a]	Physically compatible with no subvisual haze or particle formation in 4 hr at 23 °C	1758	C
Mannitol	BA	15%	SQ	40 mg/ml[a]	Physically compatible with no subvisual haze or particle formation in 4 hr at 23 °C	1758	C
Mechlorethamine HCl	MSD	1 mg/ml	SQ	40 mg/ml[a]	Physically compatible with no subvisual haze or particle formation in 4 hr at 23 °C	1758	C
Melphalan HCl	BW	0.1 mg/ml[b]	SQ	40 mg/ml[b]	Physically compatible with no change in measured turbidity or increase in particle content in 3 hr at 22 °C	1557	C
Meperidine HCl	AB	10 mg/ml	SQ	20 mg/ml[a]	Physically compatible for 4 hr at 25 °C	1397	C
	WY	4 mg/ml[a]	SQ	40 mg/ml[a]	Physically compatible with no subvisual haze or particle formation in 4 hr at 23 °C	1758	C
Mesna	MJ	10 mg/ml[a]	SQ	40 mg/ml[a]	Physically compatible with no subvisual haze or particle formation in 4 hr at 23 °C	1758	C
Methotrexate sodium	LE	15 mg/ml[a]	SQ	40 mg/ml[a]	Physically compatible with no subvisual haze or particle formation in 4 hr at 23 °C	1758	C
Methylprednisolone sodium succinate	AB	5 mg/ml[a]	SQ	40 mg/ml[a]	Physically compatible with no subvisual haze or particle formation in 4 hr at 23 °C	1758	C
Metoclopramide HCl	ES	5 mg/ml	SQ	40 mg/ml[a]	Physically compatible with no subvisual haze or particle formation in 4 hr at 23 °C	1758	C
Metronidazole	BA	5 mg/ml	SQ	40 mg/ml[a]	Color changes from colorless to orange in 4 hr	1758	I
Minocycline HCl	LE	0.2 mg/ml[a]	SQ	40 mg/ml[a]	Physically compatible with no subvisual haze or particle formation in 4 hr at 23 °C	1758	C

Y-Site Injection Compatibility (1:1 Mixture) (Cont.)

| | | Aztreonam | | | | | |
Drug	Mfr	Conc	Mfr	Conc	Remarks	Ref	C/I
Mitomycin	BMS	0.5 mg/ml	SQ	40 mg/ml[a]	Color changes from pale blue to reddish purple in 4 hr	1758	I
Mitoxantrone HCl	LE	0.5 mg/ml[a]	SQ	40 mg/ml[a]	Heavy precipitate forms in 1 hr	1758	I
Morphine sulfate	AB	1 mg/ml	SQ	20 mg/ml[a]	Physically compatible for 4 hr at 25 °C	1397	C
	AST	1 mg/ml[a]	SQ	40 mg/ml[a]	Physically compatible with no subvisual haze or particle formation in 4 hr at 23 °C	1758	C
Nalbuphine HCl	AST	10 mg/ml	SQ	40 mg/ml[a]	Physically compatible with no subvisual haze or particle formation in 4 hr at 23 °C	1758	C
Netilmicin sulfate	SC	5 mg/ml[a]	SQ	40 mg/ml[a]	Physically compatible with no subvisual haze or particle formation in 4 hr at 23 °C	1758	C
Ondansetron HCl	GL	1 mg/ml[b]	SQ	40 mg/ml[a]	Physically compatible for 4 hr at 22 °C	1365	C
	GL	0.03 and 0.3 mg/ml[a]	SQ	40 mg/ml[a]	Visually compatible with little or no loss of either drug by HPLC in 4 hr at 25 °C under fluorescent light	1732	C
	GL	1 mg/ml[a]	SQ	40 mg/ml[a]	Physically compatible with no subvisual haze or particle formation in 4 hr at 23 °C	1758	C
Piperacillin sodium	LE	40 mg/ml[a]	SQ	40 mg/ml[a]	Physically compatible with no subvisual haze or particle formation in 4 hr at 23 °C	1758	C
Piperacillin sodium–tazobactam sodium	LE	40 + 5 mg/ml[a]	SQ	40 mg/ml[a]	Physically compatible with no change in measured turbidity or increase in particle content in 4 hr at 22 °C	1688	C
Plicamycin	MI	0.01 mg/ml[a]	SQ	40 mg/ml[a]	Physically compatible with no subvisual haze or particle formation in 4 hr at 23 °C	1758	C
Potassium chloride	AB	0.1 mEq/ml[a]	SQ	40 mg/ml[a]	Physically compatible with no subvisual haze or particle formation in 4 hr at 23 °C	1758	C
Prochlorperazine edisylate	ES	0.5 mg/ml[a]	SQ	40 mg/ml[a]	Haze and tiny particles form within 4 hr	1758	I
Promethazine HCl	SCN	2 mg/ml[a]	SQ	40 mg/ml[a]	Physically compatible with no subvisual haze or particle formation in 4 hr at 23 °C	1758	C
Propofol	ZEN	10 mg/ml	SQ	40 mg/ml[a]	Physically compatible for 1 hr at 23 °C with no increase in particle content	2066	C
Ranitidine HCl	GL	1 mg/ml[b]	SQ	16.7 mg/ml[b]	No loss of either drug by HPLC in 4 hr at 22 °C under fluorescent light	1632	C
	GL	2 mg/ml[a]	SQ	40 mg/ml[a]	Physically compatible with no subvisual haze or particle formation in 4 hr at 23 °C	1758	C
Remifentanil HCl	GW	0.025 and 0.25 mg/ml[b]	SQ	40 mg/ml[a]	Physically compatible with no change in measured turbidity or increase in particle content in 4 hr at 23 °C	2075	C
Sargramostim	IMM	10 μg/ml[b]	SQ	40 mg/ml[b]	Physically compatible for 4 hr at 22 °C	1436	C

Y-Site Injection Compatibility (1:1 Mixture) (Cont.)

Drug	Mfr	Conc	Mfr	Conc	Remarks	Ref	C/I
	IMM	10 μg/ml[b]	SQ	40 mg/ml[a]	Physically compatible with no subvisual haze or particle formation in 4 hr at 23 °C	1758	C
Sodium bicarbonate	AB	1 mEq/ml	SQ	40 mg/ml[a]	Physically compatible with no subvisual haze or particle formation in 4 hr at 23 °C	1758	C
Streptozocin	UP	40 mg/ml[a]	SQ	40 mg/ml[a]	Color changes from pale gold to red in 1 hr	1758	I
Teniposide	BR	0.1 mg/ml[a]	SQ	40 mg/ml[a]	Physically compatible with no subvisual haze or particle formation in 4 hr at 23 °C	1725; 1758	C
Theophylline	TR	4 mg/ml	BV	20 mg/ml[a]	Visually compatible for 6 hr at 25 °C	1793	C
Thiotepa	LE	1 mg/ml[a]	SQ	40 mg/ml[a]	Physically compatible with no subvisual haze or particle formation in 4 hr at 23 °C	1758	C
	IMM[d]	1 mg/ml[a]	SQ	40 mg/ml[a]	Physically compatible with no change in measured turbidity or increase in particle content in 4 hr at 23 °C	1861	C
Ticarcillin disodium	BE	30 mg/ml[a]	SQ	40 mg/ml[a]	Physically compatible with no subvisual haze or particle formation in 4 hr at 23 °C	1758	C
Ticarcillin disodium–clavulanate potassium	SKB	31 mg/ml[a]	SQ	40 mg/ml[a]	Physically compatible with no subvisual haze or particle formation in 4 hr at 23 °C	1758	C
TNA #218 to #226[e]			SQ	40 mg/ml[a]	Visually compatible with no precipitate or emulsion damage apparent in 4 hr at 23 °C	2215	C
Tobramycin sulfate	LI	5 mg/ml[a]	SQ	40 mg/ml[a]	Physically compatible with no subvisual haze or particle formation in 4 hr at 23 °C	1758	C
TPN #212 to #215[e]			SQ	40 mg/ml[a]	Physically compatible with no change in measured turbidity or increase in particle content in 4 hr at 23 °C	2109	C
Trimethoprim–sulfamethoxazole	ES	0.8 + 4 mg/ml[a]	SQ	40 mg/ml[a]	Physically compatible with no subvisual haze or particle formation in 4 hr at 23 °C	1758	C
Vancomycin HCl	LI	67 mg/ml[b]	SQ	200 mg/ml[b]	White granular precipitate forms immediately in tubing when given sequentially	1364	I
	AB	10 mg/ml[a]	SQ	40 mg/ml[a]	Physically compatible with no subvisual haze or particle formation in 4 hr at 23 °C	1758	C
Vinblastine sulfate	LI	0.12 mg/ml[a]	SQ	40 mg/ml[a]	Physically compatible with no subvisual haze or particle formation in 4 hr at 23 °C	1758	C
Vincristine sulfate	LI	0.05 mg/ml[a]	SQ	40 mg/ml[a]	Physically compatible with no subvisual haze or particle formation in 4 hr at 23 °C	1758	C

Y-Site Injection Compatibility (1:1 Mixture) (Cont.)

		Aztreonam					
Drug	*Mfr*	*Conc*	*Mfr*	*Conc*	*Remarks*	*Ref*	*C/I*
Vinorelbine tartrate	BW	1 mg/ml[b]	SQ	40 mg/ml[b]	Physically compatible with no change in measured turbidity or increase in particle content in 4 hr at 22 °C	1558	C
Zidovudine	BW	4 mg/ml[a]	SQ	40 mg/ml[a]	Physically compatible for 4 hr at 25 °C under fluorescent light by visual and microscopic examination	1193	C
	BW	4 mg/ml[a]	SQ	40 mg/ml[a]	Physically compatible with no subvisual haze or particle formation in 4 hr at 23 °C	1758	C

[a]*Tested in dextrose 5% in water.*
[b]*Tested in sodium chloride 0.9%.*
[c]*Tested in both dextrose 5% in water and sodium chloride 0.9%.*
[d]*Lyophilized formulation tested.*
[e]*Refer to Appendix I for the composition of parenteral nutrition solutions. TNA indicates a 3-in-1 admixture, and TPN indicates a 2-in-1 admixture.*
[f]*Sodium carbonate–containing formulation tested.*

Additional Compatibility Information

Solutions— For intravenous infusion, the manufacturer recommends dilution of aztreonam in the following infusion solutions (2):

Dextrose 5% in Ringer's injection, lactated
Dextrose 5% in sodium chloride 0.2, 0.45, and 0.9%
Dextrose 5 and 10% in water
Invert sugar 10% in water
Invert sugar 10% in Electrolyte #1, #2, and #3
Ionosol B in dextrose 5%
Isolyte E
Isolyte E with dextrose 5%
Isolyte M with dextrose 5%
Mannitol 5 and 10%
Normosol M in dextrose 5%
Normosol R
Normosol R in dextrose 5%
Plasma-Lyte M in dextrose 5%
Ringer's injection
Ringer's injection, lactated
Sodium chloride 0.9%
Sodium lactate ⅙ M

Additives— The manufacturer states that solutions of aztreonam in sodium chloride 0.9% or dextrose 5% in water with clindamycin phosphate, gentamicin sulfate, tobramycin sulfate, or cefazolin sodium are stable for up to 48 hours at room temperature or seven days under refrigeration (2).

Aztreonam is incompatible with nafcillin sodium and metronidazole (2).

The manufacturer also states that ampicillin sodium admixtures with aztreonam in sodium chloride 0.9% are stable for 24 hours at room temperature or 48 hours under refrigeration. However, in dextrose 5% in water, the stability is reduced to two hours at room temperature or eight hours under refrigeration (2).

Peritoneal Dialysis Solutions— Aztreonam with cloxacillin sodium and aztreonam with vancomycin HCl admixtures are stable in Dianeal 137 with dextrose 4.25% for 24 hours at room temperature (2).

BACLOFEN
AHFS 12:20

Lioresal Intrathecal   **Medtronic**

Products— Baclofen injection (Medtronic) is available as a preservative-free injection in intrathecal refill kits at a concentration of 0.5 mg/ml in 20-ml ampuls and at a concentration of 2 mg/ml in 5-ml ampuls. Each milliliter of solution contains baclofen 0.5 or 2 mg (500 or 2000 μg, respectively) with sodium chloride 9 mg in water for injection (1-6/96).

pH— From 5 to 7 (1-6/96).

Sodium Content— Baclofen injection contains 0.15 mEq of sodium per milliliter (4).

Tonicity— Baclofen injection is an isotonic solution (1-6/96; 4).

Administration— For screening, baclofen injection must be diluted with sterile, preservative-free sodium chloride 0.9% injection to a concentration of 50 μg/ml. The dilution is administered by direct intrathecal injection via lumbar puncture or catheter over at least one minute using barbotage. In maintenance treatment, baclofen injection is also given by intrathecal infusion using an implantable infusion control device; concentration and rate of delivery must be carefully titrated to each patient's needs (1-6/96; 4).

Stability— Baclofen injection may be stored at controlled room temperatures not exceeding 30 °C. It should be protected from freezing (1-6/96; 4). The product is stable in implantable infusion pumps at a temperature of 37 °C (4). It should not be autoclaved. The product contains no preservatives and is intended for single-use only; unused portions must be discarded (1-6/96; 4).

Baclofen injection must be diluted only with sterile, preservative-free sodium chloride 0.9%. It is compatible with cerebrospinal fluid (1-6/96; 4).

Implantable Pump— Baclofen 0.5 mg/ml was filled into an implantable pump (Fresenius model VIP 30) and associated capillary tubing and stored at 37 °C. Samples were analyzed using an HPLC assay. No baclofen loss and no contamination from components of pump materials occurred during eight weeks of storage (1903).

Baclofen (Ciba) 0.2 mg/ml with morphine sulfate (David Bull) 1 mg/ml in an implantable pump (Infusaid) was physically compatible and exhibited little or no loss of either drug within 30 days at 37 °C (1911).

In a follow-up study at higher concentrations, baclofen (Ciba) 1 mg/ml with morphine sulfate (David Bull) 15 mg/ml in an implantable pump (Infusaid) was physically compatible, with only a slight yellowing of the solution observed. HPLC analysis found no substantial loss of either baclofen or morphine. Statistical analysis showed no significant time-dependent change in the baclofen concentration. However, a small decrease in morphine concentration of less than 4% may occur during a 30-day course of infusion at 37 °C (2170).

Compatibility Information

Additive Compatibility

Baclofen

Drug	Mfr	Conc/L	Mfr	Conc/L	Test Soln	Remarks	Ref	C/I
Morphine sulfate	DB	1 and 1.5 g	CI	200 mg	NS[a]	Physically compatible with little or no loss of either drug by HPLC in 30 days at 37 °C	1911	**C**
	DB	1 g	CI	800 mg	NS[a]	Physically compatible with little or no baclofen loss and less than 7% morphine loss by HPLC in 29 days at 37 °C	1911	**C**
	DB	1.5 g	CI	800 mg	NS[a]	Physically compatible with little or no loss of either drug by HPLC in 30 days at 37 °C	1911	**C**
	DB	7.5 g	CI	1.5 g	NS[a]	Physically compatible with little or no loss of either drug by HPLC in 30 days at 37 °C	2170	**C**
	DB	15 g	CI	1 g	NS[a]	Physically compatible with little or no loss of either drug by HPLC in 30 days at 37 °C	2170	**C**
	DB	21 g	CI	200 mg	NS[a]	Physically compatible with about 7% baclofen loss and little or no morphine loss by HPLC in 30 days at 37 °C	2170	**C**

[a]*Tested in glass containers.*

BENZTROPINE MESYLATE
AHFS 12:08.04

Cogentin   **Merck**

Products— Benztropine mesylate (Merck) is available in 2-ml ampuls containing 2 mg of drug. Each milliliter of solution contains (2):

Benztropine mesylate	1 mg
Sodium chloride	9 mg
Water for injection	qs 1 ml

pH— From 5 to 8 (4).

Osmolality— Benztropine mesylate 1 mg/ml has an osmolality of 282 mOsm/kg (1689).

Administration— Benztropine mesylate may be administered by intramuscular or, rarely, intravenous injection (2; 4).

Stability— Store the ampuls at room temperature. Avoid freezing and storing at temperatures over 40 °C (4).

Compatibility Information

Drugs in Syringe Compatibility

Benztropine mesylate

Drug (in syringe)	Mfr	Amt	Mfr	Amt	Remarks	Ref	C/I
Chlorpromazine HCl	STS	50 mg/ 2 ml	MSD	2 mg/ 2 ml	Visually compatible for 60 min	1784	C
Fluphenazine HCl	LY	5 mg/ 2 ml	MSD	2 mg/ 2 ml	Visually compatible for 60 min	1784	C
Haloperidol lactate	MN	0.25, 0.5, 1 mg	MSD	2 mg	Visually compatible for 24 hr at 21 °C	1781	C
	MN	2 mg	MSD	2 mg	Precipitate forms within 4 hr at 21 °C	1781	I
	MN	3, 4, 5 mg	MSD	2 mg	Precipitate forms within 15 min at 21 °C	1781	I
	MN	0.25 and 0.5 mg	MSD	1 mg	Visually compatible for 24 hr at 21 °C	1781	C
	MN	1 to 5 mg	MSD	1 mg	Precipitate forms within 15 min at 21 °C	1781	I
	MN	0.25 to 5 mg	MSD	0.5 mg	Precipitate forms within 15 min at 21 °C	1781	I
	MN	10 mg/ 2 ml	MSD	2 mg/ 2 ml	White precipitate forms within 5 min	1784	I
Metoclopramide HCl	RB	10 mg/ 2 ml	MSD	2 mg/ 2 ml	Physically compatible for 48 hr at room temperature	924	C
	RB	10 mg/ 2 ml	MSD	2 mg/ 2 ml	Physically compatible for 48 hr at 25 °C	1167	C
	RB	160 mg/ 32 ml	MSD	2 mg/ 2 ml	Physically compatible for 48 hr at 25 °C	1167	C
Perphenazine	SC	10 mg/ 2 ml	MSD	2 mg/ 2 ml	Visually compatible for 60 min	1784	C

Y-Site Injection Compatibility (1:1 Mixture)

Benztropine mesylate

Drug	Mfr	Conc	Mfr	Conc	Remarks	Ref	C/I
Fluconazole	RR	2 mg/ml	MSD	1 mg/ml	Physically compatible for 24 hr at 25 °C	1407	C
Tacrolimus	FUJ	1 mg/ml[a]	MSD	1 mg/ml[b]	Visually compatible for 24 hr at 25 °C	1630	C

[a]Tested in sodium chloride 0.9%.
[b]Tested in dextrose 5% in water.

BETAMETHASONE SODIUM PHOSPHATE
AHFS 68:04

Celestone Phosphate   **Schering**

Products— Betamethasone sodium phosphate (Schering) is available in 5-ml multiple-dose vials. Each milliliter of solution contains (4; 154):

Betamethasone sodium phosphate (equivalent to 3 mg of betamethasone alcohol)	4 mg
Dibasic sodium phosphate	10 mg
Edetate disodium	0.1 mg
Phenol	5 mg
Sodium bisulfite	3.2 mg
Sodium hydroxide	to adjust pH

pH— Approximately 8.5 (4).

Administration— Betamethasone sodium phosphate may be administered intravenously or intramuscularly. Intra-articular, intrasynovial, intralesional, and soft tissue injections are also recommended (4).

Stability— Betamethasone sodium phosphate should be protected from light and stored at a temperature below 40 °C, preferably between 15 and 30 °C. The injection should not be frozen (4).

Compatibility Information

Y-Site Injection Compatibility (1:1 Mixture)

Betamethasone sodium phosphate

Drug	Mfr	Conc	Mfr	Conc	Remarks	Ref	C/I
Heparin sodium	UP	1000 units/L[a]	SC	3 mg/ml	Physically compatible for at least 4 hr at room temperature by visual and microscopic examination	534	C
Hydrocortisone sodium succinate	UP	10 mg/L[a]	SC	3 mg/ml	Physically compatible for at least 4 hr at room temperature by visual and microscopic examination	534	C
Potassium chloride	AB	40 mEq/L[a]	SC	3 mg/ml	Physically compatible for at least 4 hr at room temperature by visual and microscopic examination	534	C
Vitamin B complex with C	RC	2 ml/L[a]	SC	3 mg/ml	Physically compatible for at least 4 hr at room temperature by visual and microscopic examination	534	C

[a]*Tested in dextrose 5% in water, dextrose 5% in Ringer's injection, dextrose 5% in Ringer's injection, lactated, Ringer's injection, lactated, and sodium chloride 0.9%.*

BLEOMYCIN SULFATE
AHFS 10:00

Blenoxane   **Bristol-Myers Squibb**

Products— Bleomycin sulfate (Bristol-Myers Squibb) is available in vials containing 15 and 30 units of bleomycin as the sulfate. For intramuscular or subcutaneous administration, reconstitute the 15-unit vial with 1 to 5 ml and the 30-unit vial with 2 to 10 ml of sterile water for injection, sodium chloride 0.9%, or bacteriostatic water for injection, yielding a solution containing 3 to 15 units/ml. For intravenous or intra-arterial injection, reconstitute the 15-unit vial with a minimum of 5 ml and the 30-unit vial with a minimum of 10 ml of sodium chloride 0.9%, resulting in a solution of not more than 3 units/ml. For intrapleural administration, 60 units is dissolved in 50 to 100 ml of sodium chloride 0.9% (2; 4).

Units— Bleomycin sulfate is a mixture of cytotoxic glycopeptide antibiotics. A unit of bleomycin is equal to the term milligram activity, which was formerly used (2). One unit of bleomycin is equivalent in activity to 1 mg of bleomycin A_2 reference standard (4).

pH— The pH of the reconstituted solution varies from 4.5 to 6, depending on the diluent (4).

Osmolality— Bleomycin sulfate 15 units/ml in sterile water for injection has an osmolality of 89 mOsm/kg (1689).

Administration— Bleomycin sulfate may be administered by intramuscular, subcutaneous, intravenous, intrapleural (2; 4), or intra-arterial injection (4). Intravenous and intra-arterial injections should be given slowly over a 10-minute period (2; 4).

Stability— Intact vials are stable under refrigeration and bear an expiration date (2). They are stated to be stable for 28 days at room temperature (1181; 1433). Bristol-Myers Squibb states that bleomycin sulfate is stable in sodium chloride 0.9% for 24 hours at room temperature (2). Other information indicates that solutions reconstituted with dextrose 5% in water may be less stable, with losses exceeding 10% in 24 hours at room temperature (1441). Bleomycin sulfate solutions reconstituted with sodium chloride 0.9% are reported to be stable for four weeks when stored at 2 to 8 °C (4; 1369), for two weeks (4) or longer (860; 1369) at room temperature, and for 10 days at 37 °C (1073). However, because of the risk of microbial contamination in products without preservatives, it is recommended that the solutions be used within 24 hours of reconstitution (2; 4; 860).

Bleomycin sulfate (Bristol) is stable in solution over a pH range of 4 to 10 (763).

Sorption— Koberda et al. studied the stability of bleomycin sulfate 0.3 to 3 units/ml in sodium chloride 0.9% and dextrose 5% in water in both glass and PVC containers. Contrary to a previous report (519), no loss due to sorption to PVC containers occurred. Storage for 24 hours at 23 °C resulted in similar losses in the dextrose 5% in water admixtures in both containers, while little or no loss occurred in the sodium chloride 0.9% admixtures in both containers. The authors speculated that the losses previously attributed to container sorption actually resulted from adduct formation with dextrose (1441).

DeVroe et al. confirmed this result. They compared the delivery of bleomycin sulfate 7.5 units/500 ml in dextrose 5% in water and sodium chloride 0.9% in glass, PVC, and high-density polyethylene containers and in PVC, polyethylene, and polybutadiene infusion sets. The bleomycin delivered from all of these container/set configurations was equivalent, with no evidence of sorption (1577).

Filtration— Bleomycin sulfate (Bristol) 15 units/50 ml in dextrose 5% in water and sodium chloride 0.9% filtered at a rate of about 3 ml/min through a 0.22-μm cellulose ester membrane filter

(Ivex-2) showed no significant reduction in potency due to binding to the filter (533).

Bleomycin sulfate 10 to 300 μg/ml exhibited no loss due to sorption to either cellulose nitrate/cellulose acetate ester (Millex OR) or Teflon (Millex FG) filters (1415; 1416).

Bleomycin sulfate 7.5 units/500 ml in dextrose 5% in water and sodium chloride 0.9% lost potency initially when infused over 24 hours through cellulose ester and nylon filters. However, the concentration returned to expected levels within minutes, and the total amount of drug lost was negligible (1577).

Compatibility Information

Solution Compatibility

Bleomycin sulfate

Solution	Mfr	Mfr	Conc/L	Remarks	Ref	C/I
Dextrose 5% in water	[a]		150 units	About 54% loss in 28 days at room temperature in the dark	1369	**I**
	BA[b]	BR	300 and 3000 units	About 10% loss in 8 to 10 hr and 11 to 16% loss in 24 hr at 23 °C in glass and PVC	1441	**I**
	[c]	BEL	15 units	No loss by UV spectroscopy in 24 hr at room temperature exposed to light	1577	**C**
Sodium chloride 0.9%	[a]		150 units	About 4% loss in 28 days at room temperature in the dark	1369	**C**
	BA[b]	BR	300 and 3000 units	Little or no loss in 24 hr at 23 °C in glass and PVC	1441	**C**
	[c]	BEL	15 units	No loss by UV spectroscopy in 48 hr at room temperature exposed to light	1577	**C**

[a]*Tested in PVC containers.*
[b]*Tested in both glass and PVC containers.*
[c]*Tested in glass, PVC, and high-density polyethylene containers.*

Additive Compatibility

Bleomycin sulfate

Drug	Mfr	Conc/L	Mfr	Conc/L	Test Soln	Remarks	Ref	C/I
Amikacin sulfate	BR	1.25 g	BR	20 and 30 units	NS	Physically compatible and bleomycin activity retained for 1 week at 4 °C. Amikacin not tested	763	**C**
Aminophylline	ES	250 mg	BR	20 and 30 units	NS	50% loss of bleomycin activity in 1 week at 4 °C	763	**I**
Ascorbic acid injection	PD	2.5 and 5 g	BR	20 and 30 units	NS	Loss of all bleomycin activity in 1 week at 4 °C	763	**I**
Cefazolin sodium	LI	1 g	BR	20 and 30 units	NS	43% loss of bleomycin activity in 1 week at 4 °C	763	**I**
Dexamethasone sodium phosphate	MSD	50 mg	BR	20 and 30 units	NS	Physically compatible and bleomycin activity retained for 1 week at 4 °C. Dexamethasone not tested	763	**C**

Additive Compatibility (Cont.)

Bleomycin sulfate

Drug	Mfr	Conc/L	Mfr	Conc/L	Test Soln	Remarks	Ref	C/I
Diazepam	RC	50 and 100 mg	BR	20 and 30 units	NS	Physically incompatible	763	**I**
Diphenhydramine HCl	PD	100 mg	BR	20 and 30 units	NS	Physically compatible and bleomycin activity retained for 1 week at 4 °C. Diphenhydramine not tested	763	**C**
Fluorouracil	RC	1 g	BR	20 and 30 units	NS	Physically compatible and bleomycin activity retained for 1 week at 4 °C. Fluorouracil not tested	763	**C**
Gentamicin sulfate	SC	50, 100, 300, 600 mg	BR	20 and 30 units	NS	Physically compatible and bleomycin activity retained for 1 week at 4 °C. Gentamicin not tested	763	**C**
Heparin sodium	RI	10,000 to 200,000 units	BR	20 and 30 units	NS	Physically compatible and bleomycin activity retained for 1 week at 4 °C. Heparin not tested	763	**C**
Hydrocortisone sodium phosphate	MSD	100 mg, 500 mg, 1 g, 2 g	BR	20 and 30 units	NS	Physically compatible and bleomycin activity retained for 1 week at 4 °C. Hydrocortisone not tested	763	**C**
Hydrocortisone sodium succinate	AB	300 mg, 750 mg, 1 g, 2.5 g	BR	20 and 30 units	NS	60 to 100% loss of bleomycin activity in 1 week at 4 °C	763	**I**
Methotrexate	LE	250 and 500 mg	BR	20 and 30 units	NS	About 60% loss of bleomycin activity in 1 week at 4 °C	763	**I**
Mitomycin	BR	10 mg	BR	20 and 30 units	NS	20% loss of bleomycin activity in 1 week at 4 °C	763	**I**
	BR	50 mg	BR	20 and 30 units	NS	52% loss of bleomycin activity in 1 week at 4 °C	763	**I**
Nafcillin sodium	BR	2.5 g	BR	20 and 30 units	NS	Substantial loss of bleomycin activity in 1 week at 4 °C	763	**I**
Penicillin G sodium	SQ	2 million units	BR	20 and 30 units	NS	77% loss of bleomycin activity in 1 week at 4 °C	763	**I**
	SQ	5 million units	BR	20 and 30 units	NS	41% loss of bleomycin activity in 1 week at 4 °C	763	**I**
Phenytoin sodium	PD	500 mg	BR	20 and 30 units	NS	Physically compatible and bleomycin activity retained for 1 week at 4 °C. Phenytoin not tested	763	**C**
Streptomycin sulfate	PF	4 g	BR	20 and 30 units	NS	Physically compatible and bleomycin activity retained for 1 week at 4 °C. Streptomycin not tested	763	**C**

Additive Compatibility (Cont.)

Bleomycin sulfate

Drug	Mfr	Conc/L	Mfr	Conc/L	Test Soln	Remarks	Ref	C/I
Terbutaline sulfate	GG	7.5 mg	BR	20 and 30 units	NS	36% loss of bleomycin activity in 1 week at 4 °C	763	I
Tobramycin sulfate	LI	500 mg	BR	20 and 30 units	NS	Physically compatible and bleomycin activity retained for 1 week at 4 °C	763	C
Vinblastine sulfate	LI	10 and 100 mg	BR	20 and 30 units	NS	Physically compatible and bleomycin activity retained for 1 week at 4 °C. Vinblastine not tested	763	C
Vincristine sulfate	LI	50 and 100 mg	BR	20 and 30 units	NS	Physically compatible and bleomycin activity retained for 1 week at 4 °C. Vincristine not tested	763	C

Drugs in Syringe Compatibility

Bleomycin sulfate

Drug (in syringe)	Mfr	Amt	Mfr	Amt	Remarks	Ref	C/I
Cisplatin		0.5 mg/ 0.5 ml		1.5 units/ 0.5 ml	Physically compatible for 5 min at room temperature followed by 8 min of centrifugation	980	C
Cyclophosphamide		10 mg/ 0.5 ml		1.5 units/ 0.5 ml	Physically compatible for 5 min at room temperature followed by 8 min of centrifugation	980	C
Doxorubicin HCl		1 mg/ 0.5 ml		1.5 units/ 0.5 ml	Physically compatible for 5 min at room temperature followed by 8 min of centrifugation	980	C
Droperidol		1.25 mg/ 0.5 ml		1.5 units/ 0.5 ml	Physically compatible for 5 min at room temperature followed by 8 min of centrifugation	980	C
Fluorouracil		25 mg/ 0.5 ml		1.5 units/ 0.5 ml	Physically compatible for 5 min at room temperature followed by 8 min of centrifugation	980	C
Furosemide		5 mg/ 0.5 ml		1.5 units/ 0.5 ml	Physically compatible for 5 min at room temperature followed by 8 min of centrifugation	980	C
Heparin sodium		500 units/ 0.5 ml		1.5 units/ 0.5 ml	Physically compatible for 5 min at room temperature followed by 8 min of centrifugation	980	C
Leucovorin calcium		5 mg/ 0.5 ml		1.5 units/ 0.5 ml	Physically compatible for 5 min at room temperature followed by 8 min of centrifugation	980	C
Methotrexate sodium		12.5 mg/ 0.5 ml		1.5 units/ 0.5 ml	Physically compatible for 5 min at room temperature followed by 8 min of centrifugation	980	C
Metoclopramide HCl		2.5 mg/ 0.5 ml		1.5 units/ 0.5 ml	Physically compatible for 5 min at room temperature followed by 8 min of centrifugation	980	C

Drugs in Syringe Compatibility (Cont.)

Bleomycin sulfate

Drug (in syringe)	Mfr	Amt	Mfr	Amt	Remarks	Ref	C/I
Mitomycin		0.25 mg/ 0.5 ml		1.5 units/ 0.5 ml	Physically compatible for 5 min at room temperature followed by 8 min of centrifugation	980	**C**
Vinblastine sulfate		0.5 mg/ 0.5 ml		1.5 units/ 0.5 ml	Physically compatible for 5 min at room temperature followed by 8 min of centrifugation	980	**C**
Vincristine sulfate		0.5 mg/ 0.5 ml		1.5 units/ 0.5 ml	Physically compatible for 5 min at room temperature followed by 8 min of centrifugation	980	**C**

Y-Site Injection Compatibility (1:1 Mixture)

Bleomycin sulfate

Drug	Mfr	Conc	Mfr	Conc	Remarks	Ref	C/I
Allopurinol sodium	BW	3 mg/ml[b]	BR	1 unit/ml[b]	Physically compatible with no change in measured turbidity or increase in particle content in 4 hr at 22 °C	1686	**C**
Amifostine	USB	10 mg/ml[a]	MJ	1 unit/ml[b]	Physically compatible with no change in measured turbidity or increase in particle content in 4 hr at 23 °C	1845	**C**
Aztreonam	SQ	40 mg/ml[a]	MJ	1 unit/ml[b]	Physically compatible with no subvisual haze or particle formation in 4 hr at 23 °C	1758	**C**
Cefepime HCl	BR	20 mg/ml[a]	BR	1 unit/ml[b]	Physically compatible with no change in measured turbidity or increase in particle content in 4 hr at 22 °C	1689	**C**
Cisplatin		1 mg/ml		3 units/ml	Drugs injected sequentially into Y-site with no flush between. No visually apparent precipitate forms	980	**C**
Cyclophosphamide		20 mg/ml		3 units/ml	Drugs injected sequentially into Y-site with no flush between. No visually apparent precipitate forms	980	**C**
Doxorubicin HCl		2 mg/ml		3 units/ml	Drugs injected sequentially into Y-site with no flush between. No visually apparent precipitate forms	980	**C**
Doxorubicin HCl liposome injection	SEQ	0.4 mg/ml[a]	MJ	1 unit/ml[b]	Physically compatible with little or no change in measured turbidity and no increase in particle content in 4 hr at 23 °C	2087	**C**
Droperidol		2.5 mg/ml		3 units/ml	Drugs injected sequentially into Y-site with no flush between. No visually apparent precipitate forms	980	**C**
Etoposide phosphate	BR	5 mg/ml[a]	MJ	1 unit/ml[b]	Physically compatible with no change in measured turbidity or increase in particle content in 4 hr at 23 °C	2218	**C**
Filgrastim	AMG	30 μg/ml[a]	BR	1 unit/ml[a]	Physically compatible with no change in measured turbidity or increase in particle content in 4 hr at 22 °C under fluorescent light	1687	**C**

Y-Site Injection Compatibility (1:1 Mixture) (Cont.)

Drug	Mfr	Conc	Mfr	Conc	Remarks	Ref	C/I
				Bleomycin sulfate			
Fludarabine phosphate	BX	1 mg/ml[a]	BR	1 unit/ml[b]	Physically compatible for 4 hr at room temperature under fluorescent light	1439	**C**
Fluorouracil		50 mg/ml		3 units/ml	Drugs injected sequentially into Y-site with no flush between. No visually apparent precipitate forms	980	**C**
Gemcitabine HCl	LI	10 mg/ml[b]	MJ	1 unit/ml[b]	Physically compatible with no change in measured turbidity or increase in particle content in 4 hr at 23 °C	2226	**C**
Granisetron HCl	SKB	0.05 mg/ml[a]	MJ	1 unit/ml[b]	Physically compatible with no change in measured turbidity or increase in particle content in 4 hr at 23 °C	2000	**C**
Heparin sodium		1000 units/ml		3 units/ml	Drugs injected sequentially into Y-site with no flush between. No visually apparent precipitate forms	980	**C**
Leucovorin calcium		10 mg/ml		3 units/ml	Drugs injected sequentially into Y-site with no flush between. No visually apparent precipitate forms	980	**C**
Melphalan HCl	BW	0.1 mg/ml[b]	BR	1 unit/ml[b]	Physically compatible with no change in measured turbidity or increase in particle content in 3 hr at 22 °C	1557	**C**
Methotrexate sodium		25 mg/ml		3 units/ml	Drugs injected sequentially into Y-site with no flush between. No visually apparent precipitate forms	980	**C**
Metoclopramide HCl		5 mg/ml		3 units/ml	Drugs injected sequentially into Y-site with no flush between. No visually apparent precipitate forms	980	**C**
Mitomycin		0.5 mg/ml		3 units/ml	Drugs injected sequentially into Y-site with no flush between. No visually apparent precipitate forms	980	**C**
Ondansetron HCl	GL	1 mg/ml[b]	BR	1 unit/ml[b]	Physically compatible for 4 hr at 22 °C	1365	**C**
Paclitaxel	NCI	1.2 mg/ml[a]	MJ	1 unit/ml[a]	Physically compatible with no change in measured turbidity in 4 hr at 22 °C	1556	**C**
Piperacillin sodium–tazobactam sodium	LE	40 + 5 mg/ml[a]	BR	1 unit/ml[b]	Physically compatible with no change in measured turbidity or increase in particle content in 4 hr at 22 °C	1688	**C**
Sargramostim	IMM	10 μg/ml[b]	MJ	1 unit/ml[b]	Physically compatible for 4 hr at 22 °C	1436	**C**
Teniposide	BR	0.1 mg/ml[a]	BR	1 unit/ml[b]	Physically compatible with no subvisual haze or particle formation in 4 hr at 23 °C	1725	**C**
Thiotepa	IMM[c]	1 mg/ml[a]	MJ	1 unit/ml[b]	Physically compatible with no change in measured turbidity or increase in particle content in 4 hr at 23 °C	1861	**C**
Vinblastine sulfate		1 mg/ml		3 units/ml	Drugs injected sequentially into Y-site with no flush between. No visually apparent precipitate forms	980	**C**
Vincristine sulfate		1 mg/ml		3 units/ml	Drugs injected sequentially into Y-site with no flush between. No visually apparent precipitate forms	980	**C**

Y-Site Injection Compatibility (1:1 Mixture) (Cont.)

Bleomycin sulfate

Drug	Mfr	Conc	Mfr	Conc	Remarks	Ref	C/I
Vinorelbine tartrate	BW	1 mg/ml[b]	BR	1 unit/ml[b]	Physically compatible with no change in measured turbidity or increase in particle content in 4 hr at 22 °C	1558	C

[a]*Tested in dextrose 5% in water.*
[b]*Tested in sodium chloride 0.9%.*
[c]*Lyophilized formulation tested.*

Additional Compatibility Information

Miscellaneous— The manufacturer states that bleomycin sulfate is stable for 24 hours in sodium chloride 0.9% at room temperature. (See Stability.) Diluted in sodium chloride 0.9% to concentrations of 15 units/100 ml in PVC bags and 60 units/100 ml in polypropylene syringes, bleomycin sulfate lost 4 and 6%, respectively, in 28 days at room temperature in the dark. However, at a concentration of 15 units/100 ml in dextrose 5% in water, a 54% loss occurred in PVC bags in 28 days at room temperature in the dark (1369).

Bleomycin sulfate is inactivated in vitro by agents containing sulfhydryl groups, hydrogen peroxide, and ascorbic acid (4).

No alteration in the ultraviolet/visible spectra was observed when dacarbazine was combined in solution with bleomycin sulfate (492).

Ogawa et al. reported that immersion of a needle with an aluminum component in bleomycin sulfate (Bristol) 3 units/ml resulted in no visually apparent reaction after seven days at 24 °C (988).

Inactivation— In the event of spills or leaks, Bristol-Myers recommends the use of sodium hypochlorite 5% (household bleach) or potassium permanganate 1% to inactivate bleomycin sulfate (1200).

BRETYLIUM TOSYLATE
AHFS 24:04

American Regent

Products— Bretylium tosylate (American Regent) is available at a concentration of 50 mg/ml in 10-ml single-use vials and prefilled syringes. Hydrochloric acid or sodium hydroxide may be present to adjust the pH (1-3/94; 29).

Bretylium tosylate is available premixed in dextrose 5% in water in concentrations of 2 and 4 mg/ml (4).

pH— Injection: 4.5 to 7. Premixed infusion: from 3 to 5 (4).

Osmolarity— Injection: approximately 174 mOsm/L. Premixed infusion: 2 mg/ml, 260 to 264 mOsm/L; and 4 mg/ml, 270 to 278 mOsm/L (4).

Administration— Bretylium tosylate is administered intramuscularly (not more than 5 ml per site) or intravenously by direct injection or intermittent or continuous infusion. Intramuscular injection sites should be rotated to avoid tissue damage. The patient should be recumbent or closely observed for postural hypotension during administration (1-3/94; 4).

Stability— The injection should be stored at 15 to 30 °C. The premixed infusion should be stored at room temperature and protected from freezing. Brief exposure to temperatures up to 40 °C does not adversely affect the products (4). Solutions of bretylium tosylate are stable over a pH range of 2 to 12 (607).

Compatibility Information

Solution Compatibility

Bretylium tosylate

Solution	Mfr	Mfr	Conc/L	Remarks	Ref	C/I
Dextrose 5% in Ringer's injection, lactated	MG[a], TR[b]	ACC	10 g	Physically compatible and chemically stable for 48 hr at room temperature and 7 days at 4 °C	541	C
Dextrose 5% in sodium chloride 0.45%	MG[a], TR[b]	ACC	10 g	Physically compatible and chemically stable for 48 hr at room temperature and 7 days at 4 °C	541	C
Dextrose 5% in sodium chloride 0.9%	MG[a], TR[b]	ACC	10 g	Physically compatible and chemically stable for 48 hr at room temperature and 7 days at 4 °C	541	C

Solution Compatibility (Cont.)

Bretylium tosylate

Solution	Mfr	Mfr	Conc/L	Remarks	Ref	C/I
Dextrose 5% in water	MG[a], TR[b]	ACC	10 g	Physically compatible and chemically stable for 48 hr at room temperature and 7 days at 4 °C	541	**C**
	AB[a]	ACC	1 g	Physically compatible and chemically stable for at least 48 hr (total study duration) at 25 °C	756	**C**
	AB[b]	ACC	1 g	Physically compatible and chemically stable for 30 days at 25 °C	756	**C**
	TR[b]	ES	1 g	Physically compatible with no loss in 24 hr at room temperature under fluorescent light	1358	**C**
Mannitol 20%	MG[a]	ACC	10 g	Physically compatible and chemically stable for 48 hr at room temperature. Mannitol crystallizes when refrigerated	541	**C**
Ringer's injection, lactated	MG[a], TR[b]	ACC	10 g	Physically compatible and chemically stable for 48 hr at room temperature and 7 days at 4 °C	541	**C**
	AB[a,b]	ACC	1 g	Physically compatible and chemically stable for 30 days at 25 °C	756	**C**
Sodium bicarbonate 5%	MG[a]	ACC	10 g	Physically compatible and chemically stable for 48 hr at room temperature and 7 days at 4 °C	541	**C**
Sodium chloride 0.9%	MG[a], TR[b]	ACC	10 g	Physically compatible and chemically stable for 48 hr at room temperature and 7 days at 4 °C	541	**C**
	CU[a], AB[b]	ACC	1 g	Physically compatible and chemically stable for 30 days at 25 °C	756	**C**
Sodium lactate ⅙ M	MG[a], TR[b]	ACC	10 g	Physically compatible and chemically stable for 48 hr at room temperature and 7 days at 4 °C	541	**C**

[a]Tested in glass containers.
[b]Tested in PVC containers.

Additive Compatibility

Bretylium tosylate

Drug	Mfr	Conc/L	Mfr	Conc/L	Test Soln	Remarks	Ref	C/I
Aminophylline	ES	1 g	ACC	1 g	D5W, NS	Physically compatible for 48 hr at 25 °C	756	**C**
Atracurium besylate	BW	500 mg		4 g	D5W	Physically compatible and atracurium chemically stable for 24 hr at 5 and 30 °C	1694	**C**
Calcium chloride	ES	54.4 mEq	ACC	10 g	D5W[a]	Physically compatible and bretylium chemically stable for 48 hr at room temperature and 7 days at 4 °C	541	**C**
Calcium gluconate	ES	2 g	ACC	1 g	D5W, NS	Physically compatible for 48 hr at 25 °C	756	**C**
Cibenzoline succinate		2 g	ACC	10 g	D5W, NS	Physically compatible for 24 hr at 25 °C by visual and microscopic examination	1182	**C**
Digoxin	BW	2 mg	ACC	1 g	D5W, NS	Physically compatible for 48 hr at 25 °C	756	**C**
Dobutamine HCl	LI	1 g	ACC	2 g	D5W, NS	Slightly pink in 24 hr at 25 °C	789	**I**
	LI	1 g	ACC	4 and 25 g	D5W, NS	Physically compatible for 24 hr at 21 °C	812	**C**
Dopamine HCl	ACC	800 mg	ACC	10 g	D5S[a]	Physically compatible and both drugs chemically stable for 48 hr at room temperature and 7 days at 4 °C	522	**C**

Additive Compatibility (Cont.)

			Bretylium tosylate					
Drug	*Mfr*	*Conc/L*	*Mfr*	*Conc/L*	*Test Soln*	*Remarks*	*Ref*	*C/I*
Esmolol HCl	DU	6 g	ES	1 g	D5W	Physically compatible with no loss of either drug in 24 hr at room temperature	1358	**C**
Insulin, regular	SQ	1000 units	ACC	1 g	D5W, NS	Physically compatible for 48 hr at 25 °C	756	**C**
Lidocaine HCl	AST	1 g	ACC	10 g	D5S[a]	Physically compatible and both drugs chemically stable for 48 hr at room temperature and 7 days at 4 °C	522	**C**
	AST	2 g	ACC	1 g	D5W, NS	Physically compatible for 48 hr at 25 °C	756	**C**
	AST	2 g	AS	1 g	D5W, LR, NS	Physically compatible for 24 hr at 25 °C	775	**C**
Nitroglycerin	ACC	100 mg	ACC	10 g	D5S[b]	Physically compatible and bretylium chemically stable for 48 hr at room temperature and 7 days at 4 °C. 40% loss of nitroglycerin at room temperature and 10% at 4 °C in 24 hr due to sorption to PVC	522	**I**
	ACC	100 mg	ACC	10 g	D5S[c]	Physically compatible and both drugs chemically stable for 48 hr at room temperature and 7 days at 4 °C	522	**C**
	ACC	400 mg	ACC	10 g	D5W, NS[c]	Physically compatible with little or no nitroglycerin loss in 48 hr at 23 °C. Bretylium not tested	929	**C**
Phenytoin sodium	PD	2 g	ACC	1 g	D5W, NS	Immediate precipitation	756	**I**
Potassium chloride	AB	40 mEq	ACC	10 g	D5W[a]	Physically compatible and bretylium chemically stable for 48 hr at room temperature and 7 days at 4 °C	541	**C**
Procainamide HCl	SQ	4 g	ACC	10 g	D5S[a]	Physically compatible and bretylium chemically stable for 48 hr at room temperature. Approximately 14% procainamide loss in 24 hr at room temperature	522	**I**
	SQ	4 g	ACC	10 g	D5S[a]	Physically compatible and bretylium chemically stable for 7 days at 4 °C. Approximately 7% procainamide loss in 24 hr at 4 °C	522	**C**
	SQ	1 g	ACC	1 g	D5W, NS	Physically compatible for 48 hr at 25 °C	756	**C**
Quinidine gluconate	LI	800 mg	ACC	1 g	D5W, NS	Physically compatible for 48 hr at 25 °C	756	**C**
Verapamil HCl	KN	80 mg	ACC	2 g	D5W, NS	Physically compatible for 48 hr	739	**C**

[a]Tested in both glass and PVC containers.
[b]Tested in PVC containers.
[c]Tested in glass containers.

Y-Site Injection Compatibility (1:1 Mixture)

			Bretylium tosylate				
Drug	*Mfr*	*Conc*	*Mfr*	*Conc*	*Remarks*	*Ref*	*C/I*
Amiodarone HCl	LZ	4 mg/ml[c]	ACC	8 mg/ml[c]	Physically compatible for 24 hr at 21 °C	1032	**C**
Amphotericin B cholesteryl sulfate complex	SEQ	0.83 mg/ml[a]	AST	50 mg/ml	Gross precipitate forms	2117	**I**
Amrinone lactate	WB	3 mg/ml[b]	ACC	10 mg/ml[a]	Physically compatible for at least 4 hr at 25 °C under fluorescent light	992	**C**

Y-Site Injection Compatibility (1:1 Mixture) (Cont.)

Bretylium tosylate

Drug	Mfr	Conc	Mfr	Conc	Remarks	Ref	C/I
Cisatracurium besylate	GW	0.1, 2, 5 mg/ml[a]	AST	4 mg/ml[a]	Physically compatible with no change in measured turbidity or increase in particle content in 4 hr at 23 °C	2074	C
Diltiazem HCl	MMD	5 mg/ml	DU	10[b] and 50 mg/ml	Visually compatible	1807	C
	MMD	1 mg/ml[b]	DU	50 mg/ml	Visually compatible	1807	C
Dobutamine HCl	LI	4 mg/ml[c]	LY	4 mg/ml[c]	Physically compatible for 3 hr	1316	C
Famotidine	MSD	0.2 mg/ml[a]	AB	4 mg/ml[a]	Physically compatible for 4 hr at 25 °C	1188	C
Isoproterenol HCl	ES	0.032 mg/ml[c]	LY	4 mg/ml[c]	Physically compatible for 3 hr	1316	C
Propofol	ZEN	10 mg/ml	AST	50 mg/ml	Emulsion broke and oiled out	2066	I
Ranitidine HCl	GL	0.5 mg/ml[d]	LY	4 mg/ml[a]	Physically compatible for 24 hr	1323	C
Remifentanil HCl	GW	0.025 and 0.25 mg/ml[b]	AST	4 mg/ml[a]	Physically compatible with no change in measured turbidity or increase in particle content in 4 hr at 23 °C	2075	C
Warfarin sodium	DU	2 mg/ml[e]	FAU	10 mg/ml[a]	Haze forms immediately	2010	I
	DME	2 mg/ml[e]	DU	10 mg/ml[a]	Haze forms immediately	2078	I

[a]*Tested in dextrose 5% in water.*
[b]*Tested in sodium chloride 0.9%.*
[c]*Tested in dextrose 5% in water and sodium chloride 0.9%.*
[d]*Premixed infusion solution.*
[e]*Tested in sterile water for injection.*

BUMETANIDE
AHFS 40:28

Bumex   **Roche**

Products— Bumetanide (Roche) is available as a 0.25-mg/ml solution in 2-ml ampuls and 2-, 4-, and 10-ml vials. The solution also contains sodium chloride 0.85%, ammonium acetate 0.4%, disodium edetate 0.01%, and benzyl alcohol 1% with sodium hydroxide to adjust the pH (1-9/97; 4).

pH— Adjusted to 6.8 to 7.8 (4).

Osmolality— Bumetanide 0.25 mg/ml has an osmolality of 453 mOsm/kg (1689).

Administration— Bumetanide is administered by intramuscular injection, direct intravenous injection over one to two minutes, and by intravenous infusion (1-9/97; 4). If glass ampuls are used, filtration to remove particles that may have entered the solution during ampul opening has been suggested (4).

Stability— Bumetanide discolors when exposed to light. The injection should be stored at room temperature and protected from light. Bumetanide is reported to be stable at pH 4 to 10 (4). Precipitation may occur at pH values less than 4 (1644).

Sorption— Substantial sorption to glass and PVC containers does not occur (1-9/97; 4).

Bumetanide (Roche) 0.2 mg/ml in PVC containers of dextrose 5% in water exhibited 4 to 5% loss by HPLC analysis within three hours of mixing. No further loss of drug occurred during storage for 72 hours at 24 °C under fluorescent light. A 10-fold higher concentration exhibited little or no loss under the same conditions. The authors postulated that a small amount of bumetanide loss due to sorption to the PVC might be occurring (2090).

Compatibility Information

Solution Compatibility

Bumetanide

Solution	Mfr	Mfr	Conc/L	Remarks	Ref	C/I
Dextrose 5% in water	AB[a]	RC	20 mg	4 to 5% loss by HPLC occurs within 3 hr with no further loss throughout 72 hr at 24 °C under fluorescent light	2090	C
	AB[a]	RC	200 mg	Little or no loss by HPLC occurs within 72 hr at 24 °C under fluorescent light	2090	C

[a]Tested in PVC containers.

Additive Compatibility

Bumetanide

Drug	Mfr	Conc/L	Mfr	Conc/L	Test Soln	Remarks	Ref	C/I
Dobutamine HCl	LI	1 g	RC	125 mg	D5W, NS	Immediate yellow discoloration with yellow precipitate within 6 hr at 21 °C	812	I
Floxacillin sodium	BE	20 g	LEO	6 mg	NS	Physically compatible for 72 hr at 15 and 30 °C	1479	C
Furosemide	HO	1 g	LEO	6 mg	NS	Physically compatible for 72 hr at 15 and 30 °C	1479	C

Drugs in Syringe Compatibility

Bumetanide

Drug (in syringe)	Mfr	Amt	Mfr	Amt	Remarks	Ref	C/I
Doxapram HCl	RB	400 mg/ 20 ml		0.5 mg/ 1 ml	Physically compatible with 3% doxapram loss in 24 hr	1177	C

Y-Site Injection Compatibility (1:1 Mixture)

Bumetanide

Drug	Mfr	Conc	Mfr	Conc	Remarks	Ref	C/I
Allopurinol sodium	BW	3 mg/ml[b]	RC	0.04 mg/ml[b]	Physically compatible with no change in measured turbidity or increase in particle content in 4 hr at 22 °C	1686	C
Amifostine	USB	10 mg/ml[a]	RC	0.04 mg/ml[a]	Physically compatible with no change in measured turbidity or increase in particle content in 4 hr at 23 °C	1845	C
Aztreonam	SQ	40 mg/ml[a]	RC	0.04 mg/ml[a]	Physically compatible with no subvisual haze or particle formation in 4 hr at 23 °C	1758	C
Cefepime HCl	BR	20 mg/ml[a]	RC	0.04 mg/ml[a]	Physically compatible with no change in measured turbidity or increase in particle content in 4 hr at 22 °C	1689	C
Cisatracurium besylate	GW	0.1, 2, 5 mg/ml[a]	BV	0.04 mg/ml[a]	Physically compatible with no change in measured turbidity or increase in particle content in 4 hr at 23 °C	2074	C

Y-Site Injection Compatibility (1:1 Mixture) (Cont.)

		Bumetanide					
Drug	*Mfr*	*Conc*	*Mfr*	*Conc*	*Remarks*	*Ref*	*C/I*
Cladribine	ORT	0.015[b] and 0.5[c] mg/ml	RC	0.04 mg/ml[b]	Physically compatible with no change in measured turbidity or increase in particle content in 4 hr at 23 °C	1969	**C**
Clarithromycin	AB	4 mg/ml[a]	LEO	0.5 mg/ml	Visually compatible for 72 hr at both 30 and 17 °C	2174	**C**
Diltiazem HCl	MMD	1[b] and 5 mg/ml	RC	0.25 mg/ml	Visually compatible	1563	**C**
Docetaxel	RPR	0.9 mg/ml[a]	RC	0.04 mg/ml[a]	Physically compatible with no change in measured turbidity or increase in particle content in 4 hr at 23 °C	2224	**C**
Etoposide phosphate	BR	5 mg/ml[a]	RC	0.04 mg/ml[a]	Physically compatible with no change in measured turbidity or increase in particle content in 4 hr at 23 °C	2218	**C**
Filgrastim	AMG	30 µg/ml[a]	RC	0.04 mg/ml[a]	Physically compatible with no change in measured turbidity or increase in particle content in 4 hr at 22 °C	1687	**C**
Gemcitabine HCl	LI	10 mg/ml[b]	RC	0.04 mg/ml[b]	Physically compatible with no change in measured turbidity or increase in particle content in 4 hr at 23 °C	2226	**C**
Granisetron HCl	SKB	0.05 mg/ml[a]	RC	0.04 mg/ml[a]	Physically compatible with no change in measured turbidity or increase in particle content in 4 hr at 23 °C	2000	**C**
Lorazepam	WY	0.33 mg/ml[b]	LEO	0.5 mg/ml	Visually compatible for 24 hr at 22 °C	1855	**C**
Melphalan HCl	BW	0.1 mg/ml[b]	RC	0.04 mg/ml[b]	Physically compatible with no change in measured turbidity or increase in particle content in 3 hr at 22 °C	1557	**C**
Meperidine HCl	AB	10 mg/ml	RC	0.25 mg/ml	Physically compatible for 4 hr at 25 °C	1397	**C**
Midazolam HCl	RC	5 mg/ml	LEO	0.5 mg/ml	White precipitate forms immediately	1855	**I**
Milrinone lactate	SW	0.4 mg/ml[a]	RC	0.25 mg/ml	Visually compatible with little or no loss of either drug by HPLC in 4 hr at 23 °C	2214	**C**
Morphine sulfate	AB	1 mg/ml	RC	0.25 mg/ml	Physically compatible for 4 hr at 25 °C	1397	**C**
Piperacillin sodium–tazobactam sodium	LE	40 + 5 mg/ml[a]	RC	0.04 mg/ml[a]	Physically compatible with no change in measured turbidity or increase in particle content in 4 hr at 22 °C	1688	**C**
Propofol	ZEN	10 mg/ml	RC	0.04 mg/ml[a]	Physically compatible for 1 hr at 23 °C with no increase in particle content	2066	**C**
Remifentanil HCl	GW	0.025 and 0.25 mg/ml[b]	RC	0.04 mg/ml[a]	Physically compatible with no change in measured turbidity or increase in particle content in 4 hr at 23 °C	2075	**C**
Teniposide	BR	0.1 mg/ml[a]	RC	0.04 mg/ml[a]	Physically compatible with no subvisual haze or particle formation in 4 hr at 23 °C	1725	**C**
Thiotepa	IMM[d]	1 mg/ml[a]	RC	0.04 mg/ml[a]	Physically compatible with no change in measured turbidity or increase in particle content in 4 hr at 23 °C	1861	**C**

Y-Site Injection Compatibility (1:1 Mixture) (Cont.)

Bumetanide

Drug	Mfr	Conc	Mfr	Conc	Remarks	Ref	C/I
TNA #218 to #226[e]			RC, BV	0.04 mg/ml[a]	Visually compatible with no precipitate or emulsion damage apparent in 4 hr at 23 °C	2215	C
TPN #212 to #215[e]			RC	0.04 mg/ml[a]	Physically compatible with no change in measured turbidity or increase in particle content in 4 hr at 23 °C	2109	C
Vinorelbine tartrate	BW	1 mg/ml[b]	RC	0.04 mg/ml[b]	Physically compatible with no change in measured turbidity or increase in particle content in 4 hr at 22 °C	1558	C

[a]*Tested in dextrose 5% in water.*
[b]*Tested in sodium chloride 0.9%.*
[c]*Tested in bacteriostatic sodium chloride 0.9% preserved with benzyl alcohol 0.9%.*
[d]*Lyophilized formulation tested.*
[e]*Refer to Appendix I for the composition of parenteral nutrition solutions. TNA indicates a 3-in-1 admixture, and TPN indicates a 2-in-1 admixture.*

Additional Compatibility Information

Vehicles— Bumetanide is stated to be physically and chemically compatible in glass or PVC containers of dextrose 5% in water, sodium chloride 0.9%, and Ringer's injection, lactated, for at least 24 hours (2; 4).

Milrinone— Bumetanide may precipitate if mixed with milrinone lactate infusions (1442).

BUPIVACAINE HCL
AHFS 72:00

Sensorcaine   **Astra**

Products— Bupivacaine HCl (Astra) is available in concentrations of 0.25, 0.5, and 0.75% (2.5, 5, and 7.5 mg/ml, respectively) in 10- and 30-ml single-dose vials. It also is available in 30-ml (0.25, 0.5, and 0.75%) single-dose ampuls. The 0.25 and 0.5% concentrations also come in 50-ml multiple-dose vials with methylparaben 1 mg/ml as a preservative. Sodium hydroxide or hydrochloric acid is used to adjust the pH (2).

Bupivacaine HCl is also available in concentrations of 0.25, 0.5, and 0.75% with epinephrine 1:200,000 as the bitartrate. In addition to bupivacaine HCl, each milliliter contains epinephrine bitartrate 0.005 mg, sodium metabisulfite 0.5 mg, and citric acid 0.2 mg.

Multiple-dose vials contain methylparaben 1 mg/ml as a preservative. Sodium hydroxide or hydrochloric acid is used to adjust the pH (2).

A hyperbaric solution of bupivacaine HCl is available in 2-ml ampuls. Each milliliter contains bupivacaine HCl 7.5 mg and dextrose 82.5 mg (8.25%) with sodium hydroxide or hydrochloric acid to adjust the pH (2).

pH— Bupivacaine HCl injection and the hyperbaric solution have a pH of 4 to 6.5. Bupivacaine HCl with epinephrine 1:200,000 has a pH of 3.3 to 5.5 (2; 4).

Specific Gravity— The hyperbaric solution has a specific gravity of 1.030 to 1.035 at 25 °C and 1.03 at 37 °C (4).

Administration— Bupivacaine HCl may be administered by infiltration or by epidural, spinal, or peripheral or sympathetic nerve block as a single injection or repeat injections. Injections should be made slowly, with frequent aspirations, to guard against intravascular injection. Products containing preservatives should not be used for epidural or caudal block (2; 4).

Stability— Bupivacaine HCl injections should be stored at 15 to 30 °C; freezing should be avoided (2; 4). Products containing epinephrine should be protected from light during storage (4).

Bupivacaine HCl without epinephrine and the hyperbaric solution may be autoclaved at 121 °C and 15 psi for 15 minutes. Products containing epinephrine should not be autoclaved (4).

Bupivacaine HCl with epinephrine should not be used if a pinkish color, a color darker than "slightly" yellow, or a precipitate develops (2).

Syringes— The stability of bupivacaine (salt form unspecified) 5 mg/ml repackaged in polypropylene syringes was evaluated by spectrophotometric and potentiometric methods. Little or no change in concentration was found after four weeks of storage at room temperature not exposed to direct light (2164).

Ambulatory Pump— Bupivacaine HCl (Astra) 7.5 mg/ml was filled into 50-ml ambulatory pump cassette reservoirs (Pharmacia Deltec) and stored at room temperature protected from light for 90 days. HPLC analysis found no loss of the drug. Instead, the drug concentration increased 12% during the observation period, possibly because of loss of water from the solutions (1850).

Compatibility Information

Solution Compatibility

Bupivacaine HCl

Solution	Mfr	Mfr	Conc/L	Remarks	Ref	C/I
Sodium chloride 0.9%	AB	AST	1.25 g	Visually compatible with no bupivacaine loss by HPLC in 32 days at 3 °C in the dark and 23 °C exposed to light when stored in polypropylene syringes	1718	C
	AB[a]	AB	625 mg and 1.25 g	Visually compatible with little or no bupivacaine loss by HPLC in 72 hr at 24 °C under fluorescent light	1870; 2058	C
	GRI[a]		850 mg	No change in concentration by UV spectroscopy in 28 days at 4 °C and room temperature	1910	C

[a]Tested in PVC containers.

Additive Compatibility

Bupivacaine HCl

Drug	Mfr	Conc/L	Mfr	Conc/L	Test Soln	Remarks	Ref	C/I
Buprenorphine HCl	RC	180 mg	AST	3 g	a	Little or no loss of either drug by HPLC in 30 days at 18 °C	1932	C
Diamorphine HCl		0.125 g	GL	1.25 g	NS	Visually compatible with 8% diamorphine loss and no bupivacaine loss by HPLC in 28 days at room temperature	1791	C
Fentanyl citrate	JN	20 mg	WI	1.25 g	NS[a]	Physically compatible with little or no loss of either drug in 30 days at 3 and 23 °C	1396	C
Hydromorphone HCl	KN	20 mg	AB	625 mg and 1.25 g	NS[a]	Visually compatible with little or no loss of either drug by HPLC in 72 hr at 24 °C under fluorescent light	1870	C
	KN	100 mg	AB	625 mg and 1.25 g	NS[a]	Visually compatible with little or no loss of either drug by HPLC in 72 hr at 24 °C under fluorescent light	1870	C
Morphine HCl		140 and 190 mg		850 mg	NS[a]	No change in concentration by UV spectroscopy in 28 days at 4 °C and room temperature	1910	C
Morphine sulfate		1 g	AST	3 g	a	Little or no loss of either drug by HPLC in 30 days at 18 °C	1932	C
	SCN	100 mg	AB	625 mg and 1.25 g	NS[a]	Visually compatible with no loss of either drug by HPLC in 72 hr at 24 °C under fluorescent light	2058	C
	SCN	500 mg	AB	625 mg and 1.25 g	NS[a]	Visually compatible with no loss of either drug by HPLC in 72 hr at 24 °C under fluorescent light	2058	C
Sufentanil citrate	JN	5 mg	AST	2 g	D5W[b]	9% sufentanil loss and 5% bupivacaine loss by HPLC in 30 days at 32 °C. Little or no loss of either drug in 30 days at 4 °C	1756	C
	JN	20 mg		3 g	NS[b]	5% sufentanil loss and no bupivacaine loss by HPLC in 10 days at 5, 26, and 37 °C	1751	C

[a]Tested in PVC containers.
[b]Tested in PVC/Kalex 3000 (phthalate ester) CADD pump reservoirs.

Drugs in Syringe Compatibility

Bupivacaine HCl

Drug (in syringe)	Mfr	Amt	Mfr	Amt	Remarks	Ref	*C/I*
Clonidine HCl with morphine sulfate	BI ES	0.03 mg/ ml 0.2 mg/ ml	PD	2 mg/ml	Diluted to 5 ml with NS. Visually compatible with no new GC/MS peaks appearing in 1 hr at room temperature	1956	**C**
Diamorphine HCl	EV	1 and 10 mg/ ml	AST	0.5%	10 to 11% diamorphine loss by HPLC in 5 weeks at 20 °C and 3 to 7% loss in 8 weeks at 6 °C. Little or no bupivacaine loss at 6 or 20 °C in 8 weeks	1952	**C**
Fentanyl citrate with ketamine HCl	SW PD	1.5 mg/ ml 2 mg/ml	JN	0.01 mg/ ml	Diluted to 5 ml with NS. Visually compatible with no new GC/MS peaks appearing in 1 hr at room temperature	1956	**C**
Hydromorphone HCl	KN	65 mg/ ml	AST	7.5 mg/ ml	Visually compatible for 30 days at 25 °C	1660	**C**
Iohexol		1 ml	AST	0.25 and 0.125%[a]/ 4 ml	Visually compatible with no bupivacaine loss by HPLC in 24 hr at room temperature. Iohexol not tested	1611	**C**
Morphine sulfate	MA	129 mg/ ml	AST	7.5 mg/ ml	Visually compatible for 30 days at 25 °C	1660	**C**
		1 mg/ml	AST	3 mg/ml	Little or no loss of either drug by HPLC in 30 days at 18 °C	1932	**C**
Sodium bicarbonate	AB	4%, 0.05 to 0.6 ml	AST, WI	0.25, 0.5[b], 0.75%[b], 20 ml	Precipitate forms in 1 to 2 min up to 2 hr at lowest amount of bicarbonate	1724	**I**
		1.4%, 1.5 ml	BEL	0.5%[c], 20 ml	Little or no epinephrine loss by HPLC in 7 days at room temperature. Bupivacaine not tested	1743	**C**
		4.2 and 8.4%, 1.5 ml	BEL	0.5%[c], 20 ml	5 to 7% epinephrine loss by HPLC in 7 days at room temperature. Bupivacaine not tested	1743	**C**

[a]*Diluted 1:1 in sodium chloride 0.9%.*
[b]*Tested with and without epinephrine HCl 1:200,000 added.*
[c]*Tested with epinephrine HCl 1:200,000 added.*

Additional Compatibility Information

Epinephrine and Fentanyl— A solution composed of bupivacaine HCl (Winthrop) 0.44 mg/ml, fentanyl citrate (Janssen) 1.25 µg/ml, and epinephrine HCl (Abbott) 0.69 µg/ml was stored in 100-ml portable infusion pump reservoirs (Pharmacia Deltec) for 30 days at 3 and 23 °C. The samples were then delivered through the infusion pumps over 48 hours at near-body temperature (30 °C). The samples were visually compatible throughout, and bupivacaine HCl and fentanyl citrate exhibited no loss by HPLC analysis. Epinephrine HCl sustained about a 5 to 6% loss by HPLC analysis after 20 days of storage at both temperatures and about a 9 to 10% loss after 30 days of storage and subsequent pump delivery. The authors recommended restricting storage before administration to only 20 days (1627).

Clonidine HCl— Clonidine HCl (Fujisawa) 100 µg/ml and bupivacaine HCl (Sanofi-Winthrop) 7.5 mg/ml were mixed in ratios of 1:1 and 1:8 to provide final concentrations of (1:1) clonidine HCl 50 µg/ml and bupivacaine HCl 3.75 mg/ml and (1:8) clonidine HCl 11.11 µg/ml and bupivacaine HCl 6.67 mg/ml. The combinations were transferred to flint glass vials with rubber stoppers and stored for 14 days at controlled room temperature protected from light. The solutions remained clear and colorless with no increase in particulate content. HPLC analysis found little or no change in concentration for either drug during the study period (2069).

Multiple Drugs— A seven-drug combination consisting of bupivacaine HCl (Sanofi Winthrop) 1.5 mg/ml, clonidine HCl (Boehringer Ingelheim) 0.03 mg/ml, fentanyl citrate (Janssen) 0.01 mg/ml, ketamine HCl (Parke-Davis) 2 mg/ml, lidocaine HCl (Astra) 2 mg/ml, morphine sulfate (Elkins-Sinn) 0.2 mg/ml, and tetracaine HCl (Sanofi Winthrop) 2 mg/ml mixed together in equal volumes was found to be visually compatible with no new GC/MS peaks appearing in one hour at room temperature (1956).

Clonidine HCl (Boehringer) 30 µg/ml, bupivacaine HCl (Astra) 3 mg/ml, and morphine HCl (Merck) 6.66 mg/ml were combined in 50-ml ambulatory pump cassette reservoirs (Pharmacia Deltec). The reservoirs were stored at room temperature and protected from light for 90 days. HPLC analysis found no loss of any of the drugs. Instead, drug concentrations increased 12 to 16% during the obser-

vation period, possibly because of loss of water from the solutions (1850).

BUPRENORPHINE HCL
AHFS 28:08.12

Buprenex   **Reckitt-Colman**

Products— Buprenorphine HCl (Reckitt-Colman) is available in 1-ml ampuls. Each milliliter contains buprenorphine 0.3 mg (as the hydrochloride) with anhydrous dextrose 50 mg in water for injection. The pH is adjusted with hydrochloric acid (2).

pH— From 3.5 to 5.5 (4).

Osmolality— The osmolality of buprenorphine HCl was determined to be 297 mOsm/kg by osmometer (1233).

Administration— Buprenorphine HCl is administered by deep intramuscular injection or by intravenous injection slowly over at least two minutes (2; 4). It has also been given by continuous intravenous infusion at a concentration of 15 μg/ml in sodium chloride 0.9% and by epidural injection at a concentration of 6 to 30 μg/ml (4).

Stability— The clear solution should be stored at 15 to 30 °C and protected from prolonged exposure to light and exposure to temperatures in excess of 40 °C and freezing (2; 4). Buprenorphine HCl may undergo substantial decomposition when autoclaved (4).

Compatibility Information

Additive Compatibility

Buprenorphine HCl

Drug	Mfr	Conc/L	Mfr	Conc/L	Test Soln	Remarks	Ref	C/I
Bupivacaine HCl	AST	3 g	RC	180 mg	[a]	Little or no loss of either drug by HPLC in 30 days at 18 °C	1932	**C**
Floxacillin sodium	BE	20 g		75 mg	W	Thick haze forms in 24 hr and precipitate forms in 47 hr at 30 °C. No change at 15 °C	1479	**I**
Furosemide	HO	1 g		75 mg	W	Haze for 6 hr at 30 °C. No change at 15 °C	1479	**I**

[a]*Tested in PVC containers.*

Drugs in Syringe Compatibility

Buprenorphine HCl

Drug (in syringe)	Mfr	Amt	Mfr	Amt	Remarks	Ref	C/I
Midazolam HCl	RC	5 mg/ 1 ml	NE	0.3 mg/ 1 ml	Physically compatible for 4 hr at 25 °C	1145	**C**

Y-Site Injection Compatibility (1:1 Mixture)

Buprenorphine HCl

Drug	Mfr	Conc	Mfr	Conc	Remarks	Ref	C/I
Allopurinol sodium	BW	3 mg/ml[b]	RKC	0.04 mg/ml[b]	Physically compatible with no change in measured turbidity or increase in particle content in 4 hr at 22 °C	1686	**C**
Amifostine	USB	10 mg/ml[a]	RKC	0.04 mg/ml[a]	Physically compatible with no change in measured turbidity or increase in particle content in 4 hr at 23 °C	1845	**C**

Y-Site Injection Compatibility (1:1 Mixture) (Cont.)

Buprenorphine HCl

Drug	Mfr	Conc	Mfr	Conc	Remarks	Ref	C/I
Amphotericin B cholesteryl sulfate complex	SEQ	0.83 mg/ml[a]	RKC	0.04 mg/ml[a]	Microprecipitate forms in 4 hr	2117	**I**
Aztreonam	SQ	40 mg/ml[a]	RKC	0.04 mg/ml[a]	Physically compatible with no subvisual haze or particle formation in 4 hr at 23 °C	1758	**C**
Cefepime HCl	BR	20 mg/ml[a]	RKC	0.04 mg/ml[a]	Physically compatible with no change in measured turbidity or increase in particle content in 4 hr at 22 °C	1689	**C**
Cisatracurium besylate	GW	0.1, 2, 5 mg/ml[a]	RKC	0.04 mg/ml[a]	Physically compatible with no change in measured turbidity or increase in particle content in 4 hr at 23 °C	2074	**C**
Cladribine	ORT	0.015[b] and 0.5[c] mg/ml	RKC	0.04 mg/ml[b]	Physically compatible with no change in measured turbidity or increase in particle content in 4 hr at 23 °C	1969	**C**
Docetaxel	RPR	0.9 mg/ml[a]	RKC	0.04 mg/ml[a]	Physically compatible with no change in measured turbidity or increase in particle content in 4 hr at 23 °C	2224	**C**
Doxorubicin HCl liposome injection	SEQ	0.4 mg/ml[a]	RKC	0.04 mg/ml[a]	Partial loss of measured natural turbidity	2087	**I**
Etoposide phosphate	BR	5 mg/ml[a]	RKC	0.04 mg/ml[a]	Physically compatible with no change in measured turbidity or increase in particle content in 4 hr at 23 °C	2218	**C**
Filgrastim	AMG	30 μg/ml[a]	RKC	0.04 mg/ml[a]	Physically compatible with no change in measured turbidity or increase in particle content in 4 hr at 22 °C	1687	**C**
Gemcitabine HCl	LI	10 mg/ml[b]	RKC	0.04 mg/ml[b]	Physically compatible with no change in measured turbidity or increase in particle content in 4 hr at 23 °C	2226	**C**
Granisetron HCl	SKB	0.05 mg/ml[a]	RKC	0.04 mg/ml[a]	Physically compatible with no change in measured turbidity or increase in particle content in 4 hr at 23 °C	2000	**C**
Melphalan HCl	BW	0.1 mg/ml[b]	RKC	0.04 mg/ml[b]	Physically compatible with no change in measured turbidity or increase in particle content in 3 hr at 22 °C	1557	**C**
Piperacillin sodium–tazobactam sodium	LE	40 + 5 mg/ml[a]	RKC	0.04 mg/ml[a]	Physically compatible with no change in measured turbidity or increase in particle content in 4 hr at 22 °C	1688	**C**
Propofol	ZEN	10 mg/ml	RKC	0.04 mg/ml[a]	Physically compatible for 1 hr at 23 °C with no increase in particle content	2066	**C**
Remifentanil HCl	GW	0.025 and 0.25 mg/ml[b]	RKC	0.04 mg/ml[a]	Physically compatible with no change in measured turbidity or increase in particle content in 4 hr at 23 °C	2075	**C**
Teniposide	BR	0.1 mg/ml[a]	RKC	0.04 mg/ml[a]	Physically compatible with no subvisual haze or particle formation in 4 hr at 23 °C	1725	**C**
Thiotepa	IMM[d]	1 mg/ml[a]	RKC	0.04 mg/ml[a]	Physically compatible with no change in measured turbidity or increase in particle content in 4 hr at 23 °C	1861	**C**

Y-Site Injection Compatibility (1:1 Mixture) (Cont.)

Buprenorphine HCl

Drug	Mfr	Conc	Mfr	Conc	Remarks	Ref	C/I
TNA #218 to #226[e]			RKC	0.04 mg/ml[a]	Visually compatible with no precipitate or emulsion damage apparent in 4 hr at 23 °C	2215	C
TPN #212 to #215[e]			RKC	0.04 mg/ml[a]	Physically compatible with no change in measured turbidity or increase in particle content in 4 hr at 23 °C	2109	C
Vinorelbine tartrate	BW	1 mg/ml[b]	RKC	0.04 mg/ml[b]	Physically compatible with no change in measured turbidity or increase in particle content in 4 hr at 22 °C	1558	C

[a]Tested in dextrose 5% in water.
[b]Tested in sodium chloride 0.9%.
[c]Tested in bacteriostatic sodium chloride 0.9% preserved with benzyl alcohol 0.9%.
[d]Lyophilized formulation tested.
[e]Refer to Appendix I for the composition of parenteral nutrition solutions. TNA indicates a 3-in-1 admixture, and TPN indicates a 2-in-1 admixture.

Additional Compatibility Information

Solutions—— Buprenorphine HCl is stated to be physically and chemically compatible in a 1:1 volume ratio with dextrose 5% in sodium chloride 0.9%, dextrose 5% in water, Ringer's injection, lactated, and sodium chloride 0.9% (4).

Additives—— Buprenorphine HCl is stated to be physically and chemically compatible in a 1:1 volume ratio with atropine sulfate, diphenhydramine HCl, droperidol, glycopyrrolate, haloperidol lactate, hydroxyzine HCl, promethazine HCl, and scopolamine hydrobromide (4).

The drug is stated to be incompatible with diazepam and lorazepam (4).

BUSULFAN
AHFS 10:00

Busulfex   **Orphan Medical**

Products—— Busulfan (Orphan Medical) is available as a 6-mg/ml concentrated solution dissolved in a vehicle composed of 33% w/w *N,N*-dimethylacetamide and 67% w/w polyethylene glycol 400. The product is packaged in 10-ml colorless single-use ampuls along with 25-mm 5-μm nylon membrane filters. The concentrated injection must be diluted for administration (1-2/99).

pH—— An infusion admixture of busulfan diluted for infusion in sodium chloride 0.9% or dextrose 5% in water to a concentration greater than 0.5 mg/ml has a pH of 3.4 to 3.9 (1-2/99).

Administration—— Busulfan must be diluted for administration. Sodium chloride 0.9% and dextrose 5% in water are both recommended diluents for busulfan infusion. The quantity of infusion solution should be ten times the volume of the busulfan concentrate dose to ensure that the final concentration is equal to or greater than 0.5 mg/ml. As an example, if 9.3 ml of busulfan injection provides the needed dose, then that amount should be added to 93 ml of sodium chloride 0.9% or dextrose 5% in water to yield the final admixture suitable for administration (1-2/99).

Appropriate gloves should be worn during preparation; accidental skin exposure may result in skin reactions. To prepare the infusion admixture, break open the ampul top and withdraw the contents through the 5-μm nylon filter. The filter and needle are removed and a new needle is attached. The busulfan is added into an intravenous solution bag that already contains the appropriate amount of sodium chloride 0.9% or dextrose 5% in water, making sure that the drug flows into and throughout the solution. The drug should always be added to the diluent. The solution should be mixed thoroughly by inverting several times. Other diluents should not be used. Similarly, other medications of unknown compatibility should not be infused simultaneously (1-2/99).

Busulfan admixtures should be administered intravenously through a central venous catheter as a two-hour infusion every six hours for four consecutive days (a total of 16 doses). More rapid infusion has not been tested and is not recommended. An infusion pump should be used to control the flow rate. The central venous catheter should be flushed before and after busulfan administration with about 5 ml of sodium chloride 0.9% or dextrose 5% in water (1-2/99).

Stability—— Busulfan injection in intact ampuls is a clear colorless solution and should be stored under refrigeration at 2 to 8 °C. Busulfan diluted for infusion in sodium chloride 0.9% or dextrose 5% in water is stable for up to eight hours at 25 °C; administration should be completed within that time. Admixed in sodium chloride

0.9%, the drug is stable for up to 12 hours under refrigeration at 2 to 8 °C; administration should be completed within that time (1-2/99).

Filtration— Busulfan injection is packaged with 25-mm 5-μm nylon filters for use in withdrawing the injection from the opened ampuls. The use of filters other than this type is not recommended (1-2/99).

Compatibility Information

Solution Compatibility

Busulfan

Solution	Mfr	Mfr	Conc/L	Remarks	Ref	C/I
Dextrose 5% in water	BA[a], MG[b]		0.5 g	Physically compatible with no change in measured turbidity or particulates. Less than 10% loss by HPLC in 8 hr at 23 °C but 20% or more loss in 24 hr	2183	I[c]
	BA[a], MG[b]		0.1 g	Physically compatible with no change in measured turbidity or particulates. Less than 10% loss by HPLC in 4 hr at 23 °C but up to 19% loss in 8 hr	2183	I[c]
Sodium chloride 0.9%	BA[a], MG[b]		0.5 g	Physically compatible with no change in measured turbidity or particulates. Less than 10% loss by HPLC in 8 hr at 23 °C but more than 20% loss in 24 hr	2183	I[c]
	BA[a], MG[b]		0.1 g	Physically compatible with no change in measured turbidity or particulates. Less than 10% loss by HPLC in 4 hr at 23 °C but up to 13% loss in 8 hr	2183	I[c]

[a]*Tested in PVC containers.*
[b]*Tested in polyolefin containers.*
[c]*Incompatible by conventional standards but may be used in shorter periods of time.*

BUTORPHANOL TARTRATE
AHFS 28:08.12

Stadol　　　　　　　　　　　　　**Bristol-Myers Squibb**

Products— Butorphanol tartrate (Bristol-Myers Squibb) is available in concentrations of 1 mg/ml in 1-ml vials and also 2 mg/ml in 1- and 2-ml single-use vials and 10-ml multiple-dose vials (1-8/97).

Each milliliter of solution also contains citric acid 3.3 mg, sodium citrate 6.4 mg, and sodium chloride 6.4 mg. Benzethonium chloride 0.1 mg/ml is used as a preservative in the multiple-dose vials only (1-8/97).

pH— From 3 to 5.5 (4).

Osmolality— Butorphanol tartrate 2 mg/ml has an osmolality of 284 mOsm/kg (1689).

Administration— Butorphanol tartrate may be administered by intramuscular or intravenous injection (1-8/97; 4).

Stability— Butorphanol tartrate injection should be stored at room temperature and protected from light. Freezing should be avoided (4).

Compatibility Information

Drugs in Syringe Compatibility

Butorphanol tartrate

Drug (in syringe)	Mfr	Amt	Mfr	Amt	Remarks	Ref	C/I
Atropine sulfate	ST	0.4 mg/ 1 ml	BR	4 mg/ 2 ml	Physically compatible both macroscopically and microscopically for 30 min at room temperature	566	C

Drugs in Syringe Compatibility (Cont.)

Butorphanol tartrate

Drug (in syringe)	Mfr	Amt	Mfr	Amt	Remarks	Ref	C/I
Chlorpromazine HCl	MB	25 mg/ 1 ml	BR	4 mg/ 2 ml	Physically compatible both macroscopically and microscopically for 30 min at room temperature	566	**C**
Cimetidine HCl	SKF	300 mg/ 2 ml	BR	2 mg/ 1 ml	Physically compatible for 4 hr at 25 °C	25	**C**
Dimenhydrinate	HR	50 mg/ 1 ml	BR	4 mg/ 2 ml	Gas evolves	761	**I**
Diphenhydramine HCl	PD	50 mg/ 1 ml	BR	4 mg/ 2 ml	Physically compatible both macroscopically and microscopically for 30 min at room temperature	566	**C**
Droperidol	MN	5 mg/ 2 ml	BR	4 mg/ 2 ml	Physically compatible both macroscopically and microscopically for 30 min at room temperature	566	**C**
Fentanyl citrate	MN	0.1 mg/ 2 ml	BR	4 mg/ 2 ml	Physically compatible both macroscopically and microscopically for 30 min at room temperature	566	**C**
Hydroxyzine HCl	PF	50 mg/ 1 ml	BR	2 mg/ 1 ml	Physically compatible	771	**C**
	PF	100 mg/ 2 ml	BR	1 mg/ 1 ml	Physically compatible	771	**C**
Meperidine HCl	WI	50 mg/ 1 ml	BR	4 mg/ 2 ml	Physically compatible both macroscopically and microscopically for 30 min at room temperature	566	**C**
Methotrimeprazine		25 mg/ 1 ml	BR	4 mg/ 2 ml	Physically compatible for 30 min at room temperature both macroscopically and microscopically	566	**C**
Metoclopramide HCl	NO	10 mg/ 2 ml	BR	4 mg/ 2 ml	Physically compatible for 30 min at room temperature both macroscopically and microscopically	566	**C**
Midazolam HCl	RC	5 mg/ 1 ml	BR	2 mg/ 1 ml	Physically compatible for 4 hr at 25 °C under fluorescent light	1145	**C**
Morphine sulfate	AH	15 mg/ 1 ml	BR	4 mg/ 2 ml	Physically compatible both macroscopically and microscopically for 30 min at room temperature	566	**C**
Pentazocine lactate	WI	30 mg/ 1 ml	BR	4 mg/ 2 ml	Physically compatible both macroscopically and microscopically for 30 min at room temperature	566	**C**
Pentobarbital sodium	AB	50 mg/ 1 ml	BR	4 mg/ 2 ml	Immediate precipitation	761	**I**
Perphenazine	SC	5 mg/ 1 ml	BR	4 mg/ 2 ml	Physically compatible both macroscopically and microscopically for 30 min at room temperature	761	**C**
Prochlorperazine edisylate	MB	5 mg/ 1 ml	BR	4 mg/ 2 ml	Physically compatible both macroscopically and microscopically for 30 min at room temperature	566	**C**
Promethazine HCl	WY	25 mg/ 1 ml	BR	4 mg/ 2 ml	Physically compatible both macroscopically and microscopically for 30 min at room temperature	566	**C**

Drugs in Syringe Compatibility (Cont.)

					Butorphanol tartrate		
Drug (in syringe)	Mfr	Amt	Mfr	Amt	Remarks	Ref	C/I
Scopolamine HBr	ST	0.4 mg/ 1 ml	BR	4 mg/ 2 ml	Physically compatible both macroscopically and microscopically for 30 min at room temperature	566	C
Thiethylperazine malate	BI	10 mg/ 1 ml	BR	4 mg/ 2 ml	Physically compatible both macroscopically and microscopically for 30 min at room temperature	761	C

Y-Site Injection Compatibility (1:1 Mixture)

					Butorphanol tartrate		
Drug	Mfr	Conc	Mfr	Conc	Remarks	Ref	C/I
Allopurinol sodium	BW	3 mg/ml[b]	BR	0.04 mg/ml[b]	Physically compatible with no change in measured turbidity or increase in particle content in 4 hr at 22 °C	1686	C
Amifostine	USB	10 mg/ml[a]	BR	0.04 mg/ml[a]	Physically compatible with no change in measured turbidity or increase in particle content in 4 hr at 23 °C	1845	C
Amphotericin B cholesteryl sulfate complex	SEQ	0.83 mg/ml[a]	APC	0.04 mg/ml[a]	Decreased natural turbidity occurs immediately	2117	I
Aztreonam	SQ	40 mg/ml[a]	BMS	0.04 mg/ml[a]	Physically compatible with no subvisual haze or particle formation in 4 hr at 23 °C	1758	C
Cefepime HCl	BR	20 mg/ml[a]	BR	0.04 mg/ml[a]	Physically compatible with no change in measured turbidity or increase in particle content in 4 hr at 22 °C	1689	C
Cisatracurium besylate	GW	0.1, 2, 5 mg/ml[a]	APC	0.04 mg/ml[a]	Physically compatible with no change in measured turbidity or increase in particle content in 4 hr at 23 °C	2074	C
Cladribine	ORT	0.015[b] and 0.5[c] mg/ml	APC	0.04 mg/ml[b]	Physically compatible with no change in measured turbidity or increase in particle content in 4 hr at 23 °C	1969	C
Docetaxel	RPR	0.9 mg/ml[a]	APC	0.04 mg/ml[a]	Physically compatible with no change in measured turbidity or increase in particle content in 4 hr at 23 °C	2224	C
Doxorubicin HCl liposome injection	SEQ	0.4 mg/ml[a]	APC	0.04 mg/ml[a]	Physically compatible with little or no change in measured turbidity and no increase in particle content in 4 hr at 23 °C	2087	C
Enalaprilat	MSD	0.05 mg/ml[b]	BR	0.4 mg/ml[a]	Physically compatible for 24 hr at room temperature under fluorescent light	1355	C
Esmolol HCl	DCC	10 mg/ml[a]	BR	0.04 mg/ml[a]	Physically compatible for 24 hr at 22 °C	1169	C
Etoposide phosphate	BR	5 mg/ml[a]	APC	0.04 mg/ml[a]	Physically compatible with no change in measured turbidity or increase in particle content in 4 hr at 23 °C	2218	C
Filgrastim	AMG	30 μg/ml[a]	BR	0.04 mg/ml[a]	Physically compatible with no change in measured turbidity or increase in particle content in 4 hr at 22 °C	1687	C

Y-Site Injection Compatibility (1:1 Mixture) (Cont.)

Butorphanol tartrate

Drug	Mfr	Conc	Mfr	Conc	Remarks	Ref	C/I
Fludarabine phosphate	BX	1 mg/ml[a]	BR	0.04 mg/ml[a]	Physically compatible for 4 hr at room temperature under fluorescent light	1439	C
Gemcitabine HCl	LI	10 mg/ml[b]	APC	0.04 mg/ml[b]	Physically compatible with no change in measured turbidity or increase in particle content in 4 hr at 23 °C	2226	C
Granisetron HCl	SKB	0.05 mg/ml[a]	APC	0.04 mg/ml[a]	Physically compatible with no change in measured turbidity or increase in particle content in 4 hr at 23 °C	2000	C
Labetalol HCl	SC	1 mg/ml[a]	BR	0.04 mg/ml[a]	Physically compatible for 24 hr at 18 °C	1171	C
Melphalan HCl	BW	0.1 mg/ml[b]	BR	0.04 mg/ml[b]	Physically compatible with no change in measured turbidity or increase in particle content in 3 hr at 22 °C	1557	C
Midazolam HCl	RC	[f]	BR	[f]	Crystalline precipitate identified as midazolam by HPLC formed in infusion line several hours after administration was completed	2144	I
Paclitaxel	NCI	1.2 mg/ml[a]	BR	0.04 mg/ml[a]	Physically compatible with no change in measured turbidity in 4 hr at 22 °C	1556	C
Piperacillin sodium–tazobactam sodium	LE	40 + 5 mg/ml[a]	BR	0.04 mg/ml[a]	Physically compatible with no change in measured turbidity or increase in particle content in 4 hr at 22 °C	1688	C
Propofol	ZEN	10 mg/ml	APC	0.04 mg/ml[a]	Physically compatible for 1 hr at 23 °C with no increase in particle content	2066	C
Remifentanil HCl	GW	0.025 and 0.25 mg/ml[b]	APC	0.04 mg/ml[a]	Physically compatible with no change in measured turbidity or increase in particle content in 4 hr at 23 °C	2075	C
Sargramostim	IMM	10 μg/ml[b]	BR	0.04 mg/ml[b]	Physically compatible for 4 hr at 22 °C	1436	C
Teniposide	BR	0.1 mg/ml[a]	BR	0.04 mg/ml[a]	Physically compatible with no subvisual haze or particle formation in 4 hr at 23 °C	1725	C
Thiotepa	IMM[d]	1 mg/ml[a]	APC	0.04 mg/ml[a]	Physically compatible with no change in measured turbidity or increase in particle content in 4 hr at 23 °C	1861	C
TNA #218 to #226[e]			APC	0.04 mg/ml[a]	Visually compatible with no precipitate or emulsion damage apparent in 4 hr at 23 °C	2215	C
TPN #212 to #215[e]			APC	0.04 mg/ml[a]	Physically compatible with no change in measured turbidity or increase in particle content in 4 hr at 23 °C	2109	C
Vinorelbine tartrate	BW	1 mg/ml[b]	BR	0.04 mg/ml[b]	Physically compatible with no change in measured turbidity or increase in particle content in 4 hr at 22 °C	1558	C

[a]*Tested in dextrose 5% in water.*
[b]*Tested in sodium chloride 0.9%.*
[c]*Tested in bacteriostatic sodium chloride 0.9% preserved with benzyl alcohol 0.9%.*
[d]*Lyophilized formulation tested.*
[e]*Refer to Appendix I for the composition of parenteral nutrition solutions. TNA indicates a 3-in-1 admixture, and TPN indicates a 2-in-1 admixture.*
[f]*Concentration unspecified.*

Additional Compatibility Information

Additives— Butorphanol tartrate is stated to be physically and chemically compatible with atropine sulfate, hydroxyzine HCl, and promethazine HCl for at least 24 hours (481).

Other Information

One milligram of the tartrate is equal to 0.68 mg of butorphanol base (1-8/97).

CALCITRIOL
AHFS 88:16

Calcijex   **Abbott**

Products— Calcitriol (Abbott) is available in 1-ml ampuls in two strengths. Each milliliter of the aqueous solution contains (2):

Calcitriol	1 or 2 μg
Polysorbate 20	4 mg
Sodium chloride	1.5 mg
Sodium ascorbate	10 mg
Dibasic sodium phosphate anhydrous	7.6 mg
Monobasic sodium phosphate monohydrate	1.8 mg
Edetate disodium dihydrate	1.1 mg

pH— The injection has a target pH of 7.2 with a range of 6.5 to 8 (2).

Tonicity— The injection is an isotonic solution (2).

Administration— Calcitriol is given by intravenous injection. For patients undergoing hemodialysis, it may be administered by rapid intravenous injection through the catheter after a period of hemodialysis (4).

Stability— Calcitriol injection is a clear, colorless solution. It should be stored at controlled room temperature (15 to 30 °C) and protected from light (2; 4). Freezing and excessive heat should be avoided, although brief exposure to temperatures up to 40 °C does not adversely affect the injection (4).

The product does not contain a preservative, and the manufacturer recommends discarding any unused solution (2; 4).

Calcitriol (Abbott) 1 and 2 μg/ml undiluted and 0.5 μg/ml diluted in dextrose 5% in water, sodium chloride 0.9%, and water for injection was evaluated for stability. It was stored in 1-ml polypropylene tuberculin syringes (Becton-Dickinson) for eight hours at room temperature while exposed to normal room light. HPLC analysis showed little or no loss during the study period (1662).

Sorption— Pecosky et al. evaluated the sorption potential of calcitriol (Abbott) to PVC bags and administration sets and to polypropylene syringes by determining the apparent calcitriol polymer–water partition coefficients. The mean apparent partition coefficient was 66 times greater for PVC than polypropylene. In this test, 50% of the calcitriol was lost to PVC within two hours while approximately 4% was lost to polypropylene in 20 days (1662).

CALCIUM CHLORIDE
AHFS 40:12

                              Abbott
                               Astra

Products— Calcium chloride is available in 10-ml single-dose vials and prefilled syringes containing 1 g of calcium chloride (dihydrate), providing 14 mEq (273 mg) of calcium and 14 mEq of chloride in water for injection. The pH is adjusted with hydrochloric acid (1-2/95).

pH— From 5.5 to 7.5 (1-2/95).

Osmotic Values— Both the Abbott and Astra products have an osmolarity of 2.04 mOsm/ml (1-2/95).

The osmolality of a calcium chloride 10% solution was determined by osmometer to be 1765 mOsm/kg (1233).

Administration— Calcium chloride is administered by direct intravenous injection or by continuous or intermittent intravenous infusion, usually as a 2 to 10% solution (4). Intravenous administration should be performed slowly at a rate not exceeding 1.4 mEq/min (1 ml/min). The drug may also be injected into the ventricular cavity in cardiac resuscitation. It must not be injected into the myocardium. Severe necrosis and sloughing may result if calcium chloride is injected intramuscularly or subcutaneously or leaks into the perivascular tissue (1-2/95; 4).

Compatibility Information

Solution Compatibility

Calcium chloride

Solution	Mfr	Mfr	Conc/L	Remarks	Ref	C/I
Fat emulsion 10%, intravenous	VT	UP	2 g	Physically compatible for 48 hr at 4 °C and room temperature	32	C
	CU		13.6 mEq (1 g)	Immediate flocculation with visually apparent layer in 2 hr at room temperature	656	I
	CU		6.8 mEq (500 mg)	Flocculation within 4 hr at room temperature	656	I
	VT	DB	1 g	Globule coalescence and creaming within 8 hr at 8 and 25 °C	825	I
	KV		10 and 20 mEq	Immediate flocculation, aggregation, and creaming	1018	I

Additive Compatibility

Calcium chloride

Drug	Mfr	Conc/L	Mfr	Conc/L	Test Soln	Remarks	Ref	C/I
Amikacin sulfate	BR	5 g	UP	1 g	D5LR, D5R, D5S, D5W, D10W, IS10, LR, NS, R, SL	Physically compatible and potency of both drugs retained for 24 hr at 25 °C	294	C
Amphotericin B		200 mg	BP	4 g	D5W	Haze develops over 3 hr	26	I
Ascorbic acid injection	UP	500 mg	UP	1 g	D5W	Physically compatible	15	C
Bretylium tosylate	ACC	10 g	ES	54.4 mEq	D5W[a]	Physically compatible and bretylium chemically stable for 48 hr at room temperature and 7 days at 4 °C	541	C
Chloramphenicol sodium succinate	PD	10 g	UP	1 g	D5W	Physically compatible	15	C
Chlorpheniramine maleate						Physically incompatible	9	I
	SC	100 mg	UP	1 g	D5W	Physically incompatible	15	I
Dobutamine HCl	LI	182 mg	UP	9 g	NS	Physically compatible for 20 hr. Haze forms at 24 hr	552	I
	LI	1 g	ES	2 g	D5W, NS	Deeply pink in 24 hr at 25 °C	789	I
	LI	1 g	ES	50 g	D5W, NS	Physically compatible for 24 hr at 21 °C	812	C
Dopamine HCl	AS	800 mg	UP		D5W	No dopamine decomposition in 24 hr at 25 °C	312	C
Hydrocortisone sodium succinate	UP	500 mg	UP	1 g	D5W	Physically compatible	15	C
Isoproterenol HCl	WI	4 mg	UP	1 g		Physically compatible	59	C
Lidocaine HCl	AST	2 g	UP	1 g		Physically compatible	24	C
Norepinephrine bitartrate	WI	8 mg	UP	1 g	D, D–S, S	Physically compatible	77	C
Penicillin G potassium	SQ	20 million units	UP	1 g	D5W	Physically compatible	15	C
	SQ	5 million units	UP	1 g	D	Physically compatible	47	C

Additive Compatibility (Cont.)

Calcium chloride

Drug	Mfr	Conc/L	Mfr	Conc/L	Test Soln	Remarks	Ref	C/I
Penicillin G sodium	UP	20 million units	UP	1 g	D5W	Physically compatible	15	C
Pentobarbital sodium	AB	1 g	UP	1 g	D5W	Physically compatible	15	C
Phenobarbital sodium	WI	200 mg	UP	1 g	D5W	Physically compatible	15	C
Sodium bicarbonate	AB	2.4 mEq[b]		1 g	D5W	Physically compatible for 24 hr	772	C
Verapamil HCl	KN	80 mg	ES	2 g	D5W, NS	Physically compatible for 24 hr	764	C
Vitamin B complex with C	AB	5 ml	UP	1 g	D5W	Physically compatible	15	C

[a]Tested in both glass and PVC containers.
[b]One vial of Neut added to a liter of admixture.

Drugs in Syringe Compatibility

Calcium chloride

Drug (in syringe)	Mfr	Amt	Mfr	Amt	Remarks	Ref	C/I
Milrinone lactate	WI	5.25 mg/ 5.25 ml	AB	3 g/ 30 ml	Physically compatible with no milrinone loss in 20 min at 23 °C under fluorescent light	1410	C

Y-Site Injection Compatibility (1:1 Mixture)

Calcium chloride

Drug	Mfr	Conc	Mfr	Conc	Remarks	Ref	C/I
Amphotericin B cholesteryl sulfate complex	SEQ	0.83 mg/ml[a]	AST	40 mg/ml[a]	Gross precipitate forms	2117	I
Amrinone lactate	WB	3 mg/ml[b]	AB	100 mg/ml	Physically compatible for at least 4 hr at 25 °C under fluorescent light	992	C
Dobutamine HCl	LI	4 mg/ml[c]	AB	4 mg/ml[c]	Physically compatible for 3 hr	1316	C
Epinephrine HCl	ES	0.032 mg/ml[c]	AB	4 mg/ml[c]	Physically compatible for 3 hr	1316	C
Esmolol HCl	DCC	10 mg/ml[a]	AB	20 mg/ml[a]	Physically compatible for 24 hr at 22 °C	1169	C
Morphine sulfate	WY	0.2 mg/ml[c]	AB	4 mg/ml[c]	Physically compatible for 3 hr	1316	C
Paclitaxel	NCI	1.2 mg/ml[a]	AST	20 mg/ml[a]	Physically compatible with no change in measured turbidity in 4 hr at 22 °C	1556	C
Propofol	ZEN	10 mg/ml	AST	40 mg/ml[a]	White precipitate forms in 1 hr	2066	I
Sodium bicarbonate	AB	1 mEq/ml[c]	AB	4 mg/ml[c]	Slight haze or precipitate in 1 hr	1316	I

[a]Tested in dextrose 5% in water.
[b]Tested in sodium chloride 0.9%.
[c]Tested in both dextrose 5% in water and sodium chloride 0.9%.

Additional Compatibility Information

Infusion Solutions— Calcium chloride is compatible in most common intravenous infusion solutions.

Calcium and Phosphate— UNRECOGNIZED CALCIUM PHOSPHATE PRECIPITATION IN A 3-IN-1 PARENTERAL NUTRITION MIXTURE RESULTED IN PATIENT DEATH.

The potential for the formation of a calcium phosphate precipitate in parenteral nutrition solutions is well studied and documented (1771; 1777), but the information is complex and difficult to apply to the clinical situation (1770; 1772; 1777). The incorporation of fat emulsion in 3-in-1 parenteral nutrition solutions obscures any precipitate that is present, which has led to substantial debate on the dangers associated with 3-in-1 parenteral nutrition mixtures and when or if the danger to the patient is warranted therapeutically (1770-1772; 2031-2036). Because such precipitation may be life-threatening to patients (2037), the Food and Drug Administration issued a Safety Alert containing the following recommendations (1769):

"1. The amounts of phosphorus and of calcium added to the admixture are critical. The solubility of the added calcium should be calculated from the volume at the time the calcium is added. It should not be based upon the final volume.

Some amino acid injections for TPN admixtures contain phosphate ions (as a phosphoric acid buffer). These phosphate ions and the volume at the time the phosphate is added should be considered when calculating the concentration of phosphate additives. Also, when adding calcium and phosphate to an admixture, the phosphate should be added first.

The line should be flushed between the addition of any potentially incompatible components.

2. A lipid emulsion in a three-in-one admixture obscures the presence of a precipitate. Therefore, if a lipid emulsion is needed, either (1) use a two-in-one admixture with the lipid infused separately, or (2) if a three-in-one admixture is medically necessary, then add the calcium before the lipid emulsion and according to the recommendations in number 1 above.

If the amount of calcium or phosphate which must be added is likely to cause a precipitate, some or all of the calcium should be administered separately. Such separate infusions must be properly diluted and slowly infused to avoid serious adverse events related to the calcium.

3. When using an automated compounding device, the above steps should be considered when programming the device. In addition, automated compounders should be maintained and operated according to the manufacturer's recommendations.

Any printout should be checked against the programmed admixture and weight of components.

4. During the mixing process, pharmacists who mix parenteral nutrition admixtures should periodically agitate the admixture and check for precipitates. Medical or home care personnel who start and monitor these infusions should carefully inspect for the presence of precipitates both before and during infusion. Patients and care givers should be trained to visually inspect for signs of precipitation. They also should be advised to stop the infusion and seek medical assistance if precipitates are noted.

5. A filter should be used when infusing either central or peripheral parenteral nutrition admixtures. At this time, data have not been submitted to document which size filter is most effective in trapping precipitates.

Standards of practice vary, but the following is suggested: a 1.2-μm air-eliminating filter for lipid-containing admixtures and a 0.22-μm air-eliminating filter for non-lipid-containing admixtures.

6. Parenteral nutrition admixtures should be administered within the following time frames: if stored at room temperature, the infusion should be started within 24 hours after mixing; if stored at refrigerated temperatures, the in-

fusion should be started within 24 hours of rewarming. Because warming parenteral nutrition admixtures may contribute to the formation of precipitates, once administration begins, care should be taken to avoid excessive warming of the admixture.

Persons administering home care parenteral nutrition admixtures may need to deviate from these time frames. Pharmacists who initially prepare these admixtures should check a reserve sample for precipitates over the duration and under the conditions of storage.

7. If symptoms of acute respiratory distress, pulmonary emboli, or interstitial pneumonitis develop, the infusion should be stopped immediately and thoroughly checked for precipitates. Appropriate medical interventions should be instituted. Home care personnel and patients should immediately seek medical assistance."

Calcium salts are conditionally compatible with potassium phosphate in parenteral nutrition solutions. The incompatibility is dependent on a solubility and concentration phenomenon and is not entirely predictable. Precipitation may occur during compounding or at some time after compounding is completed.

NOTE: Some amino acid solutions inherently contain calcium and phosphate, which must be considered in any projection of compatibility. See the amino acid injection monograph, Table 1.

A study by Henry et al. (608) determined the maximum concentrations of calcium (as chloride and gluconate) and phosphate that can be maintained without precipitation in a parenteral nutrition solution consisting of FreAmine II 4.25% and dextrose 25% for 24 hours at 30 °C. Their results are depicted in Figure 1.

Henry et al. noted that the amino acids in parenteral nutrition solutions form soluble complexes with calcium and phosphate, reducing the available free calcium and phosphate that can form insoluble precipitates. The concentration of calcium available for precipitation is greater with the chloride salt compared to the gluconate salt, at least in part because of differences in dissociation characteristics. This can be seen in Figure 1 by the greater concentration of calcium gluconate that can be mixed with sodium phosphate (608).

In addition to the concentrations of phosphate and calcium and the salt form of the calcium, Henry et al. noted that the concentration of amino acids and the time and temperature of storage altered

Figure 1. *Maximum solubilities of calcium chloride (○) and calcium gluconate (△) with sodium phosphate in an amino acid 4.25% – dextrose 25% solution at 30 °C*

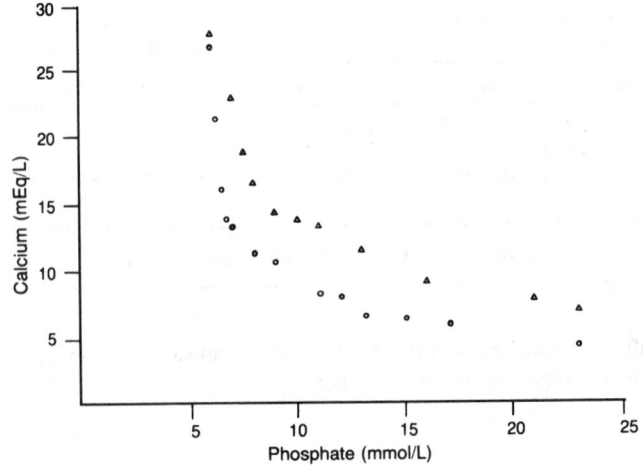

the formation of calcium phosphate in parenteral nutrition solutions. As the temperature was increased, the incidence of precipitate formation also increased. This finding was attributed, at least in part, to a greater degree of dissociation of the calcium and phosphate complexes and the decreased solubility of calcium phosphate. Therefore, it is possible for a solution to be stored at 4 °C with no precipitation, but on warming to room temperature a precipitate will form over time (608).

Koorenhof and Timmer reported the maximum allowable concentrations of calcium and phosphate in a 3-in-1 parenteral nutrition mixture for children (TNA #192 in Appendix I). Added calcium was varied from 1.5 to 150 mmol/L, while added phosphate was varied from 21 to 300 mmol/L. The mixtures were stable for 48 hours at 22 and 37 °C as long as the pH was not greater than 5.7, the calcium concentration was below 16 mmol/L, the phosphate concentration was below 52 mmol/L, and the product of the calcium and phosphate concentrations was below 250 mmol^2/L^2 (1773).

The presence of magnesium in solutions may also influence the reaction between calcium and phosphate, including the nature and extent of precipitation (158; 159).

The interaction of calcium and phosphate in parenteral nutrition solutions is a complex phenomenon. Various factors play a role in the solubility or precipitation of a given combination, including (608; 609; 1042; 1063; 1210; 1234; 1427):

1. Concentration of calcium
2. Salt form of calcium
3. Concentration of phosphate
4. Concentration of amino acids
5. Amino acids composition
6. Concentration of dextrose
7. Temperature of solution
8. pH of solution
9. Presence of other additives
10. Order of mixing

Enhanced precipitate formation would be expected from such factors as high concentrations of calcium and phosphate, increases in solution pH, decreases in amino acid concentrations, increases in temperature, addition of calcium before phosphate, lengthy standing times or slow infusion rates, and use of calcium as the chloride salt (854).

Also see the monograph on calcium gluconate.

Even if precipitation does not occur in the bottle, it has been reported that crystallization of calcium phosphate may occur in a Silastic infusion pump chamber or tubing if the rate of administration is slow, as for premature infants. Water vapor may be transmitted outward and be replaced by air rapidly enough to produce supersaturation (202). Several other cases of catheter occlusion have been reported (610; 1427–1429).

Other Ions— Calcium chloride (Upjohn) in dextrose 5% in water has been reported to be conditionally compatible with sodium bicarbonate (Abbott). The incompatibility is dependent on the concentration of the additives. Therefore, if attempting to combine calcium chloride with sodium bicarbonate, mix the solution thoroughly and observe it closely for any sign of incompatibility (15).

Calcium chloride is stated to be incompatible with soluble carbonates, phosphates, sulfates, and tartrates. Because of the presence of sodium carbonate in the cefamandole nafate (Lilly) formulation, it is incompatible with calcium ions (4; 376).

Miscellaneous— Calcium ions are stated to inhibit the activity of tobramycin sulfate (145).

CALCIUM GLUCONATE
AHFS 40:12

American Pharmaceutical Partners
American Regent

Products— Calcium gluconate is available from various manufacturers in 10-ml ampuls and 10-, 50-, and 100-ml vials as a 10% solution. Each milliliter contains 94 (American Pharmaceutical Partners) or 98 (American Regent) mg of calcium gluconate with calcium D-saccharate tetrahydrate 4.5 to 4.6 mg in water for injection, providing 9.3 mg (0.465 mEq) of elementary calcium. The pH may be adjusted with sodium hydroxide and/or hydrochloric acid (1-11/95; 1-12/98).

pH— From 6 to 8.2 (1-12/98; 4).

Osmotic Values— The osmolarity is stated to be 0.68 mOsm/ml (1-12/98).

The osmolality of a calcium gluconate 10% solution was determined by osmometer to be 276 mOsm/kg (1233).

Administration— Calcium gluconate is usually administered intravenously as a 10% solution (4), slowly by direct intravenous injection, or by continuous or intermittent intravenous infusion. A maximum administration rate of 1.5 ml/min has been recommended for direct intravenous injection (1-12/98). By intermittent infusion, a maximum of 200 mg/min has been suggested (1-11/95). Calcium gluconate has been given by intramuscular or, rarely, subcutaneous injection to adults (4), but these routes are not recommended because of possible tissue necrosis, sloughing, and abscess formation (1-11/95; 1-12/98). Numerous reports indicate that tissue irritation and necrosis may occur from intramuscular or subcutaneous injection or extravasation from intravenous administration, especially in infants and children (183-185; 359).

Stability— Calcium gluconate injection is a supersaturated solution that has been stabilized by the addition of 35 mg of calcium D-saccharate. It should be stored at room temperature. Do not use it if a precipitate is present (1-11/95; 1-12/98).

Compatibility Information

Solution Compatibility

Calcium gluconate

Solution	Mfr	Mfr	Conc/L	Remarks	Ref	C/I
Alcohol 5%, dextrose 5%	BA	PD	2 g	Physically compatible for 24 hr	315	C
Amino acids 4%, dextrose 25%	CU	PR	100 mEq	Physically compatible for 24 hr at 22 °C	313	C
Dextrose 5% in Ringer's injection, lactated	BA	PD	2 g	Physically compatible for 24 hr	315	C
Dextrose 5% in sodium chloride 0.9%			1 g	Physically compatible	74	C
	BA	PD	2 g	Physically compatible for 24 hr	315	C
Dextrose 5% in water			1 g	Physically compatible	74	C
	BA	PD	2 g	Physically compatible for 24 hr	315	C
Dextrose 10% in sodium chloride 0.18%		BP	18 g	Physically compatible for 30 hr at room temperature under fluorescent light	1347	C
Dextrose 10% in water	BA	PD	2 g	Physically compatible for 24 hr	315	C
		BP	18 g	Physically compatible for 30 hr at room temperature under fluorescent light	1347	C
Dextrose 20% in water	BA	PD	2 g	Physically compatible for 24 hr	315	C
Fat emulsion 10%, intravenous	VT	PR	2 g	Produced cracked emulsion	32	I
	KV		7.2 and 9.6 mEq	Immediate flocculation, aggregation, and creaming	1018	I
Fructose 10% in water	BA	PD	2 g	Physically compatible for 24 hr	315	C
Invert sugar 10% in Electrolyte #1	BA	PD	2 g	Physically compatible for 24 hr	315	C
Invert sugar 10% in Electrolyte #2	BA	PD	2 g	Physically compatible for 24 hr	315	C
Polysal M with dextrose 5%	CU	PD	2 g	Physically compatible for 24 hr	315	C
Ringer's injection, lactated			1 g	Physically compatible	74	C
	BA	PD	2 g	Physically compatible for 24 hr	315	C
Sodium chloride 0.9%			1 g	Physically compatible	74	C
	BA	PD	2 g	Physically compatible for 24 hr	315	C
Sodium lactate ⅙ M	BA	PD	2 g	Physically compatible for 24 hr	315	C
TPN #38 to #42[a]		PR		Physically compatible for 24 hr at 22 °C. Alterations in UV spectra in solutions containing MVI or vitamin B complex with C and TLC changes in similar solutions attributed to the vitamins	313	C
TPN #43 to #47[a]		PR		Physically compatible for 24 hr at 22 °C. TLC changes of amino acids in similar solutions attributed to MVI or vitamin B complex with C	313	C

[a]Refer to Appendix I for the composition of parenteral nutrition solutions. TPN indicates a 2-in-1 admixture.

Additive Compatibility

Calcium gluconate

Drug	Mfr	Conc/L	Mfr	Conc/L	Test Soln	Remarks	Ref	C/I
Amikacin sulfate	BR	5 g	UP	500 mg	D5LR, D5R, D5S, D5W, D10W, IS10, LR, NS, R, SL	Physically compatible and potency of both retained for 24 hr at 25 °C	294	C
Aminophylline		250 mg		1 g	D5W	Physically compatible	74	C
Amphotericin B		200 mg	BP	4 g	D5W	Haze develops over 3 hr	26	I
Ascorbic acid injection	UP	500 mg	UP	1 g	D5W	Physically compatible	15	C
Bretylium tosylate	ACC	1 g	ES	2 g	D5W, NS	Physically compatible for 48 hr at 25 °C	756	C
Cefamandole nafate	LI	2 g		200 mg	D5W, NS, W	Haze or precipitate forms	788	I
	LI	20 g		2 g	D5W, NS, W	Haze or precipitate forms	788	I
Chloramphenicol sodium succinate	PD	500 mg		1 g	D5W	Physically compatible	74	C
	PD	10 g	UP	1 g	D5W	Physically compatible	15	C
	PD	10 g	UP	1 g		Physically compatible	6	C
Corticotropin		500 units		1 g	D5W	Physically compatible	74	C
Dimenhydrinate	SE	50 mg		1 g	D5W	Physically compatible	74	C
Dobutamine HCl	LI	182 mg	VI	9 g	NS	Small particles form within 4 hr. White precipitate and haze after 15 hr	522	I
	LI	1 g	ES	2 g	D5W, NS	Deeply pink in 24 hr at 25 °C	789	I
	LI	1 g	IX	50 g	D5W, NS	Small white particles form within 24 hr at 21 °C	812	I
Floxacillin sodium	BE	20 g	ANT	2 g	NS	Thick white precipitate forms immediately	1479	I
Furosemide	HO	1 g	ANT	2 g	NS	Physically compatible for 72 hr at 15 and 30 °C	1479	C
Heparin sodium		12,000 units		1 g	D5W	Physically compatible	74	C
	UP	4000 units	UP	1 g	D5W	Physically compatible	15	C
	AB	20,000 units	UP	1 g		Physically compatible	21	C
Hydrocortisone sodium succinate	UP	100 mg		1 g	D5W	Physically compatible	74	C
	UP	500 mg	UP	1 g	D5W	Physically compatible	15	C
Lidocaine HCl	AST	2 g	ES	2 g	D5W, LR, NS	Physically compatible for 24 hr at 25 °C	775	C
Magnesium sulfate	LI	1, 2, 3, 4 mEq	PR	10, 20, 30, 40 mEq	AA 4%, D 25%	Physically compatible for 24 hr at 22 °C	313	C
	LI	4 to 100 mEq	PR	4 to 100 mEq	PH 4%, D 20%	Physically compatible for 24 hr at room temperature	464	C
Methylprednisolone sodium succinate	UP	40 mg		1 g	D5S	Physically incompatible	329	I
Norepinephrine bitartrate	WI	8 mg		1 g	D5W	Physically compatible	74	C

Additive Compatibility (Cont.)

Calcium gluconate

Drug	Mfr	Conc/L	Mfr	Conc/L	Test Soln	Remarks	Ref	C/I
Penicillin G potassium		1 million units		1 g	D5W	Physically compatible	74	C
	SQ	20 million units	UP	1 g	D5W	Physically compatible	15	C
Penicillin G sodium	UP	20 million units	UP	1 g	D5W	Physically compatible	15	C
Phenobarbital sodium	WI	200 mg	UP	1 g	D5W	Physically compatible	15	C
Potassium chloride		3 g		1 g	D5W	Physically compatible	74	C
Prochlorperazine edisylate	SKF	100 mg	UP	1 g	D5W	Physically compatible	15	C
	SKF					Physically incompatible	9	I
Tobramycin sulfate	LI	5 g		16 g	D5W	Physically compatible with no loss of tobramycin activity in 60 min at room temperature	984	C
	LI	1 g		33 g	D5W	Physically compatible with no loss of tobramycin activity in 60 min at room temperature	984	C
Vancomycin HCl	LI	1 g		1 g	D5W	Physically compatible	74	C
Verapamil HCl	KN	80 mg	IX	2 g	D5W, NS	Physically compatible for 48 hr	739	C
Vitamin B complex with C		1 vial		1 g	D5W	Physically compatible	74	C
	AB	5 ml	UP	1 g	D5W	Physically compatible	15	C

Drugs in Syringe Compatibility

Calcium gluconate

Drug (in syringe)	Mfr	Amt	Mfr	Amt	Remarks	Ref	C/I
Metoclopramide HCl	RB	10 mg/ 2 ml	ES	1 g/ 10 ml	Possible precipitate formation	924	I
	RB	10 mg/ 2 ml	ES	1 g/ 10 ml	Incompatible. If mixed, use immediately	1167	I
	RB	160 mg/ 32 ml	ES	1 g/ 10 ml	Incompatible. If mixed, use immediately	1167	I

Y-Site Injection Compatibility (1:1 Mixture)

Calcium gluconate

Drug	Mfr	Conc	Mfr	Conc	Remarks	Ref	C/I
Aldesleukin	CHI	33,800 I.U./ ml[a]	LY	100 mg/ml	Visually compatible with little or no loss of aldesleukin activity by bioassay	1857	C
Allopurinol sodium	BW	3 mg/ml[b]	AMR	40 mg/ml[b]	Physically compatible with no change in measured turbidity or increase in particle content in 4 hr at 22 °C	1686	C
Amifostine	USB	10 mg/ml[a]	AMR	40 mg/ml[a]	Physically compatible with no change in measured turbidity or increase in particle content in 4 hr at 23 °C	1845	C

Y-Site Injection Compatibility (1:1 Mixture) (Cont.)

Calcium gluconate

Drug	Mfr	Conc	Mfr	Conc	Remarks	Ref	C/I
Amphotericin B cholesteryl sulfate complex	SEQ	0.83 mg/ml[a]	AB	40 mg/ml[a]	Gross precipitate forms	2117	**I**
Ampicillin sodium	WY	40 mg/ml[b]	AST	4 mg/ml[b]	Physically compatible for 3 hr	1316	**C**
	WY	40 mg/ml[a]	AST	4 mg/ml[a]	Slight color change in 1 hr	1316	**I**
Aztreonam	SQ	40 mg/ml[a]	AMR	40 mg/ml[a]	Physically compatible with no subvisual haze or particle formation in 4 hr at 23 °C	1758	**C**
Cefazolin sodium	LI	40 mg/ml[c]	AST	4 mg/ml[c]	Physically compatible for 3 hr	1316	**C**
Cefepime HCl	BR	20 mg/ml[a]	AMR	40 mg/ml[a]	Physically compatible with no change in measured turbidity or increase in particle content in 4 hr at 22 °C	1689	**C**
Ciprofloxacin	MI	2 mg/ml[a]	LY	10%	Visually compatible for 2 hr at 25 °C	1628	**C**
Cisatracurium besylate	GW	0.1, 2, 5 mg/ml[a]	AB	40 mg/ml[a]	Physically compatible with no change in measured turbidity or increase in particle content in 4 hr at 23 °C	2074	**C**
Cladribine	ORT	0.015[b] and 0.5[d] mg/ml	AMR	40 mg/ml[b]	Physically compatible with no change in measured turbidity or increase in particle content in 4 hr at 23 °C	1969	**C**
Dobutamine HCl	LI	4 mg/ml[c]	AST	4 mg/ml[c]	Physically compatible for 3 hr	1316	**C**
Docetaxel	RPR	0.9 mg/ml[a]	FUJ	40 mg/ml[a]	Physically compatible with little or no change in measured turbidity and no increase in particle content in 4 hr at 23 °C	2224	**C**
Doxorubicin HCl liposome injection	SEQ	0.4 mg/ml[a]	AB	40 mg/ml[a]	Physically compatible with no change in measured turbidity or increase in particle content in 4 hr at 23 °C	2087	**C**
Enalaprilat	MSD	0.05 mg/ml[b]	ES	0.092 mEq/ml[a]	Physically compatible for 24 hr at room temperature under fluorescent light	1355	**C**
Epinephrine HCl	ES	0.032 mg/ml[c]	AST	4 mg/ml[c]	Physically compatible for 3 hr	1316	**C**
Etoposide phosphate	BR	5 mg/ml[a]	FUJ	40 mg/ml[a]	Physically compatible with no change in measured turbidity or increase in particle content in 4 hr at 23 °C	2218	**C**
Famotidine	MSD	0.2 mg/ml[a]	LY	0.00465 mEq/ml[b]	Physically compatible for 14 hr	1196	**C**
Filgrastim	AMG	30 μg/ml[a]	AST	40 mg/ml[a]	Physically compatible with no change in measured turbidity or increase in particle content in 4 hr at 22 °C	1687	**C**
Fluconazole	RR	2 mg/ml	ES	100 mg/ml	Cloudiness	1407	**I**
Gemcitabine HCl	LI	10 mg/ml[b]	FUJ	40 mg/ml[b]	Physically compatible with no change in measured turbidity or increase in particle content in 4 hr at 23 °C	2226	**C**
Granisetron HCl	SKB	0.05 mg/ml[a]	AB	40 mg/ml[a]	Physically compatible with no change in measured turbidity or increase in particle content in 4 hr at 23 °C	2000	**C**
Heparin sodium with hydrocortisone sodium succinate	RI UP	1000 units + 100 mg/L[e]	ES	100 mg/ml	Physically compatible for at least 4 hr at room temperature by visual and microscopic examination	322	**C**

Y-Site Injection Compatibility (1:1 Mixture) (Cont.)

				Calcium gluconate			
Drug	*Mfr*	*Conc*	*Mfr*	*Conc*	*Remarks*	*Ref*	*C/I*
Indomethacin sodium trihydrate	MSD	1 mg/ml[b]	AMR	100 mg/ml	Fine yellow precipitate forms within 1 hr	1527	**I**
Labetalol HCl	SC	1 mg/ml[a]	AMR	0.23 mEq/ml[a]	Physically compatible for 24 hr at 18 °C	1171	**C**
Melphalan HCl	BW	0.1 mg/ml[b]	AST	40 mg/ml[b]	Physically compatible with no change in measured turbidity or increase in particle content in 3 hr at 22 °C	1557	**C**
Meropenem	ZEN	1 mg/ml[b]	AMR	4 mg/ml[f]	Visually compatible for 4 hr at room temperature	1994	**C**
	ZEN	50 mg/ml[b]	AMR	4 mg/ml[f]	Yellow discoloration forms in 4 hr at room temperature	1994	**I**
Midazolam HCl	RC	1 mg/ml[a]	FUJ	100 mg/ml	Visually compatible for 24 hr at 23 °C	1847	**C**
Milrinone lactate	SW	0.4 mg/ml[a]	LY	0.465 mEq/ml	Visually compatible with no loss of milrinone by HPLC in 4 hr at 23 °C	2214	**C**
Netilmicin sulfate	SC	5 mg/ml[g]	LY	40 mg/ml[g]	Physically compatible and no netilmicin loss in 2 hr at 24 °C	1021	**C**
Piperacillin sodium–tazobactam sodium	LE	40 + 5 mg/ml[a]	AMR	40 mg/ml[a]	Physically compatible with no change in measured turbidity or increase in particle content in 4 hr at 22 °C	1688	**C**
Potassium chloride		40 mEq/L[e]	ES	100 mg/ml	Physically compatible for at least 4 hr at room temperature by visual and microscopic examination	322	**C**
Prochlorperazine edisylate	SCN	5 mg/ml	AMR	10 mg/ml[b]	Visually compatible for 24 hr at room temperature in test tubes. No precipitate found on filter from Y-site delivery	2063	**C**
Propofol	ZEN	10 mg/ml	AMR	40 mg/ml[a]	Physically compatible for 1 hr at 23 °C with no increase in particle content	2066	**C**
Remifentanil HCl	GW	0.025 and 0.25 mg/ml[b]	AB	40 mg/ml[a]	Physically compatible with no change in measured turbidity or increase in particle content in 4 hr at 23 °C	2075	**C**
Sargramostim	IMM	10 µg/ml[b]	AMR	40 mg/ml[b]	Physically compatible for 4 hr at 22 °C	1436	**C**
Tacrolimus	FUJ	1 mg/ml[b]	ES	100 mg/ml	Visually compatible for 24 hr at 25 °C	1630	**C**
Teniposide	BR	0.1 mg/ml[a]	AMR	40 mg/ml[a]	Physically compatible with no subvisual haze or particle formation in 4 hr at 23 °C	1725	**C**
Thiotepa	IMM[h]	1 mg/ml[a]	AMR	40 mg/ml[a]	Physically compatible with no change in measured turbidity or increase in particle content in 4 hr at 23 °C	1861	**C**
TNA #218 to #226[i]			AB	40 mg/ml[a]	Visually compatible with no precipitate or emulsion damage apparent in 4 hr at 23 °C	2215	**C**
Tolazoline HCl		0.1 mg/ml[a]	AMR	100 mg/ml	Physically compatible for 24 hr at 22 °C	1363	**C**
TPN #189[i]			DB	10 mg/ml[b]	Visually compatible for 24 hr at 22 °C	1767	**C**
TPN #212 to #215[i]			AB	40 mg/ml[a]	Physically compatible with no change in measured turbidity or increase in particle content in 4 hr at 23 °C	2109	**C**
Vinorelbine tartrate	BW	1 mg/ml[b]	AMR	40 mg/ml[b]	Physically compatible with no change in measured turbidity or increase in particle content in 4 hr at 22 °C	1558	**C**

Y-Site Injection Compatibility (1:1 Mixture) (Cont.)

Calcium gluconate

Drug	Mfr	Conc	Mfr	Conc	Remarks	Ref	C/I
Vitamin B complex with C	RC	2 ml/L[e]	ES	100 mg/ml	Physically compatible for at least 4 hr at room temperature by visual and microscopic examination	322	C

[a]*Tested in dextrose 5% in water.*
[b]*Tested in sodium chloride 0.9%.*
[c]*Tested in both dextrose 5% in water and sodium chloride 0.9%.*
[d]*Tested in bacteriostatic sodium chloride 0.9% preserved with benzyl alcohol 0.9%.*
[e]*Tested in dextrose 5% in water, Ringer's injection, lactated, and sodium chloride 0.9%.*
[f]*Tested in sterile water for injection.*
[g]*Tested in dextrose 5% in sodium chloride 0.9%.*
[h]*Lyophilized formulation tested.*
[i]*Refer to Appendix I for the composition of parenteral nutrition solutions. TNA indicates a 3-in-1 admixture, and TPN indicates a 2-in-1 admixture.*

Additional Compatibility Information

Calcium and Phosphate— UNRECOGNIZED CALCIUM PHOSPHATE PRECIPITATION IN A 3-IN-1 PARENTERAL NUTRITION MIXTURE RESULTED IN PATIENT DEATH.

The potential for the formation of a calcium phosphate precipitate in parenteral nutrition solutions is well studied and documented (1771; 1777), but the information is complex and difficult to apply to the clinical situation (1770; 1772; 1777). The incorporation of fat emulsion in 3-in-1 parenteral nutrition solutions obscures any precipitate that is present, which has led to substantial debate on the dangers associated with 3-in-1 parenteral nutrition mixtures and when or if the danger to the patient is warranted therapeutically (1770-1772; 2031-2036). Because such precipitation may be life-threatening to patients (2037), the Food and Drug Administration issued a Safety Alert containing the following recommendations (1769):

"1. The amounts of phosphorus and of calcium added to the admixture are critical. The solubility of the added calcium should be calculated from the volume at the time the calcium is added. It should not be based upon the final volume.

Some amino acid injections for TPN admixtures contain phosphate ions (as a phosphoric acid buffer). These phosphate ions and the volume at the time the phosphate is added should be considered when calculating the concentration of phosphate additives. Also, when adding calcium and phosphate to an admixture, the phosphate should be added first.

The line should be flushed between the addition of any potentially incompatible components.

2. A lipid emulsion in a three-in-one admixture obscures the presence of a precipitate. Therefore, if a lipid emulsion is needed, either (1) use a two-in-one admixture with the lipid infused separately, or (2) if a three-in-one admixture is medically necessary, then add the calcium before the lipid emulsion and according to the recommendations in number 1 above.

If the amount of calcium or phosphate which must be added is likely to cause a precipitate, some or all of the calcium should be administered separately. Such separate infusions must be properly diluted and slowly infused to avoid serious adverse events related to the calcium.

3. When using an automated compounding device, the above steps should be considered when programming the device. In addition, automated compounders should be maintained and operated according to the manufacturer's recommendations.

Any printout should be checked against the programmed admixture and weight of components.

4. During the mixing process, pharmacists who mix parenteral nutrition admixtures should periodically agitate the admixture and check for precipitates. Medical or home care personnel who start and monitor these infusions should carefully inspect for the presence of precipitates both before and during infusion. Patients and care givers should be trained to visually inspect for signs of precipitation. They also should be advised to stop the infusion and seek medical assistance if precipitates are noted.

5. A filter should be used when infusing either central or peripheral parenteral nutrition admixtures. At this time, data have not been submitted to document which size filter is most effective in trapping precipitates.

Standards of practice vary, but the following is suggested: a 1.2-μm air-eliminating filter for lipid-containing admixtures and a 0.22-μm air-eliminating filter for non-lipid-containing admixtures.

6. Parenteral nutrition admixtures should be administered within the following time frames: if stored at room temperature, the infusion should be started within 24 hours after mixing; if stored at refrigerated temperatures, the infusion should be started within 24 hours of rewarming. Because warming parenteral nutrition admixtures may contribute to the formation of precipitates, once administration begins, care should be taken to avoid excessive warming of the admixture.

Persons administering home care parenteral nutrition admixtures may need to deviate from these time frames. Pharmacists who initially prepare these admixtures should check a reserve sample for precipitates over the duration and under the conditions of storage.

7. If symptoms of acute respiratory distress, pulmonary emboli, or interstitial pneumonitis develop, the infusion should be stopped immediately and thoroughly checked for precipitates. Appropriate medical interventions should be

instituted. Home care personnel and patients should immediately seek medical assistance."

Calcium Phosphate Precipitation Fatalities— Hill et al. reported fatal cases of paroxysmal respiratory failure in two previously healthy women receiving peripheral vein parenteral nutrition. The patients experienced sudden cardiopulmonary arrest consistent with pulmonary emboli. The authors used in vitro simulations and an animal model to conclude that unrecognized calcium phosphate precipitation in a 3-in-1 total nutrition admixture caused the fatalities. The precipitation resulted during compounding by introducing calcium and phosphate near to one another in the compounding sequence and prior to complete fluid addition. This resulted in a temporarily high concentration of the drugs and precipitation of calcium phosphate. Observation of the precipitate was obscured by the incorporation of an intravenous 20% fat emulsion into the nutrition mixture. No filter was used during infusion of the fatal nutrition admixtures (2037).

Calcium salts are conditionally compatible with potassium phosphate in parenteral nutrition solutions. The incompatibility is dependent on a solubility and concentration phenomenon and is not entirely predictable. Precipitation may occur during compounding or at some time after compounding is completed.

NOTE: Some amino acid solutions inherently contain both calcium and phosphate, which must be considered in any projection of compatibility. See the amino acid injection monograph, Table 1.

The order of mixing of calcium gluconate and potassium phosphate may affect compatibility at elevated concentrations. Addition of potassium phosphate should precede that of calcium gluconate (313; 1210).

A study by Henry et al. (608) determined the maximum concentrations of calcium (as chloride and gluconate) and phosphate that can be maintained without precipitation in a parenteral nutrition solution consisting of FreAmine II 4.25% and dextrose 25% for 24 hours at 30 °C. Their results are depicted in Figure 1.

Henry et al. noted that the amino acids in parenteral nutrition solutions form soluble complexes with calcium and phosphate, reducing the available free calcium and phosphate that can form insoluble precipitates. The concentration of calcium available for precipitation is greater with the chloride salt compared to the gluconate salt, at least in part because of differences in dissociation charac-

Table 1. Parenteral Nutrition Solutions Used by Eggert et al. (609)

Component	Solution Number			
	#1	#2	#3	#4
FreAmine III	4%	2%	1%	1%
Dextrose	25%	20%	10%	10%
pH	6.3	6.4	6.6	7.0[a]

[a]*Adjusted with sodium hydroxide.*

teristics. This can be seen in Figure 1 by the greater concentration of calcium gluconate that can be mixed with sodium phosphate (608).

In addition to the concentrations of phosphate and calcium and the salt form of the calcium, Henry et al. noted that the concentration of amino acids and the time and temperature of storage altered the formation of calcium phosphate in parenteral nutrition solutions. As the temperature was increased, the incidence of precipitate formation also increased. This finding was attributed, at least in part, to a greater degree of dissociation of the calcium and phosphate complexes and the decreased solubility of calcium phosphate. Therefore, a solution possibly may be stored at 4 °C with no precipitation, but on warming to room temperature a precipitate will form over time (608).

Eggert et al. (609) evaluated the compatibility of calcium and phosphate in several parenteral nutrition formulas for newborn infants. Calcium gluconate 10% (Cutter) and potassium phosphate (Abbott) were used to achieve concentrations of 2.5 to 100 mEq/L of calcium and 2.5 to 100 mmol/L of phosphorus added. The parenteral nutrition solutions evaluated were as shown in Table 1. The results were reported as graphic depictions.

Eggert et al. noted the pH dependence of the phosphate–calcium precipitation. Dibasic calcium phosphate is very insoluble, while monobasic calcium phosphate is relatively soluble. At low pH, the soluble monobasic form predominates; but as the pH increases, more dibasic phosphate becomes available to bind with calcium and precipitates. Therefore, the lower the pH of the parenteral nutrition solution, the more calcium and phosphate can be solubilized. Once again, the effects of temperature were observed. As the temperature is increased, more calcium ion becomes available and more dibasic calcium phosphate is formed. Therefore, temperature increases will increase the amount of precipitate (609).

Fitzgerald and MacKay reported similar calcium and phosphate solubility curves for neonatal parenteral nutrition solutions using TrophAmine (McGaw) 2, 1.5, and 0.8% as the sources of amino acids. The solutions also contained dextrose 10%, with cysteine and pH adjustment being used in some admixtures. Calcium and phosphate solubility followed the patterns reported by Eggert et al. (609). A slightly greater concentration of phosphate could be used in some mixtures, but this finding was not consistent (1024).

Using a similar study design, Fitzgerald and MacKay also studied six neonatal parenteral nutrition solutions based on Aminosyn-PF (Abbott) 2, 1.5, and 0.8%, with and without added cysteine HCl and dextrose 10%. Calcium concentrations ranged from 2.5 to 50 mEq/L, and phosphate concentrations ranged from 2.5 to 50 mmol/L. Solutions sat for 18 hours at 25 °C and then were warmed to 37 °C in a water bath to simulate the clinical situation of warming prior to infusion into a child. Solubility curves were markedly different than those for TrophAmine in the previous study (1024). Solubilities were reported to decrease by 15 mEq/L for calcium and 15 mmol/L for phosphate. The solutions remained clear during room temperature storage, but crystals often formed on warming to 37 °C (1211).

Figure 1. *Maximum solubilities of calcium chloride (○) and calcium gluconate (△) with sodium phosphate in an amino acid 4.25% – dextrose 25% solution at 30 °C*

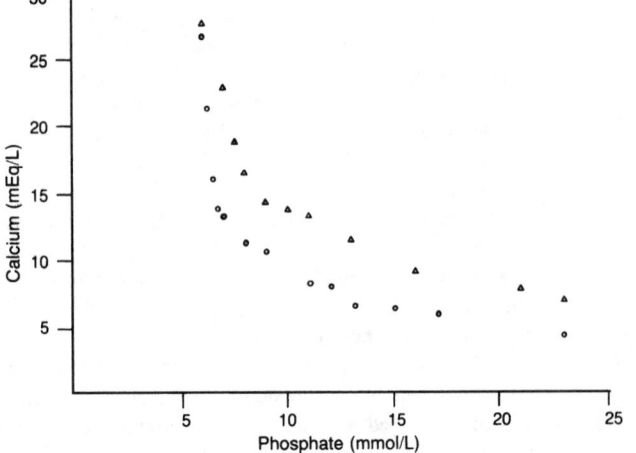

However, these data were questioned by Mikrut, who noted the similarities between the Aminosyn-PF and TrophAmine products and found little difference in calcium and phosphate solubilities in a preliminary report (1212). In the full report (1213), parenteral nutrition solutions containing Aminosyn-PF or TrophAmine 1 or 2.5% with dextrose 10 or 25%, respectively, plus electrolytes and trace metals, with or without cysteine HCl, were evaluated under the same conditions used by Fitzgerald and MacKay. Calcium concentrations ranged from 2.5 to 50 mEq/L, and phosphate concentrations ranged from 5 to 50 mmol/L. In contrast to the results of Fitzgerald and MacKay, the solubility curves were very similar for the Aminosyn-PF and TrophAmine parenteral nutrition solutions but very different from those of the previous Aminosyn-PF study (1211). The authors again showed that the solubility of calcium and phosphate is greater in solutions containing higher concentrations of amino acids and dextrose (1213).

Dunham et al. also reported calcium and phosphate solubility curves for TrophAmine 1 and 2% with dextrose 10% and electrolytes, vitamins, heparin, and trace elements. Calcium concentrations ranged from 10 to 60 mEq/L, and phosphorus concentrations ranged from 10 to 40 mmol/L. Calcium and phosphate solubilities were assessed by analysis of the calcium concentrations and followed patterns similar to those reported by Henry et al. (608). The higher percentage of amino acids (TrophAmine 2%) permitted a slightly greater solubility of calcium and phosphate, especially in the 10- to 50-mEq/L and 10- to 35-mmol/L ranges, respectively (1614).

Knight et al. reported the maximal product of the amount of calcium (as gluconate) times phosphate (as potassium) that can be added to a parenteral nutrition solution, composed of amino acids 1% (Travenol) and dextrose 10%, for preterm infants. Turbidity was observed on initial mixing when the solubility product was around 115 to 130 mM^2 or greater. After storage at 7 °C for 20 hours, visible precipitates formed at solubility products of 130 mM^2 or greater. If the solution was administered through a barium-impregnated silicone rubber catheter, crystalline precipitates obstructed the catheters in 12 hours at a solubility product of 100 mM^2 and in 10 days at 79 mM^2, much lower than the in vitro results (1041).

Poole et al. determined the solubility characteristics of calcium and phosphate in pediatric parenteral nutrition solutions composed of Aminosyn 0.5, 2, and 4% with dextrose 10 to 25%. Also present were electrolytes and vitamins. Sodium phosphate was added sequentially in phosphorus concentrations from 10 to 30 mmol/L. Calcium gluconate was added last in amounts ranging from 1 to 10 g/L. The solutions were stored at 25 °C for 30 hours and examined visually and microscopically for precipitation. The authors found that higher concentrations of Aminosyn increased the solubility of calcium and phosphate. Precipitation occurred at lower calcium and phosphate concentrations in the 0.5% solution compared to the 2 and 4% solutions. For example, at a phosphorus concentration of 30 mmol/L, precipitation occurred at calcium gluconate concentrations of about 1, 2, and 4 g/L in the 0.5, 2, and 4% Aminosyn mixtures, respectively. Similarly, at a calcium gluconate concentration of 8 g/L and above, precipitation occurred at phosphorus concentrations of about 13, 17, and 22 mmol/L in the 0.5, 2, and 4% solutions, respectively. The dextrose concentration did not appear to affect the calcium and phosphate solubility significantly (1042).

Alexander and Arena evaluated the compatibility of calcium gluconate (American Quinine) and potassium phosphate (Lyphomed) in a parenteral nutrition solution, composed of dextrose 12.5% and amino acid injection (FreAmine III, McGaw) 1.33% and having a

Table 2. Maximum Calcium and Phosphorus Concentrations Physically Compatible for 48 Hours at 4 °C (1210)

Calcium (mg/100 ml)	Phosphorus (mg/100 ml)	
	Amino Acids 1.25% + Dextrose 5%[a]	Amino Acids 2.5% + Dextrose 10%[a]
200[b]	50	75
150	50	100
100	75	100
50	100	125
25	150[b]	150[b]

[a]Plus multivitamins and trace elements.
[b]Maximum concentration tested.

pH of 6.6, for premature infants. Potassium phosphate was added in varying amounts to samples of this solution. The samples were then titrated with calcium gluconate 10%. From the resulting data, an equation was derived to predict when precipitation would occur:

$$Y = -0.455X + 2.951$$

where Y is the Log_{10} of the calcium gluconate concentration (as mg/100 ml) and X is the phosphate concentration (as mmol/100 ml). The equation can be solved to determine the maximum concentration of calcium gluconate for a given phosphate concentration or vice versa. If either additive is sufficiently dilute, then the other can be added in high concentrations without precipitation occurring, obviating the need for the equation. These lower limits were set at 60 mg/100 ml for calcium gluconate and 0.6 mmol/100 ml for phosphate (1004).

While the authors noted that this equation technically applies to the specific solution being tested and that other variables such as temperature can affect precipitation, in practice they found it applicable to a variety of parenteral nutrition solutions, having similar components and pH values, for premature infants. The equation is *not* applicable to parenteral nutrition solutions with amino acid and dextrose concentrations, other components, or pH values that are much different (1004).

Venkataraman et al. evaluated the solubility of calcium and phosphorus in neonatal parenteral nutrition solutions composed of amino acids (Abbott) 1.25 and 2.5% with dextrose 5 and 10%, respectively. Also present were multivitamins and trace elements. The solutions contained calcium (as gluconate) in amounts ranging from 25 to 200 mg/100 ml. The phosphorus (as potassium phosphate) concentrations evaluated ranged from 25 to 150 mg/100 ml. If calcium gluconate was added first, cloudiness occurred immediately. If potassium phosphate was added first, substantial quantities could be added with no precipitate formation in 48 hours at 4 °C (Table 2). However, if stored at 22 °C, the solutions were stable for only 24 hours, and all contained precipitates after 48 hours (1210).

Kirkpatrick et al. reported the physical compatibility of calcium gluconate 10 to 40 mEq/L and potassium phosphates 10 to 40 mmol/L in three neonatal parenteral nutrition solutions (TPN #123 to #125 in Appendix I), alone and with retrograde administration of aminophylline 7.5 mg diluted with 1.5 ml of sterile water for injection. Contact of the alkaline aminophylline solution with the parenteral nutrition solutions resulted in the precipitation of calcium phosphate at much lower concentrations than were compatible in the parenteral nutrition solutions alone (1404).

Koorenhof and Timmer reported the maximum allowable concentrations of calcium and phosphate in a 3-in-1 parenteral nutrition mixture for children (TNA #192 in Appendix I). Added calcium was varied from 1.5 to 150 mmol/L, while added phosphate was varied from 21 to 300 mmol/L. The mixtures were stable for 48 hours at 22 and 37 °C as long as the pH was not greater than 5.7, the calcium concentration was below 16 mmol/L, the phosphate concentration was below 52 mmol/L, and the product of the calcium and phosphate concentrations was below 250 $mmol^2/L^2$ (1773).

MacKay et al. reported additional calcium and phosphate solubility curves for specialty parenteral nutrition solutions based on NephrAmine and also HepatAmine at concentrations of 0.8, 1.5, and 2% as the sources of amino acids. The solutions also contained dextrose 10%, with cysteine and pH adjustment to simulate addition of fat emulsion used in some admixtures. Calcium and phosphate solubility followed the hyperbolic patterns reported by Eggert et al. (609). Temperature, time, and pH affected calcium and phosphate solubility, with pH having the greatest effect (2038).

Shatsky et al. reported the maximum sodium phosphate concentrations for given amounts of calcium gluconate that could be admixed in parenteral nutrition solutions containing TrophAmine in varying quantities (with cysteine HCl 40 mg/g of amino acid) and dextrose 10%. The solutions also contained magnesium sulfate 4 mEq/L, potassium acetate 24 mEq/L, sodium chloride 32 mEq/L, pediatric multivitamins, and trace elements. The presence of cysteine HCl reduces the solution pH and increases the amount of calcium and phosphate that can be incorporated before precipitation occurs. The results of this study cannot be safely extrapolated to TPN solutions with compositions other than the ones tested. The admixtures were compounded with the sodium phosphate added last after thorough mixing of all other components. The authors noted this is not the preferred order of mixing (usually phosphate is added first and thoroughly mixed before adding calcium last); however, they believed this reversed order of mixing would provide a margin of error in cases where the proper order is not followed. After compounding, the solutions were stored for 24 hours at 40 °C. The maximum calcium and phosphate amounts that could be mixed in the various solutions were reported tabularly and are shown in Table 3 (2039). However, these results are not entirely consistent with the study of Hoie and Narducci (2196). See below.

The temperature dependence of the calcium–phosphate precipitation has resulted in the occlusion of a subclavian catheter by a solution apparently free of precipitation. The parenteral nutrition solution consisted of FreAmine III 500 ml, dextrose 70% 500 ml, sodium chloride 50 mEq, sodium phosphate 40 mmol, potassium acetate 10 mEq, potassium phosphate 40 mmol, calcium gluconate 10 mEq, magnesium sulfate 10 mEq, and Shil's trace metals solution 1 ml. Although there was no evidence of precipitation in the bottle, tubing and pump cassette, and filter (all at approximately 26 °C) during administration, the occluded catheter and Vicra Loop Lock (next to the patient's body at 37 °C) had numerous crystals identified as calcium phosphate. In vitro, this parenteral nutrition solution had a precipitate in 12 hours at 37 °C but was clear for 24 hours at 26 °C (610).

Similarly, a parenteral nutrition solution that was clear and free of particulates after two weeks under refrigeration developed a precipitate in four to six hours when stored at room temperature. When the solution was warmed in a 37 °C water bath, precipitation occurred in one hour. Administration of the solution before the precipitate was noticed led to interstitial pneumonitis due to deposition of calcium phosphate crystals (1427).

A 2-ml fluid barrier of dextrose 5% in water in a microbore retrograde infusion set failed to prevent precipitation when used between calcium gluconate 200 mg/2 ml and sodium phosphate 0.3 mmol/0.1 ml (1385).

Table 3. Maximum Amount of Phosphate (as Sodium) (mmol/L) Not Resulting in Precipitation According to the Study of Shatsky et al. (2039). See CAUTION Below.[a]

Calcium (as gluconate)	Amino Acid (as TrophAmine) with Cysteine HCl 40 mg/g of Amino Acid				
	0%	0.4%	1%	2%	3%
9.8 mEq/L	0	27	42	60	66
14.7 mEq/L	0	15	18	30	36
19.6 mEq/L	0	6	15	27	30
29.4 mEq/L	0	3	6	21	24

[a]CAUTION: The results cannot be safely extrapolated to solutions with formulas other than the ones tested. See text.

Table 4. Maximum Amount of Phosphate (as Potassium) (mmol/L) Not Resulting in Precipitation According to the Study of Hoie and Narducci (2196). See CAUTION Below.[a]

Calcium (as Gluconate) (mEq/L)	Amino Acid (as TrophAmine) plus Cysteine HCl 1 g/L					
	0.5%	1%	1.5%	2%	2.5%	3%
10	22	28	38	38	38	43
14	18	18	18	38	38	43
19	18	18	18	33	33	38
24	12	18	18	22	28	28
28	12	18	18	18	18	18
33	12	12	12	12	12	12
37	12	12	12	12	12	12
41	9	9	9	12	12	12
45	0	9	9	12	12	12
49	0	9	9	9	12	12
53	0	9	9	9	9	9

[a]CAUTION: The results cannot be safely extrapolated to solutions with formulas other than the ones tested. See text.

Fausel et al. evaluated calcium phosphate precipitation phenomena in a series of parenteral nutrition admixtures composed of dextrose 22%, amino acids (FreAmine III) 2.7%, and fat emulsion (Abbott) 0, 1, and 3.2%. Incorporation of calcium gluconate 19 to 24 mEq/L and phosphate (as sodium) 22 to 28 mmol/L resulted in visible precipitation in the fat-free admixtures. New precipitate continued to form over 14 days, even after repeated filtrations of the solutions through 0.2-μm filters. The presence of the amino acids increased calcium and phosphate solubility compared with simple aqueous solutions. However, the incorporation of the fat emulsion did not result in a statistically significant increase in calcium and phosphate solubility. The authors noted that the kinetics of calcium phosphate precipitate formation do not appear to be entirely predictable; both transient and permanent precipitation can occur either during the compounding process or at some time afterward. Because calcium phosphate precipitation can be clinically very dangerous, the use of inline filters was recommended. The filters should have a porosity appropriate to the parenteral nutrition admixture—1.2 μm for fat-containing and 0.2 or 0.45 μm for fat-free nutrition mixtures (2061).

Hoie and Narducci used laser particle analysis to evaluate the formation of calcium phosphate precipitation in pediatric TPN solutions containing TrophAmine in concentrations ranging from 0.5 to 3% and also containing L-cysteine HCl 1 g/L. The solutions also contained in each liter sodium chloride 20 mEq, sodium acetate 20 mEq, magnesium sulfate 3 mEq, trace elements 3 ml, and heparin sodium 500 units. The presence of L-cysteine HCl reduces the solution pH and increases the amount of calcium and phosphate that can be incorporated before precipitation occurs. The results of this study cannot be safely extrapolated to TPN solutions with compositions other than the ones tested. The maximum amounts of phosphate that were incorporated without the appearance of a measurable increase in particulates in 24 hours at 37 °C for each of the amino acid concentrations is shown in Table 4 (2196). These results are not entirely consistent with those of Shatsky et al. See above. The use of more sensitive electronic particle measurement for the formation of subvisual particulates in this study may contribute to the differences in the results.

The presence of magnesium in solutions may also influence the reaction between calcium and phosphate, including the nature and extent of precipitation (158; 159).

The interaction of calcium and phosphate in parenteral nutrition solutions is a complex phenomenon. Various factors play a role in the solubility or precipitation of a given combination, including (608; 609; 1042; 1063; 1210; 1234; 1427):

1. Concentration of calcium
2. Salt form of calcium
3. Concentration of phosphate
4. Concentration of amino acids
5. Amino acids composition
6. Concentration of dextrose
7. Temperature of solution
8. pH of solution
9. Presence of other additives
10. Order of mixing

Enhanced precipitate formation would be expected from such factors as high concentrations of calcium and phosphate, increases in solution pH, decreases in amino acid concentrations, increases in temperature, addition of calcium before phosphate, lengthy standing times or slow infusion rates, and use of calcium as the chloride salt (854).

Even if precipitation does not occur in the bottle, it has been reported that crystallization of calcium phosphate may occur in a Silastic infusion pump chamber or tubing if the rate of administration is slow, as for premature infants. Water vapor may be transmitted outward and be replaced by air rapidly enough to produce supersaturation (202). Several other cases of catheter occlusion also have been reported (610; 1427–1429).

The UV spectrum of an equal parts mixture of amino acids 8%–dextrose 50% solution was not altered in 24 hours at 22 °C by the addition of calcium gluconate 20 mEq and potassium phosphate 25 mEq (313).

Other Incompatible Ions— Calcium gluconate (Upjohn) in dextrose 5% in water has been reported as conditionally compatible with sodium bicarbonate (Abbott). The incompatibility is dependent on the concentration of the additives. Therefore, if attempting to combine calcium gluconate with sodium bicarbonate, mix the solution thoroughly and observe it for any sign of incompatibility (15). A white precipitate and turbidity were reported in concentrated solutions (845).

Calcium gluconate is stated to be incompatible with citrates, soluble carbonates, phosphates, and sulfates. Because of the presence of sodium carbonate in the cefamandole nafate (Lilly) formulation, it is incompatible with calcium ions (4; 376).

Folic Acid— Calcium gluconate (Parke-Davis) and folic acid injection (Lederle) have been shown to interact even though a precipitate is not present. The recoverable amount of folic acid from a 10-µg/ml solution declined with increasing concentrations (0.5 to 10 µg/ml) of calcium gluconate. This interaction was reversed by the addition of edetic acid (538).

Miscellaneous— Calcium ions are stated to inhibit the activity of tobramycin sulfate (145). Clindamycin phosphate (Upjohn) is reported to be physically incompatible with calcium gluconate (2p2462). In addition, cefazolin sodium appears to be incompatible with calcium gluconate (143; 278).

CARBOPLATIN
AHFS 10:00

Paraplatin   **Bristol-Myers Squibb**

Products— Carboplatin (Bristol-Myers Squibb) is available as a lyophilized powder in vials containing 50, 150, or 450 mg with an equal amount of mannitol. Reconstitute the vials with dextrose 5% in water, sodium chloride 0.9%, or sterile water for injection in the following amounts (2):

Vial Size	Volume of Diluent
50 mg	5 ml
150 mg	15 ml
450 mg	45 ml

The reconstituted solutions have a carboplatin concentration of 10 mg/ml.

pH— A 1% solution has a pH of 5 to 7 (2).

Osmolality— Carboplatin 10 mg/ml in sterile water for injection has an osmolality of 94 mOsm/kg (1689).

Administration— Carboplatin is administered by intravenous infusion over a period of at least 15 minutes or longer. It has also been administered as a continuous intravenous infusion over 24 hours. It may be diluted with compatible diluents to a concentration as low as 0.5 mg/ml for administration (2; 4).

Stability— Intact vials should be stored at controlled room temperature and protected from light (2).

The manufacturer states that reconstituted solutions are stable for eight hours at a room temperature not exceeding 25 °C. Because no antibacterial preservative is present, the manufacturer recommends that carboplatin solutions should be discarded eight hours after dilution (2). However, other information indicates that the drug may be stable for a much longer time. At a concentration of 15 mg/ml in sterile water for injection or at concentrations of 2 and 0.5 mg/ml in dextrose 5% in water, no decomposition occurs in 24 hours at 22 to 25 °C (234). Aqueous solutions of 10 mg/ml prefilled into plastic syringes exhibited no decomposition in five days at 4 °C and only a 3% loss in 24 hours at 37 °C (1238).

Carboplatin 1 mg/ml in sterile water for injection was reported to exhibit less than a 10% loss in 14 days at room temperature (1379).

Carboplatin 7 mg/ml in sterile water for injection exhibited a 4% loss in seven days at 27 °C. At this concentration in sodium chloride 0.9%, an 8% loss occurred in 24 hours at 27 °C. In a sodium bicarbonate 200 mM solution, the carboplatin loss increased to 13% in 24 hours at 27 °C (1379).

Carboplatin (Bristol-Myers Oncology) 1 mg/ml in sterile water for injection was stable in PVC reservoirs (Parker Micropump) for 14 days at 4 and 37 °C, exhibiting no loss by HPLC analysis (1696).

pH Effects— The pH range of maximum stability has been reported to be pH 4 to 6 (1919) to 6.5 (1369). The degradation rate increases above pH 6.5 (1369).

Portable Pumps— The stability of carboplatin (Bristol-Myers Oncology) 1 mg/ml in dextrose 5% in water in drug reservoirs of three portable pumps was evaluated and compared to the stability in glass bottles and PVC bags. A PVC reservoir (Pharmacia Deltec pump), an ethylene vinyl acetate reservoir (Celsa Celinject CO1), and an elastomeric balloon (Baxter Infusor) were stored at 4, 22, and 35 °C

for 28 days. HPLC analyses for carboplatin content were performed periodically. No color changes or precipitation was observed in any sample at any time. Furthermore, little or no drug loss was found. The largest losses in 28 days were with the glass bottles (5 to 6% loss) and PVC reservoir (2 to 4% loss). However, the ethylene vinyl acetate reservoir and the elastomeric balloon showed carboplatin concentration increases of 4 and 14%, respectively, in 28 days at 35 °C due to moisture transfer through the container material (1823).

Carboplatin 10 mg/ml (Bristol-Myers Squibb) was repackaged into 30-ml polypropylene syringes for use in the Intelliject portable syringe pump. The carboplatin solution exhibited no visual changes, and HPLC analysis found no loss of carboplatin content when stored at 25 °C for eight days. No evidence of interaction between carboplatin and the syringe plastic was identified, and no impact on the functioning of the syringe pump was observed (2147).

Sorption— Comparison of the stability of carboplatin 1 mg/ml in dextrose 5% in sodium chloride 0.45% in both glass and PVC containers showed no difference, with each sustaining less than a 2% loss in 24 hours at 25 °C (1087). Simulated infusion of carboplatin 10 mg/ml through a Silastic catheter over 24 hours at 37 °C did not affect the delivered drug concentration (1238).

Compatibility Information

Solution Compatibility

Carboplatin

Solution	Mfr	Mfr	Conc/L	Remarks	Ref	C/I
Dextrose 5% in sodium chloride 0.2%	AB[a]	NCI	1 g	Physically compatible with less than 2% loss in 24 hr at 25 °C	1087	**C**
Dextrose 5% in sodium chloride 0.45%	AB[b]	NCI	1 g	Physically compatible with less than 2% loss in 24 hr at 25 °C	1087	**C**
Dextrose 5% in sodium chloride 0.9%	AB[a]	NCI	1 g	Physically compatible with 4% loss in 24 hr at 25 °C	1087	**C**
Dextrose 5% in water	[a]	NCI	500 mg and 2 g	Physically compatible with no decomposition for at least 24 hr at 25 °C	234	**C**
	AB[a]	NCI	100 mg and 1 g	Physically compatible with 1.5% or less decomposition in 6 hr at 25 °C	1087	**C**
	[c]	BR	2.4 g	No carboplatin loss by HPLC in 9 days at 23 °C when protected from light	1756	**C**
	[c]	BR	1 g	Visually compatible and little or no carboplatin loss by HPLC in 28 days at 4, 22, and 35 °C	1823	**C**
	[a]	BR	1 g	Visually compatible with 5 to 6% carboplatin loss by HPLC in 28 days at 4, 22, and 35 °C	1823	**C**
	[d]	BR	1 g	Visually compatible with no carboplatin loss by HPLC in 28 days at 4 and 22 °C. Drug concentration increased by 4% in 28 days at 35 °C due to moisture transfer through container	1823	**C**
	[e]	BR	1 g	Visually compatible with little or no carboplatin loss by HPLC in 28 days at 4 and 22 °C. Drug concentration increased by 14% in 28 days at 35 °C due to moisture transfer through container	1823	**C**
	BA[a]	BMS	500 mg and 4 g	Visually compatible with 3 to 5% loss by HPLC at 25 °C and no loss at 4 °C protected from light in 21 days	2099	**C**

Solution Compatibility (Cont.)

Carboplatin

Solution	Mfr	Mfr	Conc/L	Remarks	Ref	C/I
	BA[a]	BMS	750 mg and 2 g	Visually compatible with no loss by HPLC at 25 and 4 °C protected from light in 7 days	2099	C
Sodium bicarbonate 200 mM			7 g	13% loss in 24 hr at 27 °C	1379	I
Sodium chloride 0.9%	AB[a]	NCI	1 g	Physically compatible with 5% loss in 24 hr at 25 °C	1087	C
			7 g	8% loss in 24 hr at 27 °C	1379	C

[a]Tested in glass containers.
[b]Tested in both glass and PVC containers.
[c]Tested in PVC containers.
[d]Tested in ethylene vinyl acetate containers.
[e]Tested in elastomeric balloon reservoirs (Baxter Infusor).

Additive Compatibility

Carboplatin

Drug	Mfr	Conc/L	Mfr	Conc/L	Test Soln	Remarks	Ref	C/I
Cisplatin		200 mg		1 g	NS	Less than 10% loss of both drugs in 24 hr at 23 °C protected from light	1954	C
Etoposide		200 mg		1 g	W	Less than 10% loss of both drugs in 7 days at 23 °C protected from light	1954	C
Floxuridine		10 g		1 g	W	Less than 10% loss of both drugs in 7 days at 23 °C protected from light	1954	C
Fluorouracil		10 g		1 g	W	Greater than 20% carboplatin loss in 24 hr at room temperature	1379	I
Ifosfamide		1 g		1 g	W	Both drugs stable for 5 days at room temperature	1379	C
Ifosfamide with etoposide		2 g 200 mg		1 g	W	All drugs stable for 7 days at room temperature	1379	C
Mesna		1 g		1 g	W	Greater than 10% carboplatin loss in 24 hr at room temperature	1379	I
Paclitaxel	BMS	300 mg and 1.2 g	BMS	2 g	NS	No paclitaxel loss but carboplatin losses of less than 2, 5, and 6 to 7% at 4, 24, and 32 °C, respectively, in 24 hr by HPLC. Physically compatible for 24 hr but subvisual particulates of paclitaxel form after 3 to 5 days	2094	C
	BMS	300 mg and 1.2 g	BMS	2 g	D5W	No paclitaxel and carboplatin loss by HPLC at 4, 24, and 32 °C in 24 hr. Physically compatible for 24 hr but subvisual particulates of paclitaxel form after 3 to 5 days	2094	C

Y-Site Injection Compatibility (1:1 Mixture)

		Carboplatin					
Drug	*Mfr*	*Conc*	*Mfr*	*Conc*	*Remarks*	*Ref*	*C/I*
Allopurinol sodium	BW	3 mg/ml[b]	BR	5 mg/ml[b]	Physically compatible with no change in measured turbidity or increase in particle content in 4 hr at 22 °C	1686	**C**
Amifostine	USB	10 mg/ml[a]	BR	5 mg/ml[a]	Physically compatible with no change in measured turbidity or increase in particle content in 4 hr at 23 °C	1845	**C**
Amphotericin B cholesteryl sulfate complex	SEQ	0.83 mg/ml[a]	BR	5 mg/ml[a]	Increased turbidity forms immediately	2117	**I**
Aztreonam	SQ	40 mg/ml[a]	BMS	5 mg/ml[a]	Physically compatible with no subvisual haze or particle formation in 4 hr at 23 °C	1758	**C**
Cefepime HCl	BR	20 mg/ml[a]	BR	5 mg/ml[a]	Physically compatible with no change in measured turbidity or increase in particle content in 4 hr at 22 °C	1689	**C**
Cladribine	ORT	0.015[b] and 0.5[c] mg/ml	BR	5 mg/ml[b]	Physically compatible with no change in measured turbidity or increase in particle content in 4 hr at 23 °C	1969	**C**
Doxorubicin HCl liposome injection	SEQ	0.4 mg/ml[a]	BR	5 mg/ml[a]	Physically compatible with little or no change in measured turbidity and no increase in particle content in 4 hr at 23 °C	2087	**C**
Etoposide phosphate	BR	5 mg/ml[a]	BR	5 mg/ml[a]	Physically compatible with no change in measured turbidity or increase in particle content in 4 hr at 23 °C	2218	**C**
Filgrastim	AMG	30 μg/ml[a]	BR	5 mg/ml[a]	Physically compatible with no change in measured turbidity or increase in particle content in 4 hr at 22 °C	1687	**C**
Fludarabine phosphate	BX	1 mg/ml[a]	BR	5 mg/ml[a]	Physically compatible for 4 hr at room temperature under fluorescent light	1439	**C**
Gemcitabine HCl	LI	10 mg/ml[b]	BR	5 mg/ml[b]	Physically compatible with no change in measured turbidity or increase in particle content in 4 hr at 23 °C	2226	**C**
Granisetron HCl	SKB	1 mg/ml	BR	1 mg/ml[b]	Physically compatible with little or no loss of either drug by HPLC in 4 hr at 22 °C	1883	**C**
Melphalan HCl	BW	0.1 mg/ml[b]	BR	5 mg/ml[b]	Physically compatible with no change in measured turbidity or increase in particle content in 3 hr at 22 °C	1557	**C**
Ondansetron HCl	GL	1 mg/ml[b]	BR	5 mg/ml[a]	Physically compatible for 4 hr at 22 °C under fluorescent light	1365	**C**
	GL	16 to 160 μg/ml		0.18 to 9.9 mg/ml	Physically compatible when carboplatin given over 10 to 60 min via Y-site	1366	**C**
Paclitaxel	NCI	1.2 mg/ml[a]		5 mg/ml[a]	Physically compatible with no change in measured turbidity in 4 hr at 22 °C	1528	**C**
Piperacillin sodium–tazobactam sodium	LE	40 + 5 mg/ml[a]	BR	5 mg/ml[a]	Physically compatible with no change in measured turbidity or increase in particle content in 4 hr at 22 °C	1688	**C**
Propofol	ZEN	10 mg/ml	BR	5 mg/ml[a]	Physically compatible for 1 hr at 23 °C with no increase in particle content	2066	**C**

Y-Site Injection Compatibility (1:1 Mixture) (Cont.)

Carboplatin

Drug	Mfr	Conc	Mfr	Conc	Remarks	Ref	C/I
Sargramostim	IMM	10 μg/ml[b]	BR	5 mg/ml[b]	Physically compatible for 4 hr at 22 °C	1436	**C**
Teniposide	BR	0.1 mg/ml[a]	BR	5 mg/ml[a]	Physically compatible with no subvisual haze or particle formation in 4 hr at 23 °C	1725	**C**
Thiotepa	IMM[d]	1 mg/ml[a]	BMS	5 mg/ml[a]	Physically compatible with no change in measured turbidity or increase in particle content in 4 hr at 23 °C	1861	**C**
TNA #218 to #226[e]			BMS	5 mg/ml[a]	Visually compatible with no precipitate or emulsion damage apparent in 4 hr at 23 °C	2215	**C**
TPN #212 to #215[e]			BMS	5 mg/ml[a]	Physically compatible with no change in measured turbidity or increase in particle content in 4 hr at 23 °C	2109	**C**
Vinorelbine tartrate	BW	1 mg/ml[b]	BR	5 mg/ml[b]	Physically compatible with no change in measured turbidity or increase in particle content in 4 hr at 22 °C	1558	**C**

[a]*Tested in dextrose 5% in water.*
[b]*Tested in sodium chloride 0.9%.*
[c]*Tested in bacteriostatic sodium chloride 0.9% preserved with benzyl alcohol 0.9%.*
[d]*Lyophilized formulation tested.*
[e]*Refer to Appendix I for the composition of parenteral nutrition solutions. TNA indicates a 3-in-1 admixture, and TPN indicates a 2-in-1 admixture.*

Additional Compatibility Information

Chloride-Containing Solutions— The manufacturer states that carboplatin may be reconstituted and further diluted with sodium chloride 0.9%, along with other diluents, and used within eight hours (2). Cheung et al. noted an increased rate of carboplatin loss in sodium chloride 0.9% and dextrose 5% in sodium chloride 0.9% compared to other diluents, although they still qualify as compatible solutions. About 4 to 5% was lost in 24 hours at 25 °C (1087).

However, Perrone et al. found little conversion of carboplatin to cisplatin in sodium chloride solutions. Cisplatin formation was eval-uated by HPLC analysis of carboplatin 1 mg/ml in sodium chloride 0.9% at 25 °C with exposure to fluorescent light. Less than 0.1% of the carboplatin had converted to cisplatin in two hours, and 0.7% had converted in 24 hours. These authors do not believe that the formation of cisplatin from carboplatin is a justifiable concern (1695).

Aluminum— Because of an interaction occurring between carboplatin and the metal aluminum, resulting in precipitate formation and loss of potency, only administration equipment such as needles, syringes, catheters, and sets that contain no aluminum should be used for this drug (2).

CARMUSTINE (BCNU)
AHFS 10:00

BiCNU   **Bristol-Myers Squibb**

Products— Carmustine (Bristol-Myers Squibb) is available in vials containing 100 mg of drug, packaged with a vial containing 3 ml of dehydrated alcohol injection, USP, for use as a diluent (2).

Dissolve the contents of the vial of carmustine with 3 ml of dehydrated alcohol injection, USP. Further dilute with 27 ml of sterile water for injection. The resultant solution will contain 3.3 mg/ml of carmustine in 10% ethanol (2).

Avoid accidental contact of the reconstituted solution with the skin. Transient hyperpigmentation in the affected areas has occurred (2; 4).

pH— From 5.6 to 6 (2).

Osmolality— Carmustine (Bristol) 3.3 mg/ml, reconstituted as directed in ethanol and water, has an apparent osmolality that exceeds 2000 mOsm/kg (2043).

Administration— Carmustine is administered as an intravenous infusion over one to two hours. Shorter durations may result in pain and burning at the injection site and flushing (2; 4).

Stability— The product consists of vacuum-dried pale yellow flakes or is a congealed mass. Intact vials are stored under refrigeration and are stable for at least two years (2). The manufacturer states that intact vials are stable for seven days at room temperatures not exceeding 25 °C (1181; 1236; 1433). Room temperature storage of intact vials results in slow decomposition, with approximately 3% degradation occurring in 36 days (285).

Reconstitution as directed results in a colorless to pale yellow solution. This solution is stable for eight hours at room temperature protected from light (2; 4). Decomposition of the reconstituted solution at room temperature is linear with time. About a 6% loss occurs in three hours and about an 8% loss occurs in six hours (285). A loss of 20% in 21 hours was also reported (484).

Refrigeration of the solution significantly increases its stability. The solution is stable for 24 hours at 4 °C (4). In 24 hours at 2 to 8 °C with protection from light, approximately 4% decomposition occurs (285).

Carmustine has a melting point of approximately 30.5 to 32 °C. At this temperature, the drug liquifies, becoming an oily film on the bottom of the vial. Should this occur, the manufacturer recommends that the vials be discarded, because the melting is a sign of decomposition (2). However, one study showed that storage of the vials at 37 °C for 15 minutes followed by storage at 22 to 25 °C resulted in no decomposition in eight days and about an 8% loss in 37 days. Storage of the vials at 37 °C for seven days resulted in about 10% decomposition (862).

In 95% ethanol, carmustine 2 mg/ml is reported to be stable for at least 24 hours at 22 to 25 and 37 °C (862). Under refrigeration, carmustine 0.5 to 0.6 mg/ml in 95% ethanol or absolute ethanol is stable at 0 to 5 °C for up to three months (863).

Carmustine, reconstituted according to the manufacturer's instructions, was cultured with human lymphoblasts to determine whether its cytotoxic activity was retained. The solution retained cytotoxicity for 24 hours when stored at 4 °C (1575).

pH Effects— The degradation rate for carmustine in aqueous solution was reported to be at a minimum between pH 5.2 and 5.5 (619) and 3.3 and 4.8 (1237). Above pH 6, the degradation rate increases greatly (619). Decomposition of 10% occurred in less than two hours at pH 6.5 but in 5.5 hours at optimum pH (1237).

Light Exposure— Increased decomposition rates were reported when carmustine, in solution, was exposed to increasing intensities of light. The observed reaction rate increased sixfold when illumination rose from 500 to 4000 luxes. In this report, light protection for the infusion container was recommended (1237). However, the reconstituted drug remains stable for eight hours at 25 °C when exposed to normal fluorescent light (4).

Sorption— The manufacturer recommends the use of glass containers for carmustine administration (2; 4). The rate of loss of carmustine from infusion admixtures in dextrose 5% in water in PVC containers is substantially greater than the rate of loss in glass (519; 1658) or polyolefin (1658) containers. That observation also was confirmed in a study where the rate of loss of carmustine in dextrose 5% in water in glass containers was no more than the usual chemical degradation. A much greater loss occurred when the solution was prepared in a PVC container (1237).

Substantial loss to PVC infusion sets was also noted. In static tests, 10% of the carmustine was lost in five minutes and only 35% remained after two hours. An ethylene vinyl acetate set resulted in similar sorption; a polyurethane set was substantially worse, with only 20% remaining after two hours. Only a set lined with polyethylene proved resistant to carmustine sorption, resulting in little loss in two hours (1237).

During simulated infusion, the greatest quantity of carmustine was lost during the first few minutes, with the concentration delivered increasing with time. The drug concentration in the effluent was the lowest from the slowest flow rate because of the longer contact time. For a nominal 500-ml infusion at a flow rate of 530 ml/hr, 4.6% of the drug was lost during the first hour. At 265 ml/hr, the loss increased to 8.1% in the first hour; at a flow rate of 88 ml/hr, the loss soared to 23% in the first hour (1237).

Compatibility Information

Solution Compatibility

Carmustine

Solution	Mfr	Mfr	Conc/L	Remarks	Ref	C/I
Dextrose 5% in water	TR[a]	BR	1.25 g	10% loss of carmustine in 7.7 hr at room temperature	519	I
	TR[b]	BR	1.25 g	18.5% loss of carmustine in 1 hr at room temperature	519	I
	CU	BR	100 mg	No decomposition over 90-min study period	523	C
	MG, TR[a]		1.25 g	10% loss of carmustine by HPLC in 7.7 to 8.3 hr at room temperature exposed to light	1658	I
	MG[c]		1.25 g	10% loss of carmustine by HPLC in 7 hr at room temperature exposed to light	1658	I
	TR[b]		1.25 g	10% loss of carmustine by HPLC in 0.6 hr at room temperature exposed to light	1658	I
Sodium chloride 0.9%	CU	BR	100 mg	No decomposition over 90-min study period	523	C

[a]Tested in glass containers.
[b]Tested in PVC containers.
[c]Tested in polyolefin containers.

Additive Compatibility

Carmustine

Drug	Mfr	Conc/L	Mfr	Conc/L	Test Soln	Remarks	Ref	C/I
Sodium bicarbonate	AB	100 mEq	BR	100 mg	D5W, NS	10% carmustine decomposition in 15 min, 27% in 90 min	523	I

Y-Site Injection Compatibility (1:1 Mixture)

Carmustine

Drug	Mfr	Conc	Mfr	Conc	Remarks	Ref	C/I
Allopurinol sodium	BW	3 mg/ml[b]	BR	1.5 mg/ml[b]	Gas evolves immediately	1686	I
Amifostine	USB	10 mg/ml[a]	BR	1.5 mg/ml[a]	Physically compatible with no change in measured turbidity or increase in particle content in 4 hr at 23 °C	1845	C
Aztreonam	SQ	40 mg/ml[a]	BMS	1.5 mg/ml[a]	Physically compatible with no subvisual haze or particle formation in 4 hr at 23 °C	1758	C
Cefepime HCl	BR	20 mg/ml[a]	BR	1.5 mg/ml[a]	Physically compatible with no change in measured turbidity or increase in particle content in 4 hr at 22 °C	1689	C
Etoposide phosphate	BR	5 mg/ml[a]	BR	1.5 mg/ml[a]	Physically compatible with no change in measured turbidity or increase in particle content in 4 hr at 23 °C	2218	C
Filgrastim	AMG	30 μg/ml[a]	BR	1.5 mg/ml[a]	Physically compatible with no change in measured turbidity or increase in particle content in 4 hr at 22 °C	1687	C
Fludarabine phosphate	BX	1 mg/ml[a]	BR	1.5 mg/ml[a]	Physically compatible for 4 hr at room temperature under fluorescent light	1439	C
Gemcitabine HCl	LI	10 mg/ml[b]	BR	1.5 mg/ml[b]	Physically compatible with no change in measured turbidity or increase in particle content in 4 hr at 23 °C	2226	C
Granisetron HCl	SKB	0.05 mg/ml[a]	BMS	1.5 mg/ml[a]	Physically compatible with no change in measured turbidity or increase in particle content in 4 hr at 23 °C	2000	C
Melphalan HCl	BW	0.1 mg/ml[b]	BR	1.5 mg/ml[b]	Physically compatible with no change in measured turbidity or increase in particle content in 3 hr at 22 °C	1557	C
Ondansetron HCl	GL	1 mg/ml[b]	BR	1.5 mg/ml[a]	Physically compatible for 4 hr at 22 °C	1365	C
Piperacillin sodium–tazobactam sodium	LE	40 mg/ml[a]	BR	1.5 mg/ml[a]	Physically compatible with no change in measured turbidity or increase in particle content in 4 hr at 22 °C	1688	C
Sargramostim	IMM	10 μg/ml[b]	BR	1.5 mg/ml[b]	Physically compatible for 4 hr at room temperature under fluorescent light	1436	C
Teniposide	BR	0.1 mg/ml[a]	BR	1.5 mg/ml[a]	Physically compatible with no subvisual haze or particle formation in 4 hr at 23 °C	1725	C
Thiotepa	IMM[c]	1 mg/ml[a]	BMS	1.5 mg/ml[a]	Physically compatible with no change in measured turbidity or increase in particle content in 4 hr at 23 °C	1861	C

Y-Site Injection Compatibility (1:1 Mixture) (Cont.)

Carmustine

Drug	Mfr	Conc	Mfr	Conc	Remarks	Ref	C/I
Vinorelbine tartrate	BW	1 mg/ml[b]	BR	1.5 mg/ml[b]	Physically compatible with no change in measured turbidity or increase in particle content in 4 hr at 22 °C	1558	C

[a]*Tested in dextrose 5% in water.*
[b]*Tested in sodium chloride 0.9%.*
[c]*Lyophilized formulation tested.*

Additional Compatibility Information

Solutions— Dilution of the reconstituted solution to a 0.2-mg/ml concentration in dextrose 5% in water results in a solution that is stable for eight hours at room temperature protected from light (2).

Dacarbazine— No alteration in the ultraviolet/visible spectra was observed when dacarbazine was combined in solution with carmustine (492).

CEFAMANDOLE NAFATE
AHFS 8:12.06

Mandol   **Lilly**

Products— Cefamandole nafate (Lilly) is available in the following containers (2):

Cefamandole Content	Container
1 g	10 ml
	100-ml piggyback
2 g	20 ml
	100-ml piggyback
10 g	100-ml bulk package

The product contains 63 mg of sodium carbonate per gram of cefamandole activity (2).

For intramuscular administration, each gram of cefamandole should be reconstituted with 3 ml of sterile water for injection, bacteriostatic water for injection, sodium chloride 0.9%, or bacteriostatic sodium chloride 0.9% (2). The final concentration is approximately 285 mg/ml with a withdrawable volume of about 3.5 ml. The drug dissolves in as little as 1.2 ml of these diluents, but 3 ml yields the most acceptable solution for intramuscular administration (788). Lidocaine HCl 1% has been used to reconstitute the drug for intramuscular administration, reducing the pain upon injection. Serum concentrations and urine outputs were similar to dosing in sodium chloride 0.9% (625).

For direct intravenous administration, each gram of cefamandole should be reconstituted with 10 ml of sterile water for injection, dextrose 5% in water, or sodium chloride 0.9% (2).

When given as an intermittent intravenous infusion by means of a Y-type set or volume control set, the 1- or 2-g piggyback vials should be reconstituted with 100 ml of compatible infusion solution. (See Compatibility Information.) If sterile water for injection is to be used, about 20 ml per gram should be used for reconstitution to avoid a hypotonic solution (2).

For administration as a continuous intravenous infusion, each gram of cefamandole should be reconstituted with 10 ml of sterile water for injection. This solution may then be further diluted in an appropriate amount of a compatible infusion solution (2). (See Compatibility Information.)

Cefamandole nafate is difficult to dissolve and requires vigorous shaking. Dissolution is reportedly facilitated by keeping the powder at the stopper end of the vial while adding the diluent to the other end of the vial. Subsequent shaking tends to disperse the powder before the diluent wets the surface of a larger powder mass (620).

Because the cefamandole nafate (Lilly) formulation contains sodium carbonate, carbon dioxide gas is formed after reconstitution. The pressure may be dissipated prior to withdrawal; or it may be utilized to aid in withdrawal of the solution from the vial by inverting the vial over the syringe needle, allowing the solution to flow into the syringe (2).

pH— Freshly reconstituted solutions have a pH of 6 to 8.5 (2). Immediately after reconstitution, the pH may be near 8.5 but equilibrates near neutrality within a few minutes (376).

Storage of cefamandole nafate 2 g/100 ml in dextrose 5% in water and sodium chloride 0.9% resulted in dramatic decreases in pH from approximately 7 initially to about 4 after four days at 24 °C. The decline was less rapid at 5 °C (525).

Osmolality— A solution of cefamandole nafate 1 g/22 ml of sterile water for injection is isotonic (2).

The osmolality of cefamandole nafate 1 and 2 g was calculated for the following dilutions (1054):

Diluent	Osmolality (mOsm/kg)	
	50 ml	100 ml
1 g		
Dextrose 5% in water	314	287
Sodium chloride 0.9%	341	314
2 g		
Dextrose 5% in water	357	316
Sodium chloride 0.9%	383	343

Robinson et al. recommended the following maximum cefamandole concentrations to achieve osmolalities suitable for peripheral infusion in fluid-restricted patients (1180):

Diluent	Maximum Concentration (mg/ml)	Osmolality (mOsm/kg)
Dextrose 5% in water	54	530
Sodium chloride 0.9%	49	519
Sterile water for injection	98	466

Sodium Content— The total sodium content per gram of cefamandole activity is 3.3 mEq (77 mg) (2).

Administration— Cefamandole nafate may be administered by deep intramuscular injection, by direct intravenous injection over three to five minutes, by intermittent infusion over 15 to 30 minutes, or by continuous infusion (2; 4; 8). The manufacturer recommends temporarily discontinuing other solutions being administered at the same site (2).

Stability— Solutions of cefamandole nafate range from light yellow to amber, depending on the concentration of the drug and the diluent used (2; 471). The reconstituted solution need not be protected from light. However, light protection is recommended during storage of the vials because the powder discolors upon prolonged exposure to light (624).

Sodium carbonate is present in the formulation to prevent turbidity or precipitation when reconstituted with some intravenous solutions (471; 474; 621). This results from the precipitation of cefamandole nafate and cefamandole free acids as the pH of the solution drops from aqueous ester hydrolysis (472).

Any solutions having an unusual color or containing turbidity or a precipitate should not be used (471).

The sodium carbonate also enhances in vitro hydrolysis from the nafate to the sodium form (471; 622; 788). This occurs partially in vitro but proceeds very rapidly in vivo with a $t\frac{1}{2}$ of about 13 minutes (622). The rate of in vitro hydrolysis is greater in dextrose 5% in water than in sodium chloride 0.9% due to attack by the dextrose on the formyl ester moiety. However, this is of no clinical significance (626). The antibacterial activity of both the nafate and sodium salts is essentially the same in normal clinical situations (471; 621). In vivo, cefamandole is the major circulating species, representing 85 to 89% of the total plasma concentration (622).

After reconstitution, room temperature storage results in carbon dioxide evolution from the solution because of the sodium carbonate present in the formulation. This gas production has been reported to result in an "explosive like" reaction when cefamandole nafate is repackaged in syringes (473). The observed phenomenon was not an actual shattering of the syringe (623) but rather the separation of the plunger from the barrel of the syringe (620; 623). This phenomenon

has been described, perhaps more accurately, as "rifling" (620). The manufacturer has indicated that reconstituted solutions should be left in the original containers and should be withdrawn into syringes just prior to use (474). This carbon dioxide production is apparently of little consequence on addition to an intravenous solution (473), nor does it preclude storage of the reconstituted product for appropriate time periods in the original vial (474).

The manufacturer states that reconstituted solutions are stable for 24 hours at 25 °C or 96 hours at 5 °C (2). These time limits appear to reflect concern over possible microbiological contamination rather than drug instability (788). The drug actually appears to be stable for longer periods. At the concentrations used for intramuscular injection (approximately 285 mg/ml), the drug is stable (less than 10% decomposition) for 72 hours at 25 °C or 10 days at 5 °C in the following vehicles (788):

Bacteriostatic sodium chloride 0.9%
  (parabens or benzyl alcohol)
Bacteriostatic water for injection
  (parabens or benzyl alcohol)
Lidocaine 0.5, 1, or 2%
Sodium chloride 0.9%
Water for injection

Freezing Solutions— Cefamandole nafate (Lilly) solutions are stable in the frozen state. At the intramuscular concentration of 1 g/3 ml in the original vials using water for injection, dextrose 5% in water, or sodium chloride 0.9% as diluents, the drug exhibited 1 to 6% decomposition in 52 weeks at −20 °C. At −10 °C, the solution did not completely freeze and a transient turbidity developed when thawed to room temperature (475).

Further diluted in dextrose 5% in water or sodium chloride 0.9% to a concentration of 1 g/50 ml in glass bottles or PVC containers or a concentration of 1 g/100 ml in glass bottles, cefamandole nafate maintained stability for at least 26 weeks at −20 °C, exhibiting 7% or less decomposition. At −10 °C in sodium chloride 0.9%, the solution was acceptable after 26 weeks; but in dextrose 5% in water at −10 °C, a transient haze developed (475). At either concentration, the pH of the frozen solutions declined as a function of age (475).

In another study, cefamandole nafate (Lilly) 1 g/50 ml of dextrose 5% in water in PVC bags was frozen at −20 °C for 30 days. The bags were then thawed by exposure to ambient temperature or microwave radiation. There was no evidence of precipitation or color change and no loss of potency as determined microbiologically in the solutions thawed by either technique. Subsequent storage of the admixture at room temperature for 24 hours also yielded physically compatible solutions exhibiting little or no loss of potency (554).

Cefamandole nafate (Lilly) 1 g/3.5 ml frozen at −20 °C in glass syringes (Hy-Pod) retained potency for nine months. No gas formation was seen in the frozen syringes. It was recommended that the syringes be used in a "reasonable" time after thawing and warming to room temperature to avoid gas formation and expulsion of the plunger (532).

Minibags of cefamandole nafate in dextrose 5% in water or sodium chloride 0.9%, frozen at −20 °C for up to 35 days, were thawed at room temperature and in a microwave oven; the thawed solution temperature never exceeded 25 °C. No significant differences in cefamandole nafate concentrations occurred between the two thawing methods (1192).

If the frozen solution is to be warmed for thawing, a maximum of 37 °C should be observed. Heating after the frozen solution has thawed should be avoided. Thawed solutions should not be refrozen (2).

Compatibility Information

Solution Compatibility

Cefamandole nafate

Solution	Mfr	Mfr	Conc/L	Remarks	Ref	C/I
Acetated Ringer's injection		LI	2 g	Physically incompatible due to haze formation	788	**I**
Amino acids 3.5%	AB	LI	2 g	Physically compatible with 6% cefamandole loss in 48 hr at 25 °C and no loss in 10 days at 5 °C	788	C
Amino acids 7%	AB	LI	2 g	Physically compatible with 7% cefamandole loss in 48 hr at 25 °C and 2% loss in 10 days at 5 °C	788	C
Amino acids 8.5% (FreAmine II)	MG	LI	2 g	Physically compatible with 8% cefamandole loss in 48 hr at 25 °C and 4% loss in 10 days at 5 °C	788	C
Amino acids 8.5% with electrolytes	TR	LI	2 g	Physically compatible with 7% cefamandole loss in 48 hr at 25 °C and 1% loss in 10 days at 5 °C	788	C
Amino acids 8.5% without electrolytes	TR	LI	2 g	Physically compatible with 6% cefamandole loss in 48 hr at 25 °C and 2% loss in 10 days at 5 °C	788	C
Dextran 40 and dextrose			2 g	Physically compatible and chemically stable for 24 hr at 25 °C	596	C
Dextran 40 and sodium chloride 0.9%			2 g	Physically compatible and chemically stable for 24 hr at 25 °C	596	C
Dextran 70 and dextrose			2 g	Physically compatible with 6% cefamandole loss in 24 hr at 25 °C	596	C
Dextrose 70 and sodium chloride 0.9%			2 g	Physically compatible with 6% cefamandole loss in 24 hr at 25 °C	596	C
Dextrose 5% and potassium chloride 0.15%		LI	2 g	Physically compatible for 24 hr at 5 and 25 °C with haze formation after that time. 4% loss in 24 hr at 25 °C	788	C
Dextrose 5% in Ringer's injection, lactated		LI	2 g	Physically compatible with 6% loss in 72 hr at 25 °C and no loss in 10 days at 5 °C	788	C
Dextrose 5% in sodium chloride 0.2%		LI	2 g	Physically compatible with 5% loss in 48 hr at 25 °C and no loss in 7 days at 5 °C	376; 788	C
Dextrose 5% in sodium chloride 0.45%		LI	2 g	Physically compatible with 8% loss in 48 hr at 25 °C and 3% loss in 10 days at 5 °C	788	C
Dextrose 5% in sodium chloride 0.9%		LI	20 g	Physically compatible with 5% loss in 72 hr at 25 °C and 2% loss in 10 days at 5 °C	788	C
		LI	2 g	Physically compatible with 10% loss in 72 hr at 25 °C and no loss in 10 days at 5 °C	788	C
Dextrose 5% in water [a]		LI	20 g	Physically compatible with 3 to 5% loss in 72 hr at 25 °C and 1 to 3% loss in 10 days at 5 °C	788	C
		LI	2 g	Physically compatible with 5% loss in 48 hr (14% loss in 72 hr) at 25 °C and no loss in 10 days at 5 °C	788	C

Solution Compatibility (Cont.)

Cefamandole nafate

Solution	Mfr	Mfr	Conc/L	Remarks	Ref	C/I
	TR[b]	LI	20 g	4% decomposition in 1 day and 10% in 5 days at 24 °C. 2% loss in 4 days and 5% in 44 days at 5 °C	525	C
	TR[b]	LI	20 g	Physically compatible with little or no loss of potency in 24 hr at room temperature	554	C
			2 g	Physically compatible and chemically stable for 24 hr at 25 °C	596	C
	MG[c]	LI	10 g	Physically compatible with 4% loss in 48 hr at room temperature under fluorescent light	983	C
Dextrose 10% in water		LI	20 g	Physically compatible with 6% loss in 72 hr at 25 °C and no loss in 7 days at 5 °C	788	C
		LI	2 g	Physically compatible with 3 to 5% loss in 48 hr at 25 °C and no loss in 7 days at 5 °C	376; 788	C
			2 g	Physically compatible and chemically stable for 24 hr at 25 °C	596	C
Fat emulsion, intravenous			2 g	Physically compatible and chemically stable for 24 hr at 25 °C	596	C
Ionosol B in dextrose 5% in water	AB	LI	2 g	Physically compatible for 24 hr at 5 and 25 °C with haze formation after that time. 4% loss in 24 hr at 25 °C	788	C
Isolyte E with dextrose 5%	MG	LI	2 g	Physically compatible for 24 hr at 5 and 25 °C with haze formation after that time. 5% loss in 24 hr at 25 °C	788	C
Isolyte M with dextrose 5%	MG	LI	2 g	Physically incompatible due to haze formation	788	I
Mannitol 10% in water			2 g	Physically compatible and chemically stable for 24 hr at 25 °C	596	C
Mannitol 15% in water	TR	LI	20 g	9% cefamandole loss in 72 hr at 25 °C and 2% loss in 7 days at 5 °C	376	C
	TR	LI	20 g	Physically compatible with 9% loss in 72 hr at 25 °C and 5% loss in 10 days at 5 °C	788	C
Mannitol 20% in water			2 g	Physically compatible and chemically stable for 24 hr at 25 °C	596	C
Normosol M in dextrose 5% in water	AB	LI	2 g	Physically compatible with 6% loss in 72 hr at 25 °C and 1% loss in 10 days at 5 °C	788	C
Plasma-Lyte	TR	LI	2 g	Physically incompatible due to haze formation	788	I
Plasma-Lyte M in dextrose 5%	TR	LI	2 g	Physically compatible with 5% loss in 72 hr at 25 °C and 2% loss in 10 days at 5 °C	788	C
Ringer's injection		LI	2 g	Physically incompatible due to haze formation	788	I
Ringer's injection, lactated		LI	2 g	Physically incompatible due to haze formation	788	I
Sodium chloride 0.9%	[a]	LI	20 g	Physically compatible with 3 to 4% loss in 72 hr at 25 °C and 0 to 3% loss in 10 days at 5 °C	788	C
		LI	2 g	Physically compatible with 1% loss in 48 hr (13% loss in 72 hr) at 25 °C and no loss in 10 days at 5 °C	788	C
	TR[b]	LI	20 g	3% decomposition in 1 day and 6% in 5 days at 24 °C. 1% loss in 4 days and 6% in 44 days at 5 °C	525	C
			2 g	Physically compatible and chemically stable for 24 hr at 25 °C	596	C

Solution Compatibility (Cont.)

Cefamandole nafate

Solution	Mfr	Mfr	Conc/L	Remarks	Ref	C/I
	MG[c]	LI	10 g	Physically compatible with 4% loss in 12 hr at room temperature under fluorescent light. No further loss occurred through 48 hr	983	**C**
Sodium lactate ⅙ M		LI	2 g	Physically compatible with 9% loss in 48 hr at 25 °C and no loss in 10 days at 5 °C	788	**C**
TPN #107[d]			1.5 g	Physically compatible and cefamandole activity retained for 24 hr at 21 °C by microbiological assay	1326	**C**

[a]*Tested in glass and PVC containers.*
[b]*Tested in PVC containers.*
[c]*Tested in glass bottles.*
[d]*Refer to Appendix I for the composition of parenteral nutrition solutions. TPN indicates a 2-in-1 admixture.*

Additive Compatibility

Cefamandole nafate

Drug	Mfr	Conc/L	Mfr	Conc/L	Test Soln	Remarks	Ref	C/I
Calcium gluconate		200 mg	LI	2 g	D5W, NS, W	Haze or precipitate forms	788	**I**
		2 g	LI	20 g	D5W, NS, W	Haze or precipitate forms	788	**I**
Cimetidine HCl	SKF	3 g		10 g	D5W, NS	Cloudiness forms after 4 to 5 hr, increasing to dense precipitate in 24 hr at room temperature	516	**I**
	SKF	6 g		20 g	D5W, NS	Cloudiness forms after 4 to 5 hr, increasing to dense precipitate in 24 hr at room temperature	516	**I**
	SKF	6 g	LI	20 g	D5W	Immediate haze formation, and gelatinous precipitate observed at 24 hr at room temperature. Cimetidine loss of 7% attributed to precipitate	551	**I**
	SKF	300 mg	LI	1 g	D5W	Physically compatible and cimetidine chemically stable for 24 hr at room temperature. Cefamandole not tested	551	**C**
Clindamycin phosphate	UP	9 g	LI	10 g	D5W, NS[a]	Physically compatible with no clindamycin loss and 4 to 7% cefamandole loss in 48 hr at room temperature under fluorescent light	983	**C**
Floxacillin sodium	BE	20 g	DI	20 g	W	Physically compatible for 24 hr at 15 and 30 °C. Haze forms in 48 hr and precipitate forms in 72 hr at 30 °C. No change at 15 °C	1479	**C**
Furosemide	HO	1 g	DI	20 g	W	Physically compatible for 72 hr at 15 and 30 °C	1479	**C**
Gentamicin sulfate		80 mg	LI	2 and 20 g	D5W, NS, W	Haze or precipitate forms within 4 hr	376; 788	**I**
		100 mg		1 g	TPN #107[b]	14% gentamicin loss in 24 hr at 21 °C by microbiological assay	1326	**I**
Metronidazole	RP	5 g[c]	LI	20 g		Physically compatible with little or no pH change for at least 72 hr at 4 °C	807	**C**

Additive Compatibility (Cont.)

Cefamandole nafate

Drug	Mfr	Conc/L	Mfr	Conc/L	Test Soln	Remarks	Ref	C/I
	RP	5 g[c]	LI	20 g		Physically compatible for at least 24 hr at 23 °C, but pH changed significantly	807	?
	SE	5 g	LI	20 g		10% metronidazole loss in 2 hr at 25 °C and in 6 hr at 5 °C, with no further loss occurring up to 3 days. No cefamandole loss noted	979	I
	SE	200 mg	LI	800 mg	W	No immediate loss of potency of either drug	979	C
	BAY	4.2 g	LI	16.7 g	[d]	Visually compatible with little cefamandole loss and 8% or less metronidazole loss in 4 hr at room temperature by HPLC	1888	C
Metronidazole HCl with sodium bicarbonate	SE AB	5 g 50 mEq	LI	2 g	D5W, NS	Physically compatible for 48 hr. Gradual darkening attributed to normal cephalosporin color change with time	765	C
Ranitidine HCl	GL	50 mg and 2 g		1 g	D5W	Ranitidine chemically stable by HPLC for only 6 hr at 25 °C. Cefamandole not tested	1515	I
Tobramycin sulfate	LI	80 mg	LI	2 and 20 g	D5W, NS, W	Haze or precipitate forms within 4 hr	376; 788	I
Verapamil HCl	KN	80 mg	LI	4 g	D5W, NS	Physically compatible for 24 hr	764	C

[a]Tested in glass bottles.
[b]Refer to Appendix I for the composition of parenteral nutrition solutions. TPN indicates a 2-in-1 admixture.
[c]Minibags (100 ml) containing metronidazole 500 mg with disodium phosphate 150 mg, citric acid 44 mg, and sodium chloride 740 mg. This product differs from the Searle product.
[d]Cefamandole reconstituted with water and added to metronidazole infusion.

Drugs in Syringe Compatibility

Cefamandole nafate

Drug (in syringe)	Mfr	Amt	Mfr	Amt	Remarks	Ref	C/I
Cimetidine HCl	SKF	300 mg/ 2 ml		1 g/5 ml	Immediate precipitation	516	I
Gentamicin sulfate		80 mg/ 2 ml	LI	1 g/ 10 ml	Haze or precipitate forms within 4 hr	376; 788	I
		80 mg/ 2 ml	LI	1 g/3 ml	Haze or precipitate forms within 4 hr	376	I
Heparin sodium		2500 units/ 1 ml	LI	2 g	Physically compatible for at least 5 min	1053	C
Tobramycin sulfate	LI	80 mg/ 2 ml	LI	1 g/ 10 ml	Haze or precipitate forms within 4 hr	376; 788	I
	LI	80 mg/ 2 ml	LI	1 g/3 ml	Haze or precipitate forms within 4 hr	376	I

Y-Site Injection Compatibility (1:1 Mixture)

Cefamandole nafate

Drug	Mfr	Conc	Mfr	Conc	Remarks	Ref	C/I
Acyclovir sodium	BW	5 mg/ml[a]	LI	20 mg/ml[a]	Physically compatible for 4 hr at 25 °C	1157	C

Y-Site Injection Compatibility (1:1 Mixture) (Cont.)

Cefamandole nafate

Drug	Mfr	Conc	Mfr	Conc	Remarks	Ref	C/I
Amiodarone HCl	LZ	4 mg/ml[c]	LI	20 and 40 mg/ml[c]	Precipitate forms	1444	**I**
Cyclophosphamide	MJ	20 mg/ml[a]	LI	20 mg/ml[a]	Physically compatible for 4 hr at 25 °C	1194	**C**
Diltiazem HCl	MMD	5 mg/ml	LI	200 mg/ml[b]	Cloudiness forms but clears with swirling	1807	**?**
	MMD	5 mg/ml	LI	10[b] and 20[a] mg/ml	Cloudiness forms and persists	1807	**I**
	MMD	1 mg/ml[c]	LI	10[b], 20[a], 200[b] mg/ml	Visually compatible	1807	**C**
Hetastarch	DCC	6%	LI	20 mg/ml[a]	Small crystals formed immediately after mixing and persisted for 4 hr	1313	**I**
Hydromorphone HCl	WY	0.2 mg/ml[a]	LI	20 mg/ml[a]	Physically compatible for at least 4 hr at 25 °C under fluorescent light	987	**C**
Magnesium sulfate	IX	16.7, 33.3, 66.7, 100 mg/ml[a]	LI	20 mg/ml[a]	Physically compatible for at least 4 hr at 32 °C	813	**C**
Meperidine HCl	WY	10 mg/ml[a]	LI	20 mg/ml[a]	Physically compatible for at least 4 hr at 25 °C under fluorescent light	987	**C**
	WY	10 mg/ml[b]	LI	40 mg/ml[a]	Physically compatible for 1 hr at 25 °C	1338	**C**
Morphine sulfate	WI	1 mg/ml[a]	LI	20 mg/ml[a]	Physically compatible for at least 4 hr at 25 °C under fluorescent light	987	**C**
	ES	1 mg/ml[b]	LI	40 mg/ml[a]	Physically compatible for 1 hr at 25 °C	1338	**C**
Perphenazine	SC	0.02 mg/ml[a]	LI	20 mg/ml[a]	Physically compatible for 4 hr at 25 °C	1155	**C**
TNA #73[d]		32.5 ml[e]	LI	2 g/50 ml[a]	Physically compatible for 4 hr at 25 °C by visual observation	1008	**C**
TPN #54[d]				250 mg/ml	Physically compatible and cefamandole activity retained over 6 hr at 22 °C by microbiological assay	1045	**C**
TPN #61[d]		[f]	LI	200 mg/ 0.7 ml[g]	Physically compatible	1012	**C**
		[h]	LI	1.2 g/4.2 ml[g]	Physically compatible	1012	**C**

[a]*Tested in dextrose 5% in water.*
[b]*Tested in sodium chloride 0.9%.*
[c]*Tested in both dextrose 5% in water and sodium chloride 0.9%.*
[d]*Refer to Appendix I for the composition of parenteral nutrition solutions. TNA indicates a 3-in-1 admixture, and TPN indicates a 2-in-1 admixture.*
[e]*A 32.5-ml sample of parenteral nutrition solution combined with 50 ml of piggyback solution.*
[f]*Run at 21 ml/hr.*
[g]*Given over five minutes by syringe pump.*
[h]*Run at 94 ml/hr.*

Additional Compatibility Information

Miscellaneous— Cefamandole is compatible with lidocaine HCl 0.5, 1, and 2%. If the concentration of cefamandole nafate is less than 10%, however, turbidity, a precipitate, or both develop (376).

Because of its sodium carbonate content, cefamandole nafate has been stated to be incompatible with calcium ions (4; 788), forming a viscous gel (596). It may also be incompatible with solutions containing magnesium ions (4; 471). It is reported to be incompatible with tromethamine-containing solutions that have a high pH (596).

Aminoglycosides— The manufacturer recommends that no aminoglycoside be mixed with cefamandole nafate. If combination therapy is indicated, aminoglycosides should be administered at a different site than the cefamandole (2).

However, Teil et al. studied the stability of gentamicin 3.8 µg/ml and cefamandole 11 µg/ml in serum stored at 24, 6, and −17 °C for 24 hours. No substantial differences in the concentrations of either drug occurred, indicating that gentamicin is not inactivated in the presence of cefamandole (864).

To determine if spurious aminoglycoside levels could result from a delay in assaying blood samples, Tindula et al. evaluated the inactivation of amikacin 35 µg/ml and gentamicin and tobramycin 10 µg/ml in human serum by 400-µg/ml concentrations of several penicillins and cephalosporins. Samples were stored for 24 hours at room temperature and frozen at -20 °C. For samples at both temperatures, cefamandole caused relatively little inactivation of the aminoglycosides (824).

Spruill et al. evaluated the effect of various cephalosporins on tobramycin sulfate 7.7 µg/ml in human serum. At concentrations of 250 and 1000 µg/ml, cefazolin, cefoxitin, cefamandole, cefoperazone, and cefotaxime caused about a 10 to 15% loss of tobramycin over 48 hours at 0 and 21 °C. Moxalactam caused about a 15% loss at 0 °C and a 20 to 30% loss at 21 °C over 48 hours (1005).

Cefamandole nafate (Lilly) 125 µg/ml combined separately with the aminoglycosides amikacin sulfate (Bristol), gentamicin sulfate (Schering), and tobramycin sulfate (Lilly) at a concentration of 25 µg/ml in peritoneal dialysis solution (Dianeal 1.5%) exhibited enhanced rates of lethality to *Staphylococcus aureus*, *Escherichia coli*,

and *Pseudomonas aeruginosa* compared to any of the drugs alone (1623).

Peritoneal Dialysis Fluid— Cefamandole nafate (Lilly) 2 and 5 mg/ml in peritoneal dialysis fluid concentrates (American McGaw) with dextrose 30 and 50% was evaluated for compatibility. The 2-mg/ml concentration was physically compatible for 24 hours at 25 °C with no loss of cefamandole, but a haze formed at 5 °C. The 5-mg/ml concentration developed a haze at both 5 and 25 °C with a 5 to 6% cefamandole loss at 25 °C in 24 hours (788).

Cefamandole nafate 2 mg/ml in peritoneal dialysis solution (McGaw) containing dextrose 2.5% and electrolytes was physically compatible for three hours at room temperature. Furthermore, no significant loss of antibacterial activity was apparent by microbiological determination (142).

CEFAZOLIN SODIUM
AHFS 8:12.06

Kefzol	**Lilly**
Ancef	**SmithKline Beecham**

Products— Cefazolin as the sodium salt is available in 500-mg and 1-, 5-, and 10-g vials; 500-mg and 1-g piggyback units; and 500-mg and 1-g flexible plastic bags. For intramuscular administration, reconstitute the vials with the volumes indicated in the table below and shake well until dissolved. Sterile water for injection, bacteriostatic water for injection, or sodium chloride 0.9% may be used for reconstitution (2; 4).

Vial Size	Volume of Diluent	Approximate Solution Volume	Approximate Concentration
500 mg	2 ml	2.2 ml	225 mg/ml
1 g	2.5 ml	3 ml	330 mg/ml

For direct intravenous injection, further dilute the reconstituted cefazolin sodium with approximately 5 ml of sterile water for injection (2; 4).

For intermittent intravenous infusion, reconstituted cefazolin sodium should be diluted further in 50 to 100 ml of compatible infusion solution (2; 4). (See Compatibility Information.)

The 5- and 10-g bulk vials may be reconstituted with sterile water for injection, bacteriostatic water for injection, or sodium chloride 0.9%. The 5-g vial should be reconstituted with 23 or 48 ml to yield concentrations of 1 g/5 ml or 1 g/10 ml, respectively. The 10-g vial should be reconstituted with 45 or 96 ml to yield concentrations of 1 g/5 ml or 1 g/10 ml, respectively (2).

Cefazolin sodium (SmithKline Beecham) is also available frozen in PVC bags in concentrations of 500 mg and 1 g in 50 ml of dextrose 5% in water (4).

pH— From 4.5 to 6. The frozen premixed solutions have a pH of 4.5 to 7 (4).

Osmolality— The osmolality of a 225-mg/ml concentration in sterile

water for injection was determined to be 636 mOsm/kg by freezing-point depression (1071).

The osmolality of cefazolin sodium 1 and 2 g was calculated for the following dilutions (1054):

	Osmolality (mOsm/kg)	
Diluent	50 ml	100 ml
1 g		
Dextrose 5% in water	321	291
Sodium chloride 0.9%	344	317
2 g		
Dextrose 5% in water	379	324
Sodium chloride 0.9%	406	351

The osmolality of cefazolin sodium (Lyphomed) 20 mg/ml was determined to be 325 mOsm/kg in dextrose 5% in water and 347 mOsm/kg in sodium chloride 0.9%. At a 50-mg/ml concentration, the osmolality was determined to be 412 mOsm/kg in dextrose 5% in water and 426 mOsm/kg in sodium chloride 0.9% (1375).

The frozen premixed solutions have osmolalities of 260 to 320 mOsm/kg for the 500 mg/50-ml concentration and 310 to 380 mOsm/kg for the 1 g/50-ml concentration (4).

Robinson et al. recommended the following maximum cefazolin sodium concentrations to achieve osmolalities suitable for peripheral infusion in fluid-restricted patients (1180):

Diluent	Maximum Concentration (mg/ml)	Osmolality (mOsm/kg)
Dextrose 5% in water	77	507
Sodium chloride 0.9%	69	494
Sterile water for injection	138	404

Sodium Content— Each gram of cefazolin sodium contains 46 mg or approximately 2 mEq of sodium (2; 4).

Administration— Cefazolin sodium may be administered by deep intramuscular injection or by intravenous injection. By direct intravenous injection, it is given over three to five minutes directly into the vein or tubing of a running infusion solution. It may also be given by intermittent infusion in 50 to 100 ml of compatible diluent or by continuous infusion (2; 4; 8; 338).

Stability— Intact containers of the sterile powder should be stored at 15 to 30 °C. Reconstituted solutions of cefazolin sodium are light yellow to yellow. Protection from light is recommended for both the powder and its solutions (4).

A test of cefazolin sodium 250 mg/ml in water for injection showed that the drug lost less than 3% potency in 14 days at 5 °C. A potency loss of 8 to 10% was noted in four days at 25 °C (276). Borst et al. reported that cefazolin sodium (SKF) 1 and 2 g/10 ml in sterile water for injection, packaged in plastic syringes (Monoject), exhibited a 10% cefazolin loss in 13 days at 24 °C as determined by UV spectroscopy. At 4 °C, the drug exhibited less than a 10% loss during the 28-day study period (1178). The manufacturer recommends that solutions of cefazolin sodium be discarded after 24 hours at room temperature or 10 days under refrigeration (2). This recommendation is made to reduce the potential for the growth of microorganisms and to minimize an increase in color and a change in pH (276). Refrigeration of reconstituted solutions of cefazolin sodium may result in crystal formation (875).

Crystal formation has also been observed in reconstituted cefazolin sodium 330 mg/ml stored at room temperature after complete dissolution when sodium chloride 0.9% is the diluent. The crystals formed initially are fine and may be easily overlooked. At 330 mg/ml, cefazolin sodium is near its saturation point, and the room temperature and ionic content of the diluent are important for maintaining the drug in solution. In an evaluation of the 1-g Kefzol and Ancef products reconstituted with 2.5 ml of either sodium chloride 0.9% or sterile water for injection and stored at 24 or 26 °C, none of the vials reconstituted with sterile water for injection formed crystals within 24 hours. However, when sodium chloride 0.9% was the diluent, all Kefzol vials had crystals within 20 to 30 minutes, and two Ancef vials had crystals within 150 minutes at 24 °C. All Ancef vials had crystals within 24 hours at 24 °C. At 26 °C, all Kefzol vials had crystals within 45 minutes, but none of the Ancef vials had crystals after 24 hours. Consequently, sterile water for injection was recommended as the diluent for intramuscular doses when possible (875). The crystals of cefazolin sodium can be redissolved by hand-warming the vials or by immersion in a 35 °C water bath for two minutes. The clear solution will then be suitable for use. However, the use of sodium chloride 0.9% as a diluent for the 1-g vials was deleted from the current labeling (1075).

Exposure of cefazolin sodium (SKF) 73.2 mg/ml in sterile water for injection to 37 °C for 24 hours, to simulate the use of a portable infusion pump, did not result in a loss of cefazolin sodium (1391).

pH Effects— Cefazolin sodium solutions are relatively stable at pH 4.5 to 8.5. Above pH 8.5, rapid hydrolysis of the drug occurs. Below pH 4.5, precipitation of the insoluble free acid may occur (4; 284).

Cefazolin sodium in solutions containing dextrose, fructose, sucrose, dextran 40 or 70, mannitol, sorbitol, or glycerol in concentrations up to 15% was most stable at pH 5 to 6.5. At neutral and alkaline pH, the rate of degradation was accelerated by the carbohydrates and alcohols (820).

Cefazolin sodium 3.33 mg/ml was evaluated in several aqueous buffer solutions. The drug was most stable in pH 4.5 acetate buffer, exhibiting 10% decomposition in three days at 35 °C and in five days at 25 °C. In pH 5.7 acetate buffer, a 13% loss occurred in three

days at 35 °C and a 10% loss occurred in five days at 25 °C. No loss occurred in either acetate buffer in seven days at 4 °C (1147).

In pH 7.5 phosphate buffer, a yellow color and particulate matter developed after three to four days at 35 °C. This change was accompanied by a 6% cefazolin loss in one day and an 18% loss in three days. At 25 and 4 °C, 10 and 5% cefazolin losses occurred, respectively, in five days (1147).

Freezing Solutions— Solutions of cefazolin sodium 125, 225, and 330 mg/ml frozen in the original containers at −20 °C immediately after reconstitution with sterile water for injection, bacteriostatic water for injection, or sodium chloride 0.9% are stated to be stable for 12 weeks. Thawed solutions are stable for 24 hours at room temperature or 10 days under refrigeration; they should not be refrozen (2; 4).

When reconstituted with water for injection, dextrose 5% in water, or sodium chloride 0.9% in concentrations of 1 g/2.5 ml, 500 mg/100 ml, and 10 g/45 ml, cefazolin sodium retained more than 90% potency for up to 26 weeks when frozen within one hour after reconstitution at −10 and −20 °C. In a concentration of 500 mg/100 ml in dextrose 5% in Ringer's injection, lactated, Ionosol B in dextrose 5% in water, Normosol M in dextrose 5% in water, Plasma-Lyte in dextrose 5% in water, or Ringer's injection, lactated, cefazolin sodium was stable for up to four weeks when frozen within one hour after reconstitution at −10 °C (277).

In another study, cefazolin sodium (SKF) 1 g/50 ml of dextrose 5% in water and also sodium chloride 0.9% in PVC containers was frozen at −20 °C for 30 days. The results indicate that potency was retained for the duration of the study (299).

Cefazolin sodium (Lilly) 1 g/100 ml in dextrose 5% in water in PVC bags was frozen at −20 °C for 30 days and then thawed by exposure to ambient temperature or microwave radiation. The solutions showed no evidence of precipitation or color change and showed no loss of potency as determined microbiologically. Subsequent storage of the admixture at room temperature for 24 hours also yielded a physically compatible solution which exhibited a 3 to 6% loss of potency (554).

In an additional study, cefazolin sodium (Lilly and SKF) 10 mg/ml in 50, 100, and 250 ml of dextrose 5% in water and sodium chloride 0.9% in PVC bags was frozen at −20 °C for 48 hours. Thawing was then performed by exposure to microwave radiation carefully applied so that the solution temperature did not exceed 20 °C and so that a small amount of ice remained at the endpoint. This procedure avoids accelerated decomposition due to inadvertent excessive temperature increases. The solutions were stored for four hours at room temperature. Both brands of cefazolin sodium retained at least 90% of the initial activity as determined by microbiological assay. In addition, the solutions did not exhibit color changes or significant pH changes (627).

Miller and Pesko reported an approximate fourfold increase in particles of 2 to 60 μm produced by freezing and thawing cefazolin sodium (Lilly) 2 g/100 ml of dextrose 5% in water (Travenol). The reconstituted drug was filtered through a 0.45-μm filter into PVC bags of solution and frozen for seven days at −20 °C. Thawing was performed at room temperature (29 °C) for 12 hours. Although the total number of particles increased significantly, no particles greater than 60 μm were observed; the solution complied with USP standards for particle sizes and numbers in large volume parenteral solutions (822).

Cefazolin sodium (SKF) reconstituted with sterile water for injection to a concentration of 1 g/3 ml frozen at −20 °C in glass syringes (Hy-Pod) retained potency for nine months. However, when 0.5% lidocaine HCl (Astra) was used to constitute the cefazolin sodium, a clear solution did not result upon thawing. The solution was unsuitable for injection (532).

Borst et al. reported that cefazolin sodium (SKF) 1 and 2 g/10 ml in sterile water for injection, packaged in plastic syringes (Monoject) and frozen at −15 °C, was stable for the three-month study period, exhibiting less than a 10% loss as determined by UV spectroscopy (1178).

Stiles et al. reported no loss of cefazolin sodium (SKF) from a solution containing 73.2 mg/ml in sterile water for injection in PVC and glass containers after 30 days at −20 °C. Subsequent thawing and storage for four days at 5 °C, followed by 24 hours at 37 °C to simulate the use of a portable infusion pump, also did not result in a cefazolin loss (1391).

Cefazolin sodium (Schein) 20 mg/ml in dextrose 5% in water and sodium chloride 0.9% frozen at −20 °C for 12 weeks exhibited little or no loss of potency by HPLC analysis in latex elastomeric reservoirs (Secure Medical) and in glass containers (1970).

The manufacturer warns against continued heating of a completely thawed solution (2), which can result in accelerated drug decomposition and possibly dangerous pressure increases in the container (627).

Elastomeric Reservoir Pumps— Cefazolin sodium (Schein) 20 mg/ml in dextrose 5% in water and sodium chloride 0.9% 50 ml was packaged in elastomeric latex reservoirs (Secure Medical). Little or no loss of potency by HPLC analysis occurred in 24 hours at 25 °C and in three days at 5 °C (1970).

Filtration— Cefazolin sodium (SKF) 10 g/L in dextrose 5% in water and also in sodium chloride 0.9% was filtered through 0.45- and 0.22-μm Millipore membrane filters at time zero and at 4, 8, and 24 hours after mixing. HPLC analysis showed no significant difference in concentration between any of the filtered samples compared to unfiltered solutions at these time intervals. It was concluded that filtration of cefazolin sodium solutions through these membrane filters could be performed without adversely affecting the drug concentration (375).

Compatibility Information

Solution Compatibility

Cefazolin sodium

Solution	Mfr	Mfr	Conc/L	Remarks	Ref	C/I
Amino acids 4.25%, dextrose 25%	MG	LI	1 g	No increase in particulate matter in 24 hr at 5 °C	349	C
Dextrose 5% in Ringer's injection, lactated		LI	5 g	Potency retained for 14 days at 5 °C. 9% potency loss in 4 days at 25 °C	276	C
Dextrose 5% in water		LI	5 g	4% potency loss in 14 days at 5 °C, 6% loss in 4 days at 25 °C	276	C
	BA[a], TR	SKF	20 g	Potency retained for 24 hr at 5 and 22 °C	298	C
	TR[b]	LI	10 g	Physically compatible with approximately 3% potency loss in 24 hr at room temperature	554	C
	MG[c]	SKF	10 g	Physically compatible with no loss in 48 hr at room temperature under fluorescent light	983	C
	AB[d]	SCN	20 g	Little or no cefazolin loss by HPLC in 24 hr at 25 °C and in 7 days at 5 °C	1970	C
	BA[a]	BR	10 g	Visually compatible with about 7% loss by HPLC in 30 days at 4 °C	2142	C
Ionosol B in dextrose 5% in water		LI	5 g	2% potency loss in 14 days at 5 °C, 1 to 4% loss in 4 days at 25 °C	276	C
Normosol M in dextrose 5% in water		LI	5 g	3% potency loss in 14 days at 5 °C, 1 to 4% loss in 4 days at 25 °C	276	C
Plasma-Lyte in dextrose 5% in water		LI	5 g	Potency retained for 14 days at 5 °C. 6% potency loss in 7 days at 25 °C	276	C
Ringer's injection, lactated		LI	5 g	Potency retained for 14 days at 5 °C. 9% potency loss in 7 days at 25 °C	276	C
Sodium chloride 0.9%		LI	5 g	4% potency loss in 7 days at 5 °C, 8% loss in 4 days at 25 °C	276	C
	BA[a], TR	SKF	20 g	Potency retained for 24 hr at 5 and 22 °C	298	C
	MG[c]	SKF	10 g	Physically compatible with no loss in 48 hr at room temperature under fluorescent light	983	C
		LI	3.33 g	Physically compatible with 10% loss at 35 °C and 5% loss at 25 °C in 3 days. No loss in 7 days at 4 °C	1147	C

Solution Compatibility (Cont.)

Cefazolin sodium

Solution	Mfr	Mfr	Conc/L	Remarks	Ref	C/I
	AB[d]	SCN	20 g	4% or less cefazolin loss by HPLC in 24 hr at 25 °C and in 7 days at 5 °C	1970	C
TPN #22[e]		SKF	10 g	Physically compatible with no loss of activity by microbiological assay in 24 hr at 22 °C in the dark	837	C
TPN #107[e]			1 g	9% cefazolin loss in 24 hr at 21 °C by microbiological assay	1326	C

[a]Tested in both glass and PVC containers.
[b]Tested in PVC containers.
[c]Tested in glass bottles.
[d]Tested in glass containers and latex elastomeric reservoirs (Secure Medical).
[e]Refer to Appendix I for the composition of parenteral nutrition solutions. TPN indicates a 2-in-1 admixture.

Additive Compatibility

Cefazolin sodium

Drug	Mfr	Conc/L	Mfr	Conc/L	Test Soln	Remarks	Ref	C/I
Amikacin sulfate	BR	5 g	LI	20 g	D5LR, D5R, D5S, D5W, D10W, IS10, LR, NS, R, SL	Potency of both retained for at least 8 hr at 25 °C. Turbidity observed at 24 hr	293	I
Atracurium besylate	BW	500 mg		10 g	D5W	Atracurium chemically unstable and particles form	1694	I
Aztreonam	SQ	10 and 20 g	LI	5 and 20 g	D5W, NS[a]	Physically compatible with little or no loss of either drug in 48 hr at 25 °C and 7 days at 4 °C protected from light	1020	C
Bleomycin sulfate	BR	20 and 30 units	LI	1 g	NS	43% loss of bleomycin activity in 1 week at 4 °C	763	I
Cimetidine HCl	SKF	3 g		10 g	D5W, NS	Physically compatible for 48 hr at room temperature. Precipitate forms upon freezing	516	C
	SKF	6 g		20 g	D5W, NS	Physically compatible for 48 hr at room temperature. Precipitate forms upon freezing	516	C
	SKF	3 g	SKF	10 g	D5W	Haze observed at 24 hr at room temperature. Cimetidine chemically stable. Cefazolin not tested	551	I
	SKF	1.2 and 5 g	SKF	1 g	D5W, NS	Physically compatible and cimetidine chemically stable for 24 hr at room temperature. Cefazolin not tested	551	C
Clindamycin phosphate	UP	9 g	SKF	10 g	D5W[b]	Physically compatible with no clindamycin loss and 8% cefazolin loss in 48 hr at room temperature under fluorescent light	983	C
	UP	9 g	SKF	10 g	NS[b]	Physically compatible with no clindamycin loss and 3% cefazolin loss in 48 hr at room temperature under fluorescent light	983	C
Clindamycin phosphate with gentamicin sulfate	UP ES	9 g 800 mg	SKF	10 g	D5W[b]	10% cefazolin loss in 4 hr at 25 °C. Clindamycin and gentamicin potency retained for 24 hr	1328	I

Additive Compatibility (Cont.)

Cefazolin sodium

Drug	Mfr	Conc/L	Mfr	Conc/L	Test Soln	Remarks	Ref	C/I
Clindamycin phosphate with gentamicin sulfate	UP ES	9 g 800 mg	SKF	10 g	NS[b]	10% cefazolin loss after 12 hr at 25 °C. Clindamycin and gentamicin potency retained for 24 hr	1328	I
Famotidine	YAM	200 mg	FUJ	10 g	D5W	Visually compatible with 10% cefazolin loss and 5% famotidine loss by HPLC in 24 hr at 25 °C. 9% cefazolin loss and 5% famotidine loss in 48 hr at 4 °C	1762	C
Fluconazole	PF	1 g	SM	10 g	D5W	Visually compatible with no fluconazole loss by HPLC in 72 hr at 25 °C under fluorescent light. Cefazolin not tested	1677	C
Meperidine HCl		0.5 g	FUJ	10 g	D5W	Visually compatible with about 5% loss by HPLC of each drug in 5 days at 25 °C. 5% cefazolin loss and 7% meperidine loss in 20 days at 4 °C.	1966	C
Metronidazole	RP	5 g[c]	LI	10 g		Physically compatible with little or no pH change for at least 24 hr at 23 °C and 72 hr at 4 °C	807	C
	SE	5 g	LI	10 g		5% cefazolin loss and no metronidazole loss in 7 days at 25 °C. No loss of either drug in 12 days at 5 °C	993	C
	AB	5 g	LI	10 g		Visually compatible with no loss of either drug by HPLC in 72 hr at 8 °C	1649	C
Metronidazole HCl with sodium bicarbonate	SE AB	5 g 50 mEq	SKF	5 g	D5W, NS	Physically compatible for 48 hr. Gradual darkening attributed to normal cephalosporin color change with time	765	C
Ranitidine HCl	GL	100 mg		2 g	D5W	Color change within 24 hr at ambient temperature under fluorescent light	1151	?
	GL	50 mg and 2 g		1 g	D5W	Ranitidine chemically stable by HPLC for only 6 hr at 25 °C. Cefazolin not tested	1515	I
Verapamil HCl	KN	80 mg	SKF	2 g	D5W, NS	Physically compatible for 24 hr	764	C

[a]*Tested in PVC bags.*
[b]*Tested in glass bottles.*
[c]*Minibags (100 ml) containing metronidazole 500 mg with disodium phosphate 150 mg, citric acid 44 mg, and sodium chloride 740 mg. This product differs from the Searle product.*

Drugs in Syringe Compatibility

Cefazolin sodium

Drug (in syringe)	Mfr	Amt	Mfr	Amt	Remarks	Ref	C/I
Ascorbic acid injection	LI	1 ml	LI	1 g/3 ml	Precipitate forms within 3 min at 32 °C	766	I
Cimetidine HCl	SKF	300 mg/ 2 ml		1 g/5 ml	Immediate precipitation	516	I
Heparin sodium		2500 units/ 1 ml		2 g	Physically compatible for at least 5 min	1053	C
Hydromorphone HCl	KN	2, 10, 40 mg/ 1 ml	SKF	>200 mg/ 1 ml	Precipitate forms	2082	I

Drugs in Syringe Compatibility (Cont.)

Cefazolin sodium

Drug (in syringe)	Mfr	Amt	Mfr	Amt	Remarks	Ref	C/I
	KN	2, 10, 40 mg/ 1 ml	SKF	150 mg/ 1 ml	Visually compatible with less than 10% loss of either drug by HPLC in 24 hr at room temperature	2082	C
Lidocaine HCl	AST	0.5%/ 3 ml	SKF	1 g	Precipitate forms over 3 to 4 hr at 4 °C	532	I
Vitamin B complex (Betalin complex)	LI	1 ml	LI	1 g/3 ml	Physically compatible for 24 hr at 32 °C	766	C
Vitamin B complex with C (Berocca-C)	RC	1 ml	LI	1 g/3 ml	Crystals form below 32 °C but redissolve when warmed above 32 °C. Antibiotic activity retained for 24 hr at 4 and 32 °C	766	I
(Berocca-C)	RC	0.1 ml	LI	1 g/ 3.9 ml	Physically compatible and antibiotic activity retained for 24 hr at 4 and 32 °C	766	C
(Solu-B with ascorbic acid)	UP	1 ml	LI	1 g/3 ml	Precipitate forms within 1.5 hr at 32 °C	766	I

Y-Site Injection Compatibility (1:1 Mixture)

Cefazolin sodium

Drug	Mfr	Conc	Mfr	Conc	Remarks	Ref	C/I
Acyclovir sodium	BW	5 mg/ml[a]	SKF	20 mg/ml[a]	Physically compatible for 4 hr at 25 °C	1157	C
Allopurinol sodium	BW	3 mg/ml[b]	GEM	20 mg/ml[b]	Physically compatible with no change in measured turbidity or increase in particle content in 4 hr at 22 °C	1686	C
Amifostine	USB	10 mg/ml[a]	MAR	20 mg/ml[a]	Physically compatible with no change in measured turbidity or increase in particle content in 4 hr at 23 °C	1845	C
Amiodarone HCl	LZ	4 mg/ml[a]	LI	20 mg/ml[a]	Precipitate forms	1444	I
	LZ	4 mg/ml[b]	LI	20 mg/ml[b]	Physically compatible for 4 hr at room temperature	1444	C
Amphotericin B cholesteryl sulfate complex	SEQ	0.83 mg/ml[a]	SKB	20 mg/ml[a]	Increased turbidity forms immediately	2117	I
Atracurium besylate	BW	0.5 mg/ml[a]	LY	10 mg/ml[a]	Physically compatible for 24 hr at 28 °C	1337	C
Aztreonam	SQ	40 mg/ml[a]	MAR	20 mg/ml[a]	Physically compatible with no subvisual haze or particle formation in 4 hr at 23 °C	1758	C
Calcium gluconate	AST	4 mg/ml[c]	LI	40 mg/ml[c]	Physically compatible for 3 hr	1316	C
Cefpirome sulfate	HO	50 mg/ml[d]	LI	10 mg/ml[d]	Visually and microscopically compatible with 7% or less cefpirome loss and little or no cefazolin loss by HPLC in 8 hr at 23 °C	2044	C
Cisatracurium besylate	GW	0.1 mg/ml[a]	SKB	20 mg/ml[a]	Physically compatible with no change in measured turbidity or increase in particle content in 4 hr at 23 °C	2074	C
	GW	2 mg/ml[a]	SKB	20 mg/ml[a]	Gray subvisual haze forms immediately	2074	I
	GW	5 mg/ml[a]	SKB	20 mg/ml[a]	Gray haze forms immediately	2074	I
Cyclophosphamide	MJ	20 mg/ml[a]	SKF	20 mg/ml[a]	Physically compatible for 4 hr at 25 °C	1194	C
Diltiazem HCl	MMD	5 mg/ml	LI	20 and 200 mg/ml[b]	Visually compatible	1807	C
	MMD	1 mg/ml[b]	LI	200 mg/ml[b]	Visually compatible	1807	C

Y-Site Injection Compatibility (1:1 Mixture) (Cont.)

Cefazolin sodium

Drug	Mfr	Conc	Mfr	Conc	Remarks	Ref	C/I
Docetaxel	RPR	0.9 mg/ml[a]	APC	20 mg/ml[a]	Physically compatible with no change in measured turbidity or increase in particle content in 4 hr at 23 °C	2224	**C**
Doxorubicin HCl liposome injection	SEQ	0.4 mg/ml[a]	SKB	20 mg/ml[a]	Physically compatible with little or no change in measured turbidity and no increase in particle content in 4 hr at 23 °C	2087	**C**
Enalaprilat	MSD	0.05 mg/ml[b]	SKF	20 mg/ml[e]	Physically compatible for 24 hr at room temperature under fluorescent light	1355	**C**
Esmolol HCl	DCC	10 mg/ml[a]	LI	10 mg/ml[a]	Physically compatible for 24 hr at 22 °C	1169	**C**
Etoposide phosphate	BR	5 mg/ml[a]	APC	20 mg/ml[a]	Physically compatible with no change in measured turbidity or increase in particle content in 4 hr at 23 °C	2218	**C**
Famotidine	MSD	0.2 mg/ml[a]	LY	20 mg/ml[b]	Physically compatible for 14 hr	1196	**C**
	ME	2 mg/ml[b]		20 mg/ml[a]	Visually compatible for 4 hr at 22 °C	1936	**C**
Filgrastim	AMG	30 μg/ml[a]	LI	20 mg/ml[a]	Physically compatible with no change in measured turbidity or increase in particle content in 4 hr at 22 °C	1687	**C**
Fluconazole	RR	2 mg/ml	LY	40 mg/ml	Physically compatible for 24 hr at 25 °C	1407	**C**
Fludarabine phosphate	BX	1 mg/ml[a]	LEM	20 mg/ml[a]	Physically compatible for 4 hr at room temperature under fluorescent light	1439	**C**
Foscarnet sodium	AST	24 mg/ml	SKF	40 mg/ml	Physically compatible for 24 hr at room temperature under fluorescent light	1335	**C**
Gemcitabine HCl	LI	10 mg/ml[b]	APC	20 mg/ml[b]	Physically compatible with no change in measured turbidity or increase in particle content in 4 hr at 23 °C	2226	**C**
Granisetron HCl	SKB	0.05 mg/ml[a]	SKB	20 mg/ml[a]	Physically compatible with no change in measured turbidity or increase in particle content in 4 hr at 23 °C	2000	**C**
Heparin sodium	TR	50 units/ml	SKB	20 mg/ml[a]	Visually compatible for 6 hr at 25 °C	1793	**C**
Hetastarch	DCC	6%	SKF	20 mg/ml[a]	Physically compatible for 4 hr at room temperature by visual examination	1313	**C**
	DCC	6%	SKF	20 mg/ml[a]	Simulation in vials showed no incompatibility, but white precipitate formed in Y-site during infusion	1315	**I**
Hydromorphone HCl	WY	0.2 mg/ml[a]	SKF	20 mg/ml[a]	Physically compatible for at least 4 hr at 25 °C under fluorescent light	987	**C**
	KN	2, 10, 40 mg/ml	SKF	20[a] and 150 mg/ml	Visually compatible and potency of both drugs by HPLC retained for 24 hr	1532	**C**
	KN	2, 10, 40 mg/ml	SKF	>200 mg/ml	Precipitate forms immediately	1532	**I**
Idarubicin HCl	AD	1 mg/ml[b]	LI	20 mg/ml[a]	Precipitate forms in 1 hr	1525	**I**
Insulin, regular	LI	0.2 unit/ml[b]	LI	20 mg/ml[a]	Physically compatible for 2 hr at 25 °C	1395	**C**
Labetalol HCl	SC	1 mg/ml[a]	LI	10 mg/ml[a]	Physically compatible for 24 hr at 18 °C	1171	**C**
Lidocaine HCl	AB	8 mg/ml[c]	LI	40 mg/ml[c]	Physically compatible for 3 hr	1316	**C**

Y-Site Injection Compatibility (1:1 Mixture) (Cont.)

			Cefazolin sodium				
Drug	Mfr	Conc	Mfr	Conc	Remarks	Ref	C/I
Magnesium sulfate	IX	16.7, 33.3, 66.7, 100 mg/ml[a]	LI	20 mg/ml[a]	Physically compatible for at least 4 hr at 32 °C	813	C
Melphalan HCl	BW	0.1 mg/ml[b]	GEM	20 mg/ml[b]	Physically compatible with no change in measured turbidity or increase in particle content in 3 hr at 22 °C	1557	C
Meperidine HCl	WY	10 mg/ml[a]	SKF	20 mg/ml[a]	Physically compatible for at least 4 hr at 25 °C under fluorescent light	987	C
Midazolam HCl	RC	1 mg/ml[a]	MAR	20 mg/ml[a]	Visually compatible for 24 hr at 23 °C	1847	C
Morphine sulfate	WI	1 mg/ml[a]	SKF	20 mg/ml[a]	Physically compatible for at least 4 hr at 25 °C under fluorescent light	987	C
Multivitamins	USV	5 ml/L[a]	SKF	1 g/50 ml[a]	Physically compatible for 24 hr at room temperature	323	C
Ondansetron HCl	GL	1 mg/ml[b]	LEM	20 mg/ml[a]	Physically compatible for 4 hr at 22 °C	1365	C
	GL	0.03 and 0.3 mg/ml[a]	LI	20 mg/ml[a]	Visually compatible with little or no loss of either drug by HPLC in 4 hr at 25 °C	1732	C
Pancuronium bromide	ES	0.05 mg/ml[a]	LY	10 mg/ml[a]	Physically compatible for 24 hr at 28 °C	1337	C
Pentamidine isethionate	FUJ	3 mg/ml[a]	SKB	20 mg/ml[a]	Cloudiness and gelatin-like precipitate form immediately	1880	I
Perphenazine	SC	0.02 mg/ml[a]	SKF	20 mg/ml[e]	Physically compatible for 4 hr at 25 °C	1155	C
Promethazine HCl	ES	25 mg	LI	10 mg/ml[a]	Fine cloudy precipitate forms immediately and dissolves in seconds	1753	?
Propofol	ZEN	10 mg/ml	MAR	20 mg/ml[a]	Physically compatible for 1 hr at 23 °C with no increase in particle content	2066	C
Remifentanil HCl	GW	0.025 and 0.25 mg/ml[b]	SKB	20 mg/ml[a]	Physically compatible with no change in measured turbidity or increase in particle content in 4 hr at 23 °C	2075	C
Sargramostim	IMM	10 µg/ml[b]	LEM	20 mg/ml[b]	Physically compatible for 4 hr at 22 °C	1436	C
Tacrolimus	FUJ	1 mg/ml[b]	BR	40 mg/ml[a]	Visually compatible for 24 hr at 25 °C	1630	C
Teniposide	BR	0.1 mg/ml[a]	MAR	20 mg/ml[a]	Physically compatible with no subvisual haze or particle formation in 4 hr at 23 °C	1725	C
Theophylline	TR	4 mg/ml	SKB	20 mg/ml	Visually compatible for 6 hr at 25 °C	1793	C
Thiotepa	IMM[f]	1 mg/ml[a]	MAR	20 mg/ml[a]	Physically compatible with no change in measured turbidity or increase in particle content in 4 hr at 23 °C	1861	C
TNA #73[g]		32.5 ml[h]	SKF	1 g/50 ml[a]	Physically compatible for 4 hr at 25 °C by visual observation	1008	C
TNA #218 to #226[g]			SKB	20 mg/ml[a]	Visually compatible with no precipitate or emulsion damage apparent in 4 hr at 23 °C	2215	C
TPN #61[g]		[i]	SKF	200 mg/ 0.9 ml[j]	Physically compatible	1012	C
		[k]	SKF	1.2 g/5.3 ml[j]	Physically compatible	1012	C

Y-Site Injection Compatibility (1:1 Mixture) (Cont.)

Drug	Mfr	Conc	Mfr	Conc	Remarks	Ref	C/I
				Cefazolin sodium			
TPN #212 and #213[g]			SKB	20 mg/ml[a]	Physically compatible with no change in measured turbidity or increase in particle content in 4 hr at 23 °C	2109	C
TPN #214 and #215[g]			SKB	20 mg/ml[a]	Small amount of subvisual precipitate forms immediately	2109	I
Vancomycin HCl	AB	20 mg/ml[a]	SKB	200 mg/ml[l]	Transient precipitate forms followed by clear solution	2189	?
	AB	20 mg/ml[a]	SKB	10 and 50 mg/ml[a]	Gross white precipitate forms immediately	2189	I
	AB	20 mg/ml[a]	SKB	1 mg/ml[a]	Physically compatible with no change in measured turbidity or increase in particle content in 4 hr at 23 °C	2189	C
	AB	2 mg/ml[a]	SKB	200 mg/ml[l]	Physically compatible with no change in measured turbidity or increase in particle content in 4 hr at 23 °C	2189	C
	AB	2 mg/ml[a]	SKB	50 mg/ml[a]	Subvisual measured haze forms immediately	2189	I
	AB	2 mg/ml[a]	SKB	1 and 10 mg/ml[a]	Physically compatible with no change in measured turbidity or increase in particle content in 4 hr at 23 °C	2189	C
Vecuronium bromide	OR	0.1 mg/ml[a]	LY	10 mg/ml[a]	Physically compatible for 24 hr at 28 °C	1337	C
Vinorelbine tartrate	BW	1 mg/ml[b]	GEM	20 mg/ml[b]	Large increase in measured turbidity occurs immediately and grows over 4 hr at 22 °C	1558	I
Vitamin B complex with C (Berocca-C 500)	RC	4 ml/L[a]	SKF	1 g/50 ml[a]	Physically compatible for at least 4 hr at 25 °C under fluorescent light	323	C
(Berocca-C)	RC	20 ml/L[a]	SKF	1 g/50 ml[a]	Physically compatible for at least 4 hr at 25 °C under fluorescent light	323	C
Warfarin sodium	DU	2 mg/ml[l]	SKB	20 mg/ml[a]	Visually compatible with no warfarin loss by HPLC in 30 min	2010	C
	DME	2 mg/ml[l]	SKB	20 mg/ml[a]	Visually compatible for 24 hr at 24 °C	2078	C

[a]*Tested in dextrose 5% in water.*
[b]*Tested in sodium chloride 0.9%.*
[c]*Tested in both dextrose 5% in water and sodium chloride 0.9%.*
[d]*Tested in dextrose 5% in water, Ringer's injection, lactated, sodium chloride 0.45%, and sodium chloride 0.9%.*
[e]*Manufacturer's premixed solution.*
[f]*Lyophilized formulation tested.*
[g]*Refer to Appendix I for the composition of parenteral nutrition solutions. TNA indicates a 3-in-1 admixture, and TPN indicates a 2-in-1 admixture.*
[h]*A 32.5-ml sample of parenteral nutrition solution combined with 50 ml of antibiotic solution.*
[i]*Run at 21 ml/hr.*
[j]*Given over five minutes by syringe pump.*
[k]*Run at 94 ml/hr.*
[l]*Tested in sterile water for injection.*

Additional Compatibility Information

Solutions— The manufacturer indicates that reconstituted cefazolin sodium may be diluted in or administered into lines running the following infusion solutions (2):

Dextrose 5% in Ringer's injection, lactated
Dextrose 5% in sodium chloride 0.2%
Dextrose 5% in sodium chloride 0.45%
Dextrose 5% in sodium chloride 0.9%
Dextrose 5% in water
Dextrose 10% in water
Invert sugar 5% in water
Invert sugar 10% in water
Ionosol B with dextrose 5%
Normosol M in dextrose 5% in water
Plasma-Lyte with dextrose 5%
Ringer's injection
Ringer's injection, lactated
Sodium chloride 0.9%

Miscellaneous Additives— Cefazolin sodium is stated to be incompatible with the following drugs (278):

Amobarbital sodium
Calcium gluconate
Colistimethate sodium
Kanamycin sulfate
Pentobarbital sodium
Polymyxin B sulfate

To determine if spurious aminoglycoside levels could result from a delay in assaying blood samples, Tindula et al. evaluated the inactivation of amikacin 36 μg/ml and gentamicin and tobramycin 10 μg/ml in human serum by 400-μg/ml concentrations of several penicillins and cephalosporins. Samples were stored for 24 hours at room temperature and frozen at −20 °C. For samples at both temperatures, cefazolin caused relatively little inactivation of the aminoglycosides (824).

Spruill et al. evaluated the effect of various cephalosporins on tobramycin sulfate 7.7 μg/ml in human serum. At concentrations of 250 and 100 μg/ml, cefazolin, cefoxitin, cefamandole, cefoperazone, and cefotaxime caused about a 10 to 15% loss of tobramycin over 48 hours at 0 and 21 °C. Moxalactam caused about a 15% loss at 0 °C and a 20 to 30% loss at 21 °C over 48 hours (1005).

The inactivation of gentamicin, tobramycin, and amikacin, each 5 μg/ml, by seven β-lactam antibiotics, 250 and 500 μg/ml, in serum at 25 °C over 24 hours was studied using bioassay, enzyme-mediated immunoassay technique (EMIT), fluorescence polarization immunoassay (TDx), and radioimmunoassay. No inactivation of any aminoglycoside by the cephalosporins moxalactam, cefotaxime, and cefazolin occurred within the study period (654).

Cefazolin sodium (Lilly) 125 μg/ml combined separately with the aminoglycosides amikacin sulfate (Bristol), gentamicin sulfate (Schering), and tobramycin sulfate (Lilly) at a concentration of 25 μg/ml in peritoneal dialysis solution (Dianeal 1.5%) exhibited enhanced rates of lethality to *Staphylococcus aureus*, *Escherichia coli*, and *Pseudomonas aeruginosa* compared to any of the drugs alone (1623).

Vancomycin— The compatibility or incompatibility of vancomycin HCl mixed with or administered simultaneously with cefazolin sodium is concentration dependent (2189). See Y-Site Compatibility above. Vancomycin HCl has a low pH and is variably compatible with drugs having neutral to mildly alkaline pH, including cephalosporins and penicillins. The compatibility may depend on a number of factors, including concentration of each drug, dilution vehicle, actual pH of solutions, and completeness of mixing during administration. Combinations that are compatible when well mixed may result in precipitation if only partially mixed, presumably because of regionally different concentrations and pH values. If attempting to administer vancomycin HCl with cefazolin sodium, take care to ensure that the specific combination and the concentrations are compatible under the exact administration conditions to be used. An inline filter should be used as a final safety measure (2189).

Peritoneal Dialysis Solutions— Cefazolin sodium 2 mg/ml in peritoneal dialysis solution (McGaw) containing dextrose 2.5% and electrolytes was physically compatible for three hours at room temperature. Furthermore, no significant loss of antibacterial activity was apparent by microbiological determination (142).

The stability of cefazolin sodium 75 and 150 mg/L, alone and with gentamicin sulfate 8 mg/L, was evaluated in a peritoneal dialysis solution of dextrose 1.5% with heparin sodium 1000 units/L. Cefazolin activity was retained for 48 hours at both 4 and 26 °C at both concentrations, alone and with gentamicin. Gentamicin activity was also retained over the study period. At 37 °C, however, cefazolin losses were greater, with about a 10 to 12% loss occurring in 48 hours. Gentamicin losses ranged from 4 to 8% in this time period (1029).

Halstead et al. evaluated gentamicin 4 μg/ml in Dianeal PDS with dextrose 1.5 and 4.25% (Travenol) with cefazolin sodium 125 μg/ml, heparin 500 units, and albumin 80 mg in 2-L bags. The gentamicin content, determined by EMIT assay, was retained for 72 hours (1413).

Nahata and Ahalt studied the stability of cefazolin sodium (Lilly) 0.5 mg/ml in Dianeal PD-1 with dextrose 1.5 and 4.25% (Travenol). The drug was stable, exhibiting losses of 10.5% or less in 14 days at 4 °C, eight days at 25 °C, and 24 hours at 37 °C. However, losses of 11.7 and 14.6% occurred in the solutions containing dextrose 1.5% and dextrose 4.25%, respectively, in 11 days at 25 °C (1480).

Other Information

A study was conducted to compare Kefzol with Ancef with regard to dissolution rate, color, clarity, and particulate matter content. The only significant difference noted was a faster dissolution rate for Kefzol (373).

In contrast, a study by Janousek and Minisci reported more extensive differences. They too noted a difference in dissolution rate. Interestingly, they reported Ancef to dissolve more rapidly. Further, differences in color, clarity, and rate at which the drugs passed through a 0.45-μm filter were also noted. The authors concluded that while Kefzol took longer to dissolve, it did so more completely as reflected in less color, lower optical density (clarity), and a much greater rate of flow through a 0.45-μm filter, indicative of less particulate matter (628).

CEFEPIME HCL
AHFS 8:12.06

Maxipime   **Bristol-Myers Squibb**

Products— Cefepime HCl (Bristol-Myers Squibb) is available as 500 mg, 1 g, and 2 g of cefepime in vials and 1 and 2 g of cefepime in piggyback bottles. The products contain L-arginine in an approximate concentration of 725 mg/g of cefepime (2).

For intramuscular administration, reconstitute the vials with sterile water for injection, sodium chloride 0.9%, dextrose 5% in water, lidocaine HCl 0.5 or 1%, or bacteriostatic water for injection preserved with parabens or benzyl alcohol with the volumes indicated in Table 1 (2).

Table 1. Recommended Reconstitution of Cefepime HCl (2)

Container Size	Volume of Diluent (ml)	Approximate Solution Volume (ml)	Approximate Concentration (mg/ml)
Intramuscular			
500-mg vial	1.3	1.8	280
1-g vial	2.4	3.6	280
Intravenous			
500-mg vial	5	5.6	100
1-g vial	10	11.3	100
1-g piggyback	50 to 100	50 to 100	20 to 10
2-g vial	10	12.5	160
2-g piggyback	50 to 100	50 to 100	40 to 20

For intravenous injection, reconstitute the containers with compatible diluent in the volumes indicated in Table 1. The reconstituted solutions should be added to compatible intravenous solutions for intermittent infusion (2).

pH— From 4 to 6 (2).

Administration— Cefepime HCl is administered by deep intramuscular injection and by intermittent intravenous infusion over approximately 30 minutes (2; 4).

Stability— The intact vials should be stored between 2 and 25 °C and protected from light. Reconstituted solutions may vary from colorless to amber. Both the powder and reconstituted solutions may darken during storage like other cephalosporins. When stored as recommended, potency is not adversely affected. Reconstituted solutions of cefepime HCl in compatible diluents are stable for 24 hours at room temperatures of 20 to 25 °C and for seven days under refrigeration (2).

Cefepime HCl (Bristol-Myers Squibb) 280 mg/ml reconstituted in the following diluents is physically compatible and chemically stable by HPLC analysis for 24 hours at room temperature exposed to light and for seven days at 5 °C (1680):

    Bacteriostatic water for injection (parabens or benzyl alcohol)
    Dextrose 5% in water
    Lidocaine HCl 0.5 and 1%
    Sodium chloride 0.9%
    Sterile water for injection

At concentrations of 100 and 160 mg/ml in dextrose 5% in water, sodium chloride 0.9%, and sterile water for injection, cefepime HCl is also physically compatible and chemically stable for 24 hours at room temperature and for seven days at 5 °C (1681).

Freezing Solutions— Cefepime HCl (Bristol-Myers Squibb) 100 and 200 mg/ml in dextrose 5% in water, sodium chloride 0.9%, and sterile water for injection was packaged as 10 ml of solution in 10-ml polypropylene syringes and capped (Becton-Dickinson). The samples were stored frozen at –20 °C for 90 days. Cefepime HCl samples at both concentrations in all three diluents remained clear and had no apparent color change. HPLC analysis found little or no cefepime loss in any of the samples (2220).

Cefepime HCl (Bristol-Myers Squibb) 100 and 200 mg/ml in dextrose 5% in water, sodium chloride 0.9%, and sterile water for injection was packaged as 10 ml of solution in 10-ml polypropylene syringes and capped (Becton-Dickinson). After frozen storage for up to 90 days, the samples were thawed and stored at 4 °C for seven days. The solutions remained visually clear but exhibited a gradual darkening of color. HPLC analysis found cefepime losses of 7% or less (2220).

Samples that had been frozen for 90 days and refrigerated for three to seven days were stored for an additional one or two days at room temperature (about 23 °C). Room temperature storage for one day in the thawed samples stored under refrigeration for three or five days exhibited cefepime losses of 10% or less; cefepime losses had increased up to 11 to 19% after two days at room temperature. However, thawed samples stored under refrigeration for seven days exhibited up to 12 to 15% loss after one day at room temperature (2220).

Syringes— Cefepime HCl (Bristol-Myers Squibb) 100 and 200 mg/ml in dextrose 5% in water, sodium chloride 0.9%, and sterile water for injection packaged as 10 ml of solution in 10-ml polypropylene syringes and capped (Becton-Dickinson) was also tested without having been frozen. The solutions remained stable by HPLC analysis for up to 14 days refrigerated at 4 °C, losing 10% or less of the cefepime. In samples stored at room temperature of about 23 °C, less than 10% loss occurred in one day in most cases, but losses as high as 13% occurred in two days in some (but not all) samples that were evaluated (2220; 2221). Samples refrigerated up to five days followed by room temperature storage exhibited similar stability, exhibiting less than 10% loss in one day but higher losses after two days (2220).

Compatibility Information

Solution Compatibility

Cefepime HCl

Solution	Mfr	Mfr	Conc/L	Remarks	Ref	C/I
Amino acids 4.25%, dextrose 25% with electrolytes	AB	BR	1 and 4 g	5 to 6% cefepime loss by HPLC in 8 hr at room temperature and 3 days at 5 °C	1682	C
Dextrose 5% in Ringer's injection, lactated	a	BR	1 g	Visually compatible with 2 to 4% cefepime loss by HPLC in 24 hr at room temperature exposed to light and about 2% loss in 7 days at 5 °C	1680	C
	a	BR	40 g	Visually compatible with 6% cefepime loss by HPLC in 24 hr at room temperature exposed to light and about 1% loss in 7 days at 5 °C	1680	C

Solution Compatibility (Cont.)

Cefepime HCl

Solution	Mfr	Mfr	Conc/L	Remarks	Ref	C/I
Dextrose 5% in sodium chloride 0.9%	a	BR	1 g	Visually compatible with 3 to 4% cefepime loss by HPLC in 24 hr at room temperature exposed to light and 1% loss in 7 days at 5 °C	1680	C
	a	BR	40 g	Visually compatible with 5% cefepime loss by HPLC in 24 hr at room temperature exposed to light and 3% loss in 7 days at 5 °C	1680	C
Dextrose 5% in water	b	BR	1 g	Visually compatible with 2 to 4% cefepime loss by HPLC in 24 hr at room temperature exposed to light and 1 to 2% loss in 7 days at 5 °C	1680	C
	b	BR	40 g	Visually compatible with 4 to 7% cefepime loss by HPLC in 24 hr at room temperature exposed to light and about 2% loss in 7 days at 5 °C	1680	C
	BA[a]	BMS	20 g	6% loss by HPLC in 2 days at 25 °C and in 23 days at 5 °C. Slight increase in yellow color observed	2102	C
	BFM[c]	BMS	8 g	8 to 9% loss by HPLC in 48 hr at 24 °C and in 15 days at 4 °C. Amber discoloration observed	2150	C
Dextrose 10% in water	a	BR	1 g	Visually compatible with 3 to 5% cefepime loss by HPLC in 24 hr at room temperature exposed to light and 1% loss in 7 days at 5 °C	1680	C
	a	BR	40 g	Visually compatible with 4 to 5% cefepime loss by HPLC in 24 hr at room temperature exposed to light and 3% loss in 7 days at 5 °C	1680	C
Normosol M in dextrose 5%	AB[a]	BR	1 g	Visually compatible with 2 to 3% cefepime loss by HPLC in 24 hr at room temperature exposed to light and 2% loss in 7 days at 5 °C	1680	C
	AB[a]	BR	40 g	Visually compatible with 5% cefepime loss by HPLC in 24 hr at room temperature exposed to light and 2% loss in 7 days at 5 °C	1680	C
Normosol R	AB[a]	BR	1 g	Visually compatible with 2% cefepime loss by HPLC in 24 hr at room temperature exposed to light and 1% loss in 7 days at 5 °C	1680	C
	AB[a]	BR	40 g	Visually compatible with 5% cefepime loss by HPLC in 24 hr at room temperature exposed to light and 2% loss in 7 days at 5 °C	1680	C
Normosol R in dextrose 5%	AB[a]	BR	1 g	Visually compatible with 2% cefepime loss by HPLC in 24 hr at room temperature exposed to light	1680	C
Sodium chloride 0.9%	b	BR	1 g	Visually compatible with 2 to 5% cefepime loss by HPLC in 24 hr at room temperature exposed to light and about 1% loss in 7 days at 5 °C	1680	C
	a	BR	40 g	Visually compatible with 4 to 5% cefepime loss by HPLC in 24 hr at room temperature exposed to light and 2 to 3% loss in 7 days at 5 °C	1680	C
	BA[a]	BMS	20 g	6% loss by HPLC in 2 days at 25 °C and in 23 days at 5 °C. Slight increase in yellow color observed	2102	C

Solution Compatibility (Cont.)

	Mfr	Mfr	Conc/L	Remarks	Ref	C/I
Solution				**Cefepime HCl**		
	BFM[c]	BMS	8 g	8% loss by HPLC in 72 hr at 24 °C and in 15 days at 4 °C. Amber discoloration observed	2150	C

[a]Tested in PVC containers.
[b]Tested in both glass and PVC containers.
[c]Tested in polyethylene-lined trilayer (Clear-Flex) containers.

Additive Compatibility

Cefepime HCl

Drug	Mfr	Conc/L	Mfr	Conc/L	Test Soln	Remarks	Ref	C/I
Amikacin sulfate	BR	6 g	BR	4 g	D5W, NS	Visually compatible with 6% cefepime loss by HPLC in 24 hr at room temperature and 4% loss in 7 days at 5 °C. No amikacin loss by bioassay	1681	C
Aminophylline	LY	1 g	BR	4 g	NS	37% cefepime loss by HPLC in 18 hr at room temperature and 32% loss in 3 days at 5 °C. No aminophylline loss	1681	I
Ampicillin sodium	BR	1 g	BR	40 g	D5W	4% ampicillin loss by HPLC in 8 hr at room temperature and 5 °C. 7% cefepime loss by HPLC in 8 hr at room temperature and no loss in 8 hr at 5 °C	1682	?
	BR	1 g	BR	40 g	NS	No ampicillin loss by HPLC in 24 hr at room temperature and 9% loss in 48 hr at 5 °C. 5% cefepime loss by HPLC in 24 hr at room temperature and 2% loss in 72 hr at 5 °C	1682	C
	BR	10 g	BR	40 g	D5W	6% ampicillin loss by HPLC in 2 hr at room temperature and 2% loss in 8 hr at 5 °C. 7% cefepime loss by HPLC in 2 hr at room temperature and 8 hr at 5 °C	1682	I
	BR	10 g	BR	40 g	NS	6% ampicillin loss by HPLC in 8 hr at room temperature and 9% loss in 48 hr at 5 °C. 8% cefepime loss by HPLC in 8 hr at room temperature and 10% loss in 48 hr at 5 °C	1682	I
	BR	40 g	BR	4 g	D5W	10% ampicillin loss by HPLC in 1 hr at room temperature and 9% loss in 2 hr at 5 °C. 25% cefepime loss by HPLC in 1 hr at room temperature and 9% loss in 2 hr at 5 °C	1682	I
	BR	40 g	BR	4 g	NS	5% ampicillin loss by HPLC in 8 hr at room temperature and 4% loss in 8 hr at 5 °C. 4% cefepime loss by HPLC in 8 hr at room temperature and 6% loss in 8 hr at 5 °C	1682	?
Clindamycin phosphate	UP	0.25 g	BR	40 g	D5W, NS	7% or less cefepime loss by HPLC in 24 hr at room temperature and 10% or less loss in 7 days at 5 °C. No clindamycin loss by HPLC in 24 hr at room temperature and 8% or less loss in 7 days at 5 °C	1682	C

Additive Compatibility (Cont.)

Cefepime HCl

Drug	Mfr	Conc/L	Mfr	Conc/L	Test Soln	Remarks	Ref	C/I
	UP	6 g	BR	4 g	D5W, NS	7% or less cefepime loss by HPLC in 24 hr at room temperature and 10% or less loss in 7 days at 5 °C. No clindamycin loss by HPLC in 24 hr at room temperature and 8% or less loss in 7 days at 5 °C	1682	C
Gentamicin sulfate	ES	1.2 g	BR	4 g	D5W, NS	Cloudiness forms in 18 hr at room temperature	1681	I
Heparin sodium	MG	10,000 and 50,000 units	BR	4 g	D5W, NS	Visually compatible with 4% cefepime loss by HPLC in 24 hr at room temperature and 3% in 7 days at 5 °C. Little or no heparin loss	1681	C
Metronidazole	AB, ES, SE	5 g	BR	40 g		7% cefepime loss by HPLC in 24 hr at room temperature exposed to light and 8% loss in 5 days at 5 °C. Little or no metronidazole loss by HPLC. However, orange color develops in 18 hr at room temperature and 24 hr at 5 °C	1682	?
	AB, ES, SE	5 g	BR	4 g		6% cefepime loss by HPLC in 24 hr at room temperature exposed to light and 3% loss in 5 days at 5 °C. Little or no metronidazole loss by HPLC. However, orange color develops in 18 hr at room temperature and 24 hr at 5 °C.	1682	?
Metronidazole HCl	SE	5 g[a]	BR	40 g	D5W, NS	7% cefepime loss by HPLC in 24 hr at room temperature exposed to light and 8% loss in 5 days at 5 °C. Little or no metronidazole loss by HPLC. However, orange color develops in 18 hr at room temperature and 24 hr at 5 °C	1682	?
	SE	8 g[a]	BR	4 g	D5W, NS	6% cefepime loss by HPLC in 24 hr at room temperature exposed to light and 3% loss in 5 days at 5 °C. Little or no metronidazole loss by HPLC. However, orange color develops in 18 hr at room temperature and 24 hr at 5 °C. A precipitate forms in 48 hr at 5 °C	1682	?
Netilmicin sulfate	SC	1 g	BR	40 g	D5W, NS	Cloudiness forms immediately	1682	I
	SC	5 g	BR	2.5 g	D5W, NS	Cloudiness forms immediately	1682	I
Potassium chloride	AB	40 mEq	BR	4 g	D5W, NS	Visually compatible with 2% cefepime loss by HPLC in 24 hr at room temperature and 7 days at 5 °C	1682	C
	AB	10 mEq	BR	4 g	D5W	Visually compatible with 2% cefepime loss by HPLC in 24 hr at room temperature and 7 days at 5 °C	1682	C
Theophylline	BA	800 mg	BR	4 g	D5W	Visually compatible with 3% cefepime loss by HPLC in 24 hr at room temperature and in 7 days at 5 °C. No theophylline loss	1681	C
Tobramycin sulfate	AB	0.4 g	BR	40 g	D5W, NS	Cloudiness forms immediately	1682	I

Additive Compatibility (Cont.)

Drug	Mfr	Conc/L	Mfr	Conc/L	Test Soln	Remarks	Ref	C/I
	AB	2 g	BR	2.5 g	D5W, NS, W	Cloudiness forms immediately	1682	**I**
Vancomycin HCl	LI	5 g	BR	4 g	D5W, NS	4% cefepime loss by HPLC in 24 hr at room temperature exposed to light and 2% loss in 7 days at 5 °C. No vancomycin loss by HPLC, but cloudiness develops in 5 days at 5 °C	1682	**C**
	LI	1 g	BR	40 g	D5W, NS	4% cefepime loss by HPLC in 24 hr at room temperature exposed to light and 2% loss in 7 days at 5 °C. No vancomycin loss by HPLC and no cloudiness	1682	**C**

[a]Neutralized with sodium bicarbonate.

Y-Site Injection Compatibility (1:1 Mixture)

Cefepime HCl

Drug	Mfr	Conc	Mfr	Conc	Remarks	Ref	C/I
Acyclovir sodium	BW	7 mg/ml[a]	BR	20 mg/ml[a]	Tiny crystals form in 4 hr	1689	**I**
Amphotericin B	SQ	0.6 mg/ml[a]	BR	20 mg/ml[a]	Heavy yellow flocculent precipitate forms immediately	1689	**I**
Amphotericin B cholesteryl sulfate complex	SEQ	0.83 mg/ml[a]	BMS	20 mg/ml[a]	Gross precipitate forms	2117	**I**
Ampicillin sodium–sulbactam sodium	RR	20 + 10 mg/ml[a]	BR	20 mg/ml[a]	Physically compatible with no change in measured turbidity or increase in particle content in 4 hr at 22 °C	1689	**C**
Aztreonam	SQ	40 mg/ml[a]	BR	20 mg/ml[a]	Physically compatible with no change in measured turbidity or increase in particle content in 4 hr at 22 °C	1689	**C**
Bleomycin sulfate	BR	1 unit/ml[b]	BR	20 mg/ml[a]	Physically compatible with no change in measured turbidity or increase in particle content in 4 hr at 22 °C	1689	**C**
Bumetanide	RC	0.04 mg/ml[a]	BR	20 mg/ml[a]	Physically compatible with no change in measured turbidity or increase in particle content in 4 hr at 22 °C	1689	**C**
Buprenorphine HCl	RKC	0.04 mg/ml[a]	BR	20 mg/ml[a]	Physically compatible with no change in measured turbidity or increase in particle content in 4 hr at 22 °C	1689	**C**
Butorphanol tartrate	BR	0.04 mg/ml[a]	BR	20 mg/ml[a]	Physically compatible with no change in measured turbidity or increase in particle content in 4 hr at 22 °C	1689	**C**
Calcium gluconate	AMR	40 mg/ml[a]	BR	20 mg/ml[a]	Physically compatible with no change in measured turbidity or increase in particle content in 4 hr at 22 °C	1689	**C**
Carboplatin	BR	5 mg/ml[a]	BR	20 mg/ml[a]	Physically compatible with no change in measured turbidity or increase in particle content in 4 hr at 22 °C	1689	**C**

Y-Site Injection Compatibility (1:1 Mixture) (Cont.)

Cefepime HCl

Drug	Mfr	Conc	Mfr	Conc	Remarks	Ref	C/I
Carmustine	BR	1.5 mg/ml[a]	BR	20 mg/ml[a]	Physically compatible with no change in measured turbidity or increase in particle content in 4 hr at 22 °C	1689	C
Chlordiazepoxide HCl	RC	20 mg/ml	BR	20 mg/ml[a]	Haze forms immediately. Flocculent precipitate forms in 4 hr	1689	I
Chlorpromazine HCl	SCN	2 mg/ml[a]	BR	20 mg/ml[a]	Cloudiness forms immediately. Flocculent precipitate forms in 4 hr	1689	I
Cimetidine HCl	SKB	12 mg/ml[a]	BR	20 mg/ml[a]	Cloudiness forms immediately	1689	I
Ciprofloxacin	MI	1 mg/ml[a]	BR	20 mg/ml[a]	Cloudiness forms immediately. Flocculent precipitate forms in 4 hr	1689	I
Cisplatin	BR	1 mg/ml	BR	20 mg/ml[a]	Haze forms in 1 hr. Cloudiness and particulates form in 4 hr	1689	I
Cyclophosphamide	MJ	10 mg/ml[a]	BR	20 mg/ml[a]	Physically compatible with no change in measured turbidity or increase in particle content in 4 hr at 22 °C	1689	C
Cytarabine	CET	50 mg/ml	BR	20 mg/ml[a]	Physically compatible with no change in measured turbidity or increase in particle content in 4 hr at 22 °C	1689	C
Dacarbazine	MI	4 mg/ml[a]	BR	20 mg/ml[a]	Cloudiness forms immediately. Flocculent precipitate forms in 4 hr	1689	I
Dactinomycin	MSD	0.01 mg/ml[a]	BR	20 mg/ml[a]	Physically compatible with no change in measured turbidity or increase in particle content in 4 hr at 22 °C	1689	C
Daunorubicin HCl	WY	1 mg/ml[a]	BR	20 mg/ml[a]	Haze forms immediately. Flocculent precipitate forms in 4 hr	1689	I
Dexamethasone sodium phosphate	AMR	1 mg/ml[a]	BR	20 mg/ml[a]	Physically compatible with no change in measured turbidity or increase in particle content in 4 hr at 22 °C	1689	C
Diazepam	ES	5 mg/ml[a]	BR	20 mg/ml[a]	Cloudiness forms immediately	1689	I
Diphenhydramine HCl	WY	2 mg/ml[a]	BR	20 mg/ml[a]	Cloudy solution with precipitate forms immediately	1689	I
Dobutamine HCl	LI	4 mg/ml[a]	BR	20 mg/ml[a]	Cloudiness forms immediately. Precipitate forms in 4 hr	1689	I
Docetaxel	RPR	0.9 mg/ml[a]	BMS	20 mg/ml[a]	Physically compatible with no change in measured turbidity or increase in particle content in 4 hr at 23 °C	2224	C
Dopamine HCl	AST	3.2 mg/ml[a]	BR	20 mg/ml[a]	Haze and precipitate form in 1 hr	1689	I
Doxorubicin HCl	CET	2 mg/ml[a]	BR	20 mg/ml[a]	Haze forms immediately. Flocculent precipitate forms in 4 hr	1689	I
Doxorubicin HCl liposome injection	SEQ	0.4 mg/ml[a]	BMS	20 mg/ml[a]	Physically compatible with little or no change in measured turbidity and no increase in particle content in 4 hr at 23 °C	2087	C
Droperidol	JN	0.4 mg/ml[a]	BR	20 mg/ml[a]	Haze forms immediately. Flocculent precipitate forms in 4 hr	1689	I
Enalaprilat	MSD	0.1 mg/ml[a]	BR	20 mg/ml[a]	Tiny particles form in 4 hr	1689	I

Y-Site Injection Compatibility (1:1 Mixture) (Cont.)

		Cefepime HCl					
Drug	*Mfr*	*Conc*	*Mfr*	*Conc*	*Remarks*	*Ref*	*C/I*
Etoposide	BR	0.4 mg/ml[a]	BR	20 mg/ml[a]	Haze increases and tiny particles form in 1 hr	1689	I
Etoposide phosphate	BR	5 mg/ml[a]	BMS	20 mg/ml[a]	Increased haze and particulates form within 1 hr	2218	I
Famotidine	ME	2 mg/ml[a]	BR	20 mg/ml[a]	Haze forms immediately. Flocculent precipitate forms in 4 hr	1689	I
Filgrastim	AMG	30 μg/ml[a]	BR	20 mg/ml[a]	Hazy turbid solution forms immediately	1689	I
Floxuridine	RC	3 mg/ml[a]	BR	20 mg/ml[a]	Haze and tiny particles form immediately	1689	I
Fluconazole	RR	2 mg/ml	BR	20 mg/ml[a]	Physically compatible with no change in measured turbidity or increase in particle content in 4 hr at 22 °C	1689	C
Fludarabine phosphate	BX	1 mg/ml[a]	BR	20 mg/ml[a]	Physically compatible with no change in measured turbidity or increase in particle content in 4 hr at 22 °C	1689	C
Fluorouracil	AD	16 mg/ml[a]	BR	20 mg/ml[a]	Physically compatible with no change in measured turbidity or increase in particle content in 4 hr at 22 °C	1689	C
Furosemide	AB	3 mg/ml[a]	BR	20 mg/ml[a]	Physically compatible with no change in measured turbidity or increase in particle content in 4 hr at 22 °C	1689	C
Ganciclovir sodium	SY	20 mg/ml[a]	BR	20 mg/ml[a]	Flocculent precipitate forms immediately	1689	I
Granisetron HCl	SKB	0.05 mg/ml[a]	BMS	20 mg/ml[a]	Physically compatible with no change in measured turbidity or increase in particle content in 4 hr at 23 °C	2000	C
Haloperidol lactate	MN	0.2 mg/ml[a]	BR	20 mg/ml[a]	Haze forms immediately	1689	I
Hydrocortisone sodium phosphate	MSD	1 mg/ml[a]	BR	20 mg/ml[a]	Physically compatible with no change in measured turbidity or increase in particle content in 4 hr at 22 °C	1689	C
Hydrocortisone sodium succinate	UP	1 mg/ml[a]	BR	20 mg/ml[a]	Physically compatible with no change in measured turbidity or increase in particle content in 4 hr at 22 °C	1689	C
Hydromorphone HCl	ES	0.5 mg/ml[a]	BR	20 mg/ml[a]	Physically compatible with no change in measured turbidity or increase in particle content in 4 hr at 22 °C	1689	C
Hydroxyzine HCl	WI	4 mg/ml[a]	BR	20 mg/ml[a]	Haze forms immediately. Flocculent precipitate forms in 4 hr	1689	I
Idarubicin HCl	AD	0.5 mg/ml[a]	BR	20 mg/ml[a]	Flocculent precipitate forms in 4 hr	1689	I
Ifosfamide	MJ	25 mg/ml[a]	BR	20 mg/ml[a]	Haze and precipitate form in 1 hr	1689	I
Imipenem–cilastatin sodium	MSD	10 mg/ml[a]	BR	20 mg/ml[a]	Physically compatible with no change in measured turbidity or increase in particle content in 4 hr at 22 °C	1689	C
Leucovorin calcium	LE	2 mg/ml[a]	BR	20 mg/ml[a]	Physically compatible with no change in measured turbidity or increase in particle content in 4 hr at 22 °C	1689	C
Lorazepam	WY	0.1 mg/ml[a]	BR	20 mg/ml[a]	Physically compatible with no change in measured turbidity or increase in particle content in 4 hr at 22 °C	1689	C

Y-Site Injection Compatibility (1:1 Mixture) (Cont.)

Cefepime HCl

Drug	Mfr	Conc	Mfr	Conc	Remarks	Ref	C/I
Magnesium sulfate	AST	100 mg/ml[a]	BR	20 mg/ml[a]	Haze forms immediately	1689	I
Mannitol	BA	15%	BR	20 mg/ml[a]	Slight haze with particles forms immediately	1689	I
Mechlorethamine HCl	MSD	1 mg/ml[a]	BR	20 mg/ml[a]	Slight haze with particles forms immediately	1689	I
Melphalan	BW	0.1 mg/ml[a]	BR	20 mg/ml[a]	Physically compatible with no change in measured turbidity or increase in particle content in 4 hr at 22 °C	1689	C
Meperidine HCl	WY	4 mg/ml[a]	BR	20 mg/ml[a]	Haze forms immediately with particles in 1 hr	1689	I
Mesna	MJ	10 mg/ml[a]	BR	20 mg/ml[a]	Physically compatible with no change in measured turbidity or increase in particle content in 4 hr at 22 °C	1689	C
Methotrexate sodium	LE	15 mg/ml[a]	BR	20 mg/ml[a]	Physically compatible with no change in measured turbidity or increase in particle content in 4 hr at 22 °C	1689	C
Methylprednisolone sodium succinate	AB	5 mg/ml[a]	BR	20 mg/ml[a]	Physically compatible with no change in measured turbidity or increase in particle content in 4 hr at 22 °C	1689	C
Metoclopramide HCl	RB	5 mg/ml	BR	20 mg/ml[a]	Haze forms immediately	1689	I
Metronidazole	BA	5 mg/ml	BR	20 mg/ml[a]	Physically compatible with no change in measured turbidity or increase in particle content in 4 hr at 22 °C	1689	C
Mitomycin	BR	0.5 mg/ml[a]	BR	20 mg/ml[a]	Color changes to pinkish purple in 1 hr	1689	I
Mitoxantrone HCl	LE	0.5 mg/ml[a]	BR	20 mg/ml[a]	Haze forms immediately. Flocculent precipitate forms in 4 hr	1689	I
Morphine sulfate	AST	1 mg/ml[a]	BR	20 mg/ml[a]	Haze forms immediately with particles in 1 hr	1689	I
Nalbuphine HCl	DU	10 mg/ml[a]	BR	20 mg/ml[a]	Haze forms immediately. Flocculent precipitate forms in 4 hr	1689	I
Ofloxacin	ORT	4 mg/ml[a]	BR	20 mg/ml[a]	Haze forms immediately. Flocculent precipitate forms in 4 hr	1689	I
Ondansetron HCl	GL	1 mg/ml[a]	BR	20 mg/ml[a]	Haze forms immediately	1689	I
Paclitaxel	BR	0.6 mg/ml[a]	BR	20 mg/ml[a]	Physically compatible with no change in measured turbidity or increase in particle content in 4 hr at 22 °C	1689	C
Piperacillin sodium–tazobactam sodium	LE	40 + 5 mg/ml[a]	BR	20 mg/ml[a]	Physically compatible with no change in measured turbidity or increase in particle content in 4 hr at 22 °C	1689	C
Plicamycin	MI	0.01 mg/ml[a]	BR	20 mg/ml[a]	Haze forms immediately. Particles form in 1 hr	1689	I
Prochlorperazine edisylate	SN	0.5 mg/ml[a]	BR	20 mg/ml[a]	Haze forms immediately. Flocculent precipitate forms in 4 hr	1689	I
Promethazine HCl	WY	2 mg/ml[a]	BR	20 mg/ml[a]	Haze forms immediately. Flocculent precipitate forms in 4 hr	1689	I

Y-Site Injection Compatibility (1:1 Mixture) (Cont.)

Cefepime HCl

Drug	Mfr	Conc	Mfr	Conc	Remarks	Ref	C/I
Ranitidine HCl	GL	2 mg/ml[a]	BR	20 mg/ml[a]	Physically compatible with no change in measured turbidity or increase in particle content in 4 hr at 22 °C	1689	C
Sargramostim	IMM	10 μg/ml[b]	BR	20 mg/ml[a]	Physically compatible with no change in measured turbidity or increase in particle content in 4 hr at 22 °C	1689	C
Sodium bicarbonate	AB	1 mEq/ml	BR	20 mg/ml[a]	Physically compatible with no change in measured turbidity or increase in particle content in 4 hr at 22 °C	1689	C
Streptozocin	UP	40 mg/ml[a]	BR	20 mg/ml[a]	Haze forms immediately. Particles form in 1 hr. Deep red color forms in 4 hr	1689	I
Thiotepa	LE	1 mg/ml[a]	BR	20 mg/ml[a]	Physically compatible with no change in measured turbidity or increase in particle content in 4 hr at 22 °C	1689	C
Ticarcillin disodium–clavulanate potassium	SKB	31 mg/ml[a]	BR	20 mg/ml[a]	Physically compatible with no change in measured turbidity or increase in particle content in 4 hr at 22 °C	1689	C
Trimethoprim–sulfamethoxazole	ES	0.8 + 4 mg/ml[a]	BR	20 mg/ml[a]	Physically compatible with no change in measured turbidity or increase in particle content in 4 hr at 22 °C	1689	C
Vancomycin HCl	AB	10 mg/ml[a]	BR	20 mg/ml[a]	Haze forms immediately. Flocculent precipitate forms in 4 hr	1689	I
Vinblastine sulfate	LI	0.12 mg/ml[a]	BR	20 mg/ml[a]	Haze with particles forms immediately	1689	I
Vincristine sulfate	LI	0.05 mg/ml[a]	BR	20 mg/ml[a]	Small particles form immediately	1689	I
Zidovudine	BW	4 mg/ml[a]	BR	20 mg/ml[a]	Physically compatible with no change in measured turbidity or increase in particle content in 4 hr at 22 °C	1689	C

[a]*Tested in dextrose 5% in water.*
[b]*Tested in sodium chloride 0.9%.*

Additional Compatibility Information

Solutions— The manufacturer states that cefepime HCl 1 to 40 mg/ml is stable for 24 hours at room temperatures between 20 and 25 °C and for seven days under refrigeration at 2 to 8 °C in the following infusion solutions (2):

  Dextrose 5% in Ringer's injection, lactated
  Dextrose 5% in sodium chloride 0.9%
  Dextrose 5% in water
  Dextrose 10% in water
  Normosol M in 5% dextrose
  Normosol R
  Sodium chloride 0.9%
  Sodium lactate ⅙ M

Peritoneal Dialysis Solutions— Cefepime HCl (Bristol-Myers Squibb) 0.125 and 0.25 mg/ml in Inpersol (Abbott) peritoneal dialysis solution with dextrose 4.25% is stable, exhibiting 2 to 3% loss by HPLC analysis in seven days at 5 °C, 2% loss in 24 hours at room temperature, and 7 to 8% loss in 24 hours at 37 °C (1682).

Miscellaneous— The manufacturer states that cefepime HCl should not be mixed with aminophylline, gentamicin sulfate, metronidazole, netilmicin sulfate, tobramycin sulfate, and vancomycin HCl because of the potential for interaction. These medications should be administered separately from cefepime HCl (2).

CEFOPERAZONE SODIUM
AHFS 8:12.06

Cefobid   **Roerig**

Products— Cefoperazone sodium (Roerig) is available in vials and piggyback units containing 1 and 2 g of drug. In addition, 10-g pharmacy bulk vials are available. The vials may be reconstituted with a compatible diluent and should be allowed to stand so that any foaming may dissipate; the vials should then be inspected visually to assure complete solubilization. At concentrations above 333 mg/ml, vigorous and prolonged shaking is required to solubilize the drug. The maximum solubility is 475 mg/ml (2).

For intramuscular injection, sterile water for injection, bacteriostatic water for injection (benzyl alcohol or parabens), or another compatible solution may be used as the diluent in the dilutions listed in Table 1 (2; 4).

For concentrations above 250 mg/ml, the manufacturer recommends that a lidocaine HCl solution be used for reconstitution (2). To prepare intramuscular injections with lidocaine HCl 2%, a two-step procedure can be followed. Initially, sterile water for injection is added in the amounts indicated in Table 2. After complete dissolution of the drug, the specified volume of lidocaine HCl 2% is added. The final lidocaine HCl concentration will be about 0.5% (2).

For intravenous administration, each gram of cefoperazone is reconstituted with 5 ml of any compatible diluent except Ringer's injection, lactated, with or without dextrose 5%. (See Additional Compatibility Information.) The minimum volume of diluent is 2.8 ml per gram of cefoperazone. After dissolution is complete, the entire content of the vial is withdrawn and further diluted for intravenous administration. For intermittent infusion, further dilution in 20 to 40 ml of diluent per gram of drug is recommended. For continuous infusion, a concentration of 2 to 25 mg/ml can be used (2).

The 1- and 2-g piggyback units should be reconstituted with 20 to 40 ml of any compatible diluent per gram of drug. (See Additional Compatibility Information.) If Ringer's injection, lactated, with or without dextrose 5% is used as the vehicle, the manufacturer recommends an initial reconstitution with 2.8 to 5 ml of another compatible diluent per gram of drug prior to final dilution (2).

Table 1. Recommended Intramuscular Dilutions of Cefoperazone Sodium (2)

Vial Size	Volume of Diluent	Withdrawable Volume	Concentration
1 g	2.6 ml	3 ml	333 mg/ml
	3.8 ml	4 ml	250 mg/ml
2 g	5.0 ml	6 ml	333 mg/ml
	7.2 ml	8 ml	250 mg/ml

Table 2. Preparing Cefoperazone Sodium with Lidocaine HCl 2%

Vial Size	Step 1, Sterile Water Volume	Step 2, Lidocaine HCl 2% Volume	Cefoperazone Concentration
1 g	2.0 ml	0.6 ml	333 mg/ml
	2.8 ml	1.0 ml	250 mg/ml
2 g	3.8 ml	1.2 ml	333 mg/ml
	5.4 ml	1.8 ml	250 mg/ml

Cefoperazone sodium (Roerig) is available frozen as a premixed solution of 1 or 2 g per 50 ml of dextrose 4.6 or 3.6%, respectively (2).

The 10-g pharmacy bulk vial may be reconstituted with 95 ml of sterile water for injection in two separate, approximately equal aliquots. The resulting solution contains 100 mg/ml (2).

pH— From 4.5 to 6.5 (2; 4).

Osmotic Values— The osmolality of cefoperazone sodium 1 and 2 g was calculated for the following dilutions (1054):

Diluent	Osmolality (mOsm/kg)	
	50 ml	100 ml
1 g		
Dextrose 5% in water	302	280
Sodium chloride 0.9%	328	307
2 g		
Dextrose 5% in water	343	304
Sodium chloride 0.9%	370	330

The frozen premixed solutions have osmolalities of approximately 300 mOsm/kg (4).

Robinson et al. recommended the following maximum cefoperazone sodium concentrations to achieve osmolalities suitable for peripheral infusion in fluid-restricted patients (1180):

Diluent	Maximum Concentration (mg/ml)	Osmolality (mOsm/kg)
Dextrose 5% in water	113	461
Sodium chloride 0.9%	102	439
Sterile water for injection	202	312

Sodium Content— Cefoperazone sodium contains 1.5 mEq (34 mg) of sodium per gram (2).

Administration— Cefoperazone sodium is administered by deep intramuscular injection or by continuous intravenous infusion at a concentration of 2 to 25 mg/ml or intermittent intravenous infusion diluted in 20 to 40 ml of compatible diluent per gram of cefoperazone administered over 15 to 30 minutes (2; 4). Although not recommended by the manufacturer, cefoperazone sodium has also been given by direct intravenous injection over three to five minutes (4).

Stability— Intact vials of cefoperazone sodium should be stored at room temperatures not exceeding 25 °C and protected from light. Reconstituted solutions are colorless to straw yellow and do not need light protection. Solutions of cefoperazone sodium in compatible diluents are stable for 24 hours at room temperature and five days under refrigeration. (See Additional Compatibility Information.) Cefoperazone sodium solutions may be stored in glass or plastic syringes or in glass or PVC infusion solution containers (2; 4).

Cefoperazone (Roerig) 1 g/10 ml reconstituted with sterile water for injection or 1 g/50 ml in dextrose 5% in water in PVC bags exhibited no visible changes and no significant increases in particulate matter in 24 hours at 5 and 25 °C (986).

Freezing Solutions— Reconstitution to a concentration of 300 mg/ml with sodium chloride 0.9% or sterile water for injection yields solutions that are stable for five weeks at −20 to −10 °C. Solutions containing 50 mg/ml in dextrose 5% in water or 2 mg/ml in dextrose 5% in sodium chloride 0.2 or 0.9% are stable for three weeks at −20 to −10 °C. Frozen solutions should be thawed at room temperature; microwave techniques and heating are not recommended. Thawed solutions should not be refrozen (2; 4).

Cefoperazone sodium 40 mg/ml in both dextrose 5% in water and sodium chloride 0.9% exhibited no decomposition after 96 days at −10 °C. Thawing in a microwave oven did not affect stability (1341).

Compatibility Information

Solution Compatibility

Cefoperazone sodium

Solution	Mfr	Mfr	Conc/L	Remarks	Ref	C/I
Dextrose 5% in water	MG[a]	RR	20 g	2% loss in 48 hr at 25 °C under fluorescent light	1164	C
	TR		40 g	Physically compatible with 8% loss in 8 days at 25 °C and no loss in 80 days at 5 °C	1341	C
Sodium chloride 0.9%	MG[a]	RR	20 g	3% loss in 48 hr at 25 °C under fluorescent light	1164	C
	TR		40 g	Physically compatible with 8% loss in 8 days at 25 °C and no loss in 80 days at 5 °C	1341	C
TPN #107[b]			1 g	50% cefoperazone loss in 24 hr at 21 °C by microbiological assay	1326	I

[a]Tested in glass bottles.
[b]Refer to Appendix I for the composition of parenteral nutrition solutions. TPN indicates a 2-in-1 admixture.

Additive Compatibility

Cefoperazone sodium

Drug	Mfr	Conc/L	Mfr	Conc/L	Test Soln	Remarks	Ref	C/I
Cimetidine HCl	SKF	2 g	RR	5 g	D5W	Physically compatible. 5% cefoperazone loss at 25 °C and 3% loss at 4 °C in 48 hr. 2% or less cimetidine loss in 48 hr at 25 and 4 °C	1403	C
Clindamycin phosphate	UP	12 g	RR	20 g	D5W, NS[a]	Physically compatible with no clindamycin loss and 5% cefoperazone loss in 48 hr at 25 °C under fluorescent light	174; 1164	C
Furosemide	HO	200 mg	RR	10 g	D5W	Physically compatible. 10% loss of both drugs in 15 days at 25 °C and 20 days at 4 °C in the dark	1402	C

[a]Tested in both glass and PVC containers.

Drugs in Syringe Compatibility

Cefoperazone sodium

Drug (in syringe)	Mfr	Amt	Mfr	Amt	Remarks	Ref	C/I
Doxapram HCl	RB	400 mg/ 20 ml		500 mg/ 4 ml	Immediate precipitation	1177	I
Heparin sodium		2500 units/ 1 ml	RR	2 g	Physically compatible for at least 5 min	1053	C

Y-Site Injection Compatibility (1:1 Mixture)

Cefoperazone sodium

Drug	Mfr	Conc	Mfr	Conc	Remarks	Ref	C/I
Acyclovir sodium	BW	5 mg/ml[a]	RR	20 mg/ml[a]	Physically compatible for 4 hr at 25 °C	1157	**C**
Allopurinol sodium	BW	3 mg/ml[b]	RR	40 mg/ml[b]	Physically compatible with no change in measured turbidity or increase in particle content in 4 hr at 22 °C	1686	**C**
Amifostine	USB	10 mg/ml[a]	RR	40 mg/ml[a]	Haze forms immediately, becoming cloudy with microprecipitation in 4 hr	1845	**I**
Amphotericin B cholesteryl sulfate complex	SEQ	0.83 mg/ml[a]	RR	40 mg/ml[a]	Gross precipitate forms	2117	**I**
Aztreonam	SQ	40 mg/ml[a]	RR	40 mg/ml[a]	Physically compatible with no subvisual haze or particle formation in 4 hr at 23 °C	1758	**C**
Cisatracurium besylate	GW	0.1, 2, 5 mg/ml[a]	RR	40 mg/ml[a]	White cloudiness forms immediately	2074	**I**
Cyclophosphamide	MJ	20 mg/ml[a]	RR	20 mg/ml[a]	Physically compatible for 4 hr at 25 °C	1194	**C**
Diltiazem HCl	MMD	1[b] and 5 mg/ml	RR	20[a], 25[b], 50[b] mg/ml	Cloudiness and precipitate form	1807	**I**
	MMD	5 mg/ml	RR	10 mg/ml[b]	Precipitate forms	1807	**I**
	MMD	1 mg/ml[b]	RR	10 mg/ml[b]	Visually compatible	1807	**C**
	MMD	1[b] and 5 mg/ml	RR	2 and 5 mg/ml[b]	Visually compatible	1807	**C**
Docetaxel	RPR	0.9 mg/ml[a]	RR	40 mg/ml[a]	Physically compatible with no change in measured turbidity or increase in particle content in 4 hr at 23 °C	2224	**C**
Doxorubicin HCl liposome injection	SEQ	0.4 mg/ml[a]	RR	40 mg/ml[a]	Partial loss of measured natural turbidity	2087	**I**
Enalaprilat	MSD	0.05 mg/ml[b]	RR	10 mg/ml[a]	Physically compatible for 24 hr at room temperature under fluorescent light	1355	**C**
Esmolol HCl	DCC	10 mg/ml[a]	RR	10 mg/ml[a]	Physically compatible for 24 hr at 22 °C	1169	**C**
Etoposide phosphate	BR	5 mg/ml[a]	RR	40 mg/ml[a]	Physically compatible with no change in measured turbidity or increase in particle content in 4 hr at 23 °C	2218	**C**
Famotidine	MSD	0.2 mg/ml[a]	RR	40 mg/ml[b]	Physically compatible for 14 hr	1196	**C**
Filgrastim	AMG	30 μg/ml[a]	RR	40 mg/ml[a]	Haze and particles form immediately	1687	**I**
Fludarabine phosphate	BX	1 mg/ml[a]	RR	40 mg/ml[a]	Physically compatible for 4 hr at room temperature under fluorescent light	1439	**C**
Foscarnet sodium	AST	24 mg/ml	RR	40 mg/ml	Physically compatible for 24 hr at room temperature under fluorescent light	1335	**C**
Gemcitabine HCl	LI	10 mg/ml[b]	RR	40 mg/ml[b]	Gross precipitation occurs immediately	2226	**I**
Granisetron HCl	SKB	0.05 mg/ml[a]	RR	40 mg/ml[a]	Physically compatible with no change in measured turbidity or increase in particle content in 4 hr at 23 °C	2000	**C**
Hetastarch	DCC	6%	RR	20 mg/ml[a]	Small crystals formed immediately after mixing and persisted for 4 hr	1313	**I**
Hydromorphone HCl	WY	0.2 mg/ml[a]	RR	20 mg/ml[a]	Physically compatible for at least 4 hr at 25 °C under fluorescent light	987	**C**
Labetalol HCl	SC	1 mg/ml[a]	RR	10 mg/ml[a]	Cloudiness and fine precipitate form immediately	1171	**I**

Y-Site Injection Compatibility (1:1 Mixture) (Cont.)

			Cefoperazone sodium				
Drug	*Mfr*	*Conc*	*Mfr*	*Conc*	*Remarks*	*Ref*	*C/I*
Magnesium sulfate	IX	16.7, 33.3, 66.7, 100 mg/ml[a]	RR	20 mg/ml[a]	Physically compatible for at least 4 hr at 32 °C	813	**C**
Melphalan HCl	BW	0.1 mg/ml[b]	RR	40 mg/ml[b]	Physically compatible with no change in measured turbidity or increase in particle content in 3 hr at 22 °C	1557	**C**
Meperidine HCl	WY	10 mg/ml[a]	RR	20 mg/ml[a]	Immediate precipitation	987	**I**
Morphine sulfate	WI	1 mg/ml[a]	RR	20 mg/ml[a]	Physically compatible for at least 4 hr at 25 °C under fluorescent light	987	**C**
Ondansetron HCl	GL	1 mg/ml[b]	RR	40 mg/ml[a]	Immediate turbidity and precipitation	1365	**I**
Pentamidine isethionate	FUJ	3 mg/ml[a]	RR	20 mg/ml[c]	Heavy white precipitate forms immediately	1880	**I**
Perphenazine	SC	0.02 mg/ml[a]	RR	20 mg/ml[a]	Cloudy solution forms immediately with fine precipitate persisting for 4 hr at 25 °C	1155	**I**
Promethazine HCl		6.25 mg	RR	[d]	White precipitate forms due to ionic complex formation	1336	**I**
Propofol	ZEN	10 mg/ml	RR	40 mg/ml[a]	Physically compatible for 1 hr at 23 °C with no increase in particle content	2066	**C**
Ranitidine HCl	GL	1 mg/ml[b]	TAK	20 mg/ml[b]	Visually compatible with no loss of either drug by HPLC in 4 hr at 25 °C	2209	**C**
Remifentanil HCl	GW	0.025 mg/ml[b]	RR	40 mg/ml[a]	Physically compatible with no change in measured turbidity or increase in particle content in 4 hr at 23 °C	2075	**C**
	GW	0.25 mg/ml[b]	RR	40 mg/ml[a]	Subvisual haze forms in 1 hr	2075	**I**
Sargramostim	IMM	10 µg/ml[b]	RR	40 mg/ml[b]	Slight haze, visible with high intensity light, forms immediately	1436	**I**
Teniposide	BR	0.1 mg/ml[a]	RR	40 mg/ml[a]	Physically compatible with no subvisual haze or particle formation in 4 hr at 23 °C	1725	**C**
Thiotepa	IMM[e]	1 mg/ml[a]	RR	40 mg/ml[a]	Physically compatible with no change in measured turbidity or increase in particle content in 4 hr at 23 °C	1861	**C**
TNA #218 to #226[f]			RR	40 mg/ml[a]	Visually compatible with no precipitate or emulsion damage apparent in 4 hr at 23 °C	2215	**C**
TPN #61[f]		[g]	RR	250 mg/1 ml[h]	Physically compatible	1012	**C**
		[i]	RR	1.5 g/6 ml[h]	Physically compatible	1012	**C**
TPN #212 to #215[f]			RR	40 mg/ml[a]	Physically compatible with no change in measured turbidity or increase in particle content in 4 hr at 23 °C	2109	**C**

Y-Site Injection Compatibility (1:1 Mixture) (Cont.)

Cefoperazone sodium

Drug	Mfr	Conc	Mfr	Conc	Remarks	Ref	C/I
Vinorelbine tartrate	BW	1 mg/ml[b]	RR	40 mg/ml[b]	Heavy white flocculent precipitate forms immediately	1558	I

[a]Tested in dextrose 5% in water.
[b]Tested in sodium chloride 0.9%.
[c]Tested in dextrose 4.6% in water.
[d]Tested in dextrose 5% in water; concentration unspecified.
[e]Lyophilized formulation tested.
[f]Refer to Appendix I for the composition of parenteral nutrition solutions. TNA indicates a 3-in-1 admixture, and TPN indicates a 2-in-1 admixture.
[g]Run at 21 ml/hr.
[h]Given over five minutes by syringe pump.
[i]Run at 94 ml/hr.

Additional Compatibility Information

Solutions— The stability of cefoperazone sodium (Roerig) in various solutions, as stated by the manufacturer, is shown in Table 3 (2).

When frozen at −20 to −10 °C, cefoperazone sodium (Roerig) is stated to be stable as indicated in Table 4 (2).

Table 3. Stability of Cefoperazone Sodium in Various Solutions (2)

Solution	Cefoperazone Concentration	Stability Period 15 to 25 °C	Stability Period 2 to 8 °C
Bacteriostatic water for injection (benzyl alcohol or parabens)	300 mg/ml	24 hr	5 days
Dextrose 5% in Ringer's injection, lactated	2 to 50 mg/ml	24 hr	
Dextrose 5% in sodium chloride 0.2 or 0.9%	2 to 50 mg/ml	24 hr	5 days
Dextrose 5% in water	2 to 50 mg/ml	24 hr	5 days
Dextrose 10% in water	2 to 50 mg/ml	24 hr	
Lidocaine HCl 0.5%	300 mg/ml	24 hr	5 days
Normosol M and dextrose 5%	2 to 50 mg/ml	24 hr	5 days
Normosol R	2 to 50 mg/ml	24 hr	5 days
Ringer's injection, lactated	2 mg/ml	24 hr	5 days
Sodium chloride 0.9%	2 to 300 mg/ml	24 hr	5 days
Sterile water for injection	300 mg/ml	24 hr	5 days

Table 4. Stability of Cefoperazone Sodium Solutions Frozen at −20 to −10 °C (2)

Solution	Cefoperazone Concentration	Stability Period
Dextrose 5% in sodium chloride 0.2 or 0.9%	2 mg/ml	3 weeks
Dextrose 5% in water	50 mg/ml	3 weeks
Sodium chloride 0.9%	300 mg/ml	5 weeks
Sterile water for injection	300 mg/ml	5 weeks

Aminoglycosides— The manufacturer recommends that aminoglycosides not be mixed in the same solution because of physical incompatibility (2). When tobramycin sulfate (Lilly) 80 mg/100 ml in dextrose 5% in water was run through an administration set previously used to administer cefoperazone (Roerig) 4 g/100 ml in dextrose 5% in water, a precipitate formed immediately in the infusion tubing where the two solutions mixed. A retest, using cefoperazone 1 g/100 ml, produced the same result. Substituting gentamicin sulfate (Schering) 80 mg/100 ml for the tobramycin also yielded a precipitate immediately (831).

Spruill et al. evaluated the effect of various cephalosporins on tobramycin sulfate 7.7 µg/ml in human serum. At concentrations of 250 and 1000 µg/ml, cefazolin, cefoxitin, cefamandole, cefoperazone, and cefotaxime caused about a 10 to 15% loss of tobramycin over 48 hours at 0 and 21 °C. Moxalactam caused about a 15% loss at 0 °C and a 20 to 30% loss at 21 °C over 48 hours (1005).

Pennell et al. evaluated the potential for inactivation of tobramycin sulfate (Lilly) 9 µg/ml with 100- and 200-µg/ml concentrations of cefoperazone sodium (Roerig) in human serum. No loss of tobramycin sulfate was determined by TDx fluorescence polarization immunoassay over 48 hours when stored at 4, 24, and 37 °C (1420).

CEFOTAXIME SODIUM
AHFS 8:12.06

Claforan   **Aventis**

Products— Cefotaxime sodium (Aventis) is available in vials containing the equivalent of 500 mg and 1 and 2 g of cefotaxime and in infusion bottles containing the equivalent of 1 and 2 g of cefotaxime. It is also available in 10-g pharmacy bulk packages (2).

For intravenous administration, the contents of any size vial may be reconstituted with 10 ml of sterile water for injection. (See Table 1.) The 1- and 2-g infusion bottles may be reconstituted with 50 or 100 ml of dextrose 5% in water or sodium chloride 0.9%. For intramuscular injection, reconstitute with sterile water for injection or bacteriostatic water for injection in the amounts shown in Table 1 (2).

The 10-g pharmacy bulk package may be reconstituted with 47 or 97 ml of compatible diluent to yield a 200- or 100-mg/ml concentration, respectively. Doses from this bulk package must be diluted further for administration (2; 4).

After addition of the diluent, shake to dissolve the contents and inspect for particulate matter or discoloration (2).

For intravenous infusion, the primary solution may be diluted further to 50 to 1000 ml in a compatible diluent (2). (See Additional Compatibility Information.)

Cefotaxime sodium (Aventis) is also available as a frozen premixed infusion solution of 1 or 2 g in dextrose 5% in water (2; 4).

pH— Injectable solutions of the drug have pH values ranging from 5 to 7.5 (2).

Osmolality— A solution of cefotaxime sodium 1 g/14 ml of sterile water for injection is isotonic (2).

The osmolality of cefotaxime sodium 1, 2, and 3 g was calculated for the following dilutions (1054):

Diluent	Osmolality (mOsm/kg)	
	50 ml	100 ml
1 g		
Dextrose 5% in water	350	319
Sodium chloride 0.9%	375	344
2 g		
Dextrose 5% in water	343	327
Sodium chloride 0.9%	406	351
3 g		
Dextrose 5% in water	433	344
Sodium chloride 0.9%	458	382

The frozen premixed solutions have osmolalities of 340 to 420 mOsm/kg for the 1-g/50 ml concentration and 450 to 540 mOsm/kg for the 2-g/50 ml concentration (4).

The osmolality of cefotaxime sodium (Hoechst) 50 mg/ml was determined to be 326 mOsm/kg in dextrose 5% in water and 333 mOsm/kg in sodium chloride 0.9% (1375).

Robinson et al. recommended the following maximum cefotaxime sodium concentrations to achieve osmolalities suitable for peripheral infusion in fluid-restricted patients (1180):

Diluent	Maximum Concentration (mg/ml)	Osmolality (mOsm/kg)
Dextrose 5% in water	86	577
Sodium chloride 0.9%	73	555
Sterile water for injection	147	525

Sodium Content— Cefotaxime sodium contains approximately 2.2 mEq (50.5 mg) of sodium per gram of cefotaxime activity (2).

Administration— Cefotaxime sodium may be administered by deep intramuscular injection; doses of 2 g should be divided between different injection sites. It may also be administered by direct intravenous injection over three to five minutes directly into the vein or into the tubing of a running compatible infusion solution. In addition, cefotaxime sodium may be administered in 50 to 100 ml of compatible diluent over 20 to 30 minutes by intermittent intravenous infusion or by continuous intravenous infusion (2; 4; 8).

Stability— Intact vials of cefotaxime sodium (Aventis) should be stored below 30 °C. The dry powder is off-white to pale yellow in color. Solutions may range from light yellow to amber, depending on the diluent, concentration, and storage conditions. Both the dry material and solutions may darken and should be protected from elevated temperatures and excessive light. Discoloration of the powder or solution may indicate a loss of potency (2; 4).

Store the frozen premixed cefotaxime sodium infusions at −20 °C or below (2; 4).

Reconstituted Solutions— When reconstituted as described in the Products section, cefotaxime sodium (Aventis) is stable in the original containers as indicated in Table 2. Storage of reconstituted solutions in disposable glass or plastic syringes for five days under refrigeration is also recommended. Dilutions of cefotaxime sodium in dextrose 5% in water or sodium chloride 0.9% in PVC bags are also stable for 24 hours at room temperature or five days under refrigeration (2).

Cefotaxime sodium (Hoechst-Roussel) 1 g/10 ml reconstituted with sterile water for injection or 1 g/50 ml in dextrose 5% in water in PVC bags exhibited no visible changes in 24 hours at 5 and 25 °C. Although increased levels of particulate matter were observed in most solutions, the increases were significant only in solutions stored at 25 °C (986).

Cefotaxime sodium (Roussel) 250 mg/ml in sterile water for injection, packaged as 0.18 ml in 1-ml Injekt syringes (Braun) sealed with blind hubs and stored at about 6 °C, retained antibiotic activity against *Pseudomonas aeruginosa* for seven days. However, the yel-

Table 1. Recommended Reconstitution of Cefotaxime Sodium (2)

Vial Size	Volume of Diluent	Withdrawable Volume	Approximate Concentration
Intravenous			
500 mg	10 ml	10.2 ml	50 mg/ml
1 g	10 ml	10.4 ml	95 mg/ml
2 g	10 ml	11.0 ml	180 mg/ml
Intramuscular			
500 mg	2 ml	2.2 ml	230 mg/ml
1 g	3 ml	3.4 ml	300 mg/ml
2 g	5 ml	6.0 ml	330 mg/ml

Table 2. Manufacturer's Recommended Storage Times of Reconstituted Cefotaxime Sodium (2)

Vial Size	Concentration	Storage Temperature 22 °C	5 °C
500 mg	200 mg/ml	12 hr	7 days
	50 mg/ml	24 hr	7 days
1 g	300 mg/ml	12 hr	7 days
	95 mg/ml	24 hr	7 days
(Infusion bottle)	10 to 20 mg/ml	24 hr	10 days
2 g	330 mg/ml	12 hr	7 days
	180 mg/ml	12 hr	7 days
(Infusion bottle)	20 to 40 mg/ml	24 hr	10 days

low color of the solution became much darker over this period (1697).

Freezing Solutions— When reconstituted as recommended, cefotaxime sodium may be stored frozen in the vial or in disposable glass or plastic syringes for 13 weeks. Similarly, dilutions of cefotaxime sodium in dextrose 5% in water or sodium chloride 0.9% in PVC bags may be stored frozen for 13 weeks. Thawing at room temper-ature is recommended; frozen solutions should not be heated. Once thawed, the solutions are stable for 24 hours at room temperature or five days at less than 5 °C. Thawed solutions should not be refrozen (2; 4).

In one study, cefotaxime sodium (Hoechst-Roussel) 10 g/L in PVC bags of dextrose 5% in water and sodium chloride 0.9% (Travenol) exhibited no decomposition after 63 days of storage at −10 °C (751).

pH Effects— The primary factor in the stability of cefotaxime sodium is solution pH (792). Cefotaxime sodium in aqueous solutions is stable at pH 5 to 7 (2) or 4.3 to 6.2 (1077). The theoretical pH of minimum decomposition is 5.13 (793). However, between pH 3 and 7, the hydrolysis rate is virtually independent of pH (1072). Determination of decomposition kinetics in various aqueous buffer systems at 25 °C showed 10% decomposition occurring in 24 hours or longer over a pH range of 3.9 to 7.6. At pH 2.2 and 8.4, 10% decomposition occurred in about 13 hours (793).

The manufacturer recommends that cefotaxime sodium not be diluted in solutions with a pH greater than 7.5 (2; 4).

Compatibility Information

Solution Compatibility

Cefotaxime sodium

Solution	Mfr	Mfr	Conc/L	Remarks	Ref	C/I
Dextrose 5% in water	TR[a]	HO	10 g	Physically compatible with 3% decomposition in 24 hr at 24 °C. No decomposition in 22 days at 4 °C	751; 1077	C
	AB[b]	HO	20 g	Physically compatible with little or no cefotaxime loss in 24 hr at 25 °C	994	C
Sodium chloride 0.9%	TR[a]	HO	10 g	Physically compatible with 2% decomposition in 24 hr at 24 °C. No decomposition in 22 days at 4 °C	751; 1077	C
	AB[b]	HO	20 g	Physically compatible with little or no cefotaxime loss in 24 hr at 25 °C	994	C
TPN #107[c]			1 g	Physically compatible and cefotaxime activity retained for 24 hr at 21 °C by microbiological assay	1326	C

[a]Tested in PVC containers.
[b]Tested in both glass bottles and PVC bags.
[c]Refer to Appendix I for the composition of parenteral nutrition solutions. TPN indicates a 2-in-1 admixture.

Additive Compatibility

Cefotaxime sodium

Drug	Mfr	Conc/L	Mfr	Conc/L	Test Soln	Remarks	Ref	C/I
Clindamycin phosphate	UP	9 g	HO	20 g	D5W, NS[a]	Physically compatible with no clindamycin loss and 3% cefotaxime loss in 24 hr at 25 °C	994	C
Metronidazole	RP	5 g[b]	RS	20 g		Physically compatible with little or no pH change for at least 24 hr at 4 °C	807	C
	AB	5 g	HO	10 g		Potency of both drugs by HPLC retained for 72 hr at 8 °C	1547	C

Additive Compatibility (Cont.)

Cefotaxime sodium

Drug	Mfr	Conc/L	Mfr	Conc/L	Test Soln	Remarks	Ref	C/I
	AB	5 g	HO	10 g		Visually compatible with 10% cefotaxime loss by HPLC in 19 hr at 28 °C and 8% loss in 96 hr at 5 °C. No metronidazole loss in 96 hr at 5 or 28 °C	1754	C
Metronidazole HCl	SE	5 g	HO	10 g	NS	Visually compatible with 10% cefotaxime loss by HPLC in 24 hr at 28 °C and no loss in 96 hr at 5 °C. No metronidazole loss in 96 hr at 5 or 28 °C	1754	C
Verapamil HCl	KN	80 mg	HO	4 g	D5W, NS	Physically compatible for 24 hr	764	C

[a]*Tested in both glass and PVC containers.*
[b]*Minibags (100 ml) containing metronidazole 500 mg with disodium phosphate 150 mg, citric acid 44 mg, and sodium chloride 740 mg. This product differs from the Searle product.*

Drugs in Syringe Compatibility

Cefotaxime sodium

Drug (in syringe)	Mfr	Amt	Mfr	Amt	Remarks	Ref	C/I
Doxapram HCl	RB	400 mg/ 20 ml		500 mg/ 4 ml	Immediate precipitation	1171	I
Heparin sodium		2500 units/ 1 ml	HO	2 g	Physically compatible for at least 5 min	1053	C
Ofloxacin	HO	200 mg	HO	2 g	Visually compatible with no loss of either drug by HPLC in 4 hr at room temperature	1735	C

Y-Site Injection Compatibility (1:1 Mixture)

Cefotaxime sodium

Drug	Mfr	Conc	Mfr	Conc	Remarks	Ref	C/I
Acyclovir sodium	BW	5 mg/ml[a]	HO	20 mg/ml[a]	Physically compatible for 4 hr at 25 °C	1157	C
Allopurinol sodium	BW	3 mg/ml[b]	HO	20 mg/ml[b]	Tiny particles form immediately	1668	I
Amifostine	USB	10 mg/ml[a]	HO	20 mg/ml[a]	Physically compatible with no change in measured turbidity or increase in particle content in 4 hr at 23 °C	1845	C
Aztreonam	SQ	40 mg/ml[a]	HO	20 mg/ml[a]	Physically compatible with no subvisual haze or particle formation in 4 hr at 23 °C	1758	C
Cisatracurium besylate	GW	0.1 mg/ml[a]	HO	20 mg/ml[a]	Physically compatible with no change in measured turbidity or increase in particle content in 4 hr at 23 °C	2074	C
	GW	2 mg/ml[a]	HO	20 mg/ml[a]	Subvisual haze forms in 4 hr	2074	I
	GW	5 mg/ml[a]	HO	20 mg/ml[a]	Subvisual haze forms immediately	2074	I
Cyclophosphamide	MJ	20 mg/ml[a]	HO	20 mg/ml[a]	Physically compatible for 4 hr at 25 °C	1194	C
Diltiazem HCl	MMD	5 mg/ml	HO	10 and 180 mg/ml[b]	Visually compatible	1807	C
	MMD	1 mg/ml[b]	HO	180 mg/ml[b]	Visually compatible	1807	C

Y-Site Injection Compatibility (1:1 Mixture) (Cont.)

Cefotaxime sodium

Drug	Mfr	Conc	Mfr	Conc	Remarks	Ref	C/I
Docetaxel	RPR	0.9 mg/ml[a]	HO	20 mg/ml[a]	Physically compatible with no change in measured turbidity or increase in particle content in 4 hr at 23 °C	2224	C
Etoposide phosphate	BR	5 mg/ml[a]	HO	20 mg/ml[a]	Physically compatible with no change in measured turbidity or increase in particle content in 4 hr at 23 °C	2218	C
Famotidine	MSD	0.2 mg/ml[a]	HO	20 mg/ml[b]	Physically compatible for 14 hr	1196	C
	ME	2 mg/ml[b]		20 mg/ml[a]	Visually compatible for 4 hr at 22 °C	1936	C
Filgrastim	AMG	30 μg/ml[a]	HO	20 mg/ml[a]	Particles form in 4 hr	1687	I
Fluconazole	RR	2 mg/ml	HO	20 mg/ml	Cloudiness and amber color develop	1407	I
Fludarabine phosphate	BX	1 mg/ml[a]	HO	20 mg/ml[a]	Physically compatible for 4 hr at room temperature under fluorescent light	1439	C
Gemcitabine HCl	LI	10 mg/ml[b]	HO	20 mg/ml[b]	Slight subvisual haze forms in 1 hr with increased haze and a subvisual precipitate in 4 hr	2226	I
Granisetron HCl	SKB	0.05 mg/ml[a]	HO	20 mg/ml[a]	Physically compatible with no change in measured turbidity or increase in particle content in 4 hr at 23 °C	2000	C
Hetastarch	DCC	6%	HO	20 mg/ml[a]	Small crystals formed immediately after mixing and persisted for 4 hr	1313	I
Hydromorphone HCl	WY	0.2 mg/ml[a]	HO	20 mg/ml[a]	Physically compatible for at least 4 hr at 25 °C under fluorescent light	987	C
Lorazepam	WY	0.33 mg/ml[b]	RS	10 mg/ml	Visually compatible for 24 hr at 22 °C	1855	C
Magnesium sulfate	IX	16.7, 33.3, 66.7, 100 mg/ml[a]	HO	20 mg/ml[a]	Physically compatible for at least 4 hr at 32 °C	813	C
Melphalan HCl	BW	0.1 mg/ml[b]	HO	20 mg/ml[b]	Physically compatible with no change in measured turbidity or increase in particle content in 3 hr at 22 °C	1557	C
Meperidine HCl	WY	10 mg/ml[a]	HO	20 mg/ml[a]	Physically compatible for at least 4 hr at 25 °C under fluorescent light	987	C
Midazolam HCl	RC	1 mg/ml[a]	HO	20 mg/ml[a]	Visually compatible for 24 hr at 23 °C	1847	C
	RC	5 mg/ml	RS	10 mg/ml	Visually compatible for 24 hr at 22 °C	1855	C
Morphine sulfate	WI	1 mg/ml[a]	HO	20 mg/ml[a]	Physically compatible for at least 4 hr at 25 °C under fluorescent light	987	C
Ondansetron HCl	GL	1 mg/ml[b]	HO	20 mg/ml[a]	Physically compatible for 4 hr at 22 °C	1365	C
Pentamidine isethionate	FUJ	3 mg/ml[a]	HO	20 mg/ml[a]	Fine precipitate, difficult to see, forms immediately	1880	I
Perphenazine	SC	0.02 mg/ml[a]	HO	20 mg/ml[a]	Physically compatible for 4 hr at 25 °C	1155	C
Propofol	ZEN	10 mg/ml	HO	20 mg/ml[a]	Physically compatible for 1 hr at 23 °C with no increase in particle content	2066	C
Remifentanil HCl	GW	0.025 and 0.25 mg/ml[b]	HO	20 mg/ml[a]	Physically compatible with no change in measured turbidity or increase in particle content in 4 hr at 23 °C	2075	C
Sargramostim	IMM	10 μg/ml[b]	HO	20 mg/ml[b]	Physically compatible for 4 hr at 22 °C	1436	C

Y-Site Injection Compatibility (1:1 Mixture) (Cont.)

			Cefotaxime sodium				
Drug	*Mfr*	*Conc*	*Mfr*	*Conc*	*Remarks*	*Ref*	*C/I*
Teniposide	BR	0.1 mg/ml[a]	HO	20 mg/ml[a]	Physically compatible with no subvisual haze or particle formation in 4 hr at 23 °C	1725	**C**
Thiotepa	IMM[c]	1 mg/ml[a]	HO	20 mg/ml[a]	Physically compatible with no change in measured turbidity or increase in particle content in 4 hr at 23 °C	1861	**C**
TNA #218 to #226[d]			HO	20 mg/ml[a]	Visually compatible with no precipitate or emulsion damage apparent in 4 hr at 23 °C	2215	**C**
Tolazoline HCl		0.1 mg/ml[a]	HO	60 mg/ml[a]	Physically compatible for 24 hr at 22 °C	1363	**C**
TPN #61[d]		e	HO	200 mg/ 0.7 ml[f]	Physically compatible	1012	**C**
		g	HO	1.2 g/4 ml[f]	Physically compatible	1012	**C**
TPN #189[d]			RS	200 mg/ml[e]	Visually compatible for 24 hr at 22 °C	1767	**C**
TPN #203 and #204[d]			HO	60 mg/ml	Visually compatible for 2 hr at 23 °C	1974	**C**
TPN #212 to #215[d]			HO	20 mg/ml[a]	Physically compatible with no change in measured turbidity or increase in particle content in 4 hr at 23 °C	2109	**C**
Vancomycin HCl		12.5, 25, 30, 50 mg/ml[h]		100 mg/ml[h]	White precipitate forms immediately	1721	**I**
		5 mg/ml[h]		100 mg/ml[h]	No precipitate visually observed over 7 days at room temperature, but nonvisual incompatibility cannot be ruled out	1721	**?**
	AB	20 mg/ml[a]	HO	200 mg/ml[h]	Transient precipitate forms, followed by clear solution	2189	**?**
	AB	20 mg/ml[a]	HO	50 mg/ml[a]	White cloudiness forms immediately	2189	**I**
	AB	20 mg/ml[a]	HO	1 and 10 mg/ ml[a]	Physically compatible with no change in measured turbidity or increase in particle content in 4 hr at 23 °C	2189	**C**
	AB	2 mg/ml[a]	HO	1[a], 10[a], 50[a], and 200[h] mg/ ml	Physically compatible with no change in measured turbidity or increase in particle content in 4 hr at 23 °C	2189	**C**
Vinorelbine tartrate	BW	1 mg/ml[b]	HO	20 mg/ml[b]	Physically compatible with little change in measured turbidity or increase in particle content in 4 hr at 22 °C	1558	**C**

[a]*Tested in dextrose 5% in water.*
[b]*Tested in sodium chloride 0.9%.*
[c]*Lyophilized formulation tested.*
[d]*Refer to Appendix I for the composition of parenteral nutrition solutions. TNA indicates a 3-in-1 admixture, and TPN indicates a 2-in-1 admixture.*
[e]*Run at 21 ml/hr.*
[f]*Given over five minutes by syringe pump.*
[g]*Run at 94 ml/hr.*
[h]*Tested in sterile water for injection.*

Additional Compatibility Information

Solutions— Cefotaxime sodium (Advantis) maintains potency for 24 hours at room temperature and at least five days under refrigeration diluted in 50 to 1000 ml of the following infusion solutions (2):
  Amino acid injection 8.5%
  Dextrose 5% in sodium chloride 0.2, 0.45, and 0.9%

  Dextrose 5 and 10% in water
  Invert sugar 10% in water
  Ringer's injection, lactated
  Sodium chloride 0.9%
  Sodium lactate ⅙ M

  The manufacturer recommends that additives not be introduced into the premixed cefotaxime sodium in dextrose 5% in water infusion (2).

Peritoneal Dialysis Solutions— Cefotaxime sodium 2 mg/ml in peritoneal dialysis solution (McGaw) containing dextrose 2.5% and electrolytes was physically compatible for three hours at room temperature. Furthermore, no significant loss of antibacterial activity was apparent by microbiological determination (142).

The stability of cefotaxime sodium (Hoechst-Roussel) 125 mg/L in peritoneal dialysis solutions (Dianeal 137 and PD2) with heparin sodium 500 units/L was evaluated at 25 °C by microbiological assay. Approximately 95 ± 6% activity remained after 24 hours (1228).

Paap and Nahata studied the stability of cefotaxime sodium (Hoechst-Roussel) 1 mg/ml in Dianeal PD-1 with dextrose 1.5 and 4.25% (Travenol). At 25 °C, the drug exhibited an 8% loss in 24 hours and a 16% loss in 48 hours in both solutions. Storage at 37 °C for 12 hours resulted in 11 and 14% losses in the solutions containing dextrose 1.5% and dextrose 4.25%, respectively (1481).

Aminoglycosides— The manufacturer states that cefotaxime sodium should not be admixed with aminoglycosides (2). However, they may be administered separately to the same patient (2; 792).

No inactivation of tobramycin, gentamicin, and amikacin 10 μg/ml was caused by cefotaxime 100 and 500 μg/ml when the mixtures were stored at 37 °C for six hours. Further, no loss of cefotaxime activity was detected in any combination (973).

The inactivation of gentamicin, tobramycin, and amikacin, each 5 μg/ml, by seven β-lactam antibiotics, 250 and 500 μg/ml, in serum at 25 °C over 24 hours was studied using bioassay, enzyme-mediated immunoassay technique (EMIT), fluorescence polarization immunoassay (TDx), and radioimmunoassay. No inactivation of any aminoglycosides by the cephalosporins moxalactam, cefotaxime, and cefazolin occurred within the study period (654).

Spruill et al. evaluated the effect of various cephalosporins on tobramycin sulfate 7.7 μg/ml in human serum. At concentrations of 250 and 1000 μg/ml, cefazolin, cefoxitin, cefamandole, cefoperazone, and cefotaxime caused about a 10 to 15% loss of tobramycin over 48 hours at 0 and 21 °C. Moxalactam caused about a 15% loss at 0 °C and a 20 to 30% loss at 21 °C over 48 hours (1005).

Pennell et al. evaluated the potential for inactivation of tobramycin sulfate (Lilly) 9 μg/ml with 100- and 200-μg/ml concentrations of cefotaxime sodium (Hoechst-Roussel) in human serum. No loss of tobramycin sulfate was determined by TDx fluorescence polarization immunoassay over 48 hours when stored at 4, 24, and 37 °C (1420).

Vancomycin— The compatibility or incompatibility of vancomycin HCl mixed with or administered simultaneously with cefotaxime sodium is concentration dependent (2189). See Y-Site Compatibility above. Vancomycin HCl has a low pH and is variably compatible with drugs having neutral to mildly alkaline pH, including cephalosporins and penicillins. The compatibility may depend on a number of factors, including concentration of each drug, dilution vehicle, actual pH of solutions, and completeness of mixing during administration. Combinations that are compatible when well mixed may result in precipitation if only partially mixed, presumably because of regionally different concentrations and pH values. If attempting to administer vancomycin HCl with cefotaxime sodium, take care to ensure that the specific combination and the concentrations are compatible under the exact administration conditions to be used. An inline filter should be used as a final safety measure (2189).

Miscellaneous— Cefotaxime sodium should not be mixed in alkaline solutions such as sodium bicarbonate injection (2) or solutions containing aminophylline (792).

CEFOTETAN DISODIUM
AHFS 8:12.07

Cefotan   **Zeneca**

Products— Cefotetan disodium (Zeneca) is available in 1- and 2-g vials and infusion bottles and 10-g pharmacy bulk packages (2).

For intramuscular injection, reconstitute the vials with sterile water for injection, bacteriostatic water for injection, sodium chloride 0.9%, or lidocaine HCl 0.5 or 1%. Then shake well to dissolve and let stand until clear. Recommended volumes for reconstitution are shown in Table 1 (2).

For intravenous use, reconstitute the vials with sterile water for injection in the amounts noted in Table 1, shake well to dissolve, and let stand until clear. Piggyback infusion vials may be reconstituted with 50 to 100 ml of dextrose 5% in water or sodium chloride 0.9% (2).

Reconstitute the 10-g pharmacy bulk package with sterile water for injection, dextrose 5% in water, or sodium chloride 0.9% according to the instructions on the package label. Then shake it well to dissolve and let stand until clear (2).

Cefotetan (Zeneca) is also available as a frozen premixed infusion solution of 1 or 2 g in 50 ml of dextrose 5% in water (2).

Table 1. Recommended Dilutions of Cefotetan Disodium Vials (2; 4)

Vial Size	Volume of Diluent	Withdrawable Volume	Approximate Concentration
Intramuscular			
1 g	2 ml	2.5 ml	400 mg/ml
2 g	3 ml	4.0 ml	500 mg/ml
Intravenous			
1 g	10 ml	10.5 ml	95 mg/ml
2 g	10 to 20 ml	11 to 21 ml	182 to 95 mg/ml
Piggyback			
1 g	50 ml		20 mg/ml
	100 ml		10 mg/ml
2 g	50 ml		39 mg/ml
	100 ml		20 mg/ml

pH— Reconstituted solutions have a pH of 4.5 to 6.5 (2).

Osmolarity— Concentrations of 100 to 200 mg/ml in sterile water for injection have osmolarities of 400 to 800 mOsm/L, respectively.

The 1- and 2-g infusion bottles reconstituted with 50 to 100 ml of dextrose 5% in water or sodium chloride 0.9%, having concentrations of 10 to 39 mg/ml, have osmolarities of 340 to 480 mOsm/L. Intramuscular concentrations of 375 to 471.5 mg/ml are extremely hypertonic, with osmolarities greater than 1500 mOsm/L (4).

Sodium Content— Each gram of cefotetan disodium contains approximately 3.5 mEq (80 mg) of sodium (2).

Administration— Cefotetan disodium may be administered by deep intramuscular injection, direct intravenous injection over three to five minutes, and intermittent intravenous infusion in 50 to 100 ml of dextrose 5% in water or sodium chloride 0.9% (2; 4) infused over 20 to 60 minutes (2; 4). The manufacturer recommends temporarily discontinuing other solutions being administered at the same site (2; 4).

Stability— Intact vials should be stored at 22 °C or less and protected from light. The frozen premixed infusion solutions should be stored at −20 °C (2). Cefotetan disodium powder is white to pale yellow. Solutions may vary from colorless to yellow, depending on the concentration (2).

When reconstituted as recommended, cefotetan disodium solutions are stable for 24 hours at room temperature (25 °C) and 96 hours under refrigeration (5 °C). In disposable glass or plastic syringes, the drug also is stable for 24 hours at room temperature and 96 hours under refrigeration (2; 4).

Freezing Solutions— The manufacturer states that solutions reconstituted as recommended are stable for at least one week when frozen at −20 °C (2). The manufacturer also has stated that cefotetan disodium as the reconstituted solution in vials is stable for one year at −20 °C; in a large volume parenteral solution, it is stable for 30 weeks at −20 °C (283). Thawing should be performed at room temperature, and thawed solutions should not be refrozen (2; 4).

In one study, cefotetan disodium (Stuart) 20 mg/ml in dextrose 5% in water (Travenol) in PVC containers showed a potency loss of about 2% after two weeks at −20 °C by antimicrobial assay (966).

In another study, cefotetan disodium (Stuart) 20 mg/ml in dextrose 5% in water and sodium chloride 0.9% in PVC bags was visually clear and exhibited little or no loss by HPLC after 60 days when frozen at −10 °C (1598).

Compatibility Information

Solution Compatibility

Cefotetan disodium

Solution	Mfr	Mfr	Conc/L	Remarks	Ref	C/I
Dextrose 5% in water	TR[a]	STU	2 g	3% loss in 14 days at both 20 and 4 °C by antimicrobial assay	966	C
	[a]	AY	20 and 40 g	Visually compatible with 10% loss in 3.5 days at 23 °C and 13 days at 4 °C	1591	C
	TR[a]	STU	20 g	8% loss by HPLC in 2 days and 11% loss in 3 days at 25 °C. 6% loss in 41 days at 5 °C	1598	C
Sodium chloride 0.9%	[a]	AY	20 and 40 g	Visually compatible with 10% loss in 3.5 days at 23 °C and 14 days at 4 °C	1591	C
	TR[a]	STU	20 g	8% loss by HPLC in 2 days and 11% loss in 3 days at 25 °C. 5% loss in 41 days at 5 °C	1598	C

[a]Tested in PVC containers.

Drugs in Syringe Compatibility

Cefotetan disodium

Drug (in syringe)	Mfr	Amt	Mfr	Amt	Remarks	Ref	C/I
Doxapram HCl	RB	400 mg/ 20 ml		1 g/ 10 ml	Immediate turbidity	1177	I
Promethazine HCl	ES	25 mg/ 1 ml	ZE	10 mg/ ml[a]	White precipitate, resembling cottage cheese, forms immediately	1753	I

[a]Tested in dextrose 5% in water.

Y-Site Injection Compatibility (1:1 Mixture)

Cefotetan disodium

Drug	Mfr	Conc	Mfr	Conc	Remarks	Ref	C/I
Allopurinol sodium	BW	3 mg/ml[b]	STU	20 mg/ml[b]	Physically compatible with no change in measured turbidity or increase in particle content in 4 hr at 22 °C	1686	C

Y-Site Injection Compatibility (1:1 Mixture) (Cont.)

Cefotetan disodium

Drug	Mfr	Conc	Mfr	Conc	Remarks	Ref	C/I
Amifostine	USB	10 mg/ml[a]	STU	20 mg/ml[a]	Physically compatible with no change in measured turbidity or increase in particle content in 4 hr at 23 °C	1845	**C**
Aztreonam	SQ	40 mg/ml[b]	STU	20 mg/ml[b]	Physically compatible with no subvisual haze or particle formation in 4 hr at 23 °C	1758	**C**
Cisatracurium besylate	GW	0.1 and 2 mg/ml[a]	STU	20 mg/ml[a]	Physically compatible with no change in measured turbidity or increase in particle content in 4 hr at 23 °C	2074	**C**
	GW	5 mg/ml[a]	STU	20 mg/ml[a]	Dense turbidity forms immediately	2074	**I**
Diltiazem HCl	MMD	5 mg/ml	STU	10 and 200 mg/ml[b]	Visually compatible	1807	**C**
	MMD	1 mg/ml[b]	STU	180 mg/ml[b]	Visually compatible	1807	**C**
Docetaxel	RPR	0.9 mg/ml[a]	ZEN	20 mg/ml[a]	Physically compatible with no change in measured turbidity or increase in particle content in 4 hr at 23 °C	2224	**C**
Etoposide phosphate	BR	5 mg/ml[a]	ZEN	20 mg/ml[a]	Physically compatible with no change in measured turbidity or increase in particle content in 4 hr at 23 °C	2218	**C**
Famotidine	MSD	0.2 mg/ml[a]	STU	20 mg/ml[b]	Physically compatible for 14 hr	1196	**C**
Filgrastim	AMG	30 μg/ml[a]	STU	20 mg/ml[a]	Physically compatible with no change in measured turbidity or increase in particle content in 4 hr at 22 °C	1687	**C**
Fluconazole	RR	2 mg/ml	STU	40 mg/ml	Physically compatible for 24 hr at 25 °C	1407	**C**
Fludarabine phosphate	BX	1 mg/ml[a]	STU	20 mg/ml[a]	Physically compatible for 4 hr at room temperature under fluorescent light	1439	**C**
Gemcitabine HCl	LI	10 mg/ml[b]	ZEN	20 mg/ml[b]	Physically compatible with no change in measured turbidity or increase in particle content in 4 hr at 23 °C	2226	**C**
Granisetron HCl	SKB	0.05 mg/ml[a]	STU	20 mg/ml[a]	Physically compatible with no change in measured turbidity or increase in particle content in 4 hr at 23 °C	2000	**C**
Heparin sodium	TR	50 units/ml	STU	40 mg/ml[a]	Visually compatible for 6 hr at 25 °C	1793	**C**
Insulin, regular	LI	0.2 unit/ml[b]	STU	20 and 40 mg/ml[a]	Physically compatible for 2 hr at 25 °C	1395	**C**
Melphalan HCl	BW	0.1 mg/ml[b]	STU	20 mg/ml[b]	Physically compatible with no change in measured turbidity or increase in particle content in 3 hr at 22 °C	1557	**C**
Meperidine HCl	WY	10 mg/ml[b]	STU	20 and 40 mg/ml[a]	Physically compatible for 1 hr at 25 °C	1338	**C**
Morphine sulfate	ES	1 mg/ml[b]	STU	20 and 40 mg/ml[a]	Physically compatible for 1 hr at 25 °C	1338	**C**
Paclitaxel	NCI	1.2 mg/ml[a]	STU	20 mg/ml[a]	Physically compatible with no change in measured turbidity in 4 hr at 22 °C	1556	**C**
Promethazine HCl	ES	25 mg	ZE	10 mg/ml[a]	White lumpy precipitate forms immediately but dissipates after several minutes of agitation	1753	**I**

Y-Site Injection Compatibility (1:1 Mixture) (Cont.)

Cefotetan disodium

Drug	Mfr	Conc	Mfr	Conc	Remarks	Ref	C/I
Propofol	ZEN	10 mg/ml	STU	20 mg/ml[a]	Physically compatible for 1 hr at 23 °C with no increase in particle content	2066	**C**
Remifentanil HCl	GW	0.025 and 0.25 mg/ml[b]	ZEN	20 mg/ml[a]	Physically compatible with no change in measured turbidity or increase in particle content in 4 hr at 23 °C	2075	**C**
Sargramostim	IMM	10 µg/ml[b]	STU	20 mg/ml[b]	Physically compatible for 4 hr at 22 °C	1436	**C**
Tacrolimus	FUJ	1 mg/ml[b]	STU	40 mg/ml[a]	Visually compatible for 24 hr at 25 °C	1630	**C**
Teniposide	BR	0.1 mg/ml[a]	STU	20 mg/ml[a]	Physically compatible with no subvisual haze or particle formation in 4 hr at 23 °C	1725	**C**
Theophylline	TR	4 mg/ml	STU	40 mg/ml[a]	Visually compatible for 6 hr at 25 °C	1793	**C**
Thiotepa	IMM[c]	1 mg/ml[a]	STU	20 mg/ml[a]	Physically compatible with no change in measured turbidity or increase in particle content in 4 hr at 23 °C	1861	**C**
TNA #218 to #226[d]			ZEN	20 mg/ml[a]	Visually compatible with no precipitate or emulsion damage apparent in 4 hr at 23 °C	2215	**C**
TPN #212 to #215[d]			STU	20 mg/ml[a]	Physically compatible with no change in measured turbidity or increase in particle content in 4 hr at 23 °C	2109	**C**
Vancomycin HCl	AB	20 mg/ml[a]	ZEN	200 mg/ml[e]	Transient precipitate forms, followed by clear solution. White precipitate forms in 4 hr	2189	**I**
	AB	20 mg/ml[a]	ZEN	10 and 50 mg/ml[a]	Gross white precipitate forms immediately	2189	**I**
	AB	20 mg/ml[a]	ZEN	1 mg/ml[a]	Subvisual measured haze forms immediately, followed by white precipitate in 4 hr	2189	**I**
	AB	2 mg/ml[a]	ZEN	1[a], 10[a], 50[a], 200[e] mg/ml	Physically compatible with no change in measured turbidity or increase in particle content in 4 hr at 23 °C	2189	**C**
Vinorelbine tartrate	BW	1 mg/ml[b]	STU	20 mg/ml[b]	Tiny particles form immediately, becoming numerous in cloudy solution in 4 hr at 22 °C	1558	**I**

[a]*Tested in dextrose 5% in water.*
[b]*Tested in sodium chloride 0.9%.*
[c]*Lyophilized formulation tested.*
[d]*Refer to Appendix I for the composition of parenteral nutrition solutions. TNA indicates a 3-in-1 admixture, and TPN indicates a 2-in-1 admixture.*
[e]*Tested in sterile water for injection.*

Additional Compatibility Information

Solutions—— Cefotetan disodium (Zeneca) retains its potency for 24 hours at room temperature and 96 hours under refrigeration in concentrations of 10 to 40 mg/ml in dextrose 5% in water and sodium chloride 0.9% (4).

Miscellaneous—— Cefotetan disodium is stated to be physically incompatible with tetracyclines and heparin, possibly resulting in cloudiness and precipitation (4). The manufacturer recommends that cefotetan disodium not be mixed with aminoglycoside antibiotics (2).

However, the manufacturer has stated that cefotetan disodium is compatible with the following drugs (283):

Amikacin sulfate
Aminophylline
Ampicillin sodium
Atropine sulfate
Azlocillin sodium
Cimetidine HCl
Digoxin
Dopamine HCl
Doxycycline hyclate
Epinephrine HCl
Erythromycin lactobionate

Furosemide
Kanamycin sulfate
Mezlocillin disodium
Multivitamins
Oxytocin
Penicillin G potassium
Piperacillin sodium
Ticarcillin disodium
Tobramycin sulfate
Vitamin B complex with C

The manufacturer has also stated that cefotetan disodium is incompatible with gentamicin sulfate, heparin sodium, and netilmicin sulfate (283).

Vancomycin— The compatibility or incompatibility of vancomycin HCl mixed with or administered simultaneously with cefotetan disodium is concentration dependent (2189). See Y-Site Compatibility above. Vancomycin HCl has a low pH and is variably compatible with drugs having neutral to mildly alkaline pH, including cephalosporins and penicillins. The compatibility may depend on a number of factors, including concentration of each drug, dilution vehicle, actual pH of solutions, and completeness of mixing during administration. Combinations that are compatible when well mixed may result in precipitation if only partially mixed, presumably because of regionally different concentrations and pH values. If attempting to administer vancomycin HCl with cefotetan disodium, take care to ensure that the specific combination and the concentrations are compatible under the exact administration conditions to be used. An inline filter should be used as a final safety measure (2189).

CEFOXITIN SODIUM
AHFS 8:12.07

Mefoxin   **Merck**

Products— Cefoxitin sodium (Merck) is available in vials and infusion bottles containing the equivalent of 1 and 2 g of cefoxitin. It is also available in 10-g bulk bottles (2).

Cefoxitin sodium (Merck) is also available as a frozen premixed infusion solution of 1 or 2 g in dextrose 5% in water. Sodium bicarbonate or hydrochloric acid or both may have been added to adjust the pH (2; 4).

For intravenous administration, the vial contents may be reconstituted with sterile water for injection. The 1- and 2-g infusion bottles may be reconstituted with any compatible solution. (2; 4). (See Table 1.)

After addition of the diluent, shake the vial and allow the solution to stand until it becomes clear (2).

For intravenous infusion, the primary solution may be diluted further in 50 to 1000 ml of compatible diluent (2). (See Compatibility Information.)

Table 1. Recommended Dilutions of Cefoxitin Sodium (2)

Vial Size	Route	Volume of Diluent	Withdrawable Volume	Approximate Concentration
1 g	Intravenous	10 ml	10.5 ml	95 mg/ml
(Infusion bottle)	Intravenous	50 or 100 ml	50 or 100 ml	20 or 10 mg/ml
2 g	Intravenous	10 ml	11.1 ml	180 mg/ml
	Intravenous	20 ml	21 ml	95 mg/ml
(Infusion bottle)	Intravenous	50 or 100 ml	50 or 100 ml	40 or 20 mg/ml
10-g bulk	Intravenous	43 or 93 ml	49 or 98.5 ml	200 or 100 mg/ml

The frozen premixed infusion should be thawed at room temperature and checked for leaks by squeezing the bag (2; 4).

pH— Reconstituted solutions have a pH of 4.2 to 7. The frozen premixed infusion has a pH of about 6.5 (2; 4).

Osmolality— The osmolality of cefoxitin sodium 1 and 2 g was calculated for the following dilutions (1054):

	Osmolality (mOsm/kg)	
Diluent	50 ml	100 ml
1 g		
Dextrose 5% in water	326	293
Sodium chloride 0.9%	352	319
2 g		
Dextrose 5% in water	388	329
Sodium chloride 0.9%	415	355

The osmolality of cefoxitin sodium (MSD) 50 mg/ml was determined to be 348 mOsm/kg in dextrose 5% in water and 361 mOsm/kg in sodium chloride 0.9% (1375). At 100 mg/ml in sterile water for injection, the osmolality is 468 mOsm/kg (1689).

Robinson et al. recommended the following maximum cefoxitin sodium concentrations to achieve osmolalities suitable for peripheral infusion in fluid-restricted patients (1180):

Diluent	Maximum Concentration (mg/ml)	Osmolality (mOsm/kg)
Dextrose 5% in water	62	531
Sodium chloride 0.9%	56	508
Sterile water for injection	112	437

Sodium Content— Each gram of cefoxitin sodium contains 2.3 mEq (53.8 mg) of sodium (2).

Displacement Volume— Each gram of cefoxitin sodium displaces about 0.7 ml (865).

Administration— Cefoxitin sodium may be administered by direct intravenous injection over three to five minutes directly into the vein or slowly into the tubing of a running compatible infusion solution, or by continuous or intermittent intravenous infusion. The manufacturer recommends temporarily discontinuing other solutions being administered at the site (2; 4).

Stability— Intact vials of cefoxitin sodium (MSD) should be stored below 30 °C. Exposure to temperatures above 50 °C should be avoided. The powder is white to off-white in color. Solutions may range from colorless to light amber (2). Both the dry material and solutions may darken, depending on storage conditions. Although moisture plays a role in the rate and intensity of the darkening, exposure to oxygen is the most significant factor. However, this discoloration is stated not to affect potency or relate to any significant chemical change. The concern over color is purely aesthetic (865).

Exposure of cefoxitin sodium (MSD) 40 mg/ml in sterile water for injection to 37 °C for 24 hours, to simulate the use of a portable infusion pump, resulted in about a 3 to 4% cefoxitin loss (1391).

pH Effects— Cefoxitin sodium at 1 and 10 mg/ml in aqueous solution is stable over pH 4 to 8. The time to 10% decomposition when stored at 25 °C was essentially independent of pH, ranging from 40 to 44 hours at pH 4 to 5 to 33 hours at pH 8. Under refrigeration, a pH 7 (unbuffered) aqueous solution showed 10% decomposition in 26 days. At pH less than 4, precipitation of the free acid may occur. Above pH 8, hydrolysis of the β-lactam group may result (308).

In another study, cefoxitin sodium in aqueous solution at 25 °C exhibited minimum rates of decomposition at pH 5 to 7. The solutions in this pH range showed 10% decomposition in about two days. At pH 3, about 40 hours elapsed before 10% decomposition occurred. However, at pH 9, only 14 hours was required to incur a 10% loss (630).

Reconstituted Solutions— Cefoxitin sodium solutions reconstituted as indicated in Table 2 are stable for 48 hours at 25 °C and at least seven days and, in some cases, up to one month at 5 °C (308).

Borst et al. reported that cefoxitin sodium (MSD) 1 and 2 g/ 10 ml in sterile water for injection, packaged in plastic syringes (Monoject), exhibited a 10% cefoxitin loss in two days at 24 °C and 23 days at 4 °C as determined by UV spectroscopy (1178).

Sorption— Cefoxitin sodium (MSD) 14 mg/L in sodium chloride 0.9% (Travenol) in PVC bags did not exhibit significant sorption to the plastic during one week of storage at room temperature (15 to 20 °C) (536).

In another study, cefoxitin sodium (MSD) 14 mg/L in sodium chloride 0.9% did not exhibit any loss due to sorption during a seven-hour simulated infusion through an infusion set (Travenol) consisting of a cellulose propionate burette chamber and 170 cm of PVC tubing (606).

The drug was also tested as a simulated infusion over at least one hour by a syringe pump system. A glass syringe on a syringe pump was fitted with 20 cm of polyethylene tubing or 50 cm of Silastic tubing. No loss of drug due to sorption was observed with either tubing (606).

In a study using all-plastic syringes, a 25-ml aliquot of cefoxitin sodium (MSD) 14 mg/L in sodium chloride 0.9% stored in syringes composed of polypropylene barrels and polyethylene plungers for

Table 2. Stability of Reconstituted Cefoxitin Sodium 1 g (308)

Diluent	Volume	Remarks
Bacteriostatic water for injection (benzyl alcohol)	2 ml	9% decomposition in 48 hr at 25 °C. 4% in 7 days and 10% in 1 month at 5 °C
Bacteriostatic water for injection (parabens)	2 ml	9% decomposition in 48 hr at 25 °C. 5% in 7 days and 12% in 1 month at 5 °C
Dextrose 5% in water	10 ml	9% decomposition in 48 hr at 25 °C, 2% in 7 days at 5 °C
Lidocaine HCl 0.5% (with parabens)	2 ml	8% decomposition in 48 hr at 25 °C. 5% in 7 days and 10% in 1 month at 5 °C
Lidocaine HCl 1% (with parabens)	2 ml	7% decomposition in 48 hr at 25 °C. 2% in 7 days and 10% in 1 month at 5 °C
Sodium chloride 0.9%	10 ml	8% decomposition in 48 hr at 25 °C
Water for injection	10 ml	10% decomposition in 48 hr at 25 °C, 1% in 7 days at 5 °C
	4 ml	7% decomposition in 48 hr at 25 °C, 2% in 7 days at 5 °C
	2 ml	8% decomposition in 48 hr at 25 °C. 2% in 7 days and 10% in 1 month at 5 °C
(In plastic syringe)	10 ml	6% decomposition in 24 hr and 11% in 48 hr at 25 °C

24 hours at room temperature in the dark showed no loss of drug due to sorption (606).

Reconstituted cefoxitin sodium stored in disposable plastic syringes is stable for 24 hours at room temperature and 48 hours under refrigeration (4).

Freezing Solutions— The stability of cefoxitin sodium reconstituted with the diluents as shown in Table 3 was evaluated in the frozen state at −20 °C. The solutions retained adequate potency for at least 30 weeks (308). Thawed solutions should not be refrozen (2).

In another study, cefoxitin sodium (MSD) 1 g/50 ml of dextrose 5% in water in PVC bags frozen at −20 °C for 30 days and then thawed by exposure to ambient temperature or microwave radiation showed no evidence of precipitation or color change and showed no loss of potency as determined microbiologically. Subsequent storage of the admixture at room temperature for 24 hours yielded a physically compatible solution which exhibited a 3 to 5% loss of potency (554).

A further evaluation using an HPLC procedure was performed on frozen cefoxitin sodium solutions thawed by microwave radiation. At concentrations of 1 g/50 ml and 1 g/100 ml in both dextrose 5% in water and sodium chloride 0.9% in PVC bags, the cefoxitin sodium solutions were frozen at −20 °C for 72 hours. They were then thawed by exposure to microwave radiation and allowed to stand at room temperature for six hours. No changes were noted in the visual appearance or pH. Also, no significant differences in concentration occurred, with all solutions being at least within 97% of the initial concentration (629).

Borst et al. reported that cefoxitin sodium (MSD) 1 and 2 g/10 ml in sterile water for injection, packaged in plastic syringes (Monoject) and frozen at −15 °C, was stable for the three-month study period, exhibiting less than a 10% loss as determined by UV spectroscopy (1178).

Table 3. Stability of Reconstituted Cefoxitin Sodium 1 g Frozen at −20 °C (308)

Diluent	Volume	Remarks
Bacteriostatic water for injection (benzyl alcohol)	10 ml	2% decomposition in 30 weeks. Thawed solutions showed 6% decomposition in 24 hr at 25 °C and 1% in 7 days at 5 °C
Bacteriostatic water for injection (parabens)	10 ml	2% decomposition in 30 weeks. Thawed solutions showed no decomposition in 24 hr at 25 °C and 1% in 7 days at 5 °C
Dextrose 5% in water	10 ml	3% decomposition in 30 weeks. Thawed solutions showed 8% decomposition in 24 hr at 25 °C and 6% in 7 days at 5 °C
Lidocaine HCl 0.5%	2 ml	2% cefoxitin decomposition in 26 weeks. Thawed solutions showed 6% decomposition in 24 hr at 25 °C. HPLC demonstrated lidocaine potency
Sodium chloride 0.9%	10 ml	5% decomposition in 30 weeks. Thawed solutions showed 3% decomposition in 24 hr at 25 °C and 6% in 7 days at 5 °C
Water for injection	10 ml	1% decomposition in 30 weeks. Thawed solutions showed 3% decomposition in 24 hr at 25 °C and 5% in 7 days at 5 °C
	4 ml	No decomposition in 13 weeks

Miller and Pesko reported an approximate twofold increase in particles of 2 to 60 μm produced by freezing and thawing cefoxitin sodium (MSD) 2 g/100 ml of dextrose 5% in water (Travenol). The reconstituted drug was filtered through a 0.45-μm filter into PVC bags of solution and frozen for seven days at −20 °C. Thawing was performed at room temperature (29 °C) for 12 hours. Although the total number of particles increased significantly, no particles greater than 60 μm were observed; the solutions complied with USP standards for particle sizes and numbers in large volume parenteral solutions (822).

Stiles et al. reported a 3% or less cefoxitin sodium (MSD) loss from a solution containing 40 mg/ml in sterile water for injection in PVC and glass containers after 30 days at −20 °C. Subsequent thawing and storage for four days at 5 °C, followed by 24 hours at 37 °C to simulate the use of a portable infusion pump, resulted in an additional 3 to 4% cefoxitin loss (1391).

Cefoxitin sodium in sodium chloride 0.9%, Ringer's injection, lactated, and dextrose 5% in water in PVC bags is stable for 26 weeks if kept frozen (4).

Compatibility Information

Solution Compatibility

Cefoxitin sodium

Solution	Mfr	Mfr	Conc/L	Remarks	Ref	C/I
Dextrose 5% in Ringer's injection, lactated	a	MSD	1, 2, 10, 20 g	5 to 8% decomposition in 24 hr and 12 to 13% in 48 hr at 25 °C. 3 to 5% in 7 days at 5 °C	308	C
Dextrose 5% in sodium chloride 0.2%	a	MSD	1 g	5% decomposition in 24 hr and 11% in 48 hr at 25 °C	308	C
Dextrose 5% in sodium chloride 0.45%	a	MSD	1 g	4% decomposition in 24 hr and 10% in 48 hr at 25 °C	308	C
Dextrose 5% in sodium chloride 0.9%	a	MSD	1 g	4% decomposition in 24 hr and 10% in 48 hr at 25 °C	308	C
Dextrose 5% in water	a	MSD	1, 2, 10 g	6 to 7% decomposition in 24 hr and 11 to 13% in 48 hr at 25 °C. 3 to 6% in 7 days at 5 °C	308	C
	a	MSD	20 g	7.5% decomposition in 24 hr and 13% in 48 hr at 25 °C. 4% in 7 days at 5 °C. No decomposition noted in 13 weeks at −20 °C	308	C
	TR[b]	MSD	1 g	9% decomposition in 24 hr and 11% in 48 hr at 25 °C	308	C
	TR[b]	MSD	20 g	No decomposition noted in 24 hr but 11% loss in 48 hr at 24 °C. 3% loss in 13 days at 5 °C	525	C
	TR[b]	MSD	20 g	Physically compatible with approximately 5% potency loss in 24 hr at room temperature	554	C
	MG[a]	MSD	20 g	Physically compatible with no loss in 24 hr and 6% loss in 48 hr at room temperature under fluorescent light	983	C

Solution Compatibility (Cont.)

Cefoxitin sodium

Solution	Mfr	Mfr	Conc/L	Remarks	Ref	C/I
Dextrose 10% in water	a	MSD	1 g	6% decomposition in 24 hr and 11% in 48 hr at 25 °C	308	C
Invert sugar 10% in sodium chloride 0.9%	a	MSD	1 g	3% decomposition in 24 hr and 12% in 48 hr at 25 °C	308	C
Invert sugar 5% in water	a	MSD	1 g	4% decomposition in 24 hr and 10% in 48 hr at 25 °C	308	C
Invert sugar 10% in water	a	MSD	1 g	3% decomposition in 24 hr and 8% in 48 hr at 25 °C	308	C
Ionosol B with dextrose 5% in water	AB[a]	MSD	1, 2, 10 g	6 to 8% decomposition in 24 hr and 12 to 13% in 48 hr at 25 °C. 3 to 6% in 7 days at 5 °C	308	C
Mannitol 10% in water	a	MSD	1, 2, 10, 20 g	4 to 5% decomposition in 24 hr and 10 to 11% in 48 hr at 25 °C. 2 to 5% in 7 days at 5 °C	308	C
Normosol M in dextrose 5% in water	AB[a]	MSD	1, 2, 10, 20 g	4 to 6% decomposition in 24 hr and 11 to 12% in 48 hr at 25 °C. 3 to 5% in 7 days at 5 °C	308	C
Ringer's injection	a	MSD	1 g	2% decomposition in 24 hr and 12% in 48 hr at 25 °C	308	C
Ringer's injection, lactated	a	MSD	1, 2, 10, 20 g	5 to 7% decomposition in 24 hr and 10 to 12% in 48 hr at 25 °C. 3% in 7 days at 5 °C	308	C
	TR[b]	MSD	1 g	7% decomposition in 24 hr and 9% in 48 hr at 25 °C	308	C
Sodium bicarbonate 5%	a	MSD	1 g	6% decomposition in 24 hr and 13% in 48 hr at 25 °C	308	C
Sodium chloride 0.9%	a	MSD	1 g	5% decomposition in 24 hr and 11% in 48 hr at 25 °C	308	C
	a	MSD	10 and 20 g	8 to 10% decomposition in 24 hr and 13 and 15% in 48 hr at 25 °C. 4 to 5% in 48 hr at 5 °C	308	C
	TR[b]	MSD	20 g	No decomposition noted in 24 hr but 12% loss in 48 hr at 24 °C. 3% loss in 13 days at 5 °C	525	C
	MG[a]	MSD	20 g	Physically compatible with no loss in 24 hr and 6% loss in 48 hr at room temperature under fluorescent light	983	C
Sodium lactate ⅙ M	a	MSD	1 g	5% decomposition in 24 hr and 8% in 48 hr at 25 °C	308	C
TPN #107[c]			1 g	Physically compatible and cefoxitin activity retained for 24 hr at 21 °C by microbiological assay	1326	C

[a]Tested in glass containers.
[b]Tested in PVC containers.
[c]Refer to Appendix I for the composition of parenteral nutrition solutions. TPN indicates a 2-in-1 admixture.

Additive Compatibility

Cefoxitin sodium

Drug	Mfr	Conc/L	Mfr	Conc/L	Test Soln	Remarks	Ref	C/I
Amikacin sulfate	BR	5 g	MSD	5 g	D5S	9% cefoxitin decomposition at 25 °C and none at 5 °C in 48 hr. No amikacin decomposition at 25 °C and 1% at 5 °C in 48 hr	308	C

Additive Compatibility (Cont.)

Cefoxitin sodium

Drug	Mfr	Conc/L	Mfr	Conc/L	Test Soln	Remarks	Ref	C/I
Aztreonam	SQ	10 and 20 g	MSD	10 and 20 g	D5W, NS[a]	Both drugs stable for 12 hr at 25 °C. Yellow color accompanied 6 to 12% aztreonam loss and 9 to 15% cefoxitin loss in 48 hr at 25 °C	1023	**I**
	SQ	10 and 20 g	MSD	10 and 20 g	D5W[a]	3 to 6% cefoxitin loss and no aztreonam loss in 7 days at 4 °C	1023	**C**
	SQ	10 and 20 g	MSD	10 and 20 g	NS[a]	3 to 5% aztreonam loss and no cefoxitin loss in 7 days at 4 °C	1023	**C**
Cimetidine HCl	SKF	3 g	MSD	10 g	D5W	Physically compatible and cimetidine chemically stable for 24 hr at room temperature. Cefoxitin not tested	551	**C**
Clindamycin phosphate	UP	9 g	MSD	20 g	D5W[b]	Physically compatible with no loss of either drug in 48 hr at room temperature under fluorescent light	983	**C**
	UP	9 g	MSD	20 g	NS[b]	Physically compatible with no clindamycin loss and 7% cefoxitin loss in 48 hr at room temperature under fluorescent light	983	**C**
Gentamicin sulfate	SC	400 mg	MSD	5 g	D5S	4% cefoxitin decomposition in 24 hr and 11% in 48 hr at 25 °C. 2% in 48 hr at 5 °C. 9% gentamicin decomposition in 24 hr and 23% in 48 hr at 25 °C. 2% in 48 hr at 5 °C	308	**C**
Kanamycin sulfate	BR	5 g	MSD	5 g	D5S	9% cefoxitin decomposition at 25 °C and 1% at 5 °C in 48 hr. 6% kanamycin decomposition at 25 °C and none at 5 °C in 48 hr	308	**C**
Metronidazole	RP	5 g[c]	FC	30 g		Physically compatible with little or no pH change for at least 24 hr at 4 °C	807	**C**
	RP	5 g[c]	FC	30 g		Physically compatible but with a significant change in pH in 6 to 12 hr at 23 °C	807	**?**
	SE	5 g	MSD	30 g		9% cefoxitin loss in 48 hr at 25 °C and 3% loss in 12 days at 5 °C. No metronidazole loss occurred	993	**C**
Metronidazole HCl with sodium bicarbonate	SE AB	5 g 50 mEq	MSD	2 g	D5W, NS	Physically compatible for 48 hr	765	**C**
Multivitamins	USV	50 ml	MSD	10 g	W	5% cefoxitin decomposition in 24 hr and 10% in 48 hr at 25 °C. 3% in 48 hr at 5 °C. TLC showed no other transformation products	308	**C**
Ranitidine HCl	GL	50 mg and 2 g		10 g	D5W	Ranitidine chemically stable by HPLC for only 4 hr at 25 °C. Cefoxitin not tested	1515	**I**
Sodium bicarbonate (Neut)	AB	200 mg/g cefoxitin	MSD	1, 2, 10, 20 g	W	5 to 6% cefoxitin decomposition in 24 hr and 11 to 12% in 48 hr at 25 °C. 2 to 3% in 7 days at 5 °C	308	**C**
Tobramycin sulfate	LI	400 mg	MSD	5 g	D5S	5% cefoxitin decomposition in 24 hr and 13% in 48 hr at 25 °C. 3% in 48 hr at 5 °C. 8% tobramycin decomposition in 24 hr and 37% in 48 hr at 25 °C. 3% in 48 hr at 5 °C	308	**C**

Additive Compatibility (Cont.)

Cefoxitin sodium

Drug	Mfr	Conc/L	Mfr	Conc/L	Test Soln	Remarks	Ref	C/I
Verapamil HCl	KN	80 mg	MSD	4 g	D5W, NS	Physically compatible for 24 hr	764	C
Vitamin B complex with C	RC	50 ml	MSD	10 g	W	No cefoxitin decomposition in 24 hr and 8% in 48 hr at 25 °C. 6% in 48 hr at 5 °C. TLC showed no other transformation products	308	C

[a]Tested in PVC containers.
[b]Tested in glass bottles.
[c]Minibags (100 ml) containing metronidazole 500 mg with disodium phosphate 150 mg, citric acid 44 mg, and sodium chloride 740 mg. This product differs from the Searle product.

Drugs in Syringe Compatibility

Cefoxitin sodium

Drug (in syringe)	Mfr	Amt	Mfr	Amt	Remarks	Ref	C/I
Heparin sodium		2500 units/ 1 ml	MSD	2 g	Physically compatible for at least 5 min	1053	C

Y-Site Injection Compatibility (1:1 Mixture)

Cefoxitin sodium

Drug	Mfr	Conc	Mfr	Conc	Remarks	Ref	C/I
Acyclovir sodium	BW	5 mg/ml[a]	MSD	20 mg/ml[a]	Physically compatible for 4 hr at 25 °C	1157	C
Amifostine	USB	10 mg/ml[a]	MSD	20 mg/ml[a]	Physically compatible with no change in measured turbidity or increase in particle content in 4 hr at 23 °C	1845	C
Amphotericin B cholesteryl sulfate complex	SEQ	0.83 mg/ml[a]	ME	20 mg/ml[a]	Physically compatible with little or no change in measured turbidity or increase in particle content in 4 hr at 23 °C under fluorescent light	2117	C
Aztreonam	SQ	40 mg/ml[a]	MSD	20 mg/ml[a]	Physically compatible with no subvisual haze or particle formation in 4 hr at 23 °C	1758	C
Cisatracurium besylate	GW	0.1 mg/ml[a]	ME	20 mg/ml[a]	Physically compatible with no change in measured turbidity or increase in particle content in 4 hr 23 °C	2074	C
	GW	2 and 5 mg/ml[a]	ME	20 mg/ml[a]	Subvisual haze forms immediately	2074	I
Cyclophosphamide	MJ	20 mg/ml[a]	MSD	20 mg/ml[a]	Physically compatible for 4 hr at 25 °C	1194	C
Diltiazem HCl	MMD	5 mg/ml	MSD	10 and 200 mg/ml[b]	Visually compatible	1807	C
	MMD	1 mg/ml[b]	MSD	200 mg/ml[b]	Visually compatible	1807	C
Docetaxel	RPR	0.9 mg/ml[a]	ME	20 mg/ml[a]	Physically compatible with no change in measured turbidity or increase in particle content in 4 hr at 23 °C	2224	C
Doxorubicin HCl liposome injection	SEQ	0.4 mg/ml[a]	ME	20 mg/ml[a]	Physically compatible with little or no change in measured turbidity and no increase in particle content in 4 hr at 23 °C	2087	C

Y-Site Injection Compatibility (1:1 Mixture) (Cont.)

Cefoxitin sodium

Drug	Mfr	Conc	Mfr	Conc	Remarks	Ref	C/I
Etoposide phosphate	BR	5 mg/ml[a]	ME	20 mg/ml[a]	Physically compatible with no change in measured turbidity jor increase in particle content in 4 hr at 23 °C	2218	C
Famotidine	MSD ME	0.2 mg/ml[a] 2 mg/ml[b]	MSD	20 mg/ml[b] 20 mg/ml[a]	Physically compatible for 14 hr Visually compatible for 4 hr at 22 °C	1196 1936	C C
Filgrastim	AMG	30 μg/ml[a]	MSD	20 mg/ml[a]	Haze, particles, and filaments form immediately	1687	I
Fluconazole	RR	2 mg/ml	MSD	40 mg/ml	Physically compatible for 24 hr at 25 °C	1407	C
Foscarnet sodium	AST	24 mg/ml	MSD	40 mg/ml	Physically compatible for 24 hr at room temperature under fluorescent light	1335	C
Gemcitabine HCl	LI	10 mg/ml[b]	ME	20 mg/ml[b]	Physically compatible with no change in measured turbidity or increase in particle content in 4 hr at 23 °C	2226	C
Granisetron HCl	SKB	0.05 mg/ml[a]	ME	20 mg/ml[a]	Physically compatible with no change in measured turbidity or increase in particle content in 4 hr at 23 °C	2000	C
Hetastarch	DCC	6%	MSD	20 mg/ml[a]	Precipitate forms after 1 hr at room temperature	1313	I
Hydromorphone HCl	WY	0.2 mg/ml[a]	MSD	20 mg/ml[a]	Physically compatible for at least 4 hr at 25 °C under fluorescent light	987	C
Magnesium sulfate	IX	16.7, 33.3, 66.7, 100 mg/ml[a]	MSD	20 mg/ml[a]	Physically compatible for at least 4 hr at 32 °C	813	C
Meperidine HCl	WY WY	10 mg/ml[a] 10 mg/ml[b]	MSD MSD	20 mg/ml[a] 40 mg/ml[a]	Physically compatible for at least 4 hr at 25 °C under fluorescent light Physically compatible for 1 hr at 25 °C	987 1338	C C
Morphine sulfate	WI ES	1 mg/ml[a] 1 mg/ml[b]	MSD MSD	20 mg/ml[a] 40 mg/ml[a]	Physically compatible for at least 4 hr at 25 °C under fluorescent light Physically compatible for 1 hr at 25 °C	987 1338	C C
Ondansetron HCl	GL	1 mg/ml[b]	MSD	20 mg/ml[a]	Physically compatible for 4 hr at 22 °C	1365	C
Pentamidine isethionate	FUJ	3 mg/ml[a]	ME	20 mg/ml[c]	Cloudiness and powder-like precipitate form immediately	1880	I
Perphenazine	SC	0.02 mg/ml[a]	MSD	20 mg/ml[d]	Physically compatible for 4 hr at 25 °C	1155	C
Propofol	ZEN	10 mg/ml	ME	20 mg/ml[a]	Physically compatible for 1 hr at 23 °C with no increase in particle content	2066	C
Remifentanil HCl	GW	0.025 and 0.25 mg/ml[b]	ME	20 mg/ml[a]	Physically compatible with no change in measured turbidity or increase in particle content in 4 hr at 23 °C	2075	C
Teniposide	BR	0.1 mg/ml[a]	MSD	20 mg/ml[a]	Physically compatible with no subvisual haze or particle formation in 4 hr at 23 °C	1725	C
Thiotepa	IMM[e]	1 mg/ml[a]	ME	20 mg/ml[a]	Physically compatible with no change in measured turbidity or increase in particle content in 4 hr at 23 °C	1861	C
TNA #73[f]		32.5 ml[g]	MSD	1 g/50 ml[a]	Physically compatible for 4 hr at 25 °C by visual observation	1008	C

Y-Site Injection Compatibility (1:1 Mixture) (Cont.)

			Cefoxitin sodium				
Drug	Mfr	Conc	Mfr	Conc	Remarks	Ref	C/I
TNA #218 to #226[f]			ME	20 mg/ml[a]	Visually compatible with no precipitate or emulsion damage apparent in 4 hr at 23 °C	2215	**C**
TPN #61[f]		[h]	MSD	200 mg/2.1 ml[i]	Physically compatible	1012	**C**
		[j]	MSD	1.2 g/12.6 ml[i]	Physically compatible	1012	**C**
TPN #189[f]			MSD	200 mg/ml[k]	Visually compatible for 24 hr at 22 °C	1767	**C**
TPN #212 to #215[f]			ME	20 mg/ml[a]	Physically compatible with no change in measured turbidity or increase in particle content in 4 hr at 23 °C	2109	**C**
Vancomycin HCl	AB	20 mg/ml[a]	ME	180 mg/ml[k]	Transient precipitate forms, followed by clear solution	2189	**?**
	AB	20 mg/ml[a]	ME	50 mg/ml[a]	Gross white precipitate forms immediately	2189	**I**
	AB	20 mg/ml[a]	ME	10 mg/ml[a]	Visible haze forms in 4 hr at 23 °C	2189	**I**
	AB	20 mg/ml[a]	ME	1 mg/ml[a]	Physically compatible with no change in measured turbidity or increase in particle content in 4 hr at 23 °C	2189	**C**
	AB	2 mg/ml[a]	ME	1[a], 10[a], 50[a], 180[k] mg/ml	Physically compatible with no change in measured turbidity or increase in particle content in 4 hr at 23 °C	2189	**C**

[a]*Tested in dextrose 5% in water.*
[b]*Tested in sodium chloride 0.9%.*
[c]*Tested in dextrose 4% in water.*
[d]*Manufacturer's premixed solution.*
[e]*Lyophilized formulation tested.*
[f]*Refer to Appendix I for the composition of parenteral nutrition solutions. TNA indicates a 3-in-1 admixture, and TPN indicates a 2-in-1 admixture.*
[g]*A 32.5-ml sample of parenteral nutrition solution combined with 50 ml of antibiotic solution.*
[h]*Run at 21 ml/hr.*
[i]*Given over five minutes by syringe pump.*
[j]*Run at 94 ml/hr.*
[k]*Tested in sterile water for injection.*

Additional Compatibility Information

Peritoneal Dialysis Solutions— Cefoxitin sodium 2 mg/ml in peritoneal dialysis solution (McGaw) containing dextrose 2.5% and electrolytes was physically compatible for three hours at room temperature. Furthermore, no significant loss of antibacterial activity was apparent by microbiological determination (142).

Aminoglycosides— The manufacturer recommends that cefoxitin sodium not be mixed with aminoglycoside antibiotics such as amikacin sulfate, gentamicin sulfate, and tobramycin sulfate (2). However, compatibility studies show that such admixtures may indeed be sufficiently stable to allow combined mixture in the same solution.

To determine if spurious aminoglycoside levels could result from a delay in assaying blood samples, Tindula et al. evaluated the inactivation of amikacin 35 μg/ml and gentamicin and tobramycin 10 μg/ml in human serum by 400-μg/ml concentrations of several penicillins and cephalosporins. Samples were stored for 24 hours at room temperature and frozen at −20 °C. In the room temperature samples, cefoxitin caused moderate inactivation, 20% or less. Freezing the samples at −20 °C prevented significant inactivation of the aminoglycosides (824).

Spruill et al. evaluated the effect of various cephalosporins on tobramycin sulfate 7.7 μg/ml in human serum. At concentrations of 250 and 1000 μg/ml, cefazolin, cefoxitin, cefamandole, cefoperazone, and cefotaxime caused about a 10 to 15% loss of tobramycin over 48 hours at 0 and 21 °C. Moxalactam caused about a 15% loss at 0 °C and a 20 to 30% loss at 21 °C over 48 hours (1005).

Cefoxitin sodium (MSD) 125 μg/ml separately combined with the aminoglycosides amikacin sulfate (Bristol), gentamicin sulfate (Schering), and tobramycin sulfate (Lilly) at a concentration of 25 μg/ml in peritoneal dialysis solution (Dianeal 1.5%) exhibited enhanced rates of lethality to *Staphylococcus aureus*, *Escherichia coli*, and *Pseudomonas aeruginosa* compared to any of the drugs alone (1623).

Vancomycin— The compatibility or incompatibility of vancomycin HCl mixed with or administered simultaneously with cefoxitin sodium is concentration dependent (2189). See Y-Site Compatibility above. Vancomycin HCl has a low pH and is variably compatible with drugs having neutral to mildly alkaline pH, including cephalosporins and penicillins. The compatibility may depend on a number of factors, including concentration of each drug, dilution vehicle, actual pH of solutions, and completeness of mixing during administration. Combinations that are compatible when well mixed may result in precipitation if only partially mixed, presumably because of regionally different concentrations and pH values. If attempting to administer vancomycin HCl with cefoxitin sodium, take care to ensure that the specific combination and the concentrations are compatible under the exact administration conditions to be used. An inline filter should be used as a final safety measure (2189).

Administration Sets— Cefoxitin sodium (MSD) at a concentration of 1 g/L in sodium chloride 0.9% exhibited a 4 to 7% loss of potency in 24 hours and an 8 to 9% loss of potency in 48 hours at 25 °C in Saftiset, Soluset, and Viaflex chambers and tubing (308).

CEFTAZIDIME
AHFS 8:12.06

Ceptaz	**Glaxo Wellcome**
Fortaz	**Glaxo Wellcome**
Tazidime	**Lilly**
Tazicef	**SmithKline Beecham**

Products— Ceftazidime is available as a sodium carbonate-containing formulation (Fortaz; Tazidime; Tazicef) and an L-arginine-containing formulation (Ceptaz) (2).

Fortaz is supplied in vials containing 500 mg, 1 g, and 2 g of drug (under reduced pressure), infusion packs containing 1 and 2 g of drug, and 6-g pharmacy bulk packages. The Fortaz dosage forms contain sodium carbonate 118 mg per gram of ceftazidime. The sodium salt of ceftazidime and carbon dioxide are formed during reconstitution (2; 4). The use of a venting needle has been suggested for ease of use (1136). Spraying or leaking of the solution after needle withdrawal has been reported, especially with smaller vials (1137). The use of larger vials reduces the occurrence of such leakage (1137; 1138). Care must be taken if a multiple-additive set with a two-way valve is used for reconstitution. The negative pressure in the Glaxo Wellcome product may cause inaccuracies in the volume of diluent added to the vial. In one test, almost 3 ml extra entered the vial during reconstitution (1240). Vials have been vented prior to reconstitution, but Glaxo Wellcome recommends clamping the tubing from the supply bottle prior to adding the diluent to the vial when multiple-additive sets are used (1241).

Fortaz is also supplied in frozen solutions containing 1 and 2 g/50 ml of dextrose 4.4 and 3.2%, respectively (2; 4).

Ceptaz is available in vials containing 1 and 2 g of drug (under slightly reduced pressure), infusion packs containing 1 and 2 g of drug, and 10-g pharmacy bulk packages. The dosage forms contain L-arginine 349 mg per gram of ceftazidime. Ceptaz dissolves without gas evolution (2; 1699).

For intramuscular injection, Fortaz and Ceptaz should be reconstituted with sterile water for injection, bacteriostatic water for injection, or lidocaine HCl 0.5 or 1% in the amounts shown in Table 1. For the sodium carbonate-containing formulations, any carbon dioxide bubbles that are withdrawn into the syringe should be expelled prior to injection (2; 4).

For direct intravenous injection, Fortaz should be reconstituted with sterile water for injection and Ceptaz should be reconstituted with sterile water for injection, dextrose 5% in water, or sodium chloride 0.9% as shown in Table 2. Carbon dioxide will form during dissolution of Fortaz, but the solution will clear in about one to two minutes (2; 4).

For intravenous infusion, the reconstituted solution can be added to a compatible infusion solution (after expelling any carbon dioxide bubbles that have entered the syringe). Alternatively, the 1- or 2-g infusion packs can be reconstituted with 100 ml of compatible infusion solution, yielding a 10- or 20-mg/ml solution, respectively (2; 4). To reconstitute the Fortaz infusion packs, add the diluent in two increments. Initially, add 10 ml with shaking to dissolve the drug. To release the carbon dioxide pressure, insert a venting needle through the closure only after the drug has dissolved and become clear (about one to two minutes). Then add the remaining 90 ml and remove the venting needle. Additional pressure may develop, especially during storage, and should be released prior to use (4).

The Fortaz 6-g pharmacy bulk package should be reconstituted with 26 ml of a compatible diluent to yield 30 ml of solution containing 200 mg/ml of ceftazidime. The carbon dioxide pressure that develops should be released using a venting needle. The 200-mg/ml concentrated solution must be diluted further for intravenous use (2).

The Ceptaz 10-g pharmacy bulk package should be reconstituted with 40 ml of a compatible diluent to yield a solution containing 200 mg/ml of ceftazidime. The 200-mg/ml concentrated solution must be diluted further for intravenous use (2).

Table 1. Reconstitution for Intramuscular Injection (2)

Product	Volume of Diluent	Withdrawable Volume	Concentration
Fortaz			
500 mg	1.5 ml	1.8 ml	280 mg/ml
1 g	3.0 ml	3.6 ml	280 mg/ml
Ceptaz			
1 g	3.0 ml		250 mg/ml

Table 2. Reconstitution for Intravenous Injection (2)

Product	Volume of Diluent	Withdrawable Volume	Concentration
Fortaz			
500 mg	5 ml	5.3 ml	100 mg/ml
1 g	10 ml	10.6 ml	100 mg/ml
2 g	10 ml	11.5 ml	170 mg/ml
Ceptaz			
1 g	10 ml		90 mg/ml
2 g	10 ml		170 mg/ml

pH— Fortaz, from 5 to 8 (2; 4); Ceptaz, from 5 to 7.5 (2).

Osmolality— The osmolality of ceftazidime (Glaxo) 50 mg/ml was determined to be 321 mOsm/kg in dextrose 5% in water and 330 mOsm/kg in sodium chloride 0.9% (1375).

Robinson et al. recommended the following maximum ceftazidime concentrations to achieve osmolalities suitable for peripheral infusion in fluid-restricted patients (1180):

Diluent	Maximum Concentration (mg/ml)	Osmolality (mOsm/kg)
Dextrose 5% in water	70	503
Sodium chloride 0.9%	63	486
Sterile water for injection	126	302

Sodium Content— Each gram of ceftazidime activity in Fortaz provides 2.3 mEq (54 mg) of sodium from the sodium carbonate present in the formulation (2; 4). Ceptaz is sodium free (2).

Administration— Ceftazidime may be administered by deep intramuscular injection, by direct intravenous injection over three to five minutes directly into a vein or through the tubing of a running compatible infusion solution, or by intermittent intravenous infusion over 15 to 30 minutes (2; 4). The manufacturer recommends temporarily discontinuing other solutions being administered at the same site during ceftazidime infusion. The sodium carbonate-containing formulation may be instilled intraperitoneally in a concentration of 250 mg/2 L of compatible dialysis solution (2; 4).

Stability— Intact vials should be stored at 15 to 30 °C and protected from light (2). Approximately 2% decomposition has been reported after 12 months of storage at 37 °C with protection from light (1136).

Reconstituted ceftazidime solutions are light yellow to amber, depending on the diluent and concentration, and may darken on storage. Color changes do not necessarily indicate a potency loss (2; 4).

Solutions of Fortaz in sterile water for injection at 95 to 280 mg/ml, in lidocaine HCl 0.5 or 1% or bacteriostatic water for injection at 280 mg/ml, and in sodium chloride 0.9% or dextrose 5% in water at 10 or 20 mg/ml in piggyback infusion packs are stable for 24 hours at room temperature and seven days under refrigeration. Tazicef and Tazidime in sterile water for injection at 95 to 280 mg/ml or in sodium chloride 0.9% at 10 to 20 mg/ml is stable for 24 hours at room temperature and seven days under refrigeration (2).

One report of ceftazidime in concentrations of 1, 40, and 333 mg/ml in water indicated no loss after 24 hours at 4 °C and six hours at 25 °C. About a 4 to 6% loss was reported after 24 hours at 25 °C (1136).

Solutions of Ceptaz 250 mg/ml in sterile water for injection, bacteriostatic water for injection, or lidocaine HCl 0.5 or 1% for intramuscular injection are stable for 18 hours at room temperature or seven days under refrigeration (2).

According to the manufacturer, the stability of Ceptaz for intravenous injection in sterile water for injection, dextrose 5% in water, and sodium chloride 0.9% depends on the solution concentration. Concentrations greater than 100 mg/ml are stable for 18 hours at room temperature and seven days under refrigeration. Concentrations of 100 mg/ml or less are stable for 24 hours at room temperature and seven days under refrigeration (2).

Ambulatory Infusion Pumps— Ceftazidime (Ceptaz) 30 and 60 mg/ml in sterile water for injection in PVC portable infusion pump reservoirs (Pharmacia Deltec) exhibited a 7 to 10% loss by HPLC after 10 days at 3 °C followed by 24 hours at 30 °C (1581).

Exposure of ceftazidime (Glaxo) 36.6 mg/ml in sterile water for injection to 37 °C for 24 hours, to simulate the use of a portable infusion pump, resulted in little or no ceftazidime loss (1391).

Ceftazidime (Glaxo) containing arginine at concentrations of 3 g/50 ml and 6 g/50 ml in sodium chloride 0.9% was packaged in Singleday Infusors (Baxter) made of polyisoprene. The infusors were stored at 27 °C to simulate use with no prior storage and also at 4 °C for up to 144 hours followed by 24 hours at 27 °C to simulate storage followed by use. The 3 g/50 ml concentration exhibited 9% ceftazidime loss in 24 hours at 27 °C and in 20 hours at 27 °C if stored under refrigeration prior to use. The 6 g/50 ml concentration was slightly less stable. Ceftazidime losses of 9 to 11% were found in all samples after 16 hours at 27 °C (1860).

Ceftazidime (Glaxo) (sodium carbonate formulation) at a concentration of 60 mg/ml in water for injection was filled into PVC portable infusion pump reservoirs (Pharmacia Deltec). Storage at −20 °C resulted in less than 3% loss in 14 days. The thawed reservoirs were then stored under refrigeration at 6 °C. Losses totaled 10% after five days of refrigerated storage. Under simulated use conditions at 30 °C, ceftazidime decomposes at a rate of about 10% in 18 hours. The authors concluded prefilling of reservoirs with ceftazidime (sodium carbonate) solutions for home use was not advisable (2008).

Elastomeric Reservoir Pumps— Ceftazidime (sodium carbonate formulation) (Glaxo) 20 mg/ml in dextrose 5% in water and sodium chloride 0.9% 100 ml was packaged in latex elastomeric reservoirs (Secure Medical). A 5% loss by HPLC analysis occurred in seven days at 5 °C. Stored at 25 °C, a 9% loss in dextrose 5% in water and a 4% loss in sodium chloride 0.9% occurred in 18 hours (1970).

Ceftazidime (Glaxo) (sodium carbonate formulation) was prepared as a 60-mg/ml solution in sodium chloride 0.9% and packaged in elastomeric ambulatory pumps (Homepump, Block Medical). The solutions were visually compatible and exhibited 9% loss stored at 4 °C and no loss at –20 °C in 14 days protected from light. However, potentially toxic pyridine 0.53 mg/ml was found in the refrigerated solutions. Frozen solutions had much less pyridine. The authors recommended freezing such solutions if long-term storage is needed (2113).

Syringes— Ceftazidime (Ceptaz) 100 mg/ml in sterile water for injection in polypropylene syringes (Becton-Dickinson) exhibited a 7 to 8% loss by HPLC after 24 hours at 22 °C and little or no loss after 10 days at 4 °C (1584).

Ceftazidime (Fortaz) 100 and 200 mg/ml in sterile water for injection in polypropylene syringes (Becton-Dickinson) and glass vials exhibited a 5% or less loss by HPLC in eight hours at 22 °C and 96 hours at 4 °C (1580).

Ceftazidime (Fortaz) 100 mg/ml in sterile water for injection, packaged as 0.4 ml in 1-ml Injekt syringes (Braun) sealed with blind hubs and stored at about 6 °C, retained antibiotic activity against *Pseudomonas aeruginosa* for seven days. However, the yellow color of the solution became much darker over this period (1697).

Freezing Solutions— The various sodium carbonate-containing ceftazidime products differ in their reported stabilities, both during frozen storage of their solutions and after thawing. Table 3 summarizes the reported stabilities (4).

The commercially available frozen ceftazidime sodium solutions

Table 3. Reported Stabilities of Frozen and Thawed Solutions of Ceftazidime Sodium Carbonate-Containing Products (2; 4)

Concentration	Fortaz	Tazidime	Tazicef
280 mg/ml	3 months[a]	3 months[a]	3 months[a]
Thawed/RT[b]	8 hr	8 hr	8 hr
Thawed/4 °C[c]	4 days	4 days	4 days
100 to 180 mg/ml	6 months[a,d]	3 months[e]	3 months[e]
Thawed/RT	24 hr	8 hr	8 hr
Thawed/4 °C	7 days	4 days	4 days
10 to 20 mg/ml[f]	9 months[a]		
Thawed/RT	24 hr		
Thawed/4 °C	7 days		

[a]*In sterile water for injection.*
[b]*Thawed and stored at room temperature.*
[c]*Thawed and stored at 4 to 5 °C.*
[d]*In sodium chloride 0.9%.*
[e]*In sodium chloride 0.9% and dextrose 5% in water.*
[f]*In infusion packs.*

(Fortaz) of 1 and 2 g/50 ml of sodium chloride 0.9%, when thawed, are stable for 24 hours at room temperature or seven days under refrigeration (4).

At concentrations ranging from 10 to 250 mg/ml in the recommended diluents, Ceptaz is stable for six months when frozen at −20 °C. A precipitate may form during frozen storage, but it dissolves on warming to room temperature. Once thawed, concentrations greater than 100 mg/ml are stable for up to 12 hours at room temperature or seven days under refrigeration. Concentrations of 100 mg/ml or less are stable for up to 18 hours at room temperature or seven days under refrigeration (2; 4).

Minibags of ceftazidime in dextrose 5% in water or sodium chloride 0.9%, frozen at −20 °C for up to 35 days, were thawed at room temperature and in a microwave oven, with care taken that the thawed solution temperature never exceeded 25 °C. No significant differences in ceftazidime concentrations occurred between the two thawing methods (1192).

Ceftazidime (Lilly) 40 mg/ml in both dextrose 5% in water and sodium chloride 0.9% exhibited approximately a 4 to 6% loss after storage at −10 °C for 90 days. Thawing in a microwave oven did not affect stability (1341).

Stiles et al. reported less than a 2% ceftazidime (Glaxo) loss from a solution containing 36.6 mg/ml in sterile water for injection in PVC and glass containers after 30 days at −20 °C. Subsequent thawing and storage for four days at 5 °C, followed by 24 hours at 37 °C to simulate the use of a portable infusion pump, resulted in little additional ceftazidime loss (1391).

Ceftazidime (Ceptaz) 100 mg/ml in sterile water for injection in polypropylene syringes (Becton-Dickinson) exhibited about a 2% loss by HPLC after 91 days at −20 °C. Subsequent storage at 22 °C for 24 hours resulted in a cumulative loss of 7%; subsequent storage at 4 °C for five days resulted in a cumulative loss of 6% (1584).

Ceftazidime (Ceptaz) 30 and 60 mg/ml in sterile water for injection in PVC portable infusion pump reservoirs (Pharmacia Deltec) and glass vials exhibited no loss by HPLC after 30 days at −20 °C. Subsequent storage for four days at 3 °C resulted in about a 10% loss in the PVC bags and no loss in the glass vials (1581).

Ceftazidime (Fortaz) 100 and 200 mg/ml in sterile water for injection in glass vials and polypropylene syringes (Becton-Dickinson) was stored frozen at −20 °C for 91 days followed by eight hours at 22 °C. Losses of about 5 and 10% by HPLC occurred in the 100- and 200-mg/ml concentrations, respectively. Freezing at −20 °C for 91 days followed by refrigeration at 4 °C for four days resulted in losses of about 10 and 6% in the 100- and 200-mg/ml concentrations, respectively. Particle counts remained within USP limits throughout the study (1580).

Ceftazidime (sodium carbonate formulation) (Glaxo) 20 mg/ml in dextrose 5% in water and sodium chloride 0.9% frozen at −20 °C for 12 weeks exhibited 5% or less loss of potency by HPLC analysis in latex elastomeric reservoirs (Secure Medical) and in glass containers (1970).

Usually, frozen solutions should be thawed at room temperature. Other techniques are not recommended. Thawed solutions should not be refrozen (2; 4).

Sorption— Ceftazidime 4 mg/ml in dextrose 5% in water and sodium chloride 0.9% exhibited no loss due to sorption to PVC containers over 24 hours and to administration sets during one-hour simulated infusions (1953).

Compatibility Information

Solution Compatibility

		Ceftazidime				
Solution	*Mfr*	*Mfr*	*Conc/L*	*Remarks*	*Ref*	*C/I*
Amino acids 5%, dextrose 25%	AB	GL[c]	6 g	No substantial amino acid degradation in 48 hr at 22 °C and 10 days at 4 °C. Ceftazidime stability the determining factor	1535	**C**
Dextrose 5% in sodium chloride 0.9%		GL[c]	20 g	5% loss in 24 hr at 25 °C and no loss in 48 hr at 4 °C	1136	**C**
Dextrose 5% in water	MG[a]	GL[c]	20 g	Physically compatible with 5% drug loss in 24 hr and 9% in 48 hr at 25 °C under fluorescent light	1126	**C**
		GL[c]	20 g	6% loss in 24 hr at 25 °C. No loss in 24 hr and 3% loss in 48 hr at 4 °C	1136	**C**

Solution Compatibility (Cont.)

	Ceftazidime					
Solution	*Mfr*	*Mfr*	*Conc/L*	*Remarks*	*Ref*	*C/I*
	TR[a]		40 g	Physically compatible with 8% loss in 2 days at 25 °C and 6% loss in 21 days at 5 °C	1341	C
	[b]	GL[c]	40 g	Physically compatible with 7% loss in 1 day and 19% loss in 2 days at 23 °C; 9% loss in 10 days at 4 °C	1353	C
	BA[b]	GL[c]	20 and 60 g	Visually compatible with 7 to 9% loss by HPLC in 24 hr at room temperature	1937	C
	[b]		4 g	Visually compatible with little or no loss by HPLC in 24 hr at room temperature and 4 °C	1953	C
	AB[d]	GL[c]	20 g	6 to 9% loss by HPLC in 18 hr at 25 °C and in 7 days at 5 °C	1970	C
Sodium bicarbonate 4.2%		GL[c]	20 g	3% loss in 6 hr and 11% in 24 hr at 25 °C. 1% loss in 24 hr and 3% in 48 hr at 4 °C	1136	C
Sodium chloride 0.9%	MG[a]	GL[c]	20 g	Physically compatible with 2% drug loss in 24 hr and 5% in 48 hr at 25 °C under fluorescent light	1126	C
		GL[c]	20 g	7% loss in 24 hr at 25 °C and no loss in 48 hr at 4 °C	1136	C
	TR[a]		40 g	Physically compatible with 5% loss in 2 days and 12% loss in 3 days at 25 °C; 7% loss in 28 days at 5 °C	1341	C
	[b]	GL[c]	40 g	Physically compatible with 3% loss in 1 day and 14% loss in 3 days at 25 °C; 10% loss in 14 days at 5 °C	1353	C
	BA[e]	GL[f]	60 g	9% loss by HPLC in 24 hr stored at 27 °C	1860	C
	BA[e]	GL[f]	60 g	Stored for up to 144 hr at 4 °C followed by 27 °C; 9% loss by HPLC in 20 hr at 27 °C	1860	C
	BA[e]	GL[f]	120 g	9% loss by HPLC in 16 hr stored at 27 °C	1860	C
	BA[e]	GL[f]	120 g	Stored for up to 144 hr at 4 °C followed by 27 °C; 9 to 11% loss by HPLC in 16 hr at 27 °C	1860	C
	BA[b]	GL[c]	20 and 60 g	Visually compatible with 4 to 6% loss by HPLC in 24 hr at room temperature	1937	C
	[b]		4 g	Visually compatible with little or no loss by HPLC in 24 hr at room temperature and 4 °C	1953	C
	AB[d]	GL[c]	20 g	3 to 5% loss of drug by HPLC in 18 hr at 25 °C and 7 days at 5 °C	1970	C
	KA[h]	GL[c]	60 g	Visually compatible with little or no loss of ceftazidime by HPLC and little formation of pyridine in 14 days frozen at –20 °C protected from light	2113	C
	KA[h]	GL[c]	60 g	Visually compatible with 9% loss of ceftazidime by HPLC but formation of potentially toxic pyridine 0.53 mg/ml in 14 days at 4 °C protected from light	2113	?
Sodium lactate ⅙ M		GL[c]	20 g	6% loss in 24 hr at 25 °C and 1% in 48 hr at 4 °C	1136	C
TPN #107[g]			1 g	Physically compatible and ceftazidime activity retained for 24 hr at 21 °C by microbiological assay	1326	C
TPN #141 to #143[g]		GL[c]	1 g	Visually compatible with 8% ceftazidime loss in 6 hr and 10% loss in 24 hr by HPLC at 22 °C. 8% ceftazidime loss in 3 days at 4 °C	1535	C

Solution Compatibility (Cont.)

Ceftazidime

Solution	Mfr	Mfr	Conc/L	Remarks	Ref	C/I
		GL[c]	6 g	Visually compatible with 6% ceftazidime loss in 12 hr and 11 to 13% loss in 24 hr by HPLC at 22 °C. 7 to 9% ceftazidime loss in 3 days at 4 °C	1535	C

[a]Tested in glass containers.
[b]Tested in PVC containers.
[c]Sodium carbonate–containing formulation.
[d]Tested in glass containers and latex elastomeric reservoirs (Secure Medical).
[e]Tested in Singleday Infusors (Baxter).
[f]Arginine-containing formulation.
[g]Refer to Appendix I for the composition of parenteral nutrition solutions. TPN indicates a 2-in-1 admixture.
[h]Tested in elastomeric ambulatory pumps (Homepump, Block Medical).

Additive Compatibility

Ceftazidime

Drug	Mfr	Conc/L	Mfr	Conc/L	Test Soln	Remarks	Ref	C/I
Aminophylline	ES	1 g	GL[a]	2 g	D5W, NS	20 to 23% ceftazidime loss by HPLC in 6 hr at room temperature	1937	I
	ES	1 g	GL[a]	6 g	D5W, NS	8 to 10% ceftazidime loss and 13% theophylline loss by HPLC in 6 hr at room temperature	1937	I
	ES	2 g	GL[a]	2 g	D5W, NS	35 to 40% ceftazidime loss by HPLC in 6 hr at room temperature	1937	I
	ES	2 g	GL[a]	6 g	D5W, NS	22% ceftazidime loss by HPLC in 6 hr at room temperature	1937	I
Ciprofloxacin	MI	1 g	SKF[a]	20 g	D5W, NS	Physically compatible for 24 hr at 22 °C	1189	C
Clindamycin phosphate	UP	9 g	GL[a]	20 g	D5W[b]	Physically compatible with 9% clindamycin loss and 11% ceftazidime loss in 48 hr at 25 °C under fluorescent light	1026	C
	UP	9 g	GL[a]	20 g	NS[b]	Physically compatible with 5% clindamycin loss and 7% ceftazidime loss in 48 hr at 25 °C under fluorescent light	1026	C
Fluconazole	PF	1 g	GL	20 g	D5W	Visually compatible with no fluconazole loss by HPLC in 72 hr at 25 °C under fluorescent light. Ceftazidime not tested	1677	C
Metronidazole		5 g	GL[a]	20 g		No loss of either drug in 4 hr	1345	C
	AB	5 g	LI[a]	10 g		Visually compatible with little or no loss of either drug by HPLC in 72 hr at 8 °C	1849	C
Ofloxacin	HO	1.67 g	GL[a]	8.3 g	W	Visually compatible with little or no loss of either drug by HPLC in 48 hr	1613	C
Ranitidine HCl	GL	500 mg	GL[a]	10 g	D2.5½S	8% ranitidine loss in 4 hr and 39% loss in 24 hr by HPLC at 22 °C	1632	I

[a]Sodium carbonate–containing formulation tested.
[b]Tested in glass containers.

Drugs in Syringe Compatibility

Drug (in syringe)	Mfr	Amt	Mfr	Amt	Remarks	Ref	C/I
			Ceftazidime				
Hydromorphone HCl	KN	2, 10, 40 mg/ 1 ml	GL[a]	180 mg/ 1 ml	Visually compatible with less than 10% loss of either drug by HPLC in 24 hr at room temperature	2082	**C**

[a]*Sodium carbonate–containing formulation tested.*

Y-Site Injection Compatibility (1:1 Mixture)

Drug	Mfr	Conc	Mfr	Conc	Remarks	Ref	C/I
			Ceftazidime				
Acyclovir sodium	BW	5 mg/ml[a]	SKF[c]	20 mg/ml[a]	Physically compatible for 4 hr at 25 °C	1157	**C**
Allopurinol sodium	BW	3 mg/ml[b]	LI[c]	40 mg/ml[a]	Physically compatible with no change in measured turbidity or increase in particle content in 4 hr at 22 °C	1686	**C**
Amifostine	USB	10 mg/ml[a]	LI[c]	40 mg/ml[a]	Physically compatible with no change in measured turbidity or increase in particle content in 4 hr at 23 °C	1845	**C**
Aminophylline	ES	2 mg/ml[a]	GL[c]	40 mg/ml[a]	Visually compatible with 4% ceftazidime loss and 9% theophylline loss by HPLC in 2 hr at room temperature	1937	**C**
	ES	2 mg/ml[a]	GL[c]	40 mg/ml[b]	Visually compatible with 5% ceftazidime loss and 4% theophylline loss by HPLC in 2 hr at room temperature	1937	**C**
	ES	2 mg/ml[a]	GL[d]	40 mg/ml	Visually compatible with no ceftazidime or theophylline loss by HPLC in 2 hr at room temperature	1937	**C**
	ES	2 mg/ml[a]	GL[e]	40 mg/ml[a]	Visually compatible with 5% ceftazidime loss and 7% theophylline loss by HPLC in 2 hr at room temperature	1937	**C**
	ES	2 mg/ml[a]	GL[e]	40 mg/ml[b]	Visually compatible with 2% ceftazidime loss and no theophylline loss by HPLC in 2 hr at room temperature	1937	**C**
Amphotericin B cholesteryl sulfate complex	SEQ	0.83 mg/ml[a]	SKB[c]	40 mg/ml[a]	Increased turbidity forms in 4 hr at 23 °C under fluorescent light	2117	**I**
	SEQ	0.83 mg/ml[a]	GW[e]	40 mg/ml[a]	Gross precipitate forms	2117	**I**
Amsacrine	NCI	1 mg/ml[a]	GL[c]	40 mg/ml[a]	Light flocculent orange precipitate forms immediately, becoming heavier with time	1381	**I**
Aztreonam	SQ	40 mg/ml[a]	LI[c]	40 mg/ml[a]	Physically compatible with no subvisual haze or particle formation in 4 hr at 23 °C	1758	**C**
Ciprofloxacin	MI	1 mg/ml[a]	SKF[c]	20 mg/ml[f]	Physically compatible for 24 hr at 22 °C	1189	**C**
Cisatracurium besylate	GW	0.1 and 2 mg/ml[a]	SKB[c]	40 mg/ml[a]	Physically compatible with no change in measured turbidity or increase in particle content in 4 hr at 23 °C	2074	**C**
	GW	5 mg/ml[a]	SKB[c]	40 mg/ml[a]	Subvisual haze forms immediately	2074	**I**
	GW	0.1, 2, 5 mg/ml[a]	GW[e]	40 mg/ml[a]	Physically compatible with no change in measured turbidity or increase in particle content in 4 hr at 23 °C	2074	**C**

Y-Site Injection Compatibility (1:1 Mixture) (Cont.)

Ceftazidime

Drug	Mfr	Conc	Mfr	Conc	Remarks	Ref	C/I
Diltiazem HCl	MMD	5 mg/ml	GL[c]	10 and 170 mg/ml[b]	Visually compatible	1807	C
	MMD	1 mg/ml[b]	GL[c]	170 mg/ml[b]	Visually compatible	1807	C
Docetaxel	RPR	0.9 mg/ml[a]	SKB[c]	40 mg/ml[a]	Physically compatible with no change in measured turbidity or increase in particle content in 4 hr at 23 °C	2224	C
Doxorubicin HCl liposome injection	SEQ	0.4 mg/ml[a]	SKB[c]	40 mg/ml[a]	Partial loss of measured natural turbidity	2087	I
Enalaprilat	MSD	0.05 mg/ml[b]	GL[c]	10 mg/ml[a]	Physically compatible for 24 hr at room temperature under fluorescent light	1355	C
Esmolol HCl	DCC	10 mg/ml[a]	GL[c]	10 mg/ml[a]	Physically compatible for 24 hr at 22 °C	1169	C
Etoposide phosphate	BR	5 mg/ml[a]	SKB[c]	40 mg/ml[a]	Physically compatible with no change in measured turbidity or increase in particle content in 4 hr at 23 °C	2218	C
Famotidine	MSD	0.2 mg/ml[a]	GL[c]	20 mg/ml[b]	Physically compatible for 14 hr	1196	C
	ME	2 mg/ml[b]	[c]	20 mg/ml[a]	Visually compatible for 4 hr at 22 °C	1936	C
Filgrastim	AMG	30 μg/ml[a]	LI[c]	40 mg/ml[a]	Physically compatible with no change in measured turbidity or increase in particle content in 4 hr at 22 °C	1687	C
	AMG	10[g] and 40[a] μg/ml	LI[c]	10 mg/ml[a]	Visually compatible with little or no loss of filgrastim activity by bioassay and ceftazidime by HPLC in 4 hr at 25 °C	2060	C
Fluconazole	RR	2 mg/ml	GL	20 mg/ml	Immediate precipitation	1407	I
Fludarabine phosphate	BX	1 mg/ml[a]	GL[c]	40 mg/ml[a]	Physically compatible for 4 hr at room temperature under fluorescent light	1439	C
Foscarnet sodium	AST	24 mg/ml	GL	20 mg/ml	Physically compatible for 24 hr at room temperature under fluorescent light	1335	C
	AST	24 mg/ml	GL	20 mg/ml[f]	Physically compatible for 24 hr at 25 °C under fluorescent light by visual and microscopic examination	1393	C
Gemcitabine HCl	LI	10 mg/ml[b]	SKB[c]	40 mg/ml[b]	Physically compatible with no change in measured turbidity or increase in particle content in 4 hr at 23 °C	2226	C
Granisetron HCl	SKB	1 mg/ml	SKB[c]	16.7 mg/ml[e]	Physically compatible with little or no loss of either drug by HPLC in 4 hr at 22 °C	1883	C
Heparin sodium	TR	50 units/ml	LI[c]	20 mg/ml	Visually compatible for 6 hr at 25 °C	1793	C
Hydromorphone HCl	KN	2, 10, 40 mg/ml	GL[c]	40[a] and 180 mg/ml	Visually compatible and potency of both drugs by HPLC retained for 24 hr	1532	C
Idarubicin HCl	AD	1 mg/ml[b]	LI[c]	20 mg/ml[a]	Haze forms in 1 hr	1525	I
Labetalol HCl	SC	1 mg/ml[a]	GL[c]	10 mg/ml[a]	Physically compatible for 24 hr at 18 °C	1171	C
Melphalan HCl	BW	0.1 mg/ml[b]	LI[c]	40 mg/ml[b]	Physically compatible with no change in measured turbidity or increase in particle content in 3 hr at 22 °C	1557	C
Meperidine HCl	AB	10 mg/ml	LI[c]	20 and 40 mg/ml[a]	Physically compatible for 4 hr at 25 °C	1397	C
Midazolam HCl	RC	1 mg/ml[a]	LI[c]	20 mg/ml[a]	Haze forms in 1 hr	1847	I

Y-Site Injection Compatibility (1:1 Mixture) (Cont.)

			Ceftazidime				
Drug	*Mfr*	*Conc*	*Mfr*	*Conc*	*Remarks*	*Ref*	*C/I*
Morphine sulfate	AB	1 mg/ml	LI[c]	20 and 40 mg/ml[a]	Physically compatible for 4 hr at 25 °C	1397	**C**
Ondansetron HCl	GL	1 mg/ml[b]	GL[c]	40 mg/ml[a]	Physically compatible for 4 hr at 22 °C	1365	**C**
	GL	16 to 160 μg/ml		100 to 200 mg/ml	Physically compatible when ceftazidime given as 5-min bolus via Y-site	1366	**C**
	GL	1 mg/ml[b]	GL[e]	40 mg/ml[a]	Physically compatible for 4 hr at 22 °C	1365	**C**
	GL	0.03 and 0.3 mg/ml[a]	LI[c]	40 mg/ml[a]	Visually compatible with less than 10% loss of either drug by HPLC in 4 hr at 25 °C	1732	**C**
Paclitaxel	NCI	1.2 mg/ml[a]	LI[c]	40 mg/ml[a]	Physically compatible with no change in measured turbidity in 4 hr at 22 °C	1556	**C**
Pentamidine isethionate	FUJ	3 mg/ml[a]	LI[c]	20 mg/ml[a]	Fine precipitate, difficult to see, forms immediately	1880	**I**
Propofol	ZEN	10 mg/ml	SKB[c]	40 mg/ml[a]	Physically compatible for 1 hr at 23 °C with no increase in particle content	2066	**C**
Ranitidine HCl	GL	1 mg/ml[b]	GL[c]	20 mg/ml[a]	8% ranitidine loss and no ceftazidime loss by HPLC in 4 hr at 22 °C	1632	**C**
Remifentanil HCl	GW	0.025 and 0.25 mg/ml[b]	GW[e]	40 mg/ml[a]	Physically compatible with no change in measured turbidity or increase in particle content in 4 hr at 23 °C	2075	**C**
Sargramostim	IMM	10 μg/ml[b]	GL[c]	40 mg/ml[b]	Particles and filaments form in 4 hr	1436	**I**
	IMM	6[h] and 15 μg/ml[b]	LI[c]	40 mg/ml[f]	Visually compatible for 2 hr	1618	**C**
Tacrolimus	FUJ	1 mg/ml[b]	GL[c]	20 mg/ml[a]	Visually compatible for 24 hr at 25 °C	1630	**C**
	FUJ	10 and 40 μg/ml[a]	GW[c]	40 mg/ml[a]	Visually compatible with no loss of either drug by HPLC in 4 hr at 24 °C under fluorescent light	2216	**C**
	FUJ	10 and 40 μg/ml[a]	GW[c]	200 mg/ml[a]	Visually compatible with no loss of either drug by HPLC in 4 hr at 24 °C under fluorescent light	2216	**C**
Teniposide	BR	0.1 mg/ml[a]	LI[c]	40 mg/ml[a]	Physically compatible with no subvisual haze or particle formation in 4 hr at 23 °C	1725	**C**
Theophylline	TR	4 mg/ml	LI[c]	20 mg/ml	Visually compatible for 6 hr at 25 °C	1793	**C**
Thiotepa	IMM[i]	1 mg/ml[a]	LI[c]	40 mg/ml[a]	Physically compatible with no change in measured turbidity or increase in particle content in 4 hr at 23 °C	1861	**C**
TNA #218 to #226[j]			SKB[c]	40 mg/ml[a]	Visually compatible with no precipitate or emulsion damage apparent in 4 hr at 23 °C	2215	**C**
			GL[e]	40 mg/ml[a]	Visually compatible with no precipitate or emulsion damage apparent in 4 hr at 23 °C	2215	**C**
TPN #141 to #143[j]			GL[c]	40 mg/ml[f]	Visually compatible with 4% or less ceftazidime loss in 2 hr at 22 °C in 1:1 and 1:3 ratios	1535	**C**
TPN #189[j]			GL[c]	200 mg/ml[k]	Visually compatible for 24 hr at 22 °C	1767	**C**
TPN #203 and #204[j]			LI[c]	60 mg/ml	Visually compatible for 2 hr at 23 °C	1974	**C**

Y-Site Injection Compatibility (1:1 Mixture) (Cont.)

Drug	Mfr	Conc	Ceftazidime Mfr	Ceftazidime Conc	Remarks	Ref	C/I
TPN #212 to #215[j]			SKB[c]	40 mg/ml[a]	Physically compatible with no change in measured turbidity or increase in particle content in 4 hr at 23 °C	2109	**C**
Vancomycin HCl	AB	3 mg/ml[a]	GL[c]	25 and 60 mg/ml[a]	Physically compatible with no subvisual haze or particle formation in 4 hr at 23 °C	1563	**C**
	AB	10 mg/ml[a]	GL[c]	25 mg/ml[a]	Subvisual haze forms immediately	1563	**I**
	AB	10 mg/ml[a]	GL[c]	60 mg/ml[a]	Dense turbidity and white particles form immediately and become gross precipitate in 1 hr	1563	**I**
	AB	20 mg/ml[a]	SKB[c]	10[a], 50[a], 200[k] mg/ml	Gross white precipitate forms immediately	2189	**I**
	AB	20 mg/ml[a]	SKB[c]	1 mg/ml[a]	Physically compatible with no change in measured turbidity or increase in particle content in 4 hr at 23 °C	2189	**C**
	AB	2 mg/ml[a]	SKB[c]	1[a], 10[a], 50[a], 200[k] mg/ml	Physically compatible with no change in measured turbidity or increase in particle content in 4 hr at 23 °C	2189	**C**
Vinorelbine tartrate	BW	1 mg/ml[b]	LI[c]	40 mg/ml[b]	Physically compatible with no change in measured turbidity or increase in particle content in 4 hr at 22 °C	1558	**C**
Warfarin sodium	DME	2 mg/ml[k]	SKB[c]	20 mg/ml[a]	Haze forms in 24 hr at 24 °C	2078	**I**
Zidovudine	BW	4 mg/ml[a]	GL[c]	20 mg/ml[a]	Physically compatible for 4 hr at 25 °C under fluorescent light by visual and microscopic examination	1193	**C**

[a]*Tested in dextrose 5% in water.*
[b]*Tested in sodium chloride 0.9%.*
[c]*Sodium carbonate-containing formulation tested.*
[d]*Tested in the ceftazidime premixed infusion.*
[e]*Arginine formulation tested.*
[f]*Tested in both dextrose 5% in water and sodium chloride 0.9%.*
[g]*Tested in dextrose 5% in water with human albumin 2 mg/ml.*
[h]*With human albumin 0.1%.*
[i]*Lyophilized formulation tested.*
[j]*Refer to Appendix I for the composition of parenteral nutrition solutions. TNA indicates a 3-in-1 admixture, and TPN indicates a 2-in-1 admixture.*
[k]*Tested in sterile water for injection.*

Additional Compatibility Information

Infusion Solutions— Ceftazidime, at the concentrations and in the infusion solutions noted in Table 4, is stated to be physically compatible and chemically stable for 24 hours at room temperature and for seven days under refrigeration (2; 4).

Infusions in sodium chloride 0.9% or dextrose 5% in water are stated to be stable for six hours at room temperature in plastic tubing, drip chambers, and volume-control devices of administration sets (2; 4).

The drug is stated to be less stable in sodium bicarbonate injection, and its use as a diluent is not recommended (2; 4).

Peritoneal Dialysis Solutions— Ceftazidime 2 mg/ml in Dianeal with dextrose 1.5% is stated to be stable for 10 days under refrigeration, 24 hours at room temperature, and at least four hours at 37 °C (4).

Ceftazidime (Fortaz) 125 mg/L and tobramycin sulfate (Lilly) 8 mg/L in Dianeal PD-2 with dextrose 2.5% (Baxter) were visually compatible and chemically stable by HPLC (ceftazidime) and fluorescence polarization immunoassay (tobramycin). After 16 hours of storage at 25 °C under fluorescent light, the loss of both drugs was less than 3%. Additional storage for eight hours at 37 °C, to simulate the maximum peritoneal dwell time, showed tobramycin sulfate concentrations of 96% and ceftazidime concentrations of 92 to 96% (1652).

Ceftazidime (sodium carbonate formulation) (Glaxo) 0.1 mg/ml in Dianeal PD-2 with dextrose 1.5% in PVC containers was physically and chemically stable by HPLC analysis for 24 hours at 25 °C exposed to light, exhibiting about 9% loss; additional storage for eight hours at 37 °C resulted in additional loss of about 6%. Under refrigeration at 4 °C protected from light, no loss occurred in seven days. Additional storage for 16 hours at 25 °C followed by eight hours at 37 °C resulted in about 6% loss (1989).

Ceftazidime (sodium carbonate formulation) (Glaxo) 0.1 mg/ml

Table 4. Infusion Solutions and Concentrations for Ceftazidime Dilution

Infusion Solution	Concentration (mg/ml)		
	Ceptaz and Fortaz	Tazidime	Tazicef
Dextrose 5% in sodium chloride 0.2, 0.45, or 0.9%	1 to 40	1 to 40	1 to 40
Dextrose 5% in water	1 to 40	1 to 40	1 to 40
Dextrose 10% in water	1 to 40	1 to 40	1 to 40
Invert sugar 10%	1 to 20		
Normosol M in dextrose 5%	1 to 20		
Ringer's injection	1 to 20	1 to 40	1 to 40
Ringer's injection, lactated	1 to 20	1 to 40	1 to 40
Sodium chloride 0.9%	1 to 40	1 to 40	1 to 40
Sodium lactate ⅙ M	1 to 40		

admixed with teicoplanin (Marion Merrell Dow) 0.025 mg/ml in Dianeal PD-2 with dextrose 1.5% in PVC containers did not result in a stable mixture. Using HPLC analysis, large (but variable) teicoplanin losses generally in the 20% range were noted in as little as two hours at 25 °C exposed to light. Ceftazidime losses of about 9% occurred in 16 hours. Refrigeration and protection from light of the peritoneal dialysis admixture reduced losses of both drugs to negligible levels. Even so, the authors did not recommend admixing these two drugs because of the high levels of teicoplanin loss at room temperature (1989).

Vancomycin HCl (Lilly) 1 mg/ml admixed with ceftazidime (sodium carbonate–containing formulation) (Lilly) 0.5 mg/ml in Dianeal PD-2 (Baxter) with 1.5% and also 4.25% dextrose were evaluated for compatibility and stability. Samples were stored under fluorescent light at 4 and 24 °C for 24 hours and at 37 °C for 12 hours. No precipitation or other change was observed by visual inspection in any sample. HPLC analysis found no loss of either drug in the samples stored at 4 °C and no loss of vancomycin HCl and about 4 to 5% ceftazidime loss in the samples stored at 24 °C in 24 hours. Vancomycin HCl losses of 3% or less and ceftazidime loss of about 6% were found in the samples stored at 37 °C for 12 hours. No difference in stability was found between samples at either dextrose concentration (2217). Also see Vancomycin below.

Additives— Ceftazidime 4 mg/ml in sodium chloride 0.9% and dextrose 5% in water is stated to be stable for 24 hours at room temperature or seven (Ceptaz and Fortaz) or 10 (Tazidime) days under refrigeration when admixed with heparin 10 or 50 units/ml, potassium chloride 10 or 40 mEq/L, or cefuroxime 3 mg/ml (4).

Tazicef 20 mg/ml in sterile water for injection is stated to be stable for 18 hours at room temperature or seven days under refrigeration when admixed with cefazolin sodium 330 mg/ml, cimetidine 150 mg/ml, or heparin 1000 units/ml. At 20 mg/ml in dextrose 5% in water, Tazicef is stated to be stable for 24 hours at room temperature or seven days refrigerated when admixed with potassium chloride 40 mEq/L (4).

Ceptaz 20 mg/ml is stated to be stable for 24 hours at room temperature or seven days under refrigeration with metronidazole 5 mg/ml or clindamycin phosphate 6 mg/ml in sodium chloride 0.9% or dextrose 5% in water (2; 4).

Aminoglycosides— The manufacturers recommend that ceftazidime not be admixed with aminoglycosides because of the potential for interactions (2; 4).

Pennell et al. evaluated the potential for inactivation of tobramycin sulfate (Lilly) 9 μg/ml with 100- and 200-μg/ml concentrations of ceftazidime (Lilly) in human serum. No loss of tobramycin sulfate was determined by TDx fluorescence polarization immunoassay over 48 hours when stored at 4, 24, and 37 °C (1420).

Vancomycin— The compatibility or incompatibility of vancomycin HCl mixed with or administered simultaneously with ceftazidime is concentration dependent (2189). See Y-Site Compatibility above. Vancomycin HCl has a low pH and is variably compatible with drugs having neutral to mildly alkaline pH, including cephalosporins and penicillins. The compatibility may depend on a number of factors, including concentration of each drug, dilution vehicle, actual pH of solutions, and completeness of mixing during administration. Combinations that are compatible when well mixed may result in precipitation if only partially mixed, presumably because of regionally different concentrations and pH values. If attempting to administer vancomycin HCl with ceftazidime, take care to ensure that the specific combination and the concentrations are compatible under the exact administration conditions to be used. An inline filter should be used as a final safety measure (2189).

A precipitate formed instantaneously when ceftazidime 2 g/50 ml of sterile water for injection was added to a burette previously used to administer vancomycin HCl 1 g/100 ml of dextrose 5% in water. The authors suggested that vancomycin may have precipitated because of the alkaline pH due to the sodium carbonate in the ceftazidime formulation (873). However, the manufacturer of Ceptaz also notes precipitation with vancomycin HCl, even though no sodium carbonate is present (2).

CEFTIZOXIME SODIUM
AHFS 8:12.06

Cefizox **Fujisawa Healthcare**

Products— Ceftizoxime sodium (Fujisawa Healthcare) is available in vials and piggyback bottles containing the equivalent of 500 mg and

1 and 2 g of ceftizoxime and in 10-g pharmacy bulk vials. Reconstitute the contents of the vials with sterile water for injection in the amounts shown in Table 1 and shake well. Reconstitute the pharmacy bulk vials according to the manufacturer's label directions. Piggyback bottles should be reconstituted with sodium chloride 0.9% or any compatible solution (2). (See Additional Compatibility Information.)

Ceftizoxime sodium (Fujisawa Healthcare) is also available as a frozen pre-mixed infusion solution of 1 or 2 g. It should be thawed at room temperature and checked for leaks by squeezing the bag (2).

pH— The reconstituted solution has a pH of 6 to 8, and the frozen premixed infusion solutions have a pH of 5.5 to 8 (4).

Osmolality— Ceftizoxime 1 g in 13 ml of sterile water for injection is isotonic (2).

The frozen premixed infusion solutions have osmolalities of 330 to 405 mOsm/kg for the 1 g/50-ml concentration and 410 to 505 mOsm/kg for the 2 g/50-ml concentration (4).

Robinson et al. recommended the following maximum ceftizoxime sodium concentrations to achieve osmolalities suitable for peripheral infusion in fluid-restricted patients (1180):

Diluent	Maximum Concentration (mg/ml)	Osmolality (mOsm/kg)
Dextrose 5% in water	69	530
Sodium chloride 0.9%	62	517
Sterile water for injection	125	437

Sodium Content— Each gram of ceftizoxime sodium contains 2.6 mEq (60 mg) of sodium (2).

Administration— Ceftizoxime sodium is administered by deep intramuscular injection, by direct intravenous injection over three to five minutes directly into the vein or into the tubing of a running compatible infusion solution, as an intermittent intravenous infusion in 50 to 100 ml of diluent over 15 to 30 minutes, and as a continuous intravenous infusion. Intramuscular doses of 2 g should be divided between different large muscles (2; 4).

Stability— Intact containers should be stored at room temperature and protected from light. The freshly reconstituted solution is colorless to pale yellow but may darken on storage. Solutions may change to a yellow to amber color without a loss of potency. If a precipitate forms, the solution should be discarded. Reconstituted solutions of 95, 270, or 280 mg/ml are stable for 24 hours at room temperature and 96 hours when refrigerated at 5 °C (2; 4).

Ceftizoxime sodium 2 g/30 ml in water stored in plastic syringes exhibited a 9% loss in 24 hours at 25 °C and in five days at 5 °C (1318).

The frozen premixed infusion should be stored at or below −20 °C. After thawing, the solution is stable for 48 hours at room temperature or 21 days at 5 °C. The thawed solution should not be refrozen (4).

Ceftizoxime sodium 1 and 2 g/50 ml in sodium chloride 0.9% in both PVC bags and glass bottles was stable for 90 days when frozen at −10 °C. However, these concentrations in dextrose 5% in water in PVC bags and glass bottles were stable for only 27 days when

Table 1. Recommended Dilutions of Ceftizoxime Sodium (2)

Vial Size	Route	Volume of Diluent	Withdrawable Volume	Approximate Concentration
500 mg	Intramuscular	1.5 ml	1.8 ml	280 mg/ml
	Intravenous	5 ml	5.3 ml	95 mg/ml
1 g	Intramuscular	3 ml	3.7 ml	270 mg/ml
	Intravenous	10 ml	10.7 ml	95 mg/ml
(Piggyback)	Intravenous	50 to 100 ml	50 to 100 ml	20 to 10 mg/ml
2 g	Intramuscular	6 ml	7.4 ml	270 mg/ml
	Intravenous	20 ml	21.4 ml	95 mg/ml
(Piggyback)	Intravenous	50 to 100 ml	50 to 100 ml	40 to 20 mg/ml

frozen at −10 °C due to precipitate formation. A 2-g/30 ml concentration in water frozen at −10 °C in plastic syringes was stable for 90 days (1319).

An evaluation of ceftizoxime sodium (SKF) solutions showed significantly increased particulate levels in four and a half hours at 25 °C, with gross precipitation in eight hours at 25 °C or 24 hours at 5 °C (986). The manufacturer subsequently reformulated the product, adding sodium bicarbonate. An evaluation of the new ceftizoxime sodium formulation 1 g/10 ml in sterile water for injection or 1 g/50 ml in dextrose 5% in water in PVC bags showed that the particulate levels were not significantly different from some other cephalosporins and were acceptable for 24 hours at 5 and 25 °C (1078).

In another evaluation, the original formulation and the new formulation containing sodium bicarbonate were compared for compatibility in solution. Samples of each were reconstituted with sterile water for injection. An aliquot of 1.07 g/10.7 ml was diluted further with 9.3 ml of Ionosol MB, Ionosol T, Isolyte P, or Isolyte M and run at 40 ml/hr for 30 minutes through PVC administration sets. With the original formulation, a granular, white precipitate formed in the reservoir and tubing of all Ionosol T samples. Flushing the tubing of the Ionosol MB samples with drug-free solution failed to prevent precipitate formation in most samples within two to four hours. Precipitation did not occur with the original formulation in Isolyte P or Isolyte M. Furthermore, precipitation did not occur in any solution with the new formulation (1079).

The development of a precipitate in ceftizoxime sodium solutions seems to correlate with the solution pH; at pH values greater than 6, a precipitate did not develop. Precipitation appears to occur more readily at high concentrations, at low pH values, and when dextrose 5% in water is the vehicle (1318).

Compatibility Information

Solution Compatibility

Ceftizoxime sodium

Solution	Mfr	Mfr	Conc/L	Remarks	Ref	C/I
Dextrose 5% in water	MG[a]	SKF	20 g	Physically compatible with no loss in 24 hr and 3% in 48 hr at room temperature under fluorescent light	983	C

Solution Compatibility (Cont.)

Ceftizoxime sodium

Solution	Mfr	Mfr	Conc/L	Remarks	Ref	C/I
	b		20 and 40 g	Physically compatible and chemically stable for 48 hr at 25 °C and for 7 days at 5 °C	1319	C
	a		40 g	Physically compatible and chemically stable for 48 hr at 25 °C and for 7 days at 5 °C	1319	C
Sodium chloride 0.9%	MG[a]	SKF	20 g	Physically compatible with 3% loss in 24 hr and 10% in 48 hr at room temperature under fluorescent light	983	C
	c		20 and 40 g	Physically compatible and chemically stable for 48 hr at 25 °C and for 7 days at 5 °C	1319	C

[a]Tested in glass bottles.
[b]Tested in PVC containers.
[c]Tested in both PVC containers and glass bottles.

Additive Compatibility

Ceftizoxime sodium

Drug	Mfr	Conc/L	Mfr	Conc/L	Test Soln	Remarks	Ref	C/I
Clindamycin phosphate	UP	9 g	SKF	20 g	D5W[a]	Physically compatible with 3% clindamycin loss and 4% ceftizoxime loss in 48 hr at room temperature under fluorescent light	983	C
	UP	9 g	SKF	20 g	NS[a]	Physically compatible with 7% ceftizoxime loss in 48 hr at room temperature under fluorescent light. 10% clindamycin loss in 8 hr but no further loss through 48 hr	983	C
Metronidazole	AB	5 g	FUJ	10 g		Visually compatible with little or no loss of either drug by HPLC in 72 hr at 8 °C	1849	C
	AB	5 g	SKB	10 g		Visually compatible with 8 to 9% loss of both drugs by HPLC in 14 days at 4 °C followed by 48 hr at 25 °C. 3 to 4% loss of both drugs in 3 days and 10 to 13% in 5 days at 25 °C	1879	C

[a]Tested in glass bottles.

Y-Site Injection Compatibility (1:1 Mixture)

Ceftizoxime sodium

Drug	Mfr	Conc	Mfr	Conc	Remarks	Ref	C/I
Acyclovir sodium	BW	5 mg/ml[a]	SKF	20 mg/ml[a]	Physically compatible for 4 hr at 25 °C	1157	C
Allopurinol sodium	BW	3 mg/ml[b]	FUJ	20 mg/ml[b]	Physically compatible with no change in measured turbidity or increase in particle content in 4 hr at 22 °C	1686	C
Amifostine	USB	10 mg/ml[a]	FUJ	20 mg/ml[a]	Physically compatible with no change in measured turbidity or increase in particle content in 4 hr at 23 °C	1845	C

Y-Site Injection Compatibility (1:1 Mixture) (Cont.)

Ceftizoxime sodium

Drug	Mfr	Conc	Mfr	Conc	Remarks	Ref	C/I
Amphotericin B cholesteryl sulfate complex	SEQ	0.83 mg/ml[a]	FUJ	20 mg/ml[a]	Physically compatible with little or no change in measured turbidity or increase in particle content in 4 hr at 23 °C under fluorescent light	2117	C
Aztreonam	SQ	40 mg/ml[a]	FUJ	20 mg/ml[a]	Physically compatible with no subvisual haze or particle formation in 4 hr at 23 °C	1758	C
Cisatracurium besylate	GW	0.1 and 2 mg/ml[a]	FUJ	20 mg/ml[a]	Physically compatible with no change in measured turbidity or increase in particle content in 4 hr at 23 °C	2074	C
	GW	5 mg/ml[a]	FUJ	20 mg/ml[a]	Subvisual haze forms in 1 hr	2074	I
Docetaxel	RPR	0.9 mg/ml[a]	FUJ	20 mg/ml[a]	Physically compatible with no change in measured turbidity or increase in particle content in 4 hr at 23 °C	2224	C
Doxorubicin HCl liposome injection	SEQ	0.4 mg/ml[a]	FUJ	20 mg/ml[a]	Physically compatible with little or no change in measured turbidity and no increase in particle content in 4 hr at 23 °C	2087	C
Enalaprilat	MSD	0.05 mg/ml[b]	SKF	10 mg/ml[a]	Physically compatible for 24 hr at room temperature under fluorescent light	1355	C
Esmolol HCl	DCC	10 mg/ml[a]	SKF	10 mg/ml[a]	Physically compatible for 24 hr at 22 °C	1169	C
Etoposide phosphate	BR	5 mg/ml[a]	FUJ	20 mg/ml[a]	Physically compatible with no change in measured turbidity or increase in particle content in 4 hr at 23 °C	2218	C
Famotidine	MSD	0.2 mg/ml[a]	SKF	20 mg/ml[b]	Physically compatible for 14 hr	1196	C
Filgrastim	AMG	30 μg/ml[a]	FUJ	20 mg/ml[a]	Particles and filaments form immediately	1687	I
Fludarabine phosphate	BX	1 mg/ml[a]	SKF	20 mg/ml[a]	Physically compatible for 4 hr at room temperature under fluorescent light	1439	C
Foscarnet sodium	AST	24 mg/ml	SKF	40 mg/ml	Physically compatible for 24 hr at room temperature under fluorescent light	1335	C
Gemcitabine HCl	LI	10 mg/ml[b]	FUJ	20 mg/ml[b]	Physically compatible with no change in measured turbidity or increase in particle content in 4 hr at 23 °C	2226	C
Granisetron HCl	SKB	0.05 mg/ml[a]	FUJ	20 mg/ml[a]	Physically compatible with no change in measured turbidity or increase in particle content in 4 hr at 23 °C	2000	C
Hydromorphone HCl	WY	0.2 mg/ml[a]	SKF	20 mg/ml[a]	Physically compatible for at least 4 hr at 25 °C under fluorescent light	987	C
Labetalol HCl	SC	1 mg/ml[a]	SKF	10 mg/ml[a]	Physically compatible for 24 hr at 18 °C	1171	C
Melphalan HCl	BW	0.1 mg/ml[b]	FUJ	20 mg/ml[b]	Physically compatible with no change in measured turbidity or increase in particle content in 3 hr at 22 °C	1557	C
Meperidine HCl	WY	10 mg/ml[a]	SKF	20 mg/ml[a]	Physically compatible for at least 4 hr at 25 °C under fluorescent light	987	C
Morphine sulfate	WI	1 mg/ml[a]	SKF	20 mg/ml[a]	Physically compatible for at least 4 hr at 25 °C under fluorescent light	987	C
Ondansetron HCl	GL	1 mg/ml[b]	FUJ	20 mg/ml[a]	Physically compatible for 4 hr at 22 °C	1365	C

Y-Site Injection Compatibility (1:1 Mixture) (Cont.)

		Ceftizoxime sodium					
Drug	*Mfr*	*Conc*	*Mfr*	*Conc*	*Remarks*	*Ref*	*C/I*
Promethazine HCl	ES	25 mg	FUJ	10 mg/ml[a]	Fine cloudy precipitate forms immediately and dissolves in seconds	1753	**?**
Propofol	ZEN	10 mg/ml	FUJ	20 mg/ml[a]	Physically compatible for 1 hr at 23 °C with no increase in particle content	2066	**C**
Ranitidine HCl	GL	1 mg/ml[b]	FUJ	20 mg/ml[b]	Visually compatible with no loss of either drug by HPLC in 4 hr at 25 °C	2209	**C**
Remifentanil HCl	GW	0.025 and 0.25 mg/ml[b]	FUJ	20 mg/ml[a]	Physically compatible with no change in measured turbidity or increase in particle content in 4 hr at 23 °C	2075	**C**
Sargramostim	IMM	10 μg/ml[b]	FUJ	20 mg/ml[b]	Physically compatible for 4 hr at room temperature under fluorescent light	1436	**C**
Teniposide	BR	0.1 mg/ml[a]	FUJ	20 mg/ml[a]	Physically compatible with no subvisual haze or particle formation in 4 hr at 23 °C	1725	**C**
Thiotepa	IMM[c]	1 mg/ml[a]	FUJ	20 mg/ml[a]	Physically compatible with no change in measured turbidity or increase in particle content in 4 hr at 23 °C	1861	**C**
TNA #218 to #226[d]			FUJ	20 mg/ml[a]	Visually compatible with no precipitate or emulsion damage apparent in 4 hr at 23 °C	2215	**C**
TPN #212 to #215[d]			FUJ	20 mg/ml[a]	Physically compatible with no change in measured turbidity or increase in particle content in 4 hr at 23 °C	2109	**C**
Vancomycin HCl	AB	20 mg/ml[a]	FUJ	280 mg/ml[e]	Transient precipitate forms, followed by clear solution	2189	**?**
	AB	20 mg/ml[a]	FUJ	1, 10, and 50 mg/ml[a]	Physically compatible with no change in measured turbidity or increase in particle content in 4 hr at 23 °C	2189	**C**
	AB	2 mg/ml[a]	FUJ	1[a], 10[a], 50[a], and 280[e] mg/ml	Physically compatible with no change in measured turbidity or increase in particle content in 4 hr at 23 °C	2189	**C**
Vinorelbine tartrate	BW	1 mg/ml[b]	FUJ	20 mg/ml[b]	Physically compatible with no change in measured turbidity or increase in particle content in 4 hr at 22 °C	1558	**C**

[a]*Tested in dextrose 5% in water.*
[b]*Tested in sodium chloride 0.9%.*
[c]*Lyophilized formulation tested.*
[d]*Refer to Appendix I for the composition of parenteral nutrition solutions. TNA indicates a 3-in-1 admixture, and TPN indicates a 2-in-1 admixture.*
[e]*Tested in sterile water for injection.*

Additional Compatibility Information

Solutions— Ceftizoxime sodium is stable for 24 hours at room temperature and 96 hours when refrigerated at 5 °C in the following infusion solutions (2; 4):

Dextrose 5% in sodium chloride 0.2, 0.45, and 0.9%
Dextrose 5 and 10% in water
Invert sugar 10%
Ringer's injection
Ringer's injection, lactated
Sodium bicarbonate 5%
Sodium chloride 0.9%

The drug is similarly stable in dextrose 5% in Ringer's injection, lactated, if initially reconstituted with sodium bicarbonate 4% (2; 4).

Vancomycin— The compatibility or incompatibility of vancomycin HCl mixed with or administered simultaneously with ceftizoxime sodium may be concentration dependent (2189). See Y-Site Compatibility above. Vancomycin HCl has a low pH and is variably compatible with drugs having neutral to mildly alkaline pH, including cephalosporins and penicillins. The compatibility may depend on a number of factors, including concentration of each drug, dilution vehicle, actual pH of solutions, and completeness of mixing during administration. Combinations that are compatible when well mixed may result in precipitation if only partially mixed, presumably because of regionally different concentrations and pH values. If attempting to administer vancomycin HCl with ceftizoxime sodium, take care to ensure that the specific combination and the concentrations are compatible under the exact administration conditions to be used. An inline filter should be used as a final safety measure (2189).

CEFTRIAXONE SODIUM
AHFS 8:12.06

Rocephin　　　　　　　　　　　　　　　　**Roche**

Products— Ceftriaxone sodium (Roche) is available in vials containing the equivalent of 250 mg, 500 mg, 1 g, and 2 g of ceftriaxone. It is also available in 1- and 2-g piggyback bottles and 10-g bulk pharmacy containers (2).

For intramuscular use, reconstitute the vials with a compatible diluent in the amounts indicated (2):

Vial Size	Volume of Diluent for 250 mg/ml	Volume of Diluent for 350 mg/ml
250 mg	0.9 ml	a
500 mg	1.8 ml	1.0 ml
1 g	3.6 ml	2.1 ml
2 g	7.2 ml	4.2 ml

aThis vial size not recommended for 350-mg/ml concentration because withdrawal of the entire contents may not be possible.

More dilute solutions for intramuscular injection may be prepared if required (2).

For intermittent intravenous infusion, reconstitute the vials with a compatible diluent in the amounts indicated to yield a 100-mg/ml solution (2):

Vial Size	Volume of Diluent
250 mg	2.4 ml
500 mg	4.8 ml
1 g	9.6 ml
2 g	19.2 ml

After reconstitution, withdraw the entire vial contents and further dilute in a compatible infusion solution to the desired concentration. Concentrations between 10 and 40 mg/ml are recommended, but lower concentrations may be used (2).

The piggyback bottles should be reconstituted with 10 or 20 ml of compatible diluent for the 1- or 2-g size, respectively. After reconstitution, further dilution to 50 to 100 ml with a compatible infusion solution is recommended (2).

The bulk pharmacy container should be reconstituted with 95 ml of a compatible diluent. The solution is not for direct administration and must be diluted further before use (4).

Ceftriaxone sodium (Roche) is also available as a frozen premixed infusion solution of 1 or 2 g in 50 ml of dextrose 3.8 or 2.4%, respectively, in water. It should be thawed at room temperature (2; 4).

pH— The pH of a 1% aqueous solution is approximately 6.7 (2), and the frozen premixed infusion solutions have a pH of approximately 6.6 (range 6 to 8) (4).

Osmolality— The frozen premixed infusion solutions have osmolalities of 276 to 324 mOsm/kg (4).

The osmolality of ceftriaxone sodium (Roche) 50 mg/ml was determined to be 351 mOsm/kg in dextrose 5% in water and 364 mOsm/kg in sodium chloride 0.9% (1375).

Sodium Content— Ceftriaxone sodium contains approximately 3.6 mEq (83 mg) of sodium per gram of ceftriaxone activity (2).

Administration— Ceftriaxone sodium is administered by deep intramuscular injection or intermittent intravenous infusion over 15 to 30 minutes in adults or over 10 to 30 minutes in pediatric patients (2; 4).

Stability— Intact vials of ceftriaxone sodium should be stored at room temperature and protected from light. After reconstitution, normal exposure to light is permitted. Solutions may vary from light yellow to amber, depending on length of storage, diluent, and concentration (2).

Reconstituted solutions of ceftriaxone sodium are stable, exhibiting less than a 10% potency loss for the time periods indicated (2):

Diluent	Ceftriaxone Concentration (mg/ml)	25 °C	4 °C
Sterile water for injection	100	3 days	10 days
	250, 350	24 hr	3 days
Sodium chloride 0.9%	100	3 days	10 days
	250, 350	24 hr	3 days
Dextrose 5% in water	100	3 days	10 days
	250, 350	24 hr	3 days
Bacteriostatic water for injection (benzyl alcohol 0.9%)	100	24 hr	10 days
	250, 350	24 hr	3 days
Lidocaine HCl 1% (without epinephrine)	100	24 hr	10 days
	250, 350	24 hr	3 days

Syringes— Bailey et al. reported the stability of ceftriaxone sodium (Roche) 10 and 40 mg/ml in dextrose 5% in water and sodium chloride 0.9% packaged in polypropylene syringes. The solutions were visually compatible and lost 5% or less ceftriaxone in 48 hours at 4 and 20 °C and ten days stored frozen at −10 °C (1720).

Plumridge et al. reported on the stability of ceftriaxone sodium (Roche) 100 mg/ml in sterile water for injection packaged in polypropylene syringes (Terumo). About 9 to 10% loss of ceftriaxone by HPLC analysis occurred in five days at 20 °C and 40 days at 4 °C. However, the room temperature samples underwent color intensification that the authors found unacceptable after about 72 hours.

Little or no loss occurred during 180 days of frozen storage at −20 °C (1990).

O'Connell et al. evaluated the stability of reconstituted ceftriaxone sodium 100 mg/ml packaged in 10-ml polypropylene syringes. Stored under refrigeration at 8 °C, about 5% loss occurred in 10 days and 8% in 13 days (1999).

Elastomeric Reservoir Pumps— Ceftriaxone sodium (Roche) 20 mg/ml in dextrose 5% in water and sodium chloride 0.9% was packaged in 100-ml latex elastomeric reservoirs (Secure Medical). About 3 to 5% loss by HPLC analysis occurred in 72 hours at 25 °C and in 10 days at 5 °C (1970).

Ceftriaxone sodium (Roche) 10 mg/ml in both dextrose 5% in water and sodium chloride 0.9% was evaluated for binding potential to natural rubber elastomeric reservoirs (Baxter). No loss was found after storage for two weeks at 35 °C with gentle agitation (2014).

Freezing Solutions— The manufacturer indicates that ceftriaxone sodium 10 to 40 mg/ml in dextrose 5% in water or sodium chloride 0.9%, when frozen at −20 °C in PVC or polyolefin containers, is stable for 26 weeks. Thawing should be performed at room temperature; thawed solutions should not be refrozen (2).

The frozen premixed infusion solutions are stable for at least 90 days at −20 °C. Thawed solutions are stable for 72 hours at room temperature or 21 days at 5 °C (4).

In one study, ceftriaxone sodium (Roche) 20 mg/ml in dextrose 5% in water (Travenol) in PVC containers was evaluated by antimicrobial assay after two weeks of storage at −20 °C. The potency loss was less than 3% (966).

Ceftriaxone sodium (Roche) 10 and 50 mg/ml in dextrose 5% in water and sodium chloride 0.9% frozen at −22 °C was stable for at least 26 weeks, exhibiting no more than a 7% loss. Microwave thawing did not adversely affect stability (1245).

Ceftriaxone sodium (Roche) solutions containing 250 and 450 mg/ml in dextrose 5% in water, 250 mg/ml in bacteriostatic water

for injection, and 450 mg/ml in lidocaine HCl 1% (Lyphomed) were evaluated for stability and pharmaceutical integrity during frozen storage at −15 °C. The solutions were packaged in 10-ml polypropylene syringes with attached needles (Becton-Dickinson) and frozen for eight weeks. Some syringes were stored further at 4 °C for 10 days or at 20 °C for three days. Ceftriaxone sodium losses of 5% or less were found by HPLC analysis after eight weeks of frozen storage. However, particulate matter levels were unacceptable in most samples. Only the 250-mg/ml solution in dextrose 5% in water met USP limits for the particulate matter test. While additional storage at 4 °C for 10 days did not cause an unacceptable drug loss, storage at 20 °C for three days resulted in an 11 to 12% drug loss (1824).

Ceftriaxone sodium (Roche) 20 mg/ml in dextrose 5% in water and sodium chloride 0.9% frozen at −20 °C for 12 weeks exhibited 3 to 7% loss of potency by HPLC analysis in latex elastomeric reservoirs (Secure Medical) and in glass containers (1970).

Two studies reported little or no loss of ceftriaxone by HPLC analysis during frozen storage in syringes. At concentrations of 10 and 40 mg/ml in dextrose 5% in water and sodium chloride 0.9%, less than 5% loss was found in 10 days at −10 °C (1720). At 100 mg/ml in sterile water for injection, less than 3% loss occurred in 180 days at −20 °C (1990). Furthermore, freezing the ceftriaxone sodium solutions for 60 days at −20 °C had little adverse effect on stability when stored subsequently at 4 and 20 °C. Stability periods after thawing of 30 days at 4 °C and three days at 20 °C were recommended (1990).

Reconstituted with lidocaine HCl 1% to 250 and 450 mg/ml, ceftriaxone sodium (Roche) losses were 4 to 6% in 168 days at −20 °C (1991).

pH Effects— The pH of maximum stability for ceftriaxone sodium in solution has been variously reported as 2.5 to 4.5 (1080) and 7.2 (1244).

Compatibility Information

Solution Compatibility

Ceftriaxone sodium

Solution	Mfr	Mfr	Conc/L	Remarks	Ref	C/I
Dextrose 3.4% in sodium chloride 0.3% [a]		RC	1 g	Physically compatible with 10% loss calculated to occur in 48 hr at 20 °C	1244	C
Dextrose 5% with potassium chloride 10 mEq/L		RC	10 g	5% loss in 24 hr and 8% in 48 hr at 20 °C. 2% loss in 48 hr and 7% in 72 hr at 4 °C	965	C
Dextrose 5% in sodium chloride 0.2% with potassium chloride 20 mEq/L		RC	10 g	3% loss in 24 hr and 4% in 48 hr at 20 °C. 4% loss 72 hr and 5% in 96 hr at 4 °C	965	C
Dextrose 5% in sodium chloride 0.45%		RC	10 g	3% loss in 48 hr at 20 °C. 5% loss in 72 hr and 9% in 96 hr at 4 °C	965	C
Dextrose 5% in water		RC	10 g	No loss in 48 hr and 8% in 72 hr at 20 °C. 4% loss in 72 hr and 9% in 96 hr at 4 °C	965	C
	TR[b]	RC	2 g	Little or no loss in 14 days at 20 and 4 °C	966	C
	MG[c]	RC	20 g	Physically compatible with 5% drug loss in 24 hr and 9% in 48 hr at 25 °C under fluorescent light	1026	C
	[b]	RC	40 g	Physically compatible with 12% loss in 3 days at 23 °C and 10% loss in 14 days at 4 °C	1243	C

Solution Compatibility (Cont.)

Solution	Mfr	Mfr	Conc/L	Remarks	Ref	C/I
	[a]	RC	1 g	Physically compatible with 10% loss calculated to occur in 48 hr at 20 °C	1244	C
		RC	10 g	Physically compatible with 8% loss in 7 days at room temperature. 5 to 8% loss in 12 weeks at 5 °C	1245	C
		RC	50 g	Physically compatible with no loss in 24 hr but 12 to 17% loss in 7 days at room temperature. 5% loss in 8 weeks at 5 °C	1245	C
	MG	RC	10 and 40 g	Visually compatible with 5% or less ceftriaxone loss in 48 hr at 4 and 20 °C after 10 days storage at −15 °C in polypropylene syringes	1720	C
	AB[d]	RC	20 g	3 to 6% loss by HPLC in 72 hr at 25 °C and in 10 days at 5 °C	1970	C
Dextrose 10% in water		RC	10 g	No loss in 48 hr and 8% in 72 hr at 20 °C. 2% loss in 72 hr and 8% in 96 hr at 4 °C	965	C
Ringer's injection, lactated	[a]	RC	1 g	Physically compatible with 10% loss calculated to occur in about 3 days at 20 °C	1244	C
		RC	10 and 13 g	Precipitate forms relatively rapidly	2222	I
Sodium chloride 0.9%		RC	10 g	4% loss in 48 hr and 14% in 72 hr at 20 °C. 3% loss in 48 hr and 9% in 72 hr at 4 °C	965	C
	MG[c]	RC	20 g	Physically compatible with 10% drug loss in 24 hr and 16% in 48 hr at 25 °C under fluorescent light	1026	C
	[b]	RC	40 g	Physically compatible with 5% loss in 3 days at 23 °C and 9% loss in 30 days at 4 °C	1243	C
	[a]	RC	1 g	Physically compatible with 10% loss calculated to occur in 10 days at 20 °C	1244	C
		RC	10 g	Physically compatible with 9% loss in 7 days at room temperature. 11 to 12% loss in 6 weeks at 5 °C	1245	C
		RC	50 g	Physically compatible with 8 to 9% loss in 7 days at room temperature. 5% loss in 5 weeks and 15% in 8 weeks at 5 °C	1245	C
	BA	RC	10 and 40 g	Visually compatible with 5% or less ceftriaxone loss in 48 hr at 4 and 20 °C after 10 days storage at −15 °C in polypropylene syringes	1720	C
	AB[d]	RC	20 g	3 to 5% or less loss by HPLC in 72 hr at 25 °C and in 10 days at 5 °C	1970	C
TPN[e]		RC	10 g	7% loss in 48 hr and 12% in 72 hr at 20 °C. 2% loss in 48 hr and 10% in 72 hr at 4 °C	965	C
TPN #107[f]			1 g	Physically compatible and ceftriaxone activity retained for 24 hr at 21 °C by microbiological assay	1326	C

[a]Tested in glass, PVC, and polyethylene containers.
[b]Tested in PVC containers.
[c]Tested in glass containers.
[d]Tested in glass containers and latex elastomeric reservoirs (Secure Medical).
[e]Tested in a parenteral nutrition solution composed of amino acids 2.2%, dextrose 20%, multivitamins 10 ml, and standard electrolytes and trace elements.
[f]Refer to Appendix I for the composition of parenteral nutrition solutions. TPN indicates a 2-in-1 admixture.

Additive Compatibility

			Ceftriaxone sodium					
Drug	Mfr	Conc/L	Mfr	Conc/L	Test Soln	Remarks	Ref	C/I
Aminophylline	AMR	1 g	RC	20 g	D5W, NS[a]	Yellow color forms immediately. 3 to 6% ceftriaxone loss and 8 to 12% aminophylline loss by HPLC in 24 hr	1727	I
	AMR	4 g	RC	20 g	D5W, NS[a]	Yellow color forms immediately, 15 to 20% ceftriaxone loss and 7 to 9% aminophylline loss by HPLC in 24 hr	1727	I
	AMR	1 g	RC	40 g	D5W, NS[a]	Yellow color forms immediately, 15 to 18% ceftriaxone loss and 1 to 3% aminophylline loss by HPLC in 24 hr	1727	I
Clindamycin phosphate	UP	12 g	RC	20 g	D5W[b]	10% ceftriaxone loss in 4 hr and 17% in 24 hr at 25 °C under fluorescent light. No clindamycin loss in 48 hr	1026	I
	UP	12 g	RC	20 g	NS[b]	10% ceftriaxone loss in 1 hr and 12% in 24 hr at 25 °C under fluorescent light. 6% clindamycin loss in 48 hr	1026	I
Metronidazole	AB	5 g	RC	10 g		Visually compatible with little or no loss of either drug by HPLC in 72 hr at 8 °C	1849	C
	BA	5 g	RC	10 g		Visually compatible with no metronidazole loss by HPLC and with 6% ceftriaxone loss in 3 days and 8% in 4 days at 25 °C	2101	C
Metronidazole HCl	SCS	15 g	RC	20 g	D5W, NS	Metronidazole begins to precipitate immediately and increases with time stored at 4 and 24 °C. 22 to 50% of the metronidazole precipitates in 4 hr	2091	I
	SCS	7.5 g	RC	10 g	D5W, NS	Visually compatible with little or no loss of either drug by HPLC at 24 °C in 72 hr	2091	C
	SCS	7.5 g	RC	10 g	D5W, NS	Visually compatible with little or no loss of either drug by HPLC at 4 °C through 24 hr. Slight precipitation occurred in 48 hr	2091	C
Theophylline	BA[c]	4 g	RC	40 g		Yellow color forms immediately. 14% ceftriaxone loss and no theophylline loss by HPLC in 24 hr	1727	I

[a]Tested in polyolefin containers.
[b]Tested in glass containers.
[c]Tested in PVC containers.

Drugs in Syringe Compatibility

			Ceftriaxone sodium				
Drug (in syringe)	Mfr	Amt	Mfr	Amt	Remarks	Ref	C/I
Lidocaine HCl	LY	1%	RC	450 mg/ml	5% or less ceftriaxone loss by HPLC in 8 weeks at −15 °C but solution failed the particulate matter test	1824	I
	DW	1%	RC	250 and 450 mg/ml	10% ceftriaxone loss in 3 days at 20 °C, 7 to 8% loss in 35 days at 4 °C, and 4 to 6% loss in 168 days at −20 °C. Lidocaine not tested	1991	C

Y-Site Injection Compatibility (1:1 Mixture)

			Ceftriaxone sodium				
Drug	Mfr	Conc	Mfr	Conc	Remarks	Ref	C/I
Acyclovir sodium	BW	5 mg/ml[a]	RC	20 mg/ml[a]	Physically compatible for 4 hr at 25 °C	1157	**C**
Allopurinol sodium	BW	3 mg/ml[b]	RC	20 mg/ml[b]	Physically compatible with no change in measured turbidity or increase in particle content in 4 hr at 22 °C	1686	**C**
Amifostine	USB	10 mg/ml[a]	RC	20 mg/ml[a]	Physically compatible with no change in measured turbidity or increase in particle content in 4 hr at 23 °C	1845	**C**
Amphotericin B cholesteryl sulfate complex	SEQ	0.83 mg/ml[a]	RC	20 mg/ml[a]	Decreased natural turbidity occurs immediately	2117	**I**
Amsacrine	NCI	1 mg/ml[a]	RC	40 mg/ml[a]	Immediate orange turbidity, developing into flocculent precipitate in 4 hr	1381	**I**
Aztreonam	SQ	40 mg/ml[a]	RC	20 mg/ml[a]	Physically compatible with no subvisual haze or particle formation in 4 hr at 23 °C	1758	**C**
Cisatracurium besylate	GW	0.1, 2, 5 mg/ml[a]	RC	20 mg/ml[a]	Physically compatible with no change in measured turbidity or increase in particle content in 4 hr at 23 °C	2074	**C**
Diltiazem HCl	MMD	5 mg/ml	RC	40 mg/ml[b]	Visually compatible	1807	**C**
Docetaxel	RPR	0.9 mg/ml[a]	RC	20 mg/ml[a]	Physically compatible with no change in measured turbidity or increase in particle content in 4 hr at 23 °C	2224	**C**
Doxorubicin HCl liposome injection	SEQ	0.4 mg/ml[a]	RC	20 mg/ml[a]	Physically compatible with little or no change in measured turbidity and no increase in particle content in 4 hr at 23 °C	2087	**C**
Etoposide phosphate	BR	5 mg/ml[a]	RC	20 mg/ml[a]	Physically compatible with no change in measured turbidity or increase in particle content in 4 hr at 23 °C	2218	**C**
Famotidine	ME	2 mg/ml[b]		20 mg/ml[a]	Visually compatible for 4 hr at 22 °C	1936	**C**
Filgrastim	AMG	30 μg/ml[a]	RC	20 mg/ml[a]	Particles and filaments form in 1 hr	1687	**I**
Fluconazole	RR	2 mg/ml	RC	40 mg/ml	Immediate precipitation	1407	**I**
Fludarabine phosphate	BX	1 mg/ml[a]	RC	20 mg/ml[a]	Physically compatible for 4 hr at room temperature under fluorescent light	1439	**C**
Foscarnet sodium	AST	24 mg/ml	RC	20 mg/ml[c]	Physically compatible for 24 hr at 25 °C under fluorescent light by visual and microscopic examination	1393	**C**
Gemcitabine HCl	LI	10 mg/ml[b]	RC	20 mg/ml[b]	Physically compatible with no change in measured turbidity or increase in particle content in 4 hr at 23 °C	2226	**C**
Granisetron HCl	SKB	0.05 mg/ml[a]	RC	20 mg/ml[a]	Physically compatible with no change in measured turbidity or increase in particle content in 4 hr at 23 °C	2000	**C**
Heparin sodium	TR	50 units/ml	RC	20 mg/ml	Visually compatible for 6 hr at 25 °C	1793	**C**
Labetalol HCl	GL	2.5[d] and 5 mg/ml	RC	20[a,b] and 100[d] mg/ml	Fluffy white precipitate forms immediately	1964	**I**

Y-Site Injection Compatibility (1:1 Mixture) (Cont.)

Ceftriaxone sodium

Drug	Mfr	Conc	Mfr	Conc	Remarks	Ref	C/I
Melphalan HCl	BW	0.1 mg/ml[b]	RC	20 mg/ml[b]	Physically compatible with no change in measured turbidity or increase in particle content in 3 hr at 22 °C	1557	C
Meperidine HCl	AB	10 mg/ml	RC	20 and 40 mg/ml[a]	Physically compatible for 4 hr at 25 °C	1397	C
Methotrexate sodium		30 mg/ml	RC	100 mg/ml	Visually compatible for 4 hr at room temperature	1788	C
Morphine sulfate	AB	1 mg/ml	RC	20 and 40 mg/ml[a]	Physically compatible for 4 hr at 25 °C	1397	C
Paclitaxel	NCI	1.2 mg/ml[a]	RC	20 mg/ml[a]	Physically compatible with no change in measured turbidity in 4 hr at 22 °C	1556	C
Pentamidine isethionate	FUJ	3 mg/ml[a]	RC	20 mg/ml[a]	Heavy white precipitate forms immediately	1880	I
Propofol	ZEN	10 mg/ml	RC	20 mg/ml[a]	Physically compatible for 1 hr at 23 °C with no increase in particle content	2066	C
Remifentanil HCl	GW	0.025 and 0.25 mg/ml[b]	RC	20 mg/ml[a]	Physically compatible with no change in measured turbidity or increase in particle content in 4 hr at 23 °C	2075	C
Sargramostim	IMM	10 μg/ml[b]	RC	20 mg/ml[b]	Physically compatible for 4 hr at 22 °C	1436	C
Sodium bicarbonate		1.4%	RC	100 mg/ml	Visually compatible for 4 hr at room temperature	1788	C
Tacrolimus	FUJ	1 mg/ml[b]	RC	40 mg/ml[a]	Visually compatible for 24 hr at 25 °C	1630	C
Teniposide	BR	0.1 mg/ml[a]	RC	20 mg/ml[a]	Physically compatible with no subvisual haze or particle formation in 4 hr at 23 °C	1725	C
Theophylline	TR	4 mg/ml	RC	20 mg/ml	Visually compatible for 6 hr at 25 °C	1793	C
Thiotepa	IMM[e]	1 mg/ml[a]	RC	20 mg/ml[a]	Physically compatible with no change in measured turbidity or increase in particle content in 4 hr at 23 °C	1861	C
TNA #218 to #226[f]			RC	20 mg/ml[a]	Visually compatible with no precipitate or emulsion damage apparent in 4 hr at 23 °C	2215	C
TPN #189[f]			RC	100 mg/ml[d]	Visually compatible for 24 hr at 22 °C	1767	C
TPN #212 to #215[f]			RC	20 mg/ml[a]	Physically compatible with no change in measured turbidity or increase in particle content in 4 hr at 23 °C	2109	C
Vancomycin HCl	LI	20 mg/ml	RC	100 mg/ml	White precipitate forms immediately	1398	I
	AB	20 mg/ml[a]	RC	250 mg/ml[d]	Transient precipitate forms, followed by clear solution	2189	?
	AB	20 mg/ml[a]	RC	10 and 50 mg/ml[a]	Gross white precipitate forms immediately	2189	I
	AB	20 mg/ml[a]	RC	1 mg/ml[a]	Subvisual measured haze forms immediately	2189	I
	AB	2 mg/ml[a]	RC	1[a], 10[a], 50[a], 250[d] mg/ml	Physically compatible with no change in measured turbidity or increase in particle content in 4 hr at 23 °C	2189	C
Vinorelbine tartrate	BW	1 mg/ml[b]	RC	20 mg/ml[b]	Tiny particles form immediately, becoming more numerous in 4 hr	1558	I

Y-Site Injection Compatibility (1:1 Mixture) (Cont.)

Ceftriaxone sodium

Drug	Mfr	Conc	Mfr	Conc	Remarks	Ref	C/I
Warfarin sodium	DME	2 mg/ml[d]	RC	20 mg/ml[a]	Visually compatible for 24 hr at 24 °C	2078	C
Zidovudine	BW	4 mg/ml[a]	RC	20 mg/ml[a]	Physically compatible for 4 hr at 25 °C under fluorescent light by visual and microscopic examination	1193	C

[a]Tested in dextrose 5% in water.
[b]Tested in sodium chloride 0.9%.
[c]Tested in both dextrose 5% in water and sodium chloride 0.9%.
[d]Tested in sterile water for injection.
[e]Lyophilized formulation tested.
[f]Refer to Appendix I for the composition of parenteral nutrition solutions. TNA indicates a 3-in-1 admixture, and TPN indicates a 2-in-1 admixture.

Additional Compatibility Information

The manufacturer recommends that ceftriaxone sodium not be physically combined with other drugs (2).

Solutions— Ceftriaxone sodium (Roche) is stable, exhibiting less than a 10% potency loss in the following solutions in the time periods indicated (2):

Diluent	Concentrations (mg/ml)	25 °C	4 °C
Amino acid injection 8.5% (FreAmine III)	10 to 40[a]	24 hr	
Dextrose 5% in sodium chloride 0.45%	10[b], 20[b], 40[b], 100[a]	3 days	Incompatible
Dextrose 5% in sodium chloride 0.9%	10[c], 20[c], 40[c], 100[a]	3 days	Incompatible
Dextrose 5% in water	10[b], 20[b], 40[b], 100[a]	3 days	10 days
Dextrose 10% in water	10[b], 20[b], 40[b], 100[a]	3 days	10 days
Ionosol B in dextrose 5%	10 to 40[a]	24 hr	
Invert sugar 10% in water	10 to 40[a]	24 hr	
Mannitol 5% in water	10 to 40[a]	24 hr	
Mannitol 10% in water	10 to 40[a]	24 hr	
Normosol M in dextrose 5%	10 to 40[b]	24 hr	
Sodium bicarbonate 5%	10 to 40[a]	24 hr	
Sodium chloride 0.9%	10[b], 20[b], 40[b], 100[a]	3 days	10 days
Sodium lactate injection	10 to 40[c]	24 hr	
Sterile water for injection	10[b], 20[b], 40[b], 100[a]	3 days	10 days

[a]Tested in glass containers.
[b]Tested in both glass and PVC containers.
[c]Tested in PVC containers.

Ceftriaxone sodium at concentrations of 10 to 40 mg/ml is incompatible with calcium-containing solutions, including Ringer's injection and Ringer's injection, lactated. Precipitation has been observed to form rapidly (2222).

Vancomycin— The compatibility or incompatibility of vancomycin HCl mixed with or administered simultaneously with ceftriaxone sodium is concentration dependent (2189). See Y-Site Compatibility above. Vancomycin HCl has a low pH and is variably compatible with drugs having neutral to mildly alkaline pH, including cephalosporins and penicillins. The compatibility may depend on a number of factors, including concentration of each drug, dilution vehicle, actual pH of solutions, and completeness of mixing during administration. Combinations that are compatible when well mixed may result in precipitation if only partially mixed, presumably due to regionally different concentrations and pH values. If attempting to administer vancomycin HCl with ceftriaxone sodium, take care to ensure that the specific combination and the concentrations are compatible under the exact administration conditions to be used. An inline filter should be used as a final safety measure (2189).

Peritoneal Dialysis Solutions— Ceftriaxone sodium (Roche) 1 mg/ml in Dianeal PD-1 with dextrose 1.5 and 4.25% was stable, retaining at least 90% potency by HPLC for 14 days at 4 °C, 24 hours at 23 °C, or six hours at 37 °C (1592).

CEFUROXIME SODIUM
AHFS 8:12.06

Zinacef   **Glaxo Wellcome**

Products— Cefuroxime sodium (Glaxo Wellcome) is available in vials and infusion packs containing 750 mg and 1.5 g of drug. The drug is also available in a 7.5-g pharmacy bulk package (2).

The vials should be reconstituted with sterile water for injection. Infusion packs may be reconstituted with sterile water for injection or any compatible infusion solution. (See Additional Compatibility Information.) Recommended volumes for reconstitution are shown in Table 1 (2).

The intramuscular concentration of 220 mg/ml is a suspension. The suspension should be dispersed with shaking before the dose is withdrawn (2).

Table 1. Recommended Dilutions of Cefuroxime Sodium (2)

Vial Size	Route	Volume of Diluent	Approximate Concentration
750 mg	Intramuscular (suspension)	3 ml	220 mg/ml
	Intravenous	8 ml	90 mg/ml
(Infusion pack)	Intravenous	100 ml	7.5 mg/ml
1.5 g	Intravenous	16 ml	90 mg/ml
(Infusion pack)	Intravenous	100 ml	15 mg/ml

The 7.5-g pharmacy bulk package should be reconstituted with 77 ml of sterile water for injection to yield a 95-mg/ml concentration (2).

Previously, a significant overfill was present in the 750-mg vials of cefuroxime sodium (Glaxo) (1081). However, the manufacturer has changed the product, greatly reducing the overfill (1082).

Cefuroxime sodium is also available as a frozen premixed solution containing 750 mg or 1.5 g in 50-ml PVC bags. Approximately 1.4 g of dextrose hydrous has been added to the 750-mg bags to adjust the osmolality. Both the 750-mg and 1.5-g bags also contain sodium citrate hydrous 300 and 600 mg, respectively. The pH is adjusted with hydrochloric acid and may have been adjusted with sodium hydroxide (2).

pH— The reconstituted vials have a pH of 6 to 8.5. The frozen premixed solutions have a pH of 5 to 7.5 (2).

Osmolality— The osmolality of the frozen premixed cefuroxime sodium solutions is approximately 300 mOsm/kg (2).

The osmolality of cefuroxime sodium (Glaxo) 30 mg/ml was determined to be 315 mOsm/kg in dextrose 5% in water and 314 mOsm/kg in sodium chloride 0.9%. At a concentration of 50 mg/ml, the osmolality was determined to be 329 mOsm/kg in dextrose 5% in water and 335 mOsm/kg in sodium chloride 0.9% (1375).

Robinson et al. recommended the following maximum cefuroxime sodium concentrations to achieve osmolalities suitable for peripheral infusion in fluid-restricted patients (1180):

Diluent	Maximum Concentration (mg/ml)	Osmolality (mOsm/kg)
Dextrose 5% in water	76	568
Sodium chloride 0.9%	68	541
Sterile water for injection	137	489

Sodium Content— Cefuroxime sodium vials contain 2.4 mEq (54.2 mg) per gram of cefuroxime activity. The frozen premixed 750-mg and 1.5-g solutions contain 4.8 mEq (111 mg) and 9.7 mEq (222 mg), respectively (2).

Administration— Cefuroxime sodium is administered by deep intramuscular injection, by direct intravenous injection over three to five minutes directly into the vein or into the tubing of a running infusion solution, by intermittent intravenous infusion over 15 to 60 minutes, or by continuous intravenous infusion. The manufacturer recommends temporarily discontinuing the primary solution when giving the drug by Y-site infusion (2; 4).

Stability— Intact vials should be stored at room temperature and protected from light. The drug is present as a white to off-white powder. Solutions may range in color from light yellow to amber. Both the powder and solutions of cefuroxime sodium darken, depending on storage conditions, without affecting their potency (2; 4).

The reconstituted suspension for intramuscular injection and the 90 to 100-mg/ml intravenous solution concentrations are stable for 24 hours at room temperature and 48 hours when refrigerated at 5 °C. The bulk pharmacy vial reconstituted to a concentration of 95 mg/ml is stable for 24 hours at room temperature or seven days under refrigeration. Dilution to concentrations of 1 to 30 mg/ml in compatible diluents results in solutions that are stable for 24 hours at room temperature or seven days under refrigeration (2; 4).

Ambulatory Infusion Pumps— Cefuroxime sodium (Glaxo) 22.5 and 45 mg/ml in sterile water for injection in PVC portable infusion pump reservoirs (Pharmacia Deltec) exhibited a 4 to 6% loss by HPLC in eight hours and an 11 to 12% loss in 16 hours at 30 °C. No loss occurred in 7 days at 3 °C (1581).

Syringes— Cefuroxime sodium (Glaxo) 125 mg/ml in sterile water for injection, packaged as 0.24 ml in 1-ml Injekt syringes (Braun) sealed with blind hubs and stored at about 6 °C, retained antibiotic activity against *Escherichia coli* for seven days. However, the yellow color of the solution became much darker over this period. About a 14% loss occurred in 14 days (1697).

Freezing Solutions— Commercial, frozen, premixed cefuroxime sodium injections are stable for at least 90 days after shipment when stored at −20 °C. Frozen solutions should be thawed at room temperature or under refrigeration. Some solution components may precipitate in the frozen state, but the precipitate redissolves upon thawing and reaching room temperature. Thawed solutions are stable for 24 hours at room temperature or 28 days at 5 °C (2; 4).

Extemporaneously prepared solutions of cefuroxime sodium 750 mg or 1.5 g added to 50 to 100-ml PVC bags of dextrose 5% in water or sodium chloride 0.9% are stable for six months at −20 °C. The manufacturer does not recommend the use of water baths or microwaves for thawing. Following thawing at room temperature, the solutions are stable for 24 hours at room temperature or seven days under refrigeration. The thawed solutions should not be refrozen (2; 4).

Minibags of cefuroxime sodium in dextrose 5% in water or sodium chloride 0.9%, frozen at −20 °C for up to 35 days, were thawed at room temperature and in a microwave oven, with care taken that the thawed solution temperature never exceeded 25 °C. No significant differences in cefuroxime sodium concentrations occurred between the two thawing methods (1192).

Cefuroxime sodium (Glaxo) 30 and 60 mg/ml in sterile water for injection in PVC portable infusion pump reservoirs (Pharmacia Deltec) and glass vials exhibited a 4% loss by HPLC after 30 days at −20 °C. Subsequent storage for four days at 3 °C resulted in about a 10% loss in the PVC bags and a 4% loss in the glass vials (1581).

Sorption— Cefuroxime sodium 6 mg/ml in dextrose 5% in water and sodium chloride 0.9% exhibited no loss due to sorption to PVC containers over 24 hours and to administration sets during one-hour simulated infusions (1953).

Compatibility Information

Solution Compatibility

Cefuroxime sodium

Solution	Mfr	Mfr	Conc/L	Remarks	Ref	C/I
Dextrose 5% in water	MG[a]	GL	15 g	5% loss in 48 hr at 25 °C under fluorescent light	1164	C
	[b]		6 g	Visually compatible with little or no loss by HPLC in 24 hr at room temperature and 4 °C	1953	C
	BA[a]	GL	15 g	Visually compatible with 7% loss by HPLC in 11 days at 4 °C	2142	C
Sodium chloride 0.9%	MG[a]	GL	15 g	5% loss in 48 hr at 25 °C under fluorescent light	1164	C
	[b]		6 g	Visually compatible with little or no loss by HPLC in 24 hr at room temperature and 4 °C	1953	C
TPN #107[c]			1 g	Physically compatible and cefuroxime activity retained for 24 hr at 21 °C by microbiological assay	1326	C

[a]Tested in glass bottles.
[b]Tested in PVC containers.
[c]Refer to Appendix I for the composition of parenteral nutrition solutions. TPN indicates a 2-in-1 admixture.

Additive Compatibility

Cefuroxime sodium

Drug	Mfr	Conc/L	Mfr	Conc/L	Test Soln	Remarks	Ref	C/I
Clindamycin phosphate	UP	9 g	GL	15 g	D5W	Physically compatible with 4% clindamycin loss and 6 to 8% cefuroxime loss in 48 hr at 25 °C under fluorescent light	1164	C
	UP	9 g	GL	15 g	NS	Physically compatible with 9% clindamycin and cefuroxime loss in 48 hr at 25 °C under fluorescent light	1164	C
	UP	9 g	GL	15 g	D5W[a]	Physically compatible with 6% cefuroxime loss and 4% clindamycin loss in 48 hr at room temperature	174	C
	UP	9 g	GL	15 g	NS[a]	Physically compatible with 9% cefuroxime and clindamycin loss in 48 hr at room temperature	174	C
Floxacillin sodium	BE	20 g	GL	37.5 g	W	Physically compatible for 72 hr at 15 and 30 °C	1479	C
	BE	10 g	GL	7.5 g	D5W, NS	Physically compatible for 48 hr. Potency of both drugs retained when assayed after 1 hr at room temperature	1036	C
Furosemide	HO	1 g	GL	37.5 g	W	Physically compatible for 72 hr at 15 and 30 °C	1479	C
Gentamicin sulfate	EX	800 mg	GL	7.5 g	D5W, NS[b]	Physically compatible with no loss of either drug in 1 hr	1036	C
		100 mg		1 g	TPN #107[c]	32% gentamicin loss in 24 hr at 21 °C by microbiological assay	1326	I
Metronidazole		5 g	GL	7.5 g	[b]	Physically compatible with no loss of either drug in 1 hr	1036	C
		5 g	GL	15 g		No loss of either drug in 4 hr at 24 °C	1376	C

Additive Compatibility (Cont.)

Cefuroxime sodium

Drug	Mfr	Conc/L	Mfr	Conc/L	Test Soln	Remarks	Ref	C/I
		5 g	GL	7.5 g		10% cefuroxime loss by HPLC in 16 days at 4 °C and 35 hr at 25 °C. No metronidazole loss by HPLC in 15 days at 4 and 25 °C	1565	C
	IVX	5 g	GL	7.5 and 15 g		Physically compatible with no visible precipitation or increase in measured particulates. No loss of metronidazole and about 6% cefuroxime loss in 49 days at 5 °C	2192	C
Netilmicin sulfate	EX	1 g	GL	7.5 g	D5W, NS[b]	Physically compatible with no loss of either drug in 1 hr	1036	C
Ranitidine HCl	GL	100 mg	GL	1.5 g	D5W	Color change within 24 hr at ambient temperature under fluorescent light	1151	?
	GL	50 mg and 2 g		6 g	D5W	Ranitidine chemically stable by HPLC for only 6 hr at 25 °C. Cefuroxime not tested	1515	I

[a]Tested in both glass and PVC containers.
[b]Tested in PVC containers.
[c]Refer to Appendix I for the composition of parenteral nutrition solutions. TPN indicates a 2-in-1 admixture.

Drugs in Syringe Compatibility

Cefuroxime sodium

Drug (in syringe)	Mfr	Amt	Mfr	Amt	Remarks	Ref	C/I
Doxapram HCl	RB	400 mg/ 20 ml	GL	750 mg/ 7 ml	Immediate turbidity	1177	I

Y-Site Injection Compatibility (1:1 Mixture)

Cefuroxime sodium

Drug	Mfr	Conc	Mfr	Conc	Remarks	Ref	C/I
Acyclovir sodium	BW	5 mg/ml[a]	GL	15 mg/ml[a]	Physically compatible for 4 hr at 25 °C	1157	C
Allopurinol sodium	BW	3 mg/ml[b]	GL	20 mg/ml[b]	Physically compatible with no change in measured turbidity or increase in particle content in 4 hr at 22 °C	1686	C
Amifostine	USB	10 mg/ml[a]	GL	30 mg/ml[a]	Physically compatible with no change in measured turbidity or increase in particle content in 4 hr at 23 °C	1845	C
Atracurium besylate	BW	0.5 mg/ml[a]	GL	7.5 mg/ml[a]	Physically compatible for 24 hr at 28 °C	1337	C
Aztreonam	SQ	40 mg/ml[a]	LI	30 mg/ml[a]	Physically compatible with no subvisual haze or particle formation in 4 hr at 23 °C	1758	C
Cisatracurium besylate	GW	0.1 mg/ml[a]	LI	30 mg/ml[a]	Physically compatible with no change in measured turbidity or increase in particle content in 4 hr at 23 °C	2074	C
	GW	2 mg/ml[a]	LI	30 mg/ml[a]	White cloudiness forms immediately	2074	I
	GW	5 mg/ml[a]	LI	30 mg/ml[a]	Turbidity formed immediately	2074	I
Clarithromycin	AB	4 mg/ml[a]	GW	60 mg/ml[a]	White precipitate forms in 3 hr at 30 °C and 24 hr at 17 °C	2174	I

Y-Site Injection Compatibility (1:1 Mixture) (Cont.)

Cefuroxime sodium

Drug	Mfr	Conc	Mfr	Conc	Remarks	Ref	C/I
Cyclophosphamide	MJ	20 mg/ml[a]	GL	30 mg/ml[a]	Physically compatible for 4 hr at 25 °C	1194	**C**
Diltiazem HCl	MMD	5 mg/ml	LI	15 and 100 mg/ml[b]	Visually compatible	1807	**C**
	MMD	1 mg/ml[b]	LI	100 mg/ml[b]	Visually compatible	1807	**C**
Docetaxel	RPR	0.9 mg/ml[a]	LI	30 mg/ml[a]	Physically compatible with no change in measured turbidity or increase in particle content in 4 hr at 23 °C	2224	**C**
Etoposide phosphate	BR	5 mg/ml[a]	GW	30 mg/ml[a]	Physically compatible with no change in measured turbidity or increase in particle content in 4 hr at 23 °C	2218	**C**
Famotidine	MSD	0.2 mg/ml[a]	GL	15 mg/ml[b]	Physically compatible for 14 hr	1196	**C**
	ME	2 mg/ml[b]		20 mg/ml[a]	Visually compatible for 4 hr at 22 °C	1936	**C**
Filgrastim	AMG	30 μg/ml[a]	GL	20 mg/ml[a]	Haze, particles, and filaments form immediately	1687	**I**
Fluconazole	RR	2 mg/ml	GL	30 mg/ml	Immediate precipitation	1407	**I**
Fludarabine phosphate	BX	1 mg/ml[a]	GL	30 mg/ml[a]	Physically compatible for 4 hr at room temperature under fluorescent light	1439	**C**
Foscarnet sodium	AST	24 mg/ml	GL	30 mg/ml	Physically compatible for 24 hr at room temperature under fluorescent light	1335	**C**
Gemcitabine HCl	LI	10 mg/ml[b]	GW	30 mg/ml[b]	Physically compatible with no change in measured turbidity or increase in particle content in 4 hr at 23 °C	2226	**C**
Granisetron HCl	SKB	0.05 mg/ml[a]	LI	30 mg/ml[a]	Physically compatible with no change in measured turbidity or increase in particle content in 4 hr at 23 °C	2000	**C**
Hydromorphone HCl	WY	0.2 mg/ml[a]	GL	30 mg/ml[a]	Physically compatible for at least 4 hr at 25 °C under fluorescent light	987	**C**
Melphalan HCl	BW	0.1 mg/ml[b]	GL	20 mg/ml[b]	Physically compatible with no change in measured turbidity or increase in particle content in 3 hr at 22 °C	1557	**C**
Meperidine HCl	WY	10 mg/ml[a]	GL	30 mg/ml[a]	Physically compatible for at least 4 hr at 25 °C under fluorescent light	987	**C**
Midazolam HCl	RC	1 mg/ml[a]	LI	15 mg/ml[a]	Particles form in 8 hr	1847	**I**
Morphine sulfate	WI	1 mg/ml[a]	GL	30 mg/ml[a]	Physically compatible for at least 4 hr at 25 °C under fluorescent light	987	**C**
Ondansetron HCl	GL	1 mg/ml[b]	LI	30 mg/ml[a]	Physically compatible for 4 hr at 22 °C	1365	**C**
Pancuronium bromide	ES	0.05 mg/ml[a]	GL	7.5 mg/ml[a]	Physically compatible for 24 hr at 28 °C	1337	**C**
Perphenazine	SC	0.02 mg/ml[a]	GL	30 mg/ml[a]	Physically compatible for 4 hr at 25 °C	1155	**C**
Propofol	ZEN	10 mg/ml	LI	30 mg/ml[a]	Physically compatible for 1 hr at 23 °C with no increase in particle content	2066	**C**
Remifentanil HCl	GW	0.025 and 0.25 mg/ml[b]	LI	30 mg/ml[a]	Physically compatible with no change in measured turbidity or increase in particle content in 4 hr at 23 °C	2075	**C**
Sargramostim	IMM	10 μg/ml[b]	GL	30 mg/ml[b]	Physically compatible for 4 hr at 22 °C	1436	**C**
Tacrolimus	FUJ	1 mg/ml[b]	LI	30 mg/ml[a]	Visually compatible for 24 hr at 25 °C	1630	**C**

Y-Site Injection Compatibility (1:1 Mixture) (Cont.)

			Cefuroxime sodium				
Drug	*Mfr*	*Conc*	*Mfr*	*Conc*	*Remarks*	*Ref*	*C/I*
Teniposide	BR	0.1 mg/ml[a]	GL	20 mg/ml[a]	Physically compatible with no subvisual haze or particle formation in 4 hr at 23 °C	1725	**C**
Thiotepa	IMM[c]	1 mg/ml[a]	LI	30 mg/ml[a]	Physically compatible with no change in measured turbidity or increase in particle content in 4 hr at 23 °C	1861	**C**
TNA #218 to #226[d]			GL	30 mg/ml[a]	Visually compatible with no precipitate or emulsion damage apparent in 4 hr at 23 °C	2215	**C**
TPN #212 to #215[d]			LI	30 mg/ml[a]	Physically compatible with no change in measured turbidity or increase in particle content in 4 hr at 23 °C	2109	**C**
Vancomycin HCl	AB	20 mg/ml[a]	GW	150 mg/ml[e]	Transient precipitate forms, followed by a subvisual measured haze	2189	**I**
	AB	20 mg/ml[a]	GW	50 mg/ml[a]	Gross white precipitate forms immediately	2189	**I**
	AB	20 mg/ml[a]	GW	10 mg/ml[a]	Subvisual measured haze forms immediately	2189	**I**
	AB	20 mg/ml[a]	GW	1 mg/ml[a]	Physically compatible with no change in measured turbidity or increase in particle content in 4 hr at 23 °C	2189	**C**
	AB	2 mg/ml[a]	GW	1[a], 10[a], 50[a], 150[e] mg/ml	Physically compatible with no change in measured turbidity or increase in particle content in 4 hr at 23 °C	2189	**C**
Vecuronium bromide	OR	0.1 mg/ml[a]	GL	7.5 mg/ml[a]	Physically compatible for 24 hr at 28 °C	1337	**C**
Vinorelbine tartrate	BW	1 mg/ml[b]	GL	20 mg/ml[b]	Large increase in measured turbidity occurs immediately and grows over 4 hr at 22 °C	1558	**I**

[a]*Tested in dextrose 5% in water.*
[b]*Tested in sodium chloride 0.9%.*
[c]*Lyophilized formulation tested.*
[d]*Refer to Appendix I for the composition of parenteral nutrition solutions. TNA indicates a 3-in-1 admixture, and TPN indicates a 2-in-1 admixture.*
[e]*Tested in sterile water for injection.*

Additional Compatibility Information

Solutions— The manufacturer states that cefuroxime sodium 1 to 30 mg/ml is stable in the following infusion solutions for 24 hours at room temperature or at least seven days under refrigeration, losing not more than 10% activity (2):

Dextrose 5% in sodium chloride 0.2, 0.45, and 0.9%
Dextrose 5 and 10% in water
Invert sugar 10%
Ringer's injection
Ringer's injection, lactated
Sodium chloride 0.9%
Sodium lactate ⅙ M

Additives— The manufacturer states that cefuroxime sodium is compatible admixed with heparin sodium 10 and 50 units/ml and potassium chloride 10 and 40 mEq/L in sodium chloride 0.9% (2).

The manufacturer recommends that cefuroxime sodium not be mixed with sodium bicarbonate injection or aminoglycosides (2).

Vancomycin— The compatibility or incompatibility of vancomycin HCl mixed with or administered simultaneously with cefuroxime sodium is concentration dependent (2189). See Y-Site Compatibility above. Vancomycin HCl has a low pH and is variably compatible with drugs having neutral to mildly alkaline pH, including cephalosporins and penicillins. The compatibility may depend on a number of factors, including concentration of each drug, dilution vehicle, actual pH of solutions, and completeness of mixing during administration. Combinations that are compatible when well mixed may result in precipitation if only partially mixed, presumably because of regionally different concentrations and pH values. If attempting to administer vancomycin HCl with cefuroxime sodium, take care to ensure that the specific combination and the concentrations are compatible under the exact administration conditions to be used. An inline filter should be used as a final safety measure (2189).

CHLORAMPHENICOL SODIUM SUCCINATE
AHFS 8:12.08

Chloromycetin Sodium Succinate   **Monarch**

Products— Chloramphenicol sodium succinate (Monarch) is available in vials containing the equivalent of chloramphenicol 1 g as the sodium succinate salt. The manufacturer recommends reconstitution with 10 ml of an aqueous diluent such as water for injection or dextrose 5% in water to yield a solution containing 100 mg/ml (10%) of chloramphenicol (1-8/96; 4).

pH— From 6.4 to 7 (4; 6).

Osmolality— Chloramphenicol sodium succinate 100 mg/ml in sterile water for injection has an osmolality of 533 mOsm/kg as determined by freezing-point depression (1071).

The osmolality of chloramphenicol sodium succinate 1 g was calculated for the following dilutions (1054):

	Osmolality (mOsm/kg)	
Diluent	50 ml	100 ml
Dextrose 5% in water	341	303
Sodium chloride 0.9%	368	330

The osmolality of chloramphenicol sodium succinate (Parke-Davis) 20 mg/ml was determined to be 330 mOsm/kg in dextrose 5% in water and 344 mOsm/kg in sodium chloride 0.9%. At 50 mg/ml, the osmolality was determined to be 417 and 422 mOsm/kg, respectively (1375).

Robinson et al. recommended the following maximum chloramphenicol sodium succinate concentrations to achieve osmolalities suitable for peripheral infusion in fluid-restricted patients (1180):

Diluent	Maximum Concentration (mg/ml)	Osmolality (mOsm/kg)
Dextrose 5% in water	71	554
Sodium chloride 0.9%	64	538
Sterile water for injection	128	473

Sodium Content— Chloramphenicol sodium succinate contains 2.25 mEq (52 mg) of sodium per gram of drug (1-8/96; 4).

Administration— Chloramphenicol sodium succinate injection at a concentration not exceeding 100 mg/ml may be administered by direct intravenous injection over at least one minute (1-8/96; 4).

Stability— The commercial product is stable at room temperature until the expiration date (6). The reconstituted solution is stable for 30 days at room temperature (4; 6; 108). Cloudy solutions should not be used (4). The stability of frozen solutions of chloramphenicol sodium succinate has been stated to be six months (108).

Chloramphenicol is stable over a pH range of 2 to 7, with maximum stability at pH 6 (1072). Chloramphenicol activity was retained for 24 hours at pH 3.6 to 7.5 in dextrose 5% in water (6).

Sorption— Chloramphenicol sodium succinate (Parke-Davis) 12 mg/L in sodium chloride 0.9% (Travenol) in PVC bags did not exhibit significant sorption to the plastic during one week of storage at room temperature (15 to 20 °C) (536).

In another study, chloramphenicol sodium succinate (Parke-Davis) 12 mg/L in sodium chloride 0.9% did not exhibit any loss due to sorption during a seven-hour simulated infusion through an infusion set (Travenol) consisting of a cellulose propionate burette chamber and 170 cm of PVC tubing (606).

The drug was also tested as a simulated infusion over at least one hour by a syringe pump system. A glass syringe on a syringe pump was fitted with 20 cm of polyethylene tubing or 50 cm of Silastic tubing. No loss of drug due to sorption was observed with either tubing (606).

A 25-ml aliquot of chloramphenicol sodium succinate (Parke-Davis) 12 mg/L in sodium chloride 0.9% stored in all-plastic syringes composed of polypropylene barrels and polyethylene plungers for 24 hours at room temperature in the dark did not exhibit any loss due to sorption (606).

Compatibility Information

Solution Compatibility

Chloramphenicol sodium succinate

Solution	Mfr	Mfr	Conc/L	Remarks	Ref	C/I
Dextran 40,000	PH			Physically compatible	44	**C**
Dextran 6% in dextrose 5%	AB	PD	1 g	Physically compatible	3	**C**
Dextran 6% in sodium chloride 0.9%	AB	PD	1 g	Physically compatible	3	**C**
Dextrose–Ringer's injection combinations	AB	PD	1 g	Physically compatible	3	**C**
Dextrose–Ringer's injection, lactated, combinations	AB	PD	1 g	Physically compatible	3	**C**
Dextrose 5% in Ringer's injection, lactated	AB			Potency retained for 24 hr	6	**C**
Dextrose–saline combinations	AB	PD	1 g	Physically compatible	3	**C**
Dextrose 5% in sodium chloride 0.9%		PD	500 mg	Physically compatible	74	**C**

Solution Compatibility (Cont.)

Chloramphenicol sodium succinate

Solution	Mfr	Mfr	Conc/L	Remarks	Ref	C/I
	AB			Potency retained for 24 hr	6	**C**
		PD	2 g	Potency retained for 24 hr	109	**C**
Dextrose 2½% in water	AB	PD	1 g	Physically compatible	3	**C**
Dextrose 5% in water	AB	PD	1 g	Physically compatible	3	**C**
		PD	500 mg	Physically compatible	74	**C**
	AB			Potency retained for 24 hr	6	**C**
		PD	2 g	Potency retained for 24 hr	109	**C**
			10 g	4% loss in 24 hr at room temperature	768	**C**
Dextrose 10% in water	AB	PD	1 g	Physically compatible	3	**C**
	AB			Potency retained for 24 hr	6	**C**
		PD	2 g	Potency retained for 24 hr	109	**C**
Fat emulsion 10%, intravenous	VT	PD	2 g	Physically compatible for 48 hr at 4 °C and room temperature	32	**C**
	VT	PD	2 g	Physically compatible for 24 hr at 25 and 8 °C	825	**C**
Fructose 10% in sodium chloride 0.9%	AB	PD	1 g	Physically compatible	3	**C**
Fructose 10% in water	AB	PD	1 g	Physically compatible	3	**C**
Invert sugar 5 and 10% in sodium chloride 0.9%	AB	PD	1 g	Physically compatible	3	**C**
Invert sugar 5 and 10% in water	AB	PD	1 g	Physically compatible	3	**C**
Ionosol products	AB	PD	1 g	Physically compatible	3	**C**
Normosol M in dextrose 5% in water	AB			Potency retained for 24 hr	6	**C**
Normosol R	AB			Potency retained for 24 hr	6	**C**
Ringer's injection	AB	PD	1 g	Physically compatible	3	**C**
	AB			Potency retained for 24 hr	6	**C**
Ringer's injection, lactated	AB	PD	1 g	Physically compatible	3	**C**
		PD	500 mg	Physically compatible	74	**C**
	AB			Potency retained for 24 hr	6	**C**
Sodium chloride 0.45%	AB	PD	1 g	Physically compatible	3	**C**
Sodium chloride 0.9%	AB	PD	1 g	Physically compatible	3	**C**
		PD	500 mg	Physically compatible	74	**C**
	AB			Potency retained for 24 hr	6	**C**
		PD	2 g	Potency retained for 24 hr	109	**C**
			10 g	4% loss in 24 hr at room temperature	768	**C**
Sodium lactate ⅙ M	AB	PD	1 g	Physically compatible	3	**C**

Additive Compatibility

Chloramphenicol sodium succinate

Drug	Mfr	Conc/L	Mfr	Conc/L	Test Soln	Remarks	Ref	C/I
Amikacin sulfate	BR	5 g	PD	10 g	D5LR, D5R, D5S, D5W, D10W, IS10, LR, NS, R, SL	Physically compatible and potency of both retained for 24 hr at 25 °C	293	**C**
Aminophylline	SE	1 g	PD	10 g	D5W	Physically compatible	15	**C**
		250 mg	PD	500 mg	D5W	Physically compatible	74	**C**

Additive Compatibility (Cont.)

Chloramphenicol sodium succinate

Drug	Mfr	Conc/L	Mfr	Conc/L	Test Soln	Remarks	Ref	C/I
Ascorbic acid injection	AB	1 g	PD	1 g		Physically compatible	3	C
	AB	1 g	PD	1 g		Physically compatible	6	C
Calcium chloride	UP	1 g	PD	10 g	D5W	Physically compatible	15	C
Calcium gluconate		1 g	PD	500 mg	D5W	Physically compatible	74	C
	UP	1 g	PD	10 g	D5W	Physically compatible	15	C
	UP	1 g	PD	10 g		Physically compatible	6	C
Chlorpromazine HCl	BP	200 mg	BP	4 g	D5W	Immediate precipitation	26	I
	BP	200 mg	BP	4 g	NS	Haze develops over 3 hr	26	I
Colistimethate sodium	WC	500 mg	PD	10 g	D5W	Physically compatible	15	C
	WC	500 mg	PD	10 g		Physically compatible	6	C
Corticotropin		500 units	PD	500 mg	D5W	Physically compatible	74	C
Cyanocobalamin	AB	1000 µg	PD	1 g		Physically compatible	6	C
Dimenhydrinate	SE	50 mg	PD	500 mg	D5W	Physically compatible	74	C
Dopamine HCl	AS	800 mg	PD	4 g	D5W	Chloramphenicol and dopamine potency retained for 24 hr at 23 to 25 °C	78	C
Ephedrine sulfate	AB	50 mg	PD	1 g		Physically compatible	6	C
Heparin sodium	UP	4000 units	PD	10 g	D5W	Physically compatible	15	C
	AB	20,000 units	PD	1 g		Physically compatible	6;21	C
		12,000 units	PD	500 mg	D5W	Physically compatible	74	C
Hydrocortisone sodium succinate	UP	500 mg	PD	10 g	D5W	Physically compatible	15	C
	UP	500 mg	PD	1 g		Physically compatible	6	C
	UP	100 mg	PD	500 mg	D5W	Physically compatible	74	C
Hydroxyzine HCl	RR	250 mg	PD	10 g	D5W	Physically incompatible	15	I
Kanamycin sulfate	BR	4 g	PD	10 g	D5W	Physically compatible	15	C
	BR	4 g	PD	10 g		Physically compatible	6	C
Lidocaine HCl	AST	2 g	PD	1 g		Physically compatible	24	C
Magnesium sulfate	LI	16 mEq	PD	10 g	D5W	Physically compatible	15	C
Metaraminol bitartrate	MSD	100 mg	PD	1 g		Physically compatible	7	C
	MSD	200 mg	PD	1 g		Physically compatible	6	C
Methyldopate HCl	MSD	1 g	PD	1 g	D, D–S, S	Physically compatible	23	C
Methylprednisolone sodium succinate	UP	40 mg	PD	1 g	D5W	Clear solution for 20 hr	329	C
	UP	80 mg	PD	2 g	D5W	Clear solution for 20 hr	329	C
Metronidazole	RP	5 g[a]	PD	10 g		Physically compatible with little or no pH change for at least 72 hr at 23 °C	807	C
Metronidazole HCl with sodium bicarbonate	SE AB	5 g 50 mEq	PD	2 g	D5W, NS	Physically compatible for 48 hr	765	C
Nafcillin sodium	WY	500 mg	PD	1 g		Physically compatible	27	C
Oxacillin sodium	BR	2 g	PD	1 g		Physically compatible	6	C
	BR	500 mg	PD	500 mg	D5S, D5W	Therapeutic availability maintained	110	C
	BR	2 g	PD	1 g	D5S, D5W	Therapeutic availability maintained	110	C

Additive Compatibility (Cont.)

Chloramphenicol sodium succinate

Drug	Mfr	Conc/L	Mfr	Conc/L	Test Soln	Remarks	Ref	C/I
Oxytocin	PD	5 units	PD	1 g		Physically compatible	6	C
Penicillin G potassium		1 million units	PD	1 g		Physically compatible	3	C
	SQ	1 million units	PD	500 mg	D5S, D5W	Therapeutic availability maintained	110	C
	SQ	5 million units	PD	1 g		Physically compatible	47	C
	SQ	5 million units	PD	1 g	D5S, D5W	Therapeutic availability maintained	110	C
	SQ	10 million units	PD	1 g		Physically compatible	6	C
	SQ	10 million units	PD	1 g	D5S, D5W	Therapeutic availability maintained	110	C
	SQ	20 million units	PD	10 g	D5W	Physically compatible	15	C
Penicillin G sodium	UP	20 million units	PD	10 g	D5W	Physically compatible	15	C
Pentobarbital sodium	AB	200 mg	PD	1 g		Physically compatible	6	C
Phenylephrine HCl	WI	2.5 g	PD	500 mg	D5W, NS	Phenylephrine potency retained for over 24 hr at 22 °C	132	C
Phenylephrine HCl with sodium bicarbonate	WI AB	2.5 g 7.5 g	PD	500 mg	D5W	Phenylephrine potency retained for over 24 hr at 22 °C	132	C
Phytonadione	MSD	50 mg	PD	1 g		Physically compatible	6	C
Plasma protein fraction	CU	5 g	PD	1 g		Physically compatible	6	C
Polymyxin B sulfate	BW BW	200 mg 200 mg	PD PD	10 g 10 g	D5W	Physically incompatible Precipitate forms within 1 hr	15 6	I I
Potassium chloride		20 and 40 mEq	PD	500 mg	D5W, D2.5½S	Therapeutic availability maintained	110	C
		20 and 40 mEq	PD	1 g	D5W, D2.5½S	Therapeutic availability maintained	110	C
	AB	40 mEq	PD	1 g		Physically compatible	6	C
		3 g	PD	500 mg	D5W	Physically compatible	74	C
Prochlorperazine edisylate	SKF	100 mg	PD	10 g	D5W	Physically incompatible	15	I
Prochlorperazine mesylate	BP	100 mg	BP	4 g	NS	Haze develops over 3 hr	26	I
Promazine HCl	WY	100 mg	PD	1 g		Physically compatible	6	C
Promethazine HCl	WY	250 mg	PD	10 g	D5W	Physically incompatible	15	I
Ranitidine HCl	GL	100 mg		2 g	D5W	Physically compatible for 24 hr at ambient temperature	1151	C
Sodium bicarbonate		80 mEq	PD	1 g		Physically compatible	6	C
	AB	80 mEq	PD	1 g	D5W	Physically compatible	15	C

Additive Compatibility (Cont.)

Chloramphenicol sodium succinate

Drug	Mfr	Conc/L	Mfr	Conc/L	Test Soln	Remarks	Ref	C/I
Sodium bicarbonate with phenylephrine HCl	AB WI	7.5 g 2.5 g	PD	500 mg	D5W	Phenylephrine potency retained for over 24 hr at 22 °C	132	C
Thiopental sodium	AB	2.5 g	PD	1 g	D5W	Physically compatible	21	C
Vancomycin HCl	LI	5 g	PD	10 g	D5W	Physically incompatible	15	I
Verapamil HCl	KN	80 mg	PD	2 g	D5W, NS	Physically compatible for 24 hr	764	C
Vitamin B complex with C	AB AB	10 ml 2 ml 1 vial	PD PD PD	1 g 1 g 500 mg	D5W	Physically compatible Physically compatible Physically compatible	6 3 74	C C C

[a]*Minibags (100 ml) containing metronidazole 500 mg with disodium phosphate 150 mg, citric acid 44 mg, and sodium chloride 740 mg. This product differs from the Searle product.*

Drugs in Syringe Compatibility

Chloramphenicol sodium succinate

Drug (in syringe)	Mfr	Amt	Mfr	Amt	Remarks	Ref	C/I
Ampicillin sodium	AY	500 mg	PD	250 and 400 mg/ ml in 1.5 to 2 ml	No precipitate or color change within 1 hr at room temperature	99	C
	AY	500 mg	PD	250 and 400 mg/ 1 ml	Physically compatible for 1 hr at room temperature	300	C
Diatrizoate meglumine and diatrizoate sodium	MA	52% + 8%, 5 ml	PD	33 mg/ 1 ml	Physically compatible for at least 2 hr	1438	C
Diatrizoate sodium	WI	60%, 5 ml	PD	33 mg/ 1 ml	Physically compatible for at least 2 hr	1438	C
Glycopyrrolate	RB	0.2 mg/ 1 ml	PD	100 mg/ 1 ml	Gas evolves	331	I
	RB	0.2 mg/ 1 ml	PD	200 mg/ 2 ml	Gas evolves	331	I
	RB	0.4 mg/ 2 ml	PD	100 mg/ 1 ml	Gas evolves	331	I
Heparin sodium	AB	20,000 units/ 1 ml	PD	1 g	Physically compatible for at least 30 min	21	C
		2500 units/ 1 ml		1 g	Physically compatible for at least 5 min	1053	C
Iohexol	WI	64.7%, 5 ml	PD	33 mg/ 1 ml	Physically compatible for at least 2 hr	1438	C
Iopamidol	SQ	61%, 5 ml	PD	33 mg/ 1 ml	Physically compatible for at least 2 hr	1438	C
Iothalamate meglumine	MA	60%, 5 ml	PD	33 mg/ 1 ml	Physically compatible for at least 2 hr	1438	C
Ioxaglate meglumine and ioxaglate sodium	MA	39.3% + 19.6%, 5 ml	PD	33 mg/ 1 ml	Physically compatible for at least 2 hr	1438	C

Drugs in Syringe Compatibility (Cont.)

Chloramphenicol sodium succinate

Drug (in syringe)	Mfr	Amt	Mfr	Amt	Remarks	Ref	C/I
Metoclopramide HCl	RB	10 mg/ 2 ml	PD	250 mg/ 2.5 ml	Incompatible. Do not mix	924	I
	RB	10 mg/ 2 ml	PD	2 g/ 20 ml	Incompatible. Do not mix	924	I
	RB	10 mg/ 2 ml	PD	250 mg/ 2.5 ml	White precipitate forms within 1 hr at 25 °C	1167	I
	RB	10 mg/ 2 ml	PD	2 g/ 20 ml	White precipitate forms within 1 hr at 25 °C	1167	I
	RB	160 mg/ 32 ml	PD	2 g/ 20 ml	White precipitate forms within 1 hr at 25 °C	1167	I
Penicillin G sodium		1 million units	PD	250 and 400 mg/ ml in 1.5 to 2 ml	No precipitate or color change within 1 hr at room temperature	99	C

Y-Site Injection Compatibility (1:1 Mixture)

Chloramphenicol sodium succinate

Drug	Mfr	Conc	Mfr	Conc	Remarks	Ref	C/I
Acyclovir sodium	BW	5 mg/ml[a]	ES	20 mg/ml[a]	Physically compatible for 4 hr at 25 °C	1157	C
Cyclophosphamide	MJ	20 mg/ml[a]	ES	20 mg/ml[a]	Physically compatible for 4 hr at 25 °C	1194	C
Enalaprilat	MSD	0.05 mg/ml[b]	PD	10 mg/ml[a]	Physically compatible for 24 hr at room temperature under fluorescent light	1355	C
Esmolol HCl	DCC	10 mg/ml[a]	PD	10 mg/ml[a]	Physically compatible for 24 hr at 22 °C	1169	C
Fluconazole	RR	2 mg/ml	PD	20 mg/ml	Gas production	1407	I
Foscarnet sodium	AST	24 mg/ml	PD	20 mg/ml	Physically compatible for 24 hr at room temperature under fluorescent light	1335	C
Hydromorphone HCl	WY	0.2 mg/ml[a]	LY	20 mg/ml[a]	Physically compatible for at least 4 hr at 25 °C under fluorescent light	987	C
Labetalol HCl	SC	1 mg/ml[a]	PD	10 mg/ml[a]	Physically compatible for 24 hr at 18 °C	1171	C
Magnesium sulfate	IX	16.7, 33.3, 66.7, 100 mg/ml[a]	PD	20 mg/ml[a]	Physically compatible for at least 4 hr at 32 °C	813	C
Meperidine HCl	WY	10 mg/ml[a]	LY	20 mg/ml[a]	Physically compatible for at least 4 hr at 25 °C under fluorescent light	987	C
Morphine sulfate	WI	1 mg/ml[a]	LY	20 mg/ml[a]	Physically compatible for at least 4 hr at 25 °C under fluorescent light	987	C
Perphenazine	SC	0.02 mg/ml[a]	ES	20 mg/ml[a]	Physically compatible for 4 hr at 25 °C	1155	C
Tacrolimus	FUJ	1 mg/ml[b]	PD	20 mg/ml[a]	Visually compatible for 24 hr at 25 °C	1630	C
TPN #61[c]		[d]	PD	125 mg/ 1.25 ml[e]	Physically compatible	1012	C
		[f]	PD	750 mg/ 7.5 ml[e]	Physically compatible	1012	C

[a]Tested in dextrose 5% in water.
[b]Tested in sodium chloride 0.9%.
[c]Refer to Appendix I for the composition of parenteral nutrition solutions. TPN indicates a 2-in-1 admixture.
[d]Run at 21 ml/hr.
[e]Given over five minutes by syringe pump.
[f]Run at 94 ml/hr.

Additional Compatibility Information

Solutions— Chloramphenicol sodium succinate (Parke-Davis) 1 g/L is physically compatible with all Abbott infusion solutions. It is also compatible with benzyl alcohol–preserved bacteriostatic water for injection (6).

Additives— Chloramphenicol sodium succinate is stated to be physically compatible for 24 hours at room temperature with lincomycin HCl in infusion solutions (154).

Concentrations of chloramphenicol sodium succinate higher than 1 g/L should be used cautiously with other macromolecules (6).

Chloramphenicol sodium succinate (Parke-Davis) in dextrose 5% in water has been reported to be conditionally compatible with ascorbic acid injection (Upjohn), erythromycin lactobionate (Abbott), and vitamin B complex with C (Abbott). The incompatibility is concentration dependent. Therefore, if attempting to combine chloramphenicol sodium succinate with any of these drugs, mix the solution thoroughly and observe it closely for any sign of incompatibility (15).

Concentrated Solutions— The following incompatibility determinations were performed with concentrated solutions. The drugs in dry form were reconstituted according to the manufacturers' recommendations. One milliliter of chloramphenicol sodium succinate (Parke-Davis) was added to 5 ml of sterile distilled water along with 1 ml of each of the following drugs. Particulate matter was noted within two hours (28):

> Hydroxyzine HCl (Pfizer)
> Phenytoin sodium (Parke-Davis)
> Prochlorperazine edisylate (SKF)
> Promazine HCl (Wyeth)
> Promethazine HCl (Wyeth)
> Vancomycin HCl (Lilly)

CHLORDIAZEPOXIDE HCL
AHFS 28:24.08

Librium   **Roche**

Products— Chlordiazepoxide HCl (Roche) is available in 5-ml dry-filled ampuls containing 100 mg of drug. Accompanying the ampul of drug is a 2-ml ampul of diluent for intramuscular administration. The diluent contains (2):

Benzyl alcohol	1.5%
Polysorbate 80	4%
Propylene glycol	20%
Maleic acid	1.6%
Sodium hydroxide	to adjust pH

For intramuscular injection, the 2 ml of special intramuscular diluent should be added to the 100-mg ampul of the drug. Avoid excessive pressure in adding the diluent to preclude bubble formation. Agitate gently until a clear solution is obtained. The resultant solution has a concentration of 50 mg/ml. Do not use other diluents for intramuscular injection because of pain on injection (2; 4).

For intravenous injection, 5 ml of sterile water for injection or sodium chloride 0.9% should be added to the 100-mg ampul of chlordiazepoxide HCl. Agitate gently until dissolved. The resultant solution has a concentration of 20 mg/ml. Although the special intramuscular diluent has been given intravenously without adverse effects, this practice is not recommended because air bubbles may form during reconstitution (2; 4).

pH— The special intramuscular diluent has a pH of 2.5 to 3.5. After reconstitution of 100 mg of chlordiazepoxide HCl with 2 ml of this special diluent or 5 ml of sterile water for injection or sodium chloride 0.9%, the pH is approximately 3 (2; 4).

Administration— Chlordiazepoxide HCl is usually administered by slow direct intravenous injection over one minute. It may also be given by deep intramuscular injection slowly into the upper outer quadrant of the gluteus muscle (2; 4), but this route is rarely justified because of slow and erratic absorption (4).

Stability— Chlordiazepoxide HCl for injection is unstable in solution, and the manufacturer recommends that the solution be prepared immediately before use. Also, it is recommended that any unused solution be discarded. Heat sterilization of the solution should not be attempted (2; 4).

Hydrolysis of the polysorbate 80 in the special intramuscular diluent may occur, resulting in opalescence. Consequently, refrigerated storage is recommended. However, the diluent is stated to be stable for at least 48 hours at temperatures not exceeding 25 °C (4). Previously, Roche indicated the diluent was stable for up to one month stored at 15 to 30 °C if haziness or turbidity does not develop (853). The special intramuscular diluent should not be used if it is opalescent or hazy (2; 4).

The manufacturer recommends that the powder be protected from light (4).

Sorption— Chlordiazepoxide HCl (Roche) 1 and 2 g/L in sodium chloride 0.9% (Baxter), when transferred to PVC bags, showed about a 10 to 20% loss of drug over two hours at 22 °C in normal light. In Ringer's injection at the same concentrations and conditions, losses of about 10% occurred in four hours. Because decomposition products were well within normal USP limits and because similar losses were not observed when the admixtures were tested in glass bottles, the losses were attributed to sorption to the PVC bag. When dextrose 5% in water was the vehicle, little or no drug loss (5% or less) due to sorption to the PVC bag occurred (745).

Plasticizer Leaching— Chlordiazepoxide HCl (Roche) 2 mg/ml in dextrose 5% in water leached relatively minor amounts of diethylhexyl phthalate (DEHP) plasticizer from PVC bags. This leaching was due to the surfactant polysorbate 80 (Tween 80) in the formulation. After 24 hours at 24 °C, the DEHP concentration in 50-ml bags of infusion solution was 3.2 μg/ml. This finding is consistent with the low surfactant concentration (0.16%) in the final admixture solution. The actual amount of DEHP leached from PVC containers and administration sets may vary in clinical situations, depending on surfactant concentration, bag size, and contact time (1683).

Compatibility Information

Solution Compatibility

Chlordiazepoxide HCl

Solution	Mfr	Mfr	Conc/L	Remarks	Ref	C/I
Dextrose 5% in water	BA[a]	RC	1 and 2 g	Physically compatible and chemically stable at 22 °C for 4-hr study period	745	C
	BA[b]	RC	1 and 2 g	Physically compatible and chemically stable at 22 °C with little or no loss due to sorption during 4-hr study period	745	C
Ringer's injection	BA[a]	RC	1 and 2 g	Physically compatible and chemically stable at 22 °C for 4-hr study period	745	C
	BA[b]	RC	1 and 2 g	Physically compatible but with approximately 10% loss in 4 hr at 22 °C apparently due to sorption	745	I
Sodium chloride 0.9%	BA[a]	RC	1 and 2 g	Physically compatible and chemically stable at 22 °C for 4-hr study period	745	C
	BA[b]	RC	1 g	Approximately 10% loss in 2 hr and 20% loss in 4 hr at 22 °C apparently due to sorption	745	I
	BA[b]	RC	2 g	Approximately 20% loss in 2 hr at 22 °C apparently due to sorption	745	I

[a]Tested in glass containers.
[b]Tested in PVC containers.

Y-Site Injection Compatibility (1:1 Mixture)

Chlordiazepoxide HCl

Drug	Mfr	Conc	Mfr	Conc	Remarks	Ref	C/I
Cefepime HCl	BR	20 mg/ml[a]	RC	20 mg/ml	Haze forms immediately and becomes flocculent precipitate in 4 hr	1689	I
Heparin sodium	UP	1000 units/L[b]	RC	10 mg/ml	Physically compatible for at least 4 hr at room temperature by visual and microscopic examination	534	C
Hydrocortisone sodium succinate	UP	10 mg/L[b]	RC	10 mg/ml	Physically compatible for at least 4 hr at room temperature by visual and microscopic examination	534	C
Potassium chloride	AB	40 mEq/L[b]	RC	10 mg/ml	Physically compatible for at least 4 hr at room temperature by visual and microscopic examination	534	C
Vitamin B complex with C	RC	2 ml/L[b]	RC	10 mg/ml	Physically compatible for at least 4 hr at room temperature by visual and microscopic examination	534	C

[a]Tested in dextrose 5% in water.
[b]Tested in dextrose 5% in Ringer's injection, dextrose 5% in Ringer's injection, lactated, dextrose 5% in water, Ringer's injection, lactated, and sodium chloride 0.9%.

CHLOROQUINE HCL
CHLOROQUINE PHOSPHATE
CHLOROQUINE SULFATE
AHFS 8:20

Aralen Hydrochloride   **Sanofi Winthrop**

Products— Chloroquine HCl (Sanofi Winthrop) is available in 5-ml ampuls. Each milliliter contains 40 mg of the base as the dihydrochloride salt (2; 4).

pH— From 5.5 to 6.5 (17).

Administration— Chloroquine HCl is administered by intramuscular injection (2; 4). It has also been administered by subcutaneous or intravenous infusion (4).

Stability— Intact ampuls should be stored at room temperature and protected from freezing (4).

Sorption— Chloroquine HCl has been stated to bind to glass (877; 878). In one study, 30 or 40% of a solution of chloroquine 1×10^{-6} M or 0.32 mg/ml in various aqueous media bound to the glass of test tubes. Most of the binding took place during the first hour of contact and seemed to be independent of temperature. This binding did not occur with polycarbonate, polystyrene, or polypropylene plastic containers (877). Although concern has been expressed as to the impact of such binding on drug availability (879), the relevance of these results using a highly dilute (1×10^{-6} M) concentration compared to the clinical concentration is problematic. Of more concern is that binding to glass may lead to inaccurate conclusions of resistance during laboratory studies of chloroquine sensitivity in *Plasmodium falciparum* or to inaccurate results during pharmacokinetic studies (879).

However, Martens et al. could not confirm this result. Chloroquine sulfate 500 μg/ml in sodium chloride 0.9% in PVC bags, glass bottles, and polyethylene-lined laminated bags showed little or no loss due to sorption during storage for 24 hours at 21 °C when protected from light (1392).

Filtration— Chloroquine was also found to bind to cellulose acetate filter media. Ten milliliters of a 1×10^{-6} M solution (approximately 0.32 mg/ml) was passed through 0.45-μm cellulose acetate filters (Millipore and Nalgene). Up to 60 or 70% of the drug was removed. No drug was lost when a similar solution was filtered through a polycarbonate filter (877). Once again, the relevance of this binding phenomenon at the much greater concentrations found in clinical dosing is problematic.

Compatibility Information

Solution Compatibility

Chloroquine HCl

Solution	Mfr	Mfr	Conc/L	Remarks	Ref	C/I
Sodium chloride 0.9%	a	RP	500 mg[b]	Physically compatible with little or no drug loss in 24 hr at 21 °C in the dark	1392	C

[a]*Tested in PVC bags, glass bottles, and polyethylene-lined laminated bags.*
[b]*Tested as the sulfate salt.*

Additive Compatibility

Chloroquine phosphate

Drug	Mfr	Conc/L	Mfr	Conc/L	Test Soln	Remarks	Ref	C/I
Promethazine HCl		5 mg		5 mg	W	Visually compatible with no change in UV spectra	1745	C
		5 mg		25 mg	W	Visually compatible with no change in UV spectra	1745	C
		25 mg		5 mg	W	Visually compatible with no change in UV spectra	1745	C

Drugs in Syringe Compatibility

Chloroquine phosphate

Drug (in syringe)	Mfr	Amt	Mfr	Amt	Remarks	Ref	C/I
Promethazine HCl		50 mg/ 2 ml		250 mg/ 5 ml	Greenish-yellow discoloration becomes precipitate in 22 hr	1745	I
		50 mg/ 2 ml		50 mg/ 1 ml	Greenish-yellow discoloration becomes precipitate in 17 hr	1745	I

CHLOROTHIAZIDE SODIUM
AHFS 40:28

Sodium Diuril   **Merck**

Products— Chlorothiazide sodium (Merck) is supplied in vials containing lyophilized drug equivalent to 500 mg of chlorothiazide with mannitol 250 mg, thimerosal 0.4 mg, and sodium hydroxide to adjust the pH. Reconstitute with 18 ml of sterile water for injection to obtain an isotonic solution yielding a concentration of 28 mg/ml of drug (2; 4; 7). No less than 18 ml should be used for reconstitution (2; 4).

pH— The pH of a 2.5% solution when reconstituted with water for injection is 9.2 to 10 (4; 7).

Osmolality— Chlorothiazide sodium 28 mg/ml in sterile water for injection has an osmolality of 344 mOsm/kg (1689).

Sodium Content— Each 500-mg vial of chlorothiazide sodium (MSD) contains approximately 2.5 mEq of sodium (4).

Administration— Chlorothiazide sodium is administered intravenously by direct injection or infusion (2; 4; 8). It must not be administered intramuscularly or subcutaneously, and extravasation must be avoided (2; 4).

Stability— The lyophilized drug bears an expiration date five years from manufacture (4). The reconstituted solution is stable for 24 hours at room temperature (2; 4; 7). Depending on concentration, precipitation of chlorothiazide will occur in less than 24 hours if the pH of the reconstituted solution is less than approximately 7.4 (4; 7).

Compatibility Information

Solution Compatibility

Chlorothiazide sodium

Solution	Mfr	Mfr	Conc/L	Remarks	Ref	C/I
Dextran 6% in dextrose 5%	AB	MSD	2 g	Physically compatible	3	C
Dextran 6% in sodium chloride 0.9%	AB	MSD	1 g	Potency retained for 24 hr	7	C
	AB	MSD	2 g	Physically compatible	3	C
Dextrose–Ringer's injection combinations	AB	MSD	2 g	Physically compatible	3	C
Dextrose–Ringer's injection, lactated, combinations	AB	MSD	2 g	Physically compatible	3	C
Dextrose–saline combinations	AB	MSD	2 g	Physically compatible	3	C
Dextrose 5% in sodium chloride 0.9%	AB	MSD	1 g	Potency retained for 24 hr	7	C
Dextrose 2½% in water	AB	MSD	2 g	Physically compatible	3	C
Dextrose 5% in water	AB	MSD	1 g	Potency retained for 24 hr	7	C
	AB	MSD	2 g	Physically compatible	3	C
Dextrose 10% in water	AB	MSD	2 g	Physically compatible	3	C
Fructose 10% in sodium chloride 0.9%	AB	MSD	2 g	Physically compatible	3	C
Fructose 10% in water	AB	MSD	2 g	Physically compatible	3	C
Invert sugar 5 and 10% in sodium chloride 0.9%	AB	MSD	2 g	Physically compatible	3	C
Invert sugar 5 and 10% in water	AB	MSD	2 g	Physically compatible	3	C
Ionosol B with dextrose 5%	AB	MSD	500 mg	Physically incompatible	15	I
	AB	MSD	2 g	Precipitate forms after 6 hr	7	I
	AB	MSD	2 g	Haze or precipitate forms within 24 hr	3	I
Ionosol B with invert sugar 10%	AB	MSD	2 g	Precipitate forms after 6 hr	7	I
	AB	MSD	2 g	Haze or precipitate forms within 24 hr	3	I
Ionosol D-CM	AB	MSD	2 g	Physically compatible	3	C
Ionosol D-CM with dextrose 5%	AB	MSD	2 g	Immediate precipitation	7	I
	AB	MSD	2 g	Haze or precipitate forms within 6 hr	3	I
Ionosol D with dextrose 10%	AB	MSD	2 g	Physically compatible	3	C
Ionosol D with invert sugar 10%	AB	MSD	2 g	Precipitate forms after 6 hr	7	I
	AB	MSD	2 g	Haze or precipitate forms within 24 hr	3	I
Ionosol D modified with invert sugar 10%	AB	MSD	2 g	Precipitate forms after 6 hr	7	I
	AB	MSD	2 g	Haze or precipitate forms within 24 hr	3	I

Solution Compatibility (Cont.)

Chlorothiazide sodium

Solution	Mfr	Mfr	Conc/L	Remarks	Ref	C/I
Ionosol K with invert sugar 10%	AB	MSD	2 g	Physically compatible	3	C
Ionosol MB with dextrose 5%	AB	MSD	2 g	Physically compatible	3	C
Ionosol PSL	AB	MSD	2 g	Haze or precipitate forms within 24 hr	3	I
	AB	MSD	2 g	Precipitate forms after 6 hr	7	I
Ionosol T with dextrose 5%	AB	MSD	2 g	Physically compatible	3	C
Normosol M in dextrose 5%	AB	MSD	2 g	Precipitate forms after 6 hr	7	I
Normosol M, 900 cal	AB	MSD	2 g	Precipitate forms after 1 hr	7	I
Normosol R in dextrose 5%	AB	MSD	2 g	Precipitate forms after 6 hr	7	I
Ringer's injection	AB	MSD	1 g	Potency retained for 24 hr	7	C
	AB	MSD	2 g	Physically compatible	3	C
Ringer's injection, lactated	AB	MSD	1 g	Potency retained for 24 hr	7	C
	AB	MSD	2 g	Physically compatible	3	C
Sodium chloride 0.45%	AB	MSD	2 g	Physically compatible	3	C
Sodium chloride 0.9%	AB	MSD	1 g	Potency retained for 24 hr	7	C
	AB	MSD	2 g	Physically compatible	3	C
Sodium lactate ⅙ M	AB	MSD	2 g	Physically compatible	3	C

Additive Compatibility

Chlorothiazide sodium

Drug	Mfr	Conc/L	Mfr	Conc/L	Test Soln	Remarks	Ref	C/I
Amikacin sulfate	BR	5 g	MSD	10 mg	D5LR, D5R, D5S, D5W, D10W, IS10, LR, NS, R, SL	Precipitate forms within 4 hr at 25 °C	294	I
Chlorpromazine HCl	BP	200 mg	BP	2 g	D5W, NS	Immediate precipitation	26	I
Cimetidine HCl	SKF	3 g	MSD	5 g	D5W	Physically compatible and cimetidine chemically stable for 24 hr at room temperature. Chlorothiazide not tested	551	C
Hydralazine HCl	BP	80 mg	BP	2 g	D5W, NS	Yellow color with precipitate in 3 hr	26	I
Insulin, regular[a]			MSD			Physically incompatible	9	I
Levorphanol bitartrate	RC		MSD			Physically incompatible	9	I
Lidocaine HCl	AST	2 g	MSD	500 mg		Physically compatible	24	C
Morphine sulfate			MSD			Physically incompatible	9	I
Nafcillin sodium	WY	500 mg	MSD	500 mg		Physically compatible	27	C
Norepinephrine bitartrate	WI		MSD			Physically incompatible	9	I
Polymyxin B sulfate	BP	20 mg	BP	2 g	D5W	Yellow color	26	I
Procaine HCl			MSD			Physically incompatible	9	I
Prochlorperazine edisylate	SKF		MSD			Physically incompatible	9	I
Prochlorperazine mesylate	BP	100 mg	BP	2 g	D5W	Immediate precipitation	26	I
	BP	100 mg	BP	2 g	NS	Haze develops over 3 hr	26	I

Additive Compatibility (Cont.)

Chlorothiazide sodium

Drug	Mfr	Conc/L	Mfr	Conc/L	Test Soln	Remarks	Ref	C/I
Promazine HCl	BP	200 mg	BP	2 g	D5W, NS	Immediate precipitation	26	I
	WY		MSD			Physically incompatible	9	I
Promethazine HCl	BP	100 mg	BP	2 g	D5W, NS	Immediate precipitation	26	I
	WY		MSD			Physically incompatible	9	I
Ranitidine HCl	GL	50 mg and 2 g		5 g	D5W	Physically compatible and ranitidine chemically stable by HPLC for 24 hr at 25 °C. Chlorothiazide not tested	1515	C
Sodium bicarbonate	AB	2.4 mEq[b]	MSD	500 mg	D5W	Physically compatible for 24 hr	772	C
Streptomycin sulfate			MSD			Physically incompatible	9	I
Triflupromazine HCl	SQ					Precipitate forms	40	I
Vancomycin HCl	LI		MSD			Physically incompatible	9	I

[a]*Test performed prior to availability of neutral regular insulin.*
[b]*One vial of Neut added to a liter of admixture.*

Y-Site Injection Compatibility (1:1 Mixture)

Chlorothiazide sodium

Drug	Mfr	Conc	Mfr	Conc	Remarks	Ref	C/I
TPN #203 and #204[a]			ME	28 mg/ml	White precipitate forms immediately	1974	I

[a]*Refer to Appendix I for the composition of the parenteral nutrition solutions. TPN indicates a 2-in-1 admixture.*

Additional Compatibility Information

Chlorothiazide sodium (MSD) is stated to be physically incompatible with multivitamins (Astra) (1-4/98).

pH Effects— Chlorothiazide sodium (MSD) appears to be stable at pH 7.5 to 9.5 in dextrose 5% in water. No loss of potency was noted over a 24-hour study period (7). The solubility of chlorothiazide sodium is very pH sensitive. Depending on concentration, precipitation occurs at approximately pH 7.4 and below. Additives that result in a final pH in this range, such as vitamin B complex and ascorbic acid, should not be mixed. Chlorothiazide sodium (MSD) is sufficiently alkaline to raise the pH of unbuffered solutions such as dextrose, saline, and their combinations. But if a lactate or acetate buffer is present, the resultant pH may fall below 7.4, causing precipitation. Chlorothiazide sodium possesses some alkalizing power. Therefore, it should not be combined with drugs known to be unstable in alkaline media (7). Simultaneous administration of chlorothiazide sodium with blood or its derivatives should be avoided (2).

CHLORPROMAZINE HCL
AHFS 28:16.08

Thorazine　　　　　　　　　　**SmithKline Beecham**

Products— Chlorpromazine HCl (SmithKline Beecham) is available in 1- and 2-ml ampuls and 10-ml multiple-dose vials. Each milliliter of solution contains (2):

Component	Ampul	Vial
Chlorpromazine HCl	25 mg	25 mg
Ascorbic acid	2 mg	2 mg
Sodium bisulfite	1 mg	1 mg
Sodium sulfite	1 mg	1 mg
Sodium chloride	6 mg	1 mg
Benzyl alcohol		2%

pH— From 3 to 5 (4). A 10% solution in water has a pH of 3.5 to 5.5 (5).

Osmolality— Chlorpromazine HCl 25 mg/ml has an osmolality of 262 mOsm/kg (1689).

Administration— Chlorpromazine HCl may be administered slowly by deep intramuscular injection into the upper outer quadrant of the buttock. Dilution with sodium chloride 0.9% or procaine HCl 2% has been recommended for intramuscular injection if local irritation is a problem. Subcutaneous injection is not recommended. The drug may be diluted to 1 mg/ml with sodium chloride 0.9% and administered by direct intravenous injection at a rate of 1 mg/min to adults and 0.5 mg/min to children. For infusion, it may be diluted in 500 to 1000 ml of sodium chloride 0.9% (2; 4).

Care should be taken to avoid contact of chlorpromazine hydrochloride with skin and clothing when handling the products. Rare cases of contact dermatitis have occurred (2; 4).

Stability— Intact containers should be stored at controlled room temperature. Freezing should be avoided. Protect the solution from light or it may discolor. A slightly yellowed solution does not indicate potency loss. However, a markedly discolored solution should be discarded (2). The pH of maximum stability is 6 (67). Oxidation of chlorpromazine HCl occurs in alkaline media (4). The titration of chlorpromazine HCl in sodium chloride 0.9% with alkali resulted in precipitation of chlorpromazine base at pH 6.7 to 6.8 (138). Precipitation may occur if chlorpromazine HCl is admixed with alkaline drugs or solutions.

Diluted to a 1-mg/ml concentration with sodium chloride 0.9% and stored in 5-ml vials at 18 to 23 °C in the dark, chlorpromazine HCl (SKF) remained relatively stable for 30 days. The HPLC assay results were variable during the study, with the peak-height ratio to the internal standard being 86% on day 30. However, the authors attributed the variable results to the inherent variability of their assay method because no shifts in retention times or extra peaks on the chromatogram were observed. They concluded that the chlorpromazine HCl dilution had not undergone a significant loss of potency (1083).

Sorption— Chlorpromazine HCl (May & Baker) 9 mg/L in sodium chloride 0.9% (Travenol) in PVC bags exhibited only about 5% sorption to the plastic bag during one week of storage at room temperature (15 to 20 °C). However, when the solution was buffered from its initial pH of 5 to pH 7.4, approximately 86% of the drug was lost in one week due to sorption (536).

Chlorpromazine HCl (May & Baker) 9 mg/L in sodium chloride 0.9% exhibited a cumulative 41% loss due to sorption during a seven-hour simulated infusion through an infusion set (Travenol) consisting of a cellulose propionate burette chamber and 170 cm of PVC tubing. Both the burette chamber and the tubing contributed to the loss. The extent of sorption was found to be independent of concentration (606).

The drug was also tested as a simulated infusion over at least one hour by a syringe pump system. A glass syringe on a syringe pump was fitted with 20 cm of polyethylene tubing or 50 cm of Silastic tubing. A negligible amount of drug was lost with the polyethylene tubing, but a cumulative loss of 79% occurred during the one-hour infusion through the Silastic tubing (606).

A 25-ml aliquot of chlorpromazine HCl 9 mg/L in sodium chloride 0.9% was stored in all-plastic syringes composed of polypropylene barrels and polyethylene plungers for 24 hours at room temperature in the dark. The solution did not exhibit any loss due to sorption (606).

In a continuation of this work, chlorpromazine HCl (May & Baker) 90 mg/L in sodium chloride 0.9% in a glass bottle was delivered through a polyethylene administration set (Tridilset) over eight hours at 15 to 20 °C. The flow rate was set at 1 ml/min. No appreciable loss due to sorption occurred (769). This finding is in contrast to a 41% loss using a conventional administration set (606).

Compatibility Information

Solution Compatibility

Chlorpromazine HCl

Solution	Mfr	Mfr	Conc/L	Remarks	Ref	C/I
Dextran 6% in dextrose 5%	AB	SKF	50 mg	Physically compatible	3	C
Dextran 6% in sodium chloride 0.9%	AB	SKF	50 mg	Physically compatible	3	C
Dextrose–Ringer's injection combinations	AB	SKF	50 mg	Physically compatible	3	C
Dextrose–Ringer's injection, lactated, combinations	AB	SKF	50 mg	Physically compatible	3	C
Dextrose–saline combinations	AB	SKF	50 mg	Physically compatible	3	C
Dextrose 2½% in water	AB	SKF	50 mg	Physically compatible	3	C
Dextrose 5% in water	AB	SKF	50 mg	Physically compatible	3	C
Dextrose 10% in water	AB	SKF	50 mg	Physically compatible	3	C
Fructose 10% in sodium chloride 0.9%	AB	SKF	50 mg	Physically compatible	3	C
Fructose 10% in water	AB	SKF	50 mg	Physically compatible	3	C
Invert sugar 5 and 10% in sodium chloride 0.9%	AB	SKF	50 mg	Physically compatible	3	C
Invert sugar 5 and 10% in water	AB	SKF	50 mg	Physically compatible	3	C
Ionosol products	AB	SKF	50 mg	Physically compatible	3	C

Solution Compatibility (Cont.)

Chlorpromazine HCl

Solution	Mfr	Mfr	Conc/L	Remarks	Ref	C/I
Ringer's injection	AB	SKF	50 mg	Physically compatible	3	**C**
Ringer's injection, lactated	AB	SKF	50 mg	Physically compatible	3	**C**
Sodium chloride 0.45%	AB	SKF	50 mg	Physically compatible	3	**C**
Sodium chloride 0.9%	AB	SKF	50 mg	Physically compatible	3	**C**
Sodium lactate ⅙ M	AB	SKF	50 mg	Physically compatible	3	**C**

Additive Compatibility

Chlorpromazine HCl

Drug	Mfr	Conc/L	Mfr	Conc/L	Test Soln	Remarks	Ref	C/I
Aminophylline	BP	1 g	BP	200 mg	D5W, NS	Immediate precipitation	26	**I**
Amphotericin B		200 mg	BP	200 mg	D5W	Immediate precipitation	26	**I**
Ampicillin sodium	BP	2 g	BP	200 mg	D5W, NS	Immediate precipitation	26	**I**
Ascorbic acid injection	UP	500 mg	SKF	250 mg	D5W	Physically compatible	15	**C**
Chloramphenicol sodium succinate	BP	4 g	BP	200 mg	D5W	Immediate precipitation	26	**I**
	BP	4 g	BP	200 mg	NS	Haze develops over 3 hr	26	**I**
Chlorothiazide sodium	BP	2 g	BP	200 mg	D5W, NS	Immediate precipitation	26	**I**
Ethacrynate sodium	MSD	50 mg	SKF	50 mg	NS	Little alteration of UV spectra within 8 hr at room temperature	16	**C**
Floxacillin sodium	BE	20 g	ANT	5 g	W	Sticky yellow precipitate forms immediately	1479	**I**
Furosemide	HO	1 g	ANT	5 g	W	Immediate precipitation	1479	**I**
Methohexital sodium	BP	2 g	BP	200 mg	D5W, NS	Immediate precipitation	26	**I**
Netilmicin sulfate	SC	3 g	SKF	100 mg	D5S	Physically compatible and netilmicin chemically stable for 7 days at 25 and 4 °C. Chlorpromazine not tested	558	**C**
Penicillin G potassium or sodium	BP	10 million units	BP	200 mg	NS	Haze develops over 3 hr	26	**I**
Phenobarbital sodium	BP	800 mg	BP	200 mg	D5W, NS	Immediate precipitation	26	**I**
Theophylline		2 g		200 mg	D5W	Visually compatible with little or no theophylline loss and 7% chlorpromazine loss in 48 hr	1909	**C**
Vitamin B complex with C	AB	2 ml	SKF	50 mg		Physically compatible	3	**C**
	AB	5 ml	SKF	250 mg	D5W	Physically compatible	15	**C**

Drugs in Syringe Compatibility

Chlorpromazine HCl

Drug (in syringe)	Mfr	Amt	Mfr	Amt	Remarks	Ref	C/I
Atropine sulfate		0.6 mg/ 1.5 ml	SKF	50 mg/ 2 ml	Physically compatible for at least 15 min	14	**C**

Drugs in Syringe Compatibility (Cont.)

Chlorpromazine HCl

Drug (in syringe)	Mfr	Amt	Mfr	Amt	Remarks	Ref	C/I
	ST	0.4 mg/ 1 ml	PO	50 mg/ 2 ml	Physically compatible for at least 15 min	326	C
Benztropine mesylate	MSD	2 mg/ 2 ml	STE	50 mg/ 2 ml	Visually compatible for 60 min	1784	C
Butorphanol tartrate	BR	4 mg/ 2 ml	MB	25 mg/ 1 ml	Physically compatible for 30 min at room temperature both macroscopically and microscopically	566	C
Cimetidine HCl	SKF	300 mg/ 2 ml	WY	25 mg/ 1 ml	Haze develops immediately	25	I
Dimenhydrinate	HR	50 mg/ 1 ml	PO	50 mg/ 2 ml	Physically incompatible within 15 min	326	I
Diphenhydramine HCl	PD	50 mg/ 1 ml	PO	50 mg/ 2 ml	Physically compatible for at least 15 min	326	C
	ES	100 mg/ 2 ml	STE	50 mg/ 2 ml	Visually compatible for 60 min	1784	C
Doxapram HCl	RB	400 mg/ 20 ml		250 mg/ 5 ml	Physically compatible with no doxapram loss in 24 hr	1177	C
Droperidol	MN	2.5 mg/ 1 ml	PO	50 mg/ 2 ml	Physically compatible for at least 15 min	326	C
Fentanyl citrate	MN	0.05 mg/ 1 ml	PO	50 mg/ 2 ml	Physically compatible for at least 15 min	326	C
Glycopyrrolate	RB	0.2 mg/ 1 ml	SKF	25 mg/ 1 ml	Physically compatible and pH in stability range for glycopyrrolate for 48 hr at 25 °C	331	C
	RB	0.2 mg/ 1 ml	SKF	50 mg/ 2 ml	Physically compatible and pH in stability range for glycopyrrolate for 48 hr at 25 °C	331	C
	RB	0.4 mg/ 2 ml	SKF	25 mg/ 1 ml	Physically compatible and pH in stability range for glycopyrrolate for 48 hr at 25 °C	331	C
Heparin sodium		2500 units/ 1 ml		50 mg/ 2 ml	Turbidity or precipitate forms within 5 min	1053	I
Hydromorphone HCl	KN	4 mg/ 2 ml	ES	25 mg/ 1 ml	Physically compatible for 30 min	517	C
Hydroxyzine HCl	PF	50 mg/ 1 ml	PO	50 mg/ 2 ml	Physically compatible for at least 15 min	326	C
	ES	100 mg/ 2 ml	STE	50 mg/ 2 ml	Visually compatible for 60 min	1784	C
Meperidine HCl	WY	100 mg/ 1 ml	SKF	50 mg/ 2 ml	Physically compatible for at least 15 min	14	C
	WI	50 mg/ 1 ml	PO	50 mg/ 2 ml	Physically compatible for at least 15 min	326	C
Metoclopramide HCl	NO	10 mg/ 2 ml	MB	25 mg/ 1 ml	Physically compatible for 15 min at room temperature both macroscopically and microscopically	565	C
Midazolam HCl	RC	5 mg/ 1 ml	SKF	50 mg/ 2 ml	Physically compatible for 4 hr at 25 °C under fluorescent light	1145	C
Morphine sulfate	WY	15 mg/ 1 ml	SKF	50 mg/ 2 ml	Physically compatible for at least 15 min	14	C
	ST	15 mg/ 1 ml	PO	50 mg/ 2 ml	Physically compatible for at least 15 min	326	C

Drugs in Syringe Compatibility (Cont.)

Chlorpromazine HCl

Drug (in syringe)	Mfr	Amt	Mfr	Amt	Remarks	Ref	C/I
Morphine tartrate	DB	[a]	DB	10 mg/2 ml	Discoloration develops, although no morphine loss by HPLC in 48 hr at room temperature protected from light. Chlorpromazine not tested	1599	?
Pentazocine lactate	WI	30 mg/1 ml	SKF	50 mg/2 ml	Physically compatible for at least 15 min	14	C
	WI	30 mg/1 ml	PO	50 mg/2 ml	Physically compatible for at least 15 min	326	C
Pentobarbital sodium	WY	100 mg/2 ml	SKF	50 mg/2 ml	Precipitate forms within 15 min	14	I
	AB	500 mg/10 ml	SKF	50 mg/2 ml	Physically incompatible	55	I
	AB	50 mg/1 ml	PO	50 mg/2 ml	Physically incompatible within 15 min	326	I
Perphenazine	SC	5 mg/1 ml	MB	25 mg/1 ml	Physically compatible for 30 min at room temperature both macroscopically and microscopically	566	C
Prochlorperazine edisylate	SKF		SKF	50 mg/2 ml	Physically compatible for at least 15 min	14	C
	PO	5 mg/1 ml	PO	50 mg/2 ml	Physically compatible for at least 15 min	326	C
Promazine HCl	WY	50 mg/1 ml	PO	50 mg/2 ml	Physically compatible for at least 15 min	326	C
Promethazine HCl	PO	50 mg/2 ml	PO	50 mg/2 ml	Physically compatible for at least 15 min	326	C
Ranitidine HCl	GL	50 mg/2 ml	RP	25 mg/1 ml	Physically compatible for 1 hr at 25 °C both macroscopically and microscopically	978	C
	GL	50 mg/5 ml	RP	25 mg	Gas formation	1151	I
Scopolamine HBr		0.6 mg/1.5 ml	SKF	50 mg/2 ml	Physically compatible for at least 15 min	14	C
	ST	0.4 mg/1 ml	PO	50 mg/2 ml	Physically compatible for at least 15 min	326	C
Thiopental sodium	AB	50 mg/2 ml	SKF	75 mg/3 ml	Physically incompatible	21	I
	AB	75 mg/3 ml	SKF	50 mg/2 ml	Physically incompatible	55	I

[a]*Amount unspecified.*

Y-Site Injection Compatibility (1:1 Mixture)

Chlorpromazine HCl

Drug	Mfr	Conc	Mfr	Conc	Remarks	Ref	C/I
Allopurinol sodium	BW	3 mg/ml[b]	RU	2 mg/ml[b]	Heavy white turbidity and precipitate form immediately	1686	I
Amifostine	USB	10 mg/ml[a]	SCN	2 mg/ml[a]	Subvisual haze forms immediately	1845	I
Amphotericin B cholesteryl sulfate complex	SEQ	0.83 mg/ml[a]	ES	2 mg/ml[a]	Gross precipitate forms	2117	I

Y-Site Injection Compatibility (1:1 Mixture) (Cont.)

Chlorpromazine HCl

Drug	Mfr	Conc	Mfr	Conc	Remarks	Ref	C/I
Amsacrine	NCI	1 mg/ml[a]	ES	2 mg/ml[a]	Physically compatible for 4 hr at room temperature under fluorescent light	1381	C
Aztreonam	SQ	40 mg/ml[a]	SCN	2 mg/ml[a]	Dense white turbidity forms immediately	1758	I
Cefepime HCl	BR	20 mg/ml[a]	SCN	2 mg/ml[a]	Cloudy solution forms immediately. Flocculent precipitate forms in 4 hr	1689	I
Cisatracurium besylate	GW	0.1, 2, 5 mg/ml[a]	SCN	2 mg/ml[a]	Physically compatible with no change in measured turbidity or increase in particle content in 4 hr at 23 °C	2074	C
Cisplatin	BR	1 mg/ml	SKF	2 mg/ml[a]	Visually compatible for 4 hr at room temperature under fluorescent light	1685	C
Cladribine	ORT	0.015[b] and 0.5[c] mg/ml	SCN	2 mg/ml[b]	Physically compatible with no change in measured turbidity or increase in particle content in 4 hr at 23 °C	1969	C
Cyclophosphamide	MJ	10 mg/ml	SKF	2 mg/ml[a]	Visually compatible for 4 hr at room temperature under fluorescent light	1685	C
Cytarabine	UP	50 mg/ml	SKF	2 mg/ml[a]	Visually compatible for 4 hr at room temperature under fluorescent light	1685	C
Docetaxel	RPR	0.9 mg/ml[a]	SCN	2 mg/ml[a]	Physically compatible with no change in measured turbidity or increase in particle content in 4 hr at 23 °C	2224	C
Doxorubicin HCl	AD	0.2 mg/ml[a]	SKF	2 mg/ml[a]	Visually compatible for 4 hr at room temperature under fluorescent light	1685	C
Doxorubicin HCl liposome injection	SEQ	0.4 mg/ml[a]	ES	2 mg/ml[a]	Physically compatible with little or no change in measured turbidity and no increase in particle content in 4 hr at 23 °C	2087	C
Etoposide phosphate	BR	5 mg/ml[a]	ES	2 mg/ml[a]	White cloudy solution with brown undertones forms immediately with particulates in 4 hr	2218	I
Famotidine	ME	2 mg/ml[b]		2 mg/ml[a]	Visually compatible for 4 hr at 22 °C	1936	C
Filgrastim	AMG	30 µg/ml[a]	RU	2 mg/ml[a]	Physically compatible with no change in measured turbidity or increase in particle content in 4 hr at 22 °C	1687	C
Fluconazole	RR	2 mg/ml	ES	25 mg/ml	Physically compatible for 24 hr at 25 °C	1407	C
Fludarabine phosphate	BX	1 mg/ml[a]	ES	2 mg/ml[a]	Initial light haze intensifies within 30 min	1439	I
Gemcitabine HCl	LI	10 mg/ml[b]	ES	2 mg/ml[b]	Physically compatible with no change in measured turbidity or increase in particle content in 4 hr at 23 °C	2226	C
Granisetron HCl	SKB	0.05 mg/ml[a]	SCN	2 mg/ml[a]	Physically compatible with no change in measured turbidity or increase in particle content in 4 hr at 23 °C	2000	C
Heparin sodium	UP	1000 units/L[d]	SKF	25 mg/ml	Physically compatible for at least 4 hr at room temperature by visual and microscopic examination	534	C
Hydrocortisone sodium succinate	UP	10 mg/L[d]	SKF	25 mg/ml	Physically compatible for at least 4 hr at room temperature by visual and microscopic examination	534	C

Y-Site Injection Compatibility (1:1 Mixture) (Cont.)

Chlorpromazine HCl

Drug	Mfr	Conc	Mfr	Conc	Remarks	Ref	C/I
Melphalan HCl	BW	0.1 mg/ml[b]	ES	2 mg/ml[b]	Large increase in measured turbidity occurs within 1 hr and grows over 3 hr	1557	I
Methotrexate sodium	AD	15 mg/ml[e]	SKF	2 mg/ml[a]	Turbidity and yellow precipitate form immediately	1685	I
Ondansetron HCl	GL	1 mg/ml[b]	ES	2 mg/ml[a]	Physically compatible for 4 hr at 22 °C	1365	C
Paclitaxel	NCI	1.2 mg/ml[a]	ES	2 mg/ml[a]	Normal inherent haze from paclitaxel decreases immediately	1556	I
Piperacillin sodium–tazobactam sodium	LE	40 + 5 mg/ml[a]	RU	2 mg/ml[a]	Heavy white turbidity forms immediately. White precipitate forms in 4 hr	1688	I
Potassium chloride	AB	40 mEq/L[d]	SKF	25 mg/ml	Physically compatible for at least 4 hr at room temperature by visual and microscopic examination	534	C
Propofol	ZEN	10 mg/ml	SCN	2 mg/ml[a]	Physically compatible for 1 hr at 23 °C with no increase in particle content	2066	C
Remifentanil HCl	GW	0.025 mg/ml[b]	SCN	2 mg/ml[a]	Slight subvisual haze forms in 1 hr	2075	I
	GW	0.25 mg/ml[b]	SCN	2 mg/ml[a]	Physically compatible with no change in measured turbidity or increase in particle content in 4 hr at 23 °C	2075	C
Sargramostim	IMM	10 μg/ml[b]	ES	2 mg/ml[b]	Slight haze, visible with high intensity light, forms immediately	1436	I
Teniposide	BR	0.1 mg/ml[a]	SCN	2 mg/ml[a]	Physically compatible with no subvisual haze or particle formation in 4 hr at 23 °C	1725	C
Thiotepa	IMM[f]	1 mg/ml[a]	SCN	2 mg/ml[a]	Physically compatible with no change in measured turbidity or increase in particle content in 4 hr at 23 °C	1861	C
TNA #218 to #226[g]			SCN	2 mg/ml[a]	Visually compatible with no precipitate or emulsion damage apparent in 4 hr at 23 °C	2215	C
TPN #212 to #215[g]			SCN	2 mg/ml[a]	Physically compatible with no change in measured turbidity or increase in particle content in 4 hr at 23 °C	2109	C
Vinorelbine tartrate	BW	1 mg/ml[b]	RU	2 mg/ml[b]	Physically compatible with little change in measured turbidity or increase in particle content in 4 hr at 22 °C	1558	C
Vitamin B complex with C	RC	2 ml/L[d]	SKF	25 mg/ml	Physically compatible for at least 4 hr at room temperature by visual and microscopic examination	534	C

[a]*Tested in dextrose 5% in water.*
[b]*Tested in sodium chloride 0.9%.*
[c]*Tested in bacteriostatic sodium chloride 0.9% preserved with benzyl alcohol 0.9%.*
[d]*Tested in dextrose 5% in Ringer's injection, dextrose 5% in Ringer's injection, lactated, dextrose 5% in water, Ringer's injection, lactated, and sodium chloride 0.9%.*
[e]*Tested in dextrose 5% in water with sodium bicarbonate 0.05 mEq/ml.*
[f]*Lyophilized formulation tested.*
[g]*Refer to Appendix I for the composition of parenteral nutrition solutions. TNA indicates a 3-in-1 admixture, and TPN indicates a 2-in-1 admixture.*

Additional Compatibility Information

Miscellaneous— The formation of a precipitate was noted when chlorpromazine was mixed in a syringe with a morphine product preserved with chlorocresol 0.2%. The precipitate results from a chlorpromazine interaction with the chlorocresol rather than the morphine (467; 468).

Chlorpromazine HCl is stated to be compatible with diamorphine HCl (1442).

Hydroxyzine and Meperidine— Chlorpromazine HCl (Elkins-Sinn) 6.25 mg/ml, hydroxyzine HCl (Pfizer) 12.5 mg/ml, and meperidine HCl (Winthrop) 25 mg/ml, in both glass and plastic syringes, have been reported to be physically compatible and chemically stable for at least one year at 4 and 25 °C when protected from light. Significant discoloration, ranging from yellow to brownish yellow, occurred on storage at 44 °C (989).

Meperidine and Promethazine— Chlorpromazine HCl (Elkins-Sinn), meperidine HCl (Winthrop), and promethazine HCl (Elkins-Sinn), combined as an extemporaneous mixture for preoperative sedation, developed a brownish-yellow color after two weeks of storage with protection from light. The discoloration was attributed to the metacresol preservative content of Winthrop's meperidine HCl. Use of meperidine HCl (Wyeth) instead, which contains a different preservative, resulted in a solution that remained clear and colorless for at least three months when protected from light (1148).

Pentobarbital— Chlorpromazine HCl (SKF) 50 mg/L has been reported to be conditionally compatible with pentobarbital sodium (Abbott) 500 mg/L. The mixture is physically incompatible in most Abbott infusion solutions except as noted below (3):

Ionosol MB with dextrose 5%	Physically compatible
Ionosol T with dextrose 5%	Physically compatible

CIDOFOVIR
AHFS 8:18

Vistide   **Gilead Sciences**

Products— Cidofovir (Gilead Sciences) is available in 5-ml vials. Each milliliter contains cidofovir 75 mg with sodium hydroxide and/or hydrochloric acid to adjust pH (2). The product must be diluted in sodium chloride 0.9% for administration (2; 4).

pH— Cidofovir has a pH adjusted to 7.4 (2).

The pH values of cidofovir admixtures in three infusion solutions were (1963):

Solution	Concentration	pH
Dextrose 5% in sodium chloride 0.45%	0.085 and 3.51 mg/ml	6.7 to 7.0
Dextrose 5% in water	0.21 and 8.12 mg/ml	7.2 to 7.6
Sodium chloride 0.9%	0.21 and 8.12 mg/ml	7.1 to 7.5

Osmolality— The osmolalities of cidofovir admixtures in three infusion solutions were (1963):

Solution	Concentration	Osmolality (mOsm/kg)
Dextrose 5% in sodium chloride 0.45%	0.085 and 3.51 mg/ml	382 and 392
Dextrose 5% in water	0.21 and 8.12 mg/ml	241 and 286
Sodium chloride 0.9%	0.21 and 8.12 mg/ml	275 and 315

Administration— Cidofovir is administered by intravenous infusion in 100 ml of sodium chloride 0.9% at a constant rate over a one-hour period using an infusion-control pump. Shorter periods must not be used. Patients must be prehydrated with sodium chloride 0.9% and treated with probenecid. Intraocular administration is contraindicated (2; 4).

Stability— Cidofovir should be stored at controlled room temperature between 20 and 25 °C. The manufacturer states that, diluted in 100 ml of sodium chloride 0.9% for administration, cidofovir should be used within 24 hours of preparation. Admixtures not used immediately should be stored under refrigeration at 2 to 8 °C but should still be used within 24 hours of preparation. Refrigeration or freezing should not be used to extend beyond the 24-hour limit (2; 4).

Sorption— Cidofovir is stated to be compatible with glass, PVC, and ethylene/propylene copolymer infusion solution containers (2).

Cidofovir (Gilead Sciences) 0.21 and 8.12 mg/ml in dextrose 5% in water and sodium chloride 0.9% as well as 0.085 and 3.51 mg/ml in dextrose 5% in sodium chloride 0.45% exhibited no loss due to sorption to PVC or polyolefin containers for 24 hours at 4 and 30 °C and when run through PVC administration sets (1963). Similarly, cidofovir exhibited no losses due to sorption to PVC or polyolefin (ethylene and propylene copolymer) containers determined by HPLC analysis of 0.2 and 8.1 mg/ml solutions in sodium chloride 0.9% when stored under refrigeration at 2 to 8 °C or frozen at −20 °C over a period of five days (2076).

Freezing Solutions— Cidofovir (Gilead Sciences) 0.2 and 8.1 mg/ml in sodium chloride 0.9% was physically and chemically stable for five days when stored frozen at −20 °C in PVC or polyethylene-polypropylene containers (2076).

Compatibility Information

Solution Compatibility

Cidofovir

Solution	Mfr	Mfr	Conc/L	Remarks	Ref	C/I
Dextrose 5% in sodium chloride 0.45%	AB[a], BA[a], MG[b]	GIL	85 mg and 3.51 g	Physically compatible with no increase in subvisual particulates and no loss by HPLC in 24 hr at 4 and 30 °C	1963	C
Dextrose 5% in water	AB[a], BA[a], MG[b]	GIL	210 mg and 8.12 g	Physically compatible with no increase in subvisual particulates and no loss by HPLC in 24 hr at 4 and 30 °C	1963	C
Sodium chloride 0.9%	AB[a], BA[a], MG[b]	GIL	210 mg and 8.12 g	Physically compatible with no increase in subvisual particulates and no loss by HPLC in 24 hr at 4 and 30 °C	1963	C
	AB[a], BA[a], MG[b]	GIL	200 mg and 8.1 g	Physically compatible with no increase in subvisual particulates and no loss by HPLC in 5 days at 4 and −20 °C	2076	C

[a]Tested in PVC containers.
[b]Tested in polyolefin containers.

Additional Compatibility Information

Miscellaneous— The manufacturer states that cidofovir compatibility with Ringer's injection, lactated Ringer's injection, and solutions containing bacteriostatic agents has not been established (2; 4). Similarly, there are no data for compatibility with other drugs or supplements (2).

Other Information

Disposal— Partially used vials, diluted solutions, and materials used in admixture preparation and administration should be sealed in leak- and puncture-proof containers and incinerated at high temperature (2; 4).

Skin Contact— Appropriate safety precautions for handling mutagenic substances should be taken; preparation in a biological safety cabinet and wearing of suitable gloves and gowns with knit cuffs are recommended. If cidofovir solution contacts skin or mucosa, wash the affected area immediately with soap and water (2; 4).

CIMETIDINE HCL
AHFS 56:40

Tagamet   **SmithKline Beecham**

Products— Cimetidine HCl (SmithKline Beecham) is available in 2-ml vials and 8-ml multiple-dose vials. Each milliliter contains cimetidine HCl equivalent to cimetidine 150 mg and phenol 5 mg with sodium hydroxide to adjust pH (2).

Cimetidine HCl (SmithKline Beecham) is also available as a premixed infusion solution of 300 mg/50 ml in sodium chloride 0.9% (2).

pH— The injection has a pH range of 3.8 to 6. The premixed infusion has a pH range of 5 to 7 (2; 4).

Osmolality— The osmolality of cimetidine HCl (SKF) 6 mg/ml was determined to be 291 mOsm/kg in dextrose 5% in water and 314 mOsm/kg in sodium chloride 0.9%. At 15 mg/ml, the osmolality was determined to be 338 and 359 mOsm/kg, respectively (1375).

The osmolality of cimetidine HCl 300 mg was calculated for the following dilutions (1054):

Diluent	Osmolality (mOsm/kg)	
	50 ml	100 ml
Dextrose 5% in water	286	274
Sodium chloride 0.9%	313	301

The premixed infusion solution of 300 mg/50 ml of sodium chloride 0.9% has an osmolality of about 336 mOsm/kg (4).

Sodium Content— The premixed infusion contains about 7.7 mEq of sodium in 50 ml (4).

Administration— Cimetidine HCl is administered intramuscularly with no dilution necessary, by slow direct intravenous injection over five minutes or more after dilution to a total of 20 ml with a compatible diluent such as sodium chloride 0.9%, by intermittent intravenous infusion over 15 to 20 minutes in at least 50 ml of compatible diluent, or by continuous intravenous infusion in 100 to 1000 ml of compatible diluent over 24 hours (2; 4).

Stability— Cimetidine HCl should be stored at room temperature and protected from light. The products should be protected from excessive heat, but brief exposure of the premixed solution to temperatures up to 40 °C does not adversely affect stability (2; 4). Cimetidine HCl may precipitate from solution on exposure to cold but reportedly can be redissolved by warming without degradation (140; 854). In aqueous solution, cimetidine HCl exhibits maximum stability at pH 6 (549).

Cimetidine HCl (SmithKline Beecham) injection was diluted with sterile water for injection to a concentration of 15 mg/ml for use in minimizing measurement errors in pediatric dosing. The dilution was packaged in glass vials, and samples were stored at 22 °C in a closed cabinet and at 4 °C. The dilution remained visually free of particulate matter at both storage conditions throughout the study. HPLC analysis of the samples stored at 22 °C found cimetidine losses of 6% in 14 days and 10% in 28 days. Samples stored at 4 °C exhibited 5% loss in 28 days and 14% loss in 56 days (1714).

Freezing Solutions— Cimetidine HCl (SKF) 300 mg/50 ml of dextrose 5% in water in PVC bags (Travenol) was frozen at −20 °C for up to 30 days. The bags were then thawed for two to three hours at room temperature and subsequently stored for eight days at 4 °C in a refrigerator. The cimetidine concentration, determined by an HPLC technique, was constant over the entire study period at about 100% of the initial amount. No significant deviation from the initial concentration occurred. In addition, the admixtures remained sterile throughout the study (632).

In another study, microwave thawing of frozen cimetidine HCl admixtures was compared to room temperature thawing. Cimetidine HCl (SKF) 300 mg in 50-ml PVC bags of dextrose 5% in water and 100-ml PVC bags of sodium chloride 0.9% was frozen at −10 °C for 28 days. Samples were then thawed by microwave radiation or by standing at 27 °C. No visual changes and no loss of cimetidine occurred between the initial admixtures and the frozen solutions thawed by either means. Even overheating the 100-ml bags of sodium chloride 0.9% to allow boiling to occur for five seconds did not result in a significant loss of cimetidine (780).

Sorption— Cimetidine (SKF) 6 mg/L in sodium chloride 0.9% (Travenol) in PVC bags did not exhibit significant sorption to the plastic during one week of storage at room temperature (15 to 20 °C) (536).

In addition, a 6-mg/L admixture in sodium chloride 0.9% did not exhibit any loss due to sorption during a seven-hour simulated infusion through an infusion set (Travenol) consisting of a cellulose propionate burette chamber and 170 cm of PVC tubing (606).

The cimetidine solution was also tested as a simulated infusion over at least one hour by a syringe pump system. A glass syringe on a syringe pump was fitted with 20 cm of polyethylene tubing or 50 cm of Silastic tubing. No loss of drug due to sorption was observed with either tubing (606).

Finally, a 25-ml aliquot of the cimetidine (SKF) 6 mg/L in sodium chloride 0.9% admixture was stored in all-plastic syringes composed of polypropylene barrels and polyethylene plungers for 24 hours at room temperature in the dark. The solution did not exhibit any loss due to sorption (606).

Compatibility Information

Solution Compatibility

Cimetidine HCl

Solution	Mfr	Mfr	Conc/L	Remarks	Ref	C/I
Amino acids 3.5% with electrolytes	AB	SKF	1.2 and 5 g	Physically compatible and chemically stable for 1 week at room temperature	549	C
Amino acids 5.5%	TR	SKF	1.2 and 5 g	Physically compatible and chemically stable for 1 week at room temperature protected from light	550	C
Amino acids 5.5% with electrolytes	TR	SKF	1.2 and 5 g	Physically compatible and chemically stable for 1 week at room temperature protected from light	550	C
Amino acids 8.5%	TR	SKF	1.2 and 5 g	Physically compatible and chemically stable for 1 week at room temperature protected from light	550	C
Amino acids 8.5% with electrolytes	TR	SKF	1.2 and 5 g	Physically compatible and chemically stable for 1 week at room temperature protected from light	550	C
Dextrose 5% with Ascor-B-Sol	TR	SKF	1.2 and 5 g	Physically compatible and chemically stable for 1 week at room temperature protected from light	549	C
Dextrose 5% and Electrolyte #48	TR	SKF	1.2 and 5 g	Physically compatible and chemically stable for 1 week at room temperature	550	C

Solution Compatibility (Cont.)

Cimetidine HCl

Solution	Mfr	Mfr	Conc/L	Remarks	Ref	C/I
Dextrose 5% and Electrolyte #75	TR	SKF	1.2 and 5 g	Physically compatible and chemically stable for 1 week at room temperature	550	**C**
Dextrose 5% in Ringer's injection, lactated	TR	SKF	1.2 and 5 g	Physically compatible and chemically stable for 1 week at room temperature	549	**C**
Dextrose 5% in sodium chloride 0.2%	TR	SKF	1.2 and 5 g	Physically compatible and chemically stable for 1 week at room temperature	549	**C**
Dextrose 5% in sodium chloride 0.45%	TR	SKF	1.2 and 5 g	Physically compatible and chemically stable for 1 week at room temperature	549	**C**
Dextrose 5% in sodium chloride 0.9%	TR	SKF	1.2 and 5 g	Physically compatible and chemically stable for 1 week at room temperature	549	**C**
Dextrose 10% in sodium chloride 0.9%	TR	SKF	1.2 and 5 g	Physically compatible and chemically stable for 1 week at room temperature	549	**C**
Dextrose 5% in water	TR[a]	SKF	1.2 and 5 g	Physically compatible and chemically stable for 1 week at room temperature	549	**C**
	TR[b]	SKF	1.2 g	Physically compatible with about 3% cimetidine loss in 48 hr at room temperature	1186	**C**
	TR[b]	SKF	3 g	Physically compatible with little or no drug loss in 24 hr at 24 °C	1418	**C**
Dextrose 10% in water	TR[a]	SKF	1.2 and 5 g	Physically compatible and chemically stable for 1 week at room temperature	549	**C**
Dextrose 5% in water with vitamins	TR	SKF	1.2 and 5 g	Physically compatible and chemically stable for 1 week at room temperature	550	**C**
Fructose 5% with Electrolyte #48	TR	SKF	1.2 and 5 g	Physically compatible and chemically stable for 1 week at room temperature	550	**C**
Fructose 5% with Electrolyte #75	TR	SKF	1.2 and 5 g	Physically compatible with 4 to 7% decomposition in 1 week at room temperature	550	**C**
Invert sugar 5% in water	TR	SKF	1.2 and 5 g	Physically compatible and chemically stable for 1 week at room temperature	549	**C**
Invert sugar 10% in water	TR	SKF	1.2 and 5 g	Physically compatible and chemically stable for 1 week at room temperature	549	**C**
Ionosol B in dextrose 5% in water	AB	SKF	1.2 and 5 g	Physically compatible and chemically stable for 1 week at room temperature	549	**C**
Ionosol D-CM	AB	SKF	1.2 and 5 g	Physically compatible with 2 to 5% decomposition in 1 week at room temperature	550	**C**
Ionosol D-CM in dextrose 5% in water	AB	SKF	1.2 and 5 g	Physically compatible with 5% decomposition in 1 week at room temperature	550	**C**
Ionosol MB in dextrose 5% in water	AB	SKF	1.2 and 5 g	Physically compatible with 2 to 4% decomposition in 1 week at room temperature	550	**C**
Ionosol T in dextrose 5% in water	AB	SKF	1.2 and 5 g	Physically compatible with 4 to 6% decomposition in 1 week at room temperature	550	**C**
Mannitol 10% in water	TR	SKF	1.2 and 5 g	Physically compatible and chemically stable for 1 week at room temperature	549	**C**
Normosol M, 900 cal	AB	SKF	1.2 and 5 g	Physically compatible with 2 to 5% decomposition in 1 week at room temperature	550	**C**
Normosol M in dextrose 5% in water	AB	SKF	1.2 and 5 g	Physically compatible and chemically stable for 1 week at room temperature	549	**C**

Solution Compatibility (Cont.)

Cimetidine HCl

Solution	Mfr	Mfr	Conc/L	Remarks	Ref	C/I
Normosol M and Surbex T in dextrose 5% in water	AB	SKF	1.2 and 5 g	Physically compatible with 5 to 8% decomposition in 1 week at room temperature	550	C
Normosol R	AB	SKF	1.2 and 5 g	Physically compatible and chemically stable for 1 week at room temperature	550	C
Normosol R, pH 7.4	AB	SKF	1.2 and 5 g	Physically compatible and chemically stable for 1 week at room temperature	550	C
Normosol R in dextrose 5% in water	AB	SKF	1.2 and 5 g	Physically compatible and chemically stable for 1 week at room temperature	550	C
Plasma-Lyte 56 in dextrose 5% in water	TR	SKF	1.2 and 5 g	Physically compatible and chemically stable for 1 week at room temperature	549	C
Plasma-Lyte M in dextrose 5% in water	TR	SKF	1.2 and 5 g	Physically compatible and chemically stable for 1 week at room temperature	549	C
Ringer's injection	TR	SKF	1.2 and 5 g	Physically compatible and chemically stable for 1 week at room temperature	549	C
Ringer's injection, lactated	TR	SKF	1.2 and 5 g	Physically compatible and chemically stable for 1 week at room temperature	549	C
Sodium bicarbonate 5%	TR	SKF	1.2 and 5 g	Physically compatible and chemically stable for 1 week at room temperature	549	C
Sodium chloride 0.9%	AB	SKF	1.2 and 5 g	Physically compatible and chemically stable for 1 week at room temperature	549	C
	BA[c]	SKB	600 mg	Visually compatible with no loss by HPLC in 48 hr at 24 °C	1854	C
TNA #72[d]		SKF	400, 800, 1200 mg	Physically compatible and no cimetidine loss in 24 hr at 25 °C. Fat emulsion particle size increased in 48 hr	998	C
TNA #75[d]		SKF	1 g	Physically compatible and cimetidine chemically stable for 48 hr at room temperature	140	C
TNA #179[d]		SKF	400 and 900 mg	Visually compatible with less than 3% cimetidine loss by HPLC in 72 hr at room temperature protected from light	1622	C
TNA #197 to #200[d]		SKF	450 mg	Physically compatible with 7% or less loss by HPLC in 48 hr at 22 °C exposed to light	1921	C
TPN #34, #35, #37[d]		SKF	300 mg	Physically compatible and cimetidine chemically stable for 24 hr at room temperature and 4 °C	781	C
TPN #36[d]		SKF	300 mg	Physically compatible and cimetidine chemically stable for 24 hr at 4 °C. Room temperature sample gave spurious result	781	C
TPN #93[d]			600 mg	Physically compatible and cimetidine chemically stable for 48 hr at room temperature	1320	C
TPN #94[d]			600 mg	Physically compatible and cimetidine and copper chemically stable for 48 hr at room temperature	1320	C
TPN #196[d]		SKF	450 mg	Physically compatible with no loss by HPLC in 48 hr at 22 °C exposed to light	1921	C

[a]*Tested in both glass and PVC containers.*
[b]*Tested in PVC containers.*
[c]*Tested in glass containers.*
[d]*Refer to Appendix I for the composition of parenteral nutrition solutions. TNA indicates a 3-in-1 admixture, and TPN indicates a 2-in-1 admixture.*

Additive Compatibility

Cimetidine HCl

Drug	Mfr	Conc/L	Mfr	Conc/L	Test Soln	Remarks	Ref	C/I
Acetazolamide sodium	LE	5 g	SKF	3 g	D5W	Physically compatible and cimetidine chemically stable for 24 hr at room temperature. Acetazolamide not tested	551	C
Amikacin sulfate	BR	2.5 g	SKF	1.5 g	D5W	Physically compatible and cimetidine chemically stable for 24 hr at room temperature. Amikacin not tested	551	C
Aminophylline	IX	500 mg	SKF	1.2 g	D5W[a]	Physically compatible with about 3 to 5% cimetidine loss and little or no aminophylline loss in 48 hr at room temperature	1186	C
Amphotericin B	SQ	100 mg	SKF	600 mg	D5W	Immediate haze formation. Precipitate observed at 24 hr at room temperature	551	I
Ampicillin sodium	SKF	1 g	SKF	1.2 and 5 g	D5W, NS	Physically compatible and cimetidine chemically stable for 24 hr at room temperature. Ampicillin stability is determining factor	551	?
Atracurium besylate	BW	500 mg		5 g	D5W	Physically compatible and atracurium chemically stable for 24 hr at 5 and 30 °C	1694	C
Cefamandole nafate	LI	20 g	SKF	6 g	D5W	Immediate haze formation. Gelatinous precipitate observed at 24 hr at room temperature. Cimetidine loss of 7% attributed to precipitation	551	I
	LI	1 g	SKF	300 mg	D5W	Physically compatible and cimetidine chemically stable for 24 hr at room temperature. Cefamandole not tested	551	C
		10 g	SKF	3 g	D5W, NS	Cloudiness forms after 4 to 5 hr, increasing to a dense precipitate in 24 hr at room temperature	516	I
		20 g	SKF	6 g	D5W, NS	Cloudiness forms after 4 to 5 hr, increasing to a dense precipitate in 24 hr at room temperature	516	I
Cefazolin sodium	SKF	10 g	SKF	3 g	D5W	Haze observed at 24 hr at room temperature. Cimetidine chemically stable but cefazolin not tested	551	I
		10 g	SKF	3 g	D5W, NS	Physically compatible for 48 hr at room temperature. Precipitate forms on freezing	516	C
		20 g	SKF	6 g	D5W, NS	Physically compatible for 48 hr at room temperature. Precipitate forms on freezing	516	C
	SKF	1 g	SKF	1.2 and 5 g	D5W, NS	Physically compatible and cimetidine chemically stable for 24 hr at room temperature. Cefazolin not tested	551	C
Cefoperazone sodium	RR	5 g	SKF	2 g	D5W	Physically compatible. 5% cefoperazone loss at 25 °C and 3% at 4 °C in 48 hr. 2% or less cimetidine loss in 48 hr at 25 and 4 °C	1403	C
Cefoxitin sodium	MSD	10 g	SKF	3 g	D5W	Physically compatible and cimetidine chemically stable for 24 hr at room temperature. Cefoxitin not tested	551	C

Additive Compatibility (Cont.)

Cimetidine HCl

Drug	Mfr	Conc/L	Mfr	Conc/L	Test Soln	Remarks	Ref	C/I
Chlorothiazide sodium	MSD	5 g	SKF	3 g	D5W	Physically compatible and cimetidine chemically stable for 24 hr at room temperature. Chlorothiazide not tested	551	C
Clindamycin phosphate	UP	1.2 g	SKF	1.2 and 5 g	D5W, NS	Physically compatible and cimetidine chemically stable for 24 hr at room temperature. Clindamycin not tested	551	C
Colistimethate sodium	WC	1.5 g	SKF	3 g	D5W	Physically compatible and cimetidine chemically stable for 24 hr at room temperature. Colistimethate not tested	551	C
Cryptenamine acetate	MA	1.3 g	SKF	3 g	D5W	Physically compatible and cimetidine chemically stable for 24 hr at room temperature. Cryptenamine not tested	551	C
Dexamethasone sodium phosphate	MSD	40 mg	SKF	3 g	D5W	Physically compatible and cimetidine chemically stable for 24 hr at room temperature. Dexamethasone not tested	551	C
Digoxin	BW	2.5 mg	SKF	3 g	D5W	Physically compatible and cimetidine chemically stable for 24 hr at room temperature. Digoxin not tested	551	C
Epinephrine HCl	PD	100 mg	SKF	3 g	D5W	Physically compatible and cimetidine chemically stable for 24 hr at room temperature. Epinephrine not tested	551	C
Erythromycin lactobionate	AB	5 g	SKF	3 g	D5W	Physically compatible and cimetidine chemically stable for 24 hr at room temperature. Erythromycin not tested	551	C
Ethacrynate sodium	MSD	500 mg	SKF	3 g	D5W	Physically compatible and cimetidine chemically stable for 24 hr at room temperature. Ethacrynate not tested	551	C
Floxacillin sodium	BE	20 g	SKF	4 g	NS	Physically compatible for 72 hr at 15 and 30 °C	1479	C
Flumazenil	RC	20 mg	SKB	2.4 g	D5W[a]	Visually compatible with no flumazenil loss by HPLC in 24 hr at 23 °C under fluorescent light. Cimetidine not tested	1710	C
Furosemide	HO	400 mg	SKF	3 g	D5W	Physically compatible and cimetidine chemically stable for 24 hr at room temperature. Furosemide not tested	551	C
	HO	1 g	SKF	4 g	NS	Physically compatible for 72 hr at 15 and 30 °C	1479	C
Gentamicin sulfate	SC	800 mg	SKF	3 g	D5W	Physically compatible and cimetidine chemically stable for 24 hr at room temperature. Gentamicin not tested	551	C
	SC	800 mg	SKF	1.2 and 5 g	D5W, NS	Physically compatible and cimetidine chemically stable for 24 hr at room temperature. Gentamicin not tested	551	C
Insulin, regular	LI	100 units	SKF	1.2 and 5 g	D5W, NS	Physically compatible and cimetidine chemically stable for 24 hr at room temperature. Insulin not tested	551	C
Isoproterenol HCl	WI	20 mg	SKF	3 g	D5W	Physically compatible and cimetidine chemically stable for 24 hr at room temperature. Isoproterenol not tested	551	C

Additive Compatibility (Cont.)

Cimetidine HCl

Drug	Mfr	Conc/L	Mfr	Conc/L	Test Soln	Remarks	Ref	C/I
Lidocaine HCl	AST	2.5 g	SKF	3 g	D5W	Physically compatible and cimetidine chemically stable for 24 hr at room temperature. Lidocaine not tested	551	C
Lincomycin HCl	UP	6 g	SKF	3 g	D5W	Physically compatible and cimetidine chemically stable for 24 hr at room temperature. Lincomycin not tested	551	C
Meropenem	ZEN	1 and 20 g	SKB	3 g	NS	Visually compatible for 4 hr at room temperature	1994	C
Metaraminol bitartrate	MSD	1 g	SKF	3 g	D5W	Physically compatible and cimetidine chemically stable for 24 hr at room temperature. Metaraminol not tested	551	C
Methylprednisolone sodium succinate	UP	400 mg	SKF	3 g	D5W	Physically compatible and cimetidine chemically stable for 24 hr at room temperature. Methylprednisolone not tested	551	C
	UP	400 mg	SKF	3 g	D5W[a]	Physically compatible with no cimetidine loss and 3% methylprednisolone 21-succinate ester loss in 24 hr at 24 °C	1418	C
	UP	1.25 g	SKF	3 g	D5W[a]	Physically compatible with no cimetidine loss and 8% methylprednisolone 21-succinate ester loss in 24 hr at 24 °C	1418	C
Metoclopramide HCl	RB	100 mg	SKF	3 g	NS	Physically compatible for 48 hr at room temperature, but bioavailability of cimetidine may be reduced	924	?
	RB	100 mg and 1.6 g	SKF	3 g		Physically compatible for 48 hr at 25 °C	1167	C
Norepinephrine bitartrate	WI	40 mg	SKF	3 g	D5W	Physically compatible and cimetidine chemically stable for 24 hr at room temperature. Norepinephrine not tested	551	C
Penicillin G potassium	LI	2.4 million units	SKF	1.2 and 5 g	D5W, NS	Physically compatible and cimetidine chemically stable for 24 hr at room temperature. Penicillin not tested	551	C
Phytonadione	MSD	100 mg	SKF	3 g	D5W	Physically compatible and cimetidine chemically stable for 24 hr at room temperature. Phytonadione not tested	551	C
Polymyxin B sulfate	BW	10 million units	SKF	1.2 g	D5W	Physically compatible and cimetidine chemically stable for 24 hr at room temperature. Polymyxin B not tested	551	C
Potassium chloride	SKF	20 mEq	SKF	1.2 and 5 g	D5S, D5W, NS	Physically compatible and cimetidine chemically stable for 24 hr at room temperature. Potassium chloride not tested	551	C
	SKF	80 mEq	SKF	1.2 and 5 g	D5S, D5W, NS	Physically compatible and cimetidine chemically stable for 24 hr at room temperature. Potassium chloride not tested	551	C
Protamine sulfate	LI	500 mg	SKF	3 g	D5W	Physically compatible and cimetidine chemically stable for 24 hr at room temperature. Protamine not tested	551	C
Quinidine gluconate	LI	3.2 g	SKF	3 g	D5W	Physically compatible and cimetidine chemically stable for 24 hr at room temperature. Quinidine not tested	551	C

Additive Compatibility (Cont.)

Cimetidine HCl

Drug	Mfr	Conc/L	Mfr	Conc/L	Test Soln	Remarks	Ref	C/I
Sodium nitroprusside	RC	500 mg	SKF	3 g	D5W	Physically compatible and cimetidine chemically stable for 24 hr at room temperature. Sodium nitroprusside not tested	551	C
Tacrolimus	FUJ	10 mg	SKB	600 mg	NS[b]	Visually compatible with no cimetidine loss and 3% tacrolimus loss by HPLC in 48 hr at 24 °C	1854	C
Vancomycin HCl	LI	5 g	SKF	3 g	D5W	Physically compatible and cimetidine chemically stable for 24 hr at room temperature. Vancomycin not tested	551	C
Verapamil HCl	KN	80 mg	SKF	2.4 g	D5W, NS	Physically compatible for 24 hr	764	C
Vitamin B complex	UP	1 vial	SKF	1.2 and 5 g	D5W, NS	Physically compatible and cimetidine chemically stable for 24 hr at room temperature. Vitamins not tested	551	C
Vitamin B complex with C	TR		SKF	1.2 and 5 g	D5W	Physically compatible and stable for 48 hr	360	C

[a]*Tested in PVC containers.*
[b]*Tested in glass containers.*

Drugs in Syringe Compatibility

Cimetidine HCl

Drug (in syringe)	Mfr	Amt	Mfr	Amt	Remarks	Ref	C/I
Atropine sulfate	LI	0.6 mg/ 1.5 ml	SKF	300 mg/ 2 ml	Physically compatible and cimetidine chemically stable for 90 min at room temperature	542	C
	LI	0.4 mg/ 1 ml	SKF	300 mg/ 2 ml	Physically compatible and cimetidine chemically stable for 90 min at room temperature	542	C
Atropine sulfate with pentobarbital sodium	LI / AB	0.6 mg/ 1.5 ml / 100 mg/ 2 ml	SKF	300 mg/ 2 ml	Immediate precipitation	542	I
Butorphanol tartrate	BR	2 mg/ 1 ml	SKF	300 mg/ 2 ml	Physically compatible for 4 hr at 25 °C	25	C
Cefamandole nafate		1 g/5 ml	SKF	300 mg/ 2 ml	Immediate precipitation	516	I
Cefazolin sodium		1 g/5 ml	SKF	300 mg/ 2 ml	Immediate precipitation	516	I
Chlorpromazine HCl	WY	25 mg/ 1 ml	SKF	300 mg/ 2 ml	Immediate haze formation	25	I
Diatrizoate meglumine and diatrizoate sodium	MA	52 + 8%, 5 ml	SKF	150 mg/ 1 ml	Physically compatible for at least 2 hr	1438	C
Diatrizoate sodium	WI	60%, 5 ml	SKF	150 mg/ 1 ml	Physically compatible for at least 2 hr	1438	C
Diazepam	RC	10 mg/ 2 ml	SKF	300 mg/ 2 ml	Physically compatible for 4 hr at 25 °C	25	C
Diphenhydramine HCl	PD	50 mg/ 1 ml	SKF	300 mg/ 2 ml	Physically compatible for 4 hr at 25 °C	25	C

Drugs in Syringe Compatibility (Cont.)

Cimetidine HCl

Drug (in syringe)	Mfr	Amt	Mfr	Amt	Remarks	Ref	C/I
Doxapram HCl	RB	400 mg/ 20 ml	SKF	50 mg/ 2 ml	Physically compatible with no doxapram loss in 24 hr	1177	C
Droperidol	JN	5 mg/ 2 ml	SKF	300 mg/ 2 ml	Physically compatible for 4 hr at 25 °C	25	C
Fentanyl citrate	JN	0.1 mg/ 2 ml	SKF	300 mg/ 2 ml	Physically compatible for 4 hr at 25 °C	25	C
Glycopyrrolate	ES	0.2 mg/ 1 ml	SKF	300 mg/ 2 ml	Physically compatible for 4 hr at 25 °C	25	C
Heparin sodium		5000 units/ 5 ml	SKF	300 mg/ 2 ml	Physically compatible for 48 hr at room temperature	516	C
		2500 units/ 1 ml		200 mg/ 2 ml	Physically compatible for at least 5 min	1053	C
Hydromorphone HCl	WI	2 mg/ 1 ml	SKF	300 mg/ 2 ml	Physically compatible for 4 hr at 25 °C	25	C
Hydroxyzine HCl	ES	100 mg/ 2 ml	SKF	300 mg/ 2 ml	Physically compatible for 4 hr at 25 °C	25	C
Iohexol	WI	64.7%, 5 ml	SKF	150 mg/ 1 ml	Physically compatible for at least 2 hr	1438	C
Iopamidol	SQ	61%, 5 ml	SKF	150 mg/ 1 ml	Physically compatible for at least 2 hr	1438	C
Iothalamate meglumine	MA	60%, 5 ml	SKF	150 mg/ 1 ml	Physically compatible for at least 2 hr	1438	C
Ioxaglate meglumine and ioxaglate sodium	MA	39.3% + 19.6%, 5 ml	SKF	150 mg/ 1 ml	Precipitate forms immediately and persists for at least 2 hr	1438	I
Lorazepam	WY	2 mg/ 1 ml	SKF	300 mg/ 2 ml	Physically compatible for 4 hr at 25 °C	25	C
Meperidine HCl	WI	100 mg/ 2 ml	SKF	300 mg/ 2 ml	Physically compatible for 4 hr at 25 °C	25	C
Midazolam HCl	RC	5 mg/ 1 ml	SKF	300 mg/ 2 ml	Physically compatible for 4 hr at 25 °C under fluorescent light	1145	C
Morphine sulfate	WI	10 mg/ 1 ml	SKF	300 mg/ 2 ml	Physically compatible for 4 hr at 25 °C	25	C
Nafcillin sodium		1 g/5 ml	SKF	300 mg/ 2 ml	Physically compatible for 48 hr at room temperature	516	C
Nalbuphine HCl	EN	10 mg/ 1 ml	SKF	300 mg/ 2 ml	Physically compatible for 4 hr at 25 °C	25	C
	DU	10 mg/ 1 ml		300 mg/ 2 ml	Physically compatible for 48 hr	128	C
	DU	20 mg/ 1 ml		300 mg/ 2 ml	Physically compatible for 48 hr	128	C
Penicillin G sodium		1 million units/ 5 ml	SKF	300 mg/ 2 ml	Precipitate forms between 36 and 48 hr at room temperature	516	C
Pentazocine lactate	WI	60 mg/ 2 ml	SKF	300 mg/ 2 ml	Physically compatible for 4 hr at 25 °C	25	C

Drugs in Syringe Compatibility (Cont.)

Cimetidine HCl

Drug (in syringe)	Mfr	Amt	Mfr	Amt	Remarks	Ref	C/I
Pentobarbital sodium	AB	100 mg/ 2 ml	SKF	300 mg/ 2 ml	Immediate precipitation	542	I
Pentobarbital sodium with atropine sulfate	AB LI	100 mg/ 2 ml 0.6 mg/ 1.5 ml	SKF	300 mg/ 2 ml	Immediate precipitation	542	I
Perphenazine	SC	5 mg/ 1 ml	SKF	300 mg/ 2 ml	Physically compatible for 4 hr at 25 °C	25	C
Prochlorperazine edisylate	SKF	10 mg/ 2 ml	SKF	300 mg/ 2 ml	Physically compatible for 4 hr at 25 °C	25	C
Promazine HCl	WY	25 mg/ 1 ml	SKF	300 mg/ 2 ml	Physically compatible for 4 hr at 25 °C	25	C
Promethazine HCl	WY	25 mg/ 1 ml	SKF	300 mg/ 2 ml	Physically compatible for 4 hr at 25 °C	25	C
Scopolamine HBr	BW	0.43 mg/ 0.5 ml	SKF	300 mg/ 2 ml	Physically compatible for 4 hr at 25 °C	25	C
Secobarbital sodium	WY	100 mg/ 2 ml	SKF	300 mg/ 2 ml	Immediate precipitation	25	I
Sodium acetate		10 mEq/ 5 ml	SKF	300 mg/ 2 ml	Physically compatible for 48 hr at room temperature	516	C
Sodium chloride		12.5 mEq/ 5 ml	SKF	300 mg/ 2 ml	Precipitate forms between 36 and 48 hr at room temperature	516	C
Sodium lactate		25 mEq/ 5 ml	SKF	300 mg/ 2 ml	Physically compatible for 48 hr at room temperature	516	C

Y-Site Injection Compatibility (1:1 Mixture)

Cimetidine HCl

Drug	Mfr	Conc	Mfr	Conc	Remarks	Ref	C/I
Acyclovir sodium	BW	5 mg/ml[a]	SKF	6 mg/ml[a]	Physically compatible for 4 hr at 25 °C	1157	C
Allopurinol sodium	BW	3 mg/ml[b]	SKB	12 mg/ml[b]	Tiny crystals form in 1 hr and become large crystals in 4 hr	1686	I
Amifostine	USB	10 mg/ml[a]	SKB	12 mg/ml[a]	Physically compatible with no change in measured turbidity or increase in particle content in 4 hr at 23 °C	1845	C
Aminophylline	ES	4 mg/ml[c]	SKF	6 mg/ml[c]	Physically compatible for 3 hr	1316	C
Amphotericin B cholesteryl sulfate complex	SEQ	0.83 mg/ml[a]	AMR	12 mg/ml[a]	Gross precipitate forms	2117	I
Amrinone lactate	WB	3 mg/ml[b]	SKF	15 mg/ml[a]	Physically compatible for at least 4 hr at 25 °C under fluorescent light	992	C
Amsacrine	NCI	1 mg/ml[a]	SKF	12 mg/ml[a]	Initially clear, but yellow-orange turbidity develops in 1 hr, becoming flocculent precipitate in 4 hr	1381	I
Atracurium besylate	BW	0.5 mg/ml[a]	SKF	6 mg/ml[a]	Physically compatible for 24 hr at 28 °C	1337	C
Aztreonam	SQ	40 mg/ml[a]	SKB	12 mg/ml[a]	Physically compatible with no subvisual haze or particle formation in 4 hr at 23 °C	1758	C

Y-Site Injection Compatibility (1:1 Mixture) (Cont.)

Cimetidine HCl

Drug	Mfr	Conc	Mfr	Conc	Remarks	Ref	C/I
Cefepime HCl	BR	20 mg/ml[a]	SKB	12 mg/ml[a]	Cloudy solution forms immediately	1689	I
Cisatracurium besylate	GW	0.1, 2, 5 mg/ml[a]	SKB	12 mg/ml[a]	Physically compatible with no change in measured turbidity or increase in particle content in 4 hr at 23 °C	2074	C
Cisplatin	BR	1 mg/ml	SKF	12 mg/ml[a]	Visually compatible for 4 hr at room temperature under fluorescent light	1685	C
Cladribine	ORT	0.015[b] and 0.5[d] mg/ml	SKB	12 mg/ml[b]	Physically compatible with no change in measured turbidity or increase in particle content in 4 hr at 23 °C	1969	C
Clarithromycin	AB	4 mg/ml[a]	SKB	8 mg/ml[a]	Visually compatible for 72 hr at both 30 and 17 °C	2174	C
Cyclophosphamide	MJ	10 mg/ml	SKF	12 mg/ml[a]	Visually compatible for 4 hr at room temperature under fluorescent light	1685	C
Cytarabine	UP	50 mg/ml	SKF	12 mg/ml[a]	Visually compatible for 4 hr at room temperature under fluorescent light	1685	C
Diltiazem HCl	MMD	5 mg/ml	SKF	6[c] and 150 mg/ml	Visually compatible	1807	C
	MMD	1 mg/ml[b]	SKF	150 mg/ml	Visually compatible	1807	C
Docetaxel	RPR	0.9 mg/ml[a]	AMR	12 mg/ml[a]	Physically compatible with no change in measured turbidity or increase in particle content in 4 hr at 23 °C	2224	C
Doxorubicin HCl	AD	0.2 mg/ml[a]	SKF	12 mg/ml[a]	Visually compatible for 4 hr at room temperature under fluorescent light	1685	C
Doxorubicin HCl liposome injection	SEQ	0.4 mg/ml[a]	SKB	12 mg/ml[a]	Physically compatible with little or no change in measured turbidity and no increase in particle content in 4 hr at 23 °C	2087	C
Enalaprilat	MSD	0.05 mg/ml[b]	SKF	3 mg/ml[a]	Physically compatible for 24 hr at room temperature under fluorescent light	1355	C
Esmolol HCl	DCC	10 mg/ml[a]	SKF	6 mg/ml[a]	Physically compatible for 24 hr at 22 °C	1169	C
Etoposide phosphate	BR	5 mg/ml[a]	AMR	12 mg/ml[a]	Physically compatible with no change in measured turbidity or increase in particle content in 4 hr at 23 °C	2218	C
Filgrastim	AMG	30 μg/ml[a]	SKB	12 mg/ml[a]	Physically compatible with no change in measured turbidity or increase in particle content in 4 hr at 22 °C	1687	C
Fluconazole	RR	2 mg/ml	SKF	150 mg/ml	Physically compatible for 24 hr at 25 °C	1407	C
	RR	2 mg/ml	SKB	1 and 2 mg/ml[c]	Visually compatible for 24 hr at 28 °C	1760	C
Fludarabine phosphate	BX	1 mg/ml[a]	SKF	12 mg/ml	Physically compatible for 4 hr at room temperature under fluorescent light	1439	C
Foscarnet sodium	AST	24 mg/ml	SKF	150 mg/ml	Physically compatible for 24 hr at room temperature under fluorescent light	1335	C
Gemcitabine HCl	LI	10 mg/ml[b]	AMR	12 mg/ml[b]	Physically compatible with no change in measured turbidity or increase in particle content in 4 hr at 23 °C	2226	C

Y-Site Injection Compatibility (1:1 Mixture) (Cont.)

Cimetidine HCl

Drug	Mfr	Conc	Mfr	Conc	Remarks	Ref	C/I
Granisetron HCl	SKB	1 mg/ml	SKB	3 mg/ml[b]	Physically compatible with little or no loss of either drug by HPLC in 4 hr at 22 °C	1883	C
Haloperidol lactate	MN	0.5[a] and 5 mg/ml	SKF	6 mg/ml[a]	Visually compatible for 24 hr at 21 °C	1523	C
Heparin sodium		50 units/ml/min[b]		200 mg/2 ml[e]	Clear solution	1053	C
	TR	50 units/ml	SKB	6 mg/ml[a]	Visually compatible for 6 hr at 25 °C	1793	C
Hetastarch	DCC	6%	SKF	6 mg/ml[a]	Physically compatible for 4 hr at room temperature by visual examination	1313; 1315	C
Idarubicin HCl	AD	1 mg/ml[b]	SKF	6 mg/ml[a]	Visually compatible for 24 hr at 25 °C	1525	C
Indomethacin sodium trihydrate	MSD	1 mg/ml[b]	SKB	6 mg/ml[a]	Haze and fine precipitate form immediately	1527	I
Labetalol HCl	SC	1 mg/ml[a]	SKF	3 mg/ml[a]	Physically compatible for 24 hr at 18 °C	1171	C
Melphalan HCl	BW	0.1 mg/ml[b]	SKB	12 mg/ml[b]	Physically compatible with no change in measured turbidity or increase in particle content in 3 hr at 22 °C	1557	C
Meropenem	ZEN	1 and 50 mg/ml[b]	SKB	150 mg/ml	Visually compatible for 4 hr at room temperature	1994	C
Methotrexate sodium	AD	15 mg/ml[f]	SKF	12 mg/ml[a]	Visually compatible for 4 hr at room temperature under fluorescent light	1685	C
Midazolam HCl	RC	1 mg/ml[a]	SKB	15 mg/ml[a]	Visually compatible for 24 hr at 23 °C	1847	C
Milrinone lactate	SW	0.4 mg/ml[a]	SKB	6 mg/ml[a]	Visually compatible with little or no loss of either drug by HPLC in 4 hr at 23 °C	2214	C
Ondansetron HCl	GL	1 mg/ml[b]	SKF	12 mg/ml[a]	Physically compatible for 4 hr at 22 °C	1365	C
Paclitaxel	NCI	1.2 mg/ml[a]		12 mg/ml[a]	Physically compatible with no change in measured turbidity in 4 hr at 22 °C	1528	C
Pancuronium bromide	ES	0.05 mg/ml[a]	SKF	6 mg/ml[a]	Physically compatible for 24 hr at 28 °C	1337	C
Piperacillin sodium–tazobactam sodium	LE	40 + 5 mg/ml[a]	SKB	12 mg/ml[a]	Physically compatible with no change in measured turbidity or increase in particle content in 4 hr at 22 °C	1688	C
Propofol	ZEN	10 mg/ml	SKB	12 mg/ml[a]	Physically compatible for 1 hr at 23 °C with no increase in particle content	2066	C
Remifentanil HCl	GW	0.025 and 0.25 mg/ml[b]	SKB	12 mg/ml[a]	Physically compatible with no change in measured turbidity or increase in particle content in 4 hr at 23 °C	2075	C
Sargramostim	IMM	10 μg/ml[b]	SKF	12 mg/ml[b]	Physically compatible for 4 hr at 22 °C	1436	C
Tacrolimus	FUJ	1 mg/ml[b]	SKB	150 mg/ml[a]	Visually compatible for 24 hr at 25 °C	1630	C
Teniposide	BR	0.1 mg/ml[a]	SKB	12 mg/ml[a]	Physically compatible with no subvisual haze or particle formation in 4 hr at 23 °C	1725	C
Theophylline	TR	4 mg/ml	SKB	6 mg/ml[a]	Visually compatible for 6 hr at 25 °C	1793	C
Thiotepa	IMM[g]	1 mg/ml[a]	SKB	12 mg/ml[a]	Physically compatible with no change in measured turbidity or increase in particle content in 4 hr at 23 °C	1861	C

Y-Site Injection Compatibility (1:1 Mixture) (Cont.)

Cimetidine HCl

Drug	Mfr	Conc	Mfr	Conc	Remarks	Ref	C/I
TNA #218 to #226[h]			SKB	12 mg/ml[a]	Visually compatible with no precipitate or emulsion damage apparent in 4 hr at 23 °C	2215	C
Tolazoline HCl		0.1 mg/ml[a]	SKF	15 mg/ml[a]	Physically compatible for 24 hr at 22 °C	1363	C
TPN #189[h]			SKB	10 mg/ml[b]	Visually compatible for 24 hr at 22 °C	1767	C
TPN #212 to #215[h]			SKB	12 mg/ml[a]	Physically compatible with no change in measured turbidity or increase in particle content in 4 hr at 23 °C	2109	C
Vecuronium bromide	OR	0.1 mg/ml[a]	SKF	6 mg/ml[a]	Physically compatible for 24 hr at 28 °C	1337	C
Vinorelbine tartrate	BW	1 mg/ml[b]	SKB	12 mg/ml[b]	Physically compatible with no change in measured turbidity or increase in particle content in 4 hr at 22 °C	1558	C
Warfarin sodium	DU	2 mg/ml[i]	SKB	3.6 mg/ml[a]	Haze forms in 1 hr	2010	I
	DU	2 mg/ml[i]	EN	3.6 mg/ml[a]	Haze forms immediately	2010	I
	DME	2 mg/ml[i]	SKB	3.6 mg/ml[a]	Haze forms in 1 hr	2078	I
Zidovudine	BW	4 mg/ml[a]	SKF	6 mg/ml[a]	Physically compatible for 4 hr at 25 °C under fluorescent light by visual and microscopic examination	1193	C

[a]*Tested in dextrose 5% in water.*
[b]*Tested in sodium chloride 0.9%.*
[c]*Tested in both dextrose 5% in water and sodium chloride 0.9%.*
[d]*Tested in bacteriostatic sodium chloride 0.9% preserved with benzyl alcohol 0.9%.*
[e]*Given over three minutes via a Y-site into a running infusion solution.*
[f]*Tested in dextrose 5% in water with sodium bicarbonate 0.05 mEq/ml.*
[g]*Lyophilized formulation tested.*
[h]*Refer to Appendix I for the composition of parenteral nutrition solutions. TNA indicates a 3-in-1 admixture, and TPN indicates a 2-in-1 admixture.*
[i]*Tested in sterile water for injection.*

Additional Compatibility Information

Solutions— The manufacturer states that cimetidine HCl may be admixed in most common intravenous solutions, including sodium chloride 0.9%, dextrose 5 and 10% in water, lactated Ringer's injection, and sodium bicarbonate 5%, and used for 48 hours at room temperature (2). Other information indicates that cimetidine HCl may be stable for longer than 48 hours (549; 550). See Compatibility Information.

Miscellaneous— Cimetidine HCl is stated to be physically incompatible with barbiturates (360) as well as with amphotericin B and cephalosporins (868).

Complex formation between cimetidine and theophylline has been noted in pH 7.4 phosphate buffer solution and human plasma (1043).

Ceftazidime (Tazicef) 20 mg/ml in sterile water for injection is stated to be stable for 18 hours at room temperature or seven days under refrigeration when admixed with cimetidine HCl 150 mg/ml (4).

Cimetidine HCl (SKF) 13 to 19 mg/kg every 24 hours was administered to patients by continuous infusion in parenteral nutrition solutions composed of essential amino acids, dextrose 50% in water with varying amounts of vitamins, electrolytes, trace elements, and albumin. The admixtures were prepared within 24 hours prior to use. No physical incompatibilities were noted, and cimetidine blood levels were in the range achieved by long-term oral treatment (570). In fact, the dose required to maintain therapeutic levels may be lower than with an intermittent infusion (1084).

When compounding parenteral nutrition mixtures, cimetidine should be admixed in a sequence that separates it from the copper sulfate present in trace elements injections to avoid formation of a green-colored copper-cimetidine complex (1951).

CIPROFLOXACIN
AHFS 8:22

Cipro I.V.   **Bayer**

Products— Ciprofloxacin (Bayer) is available as a concentrate in 20-and 40-ml vials and 120-ml pharmacy bulk packages. Each milliliter of solution contains 10 mg of ciprofloxacin, with lactic acid as a solubilizer and hydrochloric acid to adjust the pH (2).

Ciprofloxacin (Bayer) is also available as a premixed, ready-to-use solution in 100- and 200-ml PVC containers. Each milliliter contains 2 mg of ciprofloxacin with dextrose 5%, lactic acid as a solubilizer, and hydrochloric acid to adjust the pH (2).

pH— Vials: from 3.3 to 3.9. PVC bags: from 3.5 to 4.6 (2).

Administration— Ciprofloxacin is administered at a concentration of 1 to 2 mg/ml by intravenous infusion into a large vein slowly over 60 minutes. When given intermittently through a Y-site, the primary solution should be discontinued temporarily (2; 4).

Stability— Ciprofloxacin is a clear, colorless to slightly yellow solution. It should be stored between 5 and 25 °C (bags) or 30 °C (vials) and protected from light, temperatures over 40 °C, and freezing (2; 4).

pH Effects— Ciprofloxacin in aqueous solution is stated to be stable for up to 14 days at room temperature in the pH range of 1.5 to 7.5 (4). However, Teraoka et al. reported substantial loss of ciprofloxacin content in admixtures with a pH over 6 (1924).

Sorption— Ciprofloxacin (Bayer) 200 mg/250 ml in dextrose 5% in water and sodium chloride 0.9% in PVC bags was infused through infusion sets at about 4 ml/min. No drug loss due to sorption was detected by HPLC (1698).

Ciprofloxacin (Bayer) 2 mg/ml in sodium chloride 0.9% exhibited no loss due to sorption to PVC administration sets including Venoset (Abbott), Ivex HP filter set (Abbott), and 9200 Accuset (IMED) during simulated administration and static studies (1934).

Compatibility Information

Solution Compatibility

Ciprofloxacin

Solution	Mfr	Mfr	Conc/L	Remarks	Ref	C/I
Dextrose 5% in Electrolyte #75		MI	0.5 and 1 g	Stable for 14 days at 5 and 25 °C	888	C
Dextrose 5% in sodium chloride 0.225%		MI	0.5 and 2 g	Stable for 14 days at 5 and 25 °C	888	C
Dextrose 5% in sodium chloride 0.45%		MI	0.5 and 2 g	Stable for 14 days at 5 and 25 °C	888	C
Dextrose 5% in water	AB[a]	MI	1.5 g	Visually compatible with no loss by HPLC in 48 hr at 25 °C under fluorescent light	1541	C
	[a]	BAY	800 mg	Visually compatible with no significant loss by HPLC in 6 hr at 22 °C exposed to light	1698	C
		MI	0.5 and 2 g	Stable for 14 days at 5 and 25 °C	888	C
	BA[a]	MI	2.86 g	Visually compatible with no loss by HPLC in 90 days at room temperature and 5 °C	1891	C
Dextrose 10% in water		MI	0.5 and 2 g	Stable for 14 days at 5 and 25 °C	888	C
Fructose 10% in water		MI	0.5 and 1 g	Stable for 14 days at 5 and 25 °C	888	C
Ringer's injection		MI	0.5 and 1 g	Stable for 14 days at 5 and 25 °C	888	C
Ringer's injection, lactated		MI	0.5 and 2 g	Stable for 14 days at 5 and 25 °C	888	C
Sodium chloride 0.9%	AB[a]	MI	1.5 g	Visually compatible with no loss by HPLC in 48 hr at 25 °C under fluorescent light	1541	C
	[a]	BAY	800 mg	Visually compatible with no significant loss by HPLC in 6 hr at 22 °C exposed to light	1698	C
		MI	0.5 and 2 g	Stable for 14 days at 5 and 25 °C	888	C
	BA[a]	MI	2.86 g	Visually compatible with no loss by HPLC in 90 days at room temperature and 5 °C	1891	C

Solution Compatibility (Cont.)

Solution		Ciprofloxacin				
Solution	Mfr	Mfr	Conc/L	Remarks	Ref	C/I
	AB	BAY	2 g	Visually compatible with no loss by HPLC in 24 hr at 25 °C	1934	C

[a]Tested in PVC containers.

Additive Compatibility

		Ciprofloxacin						
Drug	Mfr	Conc/L	Mfr	Conc/L	Test Soln	Remarks	Ref	C/I
Amikacin sulfate	BR	4.1 g	MI	1.6 g	D5W, NS	Visually compatible and ciprofloxacin potency by HPLC and amikacin potency by immunoassay retained for 48 hr at 25 °C under fluorescent light	1541	C
Aminophylline	LY	2 g	MI	1.6 g	D5W, NS	Ciprofloxacin precipitate forms in 4 hr at 4 and 25 °C	1541	I
Amoxicillin sodium		10 g		2 g	a	Immediate precipitation	1473	I
Amoxicillin sodium–clavulanate potassium		10 + 2 g		2 g	a	Immediate precipitation	1473	I
Aztreonam	SQ	20 g	MI	1 g	D5W, NS	Physically compatible for 24 hr at 22 °C	1189	C
Ceftazidime	SKF	20 g	MI	1 g	D5W, NS	Physically compatible for 24 hr at 22 °C	1189	C
Clindamycin phosphate	LY	7.1 g	MI	1.6 g	D5W, NS	Precipitate forms immediately. HPLC showed no intact clindamycin	1541	I
Cyclosporine	SZ	500 mg	BAY	2 g	NS	Visually compatible with about 8% ciprofloxacin loss by HPLC in 24 hr at 25 °C. Cyclosporine not tested	1934	C
Floxacillin sodium		10 g		2 g	a	Immediate precipitation	1473	I
Gentamicin sulfate	LY	1 g	MI	1.6 g	D5W, NS	Visually compatible and ciprofloxacin potency by HPLC and gentamicin potency by immunoassay retained for 48 hr at 25 °C under fluorescent light and 4 °C in the dark	1541	C
	SC	10 g	BAY	2 g	NS	Visually compatible with little or no ciprofloxacin loss by HPLC in 24 hr at 25 °C. Gentamicin not tested	1934	C
Heparin sodium	CP	10,000, 100,000, and 1 million units	BAY	2 g	NS	White precipitate forms immediately	1934	I
Metronidazole		5 g		2 g		No loss of either drug in 4 hr at 24 °C	1346	C
	SE	4.2 g	MI	1.6 g		Visually compatible and potency of both drugs by HPLC retained for 48 hr at 25 °C under fluorescent light and 4 °C in the dark	1541	C
Netilmicin sulfate	SC	2.5 g	BAY	2 g	NS	Visually compatible with little or no ciprofloxacin loss by HPLC in 24 hr at 25 °C. Netilmicin not tested	1934	C
Piperacillin sodium	LE	40 g	MI	1 g	D5W, NS	Physically compatible for 24 hr at 22 °C	1189	C

Additive Compatibility (Cont.)

		Ciprofloxacin						
Drug	*Mfr*	*Conc/L*	*Mfr*	*Conc/L*	*Test Soln*	*Remarks*	*Ref*	*C/I*
Potassium chloride	AB	40 mEq	BAY	2 g	NS	Visually compatible with little or no ciprofloxacin loss by HPLC in 24 hr at 25 °C	1934	**C**
Ranitidine HCl	GL	500 mg and 1 g	BAY	2 g	NS	Visually compatible with little or no ciprofloxacin loss by HPLC in 24 hr at 25 °C. Ranitidine not tested	1934	**C**
Tobramycin sulfate	LI	1.6 g	MI	1 g	D5W, NS	Physically compatible for 24 hr at 22 °C	1189	**C**
	LI	1 g	MI	1.6 g	D5W, NS	Visually compatible and ciprofloxacin potency by HPLC and tobramycin potency by immunoassay retained for 48 hr at 25 °C under fluorescent light and 4 °C in the dark	1541	**C**
Vitamin B complex	BC	2 ml	BAY	2 g	NS	Visually compatible with 8% ciprofloxacin loss by HPLC in 24 hr at 25 °C. Vitamins not tested	1934	**C**

[a]Drug added to ciprofloxacin solution.

Y-Site Injection Compatibility (1:1 Mixture)

		Ciprofloxacin					
Drug	*Mfr*	*Conc*	*Mfr*	*Conc*	*Remarks*	*Ref*	*C/I*
Amifostine	USB	10 mg/ml[a]	MI	1 mg/ml[a]	Physically compatible with no change in measured turbidity or increase in particle content in 4 hr at 23 °C	1845	**C**
Amino acids, dextrose	AB	AA 5%, D 25%	MI	2 mg/ml[a]	Visually compatible for 2 hr at 25 °C	1628	**C**
Aminophylline	AB	2 mg/ml[a,b]	MI	2 mg/ml[a,b]	Fine white crystals form in 20 min in D5W and 2 min in NS	1655	**I**
Ampicillin sodium–sulbactam sodium		3 g[c]		400 mg[c]	When administered sequentially through a Y-site into running D5S, white crystals form immediately	1887	**I**
Aztreonam	SQ	20 mg/ml[a,b]	MI	1 mg/ml[a]	Physically compatible for 24 hr at 22 °C	1189	**C**
	SQ	40 mg/ml[a]	MI	1 mg/ml[a]	Physically compatible with no subvisual haze or particle formation in 4 hr at 23 °C	1758	**C**
Calcium gluconate	LY	10%	MI	2 mg/ml[a]	Visually compatible for 2 hr at 25 °C	1628	**C**
Cefepime HCl	BR	20 mg/ml[a]	MI	1 mg/ml[b]	Cloudy solution forms immediately. Flocculent precipitate forms in 4 hr	1689	**I**
Ceftazidime	SKF[d]	20 mg/ml[a,b]	MI	1 mg/ml[a]	Physically compatible for 24 hr at 22 °C	1189	**C**
Cisatracurium besylate	GW	0.1, 2, 5 mg/ml[a]	BAY	1 mg/ml[a]	Physically compatible with no change in measured turbidity or increase in particle content in 4 hr at 23 °C	2074	**C**
Clarithromycin	AB	4 mg/ml[a]	BAY	2 mg/ml[a]	Visually compatible for 72 hr at both 30 and 17 °C	2174	**C**
Dexamethasone sodium phosphate	LY	4 mg/ml	MI	2 mg/ml[a,b]	Transient white cloudiness rapidly dissipates. White crystals and flocculence form in 1 hr at 24 °C	1655	**I**
Digoxin	ES	0.25 mg/ml	MI	2 mg/ml[a,b]	Visually compatible for 24 hr at 24 °C	1655	**C**

Y-Site Injection Compatibility (1:1 Mixture) (Cont.)

Ciprofloxacin

Drug	Mfr	Conc	Mfr	Conc	Remarks	Ref	C/I
	BW	0.25 mg/ml	BAY	2 mg/ml[b]	Visually compatible with no ciprofloxacin loss by HPLC in 15 min. Digoxin not tested	1934	C
Diltiazem HCl	MMD	5 mg/ml	MI	2 and 10 mg/ml[b]	Visually compatible	1807	C
Diphenhydramine HCl	ES	50 mg/ml	MI	2 mg/ml[a,b]	Visually compatible for 24 hr at 24 °C	1655	C
Dobutamine HCl	LI	250 μg/ml[a,b]	MI	2 mg/ml[a,b]	Visually compatible for 24 hr at 24 °C	1655	C
Docetaxel	RPR	0.9 mg/ml[a]	BAY	1 mg/ml[a]	Physically compatible with no change in measured turbidity or increase in particle content in 4 hr at 23 °C	2224	C
Dopamine HCl	AB	1.6 mg/ml[a,b]	MI	2 mg/ml[a,b]	Visually compatible for 24 hr at 24 °C	1655	C
Doxorubicin HCl liposome injection	SEQ	0.4 mg/ml[a]	BAY	1 mg/ml[a]	Physically compatible with little or no change in measured turbidity and no increase in particle content in 4 hr at 23 °C	2087	C
Etoposide phosphate	BR	5 mg/ml[a]	BAY	1 mg/ml[a]	Physically compatible with no change in measured turbidity and increase in particle content in 4 hr at 23 °C	2218	C
Furosemide	AB	10 mg/ml	MI	2 mg/ml[a,b]	Immediate precipitation	1655	I
	DMX	5 mg/ml	BAY	2 mg/ml[b]	White precipitate forms immediately	1934	I
Gemcitabine HCl	LI	10 mg/ml[b]	BAY	1 mg/ml[b]	Physically compatible with no change in measured turbidity or increase in particle content in 4 hr at 23 °C	2226	C
Gentamicin sulfate	LY	1.6 mg/ml[a,b]	MI	2 mg/ml[a,b]	Visually compatible for 24 hr at 24 °C	1655	C
Granisetron HCl	SKB	0.05 mg/ml[a]	MI	1 mg/ml[a]	Physically compatible with no change in measured turbidity or increase in particle content in 4 hr at 23 °C	2000	C
Heparin sodium		10 units/ml		2 mg/ml	Turbidity forms rapidly with subsequent white precipitate	1483	I
	LY	100 units/ml[a,b]	MI	2 mg/ml[a,b]	Immediate crystal formation	1655	I
	CP	10, 100, and 1000 units/ml[b]	BAY	2 mg/ml[b]	White precipitate forms immediately	1934	I
Hydrocortisone sodium succinate	UP	50 mg/ml	MI	2 mg/ml[a,b]	Transient white cloudiness rapidly dissipates. White crystals form in 1 hr at 24 °C	1655	I
Hydroxyzine HCl	ES	50 mg/ml	MI	2 mg/ml[a,b]	Visually compatible for 24 hr at 24 °C	1655	C
Lidocaine HCl	AB	4[a] and 20 mg/ml	MI	2 mg/ml[a,b]	Visually compatible for 24 hr at 24 °C	1655	C
Lorazepam	WY	0.33 mg/ml[b]	BAY	2 mg/ml	Visually compatible for 24 hr at 22 °C	1855	C
Magnesium sulfate	AB	4 mEq/ml	MI	2 mg/ml[a,b]	Precipitate forms in 4 hr in D5W and 1 hr in NS at 24 °C	1655	I
	LY	50%	MI	2 mg/ml[a]	Visually compatible for 2 hr at 25 °C	1628	C
Methylprednisolone sodium succinate	UP	62.5 mg/ml	MI	2 mg/ml[a,b]	Transient white cloudiness rapidly dissipates. White crystals form in 2 hr at 24 °C	1655	I
Metoclopramide HCl	DU	5 mg/ml	MI	2 mg/ml[a,b]	Visually compatible for 24 hr at 24 °C	1655	C

Y-Site Injection Compatibility (1:1 Mixture) (Cont.)

| | | | | | Ciprofloxacin | | | |
Drug	Mfr	Conc	Mfr	Conc	Remarks	Ref	C/I
		5 mg/ml	BAY	2 mg/ml[b]	Visually compatible with no ciprofloxacin loss by HPLC in 15 min. Metoclopramide not tested	1934	C
Midazolam HCl	RC	5 mg/ml	BAY	2 mg/ml	Visually compatible for 24 hr at 22 °C	1855	C
Midodrine HCl	CP	5 mg/ml	BAY	2 mg/ml[b]	Visually compatible with no ciprofloxacin loss by HPLC in 15 min. Midodrine not tested	1934	C
Phenytoin sodium	PD	50 mg/ml	MI	2 mg/ml[a,b]	Immediate crystal formation	1655	I
Piperacillin sodium	LE	40 mg/ml[a,b]	MI	1 mg/ml[a]	Physically compatible for 24 hr at 22 °C	1189	C
Potassium acetate	LY	2 mEq/ml	MI	2 mg/ml[a]	Visually compatible for 2 hr at 25 °C	1628	C
Potassium chloride	LY	0.04 mEq/ml	MI	2 mg/ml[a,b]	Visually compatible for 24 hr at 24 °C	1655	C
	AMR	2 mEq/ml	MI	2 mg/ml[a]	Visually compatible for 2 hr at 25 °C	1628	C
Potassium phosphates	LY	3 mmol/ml	MI	2 mg/ml[a]	Visually compatible for 2 hr at 25 °C	1628	C
Promethazine HCl	ES	25 mg/ml	MI	2 mg/ml[a,b]	Visually compatible for 24 hr at 24 °C	1655	C
Propofol	ZEN	10 mg/ml	MI	1 mg/ml[a]	Emulsion broke and oiled out	1916	I
Ranitidine HCl	GL	0.5 mg/ml[a,b]	MI	2 mg/ml[a,b]	Visually compatible for 24 hr at 24 °C	1655	C
Remifentanil HCl	GW	0.025 and 0.25 mg/ml[b]	BAY	1 mg/ml[a]	Physically compatible with no change in measured turbidity or increase in particle content in 4 hr at 23 °C	2075	C
Ringer's injection, lactated	AB		MI	2 mg/ml[a,b]	Visually compatible for 24 hr at 24 °C	1655	C
Sodium bicarbonate	AB	1 mEq/ml	MI	2 mg/ml[a]	Visually compatible for 24 hr at 24 °C	1655	C
	AB	1 mEq/ml	MI	2 mg/ml[b]	Very fine crystals form in 20 min in NS	1655	I
	AB	1 mEq/ml	MI	2 mg/ml[a]	Physically compatible with no change in measured turbidity or increase in particle content in 4 hr at 23 °C	1869	C
	AB	0.1 mEq/ml[a]	MI	2 mg/ml[a]	Subvisual haze forms immediately, becoming a white crystalline precipitate in 4 hr at 23 °C	1869	I
	AB	1 and 0.75[a] mEq/ml	BAY	1 and 2 mg/ml[a]	Physically compatible with no change in measured turbidity or increase in particle content in 4 hr at 23 °C	2065	C
	AB	1 and 0.75[b] mEq/ml	BAY	1 mg/ml[b]	Physically compatible with no change in measured turbidity or increase in particle content in 4 hr at 23 °C	2065	C
	AB	1 and 0.75[b] mEq/ml	BAY	2 mg/ml[b]	Small amount of particles forms immediately, becoming more numerous over 4 hr at 23 °C	2065	I
	AB	0.5, 0.25, and 0.1 mEq/ml[a]	BAY	1 and 2 mg/ml[a]	Small amount of particles forms immediately, becoming more numerous over 4 hr at 23 °C	2065	I
	AB	0.5, 0.25, and 0.1 mEq/ml[b]	BAY	1 mg/ml[b]	Small amount of particles forms in 1 hr, becoming more numerous over 4 hr at 23 °C	2065	I
	AB	0.5, 0.25, and 0.1 mEq/ml[b]	BAY	2 mg/ml[b]	Precipitate forms immediately	2065	I
Sodium chloride	AMR	4 mEq/ml	MI	2 mg/ml[a]	Visually compatible for 2 hr at 25 °C	1628	C
Sodium phosphates	AB	3 mmol/ml[a]	BAY	2 mg/ml[a]	Subvisual microcrystals form in 1 hr at 23 °C	1972	I

Y-Site Injection Compatibility (1:1 Mixture) (Cont.)

					Ciprofloxacin			
Drug	*Mfr*	*Conc*	*Mfr*	*Conc*	*Remarks*	*Ref*	*C/I*
	AB	3 mmol/ml[f]	BAY	2 mg/ml[f]	White crystalline precipitate forms immediately	1971; 1972	I
Tacrolimus	FUJ	1 mg/ml[b]	MI	1 mg/ml[a]	Visually compatible for 24 hr at 25 °C	1630	C
Teicoplanin	GRP	60 mg/ml	BAY	2 mg/ml[b]	White precipitate forms immediately but disappears with shaking	1934	?
Teniposide	BR	0.1 mg/ml[a]	MI	2 mg/ml[a]	Physically compatible with no subvisual haze or particle formation in 4 hr at 23 °C	1725	C
Thiotepa	IMM[g]	1 mg/ml[a]	MI	1 mg/ml[a]	Physically compatible with no change in measured turbidity or increase in particle content in 4 hr at 23 °C	1861	C
TNA #218 to #226[i]			BAY	1 mg/ml[a]	Visually compatible with no precipitate or emulsion damage apparent in 4 hr at 23 °C	2215	C
Tobramycin sulfate	LI	1.6 mg/ml[a,b]	MI	1 mg/ml[a]	Physically compatible for 24 hr at 22 °C	1189	C
TPN #212 to #215[i]			MI	1 mg/ml[a]	Amber discoloration forms in 1 to 4 hr	2109	I
Verapamil HCl	KN	2.5 mg/ml	MI	2 mg/ml[a,b]	Visually compatible for 24 hr at 24 °C	1655	C
Warfarin sodium	DU	2 mg/ml[a]	MI	2 mg/ml[h]	Haze forms immediately; crystals form in 1 hr	2010	I
	DME	2 mg/ml[h]	MI	2 mg/ml[a]	Haze forms immediately; crystals form in 1 hr	2078	I

[a]*Tested in dextrose 5% in water.*
[b]*Tested in sodium chloride 0.9%.*
[c]*Concentration and volume not specified.*
[d]*Sodium carbonate–containing formulation tested.*
[e]*Form unspecified.*
[f]*Tested in both sodium chloride 0.9% and 0.45%.*
[g]*Lyophilized formulation tested.*
[h]*Tested in sterile water for injection.*
[i]*Refer to Appendix 1 for the composition of parenteral nutrition solutions. TNA indicates a 3-in-1 admixture, and TPN indicates a 2-in-1 admixture.*

Additional Compatibility Information

Solutions— Ciprofloxacin in concentrations between 0.5 and 2 mg/ml in dextrose 5% in water or sodium chloride 0.9% is stable for 14 days at room temperature or under refrigeration (2; 4).

Phosphates— Admixing ciprofloxacin with sodium phosphates has resulted in reports of both compatibility and incompatibility (see table above). Combining the two drugs in sodium chloride 0.45% or 0.9% can result in a large amount of white crystalline precipitate forming (1971; 1972), while the same concentrations in dextrose 5% in water result in little or no precipitate forming (1628; 1972). This dependency of precipitation on the nature of the infusion solution may extend to potassium phosphates as well. Although ciprofloxacin has been reported compatible with potassium phosphates in dextrose 5% in water (1628), the manufacturer has had reports of precipitation of these two drugs. Unfortunately, the infusion solution vehicles involved in the precipitations were not identified (2009).

Sodium bicarbonate— Ciprofloxacin mixed with sodium bicarbonate in lower concentrations has resulted in the formation of a haze and precipitate, while 10-fold higher concentrations of sodium bi-

carbonate appear to be physically compatible with the same amount of ciprofloxacin (1869). Although not unprecedented, it is less common for high concentrations of drugs to be compatible while lower concentrations are incompatible. The differing compatibility results have been ascribed to pH-dependency of ciprofloxacin solubility (2012). However, a thorough evaluation of the compatibility of ciprofloxacin with a wide range of sodium bicarbonate concentrations found that incompatibility cannot be predicted by pH of the solutions alone; the solutions were generally in a very narrow pH range (8.0 to 8.3). Because the interaction between ciprofloxacin and sodium bicarbonate appears to be complex and variable, simultaneous administration of these drugs should be avoided (2065).

Peritoneal Dialysis Solutions— Ciprofloxacin (Bayer) 25 mg/L in peritoneal dialysis solution (Dianeal 137, Baxter) exhibited little or no loss by HPLC and bioassay after 42 days at 4, 22, and 37 °C when protected from light (1585).

The stability of ciprofloxacin (Miles) 25 mg/L in Dianeal PD-1 (Baxter) with dextrose 1.5 and 4.5% in PVC bags was evaluated by HPLC analysis during storage at 4, 25, and 37 °C. Drug losses of about 10 to 12% and 5 to 6% occurred during the first 12 hours at 4 and at 25 °C, respectively; however, concentrations were steady thereafter for two weeks at 4 °C and one week at 25 °C. Because no decomposition products were detected, the losses were attributed to sorption to the PVC containers. At 37 °C over 48 hours, losses of up to 10% occurred in the Dianeal PD-1 with dextrose 1.5%; losses of up to 7% occurred in the Dianeal PD-1 with dextrose 4.5% (1826).

CISATRACURIUM BESYLATE
AHFS 12:20

Nimbex   **Glaxo Wellcome**

Products— Cisatracurium besylate (Glaxo Wellcome) is available as a 2-mg/ml solution in 5- and 10-ml vials. The drug is also available as a 10-mg/ml solution in 20-ml vials intended for use in intensive care units only. The pH is adjusted with benzenesulfonic acid. The 2-mg/ml concentration in 10-ml vials also contains benzyl alcohol 0.9%. The other dosage forms have no preservative and are for single use only (2).

pH— From 3.25 to 3.65 (2).

Administration— Cisatracurium besylate is administered intravenously only. Both initial bolus doses and continuous intravenous infusion have been used. Rates of administration depend on the drug concentration in the solution, desired dose, and patient weight. Avoid contact with alkaline drugs during administration (2).

Stability— Cisatracurium besylate injection is a colorless to slightly yellow or greenish-yellow solution. Intact vials of cisatracurium besylate should be stored under refrigeration at 2 to 8 °C protected from light and freezing. Potency losses of 5% per year occur under refrigeration. However, at 25 °C, potency losses increase to about 5% per month. The manufacturer recommends that vials that have been warmed to room temperature be used within 21 days even if rerefrigerated (2).

In an independent study, cisatracurium besylate (Glaxo Wellcome) 2 mg/ml in the original 5- and 10-ml vials and the 10-mg/ml solution in original 20-ml vials was stored at 4 and 23 °C both protected from light and exposed to fluorescent light. All the samples remained physically stable throughout the 90-day study period. HPLC analysis found that samples stored under refrigeration exhibited little or no drug loss in 90 days whether exposed to or protected from light. At 23 °C, samples were stable through 45 days of storage with losses near 5 to 7% in most samples. However, most samples became unacceptable after 90 days of storage at 23 °C, exhibiting losses of 9 to 14% (2116).

pH Effects— The manufacturer indicates that cisatracurium besylate may not be compatible with barbiturates and other alkaline solutions having a pH greater than 8.5 (2).

Syringes— Cisatracurium besylate (Glaxo Wellcome) 2 mg/ml was repackaged in 3-ml plastic syringes (Becton Dickinson) and sealed with tip caps (Red Cap, Burron). The syringes were stored at 4 and 23 °C both protected from light and exposed to fluorescent light. All of the samples remained physically stable throughout the 30-day study period. HPLC analysis found little or no loss in the samples stored under refrigeration, whereas the samples stored at 23 °C exhibited 4 to 7% loss in 30 days (2116).

Compatibility Information

Solution Compatibility

Cisatracurium besylate

Solution	Mfr	Mfr	Conc/L	Remarks	Ref	C/I
Dextrose 5% in water	BA[a]	GW	100 mg	Physically compatible with 8% loss by HPLC in 7 days and 15% loss in 14 days at 23 °C under fluorescent light. Little or no loss in 30 days at 4 °C	2116	C
	BA[a]	GW	2 g	Physically compatible with 10% loss by HPLC in 14 days and 14% loss in 30 days at 23 °C under fluorescent light. Little or no loss in 30 days at 4 °C	2116	C
	BA[a]	GW	5 g	Physically compatible with 4% loss by HPLC in 30 days at 23 °C under fluorescent light. Little or no loss in 30 days at 4 °C	2116	C
Sodium chloride 0.9%	BA[a]	GW	100 mg	Physically compatible with 8% loss by HPLC in 14 days and 14% loss in 30 days at 23 °C under fluorescent light. Little or no loss in 30 days at 4 °C	2116	C
	BA[a]	GW	2 g	Physically compatible with 6% loss by HPLC in 30 days at 23 °C under fluorescent light. Little or no loss in 30 days at 4 °C	2116	C

Solution Compatibility (Cont.)

Cisatracurium besylate

Solution	Mfr	Mfr	Conc/L	Remarks	Ref	C/I
	BA[a]	GW	5 g	Physically compatible with 3% loss by HPLC in 30 days at 23 °C under fluorescent light. Little or no loss in 30 days at 4 °C	2116	C

[a]Tested in PVC containers.

Y-Site Injection Compatibility (1:1 Mixture)

Cisatracurium besylate

Drug	Mfr	Conc	Mfr	Conc	Remarks	Ref	C/I
Acyclovir sodium	BW	7 mg/ml[a]	GW	0.1 and 2 mg/ml[a]	Physically compatible with no change in measured turbidity or increase in particle content in 4 hr at 23 °C	2074	C
	BW	7 mg/ml[a]	GW	5 mg/ml[a]	White cloudiness forms immediately	2074	I
Alfentanil HCl	JN	0.125 mg/ml[a]	GW	0.1, 2, 5 mg/ml[a]	Physically compatible with no change in measured turbidity or increase in particle content in 4 hr at 23 °C	2074	C
Amikacin sulfate	AB	5 mg/ml[a]	GW	0.1, 2, 5 mg/ml[a]	Physically compatible with no change in measured turbidity or increase in particle content in 4 hr at 23 °C	2074	C
Aminophylline	AB	2.5 mg/ml[a]	GW	0.1 and 2 mg/ml[a]	Physically compatible with no change in measured turbidity or increase in particle content in 4 hr at 23 °C	2074	C
	AB	2.5 mg/ml[a]	GW	5 mg/ml[a]	Gray subvisual haze forms in 1 hr	2074	I
Amphotericin B	PH	0.6 mg/ml[a]	GW	0.1 mg/ml[a]	Physically compatible with no change in measured turbidity or increase in particle content in 4 hr at 23 °C	2074	C
	PH	0.6 mg/ml[a]	GW	2 mg/ml[a]	Cloudiness forms immediately; gel-like precipitate forms in 1 hr	2074	I
	PH	0.6 mg/ml[a]	GW	5 mg/ml[a]	Turbidity forms immediately	2074	I
Amphotericin B cholesteryl sulfate complex	SEQ	0.83 mg/ml[a]	GW	2 mg/ml[a]	Gross precipitate forms	2117	I
Ampicillin sodium	SKB	20 mg/ml[b]	GW	0.1 and 2 mg/ml[a]	Physically compatible with no change in measured turbidity or increase in particle content in 4 hr at 23 °C	2074	C
	SKB	20 mg/ml[b]	GW	5 mg/ml[a]	Gray subvisual haze forms in 1 hr	2074	I
Ampicillin sodium–sulbactam sodium	RR	20 + 10 mg/ml[b]	GW	0.1 and 2 mg/ml[a]	Physically compatible with no change in measured turbidity or increase in particle content in 4 hr at 23 °C	2074	C
	RR	20 + 10 mg/ml[b]	GW	5 mg/ml[a]	Subvisual haze develops in 15 min	2074	I
Amrinone lactate	SW	2.5 mg/ml[b]	GW	0.1, 2, 5 mg/ml[a]	Physically compatible with no change in measured turbidity or increase in particle content in 4 hr at 23 °C	2074	C
Aztreonam	SQ	40 mg/ml[a]	GW	0.1, 2, 5 mg/ml[a]	Physically compatible with no change in measured turbidity or increase in particle content in 4 hr at 23 °C	2074	C
Bretylium tosylate	AST	4 mg/ml[a]	GW	0.1, 2, 5 mg/ml[a]	Physically compatible with no change in measured turbidity or increase in particle content in 4 hr at 23 °C	2074	C

Y-Site Injection Compatibility (1:1 Mixture) (Cont.)

Cisatracurium besylate

Drug	Mfr	Conc	Mfr	Conc	Remarks	Ref	C/I
Bumetanide	BV	0.04 mg/ml[a]	GW	0.1, 2, 5 mg/ml[a]	Physically compatible with no change in measured turbidity or increase in particle content in 4 hr at 23 °C	2074	C
Buprenorphine HCl	RKC	0.04 mg/ml[a]	GW	0.1, 2, 5 mg/ml[a]	Physically compatible with no change in measured turbidity or increase in particle content in 4 hr at 23 °C	2074	C
Butorphanol tartrate	APC	0.04 mg/ml[a]	GW	0.1, 2, 5 mg/ml[a]	Physically compatible with no change in measured turbidity or increase in particle content in 4 hr at 23 °C	2074	C
Calcium gluconate	AB	40 mg/ml[a]	GW	0.1, 2, 5 mg/ml[a]	Physically compatible with no change in measured turbidity or increase in particle content in 4 hr at 23 °C	2074	C
Cefazolin sodium	SKB	20 mg/ml[a]	GW	0.1 mg/ml[a]	Physically compatible with no change in measured turbidity or increase in particle content in 4 hr at 23 °C	2074	C
	SKB	20 mg/ml[a]	GW	2 mg/ml[a]	Gray subvisual haze forms immediately	2074	I
	SKB	20 mg/ml[a]	GW	5 mg/ml[a]	Gray haze forms immediately	2074	I
Cefoperazone sodium	RR	40 mg/ml[a]	GW	0.1, 2, 5 mg/ml[a]	White cloudiness forms immediately	2074	I
Cefotaxime sodium	HO	20 mg/ml[a]	GW	0.1 mg/ml[a]	Physically compatible with no change in measured turbidity or increase in particle content in 4 hr at 23 °C	2074	C
	HO	20 mg/ml[a]	GW	2 mg/ml[a]	Subvisual haze forms in 4 hr	2074	I
	HO	20 mg/ml[a]	GW	5 mg/ml[a]	Subvisual haze forms immediately	2074	I
Cefotetan sodium	STU	20 mg/ml[a]	GW	0.1 and 2 mg/ml[a]	Physically compatible with no change in measured turbidity or increase in particle content in 4 hr at 23 °C	2074	C
	STU	20 mg/ml[a]	GW	5 mg/ml[a]	Dense turbidity forms immediately	2074	I
Cefoxitin sodium	ME	20 mg/ml[a]	GW	0.1 mg/ml[a]	Physically compatible with no change in measured turbidity or increase in particle content in 4 hr at 23 °C	2074	C
	ME	20 mg/ml[a]	GW	2 and 5 mg/ml[a]	Subvisual haze forms immediately	2074	I
Ceftazidime	SKB[c]	40 mg/ml[a]	GW	0.1 and 2 mg/ml[a]	Physically compatible with no change in measured turbidity or increase in particle content in 4 hr at 23 °C	2074	C
	SKB[c]	40 mg/ml[a]	GW	5 mg/ml[a]	Subvisual haze forms immediately	2074	I
	GW[d]	40 mg/ml[a]	GW	0.1, 2, 5 mg/ml[a]	Physically compatible with no change in measured turbidity or increase in particle content in 4 hr at 23 °C	2074	C
Ceftizoxime sodium	FUJ	20 mg/ml[a]	GW	0.1 and 2 mg/ml[a]	Physically compatible with no change in measured turbidity or increase in particle content in 4 hr at 23 °C	2074	C
	FUJ	20 mg/ml[a]	GW	5 mg/ml[a]	Subvisual haze forms in 1 hr	2074	I
Ceftriaxone sodium	RC	20 mg/ml[a]	GW	0.1, 2, 5 mg/ml[a]	Physically compatible with no change in measured turbidity or increase in particle content in 4 hr at 23 °C	2074	C
Cefuroxime sodium	LI	30 mg/ml[a]	GW	0.1 mg/ml[a]	Physically compatible with no change in measured turbidity or increase in particle content in 4 hr at 23 °C	2074	C

Y-Site Injection Compatibility (1:1 Mixture) (Cont.)

Drug	Mfr	Conc	Mfr	Conc	Remarks	Ref	C/I
	LI	30 mg/ml[a]	GW	2 mg/ml[a]	White cloudiness forms immediately	2074	I
	LI	30 mg/ml[a]	GW	5 mg/ml[a]	Turbidity forms immediately	2074	I
Chlorpromazine HCl	SCN	2 mg/ml[a]	GW	0.1, 2, 5 mg/ml[a]	Physically compatible with no change in measured turbidity or increase in particle content in 4 hr at 23 °C	2074	C
Cimetidine HCl	SKB	12 mg/ml[a]	GW	0.1, 2, 5 mg/ml[a]	Physically compatible with no change in measured turbidity or increase in particle content in 4 hr at 23 °C	2074	C
Ciprofloxacin	BAY	1 mg/ml[a]	GW	0.1, 2, 5 mg/ml[a]	Physically compatible with no change in measured turbidity or increase in particle content in 4 hr at 23 °C	2074	C
Clindamycin phosphate	AST	10 mg/ml[a]	GW	0.1, 2, 5 mg/ml[a]	Physically compatible with no change in measured turbidity or increase in particle content in 4 hr at 23 °C	2074	C
Dexamethasone sodium phosphate	FUJ	2 mg/ml[a]	GW	0.1, 2, 5 mg/ml[a]	Physically compatible with no change in measured turbidity or increase in particle content in 4 hr at 23 °C	2074	C
Diazepam	ES	5 mg/ml	GW	0.1, 2, 5 mg/ml[a]	White turbidity forms immediately	2074	I
	ES	0.25 mg/ml[a]	GW	0.1, 2, 5 mg/ml[a]	Physically compatible with no change in measured turbidity or increase in particle content in 4 hr at 23 °C	2074	C
Digoxin	ES	0.25 mg/ml	GW	0.1, 2, 5 mg/ml[a]	Physically compatible with no change in measured turbidity or increase in particle content in 4 hr at 23 °C	2074	C
Diphenhydramine HCl	SCN	2 mg/ml[a]	GW	0.1, 2, 5 mg/ml[a]	Physically compatible with no change in measured turbidity or increase in particle content in 4 hr at 23 °C	2074	C
Dobutamine HCl	LI	4 mg/ml[a]	GW	0.1, 2, 5 mg/ml[a]	Physically compatible with no change in measured turbidity or increase in particle content in 4 hr at 23 °C	2074	C
Dopamine HCl	AB	3.2 mg/ml[a]	GW	0.1, 2, 5 mg/ml[a]	Physically compatible with no change in measured turbidity or increase in particle content in 4 hr at 23 °C	2074	C
Doxycycline hyclate	FUJ	1 mg/ml[a]	GW	0.1, 2, 5 mg/ml[a]	Physically compatible with no change in measured turbidity or increase in particle content in 4 hr at 23 °C	2074	C
Droperidol	AB	2.5 mg/ml	GW	0.1, 2, 5 mg/ml[a]	Physically compatible with no change in measured turbidity or increase in particle content in 4 hr at 23 °C	2074	C
Enalaprilat	ME	0.1 mg/ml[a]	GW	0.1, 2, 5 mg/ml[a]	Physically compatible with no change in measured turbidity or increase in particle content in 4 hr at 23 °C	2074	C
Epinephrine HCl	AMR	0.05 mg/ml[a]	GW	0.1, 2, 5 mg/ml[a]	Physically compatible with no change in measured turbidity or increase in particle content in 4 hr at 23 °C	2074	C
Esmolol HCl	OHM	10 mg/ml[a]	GW	0.1, 2, 5 mg/ml[a]	Physically compatible with no change in measured turbidity or increase in particle content in 4 hr at 23 °C	2074	C

Y-Site Injection Compatibility (1:1 Mixture) (Cont.)

Cisatracurium besylate

Drug	Mfr	Conc	Mfr	Conc	Remarks	Ref	C/I
Famotidine	ME	2 mg/ml[a]	GW	0.1, 2, 5 mg/ml[a]	Physically compatible with no change in measured turbidity or increase in particle content in 4 hr at 23 °C	2074	C
Fentanyl citrate	AB	0.0125 mg/ml[a]	GW	0.1, 2, 5 mg/ml[a]	Physically compatible with no change in measured turbidity or increase in particle content in 4 hr at 23 °C	2074	C
Fluconazole	RR	2 mg/ml	GW	0.1, 2, 5 mg/ml[a]	Physically compatible with no change in measured turbidity or increase in particle content in 4 hr at 23 °C	2074	C
Furosemide	AB	3 mg/ml[a]	GW	0.1 mg/ml[a]	Physically compatible with no change in measured turbidity or increase in particle content in 4 hr at 23 °C	2074	C
	AB	3 mg/ml[a]	GW	2 and 5 mg/ml[a]	White cloudiness forms immediately	2074	I
Ganciclovir sodium	SY	20 mg/ml[a]	GW	0.1 and 2 mg/ml[a]	Physically compatible with no change in measured turbidity or increase in particle content in 4 hr at 23 °C	2074	C
	SY	20 mg/ml[a]	GW	5 mg/ml[a]	White cloudiness forms immediately	2074	I
Gentamicin sulfate	ES	5 mg/ml[a]	GW	0.1, 2, 5 mg/ml[a]	Physically compatible with no change in measured turbidity or increase in particle content in 4 hr at 23 °C	2074	C
Haloperidol lactate	MN	0.2 mg/ml[a]	GW	0.1, 2, 5 mg/ml[a]	Physically compatible with no change in measured turbidity or increase in particle content in 4 hr at 23 °C	2074	C
Heparin sodium	AB	100 units/ml	GW	0.1 and 2 mg/ml[a]	Physically compatible with no change in measured turbidity or increase in particle content in 4 hr at 23 °C	2074	C
	AB	100 units/ml	GW	5 mg/ml[a]	White cloudiness forms immediately	2074	I
Hydrocortisone sodium succinate	AB	1 mg/ml[a]	GW	0.1, 2, 5 mg/ml[a]	Physically compatible with no change in measured turbidity or increase in particle content in 4 hr at 23 °C	2074	C
Hydromorphone HCl	ES	0.5 mg/ml[a]	GW	0.1, 2, 5 mg/ml[a]	Physically compatible with no change in measured turbidity or increase in particle content in 4 hr at 23 °C	2074	C
Hydroxyzine HCl	ES	2 mg/ml[a]	GW	0.1, 2, 5 mg/ml[a]	Physically compatible with no change in measured turbidity or increase in particle content in 4 hr at 23 °C	2074	C
Imipenem–cilastatin sodium	ME	10 mg/ml[b]	GW	0.1, 2, 5 mg/ml[a]	Physically compatible with no change in measured turbidity or increase in particle content in 4 hr at 23 °C	2074	C
Isoproterenol HCl	AB	0.02 mg/ml[a]	GW	0.1, 2, 5 mg/ml[a]	Physically compatible with no change in measured turbidity or increase in particle content in 4 hr at 23 °C	2074	C
Ketorolac tromethamine	RC	15 mg/ml[a]	GW	0.1, 2, 5 mg/ml[a]	Physically compatible with no change in measured turbidity or increase in particle content in 4 hr at 23 °C	2074	C
Lidocaine HCl	AST	8 mg/ml[a]	GW	0.1, 2, 5 mg/ml[a]	Physically compatible with no change in measured turbidity or increase in particle content in 4 hr at 23 °C	2074	C

Y-Site Injection Compatibility (1:1 Mixture) (Cont.)

					Cisatracurium besylate		
Drug	Mfr	Conc	Mfr	Conc	Remarks	Ref	C/I
Lorazepam	WY	0.5 mg/ml[a]	GW	0.1, 2, 5 mg/ml[a]	Physically compatible with no change in measured turbidity or increase in particle content in 4 hr at 23 °C	2074	C
Magnesium sulfate	AB	100 mg/ml[a]	GW	0.1, 2, 5 mg/ml[a]	Physically compatible with no change in measured turbidity or increase in particle content in 4 hr at 23 °C	2074	C
Mannitol	BA	15%	GW	0.1, 2, 5 mg/ml[a]	Physically compatible with no change in measured turbidity or increase in particle content in 4 hr at 23 °C	2074	C
Meperidine HCl	AST	4 mg/ml[a]	GW	0.1, 2, 5 mg/ml[a]	Physically compatible with no change in measured turbidity or increase in particle content in 4 hr at 23 °C	2074	C
Methylprednisolone sodium succinate	AB	5 mg/ml[a]	GW	0.1 mg/ml[a]	Physically compatible with no change in measured turbidity or increase in particle content in 4 hr at 23 °C	2074	C
	AB	5 mg/ml[a]	GW	2 mg/ml[a]	Subvisual haze forms immediately	2074	I
	AB	5 mg/ml[a]	GW	5 mg/ml[a]	Haze forms immediately	2074	I
Metoclopramide HCl	AB	5 mg/ml	GW	0.1, 2, 5 mg/ml[a]	Physically compatible with no change in measured turbidity or increase in particle content in 4 hr at 23 °C	2074	C
Metronidazole	AB	5 mg/ml	GW	0.1, 2, 5 mg/ml[a]	Physically compatible with no change in measured turbidity or increase in particle content in 4 hr at 23 °C	2074	C
Midazolam HCl	RC	1 mg/ml[a]	GW	0.1, 2, 5 mg/ml[a]	Physically compatible with no change in measured turbidity or increase in particle content in 4 hr at 23 °C	2074	C
Minocycline HCl	LE	0.2 mg/ml[a]	GW	0.1, 2, 5 mg/ml[a]	Physically compatible with no change in measured turbidity or increase in particle content in 4 hr at 23 °C	2074	C
Morphine sulfate	AST	1 mg/ml[a]	GW	0.1, 2, 5 mg/ml[a]	Physically compatible with no change in measured turbidity or increase in particle content in 4 hr at 23 °C	2074	C
Nalbuphine HCl	AST	10 mg/ml	GW	0.1, 2, 5 mg/ml[a]	Physically compatible with no change in measured turbidity or increase in particle content in 4 hr at 23 °C	2074	C
Netilmicin sulfate	SC	5 mg/ml[a]	GW	0.1, 2, 5 mg/ml[a]	Physically compatible with no change in measured turbidity or increase in particle content in 4 hr at 23 °C	2074	C
Nitroglycerin	DU	0.4 mg/ml[a]	GW	0.1, 2, 5 mg/ml[a]	Physically compatible with no change in measured turbidity or increase in particle content in 4 hr at 23 °C	2074	C
Norepinephrine bitartrate	SW	0.12 mg/ml[a]	GW	0.1, 2, 5 mg/ml[a]	Physically compatible with no change in measured turbidity or increase in particle content in 4 hr at 23 °C	2074	C

Y-Site Injection Compatibility (1:1 Mixture) (Cont.)

Cisatracurium besylate

Drug	Mfr	Conc	Mfr	Conc	Remarks	Ref	C/I
Ofloxacin	ORT	4 mg/ml[a]	GW	0.1, 2, 5 mg/ml[a]	Physically compatible with no change in measured turbidity or increase in particle content in 4 hr at 23 °C	2074	**C**
Ondansetron HCl	CER	1 mg/ml[a]	GW	0.1, 2, 5 mg/ml[a]	Physically compatible with no change in measured turbidity or increase in particle content in 4 hr at 23 °C	2074	**C**
Phenylephrine HCl	GNS	1 mg/ml[a]	GW	0.1, 2, 5 mg/ml[a]	Physically compatible with no change in measured turbidity or increase in particle content in 4 hr at 23 °C	2074	**C**
Piperacillin sodium	LE	40 mg/ml[a]	GW	0.1 mg/ml[a]	Physically compatible with no change in measured turbidity or increase in particle content in 4 hr at 23 °C	2074	**C**
	LE	40 mg/ml[a]	GW	2 mg/ml[a]	Subvisual haze forms immediately	2074	**I**
	LE	40 mg/ml[a]	GW	5 mg/ml[a]	Haze forms immediately	2074	**I**
Piperacillin sodium–tazobactam sodium	CY	40 + 5 mg/ml[a]	GW	0.1 and 2 mg/ml[a]	Physically compatible with no change in measured turbidity or increase in particle content in 4 hr at 23 °C	2074	**C**
	CY	40 + 5 mg/ml[a]	GW	5 mg/ml[a]	Tiny particles and subvisual haze within 4 hr	2074	**I**
Potassium chloride	AB	0.1 mEq/ml[a]	GW	0.1, 2, 5 mg/ml[a]	Physically compatible with no change in measured turbidity or increase in particle content in 4 hr at 23 °C	2074	**C**
Procainamide HCl	ES	10 mg/ml[a]	GW	0.1, 2, 5 mg/ml[a]	Physically compatible with no change in measured turbidity or increase in particle content in 4 hr at 23 °C	2074	**C**
Prochlorperazine edisylate	SO	0.5 mg/ml[a]	GW	0.1, 2, 5 mg/ml[a]	Physically compatible with no change in measured turbidity or increase in particle content in 4 hr at 23 °C	2074	**C**
Promethazine HCl	ES	2 mg/ml[a]	GW	0.1, 2, 5 mg/ml[a]	Physically compatible with no change in measured turbidity or increase in particle content in 4 hr at 23 °C	2074	**C**
Ranitidine HCl	GL	2 mg/ml[a]	GW	0.1, 2, 5 mg/ml[a]	Physically compatible with no change in measured turbidity or increase in particle content in 4 hr at 23 °C	2074	**C**
Remifentanil HCl	GW	0.025 and 0.25 mg/ml[b]	GW	2 mg/ml[a]	Physically compatible with no change in measured turbidity or increase in particle content in 4 hr at 23 °C	2075	**C**
Sodium bicarbonate	AB	1 mEq/ml	GW	0.1 mg/ml[a]	Physically compatible with no change in measured turbidity or increase in particle content in 4 hr at 23 °C	2074	**C**
	AB	1 mEq/ml	GW	2 mg/ml[a]	Subvisual light brown discoloration with subvisual haze in 1 hr	2074	**I**
	AB	1 mEq/ml	GW	5 mg/ml[a]	Subvisual haze forms immediately; subvisual light brown discoloration with turbidity forms in 4 hr	2074	**I**
Sodium nitroprusside	AB	2 mg/ml[a]	GW	0.1 mg/ml[a]	Physically compatible with no change in measured turbidity or increase in particle content in 4 hr at 23 °C protected from light	2074	**C**
	AB	2 mg/ml[a]	GW	2 and 5 mg/ml[a]	White cloudiness forms immediately	2074	**I**

Y-Site Injection Compatibility (1:1 Mixture) (Cont.)

Cisatracurium besylate

Drug	Mfr	Conc	Mfr	Conc	Remarks	Ref	C/I
Sufentanil citrate	ES	0.0125 mg/ml[a]	GW	0.1, 2, 5 mg/ml[a]	Physically compatible with no change in measured turbidity or increase in particle content in 4 hr at 23 °C	2074	C
Theophylline	AB	3.2 mg/ml	GW	0.1, 2, 5 mg/ml[a]	Physically compatible with no change in measured turbidity or increase in particle content in 4 hr at 23 °C	2074	C
Thiopental sodium	AB	25 mg/ml[a]	GW	0.1 mg/ml[a]	Physically compatible with no change in measured turbidity or increase in particle content in 4 hr at 23 °C	2074	C
	AB	25 mg/ml[a]	GW	2 mg/ml[a]	White turbidity forms immediately but dissipates within 1 min; subvisual haze remains	2074	I
	AB	25 mg/ml[a]	GW	5 mg/ml[a]	White cloudiness forms immediately	2074	I
Ticarcillin disodium	SKB	30 mg/ml[a]	GW	0.1, 2, 5 mg/ml[a]	Physically compatible with no change in measured turbidity or increase in particle content in 4 hr at 23 °C	2074	C
Ticarcillin disodium–clavulanate potassium	SKB	31 mg/ml[a]	GW	0.1 and 2 mg/ml[a]	Physically compatible with no change in measured turbidity or increase in particle content in 4 hr at 23 °C	2074	C
	SKB	31 mg/ml[a]	GW	5 mg/ml[a]	Subvisual haze forms immediately	2074	I
Tobramycin sulfate	AB	5 mg/ml[a]	GW	0.1, 2, 5 mg/ml[a]	Physically compatible with no change in measured turbidity or increase in particle content in 4 hr at 23 °C	2074	C
Trimethoprim–sulfamethoxazole	ES	0.8 + 4 mg/ml[a]	GW	0.1 mg/ml[a]	Physically compatible with no change in measured turbidity or increase in particle content in 4 hr at 23 °C	2074	C
	ES	0.8 + 4 mg/ml[a]	GW	2 mg/ml[a]	Subvisual haze forms in 1 hr	2074	I
	ES	0.8 + 4 mg/ml[a]	GW	5 mg/ml[a]	Subvisual haze forms immediately	2074	I
Vancomycin HCl	AB	10 mg/ml[a]	GW	0.1, 2, 5 mg/ml[a]	Physically compatible with no change in measured turbidity or increase in particle content in 4 hr at 23 °C	2074	C
Zidovudine	BW	4 mg/ml[a]	GW	0.1, 2, 5 mg/ml[a]	Physically compatible with no change in measured turbidity or increase in particle content in 4 hr at 23 °C	2074	C

[a]Tested in dextrose 5% in water.
[b]Tested in sodium chloride 0.9%.
[c]Sodium carbonate–containing formulation tested.
[d]L-Arginine–containing formulation tested.

Additional Compatibility Information

Solutions— Cisatracurium besylate is compatible with dextrose 5% in water, sodium chloride 0.9%, and dextrose 5% in sodium chloride 0.9%. The manufacturer indicates that dilutions to concentrations down to 0.1 mg/ml may be stored under refrigeration or at room temperature for 24 hours without significant potency loss. At concentrations between 0.1 and 0.2 mg/ml, the drug may be diluted in dextrose 5% in lactated Ringer's injection and used within 24 hours if stored under refrigeration (2).

Other Drugs— The manufacturer indicates that cisatracurium besylate is compatible with alfentanil HCl, droperidol, fentanyl citrate, midazolam HCl, and sufentanil citrate (2).

Cisatracurium besylate is stated to be incompatible with propofol and ketorolac tromethamine (2).

CISPLATIN
AHFS 10:00

Platinol   **Bristol-Myers Squibb**
Platinol-AQ   **Bristol-Myers Squibb**

Products— Cisplatin (Bristol-Myers Squibb) is available in 10-mg vials with 100 mg of mannitol and 90 mg of sodium chloride and 50-mg vials with 500 mg of mannitol and 450 mg of sodium chloride. Hydrochloric acid is also present to adjust the pH. Reconstitute the 10-mg vials with 10 ml and the 50-mg vials with 50 ml of sterile water for injection to yield solutions containing 1 mg/ml (2; 4).

Cisplatin (Bristol-Myers Squibb) also is available as a sterile aqueous injection containing cisplatin 1 mg/ml and sodium chloride 9 mg/ml, with hydrochloric acid and/or sodium hydroxide to adjust the pH. This aqueous solution is available in 50-ml (50-mg) and 100-ml (100-mg) vials (2; 4).

pH— The reconstituted solution has a pH of 3.5 to 5.5, and the aqueous injection has a pH of 3.7 to 6 (4).

Osmolality— The aqueous injection has an osmolality of about 285 mOsm/kg (4).

Sodium Content— Each 10 mg of cisplatin (Bristol) contains 1.54 mEq of sodium (846; 869).

Administration— Cisplatin is administered by intravenous infusion with a regimen of hydration (with or without mannitol and/or furosemide) prior to therapy. One regimen consists of 1 to 2 L of fluid given over eight to 12 hours prior to cisplatin administration. In addition, adequate hydration and urinary output must be maintained for 24 hours after therapy. The manufacturer recommends diluting the cisplatin dose in 2 L of compatible infusion solution containing mannitol 37.5 g and infusing over six to eight hours (2; 4). Other dilutions and rates of administration have been used, including intravenous infusions over periods from 15 to 120 minutes and continuous infusion over one to five days. Intra-arterial infusion and intraperitoneal instillation have been used (4).

Stability— Intact vials of the dry product are stable for two years from manufacture when stored at room temperature (27 °C) and protected from light. The aqueous injection should be stored between 15 and 25 °C and protected from light; it should not be refrigerated (2; 4).

Reconstituted solutions of cisplatin are clear and colorless. The manufacturer states that cisplatin is stable for 20 hours after reconstitution when stored at 27 °C. The manufacturer recommends that a cisplatin solution removed from its amber vial be protected from light if it is not used within six hours (2). Reconstitution with bacteriostatic water for injection, containing benzyl alcohol or parabens, to a concentration of 1 mg/ml results in solutions that are reported to be stable for at least 72 hours at 25 °C (4).

After initial vial entry, the aqueous cisplatin injection (Platinol-AQ) in amber vials is stable for 28 days if it is protected from light or for seven days if it is exposed to fluorescent room light (2).

Concern has been expressed that storage of cisplatin solutions for several weeks might result in substantial amounts of the toxic mono- and di-aquo species (1199). However, the solution's chloride content, rather than extended storage time periods, appears to determine the extent of aquated product formation. (See Effect of Chloride Ion below.)

Kristjansson et al. evaluated the long-term stability of cisplatin 1 mg/ml in an aqueous solution containing sodium chloride 9 mg/ml and mannitol 10 mg/ml in glass vials. After 22 months at 5 °C, the 4% loss of cisplatin could be explained as the expected equilibrium between cisplatin and its aquated products. Furthermore, a precipitate formed and required sonication at 40 °C for about 20 to 30 minutes to redissolve. Storage of the cisplatin solution at 40 °C for 10 months resulted in no physical change. After an additional one year at 5 °C, these samples exhibited an average 15% loss, which the authors concluded was not the result of the formation of aquated species or the toxic and inactive oligomeric species. These proposed degradation products were not present in the 40 °C sample (1246).

Cisplatin, reconstituted according to the manufacturer's instructions, was cultured with human lymphoblasts to determine whether its cytotoxic activity was retained. The solution retained cytotoxicity for 24 hours when stored at either 4 °C or room temperature.

Theuer et al. reported little or no loss of cisplatin potency by HPLC, after 27 days at room temperature with protection from light, from a solution of cisplatin 500 µg/ml in sodium chloride 0.9% at pH 4.75 and 3.25 (1605).

pH Effects— The pH of maximum stability is 3.5 to 5.5. Alkaline media should be avoided because of increased hydrolysis (1379).

In the dark at pH 6.3, cisplatin (Bristol) 1 mg/ml in sodium chloride 0.9% reached the maximum amount of decomposition product permitted in the *USP* in 34 days. Half of that amount was formed in 96 days at pH 4.3 (1647).

Cisplatin degradation results in ammonia formation, which increases the solution pH. Thus, the initial cisplatin degradation rate may be slow but increases with time (1647).

Effect of Chloride Ion— The stability of cisplatin in solution is dependent on the chloride ion concentration present. Cisplatin is stable in solutions containing an adequate amount of chloride ion but is incompatible in solutions having a low chloride content (4; 316; 317; 634; 635; 637). In solutions with an inadequate chloride content, one or both chloride ions in the cisplatin molecule are displaced by water, forming mono- and diaquo species. The minimum acceptable chloride ion concentration is about 0.040 mol/L, the equivalent of about 0.2% sodium chloride (317; 634; 635).

At a cisplatin concentration of 200 mg/L in sodium chloride 0.9% (the chloride concentration present in the reconstituted vials) with the pH adjusted to 4, about 3% decomposition occurs in less than one hour at room temperature. An equilibrium is then reached, with the cisplatin remaining stable thereafter. At lesser concentrations of chloride ion, greater decomposition of cisplatin occurs. In sodium chloride 0.45 and 0.2%, approximately 4 and 7% decomposition occurred at equilibrium, respectively. In very low chloride-containing solutions, most of the drug may be decomposed. The decomposition appears to be reversible, with cisplatin being reformed in the presence of high chloride concentrations (317).

In another study, the stability of cisplatin 50 and 500 mg/L was evaluated in aqueous solutions containing sodium chloride 0.9, 0.45, and 0.1% and also in water over 24 hours at 25 °C exposed to light. Approximately 2 and 4% of the cisplatin were lost in the sodium chloride 0.9 and 0.45% solutions, respectively. In the 0.1% solution, about 4 to 10% decomposition occurred in four to six hours, increasing to approximately 11 to 15% at both 12 and 24 hours. In aqueous solution with no chloride content, cisplatin decomposed rapidly, with about a 30 to 35% loss in four hours increasing to a 70 to 80% loss in 24 hours (635).

Cisplatin 0.2 mg/ml in sodium chloride 0.9% has been stated to exhibit less than a 10% loss in 14 days at room temperature (1379).

Effect of Refrigeration— It is recommended that the reconstituted solution not be refrigerated because of the formation of a crystalline precipitate (2; 4; 633; 636; 1246). In a study of cisplatin at concentrations of 0.4 to 1 mg/ml in sodium chloride 0.9%, it was found that at 0.6 mg/ml or greater a precipitate formed on refrigeration at 2 to 6 °C. At 1 mg/ml (the cisplatin concentration of the reconstituted solution), the precipitation was noted in one hour. However, the 0.6-mg/ml solution did not have a precipitate until after 48 hours under refrigeration. The 0.5-mg/ml and lower solutions did not precipitate for up to 72 hours at 2 to 6 °C. In solutions where precipitate did form, redissolution occurred very slowly with warming back to room temperature (317). Sonication at 40 °C has been used to redissolve the precipitate in about 20 to 30 minutes (1246). The warming of precipitated cisplatin solutions to effect redissolution is not recommended, however. Solutions containing a precipitate should not be used (4; 633).

Freezing Solutions— If the solution is frozen, it should be thawed at room temperature until the precipitate dissolves. The manufacturer states that this thawing will not adversely affect the chemical or physical stability of the product (4).

Cisplatin (Bristol) 50 and 200 mg/L in dextrose 5% in sodium chloride 0.45% in PVC bags and admixed with either mannitol 18.75 g/L or magnesium sulfate 1 or 2 g/L is reportedly stable for 30 days when frozen at −15 °C followed by an additional 48 hours at 25 °C (1088).

Exposure to Light— Although changes in the UV spectra of cisplatin solutions on exposure to intense light have long been recognized (317), their significance was questioned (483; 635). It was reported that exposure to normal laboratory light for 72 hours had no significant effect on cisplatin's stability by HPLC (635).

More recently, however, Zieske et al. reported substantial cisplatin decomposition after exposure to typical laboratory light, a mixture of incandescent and fluorescent illumination. As much as 12% degraded to trichloroammineplatinate (II) after 25 hours. Cisplatin was most sensitive to light in the UV to blue region and had little sensitivity to yellow or red light. It was protected from light-induced degradation by low-actinic amber glass flasks but not by PVC bags, clear glass vials, or polyethylene syringes. The authors concluded that exposure to moderately intense white light for more than one hour should be avoided (1647).

The manufacturer recommends that a cisplatin solution removed from its amber vial be protected from light if it is not used within six hours. Even in the amber vial, the cisplatin solution should be discarded after seven days if exposed to fluorescent room light (2).

Filtration— Cisplatin 10 to 300 μg/ml exhibited no loss due to sorption to cellulose nitrate/cellulose acetate ester (Millex OR) or Teflon (Millex FG) filters (1415; 1416).

Portable Pumps— The stability of cisplatin (R. Bellon) 0.5 and 0.9 mg/ml in sodium chloride 0.9% was evaluated in ethylene vinyl acetate bags for use with a portable infusion pump (Celsa Celinject CO1). The bags were stored at 22 and 35 °C and protected from light for 28 days. HPLC analysis found little or no cisplatin loss and no degradation peaks at either concentration or temperature. However, about a 3% moisture loss due to permeation through the container was found in the 35 °C samples (1827).

Compatibility Information

Solution Compatibility

Cisplatin

Solution	Mfr	Mfr	Conc/L	Remarks	Ref	C/I
Dextrose 5% in sodium chloride 0.225%	AB[a]	NCI	300 mg/L	3% loss in 23 hr at 25 °C under fluorescent light	1087	C
Dextrose 5% in sodium chloride 0.45%		BV	50 and 500 mg	Less than 10% decomposition in 24 hr at room temperature	234	C
	AB[b]	NCI	300 mg/L	Less than 2% loss in 23 hr at 25 °C under fluorescent light	1087	C
Dextrose 5% in sodium chloride 0.9%		BV	50 and 500 mg	Less than 10% decomposition in 24 hr at room temperature	234	C
			500 mg	Approximately 2% decomposition in 24 hr at 25 °C	635	C
	AB[a]	NCI	300 mg/L	1% loss in 23 hr at 25 °C under fluorescent light	1087	C
Dextrose 5% in sodium chloride 0.45% with mannitol 1.875%		BR	50, 100, 200 mg	Physically compatible and cisplatin chemically stable for 72 hr at 25 and 4 °C with 2 to 10% decomposition observed after a subsequent 8-hr infusion	636	C
Dextrose 5% in sodium chloride 0.33% with mannitol 1.875%		BR	50, 100, 200 mg	Physically compatible and cisplatin chemically stable for 72 hr at 25 and 4 °C with 0 to 8% decomposition observed after a subsequent 8-hr infusion	636	C

Solution Compatibility (Cont.)

Cisplatin

Solution	Mfr	Mfr	Conc/L	Remarks	Ref	C/I
Dextrose 5% in sodium chloride 0.33% with potassium chloride 20 mEq and mannitol 1.875%		BR	50, 100, 200 mg	Physically compatible and cisplatin chemically stable for 72 hr at 25 and 4 °C	636	**C**
Dextrose 5% in water	TR	BV	100 mg	TLC indicates decomposition occurs in less than 2 hr at room temperature	316	**I**
	AB[a]	NCI	300 mg/L	4% loss in 2 hr and 6% in 23 hr at 25 °C under fluorescent light	1087	**C**
	AB[a]	NCI	75 mg/L	10% loss in 2 hr and 16% in 6 hr at 25 °C under fluorescent light	1087	**I**
Sodium bicarbonate 5%			50 and 500 mg	Bright gold precipitate forms within 8 to 24 hr at 25 °C	635	**I**
Sodium chloride 0.9%			50 and 500 mg	Approximately 2% decomposition in 24 hr at 25 °C	635	**C**
	TR	BV	100 mg	TLC indicates no decomposition in 24 hr at room temperature	316	**C**
		BV	200 mg	2 to 3% decomposition in 1 hr and no further decomposition for at least 24 hr at room temperature and pH adjusted to 4	317	**C**
	AB[a]	NCI	300 mg/L	1% loss in 23 hr at 25 °C under fluorescent light	1087	**C**
	c	BEL	600 mg	Little or no loss by HPLC in 9 days at 23 °C protected from light	1757	**C**
	d	BEL	500 and 900 mg	Little or no loss by HPLC in 28 days at 22 and 35 °C protected from light	1827	**C**
	e	WAS	167 mg	Little or no loss by HPLC in 14 days at 30 °C protected from light	1828	**C**
Sodium chloride 0.45%			50 and 500 mg	Approximately 4% decomposition in 24 hr at 25 °C	635	**C**
		BV	200 mg	4 to 5% decomposition in 1 hr and no further decomposition for at least 24 hr at room temperature and pH adjusted to 4	317	**C**
Sodium chloride 0.3%		BR	50, 100, 200 mg	Physically compatible and 2 to 3% cisplatin loss over 72 hr at 25 and 4 °C	636	**C**
Sodium chloride 0.225%		BR	50, 100, 200 mg	Physically compatible and 2 to 5% cisplatin loss over 72 hr at 25 and 4 °C	636	**C**

[a]*Tested in glass bottles.*
[b]*Tested in both glass and PVC containers.*
[c]*Tested in PVC containers.*
[d]*Tested in ethylene vinyl acetate containers.*
[e]*Tested in glass, PVC, polyethylene, and polypropylene containers.*

Additive Compatibility

Cisplatin

Drug	Mfr	Conc/L	Mfr	Conc/L	Test Soln	Remarks	Ref	C/I
Carboplatin		1 g		200 mg	NS	Less than 10% loss of both drugs in 24 hr at 23 °C protected from light	1954	**C**
Cyclophosphamide with etoposide		2 g 200 mg		200 mg	NS	All drugs stable for 7 days at room temperature	1379	**C**

Additive Compatibility (Cont.)

Cisplatin

Drug	Mfr	Conc/L	Mfr	Conc/L	Test Soln	Remarks	Ref	C/I
Etoposide	BR	400 mg	BR	200 mg	NS[a]	Physically compatible with less than 10% loss of both drugs in 48 hr at 22 °C in light and dark	1329	C
	BR	200 mg	BR	200 mg	NS[a]	Physically compatible with less than 10% loss of both drugs in 24 hr at 22 °C. Possible excess cisplatin loss in 48 hr exposed to light	1329	C
	BR	200 and 400 mg	BR	200 mg	D5½S[a]	Physically compatible with less than 10% loss of both drugs in 24 hr at 22 °C in light and dark	1329	C
		400 mg		200 mg	NS	10% etoposide loss and no cisplatin loss in 7 days at room temperature	1388	C
		200 mg		200 mg	NS	Both drugs stable for 15 days at room temperature protected from light	1379	C
Etoposide with floxuridine		300 mg 700 mg		200 mg	NS	All drugs stable for 7 days at room temperature	1379	C
Etoposide with mannitol and potassium chloride	BR LY LY	400 mg 1.875% 20 mEq	BR	200 mg	NS[a]	Physically compatible and etoposide and cisplatin chemically stable for 8 hr at 22 °C. Precipitate forms within 24 hr	1329	I
Etoposide with mannitol and potassium chloride	BR LY LY	400 mg 1.875% 20 mEq	BR	200 mg	D5½S[a]	Physically compatible and etoposide and cisplatin chemically stable for 24 hr at 22 °C. Precipitate forms within 48 hr	1329	C
Floxuridine	RC	10 g	BR	500 mg	NS	13% FUdR loss in 7 days and 18% in 14 days at room temperature protected from light	1386	C
Floxuridine with leucovorin calcium		700 mg 140 mg		200 mg	NS	All drugs stable for 7 days at room temperature	1379	C
Fluorouracil	SO	1 g	BR	200 mg	NS[b]	10% cisplatin loss in 1.5 hr and 25% loss in 4 hr at 25 °C under fluorescent light or in the dark	1339	I
	SO	10 g	BR	500 mg	NS[b]	10% cisplatin loss in 1.2 hr and 25% loss in 3 hr at 25 °C under fluorescent light or in the dark	1339	I
	AD	10 g	BR	500 mg	NS	80% cisplatin loss in 24 hr at room temperature due to low pH	1386	I
Hydroxyzine HCl	LY	500 mg	BR	200 mg	NS[c]	Physically compatible for 48 hr	1190	C
Ifosfamide		2 g		200 mg	NS	Both drugs stable for 7 days at room temperature	1379	C
Ifosfamide with etoposide		2 g 200 mg		200 mg	NS	All drugs stable for 5 days at room temperature	1379	C
Leucovorin calcium		140 mg		200 mg	NS	Both drugs stable for 15 days at room temperature protected from light	1379	C
Magnesium sulfate		1 and 2 g	BR	50 and 200 mg	D5½S[b]	Compatible for 48 hr at 25 °C and 96 hr at 4 °C followed by 48 hr at 25 °C	1088	C
Mannitol		18.75 g	BR	50 and 200 mg	D5½S[b]	Compatible for 48 hr at 25 °C and 96 hr at 4 °C followed by 48 hr at 25 °C	1088	C
Mesna		3.33 g		67 mg	NS	Cisplatin not detectable after 1 hr	1291	I
		110 mg		67 mg	NS	Cisplatin weakly detected after 1 hr	1291	I

Additive Compatibility (Cont.)

Cisplatin

Drug	Mfr	Conc/L	Mfr	Conc/L	Test Soln	Remarks	Ref	C/I
Ondansetron HCl	GL	1.031 g	BR	485 mg	NS[b]	Physically compatible with little or no loss of either drug by HPLC in 24 hr at 4 °C followed by 7 days at 30 °C	1846	C
	GL	479 mg	BR	219 mg	NS[d]	Physically compatible with little or no loss of either drug by HPLC in 24 hr at 4 °C followed by 7 days at 30 °C	1846	C
Paclitaxel	BMS	300 mg	BMS	200 mg	NS	No paclitaxel loss and cisplatin losses of 1, 4, and 5% at 4, 24, and 32 °C, respectively, in 24 hr by HPLC. Physically compatible for 24 hr but subvisual particulates of paclitaxel form after 3 to 5 days	2094	C
	BMS	1.2 g	BMS	200 mg	NS	No paclitaxel loss but cisplatin losses of 10, 19, and 22% at 4, 24, and 32 °C, respectively, in 24 hr by HPLC. Physically compatible for 24 hr but subvisual particulates of paclitaxel form after 3 to 5 days	2094	I
Thiotepa		1 g		200 mg	NS	Yellow precipitation	1379	I

[a]*Tested in both glass and PVC containers.*
[b]*Tested in PVC containers.*
[c]*Tested in glass containers.*
[d]*Tested in polyisoprene reservoirs (Travenol Infusors).*

Drugs in Syringe Compatibility

Cisplatin

Drug (in syringe)	Mfr	Amt	Mfr	Amt	Remarks	Ref	C/I
Bleomycin sulfate		1.5 units/ 0.5 ml		0.5 mg/ 0.5 ml	Physically compatible for 5 min at room temperature followed by 8 min of centrifugation	980	C
Cyclophosphamide		10 mg/ 0.5 ml		0.5 mg/ 0.5 ml	Physically compatible for 5 min at room temperature followed by 8 min of centrifugation	980	C
Doxapram HCl	RB	400 mg/ 20 ml		10 mg/ 20 ml	Physically compatible with no doxapram loss in 24 hr	1177	C
Doxorubicin HCl		1 mg/ 0.5 ml		0.5 mg/ 0.5 ml	Physically compatible for 5 min at room temperature followed by 8 min of centrifugation	980	C
Droperidol		1.25 mg/ 0.5 ml		0.5 mg/ 0.5 ml	Physically compatible for 5 min at room temperature followed by 8 min of centrifugation	980	C
Fluorouracil		25 mg/ 0.5 ml		0.5 mg/ 0.5 ml	Physically compatible for 5 min at room temperature followed by 8 min of centrifugation	980	C
Furosemide		5 mg/ 0.5 ml		0.5 mg/ 0.5 ml	Physically compatible for 5 min at room temperature followed by 8 min of centrifugation	980	C

Drugs in Syringe Compatibility (Cont.)

Drug (in syringe)	Mfr	Amt	Mfr	Amt	Remarks	Ref	C/I
		Cisplatin					
Heparin sodium		500 units/ 0.5 ml		0.5 mg/ 0.5 ml	Physically compatible for 5 min at room temperature followed by 8 min of centrifugation	980	C
Leucovorin calcium		5 mg/ 0.5 ml		0.5 mg/ 0.5 ml	Physically compatible for 5 min at room temperature followed by 8 min of centrifugation	980	C
Methotrexate sodium		12.5 mg/ 0.5 ml		0.5 mg/ 0.5 ml	Physically compatible for 5 min at room temperature followed by 8 min of centrifugation	980	C
Metoclopramide HCl		25 mg/ 0.5 ml		0.5 mg/ 0.5 ml	Physically compatible for 5 min at room temperature followed by 8 min of centrifugation	980	C
Mitomycin		0.25 mg/ 0.5 ml		0.5 mg/ 0.5 ml	Physically compatible for 5 min at room temperature followed by 8 min of centrifugation	980	C
Vinblastine sulfate		0.5 mg/ 0.5 ml		0.5 mg/ 0.5 ml	Physically compatible for 5 min at room temperature followed by 8 min of centrifugation	980	C
Vincristine sulfate		0.5 mg/ 0.5 ml		0.5 mg/ 0.5 ml	Physically compatible for 5 min at room temperature followed by 8 min of centrifugation	980	C

Y-Site Injection Compatibility (1:1 Mixture)

Drug	Mfr	Conc	Mfr	Conc	Remarks	Ref	C/I
		Cisplatin					
Allopurinol sodium	BW	3 mg/ml[b]	BR	1 mg/ml	Physically compatible with no change in measured turbidity or increase in particle content in 4 hr at 22 °C	1686	C
Amifostine	USB	10 mg/ml[a]	BR	1 mg/ml	Subvisual haze forms in 4 hr	1845	I
Amphotericin B cholesteryl sulfate complex	SEQ	0.83 mg/ml[a]	BR	1 mg/ml	Gross precipitate forms	2117	I
Aztreonam	SQ	40 mg/ml[a]	BMS	1 mg/ml	Physically compatible with no subvisual haze or particle formation in 4 hr at 23 °C	1758	C
Bleomycin sulfate		3 units/ml		1 mg/ml	Drugs injected sequentially into Y-site with no flush between. No visually apparent precipitate	980	C
Cefepime HCl	BR	20 mg/ml[a]	BR	1 mg/ml	Haze forms in 1 hr. Cloudiness and particulates form in 4 hr	1689	I
Chlorpromazine HCl	SKF	2 mg/ml[a]	BR	1 mg/ml	Visually compatible for 4 hr at room temperature under fluorescent light	1685	C
Cimetidine HCl	SKF	12 mg/ml[a]	BR	1 mg/ml	Visually compatible for 4 hr at room temperature under fluorescent light	1685	C
Cladribine	ORT	0.015[b] and 0.5[c] mg/ml	BR	1 mg/ml	Physically compatible with no change in measured turbidity or increase in particle content in 4 hr at 23 °C	1969	C

Y-Site Injection Compatibility (1:1 Mixture) (Cont.)

Drug	Mfr	Conc	Mfr	Conc	Remarks	Ref	C/I
				Cisplatin			
Cyclophosphamide		20 mg/ml		1 mg/ml	Drugs injected sequentially into Y-site with no flush between. No visually apparent precipitate	980	C
Dexamethasone sodium phosphate	QU	1 mg/ml[a]	BR	1 mg/ml	Visually compatible for 4 hr at room temperature under fluorescent light	1685	C
Diphenhydramine HCl	PD	2 mg/ml[a]	BR	1 mg/ml	Visually compatible for 4 hr at room temperature under fluorescent light	1685	C
Doxorubicin HCl		2 mg/ml		1 mg/ml	Drugs injected sequentially into Y-site with no flush between. No visually apparent precipitate	980	C
Doxorubicin HCl liposome injection	SEQ	0.4 mg/ml[a]	BR	1 mg/ml	Physically compatible with little or no change in measured turbidity and no increase in particle content in 4 hr at 23 °C	2087	C
Droperidol		2.5 mg/ml		1 mg/ml	Drugs injected sequentially into Y-site with no flush between. No visually apparent precipitate	980	C
	JN	20 µg/ml[a]	BR	1 mg/ml	Visually compatible for 4 hr at room temperature under fluorescent light	1685	C
Etoposide phosphate	BR	5 mg/ml[a]	BR	1 mg/ml	Physically compatible with no change in measured turbidity or increase in particle content in 4 hr at 23 °C	2218	C
Famotidine	MSD	2 mg/ml[a]	BR	1 mg/ml	Visually compatible for 4 hr at room temperature under fluorescent light	1685	C
Filgrastim	AMG	30 µg/ml[a]	BR	1 mg/ml	Physically compatible with no change in measured turbidity or increase in particle content in 4 hr at 22 °C	1687	C
Fludarabine phosphate	BX	1 mg/ml[a]	BR	1 mg/ml	Physically compatible for 4 hr at room temperature under fluorescent light	1439	C
Fluorouracil		50 mg/ml		1 mg/ml	Drugs injected sequentially into Y-site with no flush between. No visually apparent precipitate	980	C
Furosemide		10 mg/ml		1 mg/ml	Drugs injected sequentially into Y-site with no flush between. No visually apparent precipitate	980	C
	ES	3 mg/ml[a]	BR	1 mg/ml	Visually compatible for 4 hr at room temperature under fluorescent light	1685	C
Ganciclovir sodium	SY	20 mg/ml[a]	BR	1 mg/ml	Visually compatible for 4 hr at room temperature under fluorescent light	1685	C
Gemcitabine HCl	LI	10 mg/ml[b]	BR	1 mg/ml	Physically compatible with no change in measured turbidity or increase in particle content in 4 hr at 23 °C	2226	C
Granisetron HCl	SKB	1 mg/ml	BR	1 mg/ml	Physically compatible with little or no loss of either drug by HPLC in 4 hr at 22 °C	1883	C
	SKB	1 mg/ml	BR	0.05 mg/ml[b]	Physically compatible with little or no granisetron loss by HPLC in 4 hr at 22 °C	1883	C

Y-Site Injection Compatibility (1:1 Mixture) (Cont.)

Drug	Mfr	Conc	Mfr	Conc	Remarks	Ref	C/I
				Cisplatin			
Heparin sodium		1000 units/ml		1 mg/ml	Drugs injected sequentially into Y-site with no flush between. No visually apparent precipitate	980	C
	SO	40 units/ml[a]	BR	1 mg/ml	Visually compatible for 4 hr at room temperature under fluorescent light	1685	C
Hydromorphone HCl	ES	0.04 mg/ml[a]	BR	1 mg/ml	Visually compatible for 4 hr at room temperature under fluorescent light	1685	C
Leucovorin calcium		10 mg/ml		1 mg/ml	Drugs injected sequentially into Y-site with no flush between. No visually apparent precipitate	980	C
Lorazepam	WY	0.1 mg/ml[a]	BR	1 mg/ml	Visually compatible for 4 hr at room temperature under fluorescent light	1685	C
Melphalan HCl	BW	0.1 mg/ml[b]	BR	1 mg/ml	Physically compatible with no change in measured turbidity or increase in particle content in 3 hr at 22 °C	1557	C
Methotrexate sodium		25 mg/ml		1 mg/ml	Drugs injected sequentially into Y-site with no flush between. No visually apparent precipitate	980	C
Methylprednisolone sodium succinate	UP	0.5 mg/ml[a]	BR	1 mg/ml	Visually compatible for 4 hr at room temperature under fluorescent light	1685	C
Metoclopramide HCl		5 mg/ml		1 mg/ml	Drugs injected sequentially into Y-site with no flush between. No visually apparent precipitate	980	C
	RB	2.5 mg/ml[a]	BR	1 mg/ml	Visually compatible for 4 hr at room temperature under fluorescent light	1685	C
Mitomycin		0.5 mg/ml		1 mg/ml	Drugs injected sequentially into Y-site with no flush between. No visually apparent precipitate	980	C
Morphine sulfate	ES	0.12 mg/ml[a]	BR	1 mg/ml	Visually compatible for 4 hr at room temperature under fluorescent light	1685	C
Ondansetron HCl	GL	1 mg/ml[b]	BR	1 mg/ml	Physically compatible for 4 hr at 22 °C under fluorescent light	1365	C
	GL	16 to 160 μg/ml		0.48 mg/ml	Physically compatible when cisplatin given over 1 to 8 hr via Y-site	1366	C
Paclitaxel	NCI	1.2 mg/ml[a]		1 mg/ml	Physically compatible with no change in measured turbidity in 4 hr at 22 °C	1528	C
Piperacillin sodium–tazobactam sodium	LE	40 + 5 mg/ml[a]	BR	1 mg/ml	Haze and particles form in 1 hr	1688	I
Prochlorperazine edisylate	SKF	0.5 mg/ml[a]	BR	1 mg/ml	Visually compatible for 4 hr at room temperature under fluorescent light	1685	C
Promethazine HCl	WY	2 mg/ml[a]	BR	1 mg/ml	Visually compatible for 4 hr at room temperature under fluorescent light	1685	C
Propofol	ZEN	10 mg/ml	BR	1 mg/ml	Physically compatible for 1 hr at 23 °C with no increase in particle content	2066	C
Ranitidine HCl	GL	1 mg/ml[a]	BR	1 mg/ml	Visually compatible for 4 hr at room temperature under fluorescent light	1685	C
Sargramostim	IMM	10 μg/ml[b]	BR	1 mg/ml	Physically compatible for 4 hr at 22 °C	1436	C

Y-Site Injection Compatibility (1:1 Mixture) (Cont.)

Drug	Mfr	Conc	Cisplatin Mfr	Conc	Remarks	Ref	C/I
Teniposide	BR	0.1 mg/ml[a]	BR	1 mg/ml	Physically compatible with no subvisual haze or particle formation in 4 hr at 23 °C	1725	C
Thiotepa	IMM[d]	1 mg/ml[a]	BMS	1 mg/ml	White cloudiness appears in 4 hr at 23 °C	1861	I
TNA #218 to #226[e]			BMS	1 mg/ml	Visually compatible with no precipitate or emulsion damage apparent in 4 hr at 23 °C	2215	C
TPN #212 to #215[e]			BMS	1 mg/ml	Amber discoloration formed in 1 to 4 hr	2109	I
Vinblastine sulfate		1 mg/ml		1 mg/ml	Drugs injected sequentially into Y-site with no flush between. No visually apparent precipitate	980	C
Vincristine sulfate		1 mg/ml		1 mg/ml	Drugs injected sequentially into Y-site with no flush between. No visually apparent precipitate	980	C
Vinorelbine tartrate	BW	1 mg/ml[b]	BR	1 mg/ml	Physically compatible with no change in measured turbidity or increase in particle content in 4 hr at 22 °C	1558	C

[a]*Tested in dextrose 5% in water.*
[b]*Tested in sodium chloride 0.9%.*
[c]*Tested in bacteriostatic sodium chloride 0.9% preserved with benzyl alcohol 0.9%.*
[d]*Lyophilized formulation tested.*
[e]*Refer to Appendix I for the composition of parenteral nutrition solutions. TNA indicates a 3-in-1 admixture, and TPN indicates a 2-in-1 admixture.*

Additional Compatibility Information

Miscellaneous— In solutions containing sodium chloride 0.45 or 0.9%, the presence of mannitol 5% did not adversely affect solution stability (635). Such solutions have been reported to be compatible for 48 hours at 25 °C (1088). However, some authors believe that advanced mixing of mannitol and cisplatin should be avoided because of the formation of a mannitol–cisplatin complex over several days (524; 870).

The combination of cisplatin with bicarbonate solutions, and perhaps any alkaline solution, should be avoided because of enhanced decomposition of cisplatin. In addition, the formation of a bright gold precipitate may occur in some cases (635).

Cisplatin may react with sodium thiosulfate, sodium metabisulfite, and sodium bisulfite in solution, rapidly and completely inactivating the cisplatin (4; 1089; 1175).

The sodium metabisulfite antioxidant in the former metoclopramide HCl formulation reacted rapidly and extensively with cisplatin, displacing chloride ligands. At clinically relevant concentrations, a 10% cisplatin loss occurred in less than five minutes. A total loss of cisplatin occurred in about 30 minutes (1175). The current Reglan and Maxolon formulations contain no sulfites (4; 1247), but sulfites in other drug formulations may pose a similar stability risk.

Aluminum— Because of an interaction occurring between cisplatin and the metal aluminum, only administration equipment such as needles, syringes, catheters, and sets that contain no aluminum should be used for this drug. Aluminum in contact with cisplatin solution will result in a replacement oxidation–reduction reaction,

forcing platinum from the cisplatin molecule out of solution and appearing as a black or brown precipitate. Other metal components such as stainless steel needles and plated brass hubs do not elicit an observable reaction within 24 hours (2; 203; 204; 512; 988).

Bohart and Ogawa noted this reaction after piggybacking a 1-mg/ml cisplatin solution through an infusion line at a rate of 1 mg/min. A brownish precipitate accumulated about the inner hub of the aluminum needle. Further tests, exposing metallic aluminum, copper, and stainless steel to 1-mg/ml cisplatin solutions, showed that a brownish precipitate formed on the aluminum within a few minutes. The other two metals showed no evidence of a reaction (203).

Prestayko et al. investigated this reaction further. When metallic aluminum was placed in contact with a 1-mg/ml solution of cisplatin, microscopic examination revealed a black precipitate, accompanied by the evolution of gas bubbles, in five to 10 minutes. The black precipitate became visually apparent within 30 to 60 minutes. This precipitate contained platinum, aluminum, and oxygen (204).

When commercially marketed intravenous administration equipment such as needles, indwelling intravenous catheters, and intravenous administration sets were tested, only units containing needles with aluminum hubs were found to react. A visible black precipitate appeared in 60 to 90 minutes and increased over the 24-hour study. The extent of cisplatin loss was also determined in 1-mg/ml solutions in contact with aluminum-hubbed needles. The loss of cisplatin was approximately 29% in three hours and 50% in six hours at room temperature (204).

Bacteriostatic Properties— Cisplatin (Bristol-Myers Oncology) 20 mg/20 ml did not support the growth of several microorganisms and may impart an antimicrobial effect at this concentration. Loss of viability was observed for *Staphylococcus aureus, Escherichia coli,* *Pseudomonas aeruginosa, Pseudomonas cepacia, Candida albicans,* and *Aspergillus niger* (1187).

CLADRIBINE
AHFS 10:00

Leustatin   **Ortho Biotech**

Products— Cladribine (Ortho Biotech) is available as a solution in 10-ml single-use vials. Each milliliter of the solution contains cladribine 1 mg, sodium chloride 9 mg, and phosphoric acid and/or dibasic sodium phosphate to adjust the pH (2). The injection is a concentrate that must be diluted for administration (2; 4).

pH— From 5.5 to 8 (2).

Tonicity— Cladribine injection is isotonic (2).

Sodium Content— Each milliliter of cladribine injection contains 0.15 mEq of sodium (2).

Administration— Cladribine is administered by continuous intravenous infusion after dilution in 500 ml of sodium chloride 0.9% for repeated single daily doses. Alternatively, cladribine may be diluted in bacteriostatic sodium chloride 0.9% containing benzyl alcohol 0.9% for a seven-day continuous infusion. The seven-day solution should be prepared by adding both the drug and solution to the pump reservoir through 0.22-μm filters, bringing the final volume to 100 ml. Remove air in the reservoirs by aspiration using a syringe and filter or vent-filter assembly. The finished preserved solution is then administered continuously over seven days (2; 4).

The use of dextrose 5% in water as a diluent is not recommended because of an increased rate of cladribine degradation (2).

Stability— Cladribine vials should be stored under refrigeration and protected from light. The solution is clear and colorless. A precipitate may develop upon low-temperature storage; the precipitate may be redissolved by allowing the solution to warm to room temperature with vigorous shaking (2). Heating the solution is not recommended. However, less than 5% loss is reported to occur in seven days when the solution is stored at 37 °C (1369). Freezing does not adversely affect stability of the product. Thawing should be allowed to occur naturally by exposure to room temperature. The vials should not be heated or exposed to microwaves. After thawing, the vial contents are stable under refrigeration until expiration. Thawed vials should not be refrozen (2).

The manufacturer states that admixtures of the drug in sodium chloride 0.9% are chemically and physically stable for at least 24 hours at room temperature exposed to normal fluorescent light. Dextrose 5% in water should not be used due to increased rates of drug degradation. Cladribine diluted for administration should be used promptly; storage should be limited to no more than eight hours under refrigeration prior to administration (2). In concentrations of 0.15 to 0.3 mg/ml in bacteriostatic sodium chloride 0.9% containing benzyl alcohol, the drug is stated to be stable for at least 14 days (1369).

Prepared in bacteriostatic sodium chloride 0.9% preserved with benzyl alcohol 0.9%, cladribine exhibits both chemical and physical stability for at least seven days in Sims Deltec ambulatory infusion pump reservoirs. Preservative effectiveness may be reduced in solutions prepared for patients weighing more than 85 kg due to greater benzyl alcohol dilution (2).

Compatibility Information

Solution Compatibility

Cladribine

Solution	Mfr	Mfr	Conc/L	Remarks	Ref	C/I
Sodium chloride 0.9%	[a,b]	JC	16 mg	Visually compatible and little or no loss by HPLC in 30 days at 4 and 18 °C exposed to or protected from light	2154	C

[a]*Tested in PVC containers.*
[b]*Tested in polyethylene-lined trilayer (Clearflex) containers.*

Y-Site Injection Compatibility (1:1 Mixture)

Cladribine

Drug	Mfr	Conc	Mfr	Conc	Remarks	Ref	C/I
Aminophylline	AMR	2.5 mg/ml[a]	ORT	0.015[a] and 0.5[b] mg/ml	Physically compatible with no change in measured turbidity or increase in particle content in 4 hr at 23 °C	1969	C

Y-Site Injection Compatibility (1:1 Mixture) (Cont.)

				Cladribine			
Drug	*Mfr*	*Conc*	*Mfr*	*Conc*	*Remarks*	*Ref*	*C/I*
Bumetanide	RC	0.04 mg/ml[a]	ORT	0.015[a] and 0.5[b] mg/ml	Physically compatible with no change in measured turbidity or increase in particle content in 4 hr at 23 °C	1969	**C**
Buprenorphine HCl	RKC	0.04 mg/ml[a]	ORT	0.015[a] and 0.5[b] mg/ml	Physically compatible with no change in measured turbidity or increase in particle content in 4 hr at 23 °C	1969	**C**
Butorphanol tartrate	APC	0.04 mg/ml[a]	ORT	0.015[a] and 0.5[b] mg/ml	Physically compatible with no change in measured turbidity or increase in particle content in 4 hr at 23 °C	1969	**C**
Calcium gluconate	AMR	40 mg/ml[a]	ORT	0.015[a] and 0.5[b] mg/ml	Physically compatible with no change in measured turbidity or increase in particle content in 4 hr at 23 °C	1969	**C**
Carboplatin	BR	5 mg/ml[a]	ORT	0.015[a] and 0.5[b] mg/ml	Physically compatible with no change in measured turbidity or increase in particle content in 4 hr at 23 °C	1969	**C**
Chlorpromazine HCl	SCN	2 mg/ml[a]	ORT	0.015[a] and 0.5[b] mg/ml	Physically compatible with no change in measured turbidity or increase in particle content in 4 hr at 23 °C	1969	**C**
Cimetidine HCl	SKB	12 mg/ml[a]	ORT	0.015[a] and 0.5[b] mg/ml	Physically compatible with no change in measured turbidity or increase in particle content in 4 hr at 23 °C	1969	**C**
Cisplatin	BR	1 mg/ml	ORT	0.015[a] and 0.5[b] mg/ml	Physically compatible with no change in measured turbidity or increase in particle content in 4 hr at 23 °C	1969	**C**
Cyclophosphamide	MJ	10 mg/ml[a]	ORT	0.015[a] and 0.5[b] mg/ml	Physically compatible with no change in measured turbidity or increase in particle content in 4 hr at 23 °C	1969	**C**
Cytarabine	CHI	50 mg/ml	ORT	0.015[a] and 0.5[b] mg/ml	Physically compatible with no change in measured turbidity or increase in particle content in 4 hr at 23 °C	1969	**C**
Dexamethasone sodium phosphate	AMR	1 mg/ml[a]	ORT	0.015[a] and 0.5[b] mg/ml	Physically compatible with no change in measured turbidity or increase in particle content in 4 hr at 23 °C	1969	**C**
Diphenhydramine HCl	SCN	2 mg/ml[a]	ORT	0.015[a] and 0.5[b] mg/ml	Physically compatible with no change in measured turbidity or increase in particle content in 4 hr at 23 °C	1969	**C**
Dobutamine HCl	LI	4 mg/ml[a]	ORT	0.015[a] and 0.5[b] mg/ml	Physically compatible with no change in measured turbidity or increase in particle content in 4 hr at 23 °C	1969	**C**
Dopamine HCl	AST	3.2 mg/ml[a]	ORT	0.015[a] and 0.5[b] mg/ml	Physically compatible with no change in measured turbidity or increase in particle content in 4 hr at 23 °C	1969	**C**
Doxorubicin HCl	CHI	2 mg/ml	ORT	0.015[a] and 0.5[b] mg/ml	Physically compatible with no change in measured turbidity or increase in particle content in 4 hr at 23 °C	1969	**C**
Droperidol	JN	0.4 mg/ml[a]	ORT	0.015[a] and 0.5[b] mg/ml	Physically compatible with no change in measured turbidity or increase in particle content in 4 hr at 23 °C	1969	**C**

Y-Site Injection Compatibility (1:1 Mixture) (Cont.)

			Cladribine				
Drug	*Mfr*	*Conc*	*Mfr*	*Conc*	*Remarks*	*Ref*	*C/I*
Enalaprilat	MSD	0.1 mg/ml[a]	ORT	0.015[a] and 0.5[b] mg/ml	Physically compatible with no change in measured turbidity or increase in particle content in 4 hr at 23 °C	1969	**C**
Etoposide	BR	0.4 mg/ml[a]	ORT	0.015[a] and 0.5[b] mg/ml	Physically compatible with no change in measured turbidity or increase in particle content in 4 hr at 23 °C	1969	**C**
Famotidine	ME	2 mg/ml[a]	ORT	0.015[a] and 0.5[b] mg/ml	Physically compatible with no change in measured turbidity or increase in particle content in 4 hr at 23 °C	1969	**C**
Furosemide	AB	3 mg/ml[a]	ORT	0.015[a] and 0.5[b] mg/ml	Physically compatible with no change in measured turbidity or increase in particle content in 4 hr at 23 °C	1969	**C**
Granisetron HCl	SKB	0.05 mg/ml[a]	ORT	0.015[a] and 0.5[b] mg/ml	Physically compatible with no change in measured turbidity or increase in particle content in 4 hr at 23 °C	1969	**C**
Haloperidol lactate	MN	0.2 mg/ml[a]	ORT	0.015[a] and 0.5[b] mg/ml	Physically compatible with no change in measured turbidity or increase in particle content in 4 hr at 23 °C	1969	**C**
Heparin sodium	WY	100 units/ml[a]	ORT	0.015[a] and 0.5[b] mg/ml	Physically compatible with no change in measured turbidity or increase in particle content in 4 hr at 23 °C	1969	**C**
Hydrocortisone sodium phosphate	MSD	1 mg/ml[a]	ORT	0.015[a] and 0.5[b] mg/ml	Physically compatible with no change in measured turbidity or increase in particle content in 4 hr at 23 °C	1969	**C**
Hydrocortisone sodium succinate	UP	1 mg/ml[a]	ORT	0.015[a] and 0.5[b] mg/ml	Physically compatible with no change in measured turbidity or increase in particle content in 4 hr at 23 °C	1969	**C**
Hydromorphone HCl	KN	0.5 mg/ml[a]	ORT	0.015[a] and 0.5[b] mg/ml	Physically compatible with no change in measured turbidity or increase in particle content in 4 hr at 23 °C	1969	**C**
Hydroxyzine HCl	ES	4 mg/ml[a]	ORT	0.015[a] and 0.5[b] mg/ml	Physically compatible with no change in measured turbidity or increase in particle content in 4 hr at 23 °C	1969	**C**
Idarubicin HCl	AD	0.5 mg/ml[a]	ORT	0.015[a] and 0.5[b] mg/ml	Increase in measured turbidity no greater than simple dilution alone. No increase in particle content in 4 hr at 23 °C	1969	**C**
Leucovorin calcium	IMM	2 mg/ml[a]	ORT	0.015[a] and 0.5[b] mg/ml	Physically compatible with no change in measured turbidity or increase in particle content in 4 hr at 23 °C	1969	**C**
Lorazepam	WY	0.1 mg/ml[a]	ORT	0.015[a] and 0.5[b] mg/ml	Physically compatible with no change in measured turbidity or increase in particle content in 4 hr at 23 °C	1969	**C**
Mannitol	BA	15%	ORT	0.015[a] and 0.5[b] mg/ml	Physically compatible with no change in measured turbidity or increase in particle content in 4 hr at 23 °C	1969	**C**
Meperidine HCl	WY	4 mg/ml[a]	ORT	0.015[a] and 0.5[b] mg/ml	Physically compatible with no change in measured turbidity or increase in particle content in 4 hr at 23 °C	1969	**C**

Y-Site Injection Compatibility (1:1 Mixture) (Cont.)

Cladribine

Drug	Mfr	Conc	Mfr	Conc	Remarks	Ref	C/I
Mesna	MJ	10 mg/ml[a]	ORT	0.015[a] and 0.5[b] mg/ml	Physically compatible with no change in measured turbidity or increase in particle content in 4 hr at 23 °C	1969	**C**
Methylprednisolone sodium succinate	AB	5 mg/ml[a]	ORT	0.015[a] and 0.5[b] mg/ml	Physically compatible with no change in measured turbidity or increase in particle content in 4 hr at 23 °C	1969	**C**
Metoclopramide HCl	RB	5 mg/ml	ORT	0.015[a] and 0.5[b] mg/ml	Physically compatible with no change in measured turbidity or increase in particle content in 4 hr at 23 °C	1969	**C**
Mitoxantrone HCl	LE	0.5 mg/ml[a]	ORT	0.015[a] and 0.5[b] mg/ml	Physically compatible with no change in measured turbidity or increase in particle content in 4 hr at 23 °C	1969	**C**
Morphine sulfate	AST	1 mg/ml[a]	ORT	0.015[a] and 0.5[b] mg/ml	Physically compatible with no change in measured turbidity or increase in particle content in 4 hr at 23 °C	1969	**C**
Nalbuphine HCl	AST	10 mg/ml	ORT	0.015[a] and 0.5[b] mg/ml	Physically compatible with no change in measured turbidity or increase in particle content in 4 hr at 23 °C	1969	**C**
Ondansetron HCl	CER	1 mg/ml[a]	ORT	0.015[a] and 0.5[b] mg/ml	Physically compatible with no change in measured turbidity or increase in particle content in 4 hr at 23 °C	1969	**C**
Paclitaxel	BR	0.6 mg/ml[a]	ORT	0.015[a] and 0.5[b] mg/ml	Physically compatible with no change in measured turbidity or increase in particle content in 4 hr at 23 °C	1969	**C**
Potassium chloride	AB	0.1 mEq/ml[a]	ORT	0.015[a] and 0.5[b] mg/ml	Physically compatible with no change in measured turbidity or increase in particle content in 4 hr at 23 °C	1969	**C**
Prochlorperazine edisylate	SCN	0.5 mg/ml[a]	ORT	0.015[a] and 0.5[b] mg/ml	Physically compatible with no change in measured turbidity or increase in particle content in 4 hr at 23 °C	1969	**C**
Promethazine HCl	SCN	2 mg/ml[a]	ORT	0.015[a] and 0.5[b] mg/ml	Physically compatible with no change in measured turbidity or increase in particle content in 4 hr at 23 °C	1969	**C**
Ranitidine HCl	GL	2 mg/ml[a]	ORT	0.015[a] and 0.5[b] mg/ml	Physically compatible with no change in measured turbidity or increase in particle content in 4 hr at 23 °C	1969	**C**
Sodium bicarbonate	AB	1 mEq/ml	ORT	0.015[a] and 0.5[b] mg/ml	Physically compatible with no change in measured turbidity or increase in particle content in 4 hr at 23 °C	1969	**C**
Teniposide	BR	0.1 mg/ml[a]	ORT	0.015[a] and 0.5[b] mg/ml	Physically compatible with no change in measured turbidity or increase in particle content in 4 hr at 23 °C	1969	**C**
Vincristine sulfate	LI	0.05 mg/ml[a]	ORT	0.015[a] and 0.5[b] mg/ml	Physically compatible with no change in measured turbidity or increase in particle content in 4 hr at 23 °C	1969	**C**

[a]*Tested in sodium chloride 0.9%.*
[b]*Tested in bacteriostatic sodium chloride 0.9% preserved with benzyl alcohol 0.9%.*

Other Information

Bacterial Challenge— Cladribine (Ortho Biotech) 0.025 mg/ml diluted in sodium chloride 0.9% did not exhibit an antimicrobial effect on the growth of four organisms (*Enterococcus faecium, Staphylo-* *coccus aureus, Pseudomonas aeruginosa,* and *Candida albicans*) inoculated into the solution. Diluted solutions should be stored under refrigeration whenever possible, and the potential for microbiological growth should be considered when assigning expiration periods (2160).

CLINDAMYCIN PHOSPHATE
AHFS 8:12.28

Cleocin Phosphate   **Pharmacia & Upjohn**

Products— Clindamycin phosphate (Pharmacia & Upjohn) is available in 2-, 4-, and 6-ml vials and a 60-ml pharmacy bulk container. Each milliliter of solution contains (2; 4):

Component	Amount
Clindamycin (as phosphate)	150 mg
Benzyl alcohol	9.45 mg
Disodium edetate	0.5 mg
Sodium hydroxide and/or hydrochloric acid	to adjust pH
Water for injection	qs 1 ml

Clindamycin phosphate (Pharmacia & Upjohn) also is available in 50-ml bags containing 300, 600, or 900 mg of drug in dextrose 5% in water. Disodium edetate 0.04 mg/ml and sodium hydroxide and/or hydrochloric acid are also present to adjust the pH (2).

pH— The product pH may range from 5.5 to 7 (17) but is usually about 6 to 6.3 (102; 103).

Osmolality— Clindamycin phosphate (Upjohn) 150 mg/ml has been reported to have an osmolality of 795 mOsm/kg (50) or 835 mOsm/kg (1071) as determined by freezing-point depression. However, the manufacturer has stated that the osmolality is usually 825 to 880 mOsm/kg (1705).

The osmolality of clindamycin phosphate (Upjohn) 12 mg/ml was determined to be 293 mOsm/kg in dextrose 5% in water and 309 mOsm/kg in sodium chloride 0.9% (1375).

The osmolalities of the 300-, 600-, and 900-mg premixed infusion solutions in dextrose 5% in water are 296, 322, and 339 mOsm/kg, respectively (4).

The osmolality of clindamycin phosphate 600 mg was calculated for the following dilutions (1054):

Diluent	Osmolality (mOsm/kg)	
	50 ml	100 ml
Dextrose 5% in water	279	268
Sodium chloride 0.9%	306	294

Administration— Clindamycin phosphate is administered by intramuscular injection; single injections greater than 600 mg are not recommended. It may also be administered by intermittent intravenous infusion in concentrations not exceeding 18 mg/ml. Intermittent infusions should be infused over 10 to 60 minutes at a rate not exceeding 30 mg/min. Intravenous doses under 900 mg may be diluted in 50 ml of a compatible diluent; doses of 900 mg or more should be diluted in 100 ml of diluent. Not more than 1200 mg of clindamycin phosphate should be given in a one-hour period. The drug should not be given undiluted as a bolus (2; 4).

Alternatively, following an initial single rapid infusion, continuous intravenous infusion at rates of 0.75 to 1.25 mg/min have been suggested (2; 4).

Stability— Less than 10% decomposition occurs in two years at 25 °C at pH 3.5 to 6.5 (102; 103). Crystallization may occur on refrigeration; the crystals resolubilize on warming to room temperature, but care should be exercised to ensure that all crystals have redissolved. This would also apply if the product is frozen (102).

Clindamycin phosphate 900 mg/6 ml in polypropylene syringes (Becton-Dickinson) retained more than 95% of the initial concentration over at least 48 hours at room temperature (172). Diluted with sterile water for injection to concentrations of 20, 40, 60, and 120 mg/ml and stored in Monoject plastic syringes or glass vials, clindamycin phosphate exhibited little or no change in concentration and was free of visually apparent particulate matter over 30 days of storage at 25 °C (173).

Clindamycin phosphate (Upjohn) 900 mg/6 ml showed no more than a 4 to 5% loss when stored in polypropylene syringes (Becton-Dickinson) for 48 hours at 25 °C under fluorescent light (1159).

Clindamycin phosphate (Upjohn) 600 mg stored in polypropylene syringes (3M) at 25 °C under fluorescent light exhibited no loss in 48 hours (1164).

Dilution of clindamycin phosphate 300 and 900 mg in glass vials containing 20 ml of dextrose 10% in water resulted in no visual changes and less than a 10% loss by HPLC after 30 days of refrigeration at 10 °C (1604).

Clindamycin phosphate (Abbott) injection was diluted with sterile water for injection to a concentration of 15 mg/ml for use in minimizing measurement errors in pediatric dosing. The dilution was packaged in glass vials, and samples were stored at 22 and 4 °C. The dilution remained visually free of particulate matter at both storage conditions throughout the study. HPLC analysis of the samples found no clindamycin loss after 91 days at either 4 or 22 °C (1714).

Clindamycin phosphate is incompatible with natural rubber closures because of the extraction of crystalline particulate matter, primarily β-sitosterol and stigmasterol. Simple cleaning procedures for the closures do not effectively remove the source of contamination. It is recommended that if clindamycin phosphate is repackaged in vials or disposable syringes, storage at room temperature should be limited to a few days (102).

Freezing Solutions— Clindamycin phosphate 6, 9, and 12 mg/ml in dextrose 5% in water, sodium chloride 0.9%, or Ringer's injection, lactated, is physically and chemically stable for eight weeks when frozen at −10 °C. Solutions should be thawed at room temperature and should not be refrozen (4).

Clindamycin phosphate (Upjohn) 6, 9, and 12 g/L, in both PVC and glass containers of dextrose 5% in water, sodium chloride 0.9%, or Ringer's injection, lactated, was stored frozen at −10 °C. The drug was stable for the eight weeks of the study with only minor changes in concentration (753).

One study of clindamycin phosphate 600 mg in 100-ml PVC containers of dextrose 5% in water frozen at −20 °C showed approximately a 13% loss of potency after 23 days of storage (155).

However, in another study, clindamycin phosphate (Upjohn) 300 mg/50 ml of dextrose 5% in water in PVC bags frozen at −20 °C for 30 days and then thawed by exposure to ambient temperature or microwave radiation showed no evidence of precipitation or color change and showed little or no loss of potency determined microbiologically. Subsequent storage of the admixture at room temperature for 24 hours also yielded a physically compatible solution, which exhibited a 7 to 8% loss of activity (555; 871; 872).

Marble et al. reported that clindamycin phosphate (Upjohn) 900 mg/50 ml in dextrose 5% in water and sodium chloride 0.9% in PVC bags frozen at −20 °C lost 3 to 4% potency in 28 days (981).

Minibags of clindamycin phosphate in dextrose 5% in water or sodium chloride 0.9%, frozen at −20 °C for up to 35 days, were thawed at room temperature and in a microwave oven, with care taken that the thawed solution temperature never exceeded 25 °C. No significant differences in clindamycin phosphate concentrations occurred between the two thawing methods (1192).

At a concentration of 6 mg/ml dextrose 5% in water, clindamycin phosphate retained 97% of the initial concentration after 79 days of storage at −10 °C (174).

Clindamycin phosphate diluted with sterile water for injection to concentrations of 20, 40, 60, and 120 mg/ml was stored frozen at −15 °C in Monoject plastic syringes or glass vials. After 60 days of storage, the changes from the original concentrations ranged from −5 to +2.5%. Visual examination showed no particulate matter (173).

Clindamycin phosphate (Quad) 6 and 12 mg/ml in dextrose 5% in water and sodium chloride 0.9% exhibited no loss after 68 days when frozen at −10 °C (1351).

Clindamycin phosphate (Upjohn) 7.6 mg/ml in dextrose 5% in water was visually compatible and had no potency loss by HPLC after frozen storage (−20 °C) for 30 days followed by 14 days of refrigeration at 4 °C (1539).

pH Effects— Maximum stability occurs at pH 4, but an acceptable long-term shelf life is attained at pH 1 to 6.5 (1072).

Compatibility Information

Solution Compatibility

Clindamycin phosphate

Solution	Mfr	Mfr	Conc/L	Remarks	Ref	C/I
Amino acids 4.25%, dextrose 25%	MG	UP	600 mg	No increase in particulate matter in 24 hr at 5 °C	349	C
Dextrose 2.5% in Ringer's injection, lactated		UP	600 mg	Physically compatible and clindamycin potency retained for 24 hr at room temperature	104	C
Dextrose 5% in Ringer's injection		UP	600 mg	Physically compatible and clindamycin potency retained for 24 hr at room temperature	104	C
Dextrose 5% in sodium chloride 0.45%		UP	600 mg	Clindamycin stability maintained for 24 hr	101	C
Dextrose 5% in sodium chloride 0.9%	MG	UP	250 mg	Clindamycin potency retained for 24 hr at 4 and 25 °C	105	C
		UP	600 mg	Physically compatible and clindamycin potency retained for 24 hr at room temperature	104	C
Dextrose 5% in water	MG	UP	250 mg	Clindamycin potency retained for 24 hr at 4 and 25 °C	105	C
		UP	600 mg	Physically compatible and clindamycin potency retained for 24 hr at room temperature	104	C
		UP	6, 9, 12 g	Clindamycin stability maintained for 24 hr	101	C
	TR[a]	UP	6 g	Physically compatible and approximately 9% loss of potency in 24 hr at room temperature	555	C
	TR[b]	UP	6, 9, 12 g	Physically compatible and chemically stable for at least 16 days at 25 °C and 32 days at 4 °C	753	C
	MG[c]	UP	9 g	8 to 9% loss in 12 hr and no further loss in 48 hr at 25 °C under fluorescent light	981	C
	MG[c]	UP	9 g	9% loss in 24 hr with no further loss at 48 hr at room temperature under fluorescent light	983	C
	AB[b]	UP	9 g	Physically compatible and no clindamycin loss in 24 hr at 25 °C	994	C

Solution Compatibility (Cont.)

Clindamycin phosphate

Solution	Mfr	Mfr	Conc/L	Remarks	Ref	C/I
	MG[c]	UP	9 g	Physically compatible with about 8% loss in 8 hr and no further loss through 48 hr at 25 °C under fluorescent light	1026	C
	MG[c]	UP	12 g	Physically compatible with 3% loss in 48 hr at 25 °C under fluorescent light	1026	C
	AB[a]	UP	18 g	3% loss in 28 days frozen at −20 °C	981	C
	TR[a]	QU	6 and 12 g	Physically compatible with no loss in 22 days at 25 °C, 54 days at 5 °C, and 68 days at −10 °C	1351	C
	MG[d]	UP	7.6 g	Visually compatible with no clindamycin loss by HPLC after 30 days at −20 °C followed by 14 days at 4 °C	1539	C
Dextrose 10% in water	MG	UP	250 mg	Clindamycin potency retained for 24 hr at 4 and 25 °C	105	C
Isolyte H	MG	UP	1.2 g	Physically compatible and clindamycin potency retained for 24 hr	101	C
Isolyte M with dextrose 5%	MG	UP	250 mg	Clindamycin potency retained for 24 hr at 4 and 25 °C	105	C
Isolyte P with dextrose 5%	MG	UP	250 mg	Clindamycin potency retained for 24 hr at 4 and 25 °C	105	C
Normosol R	AB	UP	1.2 g	Clindamycin stability maintained for 24 hr	101	C
Ringer's injection, lactated	MG	UP	250 mg	Clindamycin potency retained for 24 hr at 4 and 25 °C	105	C
	TR[b]	UP	6, 9, 12 g	Physically compatible and chemically stable for at least 16 days at 25 °C and 32 days at 4 °C	753	C
Sodium chloride 0.9%		UP	600 mg	Physically compatible and clindamycin potency retained for 24 hr at room temperature	104	C
		UP	6 g	Clindamycin stability maintained for 24 hr	101	C
	MG	UP	250 mg	Clindamycin potency retained for 24 hr at 4 and 25 °C	105	C
	TR[b]	UP	6, 9, 12 g	Physically compatible and chemically stable for at least 16 days at 25 °C and 32 days at 4 °C	753	C
	MG[c]	UP	9 g	6% loss in 12 hr and 8 to 11% in 24 to 48 hr at 25 °C under fluorescent light	981	C
	MG[c]	UP	9 g	Physically compatible with 8 to 11% loss in both 24 and 48 hr at room temperature under fluorescent light	983	C
	AB[b]	UP	9 g	Physically compatible and no clindamycin loss in 24 hr at 25 °C	994	C
	MG[c]	UP	9 and 12 g	Physically compatible with 6% loss in 12 hr and 7 to 8% in 48 hr at 25 °C under fluorescent light	1026	C
	AB[a]	UP	18 g	4% loss in 28 days frozen at −20 °C	981	C
	TR[a]	QU	6 and 12 g	Physically compatible with no loss in 22 days at 25 °C, 54 days at 5 °C, and 68 days at −10 °C	1351	C
TPN #21[e]		UP	250 mg	Clindamycin potency retained for 24 hr at 4 and 25 °C	87	C
TPN #22[e]		UP	3 g	Physically compatible with no loss of activity by microbiological assay in 24 hr at 22 °C in the dark	837	C

Solution Compatibility (Cont.)

Clindamycin phosphate

Solution	Mfr	Mfr	Conc/L	Remarks	Ref	C/I
TPN #107[e]			400 mg[f]	Physically compatible and clindamycin activity retained for 24 hr at 21 °C by microbiological assay	1326	**C**

[a]Tested in PVC containers.
[b]Tested in both glass and PVC containers.
[c]Tested in glass bottles.
[d]Tested in polyolefin containers.
[e]Refer to Appendix I for the composition of parenteral nutrition solutions. TPN indicates a 2-in-1 admixture.
[f]Present as clindamycin base.

Additive Compatibility

Clindamycin phosphate

Drug	Mfr	Conc/L	Mfr	Conc/L	Test Soln	Remarks	Ref	C/I
Amikacin sulfate	BR	5 g	UP	6 g	D5LR, D5R, D5S, D5W, D10W, IS10, LR, NS, R, SL	Physically compatible and amikacin potency retained for 24 hr at 25 °C. Clindamycin not analyzed	293	**C**
	BR	4 g	UP	9 g	D5W, NS[a]	Potency of both drugs retained for 48 hr at 25 °C under fluorescent light	981	**C**
	AB	4 g	UP	9 g	D5W, NS[a]	Physically compatible and potency of both drugs retained for 48 hr at room temperature exposed to light and 1 week frozen	174	**C**
Aminophylline	SE	600 mg	UP	600 mg		Physically incompatible	101	**I**
Ampicillin sodium	WY	10 and 20 g	UP	24 g	NS	Physically compatible	1035	**C**
	WY	3.7 g	UP	3 g	NS	Physically compatible with 4% ampicillin loss in 1 day at 24 °C	1035	**C**
Aztreonam	SQ	10 and 20 g	UP	3 and 6 g	D5W, NS[b]	Physically compatible with little or no loss of either drug in 48 hr at 25 °C and 7 days at 4 °C	1002	**C**
	SQ	20 g	UP	9 g	D5W[a]	Physically compatible with 3% clindamycin loss and 5% aztreonam loss in 48 hr at 25 °C under fluorescent light	1026	**C**
	SQ	20 g	UP	9 g	NS[a]	Physically compatible with 2% clindamycin loss and no aztreonam loss in 48 hr at 25 °C under fluorescent light	1026	**C**
Cefamandole nafate	LI	10 g	UP	9 g	D5W, NS[a]	Physically compatible with no clindamycin loss and 4 to 7% cefamandole loss in 48 hr at room temperature under fluorescent light	983	**C**
Cefazolin sodium	SKF	10 g	UP	9 g	D5W[a]	Physically compatible with no clindamycin loss and 8% cefazolin loss in 48 hr at room temperature under fluorescent light	983	**C**
	SKF	10 g	UP	9 g	NS[a]	Physically compatible with no clindamycin loss and 3% cefazolin loss in 48 hr at room temperature under fluorescent light	983	**C**

Additive Compatibility (Cont.)

Clindamycin phosphate

Drug	Mfr	Conc/L	Mfr	Conc/L	Test Soln	Remarks	Ref	C/I
Cefepime HCl	BR	40 g	UP	0.25 g	D5W, NS	7% or less cefepime loss by HPLC in 24 hr at room temperature and 10% or less loss in 7 days at 5 °C. No clindamycin loss by HPLC in 24 hr at room temperature and 8% or less loss in 7 days at 5 °C	1682	C
	BR	4 g	UP	6 g	D5W, NS	7% or less cefepime loss by HPLC in 24 hr at room temperature and 10% or less loss in 7 days at 5 °C. No clindamycin loss by HPLC in 24 hr at room temperature and 8% or less loss in 7 days at 5 °C	1682	C
Cefoperazone sodium	RR	20 g	UP	12 g	D5W, NS[c]	Physically compatible with no clindamycin loss and 5% cefoperazone loss in 48 hr at 25 °C under fluorescent light	174; 1164	C
Cefotaxime sodium	HO	20 g	UP	9 g	D5W, NS[c]	Physically compatible with no clindamycin loss and 3% cefotaxime loss in 24 hr at 25 °C	994	C
Cefoxitin sodium	MSD	20 g	UP	9 g	D5W[a]	Physically compatible with no loss of either drug in 48 hr at room temperature under fluorescent light	983	C
	MSD	20 g	UP	9 g	NS[a]	Physically compatible with no clindamycin loss and 7% cefoxitin loss in 48 hr at room temperature under fluorescent light	983	C
Ceftazidime sodium	GL[g]	20 g	UP	9 g	D5W[a]	Physically compatible with 9% clindamycin loss and 11% ceftazidime loss in 48 hr at 25 °C under fluorescent light	1026	C
	GL[g]	20 g	UP	9 g	NS[a]	Physically compatible with 5% clindamycin loss and 7% ceftazidime loss in 48 hr at 25 °C under fluorescent light	1026	C
Ceftizoxime sodium	SKF	20 g	UP	9 g	D5W[a]	Physically compatible with 3% clindamycin loss and 4% ceftizoxime loss in 48 hr at room temperature under fluorescent light	983	C
	SKF	20 g	UP	9 g	NS[a]	Physically compatible with 7% ceftizoxime loss in 48 hr at room temperature under fluorescent light. 10% clindamycin loss in 8 hr with no further loss through 48 hr	983	C
Ceftriaxone sodium	RC	20 g	UP	12 g	D5W[a]	10% ceftriaxone loss in 4 hr and 17% in 24 hr at 25 °C under fluorescent light. No clindamycin loss in 48 hr	1026	I
	RC	20 g	UP	12 g	NS[a]	10% ceftriaxone loss in 1 hr and 12% in 24 hr at 25 °C under fluorescent light. 6% clindamycin loss in 48 hr	1026	I
Cefuroxime sodium	GL	15 g	UP	9 g	D5W[c]	Physically compatible with 4% clindamycin loss and 6 to 8% cefuroxime loss in 48 hr at 25 °C under fluorescent light	174	C

Additive Compatibility (Cont.)

Clindamycin phosphate

Drug	Mfr	Conc/L	Mfr	Conc/L	Test Soln	Remarks	Ref	C/I
	GL	15 g	UP	9 g	NS[c]	Physically compatible with 9% clindamycin and cefuroxime losses in 48 hr at 25 °C under fluorescent light	174	**C**
	GL	15 g	UP	9 g	D5W	Physically compatible with 4% clindamycin loss and 6 to 8% cefuroxime loss in 48 hr at 25 °C under fluorescent light	1164	**C**
	GL	15 g	UP	9 g	NS	Physically compatible with 9% clindamycin and cefuroxime losses in 48 hr at 25 °C under fluorescent light	1164	**C**
Cimetidine HCl	SKF	1.2 and 5 g	UP	1.2 g	D5W, NS	Physically compatible and cimetidine chemically stable for 24 hr at room temperature. Clindamycin not tested	551	**C**
Ciprofloxacin	MI	1.6 g	LY	7.1 g	D5W, NS	Precipitate forms immediately. HPLC showed no intact clindamycin	1541	**I**
Fluconazole	PF	1 g	AST	6 g	D5W	Visually compatible with no fluconazole loss by HPLC in 72 hr at 25 °C under fluorescent light. Clindamycin not tested	1677	**C**
Gentamicin sulfate		120 mg	UP	2.4 g	D5W	Physically compatible and clindamycin potency retained for 24 hr at room temperature	104	**C**
		60 mg	UP	1.2 g	D5W	Physically compatible and clindamycin potency retained for 24 hr at room temperature	104	**C**
		600 mg	UP	12 g	D5W	Physically compatible	101	**C**
		800 mg	UP	9 g	D5W	Clindamycin stability maintained for 24 hr	101	**C**
	AB	1 g	UP	9 g	D5W, NS[c]	Physically compatible and potency of both drugs retained for 48 hr at room temperature exposed to light and 1 week frozen	174	**C**
	LY	1.2 g	UP	9 g	D5W[a]	Physically compatible and potency of both drugs retained for 7 days at 4 and 25 °C	174	**C**
	LY	1.2 g	UP	9 g	NS[a]	Physically compatible and potency of both drugs retained for 14 days at 4 and 25 °C	174	**C**
	LY	2.4 g	UP	18 g	D5W, NS[c]	Physically compatible and potency of both drugs retained for 14 days at 4 and 25 °C	174	**C**
	ES	1.2 g	UP	9 g	D5W, NS[a]	Physically compatible and potency of both drugs retained for 28 days frozen at −20 °C	174	**C**
	ES	2.4 g	UP	18 g	D5W, NS[b]	Potency of both drugs retained for 28 days frozen at −20 °C	981	**C**
	ES	667 mg	UP	6 g	D5W[b]	Physically compatible with no clindamycin loss and 9% gentamicin loss in 24 hr at room temperature	995	**C**
		75 mg		400 mg[d]	TPN #107[e]	19% gentamicin loss and 15% clindamycin loss in 24 hr at 21 °C by microbiological assay	1326	**I**
Gentamicin sulfate with cefazolin sodium	ES SKF	800 mg 10 g	UP	9 g	D5W[a]	10% cefazolin loss in 4 hr at 25 °C. Clindamycin and gentamicin potency retained for 24 hr	1328	**I**
Gentamicin sulfate with cefazolin sodium	ES SKF	800 mg 10 g	UP	9 g	NS[a]	10% cefazolin loss after 12 hr at 25 °C. Clindamycin and gentamicin potency retained for 24 hr	1328	**I**

Additive Compatibility (Cont.)

Clindamycin phosphate

Drug	Mfr	Conc/L	Mfr	Conc/L	Test Soln	Remarks	Ref	C/I
Heparin sodium		100,000 units	UP	9 g	D5W	Clindamycin stability maintained for 24 hr	101	C
Hydrocortisone sodium succinate	UP	1 g	UP	1.2 g	W	Clindamycin stability maintained for 24 hr	101	C
Kanamycin sulfate		1 g	UP	2.4 g	D5W	Physically compatible and clindamycin potency retained for 24 hr at room temperature	104	C
		500 mg	UP	1.2 g	D5W	Physically compatible and clindamycin potency retained for 24 hr at room temperature	104	C
Methylprednisolone sodium succinate	UP	500 mg	UP	1.2 g	D5W, W	Clindamycin stability maintained for 24 hr	101	C
Metoclopramide HCl	RB	100 and 200 mg	UP	600 mg	NS	Physically compatible for 24 hr at room temperature	924	C
	RB	100 and 200 mg	UP	6 g		Physically compatible for 24 hr at 25 °C	1167	C
	RB	1.9 g	UP	3.5 g		Physically compatible for 24 hr at 25 °C	1167	C
	RB	1.2 g	UP	4.4 g		Physically compatible for 24 hr at 25 °C	1167	C
Metronidazole	RP	5 g[f]	UP	10 g		Physically compatible with little or no pH change for at least 24 hr at 23 °C	807	C
Metronidazole HCl with sodium bicarbonate	SE AB	5 g 50 mEq	UP	2.4 g	D5W, NS	Physically compatible for 48 hr	765	C
Netilmicin sulfate	SC	3 g	UP	9 g	D5W, NS[c]	Physically compatible with no clindamycin loss and 2 to 5% netilmicin loss in 24 hr at 25 °C	994	C
Ofloxacin	HO	2 g	UP	6 g	W	Visually compatible with little or no loss of either drug by HPLC in 48 hr	1613	C
Penicillin G		20 million units	UP	2.4 g	D5W	Physically compatible and clindamycin potency retained for 24 hr at room temperature	104	C
		10 million units	UP	1.2 g	D5W	Physically compatible and clindamycin potency retained for 24 hr at room temperature	104	C
Piperacillin sodium	LE	40 g	UP	9 g	D5W, NS	Physically compatible with 2% clindamycin loss and 3 to 5% piperacillin loss in 48 hr at 25 °C under fluorescent light	1026	C
Potassium chloride		40 mEq	UP	600 mg	D5½S	Physically compatible and clindamycin potency retained for 24 hr at room temperature	104	C
		100 mEq	UP	600 mg	D5W, NS	Physically compatible	101	C
		400 mEq	UP	6 g	D5½S	Clindamycin stability maintained for 24 hr	101	C
Ranitidine HCl	GL	100 mg	UP	1.2 g	D5W	Color change and gas formation	1151	I
	GL	50 mg and 2 g		1.2 g	D5W, NS	Physically compatible and ranitidine chemically stable by HPLC for 24 hr at 25 °C. Clindamycin not tested	1515	C
Sodium bicarbonate		44 mEq	UP	1.2 g	D5S, D5W	Clindamycin stability maintained for 24 hr	101	C
Tobramycin sulfate	DI	1 g	UP	9 g	D5W, NS[c]	Physically compatible and potency of both drugs retained for 48 hr at room temperature exposed to light and 1 week frozen	174	C

Additive Compatibility (Cont.)

Clindamycin phosphate

Drug	Mfr	Conc/L	Mfr	Conc/L	Test Soln	Remarks	Ref	C/I
	DI	1.2 g	UP	9 g	D5W[a]	Physically compatible and clindamycin potency retained for 28 days frozen. About 8% tobramycin loss in 14 days and 17% in 28 days	174	C
	DI	1.2 g	UP	9 g	NS[a]	Physically compatible and potency of both drugs retained for 28 days frozen	174	C
	DI	2.4 g	UP	18 g	D5W[b]	8% tobramycin activity loss in 14 days and 17% in 28 days frozen at −20 °C. Clindamycin potency retained	981	C
	DI	2.4 g	UP	18 g	NS[b]	Potency of both drugs retained for 28 days frozen at −20 °C	981	C
Verapamil HCl	KN	80 mg	UP	1.2 g	D5W, NS	Physically compatible for 24 hr	764	C
Vitamin B complex with C	UP	10 ml	UP	600 mg	D5W	Clindamycin potency retained for 24 hr	102	C

[a]*Tested in glass bottles.*
[b]*Tested in PVC containers.*
[c]*Tested in both glass and PVC containers.*
[d]*Present as clindamycin base.*
[e]*Refer to Appendix I for the composition of parenteral nutrition solutions. TPN indicates a 2-in-1 admixture.*
[f]*Minibags (100 ml) containing metronidazole 500 mg with disodium phosphate 150 mg, citric acid 44 mg, and sodium chloride 740 mg. This product differs from the Searle product.*
[g]*Sodium carbonate–containing formulation tested.*

Drugs in Syringe Compatibility

Clindamycin phosphate

Drug (in syringe)	Mfr	Amt	Mfr	Amt	Remarks	Ref	C/I
Amikacin sulfate	BR	750 mg/ 4 ml[a]	UP	900 mg/ 6 ml	Physically compatible with little or no loss of either drug in 48 hr at 25 °C in polypropylene syringes	1159	C
Aztreonam	SQ	2 g	UP	600 mg/ 4 ml	Physically compatible with 2% clindamycin loss and 8% aztreonam loss in 48 hr at 25 °C under fluorescent light in polypropylene syringes	1164	C
Gentamicin sulfate	ES	120 mg/ 4 ml[a]	UP	900 mg/ 6 ml	Physically compatible with little or no loss of either drug in 48 hr at 25 °C in polypropylene syringes	1159	C
Heparin sodium		2500 units/ 1 ml	UP	300 mg	Physically compatible for at least 5 min	1053	C
Tobramycin sulfate	DI	120 mg/ 4 ml[a]	UP	900 mg/ 6 ml	Cloudy white precipitate forms immediately and changes to gel-like precipitate	1159	I

[a]*Diluted to 4 ml with 1 ml of sodium chloride 0.9%.*

Y-Site Injection Compatibility (1:1 Mixture)

Clindamycin phosphate

Drug	Mfr	Conc	Mfr	Conc	Remarks	Ref	C/I
Allopurinol sodium	BW	3 mg/ml[b]	AB	10 mg/ml[b]	Tiny particles form immediately and become more numerous over 4 hr	1686	I

Y-Site Injection Compatibility (1:1 Mixture) (Cont.)

			Clindamycin phosphate				
Drug	*Mfr*	*Conc*	*Mfr*	*Conc*	*Remarks*	*Ref*	*C/I*
Amifostine	USB	10 mg/ml[a]	AST	10 mg/ml[a]	Physically compatible with no change in measured turbidity or increase in particle content in 4 hr at 23 °C	1845	**C**
Amiodarone HCl	LZ	4 mg/ml[c]	UP	6 mg/ml[c]	Physically compatible for 4 hr at room temperature	1444	**C**
Amphotericin B cholesteryl sulfate complex	SEQ	0.83 mg/ml[a]	UP	10 mg/ml[a]	Physically compatible with little or no change in measured turbidity or increase in particle content in 4 hr at 23 °C under fluorescent light	2117	**C**
Amsacrine	NCI	1 mg/ml[a]	UP	10 mg/ml[a]	Physically compatible for 4 hr at room temperature under fluorescent light	1381	**C**
Aztreonam	SQ	40 mg/ml[a]	AST	10 mg/ml[a]	Physically compatible with no subvisual haze or particle formation in 4 hr at 23 °C	1758	**C**
Cefpirome sulfate	HO	50 mg/ml[d]	AB	12 mg/ml[d]	Visually and microscopically compatible with 5% or less cefpirome loss and 4% or less clindamycin loss by HPLC in 8 hr at 23 °C	2044	**C**
Cisatracurium besylate	GW	0.1, 2, 5 mg/ml[a]	AST	10 mg/ml[a]	Physically compatible with no change in measured turbidity or increase in particle content in 4 hr at 23 °C	2074	**C**
Cyclophosphamide	MJ	20 mg/ml[a]	UP	12 mg/ml[a]	Physically compatible for 4 hr at 25 °C	1194	**C**
Diltiazem HCl	MMD	5 mg/ml	UP	12[b] and 150 mg/ml	Visually compatible	1807	**C**
Docetaxel	RPR	0.9 mg/ml[a]	AST	10 mg/ml[a]	Physically compatible with no change in measured turbidity or increase in particle content in 4 hr at 23 °C	2224	**C**
Doxorubicin HCl liposome injection	SEQ	0.4 mg/ml[a]	AST	10 mg/ml[a]	Physically compatible with little or no change in measured turbidity and no increase in particle content in 4 hr at 23 °C	2087	**C**
Enalaprilat	MSD	0.05 mg/ml[b]	UP	9 mg/ml[a]	Physically compatible for 24 hr at room temperature under fluorescent light	1355	**C**
Esmolol HCl	DCC	10 mg/ml[a]	UP	9 mg/ml[a]	Physically compatible for 24 hr at 22 °C	1169	**C**
Etoposide phosphate	BR	5 mg/ml[a]	AST	10 mg/ml[a]	Physically compatible with no change in measured turbidity or increase in particle content in 4 hr at 23 °C	2218	**C**
Filgrastim	AMG	30 μg/ml[a]	AB	10 mg/ml[a]	Particles and filaments form immediately	1687	**I**
Fluconazole	RR	2 mg/ml	AB	24 mg/ml	Immediate precipitation	1407	**I**
Fludarabine phosphate	BX	1 mg/ml[a]	LY	10 mg/ml[a]	Physically compatible for 4 hr at room temperature under fluorescent light	1439	**C**
Foscarnet sodium	AST	24 mg/ml	AB	24 mg/ml	Physically compatible for 24 hr at room temperature under fluorescent light	1335	**C**
	AST	24 mg/ml	UP	12 mg/ml[c]	Physically compatible for 24 hr at 25 °C under fluorescent light by visual and microscopic examination	1393	**C**

Y-Site Injection Compatibility (1:1 Mixture) (Cont.)

		Clindamycin phosphate					
Drug	Mfr	Conc	Mfr	Conc	Remarks	Ref	C/I
Gemcitabine HCl	LI	10 mg/ml[b]	AST	10 mg/ml[b]	Physically compatible with no change in measured turbidity or increase in particle content in 4 hr at 23 °C	2226	C
Granisetron HCl	SKB	0.05 mg/ml[a]	AB	10 mg/ml[a]	Physically compatible with no change in measured turbidity or increase in particle content in 4 hr at 23 °C	2000	C
Heparin sodium	TR	50 units/ml	UP	12 mg/ml[a]	Visually compatible for 6 hr at 25 °C	1793	C
Hydromorphone HCl	WY	0.2 mg/ml[a]	UP	12 mg/ml[a]	Physically compatible for at least 4 hr at 25 °C under fluorescent light	987	C
Idarubicin HCl	AD	1 mg/ml[b]	AST	12 mg/ml[a]	Haze and precipitate form immediately	1525	I
Labetalol HCl	SC	1 mg/ml[a]	UP	9 mg/ml[a]	Physically compatible for 24 hr at 18 °C	1171	C
Magnesium sulfate	IX	16.7, 33.3, 66.7, 100 mg/ml[a]	UP	12 mg/ml[a]	Physically compatible for at least 4 hr at 32 °C	813	C
Melphalan HCl	BW	0.1 mg/ml[b]	AB	10 mg/ml[b]	Physically compatible with no change in measured turbidity or increase in particle content in 3 hr at 22 °C	1557	C
Meperidine HCl	WY	10 mg/ml[a]	UP	12 mg/ml[a]	Physically compatible for at least 4 hr at 25 °C under fluorescent light	987	C
Midazolam HCl	RC	1 mg/ml[a]	UP	9 mg/ml[a]	Visually compatible for 24 hr at 23 °C	1847	C
Morphine sulfate	WI	1 mg/ml[a]	UP	12 mg/ml[a]	Physically compatible for at least 4 hr at 25 °C under fluorescent light	987	C
Multivitamins	USV	5 ml/L[a]	UP	600 mg/ 100 ml[a]	Physically compatible for 24 hr at room temperature	323	C
Ondansetron HCl	GL	1 mg/ml[b]	LY	10 mg/ml[a]	Physically compatible for 4 hr at 22 °C	1365	C
Perphenazine	SC	0.02 mg/ml[a]	UP	12 mg/ml[a]	Physically compatible for 4 hr at 25 °C	1155	C
Piperacillin sodium–tazobactam sodium	LE	40 + 5 mg/ ml[a]	AB	10 mg/ml[a]	Physically compatible with no change in measured turbidity or increase in particle content in 4 hr at 22 °C	1688	C
Propofol	ZEN	10 mg/ml	AST	10 mg/ml[a]	Physically compatible for 1 hr at 23 °C with no increase in particle content	2066	C
Remifentanil HCl	GW	0.025 and 0.25 mg/ml[b]	AST	10 mg/ml[a]	Physically compatible with no change in measured turbidity or increase in particle content in 4 hr at 23 °C	2075	C
Sargramostim	IMM	10 μg/ml[b]	LY	10 mg/ml[b]	Physically compatible for 4 hr at 22 °C	1436	C
Tacrolimus	FUJ	1 mg/ml[b]	ES	12 mg/ml[a]	Visually compatible for 24 hr at 25 °C	1630	C
Teniposide	BR	0.1 mg/ml[a]	AST	10 mg/ml[a]	Physically compatible with no subvisual haze or particle formation in 4 hr at 23 °C	1725	C
Theophylline	TR	4 mg/ml	UP	12 mg/ml[a]	Visually compatible for 6 hr at 25 °C	1793	C
Thiotepa	IMM[e]	1 mg/ml[b]	AST	10 mg/ml[b]	Physically compatible with no change in measured turbidity or increase in particle content in 4 hr at 23 °C	1861	C
TNA #73[f]		32.5 ml[g]	UP	600 mg/ 50 ml[a]	Physically compatible for 4 hr at 25 °C by visual assessment	1008	C

Y-Site Injection Compatibility (1:1 Mixture) (Cont.)

Clindamycin phosphate

Drug	Mfr	Conc	Mfr	Conc	Remarks	Ref	C/I
TNA #218 to #226[f]			AST	10 mg/ml[a]	Visually compatible with no precipitate or emulsion damage apparent in 4 hr at 23 °C	2215	C
TPN #61[f]		[h]	UP	50 mg/ 0.33 ml[i]	Physically compatible	1012	C
		[j]	UP	300 mg/2 ml[i]	Physically compatible	1012	C
TPN #212 to #215[f]			AB	10 mg/ml[a]	Physically compatible with no change in measured turbidity or increase in particle content in 4 hr at 23 °C	2109	C
Vinorelbine tartrate	BW	1 mg/ml[b]	AB	10 mg/ml[b]	Physically compatible with no change in measured turbidity or increase in particle content in 4 hr at 22 °C	1558	C
Vitamin B complex with C (Berocca-C 500)	RC	4 ml/L[a]	UP	600 mg/ 100 ml[a]	Physically compatible for 24 hr at room temperature	323	C
(Berocca-C)	RC	20 ml/L[a]	UP	600 mg/ 100 ml[a]	Physically compatible for 24 hr at room temperature	323	C
Zidovudine	BW	4 mg/ml[a]	UP	12 mg/ml[a]	Physically compatible for 4 hr at 25 °C under fluorescent light by visual and microscopic examination	1193	C

[a]*Tested in dextrose 5% in water.*
[b]*Tested in sodium chloride 0.9%.*
[c]*Tested in both dextrose 5% in water and sodium chloride 0.9%.*
[d]*Tested in dextrose 5% in water, Ringer's injection, lactated, sodium chloride 0.45%, and sodium chloride 0.9%.*
[e]*Lyophilized formulation tested.*
[f]*Refer to Appendix I for the composition of parenteral nutrition solutions. TNA indicates a 3-in-1 admixture, and TPN indicates a 2-in-1 admixture.*
[g]*A 32.5-ml sample of parenteral nutrition solution mixed with 50 ml of antibiotic solution.*
[h]*Run at 21 ml/hr.*
[i]*Given over 10 minutes by syringe pump.*
[j]*Run at 94 ml/hr.*

Additional Compatibility Information

Solutions— Clindamycin phosphate (Upjohn) 6, 9, and 12 mg/ml is physically and chemically stable for 16 days at 25 °C and 32 days at 4 °C in dextrose 5% in water, sodium chloride 0.9%, or Ringer's injection, lactated. When frozen at −10 °C, the solutions are stable for at least eight weeks (4).

Dilution of clindamycin phosphate, using the ADD-Vantage system, to concentrations of 6, 9, and 12 mg/ml in dextrose 5% in water or sodium chloride 0.9% results in solutions that are stable for 24 hours at room temperature or 14 days at 5 °C (4).

Peritoneal Dialysis Solutions— The stability of clindamycin phosphate (Upjohn) 10 mg/L in peritoneal dialysis solutions (Dianeal 137 and PD2) with heparin sodium 500 units/L was evaluated by microbiological assay. Approximately 102 ± 9% activity remained after 24 hours at 25 °C (1228).

Additives— Clindamycin phosphate (Upjohn) is stated to be physi-

cally compatible and stable for 24 hours at room temperature in intravenous infusion solutions containing potassium or vitamin B complex. Additionally, no incompatibility has been demonstrated with cephalothin, gentamicin, kanamycin, or penicillin (2).

Clindamycin phosphate (Upjohn) has been stated to be physically incompatible with aminophylline, ampicillin, barbiturates, calcium gluconate, magnesium sulfate, and phenytoin sodium (2).

Clindamycin phosphate will form a precipitate with various metals. Although it has been stated that there is no incompatibility or inactivation of clindamycin phosphate in intravenous solutions containing calcium, sufficient concentrations of this ion will result in physical instability (102).

Tobramycin sulfate 80 mg/L has been reported to be conditionally compatible with clindamycin phosphate (Upjohn) 600 mg/L. Clindamycin stability is maintained for 24 hours in sodium chloride 0.9%, but an unstable mixture results in dextrose 5% in water (101).

Ceftazidime (Ceptaz) 20 mg/ml is stated to be stable for 24 hours at room temperature or for seven days under refrigeration with clindamycin phosphate 6 mg/ml (4).

CLONIDINE HCL
AHFS 24:08

Duraclon   **Roxane**

Products— Clonidine HCl (Roxane) is available in 10-ml vials. Each milliliter of the preservative-free solution contains clonidine HCl 100 μg and sodium chloride 9 mg in water for injection. Hydrochloric acid and/or sodium hydroxide may have been added to adjust the pH (2).

pH— From 5 to 7 (2).

Administration— Clonidine HCl injection is administered by continuous epidural infusion using an appropriate epidural infusion device. Clonidine HCl injection must not be used with a preservative (2).

Stability— Intact vials containing the clear, colorless solution should be stored at controlled room temperature (2). They are stable for at least six months stored at an elevated temperature of 40 °C, remaining clear and colorless and exhibiting no loss of clonidine HCl by HPLC analysis (2069).

Clonidine HCl (Roxane) 100 μg/ml was filled into plastic syringes (Becton-Dickinson), pump medication reservoirs (Bard), and empty glass vials (Abbott) and stored at 22 to 27 °C for seven days. The solution was also filled into intravenous administration set tubing (Kendall McGaw) and stored under the same conditions. In all cases, the solution remained clear and colorless and little or no loss of potency was found by HPLC analysis (2069).

Clonidine HCl 100 μg/ml was delivered at a rate of 0.1 ml/hr for seven days through two epidural catheter sets, Epi-Cath (Abbott) and Port-A-Cath (Pharmacia Deltec). The temperature was maintained at 37 °C with a water bath to simulate internal use of the set. The delivered clonidine HCl solution remained clear and colorless throughout the study. Furthermore, the solution delivered through the Epi-Cath resulted in little or no loss by HPLC analysis. With the Port-A-Cath, a concentrating effect due to a loss of water was countered by a small clonidine HCl loss of drug (about 5%). The net effect was delivery of about 95% of the clonidine HCl dose (2069).

Drugs in Syringe Compatibility

			Clonidine HCl				
Drug (in syringe)	*Mfr*	*Amt*	*Mfr*	*Amt*	*Remarks*	*Ref*	*C/I*
Bupivacaine HCl with morphine sulfate	PD ES	2 mg/ml 0.2 mg/ml	BI	0.03 mg/ml	Diluted to 5 ml with NS. Visually compatible with no new GC/MS peaks in 1 hr at room temperature	1956	C
Fentanyl citrate with lidocaine HCl	JN AST	0.01 mg/ml 2 mg/ml	BI	0.03 mg/ml	Diluted to 5 ml with NS. Visually compatible with no new GC/MS peaks in 1 hr at room temperature	1956	C
Ketamine HCl with tetracaine HCl	PD SW	2 mg/ml 2 mg/ml	BI	0.03 mg/ml	Diluted to 5 ml with NS. Visually compatible with no new GC/MS peaks in 1 hr at room temperature	1956	C

Y-Site Injection Compatibility (1:1 Mixture)

			Clonidine HCl				
Drug	*Mfr*	*Conc*	*Mfr*	*Conc*	*Remarks*	*Ref*	*C/I*
Lorazepam	WY	0.33 mg/ml[a]	BI	0.015 mg/ml	Visually compatible for 24 hr at 22 °C	1855	C

[a]*Tested in sodium chloride 0.9%.*

Additional Compatibility Information

Bupivacaine HCl— Clonidine HCl (Fujisawa) 100 μg/ml and bupivacaine HCl (Sanofi-Winthrop) 7.5 mg/ml were mixed in ratios of 1:1 and 1:8 to provide final concentrations of (1:1) clonidine HCl 50 μg/ml and bupivacaine HCl 3.75 mg/ml and (1:8) clonidine HCl 11.11 μg/ml and bupivacaine HCl 6.67 mg/ml. The combinations were transferred to flint glass vials with rubber stoppers and stored for 14 days at controlled room temperature protected from light. The solutions remained clear and colorless with no increase in particulate content. HPLC analysis found little or no change in concentration for either drug during the study period (2069).

Morphine Sulfate— Clonidine HCl (Fujisawa) 100 μg/ml and morphine sulfate (Elkins-Sinn) 10 mg/ml were mixed in equal quantities and were transferred to flint glass vials with rubber stoppers and stored for 14 days at controlled room temperature protected from light. The solutions remained clear and colorless with no increase in particulate content. HPLC analysis found little or no change in concentration for either drug during the study period (2069).

Multiple Drugs— A seven-drug combination consisting of bupivacaine HCl (Sanofi Winthrop) 1.5 mg/ml, clonidine HCl (Boehringer Ingelheim) 0.03 mg/ml, fentanyl citrate (Janssen) 0.01 mg/ml, ketamine HCl (Parke-Davis) 2 mg/ml, lidocaine HCl (Astra) 2 mg/ml, morphine sulfate (Elkins-Sinn) 0.2 mg/ml, and tetracaine HCl (Sanofi Winthrop) 2 mg/ml mixed together in equal quantities was found to be visually compatible with no new GC/MS peaks appearing in one hour at room temperature (1956).

Clonidine HCl (Boehringer) 30 μg/ml, bupivacaine HCl (Astra) 3 mg/ml, and morphine HCl (Merck) 6.66 mg/ml were combined in 50-ml ambulatory pump cassette reservoirs (Pharmacia Deltec). The reservoirs were stored at room temperature and protected from light for 90 days. HPLC analysis found no loss of any of the drugs.

Instead, drug concentrations increased 12 to 16% during the observation period, possibly due to loss of water from the solutions (1850).

CODEINE PHOSPHATE
AHFS 28:08.08

Wyeth

Products—— Codeine phosphate is available in concentrations of 15, 30, and 60 mg/ml. The 30-mg/ml concentration is supplied in 1- and 20-ml vials and 1-ml disposable units. The 60-mg/ml concentration is supplied in 1-ml vials and disposable units (4). Each milliliter of solution contains (1-3/23/95):

Codeine phosphate	30 or 60 mg
Edetate disodium	1 mg
Sodium metabisulfite	1.5 or 2 mg
Sodium acetate buffer	present

pH—— From 3 to 6 (4).

Administration—— Codeine phosphate is usually administered by intramuscular or subcutaneous injection, but intravenous injection has also been used (4; 154).

Stability—— Store codeine phosphate injection between 15 and 30 °C and protected from light. Freezing should be avoided. Do not use the injection if it is discolored or contains a precipitate (4).

Compatibility Information

Drugs in Syringe Compatibility

Codeine phosphate

Drug (in syringe)	Mfr	Amt	Mfr	Amt	Remarks	Ref	C/I
Glycopyrrolate	RB	0.2 mg/ 1 ml	LI	30 mg/ 1 ml	Physically compatible and pH in stability range for glycopyrrolate for 48 hr at 25 °C	331	C
	RB	0.2 mg/ 1 ml	LI	60 mg/ 2 ml	Physically compatible and pH in stability range for glycopyrrolate for 48 hr at 25 °C	331	C
	RB	0.4 mg/ 2 ml	LI	30 mg/ 1 ml	Physically compatible and pH in stability range for glycopyrrolate for 48 hr at 25 °C	331	C
Hydroxyzine HCl	PF	50 mg/ 1 ml		120 mg/ 4 ml	Physically compatible	771	C
	PF	100 mg/ 2 ml		60 mg/ 2 ml	Physically compatible	771	C

COLISTIMETHATE SODIUM
AHFS 8:12.28

Coly-Mycin M Parenteral　　　　　　　　**Monarch**

Products—— Colistimethate sodium parenteral (Monarch) is available in vials containing the equivalent of 150 mg of colistin base. The 150-mg vial should be reconstituted with 2 ml of sterile water for injection to yield a solution containing 75 mg/ml of colistin base activity. During reconstitution, the contents of the vials should be gently swirled to avoid frothing (2; 4).

pH—— The pH of the reconstituted solution is 7 to 8 (4).

Administration—— Colistimethate sodium parenteral may be administered by intramuscular injection, by direct intravenous injection

injected slowly over three to five minutes, or by continuous intravenous infusion of half the daily dose at a rate of 5 to 6 mg/hr begun one to two hours after an initial half-daily dose by direct intravenous injection (4).

Stability—— Reconstituted solutions are stable for seven days when stored under refrigeration at 2 to 8 °C or at controlled room temperature (2; 4).

Filtration—— Colistimethate sodium (R. Bellon) 0.16 mg/ml in dextrose 5% in water and sodium chloride 0.9% was filtered through a 0.22-μm cellulose ester membrane filter (Ivex-HP, Millipore) over six hours. No significant drug loss due to binding to the filter was noted (1034).

Compatibility Information

Additive Compatibility

Colistimethate sodium

Drug	Mfr	Conc/L	Mfr	Conc/L	Test Soln	Remarks	Ref	C/I
Amikacin sulfate	BR	5 g	WC	500 mg	D5LR, D5R, D5S, D5W, D10W, IS10, LR, NS, R, SL	Physically compatible and amikacin potency retained for 24 hr at 25 °C. Colistimethate not analyzed	293	C
Ascorbic acid injection	UP	500 mg	WC	500 mg	D5W	Physically compatible	15	C
Chloramphenicol sodium succinate	PD	10 g	WC	500 mg	D5W	Physically compatible	15	C
	PD	10 g	WC	500 mg		Physically compatible	6	C
Cimetidine HCl	SKF	3 g	WC	1.5 g	D5W	Physically compatible and cimetidine chemically stable for 24 hr at room temperature. Colistimethate not tested	551	C
Diphenhydramine HCl	PD	80 mg	WC	500 mg	D5W	Physically compatible	15	C
Erythromycin lactobionate	AB	5 g	WC	500 mg	D5W	Physically incompatible	15	I
	AB	1 g	WC	500 mg	D	Precipitate forms within 1 hr	20	I
Heparin sodium	UP	4000 units	WC	500 mg	D5W	Physically compatible	15	C
	AB	20,000 units	WC	500 mg	D	Physically compatible	21	C
Hydrocortisone sodium succinate	UP	500 mg	WC	500 mg	D5W	Physically incompatible	15	I
Kanamycin sulfate	BR	4 g	WC	500 mg	D5W	Physically incompatible	15	I
Penicillin G potassium	SQ	20 million units	WC	500 mg	D5W	Physically compatible	15	C
	SQ	5 million units	WC	500 mg	D	Physically compatible	47	C
Penicillin G sodium	UP	20 million units	WC	500 mg	D5W	Physically compatible	15	C
Phenobarbital sodium	WI	200 mg	WC	500 mg	D5W	Physically compatible	15	C
Polymyxin B sulfate	BW	200 mg	WC	500 mg	D5W	Physically compatible	15	C
Ranitidine HCl	GL	50 mg and 2 g		1.5 g	D5W	Physically compatible and ranitidine chemically stable by HPLC for 24 hr at 25 °C. Colistimethate not tested	1515	C
Vitamin B complex with C	AB	5 ml	WC	500 mg	D5W	Physically compatible	15	C

Drugs in Syringe Compatibility

Colistimethate sodium

Drug (in syringe)	Mfr	Amt	Mfr	Amt	Remarks	Ref	C/I
Ampicillin sodium	AY	500 mg	PX	40 mg/2 ml	No precipitate or color change within 1 hr at room temperature	99	C
	AY	500 mg	PX	500 mg/2 ml	Physically compatible for 1 hr at room temperature	300	C

Drugs in Syringe Compatibility (Cont.)

Colistimethate sodium

Drug (in syringe)	Mfr	Amt	Mfr	Amt	Remarks	Ref	C/I
Penicillin G sodium		1 million units	PX	40 mg/ 2 ml	No precipitate or color change within 1 hr at room temperature	99	C

Additional Compatibility Information

Infusion Solutions— Colistimethate sodium is physically and chemically compatible with the following infusion solutions (2; 4):

Dextrose 5% in sodium chloride 0.225%
Dextrose 5% in sodium chloride 0.45%
Dextrose 5% in sodium chloride 0.9%
Dextrose 5% in water
Invert sugar 10%
Ringer's injection, lactated
Sodium chloride 0.9%

Additives— Colistimethate sodium is stated to be physically compatible for only four hours at room temperature with lincomycin HCl in infusion solutions (154).

Cefazolin sodium is stated to be incompatible with colistimethate sodium (278).

CORTICOTROPIN
(ACTH)
AHFS 36:04 and 68:28

Acthar   **Aventis**
H.P. Acthar Gel   **Aventis**

Products— Corticotropin (Aventis) is available in vials containing 25 or 40 units of drug with 9 or 14 mg, respectively, of hydrolyzed gelatin. It should be reconstituted with a sufficient quantity of sterile water for injection or sodium chloride 0.9% to yield a solution containing an individual dose in 1 to 2 ml of solution (4).

Repository corticotropin (Aventis) is available in 1- and 5-ml vials. Each milliliter of solution contains 40 or 80 units of corticotropin and 16% gelatin to provide prolonged release. Also present in the formulation are phenol 0.5%, not more than 0.1% cysteine, and sodium hydroxide and/or acetic acid to adjust the pH in water for injection (1-4/96).

Units— One USP unit of corticotropin is equivalent to 1 mg of the international standard (4).

pH— Reconstituted solutions of corticotropin have a pH of 2.5 to 6. Repository corticotropin has a pH of 3 to 7 (4).

Osmolality— Corticotropin 25 units/ml has an osmolality of 89 mOsm/kg (1689).

Administration— Corticotropin may be administered intramuscularly or subcutaneously. It may also be given by direct intravenous injection or by intravenous infusion if the label states that the specific product may be given intravenously (1-4/96; 4).

Stability— Corticotropin (Aventis) is stable for the period noted on the label when stored at room temperature (15 to 30 °C). The reconstituted solution should be refrigerated and used within 24 hours (4) or within eight hours if at room temperature (108).

Repository corticotropin (Aventis) is a colorless or light straw-colored solution. It is stable for the period noted on the label when stored under refrigeration (2 to 8 °C). The solution may be quite viscous even at room temperature (1-4/96; 4). Repository corticotropin is reported to be stable for less than 72 hours at room temperature in intact vials (1181).

Compatibility Information

Solution Compatibility

Corticotropin

Solution	Mfr	Mfr	Conc/L	Remarks	Ref	C/I
Dextrose 5% in sodium chloride 0.9%			500 units	Physically compatible	74	C
Dextrose 5% in water			500 units	Physically compatible	74	C
Ringer's injection, lactated			500 units	Physically compatible	74	C

Solution Compatibility (Cont.)

Corticotropin

Solution	Mfr	Mfr	Conc/L	Remarks	Ref	C/I
Sodium chloride 0.9%			500 units	Physically compatible	74	**C**

Additive Compatibility

Corticotropin

Drug	Mfr	Conc/L	Mfr	Conc/L	Test Soln	Remarks	Ref	C/I
Aminophylline		250 mg		500 units	D5W	Physically compatible	74	**C**
	SE	500 mg	AR, NA	40 units		Precipitate forms within 1 hr	6	**I**
Calcium gluconate		1 g		500 units	D5W	Physically compatible	74	**C**
Chloramphenicol sodium succinate	PD	500 mg		500 units	D5W	Physically compatible	74	**C**
Cytarabine	UP	100 mg	AR	25 units	D5W	Physically compatible for 8 hr	174	**C**
Dimenhydrinate	SE	50 mg		500 units	D5W	Physically compatible	74	**C**
Heparin sodium		12,000 units		500 units	D5W	Physically compatible	74	**C**
Hydrocortisone sodium succinate	UP	100 mg		500 units	D5W	Physically compatible	74	**C**
Norepinephrine bitartrate	WI	8 mg		500 units	D5W	Physically compatible	74	**C**
Oxytetracycline HCl	PF	250 mg		500 units	D5W	Physically compatible	74	**C**
Penicillin G potassium		1 million units		500 units	D5W	Physically compatible	74	**C**
Potassium chloride		3 g		500 units	D5W	Physically compatible	74	**C**
Sodium bicarbonate						Physically incompatible	9	**I**
	AB	80 mEq	AR	250 units	D5W	Physically incompatible	15	**I**
	AB	2.4 mEq[a]	AR	40 units	D5W	Physically compatible for 24 hr	772	**C**
Vancomycin HCl	LI	1 g		500 units	D5W	Physically compatible	74	**C**
Vitamin B complex with C		1 vial		500 units	D5W	Physically compatible	74	**C**

[a]One vial of Neut added to a liter of admixture.

Additional Compatibility Information

Solutions— Dextrose 5% in water (1-4/96; 4), Ringer's injection, lactated, and sodium chloride 0.9% (4) have been recommended as diluents for corticotropin administered by intravenous infusion.

CYANOCOBALAMIN
AHFS 88:08

Products— Cyanocobalamin is available in various strengths ranging from 100 µg/ml to 1 mg/ml in ampuls and vials. Also present are benzyl alcohol, sodium chloride, and either sodium hydroxide or hydrochloric acid for pH adjustment (4; 154).

pH— From 4.5 to 7 (4).

Osmolality— Cyanocobalamin 100 µg/ml has an osmolality of 446 mOsm/kg (1689).

Administration— Cyanocobalamin is administered by intramuscular or deep subcutaneous injection. The intravenous route is not recommended (4).

Stability— The clear pink to red solutions are stable at room temperature and may be autoclaved at 121 °C for short periods such as 15 to 20 minutes. Cyanocobalamin is light sensitive, so protection from light is recommended (4). Exposure to light results in the organometallic bond being cleaved, with the extent of degradation generally increasing with increasing light intensity (1072).

pH Effects— Cyanocobalamin is stable at pH 3 to 7 but is most stable at pH 4.5 to 5 (1072). It is stated to be incompatible with alkaline and strongly acidic solutions (4).

Sorption— Cyanocobalamin (Organon) 30 mg/L did not display significant sorption to a PVC plastic test strip in 24 hours (12).

Filtration— Cyanocobalamin (Wyeth) 1 mg/L in dextrose 5% in water and in sodium chloride 0.9% was filtered at a rate of 120 ml/hr for six hours through a 0.22-µm cellulose ester membrane filter (Ivex-2). No significant reduction in potency due to binding to the filter was noted (533).

Compatibility Information

Solution Compatibility

Cyanocobalamin

Solution	Mfr	Mfr	Conc/L	Remarks	Ref	C/I
Dextran 6% in dextrose 5%	AB	AB	1000 µg	Physically compatible	3	C
Dextran 6% in sodium chloride 0.9%	AB	AB	1000 µg	Physically compatible	3	C
Dextrose–Ringer's injection combinations	AB	AB	1000 µg	Physically compatible	3	C
Dextrose–Ringer's injection, lactated, combinations	AB	AB	1000 µg	Physically compatible	3	C
Dextrose–saline combinations	AB	AB	1000 µg	Physically compatible	3	C
Dextrose 2½% in water	AB	AB	1000 µg	Physically compatible	3	C
Dextrose 5% in water	AB	AB	1000 µg	Physically compatible	3	C
Dextrose 10% in water	AB	AB	1000 µg	Physically compatible	3	C
Fructose 10% in sodium chloride 0.9%	AB	AB	1000 µg	Physically compatible	3	C
Fructose 10% in water	AB	AB	1000 µg	Physically compatible	3	C
Invert sugar 5 and 10% in sodium chloride 0.9%	AB	AB	1000 µg	Physically compatible	3	C
Invert sugar 5 and 10% in water	AB	AB	1000 µg	Physically compatible	3	C
Ionosol products	AB	AB	1000 µg	Physically compatible	3	C
Ringer's injection	AB	AB	1000 µg	Physically compatible	3	C
Ringer's injection, lactated	AB	AB	1000 µg	Physically compatible	3	C
Sodium chloride 0.45%	AB	AB	1000 µg	Physically compatible	3	C
Sodium chloride 0.9%	AB	AB	1000 µg	Physically compatible	3	C
Sodium lactate ⅙ M	AB	AB	1000 µg	Physically compatible	3	C
TPN #11 to #15[a]		SQ	1 mg	Physically compatible for 24 hr at 22 °C. TLC changes of amino acids in similar solutions attributed to M.V.I. or vitamin B complex with C were observed	313	C
TPN #16 to #20[a]		SQ	0.5 and 1 mg	Physically compatible for 24 hr at 22 °C. UV spectra of amino acids solution unaltered	313	C

[a]Refer to Appendix I for the composition of parenteral nutrition solutions. TPN indicates a 2-in-1 admixture.

Additive Compatibility

Drug	Mfr	Conc/L	Mfr	Conc/L	Test Soln	Remarks	Ref	C/I
Ascorbic acid injection	AB	1 g	AB	1000 μg		Physically compatible	3	**C**
Chloramphenicol sodium succinate	PD	1 g	AB	1000 μg		Physically compatible	6	**C**
Metaraminol bitartrate	MSD	100 mg	AB	1000 μg		Physically compatible	7	**C**
Vitamin B complex with C	AB	2 ml	AB	1000 μg		Physically compatible	3	**C**

Y-Site Injection Compatibility (1:1 Mixture)

Cyanocobalamin

Drug	Mfr	Conc	Mfr	Conc	Remarks	Ref	C/I
Heparin sodium	UP	1000 units/L[a]	PD	0.1 mg/ml	Physically compatible for at least 4 hr at room temperature by visual and microscopic examination	534	**C**
Hydrocortisone sodium succinate	UP	10 mg/L[a]	PD	0.1 mg/ml	Physically compatible for at least 4 hr at room temperature by visual and microscopic examination	534	**C**
Potassium chloride	AB	40 mEq/L[a]	PD	0.1 mg/ml	Physically compatible for at least 4 hr at room temperature by visual and microscopic examination	534	**C**
Vitamin B complex with C	RC	2 ml/L[a]	PD	0.1 mg/ml	Physically compatible for at least 4 hr at room temperature by visual and microscopic examination	534	**C**

[a]*Tested in dextrose 5% in Ringer's injection, dextrose 5% in Ringer's injection, lactated, dextrose 5% in water, Ringer's injection, lactated, and sodium chloride 0.9%.*

Additional Compatibility Information

Additives—— It has been stated that cyanocobalamin with ascorbic acid can be stored for 24 hours at room temperature protected from light without loss of activity. It also has been stated that the drug is compatible with other vitamins of the B complex and with iron–dextran complex (52).

Some incompatibilities of cyanocobalamin reported in the literature were actually due to hydroxocobalamin, which was formerly present as a contaminant (52).

Cyanocobalamin (Abbott) 1000 μg/L has been reported to be conditionally compatible with hydrocortisone sodium succinate (Upjohn) 250 mg/L. The mixture is physically compatible in most Abbott infusion solutions except Ionosol D-CM with dextrose 5% with which a haze or precipitate is noted within 24 hours (3).

Cyanocobalamin injection has been reported to be incompatible with ascorbic acid, chlorpromazine HCl, dextrose, phytonadione, prochlorperazine edisylate, and warfarin sodium. It is also stated to be incompatible with heavy metals, oxidizing agents, and reducing agents (4).

CYCLOPHOSPHAMIDE
AHFS 10:00

Cytoxan **Bristol-Myers Squibb**

Products— Cyclophosphamide (Bristol-Myers Squibb) is available as a lyophilized product in vials containing cyclophosphamide 100, 200, and 500 mg and 1 and 2 g with 75 mg of mannitol per 100 mg of drug. Reconstitute the vials with sterile water for injection (2; 4) or bacteriostatic water for injection (paraben preserved only) in the following amounts (4):

Vial Size	Volume of Diluent
100 mg	5 ml
200 mg	10 ml
500 mg	20 to 25 ml
1 g	50 ml
2 g	80 to 100 ml

Shake the vials to dissolve the powder (2). The lyophilized products yield solutions with concentrations of 20 to 25 mg/ml (4).

pH— Reconstituted solutions have a pH of 3 to 9 (17). A 22-mg/ml solution was found to have a pH of 6.87 (126).

Osmolarity— The lyophilized product, reconstituted to 20 or 25 mg/ml, has an osmolarity of 172 or 219 mOsm/L, respectively (2; 4).

Administration— Cyclophosphamide may be administered intramuscularly, intraperitoneally, intrapleurally, by direct intravenous injection, or by continuous or intermittent intravenous infusion (2; 4; 8; 338).

Stability— Cyclophosphamide products should not be stored at temperatures above 25 °C, although they will withstand brief exposures to temperatures up to 30 °C. Reconstituted solutions should be used within 24 hours if stored at room temperature or within six days if stored under refrigeration (2; 4). When reconstituted with sterile water for injection or paraben-preserved bacteriostatic water for injection to a concentration of 21 mg/ml, less than 1.5% cyclophosphamide decomposition will occur within eight hours at 24 to 27 °C and within six days at 5 °C. The rate constant for decomposition of cyclophosphamide when reconstituted with benzyl alcohol-preserved bacteriostatic water for injection is significantly higher than with sterile water for injection. It was suggested that benzyl alcohol may catalyze somewhat the decomposition of cyclophosphamide (125). The rate of decomposition is independent of pH over the range of 2 to 10 (1369).

Heating cyclophosphamide solutions at a concentration of 21 mg/ml to 50 and 60 °C for 15 minutes resulted in a negligible loss of potency. However, heating to 70 and 80 °C for 15 minutes resulted in approximately 10 and 23% decomposition, respectively. The use of heat to speed dissolution is, therefore, not recommended since decomposition of cyclophosphamide may result in poorly controlled situations (126).

Kirk et al. evaluated the stability of cyclophosphamide 20 mg/ml, reconstituted with sterile water for injection and stored in various containers at several temperatures. In glass ampuls at 20 to 23 °C, approximately 13 and 35% were lost in one and four weeks, respectively. Under refrigeration at 4 °C or frozen at −20 °C, the solution lost not more than 3% over four weeks (1090).

In polypropylene syringes (Plastipak, Becton-Dickinson) sealed with blind Luer locking hubs, the 20-mg/ml cyclophosphamide solution similarly lost about 3% in four weeks at 4 °C and about 10% in 11 to 14 weeks. When frozen at −20 °C (with microwave thawing), the solution lost about 4% in 19 weeks. However, the syringe plungers contracted markedly during freezing, resulting in drug solution seeping past the plunger onto the inner surface of the barrel. This seeping poses the risk of bacterial contamination. Furthermore, cyclophosphamide precipitated during microwave thawing and required vigorous shaking for five minutes to redissolve. This precipitation during thawing appears not to occur at concentrations less than 8 mg/ml (1090).

Further diluted to a concentration of 2 g/500 ml of sodium chloride 0.9% in PVC bags, cyclophosphamide remained relatively stable at 4 °C and frozen at −20 °C (with microwave thawing), with no loss in four weeks and about an 8% loss in 19 weeks (1090).

pH Effects— Cyclophosphamide exhibits maximum solution stability over the pH range of 2 to 11; the rate of decomposition is essentially the same over this broad pH range. At pH values less than 2 and above 11, increased rates of decomposition have been observed (2002).

Compatibility Information

Solution Compatibility

Cyclophosphamide

Solution	Mfr	Mfr	Conc/L	Remarks	Ref	C/I
Amino acids 4.25%, dextrose 25%	MG	MJ	500 mg	No increase in particulate matter in 24 hr at 5 °C	349	**C**
Dextrose 5% in sodium chloride 0.9%	CU	MJ	100 mg	1.5% decomposition or less in 8 hr at 24 to 27 °C and 6 days at 5 °C	125	**C**
	CU	MJ	3.1 g	1.5% decomposition or less in 8 hr at 24 to 27 °C and 6 days at 5 °C	125	**C**
Dextrose 5% in water	CU	MJ	100 mg	1.5% decomposition or less in 8 hr at 24 to 27 °C and 6 days at 5 °C	125	**C**
	CU	MJ	3.1 g	1.5% decomposition or less in 8 hr at 24 to 27 °C and 6 days at 5 °C	125	**C**
	TR[a]	MJ	6.6 g	Less than 10% decrease in 24 hr at room temperature	519	**C**

Solution Compatibility (Cont.)

				Cyclophosphamide		
Solution	Mfr	Mfr	Conc/L	Remarks	Ref	C/I
	MG, TR[b]		6.7 g	Less than 10% cyclophosphamide loss by HPLC in 24 hr at room temperature exposed to light	1658	C
Sodium chloride 0.9%		MJ	4 g	3.5% decomposition in 24 hr at room temperature	127	C
		MJ	4 g	1% decomposition in 4 weeks under refrigeration	127	C
	TR	CE	4 g[c]	Physically compatible with no cyclophosphamide loss in 4 weeks and 8% in 19 weeks at 4 and −20 °C	1090	C

[a]Tested in both glass and PVC containers.
[b]Tested in glass, PVC, and polyolefin containers.
[c]Tested in PVC containers.

Additive Compatibility

						Cyclophosphamide		
Drug	Mfr	Conc/L	Mfr	Conc/L	Test Soln	Remarks	Ref	C/I
Cisplatin with etoposide		200 mg 200 mg		2 g	NS	All drugs stable for 7 days at room temperature	1379	C
Fluorouracil		8.3 g		1.67 g	NS	Both drugs stable for 15 days at room temperature	1389	C
Hydroxyzine HCl	LY	500 mg	AD	1 g	D5W[a]	Physically compatible for 48 hr	1190	C
Methotrexate sodium		25 mg		1.67 g	NS	6.6% cyclophosphamide loss in 14 days at room temperature	1379; 1389	C
Methotrexate sodium with fluorouracil		25 mg 8.3 g		1.67 g	NS	9.3% cyclophosphamide loss in 7 days at room temperature. No loss of other drugs observed	1389	C
Mitoxantrone HCl	LE	500 mg	AD	10 g	D5W	Visually compatible and mitoxantrone potency by HPLC retained for 24 hr at room temperature. Cyclophosphamide not tested	1531	C
Ondansetron HCl	GL	50 mg	MJ	300 mg	D5W[b], NS[b]	Visually compatible with 9 to 10% cyclophosphamide loss and no ondansetron loss by HPLC in 5 days at 24 °C. No loss of either drug in 8 days at 4 °C	1812	C
	GL	400 mg	MJ	2 g	D5W[b], NS[b]	Visually compatible with 10% cyclophosphamide loss and no ondansetron loss by HPLC in 5 days at 24 °C. No loss of either drug in 8 days at 4 °C	1812	C

[a]Tested in glass containers.
[b]Tested in PVC containers.

Drugs in Syringe Compatibility

					Cyclophosphamide		
Drug (in syringe)	Mfr	Amt	Mfr	Amt	Remarks	Ref	C/I
Bleomycin sulfate		1.5 units/ 0.5 ml		10 mg/ 0.5 ml	Physically compatible for 5 min at room temperature followed by 8 min of centrifugation	980	C

Drugs in Syringe Compatibility (Cont.)

Cyclophosphamide

Drug (in syringe)	Mfr	Amt	Mfr	Amt	Remarks	Ref	C/I
Cisplatin		0.5 mg/ 0.5 ml		10 mg/ 0.5 ml	Physically compatible for 5 min at room temperature followed by 8 min of centrifugation	980	C
Doxapram HCl	RB	400 mg/ 20 ml		100 mg/ 5 ml	Physically compatible with 2% doxapram loss in 24 hr	1177	C
Doxorubicin HCl		1 mg/ 0.5 ml		10 mg/ 0.5 ml	Physically compatible for 5 min at room temperature followed by 8 min of centrifugation	980	C
Droperidol		1.25 mg/ 0.5 ml		10 mg/ 0.5 ml	Physically compatible for 5 min at room temperature followed by 8 min of centrifugation	980	C
Fluorouracil		25 mg/ 0.5 ml		10 mg/ 0.5 ml	Physically compatible for 5 min at room temperature followed by 8 min of centrifugation	980	C
Furosemide		5 mg/ 0.5 ml		10 mg/ 0.5 ml	Physically compatible for 5 min at room temperature followed by 8 min of centrifugation	980	C
Heparin sodium		500 units/ 0.5 ml		10 mg/ 0.5 ml	Physically compatible for 5 min at room temperature followed by 8 min of centrifugation	980	C
Leucovorin calcium		5 mg/ 0.5 ml		10 mg/ 0.5 ml	Physically compatible for 5 min at room temperature followed by 8 min of centrifugation	980	C
Methotrexate sodium		12.5 mg/ 0.5 ml		10 mg/ 0.5 ml	Physically compatible for 5 min at room temperature followed by 8 min of centrifugation	980	C
Metoclopramide HCl		2.5 mg/ 0.5 ml		10 mg/ 0.5 ml	Physically compatible for 5 min at room temperature followed by 8 min of centrifugation	980	C
	RB	10 mg/ 2 ml	MJ	40 mg/ 2 ml	Physically compatible for 24 hr at room temperature	924	C
	RB	10 mg/ 2 ml	MJ	40 mg/ 2 ml	Physically compatible for 24 hr at 25 °C	1167	C
	RB	10 mg/ 2 ml	MJ	1 g/ 50 ml	Physically compatible for 24 hr at 25 °C	1167	C
	RB	160 mg/ 32 ml	MJ	1 g/ 50 ml	Physically compatible for 24 hr at 25 °C	1167	C
Mitomycin		0.25 mg/ 0.5 ml		10 mg/ 0.5 ml	Physically compatible for 5 min at room temperature followed by 8 min of centrifugation	980	C
Vinblastine sulfate		0.5 mg/ 0.5 ml		10 mg/ 0.5 ml	Physically compatible for 5 min at room temperature followed by 8 min of centrifugation	980	C
Vincristine sulfate		0.5 mg/ 0.5 ml		10 mg/ 0.5 ml	Physically compatible for 5 min at room temperature followed by 8 min of centrifugation	980	C

Y-Site Injection Compatibility (1:1 Mixture)

					Cyclophosphamide		
Drug	*Mfr*	*Conc*	*Mfr*	*Conc*	*Remarks*	*Ref*	*C/I*
Allopurinol sodium	BW	3 mg/ml[b]	MJ	10 mg/ml[b]	Physically compatible with no change in measured turbidity or increase in particle content in 4 hr at 22 °C	1686	**C**
Amifostine	USB	10 mg/ml[a]	MJ	10 mg/ml[a]	Physically compatible with no change in measured turbidity or increase in particle content in 4 hr at 23 °C	1845	**C**
Amikacin sulfate	BR	5 mg/ml[a]	MJ	20 mg/ml[a]	Physically compatible for 4 hr at 25 °C	1194	**C**
Amphotericin B cholesteryl sulfate complex	SEQ	0.83 mg/ml[a]	MJ	10 mg/ml[a]	Increased turbidity forms immediately	2117	**I**
Ampicillin sodium	BR	20 mg/ml[b]	MJ	20 mg/ml[a]	Physically compatible for 4 hr at 25 °C	1194	**C**
Azlocillin sodium	MI	20 mg/ml[a]	MJ	20 mg/ml[a]	Physically compatible for 4 hr at 25 °C	1194	**C**
Aztreonam	SQ	40 mg/ml[a]	MJ	10 mg/ml[a]	Physically compatible with no subvisual haze or particle formation in 4 hr at 23 °C	1758	**C**
Bleomycin sulfate		3 units/ml		20 mg/ml	Drugs injected sequentially into Y-site with no flush between. No visually apparent precipitate	980	**C**
Cefamandole nafate	LI	20 mg/ml[a]	MJ	20 mg/ml[a]	Physically compatible for 4 hr at 25 °C	1194	**C**
Cefazolin sodium	SKF	20 mg/ml[a]	MJ	20 mg/ml[a]	Physically compatible for 4 hr at 25 °C	1194	**C**
Cefepime HCl	BR	20 mg/ml[a]	MJ	10 mg/ml[a]	Physically compatible with no change in measured turbidity or increase in particle content in 4 hr at 22 °C	1689	**C**
Cefoperazone sodium	RR	20 mg/ml[a]	MJ	20 mg/ml[a]	Physically compatible for 4 hr at 25 °C	1194	**C**
Cefotaxime sodium	HO	20 mg/ml[a]	MJ	20 mg/ml[a]	Physically compatible for 4 hr at 25 °C	1194	**C**
Cefoxitin sodium	MSD	20 mg/ml[a]	MJ	20 mg/ml[a]	Physically compatible for 4 hr at 25 °C	1194	**C**
Cefuroxime sodium	GL	30 mg/ml[a]	MJ	20 mg/ml[a]	Physically compatible for 4 hr at 25 °C	1194	**C**
Chloramphenicol sodium succinate	ES	20 mg/ml[a]	MJ	20 mg/ml[a]	Physically compatible for 4 hr at 25 °C	1194	**C**
Chlorpromazine HCl	SKF	2 mg/ml[a]	MJ	10 mg/ml[a]	Visually compatible for 4 hr at room temperature under fluorescent light	1685	**C**
Cimetidine HCl	SKF	12 mg/ml[a]	MJ	10 mg/ml[a]	Visually compatible for 4 hr at room temperature under fluorescent light	1685	**C**
Cisplatin		1 mg/ml		20 mg/ml	Drugs injected sequentially into Y-site with no flush between. No visually apparent precipitate	980	**C**
Cladribine	ORT	0.015[b] and 0.5[c] mg/ml	MJ	10 mg/ml[b]	Physically compatible with no change in measured turbidity or increase in particle content in 4 hr at 23 °C	1969	**C**
Clindamycin phosphate	UP	12 mg/ml[a]	MJ	20 mg/ml[a]	Physically compatible for 4 hr at 25 °C	1194	**C**
Dexamethasone sodium phosphate	QU	1 mg/ml[a]	MJ	10 mg/ml[a]	Visually compatible for 4 hr at room temperature under fluorescent light	1685	**C**
Diphenhydramine HCl	PD	2 mg/ml[a]	MJ	10 mg/ml[a]	Visually compatible for 4 hr at room temperature under fluorescent light	1685	**C**
Doxorubicin HCl		2 mg/ml		20 mg/ml	Drugs injected sequentially into Y-site with no flush between. No visually apparent precipitate	980	**C**

Y-Site Injection Compatibility (1:1 Mixture) (Cont.)

Cyclophosphamide

Drug	Mfr	Conc	Mfr	Conc	Remarks	Ref	C/I
Doxorubicin HCl liposome injection	SEQ	0.4 mg/ml[a]	MJ	10 mg/ml[a]	Physically compatible with little or no change in measured turbidity and no increase in particle content in 4 hr at 23 °C	2087	C
Doxycycline hyclate	ES	1 mg/ml[a]	MJ	20 mg/ml[a]	Physically compatible for 4 hr at 25 °C	1194	C
Droperidol		2.5 mg/ml		20 mg/ml	Drugs injected sequentially into Y-site with no flush between. No visually apparent precipitate	980	C
	JN	20 µg/ml[a]	MJ	10 mg/ml[a]	Visually compatible for 4 hr at room temperature under fluorescent light	1685	C
Erythromycin lactobionate	AB	5 mg/ml[a]	MJ	20 mg/ml[a]	Physically compatible for 4 hr at 25 °C	1194	C
Etoposide phosphate	BR	5 mg/ml[a]	MJ	10 mg/ml[a]	Physically compatible with no change in measured turbidity or increase in particle content in 4 hr at 23 °C	2218	C
Famotidine	MSD	2 mg/ml[a]	MJ	10 mg/ml[a]	Visually compatible for 4 hr at room temperature under fluorescent light	1685	C
Filgrastim	AMG	30 µg/ml[a]	MJ	10 mg/ml[a]	Physically compatible with no change in measured turbidity or increase in particle content in 4 hr at 22 °C	1687	C
Fludarabine phosphate	BX	1 mg/ml[a]	MJ	10 mg/ml[a]	Physically compatible for 4 hr at room temperature under fluorescent light	1439	C
Fluorouracil		50 mg/ml		20 mg/ml	Drugs injected sequentially into Y-site with no flush between. No visually apparent precipitate	980	C
Furosemide		10 mg/ml		20 mg/ml	Drugs injected sequentially into Y-site with no flush between. No visually apparent precipitate	980	C
	ES	3 mg/ml[a]	MJ	10 mg/ml[a]	Visually compatible for 4 hr at room temperature under fluorescent light	1685	C
Ganciclovir sodium	SY	20 mg/ml[a]	MJ	10 mg/ml[a]	Visually compatible for 4 hr at room temperature under fluorescent light	1685	C
Gemcitabine HCl	LI	10 mg/ml[b]	BR	10 mg/ml[b]	Physically compatible with no change in measured turbidity or increase in particle content in 4 hr at 23 °C	2226	C
Gentamicin sulfate	TR	1.6 mg/ml[a]	MJ	20 mg/ml[a]	Physically compatible for 4 hr at 25 °C	1194	C
Granisetron HCl	SKB	1 mg/ml	MJ	2 mg/ml[b]	Physically compatible with little or no loss of either drug by HPLC in 4 hr at 22 °C	1883	C
Heparin sodium		1000 units/ml		20 mg/ml	Drugs injected sequentially into Y-site with no flush between. No visually apparent precipitate	980	C
	SO	40 units/ml[a]	MJ	10 mg/ml[a]	Visually compatible for 4 hr at room temperature under fluorescent light	1685	C
Hydromorphone HCl	ES	0.04 mg/ml[a]	MJ	10 mg/ml[a]	Visually compatible for 4 hr at room temperature under fluorescent light	1685	C
Idarubicin HCl	AD	1 mg/ml[b]	CET	4 mg/ml[a]	Visually compatible for 24 hr at 25 °C	1525	C
Kanamycin sulfate	BR	2.5 mg/ml[a]	MJ	20 mg/ml[a]	Physically compatible for 4 hr at 25 °C	1194	C

Y-Site Injection Compatibility (1:1 Mixture) (Cont.)

Drug	Mfr	Conc	Mfr	Conc	Remarks	Ref	C/I
				Cyclophosphamide			
Leucovorin calcium		10 mg/ml		20 mg/ml	Drugs injected sequentially into Y-site with no flush between. No visually apparent precipitate	980	C
Lorazepam	WY	0.1 mg/ml[a]	MJ	10 mg/ml[a]	Visually compatible for 4 hr at room temperature under fluorescent light	1685	C
Melphalan HCl	BW	0.1 mg/ml[b]	BR	10 mg/ml[b]	Physically compatible with no change in measured turbidity or increase in particle content in 3 hr at 22 °C	1557	C
Methotrexate sodium		25 mg/ml		20 mg/ml	Drugs injected sequentially into Y-site with no flush between. No visually apparent precipitate	980	C
		30 mg/ml		20 mg/ml[a]	Visually compatible for 4 hr at room temperature	1788	C
Methylprednisolone sodium succinate	UP	0.5 mg/ml[a]	MJ	10 mg/ml[a]	Visually compatible for 4 hr at room temperature under fluorescent light	1685	C
Metoclopramide HCl		5 mg/ml		20 mg/ml	Drugs injected sequentially into Y-site with no flush between. No visually apparent precipitate	980	C
	RB	2.5 mg/ml[a]	MJ	10 mg/ml[a]	Visually compatible for 4 hr at room temperature under fluorescent light	1685	C
Metronidazole	SE	5 mg/ml	MJ	20 mg/ml[a]	Physically compatible for 4 hr at 25 °C	1194	C
Minocycline HCl	LE	0.2 mg/ml[a]	MJ	20 mg/ml[a]	Physically compatible for 4 hr at 25 °C	1194	C
Mitomycin		0.5 mg/ml		20 mg/ml	Drugs injected sequentially into Y-site with no flush between. No visually apparent precipitate	980	C
Morphine sulfate	ES	0.12 mg/ml[a]	MJ	10 mg/ml[a]	Visually compatible for 4 hr at room temperature under fluorescent light	1685	C
Nafcillin sodium	WY	20 mg/ml[a]	MJ	20 mg/ml[a]	Physically compatible for 4 hr at 25 °C	1194	C
Ondansetron HCl	GL	1 mg/ml[b]	MJ	10 mg/ml[a]	Physically compatible for 4 hr at 22 °C	1365	C
	GL	16 to 160 µg/ml		20 mg/ml	Physically compatible when cyclophosphamide given as 5-min bolus via Y-site	1366	C
Oxacillin sodium	BE	20 mg/ml[a]	MJ	20 mg/ml[a]	Physically compatible for 4 hr at 25 °C	1194	C
Paclitaxel	NCI	1.2 mg/ml[a]		10 mg/ml[a]	Physically compatible with no change in measured turbidity in 4 hr at 22 °C	1528	C
Penicillin G potassium	PF	100,000 units/ml[a]	MJ	20 mg/ml[a]	Physically compatible for 4 hr at 25 °C	1194	C
Piperacillin sodium	LE	60 mg/ml[a]	MJ	20 mg/ml[a]	Physically compatible for 4 hr at 25 °C	1194	C
Piperacillin sodium–tazobactam sodium	LE	40 + 5 mg/ml[a]	MJ	10 mg/ml[a]	Physically compatible with no change in measured turbidity or increase in particle content in 4 hr at 22 °C	1688	C
Prochlorperazine edisylate	SKF	0.5 mg/ml[a]	MJ	10 mg/ml[a]	Visually compatible for 4 hr at room temperature under fluorescent light	1685	C
Promethazine HCl	WY	2 mg/ml[a]	MJ	10 mg/ml[a]	Visually compatible for 4 hr at room temperature under fluorescent light	1685	C
Propofol	ZEN	10 mg/ml	MJ	10 mg/ml[a]	Physically compatible for 1 hr at 23 °C with no increase in particle content	2066	C

Y-Site Injection Compatibility (1:1 Mixture) (Cont.)

| | | | Cyclophosphamide | | | | |
Drug	Mfr	Conc	Mfr	Conc	Remarks	Ref	C/I
Ranitidine HCl	GL	1 mg/ml[a]	MJ	10 mg/ml[a]	Visually compatible for 4 hr at room temperature under fluorescent light	1685	C
Sargramostim	IMM	10 µg/ml[b]	MJ	10 mg/ml[b]	Physically compatible for 4 hr at 22 °C	1436	C
Sodium bicarbonate		1.4%		20 mg/ml[a]	Visually compatible for 4 hr at room temperature	1788	C
Teniposide	BR	0.1 mg/ml[a]	MJ	10 mg/ml[a]	Physically compatible with no subvisual haze or particle formation in 4 hr at 23 °C	1725	C
Thiotepa	IMM[d]	1 mg/ml[a]	MJ	10 mg/ml[a]	Physically compatible with no change in measured turbidity or increase in particle content in 4 hr at 23 °C	1861	C
Ticarcillin disodium	BE	30 mg/ml[a]	MJ	20 mg/ml[a]	Physically compatible for 4 hr at 25 °C	1194	C
Ticarcillin disodium–clavulanate potassium	BE	31 mg/ml[a]	MJ	20 mg/ml[a]	Physically compatible for 4 hr at 25 °C	1194	C
TNA #218 to #226[e]			MJ	10 mg/ml[a]	Visually compatible with no precipitate or emulsion damage apparent in 4 hr at 23 °C	2215	C
Tobramycin sulfate	DI	0.8 mg/ml[a]	MJ	20 mg/ml[a]	Physically compatible for 4 hr at 25 °C	1194	C
TPN #212 to #215[e]			MJ	10 mg/ml[a]	Physically compatible with no change in measured turbidity or increase in particle content in 4 hr at 23 °C	2109	C
Trimethoprim–sulfamethoxazole	BW	0.8 + 4 mg/ml[a]	MJ	20 mg/ml[a]	Physically compatible for 4 hr at 25 °C	1194	C
Vancomycin HCl	LI	5 mg/ml[a]	MJ	20 mg/ml[a]	Physically compatible for 4 hr at 25 °C	1194	C
Vinblastine sulfate		1 mg/ml		20 mg/ml	Drugs injected sequentially into Y-site with no flush between. No visually apparent precipitate	980	C
Vincristine sulfate		1 mg/ml		20 mg/ml	Drugs injected sequentially into Y-site with no flush between. No visually apparent precipitate	980	C
Vinorelbine tartrate	BW	1 mg/ml[b]	MJ	10 mg/ml[b]	Physically compatible with no change in measured turbidity or increase in particle content in 4 hr at 22 °C	1558	C

[a]*Tested in dextrose 5% in water.*
[b]*Tested in sodium chloride 0.9%.*
[c]*Tested in bacteriostatic sodium chloride 0.9% preserved with benzyl alcohol 0.9%.*
[d]*Lyophilized formulation tested.*
[e]*Refer to Appendix I for the composition of parenteral nutrition solutions. TNA indicates a 3-in-1 admixture, and TPN indicates a 2-in-1 admixture.*

Additional Compatibility Information

Solutions— The following solutions have been recommended as diluents for intravenous infusion (2):

Dextrose 5% in Ringer's injection
Dextrose 5% in sodium chloride 0.9%
Dextrose 5% in water
Ringer's injection, lactated
Sodium chloride 0.45%
Sodium lactate ⅙ M

Dacarbazine— No alteration in the ultraviolet/visible spectra was observed when dacarbazine was combined in solution with cyclophosphamide (492).

Aluminum— Ogawa et al. reported that immersion of a needle with an aluminum component in cyclophosphamide (Adria) 20 mg/ml resulted in a slight darkening of the aluminum and gas production after a few days at 24 °C with protection from light (988).

Mesna— Cyclophosphamide is stated to be stable for 24 hours in dextrose 5% in water or Ringer's injection, lactated, when admixed with mesna (4; 1292).

CYCLOSPORINE
AHFS 92:00

Sandimmune   **Sandoz**

Products— Cyclosporine (Sandoz) is available as a concentrate in 5-ml ampuls. Each milliliter of the sterile solution contains cyclosporine 50 mg, polyoxyethylated castor oil (Cremophor EL) 650 mg, and alcohol 278 mg (32.9%) (2; 874).

Nitrogen is utilized as the atmosphere in the sealed ampuls. Cyclosporine concentrate must be diluted before administration (2; 874).

Administration— Cyclosporine concentrate for injection is administered over two to six hours by intravenous infusion after dilution. Each milliliter of concentrate should be diluted in 20 to 100 ml of dextrose 5% in water or sodium chloride 0.9% (2; 4).

Stability— Cyclosporine injection is a clear, faintly brown-yellow solution. It should be stored below 30 °C and protected from light and freezing (2; 4; 874). Light protection is not required for intravenous admixtures of cyclosporine (4; 1091).

Sorption— Simulated infusion studies of cyclosporine (Sandoz) 2 mg/ml in dextrose 5% in water and sodium chloride 0.9% were performed at a rate of 0.67 mg/ml over 75 minutes through 70-inch microdrip administration sets (Abbott). Significant amounts of cyclosporine were lost, presumably as a result of sorption to the tubing. Approximately 7% of the dose was lost from the dextrose 5% in water admixture, and about 13% was lost from the sodium chloride 0.9% admixture. The authors noted that as much as 30% of a pediatric dose could be lost (1091).

In contrast, Parr et al. did not find any significant cyclosporine loss when 2.38 and 0.495 mg/ml in dextrose 5% in water and sodium chloride 0.9%, in either glass or PVC containers, were delivered over six hours by an electronic infusion pump (1154).

Filtration— Parr et al. reported that the use of either a 0.22- or 0.45-μm filter reduced the delivered cyclosporine concentration from 2.38- and 0.495-mg/ml solutions in dextrose 5% in water and sodium chloride 0.9%. They found a significant (but unspecified) decrease in the first sample, taken at one minute. At the six-hour time point, the concentration had returned to the original concentration. The total amount of drug delivered over six hours was not quantified (1154).

Compatibility Information

Solution Compatibility

Cyclosporine

Solution	Mfr	Mfr	Conc/L	Remarks	Ref	C/I
Amino acids 5%, dextrose 25%	MG	SZ	150 mg	Visually compatible with no cyclosporine loss by HPLC in 72 hr at 21 °C	1616	C
Dextrose 5% in water	AB[a]	SZ	2 g	Physically compatible with no cyclosporine loss in 24 hr at 24 °C in the dark or light	1091	C
	AB[b]	SZ	2 g	Physically compatible with 5% cyclosporine loss in 48 hr at 24 °C under fluorescent light and refrigerated at 6 °C	1330	C
	BA	SZ	1 g	Visually compatible with no cyclosporine loss by HPLC in 72 hr at 21 °C	1616	C
Fat emulsion 10%, intravenous	AB	SZ	400 mg	No cyclosporine loss by HPLC in 72 hr at 21 °C	1616	C
Fat emulsion 10 and 20%, intravenous	KA	SZ	500 mg and 2 g	Physically compatible by visual examination and particle size assessment with no cyclosporine loss by HPLC in 48 hr at 24 °C under fluorescent light	1625	C
Sodium chloride 0.9%	AB[a]	SZ	2 g	Physically compatible with 7 to 8% cyclosporine loss in 24 hr at 24 °C in the dark or light	1091	C

[a]*Tested in both glass and PVC containers.*
[b]*Tested in glass bottles.*

Additive Compatibility

Cyclosporine

Drug	Mfr	Conc/L	Mfr	Conc/L	Test Soln	Remarks	Ref	C/I
Ciprofloxacin	BAY	2 g	SZ	500 mg	NS	Visually compatible with about 8% ciprofloxacin loss by HPLC in 24 hr at 25 °C. Cyclosporine not tested	1934	C

Additive Compatibility (Cont.)

Cyclosporine

Drug	Mfr	Conc/L	Mfr	Conc/L	Test Soln	Remarks	Ref	C/I
Magnesium sulfate	LY	30 g	SZ	2 g	D5W	Transient turbidity appears upon preparation but dissipates in 30 sec and remains clear for 36 hr at 24 °C. 5% cyclosporine loss in 6 hr and 10% loss in 12 hr by HPLC at 24 °C under fluorescent light	1629	I

Y-Site Injection Compatibility (1:1 Mixture)

Cyclosporine

Drug	Mfr	Conc	Mfr	Conc	Remarks	Ref	C/I
Amphotericin B cholesteryl sulfate complex	SEQ	0.83 mg/ml[a]	SZ	5 mg/ml[a]	Decreased natural turbidity occurs immediately	2117	I
Propofol	ZEN	10 mg/ml	SZ	5 mg/ml[a]	Physically compatible for 1 hr at 23 °C with no increase in particle content	2066	C
Sargramostim	IMM	6[c] and 15[b] μg/ml	SZ	5 mg/ml[b]	Visually compatible for 2 hr	1618	C
TNA #220 and #223[d]			SZ	5 mg/ml[a]	Small amount of precipitate forms immediately	2215	I
TNA #218, #219, #221, #222, #224 to #226[d]			SZ	5 mg/ml[a]	Visually compatible with no precipitate or emulsion damage apparent in 4 hr at 23 °C	2215	C
TPN #212 and #213[d]			SZ	5 mg/ml[a]	Physically compatible with no change in measured turbidity or increase in particle content in 4 hr at 23 °C	2109	C
TPN #214 and #215[d]			SZ	5 mg/ml[a]	Small amount of subvisual precipitate forms in 4 hr	2109	I

[a]*Tested in dextrose 5% in water.*
[b]*Tested in sodium chloride 0.9%.*
[c]*Tested in sodium chloride 0.9% with human albumin 0.1%.*
[d]*Refer to Appendix I for the composition of parenteral nutrition solutions. TNA indicates a 3-in-1 admixture, and TPN indicates a 2-in-1 admixture.*

Additional Compatibility Information

Solutions— Dextrose 5% in water and sodium chloride 0.9% are recommended for dilution of cyclosporine concentrate (2; 4). Although the drug is stable for 24 hours in these solutions (1091), it has been suggested that admixtures in sodium chloride 0.9% be considered usable for six hours in PVC containers and 12 hours in glass containers because of the combined losses from storage and sorption through PVC tubing (4). However, see Plasticizer Extraction.

Plasticizer Extraction— Polyoxyethylated castor oil (Cremophor EL), a nonionic surfactant, may leach phthalate from PVC containers such as bags of infusion solutions (2; 4). An acceptability limit of no more than 5 parts per million (5 μg/ml) for DEHP plasticizer released from PVC containers, etc. has been proposed. The limit was proposed based on a review of metabolic and toxicologic considerations (2185).

Cyclosporine (Sandoz) 3 mg/ml in dextrose 5% in water leached relatively large amounts of diethylhexyl phthalate (DEHP) plasticizer from PVC bags. This leaching was due to the surfactant Cremophor EL in the formulation. After four hours at 24 °C, the DEHP concentration in 50-ml bags of infusion solution was as much as 13 μg/ml and it increased through 24 hr to 104 μg/ml. This finding is consistent with the high surfactant concentration (3.9%) in the final admixture solution. The actual amount of DEHP leached from PVC containers and administration sets may vary in clinical situations, depending on surfactant concentration, bag size, and contact time. Non-PVC containers and administration sets should be used to administer cyclosporine solutions (1683).

Storage of cyclosporine (Sandoz) 3 mg/ml in dextrose 5% in water in PVC bags at 24 °C was shown to cause leaching of significant amounts of DEHP due to the vehicle containing Cremophor EL and alcohol. Use of glass containers and tubing that does not contain DEHP to administer cyclosporine was recommended (1092).

CYTARABINE
(CYTOSINE ARABINOSIDE)
AHFS 10:00

Cytosar-U   **Pharmacia & Upjohn**

Products— Cytarabine (Pharmacia & Upjohn) is available in 100-mg, 500-mg, 1-g, and 2-g multiple-dose vials. For intravenous or subcutaneous use, reconstitute the vials with bacteriostatic water for injection containing benzyl alcohol 0.945% in the following amounts (2):

Vial Size	Volume of Diluent	Concentration
100 mg	5 ml	20 mg/ml
500 mg	10 ml	50 mg/ml
1 g	10 ml	100 mg/ml
2 g	20 ml	100 mg/ml

For intrathecal injection, *only* a preservative-free diluent should be used (2; 4).

Hydrochloric acid and/or sodium hydroxide may be added to adjust the pH (2; 4).

pH— After reconstitution, the USP specifies a pH range of 4 to 6 for cytarabine injection (17). Pharmacia & Upjohn cite the pH of their product as about 5 (2). Cytarabine injection (Faulding) has a pH of about 7.4, with a range of 7 to 9 (4).

Sodium Content— Cytarabine injection (Faulding) contains 0.12 mEq of sodium per milliliter (4).

Osmolality— Cytarabine 20 mg/ml in sterile water for injection has an osmolality of 150 mOsm/kg (1689).

Administration— Cytarabine may be administered by subcutaneous, intrathecal, or direct intravenous injection and by continuous or intermittent intravenous infusion (2; 4). It has been administered by intramuscular injection and continuous subcutaneous infusion as well (4).

Stability— Intact vials of cytarabine (Upjohn) 100 and 500 mg have been stated to be stable at room temperatures not exceeding 25 °C (60). A study of 100- and 500-mg vials stored at 25 °C showed that potency was retained for at least 36 months (226).

The manufacturer states that cytarabine reconstituted with bacteriostatic water for injection containing benzyl alcohol 0.945% may be stored at a controlled room temperature of 20 to 25 °C for up to 48 hours. Solutions with a slight haze should be discarded (2; 4). However, a stability study of cytarabine in aqueous solution showed maximum stability in the neutral pH range. It was calculated to retain 90% potency for six and a half months at pH 6.9 at 25 °C. The rate of decomposition of cytarabine in alkaline solutions is about 10 times as great as in acid solutions (82).

The manufacturer indicates that for concentrations of 20 and 250 mg/ml in bacteriostatic water for injection, greater than 99% potency is retained after five days of storage at room temperature (174). However, cytarabine has an aqueous solubility of 100 mg/ml (4; 1369), and precipitation from more highly concentrated solutions has been observed in varying time frames. In another test, concentrations of 40 and 80 mg/ml in bacteriostatic water for injection were stored in plastic syringes (Becton-Dickinson) at 37, 25, 4, and −20 °C. Cytarabine remained stable for at least 15 days at 25 and 4 °C and for seven days at 37 °C. However, storage at −20 °C resulted in a precipitate (174).

Cytarabine (Upjohn) 50 mg/ml in polypropylene syringes containing 5, 10, and 20 ml was stable by HPLC for 29 days at 8 and 21 °C in the dark, exhibiting losses of 8.5% or less (1566).

In another report, reconstituted 100- and 500-mg vials retained between 89.2 and 92% potency at 17 days after reconstitution when stored at 25 °C (226).

Cytarabine, reconstituted according to the manufacturer's instructions, was cultured with human lymphoblasts to determine whether its cytotoxic activity was retained. The solution retained cytotoxicity for 24 hours at 4 °C and room temperature (1575).

Intrathecal Injections— Reconstituted solutions containing 20 and 50 mg/ml of cytarabine (Upjohn) were stored in plastic syringes (Pharmaseal) at 22, 8, and −10 °C. No decomposition occurred during one week of storage at these temperatures (748).

In another study, cytarabine (Upjohn) 50 mg/2.5 ml was stored at 5 and 25 °C in 5-ml plastic syringes (Becton-Dickinson) with rubber tip caps and in glass flasks covered with parafilm. After seven days, samples in the plastic syringes showed a 2 to 3% loss of cytarabine at both temperatures. The 25 °C sample in glass also showed a 2% loss, but the 5 °C sample in glass showed no loss after seven days (759).

In a study of solutions for intrathecal injection, cytarabine (Upjohn) was reconstituted to a concentration of 5 mg/ml with Elliott's B solution (artificial cerebrospinal fluid), sodium chloride 0.9%, and Ringer's injection, lactated. In Elliott's B solution and Ringer's injection, lactated, cytarabine exhibited no change in concentration by UV spectroscopy over seven days at room temperature under fluorescent light and at 30 °C. In sodium chloride 0.9%, no decomposition was noted in 24 hours, but a 3% loss was observed at room temperature and 6% at 30 °C over seven days (327).

Bacterially contaminated intrathecal solutions could pose very grave risks; consequently, such solutions should be administered as soon as possible after preparation (328).

The osmolarity and pH of cytarabine in these three solutions at a concentration of 2.5 mg/ml were as follows (327):

In Elliott's B solution	299 mOsm/kg, pH 7.3
In Ringer's injection, lactated	262 mOsm/kg, pH 5.6
In sodium chloride 0.9%	299 mOsm/kg, pH 5.3

In another study, the stability and compatibility of cytarabine (Upjohn), methotrexate (NCI), and hydrocortisone (Upjohn), mixed together in intrathecal injections, were evaluated. Two combinations were tested: (1) cytarabine 50 mg, methotrexate 12 mg (as the sodium salt), and hydrocortisone 25 mg (as the sodium succinate salt); and (2) cytarabine 30 mg, methotrexate 12 mg (as the sodium salt), and hydrocortisone 15 mg (as the sodium succinate salt). Each drug combination was added to 12 ml of Elliott's B solution (NCI), sodium chloride 0.9% (Abbott), dextrose 5% in water (Abbott), and Ringer's injection, lactated (Abbott), and stored for 24 hours at 25 °C. Cytarabine and methotrexate were both chemically stable, with no drug loss after the full 24 hours in all solutions. Hydrocortisone was also stable in the sodium chloride 0.9%, dextrose 5% in water, and Ringer's injection, lactated, with about a 2% drug loss. However, in Elliott's B solution, hydrocortisone was significantly less stable, with a 6% loss in the 25-mg concentration over 24 hours. The 15-mg concentration was worse, with a 5% loss in 10 hours and a 13% loss in 24 hours. The higher pH of Elliott's B solution and the lower concentration of hydrocortisone may have been factors in this increased decomposition. All mixtures were physically compatible during this study, but a precipitate formed after several days of storage (819).

Elliott's B solution has been recommended as a diluent for cytosine arabinoside for intrathecal administration because it is more nearly physiologic (435). The patient's own spinal fluid has been recommended also (830).

Cytarabine (Upjohn) 3 mg/ml diluted in Elliott's B solution (Orphan Medical) was packaged as 20 ml in 30-ml glass vials and 20-ml plastic syringes (Becton-Dickinson) with Red Cap (Burron) Luer-Lok syringe tip caps. The solution was physically compatible, with no change in measured turbidity or increase in particulate content and was chemically stable, exhibiting little or no loss by HPLC analysis during storage for 48 hours at 4 and 23 °C (1976).

Implantable Infusion Pump— Cytarabine (Upjohn) 1 mg/ml in Elliott's B solution was evaluated for stability in an implantable infusion pump (Infusaid model 400). In this in vitro assessment, no cytarabine loss occurred in 15 days at 37 °C with mild agitation (767).

Filtration— Cytarabine 100 mg/15 ml was injected as a bolus through a 0.2-μm nylon, air-eliminating filter (Ultipor, Pall) to evaluate the effect of filtration on simulated intravenous push delivery. Spectrophotometric evaluation showed that about 96% of the drug was delivered through the filter after flushing with 10 ml of sodium chloride 0.9% (809).

Cytarabine 10 to 100 μg/ml exhibited no loss due to sorption to either cellulose nitrate/cellulose acetate ester (Millex OR) or polytetrafluoroethylene (Millex FG) filters (1416).

Sorption— In an admixture composed of cytarabine (Upjohn) 0.157 mg/ml, daunorubicin HCl (Bellon) 15.7 μg/ml, and etoposide (Sandoz) 0.157 mg/ml in dextrose 5% in water, little or no loss of the drugs due to sorption occurred when delivered through PVC and polyethylene-lined sets and silicone central catheters (1955).

Compatibility Information

Solution Compatibility

Cytarabine

Solution	Mfr	Mfr	Conc/L	Remarks	Ref	C/I
Amino acids 4.25%, dextrose 25%	MG	UP	100 mg	No increase in particulate matter in 24 hr at 5 °C	349	C
Dextrose 5% in Ringer's injection, lactated	TR[a]	UP	500 mg	Potency retained for 24 hr at 5 °C	282	C
Dextrose 5% in sodium chloride 0.2%	[a]	UP	8, 24, 32 g	No cytarabine loss in 7 days at room temperature or 4 or −20 °C	174	C
Dextrose 5% in sodium chloride 0.9%	TR[a]	UP	500 mg	Potency retained for 24 hr at 5 °C	282	C
		UP	3.6 g	Physically compatible	174	C
Dextrose 10% in sodium chloride 0.9%		UP	3.6 g	Physically compatible	174	C
Dextrose 5% in water	TR[a]	UP	500 mg	Potency retained for 24 hr at 5 °C	282	C
	TR[a]	UP	1.87 g	Less than 10% decrease in 24 hr at room temperature	519	C
		UP	500 mg	Chemically stable for 7 days at room temperature	174	C
	[a]	UP	8, 24, 32 g	No cytarabine loss in 7 days at room temperature or 4 or −20 °C	174	
	[b]	UP	1.25 and 25 g	Visually compatible with less than 6% cytarabine loss by HPLC in 28 days at 4 and 22 °C and 7 days at 35 °C protected from light. Excessive decomposition products in 14 days at 35 °C	1548	C
	MG, TR[a]		1.83 g	Less than 10% cytarabine loss by HPLC in 24 hr at room temperature exposed to light	1658	C
		UP	157 mg	Less than 2% loss in 48 hr by HPLC at room temperature, exposed to light and in the dark, and at 4 °C	1955	C
Invert sugar 10% in Electrolyte #1	TR	UP	3.6 g	Physically compatible	174	C
Ringer's injection		UP	3.6 g	Physically compatible	174	C
Ringer's injection, lactated	TR[a]	UP	500 mg	Potency retained for 24 hr at 5 °C	282	C
Sodium chloride 0.9%	TR[a]	UP	500 mg	Potency retained for 24 hr at 5 °C	282	C
		UP	500 mg	Chemically stable for 7 days at room temperature	174	C

Solution Compatibility (Cont.)

Cytarabine

Solution	Mfr	Mfr	Conc/L	Remarks	Ref	C/I
a		UP	8, 24, 32 g	No cytarabine loss in 7 days at room temperature or 4 or −20 °C	174	**C**
		UP	3.6 g	Physically compatible	174	**C**
b		UP	1.25 and 25 g	Visually compatible with less than 6% cytarabine loss by HPLC in 28 days at 4 and 22 °C and 7 days at 35 °C protected from light. Excessive decomposition products in 14 days at 35 °C	1548	**C**
Sodium lactate ⅙ M		UP	3.6 g	Physically compatible	174	**C**
TPN #57[c]		UP	50 mg	Physically compatible with no cytarabine loss in 48 hr at 25 or 8 °C	996	**C**

[a]*Tested in both glass and PVC containers.*
[b]*Tested in ethylene vinyl acetate (EVA) containers.*
[c]*Refer to Appendix I for the composition of parenteral nutrition solutions. TPN indicates a 2-in-1 admixture.*

Additive Compatibility

Cytarabine

Drug	Mfr	Conc/L	Mfr	Conc/L	Test Soln	Remarks	Ref	C/I
Corticotropin	AR	25 units	UP	100 mg	D5W	Physically compatible for over 8 hr	174	**C**
Daunorubicin HCl with etoposide	RP BR	33 mg 400 mg	UP	267 mg	D5½S	Physically compatible with about 6% cytarabine loss and no loss of other drugs in 72 hr at 20 °C	1162	**C**
Daunorubicin HCl with etoposide	BEL SZ	15.7 mg 157 mg	UP	157 mg	D5W	Less than 10% loss of any drug in 48 hr at room temperature, exposed to light and in the dark, and at 4 °C	1955	**C**
Etoposide	BR	660 mg	CHI	1.2 g	D5W	Physically compatible with no subvisual haze or particle formation in 4 hr at 23 °C	1736	**C**
Fluorouracil	RC	250 mg	UP	400 mg	D5W	Altered UV spectra for cytarabine within 1 hr at room temperature	207	**I**
Gentamicin sulfate		80 mg	UP	100 mg	D5W	Physically compatible for 24 hr	174	**C**
		240 mg	UP	300 mg	D5W	Physically incompatible	174	**I**
Heparin sodium		10,000 units	UP	500 mg	NS	Haze formation	174	**I**
		20,000 units	UP	500 mg	D5W	Haze formation	174	**I**
Hydrocortisone sodium succinate	UP	500 mg	UP	360 mg	D5S, D10S	Physically compatible for 40 hr	174	**C**
	UP	500 mg	UP	360 mg	R, SL	Physically incompatible	174	**I**
Hydroxyzine HCl	LY	500 mg	UP	1 g	D5W[a]	Physically compatible for 48 hr	1198	**C**
Insulin, regular		40 units	UP	100 and 500 mg	D5W	Fine precipitate forms	174	**I**
Lincomycin HCl		1, 1.5, 2, 2.4, 3 g	UP	500 mg		Physically compatible for 48 hr	174	**C**
Methotrexate sodium	LE	200 mg	UP	400 mg	D5W	Physically compatible. Very little change in UV spectra in 8 hr at room temperature	207	**C**

Additive Compatibility (Cont.)

Cytarabine

Drug	Mfr	Conc/L	Mfr	Conc/L	Test Soln	Remarks	Ref	C/I
Methylprednisolone sodium succinate	UP	250 mg	UP	360 mg	D5S, D10S, NS	Clear solution for 24 hr	329	C
	UP	250 mg	UP	360 mg	R, SL	Physically incompatible	329	I
Mitoxantrone HCl	LE	500 mg	UP	500 mg	D5W	Visually compatible and mitoxantrone potency by HPLC retained for 24 hr at room temperature. Cytarabine not tested	1531	C
Nafcillin sodium		4 g	UP	100 mg	D5W	Heavy crystalline precipitate forms	174	I
Ondansetron HCl	GL	30 and 300 mg	UP	200 mg	D5W[b]	Physically compatible with little or no loss of either drug by HPLC in 48 hr at 23 °C	1876	C
	GL	30 and 300 mg	UP	40 g	D5W[b]	Physically compatible with little or no loss of either drug by HPLC in 48 hr at 23 °C	1876	C
Oxacillin sodium		2 g	UP	100 mg	D5W	pH outside stability range for oxacillin	174	I
Penicillin G sodium		2 million units	UP	200 mg	D5W	pH outside stability range for penicillin	174	I
Potassium chloride		80 mEq	UP	170 mg	D5S	Physically compatible for 24 hr	174	C
		100 mEq	UP	2 g	D5S	Physically compatible and chemically stable for 8 days	174	C
Sodium bicarbonate	AB	50 mEq	UP	200 mg and 1 g	D5W[c]	Physically compatible and no loss of cytarabine in 7 days at 8 and 22 °C	748	C
	AB	50 mEq	UP	200 mg	D5¼S[c]	Physically compatible and no loss of cytarabine in 7 days at 8 and 22 °C	748	C
Vincristine sulfate	LI	4 mg	UP	16 mg	D5W	Physically compatible. No alteration of UV spectra in 8 hr at room temperature	207	C

[a]Tested in glass containers.
[b]Tested in PVC containers.
[c]Tested in both glass and PVC containers.

Drugs in Syringe Compatibility

Cytarabine

Drug (in syringe)	Mfr	Amt	Mfr	Amt	Remarks	Ref	C/I
Metoclopramide HCl	RB	10 mg/ 2 ml	UP	50 mg/ 1 ml	Physically compatible for 48 hr at room temperature	924	C
	RB	10 mg/ 2 ml	UP	50 mg/ 1 ml	Physically compatible for 48 hr at 25 °C	1167	C
	RB	160 mg/ 32 ml	UP	500 mg/ 10 ml	Physically compatible for 48 hr at 25 °C	1167	C

Y-Site Injection Compatibility (1:1 Mixture)

Cytarabine

Drug	Mfr	Conc	Mfr	Conc	Remarks	Ref	C/I
Allopurinol sodium	BW	3 mg/ml[b]	SCN	50 mg/ml	Tiny particles form within 4 hr	1686	I
Amifostine	USB	10 mg/ml[a]	CET	50 mg/ml	Physically compatible with no change in measured turbidity or increase in particle content in 4 hr at 23 °C	1845	C

Y-Site Injection Compatibility (1:1 Mixture) (Cont.)

			Cytarabine				
Drug	*Mfr*	*Conc*	*Mfr*	*Conc*	*Remarks*	*Ref*	*C/I*
Amphotericin B cholesteryl sulfate complex	SEQ	0.83 mg/ml[a]	BED	50 mg/ml	Gross precipitate forms	2117	**I**
Amsacrine	NCI	1 mg/ml[a]	QU	50 mg/ml	Physically compatible for 4 hr at room temperature under fluorescent light	1381	**C**
Aztreonam	SQ	40 mg/ml[a]	CET	50 mg/ml	Physically compatible with no subvisual haze or particle formation in 4 hr at 23 °C	1758	**C**
Cefepime HCl	BR	20 mg/ml[a]	CET	50 mg/ml	Physically compatible with no change in measured turbidity or increase in particle content in 4 hr at 22 °C	1689	**C**
Chlorpromazine HCl	SKF	2 mg/ml[a]	UP	50 mg/ml	Visually compatible for 4 hr at room temperature under fluorescent light	1685	**C**
Cimetidine HCl	SKF	12 mg/ml[a]	UP	50 mg/ml	Visually compatible for 4 hr at room temperature under fluorescent light	1685	**C**
Cladribine	ORT	0.015[b] and 0.5[c] mg/ml	CHI	50 mg/ml	Physically compatible with no change in measured turbidity or increase in particle content in 4 hr at 23 °C	1969	**C**
Dexamethasone sodium phosphate	QU	1 mg/ml[a]	UP	50 mg/ml	Visually compatible for 4 hr at room temperature under fluorescent light	1685	**C**
Diphenhydramine HCl	PD	2 mg/ml[a]	UP	50 mg/ml	Visually compatible for 4 hr at room temperature under fluorescent light	1685	**C**
Doxorubicin HCl liposome injection	SEQ	0.4 mg/ml[a]	CHI	50 mg/ml	Physically compatible with little or no change in measured turbidity and no increase in particle content in 4 hr at 23 °C	2087	**C**
Droperidol	JN	20 μg/ml[a]	UP	50 mg/ml	Visually compatible for 4 hr at room temperature under fluorescent light	1685	**C**
Etoposide phosphate	BR	5 mg/ml[a]	BED	50 mg/ml	Physically compatible with no change in measured turbidity or increase in particle content in 4 hr at 23 °C	2218	**C**
Famotidine	MSD	2 mg/ml[a]	UP	50 mg/ml	Visually compatible for 4 hr at room temperature under fluorescent light	1685	**C**
Filgrastim	AMG	30 μg/ml[a]	CET	50 mg/ml	Physically compatible with no change in measured turbidity or increase in particle content in 4 hr at 22 °C	1687	**C**
Fludarabine phosphate	BX	1 mg/ml[a]	UP	50 mg/ml	Physically compatible for 4 hr at room temperature under fluorescent light	1439	**C**
Furosemide	ES	3 mg/ml[a]	UP	50 mg/ml	Visually compatible for 4 hr at room temperature under fluorescent light	1685	**C**
Ganciclovir sodium	SY	20 mg/ml[a]	UP	50 mg/ml	Turbidity and particles form in 30 min and become gel-like in 4 hr	1685	**I**
Gemcitabine HCl	LI	10 mg/ml[b]	BED	50 mg/ml	Physically compatible with no change in measured turbidity or increase in particle content in 4 hr at 23 °C	2226	**C**
Gentamicin sulfate	GNS	15 mg/ml[d]	UP	16 mg/ml[b]	Visually compatible for 24 hr at room temperature in test tubes. No precipitate found on filter from Y-site delivery	2063	**C**

Y-Site Injection Compatibility (1:1 Mixture) (Cont.)

				Cytarabine			
Drug	Mfr	Conc	Mfr	Conc	Remarks	Ref	C/I
Granisetron HCl	SKB	1 mg/ml	UP	2 mg/ml[b]	Physically compatible with little or no loss of either drug by HPLC in 4 hr at 22 °C	1883	C
	SKB	0.05 mg/ml[a]	UP	50 mg/ml	Physically compatible with no change in measured turbidity or increase in particle content in 4 hr at 23 °C	2000	C
Heparin sodium	SO	40 units/ml[a]	UP	50 mg/ml	Visually compatible for 4 hr at room temperature under fluorescent light	1685	C
Hydrocortisone sodium succinate	UP	125 mg/ml	UP	16 mg/ml[b]	Visually compatible for 24 hr at room temperature in test tubes. No precipitate found on filter from Y-site delivery	2063	C
Hydromorphone HCl	ES	0.04 mg/ml[a]	UP	50 mg/ml	Visually compatible for 4 hr at room temperature under fluorescent light	1685	C
Idarubicin HCl	AD	1 mg/ml[b]	CET	6 mg/ml[a]	Visually compatible for 24 hr at 25 °C	1525	C
Lorazepam	WY	0.1 mg/ml[a]	UP	50 mg/ml	Visually compatible for 4 hr at room temperature under fluorescent light	1685	C
Melphalan HCl	BW	0.1 mg/ml[b]	UP	50 mg/ml	Physically compatible with no change in measured turbidity or increase in particle content in 3 hr at 22 °C	1557	C
Methotrexate sodium		30 mg/ml	UP	0.6 mg/ml[a]	Visually compatible for 4 hr at room temperature	1788	C
Methylprednisolone sodium succinate	UP	0.5 mg/ml[a]	UP	50 mg/ml	Visually compatible for 4 hr at room temperature under fluorescent light	1685	C
	UP	5 mg/ml[a]	UP	16 mg/ml[b]	Visually compatible for 24 hr at room temperature in test tubes. No precipitate found on filter from Y-site delivery	2063	C
Metoclopramide HCl	RB	2.5 mg/ml[a]	UP	50 mg/ml	Visually compatible for 4 hr at room temperature under fluorescent light	1685	C
Morphine sulfate	ES	0.12 mg/ml[a]	UP	50 mg/ml	Visually compatible for 4 hr at room temperature under fluorescent light	1685	C
Ondansetron HCl	GL	1 mg/ml[b]	UP	50 mg/ml	Physically compatible for 4 hr at 22 °C	1365	C
Paclitaxel	NCI	1.2 mg/ml[a]		50 mg/ml	Physically compatible with no change in measured turbidity in 4 hr at 22 °C	1528	C
Piperacillin sodium–tazobactam sodium	LE	40 + 5 mg/ml[a]	SCN	50 mg/ml	Physically compatible with no change in measured turbidity or increase in particle content in 4 hr at 22 °C	1688	C
Prochlorperazine edisylate	SKF	0.5 mg/ml[a]	UP	50 mg/ml	Visually compatible for 4 hr at room temperature under fluorescent light	1685	C
Promethazine HCl	WY	2 mg/ml[a]	UP	50 mg/ml	Visually compatible for 4 hr at room temperature under fluorescent light	1685	C
Propofol	ZEN	10 mg/ml	CHI	50 mg/ml	Physically compatible for 1 hr at 23 °C with no increase in particle content	2066	C
Ranitidine HCl	GL	1 mg/ml[a]	UP	50 mg/ml	Visually compatible for 4 hr at room temperature under fluorescent light	1685	C
Sargramostim	IMM	10 μg/ml[b]	SCN	50 mg/ml	Physically compatible for 4 hr at 22 °C	1436	C
Sodium bicarbonate		1.4%	UP	0.6 mg/ml[a]	Visually compatible for 4 hr at room temperature	1788	C

Y-Site Injection Compatibility (1:1 Mixture) (Cont.)

				Cytarabine			
Drug	Mfr	Conc	Mfr	Conc	Remarks	Ref	C/I
Teniposide	BR	0.1 mg/ml[a]	CET	50 mg/ml	Physically compatible with no subvisual haze or particle formation in 4 hr at 23 °C	1725	C
Thiotepa	IMM[e]	1 mg/ml[a]	CET	50 mg/ml	Physically compatible with no change in measured turbidity or increase in particle content in 4 hr at 23 °C	1861	C
TNA #218 to #226[f]			BED	50 mg/ml	Visually compatible with no precipitate or emulsion damage apparent in 4 hr at 23 °C	2215	C
TPN #212 to #215[f]			CHI	50 mg/ml	Substantial loss of natural subvisual turbidity occurs immediately	2109	I
Vinorelbine tartrate	BW	1 mg/ml[b]	CET	50 mg/ml	Physically compatible with no change in measured turbidity or increase in particle content in 4 hr at 22 °C	1558	C

[a]*Tested in dextrose 5% in water.*
[b]*Tested in sodium chloride 0.9%.*
[c]*Tested in bacteriostatic sodium chloride 0.9% preserved with benzyl alcohol 0.9%.*
[d]*Tested in sodium chloride 0.45%.*
[e]*Lyophilized formulation tested.*
[f]*Refer to Appendix I for the composition of parenteral nutrition solutions. TNA indicates a 3-in-1 admixture, and TPN indicates a 2-in-1 admixture.*

Additional Compatibility Information

Solutions— At a concentration of 500 mg/L, 94 to 96% of the cytarabine potency is maintained for eight days at room temperature in dextrose 5% in water, sodium chloride 0.9%, and water for injection (2; 4).

Another report stated that cytarabine 0.5 to 5 mg/ml in dextrose 5% in water, sodium chloride 0.9%, Ringer's injection, and sterile water for injection exhibited less than a 10% loss in 14 days at room temperature (1379).

Dacarbazine— No alteration in the ultraviolet/visible spectra was observed when dacarbazine was combined in solution with cytarabine (492).

Aluminum— Ogawa et al. reported that immersion of a needle with an aluminum component in cytarabine (Upjohn) 20 mg/ml resulted in no visually apparent reaction after seven days at 24 °C (988).

Bacterial Challenge— Cytarabine (Quad) 12.5 mg/ml in sodium chloride 0.9% did not inhibit the growth of deliberately inoculated *Staphylococcus epidermidis* (10^6 to 10^7 CFU/ml) during 21 days at 35 °C (representing near body temperature). At a concentration of 50 mg/ml in sodium chloride 0.9%, however, viable *S. epidermidis* was reduced over the 21 days but not eliminated (1659).

DACARBAZINE
AHFS 10:00

DTIC-Dome   **Bayer**

Products— Dacarbazine (Bayer) is available in vials containing 100 and 200 mg of drug along with anhydrous citric acid and mannitol. Reconstitute the 100- and 200-mg vials with 9.9 and 19.7 ml of sterile water for injection, respectively, to yield solutions containing 10 mg/ml of dacarbazine (2).

pH— From 3 to 4 (2).

Osmolality— Dacarbazine 10 mg/ml in sterile water for injection has an osmolality of 109 mOsm/kg (1689).

Administration— Dacarbazine is administered as a direct intravenous injection over one minute and as an intravenous infusion in up to 250 ml of dextrose 5% in water or sodium chloride 0.9% over 15 to 30 minutes (4). Extravasation may result in severe pain and tissue damage (2; 4; 377).

Stability— Intact vials of dacarbazine should be stored at 2 to 8 °C and protected from light (4). Miles, the former manufacturer, indicated that the drug is stable for four weeks at controlled room temperature (1239; 1433), while Lyphomed states that its product is stable for three months at controlled room temperature (1433). Bayer also recommends storage of reconstituted solutions for up to eight hours at normal room temperatures and light or up to 72 hours at 4 °C (2). However, it has been reported that solutions are stable for at least 24 hours at room temperature (1% decomposition) and at least 96 hours under refrigeration (less than 1% decomposition) when protected from light (285). A change in color from pale yellow to pink or red is a sign of decomposition (4; 285; 1093).

Administration of dacarbazine in a room illuminated only with a red photographic light apparently reduced the incidence of disagreeable side effects. The authors attributed this result to a reduced amount of photodegradation of dacarbazine (469).

Kirk reported the effects of daylight and fluorescent light on dacarbazine (Bayer) 4 mg/ml in sodium chloride 0.9%. Exposure to direct sunlight resulted in up to a 12% loss in 30 minutes, and a pink color formed in 35 to 40 minutes. Exposure to indirect daylight resulted in less than a 2% loss in 30 minutes. Solutions protected from light or exposed to fluorescent light lost about 4% of their dacarbazine in 24 hours (1248).

The photostability of dacarbazine has been shown to increase with the addition of reduced glutathione at about 5 mg/100 ml (1829).

Dacarbazine, reconstituted according to the manufacturer's instructions, was cultured with human lymphoblasts to determine whether its cytotoxic activity was retained. The solution retained cytotoxicity for 24 hours at room temperature (1575).

Compatibility Information

Solution Compatibility

Dacarbazine

Solution	Mfr	Mfr	Conc/L	Remarks	Ref	C/I
Dextrose 5% in water	a		1.7 g	Less than 10% loss in 24 hr at room temperature	519	C
	MG, TR[b]		1.7 g	Less than 10% loss by HPLC in 24 hr at room temperature exposed to light	1658	C
	BA[c]	MI	1 and 3 g	Physically compatible with 4% loss by HPLC in 8 hr and 10 to 15% loss in 24 hr at 23 °C	1876	I

[a]Tested in both glass and PVC containers.
[b]Tested in glass, PVC, and polyolefin containers.
[c]Tested in PVC containers.

Additive Compatibility

Dacarbazine

Drug	Mfr	Conc/L	Mfr	Conc/L	Test Soln	Remarks	Ref	C/I
Ondansetron HCl	GL	30 and 300 mg	MI	1 g	D5W[a]	Physically compatible with little or no loss of ondansetron by HPLC in 48 hr at 23 °C. 8 to 12% dacarbazine loss in 24 hr and 20% loss in 48 hr at 23 °C	1876	C
	GL	30 and 300 mg	MI	3 g	D5W[a]	Physically compatible with little or no loss of ondansetron by HPLC in 48 hr at 23 °C. 8% dacarbazine loss in 24 hr and 15% loss in 48 hr at 23 °C	1876	C
Ondansetron HCl with doxorubicin HCl	GL AD	640 mg 800 mg	LY	8 g	D5W[a]	Visually compatible with >90% ondansetron and doxorubicin potency by HPLC over 24 hr at 30 °C and after 7 days at 4 °C followed by 24 hr at 30 °C. Dacarbazine stable for 8 hr but up to 13% loss in 24 hr	2092	I
Ondansetron HCl with doxorubicin HCl	GL AD	640 mg 1.5 g	LY	20 g	D5W[a]	Visually compatible with >90% potency of all drugs by HPLC over 24 hr at 30 °C and after 7 days at 4 °C followed by 24 hr at 30 °C	2092	C
Ondansetron HCl with doxorubicin HCl	GL AD	640 mg 800 mg	LY	8 g	D5W[b]	Visually compatible with >90% potency of all drugs by HPLC over 24 hr at 30 °C and after 7 days at 4 °C followed by 24 hr at 30 °C	2092	C

Additive Compatibility (Cont.)

Dacarbazine

Drug	Mfr	Conc/L	Mfr	Conc/L	Test Soln	Remarks	Ref	C/I
Ondansetron HCl with doxorubicin HCl	GL AD	640 mg 1.5 g	LY	20 g	D5W[b]	Visually compatible with >90% potency of all drugs by HPLC over 24 hr at 30 °C and after 7 days at 4 °C followed by 24 hr at 30 °C	2092	C

[a]Tested in PVC containers.
[b]Tested in polyisoprene infusion pump reservoirs.

Y-Site Injection Compatibility (1:1 Mixture)

Dacarbazine

Drug	Mfr	Conc	Mfr	Conc	Remarks	Ref	C/I
Allopurinol sodium	BW	3 mg/ml[b]	MI	4 mg/ml[b]	Small particles form within 1 hr and become large pink pellets in 24 hr	1686	I
Amifostine	USB	10 mg/ml[a]	MI	4 mg/ml[a]	Physically compatible with no change in measured turbidity or increase in particle content in 4 hr at 23 °C	1845	C
Aztreonam	SQ	40 mg/ml[a]	MI	4 mg/ml[a]	Physically compatible with no subvisual haze or particle formation in 4 hr at 23 °C	1758	C
Cefepime HCl	BR	20 mg/ml[a]	MI	4 mg/ml[a]	Cloudy solution forms immediately and develops flocculent precipitate in 4 hr	1689	I
Etoposide phosphate	BR	5 mg/ml[a]	MI	4 mg/ml[a]	Physically compatible with no change in measured turbidity or increase in particle content in 4 hr at 23 °C	2218	C
Filgrastim	AMG	30 µg/ml[a]	MI	4 mg/ml[a]	Physically compatible with no change in measured turbidity or increase in particle content in 4 hr at 22 °C	1687	C
Fludarabine phosphate	BX	1 mg/ml[a]	MI	4 mg/ml[a]	Physically compatible for 4 hr at room temperature under fluorescent light	1439	C
Granisetron HCl	SKB	1 mg/ml	MI	1.7 mg/ml[b]	Physically compatible with little or no loss of either drug by HPLC in 4 hr at 22 °C	1883	C
Heparin sodium	WY	100 units/ml	MI	25 mg/ml[b]	White flocculent precipitate forms immediately[c]	1158	I
	WY	100 units/ml	MI	10 mg/ml[b]	No observable precipitation[c]	1158	C
Melphalan HCl	BW	0.1 mg/ml[b]	MI	4 mg/ml[b]	Physically compatible with no change in measured turbidity or increase in particle content in 3 hr at 22 °C	1557	C
Ondansetron HCl	GL	1 mg/ml[b]	MI	4 mg/ml[a]	Physically compatible for 4 hr at 22 °C	1365	C
Paclitaxel	NCI	1.2 mg/ml[a]	MI	4 mg/ml[a]	Physically compatible with no change in measured turbidity in 4 hr at 22 °C	1556	C
Piperacillin sodium–tazobactam sodium	LE	40 + 5 mg/ml[a]	MI	4 mg/ml[a]	Turbidity and particles form immediately and increase over 4 hr	1688	I
Sargramostim	IMM	10 µg/ml[b]	MI	4 mg/ml[b]	Physically compatible for 4 hr at 22 °C	1436	C
Teniposide	BR	0.1 mg/ml[a]	MI	4 mg/ml[a]	Physically compatible with no subvisual haze or particle formation in 4 hr at 23 °C	1725	C

Y-Site Injection Compatibility (1:1 Mixture) (Cont.)

Dacarbazine

Drug	Mfr	Conc	Mfr	Conc	Remarks	Ref	C/I
Thiotepa	IMM[d]	1 mg/ml[a]	MI	4 mg/ml[a]	Physically compatible with no change in measured turbidity or increase in particle content in 4 hr at 23 °C	1861	C
Vinorelbine tartrate	BW	1 mg/ml[b]	MI	4 mg/ml[b]	Physically compatible with no change in measured turbidity or increase in particle content in 4 hr at 22 °C	1558	C

[a]*Tested in dextrose 5% in water.*
[b]*Tested in sodium chloride 0.9%.*
[c]*Dacarbazine in intravenous tubing flushed with heparin sodium.*
[d]*Lyophilized formulation tested.*

Additional Compatibility Information

Solutions—— Dextrose 5% in water and sodium chloride 0.9% have been recommended as diluents for dacarbazine intravenous infusions (2; 4; 285). The manufacturer indicates that dacarbazine is stable in intravenous infusion solutions for eight hours under normal room conditions and 24 hours when refrigerated at 4 °C (2). However, other reports indicated that the drug is stable for 24 hours (285; 519; 1658). One report noted that if the solutions stored at room temperature were not protected from light, they exhibited 5% decomposition in 24 hours (285). Also see Compatibility Information.

Hydrocortisone—— Dacarbazine is stated to form a pink precipitate immediately when mixed with hydrocortisone sodium succinate (Upjohn). However, a similar precipitate was not noted when mixed with hydrocortisone sodium phosphate or lidocaine HCl 1 or 2% (524).

Cytotoxic Agents—— No alteration in the ultraviolet/visible spectra was observed when dacarbazine was combined in solution with the following cytotoxic agents (492):
Bleomycin sulfate
Carmustine
Cyclophosphamide
Cytarabine
Dactinomycin
Doxorubicin HCl
Fluorouracil
Mercaptopurine sodium
Methotrexate sodium
Vinblastine sulfate

Cysteine—— Dacarbazine has been stated to couple with the thiol group of L-cysteine in the presence of light to yield an unstable azothioether (492).

Aluminum—— Ogawa et al. reported that immersion of a needle with an aluminum component in dacarbazine (Miles) 10 mg/ml resulted in no visually apparent unexpected reaction after seven days at 24 °C (988).

Other Information

Inactivation—— In the event of spills or leaks, the manufacturer recommends the use of sulfuric acid 10% in contact for 24 hours to inactivate dacarbazine (1200).

DACTINOMYCIN
(ACTINOMYCIN D)
AHFS 10:00

Cosmegen   **Merck**

Products—— Dactinomycin (Merck) is available in vials containing 0.5 mg of drug with mannitol 20 mg. Reconstitute with 1.1 ml of sterile water for injection *without* preservatives to yield a gold-colored solution containing 0.5 mg/ml of dactinomycin (2). Other solvents, especially those containing preservatives such as bacteriostatic water for injection (benzyl alcohol or parabens), may cause precipitation (2; 4).

pH— The pH of the reconstituted solution is 5.5 to 7 (4).

Osmolality— Dactinomycin 0.5 mg/ml in sterile water for injection has an osmolality of 189 mOsm/kg (1689).

Administration—— Dactinomycin may be administered by direct intravenous injection, intravenous infusion, and isolation perfusion technique. It must *not* be given intramuscularly or subcutaneously (2; 4). Extravasation should be avoided because of possible corrosion of soft tissue (2; 4; 377).

Stability—— Intact vials of dactinomycin should be stored at controlled room temperature and protected from excessive heat and humidity (2). The clear, gold-colored, reconstituted solution is stable at room temperature; however, this solution contains no preservative so it has been suggested that unused portions of the injection be discarded (2; 4). The drug is reported to be most stable at pH 5 to 7 (1369). A 30-µg/ml concentration at this pH range exhibits about a 2 to 3% loss in six hours at 25 °C; at pH 9, an 80% loss occurs under these conditions (51).

Dactinomycin, reconstituted according to the manufacturer's instructions, was cultured with human lymphoblasts to determine whether its cytotoxic activity was retained. The solution retained cytotoxicity for 24 hours at 4 °C and room temperature (1575).

Filtration— Dactinomycin may exhibit considerable binding to cellulose acetate/nitrate (Millex OR) and polytetrafluoroethylene (Millex GV) filters (1249).

Dactinomycin (MSD) 0.5 mg/L in dextrose 5% in water, sodium chloride 0.9%, and Ringer's injection, lactated, was filtered over 12 hours through a 5-µm stainless steel depth filter (Argyle Filter Connector), a 0.22-µm cellulose ester membrane filter (Ivex-2 Filter Set), and a 0.22-µm polycarbonate membrane filter (In-Sure Filter Set). No significant reduction in potency due to binding was observed with the stainless steel filter. Approximately 25% of the drug delivered through the polycarbonate filter in the first 10 ml of solution was bound, but binding decreased rapidly thereafter, resulting in only 0.3% of the total delivered dose in 12 hours being bound (320).

In contrast, filtration through the cellulose ester filter resulted in the binding of about 95 to 99% of the drug in the first 10 ml, with the total cumulative amount of drug bound in 12 hours being 13%. Approximately half of the bound drug was released by rinsing three times with 100 ml of the same intravenous solutions used in the admixtures (320).

A filter material specially treated with a proprietary agent was evaluated for a reduction in dactinomycin binding. Dactinomycin (MSD) 0.5 mg/L in dextrose 5% in water and sodium chloride 0.9% was run at a rate of 2 ml/min through an administration set with a treated 0.22-µm cellulose ester inline filter. Cumulative dactinomycin losses of less than 3% occurred from both solutions, compared to much higher losses previously reported for untreated cellulose ester filter material. Furthermore, equilibrium binding studies showed a sixfold reduction in binding from both solutions (904). All Abbott Ivex integral filter and extension sets currently use this treated filter material (1074).

In another study, dactinomycin 0.5 mg/1 ml was injected as a bolus through a 0.2-µm nylon, air-eliminating, filter (Ultipor, Pall) to evaluate the effect of filtration on simulated intravenous push delivery. Spectrophotometric evaluation showed that about 87% of the drug was delivered through the filter after flushing with 10 ml of sodium chloride 0.9% (809).

Dactinomycin 4 to 50 µg/ml exhibited a greater than 95% loss due to sorption to cellulose nitrate/cellulose acetate ester filters (Millex OR) and a 50 to 60% loss with polytetrafluoroethylene filters (Millex FG) (1415; 1416).

Compatibility Information

Solution Compatibility

Dactinomycin

Solution	Mfr	Mfr	Conc/L	Remarks	Ref	C/I
Dextrose 5% in water	[a]	MSD	9.8 mg	Less than 10% loss in 24 hr at room temperature	519	C
	MG, TR[a]	MSD	9.8 mg	Less than 10% loss by HPLC in 24 hr at room temperature exposed to light	1658	C
	MG, TR[b]	MSD	7.5 mg	Less than 10% loss by HPLC in 24 hr at room temperature exposed to light	1658	C

[a]*Tested in both glass and PVC containers.*
[b]*Tested in both glass and polyolefin containers.*

Y-Site Injection Compatibility (1:1 Mixture)

Dactinomycin

Drug	Mfr	Conc	Mfr	Conc	Remarks	Ref	C/I
Allopurinol sodium	BW	3 mg/ml[b]	MSD	0.01 mg/ml[b]	Physically compatible with no change in measured turbidity or increase in particle content in 4 hr at 22 °C	1686	C
Amifostine	USB	10 mg/ml[a]	ME	0.01 mg/ml[a]	Physically compatible with no change in measured turbidity or increase in particle content in 4 hr at 23 °C	1845	C
Aztreonam	SQ	40 mg/ml[a]	ME	0.01 mg/ml[a]	Physically compatible with no subvisual haze or particle formation in 4 hr at 23 °C	1758	C
Cefepime HCl	BR	20 mg/ml[a]	MSD	0.01 mg/ml[a]	Physically compatible with no change in measured turbidity or increase in particle content in 4 hr at 22 °C	1689	C

Y-Site Injection Compatibility (1:1 Mixture) (Cont.)

				Dactinomycin			
Drug	*Mfr*	*Conc*	*Mfr*	*Conc*	*Remarks*	*Ref*	*C/I*
Etoposide phosphate	BR	5 mg/ml[a]	ME	0.01 mg/ml[a]	Physically compatible with no change in measured turbidity or increase in particle content in 4 hr at 23 °C	2218	C
Filgrastim	AMG	30 μg/ml[a]	MSD	0.01 mg/ml[a]	Particles and filaments form immediately	1687	I
Fludarabine phosphate	BX	1 mg/ml[a]	MSD	0.01 mg/ml[a]	Physically compatible for 4 hr at room temperature under fluorescent light	1439	C
Gemcitabine HCl	LI	10 mg/ml[b]	ME	0.01 mg/ml[b]	Physically compatible with no change in measured turbidity or increase in particle content in 4 hr at 23 °C	2226	C
Granisetron HCl	SKB	0.05 mg/ml[a]	ME	0.01 mg/ml[a]	Physically compatible with no change in measured turbidity or increase in particle content in 4 hr at 23 °C	2000	C
Melphalan HCl	BW	0.1 mg/ml[b]	MSD	0.01 mg/ml[b]	Physically compatible with no change in measured turbidity or increase in particle content in 3 hr at 22 °C	1557	C
Ondansetron HCl	GL	1 mg/ml[b]	MSD	0.01 mg/ml[a]	Physically compatible for 4 hr at 22 °C	1365	C
Sargramostim	IMM	10 μg/ml[b]	MSD	0.01 mg/ml[b]	Physically compatible for 4 hr at 22 °C	1436	C
Teniposide	BR	0.1 mg/ml[a]	MSD	0.01 mg/ml[a]	Physically compatible with no subvisual haze or particle formation in 4 hr at 23 °C	1725	C
Thiotepa	IMM[c]	1 mg/ml[a]	ME	0.01 mg/ml[a]	Physically compatible with no change in measured turbidity or increase in particle content in 4 hr at 23 °C	1861	C
Vinorelbine tartrate	BW	1 mg/ml[b]	MSD	0.01 mg/ml[b]	Physically compatible with no change in measured turbidity or increase in particle content in 4 hr at 22 °C	1558	C

[a]*Tested in dextrose 5% in water.*
[b]*Tested in sodium chloride 0.9%.*
[c]*Lyophilized formulation tested.*

Additional Compatibility Information

Solutions— Dextrose 5% in water and sodium chloride 0.9% have been suggested as diluents for the reconstituted drug. It also may be injected into the tubing of a running infusion of these solutions (2; 4).

Dacarbazine— No alteration in the ultraviolet/visible spectra was observed when dacarbazine was combined in solution with dactinomycin (492).

Other Information

Inactivation— In the event of spills or leaks, MSD recommends the use of trisodium phosphate 5% to inactivate dactinomycin (1200).

DAUNORUBICIN HCL
AHFS 10:00

Cerubidine   **Bedford**

Products— Daunorubicin HCl (Bedford) is available in vials containing daunorubicin base 20 mg (21.4 mg as the hydrochloride salt) with mannitol 100 mg. Reconstitute with 4 ml of sterile water for injection to yield a solution containing 5 mg/ml of daunorubicin (2).

pH— From 4.5 to 6.5 (2; 4).

Osmolality— Daunorubicin HCl 5 mg/ml in sterile water for injection has an osmolality of 141 mOsm/kg (1689).

Administration— Daunorubicin HCl is administered intravenously *only*. Extravasation will result in severe tissue damage. The dose may be diluted with 10 to 15 ml of sodium chloride 0.9% and injected over two or three minutes into the sidearm or tubing of a rapidly flowing intravenous infusion of dextrose 5% in water or sodium chloride 0.9% (2; 4). Alternatively, the dose has been diluted in 100 ml and infused over 30 to 45 minutes (4).

Stability— Intact vials of daunorubicin HCl should be stored at controlled room temperature. The manufacturer states that the reconstituted solution is stable for 24 hours at controlled room temperature and 48 hours under refrigeration (2; 4).

Daunorubicin HCl appears to have pH-dependent stability in solution (526; 1250). Solutions of daunorubicin HCl are less stable at pH values above 8. Decomposition occurs, as indicated by a color change from red to blue-purple. The drug becomes progressively more stable as the pH of drug–infusion solution admixtures becomes more acidic from 7.4 down to 4.5 (526). The pH range of maximum stability was reported to be approximately 4.5 to 5.5. Below pH 4, decomposition increases substantially (1207).

Protection of the reconstituted solution from sunlight has been recommended (2). Photoinactivation of daunorubicin HCl exposed to radiation of 366 nm and fluorescent light has been reported (1094). One source indicates that significant losses due to light exposure for a sufficient time may occur in concentrations below 100 µg/ml. However, in clinical concentrations at or above 500 µg/ml, no special light protection is required (1369).

Wood et al. assessed the stability of daunorubicin HCl (Rhone-Poulenc) 100 mg/L in sodium chloride 0.9% (pH 6.47 and pH 5.20) and in dextrose 5% in water (pH 4.36) when stored in PVC bags at 4 and 25 °C in the dark. The drug was stable for at least 43 days at both temperatures, exhibiting not more than 7% loss by HPLC analysis (1460).

Daunorubicin HCl (Rhone-Poulenc) 2 mg/ml repackaged in polypropylene syringes exhibited little or no loss by HPLC analysis after storage for 43 days at 4 °C (1460).

Daunorubicin HCl, reconstituted according to the manufacturer's instructions, was cultured with human lymphoblasts to determine whether its cytotoxic activity was retained. The solution retained cytotoxicity for 24 hours at 4 °C and room temperature (1575).

Freezing Solutions— Wood et al. reported that daunorubicin HCl (Rhone-Poulenc) 100 mg/L in sodium chloride 0.9% and dextrose 5% in water in PVC bags (Travenol) was stable, exhibiting little or no loss by HPLC analysis after 43 days stored at −20 °C, even when subjected to 11 freeze-thaw repetitions (1460).

Sorption— Daunorubicin HCl (Roger Bellon) 16 µg/ml in dextrose 5% in water and sodium chloride 0.9% in PVC containers was infused through PVC administration sets at 21 ml/hr over 24 hours at 22 °C while exposed to light. Fluctuations in the delivered concentration by HPLC were relatively minor, with no evidence of sorption (1700).

Wood et al. reported that daunorubicin HCl was minimally adsorbed to PVC bags. After eight days of storage, HPLC analysis of solutions containing daunorubicin HCl 100 µg/ml in sodium chloride 0.9% and dextrose 5% in water stored at 4 and 25 °C indicated losses of up to 5%. At concentrations used in clinical practice, sorptive losses during storage and delivery are negligible (1460).

In an admixture composed of cytarabine (Upjohn) 0.157 mg/ml, daunorubicin HCl (Bellon) 15.7 µg/ml, and etoposide (Sandoz) 0.157 mg/ml in dextrose 5% in water, little or no loss of the drugs due to sorption occurred when delivered through PVC, PVC with polyethylene-lined sets, and a silicone central catheter (1955).

Filtration— Daunorubicin HCl (May & Baker) 10 mg/100 ml in sodium chloride 0.9% in a burette was filtered through a nylon 0.2-µm filter (ELD96LL, Pall). Little drug loss due to sorption was found spectrophotometrically (1568).

Daunorubicin HCl binds only slightly to cellulose acetate/nitrate (Millex OR) and polytetrafluoroethylene (Millex FG) filters (1249; 1415; 1416).

Compatibility Information

Solution Compatibility

Daunorubicin HCl

Solution	Mfr	Mfr	Conc/L	Remarks	Ref	C/I
Dextrose 3.3% in sodium chloride 0.3%		IV	100 mg	Drug loss of 5% or less in 4 weeks at 25 °C in the dark	1007	C
Dextrose 5% in water	AB	NCI	20 mg	Physically compatible with 2% decomposition in 24 hr at 21 °C	526	C
		IV	100 mg	Drug loss of 5% or less in 4 weeks at 25 °C in the dark	1007	C
	a	BEL	16 mg	No loss by HPLC in 7 days at 4 °C protected from light	1700	C
	TR[a]	RP	100 mg	7% or less loss by HPLC in 43 days at 4 and 25 °C in the dark	1460	C

Solution Compatibility (Cont.)

Daunorubicin HCl

Solution	Mfr	Mfr	Conc/L	Remarks	Ref	C/I
		BEL	15.7 mg	5 to 8% loss by spectroscopy in 48 hr at room temperature, exposed to light and in the dark, and at 4 °C	1955	C
Normosol R, pH 7.4	AB	NCI	20 mg	Physically compatible with 5% decomposition in 24 hr at 21 °C	526	C
Ringer's injection, lactated	AB	NCI	20 mg	Physically compatible with 5% decomposition in 24 hr at 21 °C	526	C
		IV	100 mg	Drug loss of 5% or less in 4 weeks at 25 °C in the dark	1007	C
Sodium chloride 0.9%	AB	NCI	20 mg	Physically compatible with 3% decomposition in 24 hr at 21 °C	526	C
		IV	100 mg	Drug loss of 5% or less in 4 weeks at 25 °C in the dark	1007	C
	[a]	BEL	16 mg	No loss by HPLC in 7 days at 4 °C protected from light	1700	C
	TR[a]	RP	100 mg	7% or less loss by HPLC in 43 days at 4 and 25 °C in the dark	1460	C

[a]Tested in PVC containers.

Additive Compatibility

Daunorubicin HCl

Drug	Mfr	Conc/L	Mfr	Conc/L	Test Soln	Remarks	Ref	C/I
Cytarabine with etoposide	UP BR	267 mg 400 mg	RP	33 mg	D5½S	Physically compatible with about 6% cytarabine loss and no loss of other drugs in 72 hr at 20 °C	1162	C
Cytarabine with etoposide	UP SZ	157 mg 157 mg	BEL	15.7 mg	D5W	Less than 10% loss of any drug in 48 hr at room temperature, exposed to light and in the dark, and at 4 °C	1955	C
Dexamethasone sodium phosphate						Immediate milky precipitate	524	I
Heparin sodium	UP	4000 units	FA	200 mg	D5W	Physically incompatible	15	I
Hydrocortisone sodium succinate	UP	500 mg	FA	200 mg	D5W	Physically compatible	15	C

Y-Site Injection Compatibility (1:1 Mixture)

Daunorubicin HCl

Drug	Mfr	Conc	Mfr	Conc	Remarks	Ref	C/I
Allopurinol sodium	BW	3 mg/ml[b]	WY	1 mg/ml[b]	Reddish-purple color and haze form immediately. Reddish-brown particles form within 1 hr	1686	I
Amifostine	USB	10 mg/ml[a]	WY	1 mg/ml[a]	Physically compatible with no change in measured turbidity or increase in particle content in 4 hr at 23 °C	1845	C
Aztreonam	SQ	40 mg/ml[a]	WY	1 mg/ml[a]	Haze forms immediately	1758	I
Cefepime HCl	BR	20 mg/ml[a]	WY	1 mg/ml[a]	Haze forms immediately and becomes flocculent precipitate in 4 hr	1689	I

Y-Site Injection Compatibility (1:1 Mixture) (Cont.)

Daunorubicin HCl

Drug	Mfr	Conc	Mfr	Conc	Remarks	Ref	C/I
Etoposide phosphate	BR	5 mg/ml[a]	BED	1 mg/ml[a]	Physically compatible with no change in measured turbidity or increase in particle content in 4 hr at 23 °C	2218	**C**
Filgrastim	AMG	30 µg/ml[a]	WY	1 mg/ml[a]	Physically compatible with no change in measured turbidity or increase in particle content in 4 hr at 22 °C	1687	**C**
Fludarabine phosphate	BX	1 mg/ml[a]	WY	2 mg/ml[a]	Slight haze, visible under high intensity light, forms in 4 hr at room temperature	1439	**I**
Gemcitabine HCl	LI	10 mg/ml[b]	BED	1 mg/ml[b]	Physically compatible with no change in measured turbidity or increase in particle content in 4 hr at 23 °C	2226	**C**
Granisetron HCl	SKB	0.05 mg/ml[a]	CHI	1 mg/ml[a]	Physically compatible with no change in measured turbidity or increase in particle content in 4 hr at 23 °C	2000	**C**
Melphalan HCl	BW	0.1 mg/ml[b]	WY	1 mg/ml[b]	Physically compatible with little change in measured turbidity or increase in particle content in 3 hr at 22 °C	1557	**C**
Methotrexate sodium		30 mg/ml	BEL	0.52 mg/ml[a]	Visually compatible for 4 hr at room temperature	1788	**C**
Ondansetron HCl	GL	1 mg/ml[b]	WY	2 mg/ml[a]	Physically compatible for 4 hr at 22 °C	1365	**C**
Piperacillin sodium–tazobactam sodium	LE	40 + 5 mg/ml[a]	WY	1 mg/ml[a]	Turbidity increases immediately	1688	**I**
Sodium bicarbonate		1.4%	BEL	0.52 mg/ml[a]	Visually compatible for 4 hr at room temperature	1788	**C**
Teniposide	BR	0.1 mg/ml[a]	WY	1 mg/ml[a]	Physically compatible with no subvisual haze or particle formation in 4 hr at 23 °C	1725	**C**
Thiotepa	IMM[c]	1 mg/ml[a]	WY	1 mg/ml[a]	Physically compatible with no change in measured turbidity or increase in particle content in 4 hr at 23 °C	1861	**C**
Vinorelbine tartrate	BW	1 mg/ml[b]	WY	1 mg/ml[b]	Physically compatible with little change in measured turbidity or increase in particle content in 4 hr at 22 °C	1558	**C**

[a]Tested in dextrose 5% in water.
[b]Tested in sodium chloride 0.9%.
[c]Lyophilized formulation tested.

Additional Compatibility Information

The manufacturer recommends that no other drugs be mixed with daunorubicin HCl (2).

Aluminum— Ogawa et al. reported that immersion of a needle with an aluminum component in daunorubicin HCl (Ives) 5 mg/ml resulted in a darkening of the solution, with black patches forming on the aluminum in 12 to 24 hours at 24 °C with protection from light (988).

Other Information

Inactivation— In the event of spills or leaks, Wyeth-Ayerst recommends the use of sodium hypochlorite 5% (household bleach) until a colorless liquid results to inactivate daunorubicin HCl (1200).

DEFEROXAMINE MESYLATE
AHFS 64:00

Desferal   **Novartis**

Products— Deferoxamine mesylate (Novartis) is available in vials containing 500 mg. Reconstitute with 2 ml of sterile water for injection to yield a 250-mg/ml solution (2).

Administration— Deferoxamine mesylate is administered by intramuscular injection, by slow intravenous infusion after dilution at a rate not exceeding 15 mg/kg/hr, and by subcutaneous infusion using a portable infusion control device (2).

Stability— Store the intact vials at temperatures not exceeding 25 °C. Deferoxamine mesylate is a white to off-white powder that forms a clear solution when reconstituted with sterile water for injection. The manufacturer states that reconstitution with other diluents may result in precipitation. Turbid solutions should not be used. The reconstituted solution is stable for one week at room temperature when protected from light. The solution should not be refrigerated (2; 4).

For intravenous infusion, sodium chloride 0.9%, dextrose 5% in water, or lactated Ringer's injection are recommended for use as diluents (2).

Syringes— Deferoxamine mesylate (Ciba-Geigy) 250 mg/ml in sterile water for injection was packaged as 3 ml in 10-ml polypropylene infusion pump syringes (Pharmacia Deltec). Little or no loss by HPLC analysis occurred during 14 days of storage at 30 °C (1967).

Elastomeric Reservoir Pumps— Deferoxamine mesylate (Ciba-Geigy) 5 mg/ml in both dextrose 5% in water and sodium chloride 0.9% was evaluated for binding potential to natural rubber elastomeric reservoirs (Baxter). No loss was found after storage for two weeks at 35 °C with gentle agitation (2014).

DEXAMETHASONE SODIUM PHOSPHATE
AHFS 68:04

Decadron   **Merck**

Products— Dexamethasone sodium phosphate (Merck) is available in 4- and 24-mg/ml strengths. The 4-mg/ml solution is available in 1-, 5-, and 25-ml vials. The 24-mg/ml solution is available in 5-ml vials. Each milliliter of these solutions contains (2):

Component	4 mg/ml	24 mg/ml
Dexamethasone sodium phosphate (equivalent to dexamethasone phosphate)	4 mg	24 mg
Creatinine	8 mg	8 mg
Sodium citrate	10 mg	10 mg
Sodium bisulfite	1 mg	1 mg
Methylparaben	1.5 mg	1.5 mg
Propylparaben	0.2 mg	0.2 mg
Disodium edetate		0.5 mg
Sodium hydroxide	to adjust pH	to adjust pH
Water for injection	qs	qs

Each milliliter of solution containing the equivalent of 24 mg of dexamethasone phosphate is equal to 20 mg of dexamethasone (2).

Each milliliter of solution containing the equivalent of 4 mg of dexamethasone phosphate is equal to 3.33 mg of dexamethasone (2).

Dexamethasone sodium phosphate is also available as a 10-mg/ml concentration in vials (2; 4).

pH— From 7 to 8.5 (2; 4). Dexamethasone sodium phosphate (David Bull) 0.5, 1, and 2 mg/ml in sodium chloride 0.9% for continuous subcutaneous infusion had pH values of 7.3, 7.3, and 7.5, respectively (2161).

Osmolality— The osmolality of the 4-mg/ml concentration of dexamethasone sodium phosphate (Elkins-Sinn) was determined by freezing-point depression to be 356 mOsm/kg (1071). Another study reported the osmolality of a dexamethasone injection (manufacturer not noted) to be 255 mOsm/kg (1233).

Dexamethasone sodium phosphate (David Bull) 0.5, 1, and 2 mg/ml in sodium chloride 0.9% for continuous subcutaneous infusion had osmolalities of 269, 260, and 238 mOsm/kg, respectively (2161).

Administration— Dexamethasone sodium phosphate 4- and 24-mg/ml concentrations may be administered intravenously by direct injection slowly over one to several minutes or by continuous or intermittent intravenous infusion. The 4-mg/ml concentration may be administered by intramuscular, intra-articular, intrasynovial, intralesional, or soft-tissue injection (2; 4).

Stability— The 4-mg/ml solution is clear and colorless while the 24-mg/ml solution is clear and colorless to light yellow. The solutions should be protected from light and freezing. In addition, dexamethasone sodium phosphate is heat labile and should not be autoclaved to sterilize the vial's exterior (2; 4).

Dexamethasone sodium phosphate (Lyphomed) was diluted to a concentration of 1 mg/ml with bacteriostatic sodium chloride 0.9% and packaged in 10-ml sterile glass vials. The dilutions remained clear and colorless, and little or no loss of dexamethasone was found by HPLC analysis after 28 days of storage at 4 and 22 °C (1940).

Syringes— Lau et al. reported the stability of dexamethasone sodium phosphate (Organon Teknica) 10 mg/ml repackaged into 1- and 2.5-ml Glaspak (Becton-Dickinson) and 1- and 3-ml plastic (Monoject, Sherwood) syringes. Samples in the Glaspak syringes were stored at 4 and 23 °C, unprotected from light and both shaken and unshaken during storage. Samples in plastic syringes were stored only at 23 °C. HPLC analysis for drug content showed not more than 5% loss in the Glaspak syringes after 91 days of storage at either temperature. Similarly, losses in the 3-ml plastic syringes were 7% or less after 55 days while losses in the 1-ml plastic syringes were 3% or less in 35 days; these time periods were the maximum that the plastic syringes were evaluated in this study. Furthermore, no contamination by the rubber components was found to leach into the drug solution during this time frame (1897).

These results are very different from those reported by Speaker et al. (1562). In that study, dexamethasone sodium phosphate 4 mg/ml was filled into 3-ml plastic syringes (Becton-Dickinson, Sherwood Monoject, and Terumo) and stored at −20, 4, and 25 °C in the dark. Substantial losses of UV absorbance were attributed to dexamethasone losses calculated to range from 5 to 20% in one day at all temperatures. Long-term storage for seven days at 4 °C and 30 days at −20 °C resulted in losses of 11 to 28%. The authors concluded that dexamethasone should not be prefilled and stored in plastic syringes (1562).

Speaker et al. presumed the losses in UV absorbance they observed were due to sorption to syringe surfaces and/or elastomeric plunger seals. However, the UV assay Speaker et al. used is nonspecific, and loss of absorbance could be due to loss of components other than dexamethasone. Using a more specific HPLC technique, Lau et al. did not observe this dexamethasone loss (1896).

Dexamethasone sodium phosphate (MSD) 4 mg/ml was found to retain potency for three months at room temperature when 1 ml of solution was packaged in Tubex cartridges (13). Furthermore, dexamethasone sodium phosphate exhibited no significant changes in 196 days at room temperature in glass disposable syringes (108).

Sorption— Dexamethasone sodium phosphate (MSD) 9 mg/L in sodium chloride 0.9% (Travenol) in PVC bags did not exhibit significant sorption to the plastic during one week of storage at room temperature (15 to 20 °C) (536).

In another study, dexamethasone sodium phosphate (MSD) 9 mg/L in sodium chloride 0.9% did not exhibit any loss due to sorption during a seven-hour simulated infusion through an infusion set (Travenol) consisting of a cellulose propionate burette chamber and 170 cm of PVC tubing (606).

The drug was also tested as a simulated infusion over at least one hour by a syringe pump system. A glass syringe on a syringe pump was fitted with 20 cm of polyethylene tubing or 50 cm of Silastic tubing. No loss of drug due to sorption was observed with either tubing (606).

A 25-ml aliquot of dexamethasone sodium phosphate (MSD) 9 mg/L in sodium chloride 0.9% was stored in an all-plastic syringe composed of a polypropylene barrel and a polyethylene plunger for 24 hours at room temperature in the dark. The solution did not exhibit any loss due to sorption (606).

Filtration— Dexamethasone sodium phosphate (MSD) 4 mg/L in dextrose 5% in water, sodium chloride 0.9%, and Ringer's injection, lactated, filtered over 12 hours through a 5-μm stainless steel depth filter (Argyle Filter Connector), a 0.22-μm cellulose ester membrane filter (Ivex-2 Filter Set), and a 0.22-μm polycarbonate membrane filter (In-Sure Filter Set), showed no significant reduction in potency due to binding to the filters (320).

In another study, dexamethasone sodium phosphate (MSD) 4 mg/L in dextrose 5% in water and sodium chloride 0.9% did not display significant sorption to a 0.45-μm cellulose membrane filter (Abbott S-A-I-F) during an eight-hour simulated infusion (567).

Compatibility Information

Solution Compatibility

Dexamethasone sodium phosphate

Solution	Mfr	Mfr	Conc/L	Remarks	Ref	C/I
Dextrose 5% in water	a	AMR	94 and 658 mg	Visually compatible with no loss by HPLC in 14 days stored at 24 °C protected from light	1875	C
Sodium chloride 0.9%	a	AMR	92 and 660 mg	Visually compatible with no loss by HPLC in 14 days stored at 24 °C protected from light	1875	C
	BAª	ES	200 and 400 mg	Visually compatible with no loss by HPLC in 30 days at 4 °C followed by 2 days at 25 °C	1882	C

ªTested in PVC containers.

Additive Compatibility

Dexamethasone sodium phosphate

Drug	Mfr	Conc/L	Mfr	Conc/L	Test Soln	Remarks	Ref	C/I
Amikacin sulfate	BR	5 g	MSD	40 mg	D5LR, D5R, D5S, D5W, D10W, IS10, LR, NS, R, SL	Physically compatible and potency of both retained for 24 hr at 25 °C	294	C
	BR	5 g	MSD	40 mg	D2.5S	16% dexamethasone decomposition in 4 hr at 25 °C	294	I
Aminophylline		625 mg		30 mg	D5W	Physically compatible and chemically stable for 24 hr at 4 and 30 °C	521	C

Additive Compatibility (Cont.)

Dexamethasone sodium phosphate

Drug	Mfr	Conc/L	Mfr	Conc/L	Test Soln	Remarks	Ref	C/I
Bleomycin sulfate	BR	20 and 30 units	MSD	50 mg	NS	Physically compatible and bleomycin activity retained for 1 week at 4 °C. Dexamethasone not tested	763	C
Cimetidine HCl	SKF	3 g	MSD	40 mg	D5W	Physically compatible and cimetidine chemically stable for 24 hr at room temperature. Dexamethasone not tested	551	C
Daunorubicin HCl						Immediate milky precipitation	524	I
Diphenhydramine HCl with lorazepam and metoclopramide HCl	ES WY DU	2 g 40 mg 4 g	AMR	400 mg	NS[a]	Rapid lorazepam losses of 8, 10, and 15% at 3, 23, and 30 °C, respectively, in 24 hr by HPLC. Other drugs stable for 14 days by HPLC at all three storage temperatures	1733	I
Floxacillin sodium	BE	20 g	MSD	4 g	NS	Physically compatible for 72 hr at 15 and 30 °C	1479	C
Furosemide	HO	1 g	MSD	4 g	NS	Physically compatible for 72 hr at 15 and 30 °C	1479	C
Granisetron HCl	SKB	10 and 40 mg	AMR	92 mg	D5W, NS[b]	Visually compatible with little or no loss of either drug by HPLC in 14 days at 4 and 24 °C protected from light	1875	C
	SKB	10 and 40 mg	AMR	660 mg	D5W, NS[b]	Visually compatible with little or no dexamethasone loss and up to 8% granisetron loss by HPLC in 14 days at 4 and 24 °C protected from light	1875	C
	BE	55 and 51 mg	MSD	75 and 345 mg	D5W, NS[b]	Visually compatible with little or no loss of either drug by HPLC in 72 hr at room temperature	1884	C
Lidocaine HCl	AST	2 g	MSD	4 mg		Physically compatible	24	C
Meropenem	ZEN	1 and 20 g	MSD	4 g	NS	Visually compatible for 4 hr at room temperature	1994	C
Metaraminol bitartrate	MSD	100 mg	MSD	20 mg	D5W, NS	Altered UV spectra for dexamethasone within 1 hr at room temperature	42	I
	MSD	500 mg	MSD	100 mg	D5W	Altered UV spectra for dexamethasone within 1 hr at room temperature	42	I
Mitomycin	BR	100 mg	LY	5 g	NS[c]	Visually compatible with 10% mitomycin loss calculated in 68 hr and 10% dexamethasone loss calculated in 250 hr at 25 °C	1866	C
	BR	100 mg	LY	5 g	NS[b]	Visually compatible with 10% mitomycin loss calculated in 91 hr and 10% dexamethasone loss calculated in 154 hr at 25 °C	1866	C
	BR	100 mg	LY	5 g	NS[c]	Visually compatible with 10% mitomycin loss calculated in 211 hr and 10% dexamethasone loss calculated in 98 hr at 4 °C	1866	C
	BR	100 mg	LY	5 g	NS[b]	Visually compatible with 10% mitomycin loss calculated in 238 hr and 10% dexamethasone loss calculated in 355 hr at 25 °C	1866	C
Nafcillin sodium	WY	500 mg	MSD	4 mg		Physically compatible	27	C

Additive Compatibility (Cont.)

Dexamethasone sodium phosphate

Drug	Mfr	Conc/L	Mfr	Conc/L	Test Soln	Remarks	Ref	C/I
Netilmicin sulfate	SC	3 g	MSD	80 mg	D5S	Physically compatible and netilmicin chemically stable for 7 days at 25 and 4 °C. Dexamethasone not tested	558	**C**
Ondansetron HCl	GL	48 mg		20 and 40 mg	D5W, NS	Visually compatible for 24 hr at 22 °C	1608	**C**
	GL	160 mg		200 and 400 mg	NS	Visually compatible for 24 hr at 22 °C	1608	**C**
	CER	100 mg	ES	200 mg	NS[b]	Visually compatible with no dexamethasone loss and 8% ondansetron loss by HPLC after 30 days at 4 °C followed by 2 days at 23 °C	1882	**C**
	CER	100 and 200 mg	ES	400 mg	NS[b]	Visually compatible with no dexamethasone loss and 7 to 10% ondansetron loss by HPLC after 30 days at 4 °C followed by 2 days at 23 °C	1882	**C**
	CER	200, 400, and 640 mg	ES	200 mg	NS[b]	Visually compatible with no dexamethasone loss and not more than 5% ondansetron loss by HPLC after 30 days at 4 °C followed by 2 days at 23 °C	1882	**C**
	CER	400 and 640 mg	ES	400 mg	NS[b]	Visually compatible with no dexamethasone loss and not more than 3% ondansetron loss by HPLC after 30 days at 4 °C followed by 2 days at 23 °C	1882	**C**
	CER	640 mg	ES	200 and 400 mg	D5W[d]	Visually compatible with 7% dexamethasone loss and no ondansetron loss by HPLC after 30 days at 4 °C followed by 2 days at 23 °C	1882	**C**
	GL	150 mg	MSD	400 mg	NS[a]	Visually compatible with 4% or less loss of either drug by HPLC in 28 days at 4 and 22 °C	2084	**C**
	GL	150 mg	MSD	400 mg	D5W[a]	Visually compatible with 4% or less loss of either drug by HPLC in 28 days at 4 °C. Up to 10% ondansetron loss in 3 days at 22 °C	2084	**C**
	GL	750 mg	MSD	230 mg	NS[a]	Visually compatible with 4% or less loss of either drug by HPLC in 28 days at 4 °C. Up to 10% ondansetron loss in 7 days at 22 °C	2084	**C**
	GL	750 mg	MSD	230 mg	D5W[a]	Visually compatible with up to 13% ondansetron loss by HPLC in 3 days at 4 and 22 °C	2084	**?**
Prochlorperazine edisylate	SKF	100 mg	MSD	20 mg	D5W	Physically compatible	15	**C**
Ranitidine HCl	GL	50 mg and 2 g		40 mg	D5W	Physically compatible and ranitidine chemically stable by HPLC for 24 hr at 25 °C. Dexamethasone not tested	1515	**C**
Vancomycin HCl	LI					Physically incompatible	9	**I**
Verapamil HCl	KN	80 mg	MSD	40 mg	D5W, NS	Physically compatible for 24 hr	764	**C**

[a]*Tested in Pharmacia-Deltec PVC pump reservoirs.*
[b]*Tested in PVC containers.*
[c]*Tested in glass containers.*
[d]*Tested in ondansetron HCl ready-to-use CR3 polyester bags.*

Drugs in Syringe Compatibility

Dexamethasone sodium phosphate

Drug (in syringe)	Mfr	Amt	Mfr	Amt	Remarks	Ref	C/I
Diphenhydramine HCl	PD	50 mg/ml[a]	DB, SX	4 and 10 mg/ml[a]	White turbidity and precipitate form immediately	1542	I
	PD	4.54 mg/ml[b]	DB	9.52 mg/ml[b]	Visually compatible for 24 hr at 24 °C	1542	C
	PD	4.54 to 15 mg/ml[b]	DB	5 to 9.02 mg/ml[b]	Precipitate forms	1542	I
	PD	34.8 to 40 mg/ml[b]	SX	2 mg/ml[b]	Visually compatible for 24 hr at 24 °C	1542	C
	PD	25 mg/ml[b]	SX	1 mg/ml[b]	Precipitate forms	1542	I
Doxapram HCl	RB	400 mg/20 ml	MSD	3.3 mg/1 ml	Immediate turbidity and precipitation	1177	I
Glycopyrrolate	RB	0.2 mg/1 ml	MSD	4 mg/1 ml	Physically compatible for 48 hr at 25 °C. But the pH>6. Approximately 5% glycopyrrolate decomposition may occur in 4 to 7 hr	331	I
	RB	0.2 mg/1 ml	MSD	8 mg/2 ml	Physically compatible for 48 hr at 25 °C. But the pH>6. Approximately 5% glycopyrrolate decomposition may occur in 4 to 7 hr	331	I
	RB	0.4 mg/2 ml	MSD	4 mg/1 ml	Physically compatible for 48 hr at 25 °C. But the pH>6. Approximately 5% glycopyrrolate decomposition may occur in 4 to 7 hr	331	I
	RB	0.2 mg/1 ml	MSD	24 mg/1 ml	Physically compatible for 48 hr at 25 °C. But the pH>6. Approximately 5% glycopyrrolate decomposition may occur in 4 to 7 hr	331	I
	RB	0.2 mg/1 ml	MSD	48 mg/2 ml	Physically compatible for 48 hr at 25 °C. But the pH>6. Approximately 5% glycopyrrolate decomposition may occur in 4 to 7 hr	331	I
	RB	0.4 mg/2 ml	MSD	24 mg/1 ml	Physically compatible for 48 hr at 25 °C. But the pH>6. Approximately 5% glycopyrrolate decomposition may occur in 4 to 7 hr	331	I
Granisetron HCl	BE	0.15 mg/ml[c]	MSD	0.2 and 1 mg/ml[c]	Visually compatible with little or no loss of either drug by HPLC in 72 hr at room temperature	1884	C
Hydromorphone HCl	KN	2, 10, 40 mg/ml[a]	SX	4 mg/ml[a]	Visually compatible and potency of both drugs by HPLC retained for 24 hr at 24 °C	1542	C
	KN	2 and 10 mg/ml[a]	DB	10 mg/ml[a]	Visually compatible and potency of both drugs by HPLC retained for 24 hr at 24 °C	1542	C
	KN	40 mg/ml[a]	DB	10 mg/ml[a]	White turbidity forms immediately	1542	I
	KN	11.6 mg/ml[b]	DB	7.1 mg/ml[b]	Visually compatible for 24 hr at 24 °C	1542	C

Drugs in Syringe Compatibility (Cont.)

Dexamethasone sodium phosphate

Drug (in syringe)	Mfr	Amt	Mfr	Amt	Remarks	Ref	C/I
	KN	13.3 to 17.5 mg/ml[b]	DB, SX	5.5 to 6.6 mg/ml[b]	Precipitate forms	1542	**I**
	KN	10.5 mg/ml[b]	DB	4.75 mg/ml[b]	Visually compatible for 24 hr at 24 °C	1542	**C**
	KN	14.75 to 25 mg/ml[b]	SX	3 to 4.1 mg/ml[b]	Precipitate forms	1542	**I**
	KN	26.66 mg/ml[b]	SX	3.34 mg/ml[b]	Visually compatible for 24 hr at 24 °C	1542	**C**
Metoclopramide HCl	RB	10 mg/2 ml	ES, MSD	8 mg/2 ml	Physically compatible for 48 hr at room temperature	924	**C**
	RB	10 mg/2 ml	ES, MSD	8 mg/2 ml	Physically compatible for 48 hr at 25 °C	1167	**C**
	RB	160 mg/32 ml	ES, MSD	8 mg/2 ml	Physically compatible for 48 hr at 25 °C	1167	**C**
Ondansetron HCl	CER	0.17 mg/ml[d]	ES	0.5 and 1 mg/ml[d]	Visually compatible with no loss of either drug by HPLC after 30 days at 4 °C followed by 2 days at 23 °C	1882	**C**
	CER	0.25 mg/ml[d]	ES	0.5 mg/ml[d]	Visually compatible with no loss of either drug by HPLC after 30 days at 4 °C followed by 2 days at 23 °C	1882	**C**
	CER	0.25 mg/ml[d]	ES	1 mg/ml[d]	Visually compatible for 3 days at 4 °C. Precipitation of ondansetron observed at 7 days as opaque white ring	1882	**C**
	CER	0.33 mg/ml[d]	ES	0.33 and 0.67 mg/ml[d]	Visually compatible with no loss of either drug by HPLC after 30 days at 4 °C followed by 2 days at 23 °C	1882	**C**
	CER	0.5 mg/ml[d]	ES	0.5 mg/ml[d]	Visually compatible with no loss of either drug by HPLC after 30 days at 4 °C followed by 2 days at 23 °C	1882	**C**
	CER	0.5 mg/ml[d]	ES	1 mg/ml[d]	Visually compatible for 3 days at 4 °C. Precipitation of ondansetron observed at 7 days as opaque white ring	1882	**C**
	CER	0.67 mg/ml[d]	ES	0.33 and 0.67 mg/ml[d]	Visually compatible with no loss of either drug by HPLC after 30 days at 4 °C followed by 2 days at 23 °C	1882	**C**
	CER	1.07 mg/ml[d]	ES	0.33 mg/ml[d]	Visually compatible with no loss of either drug by HPLC after 30 days at 4 °C followed by 2 days at 23 °C	1882	**C**
	CER	1.07 mg/ml[d]	ES	0.67 mg/ml[d]	Heavy white flocculent precipitate appears within 72 hr at 4 °C with 25 to 30% loss of both drugs by HPLC from solution	1882	**I**
Ranitidine HCl	GL	50 mg/5 ml	ME	4 mg	Physically compatible for 4 hr at ambient temperature under fluorescent light	1151	**C**
Sufentanil citrate	JN	50 µg/ml	AMR	4 mg/ml	Physically compatible with no subvisual haze or particle formation in 24 hr at 23 °C	1711	**C**

[a]*Mixed in equal quantities. Final concentration is one-half the indicated concentration.*
[b]*Mixed in varying quantities to yield the final concentrations noted.*
[c]*Granisetron in sodium chloride 0.9% and dextrose 5% in water. Diluted further with 17 ml of water.*
[d]*Diluted with sodium chloride 0.9% drawn into a syringe prior to drugs to yield the concentrations cited.*

Y-Site Injection Compatibility (1:1 Mixture)

			Dexamethasone sodium phosphate				
Drug	*Mfr*	*Conc*	*Mfr*	*Conc*	*Remarks*	*Ref*	*C/I*
Acyclovir sodium	BW	5 mg/ml[a]	ES	0.2 mg/ml[a]	Physically compatible for 4 hr at 25 °C	1157	C
Allopurinol sodium	BW	3 mg/ml[b]	LY	1 mg/ml[b]	Physically compatible with no change in measured turbidity or increase in particle content in 4 hr at 22 °C	1686	C
Amifostine	USB	10 mg/ml[a]	AMR	1 mg/ml[a]	Physically compatible with no change in measured turbidity or increase in particle content in 4 hr at 23 °C	1845	C
Amikacin sulfate	SQ	50 mg/ml[c]	AMR	4 mg/ml	Visually compatible for 24 hr at room temperature in test tubes. No precipitate found on filter from Y-site delivery	2063	C
Amphotericin B cholesteryl sulfate complex	SEQ	0.83 mg/ml[a]	ES	2 mg/ml[a]	Physically compatible with little or no change in measured turbidity or increase in particle content in 4 hr at 23 °C under fluorescent light	2117	C
Amsacrine	NCI	1 mg/ml[a]	QU	1 mg/ml[a]	Physically compatible for 4 hr at room temperature under fluorescent light	1381	C
Aztreonam	SQ	40 mg/ml[a]	AMR	1 mg/ml[a]	Physically compatible with no subvisual haze or particle formation in 4 hr at 23 °C	1758	C
Cefepime HCl	BR	20 mg/ml[a]	AMR	1 mg/ml[a]	Physically compatible with no change in measured turbidity or increase in particle content in 4 hr at 22 °C	1689	C
Cefpirome sulfate	HO	50 mg/ml[d]	LY	4 mg/ml[d]	Visually and microscopically compatible with 5% or less cefpirome loss and little or no dexamethasone loss by HPLC in 8 hr at 23 °C	2044	C
Ciprofloxacin	MI	2 mg/ml[e]	LY	4 mg/ml	Transient white cloudiness rapidly dissipates. White crystals and flocculation form in 1 hr at 24 °C	1655	I
Cisatracurium besylate	GW	0.1, 2, 5 mg/ml[a]	FUJ	2 mg/ml[a]	Physically compatible with no change in measured turbidity or increase in particle content in 4 hr at 23 °C	2074	C
Cisplatin	BR	1 mg/ml	QU	1 mg/ml[a]	Visually compatible for 4 hr at room temperature under fluorescent light	1685	C
Cladribine	ORT	0.015[b] and 0.5[f] mg/ml	AMR	1 mg/ml[b]	Physically compatible with no change in measured turbidity or increase in particle content in 4 hr at 23 °C	1969	C
Cyclophosphamide	MJ	10 mg/ml[a]	QU	1 mg/ml[a]	Visually compatible for 4 hr at room temperature under fluorescent light	1685	C
Cytarabine	UP	50 mg/ml	QU	1 mg/ml[a]	Visually compatible for 4 hr at room temperature under fluorescent light	1685	C
Docetaxel	RPR	0.9 mg/ml[a]	ES	2 mg/ml[a]	Physically compatible with no change in measured turbidity or increase in particle content in 4 hr at 23 °C	2224	C
Doxorubicin HCl	AD	0.2 mg/ml[a]	QU	1 mg/ml[a]	Visually compatible for 4 hr at room temperature under fluorescent light	1685	C

Y-Site Injection Compatibility (1:1 Mixture) (Cont.)

Dexamethasone sodium phosphate

Drug	Mfr	Conc	Mfr	Conc	Remarks	Ref	C/I
Doxorubicin HCl liposome injection	SEQ	0.4 mg/ml[a]	ES	2 mg/ml[a]	Physically compatible with little or no change in measured turbidity and no increase in particle content in 4 hr at 23 °C	2087	C
Etoposide phosphate	BR	5 mg/ml[a]	ES	1 mg/ml[a]	Physically compatible with no change in measured turbidity or increase in particle content in 4 hr at 23 °C	2218	C
Famotidine	MSD ME	0.2 mg/ml[a] 2 mg/ml[b]	ES	10 mg/ml 1 mg/ml[a]	Physically compatible for 14 hr Visually compatible for 4 hr at 22 °C	1196 1936	C C
Filgrastim	AMG	30 μg/ml[a]	LY	1 mg/ml[a]	Physically compatible with no change in measured turbidity or increase in particle content in 4 hr at 22 °C	1687	C
Fluconazole	RR	2 mg/ml	ES	4 mg/ml	Physically compatible for 24 hr at 25 °C	1407	C
Fludarabine phosphate	BX	1 mg/ml[a]	MSD	1 mg/ml[a]	Physically compatible for 4 hr at room temperature under fluorescent light	1439	C
Foscarnet sodium	AST	24 mg/ml	OR	10 mg/ml	Physically compatible for 24 hr at room temperature under fluorescent light	1335	C
Gemcitabine HCl	LI	10 mg/ml[b]	ES	1 mg/ml[b]	Physically compatible with no change in measured turbidity or increase in particle content in 4 hr at 23 °C	2226	C
Granisetron HCl	SKB	1 mg/ml	ME	0.24 mg/ml[b]	Physically compatible with little or no loss of either drug by HPLC in 4 hr at 22 °C	1883	C
Heparin sodium	TR	50 units/ml	LI	1 mg/ml[a]	Visually compatible for 6 hr at 25 °C	1793	C
Heparin sodium with hydrocortisone sodium succinate	RI UP	1000 units + 100 mg/L[g]	MSD	4 mg/ml	Physically compatible for at least 4 hr at room temperature by visual and microscopic examination	322	C
Idarubicin HCl	AD	1 mg/ml[b]	OR	10 mg/ml	Haze forms immediately and precipitate forms in 20 min	1525	I
	AD	1 mg/ml[b]	AMR	0.2 mg/ml[b]	Haze forms in 20 min	1525	I
Lorazepam	WY	0.33 mg/ml[b]		4 mg/ml	Visually compatible for 24 hr at 22 °C	1855	C
Melphalan HCl	BW	0.1 mg/ml[b]	LY	1 mg/ml[b]	Physically compatible with no change in measured turbidity or increase in particle content in 3 hr at 22 °C	1557	C
Meperidine HCl	AB	10 mg/ml	LY	0.2 mg/ml[a]	Physically compatible for 4 hr at 25 °C	1397	C
Meropenem	ZEN	1 and 50 mg/ml[b]	MSD	10 mg/ml[h]	Visually compatible for 4 hr at room temperature	1994	C
Methotrexate sodium	AD	15 mg/ml[i]	QU	1 mg/ml[a]	Visually compatible for 4 hr at room temperature under fluorescent light	1685	C
		30 mg/ml	MSD	4 mg/ml	Visually compatible for 2 hr at room temperature. Dark yellow precipitate forms in 4 hr	1788	I
Midazolam HCl	RC	1 mg/ml[a]	ES	4 mg/ml	Haze forms immediately. Precipitate forms in 8 hr	1847	I
	RC	5 mg/ml		4 mg/ml	White precipitate forms immediately	1855	I

Y-Site Injection Compatibility (1:1 Mixture) (Cont.)

Dexamethasone sodium phosphate

Drug	Mfr	Conc	Mfr	Conc	Remarks	Ref	C/I
Morphine sulfate	AB	1 mg/ml	LY	0.2 mg/ml[a]	Physically compatible for 4 hr at 25 °C	1397	C
Ondansetron HCl	GL	1 mg/ml[b]	MSD	1 mg/ml[a]	Physically compatible for 4 hr at 22 °C	1365	C
Paclitaxel	NCI	1.2 mg/ml[a]		1 mg/ml[a]	Physically compatible with no change in measured turbidity in 4 hr at 22 °C	1528	C
Piperacillin sodium–tazobactam sodium	LE	40 + 5 mg/ml[a]	LY	1 mg/ml[a]	Physically compatible with no change in measured turbidity or increase in particle content in 4 hr at 22 °C	1688	C
Potassium chloride		40 mEq/L[g]	MSD	4 mg/ml	Physically compatible for at least 4 hr at room temperature by visual and microscopic examination	322	C
Propofol	ZEN	10 mg/ml	AMR	1 mg/ml[a]	Physically compatible for 1 hr at 23 °C with no increase in particle content	2066	C
Remifentanil HCl	GW	0.025 and 0.25 mg/ml[b]	FUJ	2 mg/ml[a]	Physically compatible with no change in measured turbidity or increase in particle content in 4 hr at 23 °C	2075	C
Sargramostim	IMM	10 μg/ml[b]	ES	1 mg/ml[b]	Physically compatible for 4 hr at 22 °C	1436	C
Sodium bicarbonate		1.4%	MSD	4 mg/ml	Visually compatible for 4 hr at room temperature	1788	C
Sufentanil citrate	JN	12.5 μg/ml[a]	AMR	1 mg/ml[a]	Physically compatible with no subvisual haze or particle formation in 24 hr at 23 °C	1711	C
Tacrolimus	FUJ	1 mg/ml[b]	ES	4 mg/ml[a]	Visually compatible for 24 hr at 25 °C	1630	C
Teniposide	BR	0.1 mg/ml[a]	LY	1 mg/ml[a]	Physically compatible with no subvisual haze or particle formation in 4 hr at 23 °C	1725	C
Theophylline	TR	4 mg/ml	ES	0.08 mg/ml[a]	Visually compatible for 6 hr at 25 °C	1793	C
Thiotepa	IMM[j]	1 mg/ml[a]	AMR	1 mg/ml[a]	Physically compatible with no change in measured turbidity or increase in particle content in 4 hr at 23 °C	1861	C
TNA #218 to #226[k]			FUJ, ES	1 mg/ml[a]	Visually compatible with no precipitate or emulsion damage apparent in 4 hr at 23 °C	2215	C
TPN #203 and #204[k]			AMR	4 mg/ml	Visually compatible for 2 hr at 23 °C	1974	C
TPN #212 to #215[k]			AMR	1 mg/ml[a]	Physically compatible with no change in measured turbidity or increase in particle content in 4 hr at 23 °C	2109	C
Vinorelbine tartrate	BW	1 mg/ml[b]	LY	1 mg/ml[b]	Physically compatible with no change in measured turbidity or increase in particle content in 4 hr at 22 °C	1558	C
Vitamin B complex with C	RC	2 ml/L[g]	MSD	4 mg/ml	Physically compatible for at least 4 hr at room temperature by visual and microscopic examination	322	C

Y-Site Injection Compatibility (1:1 Mixture) (Cont.)

Dexamethasone sodium phosphate

Drug	Mfr	Conc	Mfr	Conc	Remarks	Ref	C/I
Zidovudine	BW	4 mg/ml[a]	ES	0.16 mg/ml[a]	Physically compatible for 4 hr at 25 °C under fluorescent light by visual and microscopic examination	1193	**C**

[a]*Tested in dextrose 5% in water.*
[b]*Tested in sodium chloride 0.9%.*
[c]*Tested in sodium chloride 0.45%.*
[d]*Tested in dextrose 5% in water, Ringer's injection, lactated, sodium chloride 0.45%, and sodium chloride 0.9%.*
[e]*Tested in both dextrose 5% in water and sodium chloride 0.9%.*
[f]*Tested in bacteriostatic sodium chloride 0.9% preserved with benzyl alcohol 0.9%.*
[g]*Tested in dextrose 5% in water, Ringer's injection, lactated, and sodium chloride 0.9%.*
[h]*Tested in sterile water for injection.*
[i]*Tested in dextrose 5% in water with sodium bicarbonate 0.05 mEq/ml.*
[j]*Lyophilized formulation tested.*
[k]*Refer to Appendix I for the composition of the parenteral nutrition solutions. TPN indicates a 2-in-1 admixture.*

Additional Compatibility Information

Dextrose 5% in water and sodium chloride 0.9% have been recommended as diluents for intravenous infusions (2; 4).

The following incompatibility determinations were performed with concentrated solutions. One milliliter of dexamethasone sodium phosphate (MSD) was added to 5 ml of sterile distilled water along with 1 ml of prochlorperazine edisylate (SKF) or vancomycin HCl (Lilly). Particulate matter was noted within two hours (28).

DEXTRAN 40
AHFS 40:12

Gentran	**Baxter**
LMD	**Abbott**
Rheomacrodex	**Medisan**

Products— Dextran 40 products are available as a 10% (10 g/100 ml) injection in dextrose 5% or sodium chloride 0.9% in 500-ml containers. The dextran products are prepared from low molecular weight dextran (average molecular weight of 40,000) with either dextrose, hydrous, 5 g/100 ml or sodium chloride 0.9 g/100 ml in water for injection (4; 154).

pH— The pH of dextran 40 10% in dextrose 5% ranges from 3 to 7. The pH of dextran 40 10% in sodium chloride 0.9% ranges from 3.5 to 7 (4).

Sodium Content— Dextran 40 10% in sodium chloride 0.9% provides 77 mEq of sodium per 500-ml bottle (4).

Administration— Dextran 40 10% injection is administered by intravenous infusion (4).

Stability— Dextran 40 products should not be administered unless they are clear. Long periods of storage or exposure to temperature fluctuations may cause the formation of dextran flakes. Therefore, solutions should be stored at a constant temperature, preferably 25 °C, and protected from freezing and extreme heat. If flakes do appear, they can be dissolved by heating in a water bath at 100 °C or autoclaving at 110 °C for 15 minutes (4; 1484; 1485).

Compatibility Information

Additive Compatibility

Dextran 40

Drug	Mfr	Conc/L	Mfr	Conc/L	Test Soln	Remarks	Ref	C/I
Amoxicillin sodium		10, 20, 50 g		10%	D5W	9, 12, and 12% amoxicillin loss at 10, 20, and 50 g/L, respectively, in 1 hr at 25 °C	1469	**I**

Additive Compatibility (Cont.)

Dextran 40

Drug	Mfr	Conc/L	Mfr	Conc/L	Test Soln	Remarks	Ref	C/I
		10, 20, 50 g		10%	NS	12, 14, and 20% amoxicillin loss at 10, 20, and 50 g/L, respectively, in 3 hr at 25 °C	1469	I

Y-Site Injection Compatibility (1:1 Mixture)

Dextran 40

Drug	Mfr	Conc	Mfr	Conc	Remarks	Ref	C/I
Enalaprilat	MSD	0.05 mg/ml[a]	TR	100 mg/ml[b]	Physically compatible for 24 hr at room temperature under fluorescent light	1355	C
Famotidine	MSD	0.2 mg/ml[b]	PH	100 mg/ml[b]	Physically compatible for 4 hr at 25 °C under fluorescent light	1188	C

[a]Tested in sodium chloride 0.9%.
[b]Tested in dextrose 5% in water.

DIATRIZOATE MEGLUMINE
AHFS 36:68

Products— Diatrizoate meglumine is available in concentrations ranging from 18 to 76%. It is also available in combination with other radiopaque contrast agents. The formulations may also contain edetate and parabens. Hydrochloric acid, diatrizoic acid, or meglumine may have been used during manufacturing to adjust pH. Some examples of single-agent products are listed in Table 1 (4; 154).

pH— From 6.5 to 7.7 (4).

Osmotic Values— Osmolarities of the various concentrations range from 640 to 1761 mOsm/L (4).

Administration— Appropriate dosage forms and concentrations of diatrizoate meglumine may be administered intravenously, intramuscularly, intra-arterially, or intra-articularly. Some products may be injected or instilled directly into selected areas to be visualized (4).

Stability— Diatrizoate meglumine solutions are colorless to pale yellow. On standing, a crystalline precipitate may form. To redissolve the crystals, place the container in hot water and shake gently. Allow the solution to cool to body temperature before administration (4).

Diatrizoate meglumine in combination with diatrizoate sodium as Renografin products is sensitive to low pH values. At about pH 3 to 4, turbidity or frank precipitation may appear (479).

Diatrizoate meglumine solutions should be protected from strong light (4).

Plastic Syringes— Plastic syringes have been stated to be unsuitable

Table 1. Some Representative Diatrizoate Meglumine Products

Diatrizoate Meglumine Content (%)	Bound Iodine (mg/ml)	Representative Trade Names
Urogenital solutions (not for intravascular use)		
18	85	Cystografin Dilute
30	141	Cystografin, Reno-M-30, Hypaque Cysto, Urovist Cysto
Parenteral solutions		
30	141	Hypaque Meglumine 30%, Reno-M-DIP, Urovist Meglumine
60	282	Hypaque Meglumine 60%, Reno-M-60, Angiovist 282
76	358	generic formulation

for accommodating radiopaque solutions for any length of time. The plastic is attacked, and the plunger tends to freeze on prolonged storage (40).

An increased incidence of adverse reactions to diatrizoate meglumine in combination with diatrizoate sodium in intravenous pyelography was attributed to extraction of phenolic compounds from the rubber plunger-stoppers when Plastipak (Becton-Dickinson) disposable syringes were used to administer the radiopaque contrast media. The use of glass syringes only was recommended (821).

Compatibility Information

Drugs in Syringe Compatibility

Diatrizoate meglumine

Drug (in syringe)	Mfr	Amt	Mfr	Amt	Remarks	Ref	C/I
Diphenhydramine HCl	PD	50 mg/ 1 ml	SQ	5 ml[a]	No precipitate observed	309	C

[a]*Percentage unspecified.*

Additional Compatibility Information

Additives— Diatrizoate meglumine products (Squibb) have been generally found to be compatible with chlorpheniramine maleate (Schering) and hyaluronidase (Wyeth) (40).

Diphenhydramine HCl (Parke-Davis) has been stated to be com-patible for short periods with diatrizoate meglumine products (Squibb) (40).

Diatrizoate meglumine products (Squibb) were found to be physically incompatible with promethazine HCl (Wyeth) (40).

Diatrizoate meglumine in combination with diatrizoate sodium as Renografin products may be physically incompatible with additives that lower the pH to 4 or below (479).

DIATRIZOATE MEGLUMINE AND DIATRIZOATE SODIUM
AHFS 36:68

Products— Diatrizoate meglumine–diatrizoate sodium is available in combined concentrations ranging from 57.6 to 76%. The formulations may also contain edetate and citrate. Hydrochloric acid, sodium hydroxide, or sodium carbonate may have been used during manufacturing to adjust pH. Some examples of representative products are listed in Table 1 (4; 154).

pH— From 6.5 to 7.7 (4).

Osmolarity— Osmolarities of the various concentrations range from 1510 to 2175 mOsm/L (4).

Administration— Appropriate dosage forms and concentrations of diatrizoate meglumine–diatrizoate sodium may be administered intravenously, intramuscularly, intra-arterially, or intra-articularly.

Table 1. Some Representative Diatrizoate Meglumine–Diatrizoate Sodium Products

Diatrizoate Meglumine Content (%)	Diatrizoate Sodium Content (%)	Bound Iodine (mg/ml)	Representative Trade Names
28.5	29.1	309	Renovist II
34.3	35	371	Renovist
52	8	290	MD-60, Renografin-60, Angiovist 292
50	25	385	Hypaque-M, 75%
66	10	370	Hypaque-76, MD-76, Renografin-76, Angiovist 370

Some products may be injected or instilled directly into selected areas to be visualized (4).

Stability— Diatrizoate meglumine–diatrizoate sodium solutions are colorless to pale yellow. They should be protected from strong light. On standing, a crystalline precipitate may form. To redissolve the crystals, place the container in hot water and shake gently. Allow the solution to cool to body temperature before administration (4).

Diatrizoate meglumine–diatrizoate sodium (Renografin) products are sensitive to low pH values. At about pH 3 to 4, turbidity or frank precipitation may appear (479).

Plastic Syringes— Plastic syringes have been stated to be unsuitable for accommodating radiopaque solutions for any length of time. The plastic is attacked, and the plunger tends to freeze on prolonged storage (40). However, when diatrizoate meglumine 52%–diatrizoate sodium 8% (Renografin-60, Squibb) and diatrizoate meglumine 34.3%–diatrizoate sodium 35% (Renovist, Squibb) were stored in polystyrene syringes (Pharmaseal) at 25 and 37 °C, no apparent changes were noted visually or spectrophotometrically over five days (530).

An increased incidence of adverse reactions to diatrizoate meglumine–diatrizoate sodium (Hypaque-M, 75%) in intravenous pyelography was attributed to extraction of phenolic compounds from the rubber plunger-stoppers when Plastipak (Becton-Dickinson) disposable syringes were used to administer the radiopaque contrast media. The use of glass syringes only was recommended (821).

Sorption— Diatrizoate meglumine–diatrizoate sodium (Squibb Diagnostics) (concentration unspecified) was filled into 3-ml plastic syringes (Becton-Dickinson, Sherwood Monoject, and Terumo) and stored at −20, 4, and 25 °C in the dark. Little or no loss occurred in one day at 25 °C, seven days at 4 °C, and 30 days at −20 °C (1562).

Compatibility Information

Drugs in Syringe Compatibility

Diatrizoate meglumine + Diatrizoate sodium

Drug (in syringe)	Mfr	Amt	Mfr	Amt	Remarks	Ref	C/I
Ampicillin sodium	BR	30 mg/ 1 ml	MA	52% + 8%, 5 ml	Physically compatible for at least 2 hr	1438	C
Chloramphenicol sodium succinate	PD	33 mg/ 1 ml	MA	52% + 8%, 5 ml	Physically compatible for at least 2 hr	1438	C
Chlorpheniramine maleate	SC	1 ml[a]	SQ	52% + 8%, 40 to 1 ml	Physically compatible for 48 hr	530	C
	SC	1 ml[a]	SQ	34% + 35%, 40 to 1 ml	Physically compatible for 48 hr	530	C
Cimetidine HCl	SKF	150 mg/ 1 ml	MA	52% + 8%, 5 ml	Physically compatible for at least 2 hr	1438	C
Dimenhydrinate	SE	50 mg/ 1 ml	SQ	52% + 8%, 40 to 1 ml	Physically compatible for 48 hr	530	C
	SE	50 mg/ 1 ml	SQ	34% + 35%, 40 to 1 ml	Physically compatible for 48 hr	530	C
Diphenhydramine HCl	PD	1 ml[a]	SQ	52% + 8%, 40 to 5 ml	Physically compatible for 48 hr	530	C
	PD	1 ml[a]	SQ	52% + 8%, 2 and 1 ml	Physically compatible for 1 hr, but precipitate forms within 48 hr	530	I
	PD	1 ml[a]	SQ	34% + 35%, 40 to 1 ml	Physically compatible for 48 hr	530	C
	PD	12.5 mg/ 0.25 ml	MA	52% + 8%, 5 ml	Transient precipitate clears and then reforms within 1 hr	1438	I
Epinephrine HCl	PD	1 mg/ 1 ml	MA	52% + 8%, 5 ml	Physically compatible for at least 2 hr	1438	C
Gentamicin sulfate	SC	0.8 mg/ 1 ml	MA	52% + 8%, 5 ml	Physically compatible for at least 2 hr	1438	C
Heparin sodium	OR	5000 units/ 0.5 ml	MA	52% + 8%, 5 ml	Physically compatible for at least 2 hr	1438	C
Hyaluronidase	WY	150 units/ 1 ml	SQ	52% + 8%, 40 to 5 ml	Physically compatible for 48 hr	530	C
	WY	150 units/ 1 ml	SQ	52% + 8%, 2 and 1 ml	Physically compatible for 1 hr, but precipitate forms within 48 hr	530	I
	WY	150 units/ 1 ml	SQ	34% + 35%, 40 to 1 ml	Physically compatible for 48 hr	530	C

Drugs in Syringe Compatibility (Cont.)

Diatrizoate meglumine + Diatrizoate sodium

Drug (in syringe)	Mfr	Amt	Mfr	Amt	Remarks	Ref	C/I
Hydrocortisone sodium succinate	UP	10 mg/ 1 ml	MA	52% + 8%, 5 ml	Physically compatible for at least 2 hr	1438	C
Methylprednisolone sodium succinate	UP	10 mg/ 1 ml	MA	52% + 8%, 5 ml	Physically compatible for at least 2 hr	1438	C
Papaverine HCl	LI	30 mg/ 1 ml	SQ	66% + 10%, 3 ml	White precipitate disappears after 1 to 2 min	1437	?
	ME	32 mg/ 1 ml	MA	52% + 8%, 5 ml	Transient precipitate clears and then reforms after 2 hr	1438	I
Promethazine HCl	WY	1 ml[a]	SQ	52% + 8%, 40 to 1 ml	Immediate precipitation	530	I
	WY	1 ml[a]	SQ	34% + 35%, 40 to 1 ml	Immediate precipitation	530	I
Protamine sulfate	LI	10 mg/ 1 ml	MA	52% + 8%, 5 ml	Precipitate forms immediately and persists for at least 2 hr	1438	I

[a]Concentration unspecified.

Additional Compatibility Information

Additives— Diatrizoate meglumine–diatrizoate sodium (Renografin) products may be physically incompatible with additives that lower the pH to 4 or below (479).

Protamine sulfate has been found to be physically incompatible with diatrizoate meglumine 66%–diatrizoate sodium 10% (Renografin-76). A thick whitish gel formed upon administration of 40 mg of protamine sulfate directly into a catheter filled with the contrast medium. The precipitate would not dissolve after heating to body temperature but dissolved slowly when further diluted 10-fold with water. Even flushing the catheter filled with contrast medium with 50 ml of sodium chloride 0.9% first did not eliminate the appearance of a precipitate upon administration of protamine sulfate through the catheter. However, the precipitate was much less dense than that formed without a saline flush (651).

DIATRIZOATE SODIUM
AHFS 36:68

Products— Diatrizoate sodium is available in concentrations ranging from 20 to 50%. It is also available in combination with other radiopaque contrast agents. The formulations may also contain edetate and benzyl alcohol. Sodium carbonate, hydrochloric acid, and/or sodium hydroxide may have been used during manufacturing to adjust pH. Some examples of single-agent products are listed in Table 1 (4; 154).

pH— From 6.5 to 7.7 (4).

Osmolarity— The 25 and 50% concentrations have osmolarities of 660 and 1270 mOsm/L, respectively (4).

Table 1. Some Representative Diatrizoate Sodium Products

Diatrizoate Sodium Content (%)	Bound Iodine (mg/ml)	Representative Trade Names
Urogenital solution (not for intravascular use)		
20	120	Hypaque Sodium 20%
Parenteral solutions		
25	150	Hypaque Sodium 25%
50	300	Hypaque Sodium 50%, Urovist Sodium 300

Sodium Content— Diatrizoate sodium contains about 1.57 mEq of sodium per gram of drug (4).

Administration— Appropriate dosage forms and concentrations of diatrizoate sodium may be administered intravenously, intramuscularly, subcutaneously, intra-arterially, or by intraosseous injection. Some products may be injected or instilled directly into selected areas to be visualized (4).

Stability— Diatrizoate sodium solutions are colorless to pale yellow. Precipitates that may form in the solutions may be redissolved by placing the container in hot water. Allow the solution to cool to body temperature before administration. The solutions may be autoclaved without adverse effects but should be protected from strong light (1-5/95; 4).

Diatrizoate sodium products, singly and in combinations, are sensitive to low pH values. At about pH 3 to 4, turbidity or frank precipitation may appear (479).

Plastic Syringes— Plastic syringes have been stated to be unsuitable for accommodating radiopaque solutions for any length of time. The plastic is attacked, and the plunger tends to freeze on prolonged storage (40). However, when diatrizoate sodium (Winthrop) 75% was stored in polystyrene syringes (Pharmaseal) at 25 and 37 °C, no apparent changes were noted visually or spectrophotometrically over five days (530).

An increased incidence of adverse reactions to diatrizoate sodium in combination with diatrizoate meglumine in intravenous pyelography was attributed to extraction of phenolic compounds from the rubber plunger-stopper when Plastipak (Becton-Dickinson) disposable syringes were used to administer the radiopaque contrast media. The use of glass syringes only was recommended (821).

Compatibility Information

Drugs in Syringe Compatibility

Diatrizoate sodium

Drug (in syringe)	Mfr	Amt	Mfr	Amt	Remarks	Ref	C/I
Ampicillin sodium	BR	30 mg/1 ml	WI	60%, 5 ml	Physically compatible for at least 2 hr	1438	C
Chloramphenicol sodium succinate	PD	33 mg/1 ml	WI	60%, 5 ml	Physically compatible for at least 2 hr	1438	C
Chlorpheniramine maleate	RB	1 ml[a]	WI	75%, 1 to 40 ml	Physically compatible for 48 hr	530	C
Cimetidine HCl	SKF	150 mg/1 ml	WI	60%, 5 ml	Physically compatible for at least 2 hr	1438	C
Dimenhydrinate	SE	50 mg/1 ml	WI	75%, 1 to 40 ml	Physically compatible for 48 hr	530	C
Diphenhydramine HCl	PD	50 mg/1 ml	WI	5 ml[a]	No precipitate observed	309	C
	PD	1 ml[a]	WI	75%, 1 to 40 ml	Physically compatible for 48 hr	530	C
	PD	12.5 mg/0.25 ml	WI	60%, 5 ml	Transient precipitate clears and then reforms after 1 hr	1438	I
Epinephrine HCl	PD	1 mg/1 ml	WI	60%, 5 ml	Physically compatible for at least 2 hr	1438	C
Gentamicin sulfate	SC	0.8 mg/1 ml	WI	60%, 5 ml	Physically compatible for at least 2 hr	1438	C
Heparin sodium	OR	5000 units/0.5 ml	WI	60%, 5 ml	Physically compatible for at least 2 hr	1438	C
Hyaluronidase	WY	150 units/1 ml	WI	75%, 5 to 40 ml	Physically compatible for 48 hr	530	C
	WY	150 units/1 ml	WI	75%, 2 and 1 ml	Physically compatible for at least 1 hr, but precipitate forms within 48 hr	530	I
Hydrocortisone sodium succinate	UP	10 mg/1 ml	WI	60%, 5 ml	Physically compatible for at least 2 hr	1438	C
Methylprednisolone sodium succinate	UP	10 mg/1 ml	WI	60%, 5 ml	Physically compatible for at least 2 hr	1438	C

Drugs in Syringe Compatibility (Cont.)

Diatrizoate sodium

Drug (in syringe)	Mfr	Amt	Mfr	Amt	Remarks	Ref	C/I
Papaverine HCl	ME	32 mg/ 1 ml	WI	60%, 5 ml	Transient precipitate clears within 5 min	1438	?
Promethazine HCl	WY	1 ml[a]	WI	75%, 1 to 40 ml	Immediate precipitation	530	I
Protamine sulfate	LI	10 mg/ 1 ml	WI	60%, 5 ml	Precipitate forms immediately and persists for at least 2 hr	1438	I

[a]*Concentration unspecified.*

Additional Compatibility Information

Additives— Diatrizoate sodium, singly or in combination, may be physically incompatible with additives that lower the pH to 4 or below (479).

DIAZEPAM
AHFS 28:24.08

Valium   **Roche**

Products— Diazepam (Roche) is available in 2-ml ampuls, 10-ml vials, and 2-ml disposable syringes. Each milliliter of solution contains (2):

Diazepam	5 mg
Propylene glycol	40%
Ethyl alcohol	10%
Sodium benzoate and benzoic acid	5%
Benzyl alcohol	1.5%

pH— From 6.2 to 6.9 (4).

Osmolality— The osmolality of diazepam (Roche) was determined to be 7775 mOsm/kg. Diazemuls (Kabi) has an osmolality of 349 mOsm/kg (1233).

Administration— Diazepam is administered by direct intravenous injection into a large vein (2; 4; 8; 338) or, if necessary, into the tubing of a running infusion solution (4). Recommended rates of administration vary from 2 (8) or 3 mg/min (31) to 5 mg/min (2; 4). Diazepam can be given by deep intramuscular injection (2; 4), but this route may yield low or erratic plasma levels (4; 121; 638). Intravenous infusion of diazepam diluted in infusion solutions has been performed but is not recommended (2; 4). See Dilution under Additional Compatibility Information.

Stability— The commercial product should be stored at controlled room temperature and protected from light (4). Diazepam (Roche) 5 mg/ml was found to retain potency for three months at room temperature when 2 ml of solution was packaged in Tubex cartridges (13).

The drug is most stable at pH 4 to 8 and is subject to acid-catalyzed hydrolysis below pH 3 (643).

In tropical climates, diazepam injection is subject to discoloration from degradation by an oxidative hydrolytic mechanism. The rate of degradation leading to discoloration is dependent on various factors including the polarity/dielectric constant of the vehicle, pH, oxygen and electrolyte content, access to light, and storage temperature (1749).

Syringes— Diazepam 5 mg/ml was filled into 3-ml plastic syringes (Becton-Dickinson, Sherwood Monoject, and Terumo) and stored at −20, 4, and 25 °C in the dark. Diazepam concentration losses, presumably due to sorption to surfaces and/or the elastomeric plunger seal, ranged from 6% at 25 °C to 2 or 3% at 4 °C to 1% or less at −20 °C in one day. Long-term storage for seven days at 4 °C and 30 days at −20 °C resulted in losses of 4 to 8% and 5 to 13%, respectively (1562).

Diazepam (Roche) 10 mg/2 ml was stored in plastic syringes composed of polypropylene and polyethylene. No loss of diazepam was detected by UV spectroscopy after four hours of storage (351).

Diazepam (Roche) 5 mg/ml was stored in 1.5-ml disposable glass syringes with slit rubber plunger-stoppers (Hy-Pod) for 90 days at 30 and 4 °C in light-resistant bags. Diazepam was gradually lost from the solution, with the disappearance being essentially complete in 60 days. At 4 °C, about 5% was lost at the 60- and 90-day intervals; about 9 to 10% was lost at 30 °C in this period. The loss was attributed to sorption to the rubber plunger-stoppers (794).

Filtration— Diazepam (Roche) 50 μg/ml in dextrose 5% in water and sodium chloride 0.9% was delivered over seven hours through four kinds of 0.2-μm membrane filters varying in size and composition. Diazepam concentration losses of 7 to 17% were found during the first 60 minutes; subsequent diazepam levels returned to the original concentration when the binding sites became saturated (1399).

Sorption— The apparent stability of diazepam in several infusion fluids in glass containers (321) does not extend to the solutions in PVC bags in which substantial sorption occurs. At concentrations of 10 mg in 100 and 200 ml, a greater than 24% loss of potency occurred in 30 minutes. The potency loss appears to be a function of drug concentration and time, with approximately 80 to 90% loss occurring in 24 hours (330). (See table.)

In another test, diazepam (David Bull Laboratories) 8 mg/L in sodium chloride 0.9% (Travenol) in PVC bags exhibited approximately 20% loss in 24 hours and 32% loss in one week at room temperature (15 to 20 °C) due to sorption (536).

Cloyd et al. also evaluated the sorption of diazepam to PVC infusion bags. At concentrations of 5 and 20 mg/100 ml in dextrose 5% in water and sodium chloride 0.9%, the diazepam content of the solutions was less than 45% in two hours and further declined to about 20 to 25% in eight hours (647).

In addition, Cloyd et al. tested the diazepam sorption that results from administration through plastic infusion sets. Dilutions of 7.5 and 30 mg in 150 ml of dextrose 5% in water and sodium chloride 0.9% were prepared in the burette chamber of a Buretrol. The solutions flowed through the tubing at 30 ml/hr for two hours. A relatively small (less than 10%) but significant decrease in diazepam content occurred in the burette chamber. However, running the solution through the tubing resulted in steep declines in potency to about 43% of the initial amount. When diazepam solutions of 25 and 100 mg/500 ml of dextrose 5% in water and sodium chloride 0.9% were prepared in glass bottles and 100-ml aliquots were run through the Buretrol over one hour, only about 60 to 70% of the diazepam was delivered. The presence of a 0.5-μm inline filter did not affect the diazepam concentration delivered (647).

MacKichan et al. reported over a 90% loss due to sorption to the administration set (Abbott) and the extension tubing (Extracorporeal) both with and without a 0.22-μm inline filter (Abbott). Solutions containing 0.02 to 0.04 mg/ml of diazepam in dextrose 5% in water had no evidence of precipitation, and solutions in glass bottles retained their initial potency over 24 hours. However, the amount delivered through the tubing was only 40 to 55% at time zero, and this amount dropped to 2 to 7% at 24 hours. No difference was noted from the inline filter (645).

Parker and MacCara also evaluated the sorption of diazepam to administration sets from solutions of diazepam 25 and 50 mg/500 ml in glass bottles of dextrose 5% in water and Ringer's injection, lactated, or 12.5 and 25 mg/250 ml of these same solutions in Soluset burette chambers. The admixtures showed no evidence of physical incompatibility by macroscopic or microscopic examination over four hours of storage at room temperature. The solutions in glass bottles were run through Venosets composed of PVC drip chambers and tubing at 2.5 and 5 mg/hr. The solutions stored in the cellulose propionate burette chambers of the Solusets were also run through their PVC tubing at the same rates. The solution delivered through the Venosets contained about 91 to 97% of the initial concentration, with the more dilute solution having slightly more drug remaining. However, the Soluset delivered only about 50 to 60% in two hours and about 35 to 45% of the initial concentration after four hours. The authors believed that most of the loss was due to sorption to the cellulose propionate burette chamber. This result was attributed to the larger surface area of the burette compared with the tubing and/or the difference in plastic composition. Almost all of the

lost diazepam could be recovered through desorption from the burettes (646). This result is in striking contrast to the results of Cloyd et al. reported above (647). The use of 0.45-μm inline filters had no effect on the drug concentration. The authors recommended that diazepam infusions be prepared only in glass bottles and be administered only through sets not having burette chambers (646).

Dasta et al. assessed a 50-mg/500 ml solution in dextrose 5% in water prepared in glass bottles and run through an administration set (Travenol) at 100 ml/hr. Only 63% of the predicted diazepam concentration was initially delivered, but this amount gradually climbed to a maximum concentration of 81% at the end of five hours (649).

Boatman and Johnson noted a 27 to 33% diazepam loss from admixtures in both dextrose 5% in water and sodium chloride 0.9% in PVC bags. The diazepam concentrations evaluated ranged from 0.05 to 0.2 mg/ml. No drug decomposition could be detected, and nearly quantitative recovery of the drug could be obtained from the PVC bags. Diazepam solutions in dextrose 5% in water were also run through a 70-inch Travenol set. A steep decline to less than 70% of the expected amount of diazepam was delivered during the first 15 minutes, after which the delivered amount increased to between 80 and 90% of the expected amount over the next 85 minutes as saturation of the tubing occurred. A quantitatively smaller, but qualitatively similar, effect was observed when diazepam was administered by intravenous push through an intravenous catheter (Abbott Venocath-18) of 11.5-inch total length. The decline in delivered diazepam reached a nadir of approximately 95% in about eight minutes before returning to 100% at 10 minutes. The smaller effect of the intravenous catheter relates to its relatively shorter length (650).

Kowaluk et al. found that diazepam (David Bull Laboratories) 8 mg/L in sodium chloride 0.9% in glass bottles exhibited a cumulative 7% loss due to sorption during a seven-hour simulated infusion through an infusion set (Travenol). The set consisted of a cellulose propionate burette chamber and 170 cm of PVC tubing. Diazepam sorption was attributed mainly to the tubing. The extent of sorption was found to be independent of concentration (606).

Diazepam was also tested as a simulated infusion over at least one hour by a syringe pump system. A glass syringe on a syringe pump was fitted with 20 cm of polyethylene tubing or 50 cm of Silastic tubing. A negligible amount of drug was lost with the polyethylene tubing, but a cumulative loss of 21% occurred during the one-hour infusion through the Silastic tubing (606).

Storage of a 25-ml aliquot of the 8-mg/L diazepam solution in all-plastic syringes composed of polypropylene barrels and polyethylene plungers for 24 hours at room temperature in the dark did not result in any drug loss due to sorption (606).

Winsnes et al. prepared a diazepam (Roche) infusion of 20 mg/500 ml in dextrose 5% in water and delivered it at 4 ml/hr through PVC tubing by means of an infusion pump. Less than 20% of this diazepam concentration was delivered at any time point over the 24-hour observation period. Increasing the concentration to 50 mg/500 ml in dextrose 5% in water and increasing the infusion rate to 20 ml/hr decreased the amount of diazepam lost from the solution. After 30 minutes of solution delivery, the diazepam in the tubing effluent was about 30% of the initial concentration. Subsequently, the delivered diazepam concentration climbed to about 60% over 24 hours, presumably due to saturation of the tubing (351).

Mason et al. determined the partition coefficients of diazepam with various plastics from intravenous containers and administration sets. It was found that PVC bags and tubings from a variety of suppliers were all similar in partitioning and hundreds of times greater than McGaw polyolefin semirigid containers. Volume-control chambers made from cellulose propionate were determined to have partition coefficients much smaller than those of PVC but still sufficient to cause serious depletion of diazepam from the chambers. Because these volume-control chambers are not essential, the authors recommended against their use (644).

It was further determined that the uptake of diazepam into PVC is absorption into the plastic matrix rather than adsorption to the surface. The absorption is independent of concentration but clearly related to contact time with the plastic. Decreasing the flow rate or increasing the tubing length increases the amount of diazepam absorbed (644).

Mason et al. found that increasing the flow rate from 10 to 264 ml/hr through 198 cm of PVC tubing decreased the amount of diazepam absorbed from a 90-ml delivered volume from 88 down to 28%. Increasing the tubing length from 100 to 350 cm increased the amount absorbed after 55 minutes at 121 ml/hr from 17 to 59%. However, it was noted that absorption is not markedly affected by tubing length within the range of lengths commercially available (644).

In a continuation of this work, diazepam (David Bull Laboratories) 50 mg/L in sodium chloride 0.9% in a glass bottle was delivered through a polyethylene administration set (Tridilset) over eight hours at 15 to 20 °C. The flow rate was set at 1 ml/min. No appreciable loss due to sorption occurred. This finding is in contrast to a 20% loss using a conventional administration set (769).

The sorption of diazepam 40 and 120 mg/L in sodium chloride 0.9% was evaluated in 100- and 500-ml PVC infusion bags (Travenol). After eight hours at 20 to 24 °C, 58 to 60% of the diazepam was lost in the 100-ml bag and 31% was lost in the 500-ml bag. The extent of sorption was independent of concentration but was greatly influenced by the size of the PVC container. This difference results from the ratio of the surface area of plastic to the volume of solution. As the volume of solution in the bag decreases, the ratio and, therefore, the extent of sorption increase (770).

Diazepam showed negligible (<3%) loss when aqueous solutions were stored in polypropylene bags (770).

Smith and Bird found extensive sorption of diazepam from dextrose 5% in water and sodium chloride 0.9% to PVC containers (Travenol and Boots). Solutions of 10 to 80 mg/L showed a 12 to 20% diazepam loss in one hour. In six hours, the potency loss was about 30% at 5 °C and about 40% at room temperature. Over 30% of the missing diazepam could be recovered by washing the PVC with methanol. This result did not extend to glass or polyethylene (Polyfusor, Boots) containers, which showed drug losses of about 6 to 8% in 24 hours (796).

Similarly, Yliruusi et al. found no loss of diazepam to glass or polyethylene containers in 200-mg/L concentrations in dextrose 5% in water or sodium chloride 0.9%. However, in PVC containers, drug losses of around 37 to 43% occurred in 24 hours at 25 °C (797).

Cossum and Roberts also investigated the administration of diazepam (Roche) with a glass syringe on an infusion pump connected with high-density polyethylene tubing, and they found negligible drug loss (795).

In another report, plastic syringes having polypropylene barrels and polyethylene plungers (Pharma-Plast, AHS Australia) and all-glass containers were compared for the possible sorption of diazepam. After 24 hours of storage of aqueous solutions of diazepam (concentration unspecified), no drug loss was found in either container. The authors indicated that these plastic syringes could be substituted for glass syringes for use with syringe pumps (782).

Kowaluk et al. evaluated the effect of several factors on the rate and extent of sorption of diazepam by PVC. The sorption proved to be independent of changes in ethanol–propylene glycol concentrations in the vehicle, pH changes in the admixtures over 4.2 to 7.5, and the initial diazepam concentration. However, the rate and extent of sorption could be minimized by decreasing the storage temperature, minimizing the storage time, and increasing the surface area to volume ratio by storing the largest possible fluid volume in a given PVC bag and using short lengths of small diameter infusion tubing. Use of glass or polyolefin solution bottles and polyolefin infusion tubing avoids the loss of diazepam (880).

The comparative sorption of diazepam (Roche) 20 mg/500 ml in sodium chloride 0.9%, run at 1 ml/min through PVC and polybutadiene (PBD) administration sets (Avon Medicals, U.K.), was reported. The delivered concentration through the PVC set was about 80% of the expected amount initially and then climbed to about 90% after four hours. For a concentration of 10 mg/120 ml prepared in a cellulose propionate burette, 10 to 15% sorption occurred in the burette. Conversely, use of the PBD set, with or without a methacrylate butadiene styrene burette chamber, resulted in no detectable loss of diazepam potency (1027).

Hancock and Black compared the delivery of diazepam (Roche) 50 and 100 mg/500 ml of dextrose 5% in water and sodium chloride 0.9% through a PVC administration set (Accuset 9210, IMED) and a set composed of ethylene–vinyl acetate with a polyethylene inner wall (Accuset 9630, IMED). The solutions were run through the sets at 50 and 100 ml/hr. The delivered diazepam concentration varied between 44 and 71% at 50 ml/hr and between 62 and 89% at 100 ml/hr, increasing from the lower to the higher percentage over the five-hour study period. The non-PVC set exhibited no sorption of diazepam, delivering essentially 100% of the diazepam at each time point measured (1096).

Yliruusi et al. found that the percentage of diazepam delivered through PVC administration sets varied with the length of the tubing; the longer the tubing, the smaller was the percentage delivered. For a 25-mg/500 ml admixture in sodium chloride 0.9%, delivery through PVC tubing in lengths from 23 to 185 cm varied from 88% of the theoretical amount for the shortest length to 53% for the 185-cm length (1097).

Yliruusi et al. also evaluated the effect of container type and flow rate on the sorption of diazepam. Glass and polyethylene containers showed 0 and 5% sorption, respectively, of the diazepam content of a 25-mg/500 ml admixture in sodium chloride 0.9% in seven days at 25 °C. However, PVC containers showed a 75% loss in this time period. Simulated infusion of this solution from glass bottles through PVC sets at flow rates of 30 to 120 ml/hr showed that a greater percentage of diazepam was lost at the slower infusion rates. At 30 ml/hr, 63% was lost after four hours, while only 23% was lost after four hours at 120 ml/hr (1098).

Martens et al. reported a rapid diazepam loss from a 40-μg/ml solution in sodium chloride 0.9% in a PVC container at 21 °C protected from light. A 15% loss occurred in two hours, and a 55% loss occurred in 24 hours. Little or no diazepam loss occurred in 24 hours in glass bottles or polyethylene-lined laminated bags (1392).

Diazepam (Orion) 100 μg/ml in sodium chloride 0.9% exhibited no loss due to sorption by UV spectroscopy and HPLC analysis in 24 hours at 21 °C in glass bottles and polypropylene trilayer bags (Softbag, Orion). However, about a 70% loss occurred due to sorption under these conditions in PVC bags (1796).

Diazepam (Takeda) 40 μg/ml in 0.9% sodium chloride and in pH 7 buffer also underwent sorption to ethylene vinyl acetate (EVA) plastic bags (Terumo). Losses exceeding 25% occurred within 24 hours stored at 30 °C in dim light. The solutions appeared to reach equilibrium after 96 hours of storage. The authors speculated that both absorption and adsorption of the diazepam to the EVA bags were occurring (1917).

Other reports support and confirm these findings (1251; 1252).

In summary, the delivery of diazepam by intravenous infusion is problematic. To minimize the sorption of diazepam, glass or polyolefin containers should be used. Alternatively, a syringe pump has been recommended since sorption to plastic syringes has not been found (1033). If PVC bags are used, the lowest possible surface-to-volume ratio should be selected and storage time should be minimized. The use of non-PVC administration sets will reduce loss. If PVC tubing is used, it should be the shortest possible length with a small diameter, and the set should not contain a burette chamber. More rapid flow rates (consistent with safe clinical use) will also reduce the loss of diazepam.

Also see Dilution under Additional Compatibility Information.

Compatibility Information

Solution Compatibility

Diazepam

Solution	Mfr	Mfr	Conc/L	Remarks	Ref	C/I
Dextrose 5% in water	BA[a]	RC	>250 mg	Immediate white precipitation	321	I
	BA[a]	RC	250 mg	No precipitate in 24 hr. 6% potency loss in 4 hr	321	I
	BA[a]	RC	100 and 125 mg	No precipitate and 8 to 10% potency loss in 24 hr	321	C
	BA[a]	RC	50 and 67 mg	No precipitate and 0 to 1% potency loss in 24 hr	321	C
	BA[b]	RC	100 mg	35% potency loss in 30 min. 90% potency loss in 24 hr at room temperature	330	I
	BA[b]	RC	50 mg	35% potency loss in 30 min. 77% potency loss in 24 hr at room temperature	330	I
		RC	370 mg	Precipitate formed. Diazepam concentration unchanged after filtration	640	I
	TR[b]	RC	50 and 200 mg	Solution initially cloudy but clears by completion of admixture. 55 to 60% potency loss within 2 hr	647	I
	[b]		50, 100, 200 mg	27 to 29% diazepam loss	650	I
	BT[b]	RC	40 mg	No precipitate but 12 to 14% potency loss in 1 hr at room temperature and 5 °C	796	I
	BT[c]	RC	40 mg	No precipitate and about 7% potency loss in 24 hr at room temperature	796	C
	ON[a,c]	ON	200 mg	No precipitate and negligible potency loss in 24 hr at 25 °C	797	C
	[b]	ON	200 mg	No precipitate but about 10% potency loss in 3.5 hr and about 37% in 24 hr at 25 °C	797	I
Ringer's injection	BA[a]	RC	>250 mg	Immediate white precipitation	321	I
	BA[a]	RC	250 mg	White precipitate formed in 6 to 8 hr. 8% potency loss in 4 hr	321	I
	BA[a]	RC	100 and 125 mg	No precipitate and 7 to 12% potency loss in 24 hr	321	C
	BA[a]	RC	50 and 67 mg	No precipitate and 0 to 3% potency loss in 24 hr	321	C
	BA[b]	RC	100 mg	38% potency loss in 30 min. 89% potency loss in 24 hr at room temperature	330	I
	BA[b]	RC	50 mg	29% potency loss in 30 min. 78% potency loss in 24 hr at room temperature	330	I
Ringer's injection, lactated	BA[a]	RC	>250 mg	Immediate white precipitation	321	I
	BA[a]	RC	250 mg	White precipitate formed in 8 to 12 hr. 5% potency loss in 4 hr	321	I
		RC	200 mg	Transient cloudiness followed by clear solution	392	C
	BA[a]	RC	100 and 125 mg	No precipitate and 8 to 10% potency loss in 24 hr	321	C

Solution Compatibility (Cont.)

Diazepam

Solution	Mfr	Mfr	Conc/L	Remarks	Ref	C/I
	BA[a]	RC	50 and 67 mg	No precipitate and 6% potency loss in 24 hr	321	**C**
	BA[b]	RC	100 mg	35% potency loss in 30 min. 89% potency loss in 24 hr at room temperature	330	**I**
	BA[b]	RC	50 mg	40% potency loss in 30 min. 78% potency loss in 24 hr at room temperature	330	**I**
Sodium chloride 0.9%	BA[a]	RC	>250 mg	Immediate white precipitation	321	**I**
	BA[a]	RC	250 mg	No precipitate in 24 hr. 6% potency loss in 4 hr	321	**I**
	BA[a]	RC	125 mg	No precipitate and 6% potency loss in 24 hr	321	**C**
	BA[a]	RC	100 mg	No precipitate and 4 to 5% potency loss in 24 hr	321; 330	**C**
	BA[a]	RC	67 mg	No precipitate and 6% potency loss in 24 hr	321	**C**
	BA[a]	RC	50 mg	No precipitate and 1 to 3% potency loss in 24 hr	321; 330	**C**
	BA[b]	RC	100 mg	29% potency loss in 30 min. 89% potency loss in 24 hr at room temperature	330	**I**
	BA[b]	RC	50 mg	24% potency loss in 30 min. 80% potency loss in 24 hr at room temperature	330	**I**
	TR[b]	RC	50 and 200 mg	Solution initially cloudy but clears by completion of admixture. 55 to 60% potency loss within 2 hr	647	**I**
	[b]		50 and 100 mg	32 to 33% diazepam loss	650	**I**
	[a]	RC	40 mg	No precipitate and about 6% potency loss in 24 hr at room temperature	796	**C**
	BT, TR[b]	RC	10 to 80 mg	No precipitate but about 12 to 20% potency loss in 1 hr at room temperature and 5 °C	796	**I**
	BT[c]	RC	10 to 80 mg	No precipitate and about 2 to 8% potency loss in 24 hr at room temperature and 5 °C	796	**C**
	ON[a,c]	ON	200 mg	No precipitate and negligible potency loss in 24 hr at 25 °C	797	**C**
	[b]	ON	200 mg	No precipitate but about 10% potency loss in 1 hr and about 43% in 24 hr at 25 °C	797	**I**
	[a]		400 mg	Precipitate forms immediately or within 1 min	1095	**I**
	[a]		333 mg	Precipitate forms after 30 min	1095	**I**
	[a]		100 and 200 mg	Remained clear for 10 days	1095	**C**
	[a]		50 mg	No diazepam loss in 7 days at 25 °C	1098	**C**
	[b]		50 mg	More than 40% loss in 1 day and 75% in 7 days at 25 °C	1098	**I**
	[c]		50 mg	About 5% loss in 7 days at 25 °C	1098	**C**
	[b]		40 mg	15% diazepam loss in 2 hr and 55% loss in 24 hr at 21 °C in the dark	1392	**I**
	[a,c]		40 mg	Little or no diazepam loss in 24 hr at 21 °C in the dark	1392	**C**
	ON[d]	ON	100 mg	Visually compatible with no loss by UV and HPLC in 24 hr at 21 °C	1796	**C**
	ON[b]	ON	100 mg	Visually compatible but 70% loss due to sorption by UV and HPLC in 24 hr at 21 °C	1796	**I**

[a]*Tested in glass containers.*
[b]*Tested in PVC containers.*
[c]*Tested in polyethylene containers.*
[d]*Tested in glass containers and polypropylene trilayer containers.*

Additive Compatibility

		Diazepam						
Drug	Mfr	Conc/L	Mfr	Conc/L	Test Soln	Remarks	Ref	C/I
Bleomycin sulfate	BR	20 and 30 units	RC	50 and 100 mg	NS	Physically incompatible	763	I
Dobutamine HCl	LI	1 g	RC	2.5 g	D5W, NS	Rapid clouding of solution with yellow precipitate in 24 hr at 21 °C	812	I
Doxorubicin HCl	AD		RC			Immediate precipitation	524	I
Floxacillin sodium	BE	20 g	PHX	1 g	D5W	Haze forms in 7 hr at 30 °C and 48 hr at 15 °C	1479	I
Fluorouracil			RC			Immediate precipitation	524	I
Furosemide	HO	20 g	PHX	1 g	D5W	Immediate precipitation	1479	I
Netilmicin sulfate	SC	3 g	RC	40 mg	D5S	Physically compatible and netilmicin chemically stable for 7 days at 25 and 4 °C. Diazepam not tested	558	C
Verapamil HCl	KN	80 mg	RC	20 mg	D5W, NS	Physically compatible for 24 hr	764	C

Drugs in Syringe Compatibility

		Diazepam					
Drug (in syringe)	Mfr	Amt	Mfr	Amt	Remarks	Ref	C/I
Cimetidine HCl	SKF	300 mg/ 2 ml	RC	10 mg/ 2 ml	Physically compatible for 4 hr at 25 °C	25	C
Doxapram HCl	RB	400 mg/ 20 ml		10 mg/ 2 ml	Immediate turbidity and precipitation	1177	I
Glycopyrrolate	RB	0.2 mg/ 1 ml	RC	5 mg/ 1 ml	Immediate precipitation	331	I
	RB	0.2 mg/ 1 ml	RC	10 mg/ 2 ml	Immediate precipitation	331	I
	RB	0.4 mg/ 2 ml	RC	5 mg/ 1 ml	Immediate precipitation	331	I
Heparin sodium		2500 units/ 1 ml		10 mg/ 2 ml	Turbidity or precipitate forms within 5 min	1053	I
Hydromorphone HCl	KN	2, 10, 40 mg/ 1 ml	SX	5 mg/ 1 ml	Diazepam precipitate forms immediately due to aqueous dilution	2082	I
Ketorolac tromethamine	SY	180 mg/ 6 ml	ES	15 mg/ 3 ml	Visually compatible for 4 hr at 24 °C under ambient light. Increase in spectrophotometric absorbance occurs immediately, persists for 30 min, and dissipates by 1 hr	1703	?
Nalbuphine HCl	EN	10 mg/ 1 ml	RC	5 mg/ 1 ml	Immediate white milky precipitate that persisted for 36 hr at 27 °C	762	I
	EN	5 mg/ 0.5 ml	RC	5 mg/ 1 ml	Immediate white milky precipitate that cleared upon vigorous shaking; remained clear for 36 hr at 27 °C	762	I
	EN	2.5 mg/ 0.25 ml	RC	5 mg/ 1 ml	Immediate white milky precipitate that cleared upon vigorous shaking; remained clear for 36 hr at 27 °C	762	I

Drugs in Syringe Compatibility (Cont.)

Diazepam

Drug (in syringe)	Mfr	Amt	Mfr	Amt	Remarks	Ref	C/I
	DU	10 mg/ 1 ml	RC	10 mg/ 2 ml	Physically incompatible	128	I
	DU	20 mg/ 1 ml	RC	10 mg/ 2 ml	Physically incompatible	128	I
Ranitidine HCl	GL	50 mg/ 2 ml	RC	10 mg/ 2 ml	Immediate white haze that disappeared following vortex mixing	978	I
	GL	50 mg/ 5 ml		10 mg	Physically compatible for 4 hr at ambient temperature under fluorescent light	1151	C
Sufentanil citrate	JN	50 μg/ml	ES	5 mg/ml	White turbidity forms immediately. Precipitate forms in 24 hr at 23 °C	1711	I

Y-Site Injection Compatibility (1:1 Mixture)

Diazepam

Drug	Mfr	Conc	Mfr	Conc	Remarks	Ref	C/I
Amphotericin B cholesteryl sulfate complex	SEQ	0.83 mg/ml[a]	SW	5 mg/ml	Gross precipitate forms	2117	I
Atracurium besylate	BW	0.5 mg/ml[a]	ES	5 mg/ml[a]	Cloudy solution forms immediately	1337	I
Cefepime HCl	BR	20 mg/ml[a]	ES	5 mg/ml[a]	Cloudy solution forms immediately	1689	I
Cisatracurium besylate	GW	0.1, 2, and 5 mg/ml[a]	ES	5 mg/ml	White turbidity forms immediately	2074	I
	GW	0.1, 2, and 5 mg/ml[a]	ES	0.25 mg/ml[a]	Physically compatible with no change in measured turbidity or increase in particle content in 4 hr at 23 °C	2074	C
Diltiazem HCl	MMD	1[b] and 5 mg/ml	ES	5 mg/ml	Cloudiness and precipitate form	1807	I
Dobutamine HCl	LI	4 mg/ml[a,b]	ES	0.2 mg/ml[a,b]	Physically compatible for 3 hr	1316	C
Fluconazole	RR	2 mg/ml	ES	5 mg/ml	Immediate precipitation	1407	I
Foscarnet sodium	AST	24 mg/ml	ES	5 mg/ml	Gas production	1335	I
Heparin sodium		50 units/ml/ min[b]		10 mg/2 ml[c]	Turbidity	1053	I
Heparin sodium with hydrocortisone sodium succinate	RI UP	1000 units + 100 mg/ L[a,b,d]	RC	5 mg/ml	Immediate haziness and globule formation	322	I
Hydromorphone HCl	KN	2, 10, 40 mg/ml	SX	5 mg/ml	Turbidity forms immediately and diazepam precipitate develops	1532	I
Meropenem	ZEN	1 and 50 mg/ml[b]	RC	5 mg/ml	White precipitate forms immediately	1994	I
Nafcillin sodium	WY	33 mg/ml[b]		5 mg/ml	No precipitation	547	C
Pancuronium bromide	ES	0.05 mg/ml[a]	ES	5 mg/ml[a]	Cloudy solution forms immediately	1337	I
Potassium chloride		40 mEq/L[a,b,d]	RC	5 mg/ml	Immediate haziness and globule formation	322	I
Propofol	ZEN	10 mg/ml	ES	5 mg/ml	Emulsion broke and oiled out	2066	I
Quinidine gluconate	LI	6 mg/ml[a,b]	ES	0.2 mg/ml[a,b]	Physically compatible for 3 hr	1316	C
Remifentanil HCl	GW	0.025 and 0.25 mg/ml[b]	ES	5 mg/ml	White turbidity forms immediately	2075	I

Y-Site Injection Compatibility (1:1 Mixture) (Cont.)

		Diazepam					
Drug	Mfr	Conc	Mfr	Conc	Remarks	Ref	C/I
	GW	0.025 and 0.25 mg/ml[b]	ES	0.25 mg/ml[a]	Physically compatible with no change in measured turbidity or increase in particle content in 4 hr at 23 °C	2075	C
Sufentanil citrate	JN	12.5 μg/ml[a]	ES	0.5 mg/ml[a]	Physically compatible with no subvisual haze or particle formation in 24 hr at 23 °C	1711	C
TPN #189[e]			DB	5 mg/ml	Visually compatible for 24 hr at 22 °C	1767	C
Vecuronium bromide	OR	0.1 mg/ml[a]	ES	5 mg/ml[a]	Cloudy solution forms immediately	1337	I
Vitamin B complex with C	RC	2 ml/L[a,b,d]		5 mg/ml	Immediate haziness and globule formation	322	I

[a]*Tested in dextrose 5% in water.*
[b]*Tested in sodium chloride 0.9%.*
[c]*Given over three minutes via a Y-site into the running heparin admixture.*
[d]*Tested in Ringer's injection, lactated.*
[e]*Refer to Appendix I for the composition of parenteral nutrition solutions. TPN indicates a 2-in-1 admixture.*

Additional Compatibility Information

Dilution— Although the package insert for diazepam (Roche) contains a caveat against dilution of the product before intravenous administration (2), interest in the intravenous administration of diluted diazepam has been expressed repeatedly in the literature.

Sillers noted that dilution of diazepam to a concentration of 1 mg/ml (diluent unspecified) decreased thrombophlebitis occurring from extravasation (378). In a reply, Roche indicated that an ampul of diazepam should be diluted in no more than 5 ml or, alternatively, all the way to 20 ml to avoid precipitation. Between these concentrations, a fine white precipitate may occur (379).

Aqueous dilution of diazepam injection in a volume of 25% or more of the diazepam volume is stated to result in the immediate precipitation of diazepam. However, no precipitation was observed if aqueous dilution was made with a volume of less than 25% of the diazepam volume (2082).

Friedenberg and Barker indicated that the dilution of diazepam may be a predisposing factor to thrombophlebitis. In contacting Roche, they were told that because diazepam has a very low solubility in aqueous systems, sodium benzoate was incorporated in the formula as a buffer. Dilution of the product, it was stated, would cause precipitation of diazepam. If the solution were then acidified, benzoic acid would precipitate and could coprecipitate with the drug (380).

Jusko et al. tried adding diazepam injection to sodium chloride 0.9% and noted the immediate formation of a light yellow to white precipitate. The maximum dilution that produced such a precipitate was 15-fold, representing a mixture of about 0.3 to 0.4 mg/ml. They noted that a precipitate also formed in human plasma. To try to identify the precipitate, they prepared a solution composed of all ingredients of diazepam injection except diazepam. Dilution yielded no precipitate. UV spectrophotometric analysis of the diazepam injection–sodium chloride 0.9% precipitate showed that the composition was almost entirely diazepam. They further estimated that injection of 5 mg/min into the tubing of an intravenous infusion of sodium chloride 0.9% would result in a precipitate unless the administration rate exceeded 17 ml/min (381).

Dam and Christiansen reported the formation of cloudiness or a precipitate upon the admixture of diazepam 370 mg/L in dextrose 5% injection, BP. A difference in the nature of the incompatibility among different manufacturers of diazepam injection was noted. The products from Roche and Dumex exhibited a precipitate. The product supplied by Apotekernes Laboratorium produced a slight cloudiness. Filtration of these solutions retained the precipitate. However, the concentration of diazepam in the filtrate was determined by a TLC method to be nearly the same in all samples and corresponded well with the calculated initial concentration. In contrast to Jusko et al., the authors concluded that the precipitate was not diazepam but was probably due to the benzoates (640).

However, this conclusion was apparently in error. Huber and Raymond, using gas chromatography–mass spectrometry, determined that the precipitate induced by adding 2 ml of sterile water for injection to 1 ml of diazepam injection is, in fact, only diazepam. No benzoate is present. The precipitate appeared to be oily and adhered to the walls of the container, leaving a clear solution. The authors postulated that this phenomenon may explain the reports of the clearing of cloudy solutions with time (641; 642).

Kortilla et al. found a similar result to that of Jusko et al. for diazepam injection in dextrose 5% in water. As little as 10 mg of diazepam in 100 ml of dextrose 5% in water resulted in a precipitate. They also found that an infusion rate of greater than 15 to 20 ml/min was required to prevent precipitation of diazepam being injected at a rate of 5 mg/min in running infusions of dextrose 5% in water and sodium chloride 0.9% (382).

Nevertheless, interest in infusing diazepam has persisted because of bioavailability problems associated with intramuscular injection (121; 383; 384; 638) and a growing belief in the utility of diazepam infusions (386–392; 1099).

Baxter et al. stated that 10 mg of diazepam in 250 ml of sodium chloride 0.9% resulted in no observable precipitate. They also tried 5 mg in 50 ml of sodium chloride 0.9% with no apparent precipitate in one hour. It was noted that diazepam has a solubility of

10 mg/4 ml of water, which should permit dilution in intravenous fluids (385).

Tehrani and Cavanaugh reported observing a transient cloudiness when 100 mg of diazepam was added to 500 ml of Ringer's injection, lactated. The solution thereafter remained clear, and the clinical response to the diazepam infusion was good (392).

More recently, a study was conducted by Morris on the compatibility and stability of diazepam in a variety of intravenous infusion solutions. Results indicate that a visible precipitate is produced in dilutions of 1:1 to 1:10. Haziness was reported at 1:15, and delayed precipitates forming after six to eight hours were seen in some solutions at 1:20. Dilutions of 1:40 to 1:100 remained clear for 24 hours. Further, the potency of the 1:40 to 1:100 dilutions was retained for 24 hours. (See table.) The author stopped short of recommending the use of diazepam infusions in clinical practice, noting that additional studies were necessary. For example, the possibility of microcrystal formation had not been evaluated (321).

Just such a possibility was raised by McLean in decrying the use of diazepam by infusion (393).

Newton et al. (643) determined the equilibrium solubilities of diazepam in water for injection, sodium chloride 0.9%, dextrose 5% in water, and Ringer's injection, lactated. The equilibrium solubilities were found to be about 0.04 to 0.05 mg/ml in all of the solutions at 25 °C. This finding corroborated the work of others which indicated the solubility to be about 0.05 to 0.06 mg/ml. It also was in general agreement with the work of Morris, which found 0.12 mg/ml (1:40) to be the lowest volume dilution to remain clear for 24 hours. Newton et al. concluded that a more conservative 1:100 dilution should be used for diazepam infusion to guarantee complete solubility for up to 24 hours (643).

Mason et al. also determined the aqueous solubility of diazepam over a pH range of approximately 3 to 8 in phosphate buffer adjusted with hydrochloric acid or sodium hydroxide as well as dextrose 5% in water, sodium chloride 0.9%, and Ringer's injection, lactated. In the pH range of 4 to 8, which included all three infusion solutions, the solubility was approximately 0.05 to 0.06 mg/ml at 25 °C. Mason et al. recommended dilution to at least 0.04 mg/ml to ensure rapid and complete re-solution upon addition to the infusion solution (644).

Maloney investigated various dilutions of diazepam in water for injection and sodium chloride 0.9%. The observations are tabulated here (1095):

Diazepam Concentration	Diluent	Observation
10 mg/5 ml	W, NS	Clear for 1 min but then precipitate forms
10 mg/10 ml	W, NS	Immediate precipitation
10 mg/20 ml	NS	Immediate precipitation
10 mg/25 ml	NS	Immediate precipitation
10 mg/30 ml	NS	Clear for 30 min but then precipitate forms
10 mg/50 ml	NS	Clear for 10 days
10 mg/100 ml	NS	Clear for 10 days

Order of Mixing— It has been reported that addition of diazepam to dextrose 5% in water and sodium chloride 0.9% to form concentrations of 50 and 200 mg/L results in an immediate and persistent yellow precipitate. However, addition of the diluent to the diazepam injection to these same concentrations results initially in a cloudy solution which clears before the completion of admixture. It was recommended that admixtures of diazepam be prepared by adding the infusion solution to the diazepam injection (647; 648).

Buprenorphine— Diazepam is stated to be incompatible with buprenorphine HCl (4).

DIAZOXIDE
AHFS 24:08

Hyperstat   **Schering**

Products— Diazoxide (Schering) is available in 20-ml ampuls containing 300 mg (15 mg/ml) of drug and sodium hydroxide to adjust the pH in aqueous solution (2).

pH— The pH is adjusted to approximately 11.6 (2; 4).

Osmolality— The osmolality of diazoxide was determined to be 130 mOsm/kg (1233).

Administration— Diazoxide should be administered intravenously undiluted and rapidly, over 30 seconds or less, into a peripheral vein via an established intravenous line. Extravasation should be avoided. It should not be injected by other routes (2; 4).

Stability— Diazoxide can be stored at controlled room temperature or in the refrigerator. The clear, colorless solution darkens on exposure to light and should be protected from light, heat, and freezing (2; 4). Darkened solutions may be subpotent and should not be administered (4).

Compatibility Information

ite Injection Compatibility (1:1 Mixture)

Diazoxide

Drug	Mfr	Conc	Mfr	Conc	Remarks	Ref	C/I
dralazine HCl	SO	1 mg/ml[a]	SC	15 mg/ml[a]	Moderate precipitate and color change in 1 hr	1316	I
pranolol HCl	AY	0.08 mg/ml[b]	SC	15 mg/ml[b]	Moderate precipitate and slight color change in 1 hr	1316	I
	AY	0.08 mg/ml[c]	SC	15 mg/ml[c]	Moderate precipitate in 3 hr	1316	I

[a]*Tested in both dextrose 5% in water and sodium chloride 0.9%.*
[b]*Tested in dextrose 5% in water.*
[c]*Tested in sodium chloride 0.9%.*

Additional Compatibility Information

Do not dilute. Diazoxide is to be administered undiluted rapidly maximum effect. Slower administration may reduce the antihyper- sive response (2).

Diazoxide 300 mg/20 ml mixed in a syringe with heparin so- dium 2500 units/1 ml has been reported to be physically compatible for at least five minutes (1053).

DIGOXIN
AHFS 24:04

noxin   **Glaxo Wellcome**

oducts— Digoxin (Glaxo Wellcome) is available in 2-ml ampuls containing 0.25 mg/ml in propylene glycol 40% and alcohol 10%, along with sodium phosphate 0.17% and citric acid 0.08% (2).

Digoxin pediatric injection is available in 1-ml ampuls containing 0.1 mg/ml in propylene glycol 40% and alcohol 10%, along with sodium phosphate 0.17% and citric acid 0.08% (2).

— From 6.8 to 7.2 (2).

molality— The osmolality of digoxin pediatric injection (Burroughs Wellcome) was determined to be 9105 mOsm/kg by freezing-point depression and 5885 mOsm/kg by vapor pressure (1071).

ministration— Digoxin is administered by direct intravenous in- ection slowly over a minimum of five minutes or longer given undiluted or diluted with a fourfold or greater volume of sterile water for injection, dextrose 5% in water, or sodium chloride 0.9% (2; 4). Deep intramuscular injection of not more than 2 ml at a single site followed by massage has been performed. However, it is painful and causes severe local irritation (4).

bility— Digoxin ampuls should be stored at controlled room tem- perature and protected from light (2).

Digoxin is hydrolyzed in acidic solutions with a pH less than 3. At pH 5 to 8, however, digoxin is not hydrolyzed in aqueous so- lutions (798–801).

Digoxin (Burroughs Wellcome) 0.25 mg/ml was found to retain potency for three months at room temperature when 1 ml of solu- tion was packaged in Tubex cartridges (13).

Filtration— Digoxin (Burroughs Wellcome) 1 mg/L in dextrose 5% in water, sodium chloride 0.9%, and Ringer's injection, lactated, filtered over 12 hours through a 5-μm stainless steel depth filter (Argyle Filter Connector), a 0.22-μm cellulose ester membrane fil- ter (Ivex-2 Filter Set), and a 0.22-μm polycarbonate membrane filter (In-Sure Filter Set), showed no significant reduction in potency due to binding to the filters (320).

In another evaluation, digoxin (Burroughs Wellcome) 3 mg/L in dextrose 5% in water and sodium chloride 0.9% did not display significant sorption to a 0.45-μm cellulose membrane filter (Abbott S-A-I-F) during an eight-hour simulated infusion (567).

Digoxin (Wellcome) 1 μg/ml in dextrose 5% in water and sodium chloride 0.9% was delivered over eight hours through four kinds of 0.2-μm membrane filters varying in size and composition. In the first 20 minutes, digoxin concentration losses were 10 to 23% through the Sterifix filter and 24 to 32% through the Pall ELD-96LL filter. However, losses of 63 to 73% occurred in the first 20 minutes with the Ivex-HP and Pall FAE-020LL filters. Subsequent digoxin levels returned to the original concentration when the binding sites became saturated (1399).

Compatibility Information

Solution Compatibility

Solution	Mfr	Mfr	Conc/L	Remarks	Ref	C/I
Dextrose 5% in sodium chloride 0.45% with potassium chloride 20 mEq	AB	BW	2.5 mg	Physically compatible with no loss of digoxin in 6-hr study period at 23 °C	778	C
Dextrose 5% in water	AB	BW	2.5 mg	Physically compatible with no loss of digoxin in 48 hr at 4 and 23 °C	778	C
Ringer's injection, lactated	AB	BW	2.5 mg	Physically compatible with no loss of digoxin in 6-hr study period at 23 °C	778	C
Sodium chloride 0.45%		ES	125 mg	Physically compatible with no loss of digoxin in 4 hr at 22 °C	1419	C
Sodium chloride 0.9%	AB	BW	2.5 mg	Physically compatible with no loss of digoxin in 48 hr at 4 and 23 °C	778	C

Additive Compatibility

Drug	Mfr	Conc/L	Mfr	Conc/L	Test Soln	Remarks	Ref	C/I
Bretylium tosylate	ACC	1 g	BW	2 mg	D5W, NS	Physically compatible for 48 hr at 25 °C	756	C
Cimetidine HCl	SKF	3 g	BW	2.5 mg	D5W	Physically compatible and cimetidine chemically stable for 24 hr at room temperature. Digoxin not tested	551	C
Dobutamine HCl	LI	1 g	BW	4 mg	D5W, NS	Slightly pink in 24 hr at 25 °C	789	I
Floxacillin sodium	BE	20 g	BW	25 mg	NS	Physically compatible for 72 hr at 15 and 30 °C	1479	C
Furosemide	HO	20 g	BW	25 mg	NS	Physically compatible for 72 hr at 15 and 30 °C	1479	C
Lidocaine HCl	AST	2 g	ES	1 mg	D5W, LR, NS	Physically compatible for 24 hr at 25 °C	775	C
Ranitidine HCl	GL	50 mg and 2 g		2.5 mg	D5W	Physically compatible and ranitidine chemically stable by HPLC for 24 hr at 25 °C. Digoxin not tested	1515	C
Verapamil HCl	KN	80 mg	BW	2 mg	D5W, NS	Physically compatible for 48 hr	739	C

Drugs in Syringe Compatibility

Drug (in syringe)	Mfr	Amt	Mfr	Amt	Remarks	Ref	C/I
Doxapram HCl	RB	400 mg/ 20 ml		0.25 mg/ 1 ml	10% doxapram loss in 9 hr and 17% in 24 hr	1177	I
Heparin sodium		2500 units/ 1 ml		0.25 mg/ 1 ml	Physically compatible for at least 5 min	1053	C
Milrinone	WI	3.5 mg/ 3.5 ml		0.5 mg/ 2 ml	Brought to 10 ml total volume with D5W. Physically compatible with no loss of either drug in 4 hr at 23 °C	1191	C

Y-Site Injection Compatibility (1:1 Mixture)

Digoxin

Drug	Mfr	Conc	Mfr	Conc	Remarks	Ref	C/I
Amphotericin B cholesteryl sulfate complex	SEQ	0.83 mg/ml[a]	WY	0.25 mg/ml	Microprecipitate forms in 4 hr at 23 °C under fluorescent light	2117	**I**
Amrinone lactate	WI	2.5 mg/ml[a]	ES	0.25 mg/ml	Physically compatible with little or no loss of either drug in 4 hr at 22 °C	1419	**C**
Ciprofloxacin	MI	2 mg/ml[c]	ES	0.25 mg/ml	Visually compatible for 24 hr at 24 °C	1655	**C**
	BAY	2 mg/ml[b]	BW	0.25 mg/ml	Visually compatible with no ciprofloxacin loss by HPLC in 15 min. Digoxin not tested	1934	**C**
Cisatracurium besylate	GW	0.1, 2, 5 mg/ml[a]	ES	0.25 mg/ml	Physically compatible with no change in measured turbidity or increase in particle content in 4 hr at 23 °C	2074	**C**
Diltiazem HCl	MMD	1[b] and 5 mg/ml	ES	0.5 mg/ml	Visually compatible	1807	**C**
Famotidine	MSD	0.2 mg/ml[a]	ES	0.25 mg/ml	Physically compatible for 14 hr	1196	**C**
Fluconazole	RR	2 mg/ml	BW	0.25 mg/ml	Gas production	1407	**I**
Foscarnet sodium	AST	24 mg/ml	WY	0.25 mg/ml	Gas production	1335	**I**
Heparin sodium with hydrocortisone sodium succinate	RI UP	1000 units + 100 mg/L[d]	BW	0.25 mg/ml	Physically compatible for at least 4 hr at room temperature by visual and microscopic examination	322	**C**
Insulin, regular (Humulin R)	LI	1 unit/ml[b]	ES	0.005 mg/ml[b]	Physically compatible for 3 hr	1316	**C**
(Humulin R)	LI	1 unit/ml[a]	ES	0.005 mg/ml[a]	Slight haze in 1 hr	1316	**I**
(beef pork)	LI	1 unit/ml[b]	ES	0.005 mg/ml[b]	Physically compatible for 3 hr	1316	**C**
(beef pork)	LI	1 unit/ml[a]	ES	0.005 mg/ml[a]	Slight haze in 1 hr	1316	**I**
Meperidine HCl	AB	10 mg/ml	BW	0.25 mg/ml	Physically compatible for 4 hr at 25 °C	1397	**C**
Meropenem	ZEN	1 and 50 mg/ml[b]	BW	0.25 mg/ml	Visually compatible for 4 hr at room temperature	1994	**C**
Midazolam HCl	RC	1 mg/ml[a]	BW	0.1 mg/ml	Visually compatible for 24 hr at 23 °C	1847	**C**
Milrinone lactate	WI	200 µg/ml[a]	BW	0.25 mg/ml	Physically compatible with no loss of either drug in 4 hr at 23 °C	1191	**C**
Morphine sulfate	AB	1 mg/ml	BW	0.25 mg/ml	Physically compatible for 4 hr at 25 °C	1397	**C**
Potassium chloride		40 mEq/L[d]	BW	0.25 mg/ml	Physically compatible for at least 4 hr at room temperature by visual and microscopic examination	322	**C**
Propofol	ZEN	10 mg/ml	ES	0.25 mg/ml	Emulsion broke and oiled out	1916	**I**
Remifentanil HCl	GW	0.025 and 0.25 mg/ml[b]	ES	0.25 mg/ml	Physically compatible with no change in measured turbidity or increase in particle content in 4 hr at 23 °C	2075	**C**
Tacrolimus	FUJ	1 mg/ml[b]	WY	0.25 mg/ml	Visually compatible for 24 hr at 25 °C	1630	**C**
TNA #73[e]			BW	0.625 mg/50 ml[c]	Physically compatible for 4 hr by visual observation	1009	**C**
TNA #218 to #226[e]			ES, WY	0.25 mg/ml	Visually compatible with no precipitate or emulsion damage apparent in 4 hr at 23 °C	2215	**C**
TPN #212 to #215[e]			BW	0.25 mg/ml	Physically compatible with no change in measured turbidity or increase in particle content in 4 hr at 23 °C	2109	**C**

Y-Site Injection Compatibility (1:1 Mixture) (Cont.)

Digoxin

Drug	Mfr	Conc	Mfr	Conc	Remarks	Ref	C/I
Vitamin B complex with C	RC	2 ml/L[d]	BW	0.25 mg/ml	Physically compatible for at least 4 hr at room temperature by visual and microscopic examination	322	C

[a]*Tested in dextrose 5% in water.*
[b]*Tested in sodium chloride 0.9%.*
[c]*Tested in both dextrose 5% in water and sodium chloride 0.9%.*
[d]*Tested in dextrose 5% in water, Ringer's injection, lactated, and sodium chloride 0.9%.*
[e]*Refer to Appendix I for the composition of parenteral nutrition solutions. TNA indicates a 3-in-1 admixture, and TPN indicates a 2-in-1 admixture.*

Additional Compatibility Information

Solutions— Digoxin is stated to be compatible with most commercially available intravenous infusion solutions (4). The manufacturer recommends dilution with at least a fourfold volume of sterile water for injection, dextrose 5% in water, or sodium chloride 0.9%. Dilution to a more concentrated solution than this fourfold volume of diluent may lead to precipitation of the digoxin (2).

Parenteral Nutrition Solution— Digoxin (Burroughs Wellcome) in doses of 0.25 and 0.125 mg/L in a parenteral nutrition solution composed of 500 ml of amino acids 5.5% with electrolytes (Travenol) and 500 ml of dextrose 50% was reported to be therapeutically available to a patient on home total parenteral nutrition, providing digoxin serum levels in the normal range (802).

In another report, digoxin 0.25 to 1 mg/L in parenteral nutrition solutions in PVC bags was reported to be stable for up to 96 hours at 4 °C when evaluated by a radioimmunoassay. Furthermore, adequate serum levels and therapeutic response were obtained in two patients. Nevertheless, the routine addition of digoxin to parenteral nutrition solutions was not recommended until additional stability testing has been conducted and pharmacologic efficacy has been documented (854).

Additives— The manufacturer recommends that digoxin not be mixed with other drugs (2).

Plasticizer Leaching— Digoxin (Elkins-Sinn) 0.04 mg/ml in dextrose 5% in water did not leach diethylhexyl phthalate (DEHP) plasticizer from 50-ml PVC bags in 24 hours at 24 °C (1683).

DILTIAZEM HCL
AHFS 24:04

Cardizem   **Aventis**

Products— Diltiazem HCl (Aventis) is available as a 5-mg/ml solution in 5-ml (25 mg) and 10-ml (50 mg) vials. Also present in each milliliter of solution are citric acid 0.75 mg, sodium citrate dihydrate 0.65 mg, sorbitol solution 71.4 mg, and water for injection. Sodium hydroxide or hydrochloric acid may be used to adjust the pH (2).

Diltiazem HCl is also available as a lyophilized powder in a 25-mg dual-chamber, single-use syringe and a 100-mg single-dose vial (called "Monovial"). The first chamber of the dual-chamber syringe contains lyophilized diltiazem HCl 25 mg and mannitol 37.5 mg. The second chamber contains 5 ml of sterile water for injection with 0.5% benzyl alcohol and sodium chloride 0.6%. The single-dose vials contain diltiazem HCl 100 mg and mannitol 75 mg. They are packaged with a transfer needle set (2; 4).

pH— From 3.7 to 4.1. The pH of the dual-chamber syringe after reconstitution is in the range of 4 to 7 (2; 4).

Administration— Diltiazem HCl is administered by direct intravenous injection over two minutes and by continuous intravenous infusion after dilution in dextrose 5% in water, sodium chloride 0.9%, or dextrose 5% in sodium chloride 0.45% (2).

The dry powder in single-dose vials is prepared for continuous administration by diluting the contents of one vial (100 mg) in 100 ml of compatible diluent to yield a 1-mg/ml solution or diluting two vials (200 mg) in 250 ml or 500 ml of compatible diluent to yield 0.8- or 0.4-mg/ml solutions, respectively (2).

The manufacturer recommends not using the product in the dual-chamber syringe on newborns because of the benzyl alcohol content (2).

See Table 1 for recommended dilutions for infusion.

Stability— Intact vials should be stored under refrigeration and protected from freezing. Diltiazem HCl may be stored for up to one month at room temperature but should then be destroyed (2).

Diltiazem HCl powder for injection in single-dose vials or in dual-chamber syringes should be stored at controlled room temperature. Freezing should be avoided. The reconstituted solutions are stable for 24 hours at controlled room temperature (2; 4).

pH Effects— Kawano et al. reported an increased rate of diltiazem HCl hydrolysis with increasing pH. Within the pH range tested, hydrolysis was lowest at pH 5 and 6 but increased substantially at pH 7 and 8. Diltiazem HCl 100 μg/ml in sodium chloride 0.9% with

Table 1. Recommended Diltiazem HCl Dilutions for Intravenous Infusion Admixtures (2)

Diluent Volume (ml)	Quantity of Diltiazem HCl Added	Final Admixture Concentration (mg/ml)	Final Admixture Volume (ml)
Liquid Dosage Forms			
100	125 mg (25 ml)	1	125
250	250 mg (50 ml)	0.83	300
500	250 mg (50 ml)	0.45	550
Lyophilized Vials			
100	100 mg (1 vial)	1	—
250	200 mg (2 vials)	0.8	—
500	200 mg (2 vials)	0.4	—

a pH between 5 and 6 exhibited no loss using HPLC analysis in 24 hours. Buffered to pH 7, losses of 3 to 4% in 24 hours were found (1915).

Sorption— Kawano et al. reported a pH-dependent loss of diltiazem HCl due to sorption to PVC containers and administration sets. Diltiazem HCl 100 µg/ml in sodium chloride 0.9% buffered to neutrality exhibited a loss of 11% in 24 hours in PVC containers but only 3 to 4% in glass and polypropylene containers (1915).

Similar results were found with PVC administration sets. Buffered to pH 8, diltiazem HCl concentration was initially reduced to about 83% when delivered at 0.52 ml/min through a 100-cm PVC administration set. At pH 6 and 7, initial losses were much less, about 1 and 5%, respectively. Delivered diltiazem HCl returned to full concentration in less than one hour at pH 6 and 7 but at pH 8 was only about 93% in two hours. The authors postulated the increased rate of hydrolysis at higher pH leads to increased sorption to PVC (1915).

Compatibility Information

Y-Site Injection Compatibility (1:1 Mixture)

Diltiazem HCl

Drug	Mfr	Conc	Mfr	Conc	Remarks	Ref	C/I
Acetazolamide sodium	LE	100 mg/ml	MMD	5 mg/ml	Precipitate forms	1807	I
	LE	100 mg/ml	MMD	1 mg/ml[b]	Visually compatible	1807	C
Acyclovir sodium	BW	5[a] and 7[b] mg/ml	MMD	5 mg/ml	Cloudiness and precipitate form	1807	I
	BW	5[a] and 7[b] mg/ml	MMD	1 mg/ml[b]	Visually compatible	1807	C
Albumin	AR, AT	5 and 25%	MMD	5 mg/ml	Visually compatible	1807	C
Amikacin sulfate	BR	5[b] and 250 mg/ml	MMD	5 mg/ml	Visually compatible	1807	C
Aminophylline	AMR	25 mg/ml[b]	MMD	5 mg/ml	Cloudiness forms	1807	I
	AMR	25 mg/ml[b]	MMD	1 mg/ml[b]	Visually compatible	1807	C
	AMR	2 mg/ml[a,b]	MMD	5 mg/ml	Visually compatible	1807	C
Amphotericin B	SQ	0.1 mg/ml[a]	MMD	5 mg/ml	Visually compatible	1807	C
Ampicillin sodium	WY	100 mg/ml[b]	MMD	5 mg/ml	Cloudiness forms	1807	I
	WY	100 mg/ml[b]	MMD	1 mg/ml[b]	Visually compatible	1807	C
	WY	10 and 20 mg/ml[b]	MMD	5 mg/ml	Visually compatible	1807	C
Ampicillin sodium–sulbactam sodium	RR	45 + 22.5 mg/ml[b]	MMD	5 mg/ml	Cloudiness forms	1807	I
	RR	45 + 22.5 mg/ml[b]	MMD	1 mg/ml[b]	Visually compatible	1807	C
	RR	2 + 1 and 15 + 7.5 mg/ml[b]	MMD	5 mg/ml	Visually compatible	1807	C
Aztreonam	SQ	20 and 333 mg/ml[b]	MMD	5 mg/ml	Visually compatible	1807	C
	SQ	333 mg/ml[b]	MMD	1 mg/ml[b]	Visually compatible	1807	C
Bretylium tosylate	DU	10[b] and 50 mg/ml	MMD	5 mg/ml	Visually compatible	1807	C
	DU	50 mg/ml	MMD	1 mg/ml[b]	Visually compatible	1807	C
Bumetanide	RC	0.25 mg/ml	MMD	1[b] and 5 mg/ml	Visually compatible	1807	C

Y-Site Injection Compatibility (1:1 Mixture) (Cont.)

Diltiazem HCl

Drug	Mfr	Conc	Mfr	Conc	Remarks	Ref	C/I
Cefamandole nafate	LI	200 mg/ml[b]	MMD	5 mg/ml	Cloudiness forms but clears with swirling	1807	?
	LI	10[b] and 20[a] mg/ml	MMD	5 mg/ml	Cloudiness forms and persists	1807	I
	LI	10[b], 20[a], 200[b] mg/ml	MMD	1 mg/ml[b]	Visually compatible	1807	C
Cefazolin sodium	LI	20 and 200 mg/ml[b]	MMD	5 mg/ml	Visually compatible	1807	C
	LI	200 mg/ml[b]	MMD	1 mg/ml[b]	Visually compatible	1807	C
Cefoperazone sodium	RR	20[a], 25[b], 50[b] mg/ml	MMD	1[b] and 5 mg/ml	Cloudiness and precipitate form	1807	I
	RR	10 mg/ml[b]	MMD	5 mg/ml	Precipitate forms	1807	I
	RR	10 mg/ml[b]	MMD	1 mg/ml[b]	Visually compatible	1807	C
	RR	2 and 5 mg/ml[b]	MMD	1[b] and 5 mg/ml	Visually compatible	1807	C
Cefotaxime sodium	HO	10 and 180 mg/ml[b]	MMD	5 mg/ml	Visually compatible	1807	C
	HO	180 mg/ml[b]	MMD	1 mg/ml[b]	Visually compatible	1807	C
Cefotetan disodium	STU	10 and 200 mg/ml[b]	MMD	5 mg/ml	Visually compatible	1807	C
	STU	200 mg/ml[b]	MMD	1 mg/ml[b]	Visually compatible	1807	C
Cefoxitin sodium	MSD	10 and 200 mg/ml[b]	MMD	5 mg/ml	Visually compatible	1807	C
	MSD	200 mg/ml[b]	MMD	1 mg/ml[b]	Visually compatible	1807	C
Ceftazidime	GL[f]	10 and 170 mg/ml[b]	MMD	5 mg/ml	Visually compatible	1807	C
	GL[f]	170 mg/ml[b]	MMD	1 mg/ml[b]	Visually compatible	1807	C
Ceftriaxone sodium	RC	40 mg/ml[b]	MMD	5 mg/ml	Visually compatible	1807	C
Cefuroxime sodium	LI	15 and 100 mg/ml[b]	MMD	5 mg/ml	Visually compatible	1807	C
	LI	100 mg/ml[b]	MMD	1 mg/ml[b]	Visually compatible	1807	C
Cimetidine HCl	SKF	6[c] and 150 mg/ml	MMD	5 mg/ml	Visually compatible	1807	C
	SKF	150 mg/ml	MMD	1 mg/ml[b]	Visually compatible	1807	C
Ciprofloxacin	MI	2 and 10 mg/ml[b]	MMD	5 mg/ml	Visually compatible	1807	C
Clindamycin phosphate	UP	12[b] and 150 mg/ml	MMD	5 mg/ml	Visually compatible	1807	C
Diazepam	ES	5 mg/ml	MMD	1[b] and 5 mg/ml	Cloudiness and precipitate form	1807	I
Digoxin	ES	0.5 mg/ml	MMD	1[b] and 5 mg/ml	Visually compatible	1807	C
Dobutamine HCl	LI	2 mg/ml[a]	MMD	1 mg/ml[a]	Visually compatible for 24 hr at 25 °C	1530	C
	LI	1 mg/ml[c]	MMD	5 mg/ml	Visually compatible	1807	C
	LI	4 mg/ml[a]	MMD	1 mg/ml[a]	Visually compatible for 4 hr at 27 °C	2062	C
Dopamine HCl	AB	1.6 mg/ml[a]	MMD	1 mg/ml[a]	Visually compatible for 24 hr at 25 °C	1530	C
	AB, SO	0.8 mg/ml[c]	MMD	5 mg/ml	Visually compatible	1807	C
	AB	3.2 mg/ml[a]	MMD	1 mg/ml[a]	Visually compatible for 4 hr at 27 °C	2062	C
Doxycycline hyclate	RR	1 and 10 mg/ml[b]	MMD	5 mg/ml	Visually compatible	1807	C

Y-Site Injection Compatibility (1:1 Mixture) (Cont.)

Diltiazem HCl

Drug	Mfr	Conc	Mfr	Conc	Remarks	Ref	C/I
Epinephrine HCl	PD	0.004 and 0.05 mg/ml[b]	MMD	5 mg/ml	Visually compatible	1807	C
	PD	0.05 mg/ml[b]	MMD	1 mg/ml[b]	Visually compatible	1807	C
	AB	0.02 mg/ml[a]	MMD	1 mg/ml[a]	Visually compatible for 4 hr at 27 °C	2062	C
Erythromycin lactobionate	ES	5 and 50 mg/ml[b]	MMD	5 mg/ml	Visually compatible	1807	C
Esmolol HCl	DU	10 mg/ml[a]	MMD	1 mg/ml[a]	Visually compatible for 24 hr at 25 °C	1530	C
Fentanyl citrate	ES	0.05 mg/ml	MMD	1 mg/ml[a]	Visually compatible for 4 hr at 27 °C	2062	C
Fluconazole	RR	2 mg/ml	MMD	5 mg/ml	Visually compatible	1807	C
Furosemide	AMR	10 mg/ml	MMD	1[b] and 5 mg/ml	Heavy precipitate forms	1807	I
	AMR	10 mg/ml	MMD	1 mg/ml[a]	Precipitate forms immediately	2062	I
Gentamicin sulfate	SC	2.4[b] and 40 mg/ml	MMD	1[b] and 5 mg/ml	Visually compatible	1807	C
Heparin sodium	LY	20,000 units/ml	MMD	5 mg/ml	Precipitate forms	1807	I
	LY	20,000 units/ml	MMD	1 mg/ml[b]	Visually compatible	1807	C
	LY, SCN	5000 and 10,000 units/ml	MMD	1[b] and 5 mg/ml	Visually compatible	1807	C
	LY, SCN	80 units/ml[c]	MMD	5 mg/ml	Visually compatible	1807	C
	ES	100 units/ml[a]	MMD	1 mg/ml[a]	Visually compatible for 4 hr at 27 °C	2062	C
Hetastarch	DU	6%[b]	MMD	5 mg/ml	Visually compatible	1807	C
Hydrocortisone sodium succinate	UP	50 and 125 mg/ml	MMD	5 mg/ml	Precipitate forms but clears with swirling	1807	?
	UP	50 and 125 mg/ml	MMD	1 mg/ml[b]	Visually compatible	1807	C
	UP	1[b] and 2[a] mg/ml	MMD	5 mg/ml	Visually compatible	1807	C
Hydromorphone HCl	KN	1 mg/ml	MMD	1 mg/ml[a]	Visually compatible for 4 hr at 27 °C	2062	C
Imipenem–cilastatin sodium	MSD	5 mg/ml[c]	MMD	5 mg/ml	Visually compatible	1807	C
Insulin, regular	NOV	100 units/ml	MMD	1[b] and 5 mg/ml	Precipitate forms and persists	1807	I
	NOV	0.4 unit/ml	MMD	5 mg/ml	Visually compatible	1807	C
Labetalol HCl	AH	2 mg/ml[a]	MMD	1 mg/ml[a]	Visually compatible for 4 hr at 27 °C	2062	C
Lidocaine HCl	AST	8 mg/ml[a]	MMD	1 mg/ml[a]	Visually compatible for 24 hr at 25 °C	1530	C
	AB	10 mg/ml[b]	MMD	1[b] and 5 mg/ml	Visually compatible	1807	C
	AB, SCN	4 and 8 mg/ml[a]	MMD	5 mg/ml	Visually compatible	1807	C
Lorazepam	WY	4 mg/ml	MMD	5 mg/ml	Visually compatible	1807	C
	WY	2 mg/ml[b]	MMD	1 mg/ml[b]	Visually compatible	1807	C
	WY	0.5 mg/ml[a]	MMD	1 mg/ml[a]	Visually compatible for 4 hr at 27 °C	2062	C
Meperidine HCl	WY	100 mg/ml	MMD	1[b] and 5 mg/ml	Visually compatible	1807	C
	WY	10 mg/ml[b]	MMD	5 mg/ml	Visually compatible	1807	C

Y-Site Injection Compatibility (1:1 Mixture) (Cont.)

Diltiazem HCl

Drug	Mfr	Conc	Mfr	Conc	Remarks	Ref	C/I
Methylprednisolone sodium succinate	UP	2.5[a], 20[b], 62.5 mg/ml	MMD	1 mg/ml[b]	Visually compatible	1807	C
	UP	2.5 mg/ml[a]	MMD	5 mg/ml	Cloudiness forms	1807	I
	UP	20 mg/ml[b]	MMD	5 mg/ml	Precipitate forms	1807	I
	UP	62.5 mg/ml	MMD	5 mg/ml	Cloudiness forms but clears with swirling	1807	?
Metoclopramide HCl	RB	5 mg/ml	MMD	1[b] and 5 mg/ml	Visually compatible	1807	C
	RB	0.2 mg/ml[b]	MMD	5 mg/ml	Visually compatible	1807	C
Metronidazole	SE	5 mg/ml	MMD	5 mg/ml	Visually compatible	1807	C
Metronidazole HCl	SE	8 mg/ml[b]	MMD	5 mg/ml	Visually compatible	1807	C
Midazolam HCl	RC	2 mg/ml[a]	MMD	1 mg/ml[a]	Visually compatible for 4 hr at 27 °C	2062	C
Milrinone lactate	SW	0.2 mg/ml[a]	MMD	1 mg/ml[a]	Visually compatible for 4 hr at 27 °C	2062	C
	SW	0.4 mg/ml[a]	MMD	1 mg/ml[a]	Visually compatible with little or no loss of either drug by HPLC in 4 hr at 23 °C	2214	C
Morphine sulfate	SCN	15 mg/ml	MMD	1[b] and 5 mg/ml	Visually compatible	1807	C
	SCN	0.4 mg/ml[b]	MMD	5 mg/ml	Visually compatible	1807	C
	SCN	2 mg/ml[a]	MMD	1 mg/ml[a]	Visually compatible for 4 hr at 27 °C	2062	C
Multivitamins (M.V.I.-12)		[d]	MMD	5 mg/ml	Visually compatible	1807	C
Nafcillin sodium	WY	10 mg/ml[b]	MMD	5 mg/ml	Cloudiness forms and persists	1807	I
	WY	200 mg/ml[b]	MMD	5 mg/ml	Cloudiness forms but clears with swirling	1807	?
	WY	10 and 200 mg/ml[b]	MMD	1 mg/ml[b]	Visually compatible	1807	C
Nicardipine HCl	WY	1 mg/ml[a]	MMD	1 mg/ml[a]	Visually compatible for 4 hr at 27 °C	2062	C
Nitroglycerin	DU	0.032 mg/ml[a]	MMD	1 mg/ml[a]	Visually compatible for 24 hr at 25 °C	1530	C
	DU	400 μg/ml[b]	MMD	1[b] and 5 mg/ml	Visually compatible	1807	C
	DU	400 μg/ml[a]	MMD	5 mg/ml	Visually compatible	1807	C
	AB	0.4 mg/ml[a]	MMD	1 mg/ml[a]	Visually compatible for 4 hr at 27 °C	2062	C
Norepinephrine bitartrate	WI	0.12 mg/ml[a]	MMD	1 mg/ml[a]	Visually compatible for 24 hr at 25 °C	1530	C
	AB	0.128 mg/ml[a]	MMD	1 mg/ml[a]	Visually compatible for 4 hr at 27 °C	2062	C
Oxacillin sodium		100 mg/ml[b]	MMD	1[b] and 5 mg/ml	Visually compatible	1807	C
		10 mg/ml[b]	MMD	5 mg/ml	Visually compatible	1807	C
Penicillin G potassium	RR	1 million units/ml	MMD	1[b] and 5 mg/ml	Visually compatible	1807	C
	RR	100,000 units/ml[b]	MMD	5 mg/ml	Visually compatible	1807	C
Pentamidine isethionate	LY	6 and 30 mg/ml[a]	MMD	5 mg/ml	Visually compatible	1807	C
Phenytoin sodium	PD	50 mg/ml	MMD	1 mg/ml[b]	Precipitate forms	1807	I
Piperacillin sodium	LE	200 mg/ml[b]	MMD	1[b] and 5 mg/ml	Visually compatible	1807	C
	LE	20 mg/ml[b]	MMD	5 mg/ml	Visually compatible	1807	C
Potassium chloride	LY	0.08[a] and 2 mEq/ml	MMD	5 mg/ml	Visually compatible	1807	C

Y-Site Injection Compatibility (1:1 Mixture) (Cont.)

Diltiazem HCl

Drug	Mfr	Conc	Mfr	Conc	Remarks	Ref	C/I
Potassium phosphates	AMR	0.015 mmol/ml	MMD	5 mg/ml	Visually compatible	1807	**C**
Procainamide HCl	ES	500 mg/ml	MMD	5 mg/ml	Cloudiness forms but clears in 2 min	1807	**?**
	ES	50 mg/ml[a]	MMD	1 mg/ml[b]	Visually compatible	1807	**C**
	ES	2 mg/ml[a]	MMD	5 mg/ml	Visually compatible	1807	**C**
Ranitidine HCl	GL	25 mg/ml	MMD	1[b] and 5 mg/ml	Visually compatible	1807	**C**
	GL	1[b] and 0.5[e] mg/ml	MMD	5 mg/ml	Visually compatible	1807	**C**
	GL	1 mg/ml[a]	MMD	1 mg/ml[a]	Visually compatible for 4 hr at 27 °C	2062	**C**
Rifampin	MMD	6 mg/ml[b]	MMD	1[b] and 5 mg/ml	Precipitate forms	1807	**I**
Sodium bicarbonate	LY	1 mEq/ml	MMD	5 mg/ml	Precipitate forms	1807	**I**
	LY	1 mEq/ml	MMD	1 mg/ml[b]	Visually compatible	1807	**C**
	AMR	0.05 mEq/ml[a]	MMD	5 mg/ml	Visually compatible	1807	**C**
Sodium nitroprusside	AB	0.2 mg/ml[a]	MMD	5 mg/ml	Visually compatible	1807	**C**
Theophylline	AB	0.8 mg/ml[a]	MMD	5 mg/ml	Visually compatible	1807	**C**
Thiopental sodium	AB	25 mg/ml[b]	MMD	1 mg/ml[a]	Precipitate forms immediately	2062	**I**
Ticarcillin disodium	BE	200 mg/ml[b]	MMD	1[b] and 5 mg/ml	Visually compatible	1807	**C**
	BE	10 mg/ml[b]	MMD	5 mg/ml	Visually compatible	1807	**C**
Ticarcillin disodium–clavulanate potassium	BE	200 mg/ml[b]	MMD	1[b] and 5 mg/ml	Visually compatible	1807	**C**
	BE	10 mg/ml[b]	MMD	5 mg/ml	Visually compatible	1807	**C**
Tobramycin sulfate	LI	2.4[b] and 40 mg/ml	MMD	5 mg/ml	Visually compatible	1807	**C**
Trimethoprim–sulfamethoxazole	BW, RC	0.21 + 1 and 0.63 + 3.2 mg/ml[a]	MMD	5 mg/ml	Visually compatible	1807	**C**
Vancomycin HCl	LI	5 and 50 mg/ml[b]	MMD	5 mg/ml	Visually compatible	1807	**C**
Vecuronium bromide	OR	1 mg/ml	MMD	1 mg/ml[a]	Visually compatible for 4 hr at 27 °C	2062	**C**

[a]*Tested in dextrose 5% in water.*
[b]*Tested in sodium chloride 0.9%.*
[c]*Tested in both dextrose 5% in water and sodium chloride 0.9%.*
[d]*Concentration not specified.*
[e]*Tested in sodium chloride 0.45%.*
[f]*Sodium carbonate–containing formulation tested.*

Additional Compatibility Information

Infusion Solutions— Dextrose 5% in water, sodium chloride 0.9%, and dextrose 5% in sodium chloride 0.45% are the recommended infusion vehicles. At concentrations up to 1 mg/ml, diltiazem HCl is physically compatible and chemically stable in these solutions in glass or PVC containers for at least 24 hours at room temperature or under refrigeration. The manufacturer recommends refrigeration storage and use within 24 hours (2).

DIMENHYDRINATE
AHFS 56:22

Products— Dimenhydrinate is available in 1-ml ampuls and 1-, 5-, and 10-ml vials containing dimenhydrinate 50 mg/ml in propylene glycol 50% and water. Sodium hydroxide and/or hydrochloric acid may be used to adjust the pH and benzyl alcohol is present in multiple-dose vials as a preservative. Dimenhydrinate contains 53 to 55.5% of diphenhydramine and 44 to 47% of 8-chlorotheophylline (4; 154).

pH— From 6.4 to 7.2 (4).

Administration— Dimenhydrinate is administered by intramuscular injection or by intravenous injection over two minutes after dilution with 10 ml of sodium chloride 0.9% (4).

Stability— Intact vials should be stored at controlled room temperature and protected from freezing (4). Dimenhydrinate (Searle) 50 mg/ml was found to retain potency for three months at room temperature when 1 ml of solution was packaged in Tubex cartridges (13).

Dilution with water for injection, sodium chloride 0.9%, or dextrose 5% in water results in a solution that is stable for at least 10 days at room temperature (279).

A test of dimenhydrinate solutions at pH 2 to 10 showed no separation or precipitation at pH 5.4 to 8.6 on extended room temperature storage. Below pH 5.4, a white powdery precipitate of 8-chlorotheophylline formed within 24 hours. Above pH 8.6, an oily liquid separated within 30 minutes (279).

Compatibility Information

Solution Compatibility

Dimenhydrinate

Solution	Mfr	Mfr	Conc/L	Remarks	Ref	C/I
Dextran 6% in dextrose 5%	AB	SE	50 mg	Physically compatible	3	C
Dextran 6% in sodium chloride 0.9%	AB	SE	50 mg	Physically compatible	3	C
Dextrose–Ringer's injection combinations	AB	SE	50 mg	Physically compatible	3	C
Dextrose–Ringer's injection, lactated, combinations	AB	SE	50 mg	Physically compatible	3	C
Dextrose–saline combinations	AB	SE	50 mg	Physically compatible	3	C
Dextrose 5% in sodium chloride 0.9%		SE	50 mg	Physically compatible	74	C
Dextrose 2½% in water	AB	SE	50 mg	Physically compatible	3	C
Dextrose 5% in water	AB	SE	50 mg	Physically compatible	3	C
		SE	50 mg	Physically compatible	74	C
Dextrose 10% in water	AB	SE	50 mg	Physically compatible	3	C
Fructose 10% in sodium chloride 0.9%	AB	SE	50 mg	Physically compatible	3	C
Fructose 10% in water	AB	SE	50 mg	Physically compatible	3	C
Invert sugar 5 and 10% in sodium chloride 0.9%	AB	SE	50 mg	Physically compatible	3	C
Invert sugar 5 and 10% in water	AB	SE	50 mg	Physically compatible	3	C
Ionosol products	AB	SE	50 mg	Physically compatible	3	C
Ringer's injection	AB	SE	50 mg	Physically compatible	3	C
Ringer's injection, lactated	AB	SE	50 mg	Physically compatible	3	C
		SE	50 mg	Physically compatible	74	C
Sodium chloride 0.45%	AB	SE	50 mg	Physically compatible	3	C
Sodium chloride 0.9%	AB	SE	50 mg	Physically compatible	3	C
		SE	50 mg	Physically compatible	74	C
Sodium lactate ⅙ M	AB	SE	50 mg	Physically compatible	3	C

Additive Compatibility

Dimenhydrinate

Drug	Mfr	Conc/L	Mfr	Conc/L	Test Soln	Remarks	Ref	C/I
Amikacin sulfate	BR	5 g	SE	100 mg	D5LR, D5R, D5S, D5W, D10W, IS10, LR, NS, R, SL	Physically compatible and potency of both retained for 24 hr at 25 °C	294	C
Aminophylline		250 mg	SE	50 mg	D5W	Physically compatible	74	C
	SE	1 g	SE	500 mg	D5W	Physically incompatible	15	I
Ammonium chloride	AB	20 g	SE	500 mg	D5W	Physically compatible	15	C
			SE			Physically incompatible	9	I
Amobarbital sodium	LI	1 g	SE	500 mg	D5W	Physically compatible	15	C
			SE			Physically incompatible	9	I
Calcium gluconate		1 g	SE	50 mg	D5W	Physically compatible	74	C
Chloramphenicol sodium succinate	PD	500 mg	SE	50 mg	D5W	Physically compatible	74	C
Corticotropin		500 units	SE	50 mg	D5W	Physically compatible	74	C
Heparin sodium		12,000 units	SE	50 mg	D5W	Physically compatible	74	C
	UP	4000 units	SE	500 mg	D5W	Physically compatible	15	C
	AB	20,000 units	SE	50 mg	D	Physically compatible	21	C
Hydrocortisone sodium succinate	UP	100 mg	SE	50 mg	D5W	Physically compatible	74	C
	UP	500 mg	SE	500 mg	D5W	Physically incompatible	15	I
Hydroxyzine HCl	RR	250 mg	SE	500 mg	D5W	Physically compatible	15	C
Norepinephrine bitartrate	WI	8 mg	SE	50 mg	D5W	Physically compatible	74	C
Penicillin G potassium		1 million units	SE	50 mg	D5W	Physically compatible	74	C
Pentobarbital sodium	AB	1 g	SE	500 mg	D5W	Physically compatible	15	C
Phenobarbital sodium	WI	200 mg	SE	500 mg	D5W	Physically compatible	15	C
Potassium chloride		3 g	SE	50 mg	D5W	Physically compatible	74	C
Prochlorperazine edisylate	SKF	100 mg	SE	500 mg	D5W	Physically compatible	15	C
Thiopental sodium	AB		SE			Physically incompatible	9	I
Vancomycin HCl	LI	1 g	SE	50 mg	D5W	Physically compatible	74	C
Vitamin B complex with C		1 vial	SE	50 mg	D5W	Physically compatible	74	C

Drugs in Syringe Compatibility

Dimenhydrinate

Drug (in syringe)	Mfr	Amt	Mfr	Amt	Remarks	Ref	C/I
Atropine sulfate	ST	0.4 mg/ 1 ml	HR	50 mg/ 1 ml	Physically compatible for at least 15 min	326	C

Drugs in Syringe Compatibility (Cont.)

Dimenhydrinate

Drug (in syringe)	Mfr	Amt	Mfr	Amt	Remarks	Ref	C/I
Butorphanol tartrate	BR	4 mg/ 2 ml	HR	50 mg/ 1 ml	Gas evolves	761	I
Chlorpromazine HCl	PO	50 mg/ 2 ml	HR	50 mg/ 1 ml	Physically incompatible within 15 min	326	I
Diatrizoate meglumine 34.3%, diatrizoate sodium 35% (Renovist)	SQ	40 to 1 ml	SE	50 mg/ 1 ml	Physically compatible for 48 hr	530	C
Diatrizoate meglumine 52%, diatrizoate sodium 8% (Renografin-60)	SQ	40 to 1 ml	SE	50 mg/ 1 ml	Physically compatible for 48 hr	530	C
Diatrizoate sodium 75% (Hypaque)	WI	40 to 1 ml	SE	50 mg/ 1 ml	Physically compatible for 48 hr	530	C
Diphenhydramine HCl	PD	50 mg/ 1 ml	HR	50 mg/ 1 ml	Physically compatible for at least 15 min	326	C
Droperidol	MN	2.5 mg/ 1 ml	HR	50 mg/ 1 ml	Physically compatible for at least 15 min	326	C
Fentanyl citrate	MN	0.05 mg/ 1 ml	HR	50 mg/ 1 ml	Physically compatible for at least 15 min	326	C
Glycopyrrolate	RB	0.2 mg/ 1 ml	SE	50 mg/ 1 ml	Immediate precipitation	331	I
	RB	0.2 mg/ 1 ml	SE	100 mg/ 2 ml	Immediate precipitation	331	I
	RB	0.4 mg/ 2 ml	SE	50 mg/ 1 ml	Immediate precipitation	331	I
Heparin sodium		2500 units/ 1 ml		65 mg/ 10 ml	Physically compatible for at least 5 min	1053	C
Hydromorphone HCl	KN	1, 10, 40 mg/ 1 ml	SQ	50 mg/ 1 ml	Visually compatible with both drugs stable by HPLC for 24 hr at 4, 23, and 37 °C. Precipitate forms after 24 hr	1776	C
Hydroxyzine HCl	PF	50 mg/ 1 ml	HR	50 mg/ 1 ml	Physically incompatible within 15 min	326	I
Iodipamide meglumine 52% (Cholografin)	SQ	40 ml	SE	50 mg/ 1 ml	Forms a precipitate initially but clears within 1 hr and remains clear for 48 hr	530	I
	SQ	20 to 1 ml	SE	50 mg/ 1 ml	Forms a precipitate initially but clears within 1 hr. Precipitate reforms upon standing	530	I
Iothalamate meglumine 60% (Conray)	MA	40 to 1 ml	SE	50 mg/ 1 ml	Physically compatible for 48 hr	530	C
Iothalamate sodium 80% (Angio-Conray)	MA	40 to 1 ml	SE	50 mg/ 1 ml	Physically compatible for 48 hr	530	C
Meperidine HCl	WI	50 mg/ 1 ml	HR	50 mg/ 1 ml	Physically compatible for at least 15 min	326	C
Metoclopramide HCl	NO	10 mg/ 2 ml	HR	50 mg/ 1 ml	Physically compatible both macroscopically and microscopically for 15 min at room temperature	565	C
Midazolam HCl	RC	5 mg/ 1 ml	SE	50 mg/ 1 ml	White precipitate forms immediately	1145	I
Morphine sulfate	ST	15 mg/ 1 ml	HR	50 mg/ 1 ml	Physically compatible for at least 15 min	326	C

Drugs in Syringe Compatibility (Cont.)

Dimenhydrinate

Drug (in syringe)	Mfr	Amt	Mfr	Amt	Remarks	Ref	C/I
Pentazocine lactate	WI	30 mg/ 1 ml	HR	50 mg/ 1 ml	Physically compatible for at least 15 min	326	C
Pentobarbital sodium	AB	500 mg/ 10 ml	SE	50 mg/ 1 ml	Physically incompatible	55	I
	AB	50 mg/ 1 ml	HR	50 mg/ 1 ml	Physically incompatible within 15 min	326	I
Perphenazine	SC	5 mg/ 1 ml	HR	50 mg/ 1 ml	Physically compatible both macroscopically and microscopically for 30 min at room temperature	761	C
Prochlorperazine edisylate	PO	5 mg/ 1 ml	HR	50 mg/ 1 ml	Physically incompatible within 15 min	326	I
Promazine HCl	WY	50 mg/ 1 ml	HR	50 mg/ 1 ml	Physically incompatible within 15 min	326	I
Promethazine HCl	PO	50 mg/ 2 ml	HR	50 mg/ 1 ml	Physically incompatible within 15 min	326	I
Ranitidine HCl	GL	50 mg/ 2 ml	HR	50 mg/ 1 ml	Physically compatible for 1 hr at 25 °C both macroscopically and microscopically	978	C
Scopolamine HBr	ST	0.4 mg/ 1 ml	HR	50 mg/ 1 ml	Physically compatible for at least 15 min	326	C
Thiopental sodium	AB	75 mg/ 3 ml	SE	50 mg/ 1 ml	Physically incompatible	21	I

Y-Site Injection Compatibility (1:1 Mixture)

Dimenhydrinate

Drug	Mfr	Conc	Mfr	Conc	Remarks	Ref	C/I
Acyclovir sodium	BW	5 mg/ml[a]	SE	1 mg/ml[a]	Physically compatible for 4 hr at 25 °C under fluorescent light	1157	C

[a]*Tested in dextrose 5% in water.*

Additional Compatibility Information

Concentrated Solutions— The following incompatibility determinations were performed with concentrated solutions. The drugs in dry form were reconstituted according to manufacturers' recommendations. One milliliter of dimenhydrinate (Searle) was added to 5 ml of sterile distilled water along with 1 ml of each of the following drugs. Particulate matter was noted within two hours (28):

Aminophylline
Heparin sodium
Hydrocortisone sodium succinate (Upjohn)
Hydroxyzine HCl (Pfizer)
Phenobarbital sodium (Winthrop)
Phenytoin sodium (Parke-Davis)
Prochlorperazine edisylate (SKF)
Promazine HCl (Wyeth)
Promethazine HCl (Wyeth)

DIPHENHYDRAMINE HCL
AHFS 4:00

Benadryl   **Parke-Davis**

Products— Diphenhydramine HCl (Parke-Davis) is available as a 50-mg/ml solution in 1-ml ampuls and disposable syringes and in 10-ml vials. Also present in the 10-ml vials is 0.1 mg/ml of benzethonium chloride. The pH may have been adjusted with sodium hydroxide or hydrochloric acid (2).

pH— From 5 to 6 (2; 4).

Osmolality— Diphenhydramine HCl 50 mg/ml has an osmolality of 240 mOsm/kg, and the osmolality of the 10-mg/ml concentration is 65 mOsm/kg (1689).

Administration— Diphenhydramine HCl is administered by deep intramuscular injection, slow direct intravenous injection, or continuous or intermittent intravenous infusion (2; 4). Subcutaneous or perivascular injection should be avoided due to irritation (4).

Stability— Diphenhydramine HCl should be stored in light-resistant containers at controlled room temperature. Freezing should be avoided (2; 4).

Compatibility Information

Solution Compatibility

Diphenhydramine HCl

Solution	Mfr	Mfr	Conc/L	Remarks	Ref	C/I
Dextran 6% in dextrose 5%	AB	PD	100 mg	Physically compatible	3	C
Dextran 6% in sodium chloride 0.9%	AB	PD	100 mg	Physically compatible	3	C
Dextrose–Ringer's injection combinations	AB	PD	100 mg	Physically compatible	3	C
Dextrose–Ringer's injection, lactated, combinations	AB	PD	100 mg	Physically compatible	3	C
Dextrose–saline combinations	AB	PD	100 mg	Physically compatible	3	C
Dextrose 2½% in water	AB	PD	100 mg	Physically compatible	3	C
Dextrose 5% in water	AB	PD	100 mg	Physically compatible	3	C
Dextrose 10% in water	AB	PD	100 mg	Physically compatible	3	C
Fat emulsion 10%, intravenous	VT	PD	200 mg	Physically compatible for 48 hr at 4 °C and room temperature	32	C
Fructose 10% in sodium chloride 0.9%	AB	PD	100 mg	Physically compatible	3	C
Fructose 10% in water	AB	PD	100 mg	Physically compatible	3	C
Invert sugar 5 and 10% in sodium chloride 0.9%	AB	PD	100 mg	Physically compatible	3	C
Invert sugar 5 and 10% in water	AB	PD	100 mg	Physically compatible	3	C
Ionosol products	AB	PD	100 mg	Physically compatible	3	C
Ringer's injection	AB	PD	100 mg	Physically compatible	3	C
Ringer's injection, lactated	AB	PD	100 mg	Physically compatible	3	C
Sodium chloride 0.45%	AB	PD	100 mg	Physically compatible	3	C
Sodium chloride 0.9%	AB	PD	100 mg	Physically compatible	3	C
Sodium lactate ⅙ M	AB	PD	100 mg	Physically compatible	3	C

Additive Compatibility

Diphenhydramine HCl

Drug	Mfr	Conc/L	Mfr	Conc/L	Test Soln	Remarks	Ref	C/I
Amikacin sulfate	BR	5 g	PD	100 mg	D5LR, D5R, D5S, D5W, IS10, LR, NS, R, SL	Physically compatible and potency of both retained for 24 hr at 25 °C	294	C

Additive Compatibility (Cont.)

Diphenhydramine HCl

Drug	Mfr	Conc/L	Mfr	Conc/L	Test Soln	Remarks	Ref	C/I
Aminophylline	SE	500 mg	PD	50 mg		Physically compatible	6	C
Amobarbital sodium			PD			Physically incompatible	9	I
	LI	1 g	PD	80 mg	D5W	Physically incompatible	15	I
Amphotericin B	SQ	100 mg	PD	80 mg	D5W	Physically incompatible	15	I
Ascorbic acid injection	UP	500 mg	PD	80 mg	D5W	Physically compatible	15	C
Bleomycin sulfate	BR	20 and 30 units	PD	100 mg	NS	Physically compatible and bleomycin activity retained for 1 week at 4 °C. Diphenhydramine not tested	763	C
Colistimethate sodium	WC	500 mg	PD	80 mg	D5W	Physically compatible	15	C
Dexamethasone sodium phosphate with lorazepam and metoclopramide HCl	AMR WY DU	400 mg 40 mg 4 g	ES	2 g	NS[a]	Rapid lorazepam losses of 8, 10, and 15% at 3, 23, and 30 °C, respectively, in 24 hr by HPLC. Other drugs stable for 14 days by HPLC at all three storage temperatures	1733	I
Erythromycin lactobionate	AB	1 g	PD	50 mg		Physically compatible. Erythromycin potency retained for 24 hr at 25 °C	20	C
	AB	1 g	PD	50 mg	D5W	Erythromycin potency retained for 24 hr at 25 °C	48	C
Hydrocortisone sodium succinate	UP	500 mg	SCN	80 mg	D5W[b]	Physically compatible with no subvisual haze or particle formation in 24 hr at 23 °C	1729	C
	UP	1 g	SCN	500 mg	D5W[b]	Physically compatible with no subvisual haze or particle formation in 24 hr at 23 °C	1729	C
Iodipamide meglumine (% unspecified)	SQ		PD	20 to 200 mg	NS	Dense putty-like white precipitate immediately forms	309	I
Lidocaine HCl	AST	2 g	PD	50 mg		Physically compatible	24	C
Methyldopate HCl	MSD	1 g	PD	50 mg	D, D–S, S	Physically compatible	23	C
Nafcillin sodium	WY	500 mg	PD	50 mg		Physically compatible	27	C
Netilmicin sulfate	SC	3 g	PD	400 mg	D5S	Physically compatible and netilmicin chemically stable for 3 days at 25 and 4 °C. 17% loss noted after 7 days at 25 °C. Diphenhydramine not tested	558	C
Penicillin G potassium	SQ	20 million units	PD	80 mg	D5W	Physically compatible	15	C
	SQ	1 million units	PD	50 mg	D5W	Physically compatible. Penicillin potency retained for 24 hr at 25 °C	47	C
Penicillin G sodium	UP	20 million units	PD	80 mg	D5W	Physically compatible	15	C
Polymyxin B sulfate	BW	200 mg	PD	80 mg	D5W	Physically compatible	15	C
Thiopental sodium	AB		PD			Physically incompatible	9	I
Vitamin B complex with C	AB	5 ml	PD	80 mg	D5W	Physically compatible	15	C

[a]Tested in Pharmacia-Deltec PVC pump reservoirs.
[b]Tested in PVC containers.

Drugs in Syringe Compatibility

Diphenhydramine HCl

Drug (in syringe)	Mfr	Amt	Mfr	Amt	Remarks	Ref	C/I
Atropine sulfate	ST	0.4 mg/ 1 ml	PD	50 mg/ 1 ml	Physically compatible for at least 15 min	326	C
Butorphanol tartrate	BR	4 mg/ 2 ml	PD	50 mg/ 1 ml	Physically compatible both macroscopically and microscopically for 30 min at room temperature	566	C
Chlorpromazine HCl	PO	50 mg/ 2 ml	PD	50 mg/ 1 ml	Physically compatible for at least 15 min	326	C
	STE	50 mg/ 2 ml	ES	100 mg/ 2 ml	Visually compatible for 60 min	1784	C
Cimetidine HCl	SKF	300 mg/ 2 ml	PD	50 mg/ 1 ml	Physically compatible for 4 hr at 25 °C	25	C
Dexamethasone sodium phosphate	DB, SX	4 and 10 mg/ ml[a]	PD	50 mg/ ml[a]	White turbidity and precipitate form immediately	1542	I
	DB	9.52 mg/ ml[b]	PD	4.54 mg/ ml[b]	Visually compatible for 24 hr at 24 °C	1542	C
	DB	5 to 9.02 mg/ ml[b]	PD	4.54 to 15 mg/ ml[b]	Precipitate forms	1542	I
	SX	2 mg/ml[b]	PD	34.8 to 40 mg/ ml[b]	Visually compatible for 24 hr at 24 °C	1542	C
	SX	1 mg/ml[b]	PD	25 mg/ ml[b]	Precipitate forms	1542	I
Diatrizoate meglumine (% unspecified)	SQ	5 ml	PD	50 mg/ 1 ml	No precipitate observed	309	C
Diatrizoate meglumine 34.3%, diatrizoate sodium 35% (Renovist)	SQ	40 to 1 ml	PD	1 ml[c]	Physically compatible for 48 hr	530	C
Diatrizoate meglumine 52%, diatrizoate sodium 8% (Renografin-60)	SQ	2 and 1 ml	PD	1 ml[c]	Physically compatible for at least 1 hr but a precipitate observed at 48 hr	530	I
	SQ	40 to 5 ml	PD	1 ml[c]	Physically compatible for 48 hr	530	C
Diatrizoate meglumine 52%, diatrizoate sodium 8%	MA	5 ml	PD	12.5 mg/ 0.25 ml	Transient precipitate clears and then reforms within 1 hr	1438	I
Diatrizoate sodium (% unspecified)	WI	5 ml	PD	50 mg/ 1 ml	No precipitate observed	309	C
Diatrizoate sodium 60%	WI	5 ml	PD	12.5 mg/ 0.25 ml	Transient precipitate clears and then reforms within 1 hr	1438	I
Diatrizoate sodium 75% (Hypaque)	WI	40 to 1 ml	PD	1 ml[c]	Physically compatible for 48 hr	530	C
Dimenhydrinate	HR	50 mg/ 1 ml	PD	50 mg/ 1 ml	Physically compatible for at least 15 min	326	C
Droperidol	MN	2.5 mg/ 1 ml	PD	50 mg/ 1 ml	Physically compatible for at least 15 min	326	C
Fentanyl citrate	MN	0.05 mg/ 1 ml	PD	50 mg/ 1 ml	Physically compatible for at least 15 min	326	C
Fluphenazine HCl	LY	5 mg/ 2 ml	ES	100 mg/ 2 ml	Visually compatible for 60 min	1784	C

Drugs in Syringe Compatibility (Cont.)

Diphenhydramine HCl

Drug (in syringe)	Mfr	Amt	Mfr	Amt	Remarks	Ref	C/I
Glycopyrrolate	RB	0.2 mg/ 1 ml	PD	10 mg/ 1 ml	Physically compatible and pH in stability range for glycopyrrolate for 48 hr at 25 °C	331	C
	RB	0.2 mg/ 1 ml	PD	20 mg/ 2 ml	Physically compatible and pH in stability range for glycopyrrolate for 48 hr at 25 °C	331	C
	RB	0.4 mg/ 2 ml	PD	10 mg/ 1 ml	Physically compatible and pH in stability range for glycopyrrolate for 48 hr at 25 °C	331	C
	RB	0.2 mg/ 1 ml	PD	50 mg/ 1 ml	Physically compatible and pH in stability range for glycopyrrolate for 48 hr at 25 °C	331	C
	RB	0.2 mg/ 1 ml	PD	100 mg/ 2 ml	Physically compatible and pH in stability range for glycopyrrolate for 48 hr at 25 °C	331	C
	RB	0.4 mg/ 2 ml	PD	50 mg/ 1 ml	Physically compatible and pH in stability range for glycopyrrolate for 48 hr at 25 °C	331	C
Haloperidol lactate	MN	10 mg/ 2 ml	ES	100 mg/ 2 ml	White precipitate forms within 5 min	1784	I
	MN	5 mg/ 1 ml	ES	50 mg/ 1 ml	White cloudy precipitate forms in 2 hr at room temperature	1886	I
Hydromorphone HCl	KN	4 mg/ 2 ml	PD	50 mg/ 1 ml	Physically compatible for 30 min	517	C
Hydroxyzine HCl	PF	50 mg/ 1 ml	PD	50 mg/ 1 ml	Physically compatible for at least 15 min	326	C
Iodipamide meglumine (% unspecified)	SQ		PD	5 mg/ 0.1 ml to 50 mg/ 1 ml	Dense putty-like white precipitate immediately forms	309	I
Iodipamide meglumine 52% (Cholografin)	SQ	40 to 1 ml	PD	1 ml[c]	Forms a precipitate initially but clears within 1 hr and remains clear for 48 hr	530	I
Iohexol	WI	64.7%, 5 ml	PD	12.5 mg/ 0.25 ml	Physically compatible for at least 2 hr	1438	C
Iopamidol	SQ	61%, 5 ml	PD	12.5 mg/ 0.25 ml	Physically compatible for at least 2 hr	1438	C
Iothalamate meglumine (% unspecified)	MA	5 ml	PD	50 mg/ 1 ml	No precipitate observed	309	C
Iothalamate meglumine 60% (Conray)	MA	40 to 1 ml	PD	1 ml[c]	Physically compatible for 48 hr	530	C
Iothalamate meglumine 60%	MA	5 ml	PD	12.5 mg/ 0.25 ml	Physically compatible for at least 2 hr	1438	C
Iothalamate sodium 80% (Angio-Conray)	MA	40 to 1 ml	PD	1 ml[c]	Physically compatible for 48 hr	530	C
Ioxaglate meglumine 39.3%, ioxaglate sodium 19.6%	MA	5 ml	PD	12.5 mg/ 0.25 ml	Precipitate forms immediately and persists for at least 2 hr	1438	I
Meperidine HCl	WY	100 mg/ 1 ml	PD	50 mg/ 1 ml	Physically compatible for at least 15 min	14	C
	WI	50 mg/ 1 ml	PD	50 mg/ 1 ml	Physically compatible for at least 15 min	309	C
Metoclopramide HCl	NO	10 mg/ 2 ml	PD	50 mg/ 1 ml	Physically compatible both macroscopically and microscopically for 15 min at room temperature	565	C
	RB	10 mg/ 2 ml	PD	50 mg/ 5 ml	Physically compatible for 48 hr at room temperature	924	C

Drugs in Syringe Compatibility (Cont.)

Diphenhydramine HCl

Drug (in syringe)	Mfr	Amt	Mfr	Amt	Remarks	Ref	C/I
	RB	10 mg/ 2 ml	PD	250 mg/ 25 ml	Physically compatible for 48 hr at room temperature	924	C
	RB	10 mg/ 2 ml	PD	50 mg/ 5 ml	Physically compatible for 48 hr at 25 °C	1167	C
	RB	10 mg/ 2 ml	PD	250 mg/ 25 ml	Physically compatible for 48 hr at 25 °C	1167	C
	RB	160 mg/ 32 ml	PD	40 mg/ 4 ml	Physically compatible for 48 hr at 25 °C	1167	C
	RB	160 mg/ 32 ml	PD	200 mg/ 20 ml	Physically compatible for 48 hr at 25 °C	1167	C
Midazolam HCl	RC	5 mg/ 1 ml	ES	50 mg/ 1 ml	Physically compatible for 4 hr at 25 °C under fluorescent light	1145	C
Morphine sulfate	WY	15 mg/ 1 ml	PD	50 mg/ 1 ml	Physically compatible for at least 15 min	14	C
	ST	15 mg/ 1 ml	PD	50 mg/ 1 ml	Physically compatible for at least 15 min	326	C
Nalbuphine HCl	DU	10 mg/ 1 ml	PD	50 mg/ 1 ml	Physically compatible for 48 hr	128	C
	DU	20 mg/ 1 ml	PD	50 mg/ 1 ml	Physically compatible for 48 hr	128	C
Pentazocine lactate	WI	30 mg/ 1 ml	PD	50 mg/ 1 ml	Physically compatible for at least 15 min	326	C
Pentobarbital sodium	WY	100 mg/ 2 ml	PD	50 mg/ 1 ml	Precipitate observed within 15 min	14	I
	AB	500 mg/ 10 ml	PD	50 mg/ 1 ml	Physically incompatible	55	I
	AB	50 mg/ 1 ml	PD	50 mg/ 1 ml	Physically incompatible within 15 min	326	I
Perphenazine	SC	5 mg/ 1 ml	PD	50 mg/ 1 ml	Physically compatible both macroscopically and microscopically for 30 min at room temperature	566	C
	SC	10 mg/ 2 ml	ES	100 mg/ 2 ml	Visually compatible for 60 min	1784	C
Prochlorperazine edisylate	PO	5 mg/ 1 ml	PD	50 mg/ 1 ml	Physically compatible for at least 15 min	326	C
Promazine HCl	WY	50 mg/ 1 ml	PD	50 mg/ 1 ml	Physically compatible for at least 15 min	326	C
Promethazine HCl	WY	50 mg/ 2 ml	PD	50 mg/ 1 ml	Physically compatible for at least 15 min	14	C
	PO	50 mg/ 2 ml	PD	50 mg/ 1 ml	Physically compatible for at least 15 min	326	C
Ranitidine HCl	GL	50 mg/ 2 ml	PD	50 mg/ 1 ml	Physically compatible for 1 hr at 25 °C both macroscopically and microscopically	978	C
Scopolamine HBr	ST	0.4 mg/ 1 ml	PD	50 mg/ 1 ml	Physically compatible for at least 15 min	326	C
Sufentanil citrate	JN	50 μg/ml	SCN	50 mg/ ml	Physically compatible with no subvisual haze or particle formation in 24 hr at 23 °C	1711	C

Drugs in Syringe Compatibility (Cont.)

Diphenhydramine HCl

Drug (in syringe)	Mfr	Amt	Mfr	Amt	Remarks	Ref	C/I
Thiopental sodium	AB	75 mg/ 3 ml	PD	50 mg/ 1 ml	Physically incompatible	21	I

[a]Mixed in equal quantities. Final concentration is one-half the indicated concentration.
[b]Mixed in varying quantities to yield the final concentrations noted.
[c]Diphenhydramine HCl concentration unspecified.

Y-Site Injection Compatibility (1:1 Mixture)

Diphenhydramine HCl

Drug	Mfr	Conc	Mfr	Conc	Remarks	Ref	C/I
Acyclovir sodium	BW	5 mg/ml[a]	ES	1 mg/ml[a]	Physically compatible for 4 hr at 25 °C	1157	C
Aldesleukin	CHI	33,800 I.U./ ml[a]	SCN	50 mg/ml	Visually compatible for 2 hr. Bioassay not possible	1857	C
Allopurinol sodium	BW	3 mg/ml[b]	PD	2 mg/ml[b]	Heavy white turbidity and precipitate form immediately	1686	I
Amifostine	USB	10 mg/ml[a]	PD	2 mg/ml[a]	Physically compatible with no change in measured turbidity or increase in particle content in 4 hr at 23 °C	1845	C
Amphotericin B cholesteryl sulfate complex	SEQ	0.83 mg/ml[a]	SCN	2 mg/ml[a]	Microprecipitate and increased turbidity form immediately	2117	I
Amsacrine	NCI	1 mg/ml[a]	PD	2 mg/ml[a]	Physically compatible for 4 hr at room temperature under fluorescent light	1381	C
Aztreonam	SQ	40 mg/ml[a]	PD	2 mg/ml[a]	Physically compatible with no subvisual haze or particle formation in 4 hr at 23 °C	1758	C
Cefepime HCl	BR	20 mg/ml[a]	WY	2 mg/ml[a]	Cloudy solution with precipitate forms immediately	1689	I
Ciprofloxacin	MI	2 mg/ml[c]	ES	50 mg/ml	Visually compatible for 24 hr at 24 °C	1655	C
Cisatracurium besylate	GW	0.1, 2, 5 mg/ ml[a]	SCN	2 mg/ml[a]	Physically compatible with no change in measured turbidity or increase in particle content in 4 hr at 23 °C	2074	C
Cisplatin	BR	1 mg/ml	PD	2 mg/ml[a]	Visually compatible for 4 hr at room temperature under fluorescent light	1685	C
Cladribine	ORT	0.015[b] and 0.5[d] mg/ml	SCN	2 mg/ml[b]	Physically compatible with no change in measured turbidity or increase in particle content in 4 hr at 23 °C	1969	C
Cyclophosphamide	MJ	10 mg/ml	PD	2 mg/ml[a]	Visually compatible for 4 hr at room temperature under fluorescent light	1685	C
Cytarabine	UP	50 mg/ml	PD	2 mg/ml[a]	Visually compatible for 4 hr at room temperature under fluorescent light	1685	C
Docetaxel	RPR	0.9 mg/ml[a]	ES	2 mg/ml[a]	Physically compatible with no change in measured turbidity or increase in particle content in 4 hr at 23 °C	2224	C
Doxorubicin HCl	AD	0.2 mg/ml[a]	PD	2 mg/ml[a]	Visually compatible for 4 hr at room temperature under fluorescent light	1685	C

Y-Site Injection Compatibility (1:1 Mixture) (Cont.)

Diphenhydramine HCl

Drug	Mfr	Conc	Mfr	Conc	Remarks	Ref	C/I
Doxorubicin HCl liposome injection	SEQ	0.4 mg/ml[a]	SCN	2 mg/ml[a]	Physically compatible with little or no change in measured turbidity and no increase in particle content in 4 hr at 23 °C	2087	**C**
Etoposide phosphate	BR	5 mg/ml[a]	ES	2 mg/ml[a]	Physically compatible with no change in measured turbidity or increase in particle content in 4 hr at 23 °C	2218	**C**
Famotidine	ME	2 mg/ml[b]		2 mg/ml[a]	Visually compatible for 4 hr at 22 °C	1936	**C**
Filgrastim	AMG	30 µg/ml[a]	ES	2 mg/ml[a]	Physically compatible with no change in measured turbidity or increase in particle content in 4 hr at 22 °C	1687	**C**
Fluconazole	RR	2 mg/ml	ES	50 mg/ml	Physically compatible for 24 hr at 25 °C	1407	**C**
Fludarabine phosphate	BX	1 mg/ml[a]	WY	2 mg/ml[a]	Physically compatible for 4 hr at room temperature under fluorescent light	1439	**C**
Foscarnet sodium	AST	24 mg/ml	PD	50 mg/ml	Cloudy solution	1335	**I**
Gemcitabine HCl	LI	10 mg/ml[b]	SCN	2 mg/ml[b]	Physically compatible with no change in measured turbidity or increase in particle content in 4 hr at 23 °C	2226	**C**
Granisetron HCl	SKB	1 mg/ml	PD	1 mg/ml[b]	Physically compatible with little or no loss of either drug by HPLC in 4 hr at 22 °C	1883	**C**
	SKB	0.05 mg/ml[a]	SCN	2 mg/ml[a]	Physically compatible with no change in measured turbidity or increase in particle content in 4 hr at 23 °C	2000	**C**
Heparin sodium	UP	1000 units/L[e]	PD	50 mg/ml	Physically compatible for at least 4 hr at room temperature by visual and microscopic examination	534	**C**
Hydrocortisone sodium succinate	UP	10 mg/L[e]	PD	50 mg/ml	Physically compatible for at least 4 hr at room temperature by visual and microscopic examination	534	**C**
	UP	1 mg/ml[a]	SCN	0.16 mg/ml[a]	Physically compatible with no subvisual haze or particle formation in 24 hr at 23 °C	1729	**C**
	UP	2 mg/ml[a]	SCN	1 mg/ml[a]	Physically compatible with no subvisual haze or particle formation in 24 hr at 23 °C	1729	**C**
Idarubicin HCl	AD	1 mg/ml[b]	ES	1[a] and 50 mg/ml	Visually compatible for 24 hr at 25 °C	1525	**C**
Melphalan HCl	BW	0.1 mg/ml[b]	WY	2 mg/ml[b]	Physically compatible with no change in measured turbidity or increase in particle content in 3 hr at 22 °C	1557	**C**
Meperidine HCl	AB	10 mg/ml	ES	1[a] and 50 mg/ml	Physically compatible for 4 hr at 25 °C	1397	**C**
Meropenem	ZEN	1 and 50 mg/ml[b]	PD	50 mg/ml	Visually compatible for 4 hr at room temperature	1994	**C**
Methotrexate sodium	AD	15 mg/ml[f]	PD	2 mg/ml[a]	Visually compatible for 4 hr at room temperature under fluorescent light	1685	**C**
Ondansetron HCl	GL	1 mg/ml[b]	PD	2 mg/ml[a]	Physically compatible for 4 hr at 22 °C	1365	**C**

Y-Site Injection Compatibility (1:1 Mixture) (Cont.)

Diphenhydramine HCl

Drug	Mfr	Conc	Mfr	Conc	Remarks	Ref	C/I
Paclitaxel	NCI	1.2 mg/ml[a]		2 mg/ml[a]	Physically compatible with no change in measured turbidity in 4 hr at 22 °C	1528	C
Piperacillin sodium–tazobactam sodium	LE	40 + 5 mg/ml[a]	WY	2 mg/ml[a]	Physically compatible with no change in measured turbidity or increase in particle content in 4 hr at 22 °C	1688	C
Potassium chloride	AB	40 mEq/L[e]	PD	50 mg/ml	Physically compatible for at least 4 hr at room temperature by visual and microscopic examination	534	C
Propofol	ZEN	10 mg/ml	SCN	2 mg/ml[a]	Physically compatible for 1 hr at 23 °C with no increase in particle content	2066	C
Remifentanil HCl	GW	0.025 and 0.25 mg/ml[b]	SCN	2 mg/ml[a]	Physically compatible with no change in measured turbidity or increase in particle content in 4 hr at 23 °C	2075	C
Sargramostim	IMM	10 μg/ml[b]	RU	1 mg/ml[b]	Physically compatible for 4 hr at 22 °C	1436	C
Sufentanil citrate	JN	12.5 μg/ml[a]	SCN	2 mg/ml[a]	Physically compatible with no subvisual haze or particle formation in 24 hr at 23 °C	1711	C
Tacrolimus	FUJ	1 mg/ml[b]	ES	1 mg/ml[a]	Visually compatible for 24 hr at 25 °C	1630	C
Teniposide	BR	0.1 mg/ml[a]	ES	2 mg/ml[a]	Physically compatible with no subvisual haze or particle formation in 4 hr at 23 °C	1725	C
Thiotepa	IMM[g]	1 mg/ml[a]	WY	2 mg/ml[a]	Physically compatible with no change in measured turbidity or increase in particle content in 4 hr at 23 °C	1861	C
TNA #218 to #226[h]			SCN, PD	2[a] and 50 mg/ml	Visually compatible with no precipitate or emulsion damage apparent in 4 hr at 23 °C	2215	C
TPN #212 to #215[h]			SCN	2 mg/ml[a]	Physically compatible with no change in measured turbidity or increase in particle content in 4 hr at 23 °C	2109	C
			SCN	50 mg/ml	Physically compatible with no change in measured turbidity or increase in particle content in 4 hr at 23 °C	2109	C
Vinorelbine tartrate	BW	1 mg/ml[b]	ES	2 mg/ml[b]	Physically compatible with no change in measured turbidity or increase in particle content in 4 hr at 22 °C	1558	C
Vitamin B complex with C	RC	2 ml/L[e]	PD	50 mg/ml	Physically compatible for at least 4 hr at room temperature by visual and microscopic examination	534	C

[a]*Tested in dextrose 5% in water.*
[b]*Tested in sodium chloride 0.9%.*
[c]*Tested in both dextrose 5% in water and sodium chloride 0.9%.*
[d]*Tested in bacteriostatic sodium chloride 0.9% preserved with benzyl alcohol 0.9%.*
[e]*Tested in dextrose 5% in Ringer's injection, dextrose 5% in Ringer's injection, lactated, dextrose 5% in water, Ringer's injection, lactated, and sodium chloride 0.9%.*
[f]*Tested in dextrose 5% in water with sodium bicarbonate 0.05 mEq/ml.*
[g]*Lyophilized formulation tested.*
[h]*Refer to Appendix I for the composition of parenteral nutrition solutions. TNA indicates a 3-in-1 admixture, and TPN indicates a 2-in-1 admixture.*

Additional Compatibility Information

Additives— Diphenhydramine HCl (Parke-Davis) has been found to be compatible with diatrizoate meglumine products (Squibb) for at least short periods (40). It is also stated to be physically and chemically compatible with buprenorphine HCl (4).

Diphenhydramine HCl has been found to be incompatible with iodipamide meglumine (Squibb) (40).

The following incompatibility determinations were performed with concentrated solutions: 1 ml of diphenhydramine HCl (Parke-Davis) was added to 5 ml of sterile distilled water along with 1 ml of either phenytoin sodium (Parke-Davis) or phenobarbital sodium (Winthrop). Particulate matter was noted within two hours (28).

DOBUTAMINE HCL
AHFS 12:12

Dobutrex   **Lilly**

Products— Dobutamine HCl (Lilly) is available in 20-ml single-dose vials as a concentrate for injection. Each milliliter contains 12.5 mg of dobutamine (as the hydrochloride), sodium bisulfite 0.24 mg, and hydrochloric acid and/or sodium hydroxide to adjust the pH. Dobutamine HCl concentrate for injection must be diluted further to a concentration not greater than 5 mg/ml before administration (2; 4).

To prepare a concentration of 250 μg/ml, dilute the contents of one vial (250 mg) with 1000 ml of a compatible infusion solution. Dilution of a vial with 500 ml will yield a 500-μg/ml solution, and dilution of a vial with 250 ml will result in a 1000-μg/ml solution (2; 4).

Dobutamine HCl is also available in plastic bags as premixed solutions in concentrations of 0.5, 1, 2, and 4 mg/ml in dextrose 5% in water. Sodium metabisulfite and edetate disodium dihydrate may also be present (2; 29).

pH— From 2.5 to 5.5 (4; 17). The premixed infusion solutions in dextrose 5% in water (Abbott) have a pH of around 3 with a range of 2.5 to 5.5 (1-7/94).

Osmolality— The osmolality of dobutamine HCl injection (Lilly) was determined to be 273 mOsm/kg by freezing-point depression and vapor pressure (1071). At a concentration of 5 mg/ml (manufacturer and diluent unstated), the osmolality was determined to be 361 mOsm/kg by freezing-point depression (1233).

The premixed infusion solutions in dextrose 5% in water (Abbott) have osmolalities ranging from 260 to 284 mOsm/kg for the four concentrations available (1-7/94).

Administration— Dobutamine HCl is administered by intravenous infusion after dilution to a concentration no greater than 5 mg/ml.

The concentration used is dependent on the patient's dosage and fluid requirements. An infusion pump or other infusion control device should be used to control the flow rate (2; 4).

Stability— Intact vials should be stored at controlled room temperature (2; 4). Solutions that are further diluted for intravenous infusion should be used within 24 hours (2; 4).

Dobutamine HCl concentrate for injection is a clear, colorless to pale straw-colored solution (4). Solutions of dobutamine HCl may have a pink discoloration. This discoloration, which will increase with time, results from a slight oxidation of the drug. However, there is no significant loss of drug potency within the recommended storage times for solutions of the drug (2; 4).

Syringes— Dobutamine HCl (Lilly) 250 mg/50 ml in dextrose 5% in water exhibited no change in appearance and no loss in potency by HPLC when stored in 60-ml plastic syringes (Becton-Dickinson) for 24 hours at 25 °C (1579).

Dobutamine HCl (Lilly) 5 mg/ml in dextrose 5% in water was packaged in 50-ml polypropylene syringes (Becton-Dickinson) and stored at 4 and 24 °C in the dark and exposed to room light for 48 hours. Dobutamine concentration losses determined by HPLC analysis were less than 10% throughout the study (1961).

Sorption— Delivering dobutamine HCl (Lilly) 5 mg/ml in dextrose 5% in water by syringe pump over 12 hours at 24 °C through PVC and polyethylene administration tubing did not result in substantial dobutamine losses determined by HPLC analysis (1961).

Filtration— Dobutamine HCl (Lilly) 0.5 mg/ml in dextrose 5% in water and sodium chloride 0.9% was filtered through a 0.22-μm cellulose ester membrane filter (Ivex-HP, Millipore) over six hours. No significant drug loss due to binding to the filter was noted (1034).

Compatibility Information

Solution Compatibility

Dobutamine HCl

Solution	Mfr	Mfr	Conc/L	Remarks	Ref	C/I
Dextrose 2.5% in half-strength Ringer's injection, lactated	MG[a]	LI	1 g	No decomposition in 48 hr at 25 °C. Slight pink color at 8 hr becoming slightly brown at 24 hr without affecting potency	789	C

Solution Compatibility (Cont.)

Dobutamine HCl

Solution	Mfr	Mfr	Conc/L	Remarks	Ref	C/I
Dextrose 5% in Ringer's injection, lactated	MG[a]	LI	1 g	No decomposition in 48 hr at 25 °C. Slight pink color at 24 hr becoming slightly brown at 48 hr without affecting potency	789	C
Dextrose 2.5% in sodium chloride 0.45%	MG[a]	LI	1 g	No decomposition in 48 hr at 25 °C. Slight pink color at 24 hr becoming slightly brown at 48 hr without affecting potency	789	C
Dextrose 5% in sodium chloride 0.45%	AB[b], CU[a]	LI	1 g	No decomposition in 48 hr at 25 °C. Slight pink color at 24 hr becoming slightly brown at 48 hr without affecting potency	749	C
Dextrose 5% in sodium chloride 0.9%	MG[b]	LI	1 g	No decomposition in 48 hr at 25 °C. Slight pink color at 24 hr becoming slightly brown at 48 hr without affecting potency	789	C
Dextrose 5% in water	CU[a], TR[b]	LI	1 g	No decomposition in 48 hr at 25 °C. Slight pink color at 24 hr becoming slightly brown in 48 hr without affecting potency	749	C
	TR[b]	LI	250 mg	Physically compatible with no loss in 48 hr at 24 °C. Transient light pink color. No decomposition after 7 days at 5 °C	811	C
	[a]		2 to 8 g	Pale pink discoloration with 4% or less dobutamine loss in 24 hr exposed to light	1412	C
	BA[b]	LI	5 g	5% loss by HPLC in 100 days at 5 °C protected from light	1610	C
	BA[b]	LI	1 g	5% loss by HPLC in 234.7 days at 5 °C protected from light	1610	C
	TR[b]	LI	0.25 and 1 g	Visually compatible with no dobutamine loss by HPLC in 48 hr at room temperature	1802	C
Ringer's injection, lactated	CU[a], TR[b]	LI	1 g	No decomposition in 48 hr at 25 °C. Slight pink color at 3 hr becoming slightly brown at 48 hr without affecting potency	749	C
Sodium bicarbonate 5%	MG[a]	LI	1 g	Cloudy brownish solution with precipitate in 3 hr at 25 °C. 18% dobutamine loss with dense precipitate in 24 hr	789	I
Sodium chloride 0.45%	MG[a]	LI	1 g	No decomposition in 48 hr at 25 °C. Slight pink color at 24 hr becoming slightly brown at 48 hr without affecting potency	789	C
Sodium chloride 0.9%	CU[a], TR[b]	LI	1 g	No decomposition in 48 hr at 25 °C. Slight pink color at 24 hr becoming slightly brown at 48 hr without affecting potency	749	C
		LI	200 mg	Physically compatible for 24 hr	552	C
	TR[b]	LI	250 mg	About 3% dobutamine loss in 48 hr at 24 °C. Initially colorless solution becomes pink with time. No decomposition after 7 days at 5 °C	811	C
	[a]		2 to 8 g	Pale pink discoloration with 3% or less dobutamine loss in 24 hr exposed to light	1412	C
	TR[a]	LI	0.25 and 1 g	Visually compatible with no dobutamine loss by HPLC in 48 hr at room temperature	1802	C

[a]*Tested in glass containers.*
[b]*Tested in PVC containers.*

Additive Compatibility

Dobutamine HCl

Drug	Mfr	Conc/L	Mfr	Conc/L	Test Soln	Remarks	Ref	C/I
Acyclovir sodium	BW	5 g	LI	1 g	D5W	Discoloration developed in 25 min and cloudiness and brown color developed in 2 hr due to dobutamine oxidation. No acyclovir loss found	1343	**I**
Alteplase	GEN	0.5 g	LI	5 g	D5W, NS	Yellow discoloration and precipitate form	1856	**I**
Aminophylline	SE	1 g	LI	1 g	D5W, NS	Cloudy in 6 hr at 25 °C	789	**I**
	ES	2.5 g	LI	1 g	D5W, NS	White precipitate forms within 12 hr at 21 °C	812	**I**
Amiodarone HCl	LZ	2.5 g	LI	1 g	D5W, NS	Physically compatible for 24 hr at 21 °C	812	**C**
Atracurium besylate	BW	500 mg		1 g	D5W	Physically compatible and atracurium chemically stable for 24 hr at 5 and 30 °C	1694	**C**
Atropine sulfate	AB	16.7 mg	LI	167 mg	NS	Physically compatible for 24 hr	552	**C**
	ES	50 mg	LI	1 g	D5W, NS	Physically compatible for 24 hr at 21 °C	812	**C**
Bretylium tosylate	ACC	2 g	LI	1 g	D5W, NS	Slightly pink in 24 hr at 25 °C	789	**I**
	ACC	4 and 25 g	LI	1 g	D5W, NS	Physically compatible for 24 hr at 21 °C	812	**C**
Bumetanide	RC	125 mg	LI	1 g	D5W, NS	Immediate yellow discoloration with yellow precipitate within 6 hr at 21 °C	812	**I**
Calcium chloride	UP	9 g	LI	182 mg	NS	Physically compatible for 20 hr. Haze formation at 24 hr	552	**I**
	ES	2 g	LI	1 g	D5W, NS	Deeply pink in 24 hr at 25 °C	789	**I**
	ES	50 g	LI	1 g	D5W, NS	Physically compatible for 24 hr at 21 °C	812	**C**
Calcium gluconate	VI	9 g	LI	182 mg	NS	Small particles form within 4 hr. White precipitate and haze after 15 hr	552	**I**
	ES	2 g	LI	1 g	D5W, NS	Deeply pink in 24 hr at 25 °C	789	**I**
	IX	50 g	LI	1 g	D5W, NS	Small white particles form within 24 hr at 21 °C	812	**I**
Cibenzoline succinate		2 g	LI	4 g	D5W, NS	Physically compatible for 24 hr at 25 °C by visual and microscopic examination	1182	**C**
Diazepam	RC	2.5 g	LI	1 g	D5W, NS	Rapid clouding of solution with yellow precipitate within 24 hr at 21 °C	812	**I**
Digoxin	BW	4 mg	LI	1 g	D5W, NS	Slightly pink in 24 hr at 25 °C	789	**I**
Dopamine HCl	AS	5.5 g	LI	172 mg	NS	Physically compatible for 24 hr	552	**C**
	ACC	1.6 g	LI	1 g	D5W, NS	Physically compatible with no color change in 24 hr at 25 °C	789	**C**
	ES	800 mg	LI	1 g	D5W, NS	Physically compatible for 24 hr at 21 °C	812	**C**
Enalaprilat	MSD	12 mg	LI	1 g	D5W[a]	Visually compatible with little or no enalaprilat loss by HPLC in 24 hr at room temperature under fluorescent light. Dobutamine not tested	1572	**C**
Epinephrine HCl	BR	50 mg	LI	1 g	D5W, NS	Physically compatible for 24 hr at 21 °C	812	**C**
Floxacillin sodium	BE	20 g	LI	500 mg	NS	Haze forms immediately and precipitate forms in 24 to 48 hr at 15 and 30 °C	1479	**I**
Flumazenil	RC	20 mg	LI	2 g	D5W[a]	Visually compatible with no flumazenil loss by HPLC in 24 hr at 23 °C under fluorescent light. Dobutamine not tested	1710	**C**

Additive Compatibility (Cont.)

Dobutamine HCl

Drug	Mfr	Conc/L	Mfr	Conc/L	Test Soln	Remarks	Ref	C/I
Furosemide	HO	1 g	LI	1 g	D5W, NS	Cloudy in 1 hr at 25 °C	789	I
	WY	5 g	LI	1 g	D5W, NS	Immediate white precipitate	812	I
	HO	1 g	LI	500 mg	NS	Haze forms immediately	1479	I
Heparin sodium	ES	40,000 units	LI	1 g	D5W, NS	Physically compatible with no color change in 24 hr at 25 °C	789	C
	LY	50,000 units	LI	1 g	D5W, NS	Physically compatible for 24 hr at 21 °C	812	C
	ES	5 million units	LI	1 g	D5W, NS	Pink discoloration within 6 hr at 21 °C	812	I
	ES	50,000 units	LI	1 g	D5W	Precipitate forms within 3 min when heparin is added to D5W and then mixed with an equal volume of dobutamine in D5W	841	I
	LY	50,000 units	LI	1.5 g	D5W, NS	Obvious precipitation	1318	I
	LY	50,000 units	LI	900 mg	D5W, W	Physically compatible for 4 hr, but heat of reaction detected by microcalorimetry	1318	I
	LY	50,000 units	LI	900 mg	NS	Physically compatible for 4 hr with no heat of reaction detected by microcalorimetry	1318	C
Hydralazine HCl	CI	200 mg	LI	200 mg	NS	Physically compatible for 24 hr	552	C
Insulin, regular	LI	1,000 units	LI	1 g	D5W, NS	Slightly pink in 24 hr at 25 °C	789	I
	LI	50,000 units	LI	1 g	D5W, NS	White precipitate forms rapidly	812	I
Isoproterenol HCl	ES	2 mg	LI	1 g	D5W, NS	Physically compatible for 24 hr at 21 °C	812	C
Lidocaine HCl	ES	4 g	LI	1 g	D5W, NS	Physically compatible with no color change in 24 hr at 25 °C	789	C
	AST	4 and 10 g	LI	1 g	D5W, NS	Physically compatible for 24 hr at 21 °C	812	C
Magnesium sulfate	TO	2 g	LI	1 g	D5W, NS	Slightly pink in 24 hr at 25 °C	789	I
	ES	83 g[b]	LI	167 mg	NS	Physically compatible for 20 hr. Haze formation at 24 hr	552	I
Meperidine HCl	ES	50 g	LI	1 g	D5W, NS	Physically compatible for 24 hr at 21 °C	812	C
Meropenem	ZEN	1 and 20 g	LI	1 g	NS	Visually compatible for 4 hr at room temperature	1994	C
Metaraminol bitartrate	MSD	100 mg	LI	1 g	D5W, NS	Physically compatible for 24 hr at 21 °C	812	C
Morphine sulfate	ES	5 g	LI	1 g	D5W, NS	Physically compatible for 24 hr at 21 °C	812	C
Nitroglycerin	AB	120 mg	LI	1 g	D5W, NS	Physically compatible for 24 hr at 21 °C	812	C
	ACC	100 mg	LI	500 mg	D5S	Chemically stable with no loss of either drug after 24 hr at 25 °C. Pale pink color after 4 hr	990	C
Nitroglycerin with sodium nitroprusside		200 to 800 mg 200 to 800 mg		2 to 8 g	D5W[c]	Pale pink discoloration with small amount of dark brown precipitate and 11 to 19% sodium nitroprusside loss in 24 hr exposed to light	1412	I

Additive Compatibility (Cont.)

Dobutamine HCl

Drug	Mfr	Conc/L	Mfr	Conc/L	Test Soln	Remarks	Ref	C/I
Nitroglycerin with sodium nitroprusside		200 to 800 mg 200 to 800 mg		2 to 8 g	NS[c]	Pale pink discoloration with all drugs stable for 24 hr exposed to light. 8% or less loss for any drug in any combination	1412	C
Norepinephrine bitartrate	BN	32 mg	LI	1 g	D5W, NS	Physically compatible for 24 hr at 21 °C	812	C
Phentolamine mesylate	CI	20 mg	LI	1 g	D5W, NS	Physically compatible for 24 hr at 21 °C	812	C
Phenylephrine HCl	WI	20 mg	LI	1 g	D5W, NS	Physically compatible for 24 hr at 21 °C	812	C
Phenytoin sodium	AHP	25 g	LI	1 g	D5W, NS	White precipitate forms rapidly with brown solution within 6 hr at 21 °C	812	I
	ES	1 g	LI	1 g	D5W, NS	White precipitate forms in 5 to 10 min	789	I
Potassium chloride	ES	160 mEq	LI	1 g	D5W, NS	Slightly pink in 24 hr at 25 °C	789	I
	AB	20 mEq	LI	1 g	D5W, NS	Physically compatible for 24 hr at 21 °C	812	C
Potassium phosphates	AB	100 mM	LI	200 mg	NS	Small particles form after 1 hr. White precipitate noted after 15 hr	552	I
Procainamide HCl	SQ	1 g	LI	1 g	D5W, NS	Physically compatible with no color change in 24 hr at 25 °C	789	C
	AHP	4 and 50 g	LI	1 g	D5W, NS	Physically compatible for 24 hr at 21 °C	812	C
Propranolol HCl	AY	50 mg	LI	1 g	D5W, NS	Physically compatible for 24 hr at 21 °C	812	C
Ranitidine HCl	GL	2 g	LI	250 mg and 1 g	D5W, NS[a]	Physically compatible with no ranitidine loss in 48 hr at room temperature under fluorescent light. Dobutamine not tested	1361	C
	GL	50 mg	LI	250 mg and 1 g	D5W[a]	Physically compatible with 5 to 7% ranitidine loss in 48 hr at room temperature under fluorescent light. Dobutamine not tested	1361	C
	GL	50 mg	LI	250 mg and 1 g	NS[a]	Physically compatible with no ranitidine loss in 48 hr at room temperature under fluorescent light. Dobutamine not tested	1361	C
	GL	50 mg and 2 g	LI	0.25 and 1 g	D5W, NS[a]	Visually compatible with little or no loss of either drug by HPLC in 48 hr at room temperature	1802	C
Sodium bicarbonate	IX	500 mEq	LI	1 g	D5W, NS	White precipitate forms within 6 hr at 21 °C	812	I
Verapamil HCl	KN	1.25 g	LI	1 g	D5W, NS	Physically compatible for 24 hr at 21 °C	812	C
	KN	160 mg	LI	250 mg	D5W	No decomposition of either drug in 48 hr at 24 °C or 7 days at 5 °C. Transient light pink color	811	C
	KN	160 mg	LI	250 mg	NS	No verapamil decomposition and 3% dobutamine loss in 48 hr at 24 °C. Initially colorless solution becomes pink with time. At 5 °C, no loss of either drug for 7 days	811	C
	KN	80 mg	LI	500 mg	D5W, NS	Slight pink color after 24 hr due to dobutamine oxidation	764	I

[a]*Tested in PVC containers.*
[b]*Tested as 1 g/12 ml final concentration.*
[c]*Tested in glass containers.*

Drugs in Syringe Compatibility

Dobutamine HCl

Drug (in syringe)	Mfr	Amt	Mfr	Amt	Remarks	Ref	C/I
Doxapram HCl	RB	400 mg/ 20 ml	LI	100 mg/ 10 ml	5% doxapram loss in 3 hr and 11% in 24 hr	1177	I
Heparin sodium		2500 units/ 1 ml	LI	250 mg/ 10 ml	Physically compatible for at least 5 min	1053	C
Ranitidine HCl	GL	50 mg/ 5 ml	LI	25 mg	Physically compatible for 4 hr at ambient temperature under fluorescent light	1151	C

Y-Site Injection Compatibility (1:1 Mixture)

Dobutamine HCl

Drug	Mfr	Conc	Mfr	Conc	Remarks	Ref	C/I
Acyclovir sodium	BW	5 mg/ml[a]	LI	1 mg/ml[a]	Solution turns cloudy and brown in 1 hr at 25 °C under fluorescent light	1157	I
Alteplase	GEN	1 mg/ml	LI	2 mg/ml[a]	Haze noted in 20 min by spectrophotometric examination and in 2 hr by visual examination	1340	I
Amifostine	USB	10 mg/ml[a]	LI	4 mg/ml[a]	Physically compatible with no change in measured turbidity or increase in particle content in 4 hr at 23 °C	1845	C
Aminophylline	ES	4 mg/ml[c]	LI	4 mg/ml[c]	Slight haze or precipitate and color change in 1 hr	1316	I
Amiodarone HCl	LZ	4 mg/ml[c]	LI	2 mg/ml[c]	Physically compatible for 24 hr at 21 °C	1032	C
Amphotericin B cholesteryl sulfate complex	SEQ	0.83 mg/ml[a]	AST	4 mg/ml[a]	Gross precipitate forms	2117	I
Amrinone lactate	WB	3 mg/ml[b]	LI	4 mg/ml[a]	Physically compatible for at least 4 hr at 25 °C under fluorescent light	992	C
Atracurium besylate	BW	0.5 mg/ml[a]	LI	1 mg/ml[a]	Physically compatible for 24 hr at 28 °C	1337	C
Aztreonam	SQ	40 mg/ml[a]	LI	4 mg/ml[a]	Physically compatible with no subvisual haze or particle formation in 4 hr at 23 °C	1758	C
Bretylium tosylate	LY	4 mg/ml[c]	LI	4 mg/ml[c]	Physically compatible for 3 hr	1316	C
Calcium chloride	AB	4 mg/ml[c]	LI	4 mg/ml[c]	Physically compatible for 3 hr	1316	C
Calcium gluconate	AST	4 mg/ml[c]	LI	4 mg/ml[c]	Physically compatible for 3 hr	1316	C
Cefepime HCl	BR	20 mg/ml[a]	LI	4 mg/ml[a]	Cloudy solution forms immediately. Precipitate forms in 4 hr	1689	I
Ciprofloxacin	MI	2 mg/ml[c]	LI	250 μg/ml[c]	Visually compatible for 24 hr at 24 °C	1655	C
Cisatracurium besylate	GW	0.1, 2, 5 mg/ml[a]	LI	4 mg/ml[a]	Physically compatible with no change in measured turbidity or increase in particle content in 4 hr at 23 °C	2074	C
Cladribine	ORT	0.015[b] and 0.5[e] mg/ml	LI	4 mg/ml[b]	Physically compatible with no change in measured turbidity or increase in particle content in 4 hr at 23 °C	1969	C
Clarithromycin	AB	4 mg/ml[a]	BI	2 mg/ml[a]	Visually compatible for 72 hr at both 30 and 17 °C	2174	C
Diazepam	ES	0.2 mg/ml[c]	LI	4 mg/ml[c]	Physically compatible for 3 hr	1316	C

Y-Site Injection Compatibility (1:1 Mixture) (Cont.)

Dobutamine HCl

Drug	Mfr	Conc	Mfr	Conc	Remarks	Ref	C/I
Diltiazem HCl	MMD	1 mg/ml[a]	LI	2 mg/ml[a]	Visually compatible for 24 hr at 25 °C	1807	C
	MMD	5 mg/ml	LI	1 mg/ml[c]	Visually compatible	1807	C
	MMD	1 mg/ml[a]	LI	4 mg/ml[a]	Visually compatible for 4 hr at 27 °C	2062	C
Docetaxel	RPR	0.9 mg/ml[a]	AST	4 mg/ml[a]	Physically compatible with no change in measured turbidity or increase in particle content in 4 hr at 23 °C	2224	C
Dopamine HCl	DCC	3.2 mg/ml[c]	LI	4 mg/ml[c]	Physically compatible for 3 hr	1316	C
	AB	3.2 mg/ml[a]	LI	4 mg/ml[a]	Visually compatible for 4 hr at 27 °C	2062	C
Dopamine HCl with lidocaine HCl	DCC AB	3.2 mg/ml[c] 8 mg/ml[c]	LI	4 mg/ml[c]	Physically compatible for 3 hr	1316	C
Dopamine HCl with nitroglycerin	DCC LY	3.2 mg/ml[c] 0.4 mg/ml[c]	LI	4 mg/ml[c]	Physically compatible for 3 hr	1316	C
Dopamine HCl with sodium nitroprusside	DCC ES	3.2 mg/ml[c] 0.4 mg/ml[c]	LI	4 mg/ml[c]	Physically compatible for 3 hr	1316	C
Doxorubicin HCl liposome injection	SEQ	0.4 mg/ml[a]	BA	4 mg/ml[a]	Physically compatible with little or no change in measured turbidity and no increase in particle content in 4 hr at 23 °C	2087	C
Enalaprilat	MSD	0.05 mg/ml[b]	LI	1 mg/ml[c]	Physically compatible for 24 hr at room temperature under fluorescent light	1355	C
Epinephrine HCl	AB	0.02 mg/ml[a]	LI	4 mg/ml[a]	Visually compatible for 4 hr at 27 °C	2062	C
Etoposide phosphate	BR	5 mg/ml[a]	AST	4 mg/ml[a]	Physically compatible with no change in measured turbidity or increase in particle content in 4 hr at 23 °C	2218	C
Famotidine	MSD	0.2 mg/ml[a]	LI	1 mg/ml[a]	Physically compatible for 4 hr at 25 °C	1188	C
	ME	2 mg/ml[b]		4 mg/ml[a]	Visually compatible for 4 hr at 22 °C	1936	C
Fentanyl citrate	ES	0.05 mg/ml	LI	4 mg/ml[a]	Visually compatible for 4 hr at 27 °C	2062	C
Fluconazole	RR	2 mg/ml	LI	2 mg/ml[a]	Visually compatible for 24 hr at 28 °C	1760	C
Foscarnet sodium	AST	24 mg/ml	LI	12.5 mg/ml	Delayed formation of muddy precipitate	1335	I
Furosemide	ES	1 mg/ml[b]	LI	4 mg/ml[b]	Physically compatible for 3 hr	1316	C
	ES	1 mg/ml[a]	LI	4 mg/ml[a]	Slight precipitate in 1 hr	1316	I
	AMR	10 mg/ml	LI	4 mg/ml[a]	Precipitate forms immediately	2062	I
Gemcitabine HCl	LI	10 mg/ml[b]	AST	4 mg/ml[b]	Physically compatible with no change in measured turbidity or increase in particle content in 4 hr at 23 °C	2226	C
Granisetron HCl	SKB	0.05 mg/ml[a]	BA	4 mg/ml[a]	Physically compatible with no change in measured turbidity or increase in particle content in 4 hr	2000	C
Haloperidol lactate	MN	0.5[a] and 5 mg/ml	DU	4 mg/ml[a]	Visually compatible for 24 hr at 21 °C	1523	C
Heparin sodium	ES	50 units/ml[b]	LI	4 mg/ml[b]	Physically compatible for 3 hr	1316	C
	ES	50 units/ml[a]	LI	4 mg/ml[a]	Immediate gross precipitation	1316	I
	OR	100 units/ml[a]	LI	4 mg/ml[a]	Haze and white precipitate form	1877	I
	ES	100 units/ml[a]	LI	4 mg/ml[a]	Precipitate forms in 4 hr at 27 °C	2062	I
Hydromorphone HCl	KN	1 mg/ml	LI	4 mg/ml[a]	Visually compatible for 4 hr at 27 °C	2062	C
Indomethacin sodium trihydrate	MSD	1 mg/ml[b]	AB	1.2 mg/ml[a]	Haze and fine precipitate form immediately	1527	I

Y-Site Injection Compatibility (1:1 Mixture) (Cont.)

Dobutamine HCl

Drug	Mfr	Conc	Mfr	Conc	Remarks	Ref	C/I
Insulin, regular (beef, pork) (Humulin R)	LI LI	1 unit/ml[c] 1 unit/ml[c]	LI LI	4 mg/ml[c] 4 mg/ml[c]	Physically compatible for 3 hr Physically compatible for 3 hr	1316 1316	C C
Labetalol HCl	GL	1 mg/ml[a]	LI	2.5 mg/ml[a]	Visually compatible with little or no loss of either drug by HPLC in 4 hr at room temperature	1762	C
	GL	5 mg/ml	LI	4 mg/ml[a]	Visually compatible for 24 hr at 23 °C	1877	C
	AH	2 mg/ml[a]	LI	4 mg/ml[a]	Visually compatible for 4 hr at 27 °C	2062	C
Lidocaine HCl	AB	8 mg/ml[c]	LI	4 mg/ml[c]	Physically compatible for 3 hr	1316	C
Lidocaine HCl with dopamine HCl	AB DCC	8 mg/ml[c] 3.2 mg/ml[c]	LI	4 mg/ml[c]	Physically compatible for 3 hr	1316	C
Lidocaine HCl with nitroglycerin	AB LY	8 mg/ml[c] 0.4 mg/ml[c]	LI	4 mg/ml[c]	Physically compatible for 3 hr	1316	C
Lidocaine HCl with sodium nitroprusside	AB ES	8 mg/ml[c] 0.4 mg/ml[c]	LI	4 mg/ml[c]	Physically compatible for 3 hr	1316	C
Lorazepam	WY	0.5 mg/ml[a]	LI	4 mg/ml[a]	Visually compatible for 4 hr at 27 °C	2062	C
Magnesium sulfate	LY	40 mg/ml[c]	LI	4 mg/ml[c]	Physically compatible for 3 hr	1316	C
Meperidine HCl	AB	10 mg/ml	LI	1 mg/ml[a]	Physically compatible for 4 hr at 25 °C	1397	C
Midazolam HCl	RC RC RC	1 mg/ml[a] 1 mg/ml[a] 2 mg/ml[a]	GNS LI LI	2 mg/ml[a] 4 mg/ml[a] 4 mg/ml[a]	Particles form in 8 hr Visually compatible for 24 hr at 23 °C Visually compatible for 4 hr at 27 °C	1847 1877 2062	I C C
Milrinone lactate	SW SW	0.2 mg/ml[a] 0.4 mg/ml[a]	LI GEN	4 mg/ml[a] 8 mg/ml[a]	Visually compatible for 4 hr at 27 °C Visually compatible with little or no loss of either drug by HPLC in 4 hr at 23 °C	2062 2214	C C
Morphine sulfate	SCN	2 mg/ml[a]	LI	4 mg/ml[a]	Visually compatible for 4 hr at 27 °C	2062	C
Nicardipine HCl	WY	1 mg/ml[a]	LI	4 mg/ml[a]	Visually compatible for 4 hr at 27 °C	2062	C
Nitroglycerin	LY AB	0.4 mg/ml[c] 0.4 mg/ml[a]	LI LI	4 mg/ml[c] 4 mg/ml[a]	Physically compatible for 3 hr Visually compatible for 4 hr at 27 °C	1316 2062	C C
Nitroglycerin with dopamine HCl	LY DCC	0.4 mg/ml[c] 3.2 mg/ml[c]	LI	4 mg/ml[c]	Physically compatible for 3 hr	1316	C
Nitroglycerin with lidocaine HCl	LY AB	0.4 mg/ml[c] 8 mg/ml[c]	LI	4 mg/ml[c]	Physically compatible for 3 hr	1316	C
Nitroglycerin with sodium nitroprusside	LY ES	0.4 mg/ml[c] 0.4 mg/ml[c]	LI	4 mg/ml[c]	Physically compatible for 3 hr	1316	C
Norepinephrine bitartrate	AB	0.128 mg/ml[a]	LI	4 mg/ml[a]	Visually compatible for 4 hr at 27 °C	2062	C
Pancuronium bromide	ES	0.05 mg/ml[a]	LI	1 mg/ml[a]	Physically compatible for 24 hr at 28 °C	1337	C
Phytonadione	MSD	0.4 mg/ml[c]	LI	4 mg/ml[c]	Slight haze in 3 hr	1316	I
Piperacillin sodium–tazobactam sodium	LE	40 + 5 mg/ml[a]	LI	4 mg/ml[a]	Heavy white turbidity forms immediately	1688	I
Potassium chloride	AB	0.06 mEq/ml[c]	LI	4 mg/ml[c]	Physically compatible for 3 hr	1316	C
Propofol	ZEN	10 mg/ml	LI	4 mg/ml[a]	Physically compatible for 1 hr at 23 °C with no increase in particle content	2066	C
Ranitidine HCl	GL GL	0.5 mg/ml[f] 1 mg/ml[a]	LI LI	1 mg/ml[a] 4 mg/ml[a]	Physically compatible for 24 hr Visually compatible for 4 hr at 27 °C	1323 2062	C C

Y-Site Injection Compatibility (1:1 Mixture) (Cont.)

Dobutamine HCl

Drug	Mfr	Conc	Mfr	Conc	Remarks	Ref	C/I
Remifentanil HCl	GW	0.025 and 0.25 mg/ml[b]	LI	4 mg/ml[a]	Physically compatible with no change in measured turbidity or increase in particle content in 4 hr at 23 °C	2075	C
Sodium nitroprusside	ES	0.4 mg/ml[c]	LI	4 mg/ml[c]	Physically compatible for 3 hr	1316	C
Sodium nitroprusside with dopamine HCl	ES DCC	0.4 mg/ml[c] 3.2 mg/ml[c]	LI	4 mg/ml[c]	Physically compatible for 3 hr	1316	C
Sodium nitroprusside with lidocaine HCl	ES AB	0.4 mg/ml[c] 8 mg/ml[c]	LI	4 mg/ml[c]	Physically compatible for 3 hr	1316	C
Sodium nitroprusside with nitroglycerin	ES LY	0.4 mg/ml[c] 0.4 mg/ml[c]	LI	4 mg/ml[c]	Physically compatible for 3 hr	1316	C
Streptokinase	HO	30,000 units/ml[a]	LI	2 mg/ml[a]	Physically compatible for at least 48 hr by spectrophotometric and visual examination	1340	C
Tacrolimus	FUJ	1 mg/ml[b]	LI	1 mg/ml[a]	Visually compatible for 24 hr at 25 °C	1630	C
Theophylline	TR	4 mg/ml	LI	1 mg/ml[a]	Visually compatible for 6 hr at 25 °C	1793	C
Thiopental sodium	AB	25 mg/ml[d]	LI	4 mg/ml[a]	Precipitate forms immediately	2062	I
Thiotepa	IMM[g]	1 mg/ml[a]	LI	4 mg/ml[a]	Physically compatible with no change in measured turbidity or increase in particle content in 4 hr at 23 °C	1861	C
TNA #91[h]		[i]	LI	1 mg/ml[j]	Physically compatible	1170	C
TNA #218 to #226[h]			AST	4 mg/ml[a]	Visually compatible with no precipitate or emulsion damage apparent in 4 hr at 23 °C	2215	C
Tolazoline HCl		0.1 mg/ml[a]	LI	1.2 mg/ml[a]	Physically compatible for 24 hr at 22 °C	1363	C
TPN #189[h]			LI	50 mg/ml[b]	Visually compatible for 24 hr at 22 °C	1767	C
TPN #203 and #204[h]			LI	5 mg/ml	Visually compatible for 4 hr at 23 °C	1974	C
TPN #212 to #215[h]			LI	4 mg/ml[a]	Physically compatible with no change in measured turbidity or increase in particle content in 4 hr at 23 °C	2109	C
Vecuronium bromide	OR OR	0.1 mg/ml[a] 1 mg/ml	LI LI	1 mg/ml[a] 4 mg/ml[a]	Physically compatible for 24 hr at 28 °C Visually compatible for 4 hr at 27 °C	1337 2062	C C
Verapamil HCl	LY	0.2 mg/ml[c]	LI	4 mg/ml[c]	Physically compatible for 3 hr	1316	C
Warfarin sodium	DU DME	2 mg/ml[d] 2 mg/ml[d]	LI LI	1 mg/ml[a] 1 mg/ml[a]	Haze and precipitate form immediately Haze and precipitate form immediately	2010 2078	I I
Zidovudine	BW	4 mg/ml[a]	LI	5 mg/ml[a]	Physically compatible for 4 hr at 25 °C under fluorescent light by visual and microscopic examination	1193	C

[a]*Tested in dextrose 5% in water.*
[b]*Tested in sodium chloride 0.9%.*
[c]*Tested in both dextrose 5% in water and sodium chloride 0.9%.*
[d]*Tested in sterile water for injection.*
[e]*Tested in bacteriostatic sodium chloride 0.9% preserved with benzyl alcohol 0.9%.*
[f]*Premixed infusion solution.*
[g]*Lyophilized formulation tested.*
[h]*Refer to Appendix I for the composition of parenteral nutrition solutions. TNA indicates a 3-in-1 admixture, and TPN indicates a 2-in-1 admixture.*
[i]*Run at 10 ml/hr.*
[j]*In dextrose 5% in water infused at 1.2 ml/hr.*

Additional Compatibility Information

Infusion Solutions— The manufacturer recommends that admixtures in the following infusion solutions be used within 24 hours (2):

    Dextrose 5% in Ringer's injection, lactated
    Dextrose 5% in sodium chloride 0.45 and 0.9%
    Dextrose 5% in water
    Dextrose 10% in water
    Isolyte M with dextrose 5%
    Mannitol 20%
    Normosol M in dextrose 5%
    Ringer's injection, lactated
    Sodium chloride 0.9%
    Sodium lactate ⅙ M

Dobutamine HCl has been stated to be incompatible with alkaline solutions and should not be mixed with sodium bicarbonate 5%, other alkaline solutions, or other drugs or diluent containing both bisulfite and ethanol (2; 4).

Peritoneal Dialysis Solutions— Dobutamine HCl (Lilly) 2.5, 5, and 7.5 μg/ml in Dianeal PD-1 (Baxter) with dextrose 1.5 and 4.25% retained at least 90% of its potency when stored for 24 hours at 4, 26, and 37 °C (1417; 1702).

Dopamine, Lidocaine, Nitroglycerin, and Nitroprusside— Dobutamine HCl (Lilly) 4 mg/ml, dopamine HCl (Dupont Critical Care) 3.2 mg/ml, lidocaine HCl (Abbott) 8 mg/ml, nitroglycerin (Lyphomed) 0.4 mg/ml, and sodium nitroprusside (Elkins-Sinn) 0.4 mg/ml, prepared in dextrose 5% in water and sodium chloride 0.9%, were combined in equal quantities in all possible combinations of two, three, four, and five drugs and then evaluated for physical compatibility. No physical incompatibility was observed in any combination within the three-hour study period (1316).

DOCETAXEL
AHFS 10:00

Taxotere   **Aventis**

Products— Docetaxel (Aventis) is available as a concentrate in polysorbate 80 in single-use vials containing 20 mg (0.5 ml) and 80 mg (2 ml). Each size vial is packaged with a vial of special diluent composed of ethanol 13% in water for injection. Both the docetaxel vials and the accompanying diluent contain an overfill. Table 1 cites the vial sizes and actual fill amounts for docetaxel products and diluents (2).

The preparation of the product is a two-step procedure. The first step is the preparation of the premix solution. The premix solution is then further diluted prior to administration (step 2).

To prepare the premix, allow the proper number of vials of docetaxel concentrate to stand at room temperature for about five minutes after taking them from the refrigerator. Then withdraw the entire contents of each of the accompanying vials of special diluent and add to each vial of docetaxel concentrate. Gently rotate each vial of premix solution for about 15 seconds to ensure thorough mixing. This final premix solution is a clear solution having a docetaxel concentration of 10 mg/ml. If foam appears from the surfactant in the formulation, allow the vials to stand until most of the foam has dissipated; it is not necessary for all of the foam to have dissipated before proceeding with the rest of the preparation steps (2).

Withdraw the necessary amount of the docetaxel 10-mg/ml premix solution using a syringe and add it into a 250-ml glass or polyolefin (polyethylene or polypropylene) container of dextrose 5% in water or sodium chloride 0.9% to produce a final concentration between 0.3 and 0.9 mg/ml. It is necessary to use a larger volume of infusion solution if the docetaxel dose exceeds 240 mg so that the concentration does not exceed 0.9 mg/ml. The infusion admixture should be mixed thoroughly by rotation (2).

The use of gloves during preparation of docetaxel doses is recommended. If the docetaxel concentrate, premix solution, or admixture comes in contact with skin, the affected area should be washed thoroughly with soap and water. Contact with mucosa requires thorough flushing with water (2).

Administration— Docetaxel is administered as a one-hour intravenous infusion at ambient temperature and light to patients adequately premedicated to control adverse effects (2).

Stability— Intact containers of docetaxel with the accompanying special diluent should be stored under refrigeration at 2 to 8 °C. Freezing of the concentrate does not adversely affect docetaxel. The vials should be left in the original packages to protect the drug from bright light (2).

It is recommended that the premix solution and the fully diluted admixture in dextrose 5% in water or sodium chloride 0.9% be used as soon as possible after preparation. However, the premix solution is stable for at least eight hours after preparation under refrigeration or at room temperatures up to 25 °C (2).

Filtration— The use of inline filters for docetaxel administration is not recommended (4).

Table 1. Docetaxel Sizes and Diluent Volumes (2)

Vial Size	Actual Vial Fill	Actual Diluent Fill
20 mg/0.5 ml	23.6 mg/0.59 ml	1.83 ml
80 mg/2 ml	94.4 mg/2.36 ml	7.33 ml

Compatibility Information

Y-Site Injection Compatibility (1:1 Mixture)

			Docetaxel				
Drug	*Mfr*	*Conc*	*Mfr*	*Conc*	*Remarks*	*Ref*	***C/I***
Acyclovir sodium	GW	7 mg/ml[a]	RPR	0.9 mg/ml[a]	Physically compatible with no change in measured turbidity or increase in particle content in 4 hr at 23 °C	2224	**C**
Amifostine	ALZ	10 mg/ml[b]	RPR	0.9 mg/ml[a]	Physically compatible with no change in measured turbidity or increase in particle content in 4 hr at 23 °C	2224	**C**
Amikacin sulfate	AB	5 mg/ml[a]	RPR	0.9 mg/ml[a]	Physically compatible with no change in measured turbidity or increase in particle content in 4 hr at 23 °C	2224	**C**
Aminophylline	AB	2.5 mg/ml[a]	RPR	0.9 mg/ml[a]	Physically compatible with no change in measured turbidity or increase in particle content in 4 hr at 23 °C	2224	**C**
Amphotericin B	PH	0.6 mg/ml[a]	RPR	0.9 mg/ml[a]	Visible turbidity forms immediately	2224	**I**
Ampicillin sodium	SKB	20 mg/ml[b]	RPR	0.9 mg/ml[a]	Physically compatible with no change in measured turbidity or increase in particle content in 4 hr at 23 °C	2224	**C**
Ampicillin sodium–sulbactam sodium	RR	20 + 10 mg/ml[b]	RPR	0.9 mg/ml[a]	Physically compatible with no change in measured turbidity or increase in particle content in 4 hr at 23 °C	2224	**C**
Aztreonam	BMS	40 mg/ml[a]	RPR	0.9 mg/ml[a]	Physically compatible with no change in measured turbidity or increase in particle content in 4 hr at 23 °C	2224	**C**
Bumetanide	RC	0.04 mg/ml[a]	RPR	0.9 mg/ml[a]	Physically compatible with no change in measured turbidity or increase in particle content in 4 hr at 23 °C	2224	**C**
Buprenorphine HCl	RKC	0.04 mg/ml[a]	RPR	0.9 mg/ml[a]	Physically compatible with no change in measured turbidity or increase in particle content in 4 hr at 23 °C	2224	**C**
Butorphanol tartrate	APC	0.04 mg/ml[a]	RPR	0.9 mg/ml[a]	Physically compatible with no change in measured turbidity or increase in particle content in 4 hr at 23 °C	2224	**C**
Calcium gluconate	FUJ	40 mg/ml[a]	RPR	0.9 mg/ml[a]	Physically compatible with no change in measured turbidity or increase in particle content in 4 hr at 23 °C	2224	**C**
Cefazolin sodium	APC	20 mg/ml[a]	RPR	0.9 mg/ml[a]	Physically compatible with no change in measured turbidity or increase in particle content in 4 hr at 23 °C	2224	**C**
Cefepime HCl	BMS	20 mg/ml[a]	RPR	0.9 mg/ml[a]	Physically compatible with no change in measured turbidity or increase in particle content in 4 hr at 23 °C	2224	**C**
Cefoperazone sodium	PF	40 mg/ml[a]	RPR	0.9 mg/ml[a]	Physically compatible with no change in measured turbidity or increase in particle content in 4 hr at 23 °C	2224	**C**
Cefotaxime sodium	HO	20 mg/ml[a]	RPR	0.9 mg/ml[a]	Physically compatible with no change in measured turbidity or increase in particle content in 4 hr at 23 °C	2224	**C**

Y-Site Injection Compatibility (1:1 Mixture) (Cont.)

			Docetaxel				
Drug	*Mfr*	*Conc*	*Mfr*	*Conc*	*Remarks*	*Ref*	*C/I*
Cefotetan sodium	ZEN	20 mg/ml[a]	RPR	0.9 mg/ml[a]	Physically compatible with no change in measured turbidity or increase in particle content in 4 hr at 23 °C	2224	**C**
Cefoxitin sodium	ME	20 mg/ml[a]	RPR	0.9 mg/ml[a]	Physically compatible with no change in measured turbidity or increase in particle content in 4 hr at 23 °C	2224	**C**
Ceftazidime	SKB[c]	40 mg/ml[a]	RPR	0.9 mg/ml[a]	Physically compatible with no change in measured turbidity or increase in particle content in 4 hr at 23 °C	2224	**C**
Ceftizoxime sodium	FUJ	20 mg/ml[a]	RPR	0.9 mg/ml[a]	Physically compatible with no change in measured turbidity or increase in particle content in 4 hr at 23 °C	2224	**C**
Ceftriaxone sodium	RC	20 mg/ml[a]	RPR	0.9 mg/ml[a]	Physically compatible with no change in measured turbidity or increase in particle content in 4 hr at 23 °C	2224	**C**
Cefuroxime sodium	LI	30 mg/ml[a]	RPR	0.9 mg/ml[a]	Physically compatible with no change in measured turbidity or increase in particle content in 4 hr at 23 °C	2224	**C**
Chlorpromazine HCl	SCN	2 mg/ml[a]	RPR	0.9 mg/ml[a]	Physically compatible with no change in measured turbidity or increase in particle content in 4 hr at 23 °C	2224	**C**
Cimetidine HCl	AMR	12 mg/ml[a]	RPR	0.9 mg/ml[a]	Physically compatible with no change in measured turbidity or increase in particle content in 4 hr at 23 °C	2224	**C**
Ciprofloxacin	BAY	1 mg/ml[a]	RPR	0.9 mg/ml[a]	Physically compatible with no change in measured turbidity or increase in particle content in 4 hr at 23 °C	2224	**C**
Clindamycin phosphate	AST	10 mg/ml[a]	RPR	0.9 mg/ml[a]	Physically compatible with no change in measured turbidity or increase in particle content in 4 hr at 23 °C	2224	**C**
Dexamethasone sodium phosphate	ES	2 mg/ml[a]	RPR	0.9 mg/ml[a]	Physically compatible with no change in measured turbidity or increase in particle content in 4 hr at 23 °C	2224	**C**
Diphenhydramine HCl	ES	2 mg/ml[a]	RPR	0.9 mg/ml[a]	Physically compatible with no change in measured turbidity or increase in particle content in 4 hr at 23 °C	2224	**C**
Dobutamine HCl	AST	4 mg/ml[a]	RPR	0.9 mg/ml[a]	Physically compatible with no change in measured turbidity or increase in particle content in 4 hr at 23 °C	2224	**C**
Dopamine HCl	AB	3.2 mg/ml[a]	RPR	0.9 mg/ml[a]	Physically compatible with no change in measured turbidity or increase in particle content in 4 hr at 23 °C	2224	**C**
Doxorubicin HCl liposome injection	SEQ	0.4 mg/ml[a]	RPR	2 mg/ml[a]	Partial loss of measured natural turbidity	2087	**I**
Doxycycline hyclate	FUJ	1 mg/ml[a]	RPR	0.9 mg/ml[a]	Physically compatible with no change in measured turbidity or increase in particle content in 4 hr at 23 °C	2224	**C**

Y-Site Injection Compatibility (1:1 Mixture) (Cont.)

		Docetaxel					
Drug	*Mfr*	*Conc*	*Mfr*	*Conc*	*Remarks*	*Ref*	*C/I*
Droperidol	AST	0.4 mg/ml[a]	RPR	0.9 mg/ml[a]	Physically compatible with no change in measured turbidity or increase in particle content in 4 hr at 23 °C	2224	**C**
Enalaprilat	ME	0.1 mg/ml[a]	RPR	0.9 mg/ml[a]	Physically compatible with no change in measured turbidity or increase in particle content in 4 hr at 23 °C	2224	**C**
Famotidine	ME	2 mg/ml[a]	RPR	0.9 mg/ml[a]	Physically compatible with no change in measured turbidity or increase in particle content in 4 hr at 23 °C	2224	**C**
Fluconazole	RR	2 mg/ml	RPR	0.9 mg/ml[a]	Physically compatible with no change in measured turbidity or increase in particle content in 4 hr at 23 °C	2224	**C**
Furosemide	AMR	3 mg/ml[a]	RPR	0.9 mg/ml[a]	Physically compatible with no change in measured turbidity or increase in particle content in 4 hr at 23 °C	2224	**C**
Ganciclovir sodium	RC	20 mg/ml[a]	RPR	0.9 mg/ml[a]	Physically compatible with no change in measured turbidity or increase in particle content in 4 hr at 23 °C	2224	**C**
Gemcitabine HCl	LI	10 mg/ml[b]	RPR	2 mg/ml[a]	Physically compatible with no change in measured turbidity or increase in particle content in 4 hr at 23 °C	2226	**C**
Gentamicin sulfate	AB	5 mg/ml[a]	RPR	0.9 mg/ml[a]	Physically compatible with no change in measured turbidity or increase in particle content in 4 hr at 23 °C	2224	**C**
Granisetron HCl	SKB	0.05 mg/ml[a]	RPR	0.9 mg/ml[a]	Physically compatible with no change in measured turbidity or increase in particle content in 4 hr at 23 °C	2224	**C**
Haloperidol lactate	MN	0.2 mg/ml[a]	RPR	0.9 mg/ml[a]	Physically compatible with no change in measured turbidity or increase in particle content in 4 hr at 23 °C	2224	**C**
Heparin sodium	ES	100 units/ml	RPR	0.9 mg/ml[a]	Physically compatible with no change in measured turbidity or increase in particle content in 4 hr at 23 °C	2224	**C**
Hydrocortisone sodium phosphate	ME	1 mg/ml[a]	RPR	0.9 mg/ml[a]	Physically compatible with no change in measured turbidity or increase in particle content in 4 hr at 23 °C	2224	**C**
Hydrocortisone sodium succinate	AB	1 mg/ml[a]	RPR	0.9 mg/ml[a]	Physically compatible with no change in measured turbidity or increase in particle content in 4 hr at 23 °C	2224	**C**
Hydromorphone HCl	AST	0.5 mg/ml[a]	RPR	0.9 mg/ml[a]	Physically compatible with no change in measured turbidity or increase in particle content in 4 hr at 23 °C	2224	**C**
Hydroxyzine HCl	ES	2 mg/ml[a]	RPR	0.9 mg/ml[a]	Physically compatible with no change in measured turbidity or increase in particle content in 4 hr at 23 °C	2224	**C**
Imipenem–cilastatin sodium	ME	10 mg/ml[b]	RPR	0.9 mg/ml[a]	Physically compatible with no change in measured turbidity or increase in particle content in 4 hr at 23 °C	2224	**C**

Y-Site Injection Compatibility (1:1 Mixture) (Cont.)

Drug	Mfr	Conc	Mfr	Conc	Remarks	Ref	C/I
				Docetaxel			
Leucovorin calcium	ES	2 mg/ml[a]	RPR	0.9 mg/ml[a]	Physically compatible with no change in measured turbidity or increase in particle content in 4 hr at 23 °C	2224	**C**
Lorazepam	WY	0.5 mg/ml[a]	RPR	0.9 mg/ml[a]	Physically compatible with no change in measured turbidity or increase in particle content in 4 hr at 23 °C	2224	**C**
Magnesium sulfate	AST	100 mg/ml[a]	RPR	0.9 mg/ml[a]	Physically compatible with no change in measured turbidity or increase in particle content in 4 hr at 23 °C	2224	**C**
Mannitol	BA	15%	RPR	0.9 mg/ml[a]	Physically compatible with no change in measured turbidity or increase in particle content in 4 hr at 23 °C	2224	**C**
Meperidine HCl	AST	4 mg/ml[a]	RPR	0.9 mg/ml[a]	Physically compatible with no change in measured turbidity or increase in particle content in 4 hr at 23 °C	2224	**C**
Meropenem	ZEN	20 mg/ml[b]	RPR	0.9 mg/ml[a]	Physically compatible with no change in measured turbidity or increase in particle content in 4 hr at 23 °C	2224	**C**
Mesna	MJ	10 mg/ml[a]	RPR	0.9 mg/ml[a]	Physically compatible with no change in measured turbidity or increase in particle content in 4 hr at 23 °C	2224	**C**
Methylprednisolone sodium succinate	PHU	5 mg/ml[a]	RPR	0.9 mg/ml[a]	Partial loss of measured natural turbidity occurs immediately	2224	**I**
Metoclopramide HCl	AB	5 mg/ml	RPR	0.9 mg/ml[a]	Physically compatible with no change in measured turbidity or increase in particle content in 4 hr at 23 °C	2224	**C**
Metronidazole	BA	5 mg/ml	RPR	0.9 mg/ml[a]	Physically compatible with no change in measured turbidity or increase in particle content in 4 hr at 23 °C	2224	**C**
Minocycline HCl	LE	0.2 mg/ml[a]	RPR	0.9 mg/ml[a]	Physically compatible with no change in measured turbidity or increase in particle content in 4 hr at 23 °C	2224	**C**
Morphine sulfate	ES	1 mg/ml[a]	RPR	0.9 mg/ml[a]	Physically compatible with no change in measured turbidity or increase in particle content in 4 hr at 23 °C	2224	**C**
Nalbuphine HCl	AST	10 mg/ml	RPR	0.9 mg/ml[a]	Increase in measured subvisual turbidity occurs immediately	2224	**I**
Netilmicin sulfate	SCH	5 mg/ml[a]	RPR	0.9 mg/ml[a]	Physically compatible with no change in measured turbidity or increase in particle content in 4 hr at 23 °C	2224	**C**
Ofloxacin	MN	4 mg/ml[a]	RPR	0.9 mg/ml[a]	Physically compatible with no change in measured turbidity or increase in particle content in 4 hr at 23 °C	2224	**C**
Ondansetron HCl	GW	1 mg/ml[a]	RPR	0.9 mg/ml[a]	Physically compatible with no change in measured turbidity or increase in particle content in 4 hr at 23 °C	2224	**C**
Piperacillin sodium	LE	40 mg/ml[a]	RPR	0.9 mg/ml[a]	Physically compatible with no change in measured turbidity or increase in particle content in 4 hr at 23 °C	2224	**C**

Y-Site Injection Compatibility (1:1 Mixture) (Cont.)

Drug	Mfr	Conc	Mfr	Conc	Remarks	Ref	C/I
				Docetaxel			
Piperacillin sodium–tazobactam sodium	CY	40 + 5 mg/ml[a]	RPR	0.9 mg/ml[a]	Physically compatible with no change in measured turbidity or increase in particle content in 4 hr at 23 °C	2224	C
Potassium chloride	AB	0.1 mEq/ml[a]	RPR	0.9 mg/ml[a]	Physically compatible with no change in measured turbidity or increase in particle content in 4 hr at 23 °C	2224	C
Prochlorperazine edisylate	SO	0.5 mg/ml[a]	RPR	0.9 mg/ml[a]	Physically compatible with no change in measured turbidity or increase in particle content in 4 hr at 23 °C	2224	C
Promethazine HCl	SCN	2 mg/ml[a]	RPR	0.9 mg/ml[a]	Physically compatible with no change in measured turbidity or increase in particle content in 4 hr at 23 °C	2224	C
Ranitidine HCl	GL	2 mg/ml[a]	RPR	0.9 mg/ml[a]	Physically compatible with no change in measured turbidity or increase in particle content in 4 hr at 23 °C	2224	C
Ringer's injection, lactated	BA		RPR	0.9 mg/ml[a]	Physically compatible with no change in measured turbidity or increase in particle content in 4 hr at 23 °C	2224	C
Sodium bicarbonate	AB	1 mEq/ml	RPR	0.9 mg/ml[a]	Physically compatible with no change in measured turbidity or increase in particle content in 4 hr at 23 °C	2224	C
Ticarcillin disodium	SKB	30 mg/ml[a]	RPR	0.9 mg/ml[a]	Physically compatible with no change in measured turbidity or increase in particle content in 4 hr at 23 °C	2224	C
Ticarcillin disodium–clavulanate potassium	SKB	31 mg/ml[a]	RPR	0.9 mg/ml[a]	Physically compatible with no change in measured turbidity or increase in particle content in 4 hr at 23 °C	2224	C
Tobramycin sulfate	LI	5 mg/ml[a]	RPR	0.9 mg/ml[a]	Physically compatible with no change in measured turbidity or increase in particle content in 4 hr at 23 °C	2224	C
Trimethoprim–sulfamethoxazole	ES	0.8 + 4 mg/ml[a]	RPR	0.9 mg/ml[a]	Physically compatible with no change in measured turbidity or increase in particle content in 4 hr at 23 °C	2224	C
Vancomycin HCl	LI	10 mg/ml[a]	RPR	0.9 mg/ml[a]	Physically compatible with no change in measured turbidity or increase in particle content in 4 hr at 23 °C	2224	C
Zidovudine	GW	4 mg/ml[a]	RPR	0.9 mg/ml[a]	Physically compatible with no change in measured turbidity or increase in particle content in 4 hr at 23 °C	2224	C

[a]*Tested in dextrose 5% in water.*
[b]*Tested in sodium chloride 0.9%.*
[c]*Sodium carbonate–containing formulation tested.*

Other Information

Bacterial Challenge— Docetaxel (Rhone Poulenc) 0.8 mg/ml diluted in sodium chloride 0.9% did not exhibit an antimicrobial effect on the growth of four organisms (*Enterococcus faecium, Staphylococcus aureus, Pseudomonas aeruginosa,* and *Candida albicans*)

inocculated into the solution. Diluted solutions should be stored under refrigeration whenever possible, and the potential for microbiological growth should be considered when assigning expiration periods (2160).

Plasticizer Extraction— The surfactant (polysorbate 80) contained in the docetaxel formulation can leach plasticizer from DEHP-plasticized PVC containers and administration sets. The amount leached is time and concentration dependent (1683). The manufacturer recommends that docetaxel concentrate not be allowed to contact such containers and equipment. To minimize the amount of plasticizer exposure to the patient, the use of glass or polyolefin (polyethylene, polypropylene, etc.) containers and polyethylene-lined administration sets is recommended for the administration of docetaxel admixtures (2).

Mazzo et al. evaluated the leaching of DEHP plasticizer by docetaxel 0.56 and 0.96 mg/ml in dextrose 5% in water and in sodium chloride 0.9%. PVC bags of the solutions were used to prepare the admixtures. The leaching of the plasticizer was found to be time and concentration dependent; however, there was little difference between the two infusion solutions. After storage for eight hours at 21 °C, HPLC analysis found leached DEHP in the range of 30 to 51 μg/ml for the 0.96 mg/ml concentration and 25 to 36 μg/ml for the 0.56 mg/ml concentration. During a simulated one-hour infusion, the amount of leached DEHP did not exceed 14 μg/ml (1825).

An acceptability limit of no more than 5 parts per million (5 μg/ml) for DEHP plasticizer released from PVC containers, etc. has been proposed. The limit was proposed based on a review of metabolic and toxicologic considerations (2185).

DOPAMINE HCL
AHFS 12:12

Abbott

Products— Dopamine HCl is available in 200-mg (40 mg/ml), 400-mg (80 mg/ml), 800-mg (80 mg/ml), and 800-mg (160 mg/ml) vials and prefilled syringes. The solutions also contain sodium metabisulfite 0.9% as an antioxidant, citric acid and sodium citrate buffer, and hydrochloric acid or sodium hydroxide to adjust the pH in water for injection (1-3/97; 4; 29).

Dopamine HCl (Abbott) is available premixed for infusion in concentrations of 0.8, 1.6, and 3.2 mg/ml in dextrose 5% in water. Also present are sodium metabisulfite 0.5 mg/ml and hydrochloric acid and/or sodium hydroxide for pH adjustment (4).

pH— Dopamine HCl (Abbott) has a pH of about 3.3 (range 2.5 to 5) (1-3/97). The premixed dopamine HCl infusions have a pH of about 3.3 (range 2.5 to 4.5) (4).

Osmotic Values— The osmolality of dopamine HCl 40 mg/ml was determined to be 619 mOsm/kg by freezing-point depression and 581 mOsm/kg by vapor pressure (1071). At a concentration of 10 mg/ml (manufacturer and diluent unspecified), the osmolality was determined to be 277 mOsm/kg (1233). The osmolarity of Abbott's premixed dopamine HCl in dextrose 5% in water is 270, 275, and 295 mOsm/L for the 0.8-, 1.6-, and 3.2-mg/ml concentrations, respectively (4).

Administration— Dopamine HCl is administered by intravenous infusion into a large vein using an infusion pump or other infusion control device. The premixed infusion solutions are suitable for administration without dilution, but the concentrated injection must be diluted for use. Often the dose of concentrate is added to 250 or 500 ml of compatible solution. The concentration used depends on the patient's requirements. Concentrations as high as 3200 μg/ml have been used (1-3/97; 4).

Stability— Intact containers of dopamine HCl should be stored at controlled room temperature (1-3/97; 4). The injections should be protected from excessive heat and from freezing (4). The commercial preparation is stable for five years from manufacture if protected from light (79). The pH of the solution is one of the most critical factors determining dopamine HCl stability. While dopamine HCl has been found to be stable over a pH range of 4 to 6.4 when mixed with other drugs in dextrose 5% in water (312), it is most stable at pH 5 or below (79). In alkaline solutions, the catechol moieties are oxidized, cyclized, and polymerized to colored materials (312), forming a pink to violet color (78). Decomposition may also be indicated by the formation of a yellow or brown discoloration of the solution (4). Discolored solutions should not be used (4; 312).

Exposure of dopamine HCl (American Critical Care) 100 mg/100 ml in dextrose 5% in water to fluorescent and blue phototherapy light for 36 hours at 25 °C, while static or flowing through tubing at 2 ml/hr, resulted in no significant difference in drug concentration compared to controls stored in the dark. Because no unacceptable potency loss occurs, protection of dopamine HCl infusions from blue phototherapy lights is not necessary (1100).

Syringes— Dopamine HCl (Abbott) 200 mg/50 ml in dextrose 5% in water exhibited no change in appearance and no loss in potency by HPLC when stored in 60-ml plastic syringes (Becton-Dickinson) for 24 hours at 25 °C (1579).

Dopamine HCl (Therabel Lucien Pharma) 4 mg/ml in dextrose 5% in water was packaged in 50-ml polypropylene syringes (Becton-Dickinson) and stored at 4 and 24 °C in the dark and exposed to room light for 48 hours. Dopamine concentration losses determined by HPLC analysis were less than 10% throughout the study (1961).

Sorption— Dopamine HCl (Sigma) 72 mg/L was added to sodium chloride 0.9% (Travenol) in PVC bags and stored for one week at room temperature (15 to 20 °C). No significant sorption of the dopamine HCl to the plastic was exhibited (536).

Dopamine HCl (Arnar-Stone) 20 mg/2 ml diluted in dextrose 5% in water or sodium chloride 0.9% was stored for 18 hours at room temperature in the following plastic syringes: Brunswick (Sherwood Medical), Plastipak (Becton-Dickinson), Steriseal (Needle Industries), and Sabre (Gillette U.K.). The first three syringes have polypropylene barrels; the Sabre has a combination polypropylene–polystyrene barrel. No significant loss of dopamine occurred due to sorption (784).

Delivering dopamine HCl (Therabel Lucien Pharma) 4 mg/ml in dextrose 5% in water by syringe pump over 12 hours at 24 °C through PVC and polyethylene administration tubing did not result in substantial dopamine concentration losses determined by HPLC analysis (1961).

Filtration— Dopamine HCl 100 μg/ml in dextrose 5% in water or sodium chloride 0.9% was delivered over five hours through four kinds of 0.2-μm membrane filters varying in size and composition. Dopamine concentration losses of 3 to 5% were found during the first 60 minutes; subsequent dopamine levels returned to the original concentration when the binding sites became saturated (1399).

Compatibility Information

Solution Compatibility

Dopamine HCl

Solution	Mfr	Mfr	Conc/L	Remarks	Ref	C/I
Amino acids 4.25%, dextrose 25%	MG	AS	400 mg	No increase in particulate matter in 24 hr at 4 °C	349	C
Dextrose 5% in Ringer's injection, lactated	MG	AS	800 mg	Less than 5% decomposition in 48 hr at 23 to 25 °C	79	C
Dextrose 5% in sodium chloride 0.45%	MG	AS	800 mg	Less than 5% decomposition in 48 hr at 23 to 25 °C	79	C
Dextrose 5% in sodium chloride 0.9%	MG	AS	800 mg	Less than 5% decomposition in 48 hr at 23 to 25 °C	79	C
Dextrose 10% in sodium chloride 0.18%	TR[a]		300 mg	Visually compatible with no loss colorimetrically in 96 hr at room temperature under fluorescent light	1569	C
Dextrose 5% in water	MG	AS	800 mg	Less than 5% decomposition in 48 hr at 23 to 25 °C	79	C
	TR[a]	AS	800 mg	Potency retained for 24 hr at 25 °C	79	C
		AS	800 mg	Potency retained for 7 days at 5 °C	79	C
	AB	ACC	800 mg	Physically compatible and chemically stable. 10% decomposition calculated to occur after 142 hr at 25 °C	527	C
	BA[a]	DB	3.2 g	5% loss by HPLC in 14.75 days at 5 °C protected from light	1610	C
	TR[a]	ES	0.4 and 3.2 g	Visually compatible with no dopamine loss by HPLC in 48 hr at room temperature	1802	C
	BA[a]	SO	6.1 g	3% dopamine loss by HPLC in 24 hr at 23 °C	2085	C
Dextrose 10% in water	TR[a]		300 mg	Visually compatible with no loss colorimetrically in 96 hr at room temperature under fluorescent light	1569	C
Mannitol 20% in water	MG	AS	800 mg	Less than 5% decomposition in 48 hr at 23 to 25 °C	79	C
Ringer's injection, lactated	MG	AS	800 mg	Less than 5% decomposition in 48 hr at 23 to 25 °C	79	C
Sodium bicarbonate 5%	MG	AS	800 mg	Color change 5 min after mixing. Also second spot appeared on TLC	79	I
Sodium chloride 0.9%	MG	AS	800 mg	Less than 5% decomposition in 48 hr at 23 to 25 °C	79	C
	TR[a]	ES	0.4 and 3.2 g	Visually compatible with 5% or less dopamine loss by HPLC in 48 hr at room temperature	1802	C
Sodium lactate ⅙ M	MG	AS	800 mg	Less than 5% decomposition in 48 hr at 23 to 25 °C	79	C

[a]Tested in PVC containers.

Additive Compatibility

		Dopamine HCl						
Drug	*Mfr*	*Conc/L*	*Mfr*	*Conc/L*	*Test Soln*	*Remarks*	*Ref*	*C/I*
Acyclovir sodium	BW	5 g	SO	1.6 g	D5W	Yellow color developed in 1.5 hr due to dopamine oxidation. No acyclovir loss	1343	**I**
Alteplase	GEN	0.5 g	ACC	5 g	D5W, NS	About 30% alteplase clot-lysis activity loss in 24 hr at 25 °C	1856	**I**
Aminophylline	SE	500 mg	ACC	800 mg	D5W	Physically compatible. 10% dopamine decomposition occurs in 111 hr at 25 °C	527	**C**
Amphotericin B	SQ	200 mg	AS	800 mg	D5W	Immediate precipitation	78	**I**
Ampicillin sodium	BR	4 g	AS	800 mg	D5W	36% ampicillin decomposition in 6 hr at 23 to 25 °C. Apparent dopamine decomposition also. Color change and second spot on TLC	78	**I**
Atracurium besylate	BW	500 mg		1.6 g	D5W	Physically compatible and atracurium chemically stable for 24 hr at 5 and 30 °C	1694	**C**
Bretylium tosylate	ACC	10 g	ACC	800 mg	D5S[a]	Physically compatible and both drugs chemically stable for 48 hr at room temperature and 7 days at 4 °C	522	**C**
Calcium chloride	UP		AS	800 mg	D5W	No dopamine decomposition in 24 hr at 25 °C	312	**C**
Chloramphenicol sodium succinate	PD	4 g	AS	800 mg	D5W	Chloramphenicol and dopamine potency retained for 24 hr at 23 to 25 °C	78	**C**
Cibenzoline succinate		2 g	ACC	3.2 g	D5W, NS	Physically compatible for 24 hr at 25 °C by visual and microscopic examination	1182	**C**
Dobutamine HCl	LI	172 mg	AS	5.5 g	NS	Physically compatible for 24 hr	552	**C**
	LI	1 g	ACC	1.6 g	D5W, NS	Physically compatible with no color change in 24 hr at 25 °C	789	**C**
	LI	1 g	ES	800 mg	D5W, NS	Physically compatible for 24 hr at 21 °C	812	**C**
Enalaprilat	MSD	12 mg	AMR	1.6 g	D5W[b]	Visually compatible with about 5% enalaprilat loss by HPLC in 24 hr at room temperature under fluorescent light. Dopamine not tested	1572	**C**
Flumazenil	RC	20 mg	AB	3.2 g	D5W[b]	Visually compatible with 7% flumazenil loss by HPLC in 24 hr at 23 °C under fluorescent light. Dopamine not tested	1710	**C**
Gentamicin sulfate	SC	2 g	AS	800 mg	D5W	No dopamine decomposition and 7% gentamicin decomposition in 24 hr at 25 °C	312	**C**
	SC	320 mg	AS	800 mg	D5W	Gentamicin potency retained only through 6 hr. 80% gentamicin decomposition in 24 hr at 23 to 25 °C. Dopamine potency retained for 24 hr	78	**I**
Heparin sodium	AB	200,000 units	AS	800 mg	D5W	No dopamine or heparin decomposition in 24 hr at 25 °C	312	**C**
Hydrocortisone sodium succinate	UP	1 g	AS	800 mg	D5W	No dopamine decomposition in 18 hr at 25 °C	312	**C**
Kanamycin sulfate	BR	2 g	AS	800 mg	D5W	Kanamycin and dopamine potency retained for 24 hr at 23 to 25 °C	78	**C**
Lidocaine HCl	AST	4 g	AS	800 mg	D5W	No dopamine or lidocaine decomposition in 24 hr at 25 °C	312	**C**

Additive Compatibility (Cont.)

Dopamine HCl

Drug	Mfr	Conc/L	Mfr	Conc/L	Test Soln	Remarks	Ref	C/I
	AST	4 g	AS	800 mg	D5W[b]	No dopamine or lidocaine decomposition in 24 hr at 25 °C	312	C
	AST	2 g	ACC	800 mg	D5W, LR, NS	Physically compatible for 24 hr at 25 °C	775	C
Meropenem	ZEN	1 and 20 g	DU	800 mg	NS	Visually compatible for 4 hr at room temperature	1994	C
Methylprednisolone sodium succinate	UP	500 mg	AS	800 mg	D5W	No dopamine decomposition in 18 hr at 25 °C	312	C
	UP	500 mg	AS	800 mg	D5W	Clear solution for 24 hr	329	C
Metronidazole HCl with sodium bicarbonate	SE AB	5 g 50 mEq	ACC	1 g	D5W, NS	Markedly discolored, turning yellow and then brown	765	I
Nitroglycerin	ACC	400 mg	ACC	800 mg	D5W, NS[c]	Physically compatible with little or no nitroglycerin loss in 48 hr at 23 °C. Dopamine not tested	929	C
Oxacillin sodium	BR	2 g	AS	800 mg	D5W	No dopamine and 2% oxacillin decomposition in 24 hr at 25 °C	312	C
Penicillin G potassium	LI	20 million units	AS	800 mg	D5W	14% penicillin decomposition in 24 hr at 23 to 25 °C. Dopamine potency retained for 24 hr	78	I
Potassium chloride	MG		AS	800 mg	D5W	No dopamine decomposition in 24 hr at 25 °C	312	C
Propafenone HCl	KN	0.54 g	DU	0.9 and 2.3 g[d]	D5W	Visually compatible with little or no propafenone loss by HPLC in 24 hr at 22 °C exposed to fluorescent light. Dopamine not tested	412	C
Ranitidine HCl	GL	50 mg and 2 g	ES	400 mg and 3.2 g	D5W, NS[b]	Physically compatible with 6% or less ranitidine loss in 48 hr at room temperature under fluorescent light. Dopamine not tested	1361	C
	GL	50 mg and 2 g	ES	0.4 and 3.2 g	D5W, NS[a]	Visually compatible with 5 to 7% ranitidine loss and little or no dopamine loss by HPLC in 48 hr at room temperature	1802	C
Verapamil HCl	KN	80 mg	ES	400 mg	D5W, NS	Physically compatible for 24 hr	764	C

[a]Tested in both glass and PVC containers.
[b]Tested in PVC containers.
[c]Tested in glass containers.
[d]Approximate concentration.

Drugs in Syringe Compatibility

Dopamine HCl

Drug (in syringe)	Mfr	Amt	Mfr	Amt	Remarks	Ref	C/I
Doxapram HCl	RB	400 mg/ 20 ml		100 mg/ 5 ml	Physically compatible with 3% doxapram loss in 24 hr	1177	C
Heparin sodium		2500 units/ 1 ml		50 mg/ 5 ml	Physically compatible for at least 5 min	1053	C
Ranitidine HCl	GL	50 mg/ 5 ml		40 mg	Physically compatible for 4 hr at ambient temperature under fluorescent light	1151	C

Y-Site Injection Compatibility (1:1 Mixture)

Drug	Mfr	Conc	Mfr	Conc	Remarks	Ref	C/I
				Dopamine HCl			
Acyclovir sodium	BW	5 mg/ml[a]	AB	1.6 mg/ml[a]	Solution turns dark brown in 2 hr at 25 °C under fluorescent light	1157	I
Aldesleukin	CHI	33,800 I.U./ml[a]	ES	1.6 mg/ml[a]	Visually compatible with little or no loss of aldesleukin activity by bioassay	1857	C
Alteplase	GEN	1 mg/ml	DU	8 mg/ml[a]	Haze noted in 4 hr by visual examination	1340	I
Amifostine	USB	10 mg/ml[a]	AST	3.2 mg/ml[a]	Physically compatible with no change in measured turbidity or increase in particle content in 4 hr at 23 °C	1845	C
Amiodarone HCl	LZ	4 mg/ml[c]	ES	1.6 mg/ml[c]	Physically compatible for 24 hr at 21 °C	1032	C
Amphotericin B cholesteryl sulfate complex	SEQ	0.83 mg/ml[a]	AB	3.2 mg/ml[a]	Gross precipitate forms	2117	I
Amrinone lactate	WB	3 mg/ml[b]	ACC	1.6 mg/ml[a]	Physically compatible for at least 4 hr at 25 °C under fluorescent light	992	C
Atracurium besylate	BW	0.5 mg/ml[a]	SO	1.6 mg/ml[a]	Physically compatible for 24 hr at 28 °C	1337	C
Aztreonam	SQ	40 mg/ml[a]	AST	3.2 mg/ml[a]	Physically compatible with no subvisual haze or particle formation in 4 hr at 23 °C	1758	C
Cefepime HCl	BR	20 mg/ml[a]	AST	3.2 mg/ml[a]	Haze and precipitate form in 1 hr	1689	I
Cefpirome sulfate	HO	50 mg/ml[e]	AB	0.8 mg/ml[e]	Visually and microscopically compatible with 7% or less cefpirome loss and 6% or less dopamine loss by HPLC in 8 hr at 23 °C	2044	C
Ciprofloxacin	MI	2 mg/ml[c]	AB	1.6 mg/ml[c]	Visually compatible for 24 hr at 24 °C	1655	C
Cisatracurium besylate	GW	0.1, 2, 5 mg/ml[a]	AB	3.2 mg/ml[a]	Physically compatible with no change in measured turbidity or increase in particle content in 4 hr at 23 °C	2074	C
Cladribine	ORT	0.015[b] and 0.5[f] mg/ml	AST	3.2 mg/ml[b]	Physically compatible with no change in measured turbidity or increase in particle content in 4 hr at 23 °C	1969	C
Clarithromycin	AB	4 mg/ml[a]	DB	3.2 mg/ml[a]	Visually compatible for 72 hr at both 30 and 17 °C	2174	C
Diltiazem HCl	MMD	1 mg/ml[a]	AB	1.6 mg/ml[a]	Visually compatible for 24 hr at 25 °C	1530	C
	MMD	5 mg/ml	AB, SO	0.8 mg/ml[c]	Visually compatible	1807	C
	MMD	1 mg/ml[a]	AB	3.2 mg/ml[a]	Visually compatible for 4 hr at 27 °C	2062	C
Dobutamine HCl	LI	4 mg/ml[b]	DCC	3.2 mg/ml[c]	Physically compatible for 3 hr	1316	C
	LI	4 mg/ml[a]	AB	3.2 mg/ml[a]	Visually compatible for 4 hr at 27 °C	2062	C
Dobutamine HCl with lidocaine HCl	LI AB	4 mg/ml[c] 8 mg/ml[c]	DCC	3.2 mg/ml[c]	Physically compatible for 3 hr	1316	C
Dobutamine HCl with nitroglycerin	LI LY	4 mg/ml[c] 0.4 mg/ml[c]	DCC	3.2 mg/ml[c]	Physically compatible for 3 hr	1316	C
Dobutamine HCl with sodium nitroprusside	LI ES	4 mg/ml[c] 0.4 mg/ml[c]	DCC	3.2 mg/ml[c]	Physically compatible for 3 hr	1316	C
Docetaxel	RPR	0.9 mg/ml[a]	AB	3.2 mg/ml[a]	Physically compatible with no change in measured turbidity or increase in particle content in 4 hr at 23 °C	2224	C

Y-Site Injection Compatibility (1:1 Mixture) (Cont.)

Dopamine HCl

Drug	Mfr	Conc	Mfr	Conc	Remarks	Ref	C/I
Doxorubicin HCl liposome injection	SEQ	0.4 mg/ml[a]	AB	3.2 mg/ml[a]	Physically compatible with little or no change in measured turbidity and no increase in particle content in 4 hr at 23 °C	2087	**C**
Enalaprilat	MSD	0.05 mg/ml[b]	IMS	1.6 mg/ml[a]	Physically compatible for 24 hr at room temperature under fluorescent light	1355	**C**
Epinephrine HCl	AB	0.02 mg/ml[a]	AB	3.2 mg/ml[a]	Visually compatible for 4 hr at 27 °C	2062	**C**
Esmolol HCl	DCC	10 mg/ml[a]	IMS	1.6 mg/ml[a]	Physically compatible for 24 hr at 22 °C	1169	**C**
Etoposide phosphate	BR	5 mg/ml[a]	AST	3.2 mg/ml[a]	Physically compatible with no change in measured turbidity or increase in particle content in 4 hr at 23 °C	2218	**C**
Famotidine	MSD	0.2 mg/ml[a]	TR	1.6 mg/ml[a]	Physically compatible for at least 4 hr at 25 °C under fluorescent light	1188	**C**
	ME	2 mg/ml[b]		1.6 mg/ml[a]	Visually compatible for 4 hr at 22 °C	1936	**C**
Fentanyl citrate	ES	0.05 mg/ml	AB	3.2 mg/ml[a]	Visually compatible for 4 hr at 27 °C	2062	**C**
Fluconazole	RR	2 mg/ml	AMR	1.6 mg/ml[a]	Visually compatible for 24 hr at 28 °C	1760	**C**
Foscarnet sodium	AST	24 mg/ml	DU	80 mg/ml	Physically compatible for 24 hr at room temperature under fluorescent light	1335	**C**
Furosemide	AB, AMR	5 mg/ml	AST, DU	12.8 mg/ml	Physically compatible for 3 hr at room temperature	1978	**C**
	AB, AMR	5 mg/ml	AB, AMR	12.8 mg/ml	White precipitate forms immediately	1978	**I**
	AMR	10 mg/ml	AB	3.2 mg/ml[a]	Precipitate forms in 4 hr at 27 °C	2062	**I**
Gemcitabine HCl	LI	10 mg/ml[b]	AB	3.2 mg/ml[b]	Physically compatible with no change in measured turbidity or increase in particle content in 4 hr at 23 °C	2226	**C**
Granisetron HCl	SKB	0.05 mg/ml[a]	AB	3.2 mg/ml[a]	Physically compatible with no change in measured turbidity or increase in particle content in 4 hr at 23 °C	2000	**C**
Haloperidol lactate	MN	0.5[a] and 5 mg/ml	DU	1.6 mg/ml[a]	Visually compatible for 24 hr at 21 °C	1523	**C**
Heparin sodium	UP	1000 units/L[g]	ACC	40 mg/ml	Physically compatible for at least 4 hr at room temperature by visual and microscopic examination	534	**C**
	ES	100 units/ml[a]	AB	3.2 mg/ml[a]	Visually compatible for 4 hr at 27 °C	2062	**C**
	TR	50 units/ml	BA	1.6 mg/ml	Visually compatible for 6 hr at 25 °C	1793	**C**
Hydrocortisone sodium succinate	UP	10 mg/L[g]	ACC	40 mg/ml	Physically compatible for at least 4 hr at room temperature by visual and microscopic examination	534	**C**
Hydromorphone HCl	KN	1 mg/ml	AB	3.2 mg/ml[a]	Visually compatible for 4 hr at 27 °C	2062	**C**
Indomethacin sodium trihydrate	MSD	1 mg/ml[b]	AB	1.2 mg/ml[a]	Haze and fine precipitate form immediately	1527	**I**
Insulin, regular	LI	1 unit/ml[a]	DU	3.2 mg/ml[a]	White precipitate forms immediately, dissolves quickly, and reforms in 24 hr at 23 °C	1877	**I**
Labetalol HCl	SC	1 mg/ml[a]	IMS	1.6 mg/ml[a]	Physically compatible for 24 hr at 18 °C	1171	**C**

Y-Site Injection Compatibility (1:1 Mixture) (Cont.)

Dopamine HCl

Drug	Mfr	Conc	Mfr	Conc	Remarks	Ref	C/I
	GL	1 mg/ml[a]	ES	1.6 mg/ml[a]	Visually compatible with little or no loss of either drug by HPLC in 4 hr at room temperature	1762	C
	AH	2 mg/ml[a]	AB	3.2 mg/ml[a]	Visually compatible for 4 hr at 27 °C	2062	C
Lidocaine HCl	AB	8 mg/ml[c]	DCC	3.2 mg/ml[c]	Physically compatible for 3 hr	1316	C
Lidocaine HCl with dobutamine HCl	AB LI	8 mg/ml[c] 4 mg/ml[c]	DCC	3.2 mg/ml[c]	Physically compatible for 3 hr	1316	C
Lidocaine HCl with nitroglycerin	AB LY	8 mg/ml[c] 0.4 mg/ml[c]	DCC	3.2 mg/ml[c]	Physically compatible for 3 hr	1316	C
Lidocaine HCl with sodium nitroprusside	AB ES	8 mg/ml[c] 0.4 mg/ml[c]	DCC	3.2 mg/ml[c]	Physically compatible for 3 hr	1316	C
Lorazepam	WY	0.5 mg/ml[a]	AB	3.2 mg/ml[a]	Visually compatible for 4 hr at 27 °C	2062	C
Meperidine HCl	AB	10 mg/ml	AB	1.6 mg/ml[a]	Physically compatible for 4 hr at 25 °C	1397	C
Methylprednisolone sodium succinate	UP	5 mg/ml[a]	AB	0.8 mg/ml[a]	Visually compatible for 24 hr at room temperature in test tubes. No precipitate found on filter from Y-site delivery	2063	C
Metronidazole	MG	5 mg/ml	AB	0.8 mg/ml[a]	Visually compatible for 24 hr at room temperature in test tubes. No precipitate found on filter from Y-site delivery	2063	C
Midazolam HCl	RC RC RC	1 mg/ml[a] 1 mg/ml[a] 2 mg/ml[a]	AB DU AB	1.6 mg/ml[a] 3.2 mg/ml[a] 3.2 mg/ml[a]	Visually compatible for 24 hr at 23 °C Visually compatible for 24 hr at 23 °C Visually compatible for 4 hr at 27 °C	1847 1877 2062	C C C
Milrinone lactate	SW SW	0.2 mg/ml[a] 0.4 mg/ml[a]	AB SO	3.2 mg/ml[a] 6.4 mg/ml[a]	Visually compatible for 4 hr at 27 °C Visually compatible with little or loss of either drug by HPLC in 4 hr at 23 °C	2062 2214	C C
Morphine sulfate	AB SCN	1 mg/ml 2 mg/ml[a]	AB AB	1.6 mg/ml[a] 3.2 mg/ml[a]	Physically compatible for 4 hr at 25 °C Visually compatible for 4 hr at 27 °C	1397 2062	C C
Nicardipine HCl	WY	1 mg/ml[a]	AB	3.2 mg/ml[a]	Visually compatible for 4 hr at 27 °C	2062	C
Nitroglycerin	LY AB	0.4 mg/ml[c] 0.4 mg/ml[a]	DCC AB	3.2 mg/ml[c] 3.2 mg/ml[a]	Physically compatible for 3 hr Visually compatible for 4 hr at 27 °C	1316 2062	C C
Nitroglycerin with dobutamine HCl	LY LI	0.4 mg/ml[c] 4 mg/ml[c]	DCC	3.2 mg/ml[c]	Physically compatible for 3 hr	1316	C
Nitroglycerin with lidocaine HCl	LY AB	0.4 mg/ml[c] 8 mg/ml[c]	DCC	3.2 mg/ml[c]	Physically compatible for 3 hr	1316	C
Nitroglycerin with sodium nitroprusside	LY ES	0.4 mg/ml[c] 0.4 mg/ml[c]	DCC	3.2 mg/ml[c]	Physically compatible for 3 hr	1316	C
Norepinephrine bitartrate	STR	0.064 mg/ml[a]	DU	3.2 mg/ml[a]	Visually compatible for 24 hr at 23 °C	1877	C
	AB	0.128 mg/ml[a]	AB	3.2 mg/ml[a]	Visually compatible for 4 hr at 27 °C	2062	C
Ondansetron HCl	GL	0.32 mg/ml[b]	AB	0.8 mg/ml[a]	Visually compatible for 24 hr at room temperature in test tubes. No precipitate found on filter from Y-site delivery	2063	C
Pancuronium bromide	ES	0.05 mg/ml[a]	SO	1.6 mg/ml[a]	Physically compatible for 24 hr at 28 °C	1337	C
Piperacillin sodium–tazobactam sodium	LE	40 + 5 mg/ml[a]	AST	3.2 mg/ml[a]	Physically compatible with no change in measured turbidity or increase in particle content in 4 hr at 22 °C	1688	C

Y-Site Injection Compatibility (1:1 Mixture) (Cont.)

Dopamine HCl

Drug	Mfr	Conc	Mfr	Conc	Remarks	Ref	C/I
Potassium chloride	AB	40 mEq/L[g]	ACC	40 mg/ml	Physically compatible for at least 4 hr at room temperature by visual and microscopic examination	534	**C**
Propofol	ZEN	10 mg/ml	AST	3.2 mg/ml[a]	Physically compatible for 1 hr at 23 °C with no increase in particle content	2066	**C**
Ranitidine HCl	GL GL	0.5 mg/ml[h] 1 mg/ml[a]	ES AB	1.6 mg/ml[a] 3.2 mg/ml[a]	Physically compatible for 24 hr Visually compatible for 4 hr at 27 °C	1323 2062	**C** **C**
Remifentanil HCl	GW	0.025 and 0.25 mg/ml[b]	AB	3.2 mg/ml[a]	Physically compatible with no change in measured turbidity or increase in particle content in 4 hr at 23 °C	2075	**C**
Sargramostim	IMM	6[b,i] and 15[b] μg/ml	DU	1.6 mg/ml[c]	Visually compatible for 2 hr	1618	**C**
Sodium nitroprusside	ES	0.4 mg/ml[c]	DCC	3.2 mg/ml[c]	Physically compatible for 3 hr	1316	**C**
Sodium nitroprusside with dobutamine HCl	ES LI	0.4 mg/ml[c] 4 mg/ml[c]	DCC	3.2 mg/ml[c]	Physically compatible for 3 hr	1316	**C**
Sodium nitroprusside with lidocaine HCl	ES AB	0.4 mg/ml[c] 8 mg/ml[c]	DCC	3.2 mg/ml[c]	Physically compatible for 3 hr	1316	**C**
Sodium nitroprusside with nitroglycerin	ES LY	0.4 mg/ml[c] 0.4 mg/ml[c]	DCC	3.2 mg/ml[c]	Physically compatible for 3 hr	1316	**C**
Streptokinase	HO	30,000 units/ml[a]	DU	8 mg/ml[a]	Physically compatible for at least 4 days by visual examination	1340	**C**
Tacrolimus	FUJ	1 mg/ml[b]	ES	1.6 mg/ml[a]	Visually compatible for 24 hr at 25 °C	1630	**C**
Theophylline	TR	4 mg/ml	BA	1.6 mg/ml	Visually compatible for 6 hr at 25 °C	1793	**C**
Thiopental sodium	AB	25 mg/ml[d]	AB	3.2 mg/ml[a]	Precipitate forms immediately	2062	**I**
Thiotepa	IMM[j]	1 mg/ml[a]	AST	3.2 mg/ml[a]	Physically compatible with no change in measured turbidity or increase in particle content in 4 hr at 23 °C	1861	**C**
TNA #73[k]			AB	80 mg/50 ml[c]	Physically compatible for 4 hr by visual observation	1009	**C**
TNA #222 and #223[k]			AB	3.2 mg/ml[a]	Precipitate forms immediately	2215	**I**
TNA #218 to #221 and #224 to #226[k]			AB	3.2 mg/ml[a]	Visually compatible with no precipitate or emulsion damage apparent in 4 hr at 23 °C	2215	**C**
Tolazoline HCl		0.1 mg/ml[a]	AB	1.2 mg/ml[a]	Physically compatible for 24 hr at 22 °C	1363	**C**
TPN #189[k]			DB	1.6 mg/ml[b]	Visually compatible for 24 hr at 22 °C	1767	**C**
TPN #203 and #204[k]			AMR	3.2 mg/ml	Visually compatible for 4 hr at 23 °C	1974	**C**
TPN #212 to #215[k]			AB	3.2 mg/ml[a]	Physically compatible with no change in measured turbidity or increase in particle content in 4 hr at 23 °C	2109	**C**
Vecuronium bromide	OR OR	0.1 mg/ml[a] 1 mg/ml	SO AB	1.6 mg/ml[a] 3.2 mg/ml[a]	Physically compatible for 24 hr at 28 °C Visually compatible for 4 hr at 27 °C	1337 2062	**C** **C**
Verapamil HCl		[l]			Physically compatible	840	**C**
Vitamin B complex with C		2 ml/L[g]	ACC	40 mg/ml	Physically compatible for at least 4 hr at room temperature by visual and microscopic examination	534	**C**

Y-Site Injection Compatibility (1:1 Mixture) (Cont.)

Dopamine HCl

Drug	Mfr	Conc	Mfr	Conc	Remarks	Ref	C/I
Warfarin sodium	DU	2 mg/ml[d]	FAU	1.6 mg/ml[a]	Visually compatible with no warfarin loss by HPLC in 30 min	2010	C
	DME	2 mg/ml[d]	DU	1.6 mg/ml[a]	Visually compatible for 24 hr at 24 °C	2078	C
Zidovudine	BW	4 mg/ml[a]	AB	1.6 mg/ml[a]	Physically compatible for 4 hr at 25 °C under fluorescent light by visual and microscopic examination	1193	C

[a]Tested in dextrose 5% in water.
[b]Tested in sodium chloride 0.9%.
[c]Tested in both dextrose 5% in water and sodium chloride 0.9%.
[d]Tested in sterile water for injection.
[e]Tested in dextrose 5% in water, Ringer's injection, lactated, sodium chloride 0.45%, and sodium chloride 0.9%.
[f]Tested in bacteriostatic sodium chloride 0.9% preserved with benzyl alcohol 0.9%.
[g]Tested in dextrose 5% in Ringer's injection, dextrose 5% in Ringer's injection, lactated, dextrose 5% in water, Ringer's injection, lactated, and sodium chloride 0.9%.
[h]Premixed infusion solution.
[i]Tested with human albumin 0.1%.
[j]Lyophilized formulation tested.
[k]Refer to Appendix I for the composition of parenteral nutrition solutions. TNA indicates a 3-in-1 admixture, and TPN indicates a 2-in-1 admixture.
[l]Injected into a line being used to infuse dopamine HCl in dextrose 5% in sodium chloride 0.3% with potassium chloride 20 mEq.

Additional Compatibility Information

Dopamine HCl is stated to be incompatible with iron salts, oxidizing agents, sodium bicarbonate, and other alkaline solutions. The drug is inactivated in alkaline solutions (1-3/97; 4; 312).

Furosemide— Furosemide has been demonstrated to be compatible or incompatible with dopamine HCl during simultaneous Y-site administration, depending on the formulation of dopamine HCl tested. Dopamine formulations supplied by Astra and DuPont have the pH adjusted with sodium hydroxide and/or hydrochloric acid and are compatible with furosemide. Formulations supplied by Abbott and American Regent contain citrate buffer and are incompatible with furosemide, forming a white precipitate immediately (1978).

Heparin— The interaction between dopamine HCl and heparin sodium in aqueous solution was evaluated by microcalorimetry. An exothermic reaction occurred in dextrose 5% in water but not sodium chloride 0.9%. Consequently, sodium chloride 0.9% was recommended as a vehicle to minimize the interaction between these two drugs (1185).

Dobutamine, Lidocaine, Nitroglycerin, and Nitroprusside— Dobutamine HCl (Lilly) 4 mg/ml, dopamine HCl (Dupont Critical Care) 3.2 mg/ml, lidocaine HCl (Abbott) 8 mg/ml, nitroglycerin (Lyphomed) 0.4 mg/ml, and sodium nitroprusside (Elkins-Sinn) 0.4 mg/ml, prepared in dextrose 5% in water and sodium chloride 0.9%, were combined in equal quantities in all possible combinations of two, three, four, and five drugs and then evaluated for physical compatibility. No physical incompatibility was observed in any combination within the three-hour study period (1316).

DOXACURIUM CHLORIDE
AHFS 12:20

Nuromax   **Glaxo Wellcome**

Products— Doxacurium chloride (Glaxo Wellcome) is available in 5-ml multiple-dose vials. Each milliliter of solution contains doxacurium (as the chloride) 1 mg, benzyl alcohol 0.9%, and hydrochloric acid to adjust the pH in water for injection (2).

pH— From 3.9 to 5 (2).

Administration— Doxacurium chloride is administered intravenously, undiluted or diluted up to 1:10 in dextrose 5% in water or sodium chloride 0.9% (2; 4).

Stability— Doxacurium chloride should be stored at controlled room temperature and protected from freezing. The drug may not be compatible with alkaline solutions having a pH greater than 8.5 (2).

Diluted 1:10 with dextrose 5% in water or sodium chloride 0.9%, doxacurium chloride is physically and chemically stable for up to 24 hours when stored in polypropylene syringes at 5 to 25 °C. Because the benzyl alcohol preservative is diluted, its effectiveness is diminished. Consequently, aseptic procedures should be followed to prepare the dilutions and they should be used within eight hours (2).

Compatibility Information

Y-Site Injection Compatibility (1:1 Mixture)

Doxacurium chloride

Drug	Mfr	Conc	Mfr	Conc	Remarks	Ref	C/I
Etomidate	AB	2 mg/ml	BW	1 mg/ml	Visually compatible for up to 7 days at 25 °C	1801	C
Propofol	STU	2 mg/ml	BW	1 mg/ml	Separates into layers within 7 days at 25 °C. No visible change in 24 hr	1801	?
Thiopental sodium	AB	25 mg/ml	BW	1 mg/ml	Visually compatible for up to 7 days at 25 °C	1801	C

Additional Compatibility Information

Doxacurium chloride is stated to be compatible with dextrose 5% in lactated Ringer's injection, dextrose 5% in sodium chloride 0.9%, dextrose 5% in water, lactated Ringer's injection, and sodium chloride 0.9% (2).

Doxacurium chloride is also stated to be compatible with alfentanil HCl, fentanyl citrate, and sufentanil citrate diluted as directed (2).

DOXAPRAM HCL
AHFS 28:20

Dopram   **Robins**

Products— Doxapram HCl (Robins) is available in 20-ml multiple-dose vials. Each milliliter of solution contains doxapram HCl 20 mg and benzyl alcohol 0.9% in water for injection (2).

pH— From 3.5 to 5 (2).

Osmolality— Doxapram HCl 20 mg/ml has an osmolality of 159 mOsm/kg (1689).

Administration— Doxapram HCl is administered by intravenous injection or infusion of a solution diluted to 1 or 2 mg/ml with a compatible diluent (2; 4).

Stability— Doxapram HCl injection should be stored at controlled room temperature and protected from freezing (2; 4).

pH Effects— Doxapram HCl in solution became turbid when the pH was adjusted from 3.8 to 5.7 with 0.1 *N* sodium hydroxide. When the pH was adjusted down to 1.9 with 0.1 *N* HCl, no visible change occurred to the clear solution (1177).

At pH 2.5 to 6.5, doxapram HCl remained chemically stable for 24 hours. At pH 7.5 and above, a 10 to 15% doxapram HCl loss occurred in about six hours (1177).

Compatibility Information

Drugs in Syringe Compatibility

Doxapram HCl

Drug (in syringe)	Mfr	Amt	Mfr	Amt	Remarks	Ref	C/I
Amikacin sulfate		100 mg/ 2 ml	RB	400 mg/ 20 ml	Physically compatible with no doxapram loss in 24 hr	1177	C
Aminophylline		250 mg/ 10 ml	RB	400 mg/ 20 ml	Immediate turbidity and precipitation	1177	I
Ascorbic acid injection		500 mg/ 2 ml	RB	400 mg/ 20 ml	Immediate turbidity changing to precipitation in 24 hr	1177	I
Bumetanide		0.5 mg/ 1 ml	RB	400 mg/ 20 ml	Physically compatible with 3% doxapram loss in 24 hr	1177	C
Cefoperazone sodium		500 mg/ 4 ml	RB	400 mg/ 20 ml	Immediate precipitation	1177	I

Drugs in Syringe Compatibility (Cont.)

Doxapram HCl

Drug (in syringe)	Mfr	Amt	Mfr	Amt	Remarks	Ref	C/I
Cefotaxime sodium		500 mg/ 4 ml	RB	400 mg/ 20 ml	Immediate precipitation	1177	I
Cefotetan disodium		1 g/ 10 ml	RB	400 mg/ 20 ml	Immediate turbidity	1177	I
Cefuroxime sodium	GL	750 mg/ 7 ml	RB	400 mg/ 20 ml	Immediate turbidity	1177	I
Chlorpromazine HCl		250 mg/ 5 ml	RB	400 mg/ 20 ml	Physically compatible with no doxapram loss in 24 hr	1177	C
Cimetidine HCl	SKF	50 mg/ 2 ml	RB	400 mg/ 20 ml	Physically compatible with no doxapram loss in 24 hr	1177	C
Cisplatin		10 mg/ 20 ml	RB	400 mg/ 20 ml	Physically compatible with no doxapram loss in 24 hr	1177	C
Cyclophosphamide		100 mg/ 5 ml	RB	400 mg/ 20 ml	Physically compatible with 2% doxapram loss in 24 hr	1177	C
Dexamethasone sodium phosphate	MSD	3.3 mg/ 1 ml	RB	400 mg/ 20 ml	Immediate turbidity and precipitation	1177	I
Diazepam		10 mg/ 2 ml	RB	400 mg/ 20 ml	Immediate turbidity and precipitation	1177	I
Digoxin		0.25 mg/ 1 ml	RB	400 mg/ 20 ml	10% doxapram loss in 9 hr and 17% in 24 hr	1177	I
Dobutamine HCl	LI	100 mg/ 10 ml	RB	400 mg/ 20 ml	5% doxapram loss in 3 hr and 11% in 24 hr	1177	I
Dopamine HCl		100 mg/ 5 ml	RB	400 mg/ 20 ml	Physically compatible with 3% doxapram loss in 24 hr	1177	C
Doxycycline hyclate		100 mg/ 5 ml	RB	400 mg/ 20 ml	Physically compatible with 3% doxapram loss in 24 hr	1177	C
Epinephrine HCl		1 mg/ 1 ml	RB	400 mg/ 20 ml	Physically compatible with no doxapram loss in 24 hr	1177	C
Folic acid		15 mg/ 1 ml	RB	400 mg/ 20 ml	Immediate turbidity	1177	I
Furosemide	HO	100 mg/ 10 ml	RB	400 mg/ 20 ml	Immediate turbidity	1177	I
Hydrocortisone sodium phosphate	MSD	100 mg/ 2 ml	RB	400 mg/ 20 ml	Immediate turbidity and precipitation	1177	I
Hydrocortisone sodium succinate	UP	500 mg/ 2 ml	RB	400 mg/ 20 ml	Immediate turbidity and precipitation	1177	I
Hydroxyzine HCl		25 mg/ 1 ml	RB	400 mg/ 20 ml	Physically compatible with no doxapram loss in 24 hr	1177	C
Isoniazid		100 mg/ 2 ml	RB	400 mg/ 20 ml	Physically compatible with 2% doxapram loss in 24 hr	1177	C
Ketamine HCl	PD	200 mg/ 20 ml	RB	400 mg/ 20 ml	Physically compatible with no doxapram loss in 9 hr and 12% loss in 24 hr	1177	I
Lincomycin HCl		300 mg/ 1 ml	RB	400 mg/ 20 ml	Physically compatible with no doxapram loss in 24 hr	1177	C
Methotrexate sodium		50 mg/ 20 ml	RB	400 mg/ 20 ml	Physically compatible with 4% doxapram loss in 24 hr	1177	C

Drugs in Syringe Compatibility (Cont.)

Doxapram HCl

Drug (in syringe)	Mfr	Amt	Mfr	Amt	Remarks	Ref	C/I
Methylprednisolone sodium succinate	UP	40 mg/ 2 ml	RB	400 mg/ 20 ml	Immediate turbidity and precipitation	1177	I
Minocycline HCl		100 mg/ 5 ml	RB	400 mg/ 20 ml	8% doxapram loss in 3 hr and 13% loss in 6 hr	1177	I
Netilmicin sulfate		100 mg/ 2 ml	RB	400 mg/ 20 ml	Physically compatible with 2% doxapram loss in 24 hr	1177	C
Phytonadione		10 mg/ 1 ml	RB	400 mg/ 20 ml	Physically compatible with no doxapram loss in 24 hr	1177	C
Pyridoxine HCl		10 mg/ 1 ml	RB	400 mg/ 20 ml	Physically compatible with 6% doxapram loss in 24 hr	1177	C
Terbutaline sulfate		0.2 mg/ 1 ml	RB	400 mg/ 20 ml	Physically compatible with 6% doxapram loss in 24 hr	1177	C
Thiamine HCl		10 mg/ 2 ml	RB	400 mg/ 20 ml	Physically compatible with 6% doxapram loss in 24 hr	1177	C
Thiopental sodium		300 mg/ 12 ml	RB	400 mg/ 20 ml	Immediate precipitation	1177	I
Ticarcillin disodium		1 g/ 20 ml	RB	400 mg/ 20 ml	18% doxapram loss in 3 hr	1177	I
Tobramycin sulfate		60 mg/ 1.5 ml	RB	400 mg/ 20 ml	Physically compatible with no doxapram loss in 24 hr	1177	C
Vincristine sulfate		1 mg/ 10 ml	RB	400 mg/ 20 ml	Physically compatible with 7% doxapram loss in 24 hr	1177	C

Additional Compatibility Information

Doxapram HCl is stated to be physically compatible with most intravenous infusion solutions (4), but sodium chloride 0.9% and dextrose 5 and 10% are recommended (2; 4).

The drug is stated to be incompatible with alkaline drugs such as aminophylline, thiopental sodium, and sodium bicarbonate (4). (See pH Effects.)

DOXORUBICIN HCL
AHFS 10:00

Adriamycin PFS and RDF   **Pharmacia & Upjohn**
Gensia

Products— Doxorubicin HCl (Adriamycin RDF, Pharmacia & Upjohn) is available as a lyophilized product in a rapid dissolution formula in 10-, 20-, and 50-mg single-dose glass vials and 150-mg multiple-dose glass vials. Also present are 50 mg of lactose and 1 mg of methylparaben for each 10 mg of doxorubicin HCl (2). The methylparaben enhances the dissolution rate by disrupting bonding between doxorubicin and other components (1253; 1254).

Reconstitution of the lyophilized products should be performed with sodium chloride 0.9%. Add 5, 10, or 25 ml to the 10-, 20-, or 50-mg vial, respectively. The 150-mg multiple-dose vials should be reconstituted with 75 ml of sodium chloride 0.9%. After the diluent is added, the vial should be shaken and the drug allowed to dissolve, forming a 2-mg/ml solution (2).

Additionally, doxorubicin HCl is available as a 2-mg/ml solution without preservatives. The solution also contains sodium chloride 0.9% and hydrochloric acid to adjust the pH in water for injection (1-5/95; 2). Doxorubicin HCl (Gensia) is provided in unbreakable plastic vials containing 5, 25, and 100 ml (1-5/95). Doxorubicin HCl (Adriamycin PFS, Pharmacia Adria) is also available in glass vials containing 5, 10, 25, 37.5, and 100 ml (2).

pH— The pH of lyophilized doxorubicin HCl reconstituted with sodium chloride 0.9% is 3.8 to 6.5 (4). The pH of the solution products is adjusted to 2.5 to 4.5 (4; 17).

Osmolality— Doxorubicin HCl 2 mg/ml in sterile water for injection has an osmolality of 280 mOsm/kg (1689).

Administration— Doxorubicin HCl is administered intravenously, preferably into the tubing of a running intravenous infusion of sodium chloride 0.9% or dextrose 5% in water over not less than three to five minutes (2; 4). The drug should not be administered intramuscularly or subcutaneously, and extravasation should be avoided because of local tissue necrosis (2; 4; 377).

Stability— Doxorubicin HCl liquid injections should be stored under refrigeration and protected from light. Intact vials should be kept in their cartons until use (2; 4).

The lyophilized products in intact vials should be stored at room temperature and protected from sunlight. The solution products, in their original cartons, should be refrigerated and protected from sunlight until ready for use (2; 4). The manufacturer states that its reconstituted lyophilized products are stable for seven days at room temperature and 15 days under refrigeration (2).

However, Vogelzang et al. reported a greater stability for 3- and 5-mg/ml concentrations in sodium chloride 0.9% in the reservoir of a Medtronic DAD implantable pump at 37 °C. With an HPLC analytical technique, approximately a 5 to 6% loss was found in one week and a 9 to 11% loss was found in two weeks. Analyses after longer periods continued to show about a 5 to 6% loss per week at 37 °C (1255).

Wood et al. assessed the stability of doxorubicin HCl (Farmitalia) 100 mg/L in sodium chloride 0.9% (pH 6.47 and pH 5.20) and in dextrose 5% in water (pH 4.36) when stored in PVC bags at 4 and 25 °C in the dark. The drug was stable for at least 43 days at both temperatures, exhibiting not more than 10 or 11% loss by HPLC analysis (1460).

Doxorubicin HCl (Farmitalia) 2 mg/ml repackaged in polypropylene syringes exhibited little or no loss by HPLC analysis after storage for 43 days at 4 °C (1460).

Doxorubicin HCl (Adria) 2 mg/ml in sodium chloride 0.9% in glass vials and plastic syringes (Monoject and Terumo) and also 1 mg/ml in sodium chloride 0.9% in plastic syringes (Monoject) exhibited no visual changes and little or no loss by HPLC analysis when stored at 4 and 23 °C while exposed to light for 142 days. Potential extractable materials from the syringes were not detected during the study period (1594).

Doxorubicin HCl is sensitive to light, especially in very dilute solutions (489; 1073; 1094). However, the photolability of dilute solutions is not observed with more concentrated solutions. A 10-fold difference in photolability half-life was found between concentrations of 0.01 and 0.1 mg/ml (1594). The manufacturers recommend that the solutions be protected from sunlight and that any unused solution be discarded (2; 4).

For 50-μg/ml and 0.5-mg/ml doxorubicin HCl solutions, Janssen et al. reported that a greater rate of decomposition occurred in the more concentrated solution (1206). However, most other studies found no concentration dependence for the degradation rate (489; 526; 1208; 1255).

Incorporation of doxorubicin HCl into liposomes did not affect the drug decomposition rate (1206).

Steam heating a doxorubicin HCl 1-mg/ml solution for one hour at 100 °C resulted in about a 26% drug loss (1256).

Freezing Solutions— The manufacturer does not recommend freezing the solutions (108).

However, Hoffman et al. found that doxorubicin HCl, constituted to 2 mg/ml with sterile water for injection and stored under refrig-

eration (4 °C), exhibited about a 1.5% loss in one month and about a 10.5% loss in six months. Freezing the solutions at −20 °C resulted in no loss of potency over 30 days. It was indicated that filtration of stored solutions through a 0.22-μm filter was appropriate to ensure sterility (652).

Karlsen et al. found that doxorubicin HCl (Farmitalia) 70 mg/50 ml in PVC bags of sodium chloride 0.9% (Travenol) could be frozen at −20 °C for at least 30 days and thawed by exposure to microwave radiation for two minutes with no significant change in concentration. However, the doxorubicin HCl concentration apparently began declining after the fourth repetition of the freeze–thaw treatment, with a loss of about 5% (818).

Keusters et al. studied the stability of doxorubicin HCl 1 mg/ml in sodium chloride 0.9% in PVC containers frozen at −20 °C. No drug loss occurred after two weeks of storage and thawing for 150 minutes at room temperature or 180 seconds in a 700-watt microwave oven. Refreezing the solutions and rethawing at room temperature or in a microwave oven three weeks later (total of five weeks of frozen storage) resulted in about a 3% doxorubicin loss (1256).

Although the thawing of frozen doxorubicin HCl solutions in microwave ovens has been suggested (818; 1256), Adria recommends only room temperature thawing because of the risks of drug decomposition from overheating and exposure if the bags burst (1257).

Wood et al. reported that doxorubicin HCl (Farmitalia) 100 mg/L in sodium chloride 0.9% and dextrose 5% in water in PVC bags (Travenol) was stable, exhibiting little or no loss by HPLC analysis after 43 days stored at −20 °C, even when subjected to 11 freeze-thaw repetitions (1460).

pH Effects— Doxorubicin HCl appears to have pH-dependent stability in solution (526; 1007; 1037). It becomes progressively more stable as the pH of drug–infusion solution admixtures becomes more acidic at 7.4 to 4.5 (526). The pH range of maximum stability has been variously stated to be about 4 to 5 (1007; 1460), 3 to 4 (1037), and about 4 (1208). At a concentration of 0.1 mg/ml in buffer solutions stored at 4 °C, no significant doxorubicin loss occurred in 60 days at pH 4, but substantial decomposition occurred at pH 7.4 (1206). Doxorubicin HCl is unstable at pH values less than 3 or greater than 7 (4). In acidic media, splitting of the glycosidic bond results in a red-colored, water-insoluble aglycone and a water-soluble amino sugar (4). In alkaline media, a color change to deep purple is indicative of decomposition. This color change also occurs with other anthracyclines (394). It is thought to reflect cleavage of the amino sugar, resulting in an ineffective moiety (524).

Portable Pump Reservoirs— Doxorubicin HCl (Cetus), reconstituted with sodium chloride 0.9% to a 2-mg/ml concentration or as the 2-mg/ml commercial solution, in portable pump reservoirs (Pharmacia Deltec) was chemically stable by HPLC analysis for 14 days at 3 and 23 °C and for an additional 28 days at 30 °C (1583).

Elastomeric Reservoir Pumps— Doxorubicin HCl (Astra) 2 mg/ml in sodium chloride 0.9% 25ml was packaged in latex elastomeric reservoirs (Secure Medical). Little or no loss by HPLC analysis occurred in 24 hours at 25 °C and in two days at 5 °C (1970).

Sorption— Doxorubicin HCl (Farmitalia) 16 μg/ml in dextrose 5% in water and sodium chloride 0.9% in PVC containers was infused through PVC infusion sets at 21 ml/hr over 24 hours at 22 °C while exposed to light. Fluctuations in the delivered concentration by HPLC analysis were relatively minor, with no evidence of sorption (1700).

Doxorubicin HCl (Farmitalia) 1 mg/ml in sodium chloride 0.9% exhibited no loss by UV spectroscopy due to sorption to PVC and polyethylene administration lines during simulated infusions at 0.875 ml/hr for 2.5 hours via a syringe pump (1795).

Wood et al. reported that doxorubicin HCl was adsorbed to PVC bags. Losses depended on temperature, concentration, and vehicle. Losses were greatest in sodium chloride 0.9% (pH 6.47), compared with dextrose 5% in water at pH 4.36. After eight days of storage, HPLC analysis of solutions containing doxorubicin HCl 100 μg/ml stored at 4 and 25 °C indicated losses of up to 7 to 8%. At concentrations used in clinical practice, sorptive losses during storage and delivery are negligible (1460).

Filtration— Although doxorubicin HCl was reported to undergo considerable binding to cellulose ester and polytetrafluoroethylene filters (1249; 1415; 1416), other studies did not confirm unacceptable losses at clinical concentrations. Doxorubicin HCl 2 mg/ml in sterile water for injection showed no loss of potency due to filtration when filtered through a 0.22-μm Millex filter (652).

In another study, doxorubicin HCl (Adria) 30 mg/15 ml was injected as a bolus through a 0.2-μm nylon, air-eliminating, filter (Ultipor, Pall) to evaluate the effect of filtration on simulated intravenous push delivery. Spectrophotometric evaluation showed that about 92% of the drug was delivered through the filter after flushing with 10 ml of sodium chloride 0.9% (809).

Doxorubicin HCl (Farmitalia) 5 mg/100 ml in sodium chloride 0.9% in a burette was filtered through a nylon 0.2-μm filter (Pall, ELD96LL). No drug loss due to sorption was found spectrophotometrically (1568).

Doxorubicin HCl (Farmitalia) 1 mg/ml in sodium chloride 0.9% exhibited little or no loss by UV spectroscopy due to sorption to cellulose acetate (Minisart 45, Sartorius), polysulfone (Acrodisc 45, Gelman), and nylon (Nylaflo, Gelman) filters. However, a 20 to 25% loss due to sorption occurred during the first 60 minutes of infusion through nylon filters (Utipore, Pall). About a 35% loss was found during the first 15 min using a nylon filter (Posidyne ELD96, Pall). The delivered concentrations gradually returned to the full concentrations within 1.5 to 2.5 hours (1795).

Compatibility Information

Solution Compatibility

Doxorubicin HCl

Solution	Mfr	Mfr	Conc/L	Remarks	Ref	C/I
Dextrose 3.3% in sodium chloride 0.3%			100 mg	5% or less drug loss in 4 weeks at 25 °C in the dark	1007	C
Dextrose 5% in water	TR[a]	AD	180 mg	10% loss of doxorubicin in 40 hr at room temperature along with a color change and an increase in pH	519	C
	TR[b]	AD	180 mg	No decrease in doxorubicin in 48 hr at room temperature	519	C
	AB[a]	AD	10 and 20 mg	Physically compatible. 2% decomposition in 24 hr at 21 °C under fluorescent light	526	C
			100 mg	5% or less drug loss in 4 weeks at 25 °C in the dark	1007	C
	c	BEL	0.5 g	Visually compatible with 5% or less doxorubicin loss by HPLC in 28 days at 4 °C and 14 days at 22 and 35 °C protected from light	1548	C
	c	BEL	1.25 g	Visually compatible with 5% or less doxorubicin loss by HPLC in 28 days at 4 and 22 °C and 7 days at 35 °C protected from light	1548	C
	MG[d], TR[b]		180 mg	Less than 10% loss by HPLC in 48 hr at room temperature exposed to light	1658	C
	b		40 mg	10% loss by HPLC in 7 days at 4 °C protected from light	1700	C
	TR[a]	FA	100 mg	10% or less loss by HPLC in 43 days at 4 and 25 °C in the dark	1460	C
Normosol R, pH 7.4	AB[a]	AD	10 and 20 mg	Physically compatible. 10% decomposition in 24 hr at 21 °C under fluorescent light	526	C
Ringer's injection, lactated	AB[a]	AD	10 and 20 mg	Physically compatible. 8% decomposition in 24 hr at 21 °C under fluorescent light	526	C
			100 mg	10% doxorubicin loss in 1.7 days at 25 °C in the dark	1007	C
Sodium chloride 0.9%	AB[a]	AD	10 and 20 mg	Physically compatible. 5% decomposition in 24 hr at 21 °C under fluorescent light	526	C

Solution Compatibility (Cont.)

Doxorubicin HCl

Solution	Mfr	Mfr	Conc/L	Remarks	Ref	C/I
			100 mg	10% doxorubicin loss in 6 days at 25 °C in the dark	1007	C
	c	BEL	0.5 g	Visually compatible with 5% or less doxorubicin loss by HPLC in 14 days at 4 and 22 °C and 7 days at 35 °C protected from light	1548	C
	c	BEL	1.25 g	Visually compatible with 5% or less doxorubicin loss by HPLC in 28 days at 4 and 22 °C and 7 days at 35 °C protected from light	1548	C
	BA[e]	CET	2 g	Chemically stable by HPLC in 14 days at 3 and 23 °C and an additional 28 days at 30 °C	1538	C
	b		40 mg	6% loss by HPLC in 7 days at 4 °C protected from light	1700	C
	TR[a]	FA	100 mg	10% or less loss by HPLC in 43 days at 4 and 25 °C in the dark	1460	C
	AB[f]	AST	2 g	Little or no loss by HPLC in 24 hr at 25 °C and in 2 days at 5 °C	1970	C

[a]Tested in glass containers.
[b]Tested in PVC containers.
[c]Tested in ethylene vinyl acetate (EVA) containers.
[d]Tested in both glass and polyolefin containers.
[e]Tested in Pharmacia Deltec reservoirs.
[f]Tested in glass containers and latex elastomeric reservoirs (Secure Medical).

Additive Compatibility

Doxorubicin HCl

Drug	Mfr	Conc/L	Mfr	Conc/L	Test Soln	Remarks	Ref	C/I
Aminophylline			AD			Solution color darkens from red to blue-purple	524	I
Dacarbazine with ondansetron HCl	LY GL	8 g 640 mg	AD	800 mg	D5W[a]	Visually compatible with >90% ondansetron and doxorubicin potency by HPLC over 24 hr at 30 °C and after 7 days at 4 °C followed by 24 hr at 30 °C. Dacarbazine stable for 8 hr but up to 13% loss in 24 hr	2092	I
Dacarbazine with ondansetron HCl	LY GL	20 g 640 mg	AD	1.5 g	D5W[a]	Visually compatible with >90% potency of all drugs by HPLC over 24 hr at 30 °C and after 7 days at 4 °C followed by 24 hr at 30 °C	2092	C
Dacarbazine with ondansetron HCl	LY GL	8 g 640 mg	AD	800 mg	D5W[b]	Visually compatible with >90% potency of all drugs by HPLC over 24 hr at 30 °C and after 7 days at 4 °C followed by 24 hr at 30 °C	2092	C
Dacarbazine with ondansetron HCl	LY GL	20 g 640 mg	AD	1.5 g	D5W[b]	Visually compatible with >90% potency of all drugs by HPLC over 24 hr at 30 °C and after 7 days at 4 °C followed by 24 hr at 30 °C	2092	C
Diazepam	RC		AD			Immediate precipitation	524	I
Fluorouracil	RC		AD			Solution color darkens from red to blue-purple	524	I
	RC	250 mg	AD	10 mg	D5W	Color change to deep purple	296	I

Additive Compatibility (Cont.)

Doxorubicin HCl

Drug	Mfr	Conc/L	Mfr	Conc/L	Test Soln	Remarks	Ref	C/I
Ondansetron HCl	GL	30 and 300 mg	MJ	100 mg	D5W[a]	Physically compatible with little or no loss of either drug by HPLC in 48 hr at 23 °C	1876	C
	GL	30 and 300 mg	MJ	2 g	D5W[a]	Physically compatible with little or no loss of either drug by HPLC in 48 hr at 23 °C	1876	C
Ondansetron HCl with vincristine sulfate	GL LI	480 mg 14 mg	AD	400 mg	D5W[b]	Visually compatible with >90% potency of all drugs by HPLC after 5 days at 4 °C followed by 24 hr at 30 °C	2092	C
Ondansetron HCl with vincristine sulfate	GL LI	960 mg 28 mg	AD	800 mg	D5W[a]	Visually compatible with >90% potency of all drugs by HPLC after 120 hr at 30 °C	2092	C
Vinblastine sulfate	LI	75 mg	AD	500 mg	NS[a]	Physically compatible for at least 10 days at 8, 25, and 32 °C. HPLC assays highly erratic	838	?
	LI	150 mg	AD	1.5 g	NS[a]	Physically compatible for at least 10 days at 8, 25, and 32 °C. HPLC assays highly erratic	838	?

[a]Tested in PVC containers.
[b]Tested in polyisoprene infusion pump reservoirs.

Drugs in Syringe Compatibility

Doxorubicin HCl

Drug (in syringe)	Mfr	Amt	Mfr	Amt	Remarks	Ref	C/I
Bleomycin sulfate		1.5 units/ 0.5 ml		1 mg/ 0.5 ml	Physically compatible for 5 min at room temperature followed by 8 min of centrifugation	980	C
Cisplatin		0.5 mg/ 0.5 ml		1 mg/ 0.5 ml	Physically compatible for 5 min at room temperature followed by 8 min of centrifugation	980	C
Cyclophosphamide		10 mg/ 0.5 ml		1 mg/ 0.5 ml	Physically compatible for 5 min at room temperature followed by 8 min of centrifugation	980	C
Droperidol		1.25 mg/ 0.5 ml		1 mg/ 0.5 ml	Physically compatible for 5 min at room temperature followed by 8 min of centrifugation	980	C
Fluorouracil		25 mg/ 0.5 ml		1 mg/ 0.5 ml	Physically compatible for 5 min at room temperature followed by 8 min of centrifugation	980	C
		500 mg/ 10 ml		5 and 10 mg/ 10 ml[a]	Precipitate forms within several hours of mixing	1564	I
Furosemide		5 mg/ 0.5 ml		1 mg/ 0.5 ml	Immediate precipitation	980	I
Heparin sodium		500 units/ 0.5 ml		1 mg/ 0.5 ml	Immediate precipitation	980	I

Drugs in Syringe Compatibility (Cont.)

Doxorubicin HCl

Drug (in syringe)	Mfr	Amt	Mfr	Amt	Remarks	Ref	C/I
Leucovorin calcium		5 mg/ 0.5 ml		1 mg/ 0.5 ml	Physically compatible for 5 min at room temperature followed by 8 min of centrifugation	980	C
Methotrexate sodium		12.5 mg/ 0.5 ml		1 mg/ 0.5 ml	Physically compatible for 5 min at room temperature followed by 8 min of centrifugation	980	C
Metoclopramide HCl		2.5 mg/ 0.5 ml		1 mg/ 0.5 ml	Physically compatible for 5 min at room temperature followed by 8 min of centrifugation	980	C
	RB	10 mg/ 2 ml	AD	40 mg/ 20 ml	Physically compatible for 48 hr at room temperature	924	C
	RB	10 mg/ 2 ml	AD	40 mg/ 20 ml	Physically compatible for 48 hr at 25 °C	1167	C
	RB	160 mg/ 32 ml	AD	90 mg/ 45 ml	Physically compatible for 48 hr at 25 °C	1167	C
Mitomycin		0.25 mg/ 0.5 ml		1 mg/ 0.5 ml	Physically compatible for 5 min at room temperature followed by 8 min of centrifugation	980	C
Vinblastine sulfate	LI	4.5 mg/ 4.5 ml	AD	45 mg/ 22.5 ml	(Brought to 30 ml total volume with NS) Physically compatible for at least 10 days at 8, 25, and 32 °C. HPLC assays highly erratic	838	?
	LI	2.25 mg/ 2.25 ml	AD	15 mg/ 7.5 ml	(Brought to 30 ml total volume with NS) Physically compatible for at least 10 days at 8, 25, and 32 °C. HPLC assays highly erratic	838	?
		0.5 mg/ 0.5 ml		1 mg/ 0.5 ml	Physically compatible for 5 min at room temperature followed by 8 min of centrifugation	980	C
Vincristine sulfate		0.5 mg/ 0.5 ml		1 mg/ 0.5 ml	Physically compatible for 5 min at room temperature followed by 8 min of centrifugation	980	C

[a]Diluted in sodium chloride 0.9%.

Y-Site Injection Compatibility (1:1 Mixture)

Doxorubicin HCl

Drug	Mfr	Conc	Mfr	Conc	Remarks	Ref	C/I
Allopurinol sodium	BW	3 mg/ml[b]	CET	2 mg/ml	Dark red color and haze form immediately. Reddish-brown particles form within 1 hr	1686	I
Amifostine	USB	10 mg/ml[a]	CET	2 mg/ml	Physically compatible with no change in measured turbidity or increase in particle content in 4 hr at 23 °C	1845	C
Amphotericin B cholesteryl sulfate complex	SEQ	0.83 mg/ml[a]	CHI	2 mg/ml	Gross precipitate forms	2117	I
Aztreonam	SQ	40 mg/ml[a]	CET	2 mg/ml	Physically compatible with no subvisual haze or particle formation in 4 hr at 23 °C	1758	C

Y-Site Injection Compatibility (1:1 Mixture) (Cont.)

Doxorubicin HCl

Drug	Mfr	Conc	Mfr	Conc	Remarks	Ref	C/I
Bleomycin sulfate		3 units/ml		2 mg/ml	Drugs injected sequentially into Y-site with no flush between. No visually apparent precipitate	980	C
Cefepime HCl	BR	20 mg/ml[a]	CET	2 mg/ml	Haze forms immediately and becomes flocculent precipitate in 4 hr	1689	I
Chlorpromazine HCl	SKF	2 mg/ml[a]	AD	0.2 mg/ml[a]	Visually compatible for 4 hr at room temperature under fluorescent light	1685	C
Cimetidine HCl	SKF	12 mg/ml[a]	AD	0.2 mg/ml[a]	Visually compatible for 4 hr at room temperature under fluorescent light	1685	C
Cisplatin		1 mg/ml		2 mg/ml	Drugs injected sequentially into Y-site with no flush between. No visually apparent precipitate	980	C
Cladribine	ORT	0.015[b] and 0.5[c] mg/ml	CHI	2 mg/ml	Physically compatible with no change in measured turbidity or increase in particle content in 4 hr at 23 °C	1969	C
Cyclophosphamide		20 mg/ml		2 mg/ml	Drugs injected sequentially into Y-site with no flush between. No visually apparent precipitate	980	C
Dexamethasone sodium phosphate	QU	1 mg/ml[a]	AD	0.2 mg/ml[a]	Visually compatible for 4 hr at room temperature under fluorescent light	1685	C
Diphenhydramine HCl	PD	2 mg/ml[a]	AD	0.2 mg/ml[a]	Visually compatible for 4 hr at room temperature under fluorescent light	1685	C
Droperidol		2.5 mg/ml		2 mg/ml	Drugs injected sequentially into Y-site with no flush between. No visually apparent precipitate	980	C
	JN	20 µg/ml[a]	AD	0.2 mg/ml[a]	Visually compatible for 4 hr at room temperature under fluorescent light	1685	C
Etoposide phosphate	BR	5 mg/ml[a]	GEN	2 mg/ml	Physically compatible with no change in measured turbidity or increase in particle content in 4 hr at 23 °C	2218	C
Famotidine	MSD	2 mg/ml[a]	AD	0.2 mg/ml[a]	Visually compatible for 4 hr at room temperature under fluorescent light	1685	C
Filgrastim	AMG	30 µg/ml[a]	CET	2 mg/ml	Physically compatible with no change in measured turbidity or increase in particle content in 4 hr at 22 °C	1687	C
Fludarabine phosphate	BX	1 mg/ml[a]	CET	2 mg/ml	Physically compatible for 4 hr at room temperature under fluorescent light	1439	C
Fluorouracil		50 mg/ml		2 mg/ml	Drugs injected sequentially into Y-site with no flush between. No visually apparent precipitate	980	C
Furosemide		10 mg/ml		2 mg/ml	Drugs injected sequentially into Y-site with no flush between. Immediate precipitation	980	I
	ES	3 mg/ml[a]	AD	0.2 mg/ml[a]	Visually compatible for 4 hr at room temperature under fluorescent light	1685	C
Ganciclovir sodium	SY	20 mg/ml[a]	AD	0.2 mg/ml[a]	Color changes to deep purple immediately	1685	I

Y-Site Injection Compatibility (1:1 Mixture) (Cont.)

Doxorubicin HCl

Drug	Mfr	Conc	Mfr	Conc	Remarks	Ref	C/I
Gemcitabine HCl	LI	10 mg/ml[b]	PH	2 mg/ml	Physically compatible with no change in measured turbidity or increase in particle content in 4 hr at 23 °C	2226	C
Granisetron HCl	SKB	1 mg/ml	AD	0.2 mg/ml[b]	Physically compatible with little or no loss of either drug by HPLC in 4 hr at 22 °C	1883	C
Heparin sodium		1000 units/ml		2 mg/ml	Drugs injected sequentially into Y-site with no flush between. Immediate precipitation	980	I
	SO	40 units/ml[a]	AD	0.2 mg/ml[a]	Visually compatible for 4 hr at room temperature under fluorescent light	1685	C
Hydromorphone HCl	ES	0.04 mg/ml[a]	AD	0.2 mg/ml[a]	Visually compatible for 4 hr at room temperature under fluorescent light	1685	C
Leucovorin calcium		10 mg/ml		2 mg/ml	Drugs injected sequentially into Y-site with no flush between. No visually apparent precipitate	980	C
Lorazepam	WY	0.1 mg/ml[a]	AD	0.2 mg/ml[a]	Visually compatible for 4 hr at room temperature under fluorescent light	1685	C
Melphalan HCl	BW	0.1 mg/ml[b]	AD	2 mg/ml	Physically compatible with no change in measured turbidity or increase in particle content in 3 hr at 22 °C	1557	C
Methotrexate sodium		25 mg/ml		2 mg/ml	Drugs injected sequentially into Y-site with no flush between. No visually apparent precipitate	980	C
		30 mg/ml	FA	0.4 mg/ml[a]	Visually compatible for 4 hr at room temperature	1788	C
Methylprednisolone sodium succinate	UP	0.5 mg/ml[a]	AD	0.2 mg/ml[a]	Visually compatible for 4 hr at room temperature under fluorescent light	1685	C
Metoclopramide HCl		5 mg/ml		2 mg/ml	Drugs injected sequentially into Y-site with no flush between. No visually apparent precipitate	980	C
	RB	2.5 mg/ml[a]	AD	0.2 mg/ml[a]	Visually compatible for 4 hr at room temperature under fluorescent light	1685	C
Mitomycin		0.5 mg/ml		2 mg/ml	Drugs injected sequentially into Y-site with no flush between. No visually apparent precipitate	980	C
Morphine sulfate	ES	0.12 mg/ml[a]	AD	0.2 mg/ml[a]	Visually compatible for 4 hr at room temperature under fluorescent light	1685	C
Ondansetron HCl	GL	1 mg/ml[b]	CET	2 mg/ml	Physically compatible for 4 hr at 22 °C	1365	C
	GL	16 to 160 μg/ml		2 mg/ml	Physically compatible when doxorubicin given as 5-min bolus via Y-site	1366	C
Paclitaxel	NCI	1.2 mg/ml[a]		2 mg/ml	Physically compatible with no change in measured turbidity in 4 hr at 22 °C	1528	C
Piperacillin sodium–tazobactam sodium	LE	40 + 5 mg/ml[a]	CET	2 mg/ml	Turbidity forms immediately	1688	I
Prochlorperazine edisylate	SKF	0.5 mg/ml[a]	AD	0.2 mg/ml[a]	Visually compatible for 4 hr at room temperature under fluorescent light	1685	C
Promethazine HCl	WY	2 mg/ml[a]	AD	0.2 mg/ml[a]	Visually compatible for 4 hr at room temperature under fluorescent light	1685	C

Y-Site Injection Compatibility (1:1 Mixture) (Cont.)

Doxorubicin HCl

Drug	Mfr	Conc	Mfr	Conc	Remarks	Ref	C/I
Propofol	ZEN	10 mg/ml	CHI	2 mg/ml	Emulsion broke and oiled out	1916	I
Ranitidine HCl	GL	1 mg/ml[a]	AD	0.2 mg/ml[a]	Visually compatible for 4 hr at room temperature under fluorescent light	1685	C
Sargramostim	IMM	10 μg/ml[b]	CET	2 mg/ml	Physically compatible for 4 hr at 22 °C	1436	C
Sodium bicarbonate		1.4%	FA	0.4 mg/ml[a]	Visually compatible for 2 hr at room temperature	1788	C
Teniposide	BR	0.1 mg/ml[a]	CET	2 mg/ml	Physically compatible with no subvisual haze or particle formation in 4 hr at 23 °C	1725	C
Thiotepa	IMM[d]	1 mg/ml[a]	CHI	2 mg/ml	Physically compatible with no change in measured turbidity or increase in particle content in 4 hr at 23 °C	1861	C
TNA #218 to #226[e]			PH, GEN	2 mg/ml	Damage to emulsion integrity occurs immediately with free oil formation possible	2215	I
TPN #212 to #215[e]			PH	2 mg/ml	Substantial loss of natural subvisual turbidity occurs immediately	2109	I
Vinblastine sulfate		1 mg/ml		2 mg/ml	Drugs injected sequentially into Y-site with no flush between. No visually apparent precipitate	980	C
Vincristine sulfate		1 mg/ml		2 mg/ml	Drugs injected sequentially into Y-site with no flush between. No visually apparent precipitate	980	C
Vinorelbine tartrate	BW	1 mg/ml[b]	CET	2 mg/ml	Physically compatible with no change in measured turbidity or increase in particle content in 4 hr at 22 °C	1558	C

[a]*Tested in dextrose 5% in water.*
[b]*Tested in sodium chloride 0.9%.*
[c]*Tested in bacteriostatic sodium chloride 0.9% preserved with benzyl alcohol 0.9%.*
[d]*Lyophilized formulation tested.*
[e]*Refer to Appendix I for the composition of parenteral nutrition solutions. TNA indicates a 3-in-1 admixture, and TPN indicates a 2-in-1 admixture.*

Additional Compatibility Information

Dacarbazine— No alteration in the ultraviolet/visible spectra was observed when dacarbazine was combined in solution with doxorubicin HCl (492).

Fluorouracil and Heparin— Doxorubicin HCl has been stated to be incompatible with fluorouracil and heparin sodium because of possible precipitate formation (2; 4).

Vincristine— The compatibility of doxorubicin HCl (Farmitalia) 1.4 mg/ml with vincristine sulfate (Lilly) 0.033 mg/ml in three infusion solutions was reported for conditions simulating prolonged infusion of the solution via an implanted device (37 °C) or a pump kept under the clothing (30 °C) as well as at 25 °C. In sodium chloride 0.9% and in dextrose 2.5% in sodium chloride 0.45%, there was no precipitate or color change; the concentrations of both drugs showed a 10% or less loss after 14 days of storage at any of the temperatures. The greatest losses of doxorubicin HCl and vincristine sulfate

were about 10 and 6 to 8%, respectively, in the 37 °C samples (1030).

However, when sodium chloride 0.45% with Ringer's acetate was used as the infusion solution, the stability of both drugs was much worse, probably because of the substantially higher solution pH. At 37 °C, a red-pink precipitate formed after two to three days, with about 40% doxorubicin HCl and 14% vincristine sulfate losses occurring in four days. The lower temperature samples showed 17 to 27% doxorubicin HCl losses in four days, followed by the eventual formation of opalescence in the solutions. Also, the degradation products of doxorubicin adsorbed extensively to the walls of the low density polyethylene–polysiloxane bags (1030).

Increasing the concentration of doxorubicin HCl from 1.4 to 1.88 and 2.37 mg/ml increased the extent of decomposition at 37 °C from 10% at the lowest concentration to 12 and 16%, respectively, after 14 days. Increasing the vincristine sulfate concentration to 0.05 mg/ml did not alter the stability of either drug (1030).

Doxorubicin HCl (Nycomed) was combined with vincristine sulfate (Lilly) in both PVC (Pharmacia-Deltec) and polyisoprene (Infusor, Baxter) infusion reservoirs. The drug solution concentrates were diluted slightly with sodium chloride 0.9% to yield a doxorubicin HCl concentration of 1.67 mg/ml and a vincristine sulfate concentration of 0.036 mg/ml. The reservoirs were stored at 4 °C for seven days. This was followed by incubation for four days at 35 °C to simulate near-body temperature during use. No visible changes occurred, and neither drug sustained any loss by HPLC analysis throughout the course of the study in either reservoir (1874).

Other Information

Aluminum— A darkening of doxorubicin HCl color has been noted when solutions of the drug contact aluminum metal. This change was initially noticed in the first small amount of drug to be injected through a needle with an aluminum hub. When solutions of doxorubicin HCl containing aluminum are allowed to stand, the color becomes much darker than the control. Precipitation may also occur. As a precautionary measure, the author recommended not using any aluminum-containing apparatus for preparing or administering doxorubicin HCl (653).

In another evaluation, stainless steel needles with steel or plastic hubs and pieces of aluminum were emersed in doxorubicin HCl 2 mg/ml in sterile water for injection or sodium chloride 0.9%. After 24 hours, the solutions containing the needles were unchanged in appearance and pH. The solution containing the aluminum was darker in color, and the pH had changed from 4.8 to 5.2. The potency of all solutions remained the same after six hours; but after three days, the solution containing aluminum was down to 91.9% while the others were only down to 94.4%. The authors concluded that doxorubicin HCl does react with aluminum but at a slow rate and without major loss of potency. They recommended not storing the drug in syringes capped with aluminum-hubbed needles but thought that doxorubicin could be injected safely through aluminum-hubbed needles (887).

Ogawa et al. reported that immersion of a needle with an aluminum component in doxorubicin HCl (Adria) 2 mg/ml resulted in a darkening of the solution, with black patches forming on the aluminum in 12 to 24 hours at 24 °C with protection from light (988).

Bacterial Challenge— At a concentration of 0.5 mg/ml in sodium chloride 0.9%, doxorubicin HCl supported the growth of several microorganisms commonly implicated in nosocomial infections, including *Escherichia coli*, *Klebsiella pneumoniae*, *Pseudomonas aeruginosa*, and *Candida albicans*. Therefore, the arbitrary application of an extended expiration date to doxorubicin HCl solutions used in ambulatory pump systems is highly questionable (827).

Inactivation— In the event of spills or leaks, Adria recommends the use of sodium hypochlorite 5% (household bleach) to inactivate doxorubicin HCl (1200).

DOXORUBICIN HCL LIPOSOME INJECTION
AHFS 10:00

Doxil   **Alza**

Products— Doxorubicin HCl liposome injection (Alza) is available as a red translucent liposomal dispersion providing 2 mg/ml of doxorubicin HCl packaged in 10-ml vials (2).

Over 90% of the doxorubicin HCl is provided inside liposome carriers composed of *N*-(carbonyl-methoxypolyethylene glycol 2000)-1,2-distearoyl-*sn*-glycero-3-phosphoethanolamine sodium, 3.19 mg/ml; fully hydrogenated soy phosphatidylcholine, 9.58 mg/ml; and cholesterol, 3.19 mg/ml. The product also contains about 2 mg/ml of ammonium sulfate, histidine as a buffer, hydrochloric acid and/or sodium hydroxide to adjust pH, and sucrose to adjust tonicity (2).

pH— Approximately 6.5 (2).

Administration— Doxorubicin HCl liposome injection is administered intravenously, usually over 30 minutes and only after dilution in 250 ml of dextrose 5% in water. The product should not be administered as a bolus injection, as the undiluted dispersion, as a rapid infusion, or by other routes. Extravasation should be avoided; the drug is extremely irritating to tissues. The manufacturer recommends the use of protective gloves during dose preparation (2).

The functional properties of a drug incorporated into a liposomal dispersion like this one may differ substantially from the functional properties of the conventional aqueous formulation (2). CAUTION: Care should be taken to ensure that the correct drug product, dose, and administration procedures are used and that no confusion with other products occurs.

Stability— Intact vials of doxorubicin HCl liposome injection should be stored under refrigeration at 2 to 8 °C. Freezing should be avoided because prolonged freezing may adversely affect liposomal products. However, short-term freezing (one month) did not adversely affect this product (2).

Filtration— Doxorubicin HCl liposome injection is a liposomal dispersion; filtration, including inline filtration, should not be performed (2).

Compatibility Information

Y-Site Injection Compatibility (1:1 Mixture)

Doxorubicin HCl liposome injection

Drug	Mfr	Conc	Mfr	Conc	Remarks	Ref	C/I
Acyclovir sodium	GW	7 mg/ml[a]	SEQ	0.4 mg/ml[a]	Physically compatible with little or no change in measured turbidity and no increase in particle content in 4 hr at 23 °C	2087	C
Allopurinol sodium	BW	3 mg/ml[a]	SEQ	0.4 mg/ml[a]	Physically compatible with little or no change in measured turbidity and no increase in particle content in 4 hr at 23 °C	2087	C
Aminophylline	AB	2.5 mg/ml[a]	SEQ	0.4 mg/ml[a]	Physically compatible with little or no change in measured turbidity and no increase in particle content in 4 hr at 23 °C	2087	C
Amphotericin B	APC	0.6 mg/ml[a]	SEQ	0.4 mg/ml[a]	Fivefold increase in measured particulates in 4 hours	2087	I
Amphotericin B cholesteryl sulfate complex	SEQ	0.83 mg/ml[a]	SEQ	2 mg/ml[a]	Gross precipitate forms	2117	I
Ampicillin sodium	SKB	20 mg/ml[b]	SEQ	0.4 mg/ml[a]	Physically compatible with little or no change in measured turbidity and no increase in particle content in 4 hr at 23 °C	2087	C
Aztreonam	SQ	40 mg/ml[a]	SEQ	0.4 mg/ml[a]	Physically compatible with little or no change in measured turbidity and no increase in particle content in 4 hr at 23 °C	2087	C
Bleomycin sulfate	MJ	1 unit/ml[b]	SEQ	0.4 mg/ml[a]	Physically compatible with little or no change in measured turbidity and no increase in particle content in 4 hr at 23 °C	2087	C
Buprenorphine HCl	RKC	0.04 mg/ml[a]	SEQ	0.4 mg/ml[a]	Partial loss of measured natural turbidity	2087	I
Butorphanol tartrate	APC	0.04 mg/ml[a]	SEQ	0.4 mg/ml[a]	Physically compatible with little or no change in measured turbidity and no increase in particle content in 4 hr at 23 °C	2087	C
Calcium gluconate	AB	40 mg/ml[a]	SEQ	0.4 mg/ml[a]	Physically compatible with little or no change in measured turbidity and no increase in particle content in 4 hr at 23 °C	2087	C
Carboplatin	BR	5 mg/ml[a]	SEQ	0.4 mg/ml[a]	Physically compatible with little or no change in measured turbidity and no increase in particle content in 4 hr at 23 °C	2087	C
Cefazolin sodium	SKB	20 mg/ml[a]	SEQ	0.4 mg/ml[a]	Physically compatible with little or no change in measured turbidity and no increase in particle content in 4 hr at 23 °C	2087	C
Cefepime HCl	BMS	20 mg/ml[a]	SEQ	0.4 mg/ml[a]	Physically compatible with little or no change in measured turbidity and no increase in particle content in 4 hr at 23 °C	2087	C

Y-Site Injection Compatibility (1:1 Mixture) (Cont.)

Doxorubicin HCl liposome injection

Drug	Mfr	Conc	Mfr	Conc	Remarks	Ref	C/I
Cefoperazone sodium	RR	40 mg/ml[a]	SEQ	0.4 mg/ml[a]	Partial loss of measured natural turbidity	2087	I
Cefoxitin sodium	ME	20 mg/ml[a]	SEQ	0.4 mg/ml[a]	Physically compatible with little or no change in measured turbidity and no increase in particle content in 4 hr at 23 °C	2087	C
Ceftazidime	SKB[c]	40 mg/ml[a]	SEQ	0.4 mg/ml[a]	Partial loss of measured natural turbidity	2087	I
Ceftizoxime sodium	FUJ	20 mg/ml[a]	SEQ	0.4 mg/ml[a]	Physically compatible with little or no change in measured turbidity and no increase in particle content in 4 hr at 23 °C	2087	C
Ceftriaxone sodium	RC	20 mg/ml[a]	SEQ	0.4 mg/ml[a]	Physically compatible with little or no change in measured turbidity and no increase in particle content in 4 hr at 23 °C	2087	C
Chlorpromazine HCl	ES	2 mg/ml[a]	SEQ	0.4 mg/ml[a]	Physically compatible with little or no change in measured turbidity and no increase in particle content in 4 hr at 23 °C	2087	C
Cimetidine HCl	SKB	12 mg/ml[a]	SEQ	0.4 mg/ml[a]	Physically compatible with little or no change in measured turbidity and no increase in particle content in 4 hr at 23 °C	2087	C
Ciprofloxacin	BAY	1 mg/ml[a]	SEQ	0.4 mg/ml[a]	Physically compatible with little or no change in measured turbidity and no increase in particle content in 4 hr at 23 °C	2087	C
Cisplatin	BR	1 mg/ml	SEQ	0.4 mg/ml[a]	Physically compatible with little or no change in measured turbidity and no increase in particle content in 4 hr at 23 °C	2087	C
Clindamycin phosphate	AST	10 mg/ml[a]	SEQ	0.4 mg/ml[a]	Physically compatible with little or no change in measured turbidity and no increase in particle content in 4 hr at 23 °C	2087	C
Cyclophosphamide	MJ	10 mg/ml[a]	SEQ	0.4 mg/ml[a]	Physically compatible with little or no change in measured turbidity and no increase in particle content in 4 hr at 23 °C	2087	C
Cytarabine	CHI	50 mg/ml	SEQ	0.4 mg/ml[a]	Physically compatible with little or no change in measured turbidity and no increase in particle content in 4 hr at 23 °C	2087	C
Dexamethasone sodium phosphate	ES	2 mg/ml[a]	SEQ	0.4 mg/ml[a]	Physically compatible with little or no change in measured turbidity and no increase in particle content in 4 hr at 23 °C	2087	C
Diphenhydramine HCl	SCN	2 mg/ml[a]	SEQ	0.4 mg/ml[a]	Physically compatible with little or no change in measured turbidity and no increase in particle content in 4 hr at 23 °C	2087	C

Y-Site Injection Compatibility (1:1 Mixture) (Cont.)

Doxorubicin HCl liposome injection

Drug	Mfr	Conc	Mfr	Conc	Remarks	Ref	C/I
Dobutamine HCl	BA	4 mg/ml[a]	SEQ	0.4 mg/ml[a]	Physically compatible with little or no change in measured turbidity and no increase in particle content in 4 hr at 23 °C	2087	**C**
Docetaxel	RP	2 mg/ml[a]	SEQ	0.4 mg/ml[a]	Partial loss of measured natural turbidity	2087	**I**
Dopamine HCl	AB	3.2 mg/ml[a]	SEQ	0.4 mg/ml[a]	Physically compatible with little or no change in measured turbidity and no increase in particle content in 4 hr at 23 °C	2087	**C**
Droperidol	AST	0.4 mg/ml[a]	SEQ	0.4 mg/ml[a]	Physically compatible with little or no change in measured turbidity and no increase in particle content in 4 hr at 23 °C	2087	**C**
Enalaprilat	MSD	0.1 mg/ml[a]	SEQ	0.4 mg/ml[a]	Physically compatible with little or no change in measured turbidity and no increase in particle content in 4 hr at 23 °C	2087	**C**
Etoposide	BR	0.4 mg/ml[a]	SEQ	0.4 mg/ml[a]	Physically compatible with little or no change in measured turbidity and no increase in particle content in 4 hr at 23 °C	2087	**C**
Famotidine	ME	2 mg/ml[a]	SEQ	0.4 mg/ml[a]	Physically compatible with little or no change in measured turbidity and no increase in particle content in 4 hr at 23 °C	2087	**C**
Fluconazole	RR	2 mg/ml	SEQ	0.4 mg/ml[a]	Physically compatible with little or no change in measured turbidity and no increase in particle content in 4 hr at 23 °C	2087	**C**
Fluorouracil	PH	16 mg/ml[a]	SEQ	0.4 mg/ml[a]	Physically compatible with little or no change in measured turbidity and no increase in particle content in 4 hr at 23 °C	2087	**C**
Furosemide	AMR	3 mg/ml[a]	SEQ	0.4 mg/ml[a]	Physically compatible with little or no change in measured turbidity and no increase in particle content in 4 hr at 23 °C	2087	**C**
Ganciclovir sodium	RC	20 mg/ml[a]	SEQ	0.4 mg/ml[a]	Physically compatible with little or no change in measured turbidity and no increase in particle content in 4 hr at 23 °C	2087	**C**
Gentamicin sulfate	ES	5 mg/ml[a]	SEQ	0.4 mg/ml[a]	Physically compatible with little or no change in measured turbidity and no increase in particle content in 4 hr at 23 °C	2087	**C**
Granisetron HCl	SKB	0.05 mg/ml[a]	SEQ	0.4 mg/ml[a]	Physically compatible with little or no change in measured turbidity and no increase in particle content in 4 hr at 23 °C	2087	**C**

Y-Site Injection Compatibility (1:1 Mixture) (Cont.)

Doxorubicin HCl liposome injection

Drug	Mfr	Conc	Mfr	Conc	Remarks	Ref	C/I
Haloperidol lactate	MN	0.2 mg/ml[a]	SEQ	0.4 mg/ml[a]	Physically compatible with little or no change in measured turbidity and no increase in particle content in 4 hr at 23 °C	2087	C
Heparin sodium	ES	1000 units/ml[a]	SEQ	0.4 mg/ml[a]	Physically compatible with little or no change in measured turbidity and no increase in particle content in 4 hr at 23 °C	2087	C
Hydrocortisone sodium succinate	AB	1 mg/ml[a]	SEQ	0.4 mg/ml[a]	Physically compatible with little or no change in measured turbidity and no increase in particle content in 4 hr at 23 °C	2087	C
Hydromorphone HCl	ES	0.5 mg/ml[a]	SEQ	0.4 mg/ml[a]	Physically compatible with little or no change in measured turbidity and no increase in particle content in 4 hr at 23 °C	2087	C
Hydroxyzine HCl	ES	2 mg/ml[a]	SEQ	0.4 mg/ml[a]	10-fold increase in particles $\geqq 10$ μm in 4 hr	2087	I
Ifosfamide	MJ	25 mg/ml[a]	SEQ	0.4 mg/ml[a]	Physically compatible with little or no change in measured turbidity and no increase in particle content in 4 hr at 23 °C	2087	C
Leucovorin calcium	IMM	2 mg/ml[a]	SEQ	0.4 mg/ml[a]	Physically compatible with little or no change in measured turbidity and no increase in particle content in 4 hr at 23 °C	2087	C
Lorazepam	WY	0.1 mg/ml[a]	SEQ	0.4 mg/ml[a]	Physically compatible with little or no change in measured turbidity and no increase in particle content in 4 hr at 23 °C	2087	C
Magnesium sulfate	AST	100 mg/ml[a]	SEQ	0.4 mg/ml[a]	Physically compatible with little or no change in measured turbidity and no increase in particle content in 4 hr at 23 °C	2087	C
Mannitol	BA	15%	SEQ	0.4 mg/ml[a]	Partial loss of measured natural turbidity	2087	I
Meperidine HCl	AST	4 mg/ml[a]	SEQ	0.4 mg/ml[a]	Increase in measured turbidity	2087	I
Mesna	MJ	10 mg/ml[a]	SEQ	0.4 mg/ml[a]	Physically compatible with little or no change in measured turbidity and no increase in particle content in 4 hr at 23 °C	2087	C
Methotrexate sodium	IMM	15 mg/ml[a]	SEQ	0.4 mg/ml[a]	Physically compatible with little or no change in measured turbidity and no increase in particle content in 4 hr at 23 °C	2087	C
Methylprednisolone sodium succinate	UP	5 mg/ml[a]	SEQ	0.4 mg/ml[a]	Physically compatible with little or no change in measured turbidity and no increase in particle content in 4 hr at 23 °C	2087	C
Metoclopramide HCl	GNS	5 mg/ml	SEQ	0.4 mg/ml[a]	Increase in measured turbidity	2087	I

Y-Site Injection Compatibility (1:1 Mixture) (Cont.)

Doxorubicin HCl liposome injection

Drug	*Mfr*	*Conc*	*Mfr*	*Conc*	*Remarks*	*Ref*	*C/I*
Metronidazole	AB	5 mg/ml	SEQ	0.4 mg/ml[a]	Physically compatible with little or no change in measured turbidity and no increase in particle content in 4 hr at 23 °C	2087	**C**
Mitoxantrone HCl	IMM	0.5 mg/ml[a]	SEQ	0.4 mg/ml[a]	Partial loss of measured natural turbidity	2087	**I**
Morphine sulfate	ES	1 mg/ml[a]	SEQ	0.4 mg/ml[a]	Partial loss of measured natural turbidity	2087	**I**
Netilmicin sulfate	SC	5 mg/ml[a]	SEQ	0.4 mg/ml[a]	Physically compatible with little or no change in measured turbidity and no increase in particle content in 4 hr at 23 °C	2087	**C**
Ofloxacin	ORT	4 mg/ml[a]	SEQ	0.4 mg/ml[a]	Increase in measured turbidity	2087	**I**
Ondansetron HCl	CER	1 mg/ml[a]	SEQ	0.4 mg/ml[a]	Physically compatible with little or no change in measured turbidity and no increase in particle content in 4 hr at 23 °C	2087	**C**
Paclitaxel	MJ	0.6 mg/ml[a]	SEQ	0.4 mg/ml[a]	Partial loss of measured natural turbidity	2087	**I**
Piperacillin disodium	LE	40 mg/ml[a]	SEQ	0.4 mg/ml[a]	Physically compatible with little or no change in measured turbidity and no increase in particle content in 4 hr at 23 °C	2087	**C**
Piperacillin sodium–tazobactam sodium	CY	40 + 5 mg/ml[a]	SEQ	0.4 mg/ml[a]	Partial loss of measured natural turbidity	2087	**I**
Potassium chloride	AB	0.1 mEq/ml[a]	SEQ	0.4 mg/ml[a]	Physically compatible with little or no change in measured turbidity and no increase in particle content in 4 hr at 23 °C	2087	**C**
Prochlorperazine edisylate	SO	0.5 mg/ml[a]	SEQ	0.4 mg/ml[a]	Physically compatible with little or no change in measured turbidity and no increase in particle content in 4 hr at 23 °C	2087	**C**
Promethazine HCl	ES	2 mg/ml[a]	SEQ	0.4 mg/ml[a]	Increase in measured turbidity	2087	**I**
Ranitidine HCl	GL	2 mg/ml[a]	SEQ	0.4 mg/ml[a]	Physically compatible with little or no change in measured turbidity and no increase in particle content in 4 hr at 23 °C	2087	**C**
Sodium bicarbonate	AB	1 mEq/ml	SEQ	0.4 mg/ml[a]	Partial loss of measured natural turbidity	2087	**I**
Ticarcillin disodium	SKB	30 mg/ml[a]	SEQ	0.4 mg/ml[a]	Physically compatible with little or no change in measured turbidity and no increase in particle content in 4 hr at 23 °C	2087	**C**
Ticarcillin disodium–clavulanate potassium	SKB	31 mg/ml[a]	SEQ	0.4 mg/ml[a]	Physically compatible with little or no change in measured turbidity and no increase in particle content in 4 hr at 23 °C	2087	**C**
Tobramycin sulfate	AB	5 mg/ml[a]	SEQ	0.4 mg/ml[a]	Physically compatible with little or no change in measured turbidity and no increase in particle content in 4 hr at 23 °C	2087	**C**

Y-Site Injection Compatibility (1:1 Mixture) (Cont.)

Doxorubicin HCl liposome injection

Drug	Mfr	Conc	Mfr	Conc	Remarks	Ref	C/I
Trimethoprim–sulfamethoxazole	ES	0.8 + 4 mg/ml[a]	SEQ	0.4 mg/ml[a]	Physically compatible with little or no change in measured turbidity and no increase in particle content in 4 hr at 23 °C	2087	C
Vancomycin HCl	AB	10 mg/ml[a]	SEQ	0.4 mg/ml[a]	Physically compatible with little or no change in measured turbidity and no increase in particle content in 4 hr at 23 °C	2087	C
Vinblastine sulfate	FAU	0.12 mg/ml[a]	SEQ	0.4 mg/ml[a]	Physically compatible with little or no change in measured turbidity and no increase in particle content in 4 hr at 23 °C	2087	C
Vincristine sulfate	FAU	0.05 mg/ml[a]	SEQ	0.4 mg/ml[a]	Physically compatible with little or no change in measured turbidity and no increase in particle content in 4 hr at 23 °C	2087	C
Vinorelbine tartrate	BW	1 mg/ml[a]	SEQ	0.4 mg/ml[a]	Physically compatible with little or no change in measured turbidity and no increase in particle content in 4 hr at 23 °C	2087	C
Zidovudine	BW	4 mg/ml[a]	SEQ	0.4 mg/ml[a]	Physically compatible with little or no change in measured turbidity and no increase in particle content in 4 hr at 23 °C	2087	C

[a]*Tested in dextrose 5% in water.*
[b]*Tested in sodium chloride 0.9%.*
[c]*Sodium carbonate–containing formulation tested.*

Additional Compatibility Information

Solutions— Doxorubicin HCl liposome injection should be diluted for infusion only with dextrose 5% in water. Other diluents, including those containing a bacteriostatic agent such as benzyl alcohol, should not be used. After dilution in dextrose 5% in water, the admixture should be stored under refrigeration at 2 to 8 °C and administered within 24 hours (2).

Other Drugs— The manufacturer recommends not mixing doxorubicin HCl liposome injection with other drugs (2).

DOXYCYCLINE HYCLATE
AHFS 8:12.24

Vibramycin Intravenous　　　　　　　　**Pfizer**
　　　　　　　　　　　　　　　　　　Elkins-Sinn

Products— Doxycycline hyclate (Pfizer) (doxycycline HCl hemiethanolate hemihydrate) is available in vials containing the equivalent of 100 and 200 mg of doxycycline with 480 and 960 mg of ascorbic acid, respectively. Mannitol is also present in products from some manufacturers (2; 4; 154).

Reconstitute the 100-mg vial with 10 ml and the 200-mg vial with 20 ml of sterile water for injection or other compatible diluent. The resultant solution contains the equivalent of 10 mg/ml of doxycycline. This solution must be further diluted to a concentration of 0.1 to 1 mg/ml with a compatible infusion solution prior to use (2; 4). (See Stability and Additional Compatibility Information.)

pH— The pH range for reconstituted solutions is 1.8 to 3.3 (4).

Osmolality— Doxycycline hyclate 10 mg/ml in sterile water for injection has an osmolality of 507 mOsm/kg (1689). The osmolality of doxycycline hyclate (Elkins-Sinn) 1 mg/ml was determined to be 292 mOsm/kg in dextrose 5% in water and 310 mOsm/kg in sodium chloride 0.9% (1375).

Administration— Doxycycline hyclate is administered by slow intravenous infusion, usually over one to four hours; rapid administration should be avoided. The reconstituted solution should be diluted further with a compatible infusion solution to a concentration of approximately 0.1 to 1 mg/ml. Other parenteral routes are not recommended, and extravasation should be avoided (2; 4).

Stability— Infusion solutions of doxycycline hyclate must be protected from direct sunlight (2).

Doxycycline hyclate 0.1- to 1-mg/ml solutions may be stored for up to 72 hours prior to starting the infusion when kept in the refrigerator and protected from both direct sunlight and artificial light and when diluted in the following infusion solutions:

> Dextrose 5% in water
> Invert sugar 10% in water
> Normosol M in dextrose 5% in water
> Normosol R in dextrose 5% in water
> Plasma-Lyte 56 in dextrose 5%
> Plasma-Lyte 148 in dextrose 5%
> Ringer's injection
> Sodium chloride 0.9%

Infusion must then be completed within 12 hours (2).

Pfizer indicates that its product is stable for 48 hours at 25 °C when diluted to 0.1 to 1 mg/ml in dextrose 5% in water or sodium chloride 0.9% (2). Elkins-Sinn states that its product should have infusion completed within 24 hours when admixed in compatible infusion solutions (4).

Freezing Solutions— The manufacturers state that at a concentration of 10 mg/ml in sterile water for injection, doxycycline hyclate is stable for eight weeks when frozen at −20 °C. Frozen solutions that have been completely thawed should not be heated. Thawed solutions should not be refrozen (2; 4).

Doxycycline hyclate (Pfizer) 10 mg/ml in sterile water for injection retained potency for eight weeks when frozen at −20 °C, as determined by both microbiological and spectrophotometric assays. At a concentration of 1 mg/ml in dextrose 5% in water, doxycycline hyclate also showed no significant decomposition over eight weeks at −20 °C when assayed by either method (310).

Portable Pumps— Stiles et al. evaluated the stability of doxycycline hyclate (Elkins-Sinn) 2 mg/ml in sterile water for injection and sodium chloride 0.9% in 100-ml portable pump reservoirs (Pharmacia Deltec) during simulated administration for 24 hours. The drug solutions were tested by HPLC analysis when administered immediately after preparation and after storage for 24 hours at 5 °C before 24-hour administration. During simulated administration, some reservoirs were kept at 30 °C; others were placed in insulated pouches with frozen (−20 °C) gel packs to keep them chilled below the ambient temperature. Freshly prepared doxycycline hyclate solutions exhibited a 5% or less loss by HPLC with or without the insulated pouch. However, solutions stored for 24 hours at 5 °C maintained adequate stability through six hours only; the presence or absence of the insulated pouch had no consistent effect on drug stability (1779).

Sorption— Doxycycline (Pfizer) 15 mg/L in sodium chloride 0.9% (Travenol) in PVC bags did not exhibit significant sorption to the plastic during one week of storage at room temperature (15 to 20 °C) (536).

In another evaluation, doxycycline (Pfizer) 15 mg/L in sodium chloride 0.9% did not exhibit any loss due to sorption during a seven-hour simulated infusion through an infusion set (Travenol) consisting of a cellulose propionate burette chamber and 170 cm of PVC tubing (606).

The drug was also tested as a simulated infusion over at least one hour by a syringe pump system. A glass syringe on a syringe pump was fitted with 20 cm of polyethylene tubing or 50 cm of Silastic tubing. No loss of drug due to sorption was observed with either tubing (606).

A 25-ml aliquot of the doxycycline (Pfizer) 15 mg/L in sodium chloride 0.9% solution was stored in all-plastic syringes composed of polypropylene barrels and polyethylene plungers for 24 hours at room temperature in the dark. No loss of drug due to sorption was observed (606).

Compatibility Information

Solution Compatibility

Doxycycline hyclate

Solution	Mfr	Mfr	Conc/L	Remarks	Ref	C/I
Dextrose 5% in water	BA[a]	PF	800 mg and 1 g	Visually compatible with 5 to 8% loss by HPLC in 96 hr at 23 °C. 2% loss in 7 days at 4 °C	1928	C
Sodium chloride 0.9%	AB[b]	ES	2 g	5% loss by HPLC for freshly prepared solutions during 24-hr simulated administration at 30 °C via portable pump	1779	C
	BA[a]	PF	800 mg and 1 g	Visually compatible with 8% loss by HPLC in 96 hr at 23 °C. 4% or less loss in 7 days at 4 °C	1928	C

[a]*Tested in PVC containers.*
[b]*Tested in portable pump reservoirs (Pharmacia Deltec).*

Additive Compatibility

Drug	Mfr	Conc/L	Mfr	Conc/L	Test Soln	Remarks	Ref	C/I
				Doxycycline hyclate				
Meropenem	ZEN	1 g	RR	200 mg	NS	Visually compatible for 4 hr at room temperature	1994	**C**
	ZEN	20 g	RR	200 mg	NS	Brown discoloration forms in 1 hr at room temperature	1994	**I**
Ranitidine HCl	GL	100 mg	PF	200 mg	D5W	Physically compatible for 24 hr at ambient temperature under fluorescent light	1151	**C**

[a]Tested in PVC containers.

Drugs in Syringe Compatibility

Drug (in syringe)	Mfr	Amt	Mfr	Amt	Remarks	Ref	C/I
				Doxycycline hyclate			
Doxapram HCl	RB	400 mg/ 20 ml		100 mg/ 5 ml	Physically compatible with 3% doxapram loss in 24 hr	1177	**C**

Y-Site Injection Compatibility (1:1 Mixture)

Drug	Mfr	Conc	Mfr	Conc	Remarks	Ref	C/I
				Doxycycline hyclate			
Acyclovir sodium	BW	5 mg/ml[a]	PF	1 mg/ml[a]	Physically compatible for 4 hr at 25 °C	1157	**C**
Allopurinol sodium	BW	3 mg/ml[b]	ES	1 mg/ml[b]	Small particles form immediately. Hazy brown solution with precipitate develops in 4 hr	1686	**I**
Amifostine	USB	10 mg/ml[a]	LY	1 mg/ml[a]	Physically compatible with no change in measured turbidity or increase in particle content in 4 hr at 23 °C	1845	**C**
Amiodarone HCl	LZ	4 mg/ml[c]	ACC	0.25 mg/ml[c]	Physically compatible for 4 hr at room temperature	1444	**C**
Aztreonam	SQ	40 mg/ml[a]	ES	1 mg/ml[a]	Physically compatible with no subvisual haze or particle formation in 4 hr at 23 °C	1758	**C**
Cisatracurium besylate	GW	0.1, 2, 5 mg/ml[a]	FUJ	1 mg/ml[a]	Physically compatible with no change in measured turbidity or increase in particle content in 4 hr at 23 °C	2074	**C**
Cyclophosphamide	MJ	20 mg/ml[a]	ES	1 mg/ml[a]	Physically compatible for 4 hr at 25 °C	1194	**C**
Diltiazem HCl	MMD	5 mg/ml	RR	1 and 10 mg/ml[b]	Visually compatible	1807	**C**
Docetaxel	RPR	0.9 mg/ml[a]	FUJ	1 mg/ml[a]	Physically compatible with no change in measured turbidity or increase in particle content in 4 hr at 23 °C	2224	**C**
Etoposide phosphate	BR	5 mg/ml[a]	FUJ	1 mg/ml[a]	Physically compatible with no change in measured turbidity or increase in particle content in 4 hr at 23 °C	2218	**C**
Filgrastim	AMG	30 μg/ml[a]	ES	1 mg/ml[a]	Physically compatible with no change in measured turbidity or increase in particle content in 4 hr at 22 °C	1687	**C**

Y-Site Injection Compatibility (1:1 Mixture) (Cont.)

			Doxycycline hyclate				
Drug	*Mfr*	*Conc*	*Mfr*	*Conc*	*Remarks*	*Ref*	*C/I*
Fludarabine phosphate	BX	1 mg/ml[a]	ES	1 mg/ml[a]	Physically compatible for 4 hr at room temperature under fluorescent light	1439	C
Gemcitabine HCl	LI	10 mg/ml[b]	FUJ	1 mg/ml[b]	Physically compatible with no change in measured turbidity or increase in particle content in 4 hr at 23 °C	2226	C
Granisetron HCl	SKB	0.05 mg/ml[a]	LY	1 mg/ml[a]	Physically compatible with no change in measured turbidity or increase in particle content in 4 hr at 23 °C	2000	C
Heparin sodium	TR	50 units/ml	ES	1 mg/ml[a]	Visually incompatible within 6 hr at 25 °C	1793	I
Hetastarch	DCC	6%	LY	1 mg/ml[a]	Physically compatible for 4 hr at room temperature by visual examination	1313	C
	DCC	6%	LY	1 mg/ml[a]	White particle in one of five vials. No evidence of incompatibility during Y-site infusion	1315	?
Hydromorphone HCl	WY	0.2 mg/ml[a]	ES	1 mg/ml[a]	Physically compatible for at least 4 hr at 25 °C under fluorescent light	987	C
Magnesium sulfate	IX	16.7, 33.3, 66.7, 100 mg/ml[a]	PF	1 mg/ml	Physically compatible for at least 4 hr at 32 °C	813	C
Melphalan HCl	BW	0.1 mg/ml[b]	LY	1 mg/ml[b]	Physically compatible with no change in measured turbidity or increase in particle content in 3 hr at 22 °C	1557	C
Meperidine HCl	WY	10 mg/ml[a]	ES	1 mg/ml[a]	Physically compatible for at least 4 hr at 25 °C under fluorescent light	987	C
Meropenem	ZEN	1 mg/ml[b]	RR	1 mg/ml[d]	Visually compatible for 4 hr at room temperature	1994	C
	ZEN	50 mg/ml[b]	RR	1 mg/ml[d]	Amber discoloration forms within 30 min	1994	I
Morphine sulfate	WI	1 mg/ml[a]	ES	1 mg/ml[a]	Physically compatible for at least 4 hr at 25 °C under fluorescent light	987	C
Ondansetron HCl	GL	1 mg/ml[b]	ES	1 mg/ml[a]	Physically compatible for 4 hr at 22 °C	1365	C
Perphenazine	SC	0.02 mg/ml[a]	ES	1 mg/ml[a]	Physically compatible for 4 hr at 25 °C	1155	C
Piperacillin sodium–tazobactam sodium	LE	40 + 5 mg/ml[a]	ES	1 mg/ml[a]	Heavy white turbidity forms immediately	1688	I
Propofol	ZEN	10 mg/ml	LY	1 mg/ml[a]	Physically compatible for 1 hr at 23 °C with no increase in particle content	2066	C
Remifentanil HCl	GW	0.025 and 0.25 mg/ml[b]	FUJ	1 mg/ml[a]	Physically compatible with no change in measured turbidity or increase in particle content in 4 hr at 23 °C	2075	C
Sargramostim	IMM	10 µg/ml[b]	LY	1 mg/ml[b]	Physically compatible for 4 hr at 22 °C	1436	C
Tacrolimus	FUJ	1 mg/ml[b]	RR	5 mg/ml[a]	Visually compatible for 24 hr at 25 °C	1630	C
Teniposide	BR	0.1 mg/ml[a]	LY	1 mg/ml[a]	Physically compatible with no subvisual haze or particle formation in 4 hr at 23 °C	1725	C
Theophylline	TR	4 mg/ml	ES	1 mg/ml[a]	Visually compatible for 6 hr at 25 °C	1793	C

Y-Site Injection Compatibility (1:1 Mixture) (Cont.)

Doxycycline hyclate

Drug	Mfr	Conc	Mfr	Conc	Remarks	Ref	C/I
Thiotepa	IMM[e]	1 mg/ml[a]	LY	1 mg/ml[a]	Physically compatible with no change in measured turbidity or increase in particle content in 4 hr at 23 °C	1861	C
TNA #218 to #226[f]			FUJ	1 mg/ml[a]	Damage to emulsion integrity occurs immediately with free oil formation possible	2215	I
TPN #61[f]		[g]	PF	10 mg/ml[h]	Physically compatible	987	C
		[i]	PF	60 mg/6 ml[h]	Physically compatible	987	C
TPN #212 to #215[f]			LY	1 mg/ml[a]	Physically compatible with no change in measured turbidity or increase in particle content in 4 hr at 23 °C	2109	C
Vinorelbine tartrate	BW	1 mg/ml[b]	ES	1 mg/ml[b]	Physically compatible with no change in measured turbidity or increase in particle content in 4 hr at 22 °C	1558	C

[a]*Tested in dextrose 5% in water.*
[b]*Tested in sodium chloride 0.9%.*
[c]*Tested in both dextrose 5% in water and sodium chloride 0.9%.*
[d]*Tested in sterile water for injection.*
[e]*Lyophilized formulation tested.*
[f]*Refer to Appendix I for the composition of parenteral nutrition solutions. TNA indicates a 3-in-1 admixture, and TPN indicates a 2-in-1 admixture.*
[g]*Run at 21 ml/hr.*
[h]*Given over 30 minutes by syringe pump.*
[i]*Run at 94 ml/hr.*

Additional Compatibility Information

Infusion Solutions— When protected from direct sunlight, the Elkins-Sinn product of doxycycline hyclate at concentrations of 0.1 to 1 mg/ml must be completely infused within 24 hours of reconstitution to ensure adequate stability in the following infusion solutions (4):

Dextrose 5% in water
Invert sugar 10% in water
Normosol M in dextrose 5% in water
Normosol R in dextrose 5% in water
Plasma-Lyte 56 in dextrose 5%
Plasma-Lyte 148 in dextrose 5%
Ringer's injection
Sodium chloride 0.9%

The Roerig product is stable at these concentrations for 48 hours at 25 °C in dextrose 5% in water and sodium chloride 0.9%. However, to ensure stability of admixtures in the other infusion solutions listed above, infusion must be completed within 12 hours (2). When stored under refrigeration and protected from light, doxycycline hyclate is stable in these same solutions for 72 hours (2; 4).

At a concentration of 0.1 to 1.0 mg/ml in Ringer's injection, lactated, or dextrose 5% in Ringer's injection, lactated, and with protection from direct sunlight, infusion of doxycycline hyclate (Roerig and Elkins-Sinn) must be completed within six hours after constitution to ensure adequate stability (2; 4).

Riboflavin— In vitro testing of riboflavin-5′-phosphate at a concentration of 0.1% with doxycycline HCl 0.025% in sterile distilled water showed significant reduction in antibiotic activity in one hour at 25 °C (314).

Acid-Sensitive Additives— Because of the acidity of the solution, doxycycline hyclate may precipitate the free acids of barbiturate salts and sulfonamide derivatives. It may also adversely affect the stability of acid-labile additives such as erythromycin lactobionate, penicillin G potassium, oxacillin sodium, methicillin sodium, and nafcillin sodium (6; 20; 22; 27).

DROPERIDOL
AHFS 28:24.92

Inapsine   **Taylor**

Products— Droperidol is available from various manufacturers in 1- and 2-ml ampuls and 2-, 5-, and 10-ml vials (29; 154). Each milliliter of solution contains droperidol 2.5 mg with lactic acid to adjust the pH. Multiple-dose vials contain methylparaben and propylparaben as preservatives. Single-dose ampuls and vials do not contain preservatives (4).

pH— From 3 to 3.8 (1-7/98; 4).

Osmolality— The osmolality of droperidol 2.5 mg/ml was determined to be 16 mOsm/kg (1233).

Administration— Droperidol may be administered intramuscularly or slowly intravenously (1-7/98; 4). Intravenous infusion has been used in high-risk patients (4).

Stability— Intact ampuls and vials of droperidol should be stored at controlled room temperature and protected from light (1-7/98; 4).

Syringes— The stability of droperidol 2.5 mg/ml repackaged in polypropylene syringes was evaluated by spectrophotometric and potentiometric methods. Little or no change in concentration was found after four weeks of storage at room temperature not exposed to direct light (2164).

Droperidol (American Regent) 1.25 mg/ml in sodium chloride injection 0.9% packaged in polypropylene syringes (Sherwood) was physically stable and exhibited little or no loss by stability-indicating HPLC analysis in 24 hours stored at 23 °C. Under refrigeration at 4 °C, droperidol precipitated within four hours (2199).

Sorption— Storage of droperidol (Janssen) 20 mg/L in PVC containers of dextrose 5% in water and sodium chloride 0.9% for seven days at 27 °C resulted in no apparent drug loss due to sorption. In fact, small increases in the droperidol concentration occurred due to permeation and evaporation of water (750).

When Ringer's injection, lactated, in PVC containers was the diluent for the 20-mg/L dilution, however, the droperidol concentration only remained constant for 24 hours at 27 °C. By 48 hours, a 15% drug loss had occurred; in seven days, a 25% loss was observed. The authors attributed the drug loss to sorption to the PVC bags. The 24-hour delay was believed to result from the use of new evacuated PVC bags that were subsequently filled for the tests, causing a delayed initial hydration of the plastic. Presumably, this sorption phenomenon can occur more rapidly if commercially prepared PVC bags of Ringer's injection, lactated, with well-hydrated plastic are used to prepare the admixture (750).

Compatibility Information

Solution Compatibility

Droperidol

Solution	Mfr	Mfr	Conc/L	Remarks	Ref	C/I
Dextrose 5% in water	AB[a], TR[b]	JN	20 mg	Physically compatible and chemically stable with no drug loss for 7 days at 27 °C	750	C
Ringer's injection, lactated	TR[a]	JN	20 mg	Physically compatible and chemically stable with no drug loss for 7 days at 27 °C	750	C
	TR[b]	JN	20 mg	Physically compatible and chemically stable with no drug loss for 24 hr at 27 °C. 15% loss in 48 hr attributed to sorption. See Sorption section	750	C
Sodium chloride 0.9%	AB[a]	JN	20 mg	Physically compatible with about 5% drug loss in 7 days at 27 °C	750	C
	TR[b]	JN	20 mg	Physically compatible and chemically stable with no drug loss for 7 days at 27 °C	750	C

[a]Tested in glass containers.
[b]Tested in PVC containers.

Drugs in Syringe Compatibility

Droperidol

Drug (in syringe)	Mfr	Amt	Mfr	Amt	Remarks	Ref	C/I
Atropine sulfate	ST	0.4 mg/ 1 ml	MN	2.5 mg/ 1 ml	Physically compatible for at least 15 min	326	C
Bleomycin sulfate		1.5 units/ 0.5 ml		1.25 mg/ 0.5 ml	Physically compatible for 5 min at room temperature followed by 8 min of centrifugation	980	C

Drugs in Syringe Compatibility (Cont.)

Droperidol

Drug (in syringe)	Mfr	Amt	Mfr	Amt	Remarks	Ref	C/I
Butorphanol tartrate	BR	4 mg/ 2 ml	MN	5 mg/ 2 ml	Physically compatible both macroscopically and microscopically for 30 min at room temperature	566	C
Chlorpromazine HCl	PO	50 mg/ 2 ml	MN	2.5 mg/ 1 ml	Physically compatible for at least 15 min	326	C
Cimetidine HCl	SKF	300 mg/ 2 ml	JN	5 mg/ 2 ml	Physically compatible for 4 hr at 25 °C	25	C
Cisplatin		0.5 mg/ 0.5 ml		1.25 mg/ 0.5 ml	Physically compatible for 5 min at room temperature followed by 8 min of centrifugation	980	C
Cyclophosphamide		10 mg/ 0.5 ml		1.25 mg/ 0.5 ml	Physically compatible for 5 min at room temperature followed by 8 min of centrifugation	980	C
Dimenhydrinate	HR	50 mg/ 1 ml	MN	2.5 mg/ 1 ml	Physically compatible for at least 15 min	326	C
Diphenhydramine HCl	PD	50 mg/ 1 ml	MN	2.5 mg/ 1 ml	Physically compatible for at least 15 min	326	C
Doxorubicin HCl		1 mg/ 0.5 ml		1.25 mg/ 0.5 ml	Physically compatible for 5 min at room temperature followed by 8 min of centrifugation	980	C
Fentanyl citrate	MN	0.05 mg/ 1 ml	MN	2.5 mg/ 1 ml	Physically compatible for at least 15 min	326	C
Fluorouracil		25 mg/ 0.5 ml		1.25 mg/ 0.5 ml	Immediate precipitation	980	I
Furosemide		5 mg/ 0.5 ml		1.25 mg/ 0.5 ml	Immediate precipitation	980	I
Glycopyrrolate	RB	0.2 mg/ 1 ml	MN	2.5 mg/ 1 ml	Physically compatible and pH in stability range for glycopyrrolate for 48 hr at 25 °C	331	C
	RB	0.2 mg/ 1 ml	MN	5 mg/ 2 ml	Physically compatible and pH in stability range for glycopyrrolate for 48 hr at 25 °C	331	C
	RB	0.4 mg/ 2 ml	MN	2.5 mg/ 1 ml	Physically compatible and pH in stability range for glycopyrrolate for 48 hr at 25 °C	331	C
Heparin sodium		500 units/ 0.5 ml		1.25 mg/ 0.5 ml	Immediate precipitation	980	I
		2500 units/ 1 ml		5 mg/ 2 ml	Turbidity or precipitate forms within 5 min	1053	I
Hydroxyzine HCl	PF	50 mg/ 1 ml	MN	2.5 mg/ 1 ml	Physically compatible for at least 15 min	326	C
Leucovorin calcium		5 mg/ 0.5 ml		1.25 mg/ 0.5 ml	Immediate precipitation	980	I
Meperidine HCl	WI	50 mg/ 1 ml	MN	2.5 mg/ 1 ml	Physically compatible for at least 15 min	326	C
Methotrexate sodium		12.5 mg/ 0.5 ml		1.25 mg/ 0.5 ml	Immediate precipitation	980	I
Metoclopramide HCl	NO	10 mg/ 2 ml	MN	2.5 mg/ 1 ml	Physically compatible both macroscopically and microscopically for 15 min at room temperature	565	C

Drugs in Syringe Compatibility (Cont.)

Droperidol

Drug (in syringe)	Mfr	Amt	Mfr	Amt	Remarks	Ref	C/I
		2.5 mg/ 0.5 ml		1.25 mg/ 0.5 ml	Physically compatible for 5 min at room temperature followed by 8 min of centrifugation	980	C
Midazolam HCl	RC	5 mg/ 1 ml	JN	2.5 mg/ 1 ml	Physically compatible for 4 hr at 25 °C under fluorescent light	1145	C
Mitomycin		0.25 mg/ 0.5 ml		1.25 mg/ 0.5 ml	Physically compatible for 5 min at room temperature followed by 8 min of centrifugation	980	C
Morphine sulfate	ST	15 mg/ 1 ml	MN	2.5 mg/ 1 ml	Physically compatible for at least 15 min	326	C
Nalbuphine HCl	EN	5 mg/ 0.5 ml	JN	5 mg/ 2 ml	Physically compatible for 36 hr at 27 °C	762	C
	EN	10 mg/ 1 ml	JN	2.5 mg/ 1 ml	Physically compatible for 36 hr at 27 °C	762	C
	EN	5 mg/ 0.5 ml	JN	2.5 mg/ 1 ml	Physically compatible for 36 hr at 27 °C	762	C
	DU	10 mg/ 1 ml	JN	5 mg/ 2 ml	Physically compatible for 48 hr	128	C
	DU	20 mg/ 1 ml	JN	5 mg/ 2 ml	Physically compatible for 48 hr	128	C
Ondansetron HCl	GW	1 mg/ml[a]	AMR	1.25 mg/ ml[a]	Droperidol precipitates in less than 4 hr at 4 °C. At 23 °C, little or no loss of either drug occurs by HPLC in 8 hr, but droperidol precipitates after that time	2199	I
Pentazocine lactate	WI	30 mg/ 1 ml	MN	2.5 mg/ 1 ml	Physically compatible for at least 15 min	326	C
Pentobarbital sodium	AB	50 mg/ 1 ml	MN	2.5 mg/ 1 ml	Physically incompatible within 15 min	326	I
Perphenazine	SC	5 mg/ 1 ml	MN	5 mg/ 2 ml	Physically compatible both macroscopically and microscopically for 30 min at room temperature	566	C
Prochlorperazine edisylate	PO	5 mg/ 1 ml	MN	2.5 mg/ 1 ml	Physically compatible for at least 15 min	326	C
Promazine HCl	WY	50 mg/ 1 ml	MN	2.5 mg/ 1 ml	Physically compatible for at least 15 min	326	C
Promethazine HCl	PO	50 mg/ 2 ml	MN	2.5 mg/ 1 ml	Physically compatible for at least 15 min	326	C
Scopolamine HBr	ST	0.4 mg/ 1 ml	MN	2.5 mg/ 1 ml	Physically compatible for at least 15 min	326	C
Vinblastine sulfate		0.5 mg/ 0.5 ml		1.25 mg/ 0.5 ml	Physically compatible for 5 min at room temperature followed by 8 min of centrifugation	980	C
Vincristine sulfate		0.5 mg/ 0.5 ml		1.25 mg/ 0.5 ml	Physically compatible for 5 min at room temperature followed by 8 min of centrifugation	980	C

[a]Tested in sodium chloride 0.9%.

Y-Site Injection Compatibility (1:1 Mixture)

Drug	Mfr	Conc	Mfr	Conc	Remarks	Ref	C/I
			Droperidol				
Allopurinol sodium	BW	3 mg/ml[b]	JN	0.4 mg/ml[b]	Heavy turbidity with particles forms immediately	1686	I
Amifostine	USB	10 mg/ml[a]	JN	0.4 mg/ml[a]	Physically compatible with no change in measured turbidity or increase in particle content in 4 hr at 23 °C	1845	C
Amphotericin B cholesteryl sulfate complex	SEQ	0.83 mg/ml[a]	AST	2.5 mg/ml	Gross precipitate forms	2117	I
Aztreonam	SQ	40 mg/ml[a]	JN	0.4 mg/ml[a]	Physically compatible with no subvisual haze or particle formation in 4 hr at 23 °C	1758	C
Bleomycin sulfate		3 units/ml		2.5 mg/ml	Drugs injected sequentially into Y-site with no flush between. No visually apparent precipitate	980	C
Cefepime HCl	BR	20 mg/ml[a]	JN	0.4 mg/ml[a]	Haze forms immediately and becomes flocculent precipitate in 4 hr	1689	I
Cisatracurium besylate	GW	0.1, 2, 5 mg/ml[a]	AB	2.5 mg/ml	Physically compatible with no change in measured turbidity or increase in particle content in 4 hr at 23 °C	2074	C
Cladribine	ORT	0.015[b] and 0.5[c] mg/ml	JN	0.4 mg/ml[b]	Physically compatible with no change in measured turbidity or increase in particle content in 4 hr at 23 °C	1969	C
Cisplatin		1 mg/ml		2.5 mg/ml	Drugs injected sequentially into Y-site with no flush between. No visually apparent precipitate	980	C
	BR	1 mg/ml	JN	20 μg/ml[a]	Visually compatible for 4 hr at room temperature under fluorescent light	1685	C
Cyclophosphamide		20 mg/ml		2.5 mg/ml	Drugs injected sequentially into Y-site with no flush between. No visually apparent precipitate	980	C
	MJ	10 mg/ml[a]	JN	20 μg/ml[a]	Visually compatible for 4 hr at room temperature under fluorescent light	1685	C
Cytarabine	UP	50 mg/ml	JN	20 μg/ml[a]	Visually compatible for 4 hr at room temperature under fluorescent light	1685	C
Docetaxel	RPR	0.9 mg/ml[a]	AST	0.4 mg/ml[a]	Physically compatible with no change in measured turbidity or increase in particle content in 4 hr at 23 °C	2224	C
Doxorubicin HCl		2 mg/ml		2.5 mg/ml	Drugs injected sequentially into Y-site with no flush between. No visually apparent precipitate	980	C
	AD	0.2 mg/ml[a]	JN	20 μg/ml[a]	Visually compatible for 4 hr at room temperature under fluorescent light	1685	C
Doxorubicin HCl liposome injection	SEQ	0.4 mg/ml[a]	AST	0.4 mg/ml[a]	Physically compatible with little or no change in measured turbidity and no increase in particle content in 4 hr at 23 °C	2087	C
Etoposide phosphate	BR	5 mg/ml[a]	AST	0.4 mg/ml[a]	Physically compatible with no change in measured turbidity or increase in particle content in 4 hr at 23 °C	2218	C
Famotidine	ME	2 mg/ml[b]		0.4 mg/ml[a]	Visually compatible for 4 hr at 22 °C	1936	C

Y-Site Injection Compatibility (1:1 Mixture) (Cont.)

Drug	Mfr	Conc	Mfr	Conc	Remarks	Ref	C/I
				Droperidol			
Filgrastim	AMG	30 µg/ml[a]	JN	0.4 mg/ml[a]	Physically compatible with no change in measured turbidity or increase in particle content in 4 hr at 22 °C	1687	C
Fluconazole	RR	2 mg/ml	DU	2.5 mg/ml	Physically compatible for 24 hr at 25 °C	1407	C
Fludarabine phosphate	BX	1 mg/ml[a]	JN	0.4 mg/ml[a]	Physically compatible for 4 hr at room temperature under fluorescent light	1439	C
Fluorouracil		50 mg/ml		2.5 mg/ml	Drugs injected sequentially into Y-site with no flush between. Immediate precipitation	980	I
Foscarnet sodium	AST	24 mg/ml	QU	2.5 mg/ml	Delayed formation of fine yellow precipitate	1335	I
Furosemide		10 mg/ml		2.5 mg/ml	Drugs injected sequentially into Y-site with no flush between. Immediate precipitation	980	I
		10 mg/ml		2.5 mg/ml	Precipitate forms	977	I
Gemcitabine HCl	LI	10 mg/ml[b]	AST	0.4 mg/ml[b]	Physically compatible with no change in measured turbidity or increase in particle content in 4 hr at 23 °C	2226	C
Granisetron HCl	SKB	0.05 mg/ml[a]	AB	0.4 mg/ml[a]	Physically compatible with no change in measured turbidity or increase in particle content in 4 hr at 23 °C	2000	C
Heparin sodium		1000 units/ml		2.5 mg/ml	Drugs injected sequentially into Y-site with no flush between. Immediate precipitation	980	I
		50 units/ml/min[b]	JN	5 mg/2 ml[d]	White turbidity	1053	I
	UP	1000 units/L[e]	CR	1.25 mg/ml	Physically compatible for at least 4 hr at room temperature by visual and microscopic examination	534	C
Hydrocortisone sodium succinate	UP	10 mg/L[e]	CR	1.25 mg/ml	Physically compatible for at least 4 hr at room temperature by visual and microscopic examination	534	C
Idarubicin HCl	AD	1 mg/ml[b]	AMR	0.04[a] and 2.5 mg/ml	Visually compatible for 24 hr at 25 °C	1525	C
Leucovorin calcium		10 mg/ml		2.5 mg/ml	Drugs injected sequentially into Y-site with no flush between. Immediate precipitation	980	I
Melphalan HCl	BW	0.1 mg/ml[b]	JN	0.4 mg/ml[b]	Physically compatible with no change in measured turbidity or increase in particle content in 3 hr at 22 °C	1557	C
Meperidine HCl	AB	10 mg/ml	AMR	2.5 mg/ml[a]	Physically compatible for 4 hr at 25 °C	1397	C
Methotrexate sodium		25 mg/ml		2.5 mg/ml	Precipitate forms	977	I
		25 mg/ml		2.5 mg/ml	Drugs injected sequentially into Y-site with no flush between. Immediate precipitation	980	I
	AD	15 mg/ml[f]	JN	20 µg/ml[a]	Visually compatible for 4 hr at room temperature under fluorescent light	1685	C

Y-Site Injection Compatibility (1:1 Mixture) (Cont.)

Droperidol

Drug	Mfr	Conc	Mfr	Conc	Remarks	Ref	C/I
Metoclopramide HCl		5 mg/ml		2.5 mg/ml	Drugs injected sequentially into Y-site with no flush between. No visually apparent precipitate	980	C
Mitomycin		0.5 mg/ml		2.5 mg/ml	Drugs injected sequentially into Y-site with no flush between. No visually apparent precipitate	980	C
Nafcillin sodium	WY	33 mg/ml[b]		2.5 mg/ml	Precipitate forms, probably free nafcillin	547	I
Ondansetron HCl	GL	1 mg/ml[b]	JN	0.4 mg/ml[a]	Physically compatible for 4 hr at 22 °C	1365	C
Paclitaxel	NCI	1.2 mg/ml[a]	JN	0.4 mg/ml[a]	Physically compatible with no change in measured turbidity in 4 hr at 22 °C	1556	C
Piperacillin sodium–tazobactam sodium	LE	40 + 5 mg/ml[a]	JN	0.4 mg/ml[a]	Heavy white turbidity with white precipitate forms immediately	1688	I
Potassium chloride	AB	40 mEq/L[e]	CR	1.25 mg/ml	Physically compatible for at least 4 hr at room temperature by visual and microscopic examination	534	C
Propofol	ZEN	10 mg/ml	JN	0.4 mg/ml[a]	Physically compatible for 1 hr at 23 °C with no increase in particle content	2066	C
Remifentanil HCl	GW	0.025 and 0.25 mg/ml[b]	AST	2.5 mg/ml	Physically compatible with no change in measured turbidity or increase in particle content in 4 hr at 23 °C	2075	C
Sargramostim	IMM	10 μg/ml[b]	DU	0.4 mg/ml[b]	Physically compatible for 4 hr at 22 °C	1436	C
Teniposide	BR	0.1 mg/ml[a]	JN	0.4 mg/ml[a]	Physically compatible with no subvisual haze or particle formation in 4 hr at 23 °C	1725	C
Thiotepa	IMM[g]	1 mg/ml[a]	JN	0.4 mg/ml[a]	Physically compatible with no change in measured turbidity or increase in particle content in 4 hr at 23 °C	1861	C
TNA #218 to #226[h]			AB	0.4 mg/ml[a]	Damage to emulsion integrity occurs in 1 to 4 hr with free oil formation possible	2215	I
TPN #212 to #215[h]			AB	0.4 mg/ml[a]	Physically compatible with no change in measured turbidity or increase in particle content in 4 hr at 23 °C	2109	C
Vinblastine sulfate		1 mg/ml		2.5 mg/ml	Drugs injected sequentially into Y-site with no flush between. No visually apparent precipitate	980	C
Vincristine sulfate		1 mg/ml		2.5 mg/ml	Drugs injected sequentially into Y-site with no flush between. No visually apparent precipitate	980	C
Vinorelbine tartrate	BW	1 mg/ml[b]	JN	0.4 mg/ml[b]	Physically compatible with no change in measured turbidity or increase in particle content in 4 hr at 22 °C	1558	C

Y-Site Injection Compatibility (1:1 Mixture) (Cont.)

Droperidol

Drug	Mfr	Conc	Mfr	Conc	Remarks	Ref	C/I
Vitamin B complex with C	RC	2 ml/L[e]	CR	1.25 mg/ml	Physically compatible for at least 4 hr at room temperature by visual and microscopic examination	534	C

[a]*Tested in dextrose 5% in water.*
[b]*Tested in sodium chloride 0.9%.*
[c]*Tested in bacteriostatic sodium chloride 0.9% preserved with benzyl alcohol 0.9%.*
[d]*Given over three minutes via a Y-site into a running infusion solution of heparin sodium in sodium chloride 0.9%.*
[e]*Tested in dextrose 5% in Ringer's injection, dextrose 5% in Ringer's injection, lactated, dextrose 5% in water, Ringer's injection, lactated, and sodium chloride 0.9%.*
[f]*Tested in dextrose 5% in water with sodium bicarbonate 0.05 mEq/ml.*
[g]*Lyophilized formulation tested.*
[h]*Refer to Appendix I for the composition of parenteral nutrition solutions. TNA indicates a 3-in-1 admixture, and TPN indicates a 2-in-1 admixture.*

Additional Compatibility Information

Dextrose 5% in water and Ringer's injection, lactated, have been recommended as diluents for intravenous infusion of droperidol (4).

Precipitation occurs if droperidol is mixed with barbiturates (4). Droperidol has been stated to be physically and chemically compatible with buprenorphine HCl (4).

EDETATE CALCIUM DISODIUM
AHFS 64:00

Calcium Disodium Versenate   3M Pharmaceuticals

Products—— Edetate calcium disodium (3M Pharmaceuticals) is available in 5-ml ampuls containing 200 mg/ml of drug (2).

pH—— From 6.5 to 8 (4).

Osmolality—— Edetate calcium disodium 200 mg/ml has an osmolality of 1514 mOsm/kg (1689).

Sodium Content—— Edetate calcium disodium contains approximately 5.3 mEq of sodium per gram of calcium EDTA (4).

Administration—— Edetate calcium disodium may be administered by slow intermittent or continuous intravenous infusion after dilution with sodium chloride 0.9% or dextrose 5% in water to a concentration of 2 to 4 mg/ml. Infusions are made over eight to 12 (2; 4) or up to 24 hours (4). Although a single, prolonged daily infusion is recommended by the manufacturer (2), the drug has been given in divided daily doses by intermittent intravenous infusions of 15 to 60 minutes in low-risk patients (4).

The total daily drug dose may also be given by intramuscular injection in equally divided doses at eight- or 12-hour intervals. To minimize pain from intramuscular injection, it should be mixed in equal quantities with procaine HCl 1% or lidocaine HCl 1% (e.g., 1 ml of local anesthetic for each milliliter of edetate calcium disodium) or 0.25 ml of lidocaine HCl 10% can be added to 5 ml of edetate calcium disodium to yield a final local anesthetic concentration of 0.5% (2; 4).

Compatibility Information

Additive Compatibility

Edetate calcium disodium

Drug	Mfr	Conc/L	Mfr	Conc/L	Test Soln	Remarks	Ref	C/I
Amphotericin B		200 mg	RI	4 g	D5W	Haze develops over 3 hr	26	I
Hydralazine HCl	BP	80 mg	RI	4 g	D5W	Yellow color produced	26	I
Netilmicin sulfate	SC	3 mg	RI	4 g	D5S	Physically compatible and netilmicin chemically stable for 7 days at 25 and 4 °C. Edetate not tested	558	C

Additional Compatibility Information

Solutions— The manufacturer recommends that dextrose 5% in water or sodium chloride 0.9% be used as a diluent for intravenous infusion (2).

Edetate calcium disodium is stated to be physically incompatible with dextrose 10% in water, invert sugar 10% in water, invert sugar 10% in sodium chloride 0.9%, Ringer's injection, lactated, Ringer's injection, and sodium lactate ⅙ M (4).

EDETATE DISODIUM
AHFS 64:00

Endrate   **Abbott**

Products— Edetate disodium (Abbott) is available in 20-ml ampuls containing 150 mg/ml of drug. The pH is adjusted with sodium hydroxide (4; 154).

pH— From 6.5 to 7.5 (4).

Sodium Content— Edetate disodium contains approximately 5.4 mEq of sodium per gram of drug (4).

Administration— Edetate disodium is administered by slow intravenous infusion over at least three hours. It must be diluted prior to administration, usually in 500 ml of sodium chloride 0.9% or dextrose 5% in water. Extravasation should be avoided because of tissue irritation (4).

Compatibility Information

Solution Compatibility

Edetate disodium

Solution	Mfr	Mfr	Conc/L	Remarks	Ref	C/I
Alcohol 5%, dextrose 5%	AB	AB	6 g	Color change	3	I
Dextran 6% in dextrose 5%	AB	AB	6 g	Physically compatible	3	C
Dextran 6% in sodium chloride 0.9%	AB	AB	6 g	Physically compatible	3	C
Dextrose–saline combinations	AB	AB	6 g	Physically compatible	3	C
Dextrose 2½% in water	AB	AB	6 g	Physically compatible	3	C
Dextrose 5% in water	AB	AB	6 g	Physically compatible	3	C
Dextrose 10% in water	AB	AB	6 g	Physically compatible	3	C
Fructose 10% in sodium chloride 0.9%	AB	AB	6 g	Physically compatible	3	C
Fructose 10% in water	AB	AB	6 g	Physically compatible	3	C
Invert sugar 5 and 10% in sodium chloride 0.9%	AB	AB	6 g	Physically compatible	3	C
Invert sugar 5 and 10% in water	AB	AB	6 g	Physically compatible	3	C
Sodium chloride 0.45%	AB	AB	6 g	Physically compatible	3	C
Sodium chloride 0.9%	AB	AB	6 g	Physically compatible	3	C
Sodium lactate ⅙ M	AB	AB	6 g	Physically compatible	3	C

Additional Compatibility Information

Solutions— Dextrose 5% in water and sodium chloride 0.9% have been recommended as diluents for intravenous infusion (4).

EDROPHONIUM CHLORIDE
AHFS 36:56

Tensilon   **ICN**

Products— Edrophonium chloride (ICN) is available in 1-ml ampuls and 10-ml multiple-dose vials. Each milliliter of solution contains edrophonium chloride 10 mg with sodium sulfite 0.2% and sodium citrate and citric acid as buffers. The multiple-dose vials also contain phenol 0.45% (2).

pH— Approximately 5.4 (2).

Osmolality— Edrophonium chloride 10 mg/ml has an osmolality of 329 mOsm/kg (1689).

Administration— Edrophonium chloride may be given intramuscularly or subcutaneously but is usually given intravenously (2; 4).

Stability— Intact containers should be stored at controlled room temperature (17).

Compatibility Information

Y-Site Injection Compatibility (1:1 Mixture)

Edrophonium chloride

Drug	Mfr	Conc	Mfr	Conc	Remarks	Ref	C/I
Heparin sodium	UP	1000 units/L[a]	RC	10 mg/ml	Physically compatible for at least 4 hr at room temperature by visual and microscopic examination	534	C
Hydrocortisone sodium succinate	UP	10 mg/L[a]	RC	10 mg/ml	Physically compatible for at least 4 hr at room temperature by visual and microscopic examination	534	C
Potassium chloride	AB	40 mEq/L[a]	RC	10 mg/ml	Physically compatible for at least 4 hr at room temperature by visual and microscopic examination	534	C
Vitamin B complex with C	RC	2 ml/L[a]	RC	10 mg/ml	Physically compatible for at least 4 hr at room temperature by visual and microscopic examination	534	C

[a]*Tested in dextrose 5% in Ringer's injection, dextrose 5% in Ringer's injection, lactated, dextrose 5% in water, Ringer's injection, lactated, and sodium chloride 0.9%.*

ENALAPRILAT
AHFS 24:04

Vasotec I.V.   **Merck**

Products— Enalaprilat (Merck) is available in 1- and 2-ml vials. Each milliliter of solution contains enalaprilat 1.25 mg with sodium chloride to adjust tonicity, sodium hydroxide to adjust pH, and benzyl alcohol 9 mg in water for injection (2).

pH— From 6.5 to 7.5 (1-1/90).

Administration— Enalaprilat is slowly injected intravenously over at least five minutes if undiluted or infused in up to 50 ml of compatible intravenous infusion solution (2; 4).

Stability— Enalaprilat is a clear, colorless solution. The product should be stored below 30 °C (2).

Compatibility Information

Solution Compatibility

Enalaprilat

Solution	Mfr	Mfr	Conc/L	Remarks	Ref	C/I
Dextran 40 10% in dextrose 5%	TR	MSD	25 mg	Physically compatible for 24 hr at room temperature under fluorescent light	1355	C

Solution Compatibility (Cont.)

Enalaprilat

Solution	Mfr	Mfr	Conc/L	Remarks	Ref	C/I
Dextrose 5% in water	TR[a]	MSD	12 mg	Visually compatible with no loss by HPLC in 24 hr at room temperature under fluorescent light	1572	C
Hetastarch 6%	DU	MSD	25 mg	Physically compatible for 24 hr at room temperature under fluorescent light	1355	C
Normosol R	AB	MSD	25 mg	Physically compatible for 24 hr at room temperature under fluorescent light	1355	C
Plasma-Lyte A	TR	MSD	25 mg	Physically compatible for 24 hr at room temperature under fluorescent light	1355	C

[a]Tested in PVC containers.

Additive Compatibility

Enalaprilat

Drug	Mfr	Conc/L	Mfr	Conc/L	Test Soln	Remarks	Ref	C/I
Dobutamine HCl	LI	1 g	MSD	12 mg	D5W[a]	Visually compatible with little or no enalaprilat loss by HPLC in 24 hr at room temperature under fluorescent light. Dobutamine not tested	1572	C
Dopamine HCl	AMR	1.6 g	MSD	12 mg	D5W[a]	Visually compatible with about 5% enalaprilat loss by HPLC in 24 hr at room temperature under fluorescent light. Dopamine not tested	1572	C
Heparin sodium	ES	50,000 units	MSD	12 mg	D5W[a]	Visually compatible with little or no enalaprilat loss by HPLC in 24 hr at room temperature under fluorescent light. Heparin not tested	1572	C
Meropenem	ZEN	1 and 20 g	MSD	50 mg	NS	Visually compatible for 4 hr at room temperature	1994	C
Nitroglycerin	DU	200 mg	MSD	12 mg	D5W[b]	Visually compatible with about 4% enalaprilat loss by HPLC in 24 hr at room temperature under fluorescent light. Nitroglycerin not tested	1572	C
Potassium chloride	AB	3 g	MSD	12 mg	D5W[a]	Visually compatible with little or no enalaprilat loss by HPLC in 24 hr at room temperature under fluorescent light. Potassium chloride not tested	1572	C
Sodium nitroprusside	ES	1 g	MSD	12 mg	D5W[a]	Visually compatible with little or no enalaprilat loss by HPLC in 24 hr at room temperature under fluorescent light. Nitroprusside not tested	1572	C

[a]Tested in PVC containers.
[b]Tested in glass containers.

Y-Site Injection Compatibility (1:1 Mixture)

Drug	Mfr	Conc	Mfr	Conc	Remarks	Ref	C/I
				Enalaprilat			
Allopurinol sodium	BW	3 mg/ml[b]	MSD	0.1 mg/ml[b]	Physically compatible with no change in measured turbidity or increase in particle content in 4 hr at 22 °C	1686	C
Amifostine	USB	10 mg/ml[a]	MSD	0.1 mg/ml[a]	Physically compatible with no change in measured turbidity or increase in particle content in 4 hr at 23 °C	1845	C
Amikacin sulfate	BR	2 mg/ml[a]	MSD	0.05 mg/ml[b]	Physically compatible for 24 hr at room temperature under fluorescent light	1355	C
Aminophylline	ES	1 mg/ml[a]	MSD	0.05 mg/ml[b]	Physically compatible for 24 hr at room temperature under fluorescent light	1355	C
Amphotericin B	SQ	0.1 mg/ml[a]	MSD	1.25 mg/ml	Layered haze develops in 4 hr at 21 °C	1409	I
Amphotericin B cholesteryl sulfate complex	SEQ	0.83 mg/ml[a]	ME	0.1 mg/ml[a]	Decreased natural turbidity occurs immediately	2117	I
Ampicillin sodium	PF	15 mg/ml[b]	MSD	0.05 mg/ml[b]	Physically compatible for 24 hr at room temperature under fluorescent light	1355	C
Ampicillin sodium–sulbactam sodium	PF	10 + 5 mg/ml[b]	MSD	0.05 mg/ml[b]	Physically compatible for 24 hr at room temperature under fluorescent light	1355	C
Aztreonam	SQ	10 mg/ml[a]	MSD	0.05 mg/ml[b]	Physically compatible for 24 hr at room temperature under fluorescent light	1355	C
	SQ	40 mg/ml[a]	MSD	0.1 mg/ml[a]	Physically compatible with no subvisual haze or particle formation in 4 hr at 23 °C	1758	C
Butorphanol tartrate	BR	0.4 mg/ml[a]	MSD	0.05 mg/ml[b]	Physically compatible for 24 hr at room temperature under fluorescent light	1355	C
Calcium gluconate	ES	0.092 mEq/ml[a]	MSD	0.05 mg/ml[b]	Physically compatible for 24 hr at room temperature under fluorescent light	1355	C
Cefazolin sodium	SKF	20 mg/ml[c]	MSD	0.05 mg/ml[b]	Physically compatible for 24 hr at room temperature under fluorescent light	1355	C
Cefepime HCl	BR	20 mg/ml[a]	MSD	0.1 mg/ml[a]	Tiny particles form in 4 hr	1689	I
Cefoperazone sodium	RR	10 mg/ml[a]	MSD	0.05 mg/ml[b]	Physically compatible for 24 hr at room temperature under fluorescent light	1355	C
Ceftazidime	GL[i]	10 mg/ml[a]	MSD	0.05 mg/ml[b]	Physically compatible for 24 hr at room temperature under fluorescent light	1355	C
Ceftizoxime sodium	SKF	10 mg/ml[a]	MSD	0.05 mg/ml[b]	Physically compatible for 24 hr at room temperature under fluorescent light	1355	C
Chloramphenicol sodium succinate	PD	10 mg/ml[a]	MSD	0.05 mg/ml[b]	Physically compatible for 24 hr at room temperature under fluorescent light	1355	C
Cimetidine HCl	SKF	3 mg/ml[a]	MSD	0.05 mg/ml[b]	Physically compatible for 24 hr at room temperature under fluorescent light	1355	C
Cisatracurium besylate	GW	0.1, 2, 5 mg/ml[a]	ME	0.1 mg/ml[a]	Physically compatible with no change in measured turbidity or increase in particle content in 4 hr at 23 °C	2074	C
Cladribine	ORT	0.015[b] and 0.5[d] mg/ml	MSD	0.1 mg/ml[b]	Physically compatible with no change in measured turbidity or increase in particle content in 4 hr at 23 °C	1969	C
Clindamycin phosphate	UP	9 mg/ml[a]	MSD	0.05 mg/ml[b]	Physically compatible for 24 hr at room temperature under fluorescent light	1355	C

Y-Site Injection Compatibility (1:1 Mixture) (Cont.)

Enalaprilat

Drug	Mfr	Conc	Mfr	Conc	Remarks	Ref	C/I
Dextran 40	TR	100 mg/ml[a]	MSD	0.05 mg/ml[b]	Physically compatible for 24 hr at room temperature under fluorescent light	1355	C
Dobutamine HCl	LI	1 mg/ml[a]	MSD	0.05 mg/ml[b]	Physically compatible for 24 hr at room temperature under fluorescent light	1355	C
Docetaxel	RPR	0.9 mg/ml[a]	ME	0.1 mg/ml[a]	Physically compatible with no change in measured turbidity or increase in particle content in 4 hr at 23 °C	2224	C
Dopamine HCl	IMS	1.6 mg/ml[a]	MSD	0.05 mg/ml[b]	Physically compatible for 24 hr at room temperature under fluorescent light	1355	C
Doxorubicin HCl liposome injection	SEQ	0.4 mg/ml[a]	MSD	0.1 mg/ml[a]	Physically compatible with little or no change in measured turbidity and no increase in particle content in 4 hr at 23 °C	2087	C
Erythromycin lactobionate	AB	5 mg/ml[a]	MSD	0.05 mg/ml[b]	Physically compatible for 24 hr at room temperature under fluorescent light	1355	C
Esmolol HCl	DU	10 mg/ml[a]	MSD	0.05 mg/ml[b]	Physically compatible for 24 hr at room temperature under fluorescent light	1355	C
Etoposide phosphate	BR	5 mg/ml[a]	ME	0.1 mg/ml[a]	Physically compatible with no change in measured turbidity or increase in particle content in 4 hr at 23 °C	2218	C
Famotidine	MSD	0.2 mg/ml[a]	MSD	0.05 mg/ml[b]	Physically compatible for 24 hr at room temperature under fluorescent light	1355	C
Fentanyl citrate	ES	2 µg/ml[a]	MSD	0.05 mg/ml[b]	Physically compatible for 24 hr at room temperature under fluorescent light	1355	C
Filgrastim	AMG	30 µg/ml[a]	MSD	0.1 mg/ml[a]	Physically compatible with no change in measured turbidity or increase in particle content in 4 hr at 22 °C	1687	C
Ganciclovir sodium	SY	5 mg/ml[e]	MSD	1.25 mg/ml	Physically compatible for 4 hr at 21 °C under fluorescent light by macroscopic and microscopic examination	1409	C
Gemcitabine HCl	LI	10 mg/ml[b]	ME	0.1 mg/ml[b]	Physically compatible with no change in measured turbidity or increase in particle content in 4 hr at 23 °C	2226	C
Gentamicin sulfate	ES	0.8 mg/ml[a]	MSD	0.05 mg/ml[b]	Physically compatible for 24 hr at room temperature under fluorescent light	1355	C
Granisetron HCl	SKB	0.05 mg/ml[a]	MSD	0.1 mg/ml[a]	Physically compatible with no change in measured turbidity or increase in particle content in 4 hr at 23 °C	2000	C
Heparin sodium	IX	40 units/ml[a]	MSD	0.05 mg/ml[b]	Physically compatible for 24 hr at room temperature under fluorescent light	1355	C
Hetastarch	DCC	6%	MSD	0.05 mg/ml[b]	Physically compatible for 24 hr at room temperature under fluorescent light	1355	C
Hydrocortisone sodium succinate	UP	2 mg/ml[a]	MSD	0.05 mg/ml[b]	Physically compatible for 24 hr at room temperature under fluorescent light	1355	C
Labetalol HCl	GL	1 mg/ml[a]	MSD	0.05 mg/ml[b]	Physically compatible for 24 hr at room temperature under fluorescent light	1355	C
Lidocaine HCl	AST	4 mg/ml[a]	MSD	0.05 mg/ml[b]	Physically compatible for 24 hr at room temperature under fluorescent light	1355	C

Y-Site Injection Compatibility (1:1 Mixture) (Cont.)

				Enalaprilat			
Drug	*Mfr*	*Conc*	*Mfr*	*Conc*	*Remarks*	*Ref*	*C/I*
Magnesium sulfate	LY	10 mEq/ml[a]	MSD	0.05 mg/ml[b]	Physically compatible for 24 hr at room temperature under fluorescent light	1355	C
Melphalan HCl	BW	0.1 mg/ml[b]	MSD	0.1 mg/ml[b]	Physically compatible with no change in measured turbidity or increase in particle content in 3 hr at 22 °C	1557	C
Meropenem	ZEN	1 and 50 mg/ml[b]	MSD	0.05 mg/ml[f]	Visually compatible for 4 hr at room temperature	1994	C
Methylprednisolone sodium succinate	UP	0.8 mg/ml[a]	MSD	0.05 mg/ml[b]	Physically compatible for 24 hr at room temperature under fluorescent light	1355	C
Metronidazole	SE	5 mg/ml	MSD	0.05 mg/ml[b]	Physically compatible for 24 hr at room temperature under fluorescent light	1355	C
Morphine sulfate	WY	0.2 mg/ml[a]	MSD	0.05 mg/ml[b]	Physically compatible for 24 hr at room temperature under fluorescent light	1355	C
Nafcillin sodium	BR	10 mg/ml[a]	MSD	0.05 mg/ml[b]	Physically compatible for 24 hr at room temperature under fluorescent light	1355	C
Nicardipine HCl	DU	0.1 mg/ml[a]	MSD	0.05 mg/ml[b]	Physically compatible for 24 hr at room temperature under fluorescent light	1355	C
Penicillin G potassium	PF	50,000 units/ml[a]	MSD	0.05 mg/ml[b]	Physically compatible for 24 hr at room temperature under fluorescent light	1355	C
Phenobarbital sodium	WY	0.32 mg/ml[e]	MSD	1.25 mg/ml	Physically compatible for 4 hr at 21 °C under fluorescent light by macroscopic and microscopic examination	1409	C
Phenytoin sodium	PD	1 mg/ml[b]	MSD	1.25 mg/ml	Crystalline precipitate forms immediately	1409	I
Piperacillin sodium	LE	12 mg/ml[a]	MSD	0.05 mg/ml[b]	Physically compatible for 24 hr at room temperature under fluorescent light	1355	C
Piperacillin sodium–tazobactam sodium	LE	40 + 5 mg/ml[a]	MSD	0.1 mg/ml[a]	Physically compatible with no change in measured turbidity or increase in particle content in 4 hr at 22 °C	1688	C
Potassium chloride	LY	0.4 mEq/ml[a]	MSD	0.05 mg/ml[b]	Physically compatible for 24 hr at room temperature under fluorescent light	1355	C
Potassium phosphates	LY	0.44 mEq/ml[a]	MSD	0.05 mg/ml[b]	Physically compatible for 24 hr at room temperature under fluorescent light	1355	C
Propofol	ZEN	10 mg/ml	MSD	0.1 mg/ml[a]	Physically compatible for 1 hr at 23 °C with no increase in particle content	2066	C
Ranitidine HCl	GL	0.5 mg/ml[a]	MSD	0.05 mg/ml[b]	Physically compatible for 24 hr at room temperature under fluorescent light	1355	C
Remifentanil HCl	GW	0.025 and 0.25 mg/ml[b]	ME	0.1 mg/ml[a]	Physically compatible with no change in measured turbidity or increase in particle content in 4 hr at 23 °C	2075	C
Sodium acetate	LY	0.4 mEq/ml[a]	MSD	0.05 mg/ml[b]	Physically compatible for 24 hr at room temperature under fluorescent light	1355	C
Sodium nitroprusside	LY	0.2 mg/ml[a]	MSD	0.05 mg/ml[b]	Physically compatible for 24 hr at room temperature under fluorescent light	1355	C
Teniposide	BR	0.1 mg/ml[a]	MSD	0.1 mg/ml[a]	Physically compatible with no subvisual haze or particle formation in 4 hr at 23 °C	1725	C

Y-Site Injection Compatibility (1:1 Mixture) (Cont.)

			Enalaprilat				
Drug	Mfr	Conc	Mfr	Conc	Remarks	Ref	C/I
Thiotepa	IMM[g]	1 mg/ml[a]	ME	0.1 mg/ml[a]	Physically compatible with no change in measured turbidity or increase in particle content in 4 hr at 23 °C	1861	C
TNA #218 to #226[h]			ME	0.1 mg/ml[a]	Visually compatible with no precipitate or emulsion damage apparent in 4 hr at 23 °C	2215	C
Tobramycin sulfate	LI	0.8 mg/ml[a]	MSD	0.05 mg/ml[b]	Physically compatible for 24 hr at room temperature under fluorescent light	1355	C
TPN #212 to #215[h]			MSD	0.1 mg/ml[a]	Physically compatible with no change in measured turbidity or increase in particle content in 4 hr at 23 °C	2109	C
Trimethoprim–sulfamethoxazole	QU	0.8 + 1.6 mg/ml[a]	MSD	0.05 mg/ml[b]	Physically compatible for 24 hr at room temperature under fluorescent light	1355	C
Vancomycin HCl	LE	5 mg/ml[a]	MSD	0.05 mg/ml[b]	Physically compatible for 24 hr at room temperature under fluorescent light	1355	C
Vinorelbine tartrate	BW	1 mg/ml[b]	MSD	0.1 mg/ml[b]	Physically compatible with no change in measured turbidity or increase in particle content in 4 hr at 22 °C	1558	C

[a]Tested in dextrose 5% in water.
[b]Tested in sodium chloride 0.9%.
[c]Premixed solution.
[d]Tested in bacteriostatic sodium chloride 0.9% preserved with benzyl alcohol 0.9%.
[e]Tested in both dextrose 5% in water and sodium chloride 0.9%.
[f]Tested in sterile water for injection.
[g]Lyophilized formulation tested.
[h]Refer to Appendix I for the composition of parenteral nutrition solutions. TNA indicates a 3-in-1 admixture, and TPN indicates a 2-in-1 admixture.
[i]Sodium carbonate–containing formulation tested.

Additional Compatibility Information

Solutions— The manufacturer states that enalaprilat is stable for 24 hours at room temperature in the following infusion solutions (2):

Dextrose 5% in Ringer's injection, lactated
Dextrose 5% in sodium chloride 0.9%
Dextrose 5% in water
Isolyte E
Sodium chloride 0.9%

ENOXAPARIN SODIUM
AHFS 20:12.04

Lovenox **Aventis**

Products— Enoxaparin sodium (Aventis) is available in prefilled syringes containing 30 mg/0.3 ml, 40 mg/0.4 ml, 60 mg/0.6 ml, 80 mg/0.8 ml, and 100 mg/1 ml in water for injection. The solution is preservative-free and is intended for use as a single-dose injection (2).

pH— From 5.5 to 7.5 (2).

Units— The approximate anti-factor Xa activity is 1000 I.U. for every 10 mg of enoxaparin sodium.

Administration— Enoxaparin sodium is administered by deep subcutaneous injection, alternating administration sites between the left and right anterolateral and left and right posterolateral abdominal wall. It must not be given intramuscularly (2; 4).

Stability— Enoxaparin sodium injection is a clear, colorless to pale yellow solution. Intact containers should be stored at controlled room temperature of 15 to 25 °C (2).

Compatibility Information

Solution Compatibility

Enoxaparin sodium

Solution	Mfr	Mfr	Conc/L	Remarks	Ref	C/I
Sodium chloride 0.9%	AB[a]	RP	1.2 g	No loss of activity by bioassay in 48 hr at 21 °C under fluorescent light	1871	C

[a]*Tested in PVC containers.*

EPHEDRINE SULFATE
AHFS 12:12

Products— Ephedrine sulfate is available in 1-ml ampuls and vials containing 50 mg of drug (154).

pH— From 4.5 to 7 (4).

Osmolarity— The osmolarity of the 50-mg/ml concentration is calculated to be 0.35 mOsm/ml (1-10/91).

Administration— Ephedrine sulfate may be administered subcutaneously, intramuscularly, or slowly intravenously (4).

Stability— Intact containers of ephedrine sulfate should be stored at controlled room temperature and protected from light (4; 17).

Syringes— The stability of ephedrine (salt form unspecified) 10 mg/ml repackaged in polypropylene syringes was evaluated by spectrophotometric and potentiometric methods. Little or no change in concentration was found after four weeks of storage at room temperature not exposed to direct light (2164).

Compatibility Information

Solution Compatibility

Ephedrine sulfate

Solution	Mfr	Mfr	Conc/L	Remarks	Ref	C/I
Dextran 6% in dextrose 5%	AB		50 mg	Physically compatible	3	C
Dextran 6% in sodium chloride 0.9%	AB		50 mg	Physically compatible	3	C
Dextrose–Ringer's injection combinations	AB		50 mg	Physically compatible	3	C
Dextrose–Ringer's injection, lactated, combinations	AB		50 mg	Physically compatible	3	C
Dextrose–saline combinations	AB		50 mg	Physically compatible	3	C
Dextrose 2½% in water	AB		50 mg	Physically compatible	3	C
Dextrose 5% in water	AB		50 mg	Physically compatible	3	C
Dextrose 10% in water	AB		50 mg	Physically compatible	3	C
Fructose 10% in sodium chloride 0.9%	AB		50 mg	Physically compatible	3	C
Fructose 10% in water	AB		50 mg	Physically compatible	3	C
Invert sugar 5 and 10% in sodium chloride 0.9%	AB		50 mg	Physically compatible	3	C
Invert sugar 5 and 10% in water	AB		50 mg	Physically compatible	3	C
Ionosol products	AB		50 mg	Physically compatible	3	C
Ringer's injection	AB		50 mg	Physically compatible	3	C
Ringer's injection, lactated	AB		50 mg	Physically compatible	3	C
Sodium chloride 0.45%	AB		50 mg	Physically compatible	3	C
Sodium chloride 0.9%	AB		50 mg	Physically compatible	3	C

Solution Compatibility (Cont.)

Ephedrine sulfate

Solution	Mfr	Mfr	Conc/L	Remarks	Ref	C/I
Sodium lactate ⅙ M	AB		50 mg	Physically compatible	3	C

Additive Compatibility

Ephedrine sulfate

Drug	Mfr	Conc/L	Mfr	Conc/L	Test Soln	Remarks	Ref	C/I
Chloramphenicol sodium succinate	PD	1 g	AB	50 mg		Physically compatible	6	C
Hydrocortisone sodium succinate						Physically incompatible	9	I
Lidocaine HCl	AST	2 g		50 mg		Physically compatible	24	C
Metaraminol bitartrate	MSD	100 mg	AB	50 mg		Physically compatible	7	C
Nafcillin sodium	WY	500 mg		50 mg		Physically compatible	27	C
Penicillin G potassium		1 million units		50 mg		Physically compatible	3	C
	SQ	5 million units	AB	50 mg		Physically compatible	47	C
Pentobarbital sodium						Physically incompatible	9	I
	AB	1 g	LI	250 mg	D5W	Physically incompatible	15	I
Phenobarbital sodium	WI					Physically incompatible	9	I
	WI	200 mg	LI	250 mg	D5W	Physically incompatible	15	I
Thiopental sodium	AB	2.5 g	AB	50 mg	D5W	Physically compatible	21	C
	AB					Physically incompatible	9	I

Drugs in Syringe Compatibility

Ephedrine sulfate

Drug (in syringe)	Mfr	Amt	Mfr	Amt	Remarks	Ref	C/I
Pentobarbital sodium	AB	500 mg/ 10 ml		50 mg/ 1 ml	Physically compatible	55	C
Thiopental sodium	AB	75 mg/ 3 ml	AB	50 mg/ 1 ml	Physically incompatible	21	I

Y-Site Injection Compatibility (1:1 Mixture)

Ephedrine sulfate

Drug	Mfr	Conc	Mfr	Conc	Remarks	Ref	C/I
Etomidate	AB	2 mg/ml	AB	50 mg/ml	Visually compatible for up to 7 days at 25 °C	1801	C
Propofol	ZEN	10 mg/ml	AB	5 mg/ml[a]	Physically compatible for 1 hr at 23 °C with no increase in particle content	2066	C
Thiopental sodium	AB	25 mg/ml	AB	50 mg/ml	White cloudiness forms immediately, followed by fine crystalline particles	1801	I

[a]Tested in dextrose 5% in water.

Additional Compatibility Information

Phenobarbital Sodium— Titration of 50 ml of a 0.5 M aqueous solution of ephedrine HCl (BP) with 30.8 ml or more of a 0.5 M aqueous solution of phenobarbital sodium (BP) resulted in precipitation of an ephedrine–phenobarbital complex. The point at which precipitation began corresponded to the point at which the pH of the ephedrine HCl solution had been increased from its initial pH of 7 to 8.5. Further additions of the phenobarbital sodium solution resulted in additional precipitation but did not alter the pH (332).

Hydrocortisone Sodium Succinate— Ephedrine sulfate 50 mg/L has been reported to be conditionally compatible with hydrocortisone sodium succinate (Upjohn) 250 mg/L. The mixture is physi-

cally compatible in most Abbott infusion solutions except as noted below (3):

Fructose 10% in sodium chloride 0.9%	Haze or precipitate within 24 hours
Ionosol B with invert sugar 10%	Haze or precipitate within 24 hours
Ionosol D-CM with dextrose 5%	Haze or precipitate within 24 hours
Ionosol D with invert sugar 10%	Haze or precipitate within six hours
Ionosol D modified with invert sugar 10%	Haze or precipitate within 24 hours

---

EPINEPHRINE HCL
AHFS 12:12

Adrenalin Chloride

Abbott

Monarch

Products— Epinephrine HCl is available in 1-ml ampuls and 30-ml vials (29). Each milliliter of solution contains epinephrine 1 mg as the hydrochloride in isotonic sodium chloride solution. The ampuls also contain sodium bisulfite 0.1%. The vials contain sodium bisulfite 0.15% and chlorobutanol 0.5% (1-7/94).

Epinephrine HCl is also available in a concentration of 0.1 mg/ml (1:10,000) in vials and prefilled syringes (1-2/93; 29). Each milliliter of solution also contains sodium chloride 8.16 mg and sodium metabisulfite 0.46 mg with citric acid 2 mg and sodium citrate 0.6 mg as buffers (1-2/93).

pH— From 2.2 to 5.0 (4; 17).

Osmolality— The osmolality of epinephrine HCl (Abbott) 0.1 mg/ml was determined to be 273 mOsm/kg by freezing-point depression (1071). A 1-mg/ml solution was determined to have an osmolality of 348 mOsm/kg (1233).

Administration— Epinephrine HCl may be administered by subcutaneous, intramuscular, intravenous, or intracardiac injection. Intramuscular injection into the buttocks should be avoided (1-7/94; 4). Intravenous infusion at a rate of 1 to 10 μg/min has also been described (4).

Stability— Epinephrine HCl is sensitive to light and air (4; 1259). Protection from light is recommended. The manufacturer recommends not removing ampuls from the carton until ready to use (1-7/94). Withdrawal of doses from multiple-dose vials introduces air, which results in oxidation. As epinephrine oxidizes, it changes from colorless to pink, as adrenochrome forms, to brown, as melanin

forms (4; 1072). Discolored solutions or solutions containing a precipitate should not be used (4). The various epinephrine preparations have varying stabilities, depending on the form and the preservatives present. The manufacturer's recommendations should be followed with regard to storage (4).

The primary determinant of catecholamine stability in intravenous admixtures is the pH of the solution (527). Epinephrine HCl is unstable in dextrose 5% in water at a pH above 5.5 (48). The pH of optimum stability is 3 to 4 (1072). In one study, the decomposition rate increased twofold (from 5 to 10% in 200 days at 30 °C) when the pH was increased from 2.5 to 4.5 (1259).

The stability of epinephrine HCl in intact ampuls subjected to resterilization to provide a sterile outer surface was evaluated. Epinephrine HCl (adrenalin injection, BP) ampuls were resterilized by the following methods:

1. Autoclaved at 121 °C for 15 minutes.
2. Autoclaved at 115 °C for 30 minutes.
3. Exposed to ethylene oxide–freon (12:88) at 55 °C for four hours followed by aeration at 50 °C for 12 hours.

No differences in epinephrine HCl concentration were detected by HPLC analysis of samples from any of these methods. However, if ampuls were resterilized twice by autoclaving two times at 121 °C for 15 minutes, approximately 8% of the drug was lost (803).

Epinephrine HCl (Parke-Davis) was diluted to concentrations of 1 and 7 mg/10 ml with sterile water for injection and repackaged into 10-ml glass vials and plastic syringes with 18-gauge needles (Becton-Dickinson). The diluted injections were stored at room temperature protected from light. Epinephrine stability was evaluated by HPLC analysis over 56 days of storage. The 1-mg/10 ml samples had an epinephrine loss of 4 to 6% in seven days and about 13% in 14 days. The 7-mg/10 ml samples lost 2% in the glass vials and 5% in the syringes in 56 days (1902).

Compatibility Information

Solution Compatibility

Epinephrine HCl

Solution	Mfr	Mfr	Conc/L	Remarks	Ref	C/I
Dextran 40,000	PH	PD		Physically compatible	44	C
Dextran 6% in dextrose 5%	AB	PD	4 mg	Physically compatible	3	C
Dextran 6% in sodium chloride 0.9%	AB	PD	4 mg	Physically compatible	3	C
Dextrose–Ringer's injection combinations	AB	PD	4 mg	Physically compatible	3	C
Dextrose–Ringer's injection, lactated, combinations	AB	PD	4 mg	Physically compatible	3	C
Dextrose 5% in Ringer's injection, lactated	TR[a]	PD	1 mg	Potency retained for 24 hr at 5 °C	282	C
Dextrose–saline combinations	AB	PD	4 mg	Physically compatible	3	C
Dextrose 5% in sodium chloride 0.9%	TR[a]	PD	1 mg	Potency retained for 24 hr at 5 °C	282	C
Dextrose 2½% in water	AB	PD	4 mg	Physically compatible	3	C
Dextrose 5% in water	AB	PD	4 mg	Physically compatible	3	C
	TR[a]	PD	1 mg	Potency retained for 24 hr at 5 °C	282	C
	AB	PD	4 mg	Physically compatible and chemically stable. At 25 °C, 10% decomposition is calculated to occur in 50 hr in light and in 1000 hr in the dark	527	C
	BA[b]	ANT	16 mg	5% loss by HPLC in 20.75 days at 5 °C protected from light	1610	C
	BA[a]	AMR	87 mg	No epinephrine loss by HPLC in 24 hr at 23 °C protected from light	2085	C
Dextrose 10% in water	AB	PD	4 mg	Physically compatible	3	C
Fructose 10% in sodium chloride 0.9%	AB	PD	4 mg	Physically compatible	3	C
Fructose 10% in water	AB	PD	4 mg	Physically compatible	3	C
Invert sugar 5 and 10% in sodium chloride 0.9%	AB	PD	4 mg	Physically compatible	3	C
Invert sugar 5 and 10% in water	AB	PD	4 mg	Physically compatible	3	C
Ionosol products (except as noted below)	AB	PD	4 mg	Physically compatible	3	C
Ionosol D-CM	AB	PD	4 mg	Color change	3	I
Ionosol PSL (Darrow's)	AB	PD	4 mg	Color change	3	I
Ionosol T with dextrose 5%	AB	PD	4 mg	Haze or precipitate within 6 to 24 hr	3	I
Ringer's injection	AB	PD	4 mg	Physically compatible	3	C
Ringer's injection, lactated	AB	PD	4 mg	Physically compatible	3	C
	TR[a]	PD	1 mg	Potency retained for 24 hr at 5 °C	282	C
Sodium bicarbonate 5%			4 mg	Epinephrine rapidly decomposes. 58% loss immediately after mixing	48	I
Sodium chloride 0.9%	TR[a]	PD	1 mg	Potency retained for 24 hr at 5 °C	282	C
Sodium lactate ⅙ M	AB	PD	4 mg	Physically compatible	3	C

[a]*Tested in both glass and PVC containers.*
[b]*Tested in PVC containers.*

Additive Compatibility

Epinephrine HCl

Drug	Mfr	Conc/L	Mfr	Conc/L	Test Soln	Remarks	Ref	C/I
Amikacin sulfate	BR	5 g	PD	2.5 mg	D5LR, D5R, D5S, D5W, D10W, IS10, LR, NS, R, SL	Physically compatible and potency of both retained for 24 hr at 25 °C	294	C
Aminophylline	SE	500 mg	PD	4 mg	D5W	At 25 °C, 10% epinephrine decomposition in 1.2 hr in the light and 3 hr in the dark	527	I
		500 mg		4 mg	D5W	Pink to brown discoloration in 8 to 24 hr at room temperature	845	I
Cimetidine HCl	SKF	3 g	PD	100 mg	D5W	Physically compatible and cimetidine chemically stable for 24 hr at room temperature. Epinephrine not tested	551	C
Dobutamine HCl	LI	1 g	BR	50 mg	D5W, NS	Physically compatible for 24 hr at 21 °C	812	C
Floxacillin sodium	BE	20 g	ANT	8 mg	W	Physically compatible for 72 hr at 15 and 30 °C	1479	C
Furosemide	HO	1 g	ANT	8 mg	W	Physically compatible for 72 hr at 15 and 30 °C	1479	C
Hyaluronidase			PD			Physically incompatible	10	I
	WY		PD			Physically incompatible	9	I
Mephentermine sulfate	WY		PD			Physically incompatible	10	I
Metaraminol bitartrate	MSD	100 mg	PD	4 mg		Physically compatible	7	C
Ranitidine HCl	GL	50 mg and 2 g		50 mg	D5W	Physically compatible and ranitidine chemically stable by HPLC for 24 hr at 25 °C. Epinephrine not tested	1515	C
Sodium bicarbonate	AB	2.4 mEq[a]		4 mg	D5W	Epinephrine inactivated	772	I
Verapamil HCl	KN	80 mg	PD	2 mg	D5W, NS	Physically compatible for 24 hr	764	C

[a] One vial of Neut added to a liter of admixture.

Drugs in Syringe Compatibility

Epinephrine HCl

Drug (in syringe)	Mfr	Amt	Mfr	Amt	Remarks	Ref	C/I
Diatrizoate meglumine 52%, diatrizoate sodium 8%	MA	5 ml	PD	1 mg/ml	Physically compatible for at least 2 hr	1438	C
Diatrizoate sodium 60%	WI	5 ml	PD	1 mg/ml	Physically compatible for at least 2 hr	1438	C
Doxapram HCl	RB	400 mg/ 20 ml		1 mg/ 1 ml	Physically compatible with no doxapram loss in 24 hr	1177	C
Heparin sodium		2500 units/ 1 ml		1 mg/ 1 ml	Physically compatible for at least 5 min	1053	C
Iohexol	WI	64.7%, 5 ml	PD	1 mg/ 1 ml	Physically compatible for at least 2 hr	1438	C
Iopamidol	SQ	61%, 5 ml	PD	1 mg/ 1 ml	Physically compatible for at least 2 hr	1438	C

Drugs in Syringe Compatibility (Cont.)

Drug (in syringe)	Mfr	Amt	Mfr	Amt	Remarks	Ref	C/I
				Epinephrine HCl			
Iothalamate meglumine 60%	MA	5 ml	PD	1 mg/ml	Physically compatible for at least 2 hr	1438	**C**
Ioxaglate meglumine 39.3%, ioxaglate sodium 19.6%	MA	5 ml	PD	1 mg/ml	Physically compatible for at least 2 hr	1438	**C**
Milrinone lactate	WI	5.25 mg/ 5.25 ml	AB	0.5 mg/ 0.5 ml	Physically compatible with no loss of either drug in 20 min at 23 °C under fluorescent light	1410	**C**
Sodium bicarbonate	AB	3 mEq/ 3 ml	ES	1:100,000[a], 30 ml	11% lidocaine loss in 1 week and 22% loss in 2 weeks at 25 °C by GC. 28% epinephrine loss by HPLC in 1 week at 25 °C	1712	**I**
	AB	3 mEq/ 3 ml	ES	1:100,000[a], 30 ml	6% lidocaine loss by GC in 4 weeks at 4 °C. 2% epinephrine loss in 1 week and 12% loss in 3 weeks at 4 °C by HPLC	1712	**C**
	LY	0.1 mEq/ml	AST	1:100,000[b]	25% epinephrine loss by HPLC in 1 week at room temperature. Lidocaine not tested	1713	**I**
	AST	8.4%, 2 ml	AST	1:200,000[c], 20 ml	Visually compatible for up to 5 hr at room temperature	1724	**C**
	AST	8.4%, 2 ml	AST	1:200,000[d], 20 ml	Haze clarifies with gentle agitation	1724	**?**
	AB	4%, 4 ml	AST	1:200,000[c], 20 ml	Visually compatible for up to 5 hr at room temperature	1724	**C**
	AB	4%, 4 ml	AST	1:200,000[d], 20 ml	Haze clarifies with gentle agitation	1724	**?**
	AB	4%, 0.05 to 0.6 ml	AST, WI	1:200,000[e], 20 ml	Precipitate forms in 1 to 2 min up to 2 hr at lowest amount of bicarbonate	1724	**I**
		1.4 and 8.4%, 1.5 ml	BEL	1:80,000[f], 20 ml	8% epinephrine loss by HPLC in 7 days at room temperature. Lidocaine not tested	1743	**C**
		4.2 and 8.4%, 1.5 ml	BEL	1:200,000[g], 20 ml	5 to 7% epinephrine loss by HPLC in 7 days at room temperature. Bupivacaine not tested	1743	**C**
		1.4%, 1.5 ml	BEL	1:200,000[g], 20 ml	Little or no epinephrine loss by HPLC in 7 days at room temperature. Bupivacaine not tested	1743	**C**

[a]*Lidocaine HCl 2% with epinephrine HCl 1:100,000.*
[b]*Lidocaine HCl 1% with epinephrine HCl 1:100,000.*
[c]*Lidocaine HCl 1 and 1.5% with epinephrine HCl 1:200,000.*
[d]*Lidocaine HCl 2% with epinephrine HCl 1:200,000.*
[e]*Bupivacaine HCl 0.5 and 0.75% with epinephrine HCl 1:200,000.*
[f]*Lidocaine HCl 2% with epinephrine HCl 1:80,000.*
[g]*Bupivacaine HCl 0.5% with epinephrine HCl 1:200,000.*

Y-Site Injection Compatibility (1:1 Mixture)

Drug	Mfr	Conc	Mfr	Conc	Remarks	Ref	C/I
				Epinephrine HCl			
Ampicillin sodium	WY	40 mg/ml[c]	ES	0.032 mg/ml[c]	Slight color change in 3 hr	1316	**I**
Amrinone lactate	WB	3 mg/ml[b]	AB	0.1 mg/ml	Physically compatible for at least 4 hr at 25 °C under fluorescent light	992	**C**
Atracurium besylate	BW	0.5 mg/ml[a]	AB	4 µg/ml[a]	Physically compatible for 24 hr at 28 °C	1337	**C**
Calcium chloride	AB	4 mg/ml[c]	ES	0.032 mg/ml[c]	Physically compatible for 3 hr	1316	**C**
Calcium gluconate	AST	4 mg/ml[c]	ES	0.032 mg/ml[c]	Physically compatible for 3 hr	1316	**C**

Y-Site Injection Compatibility (1:1 Mixture) (Cont.)

Epinephrine HCl

Drug	Mfr	Conc	Mfr	Conc	Remarks	Ref	C/I
Cisatracurium besylate	GW	0.1, 2, 5 mg/ml[a]	AMR	0.05 mg/ml[a]	Physically compatible with no change in measured turbidity or increase in particle content in 4 hr at 23 °C	2074	C
Diltiazem HCl	MMD	5 mg/ml	PD	0.004 and 0.05 mg/ml[b]	Visually compatible	1807	C
	MMD	1 mg/ml[b]	PD	0.05 mg/ml[b]	Visually compatible	1807	C
	MMD	1 mg/ml[a]	AB	0.02 mg/ml[a]	Visually compatible for 4 hr at 27 °C	2062	C
Dobutamine HCl	LI	4 mg/ml[a]	AB	0.02 mg/ml[a]	Visually compatible for 4 hr at 27 °C	2062	C
Dopamine HCl	AB	3.2 mg/ml[a]	AB	0.02 mg/ml[a]	Visually compatible for 4 hr at 27 °C	2062	C
Famotidine	MSD	0.2 mg/ml[a]	ES	0.004 mg/ml[a]	Physically compatible for 4 hr at 25 °C	1188	C
Fentanyl citrate	ES	0.05 mg/ml	AB	0.02 mg/ml[a]	Visually compatible for 4 hr at 27 °C	2062	C
Furosemide	AMR	10 mg/ml	AB	0.02 mg/ml[a]	Visually compatible for 4 hr at 27 °C	2062	C
Heparin sodium	UP	1000 units/L[d]	AB	0.1 mg/ml	Physically compatible for at least 4 hr at room temperature by visual and microscopic examination	534	C
	ES	100 units/ml[a]	AB	0.02 mg/ml[a]	Visually compatible for 4 hr at 27 °C	2062	C
Hydrocortisone sodium succinate	UP	10 mg/L[d]	AB	0.1 mg/ml	Physically compatible for at least 4 hr at room temperature by visual and microscopic examination	534	C
Hydromorphone HCl	KN	1 mg/ml	AB	0.02 mg/ml[a]	Visually compatible for 4 hr at 27 °C	2062	C
Labetalol HCl	AH	2 mg/ml[a]	AB	0.02 mg/ml[a]	Visually compatible for 4 hr at 27 °C	2062	C
Lorazepam	WY	0.5 mg/ml[a]	AB	0.02 mg/ml[a]	Visually compatible for 4 hr at 27 °C	2062	C
Midazolam HCl	RC	2 mg/ml[a]	AB	0.02 mg/ml[a]	Visually compatible for 4 hr at 27 °C	2062	C
Milrinone lactate	SW	0.2 mg/ml[a]	AB	0.02 mg/ml[a]	Visually compatible for 4 hr at 27 °C	2062	C
	SW	0.4 mg/ml[a]	AB	0.064 mg/ml[a]	Visually compatible with little or no loss of either drug by HPLC in 4 hr at 23 °C	2214	C
Morphine sulfate	SCN	2 mg/ml[a]	AB	0.02 mg/ml[a]	Visually compatible for 4 hr at 27 °C	2062	C
Nicardipine HCl	WY	1 mg/ml[a]	AB	0.02 mg/ml[a]	Visually compatible for 4 hr at 27 °C	2062	C
Nitroglycerin	AB	0.4 mg/ml[a]	AB	0.02 mg/ml[a]	Visually compatible for 4 hr at 27 °C	2062	C
Norepinephrine bitartrate	AB	0.128 mg/ml[a]	AB	0.02 mg/ml[a]	Visually compatible for 4 hr at 27 °C	2062	C
Pancuronium bromide	ES	0.05 mg/ml[a]	AB	4 μg/ml[a]	Physically compatible for 24 hr at 28 °C	1337	C
Phytonadione	MSD	0.4 mg/ml[c]	ES	0.032 mg/ml[c]	Physically compatible for 3 hr	1316	C
Potassium chloride	AB	40 mEq/L[d]	AB	0.1 mg/ml	Physically compatible for at least 4 hr at room temperature by visual and microscopic examination	534	C
Propofol	ZEN	10 mg/ml	AMR	0.1 mg/ml	Physically compatible for 1 hr at 23 °C with no increase in particle content	2066	C
Ranitidine HCl	GL	1 mg/ml[a]	AB	0.02 mg/ml[a]	Visually compatible for 4 hr at 27 °C	2062	C
Remifentanil HCl	GW	0.025 and 0.25 mg/ml[b]	AMR	0.05 mg/ml[a]	Physically compatible with no change in measured turbidity or increase in particle content in 4 hr at 23 °C	2075	C
Thiopental sodium	AB	25 mg/ml[e]	AB	0.02 mg/ml[a]	Yellow color forms in 4 hr at 27 °C	2062	I
TPN #189[f]			AST	0.2 mg/ml[b]	Visually compatible for 24 hr at 22 °C	1767	C

Y-Site Injection Compatibility (1:1 Mixture) (Cont.)

Epinephrine HCl

Drug	Mfr	Conc	Mfr	Conc	Remarks	Ref	C/I
Vecuronium bromide	OR	0.1 mg/ml[a]	AB	4 µg/ml[a]	Physically compatible for 24 hr at 28 °C	1337	C
	OR	1 mg/ml	AB	0.02 mg/ml[a]	Visually compatible for 4 hr at 27 °C	2062	C
Vitamin B complex with C	RC	2 ml/L[d]	AB	0.1 mg/ml	Physically compatible for at least 4 hr at room temperature by visual and microscopic examination	534	C
Warfarin sodium	DU	0.1[c] and 2[e] mg/ml	AMR	0.1 mg/ml[c]	Physically compatible with no change in measured turbidity or increase in particle content in 24 hr at 23 °C	2011	C

[a]*Tested in dextrose 5% in water.*
[b]*Tested in sodium chloride 0.9%.*
[c]*Tested in both dextrose 5% in water and sodium chloride 0.9%.*
[d]*Tested in dextrose 5% in Ringer's injection, dextrose 5% in Ringer's injection, lactated, dextrose 5% in water, Ringer's injection, lactated, and sodium chloride 0.9%.*
[e]*Tested in sterile water for injection.*
[f]*Refer to Appendix I for the composition of parenteral nutrition solutions. TPN indicates a 2-in-1 admixture.*

Additional Compatibility Information

Alkalies and Oxidizing Agents— Epinephrine HCl is rapidly destroyed by alkalies or oxidizing agents including sodium bicarbonate, halogens, permanganates, chromates, nitrates, nitrites, and salts of easily reducible metals such as iron, copper, and zinc (1-7/94; 4).

Drugs known to be alkali labile such as epinephrine should not be mixed in aminophylline-containing solutions because of the alkalinity of these solutions (6).

Color Changes— Visual inspection for color changes may be inadequate to assess compatibility of admixtures. In one evaluation with aminophylline stored at 25 °C, a color change was not noted until eight hours had elapsed. However, only 40% of the initial epinephrine HCl was still present in the admixture at 24 hours (527).

Lidocaine HCl— When lidocaine HCl is mixed with epinephrine HCl, the buffering capacity of the lidocaine HCl may raise the pH of intravenous admixtures above 5.5, the maximum necessary for stability of epinephrine HCl. The final pH is usually about 6. Epinephrine HCl will begin to deteriorate within several hours. Therefore, admixtures should be used promptly after preparation or the separate administration of the epinephrine HCl should be considered. This restriction does not apply to commercial lidocaine–epinephrine combinations that have had the pH adjusted to retain the maximum epinephrine potency (24).

Bupivacaine and Fentanyl— A solution composed of bupivacaine HCl (Winthrop) 0.44 mg/ml, fentanyl citrate (Janssen) 1.25 µg/ml, and epinephrine HCl (Abbott) 0.69 µg/ml was stored in 100-ml portable infusion pump reservoirs (Pharmacia Deltec) for 30 days at 3 and 23 °C. The samples were then delivered through the infusion pumps over 48 hours at near-body temperature (30 °C). The samples were visually compatible throughout, and bupivacaine HCl and fentanyl citrate exhibited no loss by HPLC analysis. Epinephrine HCl sustained about a 5 to 6% loss by HPLC analysis after 20 days of storage at both temperatures and about a 9 to 10% loss after 30 days of storage and subsequent pump delivery. The authors recommended restricting storage before administration to only 20 days (1627).

EPIRUBICIN HCL
AHFS 10:00

Ellence   **Pharmacia & Upjohn**

Products— Epirubicin HCl (Pharmacia & Upjohn) is available as a 2-mg/ml, preservative-free, ready-to-use solution in single-use polypropylene vials of 25 and 100 ml containing 50 and 200 mg of drug, respectively. The solution also contains sodium chloride and water for injection. The pH has been adjusted with hydrochloric acid (1-9/99).

pH— The solution pH has been adjusted to 3 (1-9/99).

Administration— Epirubicin HCl is administered by intravenous infusion over three to five minutes; infusion into the tubing of a freely running intravenous infusion of sodium chloride 0.9% or dextrose 5% in water is recommended. Administration by direct push is not recommended because of the risk of extravasation. Extravasation may cause pain, severe tissue lesions, and necrosis and should be avoided. Burning or stinging may indicate extravasation, requiring immediate termination of the infusion and restarting in another vein. Epirubicin HCl must *not* be given by intramuscular or subcutaneous injection (1-9/99).

Personnel preparing and administering this drug should take protective measures to avoid contact with the solution, including use of disposable gloves, gowns, masks, and eye goggles. Dose preparation should be performed in a suitable laminar airflow device on a work surface protected by plastic-backed absorbent paper. All equipment and materials used in preparing and administering doses should be disposed of safely using high-temperature incineration (1-9/99). See Inactivation below.

Stability— Epirubicin HCl in intact vials should be stored under refrigeration at 2 to 8 °C and protected from freezing and exposure to light. The manufacturer recommends discarding any unused solution from the single-dose vials within 24 hours after initial puncture of the vial stopper (1-9/99).

Beijnen et al. examined the stability of epirubicin HCl infusions. In solutions containing 100 mg/L in dextrose 5% in water (pH 4.35), the drug was stable for 28 days at 25 °C when protected from light. Epirubicin HCl was less stable in sodium chloride 0.9% or Ringer's injection, lactated, with a 10% loss in eight days under the same conditions (1007).

Wood et al. assessed the stability of epirubicin HCl 100 mg/L in sodium chloride 0.9% (pH 6.47) when stored in PVC bags at 4 and 25 °C in the dark. Epirubicin HCl was stable for at least 43 and 20 days at 4 and 25 °C, respectively. The drug admixed in dextrose 5% in water (pH 4.36) also was stable for at least 43 days at 4 °C (1460).

Epirubicin HCl was cultured with human lymphoblasts to determine whether its cytotoxic activity was retained. The solution retained cytotoxicity for 24 hours at 4 °C and room temperature (1575).

Syringes— Epirubicin HCl 2 mg/ml in sterile water for injection was stable for at least 43 days at 4 °C in Plastipak (Becton-Dickinson) plastic syringes (1460). Adams et al. reported that epirubicin HCl 0.5 mg/ml in sodium chloride 0.9% was stable for at least 28 days at 4 and 20 °C when stored in plastic syringes (1564).

Epirubicin HCl 2 mg/ml in sodium chloride 0.9% was packaged in 50-ml polypropylene syringes with blind luer hubs and stored at 25 °C both exposed to and protected from light and at 4 °C protected from light. HPLC analysis found about 2 to 4% loss in 14 days at 25 °C whether exposed to or protected from room light. No loss was found after 180 days of refrigerated storage (2081).

Freezing Solutions— Epirubicin HCl was stable for at least 43 days when stored at −20 °C at a concentration of 100 mg/L in sodium chloride 0.9% or dextrose 5% in water in PVC bags (Travenol) (1460).

Keusters et al. also reported that epirubicin HCl 1 g/L in sodium chloride 0.9% in PVC bags (Urotainer, Roussel) was stable when stored for four weeks at −20 °C and thawed by microwave or natural warming, exhibiting less than 5% degradation (1462).

pH Effects— Epirubicin HCl stability is pH dependent. It becomes progressively more stable at acid pH. Maximum stability is obtained at pH 4 to 5 (1007; 1460). Prolonged contact of epirubicin HCl with any solution having an alkaline pH should be avoided because of the resulting hydrolysis of the drug (1-9/99).

Light Effects— Although epirubicin HCl is photosensitive, no special precautions are necessary to protect solutions containing epirubicin HCl 500 μg/ml or greater during intravenous administration (1463) even over periods extending to 14 days in room light (2081).

Sorption— Wood et al. reported that epirubicin HCl was adsorbed to PVC bags. Losses depended on temperature, concentration, and vehicle. Losses were greatest in sodium chloride 0.9% at pH 6.47, compared with dextrose 5% in water at pH 4.36. After eight days of storage, examination of solutions containing epirubicin HCl 100 mg/L indicated combined losses of 4% at 4 °C and 8% at 25 °C. In clinical practice, epirubicin HCl at concentrations of at least 500 μg/ml exhibits negligible adsorptive losses during storage and delivery. Sorption to Plastipak (Becton-Dickinson) polypropylene syringes is also insignificant (1460).

DeVroe et al. compared the delivery of epirubicin HCl from 50-mg/1000 ml solutions in dextrose 5% in water and sodium chloride 0.9% in glass, PVC, and high density polyethylene containers and PVC, polyethylene, and polybutadiene infusion sets. The epirubicin HCl delivered from the container/set configurations was equivalent, with no evidence of sorption (1577).

Epirubicin HCl (Farmitalia) 20 μg/ml in dextrose 5% in water and sodium chloride 0.9% in PVC containers was infused through PVC infusion sets at 21 ml/hr over 24 hours at 22 °C while exposed to light. HPLC showed relatively minor fluctuations in delivered concentrations, with no evidence of sorption (1700).

Filtration— Epirubicin HCl 50 mg/1000 ml in dextrose 5% in water and sodium chloride 0.9% was infused over 24 hours and exhibited a potency loss during the initial period of filtration through cellulose ester and nylon filters. However, the concentrations returned to expected levels within minutes, and the total amount of drug lost was deemed negligible (1577).

Compatibility Information

Solution Compatibility

Epirubicin HCl

Solution	Mfr	Mfr	Conc/L	Remarks	Ref	C/I
Dextrose 3.3% in sodium chloride 0.3%		FA	100 mg	5% or less loss in 4 weeks at 25 °C in the dark	1007	C
Dextrose 5% in water		FA	100 mg	5% or less loss in 4 weeks at 25 °C in the dark	1007	C
	TR[a]	FA	100 mg	10% or less loss in 43 days at 4 and 25 °C in the dark	1460	C
	[b]	FA	50 mg	8 to 9% loss by HPLC in 30 days at 4 °C protected from light	1577	C
	[a]	FA	40 mg	Potency retained for 7 days at 4 °C protected from light	1700	C
Ringer's injection, lactated		FA	100 mg	5% or less loss in 4 weeks at 25 °C in the dark	1007	C

Solution Compatibility (Cont.)

Epirubicin HCl

Solution	Mfr	Mfr	Conc/L	Remarks	Ref	C/I
Sodium chloride 0.9%		FA	100 mg	5% or less loss in 4 weeks at 25 °C in the dark	1007	C
	TR[a]	FA	100 mg	10% or less loss in 43 days at 4 and 25 °C in the dark	1460	C
	[b]	FA	50 mg	6% or less loss by HPLC in 25 days at 4 °C protected from light	1577	C
	[a]	FA	40 mg	Potency retained for 7 days at 4 °C protected from light	1700	C

[a]Tested in PVC containers.
[b]Tested in glass, PVC, and high density polyethylene containers.

Drugs in Syringe Compatibility

Epirubicin HCl

Drug (in syringe)	Mfr	Amt	Mfr	Amt	Remarks	Ref	C/I
Fluorouracil		500 mg/ 10 ml		5 and 10 mg/ ml[a]	Precipitate forms within several hours	1564	I
Ifosfamide		50 mg/ ml[a]		1 mg/ml[a]	Little or no loss of either drug by HPLC in 28 days at 4 and 20 °C	1564	C
Ifosfamide with mesna		50 mg/ ml[a] 40 mg/ ml[a]		1 mg/ml[a]	50% epirubicin loss by HPLC in 7 days at 4 and 20 °C. No loss of other drugs in 7 days	1564	I

[a]Tested in sodium chloride 0.9%.

Additional Compatibility Information

The manufacturer recommends that other drugs not be mixed with epirubicin HCl. Heparin sodium and fluorouracil are incompatible with epirubicin HCl because of the potential for precipitation. Contact with any alkaline solution should be avoided because of the resulting hydrolysis of epirubicin HCl (1-9/99). See pH Effects above.

Other Information

Inactivation— Spills or leakage of epirubicin HCl solutions should be diluted with sodium hypochlorite having 1% available chlorine, preferably by soaking, and then diluted further with water (1-9/99).

Methylparaben— The methylparaben present in the lyophilized epirubicin HCl formulations available in some countries enhances the dissolution rate by disrupting bonding between epirubicin and other components (1442).

EPOETIN ALFA
AHFS 20:16

Procrit
Epogen

Ortho Biotech
Amgen

Products— Epoetin alfa is available in 1-ml single-use (unpreserved) vials containing 2000, 3000, 4000, and 10,000 units/ml. The solution also contains in each milliliter albumin (human) 2.5 mg, sodium citrate 5.8 mg, sodium chloride 5.8 mg, and citric acid 0.06 mg in water for injection (2).

Epoetin alfa is also available in 2-ml multidose (preserved) vials containing 10,000 units/ml and 1-ml multidose (preserved) vials containing 20,000 units/ml. The solution also contains in each milliliter albumin (human) 2.5 mg, sodium citrate 1.3 mg, sodium chloride 8.2 mg, citric acid 0.11 mg, and benzyl alcohol 1% in water for injection (2).

pH— Single-use vials: from 6.6 to 7.2. Multidose vials: from 5.8 to 6.4 (2).

Tonicity— The injection is isotonic (2).

Administration— Epoetin alfa is administered by intravenous or sub-cutaneous injection. For subcutaneous injection, epoetin alfa (single-dose and multidose) may be diluted at the time of administration with an equal quantity of bacteriostatic sodium chloride 0.9% containing benzyl alcohol 0.9% to help ameliorate local discomfort at the subcutaneous injection site (2; 4).

Stability— Epoetin alfa is a colorless solution. It should not be used if it contains particulate matter or is discolored. Intact vials should be stored under refrigeration and protected from freezing. To prevent foaming and inactivation, the product should not be shaken; vigorous prolonged shaking may denature the protein, inactivating it (2; 4). However, a small amount of flocculated protein in the solution does not affect potency. In addition, exposure to light for less than 24 hours does not adversely affect the product (4).

The single-dose vials have no preservative. After a single dose has been removed from this product, the vial should not be reentered and should be discarded (2). Drawn into plastic tuberculin syringes, the preservative-free products at 2000 or 10,000 units/ml are reported to be stable for two weeks at room temperature or under refrigeration. However, use shortly after drawing up in syringes is recommended because of the absence of preservative (4).

Usually, epoetin alfa should not be diluted and transferred to new containers or admixed with other drugs and solutions because of possible protein loss from adsorption to PVC containers and tubing. However, when 10,000-unit/ml single-use product is diluted in the original vial with benzyl alcohol-preserved sodium chloride 0.9% injection to a concentration of 4000 units/ml for subcutaneous use, it is stated to be stable for at least 12 weeks stored at 5 and 30 °C. Furthermore, the final benzyl alcohol concentration of 0.54% enabled the dilution to pass the USP preservative effectiveness test (1905). Restriction of this dilution to 28 days used as a multiple-dose vial has been recommended (1906). Higher concentrations of epoetin alfa (e.g., 5000 units/ml), which would have lower benzyl alcohol concentrations, were found to fail the preservative effectiveness test (1905).

The multidose vials contain a preservative and may be stored under refrigeration after initial dose removal. The vials should be discarded 21 days after initial entry (2).

Compatibility Information

Solution Compatibility

Epoetin alfa

Solution	Mfr	Mfr	Conc/L	Remarks	Ref	C/I
Dextrose 10% in water	a	ORT	100 units	Up to 40% of epoetin alfa lost by bioassay over 24-hr delivery	1878	I
Dextrose 10% in water with albumin 0.01%	a	ORT	100 units	Up to 40% of epoetin alfa lost by bioassay over 24-hr delivery	1878	I
Dextrose 10% in water with albumin 0.05%	a	ORT	100 units	98% of the epoetin alfa by bioassay delivered over 24 hr	1878	C
Dextrose 10% in water with albumin 0.1%	a	ORT	100 units	98% of the epoetin alfa by bioassay delivered over 24 hr	1878	C
Sodium chloride 0.9%	a	ORT	100 units	15% of epoetin alfa lost by bioassay over 24-hr delivery	1878	I
TPN[b]	a	ORT	100 units	98% of the epoetin alfa by bioassay delivered over 24 hr	1878	C

[a]*Delivered from a syringe through microbore tubing, T-connector, and a Teflon neonatal 24-gauge intravenous catheter.*
[b]*TPN composed of amino acids (TrophAmine) 0.5% or 2.25% with dextrose 12.5%, vitamins, trace elements, magnesium sulfate, calcium gluconate, sodium chloride, potassium acetate, and heparin sodium.*

ERGONOVINE MALEATE
AHFS 76:00

Ergotrate Maleate   **Bedford**

Products— Ergonovine maleate is available in 1-ml vials. Each milliliter of solution contains (1-6/94):

Ergonovine maleate	0.2 mg
Ethyl lactate	0.1%
Lactic acid	0.1%
Phenol	0.25%
Water for injection	qs 1 ml

pH— From 2.7 to 3.5 (4).

Administration— Ergonovine maleate may be administered by intramuscular injection or intravenous injection over at least one minute. Dilution of intravenous doses to 5 ml with sodium chloride 0.9% has been recommended (4).

Stability— Although storage of ergonovine maleate below 8 °C is recommended, intact ampuls are stable for 60 to 90 days at controlled room temperature (4; 60; 853; 1433). If discoloration occurs, the drug should not be used (4).

Filtration— Ergonovine maleate (Lilly) 0.2 mg/25 ml in dextrose 5% in water and sodium chloride 0.9%, filtered at a rate of about 3 ml/min through a 0.22-μm cellulose ester membrane filter (Ivex-2), showed no significant reduction in potency due to binding to the filter (533).

Compatibility Information

Additive Compatibility

Ergonovine maleate

Drug	Mfr	Conc/L	Mfr	Conc/L	Test Soln	Remarks	Ref	C/I
Amikacin sulfate	BR	5 g	LI	0.2 mg	D5LR, D5R, D5S, D5W, D10W, IS10, LR, NS, R, SL	Physically compatible and amikacin potency retained for 24 hr at 25 °C. Ergonovine not analyzed	294	C
Sodium bicarbonate	AB	2.4 mEq[a]		0.2 mg	D5W	Physically compatible for 24 hr	772	C

[a]*One vial of Neut added to a liter of admixture.*

ERYTHROMYCIN LACTOBIONATE
AHFS 8:12.12

Erythrocin Lactobionate-I.V.   **Abbott**
Erythrocin Piggyback   **Abbott**

Products— Erythromycin lactobionate (Abbott) is available in vials containing the equivalent of 1 g of erythromycin with benzyl alcohol 180 mg and in vials containing the equivalent of 500 mg of erythromycin with benzyl alcohol 90 mg (1-10/96). Reconstitute the 1-g vials with at least 20 ml and the 500-mg vials with at least 10 ml of sterile water for injection without preservatives (1-10/96; 4; 20). The resultant concentration is 5% (50 mg/ml) (1-10/96; 20).

Erythromycin lactobionate (Abbott) is also available in piggyback containers containing the equivalent of 500 mg of erythromycin with benzyl alcohol 90 mg. Reconstitute the 500-mg piggyback vial by adding 100 ml of sodium chloride 0.9%, Ringer's injection, lactated, or Normosol R. Alternatively, reconstitution may be made with 100 ml of the following solutions that have been buffered with 1 ml of sodium bicarbonate 4% additive solution (Neut, Abbott) (4):

    Dextrose 5% in water
    Dextrose 5% in Ringer's injection, lactated

    Dextrose 5% in sodium chloride 0.9%
    Normosol M and dextrose 5%
    Normosol R and dextrose 5%

Immediately after adding the diluent, shake the product well to decrease the time required to effect dissolution (4).

pH— Reconstitution with sterile water for injection to a 50-mg/ml concentration results in a solution with a pH of 6.5 to 7.5 (20).

One report indicated that the addition of 4% sodium bicarbonate buffer may not be necessary, even in dextrose-containing solutions. The pH of erythromycin lactobionate 500 mg/100 ml was determined to be 6.8 when dextrose 5% in water was the diluent and 7.15 when sodium chloride 0.9% was the diluent. The sodium bicarbonate buffer raised the solution pH about 0.5 to 0.7 pH unit above these values (1260).

Osmolality— Erythromycin lactobionate (Abbott) 50 mg/ml in sterile water for injection has an osmolality of 223 mOsm/kg (50).

The osmolality of erythromycin lactobionate was calculated for the following dilutions (1054):

Diluent	Osmolality (mOsm/kg)	
	50 ml	100 ml
500 mg		
Dextrose 5% in water	273	265
Sodium chloride 0.9%	299	291
1 g		
Dextrose 5% in water	287	273
Sodium chloride 0.9%	313	300

Solution pH	Approximate Time for 10% Decomposition (t_{90})
5.0	2.5 hr
5.5	8.8 hr
6.0	1 day
7.0	4.6 days
8.0	7.3 days
9.0	2.6 days
10.0	8.8 hr
11.0	53 min

Administration— Erythromycin lactobionate may be administered by continuous or intermittent intravenous infusion; it must not be given by direct intravenous injection (1-10/96; 4). To minimize venous irritation, slow continuous infusion of a 1-mg/ml concentration is recommended. By intermittent infusion, one-fourth of the daily dose at a concentration of 1 to 5 mg/ml in at least 100 ml of infusion solution may be given over 20 to 60 minutes every six hours (1-10/96; 4).

Stability— Do not use sodium chloride 0.9% or other solutions containing inorganic ions in the initial reconstitution of the regular vials. Such solutions result in the formation of a precipitate (1-10/96; 4; 20). (Note: This restriction does not apply to the drug in piggyback containers.)

The commercial vials are stable at room temperature (20) and have an expiration date four years from manufacture (4). Reconstituted (5%) solutions are stable for 14 days when stored under refrigeration at 2 to 15 °C (1-10/96; 20) or for 24 hours when kept at room temperature (1-10/96; 4).

The manufacturer indicates that the reconstituted erythromycin lactobionate in piggyback containers should be used within eight hours at room temperature or 24 hours under refrigeration (4).

pH Effects— The stability of erythromycin lactobionate is extremely pH dependent. It is most stable at pH 6 to 8 (20; 1935) or 9 (1101). Erythromycin lactobionate is unstable in acidic solutions. Decomposition occurs at an increasingly more rapid rate as the pH approaches 4 (20). A pH of at least 5.5 is recommended for the final diluted solution (1-10/96). At pH 5.5 or below and at pH 10 or above, erythromycin (both glucheptate and lactobionate) is particularly unstable, with 10% decomposition occurring in about eight or nine hours. Pluta and Morgan determined the following pH profile for erythromycin in solution (1101):

The effect of buffering erythromycin lactobionate (Abbott) solutions was evaluated by Allwood. Erythromycin lactobionate 2 mg/ml in sodium chloride 0.9% (pH 7.15 to 7.25) exhibited 5% losses by HPLC analysis in about 20 days at 5 °C. However, buffering with sodium bicarbonate to pH 7.5 to 8 extended stability, with 5% losses occurring in about 85 days at 5 °C (1587).

Freezing Solutions— Although the freezing of erythromycin lactobionate solutions was not previously recommended (108), the manufacturers indicate that freezing is acceptable for the piggyback containers and vials. The reconstituted solution should be frozen within four hours of preparation. The solution is stable for 30 days when stored frozen at −10 to −20 °C. Thawing should be performed in the refrigerator, and use of the thawed solution within eight hours is recommended. The thawed solution should not be refrozen (4).

Erythromycin lactobionate (Abbott) 500 mg/110 ml in sodium chloride 0.9% in PVC bags was frozen at −20 °C; HPLC analysis found no loss after 12 months of storage followed by microwave thawing. Furthermore, the solution was physically compatible, with no increase in subvisual particles. In addition, no erythromycin loss was found by HPLC analysis after six months at −20 °C followed by three freeze–thaw cycles (1612).

Portable Pumps— Stiles et al. evaluated the stability of erythromycin lactobionate (Elkins-Sinn) 20 mg/ml in sterile water for injection and sodium chloride 0.9% in 100-ml portable pump reservoirs (Pharmacia Deltec) during simulated administration for 24 hours. The drug solutions were tested by HPLC analysis when administered immediately after preparation and after storage for 24 hours at 5 °C before 24-hour administration. During simulated administration, some reservoirs were kept at 30 °C; others were placed in insulated pouches with frozen (−20 °C) gel packs to keep them chilled below the ambient temperature. The erythromycin lactobionate solutions exhibited little or no loss by HPLC under all study conditions. Chilling of the drug reservoirs was not necessary to complete the infusions, nor did it enhance stability substantially during the study period (1779).

Compatibility Information

Solution Compatibility

Erythromycin lactobionate

Solution	Mfr	Mfr	Conc/L	Remarks	Ref	C/I
Dextrose 2½% in half-strength Ringer's injection, lactated	AB	AB	1 g	10% decomposition in 4 hr at 25 °C	20	I
Dextrose 5% in Ringer's injection, lactated	AB	AB	1 g	10% decomposition in 3 hr at 25 °C	20	I
	TR[a]	AB	1 g	10 to 24% decomposition in 24 hr at 5 °C	282	I

Solution Compatibility (Cont.)

Erythromycin lactobionate

Solution	Mfr	Mfr	Conc/L	Remarks	Ref	C/I
Dextrose 5% in sodium chloride 0.9%	TR[a]	AB	1 g	Potency retained for 24 hr at 5 °C	282	C
	AB	AB	1 g	33% decomposition in 24 hr	46	I
	AB	AB	1 g	12% decomposition in 6 hr at 25 °C	48	I
		AB	2 g	15% decomposition in 6 hr	109	I
Dextrose 5% in water	TR[a]	AB	1 g	Potency retained for 24 hr at 5 °C	282	C
	AB	AB	1 g	15% decomposition in 24 hr	46	I
	AB	AB	1 g	10% decomposition in 10 hr at 25 °C	20	I
		AB	1 g	15% decomposition in 24 hr at 25 °C	48	I
		AB	2 g	14% decomposition in 6 hr	109	I
	TR[b]	AB	4 g	21% reduction in microbiologic inhibition in 24 hr at room temperature	518	I
	TR[b]	AB	4 g	Buffered[c]—physically compatible and potency retained for 24 hr at room temperature	518	C
Dextrose 10% in water		AB	2 g	14% decomposition in 6 hr	109	I
Multielectrolyte solution	AB	AB	1 g	14% decomposition in 24 hr	46	I
Normosol M in dextrose 5%	AB	AB	1 g	10% decomposition in 11 hr at 25 °C	20	I
Normosol R		AB	1 g	14% decomposition in 24 hr at 25 °C	48	I
Ringer's injection	AB	AB	1 g	10% decomposition in 11 hr at 25 °C	20	I
Ringer's injection, lactated	TR[a]	AB	1 g	Potency retained for 24 hr at 5 °C	282	C
	AB	AB	1 g	10% decomposition in 18 hr at 25 °C	20	I
Sodium chloride 0.9%		AB	1 g	Potency retained for 24 hr at 25 °C	48	C
		AB	2 g	Potency retained for 24 hr	109	C
	AB	AB	1 g	Potency retained for 24 hr	46	C
	AB	AB	1 g	10% decomposition in 22 hr at 25 °C	20	C
	TR[a]	AB	1 g	Potency retained for 24 hr at 5 °C	282	C
	TR[b]	AB	4 g	Physically compatible and potency retained for 24 hr at room temperature	518	C
	TR[b]	AB	4 g	Buffered[c]—physically compatible and potency retained for 24 hr at room temperature	518	C
		AB	2 g	5% loss by HPLC in about 20 days at 5 °C	1587	C
	BA[b]	AB	8.3 g	No more than 5% loss by HPLC after 60 days at 5 °C	1597	C
	AB[d]	ES	20 g	Little or no loss by HPLC with 24-hr storage at 5 °C followed by 24-hr simulated administration at 30 °C via portable pump	1779	C

[a]Tested in both glass and PVC containers.
[b]Tested in PVC containers.
[c]Buffered with sodium bicarbonate 4% (Neut, Abbott).
[d]Tested in portable pump reservoirs (Pharmacia Deltec).

Additive Compatibility

Erythromycin lactobionate

Drug	Mfr	Conc/L	Mfr	Conc/L	Test Soln	Remarks	Ref	C/I
Aminophylline	SE	500 mg	AB	1 g		Physically compatible. Erythromycin potency retained for 24 hr at 25 °C	20	C
Ampicillin sodium	WY	3.7 g	AB	3 g	NS	Physically compatible with 6% ampicillin loss in 1 day at 24 °C	1035	C
Ascorbic acid injection	AB	1 g	AB	1 g		Physically compatible	3	C
	UP	500 mg	AB	5 g	D5W	Physically incompatible	15	I

Additive Compatibility (Cont.)

Erythromycin lactobionate

Drug	Mfr	Conc/L	Mfr	Conc/L	Test Soln	Remarks	Ref	C/I
Cimetidine HCl	SKF	3 g	AB	5 g	D5W	Physically compatible and cimetidine chemically stable for 24 hr at room temperature. Erythromycin not tested	551	**C**
Colistimethate sodium	WC	500 mg	AB	5 g	D5W	Physically incompatible	15	**I**
	WC	500 mg	AB	1 g	D	Precipitate forms within 1 hr	20	**I**
Diphenhydramine HCl	PD	50 mg	AB	1 g		Physically compatible. Erythromycin potency retained for 24 hr at 25 °C	20	**C**
	PD	50 mg	AB	1 g	D5W	Erythromycin potency retained for 24 hr at 25 °C	48	**C**
Floxacillin sodium	BE	20 g	AB	5 g	NS	Immediate precipitation. Crystals form in 5 hr at 15 °C	1479	**I**
Furosemide	HO	1 g	AB	5 g	NS	Immediate precipitation. Crystals form in 12 to 24 hr at 15 and 30 °C	1479	**I**
Heparin sodium	UP	4000 units	AB	5 g	D5W	Physically incompatible	15	**I**
	AB	1500 units	AB	1 g		Precipitate forms within 1 hr	20	**I**
	AB	20,000 units	AB	1 g		Precipitate forms within 1 hr	21	**I**
	OR	20,000 units	AB	1.5 g	D5W, NS	Precipitate forms	113	**I**
Hydrocortisone sodium succinate	UP	500 mg	AB	5 g	D5W	Physically compatible	15	**C**
	UP	250 mg	AB	1 g		Physically compatible	3; 20	**C**
Lidocaine HCl	AST	2 g	AB	1 g		Physically compatible	24	**C**
Metaraminol bitartrate	MSD	100 mg	AB	750 mg	D5W	92% erythromycin decomposition in 24 hr at 25 °C	20	**I**
	MSD	100 mg	AB	1 g	D5W	44% erythromycin decomposition in 6 hr at 25 °C	48	**I**
Metoclopramide HCl	RB	400 mg	AB	4 g	NS	Incompatible. If mixed, use immediately	924	**I**
	RB	100 mg	AB	5 g	NS	Incompatible. If mixed, use immediately	924	**I**
	RB	416 mg	AB	4.1 g		Incompatible. If mixed, use immediately	1167	**I**
	RB	100 mg	AB	5 g		Incompatible. If mixed, use immediately	1167	**I**
	RB	1.1 g	AB	3.5 g		Incompatible. If mixed, use immediately	1167	**I**
Penicillin G potassium		1 million units	AB	1 g		Physically compatible	3	**C**
	SQ	20 million units	AB	5 g	D5W	Physically compatible	15	**C**
	SQ	5 million units	AB	1 g		Physically compatible	20; 47	**C**
Penicillin G sodium	UP	20 million units	AB	5 g	D5W	Physically compatible	15	**C**
Pentobarbital sodium	AB	500 mg	AB	1 g		Physically compatible. Erythromycin potency retained for 24 hr at 25 °C	20	**C**
Polymyxin B sulfate	BW	200 mg	AB	5 g	D5W	Physically compatible	15	**C**

Additive Compatibility (Cont.)

Erythromycin lactobionate

Drug	Mfr	Conc/L	Mfr	Conc/L	Test Soln	Remarks	Ref	C/I
Potassium chloride	AB	40 mEq	AB	1 g		Physically compatible	20	**C**
Prochlorperazine edisylate	SKF	10 mg	AB	1 g		Physically compatible. Erythromycin potency retained for 24 hr at 25 °C	20	**C**
Promazine HCl	WY	100 mg	AB	1 g		Physically compatible	20	**C**
Ranitidine HCl	GL	50 mg and 2 g		5 g	NS	Physically compatible and ranitidine chemically stable by HPLC for 24 hr at 25 °C. Erythromycin not tested	1515	**C**
Sodium bicarbonate	AB	3.75 g	AB	1 g		Physically compatible. Erythromycin potency retained for 24 hr at 25 °C	20	**C**
	AB	2.4 mEq[a]	AB	1 g	D5W	Physically compatible for 24 hr	772	**C**
Verapamil HCl	KN	80 mg	AB	2 g	D5W, NS	Physically compatible for 24 hr	764	**C**
Vitamin B complex with C	AB	5 ml		5 g	D5W	pH outside stability range	100	**I**
	AB	10 ml	AB	500 mg	D5W	90% erythromycin decomposition in 24 hr at 25 °C	20	**I**
		10 ml	AB	1 g	D5W	74% erythromycin decomposition in 6 hr at 25 °C	48	**I**

[a]*One vial of Neut added to a liter of admixture.*

Drugs in Syringe Compatibility

Erythromycin lactobionate

Drug (in syringe)	Mfr	Amt	Mfr	Amt	Remarks	Ref	C/I
Ampicillin sodium	AY	500 mg	AB	300 mg/6 ml	Precipitate forms in 1 hr at room temperature	300	**I**
Heparin sodium	AB	20,000 units/1 ml	AB	1 g	Physically incompatible	21	**I**
		2500 units/1 ml	SC	250 mg	Turbidity or precipitate forms within 5 min	1053	**I**

Y-Site Injection Compatibility (1:1 Mixture)

Erythromycin lactobionate

Drug	Mfr	Conc	Mfr	Conc	Remarks	Ref	C/I
Acyclovir sodium	BW	5 mg/ml[a]	AB	4 mg/ml[a]	Physically compatible for 4 hr at 25 °C	1157	**C**
Amiodarone HCl	LZ	4 mg/ml[c]	AB	2 mg/ml[c]	Physically compatible for 4 hr at room temperature	1444	**C**
Cyclophosphamide	MJ	20 mg/ml[a]	AB	5 mg/ml[a]	Physically compatible for 4 hr at 25 °C	1194	**C**
Diltiazem HCl	MMD	5 mg/ml	ES	5 and 50 mg/ml[b]	Visually compatible	1807	**C**
Enalaprilat	MSD	0.05 mg/ml[b]	AB	5 mg/ml[a]	Physically compatible for 24 hr at room temperature under fluorescent light	1355	**C**
Esmolol HCl	DCC	10 mg/ml[a]	AB	5 mg/ml[a]	Physically compatible for 24 hr at 22 °C	1169	**C**
Famotidine	MSD	0.2 mg/ml[a]	ES	2 mg/ml[b]	Physically compatible for 14 hr	1196	**C**
Fluconazole	RR	2 mg/ml	LY	20 mg/ml	Immediate precipitation	1407	**I**

Y-Site Injection Compatibility (1:1 Mixture) (Cont.)

Erythromycin lactobionate

Drug	Mfr	Conc	Mfr	Conc	Remarks	Ref	C/I
Foscarnet sodium	AST	24 mg/ml	AB	20 mg/ml	Physically compatible for 24 hr at room temperature under fluorescent light	1335	**C**
	AST	24 mg/ml	ES	20 mg/ml[c]	Physically compatible for 24 hr at 25 °C under fluorescent light by visual and microscopic examination	1393	**C**
Heparin sodium	TR	50 units/ml	AB	3.3 mg/ml[b]	Visually compatible for 6 hr at 25 °C	1793	**C**
Hydromorphone HCl	WY	0.2 mg/ml[a]	AB	5 mg/ml[a]	Physically compatible for at least 4 hr at 25 °C under fluorescent light	987	**C**
Idarubicin HCl	AD	1 mg/ml[b]	ES	2 mg/ml[b]	Visually compatible for 24 hr at 25 °C	1525	**C**
Labetalol HCl	SC	1 mg/ml[a]	AB	5 mg/ml[a]	Physically compatible for 24 hr at 18 °C	1171	**C**
Lorazepam	WY	0.33 mg/ml[b]	AB	5 mg/ml	Visually compatible for 24 hr at 22 °C	1855	**C**
Magnesium sulfate	IX	16.7, 33.3, 66.7, 100 mg/ml[a]	AB	5 mg/ml[a]	Physically compatible for at least 4 hr at 32 °C	813	**C**
Meperidine HCl	WY	10 mg/ml[a]	AB	5 mg/ml[a]	Physically compatible for at least 4 hr at 25 °C under fluorescent light	987	**C**
Midazolam HCl	RC	5 mg/ml	AB	5 mg/ml	Visually compatible for 24 hr at 22 °C	1855	**C**
Morphine sulfate	WI	1 mg/ml[a]	AB	5 mg/ml[a]	Physically compatible for at least 4 hr at 25 °C under fluorescent light	987	**C**
Multivitamins	USV	5 ml/L[a]	AB	500 mg/250 ml[b]	Physically compatible for 24 hr at room temperature	323	**C**
Perphenazine	SC	0.02 mg/ml[a]	AB	5 mg/ml[a]	Physically compatible for 4 hr at 25 °C	1155	**C**
Tacrolimus	FUJ	1 mg/ml[b]	AB	20 mg/ml[a]	Visually compatible for 24 hr at 25 °C	1630	**C**
Theophylline	TR	4 mg/ml	AB	3.3 mg/ml[b]	Visually compatible for 6 hr at 25 °C	1793	**C**
TNA #73[d]		32.5 ml[e]	AB	1 g/50 ml[b]	Physically compatible for 4 hr at 25 °C by visual assessment	1008	**C**
TPN #61[d]		[f]	AB	50 mg/1 ml[g]	Physically compatible	1012	**C**
		[h]	AB	300 mg/6 ml[g]	Physically compatible	1012	**C**
TPN #189[d]			DB	10 mg/ml[a]	Visually compatible for 24 hr at 22 °C	1767	**C**
Vitamin B complex with C (Berocca-C 500)	RC	4 ml/L[a]	AB	500 mg/250 ml[b]	Physically compatible for 24 hr at room temperature	323	**C**
(Berocca-C)	RC	20 ml/L[a]	AB	500 mg/250 ml[b]	Physically compatible for 24 hr at room temperature	323	**C**
Zidovudine	BW	4 mg/ml[a]	AB	20 mg/ml[a,i]	Physically compatible for 4 hr at 25 °C under fluorescent light by visual and microscopic examination	1193	**C**

[a]*Tested in dextrose 5% in water.*
[b]*Tested in sodium chloride 0.9%.*
[c]*Tested in both dextrose 5% in water and sodium chloride 0.9%.*
[d]*Refer to Appendix I for the composition of parenteral nutrition solutions. TNA indicates a 3-in-1 admixture, and TPN indicates a 2-in-1 admixture.*
[e]*A 32.5-ml sample of parenteral nutrition solution mixed with 50 ml of antibiotic solution.*
[f]*Run at 21 ml/hr.*
[g]*Given over 30 minutes by syringe pump.*
[h]*Run at 94 ml/hr.*
[i]*Sodium bicarbonate 2.5 mEq added to adjust pH.*

Additional Compatibility Information

Additives— Erythromycin lactobionate may exhibit physical incompatibility with sodium salts of several biologically derived macromolecules such as antibiotics (20).

In addition, additives that may result in a final admixture pH below 5.5 should not be mixed with erythromycin lactobionate. These additives include metaraminol bitartrate, ascorbic acid (but not sodium ascorbate), and vitamin B complex with C (20).

Solutions— Erythromycin lactobionate (Abbott) can alter the pH of solutions and give itself some protection against decomposition for varying periods. The length of time is dependent on the initial pH and the buffer capacity of the solution (48). The pH of unbuffered dextrose 5% in water is raised one pH unit by the addition of erythromycin lactobionate (20). The use of admixtures with a pH of less than 5 is not recommended. If the admixture pH is 5 to 6, it should be used immediately (48). (See pH Effects.)

Erythromycin lactobionate (Abbott) 1 g/L is physically compatible with all Abbott infusion solutions (20). The reconstituted drug may be added to sodium chloride 0.9%, Ringer's injection, lactated, or Normosol R for infusion. It can also be infused in dextrose 5% in water, dextrose 5% in sodium chloride 0.9%, and dextrose 5% in Ringer's injection, lactated, providing the solutions are first buffered with sodium bicarbonate 4% additive solution (Neut, Abbott). The manufacturers recommend the use of 1 ml of Neut for each 100 ml of these solutions (1-10/96).

Chloramphenicol— Erythromycin lactobionate (Abbott) in dextrose 5% in water has been reported to be conditionally compatible with chloramphenicol sodium succinate (Parke-Davis). The incompatibility is dependent on the concentration of the additives. Therefore, if attempting to combine erythromycin with chloramphenicol sodium succinate, mix the solution thoroughly and observe it closely for any sign of incompatibility (15).

Riboflavin— Erythromycin 5 mg/ml as the lactobionate in pH 8 buffer was combined with riboflavin in concentrations varying from 1 mg/ml to 20 µg/ml. On exposure to light for four hours, almost total decomposition of the erythromycin occurred, with only 4 to 12% remaining. Protection from light resulted in 12 to 25% decomposition. When no riboflavin was present, 10% or less decomposition of the erythromycin occurred. It was concluded that a photodynamic decomposition reaction was taking place (564).

ESMOLOL HCL
AHFS 24:04

Brevibloc   **Baxter**

Products— Esmolol HCl (Baxter) is available as a concentrate containing 250 mg/ml in 10-ml ampuls with propylene glycol 25% and ethanol 25% in water for injection. The product is buffered with sodium acetate 17 mg and glacial acetic acid 0.00715 ml in each milliliter and may contain sodium hydroxide and/or hydrochloric acid to adjust the pH if necessary (2; 4).

Esmolol HCl concentrate must be diluted before use. The manufacturer recommends adding the contents of two 2.5-g ampuls to 500 ml or one 2.5-g ampul to 250 ml (with prior removal of solution overage as necessary) to yield a 10-mg/ml solution (2; 4).

A ready-to-use formulation containing esmolol HCl 10 mg/ml in 10-ml single-dose vials also is available. Each milliliter of this ready-to-use product is buffered with sodium acetate 2.8 mg and glacial acetic acid 0.546 mg and may contain sodium hydroxide and/or hydrochloric acid for pH adjustment (2; 4).

pH— Concentrate: from 3.5 to 5.5. Ready-to-use: from 4.5 to 5.5 (4).

Osmolarity— Dilution of the esmolol HCl concentrate to 25 mg/ml in water results in a solution with an osmolarity of 1063 mOsm/L (4).

Administration— Esmolol HCl is administered by intravenous infusion at a concentration of 10 mg/ml, usually with an infusion control device. Concentrations exceeding 10 mg/ml are not recommended (2; 4).

Stability— Esmolol HCl is a clear, colorless to light yellow solution. It should be stored at controlled room temperature and protected from temperatures of 40 °C and above. Freezing does not affect the product adversely (2; 4). When stored appropriately, the product has an expiration date three years from manufacture (4).

pH Effects— Esmolol HCl is relatively stable at neutral pH; the optimal pH is 4.5 to 5.5. However, ester hydrolysis occurs rapidly in strongly acidic or basic solutions (1358; 1359).

Compatibility Information

Solution Compatibility

Esmolol HCl

Solution	Mfr	Mfr	Conc/L	Remarks	Ref	C/I
Dextrose 5% in Ringer's injection, lactated	BA[a], MG[b]	ACC	10 g	Visually compatible with little or no drug loss by HPLC in 7 days at 5 or 27 °C, 48 hr at 40 °C, and 24 hr under intense light	1831	C

Solution Compatibility (Cont.)

Esmolol HCl

Solution	Mfr	Mfr	Conc/L	Remarks	Ref	C/I
Dextrose 5% in sodium chloride 0.45%	BA[a], MG[b]	ACC	10 g	Visually compatible with little or no drug loss by HPLC in 7 days at 5 or 27 °C, 48 hr at 40 °C, and 24 hr under intense light	1831	**C**
Dextrose 5% in sodium chloride 0.9%	BA[a], MG[b]	ACC	10 g	Visually compatible with little or no drug loss by HPLC in 7 days at 5 or 27 °C, 48 hr at 40 °C, and 24 hr under intense light	1831	**C**
Dextrose 5% in water	TR[a]	DU	6 g	Physically compatible with no loss in 24 hr at room temperature under fluorescent light	1358	**C**
	BA[a]	DU	10, 20, 30 g	Visually compatible with little or no drug loss by HPLC in 48 hr at 23 °C	1830	**C**
	BA[a], MG[b]	ACC	10 g	Visually compatible with little or no drug loss by HPLC in 7 days at 5 or 27 °C, 48 hr at 40 °C, and 24 hr under intense light	1831	**C**
Dextrose 5% in water with potassium chloride 40 mEq/L	BA[a], MG[b]	ACC	10 g	Visually compatible with little or no drug loss by HPLC in 7 days at 5 or 27 °C, 48 hr at 40 °C, and 24 hr under intense light	1831	**C**
Ringer's injection, lactated	BA[a], MG[b]	ACC	10 g	Visually compatible with little or no drug loss by HPLC in 7 days at 5 or 27 °C, 48 hr at 40 °C, and 24 hr under intense light	1831	**C**
Sodium bicarbonate 5%	MG[b]	ACC	10 g	Visually compatible with 5 and 8% esmolol losses by HPLC in 7 days at 4 and 27 °C, respectively. 9 and 4% losses in 24 hr at 40 °C and under intense light, respectively	1831	**C**
Sodium chloride 0.45%	BA[a], MG[b]	ACC	10 g	Visually compatible with little or no drug loss by HPLC in 7 days at 5 or 27 °C, 48 hr at 40 °C, and 24 hr under intense light	1831	**C**
Sodium chloride 0.9%	BA[a], MG[b]	ACC	10 g	Visually compatible with little or no drug loss by HPLC in 7 days at 5 or 27 °C, 48 hr at 40 °C, and 24 hr under intense light	1831	**C**

[a]Tested in PVC containers.
[b]Tested in glass containers.

Additive Compatibility

Esmolol HCl

Drug	Mfr	Conc/L	Mfr	Conc/L	Test Soln	Remarks	Ref	C/I
Aminophylline	LY	1 g	DU	6 g	D5W	Physically compatible with no loss of either drug in 24 hr at room temperature under fluorescent light	1358	**C**
Atracurium besylate	BW	500 mg		10 g	D5W	Physically compatible and atracurium chemically stable for 24 hr at 5 and 30 °C	1694	**C**
Bretylium tosylate	ES	1 g	DU	6 g	D5W	Physically compatible with no loss of either drug in 24 hr at room temperature under fluorescent light	1358	**C**
Heparin sodium	LY	50,000 units	DU	6 g	D5W	Physically compatible with no esmolol loss in 24 hr at room temperature under fluorescent light. Heparin not tested	1358	**C**

Additive Compatibility (Cont.)

Esmolol HCl

Drug	Mfr	Conc/L	Mfr	Conc/L	Test Soln	Remarks	Ref	C/I
Procainamide HCl	ES	4 g	DU	6 g	D5W	43% procainamide loss in 24 hr at room temperature under fluorescent light	1358	I

Y-Site Injection Compatibility (1:1 Mixture)

Esmolol HCl

Drug	Mfr	Conc	Mfr	Conc	Remarks	Ref	C/I
Amikacin sulfate	BR	5 mg/ml[a]	DCC	10 mg/ml[a]	Physically compatible for 24 hr at 22 °C	1169	C
Aminophylline	ES	1 mg/ml[a]	DCC	10 mg/ml[a]	Physically compatible for 24 hr at 22 °C	1169	C
Amiodarone HCl	WY	4.8 mg/ml[a]	DU	40 mg/ml[a]	Visually compatible for 24 hr at 23 °C	1877	C
Amphotericin B cholesteryl sulfate complex	SEQ	0.83 mg/ml[a]	OHM	10 mg/ml[a]	Microprecipitate forms in 4 hr at 23 °C under fluorescent light	2117	I
Ampicillin sodium	WY	20 mg/ml[b]	DCC	10 mg/ml[a]	Physically compatible for 24 hr at 22 °C	1169	C
Atracurium besylate	BW	0.5 mg/ml[a]	DCC	10 mg/ml[a]	Physically compatible for 24 hr at 28 °C	1337	C
Butorphanol tartrate	BR	0.04 mg/ml[a]	DCC	10 mg/ml[a]	Physically compatible for 24 hr at 22 °C	1169	C
Calcium chloride	AB	20 mg/ml[a]	DCC	10 mg/ml[a]	Physically compatible for 24 hr at 22 °C	1169	C
Cefazolin sodium	LI	10 mg/ml[a]	DCC	10 mg/ml[a]	Physically compatible for 24 hr at 22 °C	1169	C
Cefoperazone sodium	RR	10 mg/ml[a]	DCC	10 mg/ml[a]	Physically compatible for 24 hr at 22 °C	1169	C
Ceftazidime	GL[g]	10 mg/ml[a]	DCC	10 mg/ml[a]	Physically compatible for 24 hr at 22 °C	1169	C
Ceftizoxime sodium	SKF	10 mg/ml[a]	DCC	10 mg/ml[a]	Physically compatible for 24 hr at 22 °C	1169	C
Chloramphenicol sodium succinate	PD	10 mg/ml[a]	DCC	10 mg/ml[a]	Physically compatible for 24 hr at 22 °C	1169	C
Cimetidine HCl	SKF	6 mg/ml[a]	DCC	10 mg/ml[a]	Physically compatible for 24 hr at 22 °C	1169	C
Cisatracurium besylate	GW	0.1, 2, 5 mg/ml[a]	OHM	10 mg/ml[a]	Physically compatible with no change in measured turbidity or increase in particle content in 4 hr at 23 °C	2074	C
Clindamycin phosphate	UP	9 mg/ml[a]	DCC	10 mg/ml[a]	Physically compatible for 24 hr at 22 °C	1169	C
Diltiazem HCl	MMD	1 mg/ml[a]	DU	10 mg/ml[a]	Visually compatible for 24 hr at 25 °C	1530	C
Dopamine HCl	IMS	1.6 mg/ml[a]	DCC	10 mg/ml[a]	Physically compatible for 24 hr at 22 °C	1169	C
Enalaprilat	MSD	0.05 mg/ml[b]	DU	10 mg/ml[a]	Physically compatible for 24 hr at room temperature under fluorescent light	1355	C
Erythromycin lactobionate	AB	5 mg/ml[a]	DCC	10 mg/ml[a]	Physically compatible for 24 hr at 22 °C	1169	C
Famotidine	MSD	0.2 mg/ml[a]	DU	10 mg/ml[b]	Physically compatible for 4 hr at 25 °C	1188	C
Fentanyl citrate	JN	0.05 mg/ 1 ml	DCC	1 g/100 ml[d]	Physically compatible when fentanyl is injected into Y-site of flowing admixture[e]	1168	C
	JN	0.05 mg/ml	DCC	10 mg/ml[d]	Physically compatible with no loss of either drug in 8 hr at ambient temperature exposed to light	1168	C
Furosemide	HO	10 mg/ml	ACC	10 mg/ml[f]	Cloudy white precipitate forms immediately	1146	I
Gentamicin sulfate	ES	0.8 mg/ml[a]	DCC	10 mg/ml[a]	Physically compatible for 24 hr at 22 °C	1169	C
Heparin sodium	IX	40 units/ml[a]	DCC	10 mg/ml[a]	Physically compatible for 24 hr at 22 °C	1169	C

Y-Site Injection Compatibility (1:1 Mixture) (Cont.)

Esmolol HCl

Drug	Mfr	Conc	Mfr	Conc	Remarks	Ref	C/I
Hydrocortisone sodium succinate	LY	1 mg/ml[a]	DCC	10 mg/ml[a]	Physically compatible for 24 hr at 22 °C	1169	**C**
Insulin, regular	LI	1 unit/ml[a]	DU	40 mg/ml[a]	Visually compatible for 24 hr at 23 °C	1877	**C**
Labetalol HCl	GL	5 mg/ml	DU	40 mg/ml[a]	Visually compatible for 24 hr at 23 °C	1877	**C**
Magnesium sulfate	LY	10 mg/ml[a]	DCC	10 mg/ml[a]	Physically compatible for 24 hr at 22 °C	1169	**C**
Methyldopate HCl	MSD	5 mg/ml[a]	DCC	10 mg/ml[a]	Physically compatible for 24 hr at 22 °C	1169	**C**
Metronidazole	SE	5 mg/ml	DCC	10 mg/ml[a]	Physically compatible for 24 hr at 22 °C	1169	**C**
Midazolam HCl	RC	1 mg/ml[a]	DU	40 mg/ml[a]	Visually compatible for 24 hr at 23 °C	1877	**C**
Morphine sulfate	ES	15 mg/1 ml	DCC	1 g/100 ml[d]	Physically compatible when morphine is injected into Y-site of flowing admixture[d]	1168	**C**
	ES	15 mg/ml	DCC	10 mg/ml[d]	Physically compatible with no loss of either drug in 8 hr at ambient temperature exposed to light	1168	**C**
Nafcillin sodium	BR	10 mg/ml[a]	DCC	10 mg/ml[a]	Physically compatible for 24 hr at 22 °C	1169	**C**
Nitroglycerin	OM	0.2 mg/ml[a]	DU	40 mg/ml[a]	Visually compatible for 24 hr at 23 °C	1877	**C**
Norepinephrine HCl	STR	0.064 mg/ml[a]	DU	40 mg/ml[a]	Visually compatible for 24 hr at 23 °C	1877	**C**
Pancuronium bromide	ES	0.05 mg/ml[a]	DCC	10 mg/ml[a]	Physically compatible for 24 hr at 28 °C	1337	**C**
Penicillin G potassium	PF	50,000 units/ml[a]	DCC	10 mg/ml[a]	Physically compatible for 24 hr at 22 °C	1169	**C**
Phenytoin sodium	IX	1 mg/ml[a]	DCC	10 mg/ml[a]	Physically compatible for 24 hr at 22 °C	1169	**C**
Piperacillin sodium	LE	30 mg/ml[a]	DCC	10 mg/ml[a]	Physically compatible for 24 hr at 22 °C	1169	**C**
Polymyxin B sulfate	PF	0.005 unit/ml[a]	DCC	10 mg/ml[a]	Physically compatible for 24 hr at 22 °C	1169	**C**
Potassium chloride	IX	0.4 mEq/ml[a]	DCC	10 mg/ml[a]	Physically compatible for 24 hr at 22 °C	1169	**C**
Potassium phosphates	LY	0.44 mEq/ml[a]	DCC	10 mg/ml[a]	Physically compatible for 24 hr at 22 °C	1169	**C**
Propofol	ZEN	10 mg/ml	OHM	10 mg/ml	Physically compatible for 1 hr at 23 °C with no increase in particle content	2066	**C**
Ranitidine HCl	GL	0.5 mg/ml[a]	DCC	10 mg/ml[a]	Physically compatible for 24 hr at 22 °C	1169	**C**
Remifentanil HCl	GW	0.025 and 0.25 mg/ml[b]	OHM	10 mg/ml[a]	Physically compatible with no change in measured turbidity or increase in particle content in 4 hr at 23 °C	2075	**C**
Sodium acetate	LY	0.4 mEq/ml[a]	DCC	10 mg/ml[a]	Physically compatible for 24 hr at 22 °C	1169	**C**
Sodium nitroprusside	RC	0.2 mg/ml[a]	DU	40 mg/ml[a]	Visually compatible for 24 hr at 23 °C	1877	**C**
Streptomycin sulfate	PF	10 mg/ml[a]	DCC	10 mg/ml[a]	Physically compatible for 24 hr at 22 °C	1169	**C**
Tacrolimus	FUJ	1 mg/ml[b]	DU	10 mg/ml	Visually compatible for 24 hr at 25 °C	1630	**C**
Tobramycin sulfate	LI	0.8 mg/ml[a]	DCC	10 mg/ml[a]	Physically compatible for 24 hr at 22 °C	1169	**C**
Trimethoprim–sulfamethoxazole	BW	0.64 + 3.2 mg/ml[a]	DCC	10 mg/ml[a]	Physically compatible for 24 hr at 22 °C	1169	**C**
Vancomycin HCl	LE	5 mg/ml[a]	DCC	10 mg/ml[a]	Physically compatible for 24 hr at 22 °C	1169	**C**
Vecuronium bromide	OR	0.1 mg/ml[a]	DCC	10 mg/ml[a]	Physically compatible for 24 hr at 28 °C	1337	**C**

Y-Site Injection Compatibility (1:1 Mixture) (Cont.)

Esmolol HCl

Drug	Mfr	Conc	Mfr	Conc	Remarks	Ref	C/I
Warfarin sodium	DU	2 mg/ml[c]	OH	10 mg/ml[a]	Haze forms immediately	2010	I
	DME	2 mg/ml[c]	OHM	10 mg/ml[a]	Haze forms immediately	2078	I

[a]*Tested in dextrose 5% in water.*
[b]*Tested in sodium chloride 0.9%.*
[c]*Tested in sterile water for injection.*
[d]*Tested in dextrose 5% in sodium chloride 0.9%.*
[e]*Flowing at 1.6 ml/min.*
[f]*Tested in both dextrose 5% in water and sodium chloride 0.9%.*
[g]*Sodium carbonate–containing formulation tested.*

Additional Compatibility Information

Solutions— Esmolol HCl (Baxter) is physically compatible and chemically stable at a concentration of 10 mg/ml for 24 hours at room temperature or under refrigeration in the following infusion solutions (2; 4):

Dextrose 5% in Ringer's injection
Dextrose 5% in Ringer's injection, lactated
Dextrose 5% in sodium chloride 0.45 and 0.9%
Dextrose 5% in water
Ringer's injection, lactated
Sodium chloride 0.45 and 0.9%

Additives— Although it has been stated that esmolol HCl is incompatible with sodium bicarbonate 5% and should not be admixed with it (2; 4), Baaske et al. reported little loss in an esmolol HCl 10-mg/ml solution in sodium bicarbonate 5%. By HPLC, esmolol losses were 5 and 8% in seven days at 4 and 27 °C, respectively. When the solution was stored at 40 °C, 9% esmolol loss occurred in 24 hours (1831). Esmolol HCl also is stated to be incompatible with diazepam and thiopental sodium (4).

Esmolol HCl is physically compatible and stable for at least 24 hours at room temperature or under refrigeration with potassium chloride 40 mEq/L in dextrose 5% in water (2) and is stated to be compatible with digoxin, dopamine HCl, and lidocaine HCl (4).

ESTROGENS, CONJUGATED
AHFS 68:16

Premarin Intravenous   **Wyeth-Ayerst**

Products— Estrogens, conjugated (Wyeth-Ayerst), is available in packages containing a vial with lyophilized estrogens, conjugated, 25 mg; lactose 200 mg; sodium citrate 12.2 mg; simethicone 0.2 mg; and sodium hydroxide or hydrochloric acid for pH adjustment. Also in the package is a 5-ml ampul of sterile diluent composed of water for injection and benzyl alcohol 2%. To reconstitute, withdraw the air from the vial of estrogens, conjugated; flow the sterile diluent slowly against the side of the vial, and agitate gently—not violently (2).

Osmolality— Estrogens, conjugated, 1 mg/ml in its sterile diluent has an osmolality exceeding 2000 mOsm/kg (1689).

Administration— Estrogens, conjugated may be administered by deep intramuscular injection or slow direct intravenous injection. Intravenous infusion is not recommended, but injection into the tubing of a running infusion may be performed (2; 4).

Stability— The manufacturer recommends refrigeration of the intact containers at 2 to 8 °C (2). Such storage provides a shelflife of up to 60 months. At room temperature, the product in intact vials is stable for 24 months (853). The reconstituted solution should be stored at 2 to 8 °C (2). The reconstituted drug is stable for 60 days. Do not use it, however, if precipitation or discoloration occurs (2).

Compatibility Information

Y-Site Injection Compatibility (1:1 Mixture)

Estrogens, conjugated

Drug	Mfr	Conc	Mfr	Conc	Remarks	Ref	C/I
Heparin sodium with hydrocortisone sodium succinate	RI	1000 units + 100 mg/L[a]	AY	5 mg/ml	Physically compatible for at least 4 hr at room temperature by visual and microscopic examination	322	C

Y-Site Injection Compatibility (1:1 Mixture) (Cont.)

Estrogens, conjugated

Drug	Mfr	Conc	Mfr	Conc	Remarks	Ref	C/I
Potassium chloride		40 mEq/L[a]	AY	5 mg/ml	Physically compatible for at least 4 hr at room temperature by visual and microscopic examination	322	C
Vitamin B complex with C	RC	2 ml/L[a]	AY	5 mg/ml	Physically compatible for at least 4 hr at room temperature by visual and microscopic examination	322	C

[a]*Tested in dextrose 5% in water, sodium chloride 0.9%, and Ringer's injection, lactated.*

Additional Compatibility Information

Solutions— Dextrose, saline, and invert sugar solutions have been stated to be compatible with estrogens, conjugated (2).

Additives— Estrogens, conjugated, has been stated to be incompatible with ascorbic acid or any solution with an acid pH (2; 4).

ETHACRYNATE SODIUM
AHFS 40:28

Sodium Edecrin   **Merck**

Products— Each 50-ml vial has ethacrynate sodium equivalent to ethacrynic acid 50 mg and mannitol 62.5 mg. Reconstitute with 50 ml of dextrose 5% in water or sodium chloride 0.9% to yield a 1-mg/ml solution. Some dextrose 5% in water has a pH below 5 and results in a hazy or opalescent solution, which is not recommended for use (2; 4).

pH— Reconstitution with dextrose 5% in water or sodium chloride 0.9% results in a solution having a pH of 6.3 to 7.7 (4).

Osmolality— Ethacrynate sodium 1 mg/ml in dextrose 5% in water has an osmolality of 268 mOsm/kg (1689).

Sodium Content— Ethacrynate sodium contains 0.165 mEq of sodium per 50 mg of ethacrynic acid equivalent (846).

Administration— Ethacrynate sodium may be given slowly through the tubing of a running intravenous infusion solution or directly into a vein over several minutes (2; 4). Intravenous infusion over 20 to 30 minutes has also been recommended (4). Subcutaneous or intramuscular injection should not be used because of local pain and irritation (2; 4).

Stability— Solutions of ethacrynate sodium are relatively stable for short periods at pH 7 at room temperature; but as the pH or temperature or both increase, the solutions are less stable. It is recommended that the reconstituted solution be discarded after 24 hours (2; 4).

Compatibility Information

Additive Compatibility

Ethacrynate sodium

Drug	Mfr	Conc/L	Mfr	Conc/L	Test Soln	Remarks	Ref	C/I
Chlorpromazine HCl	SKF	50 mg	MSD	50 mg	NS	Little alteration of UV spectra within 8 hr at room temperature	16	C
Cimetidine HCl	SKF	3 g	MSD	500 mg	D5W	Physically compatible and cimetidine chemically stable for 24 hr at room temperature. Ethacrynate sodium not tested	551	C
Hydralazine HCl	CI	20 mg	MSD	50 mg	NS	Altered UV spectra for both at room temperature	16	I
Procainamide HCl	SQ	1 g	MSD	50 mg	NS	Altered UV spectra for both at room temperature	16	I

Additive Compatibility (Cont.)

Ethacrynate sodium

Drug	Mfr	Conc/L	Mfr	Conc/L	Test Soln	Remarks	Ref	C/I
Prochlorperazine edisylate	SKF	20 mg	MSD	80 mg	NS	Little alteration of UV spectra within 8 hr at room temperature	16	C
Promazine HCl	WY	50 mg	MSD	50 mg	NS	Little alteration of UV spectra within 8 hr at room temperature	16	C
Ranitidine HCl	GL	50 mg and 2 g		500 mg	D5W	Ranitidine chemically stable by HPLC for only 6 hr at 25 °C. Ethacrynate not tested	1515	I
Tolazoline HCl	CI	400 mg	MSD	50 mg	NS	Altered UV spectra for both at room temperature	16	I
Triflupromazine HCl	SQ		MSD		NS	Occasional gas bubble formation	16	I

Y-Site Injection Compatibility (1:1 Mixture)

Ethacrynate sodium

Drug	Mfr	Conc	Mfr	Conc	Remarks	Ref	C/I
Heparin sodium with hydrocortisone sodium succinate	RI UP	1000 units + 100 mg/L[a]	MSD	1 mg/ml	Physically compatible for at least 4 hr at room temperature by visual and microscopic examination	322	C
Potassium chloride		40 mEq/L[a]	MSD	1 mg/ml	Physically compatible for at least 4 hr at room temperature by visual and microscopic examination	322	C
Vitamin B complex with C	RC	2 ml/L[a]	MSD	1 mg/ml	Physically compatible for at least 4 hr at room temperature by visual and microscopic examination	322	C

[a]*Tested in dextrose 5% in water, sodium chloride 0.9%, and Ringer's injection, lactated.*

Additional Compatibility Information

Infusion Solutions— Ethacrynate sodium is reported to be compatible with the following Abbott infusion solutions (4):

Dextran 75 6% in sodium chloride 0.9%
Dextrose 5% in sodium chloride 0.9%
Dextrose 5% in water
Normosol R, pH 7.4
Ringer's injection
Ringer's injection, lactated
Sodium chloride 0.9%

Ethacrynate sodium is incompatible with solutions or drugs with a final pH below 5 and with whole blood and its derivatives (2). It is also stated to be incompatible with Normosol M (4).

ETOMIDATE
AHFS 28:24.04

Bedford

Products— Etomidate (Bedford) is available at a concentration of 2 mg/ml in 10- and 20-ml single-dose vials. Each milliliter also contains propylene glycol 35% (v/v) (1-10/98).

Administration— Etomidate is administered by intravenous injection over 30 to 60 seconds (1-10/98).

Stability— Intact containers should be stored at controlled room temperature. Unused portions remaining in vials should be discarded (1-10/98).

Compatibility Information

Y-Site Injection Compatibility (1:1 Mixture)

Etomidate

Drug	Mfr	Conc	Mfr	Conc	Remarks	Ref	C/I
Alfentanil HCl	JN	0.5 mg/ml	AB	2 mg/ml	Visually compatible for up to 7 days at 25 °C	1801	C
Ascorbic acid	AB	500 mg/ml	AB	2 mg/ml	Yellow discoloration and fine precipitate form in 24 hr	1801	I
Atracurium besylate	BW	10 mg/ml	AB	2 mg/ml	Visually compatible for up to 7 days at 25 °C	1801	C
Atropine sulfate	GNS	0.4 mg/ml	AB	2 mg/ml	Visually compatible for up to 7 days at 25 °C	1801	C
Doxacurium chloride	BW	1 mg/ml	AB	2 mg/ml	Visually compatible for up to 7 days at 25 °C	1801	C
Ephedrine sulfate	AB	50 mg/ml	AB	2 mg/ml	Visually compatible for up to 7 days at 25 °C	1801	C
Fentanyl citrate	ES	0.05 mg/ml	AB	2 mg/ml	Visually compatible for up to 7 days at 25 °C	1801	C
Lidocaine HCl	AST	20 mg/ml	AB	2 mg/ml	Visually compatible for up to 7 days at 25 °C	1801	C
Lorazepam	WY	2 mg/ml	AB	2 mg/ml	Visually compatible for up to 7 days at 25 °C	1801	C
Midazolam HCl	RC	5 mg/ml	AB	2 mg/ml	Visually compatible for up to 7 days at 25 °C	1801	C
Mivacurium chloride	BW	2 mg/ml	AB	2 mg/ml	Visually compatible for up to 7 days at 25 °C	1801	C
Morphine sulfate	ES	10 mg/ml	AB	2 mg/ml	Visually compatible for up to 7 days at 25 °C	1801	C
Pancuronium bromide	GNS	2 mg/ml	AB	2 mg/ml	Visually compatible for up to 7 days at 25 °C	1801	C
Phenylephrine HCl	ES	10 mg/ml	AB	2 mg/ml	Visually compatible for up to 7 days at 25 °C	1801	C
Succinylcholine chloride	AB	20 mg/ml	AB	2 mg/ml	Visually compatible for up to 7 days at 25 °C	1801	C
Sufentanil citrate	JN	0.05 mg/ml	AB	2 mg/ml	Visually compatible for up to 7 days at 25 °C	1801	C
Vecuronium bromide	OR	1 mg/ml	AB	2 mg/ml	Slight turbidity and white particles form	1801	I

ETOPOSIDE
AHFS 10:00

VePesid　　　　　　　　　**Bristol-Myers Squibb**

Products— Etoposide (Bristol-Myers Squibb) is available in 5-, 7.5-, 25-, and 50-ml multiple-dose vials. Each milliliter contains (2):

Etoposide	20 mg
Polyethylene glycol 300	650 mg
Ethyl alcohol	30.5% (v/v)
Polysorbate 80 (Tween 80)	80 mg
Benzyl alcohol	30 mg
Citric acid	2 mg

pH— From 3 to 4 (2).

Osmolality— Etoposide 20 mg/ml has an osmolality exceeding 2000 mOsm/kg (1689).

Administration— Etoposide should be diluted for administration and given by slow intravenous infusion; concentrations of 0.2 to 0.4 mg/ml should be given over at least 30 to 60 minutes (2; 4; 915). Continuous intravenous infusion has also been used. The drug should not be given by rapid intravenous injection (4).

Stability— The clear, yellow solution is stable for 24 months in intact vials at 25 °C (2). Stability is not affected by exposure to normal room fluorescent light (1374). Also see Solutions under Additional Compatibility Information below.

Etoposide was cultured with human lymphoblasts to determine whether its cytotoxic activity was retained. The solution retained cytotoxicity for 24 hours at room temperature (1575).

pH Effects— Etoposide is most stable at a pH of about 3.5 to 6, with a calculated minimum degradation rate occurring at pH 4.8 (1262). Epimerization to the less active *cis*-etoposide may occur at pH values above 6. Hydrolysis may occur in alkaline solutions (1379).

Plastic Syringes— When etoposide 1 mg/ml in sodium chloride 0.9% was stored in plastic syringes (Gillette), seizing of the syringes occurred (1564).

Sorption— No loss of etoposide because of sorption to PVC containers has been observed (1374). At a concentration of 0.2 mg/ml in dextrose 5% in water or sodium chloride 0.9% in PVC containers, no etoposide loss due to sorption was found during 72 hours at 5 and 25 °C (1369).

In an admixture composed of cytarabine (Upjohn) 0.157 mg/ml, daunorubicin HCl (Bellon) 15.7 µg/ml, and etoposide (Sandoz) 0.157 mg/ml in dextrose 5% in water, little or no loss of the drugs due to sorption occurred when delivered through PVC, PVC with polyethylene-lined sets, and silicone central catheter (1955).

Filtration— Etoposide 0.1 to 0.4 mg/ml in dextrose 5% in water or sodium chloride 0.9% has been filtered through several commercially available filters (such as the 0.22-µm Millex-GS or Millex GV) without filter decomposition (4).

Etoposide (Sandoz) 0.2 mg/ml in dextrose 5% in water and sodium chloride 0.9% was filtered through a 0.22-µm cellulose ester membrane filter (Ivex-HP, Millipore) over six hours. No significant drug loss due to binding to the filter was noted (1034).

Precipitation— Etoposide has a very low aqueous solubility (about 0.03 mg/ml). Therefore, organic solvents and a surfactant are used in the formulation to aid in dispersing the drug in aqueous media. However, aqueous dispersion is temporary, and precipitation is inevitable even if irregular and unpredictable in terms of time. At concentrations above 0.4 mg/ml, precipitation may occur rapidly.

The rate of precipitation of a supersaturated etoposide solution depends on the presence of crystallization nuclei, agitation, contact with incompatible surfaces, and, possibly, other factors (1374).

Etoposide 1 mg/ml in sodium chloride 0.9% in polypropylene syringes (Braun Omnifix) developed a pure etoposide precipitate in about 10% of the prefilled syringes. It also precipitated at various locations in subclavian lines (1564).

Precipitation of etoposide from infusion solutions is reportedly exacerbated by the use of peristaltic pumps, especially at concentrations of 0.4 mg/ml or above. Use of volumetric pumps has been recommended to reduce this problem (1832; 1949).

Also see Solutions under Additional Compatibility Information below.

Compatibility Information

Solution Compatibility

		Etoposide				
Solution	Mfr	Mfr	Conc/L	Remarks	Ref	C/I
Dextrose 5% in water	a	BR	400 mg	Physically compatible with 3 to 4% etoposide loss in 4 days at 21 °C in the dark or exposed to fluorescent light	1374	C
		SZ	157 mg	2% or less loss in 48 hr by HPLC at room temperature, exposed to light and in the dark, and at 4 °C	1955	C
Ringer's injection, lactated	a	BR	400 mg	Physically compatible with 5% etoposide loss in 4 days at 21 °C exposed to fluorescent light	1374	C
Sodium chloride 0.9%	b	BR	400 mg	Physically compatible with 1 to 5% etoposide loss in 4 days at 21 °C in the dark or exposed to fluorescent light	1374	C
	a	BR	50 to 400 mg	Physically compatible for at least 4 days	1374	C
	a	BR	500 mg	Precipitate forms after 48 hr at 21 °C exposed to fluorescent light	1374	C
	a	BR	600 and 700 mg	Precipitate forms within 24 hr at 21 °C exposed to fluorescent light	1374	I

Solution Compatibility (Cont.)

Etoposide

Solution	Mfr	Mfr	Conc/L	Remarks	Ref	C/I
c			400 mg	Chemically stable by HPLC for 24 hr at 4 and 24 °C. Precipitation occurs at varying times after 24 hr	1833	C

[a]Tested in glass containers.
[b]Tested in both glass and PVC containers.
[c]Tested in glass, PVC, and polyethylene containers.

Additive Compatibility

Etoposide

Drug	Mfr	Conc/L	Mfr	Conc/L	Test Soln	Remarks	Ref	C/I
Carboplatin		1 g		200 mg	W	Less than 10% loss of both drugs in 7 days at 23 °C protected from light	1954	C
Cisplatin	BR	200 mg	BR	400 mg	NS[a]	Physically compatible with less than 10% loss of both drugs in 48 hr at 22 °C in light and dark	1329	C
	BR	200 mg	BR	200 mg	NS[a]	Physically compatible with less than 10% loss of both drugs in 24 hr at 22 °C. Possible excess cisplatin loss in 48 hr exposed to light	1329	C
	BR	200 mg	BR	200 and 400 mg	D5½S[a]	Physically compatible with less than 10% loss of both drugs in 24 hr at 22 °C in light and dark	1329	C
		200 mg		200 mg	NS	Both drugs stable for 15 days at room temperature protected from light	1379	C
		200 mg		400 mg	NS	10% etoposide loss and no cisplatin loss in 7 days at room temperature	1388	C
Cisplatin with cyclophosphamide		200 mg 2 g		200 mg	NS	All drugs stable for 7 days at room temperature	1379	C
Cisplatin with floxuridine		200 mg 700 mg		300 mg	NS	All drugs stable for 7 days at room temperature	1379	C
Cisplatin with mannitol and potassium chloride	BR LY LY	200 mg 1.875% 20 mEq	BR	400 mg	NS[a]	Physically compatible and etoposide and cisplatin chemically stable for 8 hr at 22 °C. Precipitate forms within 24 hr	1329	I
Cisplatin with mannitol and potassium chloride	BR LY LY	200 mg 1.875% 20 mEq	BR	400 mg	D5½S[a]	Physically compatible and etoposide and cisplatin chemically stable for 24 hr at 22 °C. Precipitate forms within 48 hr	1329	C
Cytarabine	CHI	1.2 g	BR	660 mg	D5W	Physically compatible with no subvisual haze or particle formation in 4 hr at 23 °C	1736	C
Cytarabine with daunorubicin HCl	UP RP	267 mg 33 mg	BR	400 mg	D5½S	Physically compatible with about 6% cytarabine loss and no loss of other drugs in 72 hr at 20 °C	1162	C
Cytarabine with daunorubicin HCl	UP BEL	157 mg 15.7 mg	SZ	157 mg	D5W[b]	Less than 10% loss of any drug in 48 hr at room temperature, exposed to light and in the dark, and at 4 °C	1955	C
Floxuridine		10 g		200 mg	NS	Both drugs stable for 15 days at room temperature	1379	C
Fluorouracil		10 g		200 mg	NS	Both drugs stable for 7 days at room temperature and 1 day at 35 °C	1379	C

Additive Compatibility (Cont.)

		Etoposide						
Drug	*Mfr*	*Conc/L*	*Mfr*	*Conc/L*	*Test Soln*	*Remarks*	*Ref*	*C/I*
Hydroxyzine HCl	LY	500 mg	BR	1 g	D5W[c]	Physically compatible for 48 hr	1190	C
Ifosfamide		2 g		200 mg	NS	Both drugs stable for 5 days at room temperature	1379	C
Ifosfamide with carboplatin		2 g 1 g		200 mg	W	All drugs stable for 7 days at room temperature	1379	C
Ifosfamide with cisplatin		2 g 200 mg		200 mg	NS	All drugs stable for 5 days at room temperature	1379	C
Ondansetron HCl	GL	30 and 300 mg	BR	100 mg	D5W[b]	Physically compatible with little or no loss of ondansetron by HPLC in 48 hr at 23 °C. 4% etoposide loss in 24 hr and 6% loss in 48 hr at 23 °C	1876	C
	GL	30 and 300 mg	BR	400 mg	D5W[b]	Physically compatible with little or no loss of either drug by HPLC in 48 hr at 23 °C	1876	C

[a]*Tested in both glass and PVC containers.*
[b]*Tested in PVC containers.*
[c]*Tested in glass containers.*

Y-Site Injection Compatibility (1:1 Mixture)

		Etoposide					
Drug	*Mfr*	*Conc*	*Mfr*	*Conc*	*Remarks*	*Ref*	*C/I*
Allopurinol sodium	BW	3 mg/ml[b]	BR	0.4 mg/ml[b]	Physically compatible with no change in measured turbidity or increase in particle content in 4 hr at 22 °C	1686	C
Amifostine	USB	10 mg/ml[a]	BR	0.4 mg/ml[a]	Physically compatible with no change in measured turbidity or increase in particle content in 4 hr at 23 °C	1845	C
Aztreonam	SQ	40 mg/ml[a]	BMS	0.4 mg/ml[a]	Physically compatible with no subvisual haze or particle formation in 4 hr at 23 °C	1758	C
Cefepime HCl	BR	20 mg/ml[a]	BR	0.4 mg/ml[a]	Haze increases and tiny particles form in 1 hr	1689	I
Cladribine	ORT	0.015[b] and 0.5[c] mg/ml	BR	0.4 mg/ml[b]	Physically compatible with no change in measured turbidity or increase in particle content in 4 hr at 23 °C	1969	C
Doxorubicin HCl liposome injection	SEQ	0.4 mg/ml[a]	BR	0.4 mg/ml[a]	Physically compatible with little or no change in measured turbidity and no increase in particle content in 4 hr at 23 °C	2087	C
Filgrastim	AMG	30 µg/ml[a]	BR	0.4 mg/ml[a]	Particles form immediately. Filaments form in 1 hr	1687	I
Fludarabine phosphate	BX	1 mg/ml[a]	BR	0.4 mg/ml[a]	Physically compatible for 4 hr at room temperature under fluorescent light	1439	C
Gemcitabine HCl	LI	10 mg/ml[b]	BR	0.4 mg/ml[b]	Physically compatible with no change in measured turbidity or increase in particle content in 4 hr at 23 °C	2226	C

Y-Site Injection Compatibility (1:1 Mixture) (Cont.)

		Etoposide					
Drug	*Mfr*	*Conc*	*Mfr*	*Conc*	*Remarks*	*Ref*	*C/I*
Granisetron HCl	SKB	1 mg/ml	BMS	0.4 mg/ml[b]	Physically compatible with little or no loss of either drug by HPLC in 4 hr at 22 °C	1883	**C**
	SKB	0.05 mg/ml[a]	BR	0.4 mg/ml[a]	Physically compatible with no change in measured turbidity or increase in particle content in 4 hr at 23 °C	2000	**C**
Idarubicin HCl	AD	1 mg/ml[b]	BR	0.4 mg/ml[a]	Gas forms immediately	1525	**I**
Melphalan HCl	BW	0.1 mg/ml[b]	BR	0.4 mg/ml[b]	Physically compatible with no change in measured turbidity or increase in particle content in 3 hr at 22 °C	1557	**C**
Ondansetron HCl	GL	1 mg/ml[b]	BR	0.4 mg/ml[a]	Physically compatible for 4 hr at 22 °C	1365	**C**
	GL	16 to 160 μg/ml		0.144 to 0.25 mg/ml	Physically compatible when etoposide given over 30 to 60 min via Y-site	1366	**C**
Paclitaxel	NCI	1.2 mg/ml[a]		0.4 mg/ml[a]	Physically compatible with no change in measured turbidity in 4 hr at 22 °C	1528	**C**
Piperacillin sodium–tazobactam sodium	LE	40 + 5 mg/ml[a]	BR	0.4 mg/ml[a]	Physically compatible with no change in measured turbidity or increase in particle content in 4 hr at 22 °C	1688	**C**
Sargramostim	IMM	10 μg/ml[b]	BR	0.4 mg/ml[b]	Physically compatible for 4 hr at 22 °C	1436	**C**
Sodium bicarbonate		30 mg/ml	BR	0.6 mg/ml[b]	Visually compatible for 4 hr at room temperature	1788	**C**
		1.4%	BR	0.6 mg/ml[b]	Visually compatible for 4 hr at room temperature	1788	**C**
Teniposide	BR	0.1 mg/ml[a]	BR	0.4 mg/ml[a]	Physically compatible with no subvisual haze or particle formation in 4 hr at 23 °C	1725	**C**
Thiotepa	IMM[d]	1 mg/ml[a]	BR	0.4 mg/ml[a]	Physically compatible with no change in measured turbidity or increase in particle content in 4 hr at 23 °C	1861	**C**
Vinorelbine tartrate	BW	1 mg/ml[b]	BR	0.4 mg/ml[b]	Physically compatible with no change in measured turbidity or increase in particle content in 4 hr at 22 °C	1558	**C**

[a]*Tested in dextrose 5% in water.*
[b]*Tested in sodium chloride 0.9%.*
[c]*Tested in bacteriostatic sodium chloride 0.9% preserved with benzyl alcohol 0.9%.*
[d]*Lyophilized formulation tested.*

Additional Compatibility Information

Solutions— Dextrose 5% in water and sodium chloride 0.9% have been recommended as diluents for the infusion of etoposide. The aqueous solubility of etoposide is poor (0.03 mg/ml), but the formulation temporarily increases its miscibility in an aqueous medium. Nevertheless, the drug will eventually crystallize in varying time periods, and the crystallization is reported to be exacerbated by peristaltic pumps (1949). At concentrations of 0.2 and 0.4 mg/ml in dextrose 5% in water and sodium chloride 0.9%, the solutions are stable for 96 and 24 hours, respectively, at 25 °C under normal fluorescent light in either glass or plastic containers. However, precipitation in shorter time periods has been observed. At concentra-

tions of 0.2 and 0.4 mg/ml in Ringer's injection, lactated, or mannitol 10% in glass containers under the same conditions, the solutions are stable for eight hours. Seargent et al. reported no precipitate formation in 72 hours at 20 °C in solutions of etoposide 0.4 mg/ml in dextrose 5% in water or sodium chloride 0.9% (1162). However, at 1 mg/ml, crystallization may occur in 30 minutes in a standing solution or five minutes if the solution is stirred. Occasionally, 1-mg/ml concentrations may remain in solution for extended periods (1374). Nevertheless, concentrations greater than 0.4 mg/ml are not recommended by the manufacturer. Because of the poor solubility of etoposide in aqueous media, monitor closely for precipitation before and during administration (2; 4; 915; 916).

Plastic— Devices composed of hard ABS plastic may be incompatible with undiluted etoposide. In one study, a multiport disposable infusion cassette (Omni-Flow) developed cracks within five minutes after infusion was started and leakage was evident within 15 minutes. This phenomenon did not occur when etoposide was diluted to concentrations up to 1 mg/ml. In addition, a venting pin and a connector on an extension set reportedly cracked. Exposure to the polyethylene glycol 300 content of the etoposide formulation can cause cracks in minutes. However, dehydrated alcohol did not cause any cracks within one hour (1261).

Plasticizer Leaching— Etoposide (Bristol) 0.4 mg/ml in PVC bags of dextrose 5% in water leached relatively minor amounts of diethylhexyl phthalate (DEHP) plasticizer from PVC bags. This leaching was due to the surfactant polysorbate 80 (Tween 80) in the formulation. After 24 hours at 24 °C, the DEHP concentration in 50-ml bags of infusion solution was 2.6 µg/ml. This finding is consistent with the low surfactant concentration (0.16%) in the final admixture solution. The actual amount of DEHP leached from PVC containers and administration sets may vary in clinical situations, depending on surfactant concentration, bag size, and contact time (1683).

Etoposide (Sandoz) 0.4 mg/ml in sodium chloride 0.9% in PVC containers leached DEHP plasticizer from the container material.

This leaching increased with storage time from about 12 µg/ml in eight hours to over 50 µg/ml in 96 hours at 24 °C. Refrigeration reduced, but did not eliminate, DEHP leaching (1833).

Aluminum— Ogawa et al. reported that immersion of a needle with an aluminum component in etoposide (Bristol) 20 mg/ml resulted in no visually apparent reaction after seven days at 24 °C (988).

Other Information

Skin Reactions— The manufacturer notes that accidental exposure to this potentially toxic agent may cause skin reactions. Therefore, protective gloves and syringes with Luer-Lok fittings should be used during preparation of solutions. A soap and water wash should be employed after accidental contact with the skin or mucosa (2; 4).

Inactivation— In the event of spills or leaks, Bristol-Myers Oncology recommends the use of sodium hypochlorite 5% (household bleach) or potassium permanganate 1% to inactivate etoposide (1200).

ETOPOSIDE PHOSPHATE
AHFS 10:00

Etopophos   **Bristol-Myers Squibb**

Products— Etoposide phosphate (Bristol-Myers Squibb) is available in single-dose lyophilized vials containing the equivalent of 100 mg of etoposide as the phosphate along with sodium citrate 32.7 mg and 300 mg of dextran 40 (2).

Etoposide phosphate is also available in pharmacy bulk vials containing the equivalent of 500 mg and 1 g of etoposide with sodium citrate 163.5 and 327 mg, respectively, and dextran 40 1.5 and 3 g, respectively (2).

Reconstitute the vials with the volumes of diluent cited in Table 1. Sterile water for injection, dextrose 5% in water, sodium chloride 0.9%, bacteriostatic water for injection preserved with benzyl alcohol, or bacteriostatic sodium chloride 0.9% preserved with benzyl alcohol may be used for reconstitution. The resultant solution contains the etoposide equivalent of 10 or 20 mg/ml (2).

pH— Reconstitution with sterile water for injection to a concentration of 1 mg/ml results in a pH of approximately 2.9 (4).

Table 1. Recommended Diluent Volumes for Reconstitution of Etoposide Phosphate (2)

Vial Size	Volume of Diluent	Etoposide Concentration
100 mg	5 ml	20 mg/ml
	10 ml	10 mg/ml
500 mg	25 ml	20 mg/ml
	50 ml	10 mg/ml
1 g	50 ml	20 mg/ml
	100 ml	10 mg/ml

Osmolality— Etoposide phosphate (Bristol-Myers Squibb) 10 mg/ml in sterile water for injection has an osmolality of 62 mOsm/kg (2043).

Administration— Etoposide phosphate is administered by intravenous infusion over periods from 5 to 210 minutes. The reconstituted drug may be given without further dilution or may be diluted to a concentration as low as 0.1 mg/ml with dextrose 5% in water or sodium chloride 0.9% (2; 4).

Stability— Etoposide phosphate is a white to off-white powder (4). Intact vials should be stored under refrigeration at 2 to 8 °C and protected from light (2).

The manufacturer states that etoposide phosphate reconstituted with an unpreserved diluent (such as sterile water for injection, dextrose 5% in water, or sodium chloride 0.9%) is stable for 24 hours at room temperatures of 20 to 25 °C and for seven days under refrigeration at 2 to 8 °C. If a diluent containing benzyl alcohol as a preservative (such as bacteriostatic water for injection or bacteriostatic sodium chloride 0.9%) is used to reconstitute etoposide phosphate, the solution is stable for 48 hours at room temperatures of 20 to 25 °C and for seven days under refrigeration at 2 to 8 °C (2; 4).

Unlike etoposide, the phosphate ester is highly water soluble, having a solubility over 100 mg/ml (4). Consequently, the potential for precipitation when diluted in aqueous media is reduced greatly compared with the older surfactant- and organic solvent–based formulation (2219).

Etoposide production by hydrolysis from infusion admixtures of etoposide phosphate (Bristol-Myers Squibb) was measured using HPLC. The admixtures, equivalent to etoposide 1.5 mg/ml in 66.7 ml and 1.5 mg/ml in 20 ml, were filled into PVC ambulatory infusion pump reservoirs (Pharmacia Deltec) and stored at 20 and 37 °C protected from light. Etoposide levels in the etoposide phosphate admixtures increased at both temperatures; in seven days the increase in concentration was about 2% at 20 °C and about 7% at

37 °C. The authors concluded that etoposide phosphate is suitable for multiple-day ambulatory infusion (2024).

Syringes— Etoposide phosphate (Bristol-Laboratories Oncology Products) 10 and 20 mg/ml was prepared with bacteriostatic water for injection preserved with benzyl alcohol 0.9% (Abbott). The solutions were packaged as 4 ml of solution in 5-ml polypropylene syringes (Becton-Dickinson) and sealed with tip caps (Red Cap, Burron Medical). The syringes were stored at 32 °C for seven days, 23 °C for 31 days, and 4 °C for 31 days. All samples were physically stable, with no visual change and no increase in measured haze or particle content. HPLC analysis found little loss of drug. At 32 °C, 2 to 4% loss occurred in seven days. At 23 °C, about 6 to 7% loss occurred in 31 days. Losses under refrigeration were 4% or less in 31 days (2219).

Compatibility Information

Solution Compatibility

Etoposide phosphate						
Solution	*Mfr*	*Mfr*	*Conc/L*	*Remarks*	*Ref*	*C/I*
Dextrose 5% in water	BA[a]	BR	0.1 and 10 g	Physically compatible with no increase in measured haze or particles and little or no loss by HPLC in 7 days at 32 °C and in 31 days at 23 and 4 °C	2219	**C**
Sodium chloride 0.9%	BA[a]	BR	0.1 and 10 g	Physically compatible with no increase in measured haze or particles and little or no loss by HPLC in 7 days at 32 °C and in 31 days at 23 and 4 °C	2219	**C**

[a]Tested in PVC containers.

Y-Site Injection Compatibility (1:1 Mixture)

Etoposide phosphate						
Drug	*Mfr*	*Conc*	*Mfr*	*Conc*	*Remarks*	*Ref*	*C/I*
---	---	---	---	---	---	---	---
Acyclovir sodium	GW	7 mg/ml[a]	BR	5 mg/ml[a]	Physically compatible with no change in measured turbidity or increase in particle content in 4 hr at 23 °C	2218	**C**
Amikacin sulfate	APC	5 mg/ml[a]	BR	5 mg/ml[a]	Physically compatible with no change in measured turbidity or increase in particle content in 4 hr at 23 °C	2218	**C**
Aminophylline	AB	2.5 mg/ml[a]	BR	5 mg/ml[a]	Physically compatible with no change in measured turbidity or increase in particle content in 4 hr at 23 °C	2218	**C**
Amphotericin B	GEN	0.6 mg/ml[a]	BR	5 mg/ml[a]	Yellow-orange flocculent precipitate forms immediately	2218	**I**
Ampicillin sodium	APC	20 mg/ml[b]	BR	5 mg/ml[a]	Physically compatible with no change in measured turbidity or increase in particle content in 4 hr at 23 °C	2218	**C**
Ampicillin sodium–sulbactam sodium	RR	20 + 10 mg/ml[b]	BR	5 mg/ml[a]	Physically compatible with no change in measured turbidity or increase in particle content in 4 hr at 23 °C	2218	**C**
Aztreonam	SQ	40 mg/ml[a]	BR	5 mg/ml[a]	Physically compatible with no change in measured turbidity or increase in particle content in 4 hr at 23 °C	2218	**C**
Bleomycin sulfate	MJ	1 unit/ml[b]	BR	5 mg/ml[a]	Physically compatible with no change in measured turbidity or increase in particle content in 4 hr at 23 °C	2218	**C**
Bumetanide	RC	0.04 mg/ml[a]	BR	5 mg/ml[a]	Physically compatible with no change in measured turbidity or increase in particle content in 4 hr at 23 °C	2218	**C**

Y-Site Injection Compatibility (1:1 Mixture) (Cont.)

		Etoposide phosphate					
Drug	*Mfr*	*Conc*	*Mfr*	*Conc*	*Remarks*	*Ref*	*C/I*
Buprenorphine HCl	RKC	0.04 mg/ml[a]	BR	5 mg/ml[a]	Physically compatible with no change in measured turbidity or increase in particle content in 4 hr at 23 °C	2218	C
Butorphanol tartrate	APC	0.04 mg/ml[a]	BR	5 mg/ml[a]	Physically compatible with no change in measured turbidity or increase in particle content in 4 hr at 23 °C	2218	C
Calcium gluconate	FUJ	40 mg/ml[a]	BR	5 mg/ml[a]	Physically compatible with no change in measured turbidity or increase in particle content in 4 hr at 23 °C	2218	C
Carboplatin	BR	5 mg/ml[a]	BR	5 mg/ml[a]	Physically compatible with no change in measured turbidity or increase in particle content in 4 hr at 23 °C	2218	C
Carmustine	BR	1.5 mg/ml[a]	BR	5 mg/ml[a]	Physically compatible with no change in measured turbidity or increase in particle content in 4 hr at 23 °C	2218	C
Cefazolin sodium	APC	20 mg/ml[a]	BR	5 mg/ml[a]	Physically compatible with no change in measured turbidity or increase in particle content in 4 hr at 23 °C	2218	C
Cefepime HCl	BMS	20 mg/ml[a]	BR	5 mg/ml[a]	Increased haze and particulates form within 1 hr	2218	I
Cefoperazone sodium	PF	40 mg/ml[a]	BR	5 mg/ml[a]	Physically compatible with no change in measured turbidity or increase in particle content in 4 hr at 23 °C	2218	C
Cefotaxime sodium	HO	20 mg/ml[a]	BR	5 mg/ml[a]	Physically compatible with no change in measured turbidity or increase in particle content in 4 hr at 23 °C	2218	C
Cefotetan disodium	ZEN	20 mg/ml[a]	BR	5 mg/ml[a]	Physically compatible with no change in measured turbidity or increase in particle content in 4 hr at 23 °C	2218	C
Cefoxitin sodium	ME	20 mg/ml[a]	BR	5 mg/ml[a]	Physically compatible with no change in measured turbidity or increase in particle content in 4 hr at 23 °C	2218	C
Ceftazidime	SKB[c]	40 mg/ml[a]	BR	5 mg/ml[a]	Physically compatible with no change in measured turbidity or increase in particle content in 4 hr at 23 °C	2218	C
Ceftizoxime sodium	FUJ	20 mg/ml[a]	BR	5 mg/ml[a]	Physically compatible with no change in measured turbidity or increase in particle content in 4 hr at 23 °C	2218	C
Ceftriaxone sodium	RC	20 mg/ml[a]	BR	5 mg/ml[a]	Physically compatible with no change in measured turbidity or increase in particle content in 4 hr at 23 °C	2218	C
Cefuroxime sodium	GW	30 mg/ml[a]	BR	5 mg/ml[a]	Physically compatible with no change in measured turbidity or increase in particle content in 4 hr at 23 °C	2218	C
Chlorpromazine HCl	ES	2 mg/ml[a]	BR	5 mg/ml[a]	White cloudy solution with brown undertones forms immediately with particulates in 4 hr	2218	I
Cimetidine HCl	AMR	12 mg/ml[a]	BR	5 mg/ml[a]	Physically compatible with no change in measured turbidity or increase in particle content in 4 hr at 23 °C	2218	C

Y-Site Injection Compatibility (1:1 Mixture) (Cont.)

		Etoposide phosphate					
Drug	*Mfr*	*Conc*	*Mfr*	*Conc*	*Remarks*	*Ref*	*C/I*
Ciprofloxacin	BAY	1 mg/ml[a]	BR	5 mg/ml[a]	Physically compatible with no change in measured turbidity or increase in particle content in 4 hr at 23 °C	2218	**C**
Cisplatin	BR	1 mg/ml	BR	5 mg/ml[a]	Physically compatible with no change in measured turbidity or increase in particle content in 4 hr at 23 °C	2218	**C**
Clindamycin phosphate	AST	10 mg/ml[a]	BR	5 mg/ml[a]	Physically compatible with no change in measured turbidity or increase in particle content in 4 hr at 23 °C	2218	**C**
Cyclophosphamide	MJ	10 mg/ml[a]	BR	5 mg/ml[a]	Physically compatible with no change in measured turbidity or increase in particle content in 4 hr at 23 °C	2218	**C**
Cytarabine	BED	50 mg/ml	BR	5 mg/ml[a]	Physically compatible with no change in measured turbidity or increase in particle content in 4 hr at 23 °C	2218	**C**
Dacarbazine	MI	4 mg/ml[a]	BR	5 mg/ml[a]	Physically compatible with no change in measured turbidity or increase in particle content in 4 hr at 23 °C	2218	**C**
Dactinomycin	ME	0.01 mg/ml[a]	BR	5 mg/ml[a]	Physically compatible with no change in measured turbidity or increase in particle content in 4 hr at 23 °C	2218	**C**
Daunorubicin HCl	BED	1 mg/ml[a]	BR	5 mg/ml[a]	Physically compatible with no change in measured turbidity or increase in particle content in 4 hr at 23 °C	2218	**C**
Dexamethasone sodium phosphate	ES	1 mg/ml[a]	BR	5 mg/ml[a]	Physically compatible with no change in measured turbidity or increase in particle content in 4 hr at 23 °C	2218	**C**
Diphenhydramine HCl	ES	2 mg/ml[a]	BR	5 mg/ml[a]	Physically compatible with no change in measured turbidity or increase in particle content in 4 hr at 23 °C	2218	**C**
Dobutamine HCl	AST	4 mg/ml[a]	BR	5 mg/ml[a]	Physically compatible with no change in measured turbidity or increase in particle content in 4 hr at 23 °C	2218	**C**
Dopamine HCl	AST	3.2 mg/ml[a]	BR	5 mg/ml[a]	Physically compatible with no change in measured turbidity or increase in particle content in 4 hr at 23 °C	2218	**C**
Doxorubicin HCl	GEN	2 mg/ml	BR	5 mg/ml[a]	Physically compatible with no change in measured turbidity or increase in particle content in 4 hr at 23 °C	2218	**C**
Doxycycline hyclate	FUJ	1 mg/ml[a]	BR	5 mg/ml[a]	Physically compatible with no change in measured turbidity or increase in particle content in 4 hr at 23 °C	2218	**C**
Droperidol	AST	0.4 mg/ml[a]	BR	5 mg/ml[a]	Physically compatible with no change in measured turbidity or increase in particle content in 4 hr at 23 °C	2218	**C**
Enalaprilat	ME	0.1 mg/ml[a]	BR	5 mg/ml[a]	Physically compatible with no change in measured turbidity or increase in particle content in 4 hr at 23 °C	2218	**C**

Y-Site Injection Compatibility (1:1 Mixture) (Cont.)

Etoposide phosphate

Drug	Mfr	Conc	Mfr	Conc	Remarks	Ref	C/I
Famotidine	ME	2 mg/ml[a]	BR	5 mg/ml[a]	Physically compatible with no change in measured turbidity or increase in particle content in 4 hr at 23 °C	2218	C
Floxuridine	RC	3 mg/ml[a]	BR	5 mg/ml[a]	Physically compatible with no change in measured turbidity or increase in particle content in 4 hr at 23 °C	2218	C
Fluconazole	RR	2 mg/ml	BR	5 mg/ml[a]	Physically compatible with no change in measured turbidity or increase in particle content in 4 hr at 23 °C	2218	C
Fludarabine phosphate	BX	1 mg/ml[a]	BR	5 mg/ml[a]	Physically compatible with no change in measured turbidity or increase in particle content in 4 hr at 23 °C	2218	C
Fluorouracil	PH	16 mg/ml[a]	BR	5 mg/ml[a]	Physically compatible with no change in measured turbidity or increase in particle content in 4 hr at 23 °C	2218	C
Furosemide	AMR	3 mg/ml[a]	BR	5 mg/ml[a]	Physically compatible with no change in measured turbidity or increase in particle content in 4 hr at 23 °C	2218	C
Ganciclovir sodium	RC	20 mg/ml[a]	BR	5 mg/ml[a]	Physically compatible with no change in measured turbidity or increase in particle content in 4 hr at 23 °C	2218	C
Gemcitabine HCl	LI	10 mg/ml[b]	BR	5 mg/ml[b]	Physically compatible with no change in measured turbidity or increase in particle content in 4 hr at 23 °C	2226	C
Gentamicin sulfate	AB	5 mg/ml[a]	BR	5 mg/ml[a]	Physically compatible with no change in measured turbidity or increase in particle content in 4 hr at 23 °C	2218	C
Granisetron HCl	SKB	0.05 mg/ml[a]	BR	5 mg/ml[a]	Physically compatible with no change in measured turbidity or increase in particle content in 4 hr at 23 °C	2218	C
Haloperidol lactate	MN	0.2 mg/ml[a]	BR	5 mg/ml[a]	Physically compatible with no change in measured turbidity or increase in particle content in 4 hr at 23 °C	2218	C
Heparin sodium	ES	100 units/ml[a]	BR	5 mg/ml[a]	Physically compatible with no change in measured turbidity or increase in particle content in 4 hr at 23 °C	2218	C
Hydrocortisone sodium phosphate	ME	0.5 mg/ml[a]	BR	5 mg/ml[a]	Physically compatible with no change in measured turbidity or increase in particle content in 4 hr at 23 °C	2218	C
Hydrocortisone sodium succinate	UP	1 mg/ml[a]	BR	5 mg/ml[a]	Physically compatible with no change in measured turbidity or increase in particle content in 4 hr at 23 °C	2218	C
Hydromorphone HCl	ES	0.5 mg/ml[a]	BR	5 mg/ml[a]	Physically compatible with no change in measured turbidity or increase in particle content in 4 hr at 23 °C	2218	C
Hydroxyzine HCl	ES	4 mg/ml[a]	BR	5 mg/ml[a]	Physically compatible with no change in measured turbidity or increase in particle content in 4 hr at 23 °C	2218	C

Y-Site Injection Compatibility (1:1 Mixture) (Cont.)

		Etoposide phosphate					
Drug	Mfr	Conc	Mfr	Conc	Remarks	Ref	C/I
Idarubicin HCl	AD	0.5 mg/ml[a]	BR	5 mg/ml[a]	Physically compatible with no change in measured turbidity or increase in particle content in 4 hr at 23 °C	2218	C
Ifosfamide	MJ	25 mg/ml[a]	BR	5 mg/ml[a]	Physically compatible with no change in measured turbidity or increase in particle content in 4 hr at 23 °C	2218	C
Imipenem–cilastatin sodium	ME	10 mg/ml[b]	BR	5 mg/ml[a]	Yellow discoloration forms in 4 hr at 23 °C	2218	I
Leucovorin calcium	IMM	2 mg/ml[a]	BR	5 mg/ml[a]	Physically compatible with no change in measured turbidity or increase in particle content in 4 hr at 23 °C	2218	C
Lorazepam	WY	0.5 mg/ml[a]	BR	5 mg/ml[a]	Physically compatible with no change in measured turbidity or increase in particle content in 4 hr at 23 °C	2218	C
Magnesium sulfate	AST	100 mg/ml[a]	BR	5 mg/ml[a]	Physically compatible with no change in measured turbidity or increase in particle content in 4 hr at 23 °C	2218	C
Mannitol	BA	15%	BR	5 mg/ml[a]	Physically compatible with no change in measured turbidity or increase in particle content in 4 hr at 23 °C	2218	C
Meperidine HCl	AST	4 mg/ml[a]	BR	5 mg/ml[a]	Physically compatible with no change in measured turbidity or increase in particle content in 4 hr at 23 °C	2218	C
Mesna	MJ	10 mg/ml[a]	BR	5 mg/ml[a]	Physically compatible with no change in measured turbidity or increase in particle content in 4 hr at 23 °C	2218	C
Methotrexate sodium	IMM	15 mg/ml[a]	BR	5 mg/ml[a]	Physically compatible with no change in measured turbidity or increase in particle content in 4 hr at 23 °C	2218	C
Methylprednisolone sodium succinate	AB	5 mg/ml[a]	BR	5 mg/ml[a]	Haze with small subvisual particles forms immediately. Particle content increases fivefold over 4 hr at 23 °C	2218	I
Metoclopramide HCl	FAU	5 mg/ml	BR	5 mg/ml[a]	Physically compatible with no change in measured turbidity or increase in particle content in 4 hr at 23 °C	2218	C
Metronidazole	AB	5 mg/ml	BR	5 mg/ml[a]	Physically compatible with no change in measured turbidity or increase in particle content in 4 hr at 23 °C	2218	C
Minocycline HCl	LE	0.2 mg/ml[a]	BR	5 mg/ml[a]	Physically compatible with no change in measured turbidity or increase in particle content in 4 hr at 23 °C	2218	C
Mitomycin	BR	0.5 mg/ml[a]	BR	5 mg/ml[a]	Color changed from light blue to reddish-purple in 4 hr at 23 °C	2218	I
Mitoxantrone HCl	IMM	0.5 mg/ml[a]	BR	5 mg/ml[a]	Physically compatible with no change in measured turbidity or increase in particle content in 4 hr at 23 °C	2218	C
Morphine sulfate	ES	1 mg/ml[a]	BR	5 mg/ml[a]	Physically compatible with no change in measured turbidity or increase in particle content in 4 hr at 23 °C	2218	C

Y-Site Injection Compatibility (1:1 Mixture) (Cont.)

Etoposide phosphate

Drug	Mfr	Conc	Mfr	Conc	Remarks	Ref	C/I
Nalbuphine HCl	AST	10 mg/ml	BR	5 mg/ml[a]	Physically compatible with no change in measured turbidity or increase in particle content in 4 hr at 23 °C	2218	**C**
Netilmicin sulfate	SCH	5 mg/ml[a]	BR	5 mg/ml[a]	Physically compatible with no change in measured turbidity or increase in particle content in 4 hr at 23 °C	2218	**C**
Ofloxacin	MN	4 mg/ml[a]	BR	5 mg/ml[a]	Physically compatible with no change in measured turbidity or increase in particle content in 4 hr at 23 °C	2218	**C**
Ondansetron HCl	GW	1 mg/ml[a]	BR	5 mg/ml[a]	Physically compatible with no change in measured turbidity or increase in particle content in 4 hr at 23 °C	2218	**C**
Paclitaxel	MJ	1.2 mg/ml[a]	BR	5 mg/ml[a]	Physically compatible with no change in measured turbidity or increase in particle content in 4 hr at 23 °C	2218	**C**
Piperacillin sodium	LE	40 mg/ml[a]	BR	5 mg/ml[a]	Physically compatible with no change in measured turbidity or increase in particle content in 4 hr at 23 °C	2218	**C**
Piperacillin sodium–tazobactam sodium	LE	40 + 5 mg/ml[b]	BR	5 mg/ml[a]	Physically compatible with no change in measured turbidity or increase in particle content in 4 hr at 23 °C	2218	**C**
Plicamycin	MI	0.01 mg/ml[a]	BR	5 mg/ml[a]	Physically compatible with no change in measured turbidity or increase in particle content in 4 hr at 23 °C	2218	**C**
Potassium chloride	AB	0.1 mEq/ml[a]	BR	5 mg/ml[a]	Physically compatible with no change in measured turbidity or increase in particle content in 4 hr at 23 °C	2218	**C**
Prochlorperazine edisylate	ES	0.5 mg/ml[a]	BR	5 mg/ml[a]	White cloudy solution forms immediately with precipitate in 4 hr	2218	**I**
Promethazine HCl	SCN	2 mg/ml[a]	BR	5 mg/ml[a]	Physically compatible with no change in measured turbidity or increase in particle content in 4 hr at 23 °C	2218	**C**
Ranitidine HCl	GL	2 mg/ml[a]	BR	5 mg/ml[a]	Physically compatible with no change in measured turbidity or increase in particle content in 4 hr at 23 °C	2218	**C**
Sodium bicarbonate	AB	1 mEq/ml	BR	5 mg/ml[a]	Physically compatible with no change in measured turbidity or increase in particle content in 4 hr at 23 °C	2218	**C**
Streptozocin	UP	40 mg/ml[a]	BR	5 mg/ml[a]	Physically compatible with no change in measured turbidity or increase in particle content in 4 hr at 23 °C	2218	**C**
Teniposide	BR	0.1 mg/ml[a]	BR	5 mg/ml[a]	Physically compatible with no change in measured turbidity or increase in particle content in 4 hr at 23 °C	2218	**C**
Thiotepa	IMM	1 mg/ml[a]	BR	5 mg/ml[a]	Physically compatible with no change in measured turbidity or increase in particle content in 4 hr at 23 °C	2218	**C**

Y-Site Injection Compatibility (1:1 Mixture) (Cont.)

Etoposide phosphate

Drug	Mfr	Conc	Mfr	Conc	Remarks	Ref	C/I
Ticarcillin disodium	SKB	30 mg/ml[a]	BR	5 mg/ml[a]	Physically compatible with no change in measured turbidity or increase in particle content in 4 hr at 23 °C	2218	C
Ticarcillin disodium–clavulanate potassium	SKB	31 mg/ml[a]	BR	5 mg/ml[a]	Physically compatible with no change in measured turbidity or increase in particle content in 4 hr at 23 °C	2218	C
Tobramycin sulfate	LI	5 mg/ml[a]	BR	5 mg/ml[a]	Physically compatible with no change in measured turbidity or increase in particle content in 4 hr at 23 °C	2218	C
Trimethoprim–sulfamethoxazole	ES	0.8 + 4 mg/ml[a]	BR	5 mg/ml[a]	Physically compatible with no change in measured turbidity or increase in particle content in 4 hr at 23 °C	2218	C
Vancomycin HCl	LI	10 mg/ml[a]	BR	5 mg/ml[a]	Physically compatible with no change in measured turbidity or increase in particle content in 4 hr at 23 °C	2218	C
Vinblastine sulfate	FAU	0.12 mg/ml[a]	BR	5 mg/ml[a]	Physically compatible with no change in measured turbidity or increase in particle content in 4 hr at 23 °C	2218	C
Vincristine sulfate	FAU	0.05 mg/ml[a]	BR	5 mg/ml[a]	Physically compatible with no change in measured turbidity or increase in particle content in 4 hr at 23 °C	2218	C
Zidovudine	BW	4 mg/ml[a]	BR	5 mg/ml[a]	Physically compatible with no change in measured turbidity or increase in particle content in 4 hr at 23 °C	2218	C

[a]*Tested in dextrose 5% in water.*
[b]*Tested in sodium chloride 0.9%.*
[c]*Sodium carbonate–containing formulation tested.*

Additional Compatibility Information

Solutions— Etoposide phosphate reconstituted as directed may be diluted further to concentrations as low as 0.1 mg/ml in dextrose 5% in water or sodium chloride 0.9%. The drug is stated to be stable in either glass or plastic containers for 24 hours at both room temperatures of 20 to 25 °C and under refrigeration at 2 to 8 °C (2; 4).

Other Information

Etoposide 100 mg is provided in approximately 114 mg of etoposide phosphate (2).

FAMOTIDINE
AHFS 56:40

Pepcid   **Merck**

Products— Famotidine (Merck) is available as a 10-mg/ml injection in 2-ml single-dose vials and 4- and 20-ml multiple-dose vials. Each milliliter of the solution also contains L-aspartic acid 4 mg and mannitol 20 mg. Benzyl alcohol 0.9% is present as a preservative in the multiple-dose product (2).

Famotidine (Merck) is also available premixed at a concentration of 20 mg/50 ml. Each 50 ml of solution also contains L-aspartic acid 6.8 mg and sodium chloride 450 mg in water for injection. Additional L-aspartic acid or sodium hydroxide may be added to adjust the pH (2).

pH— The injection has a pH from 5 to 5.6 (4). The premixed solution has a pH from 5.7 to 6.4 (2).

Osmolarity— The osmolarities of the single- and multiple-dose products are 217 and 290 mOsm/L, respectively (4).

Administration— Famotidine is administered by slow intravenous injection or infusion. For injection, 20 mg should be diluted to 5 to 10 ml with a compatible diluent and injected no faster than 10 mg/min. For infusion, 20 mg should be diluted in 100 ml of dextrose 5% in water or another compatible diluent and infused over 15 to 30 minutes. Alternatively, famotidine premixed solution may be administered by intravenous infusion over 15 to 30 minutes (2; 4).

Stability— Famotidine injection is a clear, colorless solution. The vials should be stored under refrigeration and protected from freezing. If freezing occurs, thaw at room temperature or by warming in a water bath or under a warm tap; make sure that all components have resolubilized (2; 4). Use of a microwave oven for thawing is not recommended because of the potential hazard of vapor pressure increases in the vials (4).

Although refrigeration is recommended, the manufacturer indicates that famotidine vials may be stored for up to 26 weeks at controlled room temperature not exceeding 25 °C (1239).

Famotidine premixed infusion solution should be stored at controlled room temperature (25 °C) and protected from excessive heat. Brief exposure to temperatures up to 35 °C does not affect the stability of the product adversely (2).

Syringes— Bullock et al. reported that famotidine (MSD) 2 mg/ml in dextrose 5% in water, sodium chloride 0.9%, or sterile water for injection stored in plastic syringes (Becton-Dickinson) exhibited no loss in 14 days at 4 °C (1487).

Keyi et al. evaluated the stability of famotidine (Merck) 0.2 mg/ml in dextrose 5% in water and in sodium chloride 0.9% packaged in PVC minibags (Abbott) and polypropylene syringes (Becton-Dickinson) and stored for 15 days at 22 °C both exposed to and protected from light. All samples were visually clear and colorless throughout the study, and famotidine concentrations remained within 95% percent of the initial values by HPLC analysis (1936).

Freezing Solutions— Famotidine (MSD) 200 μg/ml in dextrose 5% in water or sodium chloride 0.9% in PVC bags showed no loss of potency when frozen at −20 °C for 28 days followed by storage at 4 °C for 14 days (1271).

Famotidine (MSD) 2 mg/ml in dextrose 5% in water, sodium chloride 0.9%, or sterile water for injection stored in polypropylene syringes (Becton-Dickinson) exhibited a 5 to 8% loss in eight weeks when frozen at −20 °C (1486).

Compatibility Information

Solution Compatibility

Solution	Mfr	Famotidine Mfr	Conc/L	Remarks	Ref	C/I
Amino acids	[a]	MSD	20 mg	0 to 5% loss in 48 hr at 25 °C in light or dark and at 5 °C	1344	**C**
Dextrose 5% in water	AB[b]	MSD	200 mg	Physically compatible with no potency loss in 14 days at 4 °C	1271	**C**
	TR[b]		200 mg	Physically compatible with 6% loss in 15 days at 25 °C and no loss in 63 days at 5 °C	1342	**C**
		MSD	20 mg	No loss in 48 hr at 25 °C in light or dark and at 5 °C	1344	**C**
	AB[b]	ME	200 mg	Visually compatible with less than 5% loss by HPLC in 15 days at 22 °C both with and without light protection	1936	**C**
Fat emulsion 10%, intravenous		MSD	20 mg	Little or no loss in 48 hr at 25 °C in light or dark and at 5 °C	1344	**C**
Sodium chloride 0.9%	AB[b]	MSD	200 mg	Physically compatible with no potency loss in 14 days at 4 °C	1271	**C**
	TR[b]		200 mg	Physically compatible with little or no loss in 15 days at 25 °C and in 63 days at 5 °C	1342	**C**
		MSD	20 mg	No loss in 48 hr at 25 °C in light or dark and at 5 °C	1344	**C**
	AB[b]	ME	200 mg	Visually compatible with less than 5% loss by HPLC in 15 days at 22 °C both with and without light protection	1936	**C**
TNA #111 and #112[c]		MSD	20 and 50 mg	Physically compatible with little or no famotidine loss and no change in fat particle size in 48 hr at 4 and 21 °C	1332	**C**
TNA #114[c]		MSD	20 and 40 mg	Physically compatible with little or no famotidine loss and no change in fat particle size in 72 hr at 21 °C under fluorescent light	1333	**C**

Solution Compatibility (Cont.)

Famotidine

Solution	Mfr	Mfr	Conc/L	Remarks	Ref	C/I
TNA #182[c]		MSD	20 mg	Visually compatible with no famotidine loss by HPLC in 24 hr at 24 °C under fluorescent light	1576	C
TNA #197 to #200[c]		MSD	20 mg	Physically compatible with no famotidine loss by HPLC in 48 hr at 22 °C exposed to light	1921	C
TPN #109 and #110[c]		MSD	20 and 40 mg	Physically compatible with little or no famotidine loss and little change in amino acids in 48 hr at 21 °C and in 7 days at 4 °C	1331	C
TPN #113[c]		MSD	20 mg	Physically compatible with little or no famotidine loss in 35 days at 4 °C protected from light	1334	C
TPN #115 and #116[c]		MSD	16.7 and 33.3 mg	No famotidine loss in 7 days at 23 and 4 °C	1352	C
TPN #196[c]		MSD	20 mg	Physically compatible with no famotidine loss by HPLC in 48 hr at 22 °C exposed to light	1921	C

[a]Tested in Vamin 14, Vamin 18, Vamin glucose, and Vamin N.
[b]Tested in PVC containers.
[c]Refer to Appendix I for the composition of parenteral nutrition solutions. TNA indicates a 3-in-1 admixture, and TPN indicates a 2-in-1 admixture.

Additive Compatibility

Famotidine

Drug	Mfr	Conc/L	Mfr	Conc/L	Test Soln	Remarks	Ref	C/I
Cefazolin sodium	FUJ	10 g	YAM	200 mg	D5W	Visually compatible with 10% cefazolin loss and 5% famotidine loss by HPLC in 24 hr at 25 °C. 9% cefazolin loss and 5% famotidine loss in 48 hr at 4 °C	1762	C
Flumazenil	RC	20 mg	MSD	80 mg	D5W[a]	Visually compatible with 3% flumazenil loss by HPLC in 24 hr at 23 °C under fluorescent light. Famotidine not tested	1710	C
Vancomycin HCl	AB	5 g	YAM	200 mg	D5W[b]	Visually compatible with 9% vancomycin loss and 6% famotidine loss by HPLC in 14 days at 25 °C. At 4 °C, losses of 3 to 4% occurred in 14 days	2111	C

[a]Tested in PVC containers.
[b]Tested in methyl-methacrylate-butadiene-styrene plastic containers.

Y-Site Injection Compatibility (1:1 Mixture)

Famotidine

Drug	Mfr	Conc	Mfr	Conc	Remarks	Ref	C/I
Acyclovir sodium		7 mg/ml[a]	ME	2 mg/ml[b]	Visually compatible for 4 hr at 22 °C	1936	C
Allopurinol sodium	BW	3 mg/ml[b]	MSD	2 mg/ml[b]	Physically compatible with no change in measured turbidity or increase in particle content in 4 hr at 22 °C	1686	C
Amifostine	USB	10 mg/ml[a]	ME	2 mg/ml[a]	Physically compatible with no change in measured turbidity or increase in particle content in 4 hr at 23 °C	1845	C

Y-Site Injection Compatibility (1:1 Mixture) (Cont.)

		Famotidine					
Drug	*Mfr*	*Conc*	*Mfr*	*Conc*	*Remarks*	*Ref*	*C/I*
Aminophylline	LY	2.5 mg/ml[b] 2.5 mg/ml[a]	MSD ME	0.2 mg/ml[a] 2 mg/ml[b]	Physically compatible for 14 hr Visually compatible for 4 hr at 22 °C	1196 1936	**C** **C**
Amphotericin B cholesteryl sulfate complex	SEQ	0.83 mg/ml[a]	ME	2 mg/ml[a]	Microprecipitate and increased turbidity form immediately	2117	**I**
Ampicillin sodium	ES	20 mg/ml[b] 20 mg/ml[b]	MSD ME	0.2 mg/ml[a] 2 mg/ml[b]	Physically compatible for 14 hr Visually compatible for 4 hr at 22 °C	1196 1936	**C** **C**
Ampicillin sodium–sulbactam sodium	RR	20 + 10 mg/ml[b]	MSD	0.2 mg/ml[a]	Physically compatible for 14 hr	1196	**C**
Amrinone lactate	WI	2 mg/ml[b]	MSD	0.2 mg/ml[a]	Physically compatible for 4 hr at 25 °C	1188	**C**
Amsacrine	NCI	1 mg/ml[a]	MSD	2 mg/ml[a]	Physically compatible for 4 hr at room temperature under fluorescent light	1381	**C**
Atropine sulfate	AST	0.1 mg/ml[a]	MSD	0.2 mg/ml[a]	Physically compatible for 4 hr at 25 °C	1188	**C**
Aztreonam	SQ	40 mg/ml[a]	ME	2 mg/ml[a]	Physically compatible with no subvisual haze or particle formation in 4 hr at 23 °C	1758	**C**
Bretylium tosylate	AB	4 mg/ml[a]	MSD	0.2 mg/ml[a]	Physically compatible for 4 hr at 25 °C	1188	**C**
Calcium gluconate	LY	0.00465 mEq/ml[b]	MSD	0.2 mg/ml[a]	Physically compatible for 14 hr	1196	**C**
Cefazolin sodium	LY	20 mg/ml[b] 20 mg/ml[a]	MSD ME	0.2 mg/ml[a] 2 mg/ml[b]	Physically compatible for 14 hr Visually compatible for 4 hr at 22 °C	1196 1936	**C** **C**
Cefepime HCl	BR	20 mg/ml[a]	ME	2 mg/ml[a]	Haze forms immediately. Flocculent precipitate forms in 4 hr	1689	**I**
Cefoperazone sodium	RR	40 mg/ml[b]	MSD	0.2 mg/ml[a]	Physically compatible for 14 hr	1196	**C**
Cefotaxime sodium	HO	20 mg/ml[b] 20 mg/ml[a]	MSD ME	0.2 mg/ml[a] 2 mg/ml[b]	Physically compatible for 14 hr Visually compatible for 4 hr at 22 °C	1196 1936	**C** **C**
Cefotetan disodium	STU	20 mg/ml[b]	MSD	0.2 mg/ml[a]	Physically compatible for 14 hr	1196	**C**
Cefoxitin sodium	MSD	20 mg/ml[b] 20 mg/ml[a]	MSD ME	0.2 mg/ml[a] 2 mg/ml[b]	Physically compatible for 14 hr Visually compatible for 4 hr at 22 °C	1196 1936	**C** **C**
Ceftazidime	GL[c] c	20 mg/ml[b] 20 mg/ml[a]	MSD ME	0.2 mg/ml[a] 2 mg/ml[b]	Physically compatible for 14 hr Visually compatible for 4 hr at 22 °C	1196 1936	**C** **C**
Ceftizoxime sodium	FUJ	20 mg/ml[b]	MSD	0.2 mg/ml[a]	Physically compatible for 14 hr	1196	**C**
Ceftriaxone sodium		20 mg/ml[a]	ME	2 mg/ml[b]	Visually compatible for 4 hr at 22 °C	1936	**C**
Cefuroxime sodium	GL	15 mg/ml[b] 20 mg/ml[a]	MSD ME	0.2 mg/ml[a] 2 mg/ml[b]	Physically compatible for 14 hr Visually compatible for 4 hr at 22 °C	1196 1936	**C** **C**
Chlorpromazine HCl		2 mg/ml[a]	ME	2 mg/ml[b]	Visually compatible for 4 hr at 22 °C	1936	**C**
Cisatracurium besylate	GW	0.1, 2, 5 mg/ml[a]	ME	2 mg/ml[a]	Physically compatible with no change in measured turbidity or increase in particle content in 4 hr at 23 °C	2074	**C**
Cisplatin	BR	1 mg/ml	MSD	2 mg/ml[a]	Visually compatible for 4 hr at room temperature under fluorescent light	1685	**C**
Cladribine	ORT	0.015[b] and 0.5[d] mg/ml	ME	2 mg/ml[b]	Physically compatible with no change in measured turbidity or increase in particle content in 4 hr at 23 °C	1969	**C**
Cyclophosphamide	MJ	10 mg/ml[a]	MSD	2 mg/ml[a]	Visually compatible for 4 hr at room temperature under fluorescent light	1685	**C**

Y-Site Injection Compatibility (1:1 Mixture) (Cont.)

Famotidine

Drug	Mfr	Conc	Mfr	Conc	Remarks	Ref	C/I
Cytarabine	UP	50 mg/ml	MSD	2 mg/ml[a]	Visually compatible for 4 hr at room temperature under fluorescent light	1685	C
Dexamethasone sodium phosphate	ES	10 mg/ml 1 mg/ml[a]	MSD ME	0.2 mg/ml[a] 2 mg/ml[b]	Physically compatible for 14 hr Visually compatible for 4 hr at 22 °C	1196 1936	C C
Dextran 40	PH	100 mg/ml[a]	MSD	0.2 mg/ml[a]	Physically compatible for 4 hr at 25 °C	1188	C
Digoxin	ES	0.25 mg/ml	MSD	0.2 mg/ml[a]	Physically compatible for 14 hr	1196	C
Diphenhydramine HCl		2 mg/ml[a]	ME	2 mg/ml[b]	Visually compatible for 4 hr at 22 °C	1936	C
Dobutamine HCl	LI	1 mg/ml[a] 4 mg/ml[a]	MSD ME	0.2 mg/ml[a] 2 mg/ml[b]	Physically compatible for 4 hr at 25 °C Visually compatible for 4 hr at 22 °C	1188 1936	C C
Docetaxel	RPR	0.9 mg/ml[a]	ME	2 mg/ml[a]	Physically compatible with no change in measured turbidity or increase in particle content in 4 hr at 23 °C	2224	C
Dopamine HCl	TR	1.6 mg/ml[a] 1.6 mg/ml[a]	MSD ME	0.2 mg/ml[a] 2 mg/ml[b]	Physically compatible for 4 hr at 25 °C Visually compatible for 4 hr at 22 °C	1188 1936	C C
Doxorubicin HCl	AD	0.2 mg/ml[a]	MSD	2 mg/ml[a]	Visually compatible for 4 hr at room temperature under fluorescent light	1685	C
Doxorubicin HCl liposome injection	SEQ	0.4 mg/ml[a]	ME	2 mg/ml[a]	Physically compatible with little or no change in measured turbidity and no increase in particle content in 4 ,hr at 23 °C	2087	C
Droperidol		0.4 mg/ml[a]	ME	2 mg/ml[b]	Visually compatible for 4 hr at 22 °C	1936	C
Enalaprilat	MSD	0.05 mg/ml[b]	MSD	0.2 mg/ml[a]	Physically compatible for 24 hr at room temperature under fluorescent light	1355	C
Epinephrine HCl	ES	0.004 mg/ml[a]	MSD	0.2 mg/ml[a]	Physically compatible for 4 hr at 25 °C	1188	C
Erythromycin lactobionate	ES	2 mg/ml[b]	MSD	0.2 mg/ml[a]	Physically compatible for 14 hr	1196	C
Esmolol HCl	DU	10 mg/ml[b]	MSD	0.2 mg/ml[a]	Physically compatible for 4 hr at 25 °C	1188	C
Etoposide phosphate	BR	5 mg/ml[a]	ME	2 mg/ml[a]	Physically compatible with no change in measured turbidity or increase in particle content in 4 hr at 23 °C	2218	C
Filgrastim	AMG	30 μg/ml[a]	MSD	2 mg/ml[a]	Physically compatible with no change in measured turbidity or increase in particle content in 4 hr at 22 °C	1687	C
Fluconazole	RR	2 mg/ml 2 mg/ml[a]	MSD ME	10 mg/ml 2 mg/ml[b]	Physically compatible for 24 hr at 25 °C Visually compatible for 4 hr at 22 °C	1407 1936	C C
Fludarabine phosphate	BX	1 mg/ml[a]	MSD	2 mg/ml[a]	Physically compatible for 4 hr at room temperature under fluorescent light	1439	C
Folic acid	LE	5 mg/ml	MSD	0.2 mg/ml[a]	Physically compatible for 14 hr	1196	C
Furosemide	ES IMS	10 mg/ml 0.8 mg/ml[a] 3 mg/ml[a]	MSD MSD ME	0.2 mg/ml[a] 0.2 mg/ml[a] 2 mg/ml[b]	Physically compatible for 14 hr Physically compatible for 4 hr at 25 °C White precipitate forms immediately	1196 1188 1936	C C I
Gemcitabine HCl	LI	10 mg/ml[b]	ME	2 mg/ml[b]	Physically compatible with no change in measured turbidity or increase in particle content in 4 hr at 23 °C	2226	C
Gentamicin sulfate	ES	0.8 mg/ml[b] 5 mg/ml[a]	MSD ME	0.2 mg/ml[a] 2 mg/ml[b]	Physically compatible for 14 hr Visually compatible for 4 hr at 22 °C	1196 1936	C C

Y-Site Injection Compatibility (1:1 Mixture) (Cont.)

				Famotidine			
Drug	*Mfr*	*Conc*	*Mfr*	*Conc*	*Remarks*	*Ref*	*C/I*
Granisetron HCl	SKB	0.05 mg/ml[a]	ME	2 mg/ml[a]	Physically compatible with no change in measured turbidity or increase in particle content in 4 hr at 23 °C	2000	C
Haloperidol lactate	MN	0.5[a] and 5 mg/ml	MSD	0.267 mg/ml[a]	Visually compatible for 24 hr at 21 °C	1523	C
		0.2 mg/ml[a]	ME	2 mg/ml[b]	Visually compatible for 4 hr at 22 °C	1936	C
Heparin sodium	ES	40 units/ml[b]	MSD	0.2 mg/ml[a]	Physically compatible for 14 hr	1196	C
	TR	50 units/ml[a]	MSD	0.2 mg/ml[a]	Physically compatible for 4 hr at 25 °C	1188	C
		40 units/ml[a]	ME	2 mg/ml[b]	Visually compatible for 4 hr at 22 °C	1936	C
Hydrocortisone[e]		1 mg/ml[a]	ME	2 mg/ml[b]	Visually compatible for 4 hr at 22 °C	1936	C
Hydrocortisone sodium succinate	AB	1 mg/ml[a]	MSD	0.2 mg/ml[a]	Physically compatible for 4 hr at 25 °C	1188	C
	AB	125 mg/ml	MSD	0.2 mg/ml[a]	Physically compatible for 14 hr	1196	C
Hydromorphone HCl		0.5 mg/ml[a]	ME	2 mg/ml[b]	Visually compatible for 4 hr at 22 °C	1936	C
Hydroxyzine HCl		4 mg/ml[a]	ME	2 mg/ml[b]	Visually compatible for 4 hr at 22 °C	1936	C
Imipenem–cilastatin sodium	MSD	10 mg/ml[b]	MSD	0.2 mg/ml[a]	Physically compatible for 14 hr	1196	C
		5 mg/ml[b]	ME	2 mg/ml[b]	Visually compatible for 4 hr at 22 °C	1936	C
Insulin, regular	LI	0.03 unit/ml[a]	MSD	0.2 mg/ml[a]	Physically compatible for 4 hr at 25 °C	1188	C
Isoproterenol HCl	ES	0.004 mg/ml[a]	MSD	0.2 mg/ml[a]	Physically compatible for 4 hr at 25 °C	1188	C
Labetalol HCl	SC	1 mg/ml[a]	MSD	0.2 mg/ml[a]	Physically compatible for 4 hr at 25 °C	1188	C
Lidocaine HCl	LY	1 mg/ml[a]	MSD	0.2 mg/ml[a]	Physically compatible for 14 hr	1196	C
	TR	4 mg/ml[a]	MSD	0.2 mg/ml[a]	Physically compatible for 4 hr at 25 °C	1188	C
Lorazepam		0.1 mg/ml[a]	ME	2 mg/ml[b]	Visually compatible for 4 hr at 22 °C	1936	C
Magnesium sulfate	SO	100 mg/ml[b]	MSD	0.2 mg/ml[a]	Physically compatible for 14 hr	1196	C
		100 mg/ml[a]	ME	2 mg/ml[b]	Visually compatible for 4 hr at 22 °C	1936	C
Melphalan HCl	BW	0.1 mg/ml[b]	MSD	2 mg/ml[b]	Physically compatible with no change in measured turbidity or increase in particle content in 3 hr at 22 °C	1557	C
Meperidine HCl	AB	10 mg/ml	MSD	0.2 mg/ml[a]	Physically compatible for 4 hr at 25 °C	1397	C
		4 mg/ml[a]	ME	2 mg/ml[b]	Visually compatible for 4 hr at 22 °C	1936	C
Methotrexate sodium	AD	15 mg/ml[f]	MSD	2 mg/ml[a]	Visually compatible for 4 hr at room temperature under fluorescent light	1685	C
Methylprednisolone sodium succinate	QU	40 mg/ml	MSD	0.2 mg/ml[a]	Physically compatible for 14 hr	1196	C
	AB	1 mg/ml[a]	MSD	0.2 mg/ml[a]	Physically compatible for 4 hr at 25 °C	1188	C
		5 mg/ml[a]	ME	2 mg/ml[b]	Visually compatible for 4 hr at 22 °C	1936	C
Metoclopramide HCl	RB	5 mg/ml	MSD	0.2 mg/ml[a]	Physically compatible for 14 hr	1196	C
		5 mg/ml	ME	2 mg/ml[b]	Visually compatible for 4 hr at 22 °C	1936	C
Midazolam HCl	RC	0.15 mg/ml[a]	MSD	0.2 mg/ml[a]	Physically compatible for 4 hr at 25 °C	1188	C
		1.5 mg/ml[a]	ME	2 mg/ml[b]	Visually compatible for 4 hr at 22 °C	1936	C
Morphine sulfate	ES	0.2 mg/ml[a]	MSD	0.2 mg/ml[a]	Physically compatible for 4 hr at 25 °C	1188	C
	AB	1 mg/ml	MSD	0.2 mg/ml[a]	Physically compatible for 4 hr at 25 °C	1397	C
		1 mg/ml[a]	ME	2 mg/ml[b]	Visually compatible for 4 hr at 22 °C	1936	C
Nafcillin sodium	WY	15 mg/ml[b]	MSD	0.2 mg/ml[a]	Physically compatible for 14 hr	1196	C
Nitroglycerin	PD	85 μg/ml[b]	MSD	0.2 mg/ml[a]	Physically compatible for 14 hr	1196	C
	IMS	0.8 mg/ml[a]	MSD	0.2 mg/ml[a]	Physically compatible for 4 hr at 25 °C	1188	C

Y-Site Injection Compatibility (1:1 Mixture) (Cont.)

Famotidine

Drug	Mfr	Conc	Mfr	Conc	Remarks	Ref	C/I
Norepinephrine bitartrate	WI	0.004 mg/ml[a]	MSD	0.2 mg/ml[a]	Physically compatible for 4 hr at 25 °C	1188	C
Ondansetron HCl	GL	1 mg/ml[b]	MSD	2 mg/ml[a]	Physically compatible for 4 hr at 22 °C	1365	C
Oxacillin sodium	BE	20 mg/ml[b]	MSD	0.2 mg/ml[a]	Physically compatible for 14 hr	1196	C
Paclitaxel	NCI	1.2 mg/ml[a]	MSD	2 mg/ml[a]	Physically compatible with no change in measured turbidity in 4 hr at 22 °C	1556	C
Perphenazine	SC	0.04 mg/ml[a]	MSD	0.2 mg/ml[a]	Physically compatible for 4 hr at 25 °C	1188	C
Phenylephrine HCl	WI	0.02 mg/ml[a]	MSD	0.2 mg/ml[a]	Physically compatible for 4 hr at 25 °C	1188	C
Phenytoin sodium	PD	50 mg/ml	MSD	0.2 mg/ml[a]	Physically compatible for 14 hr	1196	C
Phytonadione	MSD	2 mg/ml	MSD	0.2 mg/ml[a]	Physically compatible for 14 hr	1196	C
Piperacillin sodium	LE	40 mg/ml[b]	MSD	0.2 mg/ml[a]	Physically compatible for 14 hr	1196	C
		40 mg/ml[a]	ME	2 mg/ml[b]	Visually compatible for 4 hr at 22 °C	1936	C
Piperacillin sodium–tazobactam sodium	LE	40 + 5 mg/ml[a]	MSD	2 mg/ml[a]	Particles form immediately	1688	I
Potassium chloride	AB	0.04 mEq/ml[a]	MSD	0.2 mg/ml[a]	Physically compatible for 4 hr at 25 °C	1188	C
		0.1 mEq/ml[a]	ME	2 mg/ml[b]	Visually compatible for 4 hr at 22 °C	1936	C
Potassium phosphates	LY	3 mM/ml[b]	MSD	0.2 mg/ml[a]	Physically compatible for 14 hr	1196	C
Procainamide HCl	ASC	5 mg/ml[a]	MSD	0.2 mg/ml[a]	Physically compatible for 4 hr at 25 °C	1188	C
Propofol	ZEN	10 mg/ml	ME	2 mg/ml[a]	Physically compatible with no increase in particle content in 1 hr at 23 °C	2066	C
Remifentanil HCl	GW	0.025 and 0.25 mg/ml[b]	MSD	2 mg/ml[a]	Physically compatible with no change in measured turbidity or increase in particle content in 4 hr at 23 °C	2075	C
Sargramostim	IMM	10 μg/ml[b]	MSD	2 mg/ml[b]	Physically compatible for 4 hr at 22 °C	1436	C
Sodium bicarbonate	AB	1 mEq/ml[a]	MSD	0.2 mg/ml[a]	Physically compatible for 4 hr at 25 °C	1188	C
Sodium nitroprusside	ES	0.2 mg/ml[a]	MSD	0.2 mg/ml[a]	Physically compatible for 4 hr at 25 °C protected from light	1188	C
Teniposide	BR	0.1 mg/ml[a]	MSD	2 mg/ml[a]	Physically compatible with no subvisual haze or particle formation in 4 hr at 23 °C	1725	C
Theophylline	TR	1.6 mg/ml[a]	MSD	0.2 mg/ml[a]	Physically compatible for 4 hr at 25 °C	1188	C
Thiamine HCl	ES	100 mg/ml	MSD	0.2 mg/ml[a]	Physically compatible for 14 hr	1196	C
Thiotepa	IMM[g]	1 mg/ml[a]	ME	2 mg/ml[a]	Physically compatible with no change in measured turbidity or increase in particle content in 4 hr at 23 °C	1861	C
Ticarcillin disodium	BE	30 mg/ml[b]	MSD	0.2 mg/ml[a]	Physically compatible for 14 hr	1196	C
Ticarcillin disodium–clavulanate potassium	BE	31 mg/ml[b]	MSD	0.2 mg/ml[a]	Physically compatible for 14 hr	1196	C
TNA #218 to #226[h]			ME	2 mg/ml[a]	Visually compatible with no precipitate or emulsion damage apparent in 4 hr at 23 °C	2215	C
TPN #212 to #215[h]			ME	2 mg/ml[a]	Physically compatible with no change in measured turbidity or increase in particle content in 4 hr at 23 °C	2109	C
Verapamil HCl	KN	0.1 mg/ml[a]	MSD	0.2 mg/ml[a]	Physically compatible for 4 hr at 25 °C	1188	C

Y-Site Injection Compatibility (1:1 Mixture) (Cont.)

Famotidine

Drug	Mfr	Conc	Mfr	Conc	Remarks	Ref	C/I
Vinorelbine tartrate	BW	1 mg/ml[b]	MSD	2 mg/ml[b]	Physically compatible with no change in measured turbidity or increase in particle content in 4 hr at 22 °C	1558	C

[a]*Tested in dextrose 5% in water.*
[b]*Tested in sodium chloride 0.9%.*
[c]*Sodium carbonate-containing formulation.*
[d]*Tested in bacteriostatic sodium chloride 0.9% preserved with benzyl alcohol 0.9%.*
[e]*Form not specified.*
[f]*Tested in dextrose 5% in water with sodium bicarbonate 0.05 mEq/ml.*
[g]*Lyophilized formulation tested.*
[h]*Refer to Appendix I for the composition of parenteral nutrition solutions. TNA indicates a 3-in-1 admixture, and TPN indicates a 2-in-1 admixture.*

Additional Compatibility Information

Infusion Solutions— The manufacturer states that famotidine 0.2 to 4 mg/ml is stable for 48 hours at room temperature in common infusion solutions including (2; 4):

Dextrose 5 and 10% in water
Ringer's injection, lactated
Sodium bicarbonate 5%
Sodium chloride 0.9%

FAT EMULSION, INTRAVENOUS
AHFS 40:20

Products— The compositions and characteristics of the fat emulsion products are listed in Table 1.

The pH of fat emulsion, intravenous, products is adjusted with sodium hydroxide.

Administration— Fat emulsion, intravenous, may be administered intravenously via a peripheral vein or by central venous infusion. The particle size of the emulsions may exceed the porosity of some inline filters (658; 1106). However, the use of a 1.2-μm or 5-μm filter to remove particulates has been suggested (1106; 2135).

Fat emulsion, intravenous, may also be administered intravenously in total nutrient admixtures (TNA, 3-in-1) in combination with amino acids, dextrose, and other nutrients (4; 154).

Stability— Fat emulsion, intravenous, products may be stored in the intact containers at controlled room temperature of 25 °C (Intralipid products) to 30 °C (Liposyn products) or below. They should be protected from freezing (154).

Several factors can influence the stability of fat emulsions. A two-year study of Intralipid 10% found an increase in free fatty acids and a decrease of pH on storage. Gross particles formed and toxicity to rabbits increased with time. These changes were greatest during storage at 40 °C but were measurable at 20 and even 4 °C. The toxicity of the emulsions to rabbits could be correlated to the extent of free fatty acid formation in the emulsions. The formation of free fatty acids, with a consequent lowering of pH, is the major route of degradation of fat emulsions. The rate of degradation is minimized at pH 6 to 7 (889).

The container-closure system is important for long-term stability. Plastic containers are generally permeable to oxygen, which can readily oxidize the lipid emulsions, so glass bottles are used. Furthermore, the stoppers must not be permeable to oxygen and must not soften on contact with the emulsions. Teflon-coated stoppers have been recommended. Finally, the emulsions are packed under an atmosphere of nitrogen (889).

The long-term room temperature stability of the emulsions is lost when the intact containers are entered. The integrity of the nitrogen layer in the sealed container is essential for room temperature stability. Exposure of Intralipid 10% to the atmosphere results in gradual changes in the emulsion system. No changes in the particle size distribution occurred during the first 36 hours of room temperature storage. After 48 hours at room temperature, globule coalescence was noticeable. By 72 hours, the changes had become significant. However, the visual appearance after 72 hours was unchanged. Long-term storage for 15 months at room temperature resulted in formation of a nonhomogeneous cream layer with oil globules on top (656; 657). If the pH of the emulsion is optimal and the emulsion is stored under nitrogen and not exposed to direct sunlight, oxidative degradation is not likely to be significant (889).

As mentioned previously, storage temperature may be a factor in the shelflife of fat emulsion products. Because of the increase in free fatty acid content associated with temperature increases, and because of the imprecision of shelflife stability determinations of this type of product, refrigeration was originally required for long-term storage (889). Currently, however, the restriction has been lifted to approve storage at 25 °C (Intralipid products) to 30 °C (Liposyn products) or below (154).

The emulsions should not be frozen (154). Freezing may cause physical damage. The emulsions may become coarse and coalesce, and they can undergo irreversible phase separation. If accidental freezing occurs, the products should be discarded (559).

Oscillatory movement may cause separation of some phosphatide-stabilized emulsions but does not appear to be a problem with fat emulsion, intravenous, products (889).

The manufacturers recommend that a partly used bottle should not be stored for later use, and no bottle should be used if the emulsion appears to be oiling out (513; 514; 655).

Table 1. Composition and Characteristics of Various Intravenous Fat Emulsions

Component or Characteristics	Intralipid (Clinitec)			Liposyn II (Abbott)		Liposyn III (Abbott)	
Soybean oil	10%	20%	30%[a]	5%	10%	10%	20%
Safflower oil	—	—	—	5%	10%	—	—
Egg yolk phospholipids	1.2%	1.2%	1.2%	up to 1.2%	1.2%	up to 1.2%	1.2%
Glycerin	2.25%	2.25%	1.7%	2.5%	2.5%	2.5%	2.5%
Water for Injection	qs	qs	qs	qs	qs	qs	qs
Fatty acids:							
Linoleic acid	50%	50%	44–62%	65.8%		54.5%	
Oleic acid	26%	26%	19–30%	17.7%		22.4%	
Palmitic acid	10%	10%	7–14%	8.8%		10.5%	
Linolenic acid	9%	9%	4–11%	4.2%		8.3%	
Stearic acid	3.5%	3.5%	1.4–5.5%	3.4%		4.2%	
Osmolarity (mOsm/L)	260	268	310	276	258	284	292
Approximate pH	6–8.9	6–8.9	6–8.9	6–9	6–9	6–9	6–9
Fat particle size (μm)	0.5	0.5	0.5	0.4	0.4	0.4	0.4
Caloric value (cal/ml)	1.1	2	3	1.1	2	1.1	2
Size (ml)	50, 100, 250, 500	50, 100, 250, 500	500	100, 200, 500	50, 200, 500	100, 200, 500	200, 500

[a]*Not for direct infusion. Must be diluted to 20% or less for administration (1-1/94).*

Compatibility Information

Solution Compatibility

Fat emulsion, intravenous

Solution	Mfr	Mfr	Conc/L	Remarks	Ref	C/I
Amino acids injection 8.5%	MG	VT	10%	Mixed in equal parts. Physically compatible for 48 hr at 4 °C and room temperature	32	C
	MG	CU	10%	Mixed in equal parts. Physically compatible for 72 hr at room temperature	656	C
	TR	CU	10%	Mixed in equal parts. Physically compatible for 72 hr at room temperature	656	C
Amino acids injection 7%	AB	CU	10%	Mixed in equal parts. Physically compatible for 72 hr at room temperature	656	C
Amino acids injection 10%		VT	10%	Mixed in equal parts. Changes observed in 20 min. Globule coalescence and creaming in 8 hr at 8 and 25 °C	825	I
Dextrose 5% in Ringer's injection, lactated	CU	VT	10%	Mixed in equal parts. Physically compatible for 48 hr at 4 °C and room temperature	32	C
Dextrose 10% in water	MG	CU		Mixed in equal parts. Increased globule association in 8 hr at room temperature, considered significant at 48 hr. Formation of a top cream layer by 72 hr	656	I
Dextrose 25% in water	MG	CU	10%	Mixed in equal parts. Increased globule association in 8 hr, progressing to globule coalescence at 48 hr at room temperature. Formation of a top cream layer by 72 hr	656	I
Dextrose 50% in water		VT	10%	Mixed in equal parts. Physically compatible for 48 hr at 4 °C and room temperature	32	C

Solution Compatibility (Cont.)

Fat emulsion, intravenous

Solution	Mfr	Mfr	Conc/L	Remarks	Ref	C/I
	AB	VT	10%	Mixed in equal parts. Physically compatible for 24 hr at 8 and 25 °C	825	C
Ringer's injection, lactated	CU	VT	10%	Mixed in equal parts. Physically compatible for 48 hr at 4 °C and room temperature	32	C
Sodium chloride 0.9%	CU	VT	10%	Mixed in equal parts. Physically compatible for 48 hr at 4 °C and room temperature	32	C

Additive Compatibility

Fat emulsion, intravenous

Drug	Mfr	Conc/L	Mfr	Conc/L	Test Soln	Remarks	Ref	C/I
Aminophylline	ES	1 g	VT	10%		Physically compatible for 48 hr at 4 °C and room temperature	32	C
	DB	500 mg	VT	10%		Microscopic globule coalescence in 24 hr at 8 and 25 °C	825	I
		234 and 638 mg			TNA #180[a]	Little or no theophylline loss by EMIT and no substantial increase in fat particle size in 24 hr at room temperature	1617	C
Amphotericin B	APC, PHT	0.6 g	CL	10 and 20%		Precipitate forms immediately but is concealed by opaque emulsion	1808	I
		90 mg		20%		Yellow precipitate forms in 2 hr. Cumulative delivery of only 56% of total amphotericin B dose by HPLC	1872	I
	APC	10, 50, 100, and 500 mg, 1 and 5 g	CL	20%		Emulsion separation occurred rapidly, with visible creaming within 4 hr at 27 and 8 °C	1987	I
	SQ	500 mg, 1 and 2 g	KA	20%		Precipitated amphotericin noted on bottom of containers within 4 hr	1988	I
	BMS	50 mg	CL[c]	20%		Fat emulsion separates into two phases within 8 hr. No amphotericin B loss by HPLC protected from light and 4% loss exposed to fluorescent light in 24 hr at 24 °C	2093	I
	BMS	500 mg	CL[c]	20%		Fat emulsion separates into two phases within 8 hr. No amphotericin B loss by HPLC protected from or exposed to fluorescent light in 24 hr at 24 °C	2093	I
Ampicillin sodium		20 g		10%		15% ampicillin decomposition in 24 hr. Potency retained through 6 hr at 23 °C	37	I
	BE	2 g	VT	10%		Microscopic globule coalescence in 24 hr at 8 and 25 °C	825	I
Ascorbic acid injection	VI	1 g	VT	10%		Physically compatible for 48 hr at 4 °C and room temperature	32	C
	DB	500 mg	VT	10%		Microscopic globule coalescence in 24 hr at 8 and 25 °C	825	I
Calcium chloride	UP	2 g	VT	10%		Physically compatible for 48 hr at 4 °C and room temperature	32	C

Additive Compatibility (Cont.)

Fat emulsion, intravenous

Drug	Mfr	Conc/L	Mfr	Conc/L	Test Soln	Remarks	Ref	C/I
		13.6 mEq (1 g)	CU	10%		Immediate flocculation with visually apparent layer in 2 hr at room temperature	656	I
		6.8 mEq (500 mg)	CU	10%		Flocculation within 4 hr at room temperature	656	I
	DB	1 g	VT	10%		Globule coalescence and creaming in 8 hr at 8 and 25 °C	825	I
		10 and 20 mEq	KV	10%		Immediate flocculation, aggregation, and creaming	1018	I
Calcium gluconate	PR	2 g	CU	10%		Produced cracked emulsion	32	I
		7.2 and 9.6 mEq	KV	10%		Immediate flocculation, aggregation, and creaming	1018	I
Cefamandole nafate		2 g				Physically compatible and chemically stable for 24 hr at 25 °C	596	C
Cephalothin sodium	LI	4 g	VT	10%		Physically compatible for 48 hr at 4 °C and room temperature	32	C
	GL	2 g	VT	10%		Microscopic globule coalescence in 24 hr at 8 and 25 °C	825	I
Chloramphenicol sodium succinate	PD	2 g	VT	10%		Physically compatible for 48 hr at 4 °C and room temperature	32	C
	PD	2 g	VT	10%		Physically compatible for 24 hr at 8 and 25 °C	825	C
Cimetidine HCl	SKF	400, 800, 1200 mg	TR		TNA #72[a,b]	Physically compatible with no cimetidine loss in 24 hr at 25 °C. In 48 hr, fat emulsion particle size increases noted	998	C
	SKF	450 mg	AB, KV		TNA #197 to #200[a]	Physically compatible with 7% or less cimetidine loss by HPLC in 48 hr at 22 °C exposed to light	1921	C
Cyclosporine	SZ	400 mg	AB	10%		No cyclosporine loss by HPLC in 72 hr at 21 °C	1616	C
	SZ	500 mg and 2 g	KA	10 and 20%		Physically compatible by visual examination and particle size assessment with no cyclosporine loss by HPLC in 48 hr at 24 °C under fluorescent light	1625	C
Diphenhydramine HCl	PD	200 mg	VT	10%		Physically compatible for 48 hr at 4 °C and room temperature	32	C
Famotidine	MSD	20 and 50 mg			TNA #111 and #112[a]	Physically compatible with little or no famotidine loss and no change in fat particle size in 48 hr at 4 and 21 °C	1332	C
	MSD	20 and 40 mg			TNA #114[a]	Physically compatible with little or no famotidine loss and no change in fat particle size in 72 hr at 21 °C under fluorescent light	1333	C
	MSD	20 mg	KV		TNA #182[a]	Visually compatible with no famotidine loss by HPLC in 24 hr at 24 °C under fluorescent light	1576	C
	MSD	20 mg	AB, KV		TNA #197 to #200[a]	Physically compatible with no famotidine loss by HPLC in 48 hr at 22 °C exposed to light	1921	C

Additive Compatibility (Cont.)

Fat emulsion, intravenous

Drug	Mfr	Conc/L	Mfr	Conc/L	Test Soln	Remarks	Ref	C/I
Folic acid	USP	20 and 0.2 mg	KV	10%		Physically compatible for up to 2 weeks at 4 °C and room temperature when protected from light but highly erratic radioimmunoassays	895	?
Gentamicin sulfate	RS	160 mg	VT	10%		Microscopic globule coalescence in 24 hr at 8 and 25 °C	825	I
Heparin sodium		25,000 units	VT	10%		Physically compatible for 24 hr at 8 and 25 °C	825	C
	UP	2000 units	VT	10%		Physically compatible for 48 hr at 4 °C and room temperature	32	C
		1000 and 2000 units	CU, AB	10%		Physically compatible and heparin activity retained	568	C
Hydrocortisone sodium phosphate	MSD	200 mg	VT	10%		Physically compatible for 48 hr at 4 °C and room temperature	32	C
Hydrocortisone sodium succinate	GL	200 mg	VT	10%		Physically compatible for 24 hr at 8 and 25 °C	825	C
Iron dextran	FI	50 mg			TNA #122[a]	Lipid oiling out in 18 to 19 hr with formation of yellow-brown layer on admixture surface	1383	I
	FI	2 mg			TNA #159 to #166[a]	Physically compatible with no change visually, microscopically, and in particle size distribution in 48 hr at 4 and 25 °C	1648	C
Magnesium chloride		13.6 mEq	CU	10%		Immediate flocculation with visually apparent layer in 2 hr at room temperature	656	I
Multivitamins	USV	4 ml	VT	10%		Physically compatible for 48 hr at 4 °C and room temperature	32	C
	KA		KA	10%		Physically compatible for 24 hr at 26 °C with little loss by HPLC of most vitamins; up to 52% ascorbate loss	2050	C
Nizatidine	LI	150 mg			TNA #135 to #138[a]	Physically compatible with no increase in fat particle size and 2 to 7% nizatidine loss by HPLC in 48 hr at 22 °C under fluorescent light	1534	C
Octreotide acetate	SZ	450 μg	KV		TNA #139[a,b]	Physically compatible with no change in lipid particle size in 48 hr at 22 °C under fluorescent light and 7 days at 4 °C. Octreotide activity highly variable by radioimmunoassay	1540	?
Penicillin G		2 million units	VT	10%		Microscopic globule coalescence in 24 hr at 8 and 25 °C	825	I
Penicillin G potassium	SQ	10 million units	VT	10%		Physically compatible for 48 hr at 4 °C and room temperature	32	C
Phenytoin sodium	PD	1 g	VT	10%		Phenytoin crystal precipitation	32	I
Potassium chloride		7.5 g (100 mEq)	VT	10%		Physically compatible for 48 hr at 4 °C and room temperature	32	C

Additive Compatibility (Cont.)

Fat emulsion, intravenous

Drug	Mfr	Conc/L	Mfr	Conc/L	Test Soln	Remarks	Ref	C/I
		100 mEq	CU	10%		No significant change in emulsion for 24 hr at room temperature, but significant emulsion globule coalescence in 48 hr	656	C
		200 mEq	CU	10%		Globule coalescence with noticeable surface creaming in 4 hr at room temperature. Oil globules on surface at 48 hr	656	I
	DB	4 g	VT	10%		Microscopic globule coalescence in 24 hr at 8 and 25 °C	825	I
Ranitidine HCl	GL	50 and 100 mg	KA		TNA #92[a,b]	7 to 10% ranitidine loss in 12 hr and 20 to 28% loss in 24 hr at 23 °C under fluorescent light	1183	I
	GL	50 and 100 mg			TNA #118[a]	Physically compatible with no effect on emulsion stability and about 6 to 10% ranitidine loss in 36 hr under refrigeration and at 25 °C with or without light protection	1360	C
	GL	50 mg	KV	10%		Physically compatible with no effect on emulsion stability and 2 to 4% ranitidine loss in 48 hr at 25 °C with or without light protection	1360	C
	GL	100 mg	KV	10%		Physically compatible with no effect on emulsion stability and no ranitidine loss in 48 hr under refrigeration and at 25 °C with or without light protection	1360	C
	GL	75 mg	AB, KV		TNA #197 to #200[a]	Physically compatible with 7% or less ranitidine loss by HPLC in 24 hr at 22 °C exposed to light. About 15% loss in 48 hr	1921	C
Sodium bicarbonate	BR	7.5 g	VT	10%		Physically compatible for 48 hr at 4 °C and room temperature	32	C
		3.4 g	VT	10%		Microscopic globule coalescence in 24 hr at 8 and 25 °C	825	I
		50 and 150 mEq			TNA #66 to #68[a]	Physically compatible with 10% or less carbon dioxide loss and unchanged pH in 7 days at 25 °C protected from light	1011	C
Sodium chloride		100 mEq	CU	10%		No significant change in emulsion for 24 hr at room temperature, but significant emulsion globule coalescence in 48 hr	656	C
		200 mEq	CU	10%		Globule coalescence with noticeable surface creaming in 4 hr at room temperature. Oil globules on surface at 48 hr	656	I
Vitamin B complex	DB	10 ml	VT	10%		Microscopic globule coalescence in 24 hr at 8 and 25 °C	825	I

[a]*Refer to Appendix I for the composition of parenteral nutrition solutions. TNA indicates a 3-in-1 admixture.*
[b]*Tested in ethylene vinyl acetate (EVA) containers.*
[c]*Tested in glass bottles.*

Y-Site Injection Compatibility (1:1 Mixture)

Fat emulsion, intravenous

Drug	Mfr	Conc	Mfr	Conc	Remarks	Ref	C/I
Acyclovir sodium	GW	7 mg/ml[a]		TNA #218 to #226[c]	White precipitate forms immediately	2215	**I**
Amikacin sulfate	BR	250 mg/ml		TNA #97 to #104[c]	Broken fat emulsion with oil floating in admixtures	1324	**I**
	AB	5 mg/ml[a]		TNA #218 to #226[c]	Visually compatible with no precipitate or emulsion damage apparent in 4 hr at 23 °C	2215	**C**
Aminophylline	AB	2.5 mg/ml[a]		TNA #218 to #226[c]	Visually compatible with no precipitate or emulsion damage apparent in 4 hr at 23 °C	2215	**C**
Amphotericin B	PH	0.6 mg/ml[a]		TNA #218 to #226[c]	Yellow precipitate forms immediately	2215	**I**
Ampicillin sodium	BR	2 g/50 ml[b]		TNA #73[c]	Physically compatible for 4 hr at 25 °C by visual observation	1008	**C**
	SKB	20 mg/ml[b]		TNA #218 to #226[c]	Visually compatible with no precipitate or emulsion damage apparent in 4 hr at 23 °C	2215	**C**
Ampicillin sodium–sulbactam sodium	PF	20 + 10 mg/ml[b]		TNA #218 to #226[c]	Visually compatible with no precipitate or emulsion damage apparent in 4 hr at 23 °C	2215	**C**
Aztreonam	SQ	40 mg/ml[a]		TNA #218 to #226[c]	Visually compatible with no precipitate or emulsion damage apparent in 4 hr at 23 °C	2215	**C**
Bumetanide	RC, BV	0.04 mg/ml[a]		TNA #218 to #226[c]	Visually compatible with no precipitate or emulsion damage apparent in 4 hr at 23 °C	2215	**C**
Buprenorphine HCl	RKC	0.04 mg/ml[a]		TNA #218 to #226[c]	Visually compatible with no precipitate or emulsion damage apparent in 4 hr at 23 °C	2215	**C**
Butorphanol tartrate	APC	0.04 mg/ml[a]		TNA #218 to #226[c]	Visually compatible with no precipitate or emulsion damage apparent in 4 hr at 23 °C	2215	**C**
Calcium gluconate	AB	40 mg/ml[a]		TNA #218 to #226[c]	Visually compatible with no precipitate or emulsion damage apparent in 4 hr at 23 °C	2215	**C**
Carboplatin	BMS	5 mg/ml[a]		TNA #218 to #226[c]	Visually compatible with no precipitate or emulsion damage apparent in 4 hr at 23 °C	2215	**C**
Cefamandole nafate	LI	2 g/50 ml[a]		TNA #73[c]	Physically compatible for 4 hr at 25 °C by visual observation	1008	**C**
Cefazolin sodium	SKF	1 g/50 ml[a]		TNA #73[c]	Physically compatible for 4 hr at 25 °C by visual observation	1008	**C**
	SKB	20 mg/ml[a]		TNA #218 to #226[c]	Visually compatible with no precipitate or emulsion damage apparent in 4 hr at 23 °C	2215	**C**
Cefoperazone sodium	PF	40 mg/ml[a]		TNA #218 to #226[c]	Visually compatible with no precipitate or emulsion damage apparent in 4 hr at 23 °C	2215	**C**

Y-Site Injection Compatibility (1:1 Mixture) (Cont.)

Fat emulsion, intravenous

Drug	Mfr	Conc	Mfr	Conc	Remarks	Ref	C/I
Cefotaxime sodium	HO	20 mg/ml[a]		TNA #218 to #226[c]	Visually compatible with no precipitate or emulsion damage apparent in 4 hr at 23 °C	2215	**C**
Cefotetan sodium	ZEN	20 mg/ml[a]		TNA #218 to #226[c]	Visually compatible with no precipitate or emulsion damage apparent in 4 hr at 23 °C	2215	**C**
Cefoxitin sodium	MSD	1 g/50 ml[a]		TNA #73[c]	Physically compatible for 4 hr at 25 °C by visual observation	1008	**C**
	ME	20 mg/ml[a]		TNA #218 to #226[c]	Visually compatible with no precipitate or emulsion damage apparent in 4 hr at 23 °C	2215	**C**
Ceftazidime	SKB[d]	40 mg/ml[a]		TNA #218 to #226[c]	Visually compatible with no precipitate or emulsion damage apparent in 4 hr at 23 °C	2215	**C**
	GL[e]	40 mg/ml[a]		TNA #218 to #226[c]	Visually compatible with no precipitate or emulsion damage apparent in 4 hr at 23 °C	2215	**C**
Ceftizoxime sodium	FUJ	20 mg/ml[a]		TNA #218 to #226[c]	Visually compatible with no precipitate or emulsion damage apparent in 4 hr at 23 °C	2215	**C**
Ceftriaxone sodium	RC	20 mg/ml[a]		TNA #218 to #226[c]	Visually compatible with no precipitate or emulsion damage apparent in 4 hr at 23 °C	2215	**C**
Cefuroxime sodium	GL	30 mg/ml[a]		TNA #218 to #226[c]	Visually compatible with no precipitate or emulsion damage apparent in 4 hr at 23 °C	2215	**C**
Chlorpromazine HCl	SCN	2 mg/ml[a]		TNA #218 to #226[c]	Visually compatible with no precipitate or emulsion damage apparent in 4 hr at 23 °C	2215	**C**
Cimetidine HCl	SKB	12 mg/ml[a]		TNA #218 to #226[c]	Visually compatible with no precipitate or emulsion damage apparent in 4 hr at 23 °C	2215	**C**
Ciprofloxacin	BAY	1 mg/ml[a]		TNA #218 to #226[c]	Visually compatible with no precipitate or emulsion damage apparent in 4 hr at 23 °C	2215	**C**
Cisplatin	BMS	1 mg/ml		TNA #218 to #226[c]	Visually compatible with no precipitate or emulsion damage apparent in 4 hr at 23 °C	2215	**C**
Clindamycin phosphate	UP	600 mg/ 50 ml[a]		TNA #73[c]	Physically compatible for 4 hr at 25 °C by visual observation	1008	**C**
	AST	10 mg/ml[a]		TNA #218 to #226[c]	Visually compatible with no precipitate or emulsion damage apparent in 4 hr at 23 °C	2215	**C**
Cyclophosphamide	MJ	10 mg/ml[a]		TNA #218 to #226[c]	Visually compatible with no precipitate or emulsion damage apparent in 4 hr at 23 °C	2215	**C**
Cyclosporine	SZ	5 mg/ml[a]		TNA #220 and #223[c]	Small amount of precipitate forms immediately	2215	**I**

Y-Site Injection Compatibility (1:1 Mixture) (Cont.)

Fat emulsion, intravenous

Drug	Mfr	Conc	Mfr	Conc	Remarks	Ref	C/I
	SZ	5 mg/ml[a]		TNA #218, #219, #221, #222, #224 to #226[c]	Visually compatible with no precipitate or emulsion damage apparent in 4 hr at 23 °C	2215	C
Cytarabine	BED	50 mg/ml		TNA #218 to #226[c]	Visually compatible with no precipitate or emulsion damage apparent in 4 hr at 23 °C	2215	C
Dexamethasone sodium phosphate	FUJ, ES	1 mg/ml[a]		TNA #218 to #226[c]	Visually compatible with no precipitate or emulsion damage apparent in 4 hr at 23 °C	2215	C
Digoxin	BW	0.625 mg/ 50 ml[a,b]		TNA #73[c]	Physically compatible for 4 hr by visual observation	1009	C
	ES, WY	0.25 mg/ml		TNA #218 to #226[c]	Visually compatible with no precipitate or emulsion damage apparent in 4 hr at 23 °C	2215	C
Diphenhydramine HCl	SCN, PD	2[a] and 50 mg/ml		TNA #218 to #226[c]	Visually compatible with no precipitate or emulsion damage apparent in 4 hr at 23 °C	2215	C
Dobutamine HCl	AST	4 mg/ml[a]		TNA #218 to #226[c]	Visually compatible with no precipitate or emulsion damage apparent in 4 hr at 23 °C	2215	C
Dopamine HCl	AB	80 mg/ 50 ml[a,b]		TNA #73[c]	Physically compatible for 4 hr by visual observation	1009	C
	AB	3.2 mg/ml[a]		TNA #222 and #223[c]	Precipitate forms immediately	2215	I
	AB	3.2 mg/ml[a]		TNA #218 to #221 and #224 to #226[c]	Visually compatible with no precipitate or emulsion damage apparent in 4 hr at 23 °C	2215	C
Doxorubicin HCl	PH, GEN	2 mg/ml		TNA #218 to #226[c]	Damage to emulsion integrity occurs immediately with free oil formation possible	2215	I
Doxycycline hyclate	FUJ	1 mg/ml[a]		TNA #218 to #226[c]	Damage to emulsion integrity occurs immediately with free oil formation possible	2215	I
Droperidol	AB	0.4 mg/ml[a]		TNA #218 to #226[c]	Damage to emulsion integrity occurs in 1 to 4 hr with free oil formation possible	2215	I
Enalaprilat	ME	0.1 mg/ml[a]		TNA #218 to #226[c]	Visually compatible with no precipitate or emulsion damage apparent in 4 hr at 23 °C	2215	C
Erythromycin lactobionate	AB	1 g/50 ml[b]		TNA #73[c]	Physically compatible for 4 hr at 25 °C by visual observation	1008	C
Famotidine HCl	ME	2 mg/ml[a]		TNA #218 to #226[c]	Visually compatible with no precipitate or emulsion damage apparent in 4 hr at 23 °C	2215	C
Fentanyl citrate	AB	0.0125[a] and 0.05 mg/ml		TNA #218 to #226[c]	Visually compatible with no precipitate or emulsion damage apparent in 4 hr at 23 °C	2215	C

Y-Site Injection Compatibility (1:1 Mixture) (Cont.)

Fat emulsion, intravenous

Drug	Mfr	Conc	Mfr	Conc	Remarks	Ref	C/I
Fluconazole	PF	2 mg/ml		TNA #218 to #226[c]	Visually compatible with no precipitate or emulsion damage apparent in 4 hr at 23 °C	2215	**C**
Fluorouracil	PH	16 mg/ml[a]		TNA #220 and #223[c]	Small amount of white precipitate forms immediately	2215	**I**
	PH	16 mg/ml[a]		TNA #218, #219, #221, #222, #224 to #226[c]	Visually compatible with no precipitate or emulsion damage apparent in 4 hr at 23 °C	2215	**C**
Furosemide	ES	165 mg/ 50 ml[a,b]		TNA #73[c]	Physically compatible for 4 hr by visual observation	1009	**C**
	AB	3 mg/ml[a]		TNA #218 to #226[c]	Visually compatible with no precipitate or emulsion damage apparent in 4 hr at 23 °C	2215	**C**
Ganciclovir sodium	RC	20 mg/ml[a]		TNA #218 to #226[c]	Large amount of white precipitate forms immediately	2215	**I**
Gentamicin sulfate	SC	80 mg/ 50 ml[a]		TNA #73[c]	Physically compatible for 4 hr at 25 °C by visual observation	1008	**C**
	ES	40 mg/ml		TNA #97 to #104[c]	Physically compatible and gentamicin content retained for 6 hr at 21 °C by TDx	1324	**C**
	AB, FUJ	5 mg/ml[a]		TNA #218 to #226[c]	Visually compatible with no precipitate or emulsion damage apparent in 4 hr at 23 °C	2215	**C**
Granisetron HCl	SKB	0.05 mg/ml[a]		TNA #218 to #226[c]	Visually compatible with no precipitate or emulsion damage apparent in 4 hr at 23 °C	2215	**C**
Haloperidol lactate	MN	0.2 mg/ml[a]		TNA #218 to #226[c]	Damage to emulsion integrity occurs immediately with free oil formation possible	2215	**I**
Heparin sodium	AB	100 units/ml		TNA #218 to #226[c]	Damage to emulsion integrity occurs immediately with free oil formation possible	2215	**I**
Hydrocortisone sodium phosphate	ME	1 mg/ml[a]		TNA #218 to #226[c]	Visually compatible with no precipitate or emulsion damage apparent in 4 hr at 23 °C	2215	**C**
Hydrocortisone sodium succinate	AB	1 mg/ml[a]		TNA #218 to #226[c]	Visually compatible with no precipitate or emulsion damage apparent in 4 hr at 23 °C	2215	**C**
Hydromorphone HCl	ES	0.5 mg/ml[a]		TNA #219, #222, #224 to #226[c]	Damage to emulsion integrity occurs immediately with free oil formation possible	2215	**I**
	ES	0.5 mg/ml[a]		TNA #218, #220, #221, #223[c]	Visually compatible with no precipitate or emulsion damage apparent in 4 hr at 23 °C	2215	**C**
Hydroxyzine HCl	ES	2 mg/ml[a]		TNA #218 to #226[c]	Visually compatible with no precipitate or emulsion damage apparent in 4 hr at 23 °C	2215	**C**
Ifosfamide	MJ	25 mg/ml[a]		TNA #218 to #226[c]	Visually compatible with no precipitate or emulsion damage apparent in 4 hr at 23 °C	2215	**C**

Y-Site Injection Compatibility (1:1 Mixture) (Cont.)

Fat emulsion, intravenous

Drug	Mfr	Conc	Mfr	Conc	Remarks	Ref	C/I
IL-2	RC	4800 I.U./ml[b]	KA	20%	Visually compatible and IL-2 activity by bioassay retained. Fat emulsion not tested	1552	C
Imipenem–cilastatin sodium	ME	10 mg/ml[b]		TNA #218 to #226[c]	Visually compatible with no precipitate or emulsion damage apparent in 4 hr at 23 °C	2215	C
Insulin, regular	NOV	1 unit/ml[a]		TNA #218 to #226[c]	Visually compatible with no precipitate or emulsion damage apparent in 4 hr at 23 °C	2215	C
Isoproterenol HCl	BR	0.2 mg/ 50 ml[a,b]		TNA #73[c]	Physically compatible for 4 hr by visual observation	1009	C
Kanamycin sulfate	BR	500 mg/ 50 ml[a]		TNA #73[c]	Physically compatible for 4 hr at 25 °C by visual observation	1008	C
Leucovorin calcium	IMM	2 mg/ml[a]		TNA #218 to #226[c]	Visually compatible with no precipitate or emulsion damage apparent in 4 hr at 23 °C	2215	C
Levorphanol tartrate	RC	0.5 mg/ml[a]		TNA #218 to #226[c]	Damage to emulsion integrity occurs immediately with free oil formation possible	2215	I
Lidocaine HCl	ES	200 mg/ 50 ml[a,b]		TNA #73[c]	Physically compatible for 4 hr by visual observation	1009	C
Lorazepam	WY	0.1 mg/ml[a]		TNA #218 to #226[c]	Damage to emulsion integrity occurs in 1 hr	2215	I
Magnesium sulfate	AB	100 mg/ml[a]		TNA #218 to #226[c]	Visually compatible with no precipitate or emulsion damage apparent in 4 hr at 23 °C	2215	C
Mannitol	BA	15%		TNA #218 to #226[c]	Visually compatible with no precipitate or emulsion damage apparent in 4 hr at 23 °C	2215	C
Meperidine HCl	AST	4 mg/ml[a]		TNA #218 to #226[c]	Visually compatible with no precipitate or emulsion damage apparent in 4 hr at 23 °C	2215	C
Meropenem	ZEN	20 mg/ml[a]		TNA #218 to #226[c]	Visually compatible with no precipitate or emulsion damage apparent in 4 hr at 23 °C	2215	C
Mesna	MJ	10 mg/ml[a]		TNA #218 to #226[c]	Visually compatible with no precipitate or emulsion damage apparent in 4 hr at 23 °C	2215	C
Methotrexate sodium	IMM	15 mg/ml[a]		TNA #218 to #226[c]	Visually compatible with no precipitate or emulsion damage apparent in 4 hr at 23 °C	2215	C
Methyldopate HCl	MSD	250 mg/ 50 ml[b]		TNA #73[c]	Physically compatible for 4 hr by visual observation	1009	C
	MSD	250 mg/ 50 ml[a]		TNA #73[c]	Cracked the lipid emulsion	1009	I
Methylprednisolone sodium succinate	AB	5 mg/ml[a]		TNA #218 to #226[c]	Visually compatible with no precipitate or emulsion damage apparent in 4 hr at 23 °C	2215	C

Y-Site Injection Compatibility (1:1 Mixture) (Cont.)

Fat emulsion, intravenous

Drug	Mfr	Conc	Mfr	Conc	Remarks	Ref	C/I
Metoclopramide	AB	5 mg/ml		TNA #218 to #226[c]	Visually compatible with no precipitate or emulsion damage apparent in 4 hr at 23 °C	2215	C
Metronidazole	AB	5 mg/ml		TNA #218 to #226[c]	Visually compatible with no precipitate or emulsion damage apparent in 4 hr at 23 °C	2215	C
Midazolam HCl	RC	2 mg/ml[a]		TNA #218 to #226[c]	Damage to emulsion integrity occurs immediately with free oil formation possible	2215	I
Minocycline HCl	LE	0.2 mg/ml[a]		TNA #218 to #226[c]	Damage to emulsion integrity occurs immediately with free oil formation possible	2215	I
Mitoxantrone HCl	IMM	0.5 mg/ml[a]		TNA #218 to #226[c]	Visually compatible with no precipitate or emulsion damage apparent in 4 hr at 23 °C	2215	C
Morphine sulfate	ES	1 mg/ml[a]		TNA #218 to #226[c]	Visually compatible with no precipitate or emulsion damage apparent in 4 hr at 23 °C	2215	C
	ES	15 mg/ml		TNA #218 to #226[c]	Damage to emulsion integrity occurs immediately with free oil formation possible	2215	I
Nafcillin sodium	BE, APC	20 mg/ml[a]		TNA #218 to #226[c]	Visually compatible with no precipitate or emulsion damage apparent in 4 hr at 23 °C	2215	C
Nalbuphine HCl	AB, AST	10 mg/ml		TNA #218 to #226[c]	Damage to emulsion integrity occurs immediately with free oil formation possible	2215	I
Netilmicin sulfate	SC	5 mg/ml[a]		TNA #218 to #226[c]	Visually compatible with no precipitate or emulsion damage apparent in 4 hr at 23 °C	2215	C
Nitroglycerin	DU	0.4 mg/ml[a]		TNA #218 to #226[c]	Visually compatible with no precipitate or emulsion damage apparent in 4 hr at 23 °C	2215	C
Norepinephrine bitartrate	BN	0.4 mg/ 50 ml[a,b]		TNA #73[c]	Physically compatible for 4 hr by visual observation	1009	C
Octreotide acetate	SZ	0.01 mg/ml[a]		TNA #218 to #226[c]	Visually compatible with no precipitate or emulsion damage apparent in 4 hr at 23 °C	2215	C
Ofloxacin	ORT	4 mg/ml[a]		TNA #218 to #226[c]	Visually compatible with no precipitate or emulsion damage apparent in 4 hr at 23 °C	2215	C
Ondansetron HCl	CER	1 mg/ml[a]		TNA #218 to #226[c]	Damage to emulsion integrity occurs immediately with free oil formation possible	2215	I
Oxacillin sodium	BE	1 g/50 ml[a]		TNA #73[c]	Physically compatible for 4 hr at 25 °C by visual observation	1008	C
Paclitaxel	MJ	1.2 mg/ml[a]		TNA #218 to #226[c]	Visually compatible with no precipitate or emulsion damage apparent in 4 hr at 23 °C	2215	C

Y-Site Injection Compatibility (1:1 Mixture) (Cont.)

Fat emulsion, intravenous

Drug	Mfr	Conc	Mfr	Conc	Remarks	Ref	C/I
Penicillin G potassium	SQ	2 million units/50 ml[a]		TNA #73[c]	Physically compatible for 4 hr at 25 °C by visual observation	1008	C
Pentobarbital sodium	AB	5 mg/ml[a]		TNA #218 to #226[c]	Damage to emulsion integrity occurs immediately with free oil formation possible	2215	I
Phenobarbital sodium	WY	5 mg/ml[a]		TNA #218 to #226[c]	Damage to emulsion integrity occurs immediately with free oil formation possible	2215	I
Piperacillin sodium	LE	40 mg/ml[a]		TNA #218 to #226[c]	Visually compatible with no precipitate or emulsion damage apparent in 4 hr at 23 °C	2215	C
Piperacillin sodium–tazobactam sodium	LE	40 + 5 mg/ml[a]		TNA #218 to #226[c]	Visually compatible with no precipitate or emulsion damage apparent in 4 hr at 23 °C	2215	C
Potassium chloride	AB	0.1 mEq/ml[a]		TNA #218 to #226[c]	Visually compatible with no precipitate or emulsion damage apparent in 4 hr at 23 °C	2215	C
Potassium phosphates	AB	3 mmol/ml		TNA #218 to #226[c]	Damage to emulsion integrity occurs immediately with free oil formation possible	2215	I
Prochlorperazine edisylate	SCN, SO	0.5 mg/ml[a]		TNA #218 to #226[c]	Visually compatible with no precipitate or emulsion damage apparent in 4 hr at 23 °C	2215	C
Promethazine HCl	SCN	2 mg/ml[a]		TNA #218 to #226[c]	Visually compatible with no precipitate or emulsion damage apparent in 4 hr at 23 °C	2215	C
Ranitidine HCl	GL	2 mg/ml[a]		TNA #218 to #226[c]	Visually compatible with no precipitate or emulsion damage apparent in 4 hr at 23 °C	2215	C
Sodium bicarbonate	AB	1 mEq/ml		TNA #218 to #226[c]	Visually compatible with no precipitate or emulsion damage apparent in 4 hr at 23 °C	2215	C
Sodium nitroprusside	AB	0.4 mg/ml[a]		TNA #218 to #226[c]	Visually compatible with no precipitate or emulsion damage apparent in 4 hr at 23 °C protected from light	2215	C
Sodium phosphates	AB	3 mmol/ml		TNA #218 to #226[c]	Damage to emulsion integrity occurs immediately with free oil formation possible	2215	I
Tacrolimus	FUJ	1 mg/ml[a]		TNA #218 to #226[c]	Visually compatible with no precipitate or emulsion damage apparent in 4 hr at 23 °C	2215	C
Ticarcillin disodium	BE	3 g/50 ml[a]		TNA #73[c]	Physically compatible for 4 hr at 25 °C by visual observation	1008	C
	SKB	30 mg/ml[a]		TNA #218 to #226[c]	Visually compatible with no precipitate or emulsion damage apparent in 4 hr at 23 °C	2215	C
Ticarcillin disodium–clavulanate potassium	SKB	31 mg/ml[a]		TNA #218 to #226[c]	Visually compatible with no precipitate or emulsion damage apparent in 4 hr at 23 °C	2215	C

Y-Site Injection Compatibility (1:1 Mixture) (Cont.)

Fat emulsion, intravenous

Drug	Mfr	Conc	Mfr	Conc	Remarks	Ref	C/I
Tobramycin sulfate	LI	80 mg/ 50 ml[a]		TNA #73[c]	Physically compatible for 4 hr at 25 °C by visual observation	1008	C
	LI	40 mg/ml		TNA #97 to #104[c]	Physically compatible and tobramycin content retained for 6 hr at 21 °C by TDx	1324	C
	AB	5 mg/ml[a]		TNA #218 to #226[c]	Visually compatible with no precipitate or emulsion damage apparent in 4 hr at 23 °C	2215	C
Trimethoprim–sulfamethoxazole	ES	0.8 + 4 mg/ ml[a]		TNA #218 to #226[c]	Visually compatible with no precipitate or emulsion damage apparent in 4 hr at 23 °C	2215	C
Vancomycin HCl	AB	10 mg/ml[a]		TNA #218 to #226[c]	Visually compatible with no precipitate or emulsion damage apparent in 4 hr at 23 °C	2215	C
Zidovudine	GW	4 mg/ml[a]		TNA #218 to #226[c]	Visually compatible with no precipitate or emulsion damage apparent in 4 hr at 23 °C	2215	C

[a]*Tested in dextrose 5% in water.*
[b]*Tested in sodium chloride 0.9%.*
[c]*Refer to Appendix I for the composition of parenteral nutrition solutions. TNA indicates a 3-in-1 admixture.*
[d]*Sodium carbonate–containing formulation tested.*
[e]*Arginine-containing formulation tested.*

Additional Compatibility Information

It has been recommended that no other drugs or solutions be added to fat emulsion, intravenous, because the stability of the emulsion may be disturbed (32; 37; 38p8). Further, the bioavailability of a drug from an emulsion system is uncertain (32).

More recently, however, the combining of fat emulsions with amino acids, dextrose, and certain other additives in parenteral nutrition multicomponent admixtures has been evaluated. See Multicomponent ("3-in-1") Admixtures below.

UNRECOGNIZED CALCIUM PHOSPHATE PRECIPITATION IN A 3-IN-1 PARENTERAL NUTRITION MIXTURE RESULTED IN PATIENT DEATH.

The potential for the formation of a calcium phosphate precipitate in parenteral nutrition solutions is well studied and documented (1771; 1777), but the information is complex and difficult to apply to the clinical situation (1770; 1772; 1777). The incorporation of fat emulsion in 3-in-1 parenteral nutrition solutions obscures any precipitate that is present, which has led to substantial debate on the dangers associated with 3-in-1 parenteral nutrition mixtures and when or if the danger to the patient is warranted therapeutically (1770-1772; 2031-2036). Because such precipitation may be life-threatening to patients (2037), the Food and Drug Administration issued a Safety Alert containing the following recommendations (1769):

"1. The amounts of phosphorus and of calcium added to the admixture are critical. The solubility of the added calcium should be calculated from the volume at the time the calcium is added. It should not be based upon the final volume.

Some amino acid injections for TPN admixtures contain phosphate ions (as a phosphoric acid buffer). These phosphate ions and the volume at the time the phosphate is added should be considered when calculating the concentration of phosphate additives. Also, when adding calcium and phosphate to an admixture, the phosphate should be added first.

The line should be flushed between the addition of any potentially incompatible components.

2. A lipid emulsion in a three-in-one admixture obscures the presence of a precipitate. Therefore, if a lipid emulsion is needed, either (1) use a two-in-one admixture with the lipid infused separately, or (2) if a three-in-one admixture is medically necessary, then add the calcium before the lipid emulsion and according to the recommendations in number 1 above.

If the amount of calcium or phosphate which must be added is likely to cause a precipitate, some or all of the calcium should be administered separately. Such separate infusions must be properly diluted and slowly infused to avoid serious adverse events related to the calcium.

3. When using an automated compounding device, the above steps should be considered when programming the device. In addition, automated compounders should be maintained and operated according to the manufacturer's recommendations.

Any printout should be checked against the programmed admixture and weight of components.

4. During the mixing process, pharmacists who mix parenteral nutrition admixtures should periodically agitate the admixture and check for precipitates. Medical or home care personnel who start and monitor these infusions should carefully inspect for the presence of precipitates both before

and during infusion. Patients and care givers should be trained to visually inspect for signs of precipitation. They also should be advised to stop the infusion and seek medical assistance if precipitates are noted.

5. A filter should be used when infusing either central or peripheral parenteral nutrition admixtures. At this time, data have not been submitted to document which size filter is most effective in trapping precipitates.

Standards of practice vary, but the following is suggested: a 1.2-μm air-eliminating filter for lipid-containing admixtures and a 0.22-μm air-eliminating filter for non-lipid-containing admixtures.

6. Parenteral nutrition admixtures should be administered within the following time frames: if stored at room temperature, the infusion should be started within 24 hours after mixing; if stored at refrigerated temperatures, the infusion should be started within 24 hours of rewarming. Because warming parenteral nutrition admixtures may contribute to the formation of precipitates, once administration begins, care should be taken to avoid excessive warming of the admixture.

Persons administering home care parenteral nutrition admixtures may need to deviate from these time frames. Pharmacists who initially prepare these admixtures should check a reserve sample for precipitates over the duration and under the conditions of storage.

7. If symptoms of acute respiratory distress, pulmonary emboli, or interstitial pneumonitis develop, the infusion should be stopped immediately and thoroughly checked for precipitates. Appropriate medical interventions should be instituted. Home care personnel and patients should immediately seek medical assistance."

Calcium Phosphate Precipitation Fatalities— Hill et al. reported fatal cases of paroxysmal respiratory failure in two previously healthy women receiving peripheral vein parenteral nutrition. The patients experienced sudden cardiopulmonary arrest consistent with pulmonary emboli. The authors used in vitro simulations and an animal model to conclude that unrecognized calcium phosphate precipitation in a 3-in-1 total nutrition admixture caused the fatalities. The precipitation resulted during compounding by introducing calcium and phosphate near to one another in the compounding sequence and prior to complete fluid addition. This resulted in a temporarily high concentration of the drugs and precipitation of calcium phosphate. Observation of the precipitate was obscured by the incorporation of 20% fat emulsion, intravenous, into the nutrition mixture. No filter was used during infusion of the fatal nutrition admixtures (2037).

Calcium and Phosphate Conditional Compatibility— Calcium salts are conditionally compatible with potassium phosphates in parenteral nutrition mixtures. The incompatibility is dependent on a solubility and concentration phenomenon and is not entirely predictable. Precipitation may occur during compounding or at some time after compounding is completed. See the Calcium Gluconate monograph.

NOTE: Some amino acid solutions inherently contain calcium and phosphate, which must be considered in any projection of compatibility. See Table 1 in the Amino Acid Injection monograph.

Dextrose— Dextrose in final concentrations of 5 to 12.5% has been shown to cause a progressive coalescence of the globules in Intra-

lipid 10% due to its alteration of pH from about 7 down to about 3.5 in 48 hours (656).

Monovalent Cations— Monovalent cations such as potassium and sodium also cause progressive globule coalescence in Intralipid 10 and 20%, leading to surface creaming (480; 490; 656; 890). The degree and rate of this effect are dependent on the concentration of the ions. A decreasing degree and rate of coalescence were noted as concentrations of sodium chloride or potassium chloride decreased. At 200 mEq/L, the rate is rapid and the effect is severe. In the range of 100 mEq/L or less, significant effects may not occur for over 24 hours (490; 656).

Divalent Cations— Divalent cations such as calcium and magnesium cause immediate flocculation, with a nonhomogeneous white granular layer forming at the surface of the Intralipid 10%. This is followed by a substantial, visibly distinct layer, which does not redisperse on shaking (480; 490; 656).

The creaming of Intralipid 20% when calcium chloride was admixed in concentrations from 0.25 to 5% was found to be concentration dependent, with maximum creaming occurring with the 5% additive in 30 minutes (890).

Multicomponent ("3-in-1") Admixtures— Because of the potential benefits in terms of simplicity, efficiency, time, and cost savings, the concept of mixing amino acids, carbohydrates, electrolytes, fat emulsion, and other nutritional components together in the same container has been explored. Within limits, the feasibility of preparing such "3-in-1" parenteral nutrition admixtures has been demonstrated.

However, these 3-in-1 mixtures are very complex and inherently unstable. Emulsion stability is dependent on both zeta potential and van der Waals forces, influenced by the presence of dextrose (2029). Because the ultimate stability of each mixture is the result of various complicated factors, a definitive prediction of stability is impossible. Death and injury resulted from administration of unrecognized precipitation in 3-in-1 parenteral nutrition admixtures. In addition, the use of 3-in-1 admixtures is associated with a higher rate of catheter occlusion and reduced catheter life compared with giving the fat emulsion separately from the parenteral nutrition solution (2194).

Combining an amino acids–dextrose parenteral nutrition solution containing various electrolytes with fat emulsion 20%, intravenous (Intralipid, Vitrum), resulted in a mixture that was apparently stable for a limited time. However, it ultimately exhibited a creaming phenomenon. Within 12 hours, a distinct 2-cm layer separated on the upper surface. Microscopic examination revealed aggregates believed to be clumps of fat droplets. Fewer and smaller aggregates were noted in the lower layer (560; 561).

Amino acids have been reported to have no adverse effect on the emulsion stability of Intralipid 10%. In addition, the amino acids appeared to prevent the adverse impact of dextrose and to slow the coalescence and flocculation resulting from mono- and divalent cations. However, significant coalescence did result after a somewhat longer time. Therefore, it was recommended that such cations not be mixed with fat emulsion, intravenous (656).

The compatibility and stability of parenteral nutrition solutions consisting of amino acids, dextrose, fat emulsion, and various additives, all in a single admixture, were evaluated by Cutter Laboratories (791). The study entailed combining, in glass bottles, various amino acid products with Intralipid 10 or 20% and dextrose 10 or 70% along with electrolytes, vitamins, and trace minerals. These parenteral nutrition solutions were stored at 5 °C for three days followed by 25 °C for two days. Compatibility and stability of the emulsion were evaluated initially and again after storage. Additive compatibility and stability were not evaluated. Cutter Laboratories concluded that most of the admixtures tested were compatible and stable over the test period, with minimal chemical and physical changes. (See Table 2.) The exceptions were admixtures prepared with Aminosyn 7%. In the Aminosyn 7%-containing admixtures, the emulsion broke within 24 hours at room temperature and oil globules floated on the surface. Refrigeration prevented the breaking of the emulsion, as did exclusion of the electrolytes. Presumably, the lower pH of Aminosyn 7% compared to the other amino acid products tested was associated with the disruption of the emulsion.

Although dextrose 10 and 70% were the only concentrations evaluated, Cutter Laboratories indicated that intermediate dextrose concentrations may be used as long as the amino acids–dextrose–Intralipid ratio is 1:1:1 or 1:1:0.5. Other ratios also have been recommended (703; 1068).

The disruptive effects of divalent ions are not as severe in these parenteral nutrition admixtures as they are in Intralipid alone. However, they do represent complex and somewhat unpredictable interactions. Consequently, Cutter Laboratories recommended using only combinations that have been evaluated. Concentrations of additive components may be at or below the maximum amounts indicated in Table 2.

Although some admixtures were stable over longer periods, Cutter Laboratories recommended use of these combined multicomponent admixtures within 24 hours (791).

Travenol has stated that 1:1:1 mixtures of amino acids 5.5, 8.5, or 10% (Travenol), fat emulsion 10 or 20% (Travenol), and dextrose 10 to 70% are physically stable but recommends administration within 24 hours. M.V.I.-12 3.3 ml/L and electrolytes may also be added to the admixtures up to the maximum amounts listed below (850):

Calcium	8.3 mEq/L
Magnesium	3.3 mEq/L
Sodium	23.3 mEq/L
Potassium	20 mEq/L
Chloride	23.3 mEq/L
Phosphate	20 mEq/L
Zinc	3.33 mg/L
Copper	1.33 mg/L
Manganese	0.33 mg/L
Chromium	13.33 µg/L

Knutsen et al. reported that a mixture of soybean oil emulsion 10% with amino acids 8.5%, concentrated dextrose, multivitamins, and electrolytes had good physical stability. Visual and microscopic examination of samples stored at 4 °C for one week showed the emulsion to be uniform with no flocculence (891).

Burnham et al. evaluated the stability of mixtures of Intralipid 20% 1 L, Vamin glucose (amino acids with dextrose 10%) 1.5 L, and dextrose 10% 0.5 L with various electrolytes and vitamins. Initial emulsion particle size was around 1 µm. The mixture containing only monovalent cations was stable for at least nine days at 4 °C, with little change in particle size. The mixtures containing the divalent cations, such as calcium and magnesium, demonstrated much greater particle size increases, with mean diameters of around 3.3 to 3.5 µm after nine days at 4 °C. After 48 hours of storage, however, these increases were more modest, around 1.5 to 1.85 µm. After storage at 4 °C for 48 hours followed by 24 hours at room temperature, very few particles exceeded 5 µm. It was found that the effect of particle aggregation caused by electrolytes demonstrates a critical concentration before the effect begins. For calcium and magnesium chlorides, the critical concentrations were 2.4 and 2.6 mmol/L, respectively. Sodium and potassium chloride had critical concentrations of 110 and 150 mmol/L, respectively. The rate of

Table 2. Intralipid-Containing Parenteral Nutrition Admixtures Found to be Compatible and Stable (791)

Component	FreAmine II 8.5%	FreAmine III 8.5%	Travasol 8.5% without Electrolytes	Travasol 10% without Electrolytes	Veinamine 8%
	Amount (ml)				
Amino acids	500	500	500	500	500
Dextrose 70 or 10%	500	500	500	500	500
Intralipid 20 or 10%	500 or 250	500 or 250	500 or 250	500 or 250	500 or 250
	Maximum Total Concentration				
Calcium	10 mEq	10 mEq	10 mEq	10 mEq	10 mEq
Magnesium	13 mEq	13 mEq	13 mEq	13 mEq	13 mEq
Sodium	134 mEq	134 mEq	129 mEq	129 mEq	149 mEq
Potassium	105 mEq	105 mEq	105 mEq	105 mEq	120 mEq
Chloride	244 mEq	245 mEq	261 mEq	264 mEq	279 mEq
Sulfate	13 mEq	13 mEq	13 mEq	13 mEq	13 mEq
Phosphorus	12.5 mmol	12.5 mmol	7.5 mmol	7.5 mmol	7.5 mmol
Acetate	21 mEq	37 mEq	26 mEq	44 mEq	25 mEq
Zinc	4 mg	4 mg	4 mg	4 mg	4 mg
Copper	1.5 mg	1.5 mg	1.5 mg	1.5 mg	1.5 mg
Manganese	0.8 mg	0.8 mg	0.8 mg	0.8 mg	0.8 mg
Chromium	15 µg	15 µg	15 µg	15 µg	15 µg
Multivitamin infusion concentrate (USV)	5 ml	5 ml	5 ml	5 ml	5 ml

particle aggregation increased linearly with increasing electrolyte concentration. Heparin 667 units/L had no effect on emulsion stability. The quantity of emulsion in the mixture had a relatively small influence on stability, but higher concentrations exhibited a somewhat greater coalescence (892).

Davis and Galloway noted that instability of the emulsion systems is manifested by (1) flocculation of oil droplets to form aggregates that produce a cream-like layer on top or (2) coalescence of oil droplets leading to an increase in the average droplet size and eventually to a separation of free oil. The lowering of pH and adding of electrolytes can adversely affect the mechanical and electrical properties at the oil–water interface, eventually leading to flocculation and coalescence. Amino acids act as buffering agents and provide a protective effect on emulsion stability. Addition of electrolytes, especially the divalent ions Mg^{++} and Ca^{++} in excess of 2.5 mmol/L, to simple fat emulsions causes flocculation. But in mixed parenteral nutrition solutions, the stability of the emulsion is enhanced, depending on the quantity and nature of the amino acids present. The authors recommended a careful examination of emulsion mixtures for instability prior to administration (849).

Lawrence et al. reported the stability of an amino acid 4% (Travenol), dextrose 14%, fat emulsion 4% (Pharmacia) parenteral nutrition solution to be quite good. The solution also contained electrolytes, vitamins, and heparin sodium 4000 units/L. The aqueous solution was prepared first, with the fat emulsion added subsequently. This procedure allowed visual inspection of the aqueous phase and reduced the risk of emulsion breakdown by the divalent cations. Sample mixtures were stored at 18 to 25 and 3 to 8 °C for up to five days. They were evaluated visually and with a Coulter counter for particle size measurements. Both room temperature and refrigerated mixtures were stable for 48 hours. A marked increase in particle size was noted in the room temperature sample after 72 hours, but refrigeration delayed the changes. The authors' experience with over 1400 mixtures for administration to patients resulted in one emulsion creaming and another cracking. The authors had no explanation for the failure of these particular emulsions (848).

Turner reported on six parenteral nutrition solutions having various concentrations of amino acids, dextrose, soybean oil emulsion (Kabi-Vitrum), electrolytes, and multivitamins. All of the admixtures were stable for one week under refrigeration followed by 24 hours at room temperature, with no visible changes, pH changes, or significant particle size changes (1013). However, other researchers questioned this interpretation of the results (1014; 1015).

Iliano et al. reported that the addition of trace elements to a 3-in-1 parenteral nutrition solution with electrolytes had no adverse effect on the particle size of the fat emulsion after eight days of storage at 4 °C (1017).

Harrie et al. reported on the stability of 3-in-1 parenteral nutrition solutions prepared with 500 ml of Intralipid 20% compared to Soyacal 20%, along with 500 or 1000 ml of FreAmine III 8.5% and 500 ml of dextrose 70%. Also present were relatively large amounts of electrolytes and other additives. All mixtures were similarly stable for 28 days at 4 °C followed by five days at 21 to 25 °C, with little change in the emulsion. A slight white cream layer appeared after five days at 4 °C, but it was easily dispersed with gentle agitation. The appearance of this cream layer did not statistically affect particle size distribution. The authors concluded that the emulsion mixture remained suitable for clinical use throughout the study period. The stability of other components was not evaluated (1019).

Sayeed et al. reported on the stability of 3-in-1 parenteral nutrition admixtures prepared with Liposyn II 10 and 20%, Aminosyn pH 6,

and dextrose along with electrolytes, trace metals, and vitamins. Thirty-one different combinations were evaluated. Samples were stored under the following conditions: (1) 25 °C for one day, (2) 5 °C for two days followed by 30 °C for one day, or (3) 5 °C for nine days followed by 25 °C for one day. In all cases, there was no visual evidence of creaming, free oil droplets, and other signs of emulsion instability. Furthermore, little or no change in the particle size or zeta potential (electrostatic surface charge of lipid particles) was found, indicating emulsion stability. The dextrose and amino acids remained stable over the 10-day storage period. The greatest change of an amino acid occurred with tryptophan, which lost 6% in 10 days. Vitamin stability was not tested (1025).

Hardy et al. reported on the stability of four parenteral nutrition admixtures, ranging from 1 L each of amino acids 5.5% (Travenol), dextrose 10%, and fat emulsion 10% (Travenol) up to a "worst case" of 1 L each of amino acids 10% with electrolytes (Travenol), dextrose 70%, and fat emulsion 10% (Travenol). The admixtures were stored for 48 hours at 5 to 9 °C followed by 24 hours at room temperature. There were no visible signs of creaming, flocculation, or free oil. The mean emulsion particle size remained within acceptable limits for all admixtures, and there were no significant changes in glucose, soybean oil, and amino acid concentrations. The authors noted that two factors were predominant in determining the stability of such admixtures: electrolyte concentrations and pH (1065).

Hardy and Klim reported that several parenteral nutrition solutions containing amino acids (Travenol), glucose, and lipid, with and without electrolytes and trace elements, produced no visible flocculation or any significant change in mean emulsion particle size during 24 hours at room temperature (1066).

Jeppsson and Sjoberg reported on the compatibility of 10 parenteral nutrition admixtures, evaluated over 96 hours while stored at 20 to 25 °C in both glass bottles and ethylene vinylacetate bags. A slight creaming occurred in all admixtures, but this cream layer was easily dispersed by gentle shaking. No fat globules were visually apparent. The mean drop size was larger in the cream layer, but no globules were larger than 5 µm. Analyses of the concentrations of amino acids, dextrose, and electrolytes showed no changes over the study period. The authors concluded that such parenteral nutrition admixtures can be prepared safely as long as the component concentrations are within the following ranges (1067):

Vamin glucose or Vamin N (amino acids 7%)	1000 to 2000 ml
Dextrose 10 to 30%	100 to 550 ml
Intralipid 10 or 20%	500 to 1000 ml

Electrolytes (mmol/L)	
Sodium	20 to 70
Potassium	20 to 55
Calcium	2.3 to 2.9
Magnesium	1.1 to 3.1
Phosphorus	0 to 9.2
Chloride	27 to 71
Zinc	0.005 to 0.03

Parry et al. reported on the stability of eight parenteral nutrition admixtures with various ratios of amino acids, carbohydrates, and fat. FreAmine III 8.5%, dextrose 70%, and Soyacal 10 and 20% (mixed in ratios of 2:1:1, 1:1:1, 1:1:½, and 1:1:¼, where 1 = 500 ml) were evaluated. Additive concentrations were high to stress the admixtures and represent maximum doses likely to be encountered clinically:

Sodium acetate	150 mEq
Sodium chloride	210 mEq
Potassium acetate	45 mEq
Potassium chloride	90 mEq
Potassium phosphate	15 mM
Calcium gluconate	20 mEq
Magnesium sulfate	36 mEq
Trace elements	present
Folic acid	5 mg
M.V.I.-12	10 ml

The admixtures were stored at 4 °C for 14 days followed by four days at 22 to 25 °C. After 24 hours, all admixtures developed a thin white cream layer, which was readily dispersed by gentle agitation. No free oil droplets were observed. The mean particle diameter remained near the original size of the Soyacal throughout the study. Few particles were larger than 3 μm. Osmolality and pH also remained relatively unchanged (1068).

Bettner and Stennett had somewhat less success than others in preparing stable 3-in-1 parenteral nutrition admixtures with Aminosyn and Liposyn. Standard admixtures were prepared using Aminosyn 7% 1000 ml, dextrose 50% 1000 ml, and Liposyn 10% 500 ml. Concentrated admixtures were prepared using Aminosyn 10% 500 ml, dextrose 70% 500 ml, and Liposyn 20% 500 ml. Vitamins and trace elements were added to the admixtures along with the following electrolytes:

Electrolyte	Standard Admixture	Concentrated Admixture
Sodium	125 mEq	75 mEq
Potassium	95 mEq	74 mEq
Magnesium	25 mEq	25 mEq
Calcium	28 mEq	28 mEq
Phosphate	37 mmol	36 mmol
Chloride	83 mEq	50 mEq

Samples of each admixture were (1) stored at 4 °C, (2) adjusted to pH 6.6 with sodium bicarbonate and stored at 4 °C, or (3) adjusted to pH 6.6 and stored at room temperature. Compatibility was evaluated for three weeks.

Signs of emulsion deterioration were visible by 96 hours in the standard admixture and by 48 hours in the concentrated admixture. Clear rings formed at the meniscus, becoming thicker, yellow, and oily over time. Free-floating oil was obvious in three weeks in the standard admixture and in one week in the concentrated admixture. The samples adjusted to pH 6.6 developed visible deterioration later than the others. The authors indicated that pH may play a greater role than temperature in emulsion stability. However, precipitation (probably calcium phosphate and possibly carbonate) occurred in 36 hours in the pH 6.6 concentrated admixture but not the unadjusted (pH 5.5) samples. Mean particle counts increased for all samples over time but were greatest in the concentrated admixtures. The authors concluded that the concentrated admixtures were unsatisfactory for clinical use because of the early increase in particles and precipitation. Furthermore, they recommended that the standard admixtures be prepared immediately prior to use (1069). These results do not extend to Aminosyn II as a component of 3-in-1 admixtures, as reported by Sayeed et al. below.

Barat et al. studied the physical stability of 10 parenteral nutrition admixtures with different amino acid sources. The admixtures contained 500 ml each of dextrose 70%, fat emulsion 20% (Alpha Therapeutics), and amino acids in various concentrations from each manufacturer. Also present were standard electrolytes, trace elements, and vitamins. The admixtures were stored for 14 days at 4 °C, followed by four days at 22 to 25 °C. Slight creaming was evident in all admixtures but redispersed easily with agitation. Emulsion particles were uniform in size, showing no tendency to aggregate. No cracked emulsions occurred (1217).

Cripps (1218) and Davis and Galloway (1219) described the stability of parenteral nutrition solutions containing amino acids, dextrose, and fat emulsion along with electrolytes, trace elements, and vitamins. Cripps reported that the admixtures were stable for 24 hours at room temperature and for eight days at 4 °C. The visual appearance and particle size of the fat emulsion showed little change over the observation periods (1218). Davis and Galloway reported variable stability periods, depending on electrolyte concentrations. Stability ranged from four to 25 days at room temperature (1219).

Ang et al. studied the physical stability and clinical safety of a 3-in-1 parenteral nutrition admixture composed of amino acids (Cutter), dextrose, and fat emulsion (Cutter) plus electrolytes and vitamins. The admixture was physically stable for up to six weeks at 4 °C. Furthermore, continuous infusion to 25 adult patients did not result in any adverse reaction or abnormal laboratory parameter (1220).

du Plesis et al. studied the effects of dilution, dextrose concentration, amino acids, and electrolytes on the physical stability of 3-in-1 parenteral nutrition admixtures prepared with Intralipid 10% or Travamulsion 10%. Travamulsion was affected by dilution up to 1:14, exhibiting an increase in mean particle size, while Intralipid remained virtually unchanged for 24 hours at 25 °C and for 72 hours at 4 °C. At dextrose concentrations above 15%, fat droplets larger than 5 μm formed during storage for 24 hours at either 4 °C or room temperature. The presence of amino acids increased the stability of the fat emulsions in the presence of dextrose. Fat droplets larger than 5 μm formed at a total electrolyte concentration above approximately 240 mmol/L (monovalent cation equivalent) for Travamulsion 10% and 156 mmol/L for Intralipid 10% in 24 hours at room temperature, although creaming or breaking of the emulsion was not observed visually (1221).

Sayeed et al. evaluated the stability of 43 parenteral nutrition admixtures composed of various ratios of amino acid products, dextrose 10 to 70%, and four lipid emulsions 10 and 20% with electrolytes, trace elements, and vitamins. One group of admixtures included Travasol 5.5, 8.5, and 10%, FreAmine III 8.5 and 10%, Novamine 8.5 and 11.4%, Nephramine 5.4%, and RenAmine 6.5% with Liposyn II 10 and 20%. In another group, Aminosyn II 7, 8.5, and 10% was combined with Intralipid, Travamulsion, and Soyacal 10 and 20%. A third group was comprised of Aminosyn II 7, 8.5, and 10% with electrolytes combined with the latter three lipid emulsions. The admixtures were stored for 24 hours at 25 °C and for nine days at 5 °C followed by 24 hours at 25 °C. A few admixtures containing FreAmine III and Novamine with Liposyn II developed faint yellow streaks after 10 days of storage. The streaks readily dispersed with gentle shaking, as did the creaming present in most admixtures. Other properties such as pH, zeta-potential, and osmolality underwent little change in all of the admixtures. Particle size increased fourfold in one admixture (Novamine 8.5%, dextrose 50%, and Liposyn II in a 1:1:1 ratio), which the authors noted signaled the onset of particle coalescence. Nevertheless, the authors concluded that all of the admixtures were stable for the storage conditions and time periods tested (1222).

Sayeed et al. also evaluated the stability of 24 parenteral nutrition admixtures composed of various ratios of Aminosyn II 7, 8.5, or 10%, dextrose, and Liposyn II 10 and 20% with electrolytes, trace elements, and vitamins. Four admixtures were stored for 24 hours at 25 °C, six admixtures were stored for two days at 5 °C followed by one day at 30 °C, and 14 admixtures were stored for nine days at 5 °C followed by one day at 25 °C. No visible instability was evident. Creaming was present in most admixtures but disappeared with gentle shaking. Other properties such as pH, zeta-potential, particle size, and potency of the amino acids and dextrose showed little or no change during storage (1223).

Tripp reported the emulsion stability of five parenteral nutrition formulas (TNA #126 through #130 in Appendix I) containing Liposyn II in concentrations ranging from 1.2 to 7.1%. The parenteral nutrition solutions were prepared using simultaneous pumping of the components into empty containers (as with the Nutrimix compounder) and sequential pumping of the components (as with Automix compounders). The solutions were stored for two days at 5 °C followed by 24 hours at 25 °C. Similar results were obtained for both methods of preparation using visual assessment and oil globule size distribution (1426).

Tripp et al. evaluated the stability of 24 parenteral nutrition admixtures containing various concentrations of Aminosyn II, dextrose, and Liposyn II with a variety of electrolytes, trace elements, and multivitamins in dual-chamber, flexible, Nutrimix containers. No instability was visible in the admixtures stored at 25 °C for 24 hours or in those stored for nine days at 5 °C followed by 24 hours at 25 °C. Creaming was observed, but neither particle coalescence nor free oil was noted. The pH, particle size distribution, and amino acid and dextrose concentrations remained acceptable during the observation period (1432).

Thomas reported that the lipid particle size in two parenteral nutrition solutions composed of amino acids, dextrose 50%, fat emulsion 20% (Intralipid), electrolytes, and vitamins stayed within the manufacturer's size range specifications when stored at 23 and 4 °C and when frozen at −20 °C for 72 hours (1488).

Bullock et al. evaluated the physical stability of 10 parenteral nutrition formulas (TNA #149 through #158 in Appendix I) containing TrophAmine and Intralipid 20%, Liposyn II 20%, and Nutrilipid 20% in varying concentrations with low and high electrolyte concentrations. All test formulas were prepared with an automatic compounder and protected from light. TNA #149 through #156 were stored for 48 hours at 4 °C followed by 24 hours at 21 °C; TNA #157 and #158 were stored for 24 hours at 4 °C followed by 24 hours at 21 °C. Although some minor creaming occurred in all formulas, it was completely reversible with agitation. No other changes were visible, and particle size analysis indicated little variation during the study period. The addition of cysteine HCl 1 g/25 g of amino acids, alone or with L-carnitine 16 mg/g fat, to TNA #157 and #158 did not adversely affect the physical stability of 3-in-1 admixtures within the study period (1620).

Washington and Sizer evaluated the physical stability of five 3-in-1 parenteral nutrition solutions (TNA #167 through #171 in Appendix I) by visual observation, pH and osmolality determinations, and particle size distribution analysis. All five solutions were physically stable for 90 days at 4 °C. However, some irreversible flocculation occurred in all combinations after 180 days (1651).

Tu et al. studied the stability of several parenteral nutrition formulas (TNA #159 through #166 in Appendix I), with and without

iron dextran 2 mg/L. All formulas were physically compatible both visually and microscopically for 48 hours at 4 and 25 °C, and particle size distribution remained unchanged. The order of mixing and deliberate agitation had no effect on physical compatibility (1648).

Koorenhof and Timmer reported the maximum allowable concentrations of calcium and phosphate in a 3-in-1 parenteral nutrition mixture for children (TNA #192 in Appendix I). Added calcium varied from 1.5 to 150 mmol/L, while added phosphate varied from 21 to 300 mmol/L. The mixtures were stable for 48 hours at 22 and 37 °C as long as the pH was not greater than 5.7, the calcium concentration was below 16 mmol/L, the phosphate concentration was below 52 mM/L, and the product of the calcium and phosphate concentrations was below 250 $mmol^2/L^2$ (1773).

Driscoll et al. evaluated the influence of six factors on the stability of fat emulsion in 45 different 3-in-1 parenteral nutrition mixtures. The factors were amino acid concentration (2.5 to 7%); dextrose (5 to 20%); fat emulsion, intravenous (2 to 5%); monovalent cations (0 to 150 mEq/L); divalent cations (4 to 20 mEq/L); and trivalent cations from iron dextran (0 to 10 mg elemental iron/L). Although many formulations were unstable, visual examination could identify instability in only 65% of the samples. Electronic evaluation of particle size identified the remaining unstable mixtures. Furthermore, only the concentration of trivalent ferric ions significantly and consistently affected the emulsion stability during the 30-hour test period. Of the parenteral nutrition mixtures containing iron dextran, 16% were unstable, exhibiting emulsion cracking. The authors suggested that iron dextran should not be incorporated into 3-in-1 mixtures (1814).

Shenkin et al. evaluated the vitamin and trace element status of 22 postoperative surgical patients. Twelve patients were given parenteral nutrition with the fat emulsion containing vitamins separate from amino acids and other water-soluble nutrients; 10 patients received all nutrients in one large bag. No clinically significant differences were noted after administration periods of seven to 38 days (1226).

The drop size of 3-in-1 parenteral nutrition solutions in drip chambers is variable, being altered by the constituents of the mixture. In one study, multivitamins (Multibionta, E. Merck) caused the greatest reductions in drop size, up to 37%. This change may affect the rate of delivery if flow is estimated from drops per minute (1016). Similarly, flow rates delivered by infusion controllers dependent on predictable drop size may be inaccurate. Flow rates up to 29% less than expected have been reported. Therefore, variable-pressure volumetric pumps, which are independent of drop size, should be used rather than infusion controllers (1215).

When using multicomponent, 3-in-1, parenteral nutrition admixtures, the following points should be considered (490; 703; 892; 893; 1025; 1064; 1070; 1324; 1670):

1. The order of mixing is important. The amino acid solution should be added to either the fat emulsion or the dextrose before final mixing. This practice ensures that the protective effect of the amino acids to emulsion disruption by changes in pH and the presence of electrolytes is realized.

2. Electrolytes should not be added directly to the fat emulsion. Instead, they should be added to the amino acids or dextrose before the final mixing.

3. Such 3-in-1 admixtures containing electrolytes (especially divalent cations) are unstable and will eventually aggregate. The mixed systems should be carefully examined visually before use to ensure that a uniform emulsion still exists.

4. The admixtures should be stored under refrigeration if not used immediately.

5. The ultimate stability of the admixtures will be the result of a complex interaction of pH, component concentrations, electrolyte concentrations, and, probably, storage temperature.

Furthermore, the use of a 1.2-μm filter to remove large lipid particles, electrolyte precipitates, and *Candida albicans* contaminants has been recommended (1657; 1769; 2061), although others recommend a 5-μm filter to minimize the frequency of occlusion alarms (1951).

Separate Y-Type Infusion— The simultaneous administration of fat emulsion and amino acids by a Y-type infusion set so that mixture occurs just before entering the peripheral vein has been recommended. The fat emulsion may be administered through separate lines into the same central or peripheral vein as the carbohydrate–amino acids solutions by using a Y-connector located near the infusion site (1-12/98; 35; 61). The flow rates of each solution should be controlled by infusion pumps (1-12/98). The fat emulsion line should be kept higher than the carbohydrate–amino acids line because the lower specific gravity of the fat emulsion would otherwise cause it to run up the carbohydrate–amino acids line (35). If a syringe pump is used to administer fat emulsion, intravenous, into a Y-site of a carbohydrate–amino acids line, the syringe tip should be positioned above the mixture point to avoid entry of the carbohydrate–amino acids solution into the syringe (1107).

Heparin— Heparin sodium has been stated to be compatible in fat emulsion (480; 660). The addition of heparin sodium (Abbott) 1 and 2 units/ml to Liposyn 10% and Intralipid 10% did not break the emulsion and effectively reversed the blood hypercoagulability associated with intravenous fat emulsion administration (568).

The addition of heparin 667 units/L to a multicomponent 3-in-1 admixture containing fat emulsion, amino acids, dextrose, various electrolytes, and vitamins had no effect on the emulsion stability (892).

However, Raupp et al. reported flocculation of fat emulsion (Kabi-Vitrum) during Y-site administration into a line used to infuse a parenteral nutrition solution containing both calcium gluconate and heparin sodium. Subsequent evaluation indicated that the combination of calcium gluconate (0.46 and 1.8 mmol/125 ml) and heparin sodium (25 and 100 units/125 ml) in amino acids plus dextrose induced flocculation of the fat emulsion within two to four minutes at concentrations that resulted in no visually apparent flocculation in 30 minutes with either agent alone (1214).

This result was confirmed by Johnson et al. Calcium chloride quantities of 1 to 20 mmol normally result in slow flocculation of fat emulsion 20% over several hours. When heparin sodium 5 units/ml was added, the flocculation rate was accelerated greatly and a cream layer was observed visually in a few minutes. This effect was not observed when sodium ion was substituted for the divalent calcium (1406).

Similar results were observed by Trissel et al. during simulated Y-site administration of heparin sodium into nine 3-in-1 nutrient admixtures having different compositions. Damage to the fat emulsion component was found to occur immediately, with the possible formation of free oil over time (2215).

Trace Elements— The stability of a 3-in-1 parenteral nutrition mixture (TNA #191 in Appendix I) was compared when trace elements were added as gluconate or chloride salts. TNA #191 with copper 0.24 mg/L, iron 0.5 mg/L, and zinc 2 mg/L in either salt form was physically stable for seven days at both 4 and 25 °C (1787).

Amphotericin B— In an effort to reduce toxicity, amphotericin B has been admixed in Intralipid instead of the more usual dextrose 5% in water (1809–1811; 2178). However, amphotericin B 0.75 mg/kg/day administered using this approach in 250 ml of Intralipid 20% has been associated with acute pulmonary toxicities, including sudden onset of coughing, tachypnea, agitation, cyanosis, and deterioration of oxygen saturation. The temporal relationship between the drug administration and respiratory symptoms suggested a causal relationship. Furthermore, no reduction in renal toxicity or other side effects associated with amphotericin B was observed. The authors concluded amphotericin B should not be administered to patients in Intralipid (2177).

At a concentration of 0.6 mg/ml in Intralipid 10 or 20%, amphotericin B precipitated immediately or almost immediately. The precipitate was not visible to the unaided eye because of the emulsion's dense opacity. Particle size evaluation found thousands of particles larger than 10 μm per milliliter. In dextrose 5% in water, very few particles were larger than 10 μm. Centrifuging the Intralipid admixtures resulted in rapid visualization of the precipitate as a mass at the bottom of the test tubes (1808).

However, amphotericin B precipitation is observed in fat emulsion within two to four hours without centrifuging. In concentrations ranging from 90 mg/L to 2 g/L in Intralipid 20%, amphotericin precipitate is easily seen as yellow particulate matter on the bottom of the lipid emulsion containers (1872; 1987). Damage to the emulsion integrity with creaming has also been reported (1986).

In other reports, the appearance of problems was observed in as little as 15 minutes, and actual amphotericin B precipitate formed within 20 minutes of mixing. Analysis of the precipitate confirmed its identity as amphotericin B. The authors hypothesized that amphotericin B precipitates because the excipient deoxycholic acid, an anion, attracts oppositely charged choline groups from the egg yolk components of the fat emulsion and forms a precipitate with phosphatidylcholine, leaving insufficient surfactant to keep the amphotericin B dispersed (2204; 2205).

Gentamicin— Kern et al. evaluated serum concentrations of gentamicin following intermittent 15 to 30-minute administration in piggyback infusions of 50 ml of dextrose 5% in water or 50 ml of TNA #177 (Appendix I). Gentamicin serum concentrations were equivalent using both administration methods (1573).

Plasma Expanders— Fat emulsion (Abbott) 10 and 20% were combined with the plasma expanders Macrodex 6% in sodium chloride 0.9% (Schiwa), Gelafundin (Braun), Haes Steril 10% (Fresenius), and Expafusin Sine (Pfrimmer); fat particles exceeding 5 μm resulted, as observed by microscopic examination. These combinations were incompatible (1668).

Extraction of Plasticizers— Fat emulsion tends to extract small amounts of phthalate plasticizers from PVC. Although no adverse clinical effects from small amounts of plasticizers have been reported, non-PVC administration sets and non-PVC plastic containers, such as an ethylene vinylacetate bag, may be used to avoid plasticizer exposure. If PVC tubing is used, phthalate extraction can be minimized by not storing primed sets (658; 661; 893; 1105).

Storage of fat emulsion 10 and 20% (Intralipid) for 24 hours in PVC sets resulted in phthalate contents of 64 to 70 μg/ml at 5 °C and 144 to 160 μg/ml at ambient temperature. When the fat emulsions were simply infused through PVC sets, phthalate content dropped to 3.6 to 8.5 μg/ml. A patient being administered 500 ml of fat emulsion per day would receive about 1.5 to 2.75 mg/day. Negligible levels of phthalate were delivered from a TPN solution containing fat emulsion (1264).

Mazur et al. reported that a parenteral nutrition solution containing an amino acid solution, dextrose, and electrolytes in a PVC bag did not leach measurable quantities of diethylhexylphthalate (DEHP) plasticizer during 21 days of storage at 4 and 25 °C. However, addition of fat emulsion 10 or 20% to the formula caused detectable leaching of DEHP from the PVC containers stored for 48 hours. Higher DEHP levels were found in the 25 °C samples than in the 4 °C samples. The authors recommended limiting the use of lipid-containing parenteral nutrition solutions to 24 to 36 hours. Use of non-PVC containers is another option (1430).

Microbial Contamination— Fat emulsion, intravenous, based on either soybean oil or safflower oil, has been shown to support the growth of various microbes, including both bacterial and fungal species. No visual changes occurred in the emulsions to suggest contamination (1102–1104; 1216).

The 3-in-1 parenteral nutrition solutions that have a lower pH and higher osmolality due to the presence of amino acids and dextrose do not support microbial growth as well as fat emulsion alone (1216).

FENTANYL CITRATE
AHFS 28:08.08

Sublimaze

Abbott
Taylor

Products— Fentanyl citrate is available in 2-, 5-, 10-, and 20-ml ampuls and 30- and 50-ml vials (154). Each milliliter contains fentanyl (as the citrate) 50 μg (0.05 mg) with hydrochloric acid and/or sodium hydroxide for pH adjustment (1-5/92; 4).

pH— From 4 to 7.5 (4).

Osmolality— The product osmolality was determined to be essentially 0 mOsm/kg (1233).

Administration— Fentanyl citrate is administered by intramuscular or intravenous injection (4).

Stability— Intact ampuls should be stored at controlled room temperature and protected from light. Brief exposure to temperatures up to 40 °C does not affect potency (4).

Fentanyl citrate is most stable at pH 3.5 to 7.5 (1638). Fentanyl is hydrolyzed in acidic solutions (4).

Syringes— Fentanyl citrate (Elkins Sinn) 0.0167 mg/ml in sodium chloride 0.9% packaged in polypropylene syringes (Sherwood) was physically stable and exhibited little or no loss by stability-indicating HPLC analysis in 24 hours stored at 4 and 23 °C in the dark (2199).

Fentanyl citrate (David Bull) at a concentration of 12.5 μg/ml in sodium chloride 0.9% was packaged as 8 ml in 10-ml polypropylene syringes (Terumo) with 19-gauge needles attached (Becton-Dickinson). Fentanyl citrate (David Bull) at a concentration of 33.3 μg/ml in sodium chloride 0.9% was packaged as 18 ml in 20-ml polypropylene syringes (Terumo) with 19-gauge needles attached (Becton-Dickinson). The syringes were stored refrigerated at 5 °C, at 22 °C exposed to light, and at 38 °C for seven days. The solutions were visually unchanged, and HPLC analysis found no loss at 5 and 22 °C. At 38 °C, the 12.5-μg/ml solution exhibited less than 7% loss, whereas the 33.3-μg/ml solution had no loss in seven days (2202).

Portable Infusion Pumps— Fentanyl citrate (Janssen) 20 μg/ml in sodium chloride 0.9% in PVC portable infusion pump reservoirs exhibited little or no loss after 30 days at 23 and 3 °C. Wrapping the reservoirs to prevent possible moisture loss was not necessary for storage of 30 days (1356).

Sorption— Fentanyl citrate (Janssen) 5 μg/ml in dextrose 5% in water or sodium chloride 0.9% exhibited no loss due to sorption to PVC infusion solution containers when compared to glass containers. Furthermore, use of a PCA infusion pump to deliver fentanyl citrate 4.5 μg/ml in dextrose 5% in water in a PVC bag did not result in concentration losses associated with sorption. Delivered concentrations were relatively consistent during the 30-hour evaluation period (1357).

Xu et al. reported extensive and rapid loss of fentanyl citrate due to sorption to PVC containers when the solution pH was adjusted to the alkaline range. Fentanyl citrate 12.5 μg/ml in both dextrose 5% in water and sodium chloride 0.9% at pH 9 (with added sodium hydroxide) or combined with fluorouracil with nearly the same pH lost 25% of the fentanyl content in 15 minutes and 50% in one hour by HPLC analysis. Loss of fentanyl citrate did not occur in polyethylene containers under these conditions. Sorptive loss of fentanyl citrate to PVC containers is expected to occur from any alkaline solution (2064).

Filtration— Fentanyl citrate (Janssen) 2.5 μg/ml in dextrose 5% in water or sodium chloride 0.9% was delivered over four hours through three kinds of 0.2-μm membrane filters varying in size and composition. HPLC analysis of the delivered solution showed no fentanyl loss due to sorption to the filter (1399).

Compatibility Information

Solution Compatibility

Fentanyl citrate

Solution	Mfr	Mfr	Conc/L	Remarks	Ref	C/I
Dextrose 5% in water	DB,[a] TR[b]	JA	5 mg	Physically compatible with no fentanyl loss in 48 hr at 22 °C in normal room light	1357	C
	AB	JN	20 and 40 mg	Visually compatible with 3% or less loss by HPLC in 3 hr at 24 °C	1852	C
Sodium chloride 0.9%	TR[b]	JA	20 mg	Physically compatible with little or no fentanyl loss in 30 days at 3 and 23 °C	1356	C
	DB,[a] TR[b]	JA	5 mg	Physically compatible with no fentanyl loss in 48 hr at 22 °C in normal room light	1357	C

[a]Tested in glass containers.
[b]Tested in PVC containers.

Additive Compatibility

Fentanyl citrate

Drug	Mfr	Conc/L	Mfr	Conc/L	Test Soln	Remarks	Ref	C/I
Bupivacaine HCl	WI	1.25 g	JN	20 mg	NS[a]	Physically compatible with little or no loss of either drug in 30 days at 3 and 23 °C	1396	C
Fluorouracil	AB	1 and 16 g	AB	12.5 mg	D5W, NS[a]	25% fentanyl loss in 15 min due to sorption to PVC	2064	I

[a]Tested in PVC containers.

Drugs in Syringe Compatibility

Fentanyl citrate

Drug (in syringe)	Mfr	Amt	Mfr	Amt	Remarks	Ref	C/I
Atracurium besylate	BW	10 mg/ml		50 µg/ml	Physically compatible and atracurium chemically stable for 24 hr at 5 and 25 °C	1694	C
Atropine sulfate		0.6 mg/1.5 ml	MN	100 µg/1 ml	Physically compatible for at least 15 min	14	C
	ST	0.4 mg/1 ml	MN	0.05 mg/1 ml	Physically compatible for at least 15 min	326	C
Bupivacaine HCl with ketamine HCl	SW PD	1.5 mg/ml 2 mg/ml	JN	0.01 mg/ml	Diluted to 5 ml with NS. Visually compatible with no new GC/MS peaks in 1 hr at room temperature	1956	C
Butorphanol tartrate	BR	4 mg/2 ml	MN	0.1 mg/2 ml	Physically compatible both macroscopically and microscopically for 30 min at room temperature	566	C
Chlorpromazine HCl	PO	50 mg/2 ml	MN	0.05 mg/1 ml	Physically compatible for at least 15 min	326	C
Cimetidine HCl	SKF	300 mg/2 ml	JN	0.1 mg/2 ml	Physically compatible for 4 hr at 25 °C	25	C
Clonidine HCl with lidocaine HCl	BI AST	0.03 mg/ml 2 mg/ml	JN	0.01 mg/ml	Diluted to 5 ml with NS. Visually compatible with no new GC/MS peaks in 1 hr at room temperature	1956	C
Dimenhydrinate	HR	50 mg/1 ml	MN	0.05 mg/1 ml	Physically compatible for at least 15 min	326	C

Drugs in Syringe Compatibility (Cont.)

Fentanyl citrate

Drug (in syringe)	Mfr	Amt	Mfr	Amt	Remarks	Ref	C/I
Diphenhydramine HCl	PD	50 mg/ 1 ml	MN	0.05 mg/ 1 ml	Physically compatible for at least 15 min	326	C
Droperidol	MN	2.5 mg/ 1 ml	MN	0.05 mg/ 1 ml	Physically compatible for at least 15 min	326	C
Heparin sodium		2500 units/ 1 ml	JN	0.1 mg/ 2 ml	Physically compatible for at least 5 min	1053	C
Hydromorphone HCl	KN	4 mg/ 2 ml	MN	0.05 mg/ 1 ml	Physically compatible for 30 min	517	C
Hydroxyzine HCl	PF	50 mg/ 1 ml	MN	0.05 mg/ 1 ml	Physically compatible for at least 15 min	326	C
	PF	50 mg/ 1 ml	CR	0.05 mg/ 1 ml	Physically compatible	771	C
	PF	100 mg/ 2 ml	CR	0.05 mg/ 1 ml	Physically compatible	771	C
Meperidine HCl	WI	50 mg/ 1 ml	MN	0.05 mg/ 1 ml	Physically compatible for at least 15 min	326	C
Metoclopramide HCl	NO	10 mg/ 2 ml	MN	0.05 mg/ 1 ml	Physically compatible both macroscopically and microscopically for 15 min at room temperature	565	C
Midazolam HCl	RC	5 mg/ 1 ml	ES	0.1 mg/ 2 ml	Physically compatible for 4 hr at 25 °C under fluorescent light	1145	C
	RC	0.625 and 0.938 mg/ml[a]	DB	12.5 μg/ ml[a]	Visually compatible with little fentanyl loss and 7 to 9% midazolam loss by HPLC in 7 days at 5 and 22 °C, respectively	2202	C
	RC	0.625 mg/ml[a]	DB	37.5 μg/ ml[a]	Visually compatible with no fentanyl loss and 5 to 8% midazolam loss by HPLC in 7 days at 5 and 22 °C, respectively	2202	C
	RC	0.938 mg/ml[a]	DB	37.5 μg/ ml[a]	Visually compatible with little fentanyl loss and 7 to 9% midazolam loss by HPLC in 7 days at 5 and 22 °C, respectively	2202	C
	RC	0.278 and 0.833 mg/ml[a]	DB	33.3 μg/ ml[a]	Visually compatible with no fentanyl loss and not more than 5 to 7% midazolam loss by HPLC in 7 days at 5 and 22 °C, respectively	2202	C
Morphine sulfate	ST	15 mg/ 1 ml	MN	0.05 mg/ 1 ml	Physically compatible for at least 15 min	326	C
Ondansetron HCl	GW	1.33 mg/ ml[a]	ES	0.0167 mg/ml[a]	Physically compatible with no measured increase in particulates and little or no loss of either drug by HPLC in 24 hr at 4 or 23 °C	2199	C
Pentazocine lactate	WI	30 mg/ 1 ml	MN	0.05 mg/ 1 ml	Physically compatible for at least 15 min	326	C
Pentobarbital sodium	AB	50 mg/ 1 ml	MN	0.05 mg/ 1 ml	Physically incompatible within 15 min	326	I
Perphenazine	SC	5 mg/ 1 ml	MN	0.1 mg/ 2 ml	Physically compatible both macroscopically and microscopically for 30 min at room temperature	566	C

Drugs in Syringe Compatibility (Cont.)

Fentanyl citrate

Drug (in syringe)	Mfr	Amt	Mfr	Amt	Remarks	Ref	C/I
Prochlorperazine edisylate	PO	5 mg/ 1 ml	MN	0.05 mg/ 1 ml	Physically compatible for at least 15 min	326	C
Promazine HCl	WY	50 mg/ 1 ml	MN	0.05 mg/ 1 ml	Physically compatible for at least 15 min	326	C
Promethazine HCl	PO	50 mg/ 2 ml	MN	0.05 mg/ 1 ml	Physically compatible for at least 15 min	326	C
Ranitidine HCl	GL	50 mg/ 2 ml	JN	0.1 mg/ 2 ml	Physically compatible for 1 hr at 25 °C both macroscopically and microscopically	978	C
Scopolamine HBr		0.6 mg/ 1.5 ml	MN	100 μg/ 1 ml	Physically compatible for at least 15 min	14	C
	ST	0.4 mg/ 1 ml	MN	0.05 mg/ 1 ml	Physically compatible for at least 15 min	326	C

[a]Tested in sodium chloride 0.9%.

Y-Site Injection Compatibility (1:1 Mixture)

Fentanyl citrate

Drug	Mfr	Conc	Mfr	Conc	Remarks	Ref	C/I
Amphotericin B cholesteryl sulfate complex	SEQ	0.83 mg/ml[a]	AB	0.05 mg/ml	Physically compatible with little or no change in measured turbidity or increase in particle content in 4 hr at 23 °C under fluorescent light	2117	C
Atracurium besylate	BW	0.5 mg/ml[a]	ES	10 μg/ml[a]	Physically compatible for 24 hr at 28 °C	1337	C
Cisatracurium besylate	GW	0.1, 2, 5 mg/ml[a]	AB	0.0125 mg/ ml[a]	Physically compatible with no change in measured turbidity or increase in particle content in 4 hr at 23 °C	2074	C
Diltiazem HCl	MMD	1 mg/ml[a]	ES	0.05 mg/ml	Visually compatible for 4 hr at 27 °C	2062	C
Dobutamine HCl	LI	4 mg/ml[a]	ES	0.05 mg/ml	Visually compatible for 4 hr at 27 °C	2062	C
Dopamine HCl	AB	3.2 mg/ml[a]	ES	0.05 mg/ml	Visually compatible for 4 hr at 27 °C	2062	C
Enalaprilat	MSD	0.05 mg/ml[b]	ES	2 μg/ml[a]	Physically compatible for 24 hr at room temperature under fluorescent light	1355	C
Epinephrine HCl	AB	0.02 mg/ml[a]	ES	0.05 mg/ml	Visually compatible for 4 hr at 27 °C	2062	C
Esmolol HCl	DCC	1 g/100 ml[c]	JN	0.05 mg/1 ml	Physically compatible when fentanyl is injected into Y-site of flowing admixture[d]	1168	C
	DCC	10 mg/ml[c]	JN	0.05 mg/ml	Physically compatible with no loss of either drug in 8 hr at ambient temperature exposed to light	1168	C
Etomidate	AB	2 mg/ml	ES	0.05 mg/ml	Visually compatible for up to 7 days at 25 °C	1801	C
Furosemide	AMR	10 mg/ml	ES	0.05 mg/ml	Visually compatible for 4 hr at 27 °C	2062	C
Heparin sodium	UP	1000 units/ L[e]	MN	0.05 mg/ml	Physically compatible for at least 4 hr at room temperature by visual and microscopic examination	534	C
	ES	100 units/ml[a]	ES	0.05 mg/ml	Visually compatible for 4 hr at 27 °C	2062	C
Hydrocortisone sodium succinate	UP	10 mg/L[e]	MN	0.05 mg/ml	Physically compatible for at least 4 hr at room temperature by visual and microscopic examination	534	C

Y-Site Injection Compatibility (1:1 Mixture) (Cont.)

Fentanyl citrate

Drug	Mfr	Conc	Mfr	Conc	Remarks	Ref	C/I
Hydromorphone HCl	KN	1 mg/ml	ES	0.05 mg/ml	Visually compatible for 4 hr at 27 °C	2062	C
Labetalol HCl	SC	1 mg/ml[a]	JN	10 mg/ml[a]	Physically compatible for 24 hr at 18 °C	1171	C
	AH	2 mg/ml[a]	ES	0.05 mg/ml	Visually compatible for 4 hr at 27 °C	2062	C
Lorazepam	WY	0.33 mg/ml[b]		0.05 mg/ml	Visually compatible for 24 hr at 22 °C	1855	C
	WY	0.5 mg/ml[a]	ES	0.05 mg/ml	Visually compatible for 4 hr at 27 °C	2062	C
Midazolam HCl	RC	0.1 and 0.5 mg/ml[a]	JN	40 μg/ml[a]	Visually compatible with little or no loss of either drug by HPLC in 3 hr at 24 °C	1813	C
	RC	0.1 and 0.5 mg/ml[a]	JN	20 μg/ml[a]	Visually compatible with little or no midazolam loss and 3 to 4% fentanyl loss by HPLC in 3 hr at 24 °C	1813	C
	RC	1 mg/ml[a]	ES	0.05 mg/ml	Visually compatible for 24 hr at 23 °C	1847	C
	RC	0.1 and 0.5 mg/ml[a]	JN	0.02 mg/ml[a]	Visually compatible with no midazolam loss and 3 to 4% fentanyl loss by HPLC in 3 hr at 24 °C	1852	C
	RC	0.1 and 0.5 mg/ml[a]	JN	0.04 mg/ml[a]	Visually compatible with no loss of either drug by HPLC in 3 hr at 24 °C	1852	C
	RC	5 mg/ml		0.05 mg/ml	Visually compatible for 24 hr at 22 °C	1855	C
	RC	2 mg/ml[a]	ES	0.05 mg/ml	Visually compatible for 4 hr at 27 °C	2062	C
Milrinone lactate	SW	0.2 mg/ml[a]	ES	0.05 mg/ml	Visually compatible for 4 hr at 27 °C	2062	C
	SW	0.4 mg/ml[a]	ES	50 μg/ml	Visually compatible with little or no loss of either drug by HPLC in 4 hr at 23 °C	2214	C
Morphine sulfate	SCN	2 mg/ml[a]	ES	0.05 mg/ml	Visually compatible for 4 hr at 27 °C	2062	C
Nafcillin sodium	WY	33 mg/ml[b]		0.05 mg/ml	No precipitation	547	C
Nicardipine HCl	WY	1 mg/ml[a]	ES	0.05 mg/ml	Visually compatible for 4 hr at 27 °C	2062	C
Nitroglycerin	AB	0.4 mg/ml[a]	ES	0.05 mg/ml	Visually compatible for 4 hr at 27 °C	2062	C
Norepinephrine bitartrate	AB	0.128 mg/ml[a]	ES	0.05 mg/ml	Visually compatible for 4 hr at 27 °C	2062	C
Pancuronium bromide	ES	0.05 mg/ml[a]	ES	10 μg/ml[a]	Physically compatible for 24 hr at 28 °C	1337	C
Potassium chloride	AB	40 mEq/L[e]	MN	0.05 mg/ml	Physically compatible for at least 4 hr at room temperature by visual and microscopic examination	534	C
Propofol	ZEN	10 mg/ml	AB	0.05 mg/ml	Physically compatible for 1 hr at 23 °C with no increase in particle content	2066	C
Ranitidine HCl	GL	1 mg/ml[a]	ES	0.05 mg/ml	Visually compatible for 4 hr at 27 °C	2062	C
Remifentanil HCl	GW	0.025 and 0.25 mg/ml[b]	ES	0.0125 mg/ml[a]	Physically compatible with no change in measured turbidity or increase in particle content in 4 hr at 23 °C	2075	C
Sargramostim	IMM	6[f] and 15 μg/ml[b]	ES	50 μg/ml	Visually compatible for 2 hr	1618	C
Thiopental sodium	AB	25 mg/ml	ES	0.05 mg/ml	Visually compatible for up to 7 days at 25 °C	1801	C
	AB	25 mg/ml[g]	ES	0.05 mg/ml	Visually compatible for 4 hr at 27 °C	2062	C
TNA #218 to #226[h]			AB	0.0125[a] and 0.05 mg/ml	Visually compatible with no precipitate or emulsion damage apparent in 4 hr at 23 °C	2215	C
TPN #203 and #204[h]			ES	0.05 mg/ml	Visually compatible for 4 hr at 23 °C	1974	C

Y-Site Injection Compatibility (1:1 Mixture) (Cont.)

Fentanyl citrate

Drug	Mfr	Conc	Mfr	Conc	Remarks	Ref	C/I
TPN #212 to #215[h]			AB	0.05 mg/ml	Physically compatible with no change in measured turbidity or increase in particle content in 4 hr at 23 °C	2109	**C**
			JN	0.0125 mg/ml[a]	Physically compatible with no change in measured turbidity or increase in particle content in 4 hr at 23 °C	2109	**C**
TPN #216[h]			ES	0.01 mg/ml[g]	Mixed 1 ml of fentanyl with 9 ml of TPN. Visually compatible for 24 hr	2104	**C**
Vecuronium bromide	OR	0.1 mg/ml[a]	ES	10 µg/ml[a]	Physically compatible for 24 hr at 28 °C	1337	**C**
	OR	1 mg/ml	ES	0.05 mg/ml	Visually compatible for 4 hr at 27 °C	2062	**C**
Vitamin B complex with C	RC	2 ml/L[e]	MN	0.05 mg/ml	Physically compatible for at least 4 hr at room temperature by visual and microscopic examination	534	**C**

[a]*Tested in dextrose 5% in water.*
[b]*Tested in sodium chloride 0.9%.*
[c]*Tested in dextrose 5% in sodium chloride 0.9%.*
[d]*Flowing at 1.6 ml/min.*
[e]*Tested in dextrose 5% in Ringer's injection, dextrose 5% in Ringer's injection, lactated, dextrose 5% in water, Ringer's injection, lactated, and sodium chloride 0.9%.*
[f]*Tested with human albumin 0.1%.*
[g]*Tested in sterile water for injection.*
[h]*Refer to Appendix I for the composition of parenteral nutrition solutions. TNA indicates a 3-in-1 admixture, and TPN indicates a 2-in-1 admixture.*

Additional Compatibility Information

Fentanyl citrate is stated to be physically incompatible with methohexital, pentobarbital, and thiopental (4).

Bupivacaine and Epinephrine— A solution composed of bupivacaine HCl (Winthrop) 0.44 mg/ml, fentanyl citrate (Janssen) 1.25 µg/ml, and epinephrine HCl (Abbott) 0.69 µg/ml was stored in 100-ml portable infusion pump reservoirs (Pharmacia Deltec) for 30 days at 3 and 23 °C. The samples were then delivered through the infusion pumps over 48 hours at near-body temperature (30 °C). The samples were visually compatible throughout, and bupivacaine HCl and fentanyl citrate exhibited no loss by HPLC analysis. Epinephrine HCl sustained about a 5 to 6% loss by HPLC analysis after 20 days of storage at both temperatures and about a 9 to 10% loss after 30 days of storage and subsequent pump delivery. The authors recommended restricting storage before administration to only 20 days (1627).

Multiple Drugs— A seven-drug combination consisting of bupivacaine HCl (Sanofi Winthrop) 1.5 mg/ml, clonidine HCl (Boehringer Ingelheim) 0.03 mg/ml, fentanyl citrate (Janssen) 0.01 mg/ml, ketamine (Parke-Davis) 2 mg/ml, lidocaine HCl (Astra) 2 mg/ml, morphine sulfate (Elkins-Sinn) 0.2 mg/ml, and tetracaine HCl (Sanofi Winthrop) 2 mg/ml mixed together in equal quantities was found to be visually compatible with no new GC/MS peaks appearing in one hour at room temperature (1956).

FENTANYL CITRATE AND DROPERIDOL
AHFS 28:08.08 and 28:24.92

Astra

Products— Fentanyl citrate and droperidol injection is available in 2- and 5-ml ampuls and 2-ml vials. Each milliliter contains fentanyl as the citrate 0.05 mg and droperidol 2.5 mg, with lactic acid to adjust the pH (2; 154).

pH— From 3.2 to 3.8 (17).

Administration— Fentanyl citrate and droperidol injection may be administered by intramuscular injection, intravenous injection, or intravenous infusion (4).

Stability— Intact ampuls and vials should be stored at controlled room temperature and protected from light (2; 4).

Compatibility Information

Additive Compatibility

Fentanyl citrate and droperidol

Drug	Mfr	Conc/L	Mfr	Conc/L	Test Soln	Remarks	Ref	C/I
Sodium bicarbonate	AB	2.4 mEq[a]	JN	0.05 mg + 2.5 mg	D5W	Physically compatible for 24 hr	772	**C**

[a]*One vial of Neut added to a liter of admixture.*

Drugs in Syringe Compatibility

Fentanyl citrate and droperidol

Drug (in syringe)	Mfr	Amt	Mfr	Amt	Remarks	Ref	C/I
Glycopyrrolate	RB	0.2 mg/ 1 ml	MN	0.05 mg + 2.5 mg/ 1 ml	Physically compatible and pH in stability range for glycopyrrolate for 48 hr at 25 °C	331	**C**
	RB	0.2 mg/ 1 ml	MN	0.1 mg + 5 mg/ 2 ml	Physically compatible and pH in stability range for glycopyrrolate for 48 hr at 25 °C	331	**C**
	RB	0.4 mg/ 2 ml	MN	0.05 mg + 2.5 mg/ 1 ml	Physically compatible and pH in stability range for glycopyrrolate for 48 hr at 25 °C	331	**C**
Heparin sodium		2500 units/ 1 ml	JN	0.1 mg + 5 mg/ 2 ml	Turbidity or precipitate forms within 5 min	1053	**I**

Y-Site Injection Compatibility (1:1 Mixture)

Fentanyl citrate and droperidol

Drug	Mfr	Conc	Mfr	Conc	Remarks	Ref	C/I
Heparin sodium		50 units/ml/ min[a]	JN	0.1 mg + 5 mg/2 ml[b]	Precipitate forms	1053	**I**
		1000 units/L[c]		0.05 mg + 2.5 mg/ml	Physically compatible for at least 4 hr at room temperature by visual and microscopic examination	534	**C**
Hydrocortisone sodium succinate	UP	10 mg/L[c]		0.05 mg + 2.5 mg/ml	Physically compatible for at least 4 hr at room temperature by visual and microscopic examination	534	**C**
Nafcillin sodium	WY	33 mg/ml[a]		0.05 mg + 2.5 mg/ml	Precipitate forms, probably free nafcillin	547	**I**
Potassium chloride	AB	40 mEq/L[c]	MN	0.05 mg + 2.5 mg/ml	Physically compatible for at least 4 hr at room temperature by visual and microscopic examination	534	**C**

Y-Site Injection Compatibility (1:1 Mixture) (Cont.)

Fentanyl citrate and droperidol

Drug	Mfr	Conc	Mfr	Conc	Remarks	Ref	C/I
Vitamin B complex with C	RC	2 ml/L[c]		0.05 mg + 2.5 mg/ml	Physically compatible for at least 4 hr at room temperature by visual and microscopic examination	534	C

[a]*Tested in sodium chloride 0.9%.*
[b]*Given over three minutes via a Y-site into a running infusion solution of heparin sodium in sodium chloride 0.9%.*
[c]*Tested in dextrose 5% in Ringer's injection, dextrose 5% in Ringer's injection, lactated, dextrose 5% in water, Ringer's injection, lactated, and sodium chloride 0.9%.*

Additional Compatibility Information

For additional compatibility information, also see the monographs on fentanyl citrate and droperidol.

FILGRASTIM
AHFS 20:16

Neupogen   **Amgen**

Products— Filgrastim (Amgen) is available in 1- and 1.6-ml single-dose vials. Each milliliter of solution contains (2):

Filgrastim	300 μg
Acetate	0.59 mg
Sorbitol	50 mg
Polysorbate 80 (Tween 80)	0.004%
Sodium	0.035 mg
Water for injection	qs 1 ml

pH— 4 (2).

Administration— Filgrastim is administered by subcutaneous injection undiluted or by intravenous or subcutaneous infusion. For intravenous infusion, it is diluted in 50 to 100 ml of dextrose 5% in water and given over 15 to 60 minutes or over 24 hours by continuous infusion. It may also be given over 24 hours by continuous subcutaneous infusion after diluting the dose in 10 to 50 ml of dextrose 5% in water and infusing at a rate not exceeding 10 ml/24 hours. For extended infusions by either route, a controlled-infusion device is used. For filgrastim concentrations of 5 to 15 μg/ml normal human serum albumin should be added to the solution at a final concentration of 0.2% (2 mg/ml) before the filgrastim is added. The drug should not be diluted to concentrations less than 5 μg/ml (2; 4).

Stability— Filgrastim injection is a clear, colorless solution; it should be refrigerated at 2 to 8 °C and protected from direct sunlight. The product also should be protected from freezing and temperatures above 30 °C to avoid aggregation. The solution should not be shaken since bubbles and/or foam may form. If foaming occurs, the solution should be left undisturbed for a few minutes until bubbles dissipate (2; 4).

Filgrastim is stable for 24 hours at 9 to 30 °C as long as it is clear and contains no precipitate; the manufacturer recommends discarding it after 24 hours (2; 4). The product is packaged as a single-use vial with no antibacterial preservative. The manufacturer recommends that vials not be reentered and that unused portions be discarded (2).

pH Effects— Filgrastim is stable at pH 3.8 to 4.2, but stability is limited at neutral pH (4).

Sorption— For filgrastim concentrations between 5 and 15 μg/ml, human albumin should be added before adding the filgrastim to make a final albumin concentration of 0.2% (2 mg/ml) to minimize filgrastim adsorption to infusion containers and equipment. At filgrastim concentrations above 15 μg/ml, human albumin is unnecessary. The product should not be diluted to a final concentration of less than 5 μg/ml (2; 4).

The amount of loss of filgrastim (Amgen) from the undiluted injection at a concentration of 300 μg/ml when delivered through 6.6-French, single-lumen, silicone rubber, Broviac catheters (Bard) was evaluated. The catheters were filled with dextrose 5% in water (about 0.45 ml) and flushed before and after introduction of the filgrastim. Injected amounts of filgrastim 300 μg/ml ranged from 0.17 to 1 ml. The delivered flush solution was collected and analyzed by immunoassay for filgrastim content and bioassay for maintenance of activity. The lowest volume (0.17 ml) incurred about 32% loss of filgrastim upon delivery. The other volumes incurred lower losses, ranging from 12% to none. A second repeat filgrastim injection incurred similar losses. The filgrastim that was delivered through the catheters remained active according to bioassay (2017).

Syringes— Undiluted filgrastim is stable for 24 hours at 15 to 30 °C and for seven days at 2 to 8 °C in tuberculin syringes (Becton-Dickinson). However, refrigeration and use within 24 hours are recommended because of concern for bacterial contamination (4).

In one study, filgrastim injection repackaged into 1-ml tuberculin syringes remained sterile for seven days under refrigeration (1764). However, because of the limited nature of the tests performed, the results may apply to a single institution only. Other institutions that repackage filgrastim injection need to establish specific testing results for their own sterile facilities, equipment, procedures, and personnel (1765).

Compatibility Information

Y-Site Injection Compatibility (1:1 Mixture)

	Filgrastim						
Drug	*Mfr*	*Conc*	*Mfr*	*Conc*	*Remarks*	*Ref*	*C/I*
Acyclovir sodium	BW	7 mg/ml[a]	AMG	30 μg/ml[a]	Physically compatible with no change in measured turbidity or increase in particle content in 4 hr at 22 °C	1687	**C**
Allopurinol sodium	BW	3 mg/ml[a]	AMG	30 μg/ml[a]	Physically compatible with no change in measured turbidity or increase in particle content in 4 hr at 22 °C	1687	**C**
Amikacin sulfate	ES	5 mg/ml[a]	AMG	30 μg/ml[a]	Physically compatible with no change in measured turbidity or increase in particle content in 4 hr at 22 °C	1687	**C**
	BMS	5 mg/ml[a]	AMG	10[b] and 40[a] μg/ml	Visually compatible with little or no loss of filgrastim activity by bioassay and amikacin by immunoassay in 4 hr at 25 °C	2060	**C**
Aminophylline	AB	2.5 mg/ml[a]	AMG	30 μg/ml[a]	Physically compatible with no change in measured turbidity or increase in particle content in 4 hr at 22 °C	1687	**C**
Amphotericin B	SQ	0.6 mg/ml[a]	AMG	30 μg/ml[a]	Yellow turbidity forms immediately and becomes flocculent precipitate	1687	**I**
Ampicillin sodium	WY	20 mg/ml[a]	AMG	30 μg/ml[a]	Physically compatible with no change in measured turbidity or increase in particle content in 4 hr at 22 °C	1687	**C**
Ampicillin sodium–sulbactam sodium	RR	20 + 10 mg/ml[a]	AMG	30 μg/ml[a]	Physically compatible with no change in measured turbidity or increase in particle content in 4 hr at 22 °C	1687	**C**
Aztreonam	SQ	40 mg/ml[a]	AMG	30 μg/ml[a]	Physically compatible with no change in measured turbidity or increase in particle content in 4 hr at 22 °C	1687	**C**
	SQ	40 mg/ml[a]	AMG	30 μg/ml[a]	Physically compatible with no subvisual haze or particle formation in 4 hr at 23 °C	1758	**C**
Bleomycin sulfate	BR	1 unit/ml[a]	AMG	30 μg/ml[a]	Physically compatible with no change in measured turbidity or increase in particle content in 4 hr at 22 °C	1687	**C**
Bumetanide	RC	0.04 mg/ml[a]	AMG	30 μg/ml[a]	Physically compatible with no change in measured turbidity or increase in particle content in 4 hr at 22 °C	1687	**C**
Buprenorphine HCl	RKC	0.04 mg/ml[a]	AMG	30 μg/ml[a]	Physically compatible with no change in measured turbidity or increase in particle content in 4 hr at 22 °C	1687	**C**
Butorphanol tartrate	BR	0.04 mg/ml[a]	AMG	30 μg/ml[a]	Physically compatible with no change in measured turbidity or increase in particle content in 4 hr at 22 °C	1687	**C**
Calcium gluconate	AST	40 mg/ml[a]	AMG	30 μg/ml[a]	Physically compatible with no change in measured turbidity or increase in particle content in 4 hr at 22 °C	1687	**C**
Carboplatin	BR	5 mg/ml[a]	AMG	30 μg/ml[a]	Physically compatible with no change in measured turbidity or increase in particle content in 4 hr at 22 °C	1687	**C**

Y-Site Injection Compatibility (1:1 Mixture) (Cont.)

Filgrastim

Drug	Mfr	Conc	Mfr	Conc	Remarks	Ref	C/I
Carmustine	BR	1.5 mg/ml[a]	AMG	30 μg/ml[a]	Physically compatible with no change in measured turbidity or increase in particle content in 4 hr at 22 °C	1687	**C**
Cefazolin sodium	LI	20 mg/ml[a]	AMG	30 μg/ml[a]	Physically compatible with no change in measured turbidity or increase in particle content in 4 hr at 22 °C	1687	**C**
Cefepime HCl	BR	20 mg/ml[a]	AMG	30 μg/ml[a]	Hazy turbid solution forms immediately	1689	**I**
Cefoperazone sodium	RR	40 mg/ml[a]	AMG	30 μg/ml[a]	Haze and particles form immediately	1687	**I**
Cefotaxime sodium	HO	20 mg/ml[a]	AMG	30 μg/ml[a]	Particles form in 4 hr	1687	**I**
Cefotetan disodium	STU	20 mg/ml[a]	AMG	30 μg/ml[a]	Physically compatible with no change in measured turbidity or increase in particle content in 4 hr at 22 °C	1687	**C**
Cefoxitin sodium	MSD	20 mg/ml[a]	AMG	30 μg/ml[a]	Haze, particles, and filaments form immediately	1687	**I**
Ceftazidime	LI[c]	40 mg/ml[a]	AMG	30 μg/ml[a]	Physically compatible with no change in measured turbidity or increase in particle content in 4 hr at 22 °C	1687	**C**
	LI[c]	10 mg/ml[a]	AMG	10[b] and 40[a] μg/ml	Visually compatible with little or no loss of filgrastim activity by bioassay and ceftazidime by HPLC in 4 hr at 25 °C	2060	**C**
Ceftizoxime sodium	FUJ	20 mg/ml[a]	AMG	30 μg/ml[a]	Particles and filaments form immediately	1687	**I**
Ceftriaxone sodium	RC	20 mg/ml[a]	AMG	30 μg/ml[a]	Particles and filaments form in 1 hr	1687	**I**
Cefuroxime sodium	GL	20 mg/ml[a]	AMG	30 μg/ml[a]	Haze, particles, and filaments form immediately	1687	**I**
Chlorpromazine HCl	RU	2 mg/ml[a]	AMG	30 μg/ml[a]	Physically compatible with no change in measured turbidity or increase in particle content in 4 hr at 22 °C	1687	**C**
Cimetidine HCl	SKB	12 mg/ml[a]	AMG	30 μg/ml[a]	Physically compatible with no change in measured turbidity or increase in particle content in 4 hr at 22 °C	1687	**C**
Cisplatin	BR	1 mg/ml	AMG	30 μg/ml[a]	Physically compatible with no change in measured turbidity or increase in particle content in 4 hr at 22 °C	1687	**C**
Clindamycin phosphate	AB	10 mg/ml[a]	AMG	30 μg/ml[a]	Particles and filaments form immediately	1687	**I**
Cyclophosphamide	MJ	10 mg/ml[a]	AMG	30 μg/ml[a]	Physically compatible with no change in measured turbidity or increase in particle content in 4 hr at 22 °C	1687	**C**
Cytarabine	CET	50 mg/ml	AMG	30 μg/ml[a]	Physically compatible with no change in measured turbidity or increase in particle content in 4 hr at 22 °C	1687	**C**
Dacarbazine	MI	4 mg/ml[a]	AMG	30 μg/ml[a]	Physically compatible with no change in measured turbidity or increase in particle content in 4 hr at 22 °C	1687	**C**
Dactinomycin	MSD	0.01 mg/ml[a]	AMG	30 μg/ml[a]	Particles and filaments form immediately	1687	**I**
Daunorubicin HCl	WY	1 mg/ml[a]	AMG	30 μg/ml[a]	Physically compatible with no change in measured turbidity or increase in particle content in 4 hr at 22 °C	1687	**C**

Y-Site Injection Compatibility (1:1 Mixture) (Cont.)

				Filgrastim			
Drug	*Mfr*	*Conc*	*Mfr*	*Conc*	*Remarks*	*Ref*	*C/I*
Dexamethasone sodium phosphate	LY	1 mg/ml[a]	AMG	30 μg/ml[a]	Physically compatible with no change in measured turbidity or increase in particle content in 4 hr at 22 °C	1687	**C**
Diphenhydramine HCl	ES	2 mg/ml[a]	AMG	30 μg/ml[a]	Physically compatible with no change in measured turbidity or increase in particle content in 4 hr at 22 °C	1687	**C**
Doxorubicin HCl	CET	2 mg/ml	AMG	30 μg/ml[a]	Physically compatible with no change in measured turbidity or increase in particle content in 4 hr at 22 °C	1687	**C**
Doxycycline hyclate	ES	1 mg/ml[a]	AMG	30 μg/ml[a]	Physically compatible with no change in measured turbidity or increase in particle content in 4 hr at 22 °C	1687	**C**
Droperidol	JN	0.4 mg/ml[a]	AMG	30 μg/ml[a]	Physically compatible with no change in measured turbidity or increase in particle content in 4 hr at 22 °C	1687	**C**
Enalaprilat	MSD	0.1 mg/ml[a]	AMG	30 μg/ml[a]	Physically compatible with no change in measured turbidity or increase in particle content in 4 hr at 22 °C	1687	**C**
Etoposide	BR	0.4 mg/ml[a]	AMG	30 μg/ml[a]	Particles form immediately. Filaments form in 1 hr	1687	**I**
Famotidine	MSD	2 mg/ml[a]	AMG	30 μg/ml[a]	Physically compatible with no change in measured turbidity or increase in particle content in 4 hr at 22 °C	1687	**C**
Floxuridine	RC	3 mg/ml[a]	AMG	30 μg/ml[a]	Physically compatible with no change in measured turbidity or increase in particle content in 4 hr at 22 °C	1687	**C**
Fluconazole	RR	2 mg/ml	AMG	30 μg/ml[a]	Physically compatible with no change in measured turbidity or increase in particle content in 4 hr at 22 °C	1687	**C**
	RR	2 mg/ml[a]	AMG	10[b] and 40[a] μg/ml	Visually compatible with little or no loss of filgrastim activity by bioassay and fluconazole by HPLC in 4 hr at 25 °C	2060	**C**
Fludarabine phosphate	BX	1 mg/ml[a]	AMG	30 μg/ml[a]	Physically compatible with no change in measured turbidity or increase in particle content in 4 hr at 22 °C	1687	**C**
Fluorouracil	RC	16 mg/ml[a]	AMG	30 μg/ml[a]	Particles and long filaments form in 1 hr	1687	**I**
Furosemide	AB	3 mg/ml[a]	AMG	30 μg/ml[a]	Turbidity forms immediately. Filaments and particles form in 1 hr	1687	**I**
Ganciclovir sodium	SY	20 mg/ml[a]	AMG	30 μg/ml[a]	Physically compatible with no change in measured turbidity or increase in particle content in 4 hr at 22 °C	1687	**C**
Gentamicin sulfate	LY	5 mg/ml[a]	AMG	30 μg/ml[a]	Physically compatible with no change in measured turbidity or increase in particle content in 4 hr at 22 °C	1687	**C**
	GES	1.6 mg/ml[a]	AMG	40 μg/ml[a]	Visually compatible with little or no loss of filgrastim activity by bioassay and gentamicin by immunoassay in 4 hr at 25 °C	2060	**C**

Y-Site Injection Compatibility (1:1 Mixture) (Cont.)

Drug	Mfr	Conc	Mfr	Conc	Remarks	Ref	C/I
	GES	1.6 mg/ml[a]	AMG	10 μg/ml[b]	23% loss of filgrastim activity by bioassay in 4 hr at 25 °C. Little or no gentamicin loss by immunoassay	2060	I
Granisetron HCl	SKB	0.05 mg/ml[a]	AMG	30 μg/ml[a]	Physically compatible with no change in measured turbidity or increase in particle content in 4 hr at 23 °C	2000	C
Haloperidol lactate	MN	0.2 mg/ml[a]	AMG	30 μg/ml[a]	Physically compatible with no change in measured turbidity or increase in particle content in 4 hr at 22 °C	1687	C
Heparin sodium	ES	100 units/ml[a]	AMG	30 μg/ml[a]	Particles and filaments form immediately	1687	I
Hydrocortisone sodium phosphate	MSD	1 mg/ml[a]	AMG	30 μg/ml[a]	Physically compatible with no change in measured turbidity or increase in particle content in 4 hr at 22 °C	1687	C
Hydrocortisone sodium succinate	UP	1 mg/ml[a]	AMG	30 μg/ml[a]	Physically compatible with no change in measured turbidity or increase in particle content in 4 hr at 22 °C	1687	C
Hydromorphone HCl	KN	0.5 mg/ml[a]	AMG	30 μg/ml[a]	Physically compatible with no change in measured turbidity or increase in particle content in 4 hr at 22 °C	1687	C
Hydroxyzine HCl	ES	4 mg/ml[a]	AMG	30 μg/ml[a]	Physically compatible with no change in measured turbidity or increase in particle content in 4 hr at 22 °C	1687	C
Idarubicin HCl	AD	0.5 mg/ml[a]	AMG	30 μg/ml[a]	Physically compatible with no change in measured turbidity or increase in particle content in 4 hr at 22 °C	1687	C
Ifosfamide	MJ	25 mg/ml[a]	AMG	30 μg/ml[a]	Physically compatible with no change in measured turbidity or increase in particle content in 4 hr at 22 °C	1687	C
Imipenem–cilastatin sodium	MSD	10 mg/ml[a]	AMG	30 μg/ml[a]	Physically compatible with no change in measured turbidity or increase in particle content in 4 hr at 22 °C	1687	C
	ME	5 mg/ml[a]	AMG	40 μg/ml[a]	16% loss of filgrastim activity by bioassay in 4 hr at 25 °C. Little or no imipenem and cilastatin loss by HPLC	2060	I
	ME	5 mg/ml[a]	AMG	10 μg/ml[b]	Visually compatible with little or no loss of filgrastim activity by bioassay and imipenem and cilastatin by HPLC in 4 hr at 25 °C	2060	C
Leucovorin calcium	LE	2 mg/ml[a]	AMG	30 μg/ml[a]	Physically compatible with no change in measured turbidity or increase in particle content in 4 hr at 22 °C	1687	C
Lorazepam	WY	0.1 mg/ml[a]	AMG	30 μg/ml[a]	Physically compatible with no change in measured turbidity or increase in particle content in 4 hr at 22 °C	1687	C
Mannitol	BA	15%	AMG	30 μg/ml[a]	Filaments form immediately	1687	I
Mechlorethamine HCl	MSD	1 mg/ml	AMG	30 μg/ml[a]	Physically compatible with no change in measured turbidity or increase in particle content in 4 hr at 22 °C	1687	C

Y-Site Injection Compatibility (1:1 Mixture) (Cont.)

					Filgrastim		
Drug	*Mfr*	*Conc*	*Mfr*	*Conc*	*Remarks*	*Ref*	*C/I*
Melphalan HCl	BW	0.1 mg/ml[a]	AMG	30 μg/ml[a]	Physically compatible with no change in measured turbidity or increase in particle content in 4 hr at 22 °C	1687	**C**
Meperidine HCl	WY	4 mg/ml[a]	AMG	30 μg/ml[a]	Physically compatible with no change in measured turbidity or increase in particle content in 4 hr at 22 °C	1687	**C**
Mesna	MJ	10 mg/ml[a]	AMG	30 μg/ml[a]	Physically compatible with no change in measured turbidity or increase in particle content in 4 hr at 22 °C	1687	**C**
Methotrexate sodium	LE	15 mg/ml[a]	AMG	30 μg/ml[a]	Physically compatible with no change in measured turbidity or increase in particle content in 4 hr at 22 °C	1687	**C**
Methylprednisolone sodium succinate	AB	5 mg/ml[a]	AMG	30 μg/ml[a]	Haze, particles, and filaments form immediately	1687	**I**
Metoclopramide HCl	ES	5 mg/ml	AMG	30 μg/ml[a]	Physically compatible with no change in measured turbidity or increase in particle content in 4 hr at 22 °C	1687	**C**
Metronidazole	BA	5 mg/ml	AMG	30 μg/ml[a]	Particles form immediately. Filaments form in 1 hr	1687	**I**
Minocycline HCl	LE	0.2 mg/ml[a]	AMG	30 μg/ml[a]	Physically compatible with no change in measured turbidity or increase in particle content in 4 hr at 22 °C	1687	**C**
Mitomycin	BR	0.5 mg/ml	AMG	30 μg/ml[a]	Color changes to reddish purple in 1 hr	1687	**I**
Mitoxantrone HCl	LE	0.5 mg/ml[a]	AMG	30 μg/ml[a]	Physically compatible with no change in measured turbidity or increase in particle content in 4 hr at 22 °C	1687	**C**
Morphine sulfate	WY	1 mg/ml[a]	AMG	30 μg/ml[a]	Physically compatible with no change in measured turbidity or increase in particle content in 4 hr at 22 °C	1687	**C**
Nalbuphine HCl	DU	10 mg/ml	AMG	30 μg/ml[a]	Physically compatible with no change in measured turbidity or increase in particle content in 4 hr at 22 °C	1687	**C**
Netilmicin sulfate	SC	5 mg/ml[a]	AMG	30 μg/ml[a]	Physically compatible with no change in measured turbidity or increase in particle content in 4 hr at 22 °C	1687	**C**
Ondansetron HCl	GL	1 mg/ml[a]	AMG	30 μg/ml[a]	Physically compatible with no change in measured turbidity or increase in particle content in 4 hr at 22 °C	1687	**C**
Piperacillin sodium	LE	40 mg/ml[a]	AMG	30 μg/ml[a]	Particles and filaments form immediately	1687	**I**
Plicamycin	MI	0.01 mg/ml[a]	AMG	30 μg/ml[a]	Physically compatible with no change in measured turbidity or increase in particle content in 4 hr at 22 °C	1687	**C**
Potassium chloride	AB	0.1 mEq/ml[a]	AMG	30 μg/ml[a]	Physically compatible with no change in measured turbidity or increase in particle content in 4 hr at 22 °C	1687	**C**
Prochlorperazine edisylate	SCN	0.5 mg/ml[a]	AMG	30 μg/ml[a]	Particles form immediately. Filaments form in 1 hr	1687	**I**

Y-Site Injection Compatibility (1:1 Mixture) (Cont.)

				Filgrastim			
Drug	*Mfr*	*Conc*	*Mfr*	*Conc*	*Remarks*	*Ref*	*C/I*
Promethazine HCl	SCN	2 mg/ml[a]	AMG	30 µg/ml[a]	Physically compatible with no change in measured turbidity or increase in particle content in 4 hr at 22 °C	1687	C
Ranitidine HCl	GL	2 mg/ml[a]	AMG	30 µg/ml[a]	Physically compatible with no change in measured turbidity or increase in particle content in 4 hr at 22 °C	1687	C
Sodium bicarbonate	AB	1 mEq/ml	AMG	30 µg/ml[a]	Physically compatible with no change in measured turbidity or increase in particle content in 4 hr at 22 °C	1687	C
Streptozocin	UP	40 mg/ml[a]	AMG	30 µg/ml[a]	Physically compatible with no change in measured turbidity or increase in particle content in 4 hr at 22 °C	1687	C
Thiotepa	LE	1 mg/ml[a]	AMG	30 µg/ml[a]	Particles and filaments form immediately	1687	I
Ticarcillin disodium	BE	30 mg/ml[a]	AMG	30 µg/ml[a]	Physically compatible with no change in measured turbidity or increase in particle content in 4 hr at 22 °C	1687	C
Ticarcillin disodium–clavulanate potassium	SKB	31 mg/ml[a]	AMG	30 µg/ml[a]	Physically compatible with no change in measured turbidity or increase in particle content in 4 hr at 22 °C	1687	C
Tobramycin sulfate	LI	5 mg/ml[a]	AMG	30 µg/ml[a]	Physically compatible with no change in measured turbidity or increase in particle content in 4 hr at 22 °C	1687	C
	LI	1.6 mg/ml[a]	AMG	10[b] and 40[a] µg/ml	Visually compatible with little or no loss of filgrastim activity by bioassay and tobramycin by immunoassay in 4 hr at 25 °C	2060	C
Trimethoprim–sulfamethoxazole	ES	0.8 + 4 mg/ml[a]	AMG	30 µg/ml[a]	Physically compatible with no change in measured turbidity or increase in particle content in 4 hr at 22 °C	1687	C
Vancomycin HCl	AB	10 mg/ml[a]	AMG	30 µg/ml[a]	Physically compatible with no change in measured turbidity or increase in particle content in 4 hr at 22 °C	1687	C
Vinblastine sulfate	LI	0.12 mg/ml[a]	AMG	30 µg/ml[a]	Physically compatible with no change in measured turbidity or increase in particle content in 4 hr at 22 °C	1687	C
Vincristine sulfate	LI	0.05 mg/ml[a]	AMG	30 µg/ml[a]	Physically compatible with no change in measured turbidity or increase in particle content in 4 hr at 22 °C	1687	C
Vinorelbine tartrate	BW	1 mg/ml[a]	AMG	30 µg/ml[a]	Physically compatible with no change in measured turbidity or increase in particle content in 4 hr at 22 °C	1687	C
Zidovudine	BW	4 mg/ml[a]	AMG	30 µg/ml[a]	Physically compatible with no change in measured turbidity or increase in particle content in 4 hr at 22 °C	1687	C

[a]*Tested in dextrose 5% in water.*
[b]*Tested in dextrose 5% in water with human albumin 2 mg/ml.*
[c]*Sodium carbonate–containing formulation.*

Additional Compatibility Information

Solutions— Although dilution to concentrations below 5 μg/ml is not recommended by the manufacturer, filgrastim has been stated to be stable for seven days under refrigeration when diluted with dextrose 5% in water to a concentration of at least 2 μg/ml. The manufacturer recommends use within 24 hours because of bacterial contamination concerns (4).

Filgrastim is incompatible with sodium chloride 0.9%; this solution should not be used as a diluent (4).

Plastics— Filgrastim in dextrose 5% in water at concentrations above 15 μg/ml and between 2 and 15 μg/ml with added human albumin 0.2% is compatible with common plastics used in syringes, administration sets, solution containers, and pump cassettes including PVC, polyolefin, and polypropylene (4).

Sterility— The sterility of filgrastim 300 μg/ml packaged aseptically as 0.25 ml in tuberculin syringes (Becton-Dickinson) closed with Luer Lock tip caps was evaluated. Sterility testing found no growth after seven days of storage at 4 °C (2186). However, the sterility of repackaged solutions is a function of the quality of the specific aseptic process of packaging and the quality of the environment in which the sterile product is packaged rather than a property of this unpreserved solution. Consequently, this result is valid only for the facility and operators evaluated in the study. The adequacy of such a procedure in another location and with other individuals would need to be validated independently for each (2187).

FLOXURIDINE
AHFS 10:00

FUDR **Roche**

Products— Floxuridine (Roche) is supplied in 5-ml vials containing 500 mg of drug. Reconstitute with 5 ml of sterile water for injection to yield a 100-mg/ml concentration (2; 4).

pH— From 4 to 5.5 (2; 4).

Osmolality— Floxuridine 100 mg/ml in sterile water for injection has an osmolality of 353 mOsm/kg (1689).

Administration— Floxuridine is administered by continuous arterial infusion using an appropriate infusion device after dilution in dextrose 5% in water or sodium chloride 0.9% (2; 4). Floxuridine has also been administered investigationally by intravenous injection or infusion (4).

Stability— The reconstituted solution should be stored under refrigeration at 2 to 8 °C and used within two weeks (2; 4).

The pH of optimum stability is 4 to 7. Extreme acidity or alkalinity may result in hydrolysis (1379).

Syringes— Floxuridine (Roche) 50 mg/ml and 1 mg/ml in sodium chloride 0.9% was packaged as 3 ml in 10-ml polypropylene infusion pump syringes (Pharmacia Deltec). Little or no loss by HPLC analysis occurred during 21 days of storage at 30 °C (1967).

Implantable Infusion Pumps— Floxuridine 10 mg/ml was filled into an implantable infusion pump (Fresenius VIP 30) and associated capillary tubing and stored at 37 °C. Samples were analyzed using HPLC assay. No floxuridine loss and no contamination from components of pump materials occurred during six weeks of storage. However, an unidentified additional peak on the chromatogram appeared in seven weeks, and 22% loss of floxuridine occurred by eight weeks (1903).

Floxuridine (Roche), at concentrations ranging from about 2.5 to 12 mg/ml with heparin sodium 200 units/ml in bacteriostatic sodium chloride 0.9%, was evaluated for stability in an implantable infusion pump (Infusaid model 400). In this in vivo assessment, the floxuridine concentrations were determined prior to implantation in patients and again at the time of pump refills. No appreciable floxuridine loss occurred during eight courses of therapy, from 4 to 12 days in duration, in five patients (767).

At a concentration of 5 mg/ml in sodium chloride 0.9%, floxuridine supported the growth of several microorganisms commonly implicated in nosocomial infections, including *Escherichia coli, Pseudomonas aeruginosa*, and *Candida albicans*. The arbitrary application of an extended expiration date to floxuridine solutions used in ambulatory pump systems is, therefore, highly questionable (827).

Compatibility Information

Additive Compatibility

Floxuridine

Drug	*Mfr*	*Conc/L*	*Mfr*	*Conc/L*	*Test Soln*	*Remarks*	*Ref*	*C/I*
Carboplatin		1 g		10 g	W	Both drugs stable for 7 days at room temperature	1379	C
		1 g		10 g	W	Less than 10% loss of both drugs in 7 days at 23 °C protected from light	1954	C

Additive Compatibility (Cont.)

Floxuridine

Drug	Mfr	Conc/L	Mfr	Conc/L	Test Soln	Remarks	Ref	C/I
Cisplatin	BR	500 mg	RC	10 g	NS	13% floxuridine loss in 7 days and 18% loss in 14 days at room temperature protected from light	1386	C
Cisplatin with etoposide		200 mg 300 mg		700 mg	NS	All drugs stable for 7 days at room temperature	1379	C
Cisplatin with leucovorin calcium		200 mg 140 mg		700 mg	NS	All drugs stable for 7 days at room temperature	1379	C
Etoposide		200 mg		10 g	NS	Both drugs stable for 15 days at room temperature	1379	C
Fluorouracil		10 g		10 g	NS	Both drugs stable for 15 days at room temperature	1390	C
Leucovorin calcium	QU	30 mg	QU	1 g	NS	Physically compatible and chemically stable for 48 hr at 4 and 20 °C. No floxuridine loss and 10% leucovorin loss in 48 hr at 40 °C	1317	C
	QU	240 mg	QU	2 g	NS	Physically compatible and chemically stable for 48 hr at 4 and 20 °C. No floxuridine loss and 7% leucovorin loss in 48 hr at 40 °C	1317	C
	QU	960 mg	QU	4 g	NS	Physically compatible and chemically stable for 48 hr at 4, 20, and 40 °C	1317	C
		200 mg		10 g	NS	Both drugs stable for 15 days at room temperature protected from light	1387	C

Y-Site Injection Compatibility (1:1 Mixture)

Floxuridine

Drug	Mfr	Conc	Mfr	Conc	Remarks	Ref	C/I
Allopurinol sodium	BW	3 mg/ml[b]	RC	3 mg/ml[b]	Tiny particles form in 1 to 4 hr	1686	I
Amifostine	USB	10 mg/ml[a]	RC	3 mg/ml[a]	Physically compatible with no change in measured turbidity or increase in particle content in 4 hr at 23 °C	1845	C
Aztreonam	SQ	40 mg/ml[a]	RC	3 mg/ml[a]	Physically compatible with no subvisual haze or particle formation in 4 hr at 23 °C	1758	C
Cefepime HCl	BR	20 mg/ml[a]	RC	3 mg/ml[a]	Haze and tiny particles form immediately	1689	I
Etoposide phosphate	BR	5 mg/ml[a]	RC	3 mg/ml[a]	Physically compatible with no change in measured turbidity or increase in particle content in 4 hr at 23 °C	2218	C
Filgrastim	AMG	30 μg/ml[a]	RC	3 mg/ml[a]	Physically compatible with no change in measured turbidity or increase in particle content in 4 hr at 22 °C	1687	C
Fludarabine phosphate	BX	1 mg/ml[a]	RC	3 mg/ml[a]	Physically compatible for 4 hr at room temperature under fluorescent light	1439	C
Gemcitabine HCl	LI	10 mg/ml[b]	RC	3 mg/ml[b]	Physically compatible with no change in measured turbidity or increase in particle content in 4 hr at 23 °C	2226	C

Y-Site Injection Compatibility (1:1 Mixture) (Cont.)

Floxuridine

Drug	Mfr	Conc	Mfr	Conc	Remarks	Ref	C/I
Granisetron HCl	SKB	0.05 mg/ml[a]	RC	3 mg/ml[a]	Physically compatible with no change in measured turbidity or increase in particle content in 4 hr at 23 °C	2000	C
Melphalan HCl	BW	0.1 mg/ml[b]	RC	3 mg/ml[b]	Physically compatible with no change in measured turbidity or increase in particle content in 3 hr at 22 °C	1557	C
Ondansetron HCl	GL	1 mg/ml[b]	RC	3 mg/ml[a]	Physically compatible for 4 hr at 22 °C	1365	C
Paclitaxel	NCI	1.2 mg/ml[a]	RC	3 mg/ml[a]	Physically compatible with no change in measured turbidity in 4 hr at 22 °C	1556	C
Piperacillin sodium–tazobactam sodium	LE	40 + 5 mg/ml[a]	RC	3 mg/ml[a]	Physically compatible with no change in measured turbidity or increase in particle content in 4 hr at 22 °C	1688	C
Sargramostim	IMM	10 μg/ml[b]	RC	3 mg/ml[b]	Physically compatible for 4 hr at 22 °C	1436	C
Teniposide	BR	0.1 mg/ml[a]	RC	3 mg/ml[a]	Physically compatible with no subvisual haze or particle formation in 4 hr at 23 °C	1725	C
Thiotepa	IMM[c]	1 mg/ml[a]	RC	3 mg/ml[a]	Physically compatible with no change in measured turbidity or increase in particle content in 4 hr at 23 °C	1861	C
Vinorelbine tartrate	BW	1 mg/ml[b]	RC	3 mg/ml[b]	Physically compatible with no change in measured turbidity or increase in particle content in 4 hr at 22 °C	1558	C

[a]*Tested in dextrose 5% in water.*
[b]*Tested in sodium chloride 0.9%.*
[c]*Lyophilized formulation tested.*

Additional Compatibility Information

Solutions— Floxuridine is usually diluted in dextrose 5% in water or sodium chloride 0.9% for infusion (4). At a concentration of 0.5 mg/ml in dextrose 5% in water or sodium chloride 0.9% in glass and PVC containers, floxuridine remained stable during seven days of storage at 20 and 37 °C (108).

Floxuridine 5 to 10 mg/ml in dextrose 5% in water, sodium chloride 0.9%, or sterile water for injection has been reported to exhibit less than a 10% loss in 14 days at room temperature (1379).

Leucovorin— The stability of leucovorin calcium (Quad) 30 to 960 mg/L admixed with floxuridine (Quad) 1 to 4 g/L in sodium chloride 0.9% was evaluated under a sequence of temperatures to simulate use conditions as intraperitoneal chemotherapy solutions. The admixtures were stored for 48 hours at 4 °C, followed by 12 hours at 20 °C, and finally followed by 12 hours at 40 °C (near-physiologic temperature). No floxuridine loss and about a 3 to 6% leucovorin calcium loss occurred during the study period (1317).

FLUCONAZOLE
AHFS 8:12.04

Diflucan   **Pfizer**

Products— Fluconazole (Pfizer) is available for intravenous infusion in 100- and 200-ml glass bottles and PVC bags in sodium chloride or dextrose diluents. Each milliliter of solution contains fluconazole 2 mg and either sodium chloride 9 mg or dextrose 56 mg (2).

pH— From 4 to 8 in the sodium chloride diluent and from 3.5 to 6.5 in the dextrose diluent (2).

Osmolarity— The infusion solution is iso-osmotic (2), having an osmolarity of 300 to 315 mOsm/L (4).

Administration— Fluconazole is administered by intravenous infusion at a rate not exceeding 200 mg/hr (2; 4).

Stability— Fluconazole injection in glass bottles or PVC bags should be stored between 5 and 30 °C or between 5 and 25 °C, respectively, and protected from freezing. Brief exposure to temperatures up to 40 °C does not adversely affect the product in PVC bags. The overwrap moisture barrier should not be removed from the PVC bags until ready for use. The solution should not be used if it is cloudy or precipitated (2; 4).

Elastomeric Reservoir Pumps— Fluconazole (Pfizer) 2 mg/ml in sodium chloride 0.9% was evaluated for binding potential to natural rubber elastomeric reservoirs (Baxter). Less than 2% loss was found after storage for two weeks at 35 °C with gentle agitation (2014).

Compatibility Information

Solution Compatibility

Fluconazole

Solution	Mfr	Mfr	Conc/L	Remarks	Ref	C/I
Dextrose 5% in water	BA[a]	PF	1 g	Fluconazole chemically stable by gas chromatography for at least 24 hr at 25 °C under fluorescent light	1676	C
Ringer's injection, lactated	BA[a]	PF	1 g	Fluconazole chemically stable by gas chromatography for at least 24 hr at 25 °C under fluorescent light	1676	C

[a]*Tested in PVC containers.*

Additive Compatibility

Fluconazole

Drug	Mfr	Conc/L	Mfr	Conc/L	Test Soln	Remarks	Ref	C/I
Acyclovir sodium	BW	5 g	PF	1 g	D5W	Visually compatible with no fluconazole loss by HPLC in 72 hr at 25 °C under fluorescent light. Acyclovir not tested	1677	C
Amikacin sulfate	BR	2.5 g	PF	1 g	D5W	Visually compatible with no fluconazole loss by HPLC in 72 hr at 25 °C under fluorescent light. Amikacin not tested	1677	C
Amphotericin B	LY	50 mg	PF	1 g	D5W	Visually compatible with no fluconazole loss by HPLC in 72 hr at 25 °C under fluorescent light. Amphotericin B not tested	1677	C
Cefazolin sodium	SM	10 g	PF	1 g	D5W	Visually compatible with no fluconazole loss by HPLC in 72 hr at 25 °C under fluorescent light. Cefazolin not tested	1677	C
Ceftazidime	GL	20 g	PF	1 g	D5W	Visually compatible with no fluconazole loss by HPLC in 72 hr at 25 °C under fluorescent light. Ceftazidime not tested	1677	C
Clindamycin phosphate	AST	6 g	PF	1 g	D5W	Visually compatible with no fluconazole loss by HPLC in 72 hr at 25 °C under fluorescent light. Clindamycin not tested	1677	C
Gentamicin sulfate	SO	0.5 g	PF	1 g	D5W	Visually compatible with no fluconazole loss by HPLC in 72 hr at 25 °C under fluorescent light. Gentamicin not tested	1677	C
Heparin sodium	BA	50,000 units	PF	1 g	D5W[a]	Fluconazole chemically stable by gas chromatography for at least 24 hr at 25 °C under fluorescent light. Heparin not tested	1676	C
Meropenem	ZEN	1 and 20 g	RR	2 g	NS	Visually compatible for 4 hr at room temperature	1994	C

Additive Compatibility (Cont.)

Fluconazole

Drug	Mfr	Conc/L	Mfr	Conc/L	Test Soln	Remarks	Ref	C/I
Metronidazole	AB	2.5 g	PF	1 g		Visually compatible with no fluconazole loss by HPLC in 72 hr at 25 °C under fluorescent light. Metronidazole not tested	1677	C
Morphine sulfate	ES	0.25 g	PF	1 g	D5W[a]	Fluconazole chemically stable by gas chromatography for at least 24 hr at 25 °C under fluorescent light. Morphine not tested	1676	C
Piperacillin sodium	LE	40 g	PF	1 g	D5W	Visually compatible with no fluconazole loss by HPLC in 72 hr at 25 °C under fluorescent light. Piperacillin not tested	1677	C
Potassium chloride	AB	10 mEq	PF	1 g	D5W[a]	Fluconazole chemically stable by gas chromatography for at least 24 hr at 25 °C under fluorescent light	1676	C
Ranitidine HCl with ondansetron HCl	GL GL	500 mg 100 mg	RR	2 g	[a]	Visually compatible with no loss of any drug by HPLC in 4 hr	1730	C
Theophylline	BA	0.4 g	PF	1 g	D5W[a]	Fluconazole chemically stable by gas chromatography for at least 72 hr at 25 °C under fluorescent light. Theophylline not tested	1676	C
Trimethoprim–sulfamethoxazole	ES	0.4 + 2 g	PF	1 g	D5W	Delayed cloudiness and precipitation. No fluconazole loss by HPLC in 72 hr at 25 °C under fluorescent light	1677	I

[a]*Tested in PVC containers.*

Y-Site Injection Compatibility (1:1 Mixture)

Fluconazole

Drug	Mfr	Conc	Mfr	Conc	Remarks	Ref	C/I
Acyclovir sodium	BW	10 mg/ml	RR	2 mg/ml	Physically compatible for 24 hr at 25 °C	1407	C
Aldesleukin	CHI	33,800 I.U./ml[a]	RR	2 mg/ml[a]	Visually compatible with little or no loss of aldesleukin activity by bioassay	1857	C
Allopurinol sodium	BW	3 mg/ml[b]	RR	2 mg/ml	Physically compatible with no change in measured turbidity or increase in particle content in 4 hr at 22 °C	1686	C
Amifostine	USB	10 mg/ml[a]	RR	2 mg/ml	Physically compatible with no change in measured turbidity or increase in particle content in 4 hr at 23 °C	1845	C
Amikacin sulfate	BR	20 mg/ml	RR	2 mg/ml	Physically compatible for 24 hr at 25 °C	1407	C
Aminophylline	ES AMR	25 mg/ml 0.8 and 1.5 mg/ml[c]	RR PF	2 mg/ml 0.5 and 1.5 mg/ml[c]	Physically compatible for 24 hr at 25 °C Visually compatible with no loss of either drug by HPLC in 3 hr at 24 °C	1407 1626	C C
Amphotericin B	SQ	5 mg/ml	RR	2 mg/ml	Cloudiness and yellow precipitate develop	1407	I
Amphotericin B cholesteryl sulfate complex	SEQ	0.83 mg/ml[a]	RR	2 mg/ml	Gross precipitate forms	2117	I
Ampicillin sodium	WY	20 mg/ml	RR	2 mg/ml	Cloudiness develops	1407	I

Y-Site Injection Compatibility (1:1 Mixture) (Cont.)

Fluconazole

Drug	Mfr	Conc	Mfr	Conc	Remarks	Ref	C/I
Ampicillin sodium–sulbactam sodium	PF	40 + 20 mg/ml	RR	2 mg/ml	Physically compatible for 24 hr at 25 °C	1407	**C**
Aztreonam	SQ	40 mg/ml	RR	2 mg/ml	Physically compatible for 24 hr at 25 °C	1407	**C**
	SQ	40 mg/ml[a]	RR	2 mg/ml	Physically compatible with no subvisual haze or particle formation in 4 hr at 23 °C	1758	**C**
Benztropine mesylate	MSD	1 mg/ml	RR	2 mg/ml	Physically compatible for 24 hr at 25 °C	1407	**C**
Calcium gluconate	ES	100 mg/ml	RR	2 mg/ml	Cloudiness develops	1407	**I**
Cefazolin sodium	LY	40 mg/ml	RR	2 mg/ml	Physically compatible for 24 hr at 25 °C	1407	**C**
Cefepime HCl	BR	20 mg/ml[a]	RR	2 mg/ml	Physically compatible with no change in measured turbidity or increase in particle content in 4 hr at 22 °C	1689	**C**
Cefotaxime sodium	HO	20 mg/ml	RR	2 mg/ml	Cloudiness and amber color develop	1407	**I**
Cefotetan disodium	STU	40 mg/ml	RR	2 mg/ml	Physically compatible for 24 hr at 25 °C	1407	**C**
Cefoxitin sodium	MSD	40 mg/ml	RR	2 mg/ml	Physically compatible for 24 hr at 25 °C	1407	**C**
Cefpirome sulfate	HO	50 mg/ml[d]	RR	2 mg/ml[d]	Visually and microscopically compatible with little or no cefpirome loss and 8% or less fluconazole loss by HPLC in 8 hr at 23 °C	2044	**C**
Ceftazidime	GL	20 mg/ml	RR	2 mg/ml	Immediate precipitation	1407	**I**
Ceftriaxone sodium	RC	40 mg/ml	RR	2 mg/ml	Immediate precipitation	1407	**I**
Cefuroxime sodium	GL	30 mg/ml	RR	2 mg/ml	Immediate precipitation	1407	**I**
Chloramphenicol sodium succinate	PD	20 mg/ml	RR	2 mg/ml	Gas production	1407	**I**
Chlorpromazine HCl	ES	25 mg/ml	RR	2 mg/ml	Physically compatible for 24 hr at 25 °C	1407	**C**
Cimetidine HCl	SKF	150 mg/ml	RR	2 mg/ml	Physically compatible for 24 hr at 25 °C	1407	**C**
	SKB	1 and 2 mg/ml[c]	RR	2 mg/ml	Visually compatible for 24 hr at 28 °C	1760	**C**
Cisatracurium besylate	GW	0.1, 2, 5 mg/ml[a]	RR	2 mg/ml	Physically compatible with no change in measured turbidity or increase in particle content in 4 hr at 23 °C	2074	**C**
Clindamycin phosphate	AB	24 mg/ml	RR	2 mg/ml	Immediate precipitation	1407	**I**
Dexamethasone sodium phosphate	ES	4 mg/ml	RR	2 mg/ml	Physically compatible for 24 hr at 25 °C	1407	**C**
Diazepam	ES	5 mg/ml	RR	2 mg/ml	Immediate precipitation	1407	**I**
Digoxin	BW	0.25 mg/ml	RR	2 mg/ml	Gas production	1407	**I**
Diltiazem HCl	MMD	5 mg/ml	RR	2 mg/ml	Visually compatible	1807	**C**
Diphenhydramine HCl	ES	50 mg/ml	RR	2 mg/ml	Physically compatible for 24 hr at 25 °C	1407	**C**
Dobutamine HCl	LI	2 mg/ml[a]	RR	2 mg/ml	Visually compatible for 24 hr at 28 °C under fluorescent light	1760	**C**
Docetaxel	RPR	0.9 mg/ml[a]	RR	2 mg/ml	Physically compatible with no change in measured turbidity or increase in particle content in 4 hr at 23 °C	2224	**C**
Dopamine HCl	AMR	1.6 mg/ml[a]	RR	2 mg/ml	Visually compatible for 24 hr at 28 °C under fluorescent light	1760	**C**

Y-Site Injection Compatibility (1:1 Mixture) (Cont.)

Drug	Mfr	Conc	Mfr	Conc	Remarks	Ref	C/I
				Fluconazole			
Doxorubicin HCl liposome injection	SEQ	0.4 mg/ml[a]	RR	2 mg/ml	Physically compatible with little or no change in measured turbidity and no increase in particle content in 4 hr at 23 °C	2087	C
Droperidol	DU	2.5 mg/ml	RR	2 mg/ml	Physically compatible for 24 hr at 25 °C	1407	C
Erythromycin lactobionate	LY	20 mg/ml	RR	2 mg/ml	Immediate precipitation	1407	I
Etoposide phosphate	BR	5 mg/ml[a]	RR	2 mg/ml	Physically compatible with no change in measured turbidity or increase in particle content in 4 hr at 23 °C	2218	C
Famotidine	MSD	10 mg/ml	RR	2 mg/ml	Physically compatible for 24 hr at 25 °C	1407	C
	ME	2 mg/ml[b]		2 mg/ml[a]	Visually compatible for 4 hr at 22 °C	1936	C
Filgrastim	AMG	30 μg/ml[a]	RR	2 mg/ml	Physically compatible with no change in measured turbidity or increase in particle content in 4 hr at 22 °C	1687	C
	AMG	10[e] and 40[a] μg/ml	RR	2 mg/ml[a]	Visually compatible with little or no loss of filgrastim activity by bioassay and fluconazole by HPLC in 4 hr at 25 °C	2060	C
Fludarabine phosphate	BX	1 mg/ml[a]	RR	2 mg/ml	Physically compatible for 4 hr at room temperature under fluorescent light	1439	C
Foscarnet sodium	AST	24 mg/ml	RR	2 mg/ml	Physically compatible for 24 hr at 25 °C	1407	C
Furosemide	ES	10 mg/ml	RR	2 mg/ml	Precipitate forms	1407	I
Ganciclovir sodium	SY	50 mg/ml	RR	2 mg/ml	Physically compatible for 24 hr at 25 °C	1407	C
Gemcitabine HCl	LI	10 mg/ml[b]	RR	2 mg/ml	Physically compatible with no change in measured turbidity or increase in particle content in 4 hr at 23 °C	2226	C
Gentamicin sulfate	ES	4 mg/ml	RR	2 mg/ml	Physically compatible for 24 hr at 25 °C	1407	C
Granisetron HCl	SKB	0.05 mg/ml[a]	PF	2 mg/ml	Physically compatible with no change in measured turbidity or increase in particle content in 4 hr at 23 °C	2000	C
Haloperidol lactate	MN	5 mg/ml	RR	2 mg/ml	Precipitate forms	1407	I
Heparin sodium	LY	1000 units/ml	RR	2 mg/ml	Physically compatible for 24 hr at 25 °C	1407	C
	TR	50 units/ml	PF	2 mg/ml	Visually compatible for 6 hr at 25 °C	1793	C
Hydrocortisone sodium phosphate	MSD	50 mg/ml	RR	2 mg/ml	Physically compatible for 24 hr at 25 °C	1407	C
Hydroxyzine HCl	ES	50 mg/ml	RR	2 mg/ml	Cloudiness develops	1407	I
Imipenem–cilastatin sodium	MSD	10 mg/ml	RR	2 mg/ml	Immediate precipitation	1407	I
Immune globulin intravenous	CU	50 mg/ml	RR	2 mg/ml	Physically compatible for 24 hr at 25 °C	1407	C
Leucovorin calcium	LE	10 mg/ml	RR	2 mg/ml	Physically compatible for 24 hr at 25 °C	1407	C
Lorazepam	WY	0.33 mg/ml[b]	PF	2 mg/ml	Visually compatible for 24 hr at 22 °C	1855	C
Melphalan HCl	BW	0.1 mg/ml[b]	RR	2 mg/ml	Physically compatible with no change in measured turbidity or increase in particle content in 3 hr at 22 °C	1557	C
Meperidine HCl	AB	10 mg/ml	RR	2 mg/ml	Physically compatible for 4 hr at 25 °C	1397	C
Meropenem	ZEN	1 and 50 mg/ml[b]	RR	2 mg/ml	Visually compatible for 4 hr at room temperature	1994	C

Y-Site Injection Compatibility (1:1 Mixture) (Cont.)

Fluconazole

Drug	Mfr	Conc	Mfr	Conc	Remarks	Ref	C/I
Metoclopramide HCl	RB	5 mg/ml	RR	2 mg/ml	Physically compatible for 24 hr at 25 °C	1407	C
Metronidazole	AB	5 mg/ml	RR	2 mg/ml	Physically compatible for 24 hr at 25 °C	1407	C
Midazolam HCl	RC	5 mg/ml	RR	2 mg/ml	Physically compatible for 24 hr at 25 °C	1407	C
	RC	5 mg/ml	PF	2 mg/ml	Visually compatible for 24 hr at 22 °C	1855	C
Morphine sulfate	IMS	25 mg/ml	RR	2 mg/ml	Physically compatible for 24 hr at 25 °C	1407	C
	AB	1 mg/ml	RR	2 mg/ml	Physically compatible for 4 hr at 25 °C	1397	C
Nafcillin sodium	BR	20 mg/ml	RR	2 mg/ml	Physically compatible for 24 hr at 25 °C	1407	C
Nitroglycerin	AMR	0.2 mg/ml[a]	RR	2 mg/ml	Visually compatible for 24 hr at 28 °C under fluorescent light	1760	C
Ondansetron HCl	GL	1 mg/ml[b]	PF	2 mg/ml	Physically compatible for 4 hr at 22 °C	1365	C
	GL	0.03 and 0.3 mg/ml[a]	RR	2 mg/ml[b]	Visually compatible with little or no loss of either drug by HPLC in 4 hr at 25 °C under fluorescent light	1732	C
	GL	0.03, 0.1, and 0.3 mg/ml[a,b]	RR	2 mg/ml	Visually compatible with little or no ondansetron or fluconazole loss by HPLC in 4 hr and 5% or less loss of both drugs in 12 hr at room temperature	2168	C
Oxacillin sodium	BE	40 mg/ml	RR	2 mg/ml	Physically compatible for 24 hr at 25 °C	1407	C
Paclitaxel	NCI	1.2 mg/ml[a]	RR	2 mg/ml	Physically compatible with no change in measured turbidity in 4 hr at 22 °C	1556	C
	BR	0.3 and 1.2 mg/ml[a]	PF	2 mg/ml	Visually compatible with no loss of either drug by HPLC in 4 hr at 23 °C	1790	C
Pancuronium bromide	GNS	0.5 mg/ml[b]	RR	2 mg/ml	Visually compatible for 24 hr at 28 °C under fluorescent light	1760	C
Penicillin G potassium	RR	100,000 units/ml	RR	2 mg/ml	Physically compatible for 24 hr at 25 °C	1407	C
Pentamidine isethionate	LY	6 mg/ml	RR	2 mg/ml	Cloudiness develops	1407	I
Phenytoin sodium	PD	50 mg/ml	RR	2 mg/ml	Physically compatible for 24 hr at 25 °C	1407	C
Piperacillin sodium	LE	80 mg/ml	RR	2 mg/ml	Viscous gel-like substance forms	1407	I
Piperacillin sodium–tazobactam sodium	LE	40 + 5 mg/ml[a]	RR	2 mg/ml	Physically compatible with no change in measured turbidity or increase in particle content in 4 hr at 22 °C	1688	C
Prochlorperazine edisylate	SKF	5 mg/ml	RR	2 mg/ml	Physically compatible for 24 hr at 25 °C	1407	C
Promethazine HCl	ES	50 mg/ml	RR	2 mg/ml	Physically compatible for 24 hr at 25 °C	1407	C
Propofol	ZEN	10 mg/ml	PF	2 mg/ml[a]	Physically compatible for 1 hr at 23 °C with no increase in particle content	2066	C
Ranitidine HCl	GL	0.5 and 2 mg/ml[a]	RR	2 mg/ml[b]	Visually compatible with no loss of either drug by HPLC in 4 hr	1730	C
Remifentanil HCl	GW	0.025 and 0.25 mg/ml[b]	RR	2 mg/ml	Physically compatible with no change in measured turbidity or increase in particle content in 4 hr at 23 °C	2075	C
Sargramostim	IMM	10 μg/ml[b]	RR	2 mg/ml	Physically compatible for 4 hr at 22 °C	1436	C
Tacrolimus	FUJ	1 mg/ml[b]	RR	2 mg/ml[a]	Visually compatible for 24 hr at 25 °C	1630	C
	FUJ	10 and 40 μg/ml[b]	PF	1 mg/ml[b]	Visually compatible with no loss of either drug by HPLC in 3 hr at 24 °C under fluorescent light	2225	C

Y-Site Injection Compatibility (1:1 Mixture) (Cont.)

			Fluconazole				
Drug	Mfr	Conc	Mfr	Conc	Remarks	Ref	C/I
	FUJ	50 and 200 μg/2.5 ml[b]	PF	15 mg/ 7.5 ml[b]	Mixed in the amounts indicated.[i] Visually compatible with no loss of either drug by HPLC in 3 hr at 24 °C under fluorescent light	2225	C
Teniposide	BR	0.1 mg/ml[a]	RR	2 mg/ml	Physically compatible with no subvisual haze or particle formation in 4 hr at 23 °C	1725	C
Theophylline	AMR	1.6 mg/ml[a]	RR	2 mg/ml	Visually compatible for 24 hr at 28 °C under fluorescent light	1760	C
	TR	4 mg/ml	PF	2 mg/ml	Visually compatible for 6 hr at 25 °C	1793	C
Thiotepa	IMM[f]	1 mg/ml[a]	RR	2 mg/ml	Physically compatible with no change in measured turbidity or increase in particle content in 4 hr at 23 °C	1861	C
Ticarcillin disodium	BE	15 mg/ml	RR	2 mg/ml	Viscous gel-like substance forms	1407	I
Ticarcillin disodium–clavulanate potassium	BE	60 mg/ml	RR	2 mg/ml	Physically compatible for 24 hr at 25 °C	1407	C
Tobramycin sulfate	LI	40 mg/ml	RR	2 mg/ml	Physically compatible for 24 hr at 25 °C	1407	C
TNA #218 to #226[g]			PF	2 mg/ml	Visually compatible with no precipitate or emulsion damage apparent in 4 hr at 23 °C	2215	C
TPN #146[g]		[h]	PF	0.5 and 1.75 mg/ml[h]	Visually compatible with no fluconazole loss by HPLC in 2 hr at 24 °C under fluorescent light. Amino acid concentrations by HPLC greater than 93%	1554	C
TPN #147 and #148[g]		[h]	PF	0.5 and 1.75 mg/ml[h]	Visually compatible with no fluconazole loss by HPLC in 2 hr at 24 °C under fluorescent light. Amino acids not tested	1554	C
TPN #212 to #215[g]			RR	2 mg/ml	Physically compatible with no change in measured turbidity or increase in particle content in 4 hr at 23 °C	2109	C
Trimethoprim–sulfamethoxazole	BW	16 + 80 mg/ ml	RR	2 mg/ml	Viscous gel-like substance forms	1407	I
Vancomycin HCl	LY	20 mg/ml	RR	2 mg/ml	Physically compatible for 24 hr at 25 °C	1407	C
Vecuronium bromide	OR	1 mg/ml[a]	RR	2 mg/ml	Visually compatible for 24 hr at 28 °C under fluorescent light	1760	C
Vinorelbine tartrate	BW	1 mg/ml[b]	RR	2 mg/ml	Physically compatible with no change in measured turbidity or increase in particle content in 4 hr at 22 °C	1558	C
Zidovudine	BW	10 mg/ml	RR	2 mg/ml	Physically compatible for 24 hr at 25 °C	1407	C

[a]*Tested in dextrose 5% in water.*
[b]*Tested in sodium chloride 0.9%.*
[c]*Tested in both dextrose 5% in water and sodium chloride 0.9%.*
[d]*Tested in dextrose 5% in water, Ringer's injection, lactated, sodium chloride 0.45%, and sodium chloride 0.9%.*
[e]*Tested in dextrose 5% in water with human albumin 2 mg/ml.*
[f]*Lyophilized formulation tested.*
[g]*Refer to Appendix I for the composition of parenteral nutrition solutions. TNA indicates a 3-in-1 admixture, and TPN indicates a 2-in-1 admixture.*
[h]*Varying volumes to simulate varying administration rates.*
[i]*Final concentrations were 1.5 mg/ml of fluconazole and 5 and 20 μg/ml of tacrolimus.*

Additional Compatibility Information

The manufacturer recommends that no supplementary medications be added to fluconazole injection (2).

FLUDARABINE PHOSPHATE
AHFS 10:00

Fludara   **Berlex**

Products— Fludarabine phosphate (Berlex) is supplied as a lyophilized product in 6-ml vials containing 50 mg of drug with mannitol 50 mg and sodium hydroxide for pH adjustment. Reconstitute with 2 ml of sterile water for injection to yield a 25-mg/ml concentration (2).

pH— From 7.2 to 8.2 (2).

Osmolality— Fludarabine phosphate 25 mg/ml in sterile water for injection has an osmolality of 352 mOsm/kg (1689).

Administration— Fludarabine phosphate is administered by intravenous infusion over 30 minutes in 100 or 125 ml of dextrose 5% in water or sodium chloride 0.9% (2; 4). The drug also has been administered by rapid intravenous injection and continuous infusion (4).

Stability— Intact vials should be stored under refrigeration (2). The manufacturer recommends use of the reconstituted solution within eight hours because it does not contain an antibacterial preservative. Nevertheless, the drug is chemically stable in solution, exhibiting less than 2% decomposition in 16 days when stored at room temperature and exposed to normal laboratory light (234).

pH Effects— Fludarabine phosphate is chemically stable in aqueous solution at pH 4.5 to 8. The pH of optimum stability is approximately 7.6 (234).

Sorption— Fludarabine phosphate 0.04 mg/ml in dextrose 5% in water or sodium chloride 0.9% was equally stable in either glass or PVC containers, exhibiting no loss due to sorption during 48 hours at room temperature or under refrigeration (234).

Compatibility Information

Y-Site Injection Compatibility (1:1 Mixture)

Fludarabine phosphate

Drug	Mfr	Conc	Mfr	Conc	Remarks	Ref	C/I
Acyclovir sodium	BW	7 mg/ml[a]	BX	1 mg/ml[a]	Darker color visible with high-intensity light within 4 hr	1439	I
Allopurinol sodium	BW	3 mg/ml[b]	BX	1 mg/ml[b]	Physically compatible with no change in measured turbidity or increase in particle content in 4 hr at 22 °C	1686	C
Amifostine	USB	10 mg/ml[a]	BX	1 mg/ml[a]	Physically compatible with no change in measured turbidity or increase in particle content in 4 hr at 23 °C	1845	C
Amikacin sulfate	BR	5 mg/ml[a]	BX	1 mg/ml[a]	Physically compatible for 4 hr at room temperature under fluorescent light	1439	C
Aminophylline	ES	2.5 mg/ml[a]	BX	1 mg/ml[a]	Physically compatible for 4 hr at room temperature under fluorescent light	1439	C
Amphotericin B	SQ	0.6 mg/ml[a]	BX	1 mg/ml[a]	Small amount of particulate matter develops in 4 hr at room temperature	1439	I
Ampicillin sodium	BR	20 mg/ml[b]	BX	1 mg/ml[a]	Physically compatible for 4 hr at room temperature under fluorescent light	1439	C
Ampicillin sodium–sulbactam sodium	RR	20 + 10 mg/ml[b]	BX	1 mg/ml[a]	Physically compatible for 4 hr at room temperature under fluorescent light	1439	C

Y-Site Injection Compatibility (1:1 Mixture) (Cont.)

					Fludarabine phosphate		
Drug	*Mfr*	*Conc*	*Mfr*	*Conc*	*Remarks*	*Ref*	*C/I*
Amsacrine	NCI	1 mg/ml[a]	BX	1 mg/ml[a]	Physically compatible for 4 hr at room temperature under fluorescent light	1439	**C**
Aztreonam	SQ	40 mg/ml[a]	BX	1 mg/ml[a]	Physically compatible for 4 hr at room temperature under fluorescent light	1439	**C**
	SQ	40 mg/ml[a]	BX	1 mg/ml[a]	Physically compatible with no subvisual haze or particle formation in 4 hr at 23 °C	1758	**C**
Bleomycin sulfate	BR	1 unit/ml[b]	BX	1 mg/ml[a]	Physically compatible for 4 hr at room temperature under fluorescent light	1439	**C**
Butorphanol tartrate	BR	0.04 mg/ml[a]	BX	1 mg/ml[a]	Physically compatible for 4 hr at room temperature under fluorescent light	1439	**C**
Carboplatin	BR	5 mg/ml[a]	BX	1 mg/ml[a]	Physically compatible for 4 hr at room temperature under fluorescent light	1439	**C**
Carmustine	BR	1.5 mg/ml[a]	BX	1 mg/ml[a]	Physically compatible for 4 hr at room temperature under fluorescent light	1439	**C**
Cefazolin sodium	LEM	20 mg/ml[a]	BX	1 mg/ml[a]	Physically compatible for 4 hr at room temperature under fluorescent light	1439	**C**
Cefepime HCl	BR	20 mg/ml[a]	BX	1 mg/ml[a]	Physically compatible with no change in measured turbidity or increase in particle content in 4 hr at 22 °C	1689	**C**
Cefoperazone sodium	RR	40 mg/ml[a]	BX	1 mg/ml[a]	Physically compatible for 4 hr at room temperature under fluorescent light	1439	**C**
Cefotaxime sodium	HO	20 mg/ml[a]	BX	1 mg/ml[a]	Physically compatible for 4 hr at room temperature under fluorescent light	1439	**C**
Cefotetan disodium	STU	20 mg/ml[a]	BX	1 mg/ml[a]	Physically compatible for 4 hr at room temperature under fluorescent light	1439	**C**
Ceftazidime	GL[d]	40 mg/ml[a]	BX	1 mg/ml[a]	Physically compatible for 4 hr at room temperature under fluorescent light	1439	**C**
Ceftizoxime sodium	SKF	20 mg/ml[a]	BX	1 mg/ml[a]	Physically compatible for 4 hr at room temperature under fluorescent light	1439	**C**
Ceftriaxone sodium	RC	20 mg/ml[a]	BX	1 mg/ml[a]	Physically compatible for 4 hr at room temperature under fluorescent light	1439	**C**
Cefuroxime sodium	GL	30 mg/ml[a]	BX	1 mg/ml[a]	Physically compatible for 4 hr at room temperature under fluorescent light	1439	**C**
Chlorpromazine HCl	ES	2 mg/ml[a]	BX	1 mg/ml[a]	Initial light haze intensifies within 30 min	1439	**I**
Cimetidine HCl	SKF	12 mg/ml[a]	BX	1 mg/ml[a]	Physically compatible for 4 hr at room temperature under fluorescent light	1439	**C**
Cisplatin	BR	1 mg/ml	BX	1 mg/ml[a]	Physically compatible for 4 hr at room temperature under fluorescent light	1439	**C**
Clindamycin phosphate	LY	10 mg/ml[a]	BX	1 mg/ml[a]	Physically compatible for 4 hr at room temperature under fluorescent light	1439	**C**
Cyclophosphamide	MJ	10 mg/ml[a]	BX	1 mg/ml[a]	Physically compatible for 4 hr at room temperature under fluorescent light	1439	**C**
Cytarabine	UP	50 mg/ml	BX	1 mg/ml[a]	Physically compatible for 4 hr at room temperature under fluorescent light	1439	**C**

Y-Site Injection Compatibility (1:1 Mixture) (Cont.)

Fludarabine phosphate

Drug	Mfr	Conc	Mfr	Conc	Remarks	Ref	C/I
Dacarbazine	MI	4 mg/ml[a]	BX	1 mg/ml[a]	Physically compatible for 4 hr at room temperature under fluorescent light	1439	C
Dactinomycin	MSD	0.01 mg/ml[a]	BX	1 mg/ml[a]	Physically compatible for 4 hr at room temperature under fluorescent light	1439	C
Daunorubicin HCl	WY	2 mg/ml[a]	BX	1 mg/ml[a]	Slight haze, visible with high-intensity light, forms within 4 hr at room temperature	1439	I
Dexamethasone sodium phosphate	MSD	1 mg/ml[a]	BX	1 mg/ml[a]	Physically compatible for 4 hr at room temperature under fluorescent light	1439	C
Diphenhydramine HCl	WY	2 mg/ml[a]	BX	1 mg/ml[a]	Physically compatible for 4 hr at room temperature under fluorescent light	1439	C
Doxorubicin HCl	CET	2 mg/ml	BX	1 mg/ml[a]	Physically compatible for 4 hr at room temperature under fluorescent light	1439	C
Doxycycline hyclate	ES	1 mg/ml[a]	BX	1 mg/ml[a]	Physically compatible for 4 hr at room temperature under fluorescent light	1439	C
Droperidol	JA	0.4 mg/ml[a]	BX	1 mg/ml[a]	Physically compatible for 4 hr at room temperature under fluorescent light	1439	C
Etoposide	BR	0.4 mg/ml[a]	BX	1 mg/ml[a]	Physically compatible for 4 hr at room temperature under fluorescent light	1439	C
Etoposide phosphate	BR	5 mg/ml[a]	BX	1 mg/ml[a]	Physically compatible with no change in measured turbidity or increase in particle content in 4 hr at 23 °C	2218	C
Famotidine	MSD	2 mg/ml[a]	BX	1 mg/ml[a]	Physically compatible for 4 hr at room temperature under fluorescent light	1439	C
Filgrastim	AMG	30 μg/ml[a]	BX	1 mg/ml[a]	Physically compatible with no change in measured turbidity or increase in particle content in 4 hr at 22 °C	1687	C
Floxuridine	RC	3 mg/ml[a]	BX	1 mg/ml[a]	Physically compatible for 4 hr at room temperature under fluorescent light	1439	C
Fluconazole	RR	2 mg/ml	BX	1 mg/ml[a]	Physically compatible for 4 hr at room temperature under fluorescent light	1439	C
Fluorouracil	LY	16 mg/ml[a]	BX	1 mg/ml[a]	Physically compatible for 4 hr at room temperature under fluorescent light	1439	C
Furosemide	AB	3 mg/ml[a]	BX	1 mg/ml[a]	Physically compatible for 4 hr at room temperature under fluorescent light	1439	C
Ganciclovir sodium	SY	20 mg/ml[a]	BX	1 mg/ml[a]	Darker color forms within 4 hr	1439	I
Gemcitabine HCl	LI	10 mg/ml[b]	BX	1 mg/ml[b]	Physically compatible with no change in measured turbidity or increase in particle content in 4 hr at 23 °C	2226	C
Gentamicin sulfate	ES	5 mg/ml[a]	BX	1 mg/ml[a]	Physically compatible for 4 hr at room temperature under fluorescent light	1439	C
Granisetron HCl	SKB	0.05 mg/ml[a]	BX	1 mg/ml[a]	Physically compatible with no change in measured turbidity or increase in particle content in 4 hr at 23 °C	2000	C
Haloperidol lactate	MN	0.2 mg/ml[a]	BX	1 mg/ml[a]	Physically compatible for 4 hr at room temperature under fluorescent light	1439	C

Y-Site Injection Compatibility (1:1 Mixture) (Cont.)

Fludarabine phosphate

Drug	Mfr	Conc	Mfr	Conc	Remarks	Ref	C/I
Heparin sodium	SO, WY	40, 100, 1000 units/ml[a]	BX	1 mg/ml[a]	Physically compatible for 4 hr at room temperature under fluorescent light	1439	**C**
Hydrocortisone sodium phosphate	MSD	1 mg/ml[a]	BX	1 mg/ml[a]	Physically compatible for 4 hr at room temperature under fluorescent light	1439	**C**
Hydrocortisone sodium succinate	UP	1 mg/ml[a]	BX	1 mg/ml[a]	Physically compatible for 4 hr at room temperature under fluorescent light	1439	**C**
Hydromorphone HCl	KN	0.5 mg/ml[a]	BX	1 mg/ml[a]	Physically compatible for 4 hr at room temperature under fluorescent light	1439	**C**
Hydroxyzine HCl	WI	4 mg/ml[a]	BX	1 mg/ml[a]	Slight haze, visible with high-intensity light, forms immediately	1439	**I**
Ifosfamide	MJ	25 mg/ml[a]	BX	1 mg/ml[a]	Physically compatible for 4 hr at room temperature under fluorescent light	1439	**C**
Imipenem–cilastatin sodium	MSD	5 mg/ml[b]	BX	1 mg/ml[a]	Physically compatible for 4 hr at room temperature under fluorescent light	1439	**C**
Lorazepam	WY	0.1 mg/ml[a]	BX	1 mg/ml[a]	Physically compatible for 4 hr at room temperature under fluorescent light	1439	**C**
Magnesium sulfate	SO	100 mg/ml[a]	BX	1 mg/ml[a]	Physically compatible for 4 hr at room temperature under fluorescent light	1439	**C**
Mannitol	BA	150 mg/ml	BX	1 mg/ml[a]	Physically compatible for 4 hr at room temperature under fluorescent light	1439	**C**
Mechlorethamine HCl	MSD	1 mg/ml	BX	1 mg/ml[a]	Physically compatible for 4 hr at room temperature under fluorescent light	1439	**C**
Melphalan HCl	BW	0.1 mg/ml[b]	BX	1 mg/ml[b]	Physically compatible with no change in measured turbidity or increase in particle content in 3 hr at 22 °C	1557	**C**
Meperidine HCl	WI	4 mg/ml[a]	BX	1 mg/ml[a]	Physically compatible for 4 hr at room temperature under fluorescent light	1439	**C**
Mesna	BR	10 mg/ml[a]	BX	1 mg/ml[a]	Physically compatible for 4 hr at room temperature under fluorescent light	1439	**C**
Methotrexate sodium	CET	15 mg/ml[a]	BX	1 mg/ml[a]	Physically compatible for 4 hr at room temperature under fluorescent light	1439	**C**
Methylprednisolone sodium succinate	UP	5 mg/ml[a]	BX	1 mg/ml[a]	Physically compatible for 4 hr at room temperature under fluorescent light	1439	**C**
Metoclopramide HCl	DU	5 mg/ml[a]	BX	1 mg/ml[a]	Physically compatible for 4 hr at room temperature under fluorescent light	1439	**C**
Minocycline HCl	LE	0.2 mg/ml[a]	BX	1 mg/ml[a]	Physically compatible for 4 hr at room temperature under fluorescent light	1439	**C**
Mitoxantrone HCl	LE	0.5 mg/ml[a]	BX	1 mg/ml[a]	Physically compatible for 4 hr at room temperature under fluorescent light	1439	**C**
Morphine sulfate	WI	1 mg/ml[a]	BX	1 mg/ml[a]	Physically compatible for 4 hr at room temperature under fluorescent light	1439	**C**
Multivitamins	ROR	0.01 ml/ml[a]	BX	1 mg/ml[a]	Physically compatible for 4 hr at room temperature under fluorescent light	1439	**C**
Nalbuphine HCl	DU	10 mg/ml[a]	BX	1 mg/ml[a]	Physically compatible for 4 hr at room temperature under fluorescent light	1439	**C**

Y-Site Injection Compatibility (1:1 Mixture) (Cont.)

				Fludarabine phosphate			
Drug	*Mfr*	*Conc*	*Mfr*	*Conc*	*Remarks*	*Ref*	*C/I*
Netilmicin sulfate	SC	5 mg/ml[a]	BX	1 mg/ml[a]	Physically compatible for 4 hr at room temperature under fluorescent light	1439	**C**
Ondansetron HCl	GL	0.5 mg/ml[a]	BX	1 mg/ml[a]	Physically compatible for 4 hr at room temperature under fluorescent light	1439	**C**
Pentostatin	NCI	0.4 mg/ml[b]	BX	1 mg/ml[a]	Physically compatible for 4 hr at room temperature under fluorescent light	1439	**C**
Piperacillin sodium	LE	40 mg/ml[a]	BX	1 mg/ml[a]	Physically compatible for 4 hr at room temperature under fluorescent light	1439	**C**
Piperacillin sodium–tazobactam sodium	LE	40 + 5 mg/ml[a]	BX	1 mg/ml[a]	Physically compatible with no change in measured turbidity or increase in particle content in 4 hr at 22 °C	1688	**C**
Potassium chloride	AB	0.1 mEq/ml[a]	BX	1 mg/ml[a]	Physically compatible for 4 hr at room temperature under fluorescent light	1439	**C**
Prochlorperazine edisylate	WY	0.5 mg/ml[a]	BX	1 mg/ml[a]	Slight haze forms within 30 min	1439	**I**
Promethazine HCl	WY	2 mg/ml[a]	BX	1 mg/ml[a]	Physically compatible for 4 hr at room temperature under fluorescent light	1439	**C**
Ranitidine HCl	GL	2 mg/ml[a]	BX	1 mg/ml[a]	Physically compatible for 4 hr at room temperature under fluorescent light	1439	**C**
Sodium bicarbonate	AB	1 mEq/ml	BX	1 mg/ml[a]	Physically compatible for 4 hr at room temperature under fluorescent light	1439	**C**
Teniposide	BR	0.1 mg/ml[a]	BX	1 mg/ml[a]	Physically compatible with no subvisual haze or particle formation in 4 hr at 23 °C	1725	**C**
Thiotepa	IMM[c]	1 mg/ml[a]	BX	1 mg/ml[a]	Physically compatible with no change in measured turbidity or increase in particle content in 4 hr at 23 °C	1861	**C**
Ticarcillin disodium	BE	30 mg/ml[a]	BX	1 mg/ml[a]	Physically compatible for 4 hr at room temperature under fluorescent light	1439	**C**
Ticarcillin disodium–clavulanate potassium	BE	31 mg/ml[a]	BX	1 mg/ml[a]	Physically compatible for 4 hr at room temperature under fluorescent light	1439	**C**
Tobramycin sulfate	LI	5 mg/ml[a]	BX	1 mg/ml[a]	Physically compatible for 4 hr at room temperature under fluorescent light	1439	**C**
Trimethoprim–sulfamethoxazole	ES	0.8 + 4 mg/ml[a]	BX	1 mg/ml[a]	Physically compatible for 4 hr at room temperature under fluorescent light	1439	**C**
Vancomycin HCl	LI	10 mg/ml[a]	BX	1 mg/ml[a]	Physically compatible for 4 hr at room temperature under fluorescent light	1439	**C**
Vinblastine sulfate	LY	0.12 mg/ml[a]	BX	1 mg/ml[a]	Physically compatible for 4 hr at room temperature under fluorescent light	1439	**C**
Vincristine sulfate	LY	1 mg/ml	BX	1 mg/ml[a]	Physically compatible for 4 hr at room temperature under fluorescent light	1439	**C**
Vinorelbine tartrate	BW	1 mg/ml[b]	BX	1 mg/ml[b]	Physically compatible with no change in measured turbidity or increase in particle content in 4 hr at 22 °C	1558	**C**

Y-Site Injection Compatibility (1:1 Mixture) (Cont.)

Fludarabine phosphate

Drug	Mfr	Conc	Mfr	Conc	Remarks	Ref	C/I
Zidovudine	BW	4 mg/ml[a]	BX	1 mg/ml[a]	Physically compatible for 4 hr at room temperature under fluorescent light	1439	C

[a]*Tested in dextrose 5% in water.*
[b]*Tested in sodium chloride 0.9%.*
[c]*Lyophilized formulation tested.*
[d]*Sodium carbonate–containing formulation tested.*

Additional Compatibility Information

The manufacturer recommends diluting the dose in 100 to 125 ml of dextrose 5% in water or sodium chloride 0.9% (2). At a concentration of 1 mg/ml in these solutions, less than 3% decomposition occurred in 16 days at room temperature with exposure to normal laboratory light. At a concentration of 0.04 mg/ml in dextrose 5% in water or sodium chloride 0.9%, little or no loss occurred in 48 hours at room temperature or under refrigeration (234).

Other Information

Bacterial Challenge— Fludarabine phosphate (Berlex) 0.2 mg/ml diluted in sodium chloride 0.9% and stored at 22 °C did not exhibit an antimicrobial effect on the growth of four organisms (*Enterococcus faecium, Staphylococcus aureus, Pseudomonas aeruginosa,* and *Candida albicans*) inoculated into the solution. Diluted solutions should be stored under refrigeration whenever possible, and the potential for microbiological growth should be considered when assigning expiration dates (2160).

FLUMAZENIL
AHFS 28:92

Romazicon   **Roche**

Products— Flumazenil (Roche) is available as a 0.1-mg/ml solution in 5- and 10-ml multiple-dose vials. In addition to flumazenil, each milliliter also contains methylparaben 1.8 mg, propylparaben 0.2 mg, sodium chloride 0.9%, edetate disodium 0.01%, and acetic acid 0.01%. The pH is adjusted with hydrochloric acid and, if necessary, sodium hydroxide (2).

pH— The injection has a pH of approximately 4 (2).

Administration— Flumazenil is administered intravenously over 15 to 30 seconds. To minimize pain at the injection site, flumazenil should be administered through a freely running intravenous infusion line into a large vein. Extravasation should be avoided (2; 4).

Stability— Flumazenil injection (Roche) is a stable aqueous solution; it should be stored at controlled room temperature (15 to 30 °C). The manufacturer recommends discarding the product 24 hours after removal from its original vial, whether admixed in an infusion solution or simply drawn into a syringe (2).

Compatibility Information

Solution Compatibility

Flumazenil

Solution	Mfr	Mfr	Conc/L	Remarks	Ref	C/I
Dextrose 5% in water	BA[a]	RC	20 mg	Visually compatible with no flumazenil loss by HPLC in 24 hr at 23 °C under fluorescent light	1710	C

[a]*Tested in PVC containers.*

Additive Compatibility

Flumazenil

Drug	Mfr	Conc/L	Mfr	Conc/L	Test Soln	Remarks	Ref	C/I
Aminophylline	AMR	2 g	RC	20 mg	D5W[a]	Visually compatible with no flumazenil loss by HPLC in 24 hr at 23 °C under fluorescent light. Aminophylline not tested	1710	C
Cimetidine HCl	SKB	2.4 g	RC	20 mg	D5W[a]	Visually compatible with no flumazenil loss by HPLC in 24 hr at 23 °C under fluorescent light. Cimetidine not tested	1710	C
Dobutamine HCl	LI	2 g	RC	20 mg	D5W[a]	Visually compatible with no flumazenil loss by HPLC in 24 hr at 23 °C under fluorescent light. Dobutamine not tested	1710	C
Dopamine HCl	AB	3.2 g	RC	20 mg	D5W[a]	Visually compatible with 7% flumazenil loss by HPLC in 24 hr at 23 °C under fluorescent light. Dopamine not tested	1710	C
Famotidine	MSD	80 mg	RC	20 mg	D5W[a]	Visually compatible with 3% flumazenil loss by HPLC in 24 hr at 23 °C under fluorescent light. Famotidine not tested	1710	C
Heparin sodium	ES	50,000 units	RC	20 mg	D5W[a]	Visually compatible with 4% flumazenil loss by HPLC in 24 hr at 23 °C under fluorescent light. Heparin not tested	1710	C
Lidocaine HCl	AB	4 g	RC	20 mg	D5W[a]	Visually compatible with 4% flumazenil loss by HPLC in 24 hr at 23 °C under fluorescent light. Lidocaine not tested	1710	C
Procainamide HCl	ES	4 g	RC	20 mg	D5W[a]	Visually compatible with no flumazenil loss by HPLC in 24 hr at 23 °C under fluorescent light. Procainamide not tested	1710	C
Ranitidine HCl	GL	300 mg	RC	20 mg	D5W[a]	Visually compatible with 3% flumazenil loss by HPLC in 24 hr at 23 °C under fluorescent light. Ranitidine not tested	1710	C

[a]*Tested in PVC containers.*

Additional Compatibility Information

Solutions— The manufacturer states that flumazenil is compatible with dextrose 5% in water, sodium chloride 0.9%, and Ringer's injection, lactated (2).

FLUOROURACIL
(5-FLUOROURACIL)
AHFS 10:00

Adrucil　　　　　　　　**Pharmacia & Upjohn**
　　　　　　　　　　　　　　　　　　　　Roche

Products— Fluorouracil injection is available from a variety of manufacturers in 10- and 20-ml single-use vials and ampuls and in 50-

and 100-ml bulk pharmacy vials for preparation of individual doses (4; 154). Each milliliter contains fluorouracil 50 mg with sodium hydroxide and/or hydrochloric acid for pH adjustment (1-5/97; 4).

pH— The pH is adjusted to approximately 9.2 (4) with a range of 8.6 to 9.4 (17).

Osmolality— Fluorouracil 50 mg/ml has an osmolality of 650 mOsm/kg (1689).

Administration— Fluorouracil is administered intravenously. Care should be taken to avoid extravasation. Dilution of the injection is not required for administration (2; 4). Fluorouracil has also been given by portal vein or hepatic artery infusion (4).

Stability— The solution is normally colorless to faint yellow. Its potency and safety are not affected by slight discoloration during storage. It should be stored between 15 and 30 °C and protected from light (1-5/97; 4) and freezing (4). Storing the vials in the original cartons until the time of use is recommended (1-5/97). The color of the solution results from the presence of free fluorine. A dark yellow indicates greater decomposition. Such decomposition may result from storage for several months at temperatures above room temperature. It is suggested that solutions having a darker yellow color be discarded (398). Exposure to sunlight or intense incandescent light has also caused degradation. The solutions changed in color to dark amber to brown (760). A precipitate may form from exposure to low temperatures and may be resolubilized by heating to 60 °C with vigorous shaking (1-5/97; 4). (Note: Allow the solution to cool to body temperature before administration.)

Microwave radiation also has been used to resolubilize the precipitate. Ampuls of fluorouracil (Adria) containing a precipitate were exposed to microwave radiation and shaken until clear. These ampuls were then compared to ampuls that were heated to 60 °C in a water bath and shaken until clear and also to unheated controls. The precipitate was redissolved by microwave radiation without significantly affecting the drug. No significant decrease in drug potency was observed. There was a slight change in pH. The authors concluded that microwave radiation was a suitable method for solubilizing the precipitate that may form in fluorouracil ampuls. However, they warned that extreme care should be taken to avoid overheating and the resulting explosions from excessive pressure in the ampuls (662).

Fluorouracil (Roche) 1 mg/ml in dextrose 5% in water was evaluated for stability in translucent containers (Perfupack Y, Baxter) and five opaque containers [green PVC Opafuseur (Bruneau), white EVA Perfu-opaque (Baxter), orange PVC PF170 (Cair), white PVC V86 (Codan), and white EVA Perfecran (Fandre)] when exposed to sunlight for 28 days. No photodegradation or sorption was found by HPLC analysis. However, an increase in concentration due to moisture permeation was detected after two weeks (1750).

Freezing— Fluorouracil (Abic) 5 mg/0.5 ml in sodium chloride 0.9% in polypropylene syringes (Plastipak, Becton-Dickinson) was stored frozen at −20 °C. HPLC analysis showed no fluorouracil loss after eight weeks. Refreezing and further storage at −20 °C for another two weeks (total of 10 weeks) also did not result in a fluorouracil loss (1666).

pH Effects— At a pH greater than 11, slow hydrolysis of fluorouracil occurs. At a pH less than 8, solubility is reduced and precipitation may or may not occur, depending on the concentration (1369; 1379).

Stiles et al. found that fluorouracil 50 mg/ml (Lyphomed, Roche, and SoloPak) exhibited precipitation in two to four hours at pH 8.6 to 8.68; precipitation occurred immediately at pH 8.52 or less. The precipitate consisted of needle-shaped crystals at pH 8.26 to 8.68. Cluster-shaped crystals formed at pH 8.18 and below (1489).

Syringes— Fluorouracil 25 mg/ml in polypropylene syringes (Braun Omnifix) was stable by HPLC analysis for 28 days at 4 and 20 °C (1564).

Fluorouracil (Roche) 50 mg/ml was packaged as 3 ml in 10-ml polypropylene infusion pump syringes (Pharmacia Deltec). Little or

no loss by HPLC analysis occurred during 21 days of storage at 30 °C (1967).

Fluorouracil (Roche) 12 and 40 mg/ml diluted with sodium chloride 0.9% and dextrose 5% in water was packaged in 60-ml polypropylene syringes and stored at 25 °C protected from light. Losses of 5% or less were determined by HPLC analysis of the solutions after storage for 72 hours. Furthermore, the solutions had no visually apparent precipitate or discoloration (1983).

Implantable Infusion Pumps— Fluorouracil 50 mg/ml was filled into an implantable infusion pump (Fresenius VIP 30) and associated capillary tubing and stored at 37 °C. Samples were analyzed using an HPLC assay. No fluorouracil loss and no contamination from components of pump materials occurred during eight weeks of storage (1903).

Ambulatory Infusion Pumps— The stability of fluorouracil (Roche) diluted in dextrose 5% in water was determined for use with two ambulatory infusion systems for home therapy. Fluorouracil 500 mg/50 ml was evaluated in the PVC drug reservoir used in the PL 146 MVP ambulatory pump (Travenol) at 5 and 25 °C. Fluorouracil 500 mg/60 ml was tested in the elastomeric reservoir of the Infusor (Travenol) disposable drug pump at 5 °C. No significant change occurred in samples stored at 5 °C in the PVC bags during 16 weeks of storage. However, at 25 °C, the PVC bag samples demonstrated a progressive increase in fluorouracil content over 16 weeks, presumably caused by water evaporation through the bag. During the first seven days of 25 °C storage, there appeared to be little change in fluorouracil content. In the Infusor at 5 °C, changes of less than 10% occurred after 16 weeks (894).

Stiles et al. reported the stability of undiluted fluorouracil 50 mg/ml from three manufacturers (Lyphomed, Roche, and SoloPak) in the reservoirs of four portable infusion pumps (Pharmacia Deltec CADD-1, Model 5100; Cormed II, Model 10500; Medfusion Infumed 200; and Pancretec Provider I.V., Model 2000). The fluorouracil was delivered by the pumps at a rate of 10 ml/day over a seven-day cycle at 25 and 37 °C. All fluorouracil samples in all pump reservoirs were stable over the seven-day study period, exhibiting little or no drug loss and only minimal leached plasticizer (DEHP) at either temperature (1489).

However, precipitation of the Roche fluorouracil was observed with all pumps; a fine white precipitate originated close to the connection junction and migrated in both directions until it occupied most of the tubing and was in the drug reservoir. In some cases, the pumps stopped due to the extent of precipitation. The authors noted that various factors, including solution pH, temperature, drug concentration and solubility, and the manipulative techniques used could contribute to precipitate formation (1489).

Rochard et al. reported that undiluted fluorouracil (Roche) 50 mg/ml in ethylene vinyl acetate (EVA) bags for use with portable infusion pumps remained stable, with little or no potency loss by HPLC analysis after 28 days at 4, 22, and 35 °C. The containers at 35 °C did sustain approximately a 3% water loss due to evaporation during storage, increasing the fluorouracil concentration slightly (1548).

Fluorouracil (David Bull Laboratories) 25 mg/ml was stable in PVC reservoirs (Parker Micropump) for 14 days at 4 and 37 °C, exhibiting no loss by HPLC analysis (1696).

Baud-Camus et al. packaged fluorouracil 15 and 45 mg/ml diluted in sodium chloride 0.9% in 100-ml ethylene vinyl acetate (EVA) infusion pump reservoirs and stored them at 25 °C protected from light. Little or no loss was found by HPLC analysis of the solutions after storage for 72 hours. Furthermore, the solutions had no visually apparent precipitate or discoloration (1983).

Martel et al. evaluated the stability of undiluted fluorouracil injection (Roche) 50 mg/ml in EVA reservoirs (Celsa) and PVC reservoirs (Pharmacia) for use with ambulatory infusion pumps. The filled reservoirs were stored for 14 days at 4 °C and at 33 °C to simulate the conditions of prolonged infusion from the reservoirs kept under patient's clothing. No loss of fluorouracil due to decomposition was found by HPLC analysis. However, the refrigerated samples exhibited substantial (up to 15%) loss of drug content from solution due to gross precipitation. Flocculent precipitation was observed in as little as three days. (Subvisual precipitation may occur earlier.) At the elevated temperature, substantial increases in concentration of fluorouracil occurred in the EVA reservoirs due to water loss from permeation through the plastic reservoir. Approximately 5% increase in drug concentration occurred in 14 days. No change in concentration occurred in the PVC reservoirs during this time frame (2004).

Elastomeric Reservoir Pumps— Fluorouracil (SoloPak) 5 mg/ml in sodium chloride 0.9% 100 ml was packaged in latex elastomeric reservoirs (Secure Medical). Little or no loss by HPLC analysis occurred in 24 hours at 25 °C (1970).

Sorption— Fluorouracil (Sigma) 10 mg/L in sodium chloride 0.9% (Travenol) in PVC bags did not exhibit significant sorption to the plastic during one week of storage at room temperature (15 to 20 °C) (536).

In another study, fluorouracil (Sigma) 10 mg/L in sodium chloride 0.9% did not exhibit any loss due to sorption during a seven-hour simulated infusion through an infusion set (Travenol) consisting of a cellulose propionate burette chamber and 170 cm of PVC tubing (606).

The drug was also tested as a simulated infusion over at least one hour by a syringe pump system. A glass syringe on a syringe pump was fitted with 20 cm of polyethylene tubing or 50 cm of Silastic tubing. No loss of drug due to sorption was observed with either tubing (606).

A 25-ml aliquot of fluorouracil (Sigma) 10 mg/L in sodium chloride 0.9% was stored in all-plastic syringes composed of polypropylene barrels and polyethylene plungers for 24 hours at room temperature in the dark. No loss of drug due to sorption occurred (606).

Undiluted fluorouracil (Roche) 50 mg/ml was stored for seven days at room temperature in plastic syringes (Monoject) and glass vials (Elkins-Sinn). Little or no loss of potency occurred over this period in either container (760).

Fluorouracil may be more extensively adsorbed to glass surfaces than to plastic. In one report, significant loss occurred from solutions in glass vials, but almost quantitative recovery was obtained from polyethylene and polypropylene plastic vials. The loss was ascribed to adsorption to the glass surface (663). This difference was also observed in dextrose 5% in water in glass and PVC infusion containers. A 10% loss of fluorouracil occurred in 43 hours in the PVC containers but in only seven hours in the glass containers (519).

Filtration— Fluorouracil 10 to 75 μg/ml exhibited little or no loss due to sorption to either cellulose nitrate/cellulose acetate ester (Millex OR) or Teflon (Millex FG) filters (1415; 1416).

Compatibility Information

Solution Compatibility

Fluorouracil

Solution	Mfr	Mfr	Conc/L	Remarks	Ref	C/I
Amino acids 4.25%, dextrose 25%	MG	RC	500 mg	No increase in particulate matter in 24 hr at 5 °C	349	C
Dextrose 5% in Ringer's injection, lactated	MG[a]		500 mg	No decomposition in 24 hr	399	C
Dextrose 3.3% in sodium chloride 0.3%	TR[b]	RC	1.5 g	Physically compatible and chemically stable for 8 weeks at ambient temperature both in the dark and exposed to fluorescent light	1153	C
Dextrose 5% in water		RC	10 g	No loss of fluorouracil by HPLC during 16 weeks at 5 °C. Little or no change in fluorouracil by HPLC during 7 days at 25 °C	894	C
	TR[b]	RC	1.5 g	Physically compatible and chemically stable for 8 weeks at ambient temperature both in the dark and exposed to fluorescent light	1153	C
			1 and 2 g	Physically compatible and no fluorouracil loss in 48 hr at room temperature and 7 °C by UV and TLC	1152	C
	[c]	RC	10 g	Visually compatible with little or no fluorouracil loss by HPLC in 28 days at 4, 22, and 35 °C protected from light. At 35 °C, concentration increased due to water evaporation	1548	C
	MG[a]		8.3 g	Less than 10% loss by HPLC in 48 hr at room temperature exposed to light	1658	C
	BA[d]	RC	1 and 10 g	Visually compatible with less than 3% loss by HPLC in 14 days at 4 and 21 °C	2004	C

Solution Compatibility (Cont.)

Fluorouracil

Solution	Mfr	Mfr	Conc/L	Remarks	Ref	C/I
	BA[a]	RC[g]	0.5 and 5 g	Little or no loss by HPLC in 13 days at 4 and 25 °C	2175	**C**
Plasmalyte 3G5	BA[a]	RC[g]	0.5 and 5 g	Little or no loss by HPLC in 13 days at 4 and 25 °C	2175	**C**
Sodium chloride 0.9%	TR[b]	RC	1.5 g	Physically compatible and chemically stable for 8 weeks at ambient temperature both in the dark and exposed to fluorescent light	1153	**C**
			1 and 2 g	Physically compatible and no fluorouracil loss in 48 hr at room temperature and 7 °C by UV and TLC	1152	**C**
	[c]	RC	10 g	Visually compatible with little or no fluorouracil loss by HPLC in 28 days at 4, 22, and 35 °C protected from light. At 35 °C, concentration increased due to water evaporation	1548	**C**
	[b]	FA, RC	5 and 50 g	Visually compatible with little or no loss by HPLC in 91 days at 4 °C followed by 7 days at 25 °C in the dark	1567	**C**
	AB[e]	RC	5 g	Little or no loss of drug by HPLC in 24 hr at 25 °C	1970	**C**
	[c]	RC	15 and 45 g	Visually compatible with little or no loss of drug by HPLC in 72 hr at 25 °C protected from light	1983	**C**
	BA[d]	RC	1 and 10 g	Visually compatible with less than 3% loss by HPLC in 14 days at 4 and 21 °C	2004	**C**
	BA[a]	RC[g]	0.5 and 5 g	Little or no loss by HPLC in 13 days at 4 and 25 °C	2175	**C**
TPN #23[f]		RC	1 and 4 g	Physically compatible for 42 hr at room temperature in ambient light. Results of HPLC analysis were erratic	562	**?**
		RC	1 g	Physically compatible and fluorouracil chemically stable for 48 hr at room temperature in ambient light	826	**C**

[a]Tested in both glass and polyolefin containers.
[b]Tested in both glass and PVC containers.
[c]Tested in ethylene vinyl acetate (EVA) containers.
[d]Tested in PVC containers.
[e]Tested in glass containers and latex elastomeric reservoirs (Secure Medical).
[f]Refer to Appendix I for the composition of parenteral nutrition solutions. TPN indicates a 2-in-1 admixture.
[g]A modified fluorouracil formulation containing tromethamine (TRIS, THAM, trometamol) instead of sodium hydroxide.

Additive Compatibility

Fluorouracil

Drug	Mfr	Conc/L	Mfr	Conc/L	Test Soln	Remarks	Ref	C/I
Bleomycin sulfate	BR	20 and 30 units	RC	1 g	NS	Physically compatible and bleomycin activity retained for 1 week at 4 °C. Fluorouracil not tested	763	**C**
Carboplatin		1 g		10 g	W	Greater than 20% carboplatin loss in 24 hr at room temperature	1379	**I**
Cisplatin	BR	200 mg	SO	1 g	NS[a]	10% cisplatin loss in 1.5 hr and 25% loss in 4 hr at 25 °C under fluorescent light or in the dark	1339	**I**

Additive Compatibility (Cont.)

Fluorouracil

Drug	Mfr	Conc/L	Mfr	Conc/L	Test Soln	Remarks	Ref	C/I
	BR	500 mg	SO	10 g	NS[a]	10% cisplatin loss in 1.2 hr and 25% loss in 3 hr at 25 °C under fluorescent light or in the dark	1339	I
	BR	500 mg	AD	10 g	NS	80% cisplatin loss in 24 hr at room temperature due to low pH	1386	I
Cyclophosphamide		1.67 g		8.3 g	NS	Both drugs stable for 15 days at room temperature	1389	C
Cyclophosphamide with methotrexate sodium		1.67 g 25 mg		8.3 g	NS	9.3% cyclophosphamide loss in 7 days at room temperature. No loss of other drugs observed	1389	C
Cytarabine	UP	400 mg	RC	250 mg	D5W	Altered UV spectrum for cytarabine within 1 hr at room temperature	207	I
Diazepam	RC					Immediate precipitation	524	I
Doxorubicin HCl	AD					Solution color darkens from red to blue-purple	524	I
	AD	10 mg	RC	250 mg	D5W	Color change to deep purple	296	I
Etoposide		200 mg		10 g	NS	Both drugs stable for 7 days at room temperature and 1 day at 35 °C	1379	C
Fentanyl citrate	AB	12.5 mg	AB	1 and 16 g	D5W, NS[a]	25% fentanyl loss in 15 min due to sorption to PVC	2064	I
Floxuridine		10 g		10 g	NS	Both drugs stable for 15 days at room temperature	1390	C
Hydromorphone HCl	AST	500 mg	AB	1 g	D5W, NS[a]	Physically compatible with no increase in measured turbidity or particulates and little or no loss by HPLC of either drug in 7 days at 32 °C and 35 days at 23, 4, and −20 °C	1977	C
	AST	500 mg	AB	16 g	D5W, NS[a]	Physically compatible with no increase in measured turbidity or particulates and little or no loss by HPLC of either drug in 3 days at 32 °C, 7 days at 23 °C, and 35 days at 4 and −20 °C	1977	C
Ifosfamide		2 g		10 g	NS	Both drugs stable for 5 days at room temperature	1379	C
Leucovorin calcium	LE	1.5 to 13.3 g	AD	16.7 to 46.2 g	[b]	Subvisual particulate matter forms in all combinations in variable periods from 1 to 4 days at 4, 23, and 32 °C	1816	I
Methotrexate sodium		30 mg		10 g	NS	Both drugs stable for 15 days at room temperature	1379	C
Metoclopramide HCl	FUJ	100 mg	RC	2.5 g	D5W	10% metoclopramide loss in 6 hr and 27% loss in 24 hr at 25 °C. 5% metoclopramide loss in 120 hr at 4 °C. 5 and 7% fluorouracil losses in 120 hr at 4 and 25 °C, respectively	1780	I
Mitoxantrone HCl	LE	500 mg		25 g	D5W	Visually compatible and mitoxantrone potency by HPLC retained for 24 hr at room temperature. Fluorouracil not tested	1531	C

Additive Compatibility (Cont.)

Fluorouracil

Drug	Mfr	Conc/L	Mfr	Conc/L	Test Soln	Remarks	Ref	C/I
Morphine sulfate	AST	1 g	AB	1 and 16 g	D5W, NS[a]	Subvisual morphine precipitate forms immediately, becoming grossly visible within 24 hr. Morphine losses by HPLC of 60 to 80% occur within 1 day	1977	I
Vincristine sulfate	LI	4 mg	RC	10 mg	D5W	Physically compatible. No alteration of UV spectra in 8 hr at room temperature	207	C

[a]Tested in PVC containers.
[b]Tested with both drugs undiluted and diluted by 25% with dextrose 5% in water.

Drugs in Syringe Compatibility

Fluorouracil

Drug (in syringe)	Mfr	Amt	Mfr	Amt	Remarks	Ref	C/I
Bleomycin sulfate		1.5 units/ 0.5 ml		25 mg/ 0.5 ml	Physically compatible for 5 min at room temperature followed by 8 min of centrifugation	980	C
Cisplatin		0.5 mg/ 0.5 ml		25 mg/ 0.5 ml	Physically compatible for 5 min at room temperature followed by 8 min of centrifugation	980	C
Cyclophosphamide		10 mg/ 0.5 ml		25 mg/ 0.5 ml	Physically compatible for 5 min at room temperature followed by 8 min of centrifugation	980	C
Doxorubicin HCl		1 mg/ 0.5 ml		25 mg/ 0.5 ml	Physically compatible for 5 min at room temperature followed by 8 min of centrifugation	980	C
		5 and 10 mg/ 10 ml[a]		500 mg/ 10 ml	Precipitate forms within several hours of mixing	1564	I
Droperidol		1.25 mg/ 0.5 ml		25 mg/ 0.5 ml	Immediate precipitation	980	I
Epirubicin HCl		5 and 10 mg/ 10 ml[a]		500 mg/ 10 ml	Precipitate forms within several hours of mixing	1564	I
Furosemide		5 mg/ 0.5 ml		25 mg/ 0.5 ml	Physically compatible for 5 min at room temperature followed by 8 min of centrifugation	980	C
Heparin sodium		500 units/ 0.5 ml		25 mg/ 0.5 ml	Physically compatible for 5 min at room temperature followed by 8 min of centrifugation	980	C
Leucovorin calcium		5 mg/ 0.5 ml		25 mg/ 0.5 ml	Physically compatible for 5 min at room temperature followed by 8 min of centrifugation	980	C
Methotrexate sodium		12.5 mg/ 0.5 ml		25 mg/ 0.5 ml	Physically compatible for 5 min at room temperature followed by 8 min of centrifugation	980	C
Metoclopramide HCl		2.5 mg/ 0.5 ml		25 mg/ 0.5 ml	Physically compatible for 5 min at room temperature followed by 8 min of centrifugation	980	C

Drugs in Syringe Compatibility (Cont.)

					Fluorouracil		
Drug (in syringe)	Mfr	Amt	Mfr	Amt	Remarks	Ref	C/I
Mitomycin		0.25 mg/ 0.5 ml		25 mg/ 0.5 ml	Physically compatible for 5 min at room temperature followed by 8 min of centrifugation	980	C
Vinblastine sulfate		0.5 mg/ 0.5 ml		25 mg/ 0.5 ml	Physically compatible for 5 min at room temperature followed by 8 min of centrifugation	980	C
Vincristine sulfate		0.5 mg/ 0.5 ml		25 mg/ 0.5 ml	Physically compatible for 5 min at room temperature followed by 8 min of centrifugation	980	C

[a]Diluted in sodium chloride 0.9%.

Y-Site Injection Compatibility (1:1 Mixture)

					Fluorouracil		
Drug	Mfr	Conc	Mfr	Conc	Remarks	Ref	C/I
Allopurinol sodium	BW	3 mg/ml[b]	RC	16 mg/ml[b]	Physically compatible with no change in measured turbidity or increase in particle content in 4 hr at 22 °C	1686	C
Amifostine	USB	10 mg/ml[a]	AD	16 mg/ml[b]	Physically compatible with no change in measured turbidity or increase in particle content in 4 hr at 23 °C	1845	C
Amphotericin B cholesteryl sulfate complex	SEQ	0.83 mg/ml[a]	PH	16 mg/ml[a]	Microprecipitate forms immediately	2117	I
Aztreonam	SQ	40 mg/ml[a]	AD	16 mg/ml[a]	Physically compatible with no subvisual haze or particle formation in 4 hr at 23 °C	1758	C
Bleomycin sulfate		3 units/ml		50 mg/ml	Drugs injected sequentially into Y-site with no flush between. No visually apparent precipitate	980	C
Cefepime HCl	BR	20 mg/ml[a]	AD	16 mg/ml[a]	Physically compatible with no change in measured turbidity or increase in particle content in 4 hr at 22 °C	1689	C
Cisplatin		1 mg/ml		50 mg/ml	Drugs injected sequentially into Y-site with no flush between. No visually apparent precipitate	980	C
Cyclophosphamide		20 mg/ml		50 mg/ml	Drugs injected sequentially into Y-site with no flush between. No visually apparent precipitate	980	C
Doxorubicin HCl		2 mg/ml		50 mg/ml	Drugs injected sequentially into Y-site with no flush between. No visually apparent precipitate	980	C
Doxorubicin HCl liposome injection	SEQ	0.4 mg/ml[a]	PH	16 mg/ml[a]	Physically compatible with little or no change in measured turbidity and no increase in particle content in 4 hr at 23 °C	2087	C
Droperidol		2.5 mg/ml		50 mg/ml	Drugs injected sequentially into Y-site with no flush between. Immediate precipitation	980	I

Y-Site Injection Compatibility (1:1 Mixture) (Cont.)

					Fluorouracil		
Drug	*Mfr*	*Conc*	*Mfr*	*Conc*	*Remarks*	*Ref*	*C/I*
Etoposide phosphate	BR	5 mg/ml[a]	PH	16 mg/ml[a]	Physically compatible with no change in measured turbidity or increase in particle content in 4 hr at 23 °C	2218	C
Filgrastim	AMG	30 μg/ml[a]	RC	16 mg/ml[a]	Particles and long filaments form in 1 hr	1687	I
Fludarabine phosphate	BX	1 mg/ml[a]	LY	16 mg/ml[a]	Physically compatible for 4 hr at room temperature under fluorescent light	1439	C
Furosemide		10 mg/ml		50 mg/ml	Drugs injected sequentially into Y-site with no flush between. No visually apparent precipitate	980	C
Gemcitabine HCl	LI	10 mg/ml[b]	PH	16 mg/ml[b]	Physically compatible with no change in measured turbidity or increase in particle content in 4 hr at 23 °C	2226	C
Granisetron HCl	SKB	0.05 mg/ml[b]	AD	16 mg/ml[b]	Physically compatible with no subvisual haze or particle formation in 4 hr at 23 °C	1804	C
	SKB	1 mg/ml	RC	2 mg/ml[b]	Physically compatible with little or no loss of either drug by HPLC in 4 hr at 22 °C	1883	C
	SKB	0.05 mg/ml[a]	AD	16 mg/ml[a]	Physically compatible with no change in measured turbidity or increase in particle content in 4 hr at 23 °C	2000	C
Heparin sodium		1000 units/ml		50 mg/ml	Drugs injected sequentially into Y-site with no flush between. No visually apparent precipitate	980	C
	UP	1000 units/L[c]	RC	50 mg/ml	Physically compatible for at least 4 hr at room temperature by visual and microscopic examination	534	C
Hydrocortisone sodium succinate	UP	10 mg/L[c]	RC	50 mg/ml	Physically compatible for at least 4 hr at room temperature by visual and microscopic examination	534	C
Leucovorin calcium		10 mg/ml		50 mg/ml	Drugs injected sequentially into Y-site with no flush between. No visually apparent precipitate	980	C
Mannitol		20%	SO	1 and 2 mg/ml[d]	Physically compatible both visually and microscopically and fluorouracil chemically stable by HPLC for 24 hr. Mannitol not tested	1526	C
Melphalan HCl	BW	0.1 mg/ml[b]	LY	16 mg/ml[b]	Physically compatible with no change in measured turbidity or increase in particle content in 3 hr at 22 °C	1557	C
Methotrexate sodium		25 mg/ml		50 mg/ml	Drugs injected sequentially into Y-site with no flush between. No visually apparent precipitate	980	C
Metoclopramide HCl		5 mg/ml		50 mg/ml	Drugs injected sequentially into Y-site with no flush between. No visually apparent precipitate	980	C
Mitomycin		0.5 mg/ml		50 mg/ml	Drugs injected sequentially into Y-site with no flush between. No visually apparent precipitate	980	C
Ondansetron HCl	GL	1 mg/ml[b]	SO	16 mg/ml[a]	Immediate precipitation	1365	I

Y-Site Injection Compatibility (1:1 Mixture) (Cont.)

Fluorouracil

Drug	Mfr	Conc	Mfr	Conc	Remarks	Ref	C/I
	GL	16 to 160 μg/ml		0.8 mg/ml	Physically compatible when fluorouracil given at 20 ml/hr via Y-site	1366	C
Paclitaxel	NCI	1.2 mg/ml[a]		16 mg/ml[a]	Physically compatible with no change in measured turbidity in 4 hr at 22 °C	1528	C
Piperacillin sodium–tazobactam sodium	LE	40 + 5 mg/ml[a]	LY	16 mg/ml[a]	Physically compatible with no change in measured turbidity or increase in particle content in 4 hr at 22 °C	1688	C
Potassium chloride	AB	40 mEq/L[c]	RC	50 mg/ml	Physically compatible for at least 4 hr at room temperature by visual and microscopic examination	534	C
Propofol	ZEN	10 mg/ml	AD	16 mg/ml[b]	Physically compatible for 1 hr at 23 °C with no increase in particle content	2066	C
Sargramostim	IMM	10 μg/ml[b]	SO	16 mg/ml[b]	Physically compatible for 4 hr at 22 °C	1436	C
Teniposide	BR	0.1 mg/ml[a]	AD	16 mg/ml[a]	Physically compatible with no subvisual haze or particle formation in 4 hr at 23 °C	1725	C
Thiotepa	IMM[e]	1 mg/ml[a]	AD	16 mg/ml[a]	Physically compatible with no change in measured turbidity or increase in particle content in 4 hr at 23 °C	1861	C
TNA #218, #219, #221, #222, #224 to #226[f]			PH	16 mg/ml[a]	Visually compatible with no precipitate or emulsion damage apparent in 4 hr at 23 °C	2215	C
TNA #220 and #223[f]			PH	16 mg/ml[a]	Small amount of white precipitate forms immediately	2215	I
TPN #212 and #213[f]			PH	16 mg/ml[a]	Slight subvisual haze and crystals and amber discoloration form in 1 to 4 hr	2109	I
TPN #214 and #215[f]			PH	16 mg/ml[a]	Turbidity forms immediately	2109	I
Vinblastine sulfate		1 mg/ml		50 mg/ml	Drugs injected sequentially into Y-site with no flush between. No visually apparent precipitate	980	C
Vincristine sulfate		1 mg/ml		50 mg/ml	Drugs injected sequentially into Y-site with no flush between. No visually apparent precipitate	980	C
Vinorelbine tartrate	BW	1 mg/ml[b]	RC	16 mg/ml[b]	Heavy white precipitate forms immediately	1558	I
Vitamin B complex with C	RC	2 ml/L[c]	RC	50 mg/ml	Physically compatible for at least 4 hr at room temperature by visual and microscopic examination	534	C

[a]Tested in dextrose 5% in water.

[b]Tested in sodium chloride 0.9%.

[c]Tested in dextrose 5% in Ringer's injection, dextrose 5% in Ringer's injection, lactated, dextrose 5% in water, Ringer's injected, lactated, and sodium chloride 0.9%.

[d]Tested in dextrose 5% in sodium chloride 0.45%, dextrose 5% in water, and sodium chloride 0.9%.

[e]Lyophilized formulation tested.

[f]Refer to Appendix I for the composition of parenteral nutrition solutions. TNA indicates a 3-in-1 admixture, and TPN indicates a 2-in-1 admixture.

Additional Compatibility Information

Solutions— Fluorouracil 5 to 10 mg/ml in dextrose 5% in water, sodium chloride 0.9%, or sterile water for injection exhibited less than a 10% loss in 14 days at room temperature (1379).

Miscellaneous— Admixture with acidic drugs or drugs that decompose in an alkaline environment should be avoided (524).

A color change to deep purple was reported for the mixtures of doxorubicin HCl (Adria) 10 mg/L with fluorouracil (Roche) 250 mg/L in dextrose 5% in water (296). This color change is indicative of decomposition occurring in solutions with an alkaline pH. It also occurs with other anthracyclines (394).

No alteration in the ultraviolet/visible spectra was observed when dacarbazine was combined in solution with fluorouracil (492).

Leucovorin Calcium— Several articles reported the chemical stability and physical compatibility of fluorouracil with leucovorin calcium (980; 1387; 1817). However, more recent work found substantial subvisual particles in this drug combination over numerous concentrations when stored at 4, 23, and 32 °C. Particulate formation sometimes clogged filters and disrupted multiple-day treatment. Particulate formation began in about 24 hours in most samples, and particles were found in all samples within seven days. Fluorouracil and leucovorin calcium in the same container can no longer be considered a compatible combination (1816).

Methotrexate— The reported incompatibility of fluorouracil (Roche) 250 mg/L with methotrexate sodium (Lederle) 200 mg/L in dextrose 5% in water (207) has been questioned on the grounds that the observed alteration in UV spectra for both drugs might be an artifact of the experiment, merely being a result of methotrexate's altered UV spectra at varying pH values. It was observed that the altered methotrexate spectrum could contribute to an altered spectrum for fluorouracil (318).

In reply, King noted that the pH of fluorouracil, rather than the drug itself, might be responsible for changes in methotrexate's UV spectrum. However, use of a buffered aqueous solution to simulate the admixture with a pH of approximately 8 and decrease of the pH with 0.2 M HCl back to the range of methotrexate sodium in dextrose 5% in water (pH 6.5) failed to return the UV spectrum to that of the pH 6.5 solution; in fact, it was not significantly different from the pH 8 scan. King concluded that irreversible changes were occurring that make the compatibility of the admixture suspect (319).

It is interesting to note, however, that the commercial methotrexate sodium (Lederle) used in the study is formulated in solution at a pH of approximately 8.5, not significantly different from that of the admixture suspected of incompatibility, and yet is stable for an extended period until its expiration date.

Aluminum— Ogawa et al. reported that immersion of a needle with an aluminum component in fluorouracil (Adria) 50 mg/ml resulted in no visually apparent reaction after seven days at 24 °C (988).

Other Information

Bacteriostatic Properties— Fluorouracil (Adria) 500 mg/10 ml did not support the growth of several microorganisms commonly implicated in nosocomial infections. The bacteriostatic properties were observed against *Escherichia coli, Klebsiella pneumoniae, Staphylococcus epidermidis, Pseudomonas aeruginosa, Candida albicans,* and *Clostridium perfringens* (828).

In another study, fluorouracil (Adria) 1 g/20 ml transferred to PVC containers did not support the growth of several microorganisms and may have imparted an antimicrobial effect at this concentration. Loss of viability was observed for *Staphylococcus aureus, Escherichia coli, Pseudomonas aeruginosa, Pseudomonas cepacia, Candida albicans,* and *Aspergillus niger* (1187).

Fluorouracil (Lyphomed) eliminated the viability of *Staphylococcus epidermidis* (10^6 to 10^7 CFU/ml) in varying time periods, depending on concentration and diluent, when stored at near-body temperature (35 °C). At 50 mg/ml, no viability was found after five days of incubation. At 10 mg/ml in sodium chloride 0.9% and dextrose 5% in water, no viability was found after seven and five days, respectively. Following dilution to 10 mg/ml with bacteriostatic sodium chloride 0.9%, no viability was found after two days (1659).

Inactivation— In the event of spills or leaks, Adria recommends the use of sodium hypochlorite 5% (household bleach) to inactivate fluorouracil (1200).

FLUPHENAZINE HCL
AHFS 28:16.08

Prolixin   **Apothecon**

Products— Fluphenazine HCl (Apothecon) is available in 10-ml multiple-dose vials. Each milliliter contains fluphenazine HCl 2.5 mg with sodium chloride for isotonicity, sodium hydroxide or hydrochloric acid to adjust the pH, and methylparaben 0.1% and propylparaben 0.01% as preservatives (4; 154).

pH— From 4.8 to 5.2 (4).

Administration— Fluphenazine HCl is administered by intramuscular injection (4).

Stability— Intact vials should be stored at controlled room temperature and protected from freezing and light. Parenteral solutions of fluphenazine HCl vary from colorless to light amber. Solutions that are darker than light amber, are discolored in some other way, or contain a precipitate should not be used (4).

Compatibility Information

Drugs in Syringe Compatibility

Fluphenazine HCl

Drug (in syringe)	Mfr	Amt	Mfr	Amt	Remarks	Ref	C/I
Benztropine mesylate	MSD	2 mg/ 2 ml	LY	5 mg/ 2 ml	Visually compatible for 60 min	1784	**C**
Diphenhydramine HCl	ES	100 mg/ 2 ml	LY	5 mg/ 2 ml	Visually compatible for 60 min	1784	**C**
Hydroxyzine HCl	ES	100 mg/ 2 ml	LY	5 mg/ 2 ml	Visually compatible for 60 min	1784	**C**

FOLIC ACID
AHFS 88:08

Fujisawa

Products— Folic acid injection (Fujisawa) is available in 10-ml vials. Each milliliter of solution contains (1-10/95):

Folic acid (as sodium salt)	5 mg
Edetate sodium	2 mg
Benzyl alcohol	15 mg
Hydrochloric acid and/or sodium hydroxide	to adjust pH
Water for injection	qs

pH— From 8 to 11 (1-10/95; 4).

Osmolality— Folic acid 5 mg/ml has an osmolality of 186 mOsm/kg (1689).

Administration— Folic acid injection is administered by deep intramuscular, intravenous, or subcutaneous injection (1-10/95; 4).

Stability— The yellow to orange-yellow solutions are heat sensitive and should be protected from light (4) for long-term storage. However, exposure of folic acid in parenteral nutrition solutions to fluorescent light for 48 hours did not cause any significant loss of folic acid (896).

pH Effects— Folic acid is soluble in solutions of pH 5.6 or above at room temperature to a concentration of 1 g/L. However, below about pH 4.5 to 5, folic acid may precipitate in varying time periods, depending on the acidity of the solution. In the small concentrations used for parenteral nutrition, a pH of above 5 ensures that folic acid will remain in solution. Most parenteral nutrition solutions are buffered by the amino acids to pH 5 to 6 (895).

Sorption— A parenteral nutrition solution containing 13 μg/L of folic acid injection in a 3-L PVC bag and run through an administration set delivered the full amount of folic acid, with no loss detected by radioimmunoassay (895).

Filtration— Folic acid (Lederle) 0.5 mg/L in dextrose 5% in water and sodium chloride 0.9% was filtered at 120 ml/hr for six hours through a 0.22-μm cellulose ester membrane filter (Ivex-2). No significant reduction in potency due to binding to the filter was noted (533).

Compatibility Information

Solution Compatibility

Folic acid

Solution	Mfr	Mfr	Conc/L	Remarks	Ref	C/I
Amino acids 4.25%, dextrose 25%	MG	USP	0.2 and 10 mg	Physically compatible and stable for at least 7 days at 4 °C and room temperature protected from light	895	**C**
Dextrose 20% in water		USP	0.2 and 20 mg	Physically compatible and stable for at least 7 days at 4 °C and room temperature protected from light	895	**C**

Solution Compatibility (Cont.)

Folic acid

Solution	Mfr	Mfr	Conc/L	Remarks	Ref	C/I
Dextrose 40% in water		USP	0.2 and 20 mg	Approximately 17 to 25% loss in 24 hr at 4 °C and room temperature protected from light, with precipitation at the higher concentration after 48 hr	895	I
Dextrose 50% in water		USP	20 mg	Precipitate forms within 24 hr at 4 °C and room temperature protected from light	895	I
Fat emulsion 10%, intravenous	KV	USP	0.2 and 20 mg	Physically compatible for up to 2 weeks at 4 °C and room temperature protected from light, but highly erratic assays	895	?
	KA	KA[a]	11 mg	Physically compatible for 24 hr at 26 °C with little loss of folic acid and of most other vitamins by HPLC; up to 52% ascorbate loss	2050	C
TPN #11 to #15[b]		LE	2.5 and 5 mg	Physically compatible for 24 hr at 22 °C. UV spectra of amino acids unaltered	313	C
TPN #43 to #47[b]		LE	5 mg	Physically compatible for 24 hr at 22 °C. TLC changes of amino acids in similar solutions attributed to MVI or vitamin B complex with C	313	C
TPN #69[b]		USP	0.4 mg	Physically compatible and folic acid stable for at least 7 days at 4 and 25 °C protected from light	895	C
TPN #70[b]		LE	0.25 to 1 mg	Folic acid stable for at least 48 hr at 6 and 21 °C in the light or dark	896	C
TPN #74[b]			1 mg	Folic acid stable over 8 hr at room temperature exposed to fluorescent light or sunlight	842	C
TPN #189[b]		AB	15 mg/ml	Visually compatible for 24 hr at 22 °C	1767	C

[a]*From multivitamins.*
[b]*Refer to Appendix I for the composition of parenteral nutrition solutions. TPN indicates a 2-in-1 admixture.*

Drugs in Syringe Compatibility

Folic acid

Drug (in syringe)	Mfr	Amt	Mfr	Amt	Remarks	Ref	C/I
Doxapram HCl	RB	400 mg/ 20 ml		15 mg/ 1 ml	Immediate turbidity	1177	I

Y-Site Injection Compatibility (1:1 Mixture)

Folic acid

Drug	Mfr	Conc	Mfr	Conc	Remarks	Ref	C/I
Famotidine	MSD	0.2 mg/ml[a]	LE	5 mg/ml	Physically compatible for 14 hr	1196	C

[a]*Tested in dextrose 5% in water.*

Additional Compatibility Information

Folic acid injection is stated to be incompatible with oxidizing and reducing agents and heavy metal ions (4).

Calcium— Calcium gluconate (Parke-Davis) and folic acid injection (Lederle) have been shown to interact even though a precipitate is not present. The recoverable amount of folic acid from a 10-μg/ml solution declined with increasing concentrations (0.5 to 10 μg/ml) of calcium gluconate. This interaction was reversed by the addition of edetic acid (538).

Solutions— The stability of folic acid from a multiple vitamin product in dextrose 5% in water and sodium chloride 0.9%, in both PVC and ClearFlex containers, was evaluated. HPLC analysis showed that folic acid was stable at 23 °C when either protected from or exposed to light, exhibiting little or no loss (1509).

Parenteral Nutrition Solutions— Shine and Farwell reported a 40% drop in folic acid concentration immediately after admixture in a parenteral nutrition solution composed of amino acids, dextrose, electrolytes, trace elements, and multivitamins in PVC bags. The folic acid concentration then remained relatively constant for 28 days when stored at both 4 and 25 °C (1063).

Extensive decomposition of ascorbic acid and folic acid was reported in a parenteral nutrition solution composed of amino acids 3.3%, dextrose 12.5%, electrolytes, trace elements, and M.V.I.-12 (USV) in PVC bags. Half-lives were 1.1, 2.9, and 8.9 hours for ascorbic acid and 2.7, 5.4, and 24 hours for folic acid stored at 24

°C in daylight, 24 °C protected from light, and 4 °C protected from light, respectively. The decomposition was much greater than for solutions not containing catalyzing metal ions. Also, it was greater than for the vitamins singly because of interactions with the other vitamins present (1059).

Because of these interactions, recommendations to separate the administration of vitamins and trace elements have been made (1056; 1060; 1061). Other researchers have termed such recommendations premature based on differing reports (895; 896) and the apparent absence of epidemic vitamin deficiency in parenteral nutrition patients (1062).

Smith et al. reported the stability of several vitamins from M.V.I.-12 (Armour) admixed in parenteral nutrition solutions composed of different amino acid products, with or without Intralipid 10%, in glass bottles and PVC bags at 25 and 5 °C for 48 hours. Folic acid was stable in all samples (1431).

FOSCARNET SODIUM
AHFS 8:18

Foscavir   **Astra**

Products— Foscarnet sodium (Astra) is available as a 24-mg/ml infusion solution in water for injection in 250- and 500-ml glass bottles. Hydrochloric acid and/or sodium hydroxide may be added to adjust the pH (2).

pH— Adjusted to pH 7.4 (2).

Osmolality— Foscarnet sodium 24 mg/ml has an osmolality of 271 mOsm/kg (1689).

Administration— Foscarnet sodium is administered by intravenous infusion, using an infusion pump. It should not be given by rapid injection. Recommended rates of infusion are a minimum of one hour for doses of 60 mg/kg and up to two hours for doses of 120 mg/kg. Recommended dosage, frequency, and administration rates should not be exceeded. For peripheral administration, foscarnet sodium solution must be diluted to 12 mg/ml with dextrose 5% in water or sodium chloride 0.9%. The drug may be infused without dilution through a central catheter (2; 4).

Stability— Foscarnet sodium injection is a clear, colorless solution. It should be stored at controlled room temperature and protected from temperatures above 40 °C and from freezing. The product should be used only if the seal is intact and a vacuum is present (2).

The manufacturer has stated that foscarnet sodium diluted in dextrose 5% in water or sodium chloride 0.9% and transferred to PVC containers is stable for 24 hours at room temperature or under refrigeration (71).

Autoclaving— The concentration of foscarnet sodium (Astra), diluted in sodium chloride 0.9% to 12 mg/ml and packaged in glass infusion bottles with rubber bungs, was compared before and after autoclaving at 30 psi for 15 minutes at 121 °C. HPLC analysis determined that the foscarnet sodium concentration did not change after autoclaving. Therefore, the dilution may be autoclaved to avoid limiting its shelf life due to sterility concerns (1835).

Elastomeric Reservoir Pumps— Foscarnet sodium (Astra) 24 mg/ml was evaluated for binding potential to natural rubber elastomeric reservoirs (Baxter). No loss was found after storage for two weeks at 35 °C with gentle agitation (2014).

Compatibility Information

Solution Compatibility

Foscarnet sodium

Solution	Mfr	Mfr	Conc/L	Remarks	Ref	C/I
Dextrose 5% in water	BA[a]	AST	12 g	Visually compatible and chemically stable by UV spectroscopy for 35 days at 5 and 25 °C	1834	C
Sodium chloride 0.9%	MG[a]	AST	12 g	Visually compatible and chemically stable by HPLC for 30 days at 25 °C in light or dark and at 5 °C in the dark	1726	C

Solution Compatibility (Cont.)

Foscarnet sodium

Solution	Mfr	Mfr	Conc/L	Remarks	Ref	C/I
	BA[a]	AST	12 g	Visually compatible and chemically stable by UV spectroscopy for 35 days at 5 and 25 °C	1834	C

[a]Tested in PVC containers.

Additive Compatibility

Foscarnet sodium

Drug	Mfr	Conc/L	Mfr	Conc/L	Test Soln	Remarks	Ref	C/I
Potassium chloride		20, 40, 60, 80, 120 mmol	AST	12 g	NS	Foscarnet stability was maintained for at least 65 hr. UV analysis found concentrations of 93 to 99% throughout	2156	C

Y-Site Injection Compatibility (1:1 Mixture)

Foscarnet sodium

Drug	Mfr	Conc	Mfr	Conc	Remarks	Ref	C/I
Acyclovir sodium	BW	10 mg/ml	AST	24 mg/ml	Immediate precipitation	1335	I
	BW	7 mg/ml[a,b]	AST	24 mg/ml	Acyclovir crystals form immediately	1393	I
Aldesleukin	CHI	33,800 I.U./ml[a]	AST	24 mg/ml	Visually compatible with little or no loss of aldesleukin activity by bioassay	1857	C
Amikacin sulfate	BR	20 mg/ml	AST	24 mg/ml	Physically compatible for 24 hr at room temperature under fluorescent light	1335	C
Aminophylline	LY	25 mg/ml	AST	24 mg/ml	Physically compatible for 24 hr at room temperature under fluorescent light	1335	C
Amphotericin B	SQ	5 mg/ml	AST	24 mg/ml	Delayed formation of cloudy yellow precipitate	1335	I
	SQ	0.6 mg/ml[a]	AST	24 mg/ml	Dense haze forms immediately	1393	I
Ampicillin sodium	WY	20 mg/ml	AST	24 mg/ml	Physically compatible for 24 hr at room temperature under fluorescent light	1335	C
Aztreonam	SQ	40 mg/ml	AST	24 mg/ml	Physically compatible for 24 hr at room temperature under fluorescent light	1335	C
	SQ	40 mg/ml[a,b]	AST	24 mg/ml	Physically compatible for 24 hr at 25 °C under fluorescent light by visual and microscopic examination	1393	C
Cefazolin sodium	SKF	40 mg/ml	AST	24 mg/ml	Physically compatible for 24 hr at room temperature under fluorescent light	1335	C
Cefoperazone sodium	RR	40 mg/ml	AST	24 mg/ml	Physically compatible for 24 hr at room temperature under fluorescent light	1335	C
Cefoxitin sodium	MSD	40 mg/ml	AST	24 mg/ml	Physically compatible for 24 hr at room temperature under fluorescent light	1335	C
Ceftazidime	GL	20 mg/ml	AST	24 mg/ml	Physically compatible for 24 hr at room temperature under fluorescent light	1335	C
	GL	20 mg/ml[a,b]	AST	24 mg/ml	Physically compatible for 24 hr at 25 °C under fluorescent light by visual and microscopic examination	1393	C

Y-Site Injection Compatibility (1:1 Mixture) (Cont.)

Foscarnet sodium

Drug	Mfr	Conc	Mfr	Conc	Remarks	Ref	C/I
Ceftizoxime sodium	SKF	40 mg/ml	AST	24 mg/ml	Physically compatible for 24 hr at room temperature under fluorescent light	1335	C
Ceftriaxone sodium	RC	20 mg/ml[a,b]	AST	24 mg/ml	Physically compatible for 24 hr at 25 °C under fluorescent light by visual and microscopic examination	1393	C
Cefuroxime sodium	GL	30 mg/ml	AST	24 mg/ml	Physically compatible for 24 hr at room temperature under fluorescent light	1335	C
Chloramphenicol sodium succinate	PD	20 mg/ml	AST	24 mg/ml	Physically compatible for 24 hr at room temperature under fluorescent light	1335	C
Cimetidine HCl	SKF	150 mg/ml	AST	24 mg/ml	Physically compatible for 24 hr at room temperature under fluorescent light	1335	C
Clindamycin phosphate	AB	24 mg/ml	AST	24 mg/ml	Physically compatible for 24 hr at room temperature under fluorescent light	1335	C
	UP	12 mg/ml[a,b]	AST	24 mg/ml	Physically compatible for 24 hr at 25 °C under fluorescent light by visual and microscopic examination	1393	C
Dexamethasone sodium phosphate	OR	10 mg/ml	AST	24 mg/ml	Physically compatible for 24 hr at room temperature under fluorescent light	1335	C
Diazepam	ES	5 mg/ml	AST	24 mg/ml	Gas production	1335	I
Digoxin	WY	0.25 mg/ml	AST	24 mg/ml	Gas production	1335	I
Diphenhydramine HCl	PD	50 mg/ml	AST	24 mg/ml	Cloudy solution	1335	I
Dobutamine HCl	LI	12.5 mg/ml	AST	24 mg/ml	Delayed formation of muddy precipitate	1335	I
Dopamine HCl	DU	80 mg/ml	AST	24 mg/ml	Physically compatible for 24 hr at room temperature under fluorescent light	1335	C
Droperidol	QU	2.5 mg/ml	AST	24 mg/ml	Delayed formation of fine yellow precipitate	1335	I
Erythromycin lactobionate	AB	20 mg/ml	AST	24 mg/ml	Physically compatible for 24 hr at room temperature under fluorescent light	1335	C
	ES	20 mg/ml[a,b]	AST	24 mg/ml	Physically compatible for 24 hr at 25 °C under fluorescent light by visual and microscopic examination	1393	C
Fluconazole	RR	2 mg/ml	AST	24 mg/ml	Physically compatible for 24 hr at 25 °C	1407	C
Flucytosine	RC	10 mg/ml[b]	AST	24 mg/ml	Physically compatible for 24 hr at 25 °C under fluorescent light by visual and microscopic examination	1393	C
Furosemide	AB	10 mg/ml	AST	24 mg/ml	Physically compatible for 24 hr at room temperature under fluorescent light	1335	C
Ganciclovir sodium		50 mg/ml	AST	24 mg/ml	Immediate precipitation	1335	I
Gentamicin sulfate	ES	4 mg/ml	AST	24 mg/ml	Physically compatible for 24 hr at room temperature under fluorescent light	1335	C
	ES	2 mg/ml[a,b]	AST	24 mg/ml	Physically compatible for 24 hr at 25 °C under fluorescent light by visual and microscopic examination	1393	C
Haloperidol lactate	LY	5 mg/ml	AST	24 mg/ml	Delayed formation of fine white precipitate	1335	I
Heparin sodium	ES	1000 units/ml	AST	24 mg/ml	Physically compatible for 24 hr at room temperature under fluorescent light	1335	C

Y-Site Injection Compatibility (1:1 Mixture) (Cont.)

			Foscarnet sodium				
Drug	*Mfr*	*Conc*	*Mfr*	*Conc*	*Remarks*	*Ref*	*C/I*
	LY	100 units/ml[a,b]	AST	24 mg/ml	Physically compatible for 24 hr at 25 °C under fluorescent light by visual and microscopic examination	1393	C
Hydrocortisone sodium succinate	UP	50 mg/ml	AST	24 mg/ml	Physically compatible for 24 hr at room temperature under fluorescent light	1335	C
Hydromorphone HCl	KN	10 mg/ml	AST	24 mg/ml	Physically compatible for 24 hr at room temperature under fluorescent light	1335	C
Hydroxyzine HCl	LY	50 mg/ml	AST	24 mg/ml	Physically compatible for 24 hr at room temperature under fluorescent light	1335	C
Imipenem–cilastatin sodium	MSD	10 mg/ml	AST	24 mg/ml	Physically compatible for 24 hr at room temperature under fluorescent light	1335	C
	MSD	5 mg/ml[a]	AST	24 mg/ml	Physically compatible for 24 hr at 25 °C under fluorescent light by visual and microscopic examination	1393	C
Leucovorin calcium	QU	10 mg/ml	AST	24 mg/ml	Cloudy yellow solution	1335	I
Lorazepam	WY	4 mg/ml	AST	24 mg/ml	Gas production	1335	I
	WY	0.08 mg/ml[a,b]	AST	24 mg/ml	Physically compatible for 24 hr at 25 °C under fluorescent light by visual and microscopic examination	1393	C
Metoclopramide HCl	RB	4 mg/ml	AST	24 mg/ml	Physically compatible for 24 hr at room temperature under fluorescent light	1335	C
	RB	2 mg/ml[a,b]	AST	24 mg/ml	Physically compatible for 24 hr at 25 °C under fluorescent light by visual and microscopic examination	1393	C
Metronidazole	AB	5 mg/ml	AST	24 mg/ml	Physically compatible for 24 hr at room temperature under fluorescent light	1335	C
	SE	5 mg/ml	AST	24 mg/ml	Physically compatible for 24 hr at 25 °C under fluorescent light by visual and microscopic examination	1393	C
Midazolam HCl	RC	5 mg/ml	AST	24 mg/ml	Gas production	1335	I
Morphine sulfate	IMS	1 mg/ml	AST	24 mg/ml	Physically compatible for 24 hr at room temperature under fluorescent light	1335	C
	ES	1 mg/ml[a,b]	AST	24 mg/ml	Physically compatible for 24 hr at 25 °C under fluorescent light by visual and microscopic examination	1393	C
	ES	5[b] and 15 mg/ml	AST	24 mg/ml	Visually compatible for 24 hr at 23 °C under fluorescent light	1529	C
Nafcillin sodium	BR	20 mg/ml[a,b]	AST	24 mg/ml	Physically compatible for 24 hr at 25 °C under fluorescent light by visual and microscopic examination	1393	C
Oxacillin sodium	BR	40 mg/ml	AST	24 mg/ml	Physically compatible for 24 hr at room temperature under fluorescent light	1335	C
	BE	20 mg/ml[a,b]	AST	24 mg/ml	Physically compatible for 24 hr at 25 °C under fluorescent light by visual and microscopic examination	1393	C
Penicillin G potassium	SQ	100,000 units/ml	AST	24 mg/ml	Physically compatible for 24 hr at room temperature under fluorescent light	1335	C
Pentamidine isethionate	LY	6 mg/ml	AST	24 mg/ml	Immediate precipitation	1335	I
	LY	6 mg/ml[a,b]	AST	24 mg/ml	Pentamidine crystals form immediately	1393	I

Y-Site Injection Compatibility (1:1 Mixture) (Cont.)

Foscarnet sodium

Drug	Mfr	Conc	Mfr	Conc	Remarks	Ref	C/I
Phenytoin sodium	PD	50 mg/ml	AST	24 mg/ml	Physically compatible for 24 hr at room temperature under fluorescent light	1335	C
Piperacillin sodium	LE	80 mg/ml	AST	24 mg/ml	Physically compatible for 24 hr at room temperature under fluorescent light	1335	C
Prochlorperazine edisylate	SKF	5 mg/ml	AST	24 mg/ml	Cloudy brown solution	1335	I
Promethazine HCl	ES	50 mg/ml	AST	24 mg/ml	Gas production	1335	I
Ranitidine HCl	GL	2 mg/ml[a,b]	AST	24 mg/ml	Physically compatible for 24 hr at 25 °C under fluorescent light by visual and microscopic examination	1393	C
Ticarcillin disodium–clavulanate potassium	BE	100 mg/ml[a,b]	AST	24 mg/ml	Physically compatible for 24 hr at 25 °C under fluorescent light by visual and microscopic examination	1393	C
Tobramycin sulfate	LI	40 mg/ml	AST	24 mg/ml	Physically compatible for 24 hr at room temperature under fluorescent light	1335	C
Trimethoprim–sulfamethoxazole	RC	16 + 80 mg/ml	AST	24 mg/ml	Immediate precipitation and gas production	1335	I
	BW	0.53 + 2.6 mg/ml[a]	AST	24 mg/ml	Physically compatible for 24 hr at 25 °C under fluorescent light by visual and microscopic examination	1393	C
Trimetrexate	WL	1 mg/ml[a]	AST	24 mg/ml	Trimetrexate crystals form immediately	1393	I
Vancomycin HCl	LE	20 mg/ml	AST	24 mg/ml	Immediate precipitation	1335	I
	LE	15 mg/ml[a,b]	AST	24 mg/ml	Physically compatible for 24 hr at 25 °C under fluorescent light by visual and microscopic examination	1393	C
	LE	10 mg/ml[b]	AST	24 mg/ml	Visually compatible for 24 hr at room temperature in test tubes. No precipitate found on filter from Y-site delivery	2063	C
TPN #121[d]		[c]	AST	24 mg/ml	Physically compatible for 24 hr at 25 °C under fluorescent light by visual and microscopic examination	1393	C

[a]Tested in dextrose 5% in water.
[b]Tested in sodium chloride 0.9%.
[c]Tested in equal quantities.
[d]Refer to Appendix I for the composition of parenteral nutrition solutions. TPN indicates a 2-in-1 admixture.

Additional Compatibility Information

The manufacturer recommends dextrose 5% in water or sodium chloride 0.9% for diluting foscarnet sodium for peripheral administration and the use of such dilutions within 24 hours of first opening the sealed bottle (2).

The manufacturer also recommends that no other drug or solution be administered concurrently through the same catheter as foscarnet sodium. Dextrose 30% and numerous drugs have been reported to cause physical incompatibilities with foscarnet sodium. (See Compatibility Information.) Additionally, foscarnet sodium may chelate divalent metal ions and is chemically incompatible with solutions containing calcium such as Ringer's injection, lactated, and parenteral nutrition solutions (2).

Other Information

Bacterial Challenge— Foscarnet sodium (Astra) 13 mg/ml diluted in sodium chloride 0.9% at 22 °C did not exhibit an antibacterial effect on the growth of three organisms (*Enterococcus faecium, Staphylococcus aureus,* and *Pseudomonas aeruginosa*) inoculated into the solution. Foscarnet sodium did exhibit moderate antifungal activity against *Candida albicans.* The authors recommended that ready-to-use solutions be stored under refrigeration whenever possible and that the potential for microbiological growth should be considered when assigning expiration periods (2160).

FOSPHENYTOIN SODIUM
AHFS 28:12.12

Cerebyx   **Parke-Davis**

Products— Fosphenytoin is the prodrug for its metabolite, phenytoin. Fosphenytoin sodium is available in 2- and 10-ml vials as a 75-mg/ml solution, which is the equivalent of phenytoin sodium 50 mg/ml after administration. Each milliliter also contains tromethamine (TRIS) buffer along with hydrochloric acid or sodium hydroxide to adjust pH in water for injection (2). CAUTION: Care should be taken to avoid confusion between the two different forms (fosphenytoin sodium and phenytoin sodium) to prevent dosing errors.

pH— From 8.6 to 9.0 (2).

Units— Each 75 mg of fosphenytoin sodium is metabolically converted to 50 mg of phenytoin after administration. NOTE: The amount and concentration of fosphenytoin sodium are expressed in terms of the equivalent mass of phenytoin sodium, called phenytoin sodium equivalents (PE). The manufacturer indicates that this avoids the need to perform conversions based on molecular weight between the two forms (2). However, it creates the need to express all prescribing, dispensing, and dosing consistently in PE to avoid dosing errors that could result from confusion between the two forms.

Administration— Fosphenytoin sodium is dosed in terms of phenytoin sodium equivalents (PE). (See Units section above.) CAUTION: Care should be taken to ensure that all prescribing, preparation, and dosing is performed using the correct units and that any confusion between the two forms (fosphenytoin sodium and phenytoin sodium) is avoided.

Fosphenytoin sodium is administered intravenously at a rate no greater than 150 mg PE/min. The drug may be diluted in dextrose 5% in water or sodium chloride 0.9% to a concentration of 1.5 to 25 mg PE/ml. It has also been given intramuscularly (2).

Stability— Fosphenytoin sodium injection is a clear, colorless to pale yellow solution. Intact vials should be stored under refrigeration at 2 to 8 °C. Storage at controlled room temperature should not exceed 48 hours. Any vials that develop particulate matter should not be used (2).

Syringes— Fosphenytoin sodium (Parke-Davis) 50 mg PE (phenytoin sodium equivalents) per milliliter was packaged in 3-ml polypropylene syringes with syringe caps (Becton-Dickinson) and stored at −20, 4, and 25 °C. The samples stored at 4 and 25 °C exhibited little or no loss of fosphenytoin sodium by HPLC analysis in 30 days. The samples stored at −20 °C also showed little or no loss of fosphenytoin sodium after 30 days' storage followed by seven days at 4 °C or at 25 °C. Also, stability was maintained if the thawed samples that had been stored at 25 °C were returned to the freezer for an additional seven days (2083).

Freezing Solutions — Fosphenytoin sodium (Parke-Davis) 1, 8, and 20 mg PE (phenytoin sodium equivalents) per milliliter in dextrose 5% in water (Baxter) and sodium chloride 0.9% (Baxter) in PVC containers and undiluted fosphenytoin sodium 50 mg PE per milliliter were packaged in 3-ml polypropylene syringes with syringe caps (Becton-Dickinson). The samples were frozen at −20 °C. Little or no loss of fosphenytoin sodium occurred after 30 days of frozen storage followed by seven days at 4 °C or at 25 °C. Stability was also maintained if the thawed samples that had been stored at 25 °C were returned to the freezer for an additional seven days (2083).

Sorption— No loss of fosphenytoin sodium (Parke-Davis) due to sorption to PVC containers was observed when compared to glass bottles (2083).

Compatibility Information

Solution Compatibility

Fosphenytoin sodium[a]

Solution	Mfr	Mfr	Conc/L	Remarks	Ref	C/I
Amino acid injection 10%	BA[b]	PD	1, 8, 20 mg PE/ml	Visually compatible with little or no loss of fosphenytoin by HPLC in 7 days at 25 °C under fluorescent light	2083	C
Dextrose 5% in Ringer's injection, lactated	BA[b]	PD	1, 8, 20 mg PE/ml	Visually compatible with little or no loss of fosphenytoin by HPLC in 7 days at 25 °C under fluorescent light	2083	C
Dextrose 5% in sodium chloride 0.45%	BA[b]	PD	1, 8, 20 mg PE/ml	Visually compatible with little or no loss of fosphenytoin by HPLC in 7 days at 25 °C under fluorescent light	2083	C
Dextrose 5% in water	BA[b,c]	PD	1, 8, 20 mg PE/ml	Visually compatible with little or no loss of fosphenytoin by HPLC in 30 days at 25 °C under fluorescent light	2083	C
	BA[b]	PD	1, 8, 20 mg PE/ml	Visually compatible with little or no loss of fosphenytoin by HPLC in 30 days at 4 °C under fluorescent light	2083	C

Solution Compatibility (Cont.)

Fosphenytoin sodium[a]

Solution	Mfr	Mfr	Conc/L	Remarks	Ref	C/I
Dextrose 10% in water	BA[b]	PD	1, 8, 20 mg PE/ml	Visually compatible with little or no loss of fosphenytoin by HPLC in 7 days at 25 °C under fluorescent light	2083	C
Hetastarch 6% in sodium chloride 0.9%	MG	PD	1, 8, 20 mg PE/ml	Visually compatible with little or no loss of fosphenytoin by HPLC in 7 days at 25 °C under fluorescent light	2083	C
Mannitol 20%	BA[b]	PD	1, 8, 20 mg PE/ml	Visually compatible with little or no loss of fosphenytoin by HPLC in 7 days at 25 °C under fluorescent light	2083	C
Plasma-Lyte A, pH 7.4	BA[b]	PD	1, 8, 20 mg PE/ml	Visually compatible with little or no loss of fosphenytoin by HPLC in 7 days at 25 °C under fluorescent light	2083	C
Ringer's injection, lactated	BA[b]	PD	1, 8, 20 mg PE/ml	Visually compatible with little or no loss of fosphenytoin by HPLC in 7 days at 25 °C under fluorescent light	2083	C
Sodium chloride 0.9%	BA[b,c]	PD	1, 8, 20 mg PE/ml	Visually compatible with little or no loss of fosphenytoin by HPLC in 30 days at 25 °C under fluorescent light	2083	C
	BA[b]	PD	1, 8, 20 mg PE/ml	Visually compatible with little or no loss of fosphenytoin by HPLC in 30 days at 4 °C under fluorescent light	2083	C

[a]Concentration expressed in milligrams of phenytoin sodium equivalents (PE) per milliliter.
[b]Tested in PVC containers.
[c]Tested in glass bottles.

Additive Compatibility

Fosphenytoin sodium[a]

Drug	Mfr	Conc/L	Mfr	Conc/L	Test Soln	Remarks	Ref	C/I
Potassium chloride	BA	20 and 40 mEq	PD	1, 8, 20 mg PE/ml	D5½S[b]	Visually compatible with little or no loss of fosphenytoin by HPLC in 7 days at 25 °C under fluorescent light	2083	C

[a]Concentration expressed in milligrams of phenytoin sodium equivalents (PE) per milliliter.
[b]Tested in PVC containers.

FUROSEMIDE
(FRUSEMIDE)
AHFS 40:28

Products— Furosemide is available in 2-, 4-, and 10-ml amber ampuls, single-use vials, and prefilled syringes. Each milliliter of solution contains furosemide 10 mg, with sodium chloride for isotonicity and sodium hydroxide for slight alkalinity (4; 154).

pH— From 8 to 9.3 (4).

Osmolality— Furosemide (Hoechst-Roussel) 10 mg/ml has an osmolality of 287 mOsm/kg (50). The osmolality of the Elkins-Sinn product has been determined to be 289 mOsm/kg by freezing-point depression (1071).

In another study, the osmolality of furosemide injection (manufacturer unspecified) was determined to be 291 mOsm/kg (1233).

Sodium Content— The injection contains 0.162 mEq of sodium per milliliter (4).

Administration— Furosemide may be administered by intramuscular injection, by direct intravenous injection over one to two minutes, and by intravenous infusion at a rate not exceeding 4 mg/min (1-5/97; 4).

Stability— Exposure to light may cause discoloration; protection from light for the syringes once they are removed from the package is recommended. Do not use furosemide solutions if they have a yellow color. Furosemide products should be stored at controlled room temperature (1-5/97; 4). Refrigeration may result in precipitation or crystallization. However, resolubilization at room temperature or on warming may be performed without affecting the drug's stability (593).

pH Effects— Furosemide is soluble in alkaline solutions and is prepared as a mildly buffered alkaline product (1-5/97; 4). It can usually be mixed with infusion solutions that are neutral or weakly basic (pH 7 to 10) and with some weakly acidic solutions that have a low buffer capacity (4). It should not be mixed with acidic solutions having a pH below 5.5. Solutions such as sodium chloride 0.9%, Ringer's injection, lactated, and dextrose 5% in water have been recommended. If the solution pH is below 5.5, pH adjustment has been recommended (1-5/97; 4). In addition, furosemide has been found to be unstable in acidic media but very stable in basic media (664). Also see Acidic Additives under Additional Compatibility Information below.

Syringes— Furosemide (Hoechst-Roussel) 10 mg/ml retained potency for three months at room temperature when 2 ml of solution was packaged in Tubex cartridges (13).

Furosemide (Hoechst) 10 mg/ml was filled into 25-ml polypropylene syringes (Becton-Dickinson) and stored at 25 °C while exposed to normal room light or in the dark for 24 hours. There was no detectable change in furosemide content in either light-exposed or light-protected syringes (1108).

Effects of Light— Furosemide is subject to photodegradation by several mechanisms. Photodegradation is minimized at pH 7; rates of decomposition increase as the pH becomes more acidic or basic. Photodegradation is unaffected by ionic strength and initial concentration (in the range of 10 µg/ml to 1 mg/ml), but the rate of loss may decrease at the higher concentration due to a light-filtering effect of the yellow discoloration. In pH 7 phosphate buffer, more than 60% furosemide loss occurred in transparent glass vials exposed to fluorescent light for 90 hours; little or no loss occurred if the transparent vials were covered with aluminum foil or if amber glass containers were used (2067).

Autoclaving— Autoclaving of furosemide 1 mg/ml in sodium chloride 0.9% in glass bottles at 115 °C for 34 minutes resulted in no loss of furosemide. Storage of the solution for 70 days at room temperature with protection from light also showed no detectable change in furosemide content. However, storage at room temperature with exposure to light for 70 days resulted in about a 60% loss of furosemide and the formation of a yellow-orange precipitate (1108).

Filtration— Furosemide (Hoechst) 0.04 mg/ml in dextrose 5% in water and sodium chloride 0.9% was filtered through a 0.22-µm cellulose ester membrane filter (Ivex-HP, Millipore) over six hours. No significant drug loss due to binding to the filter was noted (1034).

Compatibility Information

Solution Compatibility

Furosemide

Solution	Mfr	Mfr	Conc/L	Remarks	Ref	C/I
Alcohol 5% and dextrose 5%	BA	HO	600 mg	Physically compatible for 24 hr	315	**C**
Amino acids 4.25%, dextrose 25%	MG	HO	40 mg	No increase in particulate matter in 24 hr at 25 °C	349	**C**
Dextrose 5% in Ringer's injection, lactated	BA	HO	600 mg	Physically compatible for 24 hr	315	**C**
Dextrose 5% in sodium chloride 0.9%	BA	HO	600 mg	Physically compatible for 24 hr	315	**C**
Dextrose 5% in water	BA	HO	600 mg	Physically compatible for 24 hr	315	**C**
			200 and 400 mg	4 to 5% loss in 24 hr at 25 °C	1348	**C**
Dextrose 10% in water	BA	HO	600 mg	Physically compatible for 24 hr	315	**C**
Dextrose 20% in water	BA	HO	600 mg	Physically compatible for 24 hr	315	**C**

Solution Compatibility (Cont.)

Furosemide

Solution	Mfr	Mfr	Conc/L	Remarks	Ref	C/I
Fructose 10% in water	BA	HO	300 and 600 mg	Precipitate forms within 24 hr	315	I
Invert sugar 10% in Electrolyte #1	BA	HO	600 mg	Physically compatible for 24 hr	315	C
Invert sugar 10% in Electrolyte #2	BA	HO	300 and 600 mg	Precipitate forms within 24 hr	315	I
Mannitol 20%	BA[a]	AB	200, 400, 800 mg	Visually compatible for 72 hr at 22 °C	1803	C
Ringer's injection, lactated	BA	HO	600 mg	Physically compatible for 24 hr	315	C
	TR[a]	HO	1 g	No furosemide loss in 24 hr at 25 °C exposed to light or in the dark	1108	C
Sodium chloride 0.9%	BA	HO	600 mg	Physically compatible for 24 hr	315	C
	TR[a]	HO	1 g	No furosemide loss in 24 hr at 25 °C exposed to light or in the dark. 10% loss in 26 days at 6 °C	1108	C
			200 and 400 mg	5 to 7% loss in 24 hr at 25 °C	1348	C
Sodium lactate ⅙ M	BA	HO	600 mg	Physically compatible for 24 hr	315	C

[a]Tested in PVC containers.

Additive Compatibility

Furosemide

Drug	Mfr	Conc/L	Mfr	Conc/L	Test Soln	Remarks	Ref	C/I
Amikacin sulfate	BR	2 g	HO	160 mg	D5W, NS	Transient cloudiness during admixture but then physically compatible for 24 hr at 21 °C	876	C
Aminophylline	ANT	1 g	HO	1 g	NS	Physically compatible for 72 hr at 15 and 30 °C	1479	C
Amiodarone HCl	LZ	1.8 g	ES	200 mg	D5W, NS[a]	Physically compatible with 8% or less amiodarone loss in 24 hr at 24 °C under fluorescent light	1031	C
	LZ	4 g	HO	1 g	D5W	Haze forms in 5 hr and precipitate forms in 24 to 72 hr at 30 °C. No change at 15 °C	1479	I
Ampicillin sodium	BE	20 g	HO	1 g	NS	Physically compatible for 72 hr at 15 and 30 °C	1479	C
Atropine sulfate	ANT	60 mg	HO	1 g	W	Physically compatible for 72 hr at 15 and 30 °C	1479	C
Bumetanide	LEO	6 mg	HO	1 g	NS	Physically compatible for 72 hr at 15 and 30 °C	1479	C
Buprenorphine HCl		75 mg	HO	1 g	W	Haze for 6 hr at 30 °C. No change at 15 °C	1479	I
Calcium gluconate	ANT	2 g	HO	1 g	NS	Physically compatible for 72 hr at 15 and 30 °C	1479	C
Cefamandole nafate	DI	20 g	HO	1 g	W	Physically compatible for 72 hr at 15 and 30 °C	1479	C

Additive Compatibility (Cont.)

Furosemide

Drug	Mfr	Conc/L	Mfr	Conc/L	Test Soln	Remarks	Ref	C/I
Cefoperazone sodium	RR	10 g	HO	200 mg	D5W	Physically compatible with 10% loss of both drugs in 15 days at 25 °C and in 20 days at 4 °C in the dark	1402	**C**
Cefuroxime sodium	GL	37.5 g	HO	1 g	W	Physically compatible for 72 hr at 15 and 30 °C	1479	**C**
Chlorpromazine HCl	ANT	5 g	HO	1 g	W	Immediate precipitation	1479	**I**
Cimetidine HCl	SKF	3 g	HO	400 mg	D5W	Physically compatible and cimetidine chemically stable for 24 hr at room temperature. Furosemide not tested	551	**C**
	SKF	4 g	HO	1 g	NS	Physically compatible for 72 hr at 15 and 30 °C	1479	**C**
Dexamethasone sodium phosphate	MSD	4 g	HO	1 g	NS	Physically compatible for 72 hr at 15 and 30 °C	1479	**C**
Diamorphine HCl	EV	500 mg	HO	1 g	W	Physically compatible for 72 hr at 15 and 30 °C	1479	**C**
Diazepam	PHX	1 g	HO	1 g	D5W	Immediate precipitation	1479	**I**
Digoxin	BW	25 mg	HO	1 g	NS	Physically compatible for 72 hr at 15 and 30 °C	1479	**C**
Dobutamine HCl	LI	1 g	HO	1 g	D5W, NS	Cloudy in 1 hr at 25 °C	789	**I**
	LI	1 g	WY	5 g	D5W, NS	Immediate white precipitate	812	**I**
	LI	500 mg	HO	1 g	NS	Haze forms immediately	1479	**I**
Epinephrine HCl	ANT	8 mg	HO	1 g	W	Physically compatible for 72 hr at 15 and 30 °C	1479	**C**
Erythromycin lactobionate	AB	5 g	HO	1 g	NS	Immediate precipitation. Crystals form in 12 to 24 hr at 15 and 30 °C	1479	**I**
Gentamicin sulfate	SC	1.6 g	HO	800 mg	D5W, NS	Immediate precipitation of furosemide	876	**I**
	RS	8 g	HO	1 g	NS	Physically compatible for 24 hr at 15 and 30 °C. Slight precipitate forms in 48 to 72 hr	1479	**C**
Heparin sodium	WED	20,000 units	HO	1 g	NS	Physically compatible for 72 hr at 15 and 30 °C	1479	**C**
Hydrocortisone sodium succinate		1 g		200 and 400 mg	D5W, NS	6 to 8% hydrocortisone loss and 5 to 6% furosemide loss in 24 hr at 25 °C	1348	**C**
		300 mg		200 and 400 mg	D5W, NS	6 to 8% hydrocortisone loss in 6 hr and 10 to 14% loss in 24 hr at 25 °C. 5 to 6% furosemide loss in 24 hr	1348	**I**
	UP	50 g	HO	1 g	NS	Physically compatible for 72 hr at 15 and 30 °C	1479	**C**
Isoproterenol HCl	PX	4 mg	HO	1 g	D5W	Immediate precipitation	1479	**I**
Isosorbide dinitrate		1 g	HO	1 g		Physically compatible for 72 hr at 15 and 30 °C	1479	**C**
Kanamycin sulfate	BE	2 g	HO	160 mg	D5W, NS	Transient cloudiness during admixture, but then physically compatible for 24 hr at 21 °C	876	**C**
Lidocaine HCl	ANT	2 g	HO	1 g	NS	Physically compatible for 72 hr at 15 and 30 °C	1479	**C**
Meperidine HCl	RC	5 g	HO	1 g	W	Fine precipitate forms immediately	1479	**I**

Additive Compatibility (Cont.)

		Furosemide						
Drug	Mfr	Conc/L	Mfr	Conc/L	Test Soln	Remarks	Ref	C/I
Meropenem	ZEN	1 and 20 g	HO	1 g	NS	Visually compatible for 4 hr at room temperature	1994	C
Metoclopramide HCl	ANT	1 g	HO	1 g	NS	Immediate precipitation	1479	I
Morphine sulfate	EV	1 g	HO	1 g	W	Physically compatible for 72 hr at 15 and 30 °C	1479	C
Netilmicin sulfate	SC	1.5 g	HO	400 mg	D5W, NS	Immediate precipitation of furosemide	876	I
Nitroglycerin	ACC	400 mg	HO	1 g	D5W[b]	Physically compatible with no nitroglycerin loss in 48 hr at 23 °C. Furosemide not tested	929	C
	ACC	400 mg	HO	1 g	NS[b]	Physically compatible with 3% nitroglycerin loss in 48 hr at 23 °C. Furosemide not tested	929	C
Penicillin G	GL	12 g	HO	1 g	NS	Physically compatible for 24 hr at 15 and 30 °C. Precipitate forms in 48 to 72 hr at 30 °C. No change at 15 °C	1479	C
Potassium chloride	ANT	40 mM	HO	1 g	W	Physically compatible for 72 hr at 15 and 30 °C	1479	C
Prochlorperazine edisylate	MB	1.25 g	HO	1 g	W	Yellow globular precipitate forms immediately	1479	I
Promethazine HCl	MB	5 g	HO	1 g	W	White precipitate forms immediately	1479	I
Ranitidine HCl	GL	500 mg	HO	1 g	NS	Physically compatible for 72 hr at 15 and 30 °C	1479	C
	GL	50 mg and 2 g		400 mg	D5W	Physically compatible and ranitidine chemically stable by HPLC for 24 hr at 25 °C. Furosemide not tested	1515	C
Scopolamine butylbromide	BI	2 g	HO	1 g	W	Physically compatible for 72 hr at 15 and 30 °C	1479	C
Sodium bicarbonate	IMS	84 g	HO	1 g		Physically compatible for 72 hr at 15 and 30 °C	1479	C
Sulphadimidine	ICI	100 g	HO	1 g	W	Physically compatible for 72 hr at 15 and 30 °C	1479	C
Theophylline		2 g		330 mg	D5W	Visually compatible with little or no theophylline loss and 10% furosemide loss in 48 hr	1909	C
Tobramycin sulfate	DI	1.6 g	HO	800 mg	D5W, NS	Transient cloudiness during admixture but then physically compatible for 24 hr at 21 °C	876	C
	LI	8 g	HO	1 g	NS	Physically compatible for 72 hr at 15 and 30 °C	1479	C
Verapamil HCl	KN	80 mg	HO	200 mg	D5W, NS	Physically compatible for 24 hr	764	C
	AB	500 mg	HO	1 g	NS	Slight precipitate forms but dissipates	1479	?

[a]Tested in both polyolefin and PVC containers.
[b]Tested in glass containers.

Drugs in Syringe Compatibility

Furosemide

Drug (in syringe)	Mfr	Amt	Mfr	Amt	Remarks	Ref	C/I
Bleomycin sulfate		1.5 units/ 0.5 ml		5 mg/ 0.5 ml	Physically compatible for 5 min at room temperature followed by 8 min of centrifugation	980	C
Cisplatin		0.5 mg/ 0.5 ml		5 mg/ 0.5 ml	Physically compatible for 5 min at room temperature followed by 8 min of centrifugation	980	C
Cyclophosphamide		10 mg/ 0.5 ml		5 mg/ 0.5 ml	Physically compatible for 5 min at room temperature followed by 8 min of centrifugation	980	C
Doxapram HCl	RB	400 mg/ 20 ml	HO	100 mg/ 10 ml	Immediate turbidity	1177	I
Doxorubicin HCl		1 mg/ 0.5 ml		5 mg/ 0.5 ml	Immediate precipitation	980	I
Droperidol		1.25 mg/ 0.5 ml		5 mg/ 0.5 ml	Immediate precipitation	980	I
Fluorouracil		25 mg/ 0.5 ml		5 mg/ 0.5 ml	Physically compatible for 5 min at room temperature followed by 8 min of centrifugation	980	C
Heparin sodium		500 units/ 0.5 ml		5 mg/ 0.5 ml	Physically compatible for 5 min at room temperature followed by 8 min of centrifugation	980	C
		2500 units/ 1 ml		20 mg/ 2 ml	Physically compatible for at least 5 min	1053	C
Leucovorin calcium		5 mg/ 0.5 ml		5 mg/ 0.5 ml	Physically compatible for 5 min at room temperature followed by 8 min of centrifugation	980	C
Methotrexate sodium		12.5 mg/ 0.5 ml		5 mg/ 0.5 ml	Physically compatible for 5 min at room temperature followed by 8 min of centrifugation	980	C
Metoclopramide HCl		2.5 mg/ 0.5 ml		5 mg/ 0.5 ml	Immediate precipitation	980	I
Milrinone	WI	3.5 mg/ 3.5 ml	LY	40 mg/ 4 ml	(Brought to 10-ml total volume with D5W) Immediate precipitation	1191	I
Mitomycin		0.25 mg/ 0.5 ml		5 mg/ 0.5 ml	Physically compatible for 5 min at room temperature followed by 8 min of centrifugation	980	C
Vinblastine sulfate		0.5 mg/ 0.5 ml		5 mg/ 0.5 ml	Immediate precipitation	980	I
Vincristine sulfate		0.5 mg/ 0.5 ml		5 mg/ 0.5 ml	Immediate precipitation	980	I

Y-Site Injection Compatibility (1:1 Mixture)

		Furosemide					
Drug	*Mfr*	*Conc*	*Mfr*	*Conc*	*Remarks*	*Ref*	*C/I*
Allopurinol sodium	BW	3 mg/ml[b]	ES	3 mg/ml[b]	Physically compatible with no change in measured turbidity or increase in particle content in 4 hr at 22 °C	1686	**C**
Amifostine	USB	10 mg/ml[a]	AB	3 mg/ml[a]	Physically compatible with no change in measured turbidity or increase in particle content in 4 hr at 23 °C	1845	**C**
Amikacin sulfate	BR	2 mg/ml[c]	HO	10 mg/ml	Physically compatible for 24 hr at 21 °C	876	**C**
Amphotericin B cholesteryl sulfate complex	SEQ	0.83 mg/ml[a]	AMR	3 mg/ml[a]	Physically compatible with little or no change in measured turbidity or increase in particle content in 4 hr at 23 °C under fluorescent light	2117	**C**
Amsacrine	NCI	1 mg/ml[a]	ES	3 mg/ml[a]	Heavy yellow-orange turbidity forms initially, becoming colorless liquid with yellow precipitate	1381	**I**
Aztreonam	SQ	40 mg/ml[a]	AB	3 mg/ml[a]	Physically compatible with no subvisual haze or particle formation in 4 hr at 23 °C	1758	**C**
Bleomycin sulfate		3 units/ml		10 mg/ml	Drugs injected sequentially into Y-site with no flush between. No visually apparent precipitate	980	**C**
Cefepime HCl	BR	20 mg/ml[a]	AB	3 mg/ml[a]	Physically compatible with no change in measured turbidity or increase in particle content in 4 hr at 22 °C	1689	**C**
Ciprofloxacin	MI	2 mg/ml[c]	AB	10 mg/ml	Immediate precipitation	1655	**I**
	BAY	2 mg/ml[b]	DMX	5 mg/ml	White precipitate forms immediately	1934	**I**
Cisatracurium besylate	GW	0.1 mg/ml[a]	AB	3 mg/ml[a]	Physically compatible with no change in measured turbidity or increase in particle content in 4 hr at 23 °C	2074	**C**
	GW	2 and 5 mg/ml[a]	AB	3 mg/ml[a]	White cloudiness forms immediately	2074	**I**
Cisplatin		1 mg/ml		10 mg/ml	Drugs injected sequentially into Y-site with no flush between. No visually apparent precipitate	980	**C**
	BR	1 mg/ml	ES	3 mg/ml[a]	Visually compatible for 4 hr at room temperature under fluorescent light	1685	**C**
Cladribine	ORT	0.015[b] and 0.5[e] mg/ml	AB	3 mg/ml[b]	Physically compatible with no change in measured turbidity or increase in particle content in 4 hr at 23 °C	1969	**C**
Clarithromycin	AB	4 mg/ml[a]	ANT	10 mg/ml	White cloudiness forms immediately, becoming an obvious precipitate in 15 min	2174	**I**
Cyclophosphamide		20 mg/ml		10 mg/ml	Drugs injected sequentially into Y-site with no flush between. No visually apparent precipitate	980	**C**
	MJ	10 mg/ml[a]	ES	3 mg/ml[a]	Visually compatible for 4 hr at room temperature under fluorescent light	1685	**C**
Cytarabine	UP	50 mg/ml	ES	3 mg/ml[a]	Visually compatible for 4 hr at room temperature under fluorescent light	1685	**C**

Y-Site Injection Compatibility (1:1 Mixture) (Cont.)

Furosemide

Drug	Mfr	Conc	Mfr	Conc	Remarks	Ref	C/I
Diltiazem HCl	MMD	1[b] and 5 mg/ml	AMR	10 mg/ml	Heavy precipitate forms	1807	I
	MMD	1 mg/ml[a]	AMR	10 mg/ml	Precipitate forms immediately	2062	I
Dobutamine HCl	LI	4 mg/ml[b]	ES	1 mg/ml[b]	Physically compatible for 3 hr	1316	C
	LI	4 mg/ml[a]	ES	1 mg/ml[a]	Slight precipitate in 1 hr	1316	I
	LI	4 mg/ml[a]	AMR	10 mg/ml	Precipitate forms immediately	2062	I
Docetaxel	RPR	0.9 mg/ml[a]	AMR	3 mg/ml[a]	Physically compatible with no change in measured turbidity or increase in particle content in 4 hr at 23 °C	2224	C
Dopamine HCl	AST, DU	12.8 mg/ml	AB, AMR	5 mg/ml	Physically compatible for 3 hr at room temperature	1978	C
	AB, AMR	12.8 mg/ml	AB, AMR	5 mg/ml	White precipitate forms immediately	1978	I
	AB	3.2 mg/ml[a]	AMR	10 mg/ml	Precipitate forms in 4 hr at 27 °C	2062	I
Doxorubicin HCl		2 mg/ml		10 mg/ml	Drugs injected sequentially into Y-site with no flush between. Immediate precipitation	980	I
	AD	0.2 mg/ml[a]	ES	3 mg/ml[a]	Visually compatible for 4 hr at room temperature under fluorescent light	1685	C
Doxorubicin HCl liposome injection	SEQ	0.4 mg/ml[a]	AMR	3 mg/ml[a]	Physically compatible with little or no change in measured turbidity and no increase in particle content in 4 hr at 23 °C	2087	C
Droperidol		2.5 mg/ml		10 mg/ml	Drugs injected sequentially into Y-site with no flush between. Immediate precipitation	980	I
		2.5 mg/ml		10 mg/ml	Precipitate forms	977	I
Epinephrine HCl	AB	0.02 mg/ml[a]	AMR	10 mg/ml	Visually compatible for 4 hr at 27 °C	2062	C
Esmolol HCl	ACC	10 mg/ml[c]	HO	10 mg/ml	Cloudy white precipitate forms immediately	1146	I
Etoposide phosphate	BR	5 mg/ml[a]	AMR	3 mg/ml[a]	Physically compatible with no change in measured turbidity or increase in particle content in 4 hr at 23 °C	2218	C
Famotidine	MSD	0.2 mg/ml[a]	IMS	0.8 mg/ml[a]	Physically compatible for 4 hr at 25 °C	1188	C
	MSD	0.2 mg/ml[a]	ES	10 mg/ml	Physically compatible for 14 hr	1196	C
	ME	2 mg/ml[b]		3 mg/ml[a]	White precipitate forms immediately	1936	I
Fentanyl citrate	ES	0.05 mg/ml	AMR	10 mg/ml	Visually compatible for 4 hr at 27 °C	2062	C
Filgrastim	AMG	30 μg/ml[a]	AB	3 mg/ml[a]	Turbidity forms immediately. Filaments and particles form in 1 hr	1687	I
Fluconazole	RR	2 mg/ml	ES	10 mg/ml	Precipitate forms	1407	I
Fludarabine phosphate	BX	1 mg/ml[a]	AB	3 mg/ml[a]	Physically compatible for 4 hr at room temperature under fluorescent light	1439	C
Fluorouracil		50 mg/ml		10 mg/ml	Drugs injected sequentially into Y-site with no flush between. No visually apparent precipitate	980	C
Foscarnet sodium	AST	24 mg/ml	AB	10 mg/ml	Physically compatible for 24 hr at room temperature under fluorescent light	1335	C
Gemcitabine HCl	LI	10 mg/ml[b]	AMR	3 mg/ml[b]	Gross precipitation occurs immediately	2226	I

Y-Site Injection Compatibility (1:1 Mixture) (Cont.)

			Furosemide				
Drug	*Mfr*	*Conc*	*Mfr*	*Conc*	*Remarks*	*Ref*	*C/I*
Gentamicin sulfate	SC	1.6 mg/ml[c]	HO	10 mg/ml	White precipitate of furosemide forms immediately	876	**I**
Granisetron HCl	SKB	0.05 mg/ml[a]	AB	3 mg/ml[a]	Physically compatible with no subvisual haze or particle formation in 4 hr at 23 °C	1804	**C**
	SKB	1 mg/ml	HO	0.4 mg/ml[b]	Physically compatible with little or no loss of either drug by HPLC in 4 hr at 22 °C	1883	**C**
Heparin sodium		1000 units/ml		10 mg/ml	Drugs injected sequentially into Y-site with no flush between. No visually apparent precipitate	980	**C**
	UP	1000 units/L[f]	HO	10 mg/ml	Physically compatible for at least 4 hr at room temperature by visual and microscopic examination	534	**C**
	ES	100 units/ml[a]	AMR	10 mg/ml	Visually compatible for 4 hr at 27 °C	2062	**C**
Hydralazine HCl	SO	1 mg/ml[c]	ES	1 mg/ml[c]	Slight color change in 3 hr	1316	**I**
Hydrocortisone sodium succinate	UP	10 mg/L[f]	HO	10 mg/ml	Physically compatible for at least 4 hr at room temperature by visual and microscopic examination	534	**C**
Hydromorphone HCl	KN	1 mg/ml	AMR	10 mg/ml	Visually compatible for 4 hr at 27 °C	2062	**C**
Idarubicin HCl	AD	1 mg/ml[b]	AB	10 mg/ml	Precipitate forms immediately	1525	**I**
	AD	1 mg/ml[b]	AB	0.8 mg/ml[b]	Haze forms immediately	1525	**I**
Indomethacin sodium trihydrate	MSD	1 mg/ml[b]	AB	10 mg/ml	Visually compatible for 24 hr at 28 °C	1527	**C**
Kanamycin sulfate	BE	2 mg/ml[c]	HO	10 mg/ml	Physically compatible for 24 hr at 21 °C	876	**C**
Labetalol HCl	AB	2.5 mg/ml[a]	AB	10 mg/ml	White turbidity forms immediately. Flocculent precipitate forms in 4 hr	1704	**I**
	AB	2.5 mg/ml[a]	AB	0.5 mg/ml[a]	Physically compatible with no change in measured turbidity or increase in particle content in 4 hr at 22 °C	1704	**C**
	AB	0.25 mg/ml[a]	AB	0.5[a] and 10 mg/ml	Physically compatible with no change in measured turbidity or increase in particle content in 4 hr at 22 °C	1704	**C**
	SC	1.6 mg/ml[g]	ES	10 mg/ml[g]	White precipitate forms immediately	1714	**I**
	AH	2 mg/ml[a]	AMR	10 mg/ml	Precipitate forms immediately	2062	**I**
Leucovorin calcium		10 mg/ml		10 mg/ml	Drugs injected sequentially into Y-site with no flush between. No visually apparent precipitate	980	**C**
Lorazepam	WY	0.33 mg/ml[b]	CNF	10 mg/ml	Visually compatible for 24 hr at 22 °C	1855	**C**
	WY	0.5 mg/ml[a]	AMR	10 mg/ml	Visually compatible for 4 hr at 27 °C	2062	**C**
Melphalan HCl	BW	0.1 mg/ml[b]	AB	3 mg/ml[b]	Physically compatible with no change in measured turbidity or increase in particle content in 3 hr at 22 °C	1557	**C**
Meperidine HCl	AB	10 mg/ml	ES	0.8 mg/ml[a]	Physically compatible for 4 hr at 25 °C under fluorescent light	1397	**C**
	AB	10 mg/ml	ES	2.4 mg/ml[a]	White cloudiness forms immediately	1397	**I**
	AB	10 mg/ml	ES	10 mg/ml	White flocculent precipitate forms immediately	1397	**I**
Meropenem	ZEN	1 and 50 mg/ml[b]	HO	10 mg/ml	Visually compatible for 4 hr at room temperature	1994	**C**

Y-Site Injection Compatibility (1:1 Mixture) (Cont.)

				Furosemide			
Drug	*Mfr*	*Conc*	*Mfr*	*Conc*	*Remarks*	*Ref*	*C/I*
Methotrexate sodium		25 mg/ml		10 mg/ml	Drugs injected sequentially into Y-site with no flush between. No visually apparent precipitate	980	**C**
	AD	15 mg/ml[h]	ES	3 mg/ml[c]	Visually compatible for 4 hr at room temperature under fluorescent light	1685	**C**
Metoclopramide HCl		5 mg/ml		10 mg/ml	Drugs injected sequentially into Y-site with no flush between. Immediate precipitation	980	**I**
Midazolam HCl	RC	1 mg/ml[a]	AST	10 mg/ml[a]	Haze forms immediately. Precipitate forms in 2 hr	1847	**I**
	RC	5 mg/ml	CNF	10 mg/ml	White precipitate forms immediately	1855	**I**
	RC	2 mg/ml[a]	AMR	10 mg/ml	Precipitate forms immediately	2062	**I**
Milrinone lactate	WI	200 μg/ml[a]	LY	10 mg/ml	Immediate precipitation	1191	**I**
	SW	0.2 mg/ml[a]	AMR	10 mg/ml	Precipitate forms in 4 hr at 27 °C	2062	**I**
Mitomycin		0.5 mg/ml		10 mg/ml	Drugs injected sequentially into Y-site with no flush between. No visually apparent precipitate	980	**C**
Morphine sulfate	AB	1 mg/ml	ES	0.8[a], 2.4[a], 10 mg/ml	White precipitate forms within 1 hr at 25 °C under fluorescent light	1397	**I**
	SCN	2 mg/ml[a]	AMR	10 mg/ml	Visually compatible for 4 hr at 27 °C	2062	**C**
Netilmicin sulfate	SC	1.5 mg/ml[c]		10 mg/ml	White precipitate of furosemide forms immediately	876	**I**
Nicardipine HCl	WY	1 mg/ml[a]	AMR	10 mg/ml	Precipitate forms immediately	2062	**I**
Nitroglycerin	AB	0.4 mg/ml[a]	AMR	10 mg/ml	Visually compatible for 4 hr at 27 °C	2062	**C**
Norepinephrine bitartrate	AB	0.128 mg/ml[a]	AMR	10 mg/ml	Visually compatible for 4 hr at 27 °C	2062	**C**
Ondansetron HCl	GL	1 mg/ml[b]	AB	3 mg/ml[a]	Immediate turbidity and precipitation	1365	**I**
Paclitaxel	NCI	1.2 mg/ml[a]	AST	3 mg/ml[a]	Physically compatible with no change in measured turbidity in 4 hr at 22 °C	1556	**C**
Piperacillin sodium–tazobactam sodium	LE	40 + 5 mg/ml[a]	AB	3 mg/ml[a]	Physically compatible with no change in measured turbidity or increase in particle content in 4 hr at 22 °C	1688	**C**
Potassium chloride	AB	40 mEq/L[f]	HO	10 mg/ml	Physically compatible for at least 4 hr at room temperature by visual and microscopic examination	534	**C**
Propofol	ZEN	10 mg/ml	AB	3 mg/ml[a]	Physically compatible with no increase in particle content in 1 hr at 23 °C	2066	**C**
Ranitidine HCl	GL	1 mg/ml[a]	AMR	10 mg/ml	Visually compatible for 4 hr at 27 °C	2062	**C**
Remifentanil HCl	GW	0.025 and 0.25 mg/ml[b]	AMR	3 mg/ml[a]	Physically compatible with no change in measured turbidity or increase in particle content in 4 hr at 23 °C	2075	**C**
Quinidine gluconate	LI	6 mg/ml[c]	ES	4 mg/ml[c]	Immediate gross precipitation	1316	**I**
Sargramostim	IMM	10 μg/ml[b]	AB	3 mg/ml[b]	Physically compatible for 4 hr at 22 °C	1436	**C**
Tacrolimus	FUJ	1 mg/ml[b]	ES	10 mg/ml	Visually compatible for 24 hr at 25 °C	1630	**C**
Teniposide	BR	0.1 mg/ml[a]	AB	3 mg/ml[a]	Physically compatible with no subvisual haze or particle formation in 4 hr at 23 °C	1725	**C**
Thiopental sodium	AB	25 mg/ml[d]	AMR	10 mg/ml	Precipitate forms immediately	2062	**I**

Y-Site Injection Compatibility (1:1 Mixture) (Cont.)

			Furosemide				
Drug	*Mfr*	*Conc*	*Mfr*	*Conc*	*Remarks*	*Ref*	*C/I*
Thiotepa	IMM[i]	1 mg/ml[a]	AMR	3 mg/ml[a]	Physically compatible with no change in measured turbidity or increase in particle content in 4 hr at 23 °C	1861	**C**
TNA #73[j]			ES	165 mg/ 50 ml[c]	Physically compatible for 4 hr by visual observation	1009	**C**
TNA #218 to #226[j]			AB	3 mg/ml[a]	Visually compatible with no precipitate or emulsion damage apparent in 4 hr at 23 °C	2215	**C**
Tobramycin sulfate	DI	1.6 mg/ml	HO	10 mg/ml	Physically compatible for 24 hr at 21 °C	876	**C**
Tolazoline HCl		0.1 mg/ml[a]	AB	10 mg/ml	Physically compatible for 24 hr at 22 °C	1363	**C**
TPN #189[j]				10 mg/ml[b]	Visually compatible for 24 hr at 22 °C	1767	**C**
TPN #203 and #204[j]			AMR	10 mg/ml	Visually compatible for 2 hr at 23 °C	1974	**C**
TPN #212 to #215[j]			AB	3 mg/ml[a]	Small amount of subvisual precipitate forms immediately	2109	**I**
Vecuronium bromide	OR	1 mg/ml	AMR	10 mg/ml	Precipitate forms immediately	2062	**I**
Vinblastine sulfate		1 mg/ml		10 mg/ml	Drugs injected sequentially into Y-site with no flush between. Immediate precipitation	980	**I**
Vincristine sulfate		1 mg/ml		10 mg/ml	Drugs injected sequentially into Y-site with no flush between. Immediate precipitation	980	**I**
Vinorelbine tartrate	BW	1 mg/ml[b]	ES	3 mg/ml[b]	Heavy white precipitate forms immediately	1558	**I**
Vitamin B complex with C	RC	2 ml/L[f]	HO	10 mg/ml	Physically compatible for at least 4 hr at room temperature by visual and microscopic examination	534	**C**

[a]*Tested in dextrose 5% in water.*
[b]*Tested in sodium chloride 0.9%.*
[c]*Tested in both dextrose 5% in water and sodium chloride 0.9%.*
[d]*Tested in sterile water for injection.*
[e]*Tested in bacteriostatic sodium chloride 0.9% preserved with benzyl alcohol 0.9%.*
[f]*Tested in dextrose 5% in Ringer's injection, dextrose 5% in Ringer's injection, lactated, dextrose 5% in water, Ringer's injection, lactated, and sodium chloride 0.9%.*
[g]*Furosemide 0.5 ml injected in the Y-site port of a running infusion of labetalol HCl in dextrose 5% in water.*
[h]*Tested in dextrose 5% in water with sodium bicarbonate 0.05 mEq/ml.*
[i]*Lyophilized formulation tested.*
[j]*Refer to Appendix I for the composition of parenteral nutrition solutions. TNA indicates a 3-in-1 admixture, and TPN indicates a 2-in-1 admixture.*

Additional Compatibility Information

Acidic Additives— Furosemide may precipitate if combined with ascorbic acid, epinephrine, or norepinephrine (4).

The acidic pH of aminoglycoside admixtures may cause transient cloudiness or frank precipitation if furosemide is added, depending on which aminoglycoside is used and the concentration of the additives. Avoiding the admixture of furosemide and aminoglycosides has been recommended (876).

A 2-ml fluid barrier of dextrose 5% in water in a microbore retrograde infusion set failed to prevent precipitation when used between gentamicin sulfate 5 mg/0.5 ml and furosemide 2 mg/ 0.2 ml (1385).

Furosemide may precipitate if mixed with milrinone lactate infusions (1442).

Dopamine HCl— Furosemide has demonstrated compatibility or incompatibility with dopamine HCl during simultaneous Y-site administration, depending on the formulation of dopamine HCl tested. Dopamine formulations supplied by Astra and DuPont have the pH adjusted with sodium hydroxide and/or hydrochloric acid and are compatible with furosemide. Formulations supplied by Abbott and American Regent contain citrate buffer and are incompatible with furosemide, forming a white precipitate immediately upon contact (1978).

GANCICLOVIR SODIUM
AHFS 8:18

Cytovene-IV   **Roche**

Products— Ganciclovir sodium (Roche) is available in vials containing, in dry form, the equivalent of ganciclovir 500 mg. Reconstitute with 10 ml of sterile water for injection and shake to dissolve the drug to yield a solution containing ganciclovir 50 mg/ml. Do not use paraben-containing diluents to reconstitute ganciclovir sodium because precipitation may result (2).

pH— Approximately 11 (2).

Osmolality— Ganciclovir sodium 50 mg/ml in sterile water for injection has an osmolality of 320 mOsm/kg (1689).

Sodium Content— Each 500-mg vial contains 46 mg of sodium (2).

Administration— Ganciclovir sodium is administered by intravenous infusion. After reconstitution, the required dose may be diluted in 100 ml of compatible infusion solution and given over one hour. Concentrations greater than 10 mg/ml are not recommended. Ganciclovir sodium should not be administered by intramuscular, subcutaneous, or rapid intravenous injection or infusion (2; 4).

Stability— According to the manufacturer, intact vials should be stored at controlled room temperature and protected from temperatures above 40 °C. The reconstituted solution is stable for 12 hours at room temperature. Refrigeration of the reconstituted solution is not recommended (2). However, Heni reported that ganciclovir sodium 500 mg/10 ml in sterile water for injection was stable, with no significant loss by HPLC analysis, for 60 days when stored at 4 °C (1631).

The manufacturer recommends that admixtures of ganciclovir sodium in compatible infusion solutions be stored under refrigeration but not frozen. Ganciclovir reconstituted with sterile water for injection and diluted further in sodium chloride 0.9% in PVC bags is physically and chemically stable for up to 14 days when stored under refrigeration at 5 °C. However, because of the absence of an antibacterial preservative, use within 24 hours is recommended (2).

Syringes— Ganciclovir sodium (Syntex) 5.8 mg/ml in sodium chloride 0.9%, packaged in polypropylene infusion-pump syringes (Healthtek), exhibited 3% or less drug loss in 10 days at 4 °C and no loss in 12 hours at 25 °C by HPLC analysis (1742).

Ganciclovir sodium (Syntex) 1.4, 4, and 7 mg/ml in sodium chloride 0.9% was packaged in polypropylene syringes and stored at 20, 4, and −20 °C. HPLC analysis found 4% or less drug loss in seven days at 20 °C, in 80 days at 4 °C, and in 364 days at −20 °C (1836).

Freezing Solutions— Ganciclovir sodium (Syntex) 1.4, 4, and 7 mg/ml in sodium chloride 0.9% was packaged in polypropylene syringes, and 0.28 and 1.4 mg/ml in sodium chloride 0.9% was packaged in PVC containers. All samples exhibited 4% or less drug loss by HPLC analysis after 364 days at −20 °C (1836).

Elastomeric Reservoir Pumps— Ganciclovir sodium (Syntex) 5 mg/ml in sodium chloride 0.9% 100 ml was packaged in latex elastomeric reservoirs (Secure Medical). About 4 to 6% loss by HPLC analysis occurred in 24 hours at 25 °C and in five days at 5 °C (1970).

Sorption— During a solution stability study, no sorption to PVC containers was noted (1288).

Compatibility Information

Solution Compatibility

Ganciclovir sodium

Solution	Mfr	Mfr	Conc/L	Remarks	Ref	C/I
Dextrose 5% in water	TR[a]	SY	2.44 g	Physically compatible and chemically stable with no drug loss in 5 days at 25 °C exposed to light or in the dark and at 4 °C	1288	C
	BA[a]	SY	1, 5, 10 g	Visually compatible with 3 to 7% ganciclovir loss by HPLC in 35 days at 4 to 8 °C in the dark	1545	C
	AB[a]	SY	1 and 5 g	Visually compatible with 1% or less ganciclovir loss by HPLC in 35 days at 5 and 25 °C	1643	C
Sodium chloride 0.9%	TR[a]	SY	2.59 g	Physically compatible and chemically stable with no drug loss in 5 days at 25 °C exposed to light or in the dark and at 4 °C	1288	C
	AB[a]	SY	1 and 5 g	Visually compatible with 1% or less ganciclovir loss by HPLC in 35 days at 5 and 25 °C	1643	C
		SY	2.2 g	Little or no ganciclovir loss by HPLC in 14 days at 4 °C	1637	C
	[a]	SY	0.28 and 1.4 g	4% or less drug loss by HPLC in 7 days at 20 °C, 80 days at 4 °C, and 364 days at −20 °C	1836	C
	AB[b]	SY	5 g	4 to 6% loss of drug by HPLC in 24 hr at 25 °C and in 5 days at 5 °C	1970	C
TPN #183[c]		SY	2 g	Precipitate forms	1744	I

Solution Compatibility (Cont.)

Ganciclovir sodium

Solution	Mfr	Mfr	Conc/L	Remarks	Ref	C/I
TPN #183 to #185[c]		SY	3 and 5 g	Precipitate forms	1744	I

[a]Tested in PVC containers.
[b]Tested in glass containers and latex elastomeric reservoirs (Secure Medical).
[c]Refer to Appendix I for the composition of parenteral nutrition solutions. TPN indicates a 2-in-1 admixture.

Y-Site Injection Compatibility (1:1 Mixture)

Ganciclovir sodium

Drug	Mfr	Conc	Mfr	Conc	Remarks	Ref	C/I
Aldesleukin	CHI	33,800 I.U./ml[a]	SY	10 mg/ml[a]	Aldesleukin bioactivity inhibited	1857	I
Allopurinol sodium	BW	3 mg/ml[b]	SY	20 mg/ml[b]	Physically compatible with no change in measured turbidity or increase in particle content in 4 hr at 22 °C	1686	C
Amifostine	USB	10 mg/ml[a]	SY	20 mg/ml[a]	Subvisual needles form immediately, becoming a dense flocculent precipitate in 1 hr	1845	I
Amphotericin B cholesteryl sulfate complex	SEQ	0.83 mg/ml[a]	RC	20 mg/ml[a]	Physically compatible with little or no change in measured turbidity or increase in particle content in 4 hr at 23 °C under fluorescent light	2117	C
Amsacrine	NCI	1 mg/ml[a]	SY	20 mg/ml[a]	Immediate dark orange turbidity	1381	I
Aztreonam	SQ	40 mg/ml[a]	SY	20 mg/ml[a]	White crystalline needles form immediately and become dense flocculent precipitate in 1 hr	1758	I
Cefepime HCl	BR	20 mg/ml[a]	SY	20 mg/ml[a]	Flocculent precipitate forms immediately	1689	I
Cisatracurium besylate	GW	0.1 and 2 mg/ml[a]	SY	20 mg/ml[a]	Pysically compatible with no change in measured turbidity or increase in particle content in 4 hr at 23 °C	2074	C
	GW	5 mg/ml[a]	SY	20 mg/ml[a]	White cloudiness forms immediately	2074	I
Cisplatin	BR	1 mg/ml	SY	20 mg/ml[a]	Visually compatible for 4 hr at room temperature under fluorescent light	1685	C
Cyclophosphamide	MJ	10 mg/ml[a]	SY	20 mg/ml[a]	Visually compatible for 4 hr at room temperature under fluorescent light	1685	C
Cytarabine	UP	50 mg/ml	SY	20 mg/ml[a]	Turbidity and particles form in 30 min, becoming gel-like in 4 hr	1685	I
Docetaxel	RPR	0.9 mg/ml[a]	RC	20 mg/ml[a]	Physically compatible with no change in measured turbidity or increase in particle content in 4 hr at 23 °C	2224	C
Doxorubicin HCl	AD	0.2 mg/ml[a]	SY	20 mg/ml[a]	Color changes to deep purple immediately	1685	I
Doxorubicin HCl liposome injection	SEQ	0.4 mg/ml[a]	RC	20 mg/ml[a]	Physically compatible with little or no change in measured turbidity and no increase in particle content in 4 hr at 23 °C	2087	C
Enalaprilat	MSD	1.25 mg/ml	SY	5 mg/ml[c]	Physically compatible for 4 hr at 21 °C under fluorescent light by macroscopic and microscopic examination	1409	C

Y-Site Injection Compatibility (1:1 Mixture) (Cont.)

<table>
<tr><td></td><td colspan="4">Ganciclovir sodium</td><td></td><td></td><td></td></tr>
<tr><td>*Drug*</td><td>*Mfr*</td><td>*Conc*</td><td>*Mfr*</td><td>*Conc*</td><td>*Remarks*</td><td>*Ref*</td><td>*C/I*</td></tr>
<tr><td>Etoposide phosphate</td><td>BR</td><td>5 mg/ml[a]</td><td>RC</td><td>20 mg/ml[a]</td><td>Physically compatible with no change in measured turbidity or increase in particle content in 4 hr at 23 °C</td><td>2218</td><td>C</td></tr>
<tr><td>Filgrastim</td><td>AMG</td><td>30 μg/ml[a]</td><td>SY</td><td>20 mg/ml[a]</td><td>Physically compatible with no change in measured turbidity or increase in particle content in 4 hr at 22 °C</td><td>1687</td><td>C</td></tr>
<tr><td>Fluconazole</td><td>RR</td><td>2 mg/ml</td><td>SY</td><td>50 mg/ml</td><td>Physically compatible for 24 hr at 25 °C</td><td>1407</td><td>C</td></tr>
<tr><td>Fludarabine phosphate</td><td>BX</td><td>1 mg/ml[a]</td><td>SY</td><td>20 mg/ml[a]</td><td>Darker color visible under high intensity light within 4 hr</td><td>1439</td><td>I</td></tr>
<tr><td>Foscarnet sodium</td><td>AST</td><td>24 mg/ml</td><td></td><td>50 mg/ml</td><td>Immediate precipitation</td><td>1335</td><td>I</td></tr>
<tr><td>Gemcitabine HCl</td><td>LI</td><td>10 mg/ml[b]</td><td>RC</td><td>20 mg/ml[b]</td><td>Subvisual crystals form immediately, becoming a gross precipitate in 1 hr</td><td>2226</td><td>I</td></tr>
<tr><td>Granisetron HCl</td><td>SKB</td><td>0.05 mg/ml[a]</td><td>SY</td><td>20 mg/ml[a]</td><td>Physically compatible with no change in measured turbidity or increase in particle content in 4 hr at 23 °C</td><td>2000</td><td>C</td></tr>
<tr><td>Melphalan HCl</td><td>BW</td><td>0.1 mg/ml[b]</td><td>SY</td><td>20 mg/ml[b]</td><td>Physically compatible with no change in measured turbidity or increase in particle content in 3 hr at 22 °C</td><td>1557</td><td>C</td></tr>
<tr><td>Methotrexate sodium</td><td>AD</td><td>15 mg/ml[d]</td><td>SY</td><td>20 mg/ml[a]</td><td>Visually compatible for 4 hr at room temperature under fluorescent light</td><td>1685</td><td>C</td></tr>
<tr><td>Ondansetron HCl</td><td>GL</td><td>1 mg/ml[b]</td><td>SY</td><td>20 mg/ml[a]</td><td>Immediate turbidity and precipitation</td><td>1365</td><td>I</td></tr>
<tr><td>Paclitaxel</td><td>NCI</td><td>1.2 mg/ml[a]</td><td>SY</td><td>20 mg/ml[a]</td><td>Physically compatible with no change in measured turbidity in 4 hr at 22 °C</td><td>1556</td><td>C</td></tr>
<tr><td>Piperacillin sodium–tazobactam sodium</td><td>LE</td><td>40 + 5 mg/ml[a]</td><td>SY</td><td>20 mg/ml[a]</td><td>Large crystals form in 1 hr and become heavy white precipitate in 4 hr</td><td>1688</td><td>I</td></tr>
<tr><td>Propofol</td><td>ZEN</td><td>10 mg/ml</td><td>SY</td><td>20 mg/ml[a]</td><td>Physically compatible for 1 hr at 23 °C with no increase in particle content</td><td>2066</td><td>C</td></tr>
<tr><td>Remifentanil HCl</td><td>GW</td><td>0.025 and 0.25 mg/ml[b]</td><td>SY</td><td>20 mg/ml[a]</td><td>Physically compatible with no change in measured turbidity or increase in particle content in 4 hr at 23 °C</td><td>2075</td><td>C</td></tr>
<tr><td>Sargramostim</td><td>IMM</td><td>10 μg/ml[b]</td><td>SY</td><td>20 mg/ml[b]</td><td>Few small particles formed in 4 hr in one of two samples</td><td>1436</td><td>I</td></tr>
<tr><td>Tacrolimus</td><td>FUJ</td><td>1 mg/ml[b]</td><td>SY</td><td>50 mg/ml[a]</td><td>Visually compatible for 24 hr at 25 °C</td><td>1630</td><td>C</td></tr>
<tr><td>Teniposide</td><td>BR</td><td>0.1 mg/ml[a]</td><td>SY</td><td>20 mg/ml[a]</td><td>Physically compatible with no subvisual haze or particle formation in 4 hr at 23 °C</td><td>1725</td><td>C</td></tr>
<tr><td>Thiotepa</td><td>IMM[e]</td><td>1 mg/ml[a]</td><td>SY</td><td>20 mg/ml[a]</td><td>Physically compatible with no change in measured turbidity or increase in particle content in 4 hr at 23 °C</td><td>1861</td><td>C</td></tr>
<tr><td>TNA #218 to #226[f]</td><td></td><td></td><td>RC</td><td>20 mg/ml[a]</td><td>Large amount of white precipitate forms immediately</td><td>2215</td><td>I</td></tr>
<tr><td>TPN #144[f]</td><td></td><td></td><td>SY</td><td>1 and 5 mg/ml[a]</td><td>Visually compatible for 2 hr at 20 °C</td><td>1522</td><td>C</td></tr>
<tr><td></td><td></td><td></td><td>SY</td><td>10 mg/ml[a]</td><td>Heavy precipitate forms within 30 min</td><td>1522</td><td>I</td></tr>
<tr><td>TPN #183[f]</td><td></td><td></td><td>SY</td><td>2 mg/ml</td><td>Precipitate forms</td><td>1744</td><td>I</td></tr>
</table>

Y-Site Injection Compatibility (1:1 Mixture) (Cont.)

Ganciclovir sodium

Drug	Mfr	Conc	Mfr	Conc	Remarks	Ref	C/I
			SY	1 mg/ml[g]	Visually compatible with no ganciclovir loss by HPLC in 3 hr at 24 °C under fluorescent light. Less than 10% amino acid loss by HPLC in 2 hr	1744	**C**
TPN #183 to #185[f]			SY	3 and 5 mg/ml	Precipitate forms	1744	**I**
TPN #184 and #185[f]			SY	2 mg/ml[h]	Visually compatible with no ganciclovir loss by HPLC in 3 hr at 24 °C under fluorescent light. Less than 10% amino acid loss by HPLC in 3 hr	1744	**C**
TPN #212 to #215[f]			SY	20 mg/ml[a]	Gross white precipitate forms immediately	2109	**I**
Vinorelbine tartrate	BW	1 mg/ml[b]	SY	20 mg/ml[b]	White turbid solution with precipitate forms immediately	1558	**I**

[a]*Tested in dextrose 5% in water.*
[b]*Tested in sodium chloride 0.9%.*
[c]*Tested in both dextrose 5% in water and sodium chloride 0.9%.*
[d]*Tested in dextrose 5% in water with sodium bicarbonate 0.05 mEq/ml.*
[e]*Lyophilized formulation tested.*
[f]*Refer to Appendix I for the composition of parenteral nutrition solutions. TNA indicates a 3-in-1 admixture, and TPN indicates a 2-in-1 admixture.*
[g]*Ganciclovir sodium concentration after mixing was 0.83 mg/ml.*
[h]*Ganciclovir sodium concentration after mixing was 1.4 mg/ml.*

Additional Compatibility Information

Infusion Solutions— The manufacturer states that ganciclovir sodium is chemically and physically compatible when diluted for intravenous infusion in the following solutions (2):

    Dextrose 5% in water
    Ringer's injection
    Ringer's injection, lactated
    Sodium chloride 0.9%

The manufacturer also recommends use within 24 hours of dilution and storage under refrigeration because of the risk of bacterial contamination (2).

Parabens— Ganciclovir sodium is stated to be incompatible with paraben-containing solutions. Reconstitution with bacteriostatic water for injection containing parabens may cause precipitation (2).

Other Information

Bacterial Challenge— Ganciclovir sodium (Syntex) 0.35 mg/ml diluted in sodium chloride 0.9% and stored at 22 °C did not exhibit a substantial antimicrobial effect on the growth of four organisms (*Enterococcus faecium, Staphylococcus aureus, Pseudomonas aeruginosa,* and *Candida albicans*) inoculated into the solution. *S. aureus* and *C. albicans* remained viable for 24 hours, and the others remained viable to the end of the study at 120 hours. The author recommended that diluted solutions of ganciclovir sodium be stored under refrigeration whenever possible and that the potential for microbiological growth should be considered when assigning expiration periods (2160).

GEMCITABINE HCL
AHFS 10:00

Gemzar   **Lilly**

Products— Gemcitabine HCl (Lilly) is available as a lyophilized powder in vials containing 200 mg of drug (as the base) with mannitol 200 mg and sodium acetate 12.5 mg. Reconstitute the 200-mg vial with 5 ml of sodium chloride 0.9% (without preservatives) and shake to dissolve the powder (2).

Gemcitabine HCl is also available as a lyophilized powder in vials containing 1 g of drug (as the base) with mannitol 1 g and sodium acetate 62.5 mg. Reconstitute the 1-g vial with 25 ml of sodium chloride 0.9% (without preservatives) and shake to dissolve the powder (2).

When reconstituted as directed, the resulting solution from either size vial has a gemcitabine concentration of 38 mg/ml, which accounts for the displacement volume of the powder. The total volumes after reconstitution will be 5.26 ml for the 200-mg vial and 26.3 ml for the 1-g vial (2).

Because of the drug's aqueous solubility, reconstitution to concentrations higher than 40 mg/ml may result in incomplete dissolution and should be avoided (2).

The pH of the products may have been adjusted by the manufacturer with sodium hydroxide and/or hydrochloric acid (2).

pH— The reconstituted solution has a pH in the range of 2.7 to 3.3 (2).

Displacement Volume— The displacement volume of the powder in the 200-mg vial is 0.26 ml and in the 1-g vial is 1.3 ml (2).

Administration— Gemcitabine HCl is administered weekly by intravenous infusion over 30 minutes. It may be administered as reconstituted or diluted further in additional sodium chloride 0.9% to a concentration as low as 0.1 mg/ml. Gemcitabine HCl has not had reports of necrosis at injection sites and is not a vesicant (2).

Stability— Gemcitabine HCl in intact vials should be stored at controlled room temperatures of 20 to 25 °C. The white lyophilized powder becomes a colorless to light straw-colored solution on reconstitution. The manufacturer states that the reconstituted solution is stable for 24 hours at controlled room temperature. Unused solution should be discarded (2). However, other information indicates the reconstituted solution may be stable for longer periods (2227). See Reconstituted Solutions below. The reconstituted solution should not be refrigerated because crystallization may occur (2).

Reconstituted Solutions— Gemcitabine HCl (Lilly) 200-mg and 1-g vials reconstituted to 38 mg/ml with sterile water for injection and also sodium chloride 0.9% were evaluated over periods of 35 days at 23 °C exposed to and protected from fluorescent light and at 4 °C protected from light. The samples stored at 23 °C were physically stable with no visible particulates and no increase in electronically

measured particulates throughout the study period. HPLC analysis found less than 4% gemcitabine loss after 35 days of storage at 23 °C. Under refrigeration, the solutions remained physically and chemically stable for at least seven days, but large colorless crystals formed in some samples after that time. The crystals did not redissolve on warming to room temperature. HPLC analysis found little or no gemcitabine loss in the refrigerated solutions unless crystals formed; gemcitabine losses of 20 to 35% were determined in samples containing crystals. Exposure to or protection from fluorescent light did not affect gemcitabine stability (2227).

Syringes— Gemcitabine HCl (Lilly) 38 mg/ml in sodium chloride 0.9% was repackaged as 10 ml of solution in 20-ml polypropylene plastic syringes (Becton-Dickinson) and sealed with tip caps (Red Cap, Burron). Sample syringes were stored at 23 °C both exposed to and protected from fluorescent light and at 4 °C protected from light for 35 days. All samples were physically stable with no visible particulates and no increase in electronically measured particulates throughout the study period. Although not observed in these solutions packaged in plastic syringes, reconstituted solutions stored under refrigeration are subject to possible crystal formation. See Reconstituted Solutions above. HPLC analysis found little or no gemcitabine loss after 35 days of storage under any of the conditions (2227).

Ambulatory Infusion Pumps— Gemcitabine HCl (Lilly) 0.1, 10, and 38 mg/ml in dextrose 5% in water and in sodium chloride 0.9% in 50-ml PVC bags were evaluated over seven days for physical and chemical stability at 32 °C in the dark to simulate conditions during ambulatory infusion from a solution reservoir worn under clothes next to the body. All samples were physically stable with no visible particulates and no increase in electronically measured particulates throughout the study period. HPLC analysis found no loss of gemcitabine in any of the samples (2227).

Sorption— Gemcitabine HCl has not exhibited any incompatibilities with infusion bottles or PVC bags and administration sets (2).

Compatibility Information

Solution Compatibility

Gemcitabine HCl

Solution	Mfr	Mfr	Conc/L	Remarks	Ref	C/I
Dextrose 5% in water	BA[a]	LI	0.1 and 10 g	Physically compatible with no increase in particle content and chemically stable with no loss by HPLC in 35 days at 23 °C exposed to or protected from fluorescent light and at 4 °C in the dark	2227	C
Sodium chloride 0.9%	BA[a]	LI	0.1 and 10 g	Physically compatible with no increase in particle content and chemically stable with no loss by HPLC in 35 days at 23 °C exposed to or protected from fluorescent light and at 4 °C in the dark	2227	C

[a]*Tested in PVC containers.*

Y-Site Injection Compatibility (1:1 Mixture)

Gemcitabine HCl

Drug	Mfr	Conc	Mfr	Conc	Remarks	Ref	C/I
Acyclovir sodium	GW	7 mg/ml[b]	LI	10 mg/ml[b]	Gross precipitation occurs immediately	2226	I
Amifostine	USB	10 mg/ml[b]	LI	10 mg/ml[b]	Physically compatible with no change in measured turbidity or increase in particle content in 4 hr at 23 °C	2226	C
Amikacin sulfate	APC	5 mg/ml[b]	LI	10 mg/ml[b]	Physically compatible with no change in measured turbidity or increase in particle content in 4 hr at 23 °C	2226	C
Aminophylline	AB	2.5 mg/ml[b]	LI	10 mg/ml[b]	Physically compatible with no change in measured turbidity or increase in particle content in 4 hr at 23 °C	2226	C
Amphotericin B	PH	0.6 mg/ml[a]	LI	10 mg/ml[b]	Gross precipitation occurs immediately	2226	I
Ampicillin sodium	SKB	20 mg/ml[b]	LI	10 mg/ml[b]	Physically compatible with no change in measured turbidity or increase in particle content in 4 hr at 23 °C	2226	C
Ampicillin sodium–sulbactam sodium	RR	20 + 10 mg/ml[b]	LI	10 mg/ml[b]	Physically compatible with no change in measured turbidity or increase in particle content in 4 hr at 23 °C	2226	C
Aztreonam	SQ	40 mg/ml[b]	LI	10 mg/ml[b]	Physically compatible with no change in measured turbidity or increase in particle content in 4 hr at 23 °C	2226	C
Bleomycin sulfate	MJ	1 unit/ml[b]	LI	10 mg/ml[b]	Physically compatible with no change in measured turbidity or increase in particle content in 4 hr at 23 °C	2226	C
Bumetanide	RC	0.04 mg/ml[b]	LI	10 mg/ml[b]	Physically compatible with no change in measured turbidity or increase in particle content in 4 hr at 23 °C	2226	C
Buprenorphine HCl	RKC	0.04 mg/ml[b]	LI	10 mg/ml[b]	Physically compatible with no change in measured turbidity or increase in particle content in 4 hr at 23 °C	2226	C
Butorphanol tartrate	APC	0.04 mg/ml[b]	LI	10 mg/ml[b]	Physically compatible with no change in measured turbidity or increase in particle content in 4 hr at 23 °C	2226	C
Calcium gluconate	FUJ	40 mg/ml[b]	LI	10 mg/ml[b]	Physically compatible with no change in measured turbidity or increase in particle content in 4 hr at 23 °C	2226	C
Carboplatin	BR	5 mg/ml[b]	LI	10 mg/ml[b]	Physically compatible with no change in measured turbidity or increase in particle content in 4 hr at 23 °C	2226	C
Carmustine	BR	1.5 mg/ml[b]	LI	10 mg/ml[b]	Physically compatible with no change in measured turbidity or increase in particle content in 4 hr at 23 °C	2226	C
Cefazolin sodium	APC	20 mg/ml[b]	LI	10 mg/ml[b]	Physically compatible with no change in measured turbidity or increase in particle content in 4 hr at 23 °C	2226	C
Cefoperazone sodium	PF	40 mg/ml[b]	LI	10 mg/ml[b]	Gross precipitation occurs immediately	2226	I
Cefotaxime sodium	HO	20 mg/ml[b]	LI	10 mg/ml[b]	Slight subvisual haze forms in 1 hr with increased haze and a subvisual precipitate in 4 hr	2226	I

Y-Site Injection Compatibility (1:1 Mixture) (Cont.)

			Gemcitabine HCl				
Drug	*Mfr*	*Conc*	*Mfr*	*Conc*	*Remarks*	*Ref*	*C/I*
Cefotetan sodium	ZEN	20 mg/ml[b]	LI	10 mg/ml[b]	Physically compatible with no change in measured turbidity or increase in particle content in 4 hr at 23 °C	2226	C
Cefoxitin sodium	ME	20 mg/ml[b]	LI	10 mg/ml[b]	Physically compatible with no change in measured turbidity or increase in particle content in 4 hr at 23 °C	2226	C
Ceftazidime	SKB[c]	40 mg/ml[b]	LI	10 mg/ml[b]	Physically compatible with no change in measured turbidity or increase in particle content in 4 hr at 23 °C	2226	C
Ceftizoxime sodium	FUJ	20 mg/ml[b]	LI	10 mg/ml[b]	Physically compatible with no change in measured turbidity or increase in particle content in 4 hr at 23 °C	2226	C
Ceftriaxone sodium	RC	20 mg/ml[b]	LI	10 mg/ml[b]	Physically compatible with no change in measured turbidity or increase in particle content in 4 hr at 23 °C	2226	C
Cefuroxime sodium	GW	30 mg/ml[b]	LI	10 mg/ml[b]	Physically compatible with no change in measured turbidity or increase in particle content in 4 hr at 23 °C	2226	C
Chlorpromazine HCl	ES	2 mg/ml[b]	LI	10 mg/ml[b]	Physically compatible with no change in measured turbidity or increase in particle content in 4 hr at 23 °C	2226	C
Cimetidine HCl	AMR	12 mg/ml[b]	LI	10 mg/ml[b]	Physically compatible with no change in measured turbidity or increase in particle content in 4 hr at 23 °C	2226	C
Ciprofloxacin	BAY	1 mg/ml[b]	LI	10 mg/ml[b]	Physically compatible with no change in measured turbidity or increase in particle content in 4 hr at 23 °C	2226	C
Cisplatin	BR	1 mg/ml	LI	10 mg/ml[b]	Physically compatible with no change in measured turbidity or increase in particle content in 4 hr at 23 °C	2226	C
Clindamycin phosphate	AST	10 mg/ml[b]	LI	10 mg/ml[b]	Physically compatible with no change in measured turbidity or increase in particle content in 4 hr at 23 °C	2226	C
Cyclophosphamide	BR	10 mg/ml[b]	LI	10 mg/ml[b]	Physically compatible with no change in measured turbidity or increase in particle content in 4 hr at 23 °C	2226	C
Cytarabine	BED	50 mg/ml	LI	10 mg/ml[b]	Physically compatible with no change in measured turbidity or increase in particle content in 4 hr at 23 °C	2226	C
Dactinomycin	ME	0.01 mg/ml[b]	LI	10 mg/ml[b]	Physically compatible with no change in measured turbidity or increase in particle content in 4 hr at 23 °C	2226	C
Daunorubicin HCl	BED	1 mg/ml[b]	LI	10 mg/ml[b]	Physically compatible with no change in measured turbidity or increase in particle content in 4 hr at 23 °C	2226	C
Dexamethasone sodium phosphate	ES	1 mg/ml[b]	LI	10 mg/ml[b]	Physically compatible with no change in measured turbidity or increase in particle content in 4 hr at 23 °C	2226	C

Y-Site Injection Compatibility (1:1 Mixture) (Cont.)

Gemcitabine HCl

Drug	Mfr	Conc	Mfr	Conc	Remarks	Ref	C/I
Dexrazoxane	PH	5 mg/ml[b]	LI	10 mg/ml[b]	Physically compatible with no change in measured turbidity or increase in particle content in 4 hr at 23 °C	2226	C
Diphenhydramine HCl	SCN	2 mg/ml[b]	LI	10 mg/ml[b]	Physically compatible with no change in measured turbidity or increase in particle content in 4 hr at 23 °C	2226	C
Dobutamine HCl	AST	4 mg/ml[b]	LI	10 mg/ml[b]	Physically compatible with no change in measured turbidity or increase in particle content in 4 hr at 23 °C	2226	C
Docetaxel	RPR	2 mg/ml[a]	LI	10 mg/ml[b]	Physically compatible with no change in measured turbidity or increase in particle content in 4 hr at 23 °C	2226	C
Dopamine HCl	AB	3.2 mg/ml[b]	LI	10 mg/ml[b]	Physically compatible with no change in measured turbidity or increase in particle content in 4 hr at 23 °C	2226	C
Doxorubicin HCl	PH	2 mg/ml	LI	10 mg/ml[b]	Physically compatible with no change in measured turbidity or increase in particle content in 4 hr at 23 °C	2226	C
Doxycycline hyclate	FUJ	1 mg/ml[b]	LI	10 mg/ml[b]	Physically compatible with no change in measured turbidity or increase in particle content in 4 hr at 23 °C	2226	C
Droperidol	AST	0.4 mg/ml[b]	LI	10 mg/ml[b]	Physically compatible with no change in measured turbidity or increase in particle content in 4 hr at 23 °C	2226	C
Enalaprilat	ME	0.1 mg/ml[b]	LI	10 mg/ml[b]	Physically compatible with no change in measured turbidity or increase in particle content in 4 hr at 23 °C	2226	C
Etoposide	BR	0.4 mg/ml[b]	LI	10 mg/ml[b]	Physically compatible with no change in measured turbidity or increase in particle content in 4 hr at 23 °C	2226	C
Etoposide phosphate	BR	5 mg/ml[b]	LI	10 mg/ml[b]	Physically compatible with no change in measured turbidity or increase in particle content in 4 hr at 23 °C	2226	C
Famotidine	ME	2 mg/ml[b]	LI	10 mg/ml[b]	Physically compatible with no change in measured turbidity or increase in particle content in 4 hr at 23 °C	2226	C
Floxuridine	RC	3 mg/ml[b]	LI	10 mg/ml[b]	Physically compatible with no change in measured turbidity or increase in particle content in 4 hr at 23 °C	2226	C
Fluconazole	RR	2 mg/ml	LI	10 mg/ml[b]	Physically compatible with no change in measured turbidity or increase in particle content in 4 hr at 23 °C	2226	C
Fludarabine phosphate	BX	1 mg/ml[b]	LI	10 mg/ml[b]	Physically compatible with no change in measured turbidity or increase in particle content in 4 hr at 23 °C	2226	C
Fluorouracil	PH	16 mg/ml[b]	LI	10 mg/ml[b]	Physically compatible with no change in measured turbidity or increase in particle content in 4 hr at 23 °C	2226	C
Furosemide	AMR	3 mg/ml[b]	LI	10 mg/ml[b]	Gross precipitation occurs immediately	2226	I

Y-Site Injection Compatibility (1:1 Mixture) (Cont.)

Gemcitabine HCl

Drug	Mfr	Conc	Mfr	Conc	Remarks	Ref	C/I
Ganciclovir sodium	RC	20 mg/ml[b]	LI	10 mg/ml[b]	Subvisual crystals form immediately, becoming a gross precipitate in 1 hr	2226	**I**
Gentamicin sulfate	AB	5 mg/ml[b]	LI	10 mg/ml[b]	Physically compatible with no change in measured turbidity or increase in particle content in 4 hr at 23 °C	2226	**C**
Granisetron HCl	SKB	0.05 mg/ml[b]	LI	10 mg/ml[b]	Physically compatible with no change in measured turbidity or increase in particle content in 4 hr at 23 °C	2226	**C**
Haloperidol lactate	MN	0.2 mg/ml[b]	LI	10 mg/ml[b]	Physically compatible with no change in measured turbidity or increase in particle content in 4 hr at 23 °C	2226	**C**
Heparin sodium	ES	100 units/ml[b]	LI	10 mg/ml[b]	Physically compatible with no change in measured turbidity or increase in particle content in 4 hr at 23 °C	2226	**C**
Hydrocortisone sodium phosphate	ME	1 mg/ml[b]	LI	10 mg/ml[b]	Physically compatible with no change in measured turbidity or increase in particle content in 4 hr at 23 °C	2226	**C**
Hydrocortisone sodium succinate	UP	1 mg/ml[b]	LI	10 mg/ml[b]	Physically compatible with no change in measured turbidity or increase in particle content in 4 hr at 23 °C	2226	**C**
Hydromorphone HCl	AST	0.5 mg/ml[b]	LI	10 mg/ml[b]	Physically compatible with no change in measured turbidity or increase in particle content in 4 hr at 23 °C	2226	**C**
Hydroxyzine HCl	ES	2 mg/ml[b]	LI	10 mg/ml[b]	Physically compatible with no change in measured turbidity or increase in particle content in 4 hr at 23 °C	2226	**C**
Idarubicin HCl	AD	0.5 mg/ml[b]	LI	10 mg/ml[b]	Physically compatible with no change in measured turbidity or increase in particle content in 4 hr at 23 °C	2226	**C**
Ifosfamide	MJ	25 mg/ml[b]	LI	10 mg/ml[b]	Physically compatible with no change in measured turbidity or increase in particle content in 4 hr at 23 °C	2226	**C**
Imipenem–cilastatin sodium	ME	10 mg/ml[b]	LI	10 mg/ml[b]	Yellow-green discoloration forms in 1 hr	2226	**I**
Irinotecan	PHU	5 mg/ml[b]	LI	10 mg/ml[b]	Subvisual haze with green discoloration forms immediately	2226	**I**
Leucovorin calcium	IMM	2 mg/ml[b]	LI	10 mg/ml[b]	Physically compatible with no change in measured turbidity or increase in particle content in 4 hr at 23 °C	2226	**C**
Lorazepam	WY	0.5 mg/ml[a]	LI	10 mg/ml[b]	Physically compatible with no change in measured turbidity or increase in particle content in 4 hr at 23 °C	2226	**C**
Mannitol	BA	15%	LI	10 mg/ml[b]	Physically compatible with no change in measured turbidity or increase in particle content in 4 hr at 23 °C	2226	**C**
Meperidine HCl	AST	4 mg/ml[b]	LI	10 mg/ml[b]	Physically compatible with no change in measured turbidity or increase in particle content in 4 hr at 23 °C	2226	**C**

Y-Site Injection Compatibility (1:1 Mixture) (Cont.)

Gemcitabine HCl

Drug	Mfr	Conc	Mfr	Conc	Remarks	Ref	C/I
Mesna	MJ	10 mg/ml[b]	LI	10 mg/ml[b]	Physically compatible with no change in measured turbidity or increase in particle content in 4 hr at 23 °C	2226	C
Methotrexate sodium	IMM	15 mg/ml[b]	LI	10 mg/ml[b]	Gross precipitate forms immediately, redissolves, but reprecipitates within 15 to 20 min	2226	I
Methylprednisolone sodium succinate	AB	5 mg/ml[b]	LI	10 mg/ml[b]	Gross precipitation occurs immediately	2226	I
Metoclopramide HCl	FAU	5 mg/ml	LI	10 mg/ml[b]	Physically compatible with no change in measured turbidity or increase in particle content in 4 hr at 23 °C	2226	C
Metronidazole	AB	5 mg/ml	LI	10 mg/ml[b]	Physically compatible with no change in measured turbidity or increase in particle content in 4 hr at 23 °C	2226	C
Minocycline HCl	LE	0.2 mg/ml[b]	LI	10 mg/ml[b]	Physically compatible with no change in measured turbidity or increase in particle content in 4 hr at 23 °C	2226	C
Mitomycin	BR	0.5 mg/ml[b]	LI	10 mg/ml[b]	Reddish-purple discoloration forms in 1 hr	2226	I
Mitoxantrone HCl	IMM	0.5 mg/ml[b]	LI	10 mg/ml[b]	Physically compatible with no change in measured turbidity or increase in particle content in 4 hr at 23 °C	2226	C
Morphine sulfate	ES	1 mg/ml[b]	LI	10 mg/ml[b]	Physically compatible with no change in measured turbidity or increase in particle content in 4 hr at 23 °C	2226	C
Nalbuphine HCl	AST	10 mg/ml	LI	10 mg/ml[b]	Physically compatible with no change in measured turbidity or increase in particle content in 4 hr at 23 °C	2226	C
Netilmicin sulfate	SCH	5 mg/ml[b]	LI	10 mg/ml[b]	Physically compatible with no change in measured turbidity or increase in particle content in 4 hr at 23 °C	2226	C
Ofloxacin	MN	4 mg/ml[b]	LI	10 mg/ml[b]	Physically compatible with no change in measured turbidity or increase in particle content in 4 hr at 23 °C	2226	C
Ondansetron HCl	GW	1 mg/ml[b]	LI	10 mg/ml[b]	Physically compatible with no change in measured turbidity or increase in particle content in 4 hr at 23 °C	2226	C
Paclitaxel	MJ	1.2 mg/ml[a]	LI	10 mg/ml[b]	Physically compatible with no change in measured turbidity or increase in particle content in 4 hr at 23 °C	2226	C
Plicamycin	BAY	0.01 mg/ml[b]	LI	10 mg/ml[b]	Physically compatible with no change in measured turbidity or increase in particle content in 4 hr at 23 °C	2226	C
Piperacillin sodium	LE	40 mg/ml[b]	LI	10 mg/ml[b]	Cloudiness forms immediately, becoming precipitated clumps in 4 hr	2226	I
Piperacillin sodium–tazobactam sodium	LE	40 + 5 mg/ml[b]	LI	10 mg/ml[b]	Cloudiness forms immediately, becoming flocculent precipitate in 1 hr	2226	I

Y-Site Injection Compatibility (1:1 Mixture) (Cont.)

Gemcitabine HCl

Drug	Mfr	Conc	Mfr	Conc	Remarks	Ref	C/I
Potassium chloride	AB	0.1 mEq/ml[b]	LI	10 mg/ml[b]	Physically compatible with no change in measured turbidity or increase in particle content in 4 hr at 23 °C	2226	C
Prochlorperazine edisylate	SCN	0.5 mg/ml[b]	LI	10 mg/ml[b]	Subvisual haze forms immediately and increases over 4 hr	2226	I
Promethazine HCl	SCN	2 mg/ml[b]	LI	10 mg/ml[b]	Physically compatible with no change in measured turbidity or increase in particle content in 4 hr at 23 °C	2226	C
Ranitidine HCl	GL	2 mg/ml[b]	LI	10 mg/ml[b]	Physically compatible with no change in measured turbidity or increase in particle content in 4 hr at 23 °C	2226	C
Sodium bicarbonate	AB	1 mEq/ml	LI	10 mg/ml[b]	Physically compatible with no change in measured turbidity or increase in particle content in 4 hr at 23 °C	2226	C
Streptozocin	UP	40 mg/ml[b]	LI	10 mg/ml[b]	Physically compatible with no change in measured turbidity or increase in particle content in 4 hr at 23 °C	2226	C
Teniposide	BR	0.1 mg/ml[a]	LI	10 mg/ml[b]	Physically compatible with no change in measured turbidity or increase in particle content in 4 hr at 23 °C	2226	C
Thiotepa	IMM	1 mg/ml[b]	LI	10 mg/ml[b]	Physically compatible with no change in measured turbidity or increase in particle content in 4 hr at 23 °C	2226	C
Ticarcillin disodium	SKB	30 mg/ml[b]	LI	10 mg/ml[b]	Physically compatible with no change in measured turbidity or increase in particle content in 4 hr at 23 °C	2226	C
Ticarcillin disodium–clavulanate potassium	SKB	31 mg/ml[b]	LI	10 mg/ml[b]	Physically compatible with no change in measured turbidity or increase in particle content in 4 hr at 23 °C	2226	C
Tobramycin sulfate	LI	5 mg/ml[b]	LI	10 mg/ml[b]	Physically compatible with no change in measured turbidity or increase in particle content in 4 hr at 23 °C	2226	C
Topotecan HCl	SKB	0.1 mg/ml[b]	LI	10 mg/ml[b]	Physically compatible with no change in measured turbidity or increase in particle content in 4 hr at 23 °C	2226	C
Trimethoprim–sulfamethoxazole	ES	0.8 + 4 mg/ml[b]	LI	10 mg/ml[b]	Physically compatible with no change in measured turbidity or increase in particle content in 4 hr at 23 °C	2226	C
Vancomycin HCl	LI	10 mg/ml[b]	LI	10 mg/ml[b]	Physically compatible with no change in measured turbidity or increase in particle content in 4 hr at 23 °C	2226	C
Vinblastine sulfate	FAU	0.12 mg/ml[b]	LI	10 mg/ml[b]	Physically compatible with no change in measured turbidity or increase in particle content in 4 hr at 23 °C	2226	C
Vincristine sulfate	FAU	0.05 mg/ml[b]	LI	10 mg/ml[b]	Physically compatible with no change in measured turbidity or increase in particle content in 4 hr at 23 °C	2226	C

Y-Site Injection Compatibility (1:1 Mixture) (Cont.)

Gemcitabine HCl

Drug	Mfr	Conc	Mfr	Conc	Remarks	Ref	C/I
Vinorelbine tartrate	GW	1 mg/ml[b]	LI	10 mg/ml[b]	Physically compatible with no change in measured turbidity or increase in particle content in 4 hr at 23 °C	2226	C
Zidovudine	GW	4 mg/ml[b]	LI	10 mg/ml[b]	Physically compatible with no change in measured turbidity or increase in particle content in 4 hr at 23 °C	2226	C

[a]*Tested in dextrose 5% in water.*
[b]*Tested in sodium chloride 0.9%.*
[c]*Sodium carbonate–containing formulation tested.*

Other Information

Bacterial Challenge— Gemcitabine HCl (Lilly) 2.4 mg/ml diluted in sodium chloride 0.9% and stored at 22 °C did not exhibit a substantial antimicrobial effect on the growth of four organisms (*Enterococcus faecium, Staphylococcus aureus, Pseudomonas aerugi-* *nosa,* and *Candida albicans*) inoculated into the solution. *C. albicans* maintained viability for 120 hours, and the others were viable for 24 hours. The author recommended that diluted solutions of gemcitabine HCl be stored under refrigeration whenever possible and that the potential for microbiological growth should be considered when assigning expiration periods (2160).

GENTAMICIN SULFATE
AHFS 8:12.02

Garamycin   **Schering**

Products— Gentamicin sulfate (Schering) is available in 2-ml vials. Each milliliter contains (2):

Gentamicin (as sulfate)	40 mg
Methylparaben	1.8 mg
Propylparaben	0.2 mg
Sodium bisulfite	3.2 mg
Edetate disodium	0.1 mg

Gentamicin sulfate pediatric injection (Schering) is available in 2-ml vials. Each milliliter contains (2):

Gentamicin (as sulfate)	10 mg
Methylparaben	1.3 mg
Propylparaben	0.2 mg
Sodium bisulfite	3.2 mg
Edetate disodium	0.1 mg

Gentamicin sulfate is also available from several manufacturers premixed in various concentrations in sodium chloride 0.9% for intravenous infusion (4).

pH— The injection for intravenous or intramuscular administration has a pH of 3 to 5.5. Premixed infusions of gentamicin sulfate in sodium chloride 0.9% have a pH of around 4 to 4.5 (4).

Osmotic Values— Gentamicin sulfate (Wyeth) 40 mg/ml has a reported osmolality of 160 mOsm/kg (50). Gentamicin sulfate pediatric injection (Elkins-Sinn) 10 mg/ml has a reported osmolality of 116 mOsm/kg by freezing-point depression or 212 mOsm/kg by vapor pressure (1071).

The osmolality of gentamicin sulfate (SoloPak) 1 mg/ml was determined to be 262 mOsm/kg in dextrose 5% in water and 278 mOsm/kg in sodium chloride 0.9%. At a 2.5-mg/ml concentration, the osmolality was determined to be 278 mOsm/kg in dextrose 5% in water and 293 mOsm/kg in sodium chloride 0.9% (1375).

The osmolality of gentamicin sulfate 80 mg was calculated for the following dilutions (1054):

	Osmolality (mOsm/kg)	
Diluent	50 ml	100 ml
Dextrose 5% in water	293	285
Sodium chloride 0.9%	320	315

The osmolarity of the premixed infusions in sodium chloride 0.9% is approximately 284 to 308 mOsm/L (4).

Administration— Gentamicin sulfate is administered by intramuscular injection or intermittent intravenous infusion over 0.5 to two hours (2; 4; 8). For adults, intravenous administration after dilution in 50 to 200 ml of sodium chloride 0.9% or dextrose 5% in water is recommended, while the volume for pediatric patients should be reduced consistent with the patient's needs (2; 4).

Stability— Storage of the colorless to slightly yellow solution (4) between 2 and 30 °C is recommended, but refrigeration is not required (2). Potency loss has been determined to be unrelated to color intensity of gentamicin sulfate solutions (2139).

Freezing Solutions— Gentamicin sulfate (Schering) 50 mg in 50 ml of dextrose 5% in water and also sodium chloride 0.9% in PVC containers was frozen at −20 °C for 30 days. Potency was retained for the duration of the study (299).

In another study, gentamicin sulfate (Schering) 80 mg/100 ml of dextrose 5% in water in PVC bags was frozen at −20 °C for 30 days and then thawed by exposure to ambient temperature or microwave radiation. No evidence of precipitation or color change was observed, and no loss of potency was determined microbiologically. Subsequent storage of the admixture at room temperature for 24 hours also yielded a physically compatible solution, exhibiting little or no loss of potency (554).

Marble et al. reported that gentamicin sulfate (Elkins-Sinn) 120 mg/50 ml lost 6% activity in dextrose 5% in water and 2% activity in sodium chloride 0.9% in 28 days when frozen at −20 °C (981).

Repackaging in Syringes— Gentamicin sulfate (Schering) 40 mg/ml was found to retain potency for three months at room temperature when 1 and 2 ml of solution were packaged in Tubex cartridges (13).

In another report, the stability of gentamicin sulfate (Schering) repackaged in plastic syringes (Monoject) was significantly less than in glass syringes (Glaspak, Becton-Dickinson) at both 4 and 25 °C. The commercial concentrations were tested in the following amounts: 40 mg/ml—1, 0.75, 0.5, and 0.25 ml; and 10 mg/ml—1.5, 1, and 0.5 ml. Storage in plastic syringes resulted in an average potency loss of 16% in 30 days and in the formation of a brown precipitate. In glass syringes, the average potency loss was 7% at 30 days. The brown precipitate did not appear after 30 days but was present at 60 days. It appeared in the cannula of the needle in both glass and plastic syringes. For the 40-mg/ml concentration, the volume of the sample also affected stability. Significantly less potency loss was noted in the smaller volumes (0.25 and 0.5 ml) than in the larger volumes (0.5 and 1 ml). This volume-related phenomenon was not demonstrated in the 10-mg/ml pediatric concentration. Storage temperature had no effect on potency during the 90-day study period. The authors recommended that only glass disposable syringes be used for long-term unit dose storage of gentamicin sulfate and that storage not exceed 30 days (297).

The appearance of this report stimulated the interest of Kresel et al. They packaged gentamicin sulfate 40 mg/1 ml in polypropylene syringes (Plastipak, Becton-Dickinson) and found no significant change in potency by enzymatic assay over 30 days at 4 or 25 °C (401).

In reply, McNealy et al. noted that a different brand of polypropylene syringes had been used in the study and that plastic composition can vary considerably. Further, they disputed the applicability of the enzymatic assay to long-term plastic-stored samples (402).

The manufacturer also expressed concern about plastic packaging of gentamicin, noting a possibly inadequate oxygen and moisture barrier both through the tip and the walls of the syringe. It was indicated that gentamicin is oxygen sensitive and that depletion of the antioxidant present could result in instability. Further, loss of moisture at the tip could result in occlusion by the dried product. It was noted that disposable syringes are manufactured by Schering with a two-year expiration date (403).

Zbrozek et al. found that gentamicin sulfate (Elkins-Sinn) 120 mg, diluted with 1 ml of sodium chloride 0.9% to a final volume of 4 ml, was stable (less than 10% loss) when stored in polypropylene syringes (Becton-Dickinson) for 48 hours at 25 °C under fluorescent light (1159).

Nahata et al. studied the stability of gentamicin sulfate (Elkins-Sinn) diluted to 10 mg/ml with sodium chloride 0.9% and stored in glass syringes (Becton-Dickinson) at 4 °C. No loss of gentamicin sulfate was found by enzyme-mediated immunoassay during 12 weeks of storage (1265).

Ambulatory Pumps— Tu et al. studied the stability of gentamicin sulfate (Schering) 5.45 mg/ml in dextrose 5% in water in an ambulatory pump reservoir. The drug-filled reservoirs were stored at −20 °C for 30 days and then thawed at 5 °C for four days. This thawing was then followed by two days of drug delivery through the pump at 37 °C. No visible changes and no gentamicin loss occurred during the entire storage and delivery sequence. Furthermore, plasticizer (DEHP) levels were insignificant (1490).

Elastomeric Reservoir Pumps— Gentamicin sulfate (Lyphomed) 0.8 mg/ml in sodium chloride 0.9% 100 ml was packaged in latex elastomeric reservoirs (Secure Medical). Little or no loss by HPLC analysis occurred in 24 hours at 25 °C (1970).

Gentamicin sulfate 0.6 mg/ml in both dextrose 5% in water and sodium chloride 0.9% was evaluated for binding potential to natural rubber elastomeric reservoirs (Baxter). No loss was found after storage for two weeks at 35 °C with gentle agitation (2014).

Sorption— Gentamicin sulfate (Schering) 40 mg/L in sodium chloride 0.9% (Travenol) in PVC bags did not exhibit significant sorption to the plastic during one week of storage at room temperature (15 to 20 °C) (536).

In another study, gentamicin sulfate (Schering) 40 mg/L in sodium chloride 0.9% did not exhibit any loss due to sorption during a seven-hour simulated infusion through an infusion set (Travenol) consisting of a cellulose propionate burette chamber and 170 cm of PVC tubing (606).

The drug was also tested as a simulated infusion over at least one hour by a syringe pump system. A glass syringe on a syringe pump was fitted with 20 cm of polyethylene tubing or 50 cm of Silastic tubing. No drug loss due to sorption was observed with either tubing (606).

A 25-ml aliquot of gentamicin sulfate (Schering) 40 mg/L in sodium chloride 0.9% was stored in all-plastic syringes composed of polypropylene barrels and polyethylene plungers for 24 hours at room temperature in the dark. No loss of drug due to sorption occurred (606).

Filtration— The effect of several filters on the delivered concentration of gentamicin sulfate (Roussel) from simulated pediatric infusions was studied by Nazeravich and Otten. A syringe containing dextrose 10% in water on a syringe pump set at 8.26 ml/hr was connected by intravenous tubing to a 0.5-μm air-blocking filter set (Travenol), a 0.22-μm air-eliminating filter set (Travenol), and a 0.2-μm air-eliminating filter set (Pall). Gentamicin doses of 2.5 and 7.5 mg were injected antegrade to the filter. The effluents were sampled at 1, 1.5, 2, and 4 hours and tested using an enzyme-mediated immunoassay technique (EMIT) assay. No significant drug sorption to the plastic tubing or inline filters occurred. However, because of the difference in specific gravity of the drug (1.010) and intravenous solution (1.032), variations in delivered gentamicin did occur due to filter design and position. With the Travenol filters, gentamicin delivery was more rapid with ascending flow in both horizontal and vertical positions. Drug delivery was significantly delayed with descending flow in both positions. The Pall filter delivered gentamicin more rapidly in the horizontal position with either ascending or descending flow. The vertical filter position significantly delayed drug delivery in both flow directions (804).

However, in another study, gentamicin sulfate 60 mg/15 ml was injected as a bolus through a 0.2-μm nylon air-eliminating filter (Ultipor, Pall) to evaluate the effect of filtration on simulated intravenous push delivery. Enzyme-mediated assays showed that only about 38% of the drug was delivered through the filter after flushing with 10 ml of sodium chloride 0.9% (809).

Filtration of 30 ml of a solution of gentamicin 500 μg/ml (as the sulfate) (Schering) through Seitz sterilizing filters resulted in substantial binding of the drug to the filters. Losses ranged from 31 to 66%, depending on the filter size (823). However, this filter medium does not resemble current clinical filters. Subsequent reassay using membrane filters indicated little or no loss of activity (829).

Thompson et al. evaluated gentamicin sulfate 5 and 10 mg/55 ml of dextrose 5% in water and sodium chloride 0.9% filtered over 20 minutes through a 0.22-μm cellulose ester filter set (Ivex-2, Millipore). EMIT showed that virtually all of the drug was delivered through the filter (1003).

Kane et al. evaluated the binding of gentamicin sulfate to the filter of a set used for continuous ambulatory peritoneal dialysis (CAPD). Gentamicin sulfate (Schering) 60 mg/2 L in Dianeal 137 with dextrose 4.25 and 1.5% was filtered through a Peridex CAPD filter set (Millipore); this set has a surface area 27 times larger than an inline intravenous filter. About 25% binding occurred from the solution containing dextrose 4.25%, but only 7.5% was bound with the 1.5% solution (1112).

Gentamicin sulfate (Unicet-Unilabo) 0.32 mg/ml in dextrose 5% in water and sodium chloride 0.9% was filtered through a 0.22-μm cellulose ester membrane filter (Ivex-HP, Millipore) over six hours. No significant drug loss due to binding to the filter was noted (1034).

Compatibility Information

Solution Compatibility

| | | | | Gentamicin sulfate | | |
Solution	Mfr	Mfr	Conc/L	Remarks	Ref	C/I
Amino acids 4.25%, dextrose 25%	MG	SC	80 mg	No increase in particulate matter in 24 hr at 5 °C	349	C
Dextrose 4.3% in sodium chloride 0.18%		RS	160 mg	Potency retained for up to 48 hr at room temperature	157	C
Dextrose 5% in water		RS	160 mg	Potency retained for up to 48 hr at room temperature	157	C
	AB	SC	160 mg	Potency retained for 24 hr at 5 and 25 °C	88	C
	BA[a], TR	SC	1 g	Potency retained for 24 hr at 5 and 22 °C	298	C
	BA[b]	SC	1 g	Potency retained for 30 days at −20 °C	299	C
	TR[b]	SC	800 mg	Physically compatible with little or no loss of potency in 24 hr at room temperature	554	C
			120 mg	Physically compatible and gentamicin stable by microbiological assay for 24 hr at 25 °C	897	C
	AB[b]	UP	1.2 g	Visually compatible and potency by immunoassay retained for 48 hr at 25 °C under fluorescent light and 4 °C in the dark	1541	C
			600 mg	Formation of decomposition products found by HPLC in 48 hr at room temperature. Gentamicin not quantified	2139	?
Dextrose 10% in water	SO	SC	60 mg/ 21.5 ml[c]	Visually compatible with no gentamicin loss by TDx in 30 days at 5 °C in the dark	1731	C
	SO	SC	120 mg/ 23 ml[c]	Visually compatible with no gentamicin loss by TDx in 30 days at 5 °C in the dark	1731	C
Fat emulsion 10%, intravenous	VT	RS	160 mg	Microscopic globule coalescence within 24 hr at 8 and 25 °C	825	I
Fructose 5% in water			120 mg	Physically compatible and gentamicin stable by microbiological assay for 24 hr at 25 °C	897	C
Invert sugar 7.5% with electrolytes		SC	50 mg	Physically compatible with no gentamicin loss in 24 hr at 29 °C by microbiological assay	440	C
Mannitol 20%			120 mg	Physically compatible and gentamicin stable by microbiological assay for 24 hr at 25 °C	897	C
Ringer's injection			120 mg	Physically compatible and gentamicin stable by microbiological assay for 24 hr at 25 °C	897	C

Solution Compatibility (Cont.)

Gentamicin sulfate

Solution	Mfr	Mfr	Conc/L	Remarks	Ref	C/I
Sodium chloride 0.9%			120 mg	Physically compatible and gentamicin stable by microbiological assay for 24 hr at 25 °C	897	C
		RS	160 mg	Potency retained for up to 48 hr at room temperature	157	C
	BA[a], TR	SC	1 g	Potency retained for 24 hr at 5 and 22 °C	298	C
	BA[b]	SC	1 g	Potency retained for 30 days at −20 °C	299	C
	AB[b]	UP	1.2 g	Visually compatible and potency by immunoassay retained for 48 hr at 25 °C under fluorescent light and 4 °C in the dark	1541	C
	AB[d]	LY	800 mg	Little or no loss of drug by HPLC in 24 hr at 25 °C	1970	C
TPN #1, #4, #5, #7[e]		SC	80 mg	Physically compatible for 24 hr at 22 °C	313	C
TPN #2, #3, #6, #8, #9[e]		SC	80 mg	Physically incompatible with precipitate noted in 8 to 24 hr at 22 °C	313	I
TPN #1[e]		SC	80 mg	Antibiotic potency retained for at least 12 hr at 22 °C	313	C
TPN #10[e]		SC	80 mg	Physically compatible for 24 hr and antibiotic potency retained for at least 12 hr at 22 °C	313	C
TPN #22[e]		SC	800 mg	Physically compatible with no loss of activity by microbiological assay in 24 hr at 22 °C in the dark	837	C
TPN #52 and #53[e]		SC	50 mg	Physically compatible with no gentamicin loss in 24 hr at 29 °C by microbiological assay	440	C
TPN #107[e]			75 mg	Physically compatible and gentamicin activity retained for 24 hr at 21 °C by microbiological assay	1326	C

[a]Tested in both glass and PVC containers.
[b]Tested in PVC containers.
[c]Tested in glass vials as a concentrate.
[d]Tested in glass containers and latex elastomeric reservoirs (Secure Medical).
[e]Refer to Appendix I for the composition of parenteral nutrition solutions. TPN indicates a 2-in-1 admixture.

Additive Compatibility

Gentamicin sulfate

Drug	Mfr	Conc/L	Mfr	Conc/L	Test Soln	Remarks	Ref	C/I
Amphotericin B		200 mg		320 mg	D5W	Haze develops over 3 hr	26	I
Ampicillin sodium	BE	8 g	RS	160 mg	D5¼S, D5W, NS	50% gentamicin decomposition in 2 hr at room temperature	157	I
		1 g		100 mg	TPN #107[a]	42% gentamicin loss and 25% ampicillin loss in 24 hr at 21 °C by microbiological assay	1326	I
Atracurium besylate	BW	500 mg		2 g	D5W	Physically compatible and atracurium chemically stable for 24 hr at 5 and 30 °C	1694	C
Aztreonam	SQ	10 and 20 g	SC	200 and 800 mg	D5W, NS[b]	Little or no aztreonam loss in 48 hr at 25 °C and 7 days at 4 °C. Gentamicin potency retained for 12 hr at 25 °C and 24 hr at 4 °C, with up to 10% loss in 48 hr at 25 °C and 7 days at 4 °C	1023	C

Additive Compatibility (Cont.)

Gentamicin sulfate

Drug	Mfr	Conc/L	Mfr	Conc/L	Test Soln	Remarks	Ref	C/I
Bleomycin sulfate	BR	20 and 30 units	SC	50, 100, 300, 600 mg	NS	Physically compatible and bleomycin activity retained for 1 week at 4 °C. Gentamicin not tested	763	C
Cefamandole nafate	LI	2 and 20 g		80 mg	D5W, NS, W	Haze or precipitate forms within 4 hr	376; 788	I
		1 g		100 mg	TPN #107[a]	14% gentamicin loss in 24 hr at 21 °C by microbiological assay	1326	I
Cefazolin sodium with clindamycin phosphate	SKF UP	10 g 9 g	ES	800 mg	D5W[c]	10% cefazolin loss in 4 hr at 25 °C. Clindamycin and gentamicin potency retained for 24 hr	1328	I
Cefazolin sodium with clindamycin phosphate	SKF UP	10 g 9 g	ES	800 mg	NS[c]	10% cefazolin loss in 12 hr at 25 °C. Clindamycin and gentamicin potency retained for 24 hr	1328	I
Cefepime HCl	BR	4 g	ES	1.2 g	D5W, NS	Cloudiness forms in 18 hr at room temperature	1681	I
Cefoxitin sodium	MSD	5 g	SC	400 mg	D5S	4% cefoxitin decomposition in 24 hr and 11% in 48 hr at 25 °C. 2% in 48 hr at 5 °C. 9% gentamicin decomposition in 24 hr and 23% in 48 hr at 25 °C. 2% in 48 hr at 5 °C	308	C
Cefuroxime sodium	GL	7.5 g	EX	800 mg	D5W, NS[b]	Physically compatible with no loss of either drug in 1 hr	1036	C
		1 g		100 mg	TPN #107[a]	32% gentamicin loss in 24 hr at 21 °C by microbiological assay	1326	I
Cimetidine HCl	SKF	3 g	SC	800 mg	D5W	Physically compatible and cimetidine chemically stable for 24 hr at room temperature. Gentamicin not tested	551	C
	SKF	1.2 and 5 g	SC	80 mg	D5W, NS	Physically compatible and cimetidine chemically stable for 24 hr at room temperature. Gentamicin not tested	551	C
Ciprofloxacin	MI	1.6 g	LY	1 g	D5W, NS	Visually compatible and ciprofloxacin potency by HPLC and gentamicin potency by immunoassay retained for 48 hr at 25 °C under fluorescent light and 4 °C in the dark	1541	C
	BAY	2 g	SC	10 g	NS	Visually compatible with little or no ciprofloxacin loss by HPLC in 24 hr at 25 °C. Gentamicin not tested	1934	C
Clindamycin phosphate	UP	1.2 g		60 mg	D5W	Physically compatible. Clindamycin potency retained for 24 hr at room temperature	104	C
	UP	2.4 g		120 mg	D5W	Physically compatible. Clindamycin potency retained for 24 hr at room temperature	104	C
	UP	9 g		800 mg	D5W	Clindamycin stability maintained for 24 hr	101	C
	UP	12 g		600 mg	D5W	Physically compatible	101	C
	UP	9 g	AB	1 g	D5W, NS[d]	Physically compatible and potency of both drugs retained for 48 hr at room temperature exposed to light 1 week frozen	174	C
	UP	9 g	ES	1.2 g	D5W, NS[c]	Physically compatible and potency of both drugs retained for 28 days frozen	174	C

Additive Compatibility (Cont.)

Gentamicin sulfate

Drug	Mfr	Conc/L	Mfr	Conc/L	Test Soln	Remarks	Ref	C/I
	UP	9 g	LY	1.2 g	D5W[c]	Physically compatible and potency of both drugs retained for 7 days at 4 and 25 °C	174	C
	UP	18 g	LY	2.4 g	D5W[b]	Physically compatible and potency of both drugs retained for 14 days at 4 and 25 °C	174	C
	UP	9 g	LY	1.2 g	NS[c]	Physically compatible and potency of both drugs retained for 14 days at 4 and 25 °C	174	C
	UP	18 g	LY	2.4 g	NS[b]	Physically compatible and potency of both drugs retained for 14 days at 4 and 25 °C	174	C
	UP	18 g	ES	2.4 g	D5W, NS[b]	Potency of both drugs retained for 28 days frozen at −20 °C	981	C
	UP	6 g	ES	667 mg	D5W[b]	Physically compatible with no clindamycin loss and 9% gentamicin loss in 24 hr at room temperature	995	C
		400 mg		75 mg	TPN #107[a]	19% gentamicin loss and 15% clindamycin loss in 24 hr at 21 °C by microbiological assay	1326	I
Cytarabine	UP	100 mg		80 mg	D5W	Physically compatible for 24 hr	174	C
	UP	300 mg		240 mg	D5W	Physically incompatible	174	I
Dopamine HCl	AS	800 mg	SC	2 g	D5W	No dopamine decomposition and 7% gentamicin decomposition in 24 hr at 25 °C	312	C
	AS	800 mg	SC	320 mg	D5W	80% gentamicin decomposition in 24 hr at 23 to 25 °C. Gentamicin potency retained for 6 hr. Dopamine potency retained for 24 hr	78	I
Floxacillin sodium	BE	20 g	RS	8 g	NS	Haze forms immediately and precipitate forms in 2 hr	1479	I
	BE	10 g	EX	8 g	NS	Physically compatible for 48 hr. Potency of both drugs retained when assayed after 1 hr at room temperature	1036	C
	BE	10 g	EX	8 g	D5W	Immediate precipitation	1036	I
Fluconazole	PF	1 g	SO	0.5 g	D5W	Visually compatible with no fluconazole loss by HPLC in 72 hr at 25 °C under fluorescent light. Gentamicin not tested	1677	C
Furosemide	HO	800 mg	SC	1.6 g	D5W, NS	Immediate precipitation of furosemide	876	I
	HO	1 g	RS	8 g	NS	Physically compatible for 24 hr at 15 to 30 °C. Slight precipitate forms in 48 to 72 hr	1479	C
Heparin sodium	BP	20,000 units		320 mg	D5W, NS	Immediate precipitation	26	I
	OR	20,000 units	SC	1 g	D5W, NS	Opalescence	113	I
	BRN	1000 to 6000 units	ME	88 mg	D10W, NS	Activity of both drugs by biological assays greatly reduced	1570	I
Meropenem	ZEN	1 and 20 g	SCH	800 mg	NS	Visually compatible for 4 hr at room temperature	1994	C
Metronidazole	RP	5 g[e]	RS	800 mg		Physically compatible with little or no pH change for at least 72 hr at 23 °C	807	C

Additive Compatibility (Cont.)

Gentamicin sulfate

Drug	Mfr	Conc/L	Mfr	Conc/L	Test Soln	Remarks	Ref	C/I
		5 g	EX	800 mg	D5W, NS[b]	Physically compatible with no loss of either drug in 1 hr	1036	C
	SE	5 g	SC	800 mg and 1.2 g		Physically compatible with no loss of either drug in 2 days at 18 °C. At 4 °C, no metronidazole loss but up to 10% gentamicin loss in 7 days	1242	C
	RP	5 g		800 mg		Visually compatible with no loss of metronidazole by HPLC in 15 days at 5 and 25 °C. 10% gentamicin loss by immunoassay in 63 hr at 25 °C and 10.6 days at 5 °C	1931	C
Metronidazole HCl with sodium bicarbonate	SE AB	5 g 50 mEq	SC	320 mg	D5W, NS	Physically compatible for 48 hr	765	C
Nafcillin sodium		1 g		75 mg	TPN #107[a]	10% gentamicin loss in 24 hr at 21 °C by microbiological assay	1326	I
Ofloxacin	HO	2 g	ESX	800 mg	W	Visually compatible with little or no loss of either drug by HPLC in 48 hr	1613	C
Penicillin G sodium	GL	13 and 40 million units	RS	160 mg	D5¼S, D5W, NS	Gentamicin potency retained for 24 hr at room temperature	157	C
Ranitidine HCl	GL	100 mg		160 mg	D5W	Physically compatible for 24 hr at ambient temperature under fluorescent light	1151	C
	GL	50 mg and 2 g		80 mg	D5W, NS	Physically compatible and ranitidine chemically stable by HPLC for 24 hr at 25 °C. Gentamicin not tested	1515	C
Ticarcillin disodium		2 g		100 mg	TPN #107[a]	Over 98% gentamicin loss in 24 hr at 21 °C by microbiological assay	1326	I
Verapamil HCl	KN	80 mg	SC	160 mg	D5W, NS	Physically compatible for 24 hr	764	C

[a]*Refer to Appendix I for the composition of parenteral nutrition solutions. TPN indicates a 2-in-1 admixture.*
[b]*Tested in PVC containers.*
[c]*Tested in glass containers.*
[d]*Tested in both glass and PVC containers.*
[e]*Minibags (100 ml) containing metronidazole 500 mg with disodium phosphate 150 mg, citric acid 44 mg, and sodium chloride 740 mg. This product differs from the Searle product.*

Drugs in Syringe Compatibility

Gentamicin sulfate

Drug (in syringe)	Mfr	Amt	Mfr	Amt	Remarks	Ref	C/I
Ampicillin sodium	AY	500 mg		80 mg/ 2 ml	Physically incompatible within 1 hr at room temperature	99	I
Cefamandole nafate	LI	1 g/ 10 ml		80 mg/ 2 ml	Haze or precipitate forms within 4 hr	376; 788	I
	LI	1 g/3 ml		80 mg/ 2 ml	Haze or precipitate forms within 4 hr	376; 788	I
Clindamycin phosphate	UP	900 mg/ 6 ml	ES	120 mg/ 4 ml[a]	Physically compatible with little or no loss of either drug for 48 hr at 25 °C in polypropylene syringes	1159	C

Drugs in Syringe Compatibility (Cont.)

Gentamicin sulfate

Drug (in syringe)	Mfr	Amt	Mfr	Amt	Remarks	Ref	C/I
Diatrizoate meglumine 52%, diatrizoate sodium 8%	MA	5 ml	SC	0.8 mg/ 1 ml	Physically compatible for at least 2 hr	1438	**C**
Diatrizoate sodium 60%	MA	5 ml	SC	0.8 mg/ 1 ml	Physically compatible for at least 2 hr	1438	**C**
Heparin sodium		2500 units/ 1 ml		40 mg	Turbidity or precipitate forms within 5 min	1053	**I**
Iohexol	WI	64.7%, 5 ml	SC	0.8 mg/ 1 ml	Physically compatible for at least 2 hr	1438	**C**
Iopamidol	SQ	61%, 5 ml	SC	0.8 mg/ 1 ml	Physically compatible for at least 2 hr	1438	**C**
Iothalamate meglumine 60%	MA	5 ml	SC	0.8 mg/ 1 ml	Physically compatible for at least 2 hr	1438	**C**
Ioxaglate meglumine 39.3%, ioxaglate sodium 19.6%	MA	5 ml	SC	0.8 mg/ 1 ml	Transient precipitate clears within 5 min	1438	**?**
Penicillin G sodium		1 million units		80 mg/ 2 ml	No precipitate or color change within 1 hr at room temperature	99	**C**

[a]Diluted to 4 ml with 1 ml of sodium chloride 0.9%.

Y-Site Injection Compatibility (1:1 Mixture)

Gentamicin sulfate

Drug	Mfr	Conc	Mfr	Conc	Remarks	Ref	C/I
Acyclovir sodium	BW	5 mg/ml[a]	TR	1.6 mg/ml[a]	Physically compatible for 4 hr at 25 °C under fluorescent light	1157	**C**
Allopurinol sodium	BW	3 mg/ml[b]	ES	5 mg/ml[b]	Hazy solution with crystals forms in 1 hr	1686	**I**
Amifostine	USB	10 mg/ml[a]	ES	5 mg/ml[a]	Physically compatible with no change in measured turbidity or increase in particle content in 4 hr at 23 °C	1845	**C**
Amiodarone HCl	LZ	4 mg/ml[c]	LY	0.8 mg/ml[c]	Physically compatible for 4 hr at room temperature	1444	**C**
Amphotericin B cholesteryl sulfate complex	SEQ	0.83 mg/ml[a]	FUJ	5 mg/ml[a]	Gross precipitate forms	2117	**I**
Amsacrine	NCI	1 mg/ml[a]	SO	5 mg/ml[a]	Physically compatible for 4 hr at room temperature under fluorescent light	1381	**C**
Atracurium besylate	BW	0.5 mg/ml[a]	ES	2 mg/ml[a]	Physically compatible for 24 hr at 28 °C	1337	**C**
Aztreonam	SQ	40 mg/ml[a]	ES	5 mg/ml[a]	Physically compatible with no subvisual haze or particle formation in 4 hr at 23 °C	1758	**C**
Cefpirome sulfate	HO	50 mg/ml[d]	LY	1 mg/ml[d]	Visually and microscopically compatible with little or no cefpirome and cefazolin loss by HPLC in 8 hr at 23 °C	2044	**C**
Ciprofloxacin	MI	2 mg/ml[c]	LY	1.6 mg/ml[c]	Visually compatible for 24 hr at 24 °C	1655	**C**
Cisatracurium besylate	GW	0.1, 2, 5 mg/ml[a]	ES	5 mg/ml[a]	Physically compatible with no change in measured turbidity or increase in particle content in 4 hr at 23 °C	2074	**C**

Y-Site Injection Compatibility (1:1 Mixture) (Cont.)

				Gentamicin sulfate			
Drug	*Mfr*	*Conc*	*Mfr*	*Conc*	*Remarks*	*Ref*	*C/I*
Clarithromycin	AB	4 mg/ml[a]	RS	40 mg/ml	Visually compatible for 72 hr at both 30 and 17 °C	2174	**C**
Cyclophosphamide	MJ	20 mg/ml[a]	TR	1.6 mg/ml[a]	Physically compatible for 4 hr at 25 °C	1194	**C**
Cytarabine	UP	16 mg/ml[b]	GNS	15 mg/ml[e]	Visually compatible for 24 hr at room temperature in test tubes. No precipitate found on filter from Y-site delivery	2063	**C**
Diltiazem HCl	MMD	1[b] and 5 mg/ml	SCH	2.4[b] and 40 mg/ml	Visually compatible	1807	**C**
Docetaxel	RPR	0.9 mg/ml[a]	AB	5 mg/ml[a]	Physically compatible with no change in measured turbidity or increase in particle content in 4 hr at 23 °C	2224	**C**
Doxorubicin HCl liposome injection	SEQ	0.4 mg/ml[a]	ES	5 mg/ml[a]	Physically compatible with little or no change in measured turbidity and no increase in particle content in 4 hr at 23 °C	2087	**C**
Enalaprilat	MSD	0.05 mg/ml[b]	ES	0.8 mg/ml[a]	Physically compatible for 24 hr at room temperature under fluorescent light	1355	**C**
Esmolol HCl	DCC	10 mg/ml[a]	ES	0.8 mg/ml[a]	Physically compatible for 24 hr at 22 °C	1169	**C**
Etoposide phosphate	BR	5 mg/ml[a]	AB	5 mg/ml[a]	Physically compatible with no change in measured turbidity or increase in particle content in 4 hr at 23 °C	2218	**C**
Famotidine	MSD	0.2 mg/ml[a]	ES	0.8 mg/ml[b]	Physically compatible for 14 hr	1196	**C**
	ME	2 mg/ml[b]		5 mg/ml[a]	Visually compatible for 4 hr at 22 °C	1936	**C**
Filgrastim	AMG	30 µg/ml[a]	LY	5 mg/ml[a]	Physically compatible with no change in measured turbidity or increase in particle content in 4 hr at 22 °C	1687	**C**
	AMG	40 µg/ml[a]	GNS	1.6 mg/ml[a]	Visually compatible with little or no loss of filgrastim activity by bioassay and gentamicin by immunoassay in 4 hr at 25 °C	2060	**C**
	AMG	10 µg/ml[f]	GNS	1.6 mg/ml[a]	23% loss of filgrastim activity by bioassay in 4 hr at 25 °C. Little or no gentamicin loss by immunoassay	2060	**I**
Fluconazole	RR	2 mg/ml	ES	4 mg/ml	Physically compatible for 24 hr at 25 °C	1407	**C**
Fludarabine phosphate	BX	1 mg/ml[a]	ES	5 mg/ml[a]	Physically compatible for 4 hr at room temperature under fluorescent light	1439	**C**
Foscarnet sodium	AST	24 mg/ml	ES	4 mg/ml	Physically compatible for 24 hr at room temperature under fluorescent light	1335	**C**
	AST	24 mg/ml	ES	2 mg/ml[c]	Physically compatible for 24 hr at 25 °C under fluorescent light by visual and microscopic examination	1393	**C**
Furosemide	HO	10 mg/ml	SC	1.6 mg/ml[c]	White precipitate of furosemide forms immediately	876	**I**
Gemcitabine HCl	LI	10 mg/ml[b]	AB	5 mg/ml[b]	Physically compatible with no change in measured turbidity or increase in particle content in 4 hr at 23 °C	2226	**C**
Granisetron HCl	SKB	1 mg/ml	ES	1.5 mg/ml[b]	Physically compatible with little or no loss of either drug by HPLC in 4 hr at 22 °C	1883	**C**

Y-Site Injection Compatibility (1:1 Mixture) (Cont.)

Gentamicin sulfate

Drug	Mfr	Conc	Mfr	Conc	Remarks	Ref	C/I
Heparin sodium	ES	50 units/ml[c]	ES	3.2 mg/ml[c]	Immediate gross haze	1316	I
	TR	50 units/ml	TR	2 mg/ml	Visually incompatible within 6 hr at 25 °C	1793	I
Hetastarch	DCC	6%	TR	0.8 mg/ml[b]	Immediate precipitation which disappeared after 1 hr at room temperature	1313	I
Hydromorphone HCl	WY	0.2 mg/ml[a]	TR	0.8 mg/ml[a]	Physically compatible for at least 4 hr at 25 °C under fluorescent light	987	C
Idarubicin HCl	AD	1 mg/ml[b]	ES	3 mg/ml[a]	Color changes immediately	1525	I
IL-2	RC	4800 I.U./ml[b]	ES	40 mg/ml	Visually compatible and IL-2 activity by bioassay retained. Gentamicin not tested	1552	C
Indomethacin sodium trihydrate	MSD	0.5 and 1 mg/ml[a]		1 mg/ml[a]	White turbidity forms immediately and becomes white flakes in 1 hr	1550	I
Insulin	LI	0.2 unit/ml[b]	TR	1.2 mg/ml[b]	Physically compatible for 2 hr at 25 °C	1395	C
Iodipamide meglumine	SQ				White precipitate forms immediately downstream to Y-site when given into a set through which gentamicin was administered previously	324	I
Labetalol HCl	SC	1 mg/ml[a]	ES	0.8 mg/ml[a]	Physically compatible for 24 hr at 18 °C	1171	C
Lorazepam	WY	0.33 mg/ml[b]	CNF	3 mg/ml	Visually compatible for 24 hr at 22 °C	1855	C
Magnesium sulfate	IX	16.7, 33.3, 66.7, 100 mg/ml[a]	SC	0.8 mg/ml[a]	Physically compatible for at least 4 hr at 32 °C	813	C
Melphalan HCl	BW	0.1 mg/ml[b]	LY	5 mg/ml[b]	Physically compatible with no change in measured turbidity or increase in particle content in 3 hr at 22 °C	1557	C
Meperidine HCl	WY	10 mg/ml[a]	TR	0.8 mg/ml[a]	Physically compatible for at least 4 hr at 25 °C under fluorescent light	987	C
	WY	10 mg/ml[b]	ES	1.2 and 2 mg/ml[b]	Physically compatible for 1 hr at 25 °C	1338	C
Meropenem	ZEN	1 and 50 mg/ml[b]	SCH	4 mg/ml[g]	Visually compatible for 4 hr at room temperature	1994	C
Midazolam HCl	RC	1 mg/ml[a]	ES	10 mg/ml	Visually compatible for 24 hr at 23 °C	1847	C
	RC	5 mg/ml	CNF	3 mg/ml	Visually compatible for 24 hr at 22 °C	1855	C
Morphine sulfate	WI	1 mg/ml[a]	TR	0.8 mg/ml[a]	Physically compatible for at least 4 hr at 25 °C under fluorescent light	987	C
	ES	1 mg/ml[b]	ES	1.2 and 2 mg/ml[b]	Physically compatible for 1 hr at 25 °C	1338	C
Multivitamins	USV	5 ml/L[a]	SC	80 mg/ 100 ml[a]	Physically compatible for 24 hr at room temperature	323	C
Ondansetron HCl	GL	1 mg/ml[b]	ES	5 mg/ml[a]	Physically compatible for 4 hr at 22 °C	1365	C
Paclitaxel	NCI	1.2 mg/ml[a]	ES	5 mg/ml[a]	Physically compatible with no change in measured turbidity in 4 hr at 22 °C	1556	C
Pancuronium bromide	ES	0.05 mg/ml[a]	ES	2 mg/ml[a]	Physically compatible for 24 hr at 28 °C	1337	C
Perphenazine	SC	0.02 mg/ml[a]	TR	1.6 mg/ml[a]	Physically compatible for 4 hr at 25 °C	1155	C
Propofol	ZEN	10 mg/ml	ES	5 mg/ml[a]	White precipitate forms immediately	2066	I

Y-Site Injection Compatibility (1:1 Mixture) (Cont.)

		Gentamicin sulfate					
Drug	*Mfr*	*Conc*	*Mfr*	*Conc*	*Remarks*	*Ref*	*C/I*
Remifentanil HCl	GW	0.025 and 0.25 mg/ml[b]	ES	5 mg/ml[a]	Physically compatible with no change in measured turbidity or increase in particle content in 4 hr at 23 °C	2075	**C**
Sargramostim	IMM	10 μg/ml[a]	SO	5 mg/ml[a]	Physically compatible for 4 hr at 22 °C	1436	**C**
Tacrolimus	FUJ	1 mg/ml[b]	SCN	4 mg/ml[a]	Visually compatible for 24 hr at 25 °C	1630	**C**
Teniposide	BR	0.1 mg/ml[a]	LY	5 mg/ml[a]	Physically compatible with no subvisual haze or particle formation in 4 hr at 23 °C	1725	**C**
Theophylline	TR	4 mg/ml	TR	2 mg/ml	Visually compatible for 6 hr at 25 °C	1793	**C**
Thiotepa	IMM[h]	1 mg/ml[a]	ES	5 mg/ml[a]	Physically compatible with no change in measured turbidity or increase in particle content in 4 hr at 23 °C	1861	**C**
TNA #73[i]		32.5 ml[j]	SC	80 mg/ 50 ml[a]	Physically compatible for 4 hr at 25 °C by visual observation	1008	**C**
TNA #97 to #104[i]			ES	40 mg/ml	Physically compatible and gentamicin content retained for 6 hr at 21 °C by TDx	1324	**C**
TNA #218 to #226[i]			AB, FUJ	5 mg/ml[a]	Visually compatible with no precipitate or emulsion damage apparent in 4 hr at 23 °C	2215	**C**
Tolazoline HCl		0.1 mg/ml[a]	ES	10 mg/ml[a]	Physically compatible for 24 hr at 22 °C	1363	**C**
TPN #54[i]				13 and 20 mg/ml	Physically compatible and gentamicin activity retained over 6 hr at 22 °C by microbiological assay	1045	**C**
TPN #61[i]		[k]	IX	12.5 mg/ 1.25 ml[l]	Physically compatible	1012	**C**
		[m]	IX	75 mg/ 1.9 ml[l]	Physically compatible	1012	**C**
TPN #91[i]		[n]	IX	5 mg[o]	Physically compatible	1170	**C**
TPN #189[i]			DB	1 mg/ml[b]	Visually compatible for 24 hr at 22 °C	1767	**C**
TPN #203 and #204[i]			ES	10 mg/ml	Visually compatible for 2 hr at 23 °C	1974	**C**
TPN #212 to #215[i]			AB	5 mg/ml[a]	Physically compatible with no change in measured turbidity or increase in particle content in 4 hr at 23 °C	2109	**C**
Vecuronium bromide	OR	0.1 mg/ml[a]	ES	2 mg/ml[a]	Physically compatible for 24 hr at 28 °C	1337	**C**
Vinorelbine tartrate	BW	1 mg/ml[b]	ES	5 mg/ml[b]	Physically compatible with no change in measured turbidity or increase in particle content in 4 hr at 22 °C	1558	**C**
Vitamin B complex with C (Berocca-C 500)	RC	4 ml/L[a]	SC	80 mg/ 100 ml[a]	Physically compatible for 24 hr at room temperature	323	**C**
(Berocca-C)	RC	20 ml/L[a]	SC	80 mg/ 100 ml[a]	Physically compatible for 24 hr at room temperature	323	**C**
Warfarin sodium	DU	2 mg/ml[g]	SCH	1.6 mg/ml[a]	Haze forms immediately	2010	**I**
	DME	2 mg/ml[g]	SC	1.6 mg/ml[a]	Haze forms immediately	2078	**I**

Y-Site Injection Compatibility (1:1 Mixture) (Cont.)

Gentamicin sulfate

Drug	Mfr	Conc	Mfr	Conc	Remarks	Ref	C/I
Zidovudine	BW	4 mg/ml[a]	IMS	2 mg/ml[a]	Physically compatible for 4 hr at 25 °C under fluorescent light by visual and microscopic examination	1193	C

[a]*Tested in dextrose 5% in water.*
[b]*Tested in sodium chloride 0.9%.*
[c]*Tested in both dextrose 5% in water and sodium chloride 0.9%.*
[d]*Tested in dextrose 5% in water, Ringer's injection, lactated, sodium chloride 0.45%, and sodium chloride 0.9%.*
[e]*Tested in sodium chloride 0.45%.*
[f]*Tested in dextrose 5% in water with human albumin 2 mg/ml.*
[g]*Tested in sterile water for injection.*
[h]*Lyophilized formulation tested.*
[i]*Refer to Appendix I for the composition of parenteral nutrition solutions. TNA indicates a 3-in-1 admixture, and TPN indicates a 2-in-1 admixture.*
[j]*A 32.5-ml sample of parenteral nutrition solution mixed with 50 ml of antibiotic solution.*
[k]*Run at 21 ml/hr.*
[l]*Given over 30 minutes by syringe pump.*
[m]*Run at 94 ml/hr.*
[n]*Run at 10 ml/hr.*
[o]*Given over one hour by syringe pump.*

Additional Compatibility Information

Infusion Solutions— Gentamicin sulfate (Schering) maintains potency for 24 hours at room temperature in the following solutions (227):

Dextran 40 (Dextran 10% in dextrose 5%)
Dextrose 5% in Polysal
Dextrose 5% in Polysal M
Dextrose 5% in water
Dextrose 10% in water
Isolyte E with dextrose 5%
Isolyte M with dextrose 5%
Isolyte P with dextrose 5%
Normosol M in dextrose 5% in water
Normosol R
Normosol R in dextrose 5% in water
Normosol R, pH 7.4
Ringer's injection
Ringer's injection, lactated
Sodium chloride 0.9%
Travert 5% with Electrolyte #2
Travert 10% with Electrolyte #3

Kern et al. evaluated serum concentrations of gentamicin sulfate following intermittent 15 to 30-minute administration as piggyback infusions in 50 ml of dextrose 5% in water or 50 ml of TPN #177 (see Appendix I). Gentamicin serum concentrations were equivalent using both administration methods (1573).

Local Anesthetics— Gentamicin sulfate (Schering) 80 mg (2 ml) was physically compatible with 1 ml of each of the following local anesthetics and did not show significant loss of potency in 24 hours at room temperature or under refrigeration (227):

Chloroprocaine HCl 1 and 2% (Pennwalt)
Hexylcaine HCl 1% (MSD)
Lidocaine HCl 1 and 2% (Astra)
Lidocaine HCl 1 and 2% with epinephrine 1:100,000 (Astra)
Mepivacaine HCl 1 and 2% (Winthrop)
Piperocaine HCl 2% (Lilly)
Procaine HCl 1 and 2% (Winthrop)

β-Lactam Antibiotics— In common with other aminoglycoside antibiotics, gentamicin activity may be impaired by β-lactam antibiotics. The inactivation is dependent on concentration, temperature, and time of exposure.

In 1971, McLaughlin and Reeves first reported the inactivation of gentamicin sulfate by carbenicillin disodium. They cited two cases in which gentamicin serum levels fell when carbenicillin was subsequently added to the regimen. They further noted a decrease in gentamicin half-life in serum, distilled water, and phosphate buffer to 40 hours at 35 °C and 70 hours at 20 °C. Gentamicin alone showed no loss of activity in 140 hours under these conditions (219). Because the combined use of carbenicillin disodium and gentamicin sulfate has been reported to be additive or synergistic in its antibacterial effect against Pseudomonas and the combination has been used extensively in the clinical treatment of Pseudomonas infections, this article provoked quite a response in the literature.

Klastersky was not convinced of the result, citing the possibility that the antibacterial properties of gentamicin might have been inhibited by some other substance. It was further stated that given the success of combination therapy, even if such inhibition did occur, its clinical significance was not great (220).

Levison and Kaye were not convinced either. Their tests of carbenicillin and gentamicin in serum and trypticase soy broth did not show loss of gentamicin in 18 hours at 37 °C (221).

Eykyn et al., however, did note slow inactivation of gentamicin by carbenicillin in vitro after several hours at 37 °C (222).

Furthermore, Riff and Jackson reported that gentamicin was biologically not detectable after prolonged mixture in solution with carbenicillin. They stated that gentamicin loses potency in proportion to time, temperature, and the concentration of carbenicillin (223).

McLaughlin and Reeves combined, in vitro, 5 μg/ml of gentamicin with carbenicillin concentrations of 250, 500, and 1000 μg/ml. With incubation at 35 °C, they detected no change in gentamicin at 250 μg/ml of carbenicillin in eight hours; but in the 500-μg/ml combination, a 44% loss of gentamicin was detected at eight hours. At 1000 μg/ml of carbenicillin, 42 and 66% losses of gentamicin occurred in four and eight hours, respectively (665).

Noone and Pattison evaluated the inactivation of gentamicin by various penicillins (and cephalosporins), including carbenicillin disodium. They noted a significant loss of gentamicin activity after 30 minutes and a 50% loss of potency after eight to 12 hours when gentamicin sulfate (Roussel) 160 mg/L was combined with carbenicillin disodium (Beecham) 20 g/L in various intravenous solutions at room temperature (157).

Winters et al. confirmed that significant loss of gentamicin activity occurred in vitro when mixed with carbenicillin. Gentamicin in concentrations of 5 to 10 μg/ml was mixed with a high concentration of carbenicillin, 500 μg/ml. Within four to six hours at room temperature, significant loss of gentamicin activity had occurred. At lower concentrations, 50 to 100 μg/ml, the loss of activity was much slower. Further experiments in dogs and humans showed that gentamicin serum levels were not significantly altered by concomitant carbenicillin therapy provided the two drugs were not mixed and allowed to stand before administration (361).

In a similar in vitro experiment, Waitz et al. found the same result. Gentamicin activity dropped from 4.3 μg/ml to 2.2 μg/ml in 24 hours and to 1.4 μg/ml in 72 hours at 20 °C in the presence of carbenicillin 100 μg/ml in distilled water. The amount of inactivation was dependent on temperature and time and was slowed by the addition of pH 7.0 buffers. Tests in mice and dogs failed to reveal any effect of carbenicillin on gentamicin serum levels (362).

Zost and Yanchick failed to elucidate the situation further in their report since only the stability of carbenicillin disodium was reported (88), although they later said that the two antibiotics were stable for 24 hours (224).

Riff and Jackson, however, found a 50% inactivation of gentamicin in four to six hours at room temperature when 24 g of carbenicillin disodium was added to 240 mg of gentamicin sulfate in sodium chloride 0.9%. They also noted that the half-life of gentamicin sulfate decreased as the ratio of carbenicillin disodium increased with respect to gentamicin sulfate in distilled water at 37 °C. The authors stated that the inactivation of gentamicin by carbenicillin is dependent on the integrity of the β-lactam ring, with carbenicillin and gentamicin interacting to form a conjugate inactivating both. The higher the concentration of carbenicillin, the faster is the inactivation of gentamicin. Further, the rate of gentamicin inactivation is decreased by the presence of other solutes, especially proteins (218).

Young et al. determined the degree of gentamicin loss in vitro for combinations of gentamicin plus carbenicillin of 400 μg/ml plus 12.8 mg/ml, 40 μg/ml plus 1.28 mg/ml, and 4 μg/ml plus 0.128 mg/ml in distilled water. The solutions were incubated at 35 and 39 °C. Gentamicin levels fell to 35 to 47% of initial amounts in eight hours at 35 °C while the carbenicillin concentration was about 84 to 91% of the initial amount. At 39 °C after eight hours, gentamicin levels of 12 to 24% and carbenicillin levels of 65 to 68% were determined (666).

In vitro studies by Ervin et al. showed extensive decomposition of gentamicin by carbenicillin at 37 °C in human serum (363).

Similar inactivation effects on gentamicin sulfate occur in combination with ticarcillin (363; 365; 614), although the extent of inactivation appears to be less than with carbenicillin (574; 575).

Holt et al. found that incubation of gentamicin sulfate 10 mg/L in sodium chloride 0.9% with 500 mg/L of carbenicillin or ticarcillin at 37 °C for 24 hours resulted in about 60 to 70% reduction of gentamicin activity. When serum was substituted for the sodium chloride solution, 30 to 50% reduction in activity was reported. However, when buffered to pH 7.4 in aqueous solution, essentially all of the gentamicin activity was lost (574).

Pickering and Gearhart reported that gentamicin sulfate 5 and 10 μg/ml, dissolved in human serum and incubated with carbenicillin and ticarcillin 100 to 600 μg/ml at 37 °C, demonstrated greater rates of decomposition at the higher concentrations of the penicillins. In 24 hours, about a 9% loss of gentamicin activity occurred at 100 μg/ml and about a 60% loss occurred at 600 μg/ml of carbenicillin. Approximately a 20% loss at 100 μg/ml and an 85% loss at 600 μg/ml occurred in 72 hours with carbenicillin. Ticarcillin affected gentamicin less under these conditions. Little or no loss of gentamicin activity occurred at 100 μg/ml of ticarcillin in 72 hours. However, the gentamicin loss increased to 20% at 300 μg/ml and to 70% at 600 μg/ml of ticarcillin in 72 hours (575).

Murillo et al. determined that lower serum levels of gentamicin occurred in patients with normal renal function when concomitant ticarcillin disodium was administered compared to concomitant cephalothin sodium. The dose of ticarcillin disodium was 12 g/m²/day while cephalothin sodium was given at 7 g/m²/day. The gentamicin sulfate dose was 180 mg/m²/day. In one hour, gentamicin serum levels of 3.1 μg/ml resulted in patients receiving the cephalothin while only 2.0 μg/ml was achieved in patients on ticarcillin. Ticarcillin levels also were substantially reduced (667).

Several aminoglycosides in combination with several penicillins were evaluated. Gentamicin sulfate, netilmicin sulfate, and tobramycin sulfate 5 μg/ml were combined with carbenicillin disodium, azlocillin sodium, and mezlocillin sodium 50, 250, and 500 μg/ml in human plasma. Samples were evaluated over nine days at 27 and 37 °C. All of the aminoglycosides underwent significant inactivation during the evaluation. Aminoglycoside decomposition of 17 to 61% in 24 hours occurred at the higher two concentrations of penicillins—the highest inactivation was sustained by tobramycin and the lowest by netilmicin. Little if any aminoglycoside inactivation occurred at 50 μg/ml of penicillin. Carbenicillin caused greater aminoglycoside decomposition than did azlocillin or mezlocillin (616).

Flournoy noted the relative degree of inactivation of tobramycin, gentamicin, netilmicin, and amikacin 10 mg/L in serum when combined with carbenicillin 125 to 1000 mg/L at −20 to 42 °C. Tobramycin was more susceptible to inactivation than the others. Amikacin was the least susceptible, and gentamicin and netilmicin were similar in intermediate susceptibility to inactivation (617).

Although piperacillin sodium and aminoglycosides act synergistically and have been used successfully clinically when recommended doses of each drug have been administered, mixing piperacillin sodium directly in a syringe or infusion bottle with an aminoglycoside can substantially inactivate the aminoglycoside (740).

Hale et al. evaluated piperacillin and carbenicillin at concentrations of 62.5 to 1000 μg/ml in human serum in combination with amikacin, gentamicin, or tobramycin 10 μg/ml at 37 °C for up to 24 hours by bioassay and radioimmunoassay. Penicillin concentrations of 62.5 and 125 μg/ml had relatively little effect on the aminoglycoside concentration, even after 24 hours. However, increasing the penicillin concentration to 250 or 500 μg/ml greatly increased decomposition. After 24 hours with carbenicillin 500 μg/ml, the amounts of aminoglycosides remaining were amikacin, 82%; gentamicin, 43%; and tobramycin, 27%. After 24 hours with piperacillin 500 μg/ml, the remaining concentrations were 95, 45, and 52%, respectively. Even greater inactivation occurred at 1000 μg/ml of the penicillins, including the essentially complete loss of tobramycin in 24 hours. The authors concluded that amikacin is much more resistant to inactivation than the other aminoglycosides tested and that carbenicillin is apparently more aggressive in its inactivation than piperacillin (816).

To determine if spurious aminoglycoside levels could result from a delay in assaying blood samples, Tindula et al. evaluated the inactivation of amikacin 35 μg/ml and gentamicin and tobramycin 10 μg/ml in human serum by 400-μg/ml concentrations of several penicillins and cephalosporins. Samples were stored for 24 hours at room temperature and frozen at −20 °C. For the room temperature samples, cefazolin and cefamandole caused relatively little inactivation. Nafcillin, cephapirin, and cefoxitin caused moderate inactivation, 20% or less. Penicillin, ampicillin, carbenicillin, and ticarcillin generally caused 25% or more inactivation of gentamicin and tobramycin. Amikacin was somewhat less affected. Freezing samples at −20 °C prevented significant inactivation of amikacin and gentamicin by any of the drugs. Freezing the tobramycin samples was satisfactory for most of the drugs except penicillin, ampicillin, and carbenicillin, which still exhibited a 15 to 20% tobramycin loss in 24 hours (824).

Pickering and Rutherford evaluated several aminoglycosides combined with a number of penicillins. Gentamicin sulfate, netilmicin sulfate, and tobramycin sulfate 5 and 10 μg/ml and amikacin 10 and 20 μg/ml were combined in human serum with 125, 250, and 500 μg/ml of azlocillin, carbenicillin disodium, amdinocillin, mezlocillin, and piperacillin individually. Tobramycin and gentamicin sustained greater losses than netilmicin and amikacin at each of the penicillin concentrations. Significant decomposition of all aminoglycosides occurred in 24 hours at 37 °C at a penicillin concentration of 500 μg/ml. Tobramycin and gentamicin had losses of 40 to 60%, while 15 to 30% losses occurred for netilmicin. Amikacin sustained the least inactivation with losses of about 10 to 20%. At penicillin concentrations of 125 to 250 μg/ml, smaller losses of aminoglycosides were observed (68).

The inactivation of gentamicin 10 μg/ml in sterile distilled water by several β-lactam antibiotics stored at 37 °C was reported by Jorgensen and Crawford. Ticarcillin and carbenicillin 500 μg/ml caused 34 and 44% gentamicin losses, respectively, in six hours, but only ticarcillin caused a significant loss (about 15%) at 100 μg/ml. Cephalothin 500 μg/ml caused a 17% gentamicin loss in four hours but no significant loss at 100 μg/ml. Gentamicin was not inactivated by 500- or 100-μg/ml concentrations of penicillin G, cefotaxime, or moxalactam. No loss of β-lactam antibiotic activity was detected in any concentration (973).

The comparative inactivation of five aminoglycosides by seven β-lactam antibiotics in human serum at 37 °C was reported by Riff and Thomason. Amikacin, followed by netilmicin, had the lowest degree of inactivation; tobramycin sustained the most pronounced losses. Gentamicin and kanamycin were intermediate in the extent of losses. The six penicillins that were tested all produced aminoglycoside inactivation; the greatest extent of inactivation was caused by carbenicillin, ticarcillin, penicillin G, oxacillin, methicillin, and ampicillin, in approximate descending order. Cephalothin produced minimal inactivation (5 to 10% in 24 hours). The rate of inactivation could be reduced by storage at 4 °C and further reduced by storage at −20 °C. The authors suggested processing blood samples rapidly to avoid inaccurate serum determinations. Storage of specimens at low temperature until analysis may be helpful (1052).

Townsend reported the apparent inactivation of gentamicin sulfate

by ampicillin sodium in blood samples held for 12 hours prior to assay (1382).

Roberts et al. studied the stability of azlocillin sodium 500 mg/L combined with the aminoglycosides amikacin sulfate 20 mg/L, gentamicin sulfate 8 mg/L, and netilmicin sulfate 7.5 mg/L in peritoneal dialysis solution (Dianeal 1.36%) stored at 37 °C. No azlocillin sodium loss occurred by HPLC during the eight-hour study period. However, the aminoglycosides tested by the enzyme-multiplied immunoassay technique (EMIT) showed 10% losses in about six hours for gentamicin sulfate and netilmicin sulfate and in about 30 minutes for amikacin sulfate (1179).

Gentamicin sulfate (Schering) 25 μg/ml combined separately with the cephalosporins cefazolin sodium (Lilly), cefamandole nafate (Lilly), and cefoxitin sodium (MSD) at a concentration of 125 μg/ml in peritoneal dialysis solution (Dianeal 1.5%) exhibited enhanced rates of lethality to *Staphylococcus aureus*, *Escherichia coli*, and *Pseudomonas aeruginosa* compared to any of the drugs alone (1623).

The inactivation of gentamicin, tobramycin, and amikacin, each 5 μg/ml, by seven β-lactam antibiotics, 250 and 500 μg/ml, in serum at 25 °C over 24 hours was studied using bioassay, EMIT, fluorescence polarization immunoassay (TDx), and radioimmunoassay. No inactivation of any aminoglycoside by the cephalosporins moxalactam, cefotaxime, and cefazolin occurred within the study period. Results with the penicillins varied, depending on the assay technique used. The bioassay was the most sensitive to loss, TDx and radioimmunoassay were intermediate, and EMIT was the least sensitive. Azlocillin, carbenicillin, mezlocillin, and piperacillin all caused variable but extensive inactivation (up to 70%) of gentamicin and tobramycin in 24 hours. Amikacin, however, had only minor losses compared to the other aminoglycosides (654).

The clinical significance of these interactions in patients appears to be primarily confined to those with renal failure (218; 334; 361; 364; 616; 737; 816; 847). Literature reports of greatly reduced aminoglycoside levels in such patients have appeared frequently (363; 365–367; 614; 615; 962). In addition, the interaction may be clinically important if assays for aminoglycoside levels in serum are sufficiently delayed (576; 618; 735; 832; 847; 1052; 1382).

Most authors believe that in vitro mixing of penicillins such as ticarcillin disodium with aminoglycoside antibiotics should be avoided but that clinical use of the drugs in combination can be of great value. It is generally recommended that the drugs be given separately in such combined therapy (157; 218; 222; 224; 361; 364; 368–370).

Cephalosporins— Cefotaxime sodium (Hoechst-Roussel) should not be mixed with aminoglycosides in the same solution, but they may be administered to the same patient separately (2; 792).

Cefotetan disodium is stated to be physically incompatible with aminoglycosides (4; 283).

When gentamicin sulfate (Schering) 80 mg/100 ml in dextrose 5% in water was run through an administration set previously used to administer cefoperazone (Roerig) 1 g/100 ml in dextrose 5% in water, an immediate precipitate formed in the infusion tubing where the two solutions mixed (831).

Teil et al. studied the stability of gentamicin 3.8 μg/ml and cefamandole 11 μg/ml in serum stored at 24, 6, and −17 °C for 24 hours. No substantial differences in the concentration of either drug occurred, indicating that gentamicin is not inactivated in the presence of cefamandole (864). (Also see the section on β-Lactam Antibiotics.)

Heparin—— Addition of gentamicin sulfate (Roussel) 80 mg to the tubing of an infusion solution of sodium chloride 0.9% containing heparin resulted in immediate precipitation (528).

Gentamicin sulfate 10 mg/L with heparin sodium 1000 units/L in Dianeal with dextrose 5% peritoneal dialysis solution was reported to be conditionally compatible. Koup and Gerbracht reported no significant reduction in gentamicin sulfate concentration or in the UV absorbance of heparin sodium in four to six hours (228). However, a clarifying communication noted a marked reduction in the anticoagulant activity of heparin sodium if opalescence or a precipitate formed (which results if the undiluted drugs are combined), even if the precipitate redissolved. Heparin activity was retained if one drug was added to a dilute solution of the other and no precipitate formed (295).

The incompatibility of heparin sodium with gentamicin sulfate is said to result from coprecipitation (230).

A white precipitate may result from the administration of gentamicin sulfate through a heparinized intravenous cannula (976). Flushing heparin locks with sodium chloride 0.9% before and after administering drugs incompatible with heparin has been recommended (4).

Phenytoin and Furosemide—— A 2-ml fluid barrier of dextrose 5% in water in a microbore retrograde infusion set failed to prevent precipitation when used between gentamicin sulfate 5 mg/0.5 ml and phenytoin sodium 5 mg/0.1 ml or furosemide 2 mg/0.2 ml (1385).

Peritoneal Dialysis Solutions—— The activity of gentamicin 10 mg/L was evaluated in peritoneal dialysis fluids containing 1.5 or 4.25% dextrose (Dianeal 137, Travenol). Storage at 25 °C resulted in no loss of antimicrobial activity in 24 hours (515).

Gentamicin sulfate (Schering) 3 and 10 mg/L in peritoneal dialysis concentrate with 50% dextrose (McGaw) retained about 90% of initial activity in seven hours and about 50 to 70% in 24 hours at room temperature as determined by microbiological assay (1044).

The stability of gentamicin sulfate 8 mg/L, alone and with cefazolin sodium 75 and 150 mg/L, was evaluated in a peritoneal dialysis solution of dextrose 1.5% with heparin sodium 1000 units/L. Gentamicin activity was retained for 48 hours at both 4 and 26 °C, alone and with both concentrations of cefazolin. Cefazolin activity was also retained over the study period. At 37 °C, gentamicin losses ranged from 4 to 8% and cefazolin losses ranged from 10 to 12% in 48 hours (1029).

In another study, the stability of gentamicin sulfate (Schering) was evaluated in peritoneal dialysate concentrates containing dextrose 30 and 50% (Dianeal) as well as in a diluted solution containing dextrose 2.5%. The gentamicin sulfate concentrations were 100 and 160 mg/L in the peritoneal dialysate concentrates and 5 and 8 mg/L in the diluted solutions. By immunoassay techniques, gentamicin sulfate was found to be stable in all of these solutions for at least 24 hours at 23 °C (1229).

Halstead et al. evaluated gentamicin 4 μg/ml in Dianeal PDS with dextrose 1.5 and 4.25% (Travenol) with cefazolin 125 μg/ml, heparin 500 units, and albumin 80 mg in 2-L bags. The gentamicin content, determined by EMIT assay, was retained for 72 hours (1413).

Drake et al. evaluated the retention of antimicrobial activity, using a disc diffusion bioassay, of gentamicin sulfate (SoloPak) 120 mg/L alone and with vancomycin HCl (Lilly) 1 g/L in Dianeal PD-2 (Travenol) with dextrose 1.5%. Little or no loss of either antibiotic occurred in eight hours at 37 °C. Gentamicin sulfate alone retained activity for at least 48 hours at 4 and 25 °C. In combination with vancomycin HCl, antimicrobial activity of both antibiotics was retained for up to 48 hours. However, the authors recommended refrigeration at 4 °C for storage periods greater than 24 hours (1414).

Other Information

Heating Plasma—— Heating plasma samples to 56 °C for one hour to inactivate potential HIV content resulted in no gentamicin loss as determined by TDx (1615).

GLYCOPYRROLATE
AHFS 12:08.08

Robinul   **Robins**

Products—— Glycopyrrolate (Robins) is available in 1- and 2-ml single-dose vials and 5- and 20-ml multiple-dose vials. Each milliliter of solution contains glycopyrrolate 0.2 mg, sodium hydroxide and/or hydrochloric acid to adjust the pH, and benzyl alcohol 0.9% in water for injection (2).

pH—— From 2 to 3 (2).

Osmolality—— Glycopyrrolate 0.2 mg/ml has an osmolality of 91 mOsm/kg (1689).

Administration—— Glycopyrrolate may be administered by intravenous or intramuscular injection without dilution (2; 4). The drug may also be given via the tubing of a running intravenous infusion (2; 4; 8).

Stability—— Glycopyrrolate (Robins) is a clear, colorless solution; intact vials should be stored at controlled room temperature (2).

pH Effects—— The stability of glycopyrrolate in solution is pH dependent. At pH 2 to 3, the drug is very stable. Above pH 6, the stability becomes questionable because of ester hydrolysis. The speed of this hydrolysis is increased with increasing pH (331).

Table 1. Stability of Glycopyrrolate 0.8 mg/L in Dextrose 5% in Water Adjusted to Various pH Values (25 °C)

Admixture pH	Approximate Time for 5% Decomposition (hr)
4.0	>48
5.0	>48
6.0	30
6.5	7
7.0	4
8.0	2

The effect of increasing pH on stability can be seen in Table 1. Ingallinera et al. showed a significant decline in stability as the pH was increased above 6 (331).

Also see Alkaline Drugs in Additional Compatibility Information below.

Syringes— Glycopyrrolate (American Regent) 0.1 mg/ml in sodium chloride 0.9% packaged in polypropylene syringes (Sherwood) was physically stable and exhibited little or no loss by stability-indicating HPLC analysis in 24 hours stored at 4 and 23 °C (2199).

Compatibility Information

Solution Compatibility

Glycopyrrolate

Solution	Mfr	Mfr	Conc/L	Remarks	Ref	C/I
Dextrose 5% in sodium chloride 0.45%	MG	RB	0.8 mg	Physically compatible and pH in stability range for glycopyrrolate for 48 hr at 25 °C	331	C
Dextrose 5% in water	AB	RB	0.8 mg	Physically compatible and pH in stability range for glycopyrrolate for 48 hr at 25 °C	331	C
Ringer's injection	AB	RB	0.8 mg	Physically compatible and pH in stability range for glycopyrrolate for 48 hr at 25 °C	331	C
Sodium chloride 0.9%	CU	RB	0.8 mg	Physically compatible and pH in stability range for glycopyrrolate for 48 hr at 25 °C	331	C

Additive Compatibility

Glycopyrrolate

Drug	Mfr	Conc/L	Mfr	Conc/L	Test Soln	Remarks	Ref	C/I
Methylprednisolone sodium succinate	UP	250 mg	RB	Up to 1.33 mg	D5½S	Physically incompatible	329	I

Drugs in Syringe Compatibility

Glycopyrrolate

Drug (in syringe)	Mfr	Amt	Mfr	Amt	Remarks	Ref	C/I
Atropine sulfate	ES	0.4 mg/ 1 ml	RB	0.2 mg/ 1 ml	[a]	331	C
	ES	0.8 mg/ 2 ml	RB	0.2 mg/ 1 ml	[a]	331	C
	ES	0.4 mg/ 1 ml	RB	0.4 mg/ 2 ml	[a]	331	C
Chloramphenicol sodium succinate	PD	100 mg/ 1 ml	RB	0.2 mg/ 1 ml	Gas evolves	331	I
	PD	200 mg/ 2 ml	RB	0.2 mg/ 1 ml	Gas evolves	331	I
	PD	100 mg/ 1 ml	RB	0.4 mg/ 2 ml	Gas evolves	331	I
Chlorpromazine HCl	SKF	25 mg/ 1 ml	RB	0.2 mg/ 1 ml	[a]	331	C
	SKF	50 mg/ 2 ml	RB	0.2 mg/ 1 ml	[a]	331	C
	SKF	25 mg/ 1 ml	RB	0.4 mg/ 2 ml	[a]	331	C
Cimetidine HCl	SKF	300 mg/ 2 ml	ES	0.2 mg/ 1 ml	Physically compatible for 4 hr at 25 °C	25	C
Codeine phosphate	LI	30 mg/ 1 ml	RB	0.2 mg/ 1 ml	[a]	331	C

Drugs in Syringe Compatibility (Cont.)

Glycopyrrolate

Drug (in syringe)	Mfr	Amt	Mfr	Amt	Remarks	Ref	C/I
	LI	60 mg/ 2 ml	RB	0.2 mg/ 1 ml	a	331	**C**
	LI	30 mg/ 1 ml	RB	0.4 mg/ 2 ml	a	331	**C**
Dexamethasone sodium phosphate	MSD	4 mg/ 1 ml	RB	0.2 mg/ 1 ml	Physically compatible for 48 hr at 25 °C but pH >6.0. 5% glycopyrrolate decomposition may occur in 4 to 7 hr	331	**I**
	MSD	8 mg/ 2 ml	RB	0.2 mg/ 1 ml	Physically compatible for 48 hr at 25 °C but pH >6.0. 5% glycopyrrolate decomposition may occur in 4 to 7 hr	331	**I**
	MSD	4 mg/ 1 ml	RB	0.4 mg/ 2 ml	Physically compatible for 48 hr at 25 °C but pH >6.0. 5% glycopyrrolate decomposition may occur in 4 to 7 hr	331	**I**
	MSD	24 mg/ 1 ml	RB	0.2 mg/ 1 ml	Physically compatible for 48 hr at 25 °C but pH >6.0. 5% glycopyrrolate decomposition may occur in 4 to 7 hr	331	**I**
	MSD	48 mg/ 2 ml	RB	0.2 mg/ 1 ml	Physically compatible for 48 hr at 25 °C but pH >6.0. 5% glycopyrrolate decomposition may occur in 4 to 7 hr	331	**I**
	MSD	24 mg/ 1 ml	RB	0.4 mg/ 2 ml	Physically compatible for 48 hr at 25 °C but pH >6.0. 5% glycopyrrolate decomposition may occur in 4 to 7 hr	331	**I**
Diazepam	RC	5 mg/ 1 ml	RB	0.2 mg/ 1 ml	Immediate precipitation	331	**I**
	RC	10 mg/ 2 ml	RB	0.2 mg/ 1 ml	Immediate precipitation	331	**I**
	RC	5 mg/ 1 ml	RB	0.4 mg/ 2 ml	Immediate precipitation	331	**I**
Dimenhydrinate	SE	50 mg/ 1 ml	RB	0.2 mg/ 1 ml	Immediate precipitation	331	**I**
	SE	100 mg/ 2 ml	RB	0.2 mg/ 1 ml	Immediate precipitation	331	**I**
	SE	50 mg/ 1 ml	RB	0.4 mg/ 2 ml	Immediate precipitation	331	**I**
Diphenhydramine HCl	PD	10 mg/ 1 ml	RB	0.2 mg/ 1 ml	a	331	**C**
	PD	20 mg/ 2 ml	RB	0.2 mg/ 1 ml	a	331	**C**
	PD	10 mg/ 1 ml	RB	0.4 mg/ 2 ml	a	331	**C**
	PD	50 mg/ 1 ml	RB	0.2 mg/ 1 ml	a	331	**C**
	PD	100 mg/ 2 ml	RB	0.2 mg/ 1 ml	a	331	**C**
	PD	50 mg/ 1 ml	RB	0.4 mg/ 2 ml	a	331	**C**
Droperidol	MN	2.5 mg/ 1 ml	RB	0.2 mg/ 1 ml	a	331	**C**
	MN	5 mg/ 2 ml	RB	0.2 mg/ 1 ml	a	331	**C**
	MN	2.5 mg/ 1 ml	RB	0.4 mg/ 2 ml	a	331	**C**

Drugs in Syringe Compatibility (Cont.)

Glycopyrrolate

Drug (in syringe)	Mfr	Amt	Mfr	Amt	Remarks	Ref	C/I
Droperidol and fentanyl citrate (Innovar)	MN	2.5 mg + 0.05 mg/ 1 ml	RB	0.2 mg/ 1 ml	a	331	C
	MN	5 mg + 0.1 mg/ 2 ml	RB	0.2 mg/ 1 ml	a	331	C
	MN	2.5 mg + 0.05 mg/ 1 ml	RB	0.4 mg/ 2 ml	a	331	C
Hydromorphone HCl	KN	2 mg/ 1 ml	RB	0.2 mg/ 1 ml	a	331	C
	KN	4 mg/ 2 ml	RB	0.2 mg/ 1 ml	a	331	C
	KN	2 mg/ 1 ml	RB	0.4 mg/ 2 ml	a	331	C
Hydroxyzine HCl	PF	25 mg/ 1 ml	RB	0.2 mg/ 1 ml	a	331	C
	PF	50 mg/ 2 ml	RB	0.2 mg/ 1 ml	a	331	C
	PF	25 mg/ 1 ml	RB	0.4 mg/ 2 ml	a	331	C
Levorphanol tartrate	RC	2 mg/ 1 ml	RB	0.2 mg/ 1 ml	a	331	C
	RC	4 mg/ 2 ml	RB	0.2 mg/ 1 ml	a	331	C
	RC	2 mg/ 1 ml	RB	0.4 mg/ 2 ml	a	331	C
Lidocaine HCl	ES	10 mg/ 1 ml	RB	0.2 mg/ 1 ml	a	331	C
	ES	20 mg/ 2 ml	RB	0.2 mg/ 1 ml	a	331	C
	ES	10 mg/ 1 ml	RB	0.4 mg/ 2 ml	a	331	C
	ES	20 mg/ 1 ml	RB	0.2 mg/ 1 ml	a	331	C
	ES	40 mg/ 2 ml	RB	0.2 mg/ 1 ml	a	331	C
	ES	20 mg/ 1 ml	RB	0.4 mg/ 2 ml	a	331	C
Meperidine HCl	WI	50 mg/ 1 ml	RB	0.2 mg/ 1 ml	a	331	C
	WI	100 mg/ 2 ml	RB	0.2 mg/ 1 ml	a	331	C
	WI	50 mg/ 1 ml	RB	0.4 mg/ 2 ml	a	331	C
Meperidine HCl and promethazine HCl (Mepergan)	WY	25 mg + 25 mg/ 1 ml	RB	0.2 mg/ 1 ml	a	331	C
	WY	50 mg + 50 mg/ 2 ml	RB	0.2 mg/ 1 ml	a	331	C

Drugs in Syringe Compatibility (Cont.)

Glycopyrrolate

Drug (in syringe)	Mfr	Amt	Mfr	Amt	Remarks	Ref	C/I
	WY	25 mg + 25 mg/ 1 ml	RB	0.4 mg/ 2 ml	a	331	C
Methohexital sodium	LI	10 mg/ 1 ml	RB	0.2 mg/ 1 ml	Immediate precipitation	331	I
	LI	20 mg/ 2 ml	RB	0.2 mg/ 1 ml	Immediate precipitation	331	I
	LI	10 mg/ 1 ml	RB	0.4 mg/ 2 ml	Immediate precipitation	331	I
Midazolam HCl	RC	5 mg/ 1 ml	RB	0.2 mg/ 1 ml	Physically compatible for 4 hr at 25 °C under fluorescent light	1145	C
Morphine sulfate	LI	15 mg/ 1 ml	RB	0.2 mg/ 1 ml	a	331	C
	LI	30 mg/ 2 ml	RB	0.2 mg/ 1 ml	a	331	C
	LI	15 mg/ 1 ml	RB	0.4 mg/ 2 ml	a	331	C
Nalbuphine HCl	DU	10 mg/ 1 ml	RB	0.2 mg/ 1 ml	Physically compatible for 48 hr	128	C
	DU	20 mg/ 1 ml	RB	0.2 mg/ 1 ml	Physically compatible for 48 hr	128	C
Neostigmine methylsulfate	RC	0.5 mg/ 1 ml	RB	0.2 mg/ 1 ml	a	331	C
	RC	1 mg/ 2 ml	RB	0.2 mg/ 1 ml	a	331	C
	RC	0.5 mg/ 1 ml	RB	0.4 mg/ 2 ml	a	331	C
Ondansetron HCl	GW	1 mg/ml[b]	AMR	0.1 mg/ ml[b]	Physically compatible with no measured increase in particulates and little or no loss of either drug by HPLC in 24 hr at 4 or 23 °C	2199	C
Oxymorphone HCl	EN	1 mg/ 1 ml	RB	0.2 mg/ 1 ml	a	331	C
	EN	2 mg/ 2 ml	RB	0.2 mg/ 1 ml	a	331	C
	EN	1 mg/ 1 ml	RB	0.4 mg/ 2 ml	a	331	C
	EN	1.5 mg/ 1 ml	RB	0.2 mg/ 1 ml	a	331	C
	EN	3 mg/ 2 ml	RB	0.2 mg/ 1 ml	a	331	C
	EN	1.5 mg/ 1 ml	RB	0.4 mg/ 2 ml	a	331	C
Pentazocine lactate	WI	30 mg/ 1 ml	RB	0.2 mg/ 1 ml	Immediate precipitation	331	I
	WI	60 mg/ 2 ml	RB	0.2 mg/ 1 ml	Immediate precipitation	331	I
	WI	30 mg/ 1 ml	RB	0.4 mg/ 2 ml	Immediate precipitation	331	I
Pentobarbital sodium	AB	50 mg/ 1 ml	RB	0.2 mg/ 1 ml	Immediate precipitation	331	I

Drugs in Syringe Compatibility (Cont.)

Glycopyrrolate

Drug (in syringe)	Mfr	Amt	Mfr	Amt	Remarks	Ref	C/I
	AB	100 mg/ 2 ml	RB	0.2 mg/ 1 ml	Immediate precipitation	331	**I**
	AB	50 mg/ 1 ml	RB	0.4 mg/ 2 ml	Immediate precipitation	331	**I**
Procaine HCl	ES	10 mg/ 1 ml	RB	0.2 mg/ 1 ml	a	331	**C**
	ES	20 mg/ 2 ml	RB	0.2 mg/ 1 ml	a	331	**C**
	ES	10 mg/ 1 ml	RB	0.4 mg/ 2 ml	a	331	**C**
	ES	20 mg/ 1 ml	RB	0.2 mg/ 1 ml	a	331	**C**
	ES	40 mg/ 2 ml	RB	0.2 mg/ 1 ml	a	331	**C**
	ES	20 mg/ 1 ml	RB	0.4 mg/ 2 ml	a	331	**C**
Prochlorperazine edisylate	SKF	5 mg/ 1 ml	RB	0.2 mg/ 1 ml	a	331	**C**
	SKF	10 mg/ 2 ml	RB	0.2 mg/ 1 ml	a	331	**C**
	SKF	5 mg/ 1 ml	RB	0.4 mg/ 2 ml	a	331	**C**
Promazine HCl	WY	50 mg/ 1 ml	RB	0.2 mg/ 1 ml	a	331	**C**
	WY	100 mg/ 2 ml	RB	0.2 mg/ 1 ml	a	331	**C**
	WY	50 mg/ 1 ml	RB	0.4 mg/ 2 ml	a	331	**C**
Promethazine HCl	WY	25 mg/ 1 ml	RB	0.2 mg/ 1 ml	a	331	**C**
	WY	50 mg/ 2 ml	RB	0.2 mg/ 1 ml	a	331	**C**
	WY	25 mg/ 1 ml	RB	0.4 mg/ 2 ml	a	331	**C**
Promethazine HCl and meperidine HCl (Mepergan)	WY	25 mg + 25 mg/ 1 ml	RB	0.2 mg/ 1 ml	a	331	**C**
	WY	50 mg + 50 mg/ 2 ml	RB	0.2 mg/ 1 ml	a	331	**C**
	WY	25 mg + 25 mg/ 1 ml	RB	0.4 mg/ 2 ml	a	331	**C**
Propiomazine HCl	WY	20 mg/ 1 ml	RB	0.2 mg/ 1 ml	a	331	**C**
	WY	40 mg/ 2 ml	RB	0.2 mg/ 1 ml	a	331	**C**
	WY	20 mg/ 1 ml	RB	0.4 mg/ 2 ml	a	331	**C**
Pyridostigmine bromide	RC	5 mg/ 1 ml	RB	0.2 mg/ 1 ml	a	331	**C**
	RC	10 mg/ 2 ml	RB	0.2 mg/ 1 ml	a	331	**C**

Drugs in Syringe Compatibility (Cont.)

Glycopyrrolate

Drug (in syringe)	Mfr	Amt	Mfr	Amt	Remarks	Ref	C/I
	RC	5 mg/ 1 ml	RB	0.4 mg/ 2 ml	a	331	C
Ranitidine HCl	GL	50 mg/ 2 ml	RB	0.2 mg/ 1 ml	Physically compatible for 1 hr at 25 °C both macroscopically and microscopically	978	C
Scopolamine HBr	ES	0.4 mg/ 1 ml	RB	0.2 mg/ 1 ml	a	331	C
	ES	0.8 mg/ 2 ml	RB	0.2 mg/ 1 ml	a	331	C
	ES	0.4 mg/ 1 ml	RB	0.4 mg/ 2 ml	a	331	C
Secobarbital sodium	LI	50 mg/ 1 ml	RB	0.2 mg/ 1 ml	Immediate precipitation	331	I
	LI	100 mg/ 2 ml	RB	0.2 mg/ 1 ml	Immediate precipitation	331	I
	LI	50 mg/ 1 ml	RB	0.4 mg/ 2 ml	Immediate precipitation	331	I
Sodium bicarbonate	AB	75 mg/ 1 ml	RB	0.2 mg/ 1 ml	Gas evolves	331	I
	AB	150 mg/ 2 ml	RB	0.2 mg/ 1 ml	Gas evolves	331	I
	AB	75 mg/ 1 ml	RB	0.4 mg/ 2 ml	Gas evolves	331	I
Thiopental sodium	AB	25 mg/ 1 ml	RB	0.2 mg/ 1 ml	Immediate precipitation	331	I
	AB	50 mg/ 2 ml	RB	0.2 mg/ 1 ml	Immediate precipitation	331	I
	AB	25 mg/ 1 ml	RB	0.4 mg/ 2 ml	Immediate precipitation	331	I
Triflupromazine HCl	SQ	10 mg/ 1 ml	RB	0.2 mg/ 1 ml	a	331	C
	SQ	20 mg/ 2 ml	RB	0.2 mg/ 1 ml	a	331	C
	SQ	10 mg/ 1 ml	RB	0.4 mg/ 2 ml	a	331	C
	SQ	20 mg/ 1 ml	RB	0.2 mg/ 1 ml	a	331	C
	SQ	40 mg/ 2 ml	RB	0.2 mg/ 1 ml	a	331	C
	SQ	20 mg/ 1 ml	RB	0.4 mg/ 2 ml	a	331	C
Trimethobenzamide HCl	BE	100 mg/ 1 ml	RB	0.2 mg/ 1 ml	a	331	C
	BE	200 mg/ 2 ml	RB	0.2 mg/ 1 ml	a	331	C
	BE	100 mg/ 1 ml	RB	0.4 mg/ 2 ml	a	331	C

[a]*Physically compatible for 48 hours at 25 °C. The pH of the mixture was within the stability range of glycopyrrolate (2 to 6) for 48 hours at 25 °C.*
[b]*Tested in sodium chloride 0.9%.*

Y-Site Injection Compatibility (1:1 Mixture)

Glycopyrrolate

Drug	Mfr	Conc	Mfr	Conc	Remarks	Ref	C/I
Propofol	ZEN	10 mg/ml	RB	0.2 mg/ml	Physically compatible for 1 hr at 23 °C with no increase in particle content	2066	C

Additional Compatibility Information

Glycopyrrolate is stated to be physically and chemically compatible with buprenorphine HCl (4).

Alkaline Drugs— Because of the low pH of glycopyrrolate (Robins), mixtures with alkaline drugs such as barbiturates result in precipitation of the free acid. If the pH of the admixture is increased above 6 by an alkaline additive or solution, rapid ester hydrolysis of the glycopyrrolate results (331).

Infusion Solutions— Glycopyrrolate (Robins) is stated to be physically compatible with dextrose 5% in water, dextrose 10% in water, and sodium chloride 0.9% (2). Glycopyrrolate 0.8 mg/L in Ringer's injection, lactated, is physically compatible for 48 hours at 25 °C. The pH of the solution (6.1) is slightly higher than the pH range yielding acceptable glycopyrrolate stability (2 to 6). In dextrose 5% in water with the pH adjusted to 6, less than 5% decomposition occurred in 30 hours at 25 °C. With the pH adjusted to 6.5, 5% decomposition resulted in only seven hours (331). However, the drug can be administered via the tubing of a running intravenous infusion of lactated Ringer's injection (2; 4).

GRANISETRON HCL
AHFS 56:22

Kytril   **SmithKline Beecham**

Products— Granisetron HCl (SmithKline Beecham) is available in 1-ml single-use vials containing granisetron 1 mg and sodium chloride 9 mg. Granisetron HCl is also available in 4-ml multiple-dose vials providing in each milliliter granisetron 1 mg, sodium chloride 9 mg, citric acid 2 mg, and benzyl alcohol 10 mg as a preservative (2).

pH— Single-use vials: from 4.7 to 7.3. Multiple-dose vials: from 4 to 6 (2).

Equivalency— Granisetron HCl 1.12 mg provides 1 mg of granisetron (2).

Osmolality— Granisetron HCl (SmithKline Beecham) 1 mg/ml has an osmolality of 290 mOsm/kg (2043).

Administration— Granisetron HCl may be administered intravenously undiluted over 30 seconds or by intravenous infusion over five minutes after dilution to 20 to 50 ml with dextrose 5% in water or sodium chloride 0.9% (2; 4).

Stability— Granisetron HCl is a clear, colorless injection. Intact single-use vials should be stored at 30 °C or less and protected from freezing and light. Multiple-dose vials should be stored at 20 to 25 °C. The drug is stable for at least 24 hours when diluted as directed in dextrose 5% in water or sodium chloride 0.9% and stored at room temperature under normal lighting conditions (2).

Syringes— Granisetron HCl (SmithKline Beecham) 0.05, 0.07, and 0.1 mg/ml (as granisetron) in sodium chloride 0.9% and in dextrose 5% in water was repackaged in polypropylene syringes (Sherwood Medical) (closure used not cited). Little or no granisetron HCl loss occurred by HPLC analysis after 14 days at 5 and 24 °C (1968).

Granisetron HCl (SmithKline Beecham) 1 mg/ml was repackaged into Plastipak (Becton Dickinson) polypropylene syringes and stored at room temperature exposed to or protected from light and refrigerated at 4 °C. HPLC analysis found little or no granisetron HCl loss in 15 days under any of these storage conditions (2149).

Granisetron HCl (Beecham) 0.15 mg/ml in dextrose 5% in water or sodium chloride 0.9% packaged in polypropylene syringes (Becton-Dickinson) was stored for three days at 20 °C, for seven days at 4 °C followed by three days at 20 °C, and frozen at –20 °C for 30 days, followed by seven days at 4 °C and then three more days at 20 °C. All the solutions remained visually clear and without color change, and HPLC analysis found little or no loss of granisetron HCl (1884).

Portable Pumps— The stability of granisetron HCl (SmithKline Beecham) 0.02 mg/ml in dextrose 5% in water and sodium chloride 0.9% in elastomeric balloons, composed of the polymer Krayton (Shell), for a portable pump (Homepump, 100 ml/hr, Block Medical) was evaluated. The disposable balloons were stored at 4 °C for 14 days and assayed periodically by HPLC analysis. Granisetron losses of 5% or less were found during seven days in sodium chloride 0.9% and during 14 days in dextrose 5% in water. However, after 14 days, a granisetron sample in sodium chloride 0.9% exhibited a 13% loss and could not be considered stable for this time period (1837).

Compatibility Information

Solution Compatibility

Granisetron HCl

Solution	Mfr	Mfr	Conc/L	Remarks	Ref	C/I
Bacteriostatic water for injection	ES[a]	SKB	200 mg	Physically compatible with little or no loss by HPLC in 24 hr at 20 °C under fluorescent light	1883	**C**
Dextrose 5% in sodium chloride 0.45%	BA[b]	SKB	20 mg	Physically compatible with little or no loss by HPLC in 24 hr at 20 °C under fluorescent light	1883	**C**
Dextrose 5% in sodium chloride 0.9%	BA[b]	SKB	20 mg	Physically compatible with little or no loss by HPLC in 24 hr at 20 °C under fluorescent light	1883	**C**
Dextrose 5% in water	BA[b]	SKB	20 mg	Physically compatible with little or no loss by HPLC in 24 hr at 20 °C under fluorescent light	1883	**C**
	BA[a]	SKB	200 mg	Physically compatible with little or no loss by HPLC in 24 hr at 20 °C under fluorescent light	1883	**C**
		BE	56[a] and 150[b] mg	Visually compatible with little or no loss by HPLC in 30 days at −20 °C followed by 7 days at 4 °C followed by 3 days at 20 °C	1884	**C**
Sodium chloride 0.9%	BA[b]	SKB	20 mg	Physically compatible with little or no loss by HPLC in 24 hr at 20 °C under fluorescent light	1883	**C**
	BA[a]	SKB	200 mg	Physically compatible with little or no loss by HPLC in 24 hr at 20 °C under fluorescent light	1883	**C**
		BE	56[a] and 150[b] mg	Visually compatible with little or no loss by HPLC in 30 days at −20 °C followed by 7 days at 4 °C followed by 3 days at 20 °C	1884	**C**

[a]Tested in polypropylene syringes.
[b]Tested in PVC containers.

Additive Compatibility

Granisetron HCl

Drug	Mfr	Conc/L	Mfr	Conc/L	Test Soln	Remarks	Ref	C/I
Dexamethasone sodium phosphate	AMR	92 mg	SKB	10 and 40 mg	D5W, NS[a]	Visually compatible with little or no loss of either drug by HPLC in 14 days at 4 and 24 °C protected from light	1875	**C**
	AMR	660 mg	SKB	10 and 40 mg	D5W, NS[a]	Visually compatible with little or no dexamethasone loss and up to 8% granisetron loss by HPLC in 14 days at 4 and 24 °C protected from light	1875	**C**
	MSD	75 and 345 mg	BE	55 and 51 mg	D5W, NS[a]	Visually compatible with little or no loss of either drug by HPLC in 72 hr at room temperature	1884	**C**
Methylprednisolone sodium succinate	DAK	2.26 g	BE	56 mg	D5W, NS[a]	Visually compatible with little or no loss of either drug by HPLC in 72 hr at room temperature	1884	**C**

[a]Tested in PVC containers.

Drugs in Syringe Compatibility

Granisetron HCl

Drug (in syringe)	Mfr	Amt	Mfr	Amt	Remarks	Ref	C/I
Dexamethasone sodium phosphate	MSD	0.2 and 1 mg/ml[a]	BE	0.15 mg/ml[a]	Visually compatible with little or no loss of either drug by HPLC in 72 hr at room temperature	1884	C
Methylprednisolone sodium succinate	DAK	6 mg/ml[a]	BE	0.15 mg/ml[a]	Visually compatible with little or no loss of either drug by HPLC in 72 hr at room temperature	1884	C

[a]*Granisetron HCl in sodium chloride 0.9% and dextrose 5% in water. Diluted further with 17 ml of water.*

Y-Site Injection Compatibility (1:1 Mixture)

Granisetron HCl

Drug	Mfr	Conc	Mfr	Conc	Remarks	Ref	C/I
Acyclovir sodium	BW	7 mg/ml[a]	SKB	0.05 mg/ml[a]	Physically compatible with no change in measured turbidity or increase in particle content in 4 hr at 23 °C	2000	C
Allopurinol sodium	BW	3 mg/ml[a]	SKB	0.05 mg/ml[a]	Physically compatible with no change in measured turbidity or increase in particle content in 4 hr at 23 °C	2000	C
Amifostine	USB	10 mg/ml[a]	SKB	0.05 mg/ml[a]	Physically compatible with no change in measured turbidity or increase in particle content in 4 hr at 23 °C	2000	C
Amikacin sulfate	AB	5 mg/ml[a]	SKB	0.05 mg/ml[a]	Physically compatible with no change in measured turbidity or increase in particle content in 4 hr at 23 °C	2000	C
Aminophylline	AB	2.5 mg/ml[a]	SKB	0.05 mg/ml[a]	Physically compatible with no change in measured turbidity or increase in particle content in 4 hr at 23 °C	2000	C
Amphotericin B	PH	0.6 mg/ml[a]	SKB	0.05 mg/ml[a]	Large increase in measured turbidity occurs immediately	2000	I
Amphotericin B cholesteryl sulfate complex	SEQ	0.83 mg/ml[a]	SKB	0.05 mg/ml[a]	Physically compatible with little or no change in measured turbidity or increase in particle content in 4 hr at 23 °C under fluorescent light	2117	C
Ampicillin sodium	MAR	20 mg/ml[b]	SKB	0.05 mg/ml[a]	Physically compatible with no change in measured turbidity or increase in particle content in 4 hr at 23 °C	2000	C
Ampicillin sodium–sulbactam sodium	RR	20 + 10 mg/ml[b]	SKB	0.05 mg/ml[a]	Physically compatible with no change in measured turbidity or increase in particle content in 4 hr at 23 °C	2000	C
Amsacrine	NCI	1 mg/ml[a]	SKB	0.05 mg/ml[a]	Physically compatible with no change in measured turbidity or increase in particle content in 4 hr at 23 °C. Precipitate forms in 24 hr	2000	C
Aztreonam	SQ	40 mg/ml[a]	SKB	0.05 mg/ml[a]	Physically compatible with no change in measured turbidity or increase in particle content in 4 hr at 23 °C	2000	C
Bleomycin	MJ	1 unit/ml[b]	SKB	0.05 mg/ml[a]	Physically compatible with no change in measured turbidity or increase in particle content in 4 hr at 23 °C	2000	C

Y-Site Injection Compatibility (1:1 Mixture) (Cont.)

Granisetron HCl

Drug	Mfr	Conc	Mfr	Conc	Remarks	Ref	C/I
Bumetanide	RC	0.04 mg/ml[a]	SKB	0.05 mg/ml[a]	Physically compatible with no change in measured turbidity or increase in particle content in 4 hr at 23 °C	2000	**C**
Buprenorphine HCl	RKC	0.04 mg/ml[a]	SKB	0.05 mg/ml[a]	Physically compatible with no change in measured turbidity or increase in particle content in 4 hr at 23 °C	2000	**C**
Butorphanol tartrate	APC	0.04 mg/ml[a]	SKB	0.05 mg/ml[a]	Physically compatible with no change in measured turbidity or increase in particle content in 4 hr at 23 °C	2000	**C**
Calcium gluconate	AB	40 mg/ml[a]	SKB	0.05 mg/ml[a]	Physically compatible with no change in measured turbidity or increase in particle content in 4 hr at 23 °C	2000	**C**
Carboplatin	BR	1 mg/ml[b]	SKB	1 mg/ml	Physically compatible with little or no loss of either drug by HPLC in 4 hr at 22 °C	1883	**C**
Carmustine	BMS	1.5 mg/ml[a]	SKB	0.05 mg/ml[a]	Physically compatible with no change in measured turbidity or increase in particle content in 4 hr at 23 °C	2000	**C**
Cefazolin sodium	SKB	20 mg/ml[a]	SKB	0.05 mg/ml[a]	Physically compatible with no change in measured turbidity or increase in particle content in 4 hr at 23 °C	2000	**C**
Cefepime HCl	BMS	20 mg/ml[a]	SKB	0.05 mg/ml[a]	Physically compatible with no change in measured turbidity or increase in particle content in 4 hr at 23 °C	2000	**C**
Cefoperazone sodium	RR	40 mg/ml[a]	SKB	0.05 mg/ml[a]	Physically compatible with no change in measured turbidity or increase in particle content in 4 hr at 23 °C	2000	**C**
Cefotaxime sodium	HO	20 mg/ml[a]	SKB	0.05 mg/ml[a]	Physically compatible with no change in measured turbidity or increase in particle content in 4 hr at 23 °C	2000	**C**
Cefotetan sodium	STU	20 mg/ml[a]	SKB	0.05 mg/ml[a]	Physically compatible with no change in measured turbidity or increase in particle content in 4 hr at 23 °C	2000	**C**
Cefoxitin sodium	ME	20 mg/ml[a]	SKB	0.05 mg/ml[a]	Physically compatible with no change in measured turbidity or increase in particle content in 4 hr at 23 °C	2000	**C**
Ceftazidime[c]	SKB	16.7 mg/ml[b]	SKB	1 mg/ml	Physically compatible with little or no loss of either drug by HPLC in 4 hr at 22 °C	1883	**C**
Ceftizoxime sodium	FUJ	20 mg/ml[a]	SKB	0.05 mg/ml[a]	Physically compatible with no change in measured turbidity or increase in particle content in 4 hr at 23 °C	2000	**C**
Ceftriaxone sodium	RC	20 mg/ml[a]	SKB	0.05 mg/ml[a]	Physically compatible with no change in measured turbidity or increase in particle content in 4 hr at 23 °C	2000	**C**
Cefuroxime sodium	LI	30 mg/ml[a]	SKB	0.05 mg/ml[a]	Physically compatible with no change in measured turbidity or increase in particle content in 4 hr at 23 °C	2000	**C**

Y-Site Injection Compatibility (1:1 Mixture) (Cont.)

Granisetron HCl

Drug	Mfr	Conc	Mfr	Conc	Remarks	Ref	C/I
Chlorpromazine HCl	SCN	2 mg/ml[a]	SKB	0.05 mg/ml[a]	Physically compatible with no change in measured turbidity or increase in particle content in 4 hr at 23 °C	2000	C
Cimetidine HCl	SKB	3 mg/ml[b]	SKB	1 mg/ml	Physically compatible with little or no loss of either drug by HPLC in 4 hr at 22 °C	1883	C
Ciprofloxacin	MI	1 mg/ml[a]	SKB	0.05 mg/ml[a]	Physically compatible with no change in measured turbidity or increase in particle content in 4 hr at 23 °C	2000	C
Cisplatin	BR	1 mg/ml	SKB	1 mg/ml	Physically compatible with little or no loss of either drug by HPLC in 4 hr at 22 °C	1883	C
	BR	0.05 mg/ml[b]	SKB	1 mg/ml	Physically compatible with little or no granisetron loss by HPLC in 4 hr at 22 °C	1883	C
Cladribine	ORT	0.015[b] and 0.5[d] mg/ml	SKB	0.05 mg/ml[b]	Physically compatible with no change in measured turbidity or increase in particle content in 4 hr at 23 °C	1969	C
Clindamycin phosphate	AB	10 mg/ml[a]	SKB	0.05 mg/ml[a]	Physically compatible with no change in measured turbidity or increase in particle content in 4 hr at 23 °C	2000	C
Cyclophosphamide	MJ	2 mg/ml[b]	SKB	1 mg/ml	Physically compatible with little or no loss of either drug by HPLC in 4 hr at 22 °C	1883	C
Cytarabine	UP	2 mg/ml[b]	SKB	1 mg/ml	Physically compatible with little or no loss of either drug by HPLC in 4 hr at 22 °C	1883	C
	UP	50 mg/ml	SKB	0.05 mg/ml[a]	Physically compatible with no change in measured turbidity or increase in particle content in 4 hr at 23 °C	2000	C
Dacarbazine	MI	1.7 mg/ml[b]	SKB	1 mg/ml	Physically compatible with little or no loss of either drug by HPLC in 4 hr at 22 °C	1883	C
Dactinomycin	ME	0.01 mg/ml[a]	SKB	0.05 mg/ml[a]	Physically compatible with no change in measured turbidity or increase in particle content in 4 hr at 23 °C	2000	C
Daunorubicin HCl	CHI	1 mg/ml[a]	SKB	0.05 mg/ml[a]	Physically compatible with no change in measured turbidity or increase in particle content in 4 hr at 23 °C	2000	C
Dexamethasone sodium phosphate	ME	0.24 mg/ml[b]	SKB	1 mg/ml	Physically compatible with little or no loss of either drug by HPLC in 4 hr at 22 °C	1883	C
	MSD	0.2 and 1 mg/ml[e]	BE	0.15 mg/ml[e]	Visually compatible with little or no loss of either drug by HPLC in 72 hr at room temperature	1884	C
Diphenhydramine HCl	PD	1 mg/ml[b]	SKB	1 mg/ml	Physically compatible with little or no loss of either drug by HPLC in 4 hr at 22 °C	1883	C
	SCN	2 mg/ml[a]	SKB	0.05 mg/ml[a]	Physically compatible with no change in measured turbidity or increase in particle content in 4 hr at 23 °	2000	C

Y-Site Injection Compatibility (1:1 Mixture) (Cont.)

Granisetron HCl

Drug	Mfr	Conc	Mfr	Conc	Remarks	Ref	C/I
Dobutamine HCl	BA	4 mg/ml[a]	SKB	0.05 mg/ml[a]	Physically compatible with no change in measured turbidity or increase in particle content in 4 hr at 23 °C	2000	C
Docetaxel	RPR	0.9 mg/ml[a]	SKB	0.05 mg/ml[a]	Physically compatible with no change in measured turbidity or increase in particle content in 4 hr at 23 °C	2224	C
Dopamine HCl	AB	3.2 mg/ml[a]	SKB	0.05 mg/ml[a]	Physically compatible with no change in measured turbidity or increase in particle content in 4 hr at 23 °C	2000	C
Doxorubicin HCl	AD	0.2 mg/ml[b]	SKB	1 mg/ml	Physically compatible with little or no loss of either drug by HPLC in 4 hr at 22 °C	1883	C
Doxorubicin HCl liposome injection	SEQ	0.4 mg/ml[a]	SKB	0.05 mg/ml[a]	Physically compatible with little or no change in measured turbidity and no increase in particle content in 4 hr at 23 °C	2087	C
Doxycycline hyclate	LY	1 mg/ml[a]	SKB	0.05 mg/ml[a]	Physically compatible with no change in measured turbidity or increase in particle content in 4 hr at 23 °C	2000	C
Droperidol	AB	0.4 mg/ml[a]	SKB	0.05 mg/ml[a]	Physically compatible with no change in measured turbidity or increase in particle content in 4 hr at 23 °C	2000	C
Enalaprilat	MSD	0.1 mg/ml[a]	SKB	0.05 mg/ml[a]	Physically compatible with no change in measured turbidity or increase in particle content in 4 hr at 23 °C	2000	C
Etoposide	BMS	0.4 mg/ml[b]	SKB	1 mg/ml	Physically compatible with little or no loss of either drug by HPLC in 4 hr at 22 °C	1883	C
	BR	0.4 mg/ml[a]	SKB	0.05 mg/ml[a]	Physically compatible with no change in measured turbidity or increase in particle content in 4 hr at 23 °C	2000	C
Etoposide phosphate	BR	5 mg/ml[a]	SKB	0.05 mg/ml[a]	Physically compatible with no change in measured turbidity or increase in particle content in 4 hr at 23 °C	2218	C
Famotidine	ME	2 mg/ml[a]	SKB	0.05 mg/ml[a]	Physically compatible with no change in measured turbidity or increase in particle content in 4 hr at 23 °C	2000	C
Filgrastim	AMG	30 μg/ml[a]	SKB	0.05 mg/ml[a]	Physically compatible with no change in measured turbidity or increase in particle content in 4 hr at 23 °C	2000	C
Floxuridine	RC	3 mg/ml[a]	SKB	0.05 mg/ml[a]	Physically compatible with no change in measured turbidity or increase in particle content in 4 hr at 23 °C	2000	C
Fluconazole	PF	2 mg/ml	SKB	0.05 mg/ml[a]	Physically compatible with no change in measured turbidity or increase in particle content in 4 hr at 23 °C	2000	C
Fludarabine phosphate	BX	1 mg/ml[a]	SKB	0.05 mg/ml[a]	Physically compatible with no change in measured turbidity or increase in particle content in 4 hr at 23 °C	2000	C

Y-Site Injection Compatibility (1:1 Mixture) (Cont.)

Granisetron HCl

Drug	Mfr	Conc	Mfr	Conc	Remarks	Ref	C/I
Fluorouracil	AD	16 mg/ml[a]	SKB	0.05 mg/ml[a]	Physically compatible with no subvisual haze or particle formation in 4 hr at 23 °C	1804	C
	RC	2 mg/ml[b]	SKB	1 mg/ml	Physically compatible with little or no loss of either drug by HPLC in 4 hr at 22 °C	1883	C
	AD	16 mg/ml[a]	SKB	0.05 mg/ml[a]	Physically compatible with no change in measured turbidity or increase in particle content in 4 hr at 23 °C	2000	C
Furosemide	AB	3 mg/ml[a]	SKB	0.05 mg/ml[a]	Physically compatible with no subvisual haze or particle formation in 4 hr at 23 °C	1804	C
	HO	0.4 mg/ml[b]	SKB	1 mg/ml	Physically compatible with little or no loss of either drug by HPLC in 4 hr at 22 °C	1883	C
Ganciclovir sodium	SY	20 mg/ml[a]	SKB	0.05 mg/ml[a]	Physically compatible with no change in measured turbidity or increase in particle content in 4 hr at 23 °C	2000	C
Gemcitabine HCl	LI	10 mg/ml[b]	SKB	0.05 mg/ml[b]	Physically compatible with no change in measured turbidity or increase in particle content in 4 hr at 23 °C	2226	C
Gentamicin sulfate	ES	1.5 mg/ml[b]	SKB	1 mg/ml	Physically compatible with little or no loss of either drug by HPLC in 4 hr at 22 °C	1883	C
Haloperidol lactate	MN	0.2 mg/ml[a]	SKB	0.05 mg/ml[a]	Physically compatible with no change in measured turbidity or increase in particle content in 4 hr at 23 °C	2000	C
Heparin sodium	AB	100 units/ml[a]	SKB	0.05 mg/ml[a]	Physically compatible with no change in measured turbidity or increase in particle content in 4 hr at 23 °C	2000	C
Hydrocortisone sodium phosphate	MSD	1 mg/ml[a]	SKB	0.05 mg/ml[a]	Physically compatible with no change in measured turbidity or increase in particle content in 4 hr at 23 °C	2000	C
Hydrocortisone sodium succinate	AB	1 mg/ml[a]	SKB	0.05 mg/ml[a]	Physically compatible with no change in measured turbidity or increase in particle content in 4 hr at 23 °C	2000	C
Hydromorphone HCl	KN	0.5 mg/ml[b]	SKB	1 mg/ml	Physically compatible with little or no loss of either drug by HPLC in 4 hr at 22 °C	1883	C
	ES	0.5 mg/ml[a]	SKB	0.05 mg/ml[a]	Physically compatible with no change in measured turbidity or increase in particle content in 4 hr at 23 °C	2000	C
Hydroxyzine HCl	ES	2 mg/ml[a]	SKB	0.05 mg/ml[a]	Physically compatible with no change in measured turbidity or increase in particle content in 4 hr at 23 °C	2000	C
Idarubicin HCl	AD	0.5 mg/ml[a]	SKB	0.05 mg/ml[a]	Increase in turbidity no greater than dilution with D5W alone. No increase in particle content in 4 hr at 23 °C	2000	C
Ifosfamide	MJ	4 mg/ml[b]	SKB	1 mg/ml	Physically compatible with little or no loss of either drug by HPLC in 4 hr at 22 °C	1883	C

Y-Site Injection Compatibility (1:1 Mixture) (Cont.)

Granisetron HCl

Drug	Mfr	Conc	Mfr	Conc	Remarks	Ref	C/I
Imipenem–cilastatin sodium	ME	10 mg/ml[a]	SKB	0.05 mg/ml[a]	Physically compatible with no change in measured turbidity or increase in particle content in 4 hr at 23 °C	2000	**C**
Leucovorin calcium	IMM	2 mg/ml[a]	SKB	0.05 mg/ml[a]	Physically compatible with no change in measured turbidity or increase in particle content in 4 hr at 23 °C	2000	**C**
Levoleucovorin calcium	LE	2 mg/ml[a]	SKB	0.05 mg/ml[a]	Physically compatible with no change in measured turbidity or increase in particle content in 4 hr at 23 °C	2000	**C**
Lorazepam	WY	0.1 mg/ml[b]	SKB	1 mg/ml	Physically compatible with little or no loss of either drug by HPLC in 4 hr at 22 °C	1883	**C**
	WY	0.1 mg/ml[a]	SKB	0.05 mg/ml[a]	Physically compatible with no change in measured turbidity or increase in particle content in 4 hr at 23 °C	2000	**C**
Magnesium sulfate	AB	16 mg/ml[b]	SKB	1 mg/ml	Physically compatible with little or no loss of granisetron by HPLC in 4 hr at 22 °C	1883	**C**
	AB	100 mg/ml[a]	SKB	0.05 mg/ml[a]	Physically compatible with no change in measured turbidity or increase in particle content in 4 hr at 23 °C	2000	**C**
Mechlorethamine HCl	MSD	0.5 mg/ml[b]	SKB	1 mg/ml	Physically compatible with little or no loss of either drug by HPLC in 4 hr at 22 °C	1883	**C**
Melphalan	BW	0.1 mg/ml[b]	SKB	0.05 mg/ml[a]	Physically compatible with no change in measured turbidity or increase in particle content in 4 hr at 23 °C	2000	**C**
Meperidine HCl	WY	4 mg/ml[a]	SKB	0.05 mg/ml[a]	Physically compatible with no change in measured turbidity or increase in particle content in 4 hr at 23 °C	2000	**C**
Mesna	MJ	4 mg/ml[b]	SKB	1 mg/ml	Physically compatible with little or no loss of either drug by HPLC in 4 hr at 22 °C	1883	**C**
Methotrexate sodium	CET	12.5 mg/ml[b]	SKB	1 mg/ml	Physically compatible with little or no loss of either drug by HPLC in 4 hr at 22 °C	1883	**C**
Methylprednisolone sodium succinate	DAK	6 mg/ml[e]	BE	0.15 mg/ml[e]	Visually compatible with little or no loss of either drug by HPLC in 72 hr at room temperature	1884	**C**
	WY	5 mg/ml[a]	SKB	0.05 mg/ml[a]	Physically compatible with no change in measured turbidity or increase in particle content in 4 hr at 23 °C	2000	**C**
Metoclopramide HCl	AB	5 mg/ml	SKB	0.05 mg/ml[a]	Physically compatible with no change in measured turbidity or increase in particle content in 4 hr at 23 °C	2000	**C**
Metronidazole	BA	5 mg/ml	SKB	0.05 mg/ml[a]	Physically compatible with no change in measured turbidity or increase in particle content in 4 hr at 23 °C	2000	**C**

Y-Site Injection Compatibility (1:1 Mixture) (Cont.)

Granisetron HCl

Drug	Mfr	Conc	Mfr	Conc	Remarks	Ref	C/I
Minocycline HCl	LE	0.2 mg/ml[a]	SKB	0.05 mg/ml[a]	Physically compatible with no change in measured turbidity or increase in particle content in 4 hr at 23 °C	2000	C
Mitomycin	BMS	0.5 mg/ml	SKB	0.05 mg/ml[a]	Physically compatible with no change in measured turbidity or increase in particle content in 4 hr at 23 °C	2000	C
Mitoxantrone HCl	IMM	0.5 mg/ml[a]	SKB	0.05 mg/ml[a]	Physically compatible with no change in measured turbidity or increase in particle content in 4 hr at 23 °C	2000	C
Morphine sulfate	AST	1 mg/ml[b]	SKB	1 mg/ml	Physically compatible with little or no loss of either drug by HPLC in 4 hr at 22 °C	1883	C
	AST	1 mg/ml[a]	SKB	0.05 mg/ml[a]	Physically compatible with no change in measured turbidity or increase in particle content in 4 hr at 23 °C	2000	C
Nalbuphine HCl	AB	10 mg/ml	SKB	0.05 mg/ml[a]	Physically compatible with no change in measured turbidity or increase in particle content in 4 hr at 23 °C	2000	C
Netilmicin sulfate	SCH	5 mg/ml[a]	SKB	0.05 mg/ml[a]	Physically compatible with no change in measured turbidity or increase in particle content in 4 hr at 23 °C	2000	C
Ofloxacin	ORT	4 mg/ml[a]	SKB	0.05 mg/ml[a]	Physically compatible with no change in measured turbidity or increase in particle content in 4 hr at 23 °C	2000	C
Paclitaxel	MJ	0.3 mg/ml[b]	SKB	1 mg/ml	Physically compatible with little or no loss of either drug by HPLC in 4 hr at 22 °C	1883	C
	MJ	1.2 mg/ml[a]	SKB	0.05 mg/ml[a]	Physically compatible with no change in measured turbidity or increase in particle content in 4 hr at 23 °C	2000	C
Piperacillin sodium	LE	40 mg/ml[a]	SKB	0.05 mg/ml[a]	Physically compatible with no change in measured turbidity or increase in particle content in 4 hr at 23 °C	2000	C
Piperacillin sodium–tazobactam sodium	CY	40 + 5 mg/ml[a]	SKB	0.05 mg/ml[a]	Physically compatible with no change in measured turbidity or increase in particle content in 4 hr at 23 °C	2000	C
Plicamycin	BAY	0.01 mg/ml[a]	SKB	0.05 mg/ml[a]	Physically compatible with no change in measured turbidity or increase in particle content in 4 hr at 23 °C	2000	C
Potassium chloride	LY	0.04 mEq/ml[b]	SKB	1 mg/ml	Physically compatible with little or no loss of granisetron by HPLC in 4 hr at 22 °C	1883	C
Prochlorperazine edisylate	SCN	0.5 mg/ml[a]	SKB	0.05 mg/ml[a]	Physically compatible with no change in measured turbidity or increase in particle content in 4 hr at 23 °C	2000	C
Promethazine HCl	WY	2 mg/ml[a]	SKB	0.05 mg/ml[a]	Physically compatible with no change in measured turbidity or increase in particle content in 4 hr at 23 °C	2000	C
Propofol	ZEN	10 mg/ml	SKB	0.05 mg/ml[a]	Physically compatible for 1 hr at 23 °C with no increase in particle content	2066	C

Y-Site Injection Compatibility (1:1 Mixture) (Cont.)

Granisetron HCl

Drug	Mfr	Conc	Mfr	Conc	Remarks	Ref	C/I
Ranitidine HCl	GL	2 mg/ml[a]	SKB	0.05 mg/ml[a]	Physically compatible with no change in measured turbidity or increase in particle content in 4 hr at 23 °C	2000	C
Sargramostim	IMM	10 μg/ml[b]	SKB	0.05 mg/ml[a]	Physically compatible with no change in measured turbidity or increase in particle content in 4 hr at 23 °C	2000	C
Sodium bicarbonate	AB	1 mEq/ml	SKB	0.05 mg/ml[a]	Physically compatible with no subvisual haze or particle formation in 4 hr at 23 °C	1804	C
	AB	0.33 mEq/ml[b]	SKB	1 mg/ml	Physically compatible with 8% loss of granisetron by HPLC in 4 hr at 22 °C	1883	C
	AB	1 mEq/ml	SKB	0.05 mg/ml[a]	Physically compatible with no change in measured turbidity or increase in particle content in 4 hr at 23 °C	2000	C
Streptozocin	UP	9.1 mg/ml[b]	SKB	1 mg/ml	Physically compatible with little or no loss of either drug by HPLC in 4 hr at 22 °C	1883	C
Teniposide	BMS	0.1 mg/ml[a]	SKB	0.05 mg/ml[a]	Physically compatible with no change in measured turbidity or increase in particle content in 4 hr at 23 °C	2000	C
Thiotepa	IMM[f]	1 mg/ml[a]	SKB	0.05 mg/ml[a]	Physically compatible with no change in measured turbidity or increase in particle content in 4 hr at 23 °C	1861; 2000	C
Ticarcillin disodium	SKB	30 mg/ml[a]	SKB	0.05 mg/ml[a]	Physically compatible with no change in measured turbidity or increase in particle content in 4 hr at 23 °C	2000	C
Ticarcillin disodium–clavulanate potassium	SKB	27 mg/ml[b]	SKB	1 mg/ml	Physically compatible with little or no loss of either drug by HPLC in 4 hr at 22 °C	1883	C
	SKB	31 mg/ml[a]	SKB	0.05 mg/ml[a]	Physically compatible with no change in measured turbidity or increase in particle content in 4 hr at 23 °C	2000	C
TNA #218 to #226[g]			SKB	0.05 mg/ml[a]	Visually compatible with no precipitate or emulsion damage apparent in 4 hr at 23 °C	2215	C
Tobramycin sulfate	AB	5 mg/ml[a]	SKB	0.05 mg/ml[a]	Physically compatible with no change in measured turbidity or increase in particle content in 4 hr at 23 °C	2000	C
TPN #212 to #215[g]			SKB	0.05 mg/ml[a]	Physically compatible with no change in measured turbidity or increase in particle content in 4 hr at 23 °C	2109	C
Trimethoprim–sulfamethoxazole	ES	0.8 + 4 mg/ml[a]	SKB	0.05 mg/ml[a]	Physically compatible with no change in measured turbidity or increase in particle content in 4 hr at 23 °C	2000	C
Vancomycin HCl	AB	10 mg/ml[a]	SKB	0.05 mg/ml[a]	Physically compatible with no change in measured turbidity or increase in particle content in 4 hr at 23 °C	2000	C
Vinblastine sulfate	LI	0.12 mg/ml[a]	SKB	0.05 mg/ml[a]	Physically compatible with no change in measured turbidity or increase in particle content in 4 hr at 23 °C	2000	C

Y-Site Injection Compatibility (1:1 Mixture) (Cont.)

Granisetron HCl

Drug	Mfr	Conc	Mfr	Conc	Remarks	Ref	C/I
Vincristine sulfate	LI	0.34 mg/ml[b]	SKB	1 mg/ml	Physically compatible with little or no loss of either drug by HPLC in 4 hr at 22 °C	1883	C
	LI	0.01 mg/ml[b]	SKB	1 mg/ml	Physically compatible with little or no loss of granisetron by HPLC in 4 hr at 22 °C	1883	C
Vinorelbine tartrate	BW	1 mg/ml[a]	SKB	0.05 mg/ml[a]	Physically compatible with no change in measured turbidity or increase in particle content in 4 hr at 23 °C	2000	C
Zidovudine	BW	4 mg/ml[a]	SKB	0.05 mg/ml[a]	Physically compatible with no change in measured turbidity or increase in particle content in 4 hr at 23 °C	2000	C

[a]*Tested in dextrose 5% in water.*
[b]*Tested in sodium chloride 0.9%.*
[c]*Sodium carbonate–containing formulation tested.*
[d]*Tested in bacteriostatic sodium chloride 0.9% preserved with benzyl alcohol 0.9%.*
[e]*Granisetron in sodium chloride 0.9% and dextrose 5% in water. Diluted further with 17 ml of water.*
[f]*Lyophilized formulation tested.*
[g]*Refer to Appendix I for the composition of parenteral nutrition solutions. TNA indicates a 3-in-1 admixture, and TPN indicates a 2-in-1 admixture.*

Additional Compatibility Information

Dextrose 5% in water and sodium chloride 0.9% are recommended for dilution of granisetron HCl (2).

HALOPERIDOL LACTATE
AHFS 28:16.08

Haldol   **Ortho-McNeil**

Products— Haloperidol lactate (Ortho-McNeil) is available in 1-ml ampuls and disposable syringes and 10-ml multiple-dose vials. Each milliliter of solution contains haloperidol 5 mg (as the lactate), methylparaben 1.8 mg, propylparaben 0.2 mg, and lactic acid for pH adjustment (2).

pH— From 3 to 3.6 (2).

Administration— Haloperidol lactate should be administered intramuscularly (2; 4), although intravenous administration has been performed (571; 1258).

Stability— Haloperidol lactate should be stored at controlled room temperature and protected from light; freezing and temperatures above 40 °C should be avoided (2; 4).

Compatibility Information

Solution Compatibility

Haloperidol lactate

Solution	Mfr	Mfr	Conc/L	Remarks	Ref	C/I
Dextrose 5% in sodium chloride 0.2%	AB	MN	0.1 to 1 g	Visually compatible for 7 days at 21 °C	1740	C
	AB	MN	2 and 3 g	Precipitate forms in 30 to 60 min	1740	I

Solution Compatibility (Cont.)

Haloperidol lactate

Solution	Mfr	Mfr	Conc/L	Remarks	Ref	C/I
Dextrose 5% in water	TR[a]	MN	100 mg	Physically compatible and potency retained for 38 days at 24 °C	571	**C**
	AB	MN	0.1 to 3 g	Visually compatible for 7 days at 21 °C	1740	**C**
Ringer's injection, lactated	AB	MN	0.1 to 1 g	Visually compatible for 7 days at 21 °C	1740	**C**
	AB	MN	2 g	Precipitate forms within 15 min	1740	**I**
	AB	MN	3 g	Precipitate forms immediately	1740	**I**
Sodium chloride 0.45%	AB	MN	0.1 to 1 g	Visually compatible for 7 days at 21 °C	1740	**C**
	AB	MN	2 g	Precipitate forms within 15 min	1740	**I**
	AB	MN	3 g	Precipitate forms immediately	1740	**I**
Sodium chloride 0.9%	AB[b]	MN	2 and 3 g	Slight precipitate forms immediately and becomes much heavier within 15 to 30 min	1523	**I**
	AB[b]	MN	1 g	Slight precipitate forms immediately and persists through 8 hr of observation	1523	**I**
	AB[b]	MN	100 and 500 mg	Visually compatible for 8 hr at 21 °C under fluorescent light	1523	**C**
	AB	MN	0.1 to 0.75 g	Visually compatible for 7 days at 21 °C	1740	**C**
	AB	MN	1 to 3 g	Precipitate forms immediately	1740	**I**

[a]Tested in both glass and PVC containers.
[b]Tested in glass containers.

Drugs in Syringe Compatibility

Haloperidol lactate

Drug (in syringe)	Mfr	Amt	Mfr	Amt	Remarks	Ref	C/I
Benztropine mesylate	MSD	2 mg	MN	0.25, 0.5, 1 mg	Visually compatible for 24 hr at 21 °C	1781	**C**
	MSD	2 mg	MN	2 mg	Precipitate forms within 4 hr at 21 °C	1781	**I**
	MSD	2 mg	MN	3, 4, 5 mg	Precipitate forms within 15 min at 21 °C	1781	**I**
	MSD	1 mg	MN	0.25 and 0.5 mg	Visually compatible for 24 hr at 21 °C	1781	**C**
	MSD	1 mg	MN	1 to 5 mg	Precipitate forms within 15 min at 21 °C	1781	**I**
	MSD	0.5 mg	MN	0.25 to 5 mg	Precipitate forms within 15 min at 21 °C	1781	**I**
	MSD	2 mg/ 2 ml	MN	10 mg/ 2 ml	White precipitate forms within 5 min	1784	**I**
Cyclizine lactate	WEL	150 mg/ 3 ml	SE	1.5 mg/ 0.3 ml	Diluted with 17 ml of NS. Crystals of cyclizine form within 24 hr at 25 °C	1761	**I**
	WEL	150 mg/ 3 ml	SE	1.5 mg/ 0.3 ml	Diluted with 17 ml of D5W or W. Visually compatible for 24 hr at 25 °C	1761	**C**
Diamorphine HCl	MB	10, 25, 50 mg/ 1 ml	SE	1.5 mg/ 1 ml[a]	Physically compatible and diamorphine content retained for 24 hr at room temperature	1454	**C**
	EV	20 mg/ 1 ml	SE	2 mg/ 1 ml	Crystallization with 58% haloperidol loss in 7 days at room temperature	1455	**I**

Drugs in Syringe Compatibility (Cont.)

Haloperidol lactate

Drug (in syringe)	Mfr	Amt	Mfr	Amt	Remarks	Ref	C/I
	EV	50 and 150 mg/ 1 ml	SE	5 mg/ 1 ml	Immediate precipitation	1455	**I**
	EV	100 mg/ 8 ml	SE	2.5 mg/ 8 ml	Physically compatible for 24 hr at room temperature and 7 days at 6 °C	1456	**C**
	HC	20 to 100 mg/ ml	SE	0.75 mg/ ml	Visually compatible for 48 hr at 5 and 20 °C	1672	**C**
	HC	2 mg/ml	SE	0.75 mg/ ml	5% diamorphine loss by HPLC in 14.8 days at 20 °C. Haloperidol potency by HPLC retained for at least 45 days	1672	**C**
	HC	20 mg/ ml	SE	0.75 mg/ ml	5% diamorphine loss by HPLC in 20.7 days at 20 °C. Haloperidol potency by HPLC retained for at least 45 days	1672	**C**
Diphenhydramine HCl	ES	100 mg/ 2 ml	MN	10 mg/ 2 ml	White precipitate forms within 5 min	1784	**I**
	ES	50 mg/ 1 ml	MN	5 mg/ 1 ml	White cloudy precipitate forms in 2 hr at room temperature	1886	**I**
Heparin sodium		2500 units/ 1 ml	JN	5 mg/ 1 ml	Turbidity or precipitate forms within 5 min	1053	**I**
Hydromorphone HCl	KN	1[a] and 10 mg/ 1 ml	MN	1[a], 2[a], 5 mg/ 1 ml	Visually compatible for 24 hr at 25 °C under fluorescent light	1785	**C**
Hydroxyzine HCl	ES	100 mg/ 2 ml	MN	10 mg/ 2 ml	White precipitate forms within 5 min	1784	**I**
Ketorolac tromethamine	SY	30 mg/ 1 ml	SO	5 mg/ 1 ml	White crystalline precipitate forms immediately	1786	**I**
Morphine sulfate		5 and 10 mg/ 1 ml[b,c]	MN	5 mg/ 1 ml	Cloudiness forms immediately, becoming a crystalline precipitate of haloperidol and parabens	1901	**I**
Sufentanil citrate	JN	50 μg/ml	MN	5 mg/ml	Physically compatible with no subvisual haze or particle formation in 24 hr at 23 °C	1711	**C**

[a]Diluted with sterile water for injection.
[b]Morphine sulfate powder dissolved in dextrose 5% in water.
[c]Morphine sulfate powder dissolved in water and sodium chloride 0.9%.

Y-Site Injection Compatibility (1:1 Mixture)

Haloperidol lactate

Drug	Mfr	Conc	Mfr	Conc	Remarks	Ref	C/I
Allopurinol sodium	BW	3 mg/ml[b]	MN	0.2 mg/ml[b]	Heavy turbidity forms immediately. Crystals form within 1 hr	1686	**I**
Amifostine	USB	10 mg/ml[a]	MN	0.2 mg/ml[a]	Physically compatible with no change in measured turbidity or increase in particle content in 4 hr at 23 °C	1845	**C**
Amphotericin B cholesteryl sulfate complex	SEQ	0.83 mg/ml[a]	MN	0.2 mg/ml[a]	Gross precipitate forms	2117	**I**
Amsacrine	NCI	1 mg/ml[a]	MN	0.2 mg/ml[a]	Physically compatible for 4 hr at room temperature under fluorescent light	1381	**C**

Y-Site Injection Compatibility (1:1 Mixture) (Cont.)

Haloperidol lactate

Drug	Mfr	Conc	Mfr	Conc	Remarks	Ref	C/I
Aztreonam	SQ	40 mg/ml[a]	MN	0.2 mg/ml[a]	Physically compatible with no subvisual haze or particle formation in 4 hr at 23 °C	1758	C
Cefepime HCl	BR	20 mg/ml[a]	MN	0.2 mg/ml[a]	Haze forms immediately	1689	I
Cimetidine HCl	SKF	6 mg/ml[a]	MN	0.5[a] and 5 mg/ml	Visually compatible for 24 hr at 21 °C	1523	C
Cisatracurium besylate	GW	0.1, 2, and 5 mg/ml[a]	MN	0.2 mg/ml[a]	Physically compatible with no change in measured turbidity or increase in particle content in 4 hr at 23 °C	2074	C
Cladribine	ORT	0.015[b] and 0.5[c] mg/ml	MN	0.2 mg/ml[b]	Physically compatible with no change in measured turbidity or increase in particle content in 4 hr at 23 °C	1969	C
Dobutamine HCl	LI	4 mg/ml[a]	MN	0.5[a] and 5 mg/ml	Visually compatible for 24 hr at 21 °C	1523	C
Docetaxel	RPR	0.9 mg/ml[a]	MN	0.2 mg/ml[a]	Physically compatible with no change in measured turbidity or increase in particle content in 4 hr at 23 °C	2224	C
Dopamine HCl	DU	1.6 mg/ml[a]	MN	0.5[a] and 5 mg/ml	Visually compatible for 24 hr at 21 °C	1523	C
Doxorubicin HCl liposome injection	SEQ	0.4 mg/ml[a]	MN	0.2 mg/ml[a]	Physically compatible with little or no change in measured turbidity and no increase in particle content in 4 hr at 23 °C	2087	C
Etoposide phosphate	BR	5 mg/ml[a]	MN	0.2 mg/ml[a]	Physically compatible with no change in measured turbidity or increase in particle content in 4 hr at 23 °C	2218	C
Famotidine	MSD	0.267 mg/ml[a]	MN	0.5[a] and 5 mg/ml	Visually compatible for 24 hr at 21 °C	1523	C
	ME	2 mg/ml[b]		0.2 mg/ml[a]	Visually compatible for 4 hr at 22 °C	1936	C
Filgrastim	AMG	30 μg/ml[a]	MN	0.2 mg/ml[a]	Physically compatible with no change in measured turbidity or increase in particle content in 4 hr at 22 °C	1687	C
Fluconazole	RR	2 mg/ml	MN	5 mg/ml	Precipitate forms	1407	I
Fludarabine phosphate	BX	1 mg/ml[a]	MN	0.2 mg/ml[a]	Physically compatible for 4 hr at room temperature under fluorescent light	1439	C
Foscarnet sodium	AST	24 mg/ml	LY	5 mg/ml	Delayed formation of fine white precipitate	1335	I
Gemcitabine HCl	LI	10 mg/ml[b]	MN	0.2 mg/ml[b]	Physically compatible with no change in measured turbidity or increase in particle content in 4 hr at 23 °C	2226	C
Granisetron HCl	SKB	0.05 mg/ml[a]	MN	0.2 mg/ml[a]	Physically compatible with no change in measured turbidity or increase in particle content in 4 hr at 23 °C	2000	C
Heparin sodium	OR	25,000 and 50,000 units/250 ml[e]	MN	5 mg/1 ml[d]	White precipitate forms immediately	779	I
		50 units/ml[b,f]	JN	5 mg/1 ml[g]	White turbidity	1053	I

Y-Site Injection Compatibility (1:1 Mixture) (Cont.)

Haloperidol lactate

Drug	Mfr	Conc	Mfr	Conc	Remarks	Ref	C/I
Lidocaine HCl	AB	4 mg/ml[a]	MN	0.5[a] and 5 mg/ml	Visually compatible for 24 hr at 21 °C	1523	**C**
Lorazepam	WY	2 mg/ml	MN	5 mg/ml	Physically compatible and chemically stable for 16 hr at room temperature	1838	**C**
	WY	0.33 mg/ml[b]	JN	0.5 and 5 mg/ml	Visually compatible for 24 hr at 22 °C	1855	**C**
Melphalan HCl	BW	0.1 mg/ml[b]	MN	0.2 mg/ml[b]	Physically compatible with no change in measured turbidity or increase in particle content in 3 hr at 22 °C	1557	**C**
Midazolam HCl	RC	5 mg/ml	JN	0.5 and 5 mg/ml	Visually compatible for 24 hr at 22 °C	1855	**C**
Nitroglycerin	DU	0.4 mg/ml[a]	MN	0.5[a] and 5 mg/ml	Visually compatible for 24 hr at 21 °C	1523	**C**
Norepinephrine bitartrate	WI	0.032 mg/ml[a]	MN	0.5[a] and 5 mg/ml	Visually compatible for 24 hr at 21 °C	1523	**C**
Ondansetron HCl	GL	1 mg/ml[b]	LY	0.2 mg/ml[a]	Physically compatible for 4 hr at 22 °C	1365	**C**
Paclitaxel	NCI	1.2 mg/ml[a]		0.2 mg/ml[a]	Physically compatible with no change in measured turbidity in 4 hr at 22 °C	1528	**C**
Phenylephrine HCl	WB	0.02 mg/ml[a]	MN	0.5[a] and 5 mg/ml	Visually compatible for 24 hr at 21 °C	1523	**C**
Piperacillin sodium–tazobactam sodium	LE	40 + 5 mg/ml[a]	MN	0.2 mg/ml[a]	White turbidity and particles form immediately	1688	**I**
Propofol	ZEN	10 mg/ml	MN	0.2 mg/ml[a]	Physically compatible for 1 hr at 23 °C with no increase in particle content	2066	**C**
Remifentanil HCl	GW	0.025 and 0.25 mg/ml[b]	MN	0.2 mg/ml[a]	Physically compatible with no change in measured turbidity or increase in particle content in 4 hr at 23 °C	2075	**C**
Sargramostim	IMM	10 μg/ml[b]	LY	0.2 mg/ml[b]	Small particles formed in 4 hr in one of two samples	1436	**I**
Sodium nitroprusside	AB	0.2 mg/ml[h]	MN	5 mg/ml	Turbidity forms immediately and persists, developing fine precipitate in 24 hr at 21 °C under fluorescent light	1523	**I**
	AB	0.2 mg/ml[h]	MN	0.5 mg/ml[a]	Visually compatible for 24 hr at 21 °C	1523	**C**
Sufentanil citrate	JN	12.5 μg/ml[a]	MN	0.2 mg/ml[a]	Physically compatible with no subvisual haze or particle formation in 24 hr at 23 °C	1711	**C**
Tacrolimus	FUJ	1 mg/ml[b]	SO	2.5 mg/ml[a]	Visually compatible for 24 hr at 25 °C	1630	**C**
Teniposide	BR	0.1 mg/ml[a]	MN	0.2 mg/ml[a]	Physically compatible with no subvisual haze or particle formation in 4 hr at 23 °C	1725	**C**
Theophylline	TR	1.6 mg/ml[a]	MN	0.5[a] and 5 mg/ml	Visually compatible for 24 hr at 21 °C	1523	**C**
Thiotepa	IMM[i]	1 mg/ml[b]	MN	0.2 mg/ml[b]	Physically compatible with no change in measured turbidity or increase in particle content in 4 hr at 23 °C	1861	**C**
TNA #218 to #226[j]			MN	0.2 mg/ml[a]	Damage to emulsion integrity occurs immediately with free oil formation possible	2215	**I**

Y-Site Injection Compatibility (1:1 Mixture) (Cont.)

Haloperidol lactate

Drug	Mfr	Conc	Mfr	Conc	Remarks	Ref	C/I
TPN #189[j]			SE	10 mg/ml	Visually compatible for 24 hr at 22 °C	1767	**C**
TPN #212 to #215[j]			MN	0.2 mg/ml[a]	Physically compatible with no change in measured turbidity or increase in particle content in 4 hr at 23 °C	2109	**C**
Vinorelbine tartrate	BW	1 mg/ml[b]	MN	0.2 mg/ml[b]	Physically compatible with no change in measured turbidity or increase in particle content in 4 hr at 22 °C	1558	**C**

[a]*Tested in dextrose 5% in water.*
[b]*Tested in sodium chloride 0.9%.*
[c]*Tested in bacteriostatic sodium chloride 0.9% preserved with benzyl alcohol 0.9%.*
[d]*Injected over one minute.*
[e]*Tested in both dextrose 5% in water and sodium chloride 0.9%. Run at 1000 units/hr.*
[f]*Run at 1 ml/min.*
[g]*Given over three minutes.*
[h]*Tested in sterile water for injection.*
[i]*Lyophilized formulation tested.*
[j]*Refer to Appendix I for the composition of parenteral nutrition solutions. TNA indicates a 3-in-1 admixture, and TPN indicates a 2-in-1 admixture.*

Additional Compatibility Information

Haloperidol lactate is stated to be physically and chemically compatible with buprenorphine HCl (4).

Heparin—— Heparin sodium forms a precipitate when combined with haloperidol lactate (779; 1053). It has been recommended that heparin infusions be stopped and that lines be flushed with sodium chloride 0.9% or dextrose 5% in water before and after injecting haloperidol lactate into an injection port. Administration of haloperidol lactate through a heparin lock would require a similar flushing procedure (779).

HEPARIN SODIUM
AHFS 20:12.04

Products—— Heparin sodium derived from beef lung or porcine intestinal mucosa is available from various manufacturers in concentrations ranging from 1000 to 20,000 units/ml, packaged in sizes ranging from 0.5- to 1-ml ampuls, vials, or prefilled syringes to 30-ml multiple-dose vials. Benzyl alcohol or parabens may also be present as preservatives, and hydrochloric acid and/or sodium hydroxide may have been added to adjust pH. In addition, dilute solutions of 10 and 100 units/ml in 1- to 5-ml disposable syringes and 1- to 30-ml vials are available for use in flushing heparin locks (4; 29).

Heparin sodium is also available premixed in various concentrations in sodium chloride 0.45 and 0.9% and dextrose 5% in water (4; 154).

pH— From 5 to 8 (4).

Osmolality— The osmolality of heparin sodium (Elkins-Sinn) 1000 units/ml was determined to be 384 mOsm/kg by freezing-point depression and 283 mOsm/kg by vapor pressure (1071).

Commercial heparin sodium infusion solutions in sodium chloride 0.9% and dextrose 5% in water have osmolalities of 322 and 270 mOsm/kg, respectively (4).

Administration—— Heparin sodium may be administered by deep subcutaneous injection, by intermittent intravenous injection undiluted or diluted in 50 to 100 ml of dextrose 5% in water or sodium chloride 0.9%, or by continuous intravenous infusion in a liter of compatible solution, preferably using an electronic rate-control device. The container should be inverted at least six times after heparin sodium addition to prevent pooling of the heparin. Intramuscular injection should not be used because of pain and hematoma formation (2; 4).

Stability—— Heparin sodium solutions are colorless to slightly yellow (4). Minor color variations do not affect therapeutic efficacy. Heparin sodium should be stored at controlled room temperature (2; 4) and protected from freezing and temperatures exceeding 40 °C (2; 4; 21). Heparin sodium retains its activity during autoclaving (1492). In a study of hospital-manufactured heparin sodium 1 unit/ml in sodium chloride 0.9%, full anticoagulant activity was retained for at least 12 months after sterilization by autoclaving and subsequent storage at room temperature exposed to daylight (675).

In another study, heparin sodium solutions of 10 to 35,000 units/ml in distilled water at pH 7 to 8 were stable for 15 years at 4 °C and for seven years at 18 °C (243).

pH Effects— A pH profile of heparin sodium (Abbott) 20,000 units/L in dextrose 5% in water over a pH range of 3.8 to 7.6 did not reveal a potency loss during the 24-hour study (21). In another report, heparin sodium in sodium chloride 0.9% was tested at pH 3.2 (adjusted with hydrochloric acid) and 9.2 (adjusted with sodium hydroxide). No loss of potency was noted in 24 hours (57). However, a pH profile of heparin sodium 660 units/ml, when autoclaved for 10 minutes at 10 pounds/inch^2 at 115 °C, showed loss of activity at pH values above 8.5 and especially below 5 (243).

Syringes— The stability of 50 ml of a 500-unit/ml heparin sodium solution in sodium chloride 0.9% packaged in 50-ml polypropylene syringes was studied. Storage both at room temperature and at 0 to 4 °C showed an overall trend to lower activity by about 8% after three weeks.

When glass containers were compared to plastic syringes, the glass containers consistently showed lower retained activity in as little as two hours after preparation. The possibility of adsorption to glass surfaces was noted (676) but has not been demonstrated. (See Sorption below.)

Heparin sodium 1 unit/ml, prefilled into Injekt (Braun) all-plastic syringes having polyethylene barrels and polypropylene plungers, showed no significant activity loss over 52 weeks at 37 °C due to decomposition or sorption. However, plastic syringes with rubber-tipped plungers, such as Plastipak (Becton-Dickinson) and Perfusor (Braun), exhibited extra ultraviolet peaks, presumably due to leaching of rubber components (1491).

Heparin sodium (Leo) 300 units/ml in dextrose 5% in water or water for injection was drawn into 50-ml polypropylene syringes (Plastipak, Becton-Dickinson) and stored for eight hours at room temperature and 4 °C. HPLC analysis found no loss in either solvent (1799).

Sorption— No measurable adsorption of heparin sodium to the surface of glass containers occurred during a study of admixture compatibility (407).

Heparin sodium, BP, 2000 units/2 ml was stored for 18 hours at room temperature in the following plastic syringes: Brunswick (Sherwood Medical), Plastipak (Becton-Dickinson), Steriseal (Needle Industries), and Sabre (Gillette U.K.). The first three syringes have polypropylene barrels; the Sabre has a combination polypropylene–polystyrene barrel. No significant loss of heparin occurred due to sorption (784).

Heparin sodium (Leo) 300 units/ml in dextrose 5% in water or water for injection was delivered at 4 ml/hr by syringe pump through PVC and polyethylene-lined PVC infusion tubing for 12 hours at room temperature. HPLC analysis found no loss due to sorption to the polyethylene-lined tubing. However, losses of about 15 to 25% occurred with the PVC tubing and were especially high during the first 15 minutes of infusion (1799).

Filtration— Heparin sodium (Abbott) 10,000 units/L in dextrose 5% in water and sodium chloride 0.9% was filtered at 120 ml/hr for six hours through a 0.22-μm cellulose ester membrane filter (Ivex-2). No significant reduction in potency due to binding to the filter was noted (533).

Compatibility Information

Solution Compatibility

Heparin sodium

Solution	Mfr	Mfr	Conc/L	Remarks	Ref	C/I
Amino acids 4.25%, dextrose 25%	MG	RI	20,000 units	No increase in particulate matter in 24 hr at 5 °C	349	C
Dextran 40,000	PH			Physically compatible	44	C
Dextran 6% in dextrose 5%	AB	AB	1000 and 4000 units	Physically compatible	3	C
Dextran 6% in sodium chloride 0.9%	AB	AB	1000 and 4000 units	Physically compatible	3	C
Dextrose–Ringer's injection combinations	AB	AB	1000 and 4000 units	Physically compatible	3	C
Dextrose–Ringer's injection, lactated, combinations	AB	AB	1000 and 4000 units	Physically compatible	3	C
Dextrose 5% in Ringer's injection, lactated	TR[a]	UP	10,000 units	Potency retained for 24 hr at 5 °C	282	C

Solution Compatibility (Cont.)

Heparin sodium

Solution	Mfr	Mfr	Conc/L	Remarks	Ref	C/I
Dextrose–saline combinations	AB	AB	1000 and 4000 units	Physically compatible	3	**C**
Dextrose 2.5% in sodium chloride 0.45%	BA	DB	1000 units	Heparin activity retained for 12 months at 4 °C	1914	**C**
Dextrose 3.75% in sodium chloride 0.2%	BA	DB	1000 units	Heparin activity retained for 12 months at 4 and 22 °C	1914	**C**
Dextrose 4.3% in sodium chloride 0.18%		OR	20,000 units	40% potency loss within 1 hr at 23 °C	113	**I**
		AH	35,000 units	Apparent temporary 50% loss of heparin activity in 4 to 6 hr with recovery in 8 hr at 25 °C. Heparin activity then maintained for 14 days at 4 °C	900	**?**
Dextrose 5% in sodium chloride 0.45%	TR	AB	20,000 units	No decrease in activity in 24 hr at room temperature	407	**C**
Dextrose 5% in sodium chloride 0.9%			12,000 units	Physically compatible	74	**C**
			32,000 units	Potency retained for 24 hr	57	**C**
	AB	AB	20,000 units	Potency retained for 24 hr	21	**C**
	AB		20,000 units	Potency retained for 72 hr	46	**C**
	TR[a]	UP	10,000 units	Potency retained for 24 hr at 5 °C	282	**C**
	BA		30,000 units	40% potency loss in 5 hr at 15, 25, and 35 °C. Activity recovered 5 to 7 hr later	674	**I**
Dextrose 2½% in water	AB	AB	1000 and 4000 units	Physically compatible	3	**C**
Dextrose 5% in water			12,000 units	Physically compatible	74	**C**
	AB	AB	1000 and 4000 units	Physically compatible	3	**C**
	BP		40,000 units	Potency retained for 24 hr at 23 °C	252	**C**
			32,000 units	Potency retained for 24 hr	57	**C**
	AB	AB	20,000 units	Potency retained for 24 hr	21	**C**
	AB		20,000 units	Potency retained for 72 hr	46	**C**
	TR[b]	OR	20,000 and 40,000 units	Potency retained for 48 hr at 27 °C	254	**C**
	TR[a]	UP	10,000 units	Potency retained for 24 hr at 5 °C	282	**C**

Solution Compatibility (Cont.)

Heparin sodium

Solution	Mfr	Mfr	Conc/L	Remarks	Ref	C/I
	TR	AS	20,000 units	No decrease in activity in 24 hr at room temperature	407	**C**
		OR	20,000 units	50% potency loss within 1 hr at 23 °C	113	**I**
	MG	UP	10,000 units	30 to 50% activity loss in 6 hr at room temperature. Partial rebound in 24 hr	406	**I**
	BA		30,000 units	65% potency loss in 5 hr at 15, 25, and 35 °C. Activity recovered in 24 to 48 hr	674	**I**
		AH	35,000 units	Apparent temporary 50% loss of heparin activity in 4 hr with recovery in 6 hr at 25 °C. Heparin activity then maintained for 14 days at 4 °C	900	**?**
	BA	DB	1000 units	Heparin activity retained for 7 days at 22 °C	1914	**C**
	BA	DB	10,000 units	Heparin activity retained for 12 months at 22 °C	1914	**C**
Dextrose 10% in water	AB	AB	1000 and 4000 units	Physically compatible	3	**C**
	MG	UP	10,000 units	40% activity loss in 6 hr at room temperature. Partial rebound at 24 hr	406	**I**
Dextrose 25% in water		LY	5000 units	About 6% heparin activity loss in 21 days and 11% loss in 28 days at 4 °C	2025	**C**
Fat emulsion 10%, intravenous	VT	UP	2000 units	Physically compatible for 48 hr at 4 °C and room temperature	32	**C**
	AB, CU		1000 and 2000 units	Physically compatible and heparin activity retained	568	**C**
	VT		25,000 units	Physically compatible for 24 hr at 8 and 25 °C	825	**C**
Fructose 10% in sodium chloride 0.9%	AB	AB	1000 and 4000 units	Physically compatible	3	**C**
Fructose 10% in water	AB	AB	1000 and 4000 units	Physically compatible	3	**C**
Invert sugar 5 and 10% in sodium chloride 0.9%	AB	AB	1000 and 4000 units	Physically compatible	3	**C**
Invert sugar 5 and 10% in water	AB	AB	1000 and 4000 units	Physically compatible	3	**C**
Ionosol products	AB	AB	1000 and 4000 units	Physically compatible	3	**C**

Solution Compatibility (Cont.)

Solution Compatibility (Cont.)

Heparin sodium

Solution	Mfr	Mfr	Conc/L	Remarks	Ref	C/I
Normosol R	AB	AB	20,000 units	Potency retained for 24 hr	21	**C**
Ringer's injection	AB	AB	1000 and 4000 units	Physically compatible	3	**C**
Ringer's injection, lactated	AB	AB	1000 and 4000 units	Physically compatible	3	**C**
			12,000 units	Physically compatible	74	**C**
	TR[a]	UP	10,000 units	Potency retained for 24 hr at 5 °C	282	**C**
	OR		20,000 units	40% potency loss within 1 hr at 23 °C	113	**I**
	MG	UP	10,000 units	50 to 60% activity loss in 6 hr at room temperature. Partial rebound at 24 hr	406	**I**
		AH	35,000 units	Apparent temporary 50% loss of heparin activity in 4 hr with recovery in 6 hr at 25 °C. Heparin activity gradually lost over 14 days	900	**?**
Sodium chloride 0.45%	AB	AB	1000 and 4000 units	Physically compatible	3	**C**
Sodium chloride 0.9%			12,000 units	Physically compatible	74	**C**
	AB	AB	1000 and 4000 units	Physically compatible	3	**C**
			32,000 units	Potency retained for 24 hr	57	**C**
	AB	AB	20,000 units	Potency retained for 24 hr	21	**C**
	AB		20,000 units	Potency retained for 72 hr	46	**C**
	TR[a]	UP	10,000 units	Potency retained for 24 hr at 5 °C	282	**C**
	TR[b]	OR	20,000 and 40,000 units	Potency retained for 48 hr at 27 °C	254	**C**
		AH	35,000 units	Heparin activity stable for 24 hr at 25 °C followed by 14 days at 4 °C	900	**C**
	MG	UP	10,000 units	30 to 50% activity loss in 6 hr at room temperature. Partial rebound at 24 hr	406	**I**
	BA	DB	1000 units	Heparin activity retained for 12 months at 22 °C	1914	**C**
	BA	DB	10,000 units	Heparin activity retained for 12 months at 4 and 22 °C	1914	**C**
		LY	5000 units	Heparin activity retained for 28 days at 4 °C	2025	**C**

Solution Compatibility (Cont.)

Heparin sodium

Solution	Mfr	Mfr	Conc/L	Remarks	Ref	C/I
Sodium lactate ⅙ M		OR	20,000 units	50% potency loss within 1 hr at 23 °C	113	**I**
TPN #48 to #51[c]		AH	35,000 units	Heparin activity retained for 24 hr at 25 °C but significantly decreased after 24 hr	900	**C**
TPN #205[c]		LY	3000 to 20,000 units	Heparin activity retained for 28 days at 4 °C	2025	**C**

[a]Tested in both glass and PVC containers.
[b]Tested in PVC containers.
[c]Refer to Appendix I for the composition of parenteral nutrition solutions. TPN indicates a 2-in-1 admixture.

Additive Compatibility

Heparin sodium

Drug	Mfr	Conc/L	Mfr	Conc/L	Test Soln	Remarks	Ref	C/I
Alteplase	GEN	0.5 g	ES	40,000 units	NS	Heparin interacts with alteplase. Opalescence forms within 5 min with peak intensity at 4 hr at 25 °C. Alteplase activity reduced slightly	1856	**I**
Amikacin sulfate	BR	5 g	AB	30,000 units	D5LR, D5R, D5S, D5W, D10W, IS10, LR, NS, R, SL	Immediate precipitation	294	**I**
Aminophylline		250 mg		12,000 units	D5W	Physically compatible	74	**C**
	SE	1 g	UP	4000 units	D5W	Physically compatible	15	**C**
Amphotericin B	SQ	100 mg	AB	4000 units	D	Physically compatible	21	**C**
	SQ	100 mg	AB	4000 units	D5W	Physically compatible	15	**C**
Amphotericin B with hydrocortisone sodium phosphate	SQ MSD	50 mg 50 and 100 mg	AB	1500 units	D5W	Physically compatible and amphotericin B bioactivity retained in normal light at 25 °C for 24 hr. Hydrocortisone and heparin activity not tested	540	**C**
Amphotericin B with hydrocortisone sodium phosphate	SQ MSD	100 mg 50 and 100 mg	AB	1500 units	D5W	Physically compatible and amphotericin B bioactivity retained in normal light at 25 °C for 24 hr. Hydrocortisone and heparin activity not tested	540	**C**
Ampicillin sodium		2 g		32,000 units	NS	Physically compatible and heparin activity retained for 24 hr	57	**C**
	BE	10 g	OR	20,000 units	NS	Potency of both retained for 24 hr at 25 °C	113	**C**
	BR	1 g		12,000 units	D5W, D10W, IM, IP, LR, NS	Ampicillin potency retained for 24 hr at 4 °C	87	**C**

Additive Compatibility (Cont.)

Heparin sodium

Drug	Mfr	Conc/L	Mfr	Conc/L	Test Soln	Remarks	Ref	C/I
	BR	1 g		12,000 units	D5S	15% ampicillin decomposition in 24 hr at 4 °C	87	I
	BR	1 g		12,000 units	D5W, D10W, LR	20 to 25% ampicillin decomposition in 24 hr at 25 °C	87	I
Ascorbic acid injection	UP	500 mg	UP	4000 units	D5W	Physically compatible	15	C
Atracurium besylate	BW	500 mg		40,000 units	D5W	Particles form at 5 and 30 °C	1694	I
Bleomycin sulfate	BR	20 and 30 units	RI	10,000 to 200,000 units	NS	Physically compatible and bleomycin activity retained for 1 week at 4 °C. Heparin not tested	763	C
Calcium gluconate		1 g		12,000 units	D5W	Physically compatible	74	C
	UP	1 g	UP	4000 units	D5W	Physically compatible	15	C
	UP	1 g	AB	20,000 units		Physically compatible	21	C
Cefepime HCl	BR	4 g	MG	10,000 and 50,000 units	D5W, NS	Visually compatible with 4% cefepime loss by HPLC in 24 hr at room temperature and 3% loss in 7 days at 5 °C. Little or no heparin loss	1681	C
Chloramphenicol sodium succinate	PD	500 mg		12,000 units	D5W	Physically compatible	74	C
	PD	10 g	UP	4000 units	D5W	Physically compatible	15	C
	PD	1 g	AB	20,000 units		Physically compatible	6; 21	C
Cibenzoline succinate		2 g	ES	40,000 units	D5W, NS	Physically compatible for 24 hr at 25 °C by visual and microscopic examination	1182	C
Ciprofloxacin	BAY	2 g	CP	10,000, 100,000, and 1 million units	NS	White precipitate forms immediately	1934	I
Clindamycin phosphate	UP	9 g		100,000 units	D5W	Clindamycin stability maintained for 24 hr	101	C
Colistimethate sodium	WC	500 mg	AB	20,000 units	D	Physically compatible	21	C
	WC	500 mg	UP	4000 units	D5W	Physically compatible	15	C
Cytarabine	UP	500 mg		10,000 units	NS	Haze formation	174	I
	UP	500 mg		20,000 units	D5W	Haze formation	174	I
Daunorubicin HCl	FA	200 mg	UP	4000 units	D5W	Physically incompatible	15	I
Dimenhydrinate	SE	50 mg		12,000 units	D5W	Physically compatible	74	C

Additive Compatibility (Cont.)

Heparin sodium

Drug	Mfr	Conc/L	Mfr	Conc/L	Test Soln	Remarks	Ref	C/I
	SE	500 mg	UP	4000 units	D5W	Physically compatible	15	**C**
	SE	50 mg	AB	20,000 units	D	Physically compatible	21	**C**
Dobutamine HCl	LI	1 g	ES	40,000 units	D5W, NS	Physically compatible with no color change in 24 hr at 25 °C	789	**C**
	LI	1 g	LY	50,000 units	D5W, NS	Physically compatible for 24 hr at 21 °C	812	**C**
	LI	1 g	ES	5 million units	D5W, NS	Pink discoloration within 6 hr at 21 °C	812	**I**
	LI	1 g	ES	50,000 units	D5W	Heparin added to D5W and then mixed with an equal volume of dobutamine in D5W. Precipitate forms within 3 min	841	**I**
	LI	1.5 g	LY	50,000 units	D5W, NS	Obvious precipitation	1318	**I**
	LI	900 mg	LY	50,000 units	D5W, W	Physically compatible for 4 hr, but heat of reaction detected by microcalorimetry	1318	**I**
	LI	900 mg	LY	50,000 units	NS	Physically compatible for 4 hr with no heat of reaction detected by microcalorimetry	1318	**C**
Dopamine HCl	AS	800 mg	AB	200,000 units	D5W	No dopamine or heparin decomposition in 24 hr at 25 °C	312	**C**
Enalaprilat	MSD	12 mg	ES	50,000 units	D5W[a]	Visually compatible with little or no enalaprilat loss by HPLC in 24 hr at room temperature under fluorescent light. Heparin not tested	1572	**C**
Erythromycin lactobionate	AB	1 g	AB	1500 units		Precipitate forms within 1 hr	20	**I**
	AB	5 g	UP	4000 units	D5W	Physically incompatible	15	**I**
	AB	1.5 g	OR	20,000 units	D5W, NS	Precipitate forms	113	**I**
	AB	1 g	AB	20,000 units		Precipitate forms within 1 hr	21	**I**
Esmolol HCl	DU	6 g	LY	50,000 units	D5W	Physically compatible with no esmolol loss in 24 hr at room temperature under fluorescent light. Heparin not tested	1358	**C**
Floxacillin sodium	BE	20 g	WED	20,000 units	NS	Physically compatible for 24 hr at 15 and 30 °C. Haze forms in 48 hr at 30 °C. No change at 15 °C	1479	**C**
Fluconazole	PF	1 g	BA	50,000 units	D5W	Fluconazole chemically stable by gas chromatography for at least 24 hr at 25 °C under fluorescent light. Heparin not tested	1676	**C**
Flumazenil	RC	20 mg	ES	50,000 units	D5W[a]	Visually compatible with 4% flumazenil loss by HPLC in 24 hr at 23 °C under fluorescent light. Heparin not tested	1710	**C**
Furosemide	HO	1 g	WED	20,000 units	NS	Physically compatible for 72 hr at 15 and 30 °C	1479	**C**
Gentamicin sulfate		320 mg	BP	20,000 units	D5W, NS	Immediate precipitation	26	**I**

Additive Compatibility (Cont.)

Heparin sodium

Drug	Mfr	Conc/L	Mfr	Conc/L	Test Soln	Remarks	Ref	C/I
	SC	1 g	OR	20,000 units	D5W, NS	Opalescence	113	I
	ME	88 mg	BRN	1000 to 6000 units	D10W, NS	Activity of both drugs by biological assays greatly reduced	1570	I
Hyaluronidase						Physically incompatible	10	I
	WY					Physically incompatible	9	I
Hydrocortisone sodium phosphate with amphotericin B	MSD SQ	50 and 100 mg 50 mg	AB	1500 units	D5W	Physically compatible and amphotericin B bioactivity retained in normal light at 25 °C for 24 hr. Hydrocortisone and heparin activity not tested	540	C
Hydrocortisone sodium phosphate with amphotericin B	MSD SQ	50 and 100 mg 100 mg	AB	1500 units	D5W	Physically compatible and amphotericin B bioactivity retained in normal light at 25 °C for 24 hr. Hydrocortisone and heparin activity not tested	540	C
Hydrocortisone sodium succinate		800 mg		32,000 units	NS	Physically compatible and heparin activity retained for 24 hr	57	C
						Physically incompatible	9	I
	UP	500 mg	UP	4000 units	D5W	Physically incompatible	15	I
Isoproterenol HCl		2 mg		32,000 units	NS	Physically compatible and heparin activity retained for 24 hr	57	C
	WI	4 mg	AB	20,000 units		Physically compatible	59	C
Kanamycin sulfate	BR	4 g	UP	4000 units	D5W	Physically incompatible	15	I
	BR	500 mg	AB	20,000 units		Precipitate forms within 1 hr	21	I
	TE	2 g	OR	20,000 units	D5W, NS	Precipitate forms	113	I
	BR	250 mg		12,000 units	D5S, D5W, D10W, IM, IP, LR, NS	Immediate precipitation	87	I
	BPC	4 g	BP	20,000 units	D5W, NS	Immediate precipitation	26	I
Levorphanol bitartrate	RC					Physically incompatible	9	I
Lidocaine HCl		4 g		32,000 units	NS	Physically compatible and heparin activity retained for 24 hr	57	C
	AST	2 g	AB	20,000 units		Physically compatible	24	C
Lincomycin HCl	UP	600 mg	AB	20,000 units		Physically compatible	21	C
Magnesium sulfate		130 mEq		50,000 units	NS[b]	Visually compatible with heparin activity retained for 14 days at 24 °C under fluorescent light	1908	C
Meperidine HCl	WI					Physically incompatible	9	I

Additive Compatibility (Cont.)

Heparin sodium

Drug	Mfr	Conc/L	Mfr	Conc/L	Test Soln	Remarks	Ref	C/I
Meropenem	ZEN	1 and 20 g	ES	20,000 units	NS	Visually compatible for 4 hr at room temperature	1994	C
Methyldopa HCl	MSD	1 g	AB	20,000 units	D, D–S, S	Physically compatible	23	C
Methylprednisolone sodium succinate	UP	40 mg		10,000 units	D5S	Clear solution for 24 hr	329	C
	UP	125 mg		5000 units	D5S, D5W, LR, R	Clear solution for 24 hr	329	C
	UP	25 g		40,000 units	NS	Clear solution for 24 hr	329	C
Metronidazole HCl with sodium bicarbonate	SE AB	5 g 50 mEq	UP	30,000 units	D5W, NS	Physically compatible for 48 hr	765	C
Mitomycin	BR	167 mg	ES	33,300 units	NS[b]	Visually compatible with 10% mitomycin loss calculated in 21 hr and no decrease in heparin bioactivity at 25 °C	1866	I
	BR	167 mg	ES	33,300 units	NS[a]	Visually compatible with 10% mitomycin loss calculated in 25 hr and no decrease in heparin bioactivity at 25 °C	1866	C
	BR	500 mg	ES	33,300 units	NS[b]	Visually compatible with 10% mitomycin loss calculated in 42 hr and no decrease in heparin bioactivity at 25 °C	1866	C
	BR	500 mg	ES	33,300 units	NS[a]	Visually compatible with 10% mitomycin loss calculated in 61 hr and no decrease in heparin bioactivity at 25 °C	1866	C
Morphine sulfate						Physically incompatible	9	I
Nafcillin sodium	WY	500 mg	AB, WY	20,000 units		Physically compatible	27	C
	WY	500 mg	AB	20,000 units		Physically compatible	21	C
Norepinephrine bitartrate	WI	8 mg		12,000 units	D5W	Physically compatible	74	C
	WI	8 mg	AB	20,000 units	D, D–S, S	Physically compatible	77	C
Octreotide acetate	SZ	1.5 mg	ES	1000 units	TPN #120[c]	Little octreotide loss over 48 hr at room temperature in ambient light	1373	C
Penicillin G[d]		20 million units		32,000 units	NS	Physically compatible and heparin activity retained for 24 hr	57	C
Penicillin G potassium		1 million units		12,000 units	D5W	Physically compatible	74	C
	SQ	1 million units	AB	20,000 units	D5W	Penicillin potency retained for 24 hr at 25 °C	47	C
		20 million units		32,000 units	NS	Physically compatible and heparin activity retained for 24 hr	57	C
	SQ	20 million units		4000 units	D5W	Physically incompatible	15	I

Additive Compatibility (Cont.)

Heparin sodium

Drug	Mfr	Conc/L	Mfr	Conc/L	Test Soln	Remarks	Ref	C/I
Penicillin G sodium	BE	20 million units	OR	20,000 units	NS	Potency of both retained for 24 hr at 25 °C	113	**C**
	UP	20 million units	UP	4000 units	D5W	Physically incompatible	15	**I**
Polymyxin B sulfate	BP	20 mg	BP	20,000 units	D5W	Immediate precipitation	26	**I**
	BP	20 mg	BP	20,000 units	NS	Haze develops over 3 hr	26	**I**
Potassium chloride		3 g		12,000 units	D5W	Physically compatible	74	**C**
	AB	40 mEq	AB	20,000 units		Physically compatible	21	**C**
		80 mEq		32,000 units	NS	Physically compatible and heparin activity retained for 24 hr	57	**C**
Promazine HCl	WY	100 mg	AB	20,000 units		Physically compatible	21	**C**
Promethazine HCl	WY	250 mg	UP	4000 units	D5W	Physically incompatible	15	**I**
Ranitidine HCl	GL	2 g	ES	10,000 and 40,000 units	D5W, NS[a]	Physically compatible with 2% or less ranitidine loss in 48 hr at room temperature under fluorescent light. Heparin not tested	1361	**C**
	GL	50 mg	ES	10,000 and 40,000 units	NS[a]	Physically compatible with no ranitidine loss in 48 hr at room temperature under fluorescent light. Heparin not tested	1361	**C**
	GL	50 mg	ES	10,000 and 40,000 units	D5W[a]	Physically compatible with 7% ranitidine loss in 24 hr and about 12% loss in 48 hr at room temperature under fluorescent light. Heparin not tested	1361	**C**
Sodium bicarbonate	AB	2.4 mEq[e]	AB	20,000 units	D5W	Physically compatible for 24 hr	772	**C**
Streptomycin sulfate						Physically incompatible	9	**I**
		1 g	AB	20,000 units		Precipitate forms within 1 hr	21	**I**
	BP	4 g	BP	20,000 units	D5W, NS	Immediate precipitation	26	**I**
Teicoplanin	HO	2 g	CPP	20,000 and 40,000 units	D5W, NS	Visually compatible with no loss of teicoplanin by HPLC and microbiological assay and no loss of heparin activity in 24 hr at 25 °C	2165	**C**
Vancomycin HCl	LI	1 g		12,000 units	D5W	Immediate precipitation	74	**I**
	LE	400 mg	IX	1000 units	TPN #95[c]	Physically compatible and vancomycin content retained for 8 days at room temperature and under refrigeration by TDx	1321	**C**
	LI	15 mg to 5.3 g	OR	500 to 14,300 units	[f]	Physically compatible for 24 hr at 25 °C	1322	**C**

Additive Compatibility (Cont.)

Heparin sodium

Drug	Mfr	Conc/L	Mfr	Conc/L	Test Soln	Remarks	Ref	C/I
	LI	6.9 to 14.3 g	OR	500 to 14,300 units	f	Immediate white precipitation	1322	**I**
Verapamil HCl	KN	80 mg	ES	20,000 units	D5W, NS	Physically compatible for 24 hr	764	**C**
Vitamin B complex	WY	20 ml		32,000 units	NS	Physically compatible and heparin activity retained for 24 hr	57	**C**
Vitamin B complex with C		1 vial		12,000 units	D5W	Physically compatible	74	**C**
	AB	5 ml	UP	4000 units	D5W	Physically compatible	15	**C**
	AB	10 ml	AB	20,000 units		Physically compatible	21	**C**
	WY	4 ampuls		32,000 units	NS	Physically compatible and heparin activity retained for 24 hr	57	**C**

[a]*Tested in PVC containers.*
[b]*Tested in glass containers.*
[c]*Refer to Appendix I for the composition of parenteral nutrition solutions. TPN indicates a 2-in-1 admixture.*
[d]*Salt form unspecified.*
[e]*One vial of Neut added to a liter of admixture.*
[f]*Tested in Dianeal with dextrose 2.5 and 4.25%.*

Drugs in Syringe Compatibility

Heparin sodium

Drug (in syringe)	Mfr	Amt	Mfr	Amt	Remarks	Ref	C/I
Amikacin sulfate		100 mg		2500 units/ 1 ml	Turbidity or precipitate forms within 5 min	1053	**I**
Aminophylline		240 mg/ 10 ml		2500 units/ 1 ml	Physically compatible for at least 5 min	1053	**C**
Amiodarone HCl	LZ	150 mg/ 3 ml		2500 units/ 1 ml	Turbidity or precipitate forms within 5 min	1053	**I**
Amphotericin B		50 mg		2500 units/ 1 ml	Physically compatible for at least 5 min	1053	**C**
Ampicillin sodium		2 g		2500 units/ 1 ml	Physically compatible for at least 5 min	1053	**C**
Atropine sulfate		0.5 mg/ 1 ml		2500 units/ 1 ml	Physically compatible for at least 5 min	1053	**C**
Azlocillin sodium		2 g		2500 units/ 1 ml	Physically compatible for at least 5 min	1053	**C**
Bleomycin sulfate		1.5 units/ 0.5 ml		500 units/ 0.5 ml	Physically compatible for 5 min at room temperature followed by 8 min of centrifugation	980	**C**

Drugs in Syringe Compatibility (Cont.)

Heparin sodium

Drug (in syringe)	Mfr	Amt	Mfr	Amt	Remarks	Ref	C/I
Cefamandole nafate	LI	2 g		2500 units/ 1 ml	Physically compatible for at least 5 min	1053	C
Cefazolin sodium		2 g		2500 units/ 1 ml	Physically compatible for at least 5 min	1053	C
Cefoperazone sodium	RR	2 g		2500 units/ 1 ml	Physically compatible for at least 5 min	1053	C
Cefotaxime sodium	HO	2 g		2500 units/ 1 ml	Physically compatible for at least 5 min	1053	C
Cefoxitin sodium	MSD	2 g		2500 units/ 1 ml	Physically compatible for at least 5 min	1053	C
Chloramphenicol sodium succinate	PD	1 g	AB	20,000 units/ 1 ml	Physically compatible for at least 30 min	21	C
		1 g		2500 units/ 1 ml	Physically compatible for at least 5 min	1053	C
Chlorpromazine HCl		50 mg/ 2 ml		2500 units/ 1 ml	Turbidity or precipitate forms within 5 min	1053	I
Cimetidine HCl	SKF	300 mg/ 2 ml		5000 units/ 5 ml	Physically compatible for 48 hr at room temperature	516	C
		200 mg/ 2 ml		2500 units/ 1 ml	Physically compatible for at least 5 min	1053	C
Cisplatin		0.5 mg/ 0.5 ml		500 units/ 0.5 ml	Physically compatible for 5 min at room temperature followed by 8 min of centrifugation	980	C
Clindamycin phosphate	UP	300 mg		2500 units/ 1 ml	Physically compatible for at least 5 min	1053	C
Cyclophosphamide		10 mg/ 0.5 ml		500 units/ 0.5 ml	Physically compatible for 5 min at room temperature followed by 8 min of centrifugation	980	C
Diatrizoate meglumine 52%, diatrizoate sodium 8%	MA	5 ml	OR	5000 units/ 0.5 ml	Physically compatible for at least 2 hr	1438	C
Diatrizoate sodium 60%	WI	5 ml	OR	5000 units/ 0.5 ml	Physically compatible for at least 2 hr	1438	C
Diazepam		10 mg/ 2 ml		2500 units/ 1 ml	Turbidity or precipitate forms within 5 min	1053	I

Drugs in Syringe Compatibility (Cont.)

Heparin sodium

Drug (in syringe)	Mfr	Amt	Mfr	Amt	Remarks	Ref	C/I
Diazoxide		300 mg/ 20 ml		2500 units/ 1 ml	Physically compatible for at least 5 min	1053	C
Digoxin		0.25 mg/ 1 ml		2500 units/ 1 ml	Physically compatible for at least 5 min	1053	C
Dimenhydrinate		65 mg/ 10 ml		2500 units/ 1 ml	Physically compatible for at least 5 min	1053	C
Dobutamine HCl	LI	250 mg/ 10 ml		2500 units/ 1 ml	Physically compatible for at least 5 min	1053	C
Dopamine HCl		50 mg/ 5 ml		2500 units/ 1 ml	Physically compatible for at least 5 min	1053	C
Doxorubicin HCl		1 mg/ 0.5 ml		500 units/ 0.5 ml	Immediate precipitation	980	I
Droperidol		1.25 mg/ 0.5 ml		500 units/ 0.5 ml	Immediate precipitation	980	I
	JN	5 mg/ 2 ml		2500 units/ 1 ml	Turbidity or precipitate forms within 5 min	1053	I
Epinephrine HCl		1 mg/ 1 ml		2500 units/ 1 ml	Physically compatible for at least 5 min	1053	C
Erythromycin lactobionate	AB	1 g	AB	20,000 units/ 1 ml	Physically incompatible	21	I
Erythromycin (form unspecified)	SC	250 mg		2500 units/ 1 ml	Turbidity or precipitate forms within 5 min	1053	I
Fentanyl citrate	JN	0.1 mg/ 2 ml		2500 units/ 1 ml	Physically compatible for at least 5 min	1053	C
Fentanyl citrate and droperidol (Innovar)	JN	0.1 mg + 5 mg/ 2 ml		2500 units/ 1 ml	Turbidity or precipitate forms within 5 min	1053	I
Fluorouracil		25 mg/ 0.5 ml		500 units/ 0.5 ml	Physically compatible for 5 min at room temperature followed by 8 min of centrifugation	980	C
Furosemide		5 mg/ 0.5 ml		500 units/ 0.5 ml	Physically compatible for 5 min at room temperature followed by 8 min of centrifugation	980	C
		20 mg/ 2 ml		2500 units/ 1 ml	Physically compatible for at least 5 min	1053	C

Drugs in Syringe Compatibility (Cont.)

Heparin sodium

Drug (in syringe)	Mfr	Amt	Mfr	Amt	Remarks	Ref	C/I
Gentamicin sulfate		40 mg		2500 units/ 1 ml	Turbidity or precipitate forms within 5 min	1053	I
Haloperidol lactate	JN	5 mg/ 1 ml		2500 units/ 1 ml	Turbidity or precipitate forms within 5 min	1053	I
Iohexol	WI	64.7%, 5 ml	OR	5000 units/ 0.5 ml	Physically compatible for at least 2 hr	1438	C
Iopamidol	SQ	61%, 5 ml	OR	5000 units/ 0.5 ml	Physically compatible for at least 2 hr	1438	C
Iothalamate meglumine 60%	MA	5 ml	OR	5000 units/ 0.5 ml	Physically compatible for at least 2 hr	1438	C
Ioxaglate meglumine 39.3%, ioxaglate sodium 19.6%	MA	5 ml	OR	5000 units/ 0.5 ml	Physically compatible for at least 2 hr	1438	C
Kanamycin sulfate	BR	500 mg	AB	20,000 units/ 1 ml	Physically incompatible	21	I
Leucovorin calcium		5 mg/ 0.5 ml		500 units/ 0.5 ml	Physically compatible for 5 min at room temperature followed by 8 min of centrifugation	980	C
Lidocaine HCl	AST	100 mg/ 5 ml		2500 units/ 1 ml	Physically compatible for at least 5 min	1053	C
Lincomycin HCl	UP	600 mg	AB	20,000 units/ 1 ml	Physically compatible for at least 30 min	21	C
Meperidine HCl	HO	100 mg/ 2 ml		2500 units/ 1 ml	Turbidity or precipitate forms within 5 min	1053	I
Methotrexate sodium		12.5 mg/ 0.5 ml		500 units/ 0.5 ml	Physically compatible for 5 min at room temperature followed by 8 min of centrifugation	980	C
Methotrimeprazine		25 mg/ 1 ml		2500 units/ 1 ml	Turbidity or precipitate forms within 5 min	1053	I
Metoclopramide HCl		2.5 mg/ 0.5 ml		500 units/ 0.5 ml	Physically compatible for 5 min at room temperature followed by 8 min of centrifugation	980	C
		10 mg/ 2 ml		2500 units/ 1 ml	Physically compatible for at least 5 min	1053	C
	RB	10 mg/ 2 ml	ES	2000 units/ 2 ml	Physically compatible for 48 hr at room temperature	924	C

Drugs in Syringe Compatibility (Cont.)

Heparin sodium

Drug (in syringe)	Mfr	Amt	Mfr	Amt	Remarks	Ref	C/I
	RB	10 mg/ 2 ml	ES	4000 units/ 4 ml	Physically compatible for 48 hr at room temperature	924	C
	RB	10 mg/ 2 ml	ES	2000 units/ 2 ml	Physically compatible for 48 hr at 25 °C	1167	C
	RB	10 mg/ 2 ml	ES	4000 units/ 4 ml	Physically compatible for 48 hr at 25 °C	1167	C
	RB	160 mg/ 32 ml	ES	16,000 units/ 16 ml	Physically compatible for 48 hr at 25 °C	1167	C
Mitomycin		0.25 mg/ 0.5 ml		500 units/ 0.5 ml	Physically compatible for 5 min at room temperature followed by 8 min of centrifugation	980	C
Morphine sulfate		1, 2, 5, 10 mg	WY	100 and 200 units	Brought to 5 ml with NS. Physically compatible with no morphine loss in 24 hr at 23 °C	985	C
		1, 2, 5 mg	WY	100 and 200 units	Brought to 5 ml with W. Physically compatible with no morphine loss in 24 hr at 23 °C	985	C
		10 mg	WY	100 and 200 units	Brought to 5 ml with W. Immediate haze with white precipitate and 5 to 7% loss of morphine potency	985	I
Nafcillin sodium	WY	500 mg	AB	20,000 units/ 1 ml	Physically compatible for at least 30 min	21	C
Naloxone HCl	DU	0.4 mg/ 1 ml		2500 units/ 1 ml	Physically compatible for at least 5 min	1053	C
Neostigmine methylsulfate	RC	0.5 mg/ 1 ml		2500 units/ 1 ml	Physically compatible for at least 5 min	1053	C
Netilmicin sulfate		150 mg		2500 units/ 1 ml	Turbidity or precipitate forms within 5 min	1053	I
Nitroglycerin		25 mg/ 25 ml		2500 units/ 1 ml	Physically compatible for at least 5 min	1053	C
Norepinephrine HCl	HO	1 mg/ 1 ml		2500 units/ 1 ml	Physically compatible for at least 5 min	1053	C
Pancuronium bromide		4 mg/ 2 ml		2500 units/ 1 ml	Physically compatible for at least 5 min	1053	C
Penicillin G		10 million units		2500 units/ 1 ml	Physically compatible for at least 5 min	1053	C
Pentazocine lactate	WI	30 mg/ 1 ml		2500 units/ 1 ml	Turbidity or precipitate forms within 5 min	1053	I

Drugs in Syringe Compatibility (Cont.)

				Heparin sodium			
Drug (in syringe)	*Mfr*	*Amt*	*Mfr*	*Amt*	*Remarks*	*Ref*	*C/I*
Phenobarbital sodium		200 mg/ 1 ml		2500 units/ 1 ml	Physically compatible for at least 5 min	1053	**C**
Piperacillin sodium	LE	2 g		2500 units/ 1 ml	Physically compatible for at least 5 min	1053	**C**
Promethazine HCl		50 mg/ 2 ml		2500 units/ 1 ml	Turbidity or precipitate forms within 5 min	1053	**I**
Sodium nitroprusside		60 mg/ 5 ml		2500 units/ 1 ml	Physically compatible for at least 5 min	1053	**C**
Streptomycin sulfate		1 g	AB	20,000 units/ 1 ml	Physically incompatible	21	**I**
Succinylcholine chloride		100 mg/ 5 ml		2500 units/ 1 ml	Physically compatible for at least 5 min	1053	**C**
Tobramycin sulfate		80 mg/ 2 ml		10 units/ 1 ml	Turbidity or fine white precipitate due to formation of insoluble salt	845	**I**
	LI	40 mg		2500 units/ 1 ml	Turbidity or precipitate forms within 5 min	1053	**I**
Triflupromazine HCl		10 mg/ 1 ml		2500 units/ 1 ml	Turbidity or precipitate forms within 5 min	1053	**I**
Trimethoprim–sulfamethoxazole		80 + 400 mg/ 5 ml		2500 units/ 1 ml	Physically compatible for at least 5 min	1053	**C**
Vancomycin HCl	LI	500 mg		2500 units/ 1 ml	Turbidity or precipitate forms within 5 min	1053	**I**
Verapamil HCl	KN	5 mg/ 2 ml		2500 units/ 1 ml	Physically compatible for at least 5 min	1053	**C**
Vinblastine sulfate		0.5 mg/ 0.5 ml		500 units/ 0.5 ml	Physically compatible for 5 min at room temperature followed by 8 min of centrifugation	980	**C**
	LI	1 mg/ml		200 units/ml[a]	Turbidity appears in 2 to 3 min	767	**I**
Vincristine sulfate		0.5 mg/ 0.5 ml		500 units/ 0.5 ml	Physically compatible for 5 min at room temperature followed by 8 min of centrifugation	980	**C**
Warfarin sodium	DU	2 mg/ 1 ml[b]	ES	5000 units/ 1 ml	Low-level haze forms immediately and becomes visible in ambient light in 1 hr	2010	**I**

[a]*Tested in bacteriostatic sodium chloride 0.9%.*
[b]*Tested in sterile water for injection.*

Y-Site Injection Compatibility (1:1 Mixture)

Heparin sodium

Drug	Mfr	Conc	Mfr	Conc	Remarks	Ref	C/I
Acyclovir sodium	BW	5 mg/ml[a]	ES	50 units/ml[a]	Physically compatible for 4 hr at 25 °C	1157	**C**
Aldesleukin	CHI	33,800 I.U./ml[a]	BA	100 units/ml	Visually compatible with little or no loss of aldesleukin activity by bioassay	1857	**C**
Allopurinol sodium	BW	3 mg/ml[b]	ES	100 units/ml[b]	Physically compatible with no change in measured turbidity or increase in particle content in 4 hr at 22 °C	1686	**C**
Alteplase	GEN	1 mg/ml	ES	100 units/ml[a]	Haze noted in 24 hr by visual examination. Erratic spectrophotometer readings	1340	**I**
Amifostine	USB	10 mg/ml[a]	ES	100 units/ml[a]	Physically compatible with no change in measured turbidity or increase in particle content in 4 hr at 23 °C	1845	**C**
Aminophylline	SE	25 mg/ml	RI	1000 units/L[c]	Physically compatible for at least 4 hr at room temperature by visual and microscopic examination	322	**C**
Amiodarone HCl	LZ	150 mg/3 ml[d]		50 units/ml/min[b]	Yellow solution with opalescence	1053	**I**
Amphotericin B cholesteryl sulfate complex	SEQ	0.83 mg/ml[a]	WY	1000 units/ml[a]	Gross precipitate forms	2117	**I**
Ampicillin sodium	BR	25, 50, 100, 135 mg/ml	RI	1000 units/L[c]	Physically compatible for at least 4 hr at room temperature by visual and microscopic examination	322	**C**
	WY	20 mg/ml[b]	TR	50 units/ml	Visually compatible for 6 hr at 25 °C	1793	**C**
Ampicillin sodium–sulbactam sodium	PF	20 + 10 mg/ml[b]	TR	50 units/ml	Visually compatible for 6 hr at 25 °C	1793	**C**
Amsacrine	NCI	1 mg/ml[a]	SO	40 units/ml[a]	Light flocculent orange precipitate forms immediately	1381	**I**
Atracurium besylate	BW	0.5 mg/ml[a]	SO	40 units/ml[a]	Physically compatible for 24 hr at 28 °C	1337	**C**
Atropine sulfate	BW	0.5 mg/ml	UP	1000 units/L[e]	Physically compatible for at least 4 hr at room temperature by visual and microscopic examination	534	**C**
Aztreonam	SQ	40 mg/ml[a]	ES	100 units/ml[a]	Physically compatible with no subvisual haze or particle formation in 4 hr at 23 °C	1758	**C**
	BV	20 mg/ml[a]	TR	50 units/ml	Visually compatible for 6 hr at 25 °C	1793	**C**
Betamethasone sodium phosphate	SC	3 mg/ml	UP	1000 units/L[e]	Physically compatible for at least 4 hr at room temperature by visual and microscopic examination	534	**C**
Bleomycin sulfate		3 units/ml		1000 units/ml	Drugs injected sequentially into Y-site with no flush between. No visually apparent precipitate	980	**C**
Calcium gluconate	ES	100 mg/ml	RI	1000 units/L[c]	Physically compatible for at least 4 hr at room temperature by visual and microscopic examination	322	**C**
Cefazolin sodium	SKB	20 mg/ml	TR	50 units/ml	Visually compatible for 6 hr at 25 °C	1793	**C**
Cefotetan disodium	STU	40 mg/ml[a]	TR	50 units/ml	Visually compatible for 6 hr at 25 °C	1793	**C**
Cefotiam	GRU	8 mg/ml	RC	333 and 666 units/ml	Little cefotiam loss in 1 hr by HPLC	1889	**C**

Y-Site Injection Compatibility (1:1 Mixture) (Cont.)

Heparin sodium

Drug	Mfr	Conc	Mfr	Conc	Remarks	Ref	C/I
Ceftazidime	LI[p]	20 mg/ml	TR	50 units/ml	Visually compatible for 6 hr at 25 °C	1793	C
Ceftriaxone sodium	RC	20 mg/ml	TR	50 units/ml	Visually compatible for 6 hr at 25 °C	1793	C
Chlordiazepoxide HCl	RC	10 mg/ml	UP	1000 units/L[e]	Physically compatible for at least 4 hr at room temperature by visual and microscopic examination	534	C
Chlorpromazine HCl	SKF	25 mg/ml	UP	1000 units/L[e]	Physically compatible for at least 4 hr at room temperature by visual and microscopic examination	534	C
Cimetidine HCl		200 mg/ 2 ml[d]		50 units/ml/ min[b]	Clear solution	1053	C
	SKB	6 mg/ml[a]	TR	50 units/ml	Visually compatible for 6 hr at 25 °C	1793	C
Ciprofloxacin		2 mg/ml		10 units/ml	Turbidity forms rapidly with subsequent white precipitate	1483	I
	MI	2 mg/ml[f]	LY	100 units/ml	Crystals form immediately	1655	I
	BAY	2 mg/ml[b]	CP	10, 100, and 1000 units/ ml[b]	White precipitate forms immediately	1934	I
Cisatracurium besylate	GW	0.1 and 2 mg/ml[a]	AB	100 units/ml	Physically compatible with no change in measured turbidity or increase in particle content in 4 hr at 23 °C	2074	C
	GW	5 mg/ml[a]	AB	100 units/ml	White cloudiness forms immediately	2074	I
Cisplatin		1 mg/ml		1000 units/ml	Drugs injected sequentially into Y-site with no flush between. No visually apparent precipitate	980	C
	BR	1 mg/ml	SO	40 units/ml[a]	Visually compatible for 4 hr at room temperature under fluorescent light	1685	C
Cladribine	ORT	0.015[b] and 0.5[g] mg/ml	WY	100 units/ml[b]	Physically compatible with no change in measured turbidity or increase in particle content in 4 hr at 23 °C	1969	C
Clarithromycin	AB	4 mg/ml[a]	CPP	1000 units/ ml[a]	White cloudiness forms immediately	2174	I
Clindamycin phosphate	UP	12 mg/ml[a]	TR	50 units/ml	Visually compatible for 6 hr at 25 °C	1793	C
Cyanocobalamin	PD	0.1 mg/ml	UP	1000 units/L[e]	Physically compatible for at least 4 hr at room temperature by visual and microscopic examination	534	C
Cyclophosphamide		20 mg/ml		1000 units/ml	Drugs injected sequentially into Y-site with no flush between. No visually apparent precipitate	980	C
	MJ	10 mg/ml[a]	SO	40 units/ml[a]	Visually compatible for 4 hr at room temperature under fluorescent light	1685	C
Cytarabine	UP	50 mg/ml	SO	40 units/ml[a]	Visually compatible for 4 hr at room temperature under fluorescent light	1685	C
Dacarbazine	MI	25 mg/ml[b]	WY	100 units/ml	White flocculent precipitate forms immediately[h]	1158	I
	MI	10 mg/ml[b]	WY	100 units/ml	No observable precipitation[g]	1158	C
Dexamethasone sodium phosphate	MSD	4 mg/ml	RI	1000 units/L[c]	Physically compatible for at least 4 hr at room temperature by visual and microscopic examination	322	C
	ES	0.08 mg/ml[a]	TR	50 units/ml	Visually compatible for 6 hr at 25 °C	1793	C

Y-Site Injection Compatibility (1:1 Mixture) (Cont.)

				Heparin sodium			
Drug	*Mfr*	*Conc*	*Mfr*	*Conc*	*Remarks*	*Ref*	*C/I*
Diazepam		10 mg/2 ml[d]		50 units/ml/min[b]	Turbidity	1053	I
	RC	5 mg/ml	RI	1000 units/L[c]	Immediate haziness and globule formation	322	I
Digoxin	BW	0.25 mg/ml	RI	1000 units/L[c]	Physically compatible for at least 4 hr at room temperature by visual and microscopic examination	322	C
Diltiazem HCl	MMD	5 mg/ml	LY	20,000 units/ml	Precipitate forms	1807	I
	MMD	1 mg/ml[b]	LY	20,000 units/ml	Visually compatible	1807	C
	MMD	1[b] and 5 mg/ml	LY, SCN	5000 and 10,000 units/ml	Visually compatible	1807	C
	MMD	5 mg/ml	LY, SCN	80 units/ml[f]	Visually compatible	1807	C
	MMD	1 mg/ml[a]	ES	100 units/ml[a]	Visually compatible for 4 hr at 27 °C	2062	C
Diphenhydramine HCl	PD	50 mg/ml	UP	1000 units/L[e]	Physically compatible for at least 4 hr at room temperature by visual and microscopic examination	534	C
Dobutamine HCl	LI	4 mg/ml[b]	ES	50 units/ml[b]	Physically compatible for 3 hr	1316	C
	LI	4 mg/ml[a]	ES	50 units/ml[a]	Immediate gross precipitation	1316	I
	LI	1 mg/ml[a]	TR	50 units/ml	Visually compatible for 6 hr at 25 °C	1793	C
	LI	4 mg/ml[a]	OR	100 units/ml[a]	Haze and white precipitate form	1877	I
	LI	4 mg/ml[a]	ES	100 units/ml[a]	Precipitate forms in 4 hr at 27 °C	2062	I
Docetaxel	RPR	0.9 mg/ml[a]	ES	100 units/ml	Physically compatible with no change in measured turbidity or increase in particle content in 4 hr at 23 °C	2224	C
Dopamine HCl	ACC	40 mg/ml	UP	1000 units/L[e]	Physically compatible for at least 4 hr at room temperature by visual and microscopic examination	534	C
	BA	1.6 mg/ml	TR	50 units/ml	Visually compatible for 6 hr at 25 °C	1793	C
	AB	3.2 mg/ml[a]	ES	100 units/ml[a]	Visually compatible for 4 hr at 27 °C	2062	C
Doxorubicin HCl		2 mg/ml		1000 units/ml	Drugs injected sequentially into Y-site with no flush between. Immediate precipitation	980	I
	AD	0.2 mg/ml[a]	SO	40 units/ml[a]	Visually compatible for 4 hr at room temperature under fluorescent light	1685	C
Doxorubicin HCl liposome injection	SEQ	0.4 mg/ml[a]	ES	1000 units/ml[a]	Physically compatible with little or no change in measured turbidity and no increase in particle content in 4 hr at 23 °C	2087	C
Doxycycline hyclate	ES	1 mg/ml[a]	TR	50 units/ml	Visually incompatible within 6 hr at 25 °C	1793	I
Droperidol		2.5 mg/ml		1000 units/ml	Drugs injected sequentially into Y-site with no flush between. Immediate precipitation	980	I
	CR	1.25 mg/ml	UP	1000 units/L[e]	Physically compatible for at least 4 hr at room temperature by visual and microscopic examination	534	C

Y-Site Injection Compatibility (1:1 Mixture) (Cont.)

Drug	Mfr	Conc	Mfr	Conc	Remarks	Ref	C/I
	JN	5 mg/2 ml[d]		50 units/ml/min[b]	White turbidity	1053	**I**
Edrophonium chloride	RC	10 mg/ml	UP	1000 units/L[e]	Physically compatible for at least 4 hr at room temperature by visual and microscopic examination	534	**C**
Enalaprilat	MSD	0.05 mg/ml[c]	IX	40 units/ml[a]	Physically compatible for 24 hr at room temperature under fluorescent light	1355	**C**
Epinephrine HCl	AB	0.1 mg/ml	UP	1000 units/L[e]	Physically compatible for at least 4 hr at room temperature by visual and microscopic examination	534	**C**
	AB	0.02 mg/ml[a]	ES	100 units/ml[a]	Visually compatible for 4 hr at 27 °C	2062	**C**
Ergotamine tartrate	SZ	0.5 mg/ml	UP	1000 units/L[e]	Crystal formation and brown discoloration in 4 hr at room temperature	534	**I**
Erythromycin lactobionate	AB	3.3 mg/ml[b]	TR	50 units/ml	Visually compatible for 6 hr at 25 °C	1793	**C**
Esmolol HCl	DCC	10 mg/ml[a]	IX	40 units/ml[a]	Physically compatible for 24 hr at 22 °C	1169	**C**
Estrogens, conjugated	AY	5 mg/ml	RI	1000 units/L[c]	Physically compatible for at least 4 hr at room temperature by visual and microscopic examination	322	**C**
Ethacrynate sodium	MSD	1 mg/ml	RI	1000 units/L[c]	Physically compatible for at least 4 hr at room temperature by visual and microscopic examination	322	**C**
Etoposide phosphate	BR	5 mg/ml[a]	ES	100 units/ml[a]	Physically compatible with no change in measured turbidity or increase in particle content in 4 hr at 23 °C	2218	**C**
Famotidine	MSD	0.2 mg/ml[a]	ES	40 units/ml[b]	Physically compatible for 14 hr	1196	**C**
	MSD	0.2 mg/ml[a]	TR	50 units/ml[a]	Physically compatible for 4 hr at 25 °C	1188	**C**
	ME	2 mg/ml[b]		40 units/ml[a]	Visually compatible for 4 hr at 22 °C	1936	**C**
Fentanyl citrate	MN	0.05 mg/ml	UP	1000 units/L[e]	Physically compatible for at least 4 hr at room temperature by visual and microscopic examination	534	**C**
	ES	0.05 mg/ml	ES	100 units/ml[a]	Visually compatible for 4 hr at 27 °C	2062	**C**
Fentanyl citrate and droperidol (Innovar)	MN	0.05 mg + 2.5 mg/ml	UP	1000 units/L[e]	Physically compatible for at least 4 hr at room temperature by visual and microscopic examination	534	**C**
	JN	0.1 mg + 5 mg/2 ml[d]		50 units/ml/min[b]	Precipitate forms	1053	**I**
Filgrastim	AMG	30 μg/ml[a]	ES	100 units/ml[a]	Particles and filaments form immediately	1687	**I**
Fluconazole	RR	2 mg/ml	LY	1000 units/ml	Physically compatible for 24 hr at 25 °C	1407	**C**
	PF	2 mg/ml	TR	50 units/ml	Visually compatible for 6 hr at 25 °C	1793	**C**
Fludarabine phosphate	BX	1 mg/ml[a]	SO, WY	40, 100, 1000 units/ml	Physically compatible for 4 hr at room temperature under fluorescent light	1439	**C**
Fluorouracil	RC	50 mg/ml	UP	1000 units/L[e]	Physically compatible for at least 4 hr at room temperature by visual and microscopic examination	534	**C**
		50 mg/ml		1000 units/ml	Drugs injected sequentially into Y-site with no flush between. No visually apparent precipitate	980	**C**
Foscarnet sodium	AST	24 mg/ml	ES	1000 units/ml	Physically compatible for 24 hr at room temperature under fluorescent light	1335	**C**

Y-Site Injection Compatibility (1:1 Mixture) (Cont.)

Drug	Mfr	Conc	Mfr	Conc	Remarks	Ref	C/I
	AST	24 mg/ml	LY	100 units/ml[f]	Physically compatible for 24 hr at 25 °C under fluorescent light by visual and microscopic examination	1393	C
Furosemide		10 mg/ml		1000 units/ml	Drugs injected sequentially into Y-site with no flush between. No visually apparent precipitate	980	C
	HO	10 mg/ml	UP	1000 units/L[e]	Physically compatible for at least 4 hr at room temperature by visual and microscopic examination	534	C
	AMR	10 mg/ml	ES	100 units/ml[a]	Visually compatible for 4 hr at 27 °C	2062	C
Gemcitabine HCl	LI	10 mg/ml[b]	ES	100 units/ml[b]	Physically compatible with no change in measured turbidity or increase in particle content in 4 hr at 23 °C	2226	C
Gentamicin sulfate	ES	3.2 mg/ml[f]	ES	50 units/ml[f]	Immediate gross haze	1316	I
	TR	2 mg/ml	TR	50 units/ml	Visually incompatible within 6 hr at 25 °C	1793	I
Granisetron HCl	SKB	0.05 mg/ml[a]	AB	100 units/ml[a]	Physically compatible with no change in measured turbidity or increase in particle content in 4 hr at 23 °C	2000	C
Haloperidol lactate	JN	5 mg/1 ml[d]		50 units/ml/min[b]	White turbidity	1053	I
	MN	5 mg/1 ml[i]	OR	25,000 and 50,000 units/250 ml[f]	White precipitate forms immediately	1436	I
Hydralazine HCl	CI	20 mg/ml	UP	1000 units/L[e]	Physically compatible for at least 4 hr at room temperature by visual and microscopic examination	534	C
Hydrocortisone sodium succinate	UP	2 mg/ml[a]	TR	50 units/ml	Visually compatible for 6 hr at 25 °C	1793	C
	UP	125 mg/ml	ES	100 units/ml[f]	Visually compatible for 24 hr at room temperature in test tubes. No precipitate found on filter from Y-site delivery	2063	C
Hydromorphone HCl	KN	1 mg/ml	ES	100 units/ml[a]	Visually compatible for 4 hr at 27 °C	2062	C
Idarubicin HCl	AD	1 mg/ml[b]	ES	1000 units/ml	Haze forms immediately and precipitate forms in 20 min	1525	I
	AD	1 mg/ml[b]	SO	100 units/ml	Haze forms immediately and precipitate forms in 12 min	1525	I
Insulin, regular	LI	40 units/ml	RI	1000 units/L[c]	Physically compatible for at least 4 hr at room temperature by visual and microscopic examination	322	C
	LI	0.2 unit/ml[b]	ES	60 units/ml[a]	Physically compatible for 2 hr at 25 °C	1395	C
Isoproterenol HCl	WI	0.2 mg/ml	UP	1000 units/L[e]	Physically compatible for at least 4 hr at room temperature by visual and microscopic examination	534	C
Isosorbide dinitrate	RP	10 mg/ml[a]	LEO	300 units/ml[a]	Erratic availability of both drugs delivered through PVC tubing	1799	I
Kanamycin sulfate	BR	250 mg/ml	RI	1000 units/L[c]	Physically compatible for at least 4 hr at room temperature by visual and microscopic examination	322	C
Labetalol HCl	SC	1 mg/ml[a]	IX	40 units/ml[a]	Physically compatible for 24 hr at 18 °C	1171	C

Y-Site Injection Compatibility (1:1 Mixture) (Cont.)

Heparin sodium

Drug	Mfr	Conc	Mfr	Conc	Remarks	Ref	C/I
	GL	5 mg/ml	OR	100 units/ml[a]	Cloudiness with particles forms immediately	1877	I
	AH	2 mg/ml[a]	ES	100 units/ml[a]	Visually compatible for 4 hr at 27 °C	2062	C
Leucovorin calcium		10 mg/ml		1000 units/ml	Drugs injected sequentially into Y-site with no flush between. No visually apparent precipitate	980	C
Lidocaine HCl	AST	20 mg/ml	RI	1000 units/L[c]	Physically compatible for at least 4 hr at room temperature by visual and microscopic examination	322	C
	TR	4 mg/ml	TR	50 units/ml	Visually compatible for 6 hr at 25 °C	1793	C
Lorazepam	WY	0.33 mg/ml[b]		417 units/ml	Visually compatible for 24 hr at 22 °C	1855	C
	WY	0.5 mg/ml[a]	ES	100 units/ml[a]	Visually compatible for 4 hr at 27 °C	2062	C
Magnesium sulfate	AB	500 mg/ml	UP	1000 units/L[c]	Physically compatible for at least 4 hr at room temperature by visual and microscopic examination	534	C
Melphalan HCl	BW	0.1 mg/ml[b]	WY	100 units/ml[b]	Physically compatible with no change in measured turbidity or increase in particle content in 3 hr at 22 °C	1557	C
Menadiol sodium diphosphate	RC	5 mg/ml	UP	1000 units/L[e]	Physically compatible for at least 4 hr at room temperature by visual and microscopic examination	534	C
Meperidine HCl	HO	100 mg/2 ml[d]		50 units/ml/min[b]	Clear solution	1053	C
	WY	10 mg/ml[c]	ES	60 units/ml[a]	Physically compatible for 1 hr at 25 °C	1338	C
Meropenem	ZEN	1 and 50 mg/ml[b]	ES	1 unit/ml[j]	Visually compatible for 4 hr at room temperature	1994	C
Methotrexate sodium		25 mg/ml		1000 units/ml	Drugs injected sequentially into Y-site with no flush between. No visually apparent precipitate	980	C
	AD	15 mg/ml[k]	SO	40 units/ml[a]	Visually compatible for 4 hr at room temperature under fluorescent light	1685	C
		30 mg/ml	CH	500 units/ml[b]	Visually compatible for 4 hr at room temperature	1788	C
Methotrimeprazine		25 mg/ml[d]		50 units/ml/min[b]	White precipitate	1053	I
Methoxamine HCl	BW	10 mg/ml	UP	1000 units/L[e]	Physically compatible for at least 4 hr at room temperature by visual and microscopic examination	534	C
Methyldopate HCl	ES	5 mg/ml[a]	TR	50 units/ml	Visually compatible for 6 hr at 25 °C	1793	C
Methylergonovine maleate	SZ	0.2 mg/ml	UP	1000 units/L[e]	Physically compatible for at least 4 hr at room temperature by visual and microscopic examination	534	C
Methylprednisolone sodium succinate	UP	40 mg/ml	RI	1000 units/L[l]	In D5W. Physically compatible for at least 4 hr at room temperature by visual and microscopic examination	322	C
	UP	40 mg/ml	RI	1000 units/L[l]	In RL and NS. Physically compatible initially but haziness in 4 hr at room temperature	322	I
	UP	2.5 mg/ml[a]	TR	50 units/ml	Visually compatible for 6 hr at 25 °C	1793	C

Y-Site Injection Compatibility (1:1 Mixture) (Cont.)

Heparin sodium

Drug	Mfr	Conc	Mfr	Conc	Remarks	Ref	C/I
	UP	5 mg/ml[b]	ES	100 units/ml[f]	Visually compatible for 24 hr at room temperature in test tubes. No precipitate found on filter from Y-site delivery	2063	C
Metoclopramide HCl		5 mg/ml		1000 units/ml	Drugs injected sequentially into Y-site with no flush between. No visually apparent precipitate	980	C
Metronidazole	MG	5 mg/ml	TR	50 units/ml	Visually compatible for 6 hr at 25 °C	1793	C
Midazolam HCl	RC	5 mg/ml		417 units/ml	Visually compatible for 24 hr at 22 °C	1855	C
	RC	2 mg/ml[a]	ES	100 units/ml[a]	Visually compatible for 4 hr at 27 °C	2062	C
Milrinone lactate	SW	0.2 mg/ml[a]	ES	100 units/ml[a]	Visually compatible for 4 hr at 27 °C	2062	C
	SW	0.4 mg/ml[a]	ES	100 units/ml[a]	Visually compatible with little or no loss of milrinone by HPLC and heparin by immunoassay in 4 hr at 23 °C	2214	C
Minocycline HCl	LE	50 mg/ml	UP	1000 units/L[e]	Physically compatible for at least 4 hr at room temperature by visual and microscopic examination	534	C
Mitomycin		0.5 mg/ml		1000 units/ml	Drugs injected sequentially into Y-site with no flush between. No visually apparent precipitate	980	C
Morphine sulfate	WY	15 mg/ml	UP	1000 units/L[e]	Physically compatible for at least 4 hr at room temperature by visual and microscopic examination	534	C
	WY	0.2 mg/ml[f]	ES	50 units/ml[f]	Physically compatible for 3 hr	1316	C
	ES	1 mg/ml[c]	ES	60 units/ml[a]	Physically compatible for 1 hr at 25 °C	1338	C
	SCN	2 mg/ml[a]	ES	100 units/ml[a]	Visually compatible for 4 hr at 27 °C	2062	C
Nafcillin sodium	WY	20 mg/ml[a]	TR	50 units/ml	Visually compatible for 6 hr at 25 °C	1793	C
Neostigmine methylsulfate	RC	0.5 mg/ml	UP	1000 units/L[e]	Physically compatible for at least 4 hr at room temperature by visual and microscopic examination	534	C
Nicardipine HCl	WY	1 mg/ml[a]	ES	100 units/ml[a]	Precipitate forms immediately	2062	I
Nitroglycerin	BA	0.2 mg/ml	ES	50 units/ml	Visually compatible for 24 hr at 23 °C	1794	C
	OM	0.2 mg/ml[a]	OR	100 units/ml[a]	Visually compatible for 24 hr at 23 °C	1877	C
	AB	0.4 mg/ml[a]	ES	100 units/ml[a]	Visually compatible for 4 hr at 27 °C	2062	C
Norepinephrine bitartrate	WI	1 mg/ml	UP	1000 units/L[e]	Physically compatible for at least 4 hr at room temperature by visual and microscopic examination	534	C
	AB	0.128 mg/ml[a]	ES	100 units/ml[a]	Visually compatible for 4 hr at 27 °C	2062	C
Ondansetron HCl	GL	1 mg/ml[b]	SO	40 units/ml[a]	Physically compatible for 4 hr at 22 °C	1365	C
Oxacillin sodium	BR	100 mg/ml	UP	1000 units/L[e]	Physically compatible for at least 4 hr at room temperature by visual and microscopic examination	534	C
Oxytocin	SZ	1 mg/ml	UP	1000 units/L[e]	Physically compatible for at least 4 hr at room temperature by visual and microscopic examination	534	C
Paclitaxel	NCI	1.2 mg/ml[a]	WY	100 units/ml[a]	Physically compatible with no change in measured turbidity in 4 hr at 22 °C	1556	C
Pancuronium bromide	ES	0.05 mg/ml[a]	SO	40 units/ml[a]	Physically compatible for 24 hr at 28 °C	1337	C

Y-Site Injection Compatibility (1:1 Mixture) (Cont.)

Heparin sodium

Drug	Mfr	Conc	Mfr	Conc	Remarks	Ref	C/I
Penicillin G potassium	LI	200,000 units/ml	RI	1000 units/L[c]	Physically compatible for at least 4 hr at room temperature by visual and microscopic examination	322	C
	RR	40,000 units/ml[a]	TR	50 units/ml	Visually compatible for 6 hr at 25 °C	1793	C
Pentazocine lactate	WI	30 mg/ml	UP	1000 units/L[c]	Physically compatible for at least 4 hr at room temperature by visual and microscopic examination	534	C
Phenytoin sodium	PD	50 mg/ml	RI	1000 units/L[c]	Immediate crystal formation	322	I
	ES	2 mg/ml[b]	TR	50 units/ml	Cloudiness forms immediately and becomes dense, white, flocculent precipitate in 6 hr at 25 °C	1793	I
Phytonadione	RC	10 mg/ml	UP	1000 units/L[c]	Physically compatible for at least 4 hr at room temperature by visual and microscopic examination	534	C
Piperacillin sodium	LE	60 mg/ml[a]	TR	50 units/ml	Visually compatible for 6 hr at 25 °C	1793	C
Piperacillin sodium–tazobactam sodium	LE	40 + 5 mg/ml[a]	ES	100 units/ml[a]	Physically compatible with no change in measured turbidity or increase in particle content in 4 hr at 22 °C	1688	C
Potassium chloride	AB	0.2 mEq/ml[a]	TR	50 units/ml	Visually compatible for 6 hr at 25 °C	1793	C
Procainamide HCl	SQ	100 mg/ml	UP	1000 units/L[c]	Physically compatible for at least 4 hr at room temperature by visual and microscopic examination	534	C
Prochlorperazine edisylate	SKF	5 mg/ml	UP	1000 units/L[c]	Physically compatible for at least 4 hr at room temperature by visual and microscopic examination	534	C
Promethazine HCl	SV	50 mg/ml	UP	1000 units/L	In D5LR, D5W, LR, and NS. Physically compatible for at least 4 hr at room temperature by visual and microscopic examination	534	C
	SV	50 mg/ml	UP	1000 units/L	In D5R. Physically compatible initially but cloudiness in 4 hr at room temperature	534	I
		50 mg/2 ml[d]		50 units/ml/min[b]	Distinctly turbid	1053	I
Propofol	ZEN	10 mg/ml	ES	100 units/ml[a]	Physically compatible for 1 hr at 23 °C with no increase in particle content	2066	C
Propranolol HCl	AY	1 mg/ml	UP	1000 units/L[c]	Physically compatible for at least 4 hr at room temperature by visual and microscopic examination	534	C
Pyridostigmine bromide	RC	5 mg/ml	UP	1000 units/L[c]	Physically compatible for at least 4 hr at room temperature by visual and microscopic examination	534	C
Quinidine gluconate	LI	6 mg/ml[c]	ES	50 units/ml[c]	Physically compatible for 3 hr	1316	C
	LI	6 mg/ml[a]	ES	50 units/ml[a]	Immediate gross haze	1316	I
Ranitidine HCl	GL	0.5 mg/ml[m]	LY	50 units/ml[a]	Physically compatible for 24 hr	1323	C
	GL	1 mg/ml	TR	50 units/ml	Visually compatible for 6 hr at 25 °C	1793	C
	GL	1 mg/ml[a]	ES	100 units/ml[a]	Visually compatible for 4 hr at 27 °C	2062	C

Y-Site Injection Compatibility (1:1 Mixture) (Cont.)

Heparin sodium

Drug	Mfr	Conc	Mfr	Conc	Remarks	Ref	C/I
Remifentanil HCl	GW	0.025 and 0.25 mg/ml[b]	AB	100 units/ml	Physically compatible with no change in measured turbidity or increase in particle content in 4 hr at 23 °C	2075	C
Sargramostim	IMM	10 μg/ml[b]	WY	100 units/ml	Physically compatible for 4 hr at 22 °C	1436	C
Scopolamine HBr	BW	0.86 mg/ml	UP	1000 units/L[e]	Physically compatible for at least 4 hr at room temperature by visual and microscopic examination	534	C
Sodium bicarbonate	BR	75 mg/ml	RI	1000 units/L[c]	Physically compatible for at least 4 hr at room temperature by visual and microscopic examination	322	C
		1.4%	CH	500 units/ml[b]	Visually compatible for 4 hr at room temperature	1788	C
Sodium nitroprusside	ES	0.2 mg/ml[a]	TR	50 units/ml	Visually compatible for 6 hr at 25 °C protected from light	1793	C
	RC	0.2 mg/ml[a]	OR	100 units/ml[a]	Visually compatible for 24 hr at 23 °C	1877	C
Streptokinase	HO	30,000 units/ml[a]	ES	100 units/ml[a]	Physically compatible for at least 5 days by visual examination	1340	C
Succinylcholine chloride	BW	20 mg/ml	RI	1000 units/L[c]	Physically compatible for at least 4 hr at room temperature by visual and microscopic examination	322	C
Tacrolimus	FUJ	1 mg/ml[b]	ES	10 units/ml[a]	Visually compatible for 24 hr at 25 °C	1630	C
Theophylline	TR	4 mg/ml	TR	50 units/ml	Visually compatible for 6 hr at 25 °C	1793	C
Thiopental sodium	AB	25 mg/ml[j]	ES	100 units/ml[a]	Visually compatible for 4 hr at 27 °C	2062	C
Thiotepa	IMM[n]	1 mg/ml[a]	ES	100 units/ml[a]	Physically compatible with no change in measured turbidity or increase in particle content in 4 hr at 23 °C	1861	C
Ticarcillin disodium	BE	20 mg/ml[a]	TR	50 units/ml	Visually compatible for 6 hr at 25 °C	1793	C
Ticarcillin disodium–clavulanate potassium	BE	31 mg/ml[a]	TR	50 units/ml	Visually compatible for 6 hr at 25 °C	1793	C
TNA #218 to #226[o]			AB	100 units/ml	Damage to emulsion integrity occurs immediately with free oil formation possible	2215	I
Tobramycin sulfate	LI	3.2 mg/ml[f]	ES	50 units/ml[f]	Immediate gross haze	1316	I
	LI	0.8 mg/ml[a]	TR	50 units/ml	Visually incompatible within 6 hr at 25 °C	1793	I
TPN #189[o]			DB	500 units/ml[b]	Visually compatible for 24 hr at 22 °C	1767	C
TPN #212 to #215[o]			AB	100 units/ml	Physically compatible with no change in measured turbidity or increase in particle content in 4 hr at 23 °C	2109	C
Triflupromazine HCl	SQ	10 mg/1 ml[d]		50 units/ml/min[b]	White precipitate forms	1053	I
Trimethobenzamide HCl	RC	100 mg/ml	UP	1000 units/L[e]	Physically compatible for at least 4 hr at room temperature by visual and microscopic examination	534	C
Trimethophan camsylate	RC	50 mg/1 ml	UP	1000 units/L[e]	Physically compatible for at least 4 hr at room temperature by visual and microscopic examination	534	C

Y-Site Injection Compatibility (1:1 Mixture) (Cont.)

Heparin sodium

Drug	Mfr	Conc	Mfr	Conc	Remarks	Ref	C/I
Vancomycin HCl	LI	6.6 mg/ml[a]	TR	50 units/ml	Visually incompatible within 6 hr at 25 °C	1793	**I**
	LE	10 mg/ml[b]	ES	100 units/ml[f]	Precipitate forms	2063	**I**
Vecuronium bromide	OR	0.1 mg/ml[a]	SO	40 units/ml[a]	Physically compatible for 24 hr at 28 °C	1337	**C**
	OR	1 mg/ml	ES	100 units/ml[a]	Visually compatible for 4 hr at 27 °C	2062	**C**
Vinblastine sulfate		1 mg/ml		1000 units/ml	Drugs injected sequentially into Y-site with no flush between. No visually apparent precipitate	980	**C**
Vincristine sulfate		1 mg/ml		1000 units/ml	Drugs injected sequentially into Y-site with no flush between. No visually apparent precipitate	980	**C**
Vinorelbine tartrate	BW	1 mg/ml[b]	ES	100 units/ml[b]	Physically compatible with no change in measured turbidity or increase in particle content in 4 hr at 22 °C	1558	**C**
Warfarin sodium	DU	2 mg/ml[j]	AB	100 units/ml[a]	Visually compatible with no warfarin loss by HPLC in 30 min	2010	**C**
	DME	2 mg/ml[j]	AB	100 units/ml[a]	Visually compatible for 24 hr at 24 °C	2078	**C**
Zidovudine	BW	4 mg/ml[a]	LY	100 units/ml[a]	Physically compatible for 4 hr at 25 °C under fluorescent light by visual and microscopic examination	1193	**C**

[a]*Tested in dextrose 5% in water.*
[b]*Tested in sodium chloride 0.9%.*
[c]*Tested in combination with hydrocortisone sodium succinate (Upjohn) 100 mg/L in dextrose 5% in water, sodium chloride 0.9%, and Ringer's injection, lactated.*
[d]*Given over three minutes into a heparin infusion run at 1 ml/min.*
[e]*Tested in dextrose 5% in Ringer's injection, dextrose 5% in Ringer's injection, lactated, dextrose 5% in water, Ringer's injection, lactated, and sodium chloride 0.9%.*
[f]*Tested in both dextrose 5% in water and sodium chloride 0.9%.*
[g]*Tested in bacteriostatic sodium chloride 0.9% preserved with benzyl alcohol 0.9%.*
[h]*Dacarbazine in intravenous tubing flushed with heparin sodium.*
[i]*Injected over one minute.*
[j]*Tested in sterile water for injection.*
[k]*Tested in dextrose 5% in water with sodium bicarbonate 0.05 mEq/ml.*
[l]*Also contained hydrocortisone sodium succinate (Upjohn) 100 mg/ml.*
[m]*Premixed infusion solution.*
[n]*Lyophilized formulation tested.*
[o]*Refer to Appendix I for the composition of parenteral nutrition solutions. TNA indicates a 3-in-1 admixture, and TPN indicates a 2-in-1 admixture.*
[p]*Sodium carbonate–containing formulation.*

Additional Compatibility Information

Miscellaneous— Amphotericin B infusions appear to be compatible with limited amounts of heparin sodium (4). Also, epirubicin HCl (1442), ceftazidime (4), and cefotetan disodium (283) have been stated to be compatible with heparin sodium.

Heparin is strongly acidic, reacting with certain basic compounds and losing activity (4). Solutions containing heparin sodium have been reported to be incompatible with tobramycin sulfate and gentamicin sulfate (4; 147; 230). A precipitate resulted when heparin sodium was added to an infusion solution containing antihuman lymphocyte globulin (Pressimmune, Hoechst) (408). Heparin is reported to decrease the antibacterial activity of neomycin (409). Ciprofloxacin, doxorubicin HCl, droperidol, mitoxantrone (4), and idarubicin HCl (2p2495) have been reported to be incompatible with

heparin sodium because of possible precipitate formation. Immunex also recommends not combining heparin sodium with mitoxantrone HCl in the same admixture because of possible precipitate formation (2p1404; 1293).

Dextrose Solutions— Evaluations of the stability of heparin sodium in dextrose-containing solutions have appeared frequently in the literature, but the results are conflicting.

Pritchard found that heparin sodium solutions, autoclaved for 10 minutes at 10 pounds/inch^2 at 115 °C, exhibited rapid loss of activity at pH values less than 5. It was speculated that a 50% loss of activity could occur if heparin sodium in dextrose 5% in water was autoclaved. The author suggested that heparin sodium should be added to the dextrose solution immediately before use (243).

Jacobs et al. noted a 50% reduction of activity within one hour at 23 °C when heparin sodium 10,000 units was added to 500 ml of dextrose 5% in water. A 40% reduction of activity occurred when dextrose 4.3% in sodium chloride 0.18% was used as the diluent. The pH of both solutions initially was 3.9, but the addition of heparin sodium raised the pH to approximately 6. After the initial fall in activity, the levels remained constant for the duration of the 24-hour test. The authors had no explanation for this phenomenon (113).

Okuno and Nelson, using two different assay methods, noted a similar result. A 25 to 60% reduction in heparin activity was observed when heparin sodium was added to several intravenous infusion solutions, including dextrose 5 and 10% in water, at a concentration of 10,000 units/L at room temperature. The nadir of activity was reached at six hours, although substantial loss occurred as early as two hours after mixing. This loss of activity extended to the non-dextrose-containing solutions sodium chloride 0.9% and Ringer's injection, lactated. Surprisingly, a partial rebound in activity was noted at the 24-hour observation period by one method. As an explanation of the rebound of activity, the authors speculated that heparin might transiently undergo molecular alteration in fluids or that the fluids could interfere in the coagulation process (406).

Anderson et al. reported a 65% loss of activity in five hours in a heparin sodium solution of 30 units/ml in dextrose 5% in water stored at 15, 25, and 35 °C. A total recovery of activity occurred in 24 to 48 hours, however. In dextrose 5% in sodium chloride 0.9%, 40% of the activity was lost in five hours, but only five to seven hours elapsed before complete recovery of activity was noted. If the sodium chloride content of the solution was increased up to 2% or if the dextrose concentration was decreased, no fall in activity was observed. Because of the eventual recovery of full activity and the lack of temperature effect, the authors concluded that degradation was not occurring. They speculated that a molecular rearrangement or interaction might be occurring (674).

Matthews noted a 50% loss of heparin activity in four hours at 25 °C in a concentration of 35,000 units/L in dextrose 5% in water and dextrose 4.3% in sodium chloride 0.9%. The activity recovered to initial levels by six hours after mixing and remained stable through 24 hours. Subsequent storage at 4 °C for 14 days resulted in no further loss in potency (900).

Parker's work did not support these results. No loss of potency was found in 24 hours when heparin sodium 20,000 units/L in dextrose 5% in water was tested at pH 3.8 to 7.6 (21). In another study, he found that heparin sodium 20,000 units/L was stable for 72 hours in several solutions, including dextrose 5% in water and dextrose 5% in sodium chloride 0.9% (46).

Hadgraft noted that both dextrose 5% in water and fructose 5% in water have little buffer capacity. A sample of dextrose 5% in water with a pH of 4.1 was mixed with 10,000 units of heparin sodium. The pH of the resultant solution was 5.95. Use of fructose 5% in water with a pH of 3.67 resulted in a final pH of 4.14 with the addition of heparin sodium 10,000 units. The author stated that at either of these pH values, heparin sodium would remain stable at room temperature (251).

Stock and Warner added heparin sodium to dextrose 5% in water having a pH of 4.4. The concentrations tested were 40, 200, and 964 units/ml having pH values of 6.6, 6.8, and 7, respectively, after addition of heparin sodium. No loss of potency was observed within 24 hours at 23 °C. The authors observed deterioration only after 60 hours at a minimum concentration of 1000 units/ml (252).

Hodby et al. found no significant loss of heparin activity in 24 hours when heparin sodium 8000 units was added to dextrose 5% in water or dextrose 5% in sodium chloride 0.9%. Additionally, they found no loss of activity in 24 hours of heparin sodium in sodium

chloride 0.9% adjusted to pH 3.2 with hydrochloric acid or to pH 9.2 with sodium hydroxide (57).

Chessels et al. found that, in 10 male patients, the effectiveness of heparin sodium 20,000 units in 500 ml of dextrose 5% administered as a 12-hour infusion was not impaired (253).

Mitchell et al. reported on heparin sodium 10,000 and 20,000 units in PVC containers of dextrose 5% in water and sodium chloride 0.9%. They found that the heparin activity remained stable for 48 hours at 27 °C. Additionally, they found that the mean pH was 6.17 for the dextrose admixtures and 5.97 for the sodium chloride admixtures. They did note a decrease in pH at four hours, which rose again at eight hours (254).

Turco reported the results of two tests of heparin stability, obtained as personal communications from a second party. In the first, heparin was stable for 24 hours in dextrose solutions containing heparin sodium 40,000 units/L. The second indicated that heparin stability was maintained for 48 hours at concentrations of 10,000 units/L in dextrose–saline solutions (244).

Joy et al. studied heparin sodium 20,000 units/L in dextrose 5% in water at pH 2, 5.4, and 9 at room temperature. No decrease in anticoagulant effectiveness was observed at any point over the 24-hour test period at any of the pH values. In an analogous manner, heparin activity was evaluated in dextrose 5% in sodium chloride 0.45%. Again, no change in anticoagulant effectiveness was observed in 24 hours (407).

Anderson and Harthill described a fluctuating effect of dextrose-containing solutions on heparin activity, which they termed the "dextrose effect." They noted that no evidence supports the degradation of heparin; the reversible nature of the activity reduction rules it out. In fact, they observed both decreased and increased heparin activity, presumably fluctuating in response to certain variables. Although pH may be a factor, it is not the determining one. Other factors may include heparin concentration, salt concentration, dextrose degradation products from autoclaving, heparin molecular weight distribution in the product, differences in proprietary dextrose products, and container effects. The authors attributed the variable activity results to reversible conformational changes in the heparin molecule itself, such as chain extension or, possibly, folding (905).

Wright and Hecker evaluated the activity of heparin sodium by activated partial thromboplastin time and by thrombin time in several dextrose-containing infusion solutions over periods up to one year. At a concentration of 1 unit/ml in dextrose 5% in water, heparin activity was retained for up to seven days at room temperature but fell substantially after that time. At 10 units/ml in dextrose 5% in water, no loss of activity was observed after 12 months of storage at either 4 °C or room temperature. At both 1 and 10 units/ml in several dextrose-containing solutions that also contained sodium chloride, no loss of heparin activity was found after 12 months of storage at either 4 °C or room temperature (1914).

Although conflicting information exists (113; 243; 406; 674; 900), most authors believe that heparin sodium may be administered in dextrose-containing solutions (21; 46; 57; 244; 251–254; 407; 1914).

Peritoneal Dialysis Fluids— The activity of heparin 35,000 units/L was evaluated in peritoneal dialysis fluids containing 1.5 and 2.5% dextrose (Dianeal, Travenol). Storage at 25 °C resulted in an apparent temporary 50% loss of heparin activity in four hours with recovery in six hours. Heparin activity was then retained for 14 days at 4 °C (900).

Parenteral Nutrition Solutions— It has been stated that heparin sodium is physically and chemically compatible in amino acid injection (McGaw) (189).

The addition of heparin sodium (Abbott) 1 and 2 units/ml to fat emulsion 10%, intravenous, from both Abbott (Liposyn) and Cutter (Intralipid) did not break the emulsion and effectively reversed the blood hypercoagulability associated with intravenous fat emulsion administration (568).

In solutions of amino acids 5% and dextrose 5 or 25% with vitamins or trace elements, heparin activity was retained for 24 hours at 25 °C. However, the activity fell significantly after 24 hours (900).

However, Raupp et al. reported flocculation of fat emulsion (Kabi-Vitrum) during Y-site administration into a line being used to infuse a parenteral nutrition solution containing both calcium gluconate and heparin sodium. Subsequent evaluation indicated that the combination of calcium gluconate (0.46 and 1.8 mM/125 ml) plus heparin sodium (25 and 100 units/125 ml) in amino acids plus dextrose would induce flocculation of the fat emulsion within two to four minutes at concentrations that resulted in no visually apparent flocculation in 30 minutes with either agent alone (1214).

This result was confirmed by Johnson et al. Calcium chloride concentrations of 1 to 20 mM normally result in slow flocculation of fat emulsion 20%, intravenous, over a period of hours. When heparin sodium 5 units/ml was added, the flocculation rate accelerated greatly; a cream layer was observed visually in a few minutes. This effect was not observed when sodium ion was substituted for the divalent calcium (1406).

Dobutamine— Several studies (789; 812; 841) have concerned the physical compatibility of dobutamine HCl in admixture with heparin sodium. The results have not been entirely consistent. Most reports indicate that the combinations tested were physically compatible. However, Hasegawa and Eder reported the formation of a precipitate with this combination. Heparin sodium (Elkins-Sinn) was diluted to a concentration of 100 units/ml with dextrose 5% in water and added to an equal volume of dobutamine HCl (Lilly), which had been diluted to 2 mg/ml with dextrose 5% in water. The precipitate formed within three minutes of combining the two drug dilutions. However, if the same heparin sodium lot or other lots (Elkins-Sinn and Invenex) were added undiluted to the dobutamine HCl in dextrose 5% in water, no visible precipitate resulted in 24 hours. Furthermore, no precipitate formed using either dilution method or any lot of heparin sodium tested when sodium chloride 0.9% was the diluent. The authors thought that precipitation may occur unpredictably. Because of this possibility plus Eli Lilly's consideration that the drugs are incompatible, the authors recommended not mixing the two drugs or infusing them through the same line (841).

Dopamine— The interaction between dopamine HCl and heparin sodium in aqueous solution was evaluated by microcalorimetry. An exothermic reaction occurred in dextrose 5% in water but not sodium chloride 0.9%. Consequently, sodium chloride 0.9% was recommended as a vehicle to minimize the interaction between the two drugs (1185).

Urokinase— To simulate an admixture used to maintain patency in implantable vascular-access devices, heparin (Burgess) 100 units/ml was used to constitute urokinase (Leo) to a concentration of 6250 units/ml. The mixture was stored for 21 days at 37 °C. No visible precipitation and no loss of anticoagulant activity occurred. An apparent decline in urokinase thrombolytic activity was noted, however. Nevertheless, marked fibrinolytic activity still remained after 24 days of incubation. The authors concluded that the mixture could be used in implantable vascular-access devices for up to three weeks (1174).

Vancomycin— Heparin sodium 5000 units/L (approximately) has been reported to be conditionally compatible with vancomycin HCl 2 g/L. A satisfactory solution is obtained if the infusion solution used is sodium chloride 0.9%. However, if dextrose 5% in water is used, a precipitate may form (143).

Vancomycin HCl (Lilly) 25 µg/ml and heparin sodium (Elkins-Sinn) 100 units/ml in 0.9% sodium chloride injection as a catheter flush solution was evaluated for stability when stored at 4 °C for 14 days. The flush solution was visually clear, and vancomycin activity (by bioassay and immunoassay) and heparin activity (by colorimetric assay) were retained throughout the storage period. However, an additional 24 hours at 37 °C to simulate use conditions resulted in losses of both agents ranging from 20 to 37% (1933).

Aminoglycosides— Gentamicin sulfate 10 mg/L with heparin sodium 1000 units/L in Dianeal with dextrose 5% peritoneal dialysis solution has been reported conditionally compatible. Koup and Gerbracht reported no significant reduction in gentamicin sulfate concentration or in the UV absorbance of heparin sodium in four to six hours (228). However, a clarifying communication noted a marked reduction in the anticoagulant activity of heparin sodium if opalescence or a precipitate is formed (which results if the undiluted drugs are combined), even if the precipitate redissolves. Heparin activity was retained if one drug was added to a dilute solution of the other and no precipitate formed (295).

Addition of gentamicin sulfate (Roussel) 80 mg to the tubing of an infusion solution of sodium chloride 0.9% containing heparin resulted in immediate precipitation (528).

The incompatibility of heparin sodium with gentamicin sulfate is said to result from coprecipitation (230). Similar precipitation may result from the administration of tobramycin sulfate (4; 147; 976), netilmicin sulfate, and amikacin sulfate through heparinized intravenous cannulas (976).

Methylprednisolone— The compatibility of methylprednisolone sodium succinate (Upjohn) with heparin sodium added to an auxiliary medication infusion unit has been studied. Primary admixtures were prepared by adding heparin sodium 10,000 units/L to dextrose 5% in water, dextrose 5% in sodium chloride 0.9%, and Ringer's injection, lactated. Up to 100 ml of the primary admixture was added along with methylprednisolone sodium succinate (Upjohn) to the auxiliary medication infusion unit with the following results (329):

Methylprednisolone Sodium Succinate	Heparin Sodium 10,000 units/L of Primary Solution	Results
500 mg	D5S, D5W qs 100 ml	Clear solution for 24 hr
	LR qs 100 ml or added to 100 ml LR	Clear solution for 6 hr
1000 mg	D5S, D5W qs 100 ml	Clear solution for 6 hr
	Added to 100 ml D5W	Clear solution for 24 hr
	LR qs 100 ml or added to 100 ml LR	Clear solution for 4 to 6 hr
2000 mg	D5W qs 100 ml	Clear solution for 6 hr
	D5S, LR qs 100 ml	Clear solution for 24 hr

Haloperidol— Heparin sodium (Organon) 25,000 and 50,000 units/ 250 ml of dextrose 5% in water and sodium chloride 0.9% was delivered through an administration set at a rate of 1000 units/hr. Haloperidol lactate (McNeil) 5 mg/1 ml was injected undiluted over one minute through an injection site on the set. In all cases, a precipitate formed immediately. The sodium chloride 0.9% admixtures developed a hazy milky white precipitate, while the dextrose 5% in water admixtures formed an opaque milky white precipitate with solid white particles of varying size. Injecting haloperidol lactate through sets with the infusion solutions and no heparin sodium did not yield a precipitate, ruling out incompatibility with the sets or solutions. The haloperidol lactate lowered the pH of the heparin sodium admixtures by 2 to 3 pH units, resulting in the unidentified precipitate. It was recommended that heparin infusions be stopped and that lines be flushed with sodium chloride 0.9% or dextrose 5% in water before and after injecting haloperidol lactate into the injection port. Administration of haloperidol lactate through a heparin lock would require a similar flushing procedure (779).

Concentrated Solutions— The following incompatibility determinations were performed with concentrated solutions. The drugs in dry form were reconstituted according to manufacturers' recommendations. One milliliter of heparin sodium was added to 5 ml of sterile distilled water along with 1 ml of each of the following drugs. Particulate matter was noted within two hours (28):

Dimenhydrinate (Searle)
Hydroxyzine HCl (Pfizer)
Kanamycin sulfate (Bristol)
Prochlorperazine edisylate (SKF)
Promazine HCl (Wyeth)
Promethazine HCl (Wyeth)
Vancomycin HCl (Lilly)

Heparin Locks— Heparin locks, weak heparin solutions instilled or "locked" into infusion ports or sets through a resealing latex diaphragm, are useful in providing an established intravenous route for intermittent intravenous injections. To maintain patency, a weak heparin solution is left in the tubing. Concentrations of heparin sodium used have varied from about 10 to 1000 units/ml of sodium chloride 0.9%, with 10 and 100 units/ml being the most common. The volume of dilute heparin sodium in sodium chloride 0.9% usu-ally used to flush the set is 0.2 to 1 ml (255-258; 405; 677; 678; 901; 2119). However, the use of sodium chloride 0.9% instead of a solution containing heparin has been suggested to maintain patency. Studies have found sodium chloride 0.9% to be as effective in maintaining patency as 10- and 100-unit/ml solutions of heparin (902; 903; 1109; 1266-1269; 1639-1641; 1656; 1839; 1959; 2003; 2119). Other investigators reported that even small amounts of heparin solution are more effective than sodium chloride 0.9% alone (678; 1270; 2120; 2121).

Evaluations of the use of heparinized solutions as locks or continuous flow solutions to help maintain patency in central venous catheters and arterial catheters have resulted in similarly variable results and recommendations (2122–2126). Although use of such heparinized solutions has been generally considered a benign technique causing minimal problems, a number of adverse effects have been reported, especially from solutions with a high heparin concentration and/or numerous heparin flushes (2127–2132).

It has been noted that if drugs such as meperidine HCl, promethazine HCl, and hydroxyzine HCl are injected into a heparinized scalp vein infusion set, a precipitate forms (97). It has been suggested that the venipuncture device be flushed with sterile water for injection or sodium chloride 0.9% prior to and immediately after drug administration. Heparin lock flush solution may then be reinjected into the device (4; 97).

Precipitation during the administration of aminoglycosides, such as gentamicin sulfate, tobramycin sulfate, netilmicin sulfate, and amikacin sulfate, through heparinized intravenous cannulas also may occur (976).

Other Information

Care is required when adding heparin sodium to infusion solutions, especially in flexible containers. When heparin sodium was added to a flexible PVC container of sodium chloride 0.9% hanging in the use position, pooling of the heparin resulted; 97% of the heparin was delivered in the first 30% of the solution. Repeated inversion and agitation of the containers to effect thorough mixing eliminates this pooling (and the danger of overdosage), yielding an even distribution and a constant delivery concentration (85).

HETASTARCH
AHFS 40:12

Hespan   **DuPont Pharma**

Products— Hetastarch (DuPont Pharma) is available as a 6% (6 g/100 ml) injection in sodium chloride 0.9% in 250- and 500-ml plastic containers. The solution also contains sodium hydroxide for pH adjustment (2).

pH— From 3.5 to 7 (2).

Osmolarity— The product has an osmolarity of 310 mOsm/L (2).

Sodium Content— Hetastarch 6% in sodium chloride 0.9% provides 77 mEq of sodium per 500-ml container or 38.5 mEq of sodium per 250-ml container (2).

Administration— Hetastarch is given only by intravenous infusion; discard any remaining solution in partially used containers. The dosage and rate of infusion must be individualized to the patient's condition and response (2; 4).

Stability— Hetastarch injection is a clear, pale yellow to amber colloidal solution. The product should be stored at controlled room temperature and protected from freezing and excessive heat. Brief exposure to temperatures up to 40 °C does not affect potency. However, prolonged storage under adverse conditions may result in a crystalline precipitate or a deep brown turbid appearance. Such solutions should not be administered (2; 4).

Before hetastarch is used, the colloidal solution should be checked for clarity and particulates and the flexible plastic containers should be squeezed to check for small leaks (2).

Compatibility Information

Additive Compatibility

Hetastarch

Drug	Mfr	Conc/L	Mfr	Conc/L	Test Soln	Remarks	Ref	C/I
Fosphenytoin sodium	PD	1, 8, 20 mg PE/ml[a]	MG	6%[b]		Visually compatible with little or no loss of fosphenytoin by HPLC in 7 days at 25 °C under fluorescent light	2083	C

[a]Concentration expressed in milligrams of phenytoin sodium equivalents (PE) per milliliter.
[b]In sodium chloride 0.9%.

Y-Site Injection Compatibility (1:1 Mixture)

Hetastarch

Drug	Mfr	Conc	Mfr	Conc	Remarks	Ref	C/I
Amikacin sulfate	BR	5 mg/ml[a]	DCC	6%	Small crystals formed immediately after mixing and persisted for 4 hr	1313	I
Ampicillin sodium	BR	20 mg/ml[a]	DCC	6%	Physically compatible for 4 hr at room temperature by visual examination	1313	C
	BR	20 mg/ml[a]	DCC	6%	One or two particles in one of five vials. Fine white strands appeared immediately during Y-site infusion	1315	I
Cefamandole nafate	LI	20 mg/ml[a]	DCC	6%	Small crystals formed immediately after mixing and persisted for 4 hr	1313	I
Cefazolin sodium	SKF	20 mg/ml[a]	DCC	6%	Physically compatible for 4 hr at room temperature by visual examination	1313	C
	SKF	20 mg/ml[a]	DCC	6%	Simulation in vials showed no incompatibility, but white precipitate formed in Y-site during infusion	1315	I
Cefoperazone sodium	RR	20 mg/ml[a]	DCC	6%	Small crystals formed immediately after mixing and persisted for 4 hr	1313	I
Cefotaxime sodium	HO	20 mg/ml[a]	DCC	6%	Small crystals formed immediately after mixing and persisted for 4 hr	1313	I
Cefoxitin sodium	MSD	20 mg/ml[a]	DCC	6%	Precipitate forms after 1 hr at room temperature	1313	I
Cimetidine HCl	SKF	6 mg/ml[a]	DCC	6%	Physically compatible for 4 hr at room temperature by visual examination	1313; 1315	C
Diltiazem HCl	MMD	5 mg/ml	DU	6%	Visually compatible	1807	C
Doxycycline hyclate	LY	1 mg/ml[a]	DCC	6%	Physically compatible for 4 hr at room temperature by visual examination	1313	C
	LY	1 mg/ml[a]	DCC	6%	White particle in one of five vials. No evidence of incompatibility during Y-site infusion	1315	?
Enalaprilat	MSD	0.05 mg/ml[b]	DCC	6%	Physically compatible for 24 hr at room temperature under fluorescent light	1355	C
Gentamicin sulfate	TR	0.8 mg/ml[c]	DCC	6%	Immediate precipitation which disappeared after 1 hr at room temperature	1313	I

Y-Site Injection Compatibility (1:1 Mixture) (Cont.)

			Hetastarch				
Drug	*Mfr*	*Conc*	*Mfr*	*Conc*	*Remarks*	*Ref*	*C/I*
Ranitidine HCl	GL	0.5 mg/ml[c]	DCC	6%	Barely visible single particle appeared after 1 hr but disappeared when vial was rotated	1313	?
	GL	0.5 mg/ml[c]	DCC	6%	Barely visible particles appeared and disappeared in three of five vials	1314	I
	GL	0.5 mg/ml[c]	DCC	6%	Small white particle in two of five vials. Small white fiber formed on needle during Y-site infusion	1315	I
Theophylline	TR	4 mg/ml[c]	DCC	6%	Precipitation after 2 hr at room temperature	1313	I
Tobramycin sulfate	LI	0.8 mg/ml[c]	DCC	6%	Small crystals formed immediately after mixing and persisted for 4 hr	1313	I

[a]Tested in dextrose 5% in water.
[b]Tested in sodium chloride 0.9%.
[c]Premixed infusion solution.

HYALURONIDASE
AHFS 44:00

Wydase   **Wyeth-Ayerst**

Products— Hyaluronidase (Wyeth-Ayerst) is supplied as a stabilized solution and a lyophilized product. The stabilized solution is available in 1- and 10-ml vials, providing 150 and 1500 USP units of hyaluronidase, respectively. Each milliliter of solution contains (1-2/8/94):

Hyaluronidase	150 USP units
Sodium chloride	8.5 mg
Disodium edetate	1 mg
Calcium chloride	0.4 mg
Sodium phosphate buffer	
Thimerosal	0.1 mg

The lyophilized product is available in 1- and 10-ml vials, also providing 150 and 1500 USP units of hyaluronidase, respectively. Reconstitution should be performed with sodium chloride 0.9%, 1 ml for the 1-ml vial and 10 ml for the 10-ml vial. Each milliliter of the resultant solution contains (1-2/8/94):

	Quantity/ml	
Component	1-ml Vial	10-ml Vial
Hyaluronidase	150 USP units	150 USP units
Lactose	2.66 mg	1.33 mg
Thimerosal	0.075 mg	0.1 mg

pH— From 6.4 to 7.4 (4).

Osmolality— Hyaluronidase 150 units/ml has an osmolality of 300 mOsm/kg (1689).

Units— The USP hyaluronidase unit is equivalent to the turbidity-reducing (TR) unit and the International Unit (1-2/8/94).

Administration— Hyaluronidase is administered subcutaneously, intradermally, or intramuscularly along with other drugs or solutions. It should not be administered intravenously (1-2/8/94; 4).

Stability— Hyaluronidase stabilized solution is stable for three years when stored at 2 to 8 °C (4). Although refrigeration is recommended, intact vials of hyaluronidase solution (Wyeth) are reported to be stable for three months at room temperatures not exceeding 25 °C (60). The injection should not be used if it is discolored or contains a precipitate (4).

Lyophilized hyaluronidase 1500 units/vial is reported to be stable after reconstitution with sodium chloride 0.9% for up to two weeks at temperatures below 30 °C. However, lyophilized hyaluronidase 150 units/vial is stated to be stable after reconstitution with sodium chloride 0.9% for only 24 hours when stored below 30 °C (4).

Hyaluronidase solutions should not be used if they are discolored or contain a precipitate (4).

Hyaluronidase (Wyeth) 75 units/ml in citric acid/sodium citrate buffer (pH ≈ 4.5) was found to lose about 7 to 8% activity in 24 hours at 4 and 23 °C. Hyaluronidase activity decreased by 25 to 33% in 48 hours (1907).

Compatibility Information

Solution Compatibility

Hyaluronidase

Solution	Mfr	Mfr	Conc/L	Remarks	Ref	C/I
Dextran 6% in dextrose 5%	AB	AB	150 units	Physically compatible	3	**C**
Dextran 6% in sodium chloride 0.9%	AB	AB	150 units	Physically compatible	3	**C**
Dextrose–Ringer's injection combinations	AB	AB	150 units	Physically compatible	3	**C**
Dextrose–Ringer's injection, lactated, combinations	AB	AB	150 units	Physically compatible	3	**C**
Dextrose–saline combinations	AB	AB	150 units	Physically compatible	3	**C**
Dextrose 2½% in water	AB	AB	150 units	Physically compatible	3	**C**
Dextrose 5% in water	AB	AB	150 units	Physically compatible	3	**C**
Dextrose 10% in water	AB	AB	150 units	Physically compatible	3	**C**
Fructose 10% in sodium chloride 0.9%	AB	AB	150 units	Physically compatible	3	**C**
Fructose 10% in water	AB	AB	150 units	Physically compatible	3	**C**
Invert sugar 5 and 10% in sodium chloride 0.9%	AB	AB	150 units	Physically compatible	3	**C**
Invert sugar 5 and 10% in water	AB	AB	150 units	Physically compatible	3	**C**
Ionosol products	AB	AB	150 units	Physically compatible	3	**C**
Ringer's injection	AB	AB	150 units	Physically compatible	3	**C**
Ringer's injection, lactated	AB	AB	150 units	Physically compatible	3	**C**
Sodium chloride 0.45%	AB	AB	150 units	Physically compatible	3	**C**
Sodium chloride 0.9%	AB	AB	150 units	Physically compatible	3	**C**
Sodium lactate ⅙ M	AB	AB	150 units	Physically compatible	3	**C**

Additive Compatibility

			Hyaluronidase					
Drug	*Mfr*	*Conc/L*	*Mfr*	*Conc/L*	*Test Soln*	*Remarks*	*Ref*	*C/I*
Amikacin sulfate	BR	5 g	SE	150 units	D5LR, D5R, D5S, D5W, D10W, IS10, LR, NS, R, SL	Physically compatible and amikacin potency retained for 24 hr at 25 °C. Hyaluronidase not analyzed	294	**C**
Epinephrine HCl	PD					Physically incompatible	10	**I**
	PD		WY			Physically incompatible	9	**I**
Heparin sodium						Physically incompatible	10	**I**
			WY			Physically incompatible	9	**I**
Sodium bicarbonate	AB	2.4 mEq[a]	WY	150 units	D5W	Physically compatible for 24 hr	772	**C**

[a]*One vial of Neut added to a liter of admixture.*

Drugs in Syringe Compatibility

			Hyaluronidase				
Drug (in syringe)	*Mfr*	*Amt*	*Mfr*	*Amt*	*Remarks*	*Ref*	*C/I*
Diatrizoate meglumine 52%, diatrizoate sodium 8% (Renografin-60)	SQ	40 to 5 ml	WY	150 units/ 1 ml	Physically compatible for 48 hr	530	**C**
	SQ	2 and 1 ml	WY	150 units/ 1 ml	Physically compatible for at least 1 hr but a precipitate forms within 48 hr	530	**I**
Diatrizoate meglumine 34.3%, diatrizoate sodium 35% (Renovist)	SQ	40 to 1 ml	WY	150 units/ 1 ml	Physically compatible for 48 hr	530	**C**
Diatrizoate sodium 75% (Hypaque)	WI	40 to 5 ml	WY	150 units/ 1 ml	Physically compatible for 48 hr	530	**C**
	WI	2 and 1 ml	WY	150 units/ 1 ml	Physically compatible for at least 1 hr but a precipitate forms within 48 hr	530	**I**
Hydromorphone HCl	KN	2 mg/ml[a]	WY	150 units/ml[a]	43 and 56% hyaluronidase loss in 24 hr at 4 and 23 °C, respectively	1907	**I**
	KN	10 and 40 mg/ ml[a]	WY	150 units/ml[a]	70 to 82% hyaluronidase loss in 24 hr at 4 and 23 °C	1907	**I**
Iodipamide meglumine 52% (Cholografin)	SQ	40 to 2 ml	WY	150 units/ 1 ml	Physically compatible for 48 hr	530	**C**
	SQ	1 ml	WY	150 units/ 1 ml	Physically compatible for at least 1 hr but a precipitate forms within 48 hr	530	**I**
Iothalamate meglumine 60% (Conray)	MA	40 to 1 ml	WY	150 units/ 1 ml	Physically compatible for 48 hr	530	**C**

Drugs in Syringe Compatibility (Cont.)

Hyaluronidase

Drug (in syringe)	Mfr	Amt	Mfr	Amt	Remarks	Ref	C/I
Iothalamate sodium 80% (Angio-Conray)	MA	40 to 1 ml	WY	150 units/ 1 ml	Physically compatible for 48 hr	530	C
Pentobarbital sodium	AB	500 mg/ 10 ml	AB	150 units	Physically compatible	55	C
Thiopental sodium	AB	75 mg/ 3 ml	AB	150 units	Physically compatible	55	C

ᵃ*Mixed in equal quantities.*

Additional Compatibility Information

Hyaluronidase has been found to be compatible with diatrizoate meglumine products (Squibb) (40).

HYDRALAZINE HCL
AHFS 24:08

American Regent

Products— Hydralazine HCl (American Regent) is available in 1-ml vials. Each milliliter of solution contains (2):

Hydralazine HCl	20 mg
Propylene glycol	103.6 mg
Methylparaben	0.65 mg
Propylparaben	0.35 mg
Water	qs

The pH may have been adjusted with hydrochloric acid and/or sodium hydroxide (1-4/96).

pH— From 3.4 to 4.4 (1-4/96).

Administration— Hydralazine HCl may be administered intramuscularly or as a rapid intravenous injection directly into the vein; the manufacturer does not recommend adding the drug to infusion solutions (1-4/96; 4).

Stability— Hydralazine HCl in intact vials should be stored at controlled room temperature (1-4/96). It is recommended that hydralazine HCl (Ciba) in intact ampuls not be stored under refrigeration because of possible precipitation or crystallization (593).

Hydralazine HCl undergoes color changes in most infusion solutions. However, it has been stated that color changes within eight to 12 hours of admixture preparation in solutions stored at 30 °C are not indicative of potency losses (4). The manufacturer does not recommend admixture in infusion solutions (1-4/96).

Hydralazine HCl (Ciba) at a concentration of 40 mg/L in dextrose 5% in water, with the pH varied by the addition of hydrochloric acid, was stable at pH 3 to 5 by UV spectroscopy (466).

Effects of Light— Exposure to light increases the rate of hydralazine HCl decomposition during long-term storage. At a hydralazine HCl concentration of 0.35 mg/ml in sodium chloride 0.9% in glass bottles, 10% decomposition was calculated to occur in 14.4 weeks in the dark and 12.3 weeks under fluorescent light. In PVC containers, decomposition occurs more rapidly; a 10% loss was calculated to occur in 12.8 weeks in the dark and 9.9 weeks under fluorescent light (1561).

Sorption— Hydralazine HCl (Sigma) 27 mg/L in sodium chloride 0.9% (Travenol) in PVC bags exhibited approximately 10% loss in one week at room temperature (15 to 20 °C) due to sorption (536).

However, hydralazine HCl (Sigma) 27 mg/L in sodium chloride 0.9% did not exhibit any loss due to sorption during a seven-hour simulated infusion through an infusion set (Travenol) consisting of a cellulose propionate burette chamber and 170 cm of PVC tubing (606).

The drug also was tested as a simulated infusion over at least one hour by a syringe pump system. A glass syringe on a syringe pump was fitted with 20 cm of polyethylene tubing or 50 cm of Silastic tubing. No loss of drug due to sorption was observed with either tubing (606).

In addition, a 25-ml aliquot of hydralazine HCl (Sigma) 27 mg/L in sodium chloride 0.9% was stored in all-plastic syringes composed of polypropylene barrels and polyethylene plungers for 24 hours at room temperature in the dark. No loss due to sorption occurred (606).

Compatibility Information

Solution Compatibility

Hydralazine HCl

Solution	Mfr	Mfr	Conc/L	Remarks	Ref	C/I
Dextran 6% in dextrose 5%	AB	CI	400 mg	Physically compatible	3	**C**
Dextran 6% in sodium chloride 0.9%	AB	CI	400 mg	Physically compatible	3	**C**
Dextrose–Ringer's injection combinations	AB	CI	400 mg	Physically compatible	3	**C**
Dextrose 5% in Ringer's injection, lactated	AB	CI	400 mg	Physically compatible	3	**C**
Dextrose 2½% in half-strength Ringer's injection, lactated	AB	CI	400 mg	Physically compatible	3	**C**
Dextrose–saline combinations	AB	CI	400 mg	Physically compatible	3	**C**
Dextrose 2½% in water	AB	CI	400 mg	Physically compatible	3	**C**
Dextrose 5% in water		CI	40 mg	Yellow color within 1 hr. 4% decomposition in 2 hr and 8% in 3.5 hr by UV	466	**I**
			200 to 400 mg	Progressive yellow discoloration due to hydralazine reaction with dextrose	845	**I**
		TRª	350 mg	10% loss by HPLC in 1 hr at 21 °C under fluorescent light. Approximately 11 to 12% loss in 1.5 hr at 21 °C in the dark	1561	**I**
Dextrose 10% in water	AB	CI	400 mg	Physically compatible	3	**C**
Dextrose 10% in Ringer's injection, lactated	AB	CI	400 mg	Color change	3	**I**
Fructose 10% in sodium chloride 0.9%	AB	CI	400 mg	Color change	3	**I**
Fructose 10% in water	AB	CI	400 mg	Color change	3	**I**
Invert sugar 5 and 10% in sodium chloride 0.9%	AB	CI	400 mg	Physically compatible	3	**C**
Invert sugar 5 and 10% in water	AB	CI	400 mg	Physically compatible	3	**C**
Ionosol products	AB	CI	400 mg	Physically compatible	3	**C**
Ringer's injection	AB	CI	400 mg	Physically compatible	3	**C**
Ringer's injection, lactated	AB	CI	400 mg	Physically compatible	3	**C**
		CI	40 mg	No decomposition in 2.5 hr	466	**C**
Sodium chloride 0.45%	AB	CI	400 mg	Physically compatible	3	**C**
Sodium chloride 0.9%	AB	CI	400 mg	Physically compatible	3	**C**
		CI	40 mg	No decomposition in 4 days by UV	466	**C**
		CI	200 to 400 mg	Physically compatible	845	**C**
		TRª	350 mg	6 to 8% loss by HPLC in 52 days at 21 °C under fluorescent light	1561	**C**
Sodium lactate ⅙ M	AB	CI	400 mg	Physically compatible	3	**C**

ªTested in both glass and PVC containers.

Additive Compatibility

Hydralazine HCl

Drug	Mfr	Conc/L	Mfr	Conc/L	Test Soln	Remarks	Ref	C/I
Aminophylline	BP	1 g	BP	80 mg	D5W	Yellow color produced	26	**I**
Ampicillin sodium	BP	2 g	BP	80 mg	D5W	Yellow color produced	26	**I**

Additive Compatibility (Cont.)

Hydralazine HCl

Drug	Mfr	Conc/L	Mfr	Conc/L	Test Soln	Remarks	Ref	C/I
Chlorothiazide sodium	BP	2 g	BP	80 mg	D5W, NS	Yellow color produced with precipitate in 3 hr	26	I
Dobutamine HCl	LI	200 mg	CI	200 mg	NS	Physically compatible for 24 hr	552	C
Edetate calcium disodium	RI	4 g	BP	80 mg	D5W	Yellow color produced	26	I
Ethacrynate sodium	MSD	50 mg	CI	20 mg	NS	Altered UV spectra for both at room temperature	16	I
Hydrocortisone sodium succinate	BP	400 mg	BP	80 mg	D5W	Yellow color produced	26	I
Mephentermine sulfate	BP	120 mg	BP	80 mg	D5W	Yellow color produced	26	I
Methohexital sodium	BP	2 g	BP	80 mg	D5W, NS	Yellow color produced with precipitate in 3 hr	26	I
Nitroglycerin	ACC	400 mg	CI	1 g	D5W[a]	Deep yellow color produced. 4% nitroglycerin loss in 48 hr at 23 °C. Hydralazine not tested	929	I
	ACC	400 mg	CI	1 g	NS[a]	Pale yellow color produced. No nitroglycerin loss in 48 hr at 23 °C. Hydralazine not tested	929	I
Phenobarbital sodium	BP	800 mg	BP	80 mg	D5W	Yellow color produced with precipitate in 3 hr	26	I
Verapamil HCl	KN	80 mg	CI	40 mg	D5W, NS	Yellow color produced	764	I

[a]*Tested in glass containers.*

Y-Site Injection Compatibility (1:1 Mixture)

Hydralazine HCl

Drug	Mfr	Conc	Mfr	Conc	Remarks	Ref	C/I
Aminophylline	ES	4 mg/ml[a]	SO	1 mg/ml[a]	Gross color change in 1 hr	1316	I
	ES	4 mg/ml[b]	SO	1 mg/ml[b]	Moderate color change in 1 hr and slight haze in 3 hr	1316	I
Ampicillin sodium	WY	40 mg/ml[a]	SO	1 mg/ml[a]	Moderate color change in 1 hr	1316	I
	WY	40 mg/ml[b]	SO	1 mg/ml[b]	Moderate color change in 3 hr	1316	I
Diazoxide	SC	15 mg/ml[c]	SO	1 mg/ml[c]	Moderate precipitate and color change in 1 hr	1316	I
Furosemide	ES	1 mg/ml[c]	SO	1 mg/ml[c]	Slight color change in 3 hr	1316	I
Heparin sodium	UP	1000 units/L[d]	CI	20 mg/ml	Physically compatible for at least 4 hr at room temperature by visual and microscopic examination	534	C
Hydrocortisone sodium succinate	UP	10 mg/L[d]	CI	20 mg/ml	Physically compatible for at least 4 hr at room temperature by visual and microscopic examination	534	C
Nitroglycerin	LY	0.4 mg/ml[a]	SO	1 mg/ml[a]	Physically compatible for 3 hr	1316	C
	LY	0.4 mg/ml[b]	SO	1 mg/ml[b]	Slight precipitate in 3 hr	1316	I
Potassium chloride	AB	40 mEq/L[d]	CI	20 mg/ml	Physically compatible for at least 4 hr at room temperature by visual and microscopic examination	534	C
Verapamil HCl	LY	0.2 mg/ml[c]	SO	1 mg/ml[c]	Physically compatible for 3 hr	1316	C

Y-Site Injection Compatibility (1:1 Mixture) (Cont.)

Hydralazine HCl

Drug	Mfr	Conc	Mfr	Conc	Remarks	Ref	C/I
Vitamin B complex with C	RC	2 ml/L[d]	CI	20 mg/ml	Physically compatible for at least 4 hr at room temperature by visual and microscopic examination	534	C

[a]*Tested in dextrose 5% in water.*
[b]*Tested in sodium chloride 0.9%.*
[c]*Tested in both dextrose 5% in water and sodium chloride 0.9%.*
[d]*Tested in dextrose 5% in Ringer's injection, dextrose 5% in Ringer's injection, lactated, dextrose 5% in water, Ringer's injection, lactated, and sodium chloride 0.9%.*

Additional Compatibility Information

Metals— Hydralazine HCl may react with various metals (1-4/96) to yield discolored solutions, often yellow or pink. One report indicated a pink discoloration in prefilled syringes when the hydralazine HCl had been drawn up through filter needles (Monoject) with a stainless steel filter and stored for up to 12 hours. The reaction is not specific to any one metal. Consequently, contact with metal parts should be minimized, and hydralazine HCl should be prepared just prior to use (906).

HYDROCORTISONE SODIUM PHOSPHATE
AHFS 68:04

Hydrocortone Phosphate   **Merck**

Products— Hydrocortisone sodium phosphate (Merck) is available in 2-ml single-dose vials. Each milliliter of solution contains (2):

Hydrocortisone (as sodium phosphate)	50 mg
Creatinine	8 mg
Sodium citrate	10 mg
Sodium bisulfite	3.2 mg
Methylparaben	1.5 mg
Propylparaben	0.2 mg
Sodium hydroxide	to adjust pH
Water for injection	qs 1 ml

pH— From 7.5 to 8.5 (2).

Osmolality— Hydrocortisone sodium phosphate 50 mg/ml has an osmolality of 533 mOsm/kg (1689).

Administration— Hydrocortisone sodium phosphate may be administered by subcutaneous, intramuscular, or direct intravenous injection or by continuous or intermittent intravenous infusion after addition to dextrose or sodium chloride injections. It is usually given at 12-hour intervals (2; 4).

Stability— Hydrocortisone sodium phosphate (MSD) in intact vials should be stored at controlled room temperature and protected from freezing and temperatures above 40 °C (4). The drug is a clear, light yellow solution which is heat labile and should not be autoclaved to sterilize the outside of the vial (2; 4).

Solutions of hydrocortisone buffered to pH 9.1 showed oxidation to 21-dehydrocortisone at rates of 1.6 to 2.8%/hr at 26 °C. This rate is four or five times greater than that observed at pH 6.9 to 7.9 (531).

Sorption— Hydrocortisone sodium phosphate (Glaxo) 16 mg/2 ml diluted in dextrose 5% in water or sodium chloride 0.9% was stored for 18 hours at room temperature in the following plastic syringes: Brunswick (Sherwood Medical), Plastipak (Becton-Dickinson), Steriseal (Needle Industries), and Sabre (Gillette U.K.). The first three syringes have polypropylene barrels; the Sabre has a combination polypropylene–polystyrene barrel. No significant loss of hydrocortisone occurred due to sorption (784).

Compatibility Information

Solution Compatibility

Hydrocortisone sodium phosphate

Solution	Mfr	Mfr	Conc/L	Remarks	Ref	C/I
Fat emulsion 10%, intravenous	VT		200 mg	Physically compatible for 48 hr at 4 °C and room temperature	32	C

Additive Compatibility

Hydrocortisone sodium phosphate

Drug	Mfr	Conc/L	Mfr	Conc/L	Test Soln	Remarks	Ref	C/I
Amikacin sulfate	BR	5 g	MSD	250 mg	D5LR, D5R, D5S, D5W, D10W, IS10, LR, NS, R, SL	Physically compatible and potency of both retained for 24 hr at 25 °C	294	C
Amphotericin B	SQ	50 mg	MSD	50 and 100 mg	D5W	Physically compatible and amphotericin B bioactivity retained in normal light at 25 °C for 24 hr. Hydrocortisone activity not tested	540	C
	SQ	100 mg	MSD	50 and 100 mg	D5W	Physically compatible and amphotericin B bioactivity retained in normal light at 25 °C for 24 hr. Hydrocortisone activity not tested	540	C
Amphotericin B with heparin sodium	SQ AB	50 mg 1500 units	MSD	50 and 100 mg	D5W	Physically compatible and amphotericin B bioactivity retained in normal light at 25 °C for 24 hr. Heparin and hydrocortisone activity not tested	540	C
Amphotericin B with heparin sodium	SQ AB	100 mg 1500 units	MSD	50 and 100 mg	D5W	Physically compatible and amphotericin B bioactivity retained in normal light at 25 °C for 24 hr. Heparin and hydrocortisone activity not tested	540	C
Bleomycin sulfate	BR	20 and 30 units	MSD	100 mg, 500 mg, 1 g, 2 g	NS	Physically compatible and bleomycin activity retained for 1 week at 4 °C. Hydrocortisone not tested	763	C
Metaraminol bitartrate	MSD	500 mg	MSD	250 mg	D5W, NS	UV spectra of both not altered in 8 hr at room temperature	42	C
Mitoxantrone HCl	LE	50 to 200 mg		100 mg to 2 g	NS[a]	Physically compatible and potency of both drugs retained for 24 hr at room temperature	1293	C
	LE	50 to 200 mg		100 mg to 2 g	D5W[a]	Small blue particles on inner surface of bag	1293	I
	LE	50 to 200 mg		100 mg to 2 g	D5W[b]	Physically compatible	1293	C
Sodium bicarbonate	AB	2.4 mEq[c]	MSD	100 mg	D5W	Physically compatible for 24 hr	772	C
Verapamil HCl	KN	80 mg	MSD	200 mg	D5W, NS	Physically compatible for 24 hr	764	C

[a]Tested in PVC containers.
[b]Tested in glass containers.
[c]One vial of Neut added to a liter of admixture.

Drugs in Syringe Compatibility

Hydrocortisone sodium phosphate

Drug (in syringe)	Mfr	Amt	Mfr	Amt	Remarks	Ref	C/I
Doxapram HCl	RB	400 mg/ 20 ml	MSD	100 mg/ 2 ml	Immediate turbidity and precipitation	1177	I
Metoclopramide HCl	RB	10 mg/ 2 ml	MSD	10 mg/ 2 ml	Physically compatible for 48 hr at 25 °C	1167	C

Drugs in Syringe Compatibility (Cont.)

Hydrocortisone sodium phosphate

Drug (in syringe)	Mfr	Amt	Mfr	Amt	Remarks	Ref	C/I
	RB	10 mg/ 2 ml	MSD	20 mg/ 4 ml	Physically compatible for 48 hr at 25 °C	1167	C
	RB	160 mg/ 32 ml	MSD	80 mg/ 16 ml	Physically compatible for 48 hr at 25 °C	1167	C

Y-Site Injection Compatibility (1:1 Mixture)

Hydrocortisone sodium phosphate

Drug	Mfr	Conc	Mfr	Conc	Remarks	Ref	C/I
Allopurinol sodium	BW	3 mg/ml[b]	MSD	1 mg/ml[b]	Physically compatible with no change in measured turbidity or increase in particle content in 4 hr at 22 °C	1686	C
Amifostine	USB	10 mg/ml[a]	MSD	1 mg/ml[a]	Physically compatible with no change in measured turbidity or increase in particle content in 4 hr at 23 °C	1845	C
Aztreonam	SQ	40 mg/ml[a]	MSD	1 mg/ml[a]	Physically compatible with no subvisual haze or particle formation in 4 hr at 23 °C	1758	C
Cefepime HCl	BR	20 mg/ml[a]	MSD	1 mg/ml[a]	Physically compatible with no change in measured turbidity or increase in particle content in 4 hr at 22 °C	1689	C
Cladribine	ORT	0.015[b] and 0.5[c] mg/ml	MSD	1 mg/ml[b]	Physically compatible with no change in measured turbidity or increase in particle content in 4 hr at 23 °C	1969	C
Clarithromycin	AB	4 mg/ml[a]	GL	100 mg/ml	Visually compatible for 72 hr at both 30 and 17 °C	2174	C
Docetaxel	RPR	0.9 mg/ml[a]	ME	1 mg/ml[a]	Physically compatible with no change in measured turbidity or increase in particle content in 4 hr at 23 °C	2224	C
Etoposide phosphate	BR	5 mg/ml[a]	ME	0.5 mg/ml[a]	Physically compatible with no change in measured turbidity or increase in particle content in 4 hr at 23 °C	2218	C
Famotidine	ME	2 mg/ml[b]	[d]	1 mg/ml[a]	Visually compatible for 4 hr at 22 °C	1936	C
Filgrastim	AMG	30 μg/ml[a]	MSD	1 mg/ml[a]	Physically compatible with no change in measured turbidity or increase in particle content in 4 hr at 22 °C	1687	C
Fluconazole	RR	2 mg/ml	MSD	50 mg/ml	Physically compatible for 24 hr at 25 °C	1407	C
Fludarabine phosphate	BX	1 mg/ml[a]	MSD	1 mg/ml[a]	Physically compatible for 4 hr at room temperature under fluorescent light	1439	C
Gemcitabine HCl	LI	10 mg/ml[b]	ME	1 mg/ml[b]	Physically compatible with no change in measured turbidity or increase in particle content in 4 hr at 23 °C	2226	C
Granisetron HCl	SKB	0.05 mg/ml[a]	MSD	1 mg/ml[a]	Physically compatible with no change in measured turbidity or increase in particle content in 4 hr at 23 °C	2000	C
Melphalan HCl	BW	0.1 mg/ml[b]	MSD	1 mg/ml[b]	Physically compatible with no change in measured turbidity or increase in particle content in 3 hr at 22 °C	1557	C

Y-Site Injection Compatibility (1:1 Mixture) (Cont.)

Hydrocortisone sodium phosphate

Drug	Mfr	Conc	Mfr	Conc	Remarks	Ref	C/I
Ondansetron HCl	GL	1 mg/ml[b]	MSD	1 mg/ml[a]	Physically compatible for 4 hr at 22 °C	1365	C
Paclitaxel	NCI	1.2 mg/ml[a]	MSD	1 mg/ml[a]	Physically compatible with no change in measured turbidity in 4 hr at 22 °C	1556	C
Piperacillin sodium–tazobactam sodium	LE	40 + 5 mg/ml[a]	MSD	1 mg/ml[a]	Physically compatible with no change in measured turbidity or increase in particle content in 4 hr at 22 °C	1688	C
Sargramostim	IMM	10 μg/ml[b]	MSD	1 mg/ml[b]	Filament formation in 4 hr in one of two samples	1436	I
Teniposide	BR	0.1 mg/ml[a]	MSD	1 mg/ml[a]	Physically compatible with no subvisual haze or particle formation in 4 hr at 23 °C	1725	C
Thiotepa	IMM[e]	1 mg/ml[a]	MSD	1 mg/ml[a]	Physically compatible with no change in measured turbidity or increase in particle content in 4 hr at 23 °C	1861	C
TNA #218 to #226[f]			ME	1 mg/ml[a]	Visually compatible with no precipitate or emulsion damage apparent in 4 hr at 23 °C	2215	C
TPN #212 to #215[f]			ME	1 mg/ml[a]	Physically compatible with no change in measured turbidity or increase in particle content in 4 hr at 23 °C	2109	C
Vinorelbine tartrate	BW	1 mg/ml[b]	MSD	1 mg/ml[b]	Physically compatible with no change in measured turbidity or increase in particle content in 4 hr at 22 °C	1558	C

[a]Tested in dextrose 5% in water.
[b]Tested in sodium chloride 0.9%.
[c]Tested in bacteriostatic sodium chloride 0.9% preserved with benzyl alcohol 0.9%.
[d]Form not specified.
[e]Lyophilized formulation tested.
[f]Refer to Appendix I for the composition of parenteral nutrition solutions. TNA indicates a 3-in-1 admixture, and TPN indicates a 2-in-1 admixture.

Additional Compatibility Information

Infusion Solutions— Dextrose injections and sodium chloride injections have been recommended as diluents for the intravenous infusion of hydrocortisone sodium phosphate (2; 4).

Additives— Dacarbazine is stated to be physically compatible when mixed with hydrocortisone sodium phosphate (524).

HYDROCORTISONE SODIUM SUCCINATE
AHFS 68:04

Solu-Cortef   **Pharmacia & Upjohn**

Products— Hydrocortisone sodium succinate is available in a variety of sizes and containers (4; 154). Pharmacia & Upjohn supplies the drug in 100-mg conventional vials containing hydrocortisone sodium succinate equivalent to hydrocortisone 100 mg with monobasic sodium phosphate anhydrous 0.8 mg and dibasic sodium phosphate dried 8.73 mg. Reconstitute the vial by adding not more than 2 ml of bacteriostatic water for injection or bacteriostatic sodium chloride injection (1-2/98).

Hydrocortisone sodium succinate (Pharmacia & Upjohn) is also supplied in "Act-O-Vial" containers of 100, 250, 500, and 1000 mg. For the "Act-O-Vial" containers, press the plastic activator down to force the diluent into the lower chamber. Agitate gently to dissolve the drug. When reconstituted, each milliliter of solution contains (1-2/98):

Component	100 mg	250, 500, 1000 mg
Hydrocortisone equivalent (as sodium succinate)	50 mg	125 mg
Monobasic sodium phosphate anhydrous	0.4 mg	1 mg
Dibasic sodium phosphate dried	4.38 mg	11 mg
Benzyl alcohol	~9 mg	~8.3 mg
Water for injection	qs	qs

The pH has been adjusted when necessary with sodium hydroxide.

pH— From 7 to 8 (4).

Osmotic Values— The osmolality of hydrocortisone sodium succinate (Abbott) 50 mg/ml was determined to be 292 mOsm/kg by freezing-point depression and 260 mOsm/kg by vapor pressure (1071).

Pharmacia & Upjohn states that the osmolarities of the constituted products are 360 mOsm/L for the 100-mg vials and 570 mOsm/L for the other sizes.

Sodium Content— Hydrocortisone sodium succinate contains 2.066 mEq of sodium per gram of drug (846).

Administration— Hydrocortisone sodium succinate may be administered by intramuscular injection, direct intravenous injection over 30 seconds to several minutes, or continuous or intermittent intravenous infusion at a concentration of 0.1 to 1 mg/ml in a compatible infusion solution (1-2/98; 4).

Stability— Hydrocortisone sodium succinate in intact containers should be stored at controlled room temperatures of 20 to 25 °C (1-2/98). After reconstitution, solutions are stable at controlled room temperature or below if protected from light. The solution should only be used if it is clear. Unused solutions should be discarded after three days. Hydrocortisone sodium succinate is heat labile and must not be autoclaved (1-2/98; 4).

pH Effects— Hydrocortisone sodium succinate is optimally stable at pH 7 to 8. It is stable for 72 hours at pH 6 and for 12 hours at pH 5. More acidic solutions cause precipitation (41).

Solutions of hydrocortisone buffered to pH 9.1 showed oxidation to 21-dehydrocortisone at rates of 1.6 to 2.8%/hr at 26 °C. This rate is four or five times greater than that observed at pH 6.9 to 7.9 (531).

Freezing Solutions— Hydrocortisone sodium succinate (Upjohn) 500-mg/4 ml reconstituted solution exhibited no loss of potency over four weeks when stored frozen (69).

Intrathecal Solutions— In a study of solutions for intrathecal injection, hydrocortisone sodium succinate (Upjohn) was reconstituted to a concentration of 1 mg/ml with Elliott's B solution (295 mOsm/kg, pH 7.3), sodium chloride 0.9% injection (296 mOsm/kg, pH 7), and Ringer's injection, lactated (258 mOsm/kg, pH 7). In Ringer's injection, lactated, and sodium chloride 0.9% injection, no decomposition was observed by UV spectroscopy in 24 hours at room temperature under fluorescent light or at 30 °C. However, in seven days, approximately 10% decomposition occurred at room temperature and about 15% was noted at 30 °C. In Elliott's B solution,

hydrocortisone sodium succinate is much less stable. In 24 hours, a 7% loss occurred at room temperature and a 12% loss occurred at 30 °C, increasing to 21 and 32%, respectively, at 72 hours. The authors noted that less than 10% decomposition of this combination occurred in four to eight hours (327).

In another study, the stability and compatibility of cytarabine (Upjohn), methotrexate (NCI), and hydrocortisone (Upjohn), mixed together in intrathecal injections, were evaluated. Two combinations were tested: (1) cytarabine 50 mg, methotrexate 12 mg (as the sodium salt), and hydrocortisone 25 mg (as the sodium succinate salt); and (2) cytarabine 30 mg, methotrexate 12 mg (as the sodium salt), and hydrocortisone 15 mg (as the sodium succinate salt). Each drug combination was added to 12 ml of Elliott's B solution (NCI), sodium chloride 0.9% (Abbott), dextrose 5% in water (Abbott), and Ringer's injection, lactated (Abbott), and stored for 24 hours at 25 °C. Cytarabine and methotrexate were both chemically stable, with no drug loss after the full 24 hours in all solutions. Hydrocortisone was also stable in the sodium chloride 0.9%, dextrose 5% in water, and Ringer's injection, lactated, with about a 2% drug loss. However, in Elliott's B solution, hydrocortisone was significantly less stable, with a 6% loss in the 25-mg concentration over 24 hours. The 15-mg concentration was worse, with a 5% loss in 10 hours and a 13% loss in 24 hours. The higher pH of Elliott's B solution and the lower concentration of hydrocortisone may have been factors in this increased decomposition. All mixtures were physically compatible during this study, but a precipitate formed after several days of storage (819).

Hydrocortisone sodium succinate (Upjohn) 2 mg/ml diluted in Elliott's B solution (Orphan Medical) was packaged as 20 ml in 30-ml glass vials and 20-ml plastic syringes (Becton-Dickinson) with Red Cap (Burron) Luer-lok syringe tip caps. The solution was physically compatible with no increase in measured turbidity or particulates and was chemically stable exhibiting about 9% or less loss by HPLC analysis during storage for 24 hours at 23 °C and 7% or less loss in 48 hours at 4 °C (1976).

Bacterially contaminated intrathecal solutions could pose grave risks and, consequently, such solutions should be administered as soon as possible after preparation (328).

Sorption— Hydrocortisone sodium succinate (Upjohn) 25 mg/L did not display significant sorption to a PVC plastic test strip in 24 hours (12).

Hydrocortisone sodium succinate (Upjohn) 9 mg/L in sodium chloride 0.9% (Travenol) in PVC bags did not exhibit significant sorption to the plastic during one week of storage at room temperature (15 to 20 °C) (536).

In another study, hydrocortisone sodium succinate (Upjohn) 9 mg/L in sodium chloride 0.9% did not exhibit any loss due to sorption during a seven-hour simulated infusion through an infusion set (Travenol) consisting of a cellulose propionate burette chamber and 170 cm of PVC tubing (606).

The drug also was tested as a simulated infusion over at least one hour by a syringe pump system. A glass syringe on a syringe pump was fitted with 20 cm of polyethylene tubing or 50 cm of Silastic tubing. No loss of drug due to sorption was observed with either tubing (606).

A 25-ml aliquot of hydrocortisone sodium succinate (Upjohn) 9 mg/L in sodium chloride 0.9% was stored in all-plastic syringes composed of polypropylene barrels and polyethylene plungers for 24 hours at room temperature in the dark. No loss due to sorption occurred (606).

Filtration— Hydrocortisone sodium succinate (Upjohn) 10 mg/L in dextrose 5% in water and sodium chloride 0.9% did not display significant sorption to a 0.45-μm cellulose membrane filter (Abbott S-A-I-F) during an eight-hour simulated infusion (567).

Compatibility Information

Solution Compatibility

Hydrocortisone sodium succinate

Solution	Mfr	Mfr	Conc/L	Remarks	Ref	C/I
Alcohol 5%, dextrose 5%	BA	UP	600 mg	Physically compatible for 24 hr	315	C
Dextran 40,000	PH			Physically compatible	44	C
Dextran 6% in dextrose 5%	AB	UP	250 mg	Physically compatible	3	C
Dextran 6% in sodium chloride 0.9%	AB	UP	250 mg	Physically compatible	3	C
Dextrose–Ringer's injection combinations	AB	UP	250 mg	Physically compatible	3	C
Dextrose–Ringer's injection, lactated, combinations	AB	UP	250 mg	Physically compatible	3	C
Dextrose 5% in Ringer's injection, lactated	TR[a]	UP	500 mg	Potency retained for 24 hr at 5 °C	282	C
	BA	UP	600 mg	Physically compatible for 24 hr	315	C
Dextrose–saline combinations	AB	UP	250 mg	Physically compatible	3	C
Dextrose 5% in sodium chloride 0.9%		UP	100, 200, 300 mg	Potency retained for 48 hr	43	C
	AB	UP	250 mg	Potency retained for 48 hr	46	C
		UP	100 mg	Physically compatible	74	C
	TR[a]	UP	500 mg	Potency retained for 24 hr at 5 °C	282	C
	BA	UP	600 mg	Physically compatible for 24 hr	315	C
Dextrose 2½% in water	AB	UP	250 mg	Physically compatible	3	C
Dextrose 5% in water	AB	UP	250 mg	Physically compatible	3	C
	AB	UP	250 mg	Potency retained for 48 hr	46	C
		UP	100 mg	Physically compatible	74	C
	TR[a]	UP	500 mg	Potency retained for 24 hr at 5 °C	282	C
	BA	UP	600 mg	Physically compatible for 24 hr	315	C
Dextrose 10% in water	AB	UP	250 mg	Physically compatible	3	C
	BA	UP	600 mg	Physically compatible for 24 hr	315	C
Dextrose 20% in water	BA	UP	600 mg	Physically compatible for 24 hr	315	C
Fat emulsion 10%, intravenous	VT	GL	200 mg	Physically compatible for 24 hr at 8 and 25 °C	825	C
Fructose 10% in sodium chloride 0.9%	AB	UP	250 mg	Physically compatible	3	C
Fructose 10% in water	AB	UP	250 mg	Physically compatible	3	C
	BA	UP	600 mg	Physically compatible for 24 hr	315	C
Invert sugar 10% in Electrolyte #1	BA	UP	600 mg	Physically compatible for 24 hr	315	C
Invert sugar 10% in Electrolyte #2	BA	UP	600 mg	Physically compatible for 24 hr	315	C
Invert sugar 5 and 10% in sodium chloride 0.9%	AB	UP	250 mg	Physically compatible	3	C
Invert sugar 5 and 10% in water	AB	UP	250 mg	Physically compatible	3	C
Ionosol products (except as noted below)	AB	UP	250 mg	Physically compatible	3	C
Ionosol B with invert sugar 10%	AB	UP	250 mg	Haze or precipitate forms within 24 hr	3	I
Polysal M with dextrose 5%	CU	UP	600 mg	Physically compatible for 24 hr	315	C
Ringer's injection	AB	UP	250 mg	Physically compatible	3	C
Ringer's injection, lactated	AB	UP	250 mg	Physically compatible	3	C
		UP	100 mg	Physically compatible	74	C

Solution Compatibility (Cont.)

Hydrocortisone sodium succinate

Solution	Mfr	Mfr	Conc/L	Remarks	Ref	C/I
	TR[a]	UP	500 mg	Potency retained for 24 hr at 5 °C	282	C
	BA	UP	600 mg	Physically compatible for 24 hr	315	C
Sodium chloride 0.45%	AB	UP	250 mg	Physically compatible	74	C
Sodium chloride 0.9%	AB	UP	250 mg	Physically compatible	3	C
	AB	UP	250 mg	Potency retained for 48 hr	46	C
		UP	100 mg	Physically compatible	74	C
	TR[a]	UP	500 mg	Potency retained for 24 hr at 5 °C	282	C
	BA	UP	600 mg	Physically compatible for 24 hr	315	C
Sodium lactate ⅙ M	AB	UP	250 mg	Physically compatible	3	C
	BA	UP	600 mg	Physically compatible for 24 hr	315	C

[a]Tested in both glass and PVC containers.

Additive Compatibility

Hydrocortisone sodium succinate

Drug	Mfr	Conc/L	Mfr	Conc/L	Test Soln	Remarks	Ref	C/I
Amikacin sulfate	BR	5 g	UP	200 mg	D5LR, D5R, D5S, D5W, D10W, IS10, LR, NS, R, SL	Physically compatible and potency of both retained for 24 hr at 25 °C	294	C
Aminophylline		250 mg	UP	100 mg	D5W	Physically compatible	74	C
	SE	1 g	UP	500 mg	D5W	Physically compatible	15	C
	SE	500 mg	UP	100 mg		Physically compatible	6	C
		625 mg		250 mg	D5W	Physically compatible and aminophylline chemically stable for 24 hr at 4 and 30 °C. Total hydrocortisone content changed little but substantial ester hydrolysis noted	521	C
Aminophylline with cephalothin sodium	SE LI	1 g 1 g	UP	100 mg	D5S	pH outside stability range for cephalothin. Precipitate forms within 12 hr	41	I
Amobarbital sodium						Physically incompatible	9	I
	LI	1 g	UP	500 mg	D5W	Physically compatible	15	C
Amphotericin B	SQ	100 mg	UP	500 mg	D5W	Physically compatible	15	C
Ampicillin sodium	BR	1 g		200 and 400 mg	LR	Ampicillin potency retained for 24 hr at 25 °C	87	C
	BR	1 g		1.8 g	D5S, D5W, D10W, IM, IP, LR, NS	Ampicillin potency retained for 24 hr at 4 °C	87	C
	BR	1 g		100 mg	LR	14% ampicillin decomposition in 12 hr at 25 °C	87	I
	BR	1 g		50 mg	LR	14% ampicillin decomposition in 12 hr at 25 °C	87	I
	BR	1 g		1.8 g	D5S, D10W, IP, IM, LR	11 to 28% ampicillin decomposition in 24 hr at 25 °C	87	I

Additive Compatibility (Cont.)

Hydrocortisone sodium succinate

Drug	Mfr	Conc/L	Mfr	Conc/L	Test Soln	Remarks	Ref	C/I
	BE	20 g		200 mg	NS	18% ampicillin decomposition in 6 hr at 25 °C	89	I
	BE	20 g		200 mg	D5W	23% ampicillin decomposition in 6 hr at 25 °C	89	I
	BE	20 g		200 mg	D–S	32% ampicillin decomposition in 6 hr at 25 °C	89	I
Bleomycin sulfate	BR	20 and 30 units	AB	300 mg, 750 mg, 1 g, 2.5 g	NS	60 to 100% bleomycin activity lost in 1 week at 4 °C	763	I
Calcium chloride	UP	1 g	UP	500 mg	D5W	Physically compatible	15	C
Calcium gluconate		1 g	UP	100 mg	D5W	Physically compatible	74	C
	UP	1 g	UP	500 mg	D5W	Physically compatible	15	C
Chloramphenicol sodium succinate	PD	500 mg	UP	100 mg	D5W	Physically compatible	74	C
	PD	10 g	UP	500 mg	D5W	Physically compatible	15	C
	PD	1 g	UP	500 mg		Physically compatible	6	C
Clindamycin phosphate	UP	1.2 g	UP	1 g	W	Clindamycin stability maintained for 24 hr	101	C
Colistimethate sodium	WC	500 mg	UP	500 mg	D5W	Physically incompatible	15	I
Corticotropin		500 units	UP	100 mg	D5W	Physically compatible	74	C
Cytarabine	UP	360 mg	UP	500 mg	D5S, D10S	Physically compatible for 40 hr	174	C
	UP	360 mg	UP	500 mg	R, SL	Physically incompatible	174	I
Daunorubicin HCl	FA	200 mg	UP	500 mg	D5W	Physically compatible	¨	C
Dimenhydrinate	SE	50 mg	UP	100 mg	D5W	Physically compatible	·+	C
	SE	500 mg	UP	500 mg	D5W	Physically incompatible	15	I
Diphenhydramine HCl	SCN	80 mg	UP	500 mg	D5W[a]	Physically compatible with no subvisual haze or particle formation in 24 hr at 23 °C	1729	C
	SCN	500 mg	UP	1 g	D5W[a]	Physically compatible with no subvisual haze or particle formation in 24 hr at 23 °C	1729	C
Dopamine HCl	AS	800 mg	UP	1 g	D5W	No dopamine decomposition in 18 hr at 25 °C	312	C
Ephedrine sulfate						Physically incompatible	9	I
Erythromycin lactobionate	AB	5 g	UP	500 mg	D5W	Physically compatible	15	C
	AB	1 g	UP	250 mg		Physically compatible	3; 20	C
Floxacillin sodium	BE	20 g	UP	50 g	NS	Physically compatible for 72 hr at 15 and 30 °C	1479	C
Furosemide		200 and 400 mg		1 g	D5W, NS	6 to 8% hydrocortisone loss and 5 to 6% furosemide loss in 24 hr at 25 °C	1348	C
		200 and 400 mg		300 mg	D5W, NS	6 to 8% hydrocortisone loss in 6 hr and 10 to 14% loss in 24 hr at 25 °C. 5 to 6% furosemide loss in 24 hr	1348	I
	HO	1 g	UP	50 g	NS	Physically compatible for 72 hr at 15 and 30 °C	1479	C

Additive Compatibility (Cont.)

Hydrocortisone sodium succinate

Drug	Mfr	Conc/L	Mfr	Conc/L	Test Soln	Remarks	Ref	C/I
Heparin sodium		32,000 units		800 mg	NS	Physically compatible and heparin activity retained for 24 hr	57	**C**
						Physically incompatible	9	**I**
	UP	4000 units	UP	500 mg	D5W	Physically incompatible	15	**I**
		12,000 units	UP	100 mg	D5W	Immediate precipitation	74	**I**
Hydralazine HCl	BP	80 mg	BP	400 mg	D5W	Yellow color produced	26	**I**
Kanamycin sulfate	BR	250 mg		1.8 g	D5S, D5W, D10W, IM, IP, LR, NS	Kanamycin potency retained for 24 hr at 4 and 25 °C	87	**C**
	BR	4 g	UP	500 mg	D5W	Physically incompatible	15	**I**
Lidocaine HCl	AST	2 g	UP	250 mg		Physically compatible	24	**C**
Magnesium sulfate	ES	750 mg	UP	100 g	AA 3.5%, D 25%	Physically compatible	302	**C**
Mephentermine sulfate		750 mg		250 mg	D5W	Physically compatible and chemically stable for 24 hr at 3 and 30 °C	520	**C**
Metaraminol bitartrate	MSD	100 mg	UP	100 mg	D5S	Potency of both retained for 24 hr	43	**C**
	MSD					Physically incompatible	9	**I**
	MSD	100, 200, 300 mg	UP	200 and 300 mg	D5S	Precipitate forms and chemical decomposition of hydrocortisone occurs	43	**I**
	MSD	500 mg		250 mg	D5W, NS	Precipitate forms within 1 hr	42	**I**
	MSD	100 mg	UP	250 mg		Precipitate forms within 1 hr	7	**I**
Metronidazole	RP	5 g[b]	UP	10 g		Physically compatible for at least 72 hr at 23 °C, but a significant change in pH	807	**?**
	SE	5 g	UP	10 g		No loss of either drug in 7 days at 25 °C and 12 days at 5 °C	993	**C**
Metronidazole HCl with sodium bicarbonate	SE AB	5 g 50 mEq	UP	1 g	D5W, NS	Physically compatible for 48 hr	765	**C**
Mitomycin	BR	1 g	AB	33.3 g	W[c]	Visually compatible with 10% mitomycin loss calculated in 172 hr and 10% hydrocortisone loss calculated in 212 hr at 25 °C	1866	**C**
	BR	1 g	AB	33.3 g	W[a]	Visually compatible with 10% mitomycin loss calculated in 206 hr and 10% hydrocortisone loss calculated in 218 hr at 25 °C	1866	**C**
	BR	1 g	AB	33.3 g	W[c]	Visually compatible with 10% mitomycin loss calculated in 1423 hr and 10% hydrocortisone loss calculated in 176 hr at 4 °C	1866	**C**
	BR	1 g	AB	33.3 g	W[a]	Visually compatible with 10% mitomycin loss calculated in 820 hr and 10% hydrocortisone loss calculated in 807 hr at 4 °C	1866	**C**
Mitoxantrone HCl	LE	50 to 200 mg		100 mg to 2 g	D5W, NS[a]	Physically compatible and potency of both drugs retained for 24 hr at room temperature	1293	**C**

Additive Compatibility (Cont.)

Hydrocortisone sodium succinate

Drug	Mfr	Conc/L	Mfr	Conc/L	Test Soln	Remarks	Ref	C/I
Nafcillin sodium	WY	500 mg	UP	250 mg		Precipitate forms within 1 hr	27	I
Netilmicin sulfate	SC	3 g	UP	400 mg	D5S	Physically compatible and netilmicin chemically stable for 7 days at 4 and 25 °C. Hydrocortisone not tested	558	C
Netilmicin sulfate with potassium chloride	SC AB	3 g 160 mEq	UP	400 mg	D5S	Physically compatible and netilmicin chemically stable for 7 days at 4 and 25 °C. Other drugs not tested	558	C
Norepinephrine bitartrate	WI	8 mg	UP	100 mg	D5W	Physically compatible	74	C
Penicillin G potassium		1 million units	UP	100 mg	D5W	Physically compatible	74	C
	SQ	20 million units	UP	500 mg	D5W	Physically compatible	15	C
	SQ	5 million units	UP	250 mg	D	Physically compatible	47	C
Penicillin G sodium	UP	20 million units	UP	500 mg	D5W	Physically compatible	15	C
Pentobarbital sodium						Physically incompatible	9	I
	AB	1 g	UP	500 mg	D5W	Physically incompatible	15	I
Phenobarbital sodium	WI					Physically incompatible	9	I
	WI	200 mg	UP	500 mg	D5W	Physically incompatible	15	I
Piperacillin sodium	LE	40 g	UP	40 mg	D5S[a]	Physically compatible and piperacillin chemically stable for 24 hr at room temperature and 1 week under refrigeration. Hydrocortisone not tested	740	C
Polymyxin B sulfate	BW	200 mg	UP	500 mg	D5W	Physically compatible	15	C
Potassium chloride		3 g	UP	100 mg	D5W	Physically compatible	74	C
Potassium chloride with netilmicin sulfate	AB SC	160 mEq 3 g	UP	400 mg	D5S	Physically compatible and netilmicin chemically stable for 7 days at 4 and 25 °C. Other drugs not tested	558	C
Procaine HCl	WI	1 g	UP	500 mg	D5W	Physically compatible	15	C
Prochlorperazine edisylate	SKF					Physically incompatible	9	I
Promethazine HCl	WY	250 mg	UP	500 mg	D5W	Physically incompatible	15	I
Sodium bicarbonate	AB	2.4 mEq[d]	UP	250 mg	D5W	Physically compatible for 24 hr	772	C
Theophylline		2 g		390 mg[e]	D5W	Visually compatible with little or no loss of either drug in 48 hr	1909	C
Thiopental sodium	AB	2.5 g	UP	100 mg	D5W	Physically compatible	21	C
Vancomycin HCl	LI	1 g	UP	100 mg	D5W	Physically compatible	74	C
Verapamil HCl	KN	80 mg	UP	200 mg	D5W, NS	Physically compatible for 24 hr	764	C

Additive Compatibility (Cont.)

Hydrocortisone sodium succinate

Drug	Mfr	Conc/L	Mfr	Conc/L	Test Soln	Remarks	Ref	C/I
Vitamin B complex with C		1 vial	UP	100 mg	D5W	Physically compatible	74	C
	RC	2 ml	UP	100 mg	D5W, LR	pH within stability range for both	41	C

[a]Tested in PVC containers.

[b]Minibags (100 ml) containing metronidazole 500 mg with disodium phosphate 150 mg, citric acid 44 mg, and sodium chloride 740 mg. This product differs from the Searle product.

[c]Tested in glass containers.

[d]One vial of Neut added to a liter of admixture.

[e]Tested as the hemisuccinate.

Drugs in Syringe Compatibility

Hydrocortisone sodium succinate

Drug (in syringe)	Mfr	Amt	Mfr	Amt	Remarks	Ref	C/I
Diatrizoate meglumine 52%, diatrizoate sodium 8%	MA	5 ml	UP	10 mg/1 ml	Physically compatible for at least 2 hr	1438	C
Diatrizoate sodium 60%	MA	5 ml	UP	10 mg/1 ml	Physically compatible for at least 2 hr	1438	C
Doxapram HCl	RB	400 mg/20 ml	UP	500 mg/2 ml	Immediate turbidity and precipitation	1177	I
Iohexol	WI	64.7%, 5 ml	UP	10 mg/1 ml	Physically compatible for at least 2 hr	1438	C
Iopamidol	SQ	61%, 5 ml	UP	10 mg/1 ml	Physically compatible for at least 2 hr	1438	C
Iothalamate meglumine 60%	MA	5 ml	UP	10 mg/1 ml	Physically compatible for at least 2 hr	1438	C
Ioxaglate meglumine 39.3%, ioxaglate sodium 19.6%	MA	5 ml	UP	10 mg/1 ml	Physically compatible for at least 2 hr	1438	C
Metoclopramide HCl	RB	10 mg/2 ml	MSD	10 mg/2 ml[a]	Physically compatible for 48 hr at room temperature	924	C
	RB	10 mg/2 ml	MSD	20 mg/4 ml[a]	Physically compatible for 48 hr at room temperature	924	C
Thiopental sodium	AB	75 mg/3 ml	UP	250 mg/2 ml	Physically compatible for at least 30 min	21	C

[a]Brought to volume with distilled water.

Y-Site Injection Compatibility (1:1 Mixture)

Hydrocortisone sodium succinate

Drug	Mfr	Conc	Mfr	Conc	Remarks	Ref	C/I
Acyclovir sodium	BW	5 mg/ml[a]	LY	1 mg/ml[a]	Physically compatible for 4 hr at 25 °C	1157	C
Allopurinol sodium	BW	3 mg/ml[b]	UP	1 mg/ml[b]	Physically compatible with no change in measured turbidity or increase in particle content in 4 hr at 22 °C	1686	C
Amifostine	USB	10 mg/ml[a]	UP	1 mg/ml[a]	Physically compatible with no change in measured turbidity or increase in particle content in 4 hr at 23 °C	1845	C

Y-Site Injection Compatibility (1:1 Mixture) (Cont.)

Hydrocortisone sodium succinate

Drug	Mfr	Conc	Mfr	Conc	Remarks	Ref	C/I
Aminophylline	SE	25 mg/ml	UP	100 mg/L[c]	Physically compatible for at least 4 hr at room temperature by visual and microscopic examination	322	C
Amphotericin B cholesteryl sulfate complex	SEQ	0.83 mg/ml[a]	AB	1 mg/ml[a]	Physically compatible with little or no change in measured turbidity or increase in particle content in 4 hr at 23 °C under fluorescent light	2117	C
Ampicillin sodium	BR	25, 50, 100, 135 mg/ml	UP	100 mg/L[c]	Physically compatible for at least 4 hr at room temperature by visual and microscopic examination	322	C
Amrinone lactate	WB	3 mg/ml[b]	ES	1 mg/ml[a]	Physically compatible for at least 4 hr at 25 °C under fluorescent light	992	C
Amsacrine	NCI	1 mg/ml[a]	UP	1 mg/ml[a]	Physically compatible for 4 hr at room temperature under fluorescent light	1381	C
Atracurium besylate	BW	0.5 mg/ml[a]	AB	1 mg/ml[a]	Physically compatible for 24 hr at 28 °C	1337	C
Atropine sulfate	BW	0.5 mg/ml	UP	10 mg/L[d]	Physically compatible for at least 4 hr at room temperature by visual and microscopic examination	534	C
Aztreonam	SQ	40 mg/ml[a]	UP	1 mg/ml[a]	Physically compatible with no subvisual haze or particle formation in 4 hr at 23 °C	1758	C
Betamethasone sodium phosphate	SC	3 mg/ml	UP	10 mg/L[d]	Physically compatible for at least 4 hr at room temperature by visual and microscopic examination	534	C
Calcium gluconate	ES	100 mg/ml	UP	100 mg/L[c]	Physically compatible for at least 4 hr at room temperature by visual and microscopic examination	322	C
Cefepime HCl	BR	20 mg/ml[a]	UP	1 mg/ml[a]	Physically compatible with no change in measured turbidity or increase in particle content in 4 hr at 22 °C	1689	C
Chlordiazepoxide HCl	RC	10 mg/ml	UP	10 mg/L[d]	Physically compatible for at least 4 hr at room temperature by visual and microscopic examination	534	C
Chlorpromazine HCl	SKF	25 mg/ml	UP	10 mg/L[d]	Physically compatible for at least 4 hr at room temperature by visual and microscopic examination	534	C
Ciprofloxacin	MI	2 mg/ml[e]	UP	50 mg/ml	Transient white cloudiness rapidly dissipates. White crystals form in 1 hr at 24 °C	1655	I
Cisatracurium besylate	GW	0.1, 2, 5 mg/ml[a]	AB	1 mg/ml[a]	Physically compatible with no change in measured turbidity or increase in particle content in 4 hr at 23 °C	2074	C
Cladribine	ORT	0.015[b] and 0.5[f] mg/ml	UP	1 mg/ml[b]	Physically compatible with no change in measured turbidity or increase in particle content in 4 hr at 23 °C	1969	C
Cyanocobalamin	PD	0.1 mg/ml	UP	10 mg/L[d]	Physically compatible for at least 4 hr at room temperature by visual and microscopic examination	534	C

Y-Site Injection Compatibility (1:1 Mixture) (Cont.)

Hydrocortisone sodium succinate

Drug	Mfr	Conc	Mfr	Conc	Remarks	Ref	C/I
Cytarabine	UP	16 mg/ml[b]	UP	125 mg/ml	Visually compatible for 24 hr at room temperature in test tubes. No precipitate found on filter from Y-site delivery	2063	C
Dexamethasone sodium phosphate	MSD	4 mg/ml	UP	100 mg/L[c]	Physically compatible for at least 4 hr at room temperature by visual and microscopic examination	322	C
Diazepam	RC	5 mg/ml	UP	100 mg/L[c]	Immediate haziness with globule formation	322	I
Digoxin	BW	0.25 mg/ml	UP	100 mg/L[c]	Physically compatible for at least 4 hr at room temperature by visual and microscopic examination	322	C
Diltiazem HCl	MMD	5 mg/ml	UP	50 and 125 mg/ml	Precipitate forms but clears with swirling	1807	?
	MMD	1 mg/ml[b]	UP	50 and 125 mg/ml	Visually compatible	1807	C
	MMD	5 mg/ml	UP	1[b] and 2[a] mg/ml	Visually compatible	1807	C
Diphenhydramine HCl	PD	50 mg/ml	UP	10 mg/L[d]	Physically compatible for at least 4 hr at room temperature by visual and microscopic examination	534	C
	SCN	0.16 mg/ml[a]	UP	1 mg/ml[a]	Physically compatible with no subvisual haze or particle formation in 4 hr at 23 °C	1729	C
	SCN	1 mg/ml[a]	UP	2 mg/ml[a]	Physically compatible with no subvisual haze or particle formation in 4 hr at 23 °C	1729	C
Docetaxel	RPR	0.9 mg/ml[a]	AB	1 mg/ml[a]	Physically compatible with no change in measured turbidity or increase in particle content in 4 hr at 23 °C	2224	C
Dopamine HCl	ACC	40 mg/ml	UP	10 mg/L[d]	Physically compatible for at least 4 hr at room temperature by visual and microscopic examination	534	C
Doxorubicin HCl liposome injection	SEQ	0.4 mg/ml[a]	AB	1 mg/ml[a]	Physically compatible with little or no change in measured turbidity and no increase in particle content in 4 hr at 23 °C	2087	C
Droperidol	CR	1.25 mg/ml	UP	10 mg/L[d]	Physically compatible for at least 4 hr at room temperature by visual and microscopic examination	534	C
Edrophonium chloride	RC	10 mg/ml	UP	10 mg/L[d]	Physically compatible for at least 4 hr at room temperature by visual and microscopic examination	534	C
Enalaprilat	MSD	0.05 mg/ml[b]	UP	2 mg/ml[a]	Physically compatible for 24 hr at room temperature under fluorescent light	1355	C
Epinephrine HCl	AB	0.1 mg/ml	UP	10 mg/L[d]	Physically compatible for at least 4 hr at room temperature by visual and microscopic examination	534	C
Ergotamine tartrate	SZ	0.5 mg/ml	UP	10 mg/L[d]	Crystal formation and brown discoloration after 4 hr at room temperature	534	I
Esmolol HCl	DCC	10 mg/ml[a]	LY	1 mg/ml[a]	Physically compatible for 24 hr at 22 °C	1169	C

Y-Site Injection Compatibility (1:1 Mixture) (Cont.)

Hydrocortisone sodium succinate

Drug	Mfr	Conc	Mfr	Conc	Remarks	Ref	C/I
Estrogens, conjugated	AY	5 mg/ml	UP	100 mg/L[c]	Physically compatible for at least 4 hr at room temperature by visual and microscopic examination	322	C
Ethacrynate sodium	MSD	1 mg/ml	UP	100 mg/L[c]	Physically compatible for at least 4 hr at room temperature by visual and microscopic examination	322	C
Etoposide phosphate	BR	5 mg/ml[a]	UP	1 mg/ml[a]	Physically compatible with no change in measured turbidity or increase in particle content in 4 hr at 23 °C	2218	C
Famotidine	MSD	0.2 mg/ml[a]	AB	1 mg/ml[a]	Physically compatible for 4 hr at 25 °C under fluorescent light	1188	C
	MSD	0.2 mg/ml[a]	AB	125 mg/ml	Physically compatible for 14 hr	1196	C
	ME	2 mg/ml[b]	[g]	1 mg/ml[a]	Visually compatible for 4 hr at 22 °C	1936	C
Fentanyl citrate	MN	0.05 mg/ml	UP	10 mg/L[d]	Physically compatible for at least 4 hr at room temperature by visual and microscopic examination	322	C
Fentanyl citrate and droperidol	MN	0.05 mg + 2.5 mg/ml	UP	10 mg/L[d]	Physically compatible for at least 4 hr at room temperature by visual and microscopic examination	322	C
Filgrastim	AMG	30 μg/ml[a]	UP	1 mg/ml[a]	Physically compatible with no change in measured turbidity or increase in particle content in 4 hr at 22 °C	1687	C
Fludarabine phosphate	UP	1 mg/ml[a]	UP	1 mg/ml[a]	Physically compatible for 4 hr at room temperature under fluorescent light	1439	C
Fluorouracil	RC	50 mg/ml	UP	10 mg/L[d]	Physically compatible for at least 4 hr at room temperature by visual and microscopic examination	534	C
Foscarnet sodium	AST	24 mg/ml	UP	50 mg/ml	Physically compatible for 24 hr at room temperature under fluorescent light	1335	C
Furosemide	HO	10 mg/ml	UP	10 mg/L[d]	Physically compatible for at least 4 hr at room temperature by visual and microscopic examination	534	C
Gemcitabine HCl	LI	10 mg/ml[b]	UP	1 mg/ml[b]	Physically compatible with no change in measured turbidity or increase in particle content in 4 hr at 23 °C	2226	C
Granisetron HCl	SKB	0.05 mg/ml[a]	AB	1 mg/ml[a]	Physically compatible with no change in measured turbidity or increase in particle content in 4 hr at 23 °C	2000	C
Heparin sodium	TR	50 units/ml	UP	2 mg/ml[b]	Visually compatible for 6 hr at 25 °C	1793	C
	ES	100 units/ml[e]	UP	125 mg/ml	Visually compatible for 24 hr at room temperature in test tubes. No precipitate found on filter from Y-site delivery	2063	C
Hydralazine HCl	CI	20 mg/ml	UP	10 mg/L[d]	Physically compatible for at least 4 hr at room temperature by visual and microscopic examination	534	C
Idarubicin HCl	AD	1 mg/ml[b]	UP	2[a] and 50 mg/ml	Haze forms immediately and precipitate forms in 20 min	1525	I

Y-Site Injection Compatibility (1:1 Mixture) (Cont.)

Hydrocortisone sodium succinate

Drug	Mfr	Conc	Mfr	Conc	Remarks	Ref	C/I
Insulin, regular	LI	40 units/ml	UP	100 mg/L[c]	Physically compatible for at least 4 hr at room temperature by visual and micro-scopic examination	322	**C**
Isoproterenol HCl	WI	0.2 mg/ml	UP	10 mg/L[d]	Physically compatible for at least 4 hr at room temperature by visual and micro-scopic examination	534	**C**
Kanamycin sulfate	BR	250 mg/ml	UP	100 mg/L[c]	Physically compatible for at least 4 hr at room temperature by visual and micro-scopic examination	322	**C**
Lidocaine HCl	AST	20 mg/ml	UP	100 mg/L[c]	Physically compatible for at least 4 hr at room temperature by visual and micro-scopic examination	322	**C**
Lorazepam	WY	0.33 mg/ml[b]	UP	50 mg/ml	Visually compatible for 24 hr at 22 °C	1855	**C**
Magnesium sulfate	AB	500 mg/ml	UP	10 mg/L[d]	Physically compatible for at least 4 hr at room temperature by visual and micro-scopic examination	534	**C**
Melphalan HCl	BW	0.1 mg/ml[b]	UP	1 mg/ml[b]	Physically compatible with no change in measured turbidity or increase in parti-cle content in 3 hr at 22 °C	1557	**C**
Menadiol sodium diphosphate	RC	5 mg/ml	UP	10 mg/L[d]	Physically compatible for at least 4 hr at room temperature by visual and micro-scopic examination	534	**C**
Meperidine HCl	AB	10 mg/ml	AB	2 mg/ml[a]	Physically compatible for 4 hr at 25 °C	1397	**C**
Methoxamine HCl	BW	10 mg/ml	UP	10 mg/L[d]	Physically compatible for at least 4 hr at room temperature by visual and micro-scopic examination	534	**C**
Methylergonovine maleate	SZ	0.2 mg/ml	UP	10 mg/L[d]	Physically compatible for at least 4 hr at room temperature by visual and micro-scopic examination	534	**C**
Methylprednisolone sodium succinate	UP	40 mg/ml	UP	100 mg/L[h]	In D5W. Physically compatible for at least 4 hr at room temperature by visu-al and microscopic examination	322	**C**
	UP	40 mg/ml	UP	100 mg/L[h]	In NS and RL. Physically compatible initially but haziness in 4 hr at room temperature	322	**I**
Midazolam HCl	RC	5 mg/ml	UP	50 mg/ml	White precipitate forms immediately	1855	**I**
Minocycline HCl	LE	50 mg/ml	UP	10 mg/L[d]	Physically compatible for at least 4 hr at room temperature by visual and micro-scopic examination	534	**C**
Morphine sulfate	WY	15 mg/ml	UP	10 mg/L[d]	Physically compatible for at least 4 hr at room temperature by visual and micro-scopic examination	534	**C**
Neostigmine methylsulfate	RC	0.5 mg/ml	UP	10 mg/L[d]	Physically compatible for at least 4 hr at room temperature by visual and micro-scopic examination	534	**C**
Norepinephrine bitartrate	WI	1 mg/ml	UP	10 mg/L[d]	Physically compatible for at least 4 hr at room temperature by visual and micro-scopic examination	534	**C**
Ondansetron HCl	GL	1 mg/ml[b]	UP	1 mg/ml[a]	Physically compatible for 4 hr at 22 °C	1365	**C**

Y-Site Injection Compatibility (1:1 Mixture) (Cont.)

Hydrocortisone sodium succinate

Drug	Mfr	Conc	Mfr	Conc	Remarks	Ref	C/I
Oxacillin sodium	BR	100 mg/ml	UP	10 mg/L[d]	Physically compatible for at least 4 hr at room temperature by visual and microscopic examination	534	C
Oxytocin	SZ	1 mg/ml	UP	10 mg/L[d]	Physically compatible for at least 4 hr at room temperature by visual and microscopic examination	534	C
Paclitaxel	NCI	1.2 mg/ml[a]	AB	1 mg/ml[a]	Physically compatible with no change in measured turbidity in 4 hr at 22 °C	1556	C
Pancuronium bromide	ES	0.05 mg/ml[a]	AB	1 mg/ml[a]	Physically compatible for 24 hr at 28 °C	1337	C
Penicillin G potassium	LI	200,000 units/ml	UP	100 mg/L[c]	Physically compatible for at least 4 hr at room temperature by visual and microscopic examination	322	C
Pentazocine lactate	WI	30 mg/ml	UP	10 mg/L[d]	Physically compatible for at least 4 hr at room temperature by visual and microscopic examination	534	C
Phenytoin sodium	PD	50 mg/ml	UP	100 mg/L[c]	Immediate crystal formation	322	I
Phytonadione	RC	10 mg/ml	UP	10 mg/L[d]	Physically compatible for at least 4 hr at room temperature by visual and microscopic examination	534	C
Piperacillin sodium–tazobactam sodium	LE	40 + 5 mg/ml[a]	UP	1 mg/ml[a]	Physically compatible with no change in measured turbidity or increase in particle content in 4 hr at 22 °C	1688	C
Procainamide HCl	SQ	100 mg/ml	UP	10 mg/L[d]	Physically compatible for at least 4 hr at room temperature by visual and microscopic examination	534	C
Prochlorperazine edisylate	SKF	5 mg/ml	UP	10 mg/L[d]	Physically compatible for at least 4 hr at room temperature by visual and microscopic examination	534	C
Promethazine HCl	SV	50 mg/ml	UP	10 mg/L	In D5LR, D5W, NS, and LR. Physically compatible for at least 4 hr at room temperature by visual and microscopic examination	534	C
	SV	50 mg/ml	UP	10 mg/L	In D5R. Physically compatible initially but cloudiness in 4 hr at room temperature	534	I
Propofol	ZEN	10 mg/ml	UP	1 mg/ml[a]	Physically compatible for 1 hr at 23 °C with no increase in particle content	2066	C
Propranolol HCl	AY	1 mg/ml	UP	10 mg/L[d]	Physically compatible for at least 4 hr at room temperature by visual and microscopic examination	534	C
Pyridostigmine bromide	RC	5 mg/ml	UP	10 mg/L[d]	Physically compatible for at least 4 hr at room temperature by visual and microscopic examination	534	C
Remifentanil HCl	GW	0.025 and 0.25 mg/ml[b]	AB	1 mg/ml[a]	Physically compatible with no change in measured turbidity or increase in particle content in 4 hr at 23 °C	2075	C
Sargramostim	IMM	10 μg/ml[b]	UP	1 mg/ml[b]	Few small particles form in 1 hr	1436	I

Y-Site Injection Compatibility (1:1 Mixture) (Cont.)

Hydrocortisone sodium succinate

Drug	Mfr	Conc	Mfr	Conc	Remarks	Ref	C/I
Scopolamine HBr	BW	0.86 mg/ml	UP	10 mg/L[d]	Physically compatible for at least 4 hr at room temperature by visual and microscopic examination	534	C
Sodium bicarbonate	BR	75 mg/ml	UP	100 mg/L[c]	Physically compatible for at least 4 hr at room temperature by visual and microscopic examination	322	C
Succinylcholine chloride	BW	20 mg/ml	UP	100 mg/L[c]	Physically compatible for at least 4 hr at room temperature by visual and microscopic examination	322	C
Tacrolimus	FUJ	1 mg/ml[b]	AB	50 mg/ml[a]	Visually compatible for 24 hr at 25 °C	1630	C
Teniposide	BR	0.1 mg/ml[a]	UP	1 mg/ml[a]	Physically compatible with no subvisual haze or particle formation in 4 hr at 23 °C	1725	C
Theophylline	TR	4 mg/ml	UP	2 mg/ml[a]	Visually compatible for 6 hr at 25 °C	1793	C
Thiotepa	IMM[i]	1 mg/ml[a]	UP	1 mg/ml[a]	Physically compatible with no change in measured turbidity or increase in particle content in 4 hr at 23 °C	1861	C
TNA #218 to #226[j]			AB	1 mg/ml[a]	Visually compatible with no precipitate or emulsion damage apparent in 4 hr at 23 °C	2215	C
TPN #189[j]			UP	50 mg/ml[b]	Visually compatible for 24 hr at 22 °C	1767	C
TPN #212 to #215[j]			AB	1 mg/ml[a]	Physically compatible with no change in measured turbidity or increase in particle content in 4 hr at 23 °C	2109	C
Trimethaphan camsylate	RC	50 mg/ml	UP	10 mg/L[d]	Physically compatible for at least 4 hr at room temperature by visual and microscopic examination	534	C
Trimethobenzamide HCl	RC	100 mg/ml	UP	10 mg/L[d]	Physically compatible for at least 4 hr at room temperature by visual and microscopic examination	534	C
Vecuronium bromide	OR	0.1 mg/ml[a]	AB	1 mg/ml[a]	Physically compatible for 24 hr at 28 °C	1337	C
Vinorelbine tartrate	BW	1 mg/ml[b]	UP	1 mg/ml[b]	Physically compatible with no change in measured turbidity or increase in particle content in 4 hr at 22 °C	1558	C

[a]*Tested in dextrose 5% in water.*
[b]*Tested in sodium chloride 0.9%.*
[c]*Tested in combination with heparin sodium (Riker) 1000 units/L in dextrose 5% in water, sodium chloride 0.9%, and Ringer's injection, lactated.*
[d]*Tested in dextrose 5% in Ringer's injection, dextrose 5% in Ringer's injection, lactated, dextrose 5% in water, Ringer's injection, lactated, and sodium chloride 0.9%.*
[e]*Tested in both dextrose 5% in water and sodium chloride 0.9%.*
[f]*Tested in bacteriostatic sodium chloride 0.9% preserved with benzyl alcohol 0.9%.*
[g]*Form not specified.*
[h]*Also contained heparin sodium (Riker) 1000 units/L.*
[i]*Lyophilized formulation tested.*
[j]*Refer to Appendix I for the composition of parenteral nutrition solutions. TNA indicates a 3-in-1 admixture, and TPN indicates a 2-in-1 admixture.*

Additional Compatibility Information

Infusion Solutions— Dextrose 5% in water, sodium chloride 0.9%, and dextrose 5% in sodium chloride 0.9% have been recommended as diluents for the administration of hydrocortisone sodium succinate as an intravenous infusion. In concentrations of 100 mg to 3 g/50 ml of these diluents for piggyback administration, the drug is stated by the manufacturer to be stable for at least four hours (2). In addition, hydrocortisone sodium succinate is stated to be physically and chemically compatible in amino acid injection (McGaw) (189).

Miscellaneous— Amphotericin B in infusions appears to be compatible with limited amounts of hydrocortisone sodium succinate (4).

However, dacarbazine forms a pink precipitate immediately when mixed with hydrocortisone sodium succinate (Upjohn) (524).

Magnesium Sulfate— A white flocculent precipitate was observed when hydrocortisone sodium succinate (Upjohn) 100 mg in 2 ml was drawn up into a syringe previously used to add magnesium sulfate 50% (Elkins-Sinn) 1.5 ml to a parenteral nutrition solution. Hydrocortisone sodium succinate (Upjohn) contains phosphate buffers, and it was postulated that insoluble magnesium phosphate was formed. This finding indicates that magnesium sulfate and hydrocortisone sodium succinate should not be admixed as concentrated solutions and should be added separately to large volume parenteral solutions, with thorough mixing after each addition (302).

Vitamins— The following conditional compatibilities have been reported:

Hydrocortisone sodium succinate (Upjohn) in dextrose 5% in water with ascorbic acid injection (Upjohn) and vitamin B complex with C (Abbott); the compatibility is dependent on the concentration of the additives. Therefore, if attempting to combine hydrocortisone sodium succinate with either of these drugs, mix the solution thoroughly and observe it closely for any sign of incompatibility (15).

Hydrocortisone sodium succinate (Upjohn) 250 mg/L with vitamin B complex with C (Abbott) 2 ml/L; the mixture is physically compatible in most Abbott infusion solutions except Beclysyl 5 and 10% (3).

Hydrocortisone sodium succinate (Upjohn) 250 mg/L with cyanocobalamin (Abbott) 1000 μg/L; the mixture is physically compatible in most Abbott infusion solutions except Ionosol D-CM with dextrose 5%. A haze or precipitate forms within 24 hours (3).

Ephedrine Sulfate— Hydrocortisone sodium succinate (Upjohn) 250 mg/L with ephedrine sulfate 50 mg/L; the mixture is physically compatible in most Abbott infusion solutions except as noted below (3):

Fructose 10% in sodium chloride 0.9%	Haze or precipitate forms within 24 hr
Ionosol B with invert sugar 10%	Haze or precipitate forms within 24 hr

Ionosol D-CM with dextrose 5%	Haze or precipitate forms within 24 hr
Ionosol D with invert sugar 10%	Haze or precipitate forms within 6 hr
Ionosol D modified with invert sugar 10%	Haze or precipitate forms within 24 hr

Pentobarbital— Hydrocortisone sodium succinate (Upjohn) 250 mg/L with pentobarbital sodium (Abbott) 500 mg/L; the mixture is physically compatible in most Abbott infusion solutions except Ionosol G with invert sugar 10%. A haze or precipitate forms within six hours (3).

Penicillin G— Hydrocortisone sodium succinate (Upjohn) 250 mg/L with penicillin G potassium 1 million units/L; the mixture is physically compatible in most Abbott infusion solutions except as noted below (3):

Ionosol B with invert sugar 10%	Haze or precipitate forms within 24 hr
Ionosol D-CM with dextrose 5%	Haze or precipitate forms within 24 hr
Ionosol D with invert sugar 10%	Haze or precipitate forms within 24 hr

Procaine HCl— Hydrocortisone sodium succinate (Upjohn) 250 mg/L with procaine HCl 1 g/L; the mixture is physically compatible in most Abbott infusion solutions except as noted below (3):

Ionosol B with invert sugar 10%	Haze or precipitate forms within 24 hr

Concentrated Solutions— The following incompatibility determinations were performed with concentrated solutions. The drugs in dry form were reconstituted according to manufacturers' recommendations. One milliliter of hydrocortisone sodium succinate (Upjohn) was added to 5 ml of sterile distilled water along with 1 ml of each of the following drugs. Particulate matter was noted within two hours (28):

Dimenhydrinate (Searle)
Kanamycin sulfate (Bristol)
Promazine HCl (Wyeth)
Promethazine HCl (Wyeth)
Vancomycin HCl (Lilly)
Vitamin B complex with C (Lederle)

HYDROMORPHONE HCL
AHFS 28:08.08

Dilaudid HCl   **Knoll**

Products— Hydromorphone HCl (Knoll) is available in 1-ml ampuls and 20-ml multiple-dose vials. Each milliliter of the solution contains (2):

Component	Ampul	Vial
Hydromorphone HCl	1, 2, or 4 mg	2 mg
Sodium citrate	0.2%	
Citric acid	0.2%	
Edetate disodium		0.5 mg
Methylparaben		1.8 mg
Propylparaben		0.2 mg

Sodium hydroxide or hydrochloric acid may have been used to adjust the pH of the solutions in vials (2).

Hydromorphone HCl (Knoll) is also available in 1- and 5-ml amber ampuls and 50-ml single-dose vials as a high potency form (Dilaudid-HP). Each milliliter of the solution contains 10 mg of hydromorphone HCl with citric acid 0.2% and sodium citrate 0.2% (2).

In addition to the liquid dosage forms, high potency hydromorphone HCl (Dilaudid-HP, Knoll) is available as a 250-mg single-dose vial as a lyophilized powder. Reconstitute with 25 ml of sterile water for injection to yield a 10-mg/ml solution (2).

pH— From 4 to 5.5 (4).

Administration— Hydromorphone HCl may be administered by subcutaneous, intramuscular, or slow direct intravenous injection over at least two to three minutes (2; 4).

Stability— Hydromorphone HCl (Knoll) products should be stored at controlled room temperature and protected from light (2). The liquid dosage forms in intact ampuls or vials should not be stored under refrigeration because of possible precipitation or crystallization. Resolubilization at room temperature or on warming may be performed without affecting the stability of the drug (593). The manufacturer recommends inspecting for particulate matter or discoloration. A slight yellowish discoloration may develop in both the ampuls and vials, but it has not been associated with a loss of potency (2; 4).

Extemporaneously prepared hydromorphone HCl 10 and 50 mg/ml, stored in 100-ml glass vials or PVC bags, exhibited no loss in 42 days at 4 and 23 °C (1394).

Syringes— Hydromorphone HCl (Knoll) 10 mg/ml undiluted and diluted to 0.1 mg/ml in sodium chloride 0.9% was packaged as 3 ml in 10-ml polypropylene infusion pump syringes (Pharmacia Deltec). No loss by HPLC analysis occurred during 30 days storage at 30 °C (1967).

Compatibility Information

Solution Compatibility

Hydromorphone HCl

Solution	Mfr	Mfr	Conc/L	Remarks	Ref	C/I
Amino acids 7%	AB	KN[a]	80 mg	Physically compatible and TLC indicates no decomposition in 24 hr at 25 °C	572	**C**
Amino acids 8%	CU	KN[a]	80 mg	Physically compatible and TLC indicates no decomposition in 24 hr at 25 °C	572	**C**
Amino acids 8.5%	MG	KN[a]	80 mg	Physically compatible and TLC indicates no decomposition in 24 hr at 25 °C	572	**C**
	TR	KN[a]	80 mg	Physically compatible and TLC indicates no decomposition in 24 hr at 25 °C	572	**C**
Amino acids 8.5% with electrolytes	TR	KN[a]	80 mg	Physically compatible and TLC indicates no decomposition in 24 hr at 25 °C	572	**C**
Amino acids, essential, 5.4%	MG	KN[a]	80 mg	Physically compatible and TLC indicates no decomposition in 24 hr at 25 °C	572	**C**
Dextrose 5% in Ringer's injection	CU	KN[a]	80 mg	Physically compatible and TLC indicates no decomposition in 24 hr at 25 °C	572	**C**
Dextrose 5% in Ringer's injection, lactated	MG	KN[a]	80 mg	Physically compatible and TLC indicates no decomposition in 24 hr at 25 °C	572	**C**
Dextrose 5% in water	CU	KN[a]	80 mg	Physically compatible and TLC indicates no decomposition in 24 hr at 25 °C	572	**C**
	TR[b]	KN[a]	80 mg	Physically compatible and TLC indicates no decomposition in 24 hr at 25 °C	572	**C**
	MG[c]	KN[a]	80 mg	Physically compatible and TLC indicates no decomposition in 24 hr at 25 °C	572	**C**
	[b]	KN	1 and 5 g	No hydromorphone loss in 42 days at 4 and 23 °C	1394	**C**
Dextrose 5% in sodium chloride 0.45%	MG	KN[a]	80 mg	Physically compatible and TLC indicates no decomposition in 24 hr at 25 °C	572	**C**
Dextrose 5% in sodium chloride 0.9%	MG	KN[a]	80 mg	Physically compatible and TLC indicates no decomposition in 24 hr at 25 °C	572	**C**
Fructose 10% in water	CU	KN[a]	80 mg	Physically compatible and TLC indicates no decomposition in 24 hr at 25 °C	572	**C**

Solution Compatibility (Cont.)

Hydromorphone HCl

Solution	Mfr	Mfr	Conc/L	Remarks	Ref	C/I
Ringer's injection	MG	KN[a]	80 mg	Physically compatible and TLC indicates no decomposition in 24 hr at 25 °C	572	C
Ringer's injection, lactated	MG	KN[a]	80 mg	Physically compatible and TLC indicates no decomposition in 24 hr at 25 °C	572	C
Sodium chloride 0.45%	MG	KN[a]	80 mg	Physically compatible and TLC indicates no decomposition in 24 hr at 25 °C	572	C
Sodium chloride 0.9%	CU	KN[a]	80 mg	Physically compatible and TLC indicates no decomposition in 24 hr at 25 °C	572	C
	TR[b]	KN[a]	80 mg	Physically compatible and TLC indicates no decomposition in 24 hr at 25 °C	572	C
	MG[c]	KN[a]	80 mg	Physically compatible and TLC indicates no decomposition in 24 hr at 25 °C	572	C
	[b]	KN	1 and 5 g	No hydromorphone loss in 42 days at 4 and 23 °C	1394	C
	AB[b]	KN	20 and 100 mg	Visually compatible with little or no loss by HPLC in 72 hr at 24 °C under fluorescent light	1870	C
Sodium lactate 1/6 M	CU	KN[a]	80 mg	Physically compatible and TLC indicates no decomposition in 24 hr at 25 °C	572	C

[a]Both ampul and vial formulations tested.
[b]Tested in PVC containers.
[c]Tested in polyolefin containers.

Additive Compatibility

Hydromorphone HCl

Drug	Mfr	Conc/L	Mfr	Conc/L	Test Soln	Remarks	Ref	C/I
Bupivacaine HCl	AB	625 mg and 1.25 g	KN	20 mg	NS[a]	Visually compatible with little or no loss of either drug by HPLC in 72 hr at 24 °C under fluorescent light	1870	C
	AB	625 mg and 1.25 g	KN	100 mg	NS[a]	Visually compatible with little or no loss of either drug by HPLC in 72 hr at 24 °C under fluorescent light	1870	C
Fluorouracil	AB	1 g	AST	500 mg	D5W, NS[a]	Physically compatible with no increase in measured turbidity or particulates and little or no loss of either drug by HPLC in 7 days at 32 °C and 35 days at 23, 4, and −20 °C	1977	C
	AB	16 g	AST	500 mg	D5W, NS[a]	Physically compatible with no increase in measured turbidity or particulates and little or no loss of either drug by HPLC in 3 days at 32 °C, 7 days at 23 °C, and 35 days at 4 and −20 °C	1977	C
Midazolam HCl	RC	0.1 to 4.5 g	KN	0.5 to 45 g	D5W, NS	Visually compatible for 24 hr at room temperature	2086	C
	RC	100 mg	KN	2 and 20 g	D5W, NS	Visually compatible with less than 7% hydromorphone loss and less than 3% midazolam loss by HPLC in 23 days at 4 and 23 °C	2086	C

Additive Compatibility (Cont.)

Hydromorphone HCl

Drug	Mfr	Conc/L	Mfr	Conc/L	Test Soln	Remarks	Ref	C/I
	RC	500 mg	KN	2 and 20 g	D5W, NS	Visually compatible with less than 6% hydromorphone loss and less than 7% midazolam loss by HPLC in 23 days at 4 and 23 °C	2086	**C**
Ondansetron HCl	GL	100 mg and 1 g	ES	500 mg	NS	Physically compatible with no loss of either drug by HPLC in 7 days at 32 °C or 31 days at 4 and 22 °C protected from light	1690	**C**
Promethazine HCl	ES	300 mg	KN	1 g	NS[a]	Visually compatible for 21 days at 4 and 25 °C	1992	**C**
Sodium bicarbonate						Physically incompatible	9	**I**
Thiopental sodium	AB					Physically incompatible	9	**I**
Verapamil HCl	KN	80 mg	KN	16 mg	D5W, NS	Physically compatible for 24 hr	764	**C**

[a]Tested in PVC containers.

Drugs in Syringe Compatibility

Hydromorphone HCl

Drug (in syringe)	Mfr	Amt	Mfr	Amt	Remarks	Ref	C/I
Ampicillin sodium	AY	250 mg/ 1 ml	KN	2, 10, 40 mg/ 1 ml	Visually compatible but 10% loss of ampicillin by HPLC in 5 hr at room temperature	2082	**I**
Atropine sulfate	ES	0.4 mg/ 0.5 ml	KN	4 mg/ 2 ml[a]	Physically compatible for 30 min	517	**C**
Bupivacaine HCl	AST	7.5 mg/ ml	KN	65 mg/ ml	Visually compatible for 30 days at 25 °C	1660	**C**
Cefazolin sodium	SKF	>200 mg/1 ml	KN	2, 10, 40 mg/ 1 ml	Precipitate forms	2082	**I**
	SKF	150 mg/ 1 ml	KN	2, 10, 40 mg/ 1 ml	Visually compatible with less than 10% loss of either drug by HPLC in 24 hr at room temperature	2082	**C**
Ceftazidime	GL[i]	180 mg/ 1 ml	KN	2, 10, 40 mg/ 1 ml	Visually compatible with less than 10% loss of either drug by HPLC in 24 hr at room temperature	2082	**C**
Chlorpromazine HCl	ES	25 mg/ 1 ml	KN	4 mg/ 2 ml[a]	Physically compatible for 30 min	517	**C**
Cimetidine HCl	SKF	300 mg/ 2 ml	WI	2 mg/ 1 ml	Physically compatible for 4 hr at 25 °C	25	**C**
Dexamethasone sodium phosphate	SX	4 mg/ml[b]	KN	2, 10, 40 mg/ ml[b]	Visually compatible and potency of both drugs by HPLC retained for 24 hr at 24 °C	1542	**C**

Drugs in Syringe Compatibility (Cont.)

Hydromorphone HCl

Drug (in syringe)	Mfr	Amt	Mfr	Amt	Remarks	Ref	C/I
	DB	10 mg/ ml[b]	KN	2 and 10 mg/ ml[b]	Visually compatible and potency of both drugs by HPLC retained for 24 hr at 24 °C	1542	C
	DB	10 mg/ ml[b]	KN	40 mg/ ml[b]	White turbidity forms immediately	1542	I
	DB	7.1 mg/ ml[c]	KN	11.6 mg/ ml[c]	Visually compatible for 24 hr at 24 °C	1542	C
	DB, SX	5.5 to 6.6 mg/ ml[c]	KN	13.3 to 17.5 mg/ ml[c]	Precipitate forms	1542	I
	DB	4.75 mg/ ml[c]	KN	10.5 mg/ ml[c]	Visually compatible for 24 hr at 24 °C	1542	C
	SX	3 to 4.1 mg/ ml[c]	KN	14.75 to 25 mg/ ml[c]	Precipitate forms	1542	I
	SX	3.34 mg/ ml[c]	KN	26.66 mg/ ml[c]	Visually compatible for 24 hr at 24 °C	1542	C
Diazepam	SX	5 mg/ 1 ml	KN	2, 10, 40 mg/ 1 ml	Diazepam precipitate forms immediately due to aqueous dilution	2082	I
Dimenhydrinate	SQ	50 mg/ 1 ml	KN	1, 10, 40 mg/ 1 ml	Visually compatible with both drugs stable by HPLC for 24 hr at 4, 23, and 37 °C. Precipitate forms after 24 hr	1776	C
Diphenhydramine HCl	PD	50 mg/ 1 ml	KN	4 mg/ 2 ml[a]	Physically compatible for 30 min	517	C
Fentanyl citrate	MN	0.05 mg/ 1 ml	KN	4 mg/ 2 ml[a]	Physically compatible for 30 min	517	C
Glycopyrrolate	RB	0.2 mg/ 1 ml	KN	2 mg/ 1 ml	Physically compatible and pH in stability range for glycopyrrolate for 48 hr at 25 °C	331	C
	RB	0.2 mg/ 1 ml	KN	4 mg/ 2 ml	Physically compatible and pH in stability range for glycopyrrolate for 48 hr at 25 °C	331	C
	RB	0.4 mg/ 2 ml	KN	2 mg/ 1 ml	Physically compatible and pH in stability range for glycopyrrolate for 48 hr at 25 °C	331	C
Haloperidol lactate	MN	1[d], 2[d], 5 mg/ 1 ml	KN	1[d] and 10 mg/ 1 ml	Visually compatible for 24 hr at 25 °C under fluorescent light	1785	C
Hyaluronidase	WY	150 units/ml[e]	KN	2 mg/ml[e]	43 and 56% hyaluronidase loss in 24 hr at 4 and 23 °C, respectively	1907	I
	WY	150 units/ml[e]	KN	10 and 40 mg/ ml[e]	70 to 82% hyaluronidase loss in 24 hr at 4 and 23 °C	1907	I
Hydroxyzine HCl	PF	50 mg/ 1 ml	KN	4 mg/ 2 ml[a]	Physically compatible for 30 min	517	C
	PF	100 mg/ 2 ml	KN	0.75 mg/ 0.8 ml	Physically compatible	771	C
Ketorolac tromethamine	SY	30 mg/ 1 ml	KN	10 mg/ 1 ml	Cloudiness forms immediately but clears with swirling	1785	?
	SY	30 mg/ 1 ml	KN	1 mg/ 1 ml[d]	Visually compatible for 24 hr at 25 °C under fluorescent light	1785	C

Drugs in Syringe Compatibility (Cont.)

Hydromorphone HCl

Drug (in syringe)	Mfr	Amt	Mfr	Amt	Remarks	Ref	C/I
	SY	15 mg/ 1 ml[d]	KN	1[d] and 10 mg/ 1 ml	Visually compatible for 24 hr at 25 °C under fluorescent light	1785	C
Lorazepam	WY	4 mg/ 1 ml	KN	1, 10, 40 mg/ 1 ml	Visually compatible with 10% lorazepam loss by HPLC in 6 days at 4 °C, 4 days at 23 °C, and 24 hr at 37 °C. Little or no hydromorphone loss in 7 days at all three temperatures	1776	C
Midazolam HCl	RC	5 mg/ 1 ml	WB	2 mg/ 0.5 ml	Physically compatible for 4 hr at 25 °C under fluorescent light	1145	C
Pentazocine lactate	WI	30 mg/ 1 ml	KN	4 mg/ 2 ml[a]	Physically compatible for 30 min	517	C
Pentobarbital sodium	AB	50 mg/ 1 ml	KN	4 mg/ 2 ml[f]	Physically compatible for 30 min	517	C
	AB	50 mg/ 1 ml	KN	4 mg/ 2 ml[g]	Transient precipitate that dissipates after mixing. Physically compatible for 30 min	517	C
Phenobarbital sodium	AB	120 mg/ 1 ml	KN	2, 10, 40 mg/ 1 ml	Precipitate forms immediately but dissipates with shaking. A white precipitate of phenobarbital reforms after 6 hr at room temperature	2082	I
Phenytoin sodium	AB	50 mg/ 1 ml	KN	2, 10, 40 mg/ 1 ml	White precipitate of phenytoin forms immediately	2082	I
Prochlorperazine edisylate	SKF	5 mg/ 1 ml	KN	4 mg/ 2 ml[f]	Immediate precipitation	517	I
	SKF	5 mg/ 1 ml	KN	4 mg/ 2 ml[g]	Physically compatible for 30 min	517	C
Prochlorperazine mesylate	RP	5 mg/ 1 ml	KN	1, 10, 40 mg/ 1 ml	Visually compatible with little or no loss of either drug by HPLC in 7 days at 4, 23, and 37 °C	1776	C
	RP	1.5 mg/ ml[j]	SX	0.5 mg/ ml[j]	Visually and microscopically compatible for 96 hr at room temperature exposed to light	2171	C
Promethazine HCl	WY	50 mg/ 1 ml	KN	4 mg/ 2 ml[a]	Physically compatible for 30 min	517	C
	WY	25 mg/ 1 ml	KN	4 mg/ 2 ml[a]	Physically compatible for 30 min	517	C
Ranitidine HCl	GL	50 mg/ 2 ml	PE	2 mg/ 1 ml	Physically compatible for 1 hr at 25 °C both macroscopically and microscopically	978	C
Salbutamol	GL	2.5 mg/ 2.5 ml[h]	KN	1 mg/ 0.5 ml	Visually compatible for one hour both macroscopically and microscopically	1904	C
Scopolamine HBr	BW	0.43 mg/ 0.5 ml	KN	4 mg/ 2 ml[a]	Physically compatible for 30 min	517	C
Thiethylperazine malate	SZ	5 mg/ 1 ml	KN	4 mg/ 2 ml[a]	Physically compatible for 30 min	517	C

Drugs in Syringe Compatibility (Cont.)

Hydromorphone HCl

Drug (in syringe)	Mfr	Amt	Mfr	Amt	Remarks	Ref	C/I
Trimethobenzamide HCl	BE	100 mg/ 1 ml	KN	4 mg/ 2 ml[a]	Physically compatible for 30 min	517	**C**

[a]*Both ampul and vial formulations tested.*
[b]*Mixed in equal quantities. Final concentration is one-half the indicated concentration.*
[c]*Mixed in varying quantities to yield the final concentrations noted.*
[d]*Dilution prepared in sterile water for injection.*
[e]*Mixed in equal quantities for testing.*
[f]*Vial formulation tested.*
[g]*Ampul formulation tested.*
[h]*Both preserved (benzyl alcohol 0.9%; benzalkonium chloride 0.01%) and unpreserved sodium chloride 0.9% were used as a diluent.*
[i]*Sodium carbonate–containing formulation.*
[j]*Diluted in sodium chloride 0.9%.*

Y-Site Injection Compatibility (1:1 Mixture)

Hydromorphone HCl

Drug	Mfr	Conc	Mfr	Conc	Remarks	Ref	C/I
Acyclovir sodium	BW	5 mg/ml[a]	WB	0.04 mg/ml[a]	Physically compatible for 4 hr at 25 °C	1157	**C**
Allopurinol sodium	BW	3 mg/ml[b]	KN	0.5 mg/ml[b]	Physically compatible with no change in measured turbidity or increase in particle content in 4 hr at 22 °C	1686	**C**
Amifostine	USB	10 mg/ml[a]	AST	0.5 mg/ml[a]	Physically compatible with no change in measured turbidity or increase in particle content in 4 hr at 23 °C	1845	**C**
Amikacin sulfate	BR	5 mg/ml[a]	WY	0.2 mg/ml[a]	Physically compatible for at least 4 hr at 25 °C under fluorescent light	987	**C**
Amphotericin B cholesteryl sulfate complex	SEQ	0.83 mg/ml[a]	ES	0.5 mg/ml[a]	Decreased natural turbidity occurs immediately	2117	**I**
Ampicillin sodium	BR	20 mg/ml[b]	WY	0.2 mg/ml[a]	Physically compatible for at least 4 hr at 25 °C under fluorescent light	987	**C**
	AY	20[a] and 250 mg/ml	KN	2, 10, 40 mg/ ml	Visually compatible and hydromorphone potency by HPLC retained for 24 hr. 10% ampicillin loss by HPLC in 5 hr with or without hydromorphone	1532	**I**
Amsacrine	NCI	1 mg/ml[a]	AST	0.5 mg/ml[a]	Physically compatible for 4 hr at room temperature under fluorescent light	1381	**C**
Aztreonam	SQ	40 mg/ml[a]	KN	0.5 mg/ml[a]	Physically compatible with no subvisual haze or particle formation in 4 hr at 23 °C	1758	**C**
Cefamandole nafate	LI	20 mg/ml[a]	WY	0.2 mg/ml[a]	Physically compatible for at least 4 hr at 25 °C under fluorescent light	987	**C**
Cefazolin sodium	SKF	20 mg/ml[a]	WY	0.2 mg/ml[a]	Physically compatible for at least 4 hr at 25 °C under fluorescent light	987	**C**
	SKF	20[a] and 150 mg/ml	KN	2, 10, 40 mg/ ml	Visually compatible and potency of both drugs by HPLC retained for 24 hr	1532	**C**
	SKF	>200 mg/ml	KN	2, 10, 40 mg/ ml	Precipitate forms immediately	1532	**I**
Cefepime HCl	BR	20 mg/ml[a]	ES	0.5 mg/ml[a]	Physically compatible with no change in measured turbidity or increase in particle content in 4 hr at 22 °C	1689	**C**

Y-Site Injection Compatibility (1:1 Mixture) (Cont.)

Hydromorphone HCl

Drug	Mfr	Conc	Mfr	Conc	Remarks	Ref	C/I
Cefoperazone sodium	RR	20 mg/ml[a]	WY	0.2 mg/ml[a]	Physically compatible for at least 4 hr at 25 °C under fluorescent light	987	**C**
Cefotaxime sodium	HO	20 mg/ml[a]	WY	0.2 mg/ml[a]	Physically compatible for at least 4 hr at 25 °C under fluorescent light	987	**C**
Cefoxitin sodium	MSD	20 mg/ml[a]	WY	0.2 mg/ml[a]	Physically compatible for at least 4 hr at 25 °C under fluorescent light	987	**C**
Ceftazidime	GL[f]	40[a] and 180 mg/ml	KN	2, 10, 40 mg/ml	Visually compatible and potency of both drugs by HPLC retained for 24 hr	1532	**C**
Ceftizoxime sodium	SKF	20 mg/ml[a]	WY	0.2 mg/ml[a]	Physically compatible for at least 4 hr at 25 °C under fluorescent light	987	**C**
Cefuroxime sodium	GL	30 mg/ml[a]	WY	0.2 mg/ml[a]	Physically compatible for at least 4 hr at 25 °C under fluorescent light	987	**C**
Chloramphenicol sodium succinate	LY	20 mg/ml[a]	WY	0.2 mg/ml[a]	Physically compatible for at least 4 hr at 25 °C under fluorescent light	987	**C**
Cisatracurium besylate	GW	0.1, 2, 5 mg/ml[a]	ES	0.5 mg/ml[a]	Physically compatible with no change in measured turbidity or increase in particle content in 4 hr at 23 °C	2074	**C**
Cisplatin	BR	1 mg/ml	ES	0.04 mg/ml[a]	Visually compatible for 4 hr at room temperature under fluorescent light	1685	**C**
Cladribine	ORT	0.015[b] and 0.5[d] mg/ml	KN	0.5 mg/ml[b]	Physically compatible with no change in measured turbidity or increase in particle content in 4 hr at 23 °C	1969	**C**
Clindamycin phosphate	UP	12 mg/ml[a]	WY	0.2 mg/ml[a]	Physically compatible for at least 4 hr at 25 °C under fluorescent light	987	**C**
Cyclophosphamide	MJ	10 mg/ml	ES	0.04 mg/ml[a]	Visually compatible for 4 hr at room temperature under fluorescent light	1685	**C**
Cytarabine	UP	50 mg/ml	ES	0.04 mg/ml[a]	Visually compatible for 4 hr at room temperature under fluorescent light	1685	**C**
Diazepam	SX	5 mg/ml	KN	2, 10, 40 mg/ml	Turbidity forms immediately and diazepam precipitate develops	1532	**I**
Diltiazem HCl	MMD	1 mg/ml[a]	KN	1 mg/ml	Visually compatible for 4 hr at 27 °C	2062	**C**
Dobutamine HCl	LI	4 mg/ml[a]	KN	1 mg/ml	Visually compatible for 4 hr at 27 °C	2062	**C**
Docetaxel	RPR	0.9 mg/ml[a]	AST	0.5 mg/ml[a]	Physically compatible with no change in measured turbidity or increase in particle content in 4 hr at 23 °C	2224	**C**
Dopamine HCl	AB	3.2 mg/ml[a]	KN	1 mg/ml	Visually compatible for 4 hr at 27 °C	2062	**C**
Doxorubicin HCl	AD	0.2 mg/ml[a]	ES	0.04 mg/ml[a]	Visually compatible for 4 hr at room temperature under fluorescent light	1685	**C**
Doxorubicin HCl liposome injection	SEQ	0.4 mg/ml[a]	ES	0.5 mg/ml[a]	Physically compatible with little or no change in measured turbidity and no increase in particle content in 4 hr at 23 °C	2087	**C**
Doxycycline hyclate	ES	1 mg/ml[a]	WY	0.2 mg/ml[a]	Physically compatible for at least 4 hr at 25 °C under fluorescent light	987	**C**
Epinephrine HCl	AB	0.02 mg/ml[a]	KN	1 mg/ml	Visually compatible for 4 hr at 27 °C	2062	**C**

Y-Site Injection Compatibility (1:1 Mixture) (Cont.)

Hydromorphone HCl

Drug	Mfr	Conc	Mfr	Conc	Remarks	Ref	C/I
Erythromycin lactobionate	AB	5 mg/ml[a]	WY	0.2 mg/ml[a]	Physically compatible for at least 4 hr at 25 °C under fluorescent light	987	C
Etoposide phosphate	BR	5 mg/ml[a]	ES	0.5 mg/ml[a]	Physically compatible with no change in measured turbidity or increase in particle content in 4 hr at 23 °C	2218	C
Famotidine	ME	2 mg/ml[b]		0.5 mg/ml[a]	Visually compatible for 4 hr at 22 °C	1936	C
Fentanyl citrate	ES	0.05 mg/ml	KN	1 mg/ml	Visually compatible for 4 hr at 27 °C	2062	C
Filgrastim	AMG	30 µg/ml[a]	KN	0.5 mg/ml[a]	Physically compatible with no change in measured turbidity or increase in particle content in 4 hr at 22 °C	1687	C
Fludarabine phosphate	BX	1 mg/ml[a]	KN	0.5 mg/ml[a]	Physically compatible for 4 hr at room temperature under fluorescent light	1439	C
Foscarnet sodium	AST	24 mg/ml	KN	10 mg/ml	Physically compatible for 24 hr at room temperature under fluorescent light	1335	C
Furosemide	AMR	10 mg/ml	KN	1 mg/ml	Visually compatible for 4 hr at 27 °C	2062	C
Gemcitabine HCl	LI	10 mg/ml[b]	AST	0.5 mg/ml[b]	Physically compatible with no change in measured turbidity or increase in particle content in 4 hr at 23 °C	2226	C
Gentamicin sulfate	TR	0.8 mg/ml[a]	WY	0.2 mg/ml[a]	Physically compatible for at least 4 hr at 25 °C under fluorescent light	987	C
Granisetron HCl	SKB	1 mg/ml	KN	0.5 mg/ml[b]	Physically compatible with little or no loss of either drug by HPLC in 4 hr at 22 °C	1883	C
	SKB	0.05 mg/ml[a]	ES	0.5 mg/ml[a]	Physically compatible with no change in measured turbidity or increase in particle content in 4 hr at 23 °C	2000	C
Heparin sodium	ES	100 units/ml[a]	KN	1 mg/ml	Visually compatible for 4 hr at 27 °C	2062	C
Kanamycin sulfate	BR	2.5 mg/ml[a]	WY	0.2 mg/ml[a]	Physically compatible for at least 4 hr at 25 °C under fluorescent light	987	C
Labetalol HCl	AH	2 mg/ml[a]	KN	1 mg/ml	Visually compatible for 4 hr at 27 °C	2062	C
Lorazepam	WY	0.5 mg/ml[a]	KN	1 mg/ml	Visually compatible for 4 hr at 27 °C	2062	C
Magnesium sulfate	LY	16.7, 33.3, 50, 100 mg/ml[a]	KN	2 mg/ml[a]	Visually compatible for 4 hr at 25 °C under fluorescent light	1549	C
Melphalan HCl	BW	0.1 mg/ml[b]	KN	0.5 mg/ml[b]	Physically compatible with no change in measured turbidity or increase in particle content in 3 hr at 22 °C	1557	C
Methotrexate sodium	AD	15 mg/ml[e]	ES	0.04 mg/ml[a]	Visually compatible for 4 hr at room temperature under fluorescent light	1685	C
Metronidazole	SE	5 mg/ml	WY	0.2 mg/ml[a]	Physically compatible for at least 4 hr at 25 °C under fluorescent light	987	C
Midazolam HCl	RC	2 mg/ml[a]	KN	1 mg/ml	Visually compatible for 4 hr at 27 °C	2062	C
Milrinone lactate	SW	0.2 mg/ml[a]	KN	1 mg/ml	Visually compatible for 4 hr at 27 °C	2062	C
Minocycline HCl	LE	0.2 mg/ml[a]	WY	0.2 mg/ml[a]	Color changed from pale yellow to light green within 1 hr at 25 °C	987	I
Morphine sulfate	SCN	2 mg/ml[a]	KN	1 mg/ml	Visually compatible for 4 hr at 27 °C	2062	C

Y-Site Injection Compatibility (1:1 Mixture) (Cont.)

Hydromorphone HCl

Drug	Mfr	Conc	Mfr	Conc	Remarks	Ref	C/I
Nafcillin sodium	WY	20 mg/ml[a]	WY	0.2 mg/ml[a]	Physically compatible for at least 4 hr at 25 °C under fluorescent light	987	**C**
Nicardipine HCl	WY	1 mg/ml[a]	KN	1 mg/ml	Visually compatible for 4 hr at 27 °C	2062	**C**
Nitroglycerin	AB	0.4 mg/ml[a]	KN	1 mg/ml	Visually compatible for 4 hr at 27 °C	2062	**C**
Norepinephrine bitartrate	AB	0.128 mg/ml[a]	KN	1 mg/ml	Visually compatible for 4 hr at 27 °C	2062	**C**
Ondansetron HCl	GL	1 mg/ml[b]	KN	0.5 mg/ml[a]	Physically compatible for 4 hr at 22 °C	1365	**C**
Oxacillin sodium	BE	20 mg/ml[a]	WY	0.2 mg/ml[a]	Physically compatible for at least 4 hr at 25 °C under fluorescent light	987	**C**
Paclitaxel	NCI	1.2 mg/ml[a]	KN	0.5 mg/ml[a]	Physically compatible with no change in measured turbidity in 4 hr at 22 °C	1556	**C**
Penicillin G potassium	PF	100,000 units/ml[a]	WY	0.2 mg/ml[a]	Physically compatible for at least 4 hr at 25 °C under fluorescent light	987	**C**
Phenobarbital sodium	AB	120 mg/ml	KN	2, 10, 40 mg/ml	Turbidity forms immediately but dissipates; phenobarbital precipitate develops in 6 hr	1532	**I**
Phenytoin sodium	AB	50 mg/ml	KN	2, 10, 40 mg/ml	Turbidity forms immediately and phenytoin precipitate develops	1532	**I**
Piperacillin sodium	LE	60 mg/ml[a]	WY	0.2 mg/ml[a]	Physically compatible for at least 4 hr at 25 °C under fluorescent light	987	**C**
Piperacillin sodium–tazobactam sodium	LE	40 + 5 mg/ml[a]	KN	0.5 mg/ml[a]	Physically compatible with no change in measured turbidity or increase in particle content in 4 hr at 22 °C	1688	**C**
Propofol	ZEN	10 mg/ml	AST	0.5 mg/ml[a]	Physically compatible for 1 hr at 23 °C with no increase in particle content	2066	**C**
Ranitidine HCl	GL	1 mg/ml[a]	KN	1 mg/ml	Visually compatible for 4 hr at 27 °C	2062	**C**
Remifentanil HCl	GW	0.025 and 0.25 mg/ml[b]	ES	0.5 mg/ml[a]	Physically compatible with no change in measured turbidity or increase in particle content in 4 hr at 23 °C	2075	**C**
Sargramostim	IMM	10 μg/ml[b]	KN	0.5 mg/ml[b]	Few small particles form in 30 min	1436	**I**
Tacrolimus	FUJ	10 and 40 μg/ml[a]	KN	200 μg/ml[a]	Visually compatible with no loss of either drug by HPLC in 4 hr at 24 °C under fluorescent light	2216	**C**
	FUJ	10 and 40 μg/ml[a]	KN	2 mg/ml[a]	Visually compatible with no loss of either drug by HPLC in 4 hr at 24 °C under fluorescent light	2216	**C**
Teniposide	BR	0.1 mg/ml[a]	KN	0.5 mg/ml[a]	Physically compatible with no subvisual haze or particle formation in 4 hr at 23 °C	1725	**C**
Thiopental sodium	AB	25 mg/ml[c]	KN	1 mg/ml	Precipitate forms in 4 hr at 27 °C	2062	**I**
Thiotepa	IMM[g]	1 mg/ml[a]	AST	0.5 mg/ml[a]	Physically compatible with no change in measured turbidity or increase in particle content in 4 hr at 23 °C	1861	**C**
Ticarcillin disodium	BE	60 mg/ml[a]	WY	0.2 mg/ml[a]	Physically compatible for at least 4 hr at 25 °C under fluorescent light	987	**C**

Y-Site Injection Compatibility (1:1 Mixture) (Cont.)

Hydromorphone HCl

Drug	Mfr	Conc	Mfr	Conc	Remarks	Ref	C/I
TNA #219, #222, #224 to #226[h]			ES	0.5 mg/ml[a]	Damage to emulsion integrity occurs immediately with free oil formation possible	2215	I
TNA #218, #220, #221, #223[h]			ES	0.5 mg/ml[a]	Visually compatible with no precipitate or emulsion damage apparent in 4 hr at 23 °C	2215	C
Tobramycin sulfate	DI	0.8 mg/ml[a]	WY	0.2 mg/ml[a]	Physically compatible for at least 4 hr at 25 °C under fluorescent light	987	C
TPN #212 to #215[h]			ES	0.5 mg/ml[a]	Physically compatible with no change in measured turbidity or increase in particle content in 4 hr at 23 °C	2109	C
Trimethoprim–sulfamethoxazole	BW	0.8 + 4 mg/ml	WY	0.2 mg/ml[a]	Physically compatible for at least 4 hr at 25 °C under fluorescent light	987	C
Vancomycin HCl	LI	5 mg/ml[a]	WY	0.2 mg/ml[a]	Physically compatible for at least 4 hr at 25 °C under fluorescent light	987	C
Vecuronium bromide	OR	1 mg/ml	KN	1 mg/ml	Visually compatible for 4 hr at 27 °C	2062	C
Vinorelbine tartrate	BW	1 mg/ml[b]	KN	0.5 mg/ml[b]	Physically compatible with no change in measured turbidity or increase in particle content in 4 hr at 22 °C	1558	C

[a]*Tested in dextrose 5% in water.*
[b]*Tested in sodium chloride 0.9%.*
[c]*Tested in sterile water for injection.*
[d]*Tested in bacteriostatic sodium chloride 0.9% preserved with benzyl alcohol 0.9%.*
[e]*Tested in dextrose 5% in water with sodium bicarbonate 0.05 mEq/ml.*
[f]*Sodium carbonate–containing formulation.*
[g]*Lyophilized formulation tested.*
[h]*Refer to Appendix I for the composition of parenteral nutrition solutions. TNA indicates a 3-in-1 admixture, and TPN indicates a 2-in-1 admixture.*

Additional Compatibility Information

Solutions— Hydromorphone HCl reportedly is physically and chemically stable for at least 24 hours in most common intravenous infusion solutions when stored protected from light at 25 °C. However, it is reported to be physically or chemically incompatible with sodium bicarbonate–containing solutions (4).

Tetracaine HCl— Hydromorphone HCl (Winthrop) 4.38 mg/ml with tetracaine HCl (Winthrop) 1.25 mg/ml in sodium chloride 0.9% in an implantable pump controlled pain through 18 days of use. After that time, supplementary medication was needed. The authors speculated that a potency loss after 18 days at 37 °C caused the inadequate pain control, but this speculation was not verified (1524).

HYDROXYZINE HCL
AHFS 28:24.92

Vistaril   **Pfizer**

Products— Hydroxyzine HCl (Pfizer) is available as a 25-mg/ml solution in 10-ml multiple-dose vials. It is also available as a 50-mg/ml solution in 1- and 2-ml single-dose vials and 10-ml multiple-dose vials. Also present in the solutions are benzyl alcohol 0.9% and sodium hydroxide to adjust the pH (2).

pH— From 3.5 to 6 (4).

Osmolality— Hydroxyzine HCl (Elkins-Sinn) 50 mg/ml has an osmolality of 345 mOsm/kg (2043).

Administration— Hydroxyzine HCl may be administered undiluted by intramuscular injection only, preferably into the upper outer quadrant of the buttock or the midlateral muscles of the thigh in adults. In children, the midlateral muscles of the thigh are preferred (2; 4).

Stability— Hydroxyzine injection should be stored at 15 to 30 °C and protected from freezing (2; 4). Hydroxyzine HCl (Pfizer) 50 mg/ml retained its potency for three months at room temperature when 1 and 2 ml of solution were packaged in Tubex cartridges (13).

Compatibility Information

Additive Compatibility

Hydroxyzine HCl

Drug	Mfr	Conc/L	Mfr	Conc/L	Test Soln	Remarks	Ref	C/I
Aminophylline	SE	1 g	RR	250 mg	D5W	Physically incompatible	15	I
Amobarbital sodium			PF			Physically incompatible	9	I
	LI	1 g	RR	250 mg	D5W	Physically incompatible	15	I
Chloramphenicol sodium succinate	PD	10 g	RR	250 mg	D5W	Physically incompatible	15	I
Cisplatin	BR	200 mg	LY	500 mg	NS[a]	Physically compatible for 48 hr	1190	C
Cyclophosphamide	AD	1 g	LY	500 mg	D5W[a]	Physically compatible for 48 hr	1190	C
Cytarabine	UP	1 g	LY	500 mg	D5W[a]	Physically compatible for 48 hr	1190	C
Dimenhydrinate	SE	500 mg	RR	250 mg	D5W	Physically compatible	15	C
Etoposide	BR	1 g	LY	500 mg	D5W[a]	Physically compatible for 48 hr	1190	C
Lidocaine HCl	AST	2 g	PF	100 mg		Physically compatible	24	C
Mesna	AW	3 g	LY	500 mg	D5W[a]	Physically compatible for 48 hr	1190	C
Methotrexate sodium	BV	1 and 3 g	LY	500 mg	D5W[a]	Physically compatible for 48 hr	1190	C
Nafcillin sodium	WY	500 mg	PF	100 mg		Physically compatible	27	C
Penicillin G potassium	SQ	20 million units	RR	250 mg	D5W	Physically incompatible	15	I
Penicillin G sodium	UP	20 million units	RR	250 mg	D5W	Physically incompatible	15	I
Pentobarbital sodium			PF			Physically incompatible	9	I
	AB	1 g	RR	250 mg	D5W	Physically incompatible	15	I
Phenobarbital sodium	WI	200 mg	RR	250 mg	D5W	Physically incompatible	15	I

[a]Tested in glass containers.

Drugs in Syringe Compatibility

Hydroxyzine HCl

Drug (in syringe)	Mfr	Amt	Mfr	Amt	Remarks	Ref	C/I
Atropine sulfate		0.4 mg/ 1 ml	PF	100 mg/ 2 ml	Physically compatible	771	C
		0.4 mg/ 1 ml	PF	50 mg/ 1 ml	Physically compatible	771	C
		0.6 mg/ 1.5 ml	PF	100 mg/ 4 ml	Physically compatible for at least 15 min	14	C
	USP	0.4 mg/ 0.4 ml	NF	50 mg/ 1 ml	Hydroxyzine potency retained for at least 10 days at 3 and 25 °C	49	C
	ST	0.4 mg/ 1 ml	PF	50 mg/ 1 ml	Physically compatible for at least 15 min	326	C

Drugs in Syringe Compatibility (Cont.)

Hydroxyzine HCl

Drug (in syringe)	Mfr	Amt	Mfr	Amt	Remarks	Ref	C/I
Atropine sulfate with meperidine HCl[a]	ES WI	0.4 mg 50 mg	PF	50 mg/ 2.5 ml	No alteration of UV spectra in 10 days at 3 and 25 °C	301	C
Butorphanol tartrate	BR	2 mg/ 1 ml	PF	50 mg/ 1 ml	Physically compatible	771	C
	BR	1 mg/ 1 ml	PF	100 mg/ 2 ml	Physically compatible	771	C
Chlorpromazine HCl	PO	50 mg/ 2 ml	PF	50 mg/ 1 ml	Physically compatible for at least 15 min	326	C
	STE	50 mg/ 2 ml	ES	100 mg/ 2 ml	Visually compatible for 60 min	1784	C
Cimetidine HCl	SKF	300 mg/ 2 ml	ES	100 mg/ 2 ml	Physically compatible for 4 hr at 25 °C	25	C
Codeine phosphate		120 mg/ 4 ml	PF	50 mg/ 1 ml	Physically compatible	771	C
		60 mg/ 2 ml	PF	100 mg/ 2 ml	Physically compatible	771	C
Dimenhydrinate	HR	50 mg/ 1 ml	PF	50 mg/ 1 ml	Physically incompatible within 15 min	326	I
Diphenhydramine HCl	PD	50 mg/ 1 ml	PF	50 mg/ 1 ml	Physically compatible for at least 15 min	326	C
Doxapram HCl	RB	400 mg/ 20 ml		25 mg/ 1 ml	Physically compatible with no doxapram loss in 24 hr	1177	C
Droperidol	MN	2.5 mg/ 1 ml	PF	50 mg/ 1 ml	Physically compatible for at least 15 min	326	C
Fentanyl citrate	MN	0.05 mg/ 1 ml	PF	50 mg/ 1 ml	Physically compatible for at least 15 min	326	C
	CR	0.05 mg/ 1 ml	PF	50 mg/ 1 ml	Physically compatible	771	C
	CR	0.05 mg/ 1 ml	PF	100 mg/ 2 ml	Physically compatible	771	C
Fluphenazine HCl	LY	5 mg/ 2 ml	ES	100 mg/ 2 ml	Visually compatible for 60 min	1784	C
Glycopyrrolate	RB	0.2 mg/ 1 ml	PF	25 mg/ 1 ml	Physically compatible and pH in stability range for glycopyrrolate for 48 hr at 25 °C	331	C
	RB	0.2 mg/ 1 ml	PF	50 mg/ 2 ml	Physically compatible and pH in stability range for glycopyrrolate for 48 hr at 25 °C	331	C
	RB	0.4 mg/ 2 ml	PF	25 mg/ 1 ml	Physically compatible and pH in stability range for glycopyrrolate for 48 hr at 25 °C	331	C
Haloperidol lactate	MN	10 mg/ 2 ml	ES	100 mg/ 2 ml	White precipitate forms within 5 min	1784	I
Hydromorphone HCl	KN	4 mg/ 2 ml	PF	50 mg/ 1 ml	Physically compatible for 30 min	517	C
	KN	0.75 mg/ 0.8 ml	PF	100 mg/ 2 ml	Physically compatible	771	C
Ketorolac tromethamine	SY	180 mg/ 6 ml	SO	150 mg/ 3 ml	Heavy white precipitate forms immediately, separating into two layers over time	1703	I
Lidocaine HCl	AST	2%/2 ml	PF	50 mg/ 2 ml	Physically compatible	771	C

Drugs in Syringe Compatibility (Cont.)

Hydroxyzine HCl

Drug (in syringe)	Mfr	Amt	Mfr	Amt	Remarks	Ref	C/I
	AST	2%/2 ml	PF	100 mg/ 2 ml	Physically compatible	771	**C**
Meperidine HCl	WI	100 mg/ 2 ml	PF	50 mg/ 1 ml	Physically compatible	771	**C**
	WI	50 mg/ 1 ml	PF	100 mg/ 2 ml	Physically compatible	771	**C**
	WY	100 mg/ 1 ml	PF	100 mg/ 4 ml	Physically compatible for at least 15 min	14	**C**
	WI	50 mg/ 1 ml	PF	50 mg/ 1 ml	Physically compatible for at least 15 min	326	**C**
Meperidine HCl with atropine sulfate[a]	WI ES	50 mg 0.4 mg	PF	50 mg/ 2.5 ml	No alteration of UV spectra in 10 days at 3 and 25 °C	301	**C**
Methotrimeprazine	LE	20 mg/ 1 ml	PF	50 mg/ 1 ml	Physically compatible	771	**C**
	LE	10 mg/ 0.5 ml	PF	100 mg/ 2 ml	Physically compatible	771	**C**
Metoclopramide HCl	NO	10 mg/ 2 ml	PF	50 mg/ 1 ml	Physically compatible both macroscopically and microscopically for 15 min at room temperature	565	**C**
Midazolam HCl	RC	5 mg/ 1 ml	ES	100 mg/ 2 ml	Physically compatible for 4 hr at 25 °C under fluorescent light	1145	**C**
Morphine sulfate	WY	15 mg/ 1 ml	PF	100 mg/ 4 ml	Physically compatible for at least 15 min	14	**C**
	ST	15 mg/ 1 ml	PF	50 mg/ 1 ml	Physically compatible for at least 15 min	326	**C**
		10 mg/ 0.7 ml	PF	50 mg/ 1 ml	Physically compatible	771	**C**
		5 mg/ 0.3 ml	PF	100 mg/ 2 ml	Physically compatible	771	**C**
Nalbuphine HCl	EN	10 mg/ 1 ml	PF	50 mg	Physically compatible for 36 hr at 27 °C	762	**C**
	EN	5 mg/ 0.5 ml	PF	50 mg	Physically compatible for 36 hr at 27 °C	762	**C**
	EN	2.5 mg/ 0.25 ml	PF	50 mg	Physically compatible for 36 hr at 27 °C	762	**C**
	DU	10 mg/ 1 ml	PF	25 mg/ 1 ml	Physically compatible for 48 hr	128	**C**
	DU	20 mg/ 1 ml	PF	25 mg/ 1 ml	Physically compatible for 48 hr	128	**C**
Oxymorphone HCl	EN	0.75 mg/ 0.5 ml	PF	100 mg/ 2 ml	Physically compatible	771	**C**
Pentazocine lactate	WI	60 mg/ 2 ml	PF	50 mg/ 1 ml	Physically compatible	771	**C**
	WI	30 mg/ 1 ml	PF	100 mg/ 2 ml	Physically compatible	771	**C**
	WI	30 mg/ 1 ml	PF	100 mg/ 4 ml	Physically compatible for at least 15 min	14	**C**
	WI	30 mg/ 1 ml	PF	50 mg/ 1 ml	Physically compatible for at least 15 min	326	**C**
Pentobarbital sodium	WY	100 mg/ 2 ml	PF	100 mg/ 4 ml	Precipitate forms within 15 min	14	**I**

Drugs in Syringe Compatibility (Cont.)

Hydroxyzine HCl

Drug (in syringe)	Mfr	Amt	Mfr	Amt	Remarks	Ref	C/I
	AB	50 mg/ 1 ml	PF	50 mg/ 1 ml	Physically incompatible within 15 min	326	I
Perphenazine	SC	10 mg/ 2 ml	ES	100 mg/ 2 ml	Visually compatible for 60 min	1784	C
Procaine HCl	WI	2%/2 ml	PF	50 mg/ 2 ml	Physically compatible	771	C
	WI	2%/2 ml	PF	100 mg/ 2 ml	Physically compatible	771	C
Prochlorperazine edisylate	PO	5 mg/ 1 ml	PF	50 mg/ 1 ml	Physically compatible for at least 15 min	326	C
Promazine HCl	WY	50 mg/ 1 ml	PF	50 mg/ 1 ml	Physically compatible for at least 15 min	326	C
Promethazine HCl	WY	50 mg/ 2 ml	PF	100 mg/ 4 ml	Physically compatible for at least 15 min	14	C
	PO	50 mg/ 2 ml	PF	50 mg/ 1 ml	Physically compatible for at least 15 min	326	C
Ranitidine HCl	GL	50 mg/ 2 ml	PF	50 mg/ 1 ml	Immediate white haze that disappeared following vortex mixing	978	I
Scopolamine HBr		0.6 mg/ 1.5 ml	PF	100 mg/ 4 ml	Physically compatible for at least 15 min	14	C
	ST	0.4 mg/ 1 ml	PF	50 mg/ 1 ml	Physically compatible for at least 15 min	326	C
		0.65 mg/ 1 ml	PF	100 mg/ 2 ml	Physically compatible	771	C
		0.65 mg/ 1 ml	PF	50 mg/ 1 ml	Physically compatible	771	C
Sufentanil citrate	JN	50 µg/ml	ES	50 mg/ ml	Physically compatible with no subvisual haze or particle formation in 24 hr at 23 °C	1711	C

[a]*Tested in both glass and plastic syringes.*

Y-Site Injection Compatibility (1:1 Mixture)

Hydroxyzine HCl

Drug	Mfr	Conc	Mfr	Conc	Remarks	Ref	C/I
Allopurinol sodium	BW	3 mg/ml[b]	ES	4 mg/ml[b]	Heavy white turbidity and precipitate form immediately	1686	I
Amifostine	USB	10 mg/ml[a]	WI	4 mg/ml[a]	Subvisual haze forms immediately	1845	I
Amphotericin B cholesteryl sulfate complex	SEQ	0.83 mg/ml[a]	ES	2 mg/ml[a]	Gross precipitate forms	2117	I
Aztreonam	SQ	40 mg/ml[a]	WI	4 mg/ml[a]	Physically compatible with no subvisual haze or particle formation in 4 hr at 23 °C	1758	C
Cefepime HCl	BR	20 mg/ml[a]	WI	4 mg/ml[a]	Haze forms immediately and becomes flocculent precipitate in 4 hr	1689	I
Ciprofloxacin	MI	2 mg/ml[c]	ES	50 mg/ml	Visually compatible for 24 hr at 24 °C	1655	C
Cisatracurium besylate	GW	0.1, 2, 5 mg/ml[a]	ES	2 mg/ml[a]	Physically compatible with no change in measured turbidity or increase in particle content in 4 hr at 23 °C	2074	C

Y-Site Injection Compatibility (1:1 Mixture) (Cont.)

			Hydroxyzine HCl				
Drug	Mfr	Conc	Mfr	Conc	Remarks	Ref	C/I
Cladribine	ORT	0.015[b] and 0.5[d] mg/ml	ES	4 mg/ml[b]	Physically compatible with no change in measured turbidity or increase in particle content in 4 hr at 23 °C	1969	C
Docetaxel	RPR	0.9 mg/ml[a]	ES	2 mg/ml[a]	Physically compatible with no change in measured turbidity or increase in particle content in 4 hr at 23 °C	2224	C
Doxorubicin HCl liposome injection	SEQ	0.4 mg/ml[a]	ES	2 mg/ml[a]	10-fold increase in particles ≥10 μm in 4 hr	2087	I
Etoposide phosphate	BR	5 mg/ml[a]	ES	4 mg/ml[a]	Physically compatible with no change in measured turbidity or increase in particle content in 4 hr at 23 °C	2218	C
Famotidine	ME	2 mg/ml[b]		4 mg/ml[a]	Visually compatible for 4 hr at 22 °C	1936	C
Filgrastim	AMG	30 μg/ml[a]	ES	4 mg/ml[a]	Physically compatible with no change in measured turbidity or increase in particle content in 4 hr at 22 °C	1687	C
Fluconazole	RR	2 mg/ml	ES	50 mg/ml	Cloudiness develops	1407	I
Fludarabine phosphate	BX	1 mg/ml[a]	WI	4 mg/ml[a]	Slight haze, visible with high intensity light, forms immediately	1439	I
Foscarnet sodium	AST	24 mg/ml	LY	50 mg/ml	Physically compatible for 24 hr at room temperature under fluorescent light	1335	C
Gemcitabine HCl	LI	10 mg/ml[b]	ES	2 mg/ml[b]	Physically compatible with no change in measured turbidity or increase in particle content in 4 hr at 23 °C	2226	C
Granisetron HCl	SKB	0.05 mg/ml[a]	ES	2 mg/ml[a]	Physically compatible with no change in measured turbidity or increase in particle content in 4 hr at 23 °C	2000	C
Melphalan HCl	BW	0.1 mg/ml[b]	WI	4 mg/ml[b]	Physically compatible with no change in measured turbidity or increase in particle content in 3 hr at 22 °C	1557	C
Ondansetron HCl	GL	1 mg/ml[b]	WI	4 mg/ml[a]	Physically compatible for 4 hr at 22 °C	1365	C
Paclitaxel	NCI	1.2 mg/ml[a]	ES	4 mg/ml[a]	Normal inherent haze from paclitaxel decreases immediately	1556	I
Piperacillin sodium–tazobactam sodium	LE	40 + 5 mg/ml[a]	WI	4 mg/ml[a]	Haze and particles form immediately	1688	I
Propofol	ZEN	10 mg/ml	ES	2 mg/ml[a]	Physically compatible for 1 hr at 23 °C with no increase in particle content	2066	C
Remifentanil HCl	GW	0.025 and 0.25 mg/ml[b]	ES	2 mg/ml[a]	Physically compatible with no change in measured turbidity or increase in particle content in 4 hr at 23 °C	2075	C
Sargramostim	IMM	10 μg/ml[b]	ES	4 mg/ml[b]	Slight haze, visible with high intensity light, and small flake-like particles formed in 4 hr in one of two samples	1436	I
Sufentanil citrate	JN	12.5 μg/ml[a]	ES	4 mg/ml[a]	Physically compatible with little subvisual haze or particle formation in 24 hr at 23 °C	1711	C
Teniposide	BR	0.1 mg/ml[a]	WI	4 mg/ml[a]	Physically compatible with no subvisual haze or particle formation in 4 hr at 23 °C	1725	C

Y-Site Injection Compatibility (1:1 Mixture) (Cont.)

Hydroxyzine HCl

Drug	Mfr	Conc	Mfr	Conc	Remarks	Ref	C/I
Thiotepa	IMM[e]	1 mg/ml[a]	ES	4 mg/ml[a]	Physically compatible with no change in measured turbidity or increase in particle content in 4 hr at 23 °C	1861	C
TNA #218 to #226[f]			ES	2 mg/ml[a]	Visually compatible with no precipitate or emulsion damage apparent in 4 hr at 23 °C	2215	C
TPN #212 to #215[f]			ES	2 mg/ml[a]	Physically compatible with no change in measured turbidity or increase in particle content in 4 hr at 23 °C	2109	C
Vinorelbine tartrate	BW	1 mg/ml[b]	ES	4 mg/ml[b]	Physically compatible with no change in measured turbidity or increase in particle content in 4 hr at 22 °C	1558	C

[a]*Tested in dextrose 5% in water.*
[b]*Tested in sodium chloride 0.9%.*
[c]*Tested in both dextrose 5% in water and sodium chloride 0.9%.*
[d]*Tested in bacteriostatic sodium chloride 0.9% preserved with benzyl alcohol 0.9%.*
[e]*Lyophilized formulation tested.*
[f]*Refer to Appendix I for the composition of parenteral nutrition solutions. TNA indicates a 3-in-1 admixture, and TPN indicates a 2-in-1 admixture.*

Additional Compatibility Information

Miscellaneous— Hydroxyzine HCl is stated to be physically and chemically compatible with butorphanol tartrate (Bristol) (481) and buprenorphine HCl (4).

Chlorpromazine and Meperidine— Chlorpromazine HCl (Elkins-Sinn) 6.25 mg/ml, hydroxyzine HCl (Pfizer) 12.5 mg/ml, and meperidine HCl (Winthrop) 25 mg/ml, in both glass and plastic syringes, were reported to be physically compatible and chemically stable for at least one year at 4 and 25 °C when protected from light. Significant discoloration, ranging from yellow to brownish yellow, occurred on storage at 44 °C (989).

Heparin— It has been stated that if hydroxyzine HCl is injected into a heparinized scalp vein infusion set, a precipitate will form. It has been suggested that these heparinized sets be flushed with sterile water for injection or sodium chloride 0.9% before and after ad-ministering a drug. Heparin lock flush solution may then be reinjected into the device (97).

Concentrated Solutions— The following incompatibility determinations were performed with concentrated solutions. The drugs in dry form were constituted according to the manufacturers' recommendations. One milliliter of hydroxyzine HCl (Pfizer) was added to 5 ml of sterile distilled water along with 1 ml of each of the following drugs. Particulate matter was noted within two hours (28):

> Aminophylline
> Chloramphenicol sodium succinate (Parke-Davis)
> Dimenhydrinate (Searle)
> Heparin sodium
> Penicillin G potassium
> Phenobarbital sodium (Winthrop)
> Phenytoin sodium (Parke-Davis)
> Vitamin B complex with C (Lederle)

IDARUBICIN HCL
AHFS 10:00

Idamycin   **Pharmacia & Upjohn**
Idamycin PFS   **Pharmacia & Upjohn**

Products— Idarubicin HCl (Pharmacia & Upjohn) is available as an orange-red lyophilized powder in single-use vials containing 5, 10, and 20 mg. Also present is lactose NF (hydrous) 50, 100, and 200 mg, respectively (1-8/98).

The 5-, 10-, and 20-mg vials should be reconstituted with 5, 10, and 20 ml, respectively, of water for injection to yield a 1-mg/ml concentration. Bacteriostatic diluents are not recommended by the manufacturer. The vial contents are under negative pressure to minimize aerosolization (1-8/98).

Idarubicin HCl (Idamycin PFS, Pharmacia & Upjohn) is also available as a 1-mg/ml orange-red solution in single-use vials containing 5, 10, and 20 ml. In addition to the drug, each milliliter also contains glycerin 25 mg and hydrochloric acid to adjust pH in water for injection (2).

pH— The reconstituted lyophilized idarubicin HCl (Idamycin) has a pH in the range of 5 to 7 (1368). The idarubicin HCl solution (Idamycin PFS) has been adjusted with hydrochloric acid to a target pH of 3.5 (2).

Administration— Idarubicin HCl should be administered by slow intravenous injection over 10 to 15 minutes into the tubing of a running infusion of sodium chloride 0.9% or dextrose 5% in water. The drug should not be given subcutaneously or intramuscularly, and extravasation should be avoided to prevent severe tissue necrosis. Care should be exercised during dose preparation to avoid inadvertent skin contact with the drug (1-8/98; 2).

Stability— Idarubicin HCl in intact lyophilized vials should be stored at room temperature and protected from light. The reconstituted solution is physically and chemically stable for at least 72 hours under refrigeration or at room temperature (1-8/98).

Idarubicin HCl solution (Idamycin PFS) in intact vials should be stored under refrigeration at 2 to 8 °C and protected from light. Leaving the vials in the carton until the time of use is recommended (2).

Idarubicin HCl in prolonged contact with alkaline solutions will undergo decomposition (1-8/98; 2).

Dilute solutions (0.01 mg/ml) of idarubicin HCl are light sensitive, undergoing some degradation with exposure to light over periods greater than six hours (1368). However, the manufacturer indicates that no special precautions are necessary to protect freshly prepared solutions for administration (1369). The drug is unstable in alkaline solutions, resulting in degradation after prolonged contact (1-8/98; 2; 1368).

Idarubicin HCl is compatible with PVC, glass, and polypropylene (1369).

Haze Formation— Idarubicin HCl solutions in sodium chloride 0.9% exhibit a low level haze that is visible under high intensity light and measurable with a turbidimeter. Dilution of the drug from concentrations of 0.5 to 1 mg/ml increases this haze until a maximum is reached at about 0.05 mg/ml. This haze increase appears to be normal for idarubicin HCl in solution and is not an incompatibility (1675).

Compatibility Information

Solution Compatibility

Idarubicin HCl

Solution	Mfr	Conc/L	Remarks	Ref	C/I
Dextrose 3.3% in sodium chloride 0.3%	FA	100 mg	5% or less drug loss in 4 weeks at 25 °C in the dark	1007	**C**
Dextrose 5% in sodium chloride 0.9%	FA	10 mg	No drug loss in 72 hr at room temperature protected from light. Less than 10% loss in 6 hr at room temperature exposed to light	1493	**C**
Dextrose 5% in water	FA	100 mg	5% or less drug loss in 4 weeks at 25 °C in the dark	1007	**C**
	FA	10 mg	No drug loss in 72 hr at room temperature protected from light. Less than 10% loss in 6 hr at room temperature exposed to light	1493	**C**
Ringer's injection, lactated	FA	100 mg	5% or less drug loss in 4 weeks at 25 °C in the dark	1007	**C**
Sodium chloride 0.9%	FA	100 mg	5% or less drug loss in 4 weeks at 25 °C in the dark	1007	**C**
	FA	10 mg	No drug loss in 72 hr at room temperature protected from light. Less than 10% loss in 6 hr at room temperature exposed to light	1493	**C**

Y-Site Injection Compatibility (1:1 Mixture)

Idarubicin HCl

Drug	Mfr	Conc	Mfr	Conc	Remarks	Ref	C/I
Acyclovir sodium	BW	5 mg/ml[b]	AD	1 mg/ml[b]	Haze forms and color changes immediately. Precipitate forms in 12 min	1525	**I**
Allopurinol sodium	BW	3 mg/ml[b]	AD	0.5 mg/ml[b]	Reddish-purple color forms immediately. Particles form within 1 hr. Complete color loss in 24 hr	1686	**I**
Amifostine	USB	10 mg/ml[a]	AD	0.5 mg/ml[a]	Increase in turbidity no greater than dilution with D5W alone. No increase in particle content in 4 hr at 23 °C	1845	**C**

Y-Site Injection Compatibility (1:1 Mixture) (Cont.)

Idarubicin HCl

Drug	Mfr	Conc	Mfr	Conc	Remarks	Ref	C/I
Amikacin sulfate	BR	5 mg/ml[a]	AD	1 mg/ml[b]	Visually compatible for 24 hr at 25 °C	1525	C
Ampicillin sodium–sulbactam sodium	RR	20 + 10 mg/ml[b]	AD	1 mg/ml[b]	Haze forms and color changes immediately. Precipitate forms in 20 min	1525	I
Aztreonam	SQ	40 mg/ml[a]	AD	0.5 mg/ml[a]	Increase in measured turbidity no greater than dilution of idarubicin with NS. No increase in particle content in 4 hr at 23 °C	1758	C
Cefazolin sodium	LI	20 mg/ml[a]	AD	1 mg/ml[b]	Precipitate forms in 1 hr	1525	I
Cefepime HCl	BR	20 mg/ml[a]	AD	0.5 mg/ml[a]	Flocculent precipitate forms in 4 hr	1689	I
Ceftazidime	LI[f]	20 mg/ml[a]	AD	1 mg/ml[b]	Haze forms in 1 hr	1525	I
Cimetidine HCl	SKF	6 mg/ml[a]	AD	1 mg/ml[b]	Visually compatible for 24 hr at 25 °C	1525	C
Cladribine	ORT	0.015[b] and 0.5[c] mg/ml	AD	0.5 mg/ml[b]	Increase in measured turbidity no greater than simple dilution alone. No increase in particle content in 4 hr at 23 °C	1969	C
Clindamycin phosphate	AST	12 mg/ml[a]	AD	1 mg/ml[b]	Haze and precipitate form immediately	1525	I
Cyclophosphamide	AD	4 mg/ml[a]	AD	1 mg/ml[b]	Visually compatible for 24 hr at 25 °C	1525	C
Cytarabine	CET	6 mg/ml[a]	AD	1 mg/ml[b]	Visually compatible for 24 hr at 25 °C	1525	C
Dexamethasone sodium phosphate	OR	10 mg/ml	AD	1 mg/ml[b]	Haze forms immediately and precipitate forms in 20 min	1525	I
	AMR	0.2 mg/ml[b]	AD	1 mg/ml[b]	Haze forms in 20 min	1525	I
Diphenhydramine HCl	ES	1[a] and 50 mg/ml	AD	1 mg/ml[b]	Visually compatible for 24 hr at 25 °C	1525	C
Droperidol	AMR	0.04[a] and 2.5 mg/ml	AD	1 mg/ml[b]	Visually compatible for 24 hr at 25 °C	1525	C
Erythromycin lactobionate	ES	2 mg/ml[b]	AD	1 mg/ml[b]	Visually compatible for 24 hr at 25 °C	1525	C
Etoposide	BR	0.4 mg/ml[a]	AD	1 mg/ml[b]	Gas forms immediately	1525	I
Etoposide phosphate	BR	5 mg/ml[a]	AD	0.5 mg/ml[a]	Physically compatible with no change in measured turbidity or increase in particle content in 4 hr at 23 °C	2218	C
Filgrastim	AMG	30 μg/ml[a]	AD	0.5 mg/ml[a]	Physically compatible with no change in measured turbidity or increase in particle content in 4 hr at 22 °C	1687	C
Furosemide	AB	10 mg/ml	AD	1 mg/ml[b]	Precipitate forms immediately	1525	I
	AB	0.8 mg/ml[b]	AD	1 mg/ml[b]	Haze forms immediately	1525	I
Gemcitabine HCl	LI	10 mg/ml[b]	AD	0.5 mg/ml[b]	Physically compatible with no change in measured turbidity or increase in particle content in 4 hr at 23 °C	2226	C
Gentamicin sulfate	ES	3 mg/ml[a]	AD	1 mg/ml[b]	Color changes immediately	1525	I
Granisetron HCl	SKB	0.05 mg/ml[a]	AD	0.5 mg/ml[a]	Increase in turbidity no greater than dilution with D5W alone. No increase in particle content in 4 hr at 23 °C	2000	C
Heparin sodium	ES	1000 units/ml	AD	1 mg/ml[b]	Haze forms immediately and precipitate forms in 20 min	1525	I
	SO	100 units/ml	AD	1 mg/ml[b]	Haze forms immediately and precipitate forms in 12 min	1525	I

Y-Site Injection Compatibility (1:1 Mixture) (Cont.)

Idarubicin HCl

Drug	Mfr	Conc	Mfr	Conc	Remarks	Ref	C/I
Hydrocortisone sodium succinate	UP	2[a] and 50 mg/ml	AD	1 mg/ml[b]	Haze forms immediately and precipitate forms in 20 min	1525	I
Imipenem–cilastatin sodium	MSD	5 mg/ml[b]	AD	1 mg/ml[b]	Visually compatible for 12 hr at 25 °C under fluorescent light. Precipitate forms in 24 hr	1525	C
Lorazepam	WY	2 mg/ml	AD	1 mg/ml[b]	Color changes immediately	1525	I
Magnesium sulfate	SO	2 mg/ml[b]	AD	1 mg/ml[b]	Visually compatible for 24 hr at 25 °C	1525	C
Mannitol	AB	12.5 mg/ml[a]	AD	1 mg/ml[b]	Visually compatible for 24 hr at 25 °C	1525	C
Melphalan HCl	BW	0.1 mg/ml[b]	AD	0.5 mg/ml[b]	Increase in measured turbidity no greater than dilution of idarubicin with sodium chloride 0.9%. No increase in particle content in 4 hr at 22 °C	1557; 1675	C
Meperidine HCl	WY	1[a] and 50 mg/ml	AD	1 mg/ml[b]	Color changes immediately	1525	I
Methotrexate sodium	LE	25 mg/ml	AD	1 mg/ml[b]	Color changes immediately	1525	I
Metoclopramide HCl	SO	5 mg/ml	AD	1 mg/ml[b]	Visually compatible for 24 hr at 25 °C	1525	C
Piperacillin sodium–tazobactam sodium	LE	40 + 5 mg/ml[a]	AD	0.5 mg/ml[a]	Immediate increase in haze much larger than from simple dilution alone	1688	I
Potassium chloride	AB	0.03 mEq/ml[b]	AD	1 mg/ml[b]	Visually compatible for 24 hr at 25 °C	1525	C
Ranitidine HCl	GL	1 mg/ml[a]	AD	1 mg/ml[b]	Visually compatible for 24 hr at 25 °C	1525	C
Sargramostim	IMM	10 μg/ml[b]	AD	0.5 mg/ml[b]	Increase in measured turbidity no greater than dilution of idarubicin with sodium chloride 0.9%	1675	C
Sodium bicarbonate	AB	0.09 mEq/ml[a]	AD	1 mg/ml[b]	Haze forms and color changes immediately. Precipitate forms in 20 min	1525	I
Teniposide	BR	0.1 mg/ml[a]	AD	0.5 mg/ml[a]	Unacceptable increase in turbidity occurs immediately	1725	I
Thiotepa	IMM[d]	1 mg/ml[a]	AD	0.5 mg/ml[a]	Increase in measured turbidity no greater than simple dilution alone. No increase in particle content in 4 hr at 23 °C	1861	C
TPN #140[e]			AD	1 mg/ml[b]	Visually compatible for 24 hr at 25 °C	1525	C
Vancomycin HCl	AD	4 mg/ml[a]	AD	1 mg/ml[b]	Color changes immediately	1525	I
Vincristine sulfate	AD	1 mg/ml	AD	1 mg/ml[b]	Color changes immediately	1525	I
Vinorelbine tartrate	BW	1 mg/ml[b]	AD	0.5 mg/ml[b]	Increase in measured turbidity no greater than dilution of idarubicin with sodium chloride 0.9%. No increase in particle content in 4 hr at 22 °C	1558; 1675	C

[a]Tested in dextrose 5% in water.
[b]Tested in sodium chloride 0.9%.
[c]Tested in bacteriostatic sodium chloride 0.9% preserved with benzyl alcohol 0.9%.
[d]Lyophilized formulation tested.
[e]Refer to Appendix I for the composition of parenteral nutrition solutions. TPN indicates a 2-in-1 admixture.
[f]Sodium carbonate–containing formulation tested.

Additional Compatibility Information

Heparin— According to the manufacturer, idarubicin HCl is physically incompatible with heparin due to precipitate formation (1-8/98; 2; 1368).

Other Information

Bacterial Challenge— Idarubicin HCl (Farmitalia) 0.07 mg/ml diluted in sodium chloride 0.9% and stored at 22 °C did not exhibit an antimicrobial effect on the growth of four organisms (*Enterococcus faecium*, *Staphylococcus aureus*, *Pseudomonas aeruginosa*, and *Candida albicans*) inoculated into the solution. Viability was maintained for periods of 48 to 120 hours. The author recommended that diluted solutions of idarubicin HCl be stored under refrigeration whenever possible and that the potential for microbiological growth should be considered when assigning expiration periods (2160).

IFOSFAMIDE
AHFS 10:00

Ifex　　　　　　　　　　　　　　**Bristol-Myers Squibb**

Products— Ifosfamide (Bristol-Myers Squibb) is available in vials containing 1 or 3 g of drug in combination packages with mesna injection. Reconstitute the ifosfamide with 20 or 60 ml of sterile water for injection or bacteriostatic water for injection (parabens or benzyl alcohol), respectively, to yield a 50-mg/ml solution (2).

pH— Approximately 6 (72).

Administration— Ifosfamide is administered by slow intravenous infusion over a minimum of 30 minutes diluted to a concentration between 0.6 and 20 mg/ml. To prevent bladder toxicity, mesna and at least 2 L/day of fluid should also be given (2).

Stability— Intact vials of ifosfamide should be stored at controlled room temperature and protected from temperatures above 30 °C (2). Ifosfamide may liquify at temperatures above 35 °C (72).

The reconstituted solution is stated to be chemically and physically stable for seven days at 30 °C and for three (4) to six (72) weeks under refrigeration. Because of microbiological concerns, the manufacturer recommends storage under refrigeration and use in 24 hours for reconstituted or diluted ifosfamide solutions (2).

Radford et al. reported that ifosfamide (Boehringer-Ingelheim) 80 mg/ml in sodium chloride 0.9% is chemically stable, exhibiting about a 7% loss in nine days at 37 °C in the dark (1494).

Ifosfamide 0.6 and 20 mg/ml in dextrose 5% in water, Ringer's injection, lactated, sodium chloride 0.9%, or sterile water for injection, in polypropylene syringes (Becton-Dickinson), is physically and chemically stable for at least 24 hours at 30 °C (1496).

Reconstitution to an ifosfamide concentration of 100 mg/ml with benzyl alcohol-preserved bacteriostatic water for injection resulted in a turbid mixture, separating into two distinct liquid phases. The separate phases dissolved completely, with no loss of drug or preservative, when diluted to about 60 mg/ml or less (1289).

Ifosfamide, reconstituted according to the manufacturer's instructions, was cultured with human lymphoblasts to determine whether its cytotoxic activity was retained. The solution retained cytotoxicity for 24 hours at 4 °C and room temperature (1575).

pH Effects— Ifosfamide exhibits maximum solution stability in the pH range of 4 to 10; the rate of decomposition is essentially the same over this pH range. At pH values less than 4 and above 10, increased rates of decomposition have been observed (2002).

Compatibility Information

Solution Compatibility

Ifosfamide

Solution	Mfr	Mfr	Conc/L	Remarks	Ref	C/I
Dextrose 5% in Ringer's injection			600 mg and 16 g	Physically compatible with less than 5% loss in 7 days at room temperature and no loss in 6 weeks under refrigeration	72	**C**
Dextrose 5% in sodium chloride 0.9%			600 mg and 16 g	Physically compatible with less than 5% loss in 7 days at room temperature and no loss in 6 weeks under refrigeration	72	**C**
Dextrose 5% in water			600 mg and 16 g	Physically compatible with less than 5% loss in 7 days at room temperature and no loss in 6 weeks under refrigeration	72	**C**

Solution Compatibility (Cont.)

Ifosfamide

Solution	Mfr	Mfr	Conc/L	Remarks	Ref	C/I
Ringer's injection, lactated			600 mg and 16 g	Physically compatible with less than 5% loss in 7 days at room temperature and no loss in 6 weeks under refrigeration	72	**C**
Sodium chloride 0.45%			600 mg and 16 g	Physically compatible with less than 5% loss in 7 days at room temperature and no loss in 6 weeks under refrigeration	72	**C**
Sodium chloride 0.9%			600 mg and 16 g	Physically compatible with less than 5% loss in 7 days at room temperature and no loss in 6 weeks under refrigeration	72	**C**
	a		10 g	No ifosfamide loss by HPLC in 8 days at 4 and 25 °C protected from light and at 25 °C exposed to light	1551	**C**
	a		20, 40, 80 g	No ifosfamide loss by HPLC in 8 days at 35 °C	1551	**C**
Sodium lactate ⅙ M			600 mg and 16 g	Physically compatible with less than 5% loss in 7 days at room temperature and no loss in 6 weeks under refrigeration	72	**C**

[a] Tested in PVC containers.

Additive Compatibility

Ifosfamide

Drug	Mfr	Conc/L	Mfr	Conc/L	Test Soln	Remarks	Ref	C/I
Carboplatin		1 g		1 g	W	Both drugs stable for 5 days at room temperature	1379	**C**
Carboplatin with etoposide		1 g 200 mg		2 g	W	Both drugs stable for 7 days at room temperature	1379	**C**
Cisplatin		200 mg		2 g	NS	Both drugs stable for 7 days at room temperature	1379	**C**
Cisplatin with etoposide		200 mg 200 mg		2 g	NS	All drugs stable for 5 days at room temperature	1379	**C**
Epirubicin HCl		1 g		50 g	NS	Both drugs stable for 14 days at room temperature	1380	**C**
Etoposide		200 mg		2 g	NS	Both drugs stable for 5 days at room temperature	1379	**C**
Fluorouracil		10 g		2 g	NS	Both drugs stable for 5 days at room temperature	1379	**C**
Mesna	AW	3.3 g	MJ	3.3 g	D5W, LR	Physically compatible with no ifosfamide loss and about 5% mesna loss in 24 hr at 21 °C exposed to light	72	**C**
	AW	5 g	MJ	5 g	D5W, LR	Physically compatible with no ifosfamide loss and about 5% mesna loss in 24 hr at 21 °C exposed to light	72	**C**
		40 g		50 g	NS	Both drugs stable for 14 days at room temperature	1380	**C**
	BI	79 g	BI	83.3 g	NS	Little or no ifosfamide loss in 9 days at room temperature and 7% ifosfamide loss in 9 days at 37 °C. Mesna not tested	1494	**C**

Additive Compatibility (Cont.)

		Ifosfamide					
Drug	Mfr	Conc/L	Mfr	Conc/L	Test Soln	Remarks	Ref	C/I
		1.6 g		2.6 g	D5S[a]	No increase in decomposition products in 8 hr at room temperature	1495	**C**
	BR	600 mg	BR	600 mg	D5½S, D5W, LR, NS[b]	Both drugs chemically stable for at least 24 hr at room temperature	1496	**C**
Mesna with epirubicin HCl		80 g 500 mg		50 g	NS	Over 50% epirubicin loss in 7 days at room temperature	1380	**I**

[a]Tested in polyethylene containers.
[b]Tested in PVC containers.

Drugs in Syringe Compatibility

		Ifosfamide				
Drug (in syringe)	Mfr	Amt	Mfr	Amt	Remarks	Ref	C/I
Epirubicin HCl		1 mg/ml[a]		50 mg/ml[a]	Little or no loss of either drug by HPLC in 28 days at 4 and 20 °C	1564	**C**
Mesna		400 mg/ 10 ml		500 mg/ 10 ml	3% ifosfamide loss in 7 days and 12% in 4 weeks at 4 °C and room temperature. No mesna loss	1290	**C**
		40 mg/ ml[a]		50 mg/ ml[a]	Little or no loss of either drug by HPLC in 28 days at 4 and 20 °C	1564	**C**
Mesna with epirubicin HCl		40 mg/ ml[a] 1 mg/ml		50 mg/ ml[a]	50% epirubicin loss by HPLC in 7 days at 4 and 20 °C. No loss of other drugs in 7 days	1564	**I**

[a]Diluted in sodium chloride 0.9%.

Y-Site Injection Compatibility (1:1 Mixture)

		Ifosfamide				
Drug	Mfr	Conc	Mfr	Conc	Remarks	Ref	C/I
Allopurinol sodium	BW	3 mg/ml[b]	MJ	25 mg/ml[b]	Physically compatible with no change in measured turbidity or increase in particle content in 4 hr at 22 °C	1686	**C**
Amifostine	USB	10 mg/ml[a]	MJ	25 mg/ml[a]	Physically compatible with no change in measured turbidity or increase in particle content in 4 hr at 23 °C	1845	**C**
Amphotericin B cholesteryl sulfate complex	SEQ	0.83 mg/ml[a]	MJ	25 mg/ml[a]	Physically compatible with little or no change in measured turbidity or increase in particle content in 4 hr at 23 °C under fluorescent light	2117	**C**
Aztreonam	SQ	40 mg/ml[a]	MJ	25 mg/ml[a]	Physically compatible with no subvisual haze or particle formation in 4 hr at 23 °C	1758	**C**
Cefepime HCl	BR	20 mg/ml[a]	MJ	25 mg/ml[a]	Haze and precipitate form in 1 hr	1689	**I**

Y-Site Injection Compatibility (1:1 Mixture) (Cont.)

Ifosfamide

Drug	Mfr	Conc	Mfr	Conc	Remarks	Ref	C/I
Doxorubicin HCl liposome injection	SEQ	0.4 mg/ml[a]	MJ	25 mg/ml[a]	Physically compatible with little or no change in measured turbidity and no increase in particle content in 4 hr at 23 °C	2087	C
Etoposide phosphate	BR	5 mg/ml[a]	MJ	25 mg/ml[a]	Physically compatible with no change in measured turbidity or increase in particle content in 4 hr at 23 °C	2118	C
Filgrastim	AMG	30 μg/ml[a]	MJ	25 mg/ml[a]	Physically compatible with no change in measured turbidity or increase in particle content in 4 hr at 22 °C	1687	C
Fludarabine phosphate	BX	1 mg/ml[a]	MJ	25 mg/ml[a]	Physically compatible for 4 hr at room temperature under fluorescent light	1439	C
Gemcitabine HCl	LI	10 mg/ml[b]	MJ	25 mg/ml[b]	Physically compatible with no change in measured turbidity or increase in particle content in 4 hr at 23 °C	2226	C
Granisetron HCl	SKB	1 mg/ml	MJ	4 mg/ml[b]	Physically compatible with little or no loss of either drug by HPLC in 4 hr at 22 °C	1883	C
Melphalan HCl	BW	0.1 mg/ml[b]	BR	25 mg/ml[b]	Physically compatible with no change in measured turbidity or increase in particle content in 3 hr at 22 °C	1557	C
Methotrexate sodium		30 mg/ml		36 mg/ml[a]	Visually compatible for 2 hr at room temperature. Dark yellow precipitate forms in 4 hr	1788	I
Ondansetron HCl	GL	1 mg/ml[b]	MJ	25 mg/ml[a]	Physically compatible for 4 hr at 22 °C	1365	C
Paclitaxel	NCI	1.2 mg/ml[a]	BR	25 mg/ml[a]	Physically compatible with no change in measured turbidity in 4 hr at 22 °C	1556	C
Piperacillin sodium–tazobactam sodium	LE	40 + 5 mg/ml[a]	MJ	25 mg/ml[a]	Physically compatible with no change in measured turbidity or increase in particle content in 4 hr at 22 °C	1688	C
Propofol	ZEN	10 mg/ml	MJ	25 mg/ml[a]	Physically compatible for 1 hr at 23 °C with no increase in particle content	2066	C
Sargramostim	IMM	10 μg/ml[b]	MJ	25 mg/ml[b]	Physically compatible for 4 hr at 22 °C	1436	C
Sodium bicarbonate		1.4%		36 mg/ml[a]	Visually compatible for 4 hr at room temperature	1788	C
Teniposide	BR	0.1 mg/ml[a]	MJ	25 mg/ml[a]	Physically compatible with no subvisual haze or particle formation in 4 hr at 23 °C	1725	C
Thiotepa	IMM[c]	1 mg/ml[a]	MJ	25 mg/ml[a]	Physically compatible with no change in measured turbidity or increase in particle content in 4 hr at 23 °C	1861	C
TNA #218 to #226[d]			MJ	25 mg/ml[a]	Visually compatible with no precipitate or emulsion damage apparent in 4 hr at 23 °C	2215	C
TPN #212 to #215[d]			MJ	25 mg/ml[a]	Physically compatible with no change in measured turbidity or increase in particle content in 4 hr at 23 °C	2109	C

Y-Site Injection Compatibility (1:1 Mixture) (Cont.)

Ifosfamide

Drug	Mfr	Conc	Mfr	Conc	Remarks	Ref	C/I
Vinorelbine tartrate	BW	1 mg/ml[b]	MJ	25 mg/ml[b]	Physically compatible with no change in measured turbidity or increase in particle content in 4 hr at 22 °C	1558	C

[a]*Tested in dextrose 5% in water.*
[b]*Tested in sodium chloride 0.9%.*
[c]*Lyophilized formulation tested.*
[d]*Refer to Appendix I for the composition of parenteral nutrition solutions. TNA indicates a 3-in-1 admixture, and TPN indicates a 2-in-1 admixture.*

Additional Compatibility Information

Solutions— The manufacturer states that ifosfamide may be diluted to concentrations between 0.6 and 20 mg/ml in the following solutions (2):

> Dextrose 5% in water
> Ringer's injection, lactated
> Sodium chloride 0.9%

Intermediate concentrations and mixtures of these diluents (e.g., dextrose 2.5% in water, dextrose 5% in sodium chloride 0.9%, etc.) are also acceptable as infusion solutions for the dilution of ifosfamide (2).

Reconstituted solutions of ifosfamide that are diluted for administration in one of the compatible infusion solutions are stated to be physically and chemically stable in glass, polyolefin, or PVC containers for at least a week at 30 °C and six weeks at 5 °C (4).

Mesna— Ifosfamide is stated to be physically and chemically stable for 24 hours in dextrose 5% in water or Ringer's injection, lactated, when admixed with mesna (4).

IMIPENEM–CILASTATIN SODIUM
AHFS 8:12.07

Primaxin I.V.   **Merck**
Primaxin I.M.   **Merck**

Products— Imipenem–cilastatin sodium (Merck) for intravenous use is available as a fixed combination of equal quantities of both drugs. The combination is provided in vials and infusion bottles containing 250 and 500 mg of each drug with sodium bicarbonate 10 and 20 mg, respectively (2).

The vials should be reconstituted with about 10 ml of a compatible diluent from a 100-ml infusion container and shaken well to form a suspension. Diluents containing benzyl alcohol should not be used to reconstitute the drug for use in neonates and small pediatric patients. The suspension must be transferred to the remaining solution in the infusion container for dilution. The suspension is *not* for direct injection. The procedure is then repeated: a 10-ml aliquot from the admixture is added to the vial and, once again, returned to the infusion admixture. This procedure ensures that all of the vial contents are transferred. The admixture should be agitated until it is clear to yield either a 2.5- or 5-mg/ml concentration, depending on the vial content. The admixture should *not* be heated to aid dissolution (2; 4).

ADD-Vantage vials of imipenem–cilastatin sodium should be prepared with 100 ml of dextrose 5% in water or sodium chloride 0.9% in ADD-Vantage diluent bags (2; 4).

The 250- and 500-mg piggyback infusion bottles should be reconstituted with 100 ml of compatible diluent and shaken until clear to yield 2.5- and 5-mg/ml concentrations, respectively (2; 4).

Imipenem–cilastatin sodium (Merck) for intramuscular use is available in vials containing 500 or 750 mg of each component. The vials should be reconstituted with 2 or 3 ml, respectively, of lidocaine HCl 1% (without epinephrine) and agitated to form a suspension. This intramuscular formulation is not for intravenous use (2; 4).

pH— The intravenous product is buffered to pH 6.5 to 7.5 (2; 4).

Osmolarity— When reconstituted and diluted as directed by the manufacturer, the osmolarity of the intravenous admixture approximates that of the diluent (4).

Sodium Content— The 250- and 500-mg intravenous vials contain 0.8 mEq (18.8 mg) and 1.6 mEq (37.5 mg) of sodium, respectively. The 500- and 750-mg intramuscular vials contain 1.4 mEq (32 mg) and 2.1 mEq (48 mg) of sodium, respectively (2; 4).

Administration— Imipenem–cilastatin sodium for intravenous use is given by intermittent intravenous infusion, usually in sodium chloride 0.9%, at a concentration not exceeding 5 mg/ml. Infusion periods vary from 20 to 30 minutes up to 40 to 60 minutes, depending on the dose. The intramuscular formulation reconstituted as directed should be injected deeply into a large muscle mass. Suspensions of either formulation should not be given intravenously (2; 4).

Stability— The sterile powder for injection should be stored below 25 °C (2; 4).

Reconstituted as directed, intravenous solutions are colorless to yellow but may become a deeper yellow over time. Intramuscular suspensions are white to light tan. The manufacturer indicates that potency is not affected by color variations within this range (2), but the solutions should be discarded if they darken to brown (4). Intramuscular suspensions should be used within one hour of preparation (2; 4).

In solution, imipenem is substantially less stable than cilastatin and is the determining factor in the overall stability of the combination product. Reconstitution with most recommended infusion solutions (see Additional Compatibility Information) results in solutions that are stable for four hours at room temperature or 24 hours under refrigeration at 4 °C (2).

Imipenem degradation kinetics were determined for a 2.5-mg/ml solution in sodium chloride 0.9%. The degradation rates were temperature dependent, with a half-life of over 44 hours at 2 °C dropping to six hours at 25 °C and to two hours at 37 °C. The decomposition was consistent with hydrolysis, and the loss of antimicrobial activity suggests cleavage of the β-lactam ring (1272).

The decomposition of imipenem as a 5-mg/ml solution in dextrose 5% in water in the presence of cilastatin was estimated to occur at a rate of about 1.4% per hour at room temperature. At this rate, the time to 10% decomposition will be reached in 6 to 7 hours (2166).

pH Effects— Imipenem is inactivated at acidic or alkaline pH but is more stable at neutral pH (4). The pH range of maximum stability appears to be 6.5 to 7.5, with increasing rates of decomposition occurring as the pH moves away from this range (1273). At a pH of about 4, the half-life of imipenem is about 35 minutes (2166).

Freezing Solutions— The manufacturer recommends that imipenem–cilastatin solutions not be frozen (2). At concentrations of 250 and 500 mg/100 ml in sodium chloride 0.9%, imipenem losses of around 15% occurred in one week when frozen at −20 and −10 °C (1141). Freezing solutions at temperatures above −70 °C offers no stability advantage over refrigerated storage (1141) and results in decomposition of imipenem in a manner similar to ampicillin (4).

Effects of Solution Components— Dextrose exerts an adverse effect on the stability of imipenem. Dextrose 5 and 10% reduced the time to 10% decomposition by about one-half compared to sterile water. Similarly, increasing mannitol concentrations reduce imipenem stability. Sodium chloride content increases imipenem stability because of a positive kinetic salt effect similar to other β-lactam antibiotics. Both lactate and bicarbonate anions attack the β-lactam ring and decrease imipenem stability (1141). (See Additional Compatibility Information.)

Elastomeric Reservoir Pumps— Imipenem–cilastatin sodium (Merck) 5 mg/ml in dextrose 5% in water and sodium chloride 0.9% 100 ml was packaged in latex elastomeric reservoirs (Secure Medical). Little or no loss by HPLC analysis occurred in 4 hours at 25 °C and in 24 hr at 5 °C (1970).

Imipenem–cilastatin sodium (Merck) 5 mg/ml in both dextrose 5% in water and sodium chloride 0.9% was evaluated for binding potential to natural rubber elastomeric reservoirs (Baxter). Less than 1% loss was found after storage for two weeks at 35 °C with gentle agitation (2014).

Compatibility Information

Solution Compatibility

Imipenem–cilastatin sodium

Solution	Mfr	Mfr	Conc/L	Remarks	Ref	C/I
Dextrose 5% with potassium chloride 0.15%	AB[a]	MSD	2.5 g	9% imipenem loss in 6 hr and 15% in 9 hr at 25 °C. 8% loss in 48 hr and 14% in 72 hr at 4 °C	1141	I[b]
	AB[a]	MSD	5 g	8% imipenem loss in 3 hr and 15% in 6 hr at 25 °C. 8% loss in 24 hr and 13% in 48 hr at 4 °C	1141	I[b]
Dextrose 5% in Ringer's injection, lactated	AB[a]	MSD	2.5 g	8% imipenem loss in 3 hr and 15% in 6 hr at 25 °C. 9% loss in 24 hr and 15% in 48 hr at 4 °C	1141	I
	AB[a]	MSD	5 g	14% imipenem loss in 3 hr at 25 °C and 13% in 24 hr at 4 °C	1141	I
Dextrose 5% with sodium bicarbonate 0.02%	AB[a]	MSD	2.5 g	7% imipenem loss in 3 hr and 13% in 6 hr at 25 °C. 9% loss in 24 hr and 13% in 48 hr at 4 °C	1141	I[b]
	AB[a]	MSD	5 g	5% imipenem loss in 3 hr and 11% in 6 hr at 25 °C. 9% loss in 24 hr and 15% in 48 hr at 4 °C	1141	I[b]
Dextrose 5% in sodium chloride 0.225%	AB[a]	MSD	2.5 g	8% imipenem loss in 6 hr and 12% in 9 hr at 25 °C. 10% loss in 48 hr at 4 °C	1141	I[b]
	AB[a]	MSD	5 g	5% imipenem loss in 3 hr and 13% in 6 hr at 25 °C. 7% loss in 24 hr and 13% in 48 hr at 4 °C	1141	I[b]

Solution Compatibility (Cont.)

Imipenem–cilastatin sodium

Solution	Mfr	Mfr	Conc/L	Remarks	Ref	C/I
Dextrose 5% in sodium chloride 0.45%	AB[a]	MSD	2.5 g	8% imipenem loss in 6 hr and 11% in 9 hr at 25 °C. 9% loss in 48 hr and 13% in 72 hr at 4 °C	1141	I[b]
	AB[a]	MSD	5 g	5% imipenem loss in 3 hr and 11% in 6 hr at 25 °C. 6% loss in 24 hr and 13% in 48 hr at 4 °C	1141	I[b]
Dextrose 5% in sodium chloride 0.9%	AB[a]	MSD	2.5 g	6% imipenem loss in 6 hr and 10% in 9 hr at 25 °C. 6% loss in 24 hr and 11% in 48 hr at 4 °C	1141	I[b]
	AB[a]	MSD	5 g	6% imipenem loss in 3 hr and 11% in 6 hr at 25 °C. 6% loss in 24 hr and 13% in 48 hr at 4 °C	1141	I[b]
Dextrose 5% in water	AB[a]	MSD	2.5 g	5% imipenem loss in 3 hr and 10% in 6 hr at 25 °C. 8% loss in 24 hr and 14% in 48 hr at 4 °C	1141	I[b]
	AB[a]	MSD	5 g	6% imipenem loss in 3 hr and 15% in 6 hr at 25 °C. 8% loss in 24 hr and 14% in 48 hr at 4 °C	1141	I[b]
	AB[c]	ME	5 g	Little or no loss of drug by HPLC in 4 hr at 25 °C and in 24 hr at 5 °C	1970	C
	BA	MSD	5 g	Visually compatible with 10% imipenem loss by HPLC in about 6 hr at 23 °C and in 48 hr at 4 °C	2166	I[b]
Dextrose 10% in water	AB[a]	MSD	2.5 g	6% imipenem loss in 3 hr and 10% in 6 hr at 25 °C. 8% loss in 24 hr and 13% in 48 hr at 4 °C	1141	I[b]
	AB[a]	MSD	5 g	8% imipenem loss in 3 hr and 13% in 6 hr at 25 °C. 10% loss in 24 hr at 4 °C	1141	I[b]
Mannitol 2.5% in water	AB[a]	MSD	2.5 g	9% imipenem loss in 9 hr at 25 °C. 7% loss in 48 hr and 11% in 72 hr at 4 °C	1141	I[b]
	AB[a]	MSD	5 g	6% imipenem loss in 3 hr and 12% in 6 hr at 25 °C. 7% loss in 24 hr and 10% in 48 hr at 4 °C	1141	I[b]
Mannitol 5% in water	AB[a]	MSD	2.5 g	6% imipenem loss in 3 hr and 10% in 6 hr at 25 °C. 9% loss in 48 hr and 13% in 72 hr at 4 °C	1141	I[b]
	AB[a]	MSD	5 g	7% imipenem loss in 3 hr and 12% in 6 hr at 25 °C. 12% loss in 48 hr at 4 °C	1141	I[b]
Mannitol 10% in water	AB[a]	MSD	2.5 g	6% imipenem loss in 3 hr and 10% in 6 hr at 25 °C. 7% loss in 24 hr and 12% in 48 hr at 4 °C	1141	I[b]
	AB[a]	MSD	5 g	12% imipenem loss in 3 hr at 25 °C. 13% loss in 48 hr at 4 °C	1141	I[b]
Normosol M in dextrose 5%	AB[a]	MSD	2.5 g	7% imipenem loss in 3 hr and 11% in 6 hr at 25 °C. 9% loss in 24 hr and 19% in 48 hr at 4 °C	1141	I[b]
	AB[a]	MSD	5 g	8% imipenem loss in 3 hr and 14% in 6 hr at 25 °C. 10% loss in 24 hr at 4 °C	1141	I[b]
Ringer's injection, lactated	AB[a]	MSD	2.5 g	9% imipenem loss in 6 hr and 12% in 9 hr at 25 °C. 4% loss in 24 hr and 10% in 48 hr at 4 °C	1141	I

Solution Compatibility (Cont.)

Imipenem–cilastatin sodium

Solution	Mfr	Mfr	Conc/L	Remarks	Ref	C/I
	AB[a]	MSD	5 g	6% imipenem loss in 3 hr and 12% in 6 hr at 25 °C. 7% loss in 24 hr and 12% in 48 hr at 4 °C	1141	I
Sodium bicarbonate 5%	AB[a]	MSD	2.5 g	43% imipenem loss in 3 hr at 25 °C. 52% loss in 24 hr at 4 °C	1141	I
	AB[a]	MSD	5 g	45% imipenem loss in 3 hr at 25 °C. 50% loss in 24 hr at 4 °C	1141	I
Sodium chloride 0.9%	AB[a]	MSD	2.5 g	6% imipenem loss in 9 hr at 25 °C. 7% loss in 72 hr at 4 °C	1141	I[b]
	AB[a]	MSD	5 g	8% imipenem loss in 9 hr at 25 °C. 7% loss in 48 hr and 11% in 72 hr at 4 °C	1141	I[b]
	AB[c]	ME	5 g	Little or no loss of drug by HPLC in 4 hr at 25 °C and in 24 hr at 5 °C	1970	C
Sodium lactate ⅙ M	AB[a]	MSD	2.5 g	13% imipenem loss in 3 hr at 25 °C. 8% loss in 24 hr and 15% in 48 hr at 4 °C	1141	I
	AB[a]	MSD	5 g	18% imipenem loss in 3 hr at 25 °C. 14% loss in 24 hr at 4 °C	1141	I
TPN #107[d]			500 mg	57% imipenem loss in 24 hr at 21 °C by micro-biological assay	1326	I

[a]Tested in glass containers.
[b]Incompatible by conventional standards but recommended for dilution of imipenem–cilastatin with use in shorter periods of time.
[c]Tested in glass containers and latex elastomeric reservoirs (Secure Medical).
[d]Refer to Appendix I for the composition of parenteral nutrition solutions. TPN indicates a 2-in-1 admixture.

Y-Site Injection Compatibility (1:1 Mixture)

Imipenem–cilastatin sodium

Drug	Mfr	Conc	Mfr	Conc	Remarks	Ref	C/I
Acyclovir sodium	BW	5 mg/ml[a]	MSD	5 mg/ml[b]	Physically compatible for 4 hr at 25 °C	1157	C
Allopurinol sodium	BW	3 mg/ml[b]	MSD	10 mg/ml[b]	Haze and particles form in 1 hr	1686	I
Amifostine	USB	10 mg/ml[a]	MSD	10 mg/ml[a]	Physically compatible with no change in measured turbidity or increase in particle content in 4 hr at 23 °C	1845	C
Amphotericin B cholesteryl sulfate complex	SEQ	0.83 mg/ml[a]	ME	10 mg/ml[b]	Gross precipitate forms	2117	I
Aztreonam	SQ	40 mg/ml[a]	MSD	10 mg/ml[a]	Physically compatible with no subvisual haze or particle formation in 4 hr at 23 °C	1758	C
Cefepime HCl	BR	20 mg/ml[a]	MSD	10 mg/ml[a]	Physically compatible with no change in measured turbidity or increase in particle content in 4 hr at 22 °C	1689	C
Cisatracurium besylate	GW	0.1, 2, 5 mg/ml[a]	ME	10 mg/ml[b]	Physically compatible with no change in measured turbidity or increase in particle content in 4 hr at 23 °C	2074	C
Diltiazem HCl	MMD	5 mg/ml	MSD	5 mg/ml[c]	Visually compatible	1807	C
Docetaxel	RPR	0.9 mg/ml[a]	ME	10 mg/ml[b]	Physically compatible with no change in measured turbidity or increase in particle content in 4 hr at 23 °C	2224	C

Y-Site Injection Compatibility (1:1 Mixture) (Cont.)

Imipenem–cilastatin sodium

Drug	Mfr	Conc	Mfr	Conc	Remarks	Ref	C/I
Etoposide phosphate	BR	5 mg/ml[a]	ME	10 mg/ml[b]	Yellow discoloration forms in 4 hr at 23 °C	2218	I
Famotidine	MSD	0.2 mg/ml[a]	MSD	10 mg/ml[b]	Physically compatible for 14 hr	1196	C
	ME	2 mg/ml[b]		5 mg/ml[b]	Visually compatible for 4 hr at 22 °C	1936	C
Filgrastim	AMG	30 μg/ml[a]	MSD	10 mg/ml[a]	Physically compatible with no change in measured turbidity or increase in particle content in 4 hr at 22 °C	1687	C
	AMG	40 μg/ml[a]	ME	5 mg/ml[a]	16% loss of filgrastim activity by bioassay in 4 hr at 25 °C. Little or no imipenem and cilastatin loss by HPLC	2060	I
	AMG	10 μg/ml[d]	ME	5 mg/ml[a]	Visually compatible with little or no loss of filgrastim activity by bioassay and imipenem and cilastatin by HPLC in 4 hr at 25 °C	2060	C
Fluconazole	RR	2 mg/ml	MSD	10 mg/ml	Immediate precipitation	1407	I
Fludarabine phosphate	BX	1 mg/ml[a]	MSD	5 mg/ml[a]	Physically compatible for 4 hr at room temperature under fluorescent light	1439	C
Foscarnet sodium	AST	24 mg/ml	MSD	10 mg/ml	Physically compatible for 24 hr at room temperature under fluorescent light	1335	C
	AST	24 mg/ml	MSD	5 mg/ml[a]	Physically compatible for 24 hr at 25 °C under fluorescent light by visual and microscopic examination	1393	C
Gemcitabine HCl	LI	10 mg/ml[b]	ME	10 mg/ml[b]	Yellow-green discoloration forms in 1 hr	2226	I
Granisetron HCl	SKB	0.05 mg/ml[a]	ME	10 mg/ml[a]	Physically compatible with no change in measured turbidity or increase in particle content in 4 hr at 23 °C	2000	C
Idarubicin HCl	AD	1 mg/ml[b]	MSD	5 mg/ml[b]	Visually compatible for 12 hr at 25 °C under fluorescent light. Precipitate forms in 24 hr	1525	C
Insulin, regular	LI	0.2 unit/ml[b]	MSD	4 and 5 mg/ml[b]	Physically compatible for 2 hr at 25 °C	1395	C
Lorazepam	WY	0.33 mg/ml[b]	MSD	5 mg/ml	Yellow precipitate forms in 24 hr	1855	I
Melphalan HCl	BW	0.1 mg/ml[b]	MSD	10 mg/ml[b]	Physically compatible with no change in measured turbidity or increase in particle content in 3 hr at 22 °C	1557	C
Meperidine HCl	AB	10 mg/ml	MSD	5 mg/ml[a]	Yellow discoloration forms within 2 hr at 25 °C under fluorescent light	1397	I
Methotrexate sodium		30 mg/ml	MSD	5 mg/ml	Visually compatible for 4 hr at room temperature	1788	C
Midazolam HCl	RC	5 mg/ml	MSD	5 mg/ml	Haze forms in 24 hr	1855	I
Ondansetron HCl	GL	1 mg/ml[b]	MSD	5 mg/ml[b]	Physically compatible for 4 hr at 22 °C	1365	C
Propofol	ZEN	10 mg/ml	ME	10 mg/ml[b]	Physically compatible for 1 hr at 23 °C with no increase in particle content	2066	C
Remifentanil HCl	GW	0.025 and 0.25 mg/ml[b]	ME	10 mg/ml[a]	Physically compatible with no change in measured turbidity or increase in particle content in 4 hr at 23 °C	2075	C

Y-Site Injection Compatibility (1:1 Mixture) (Cont.)

Imipenem–cilastatin sodium

Drug	Mfr	Conc	Mfr	Conc	Remarks	Ref	C/I
Sargramostim	IMM	10 μg/ml[b]	MSD	5 mg/ml[b]	Large particle and fibrous clump form in 4 hr	1436	I
Sodium bicarbonate		1.4%		5 mg/ml[a]	Pale yellow precipitate forms in 1 hr at room temperature	1788	I
Tacrolimus	FUJ	1 mg/ml[b]	MSD	10 mg/ml[b]	Visually compatible for 24 hr at 25 °C	1630	C
Teniposide	BR	0.1 mg/ml[a]	MSD	10 mg/ml[b]	Physically compatible with no subvisual haze or particle formation in 4 hr at 23 °C	1725	C
Thiotepa	IMM[e]	1 mg/ml[a]	ME	10 mg/ml[a]	Physically compatible with no change in measured turbidity or increase in particle content in 4 hr at 23 °C	1861	C
TNA #218 to #226[f]			ME	10 mg/ml[b]	Visually compatible with no precipitate or emulsion damage apparent in 4 hr at 23 °C	2215	C
TPN #212 to #215[f]			ME	10 mg/ml[b]	Physically compatible with no change in measured turbidity or increase in particle content in 4 hr at 23 °C	2109	C
Vinorelbine tartrate	BW	1 mg/ml[b]	MSD	10 mg/ml[b]	Physically compatible with no change in measured turbidity or increase in particle content in 4 hr at 22 °C	1558	C
Zidovudine	BW	4 mg/ml[a]	MSD	5 mg/ml[a]	Physically compatible for 4 hr at 25 °C under fluorescent light by visual and microscopic examination	1193	C

[a]*Tested in dextrose 5% in water.*
[b]*Tested in sodium chloride 0.9%.*
[c]*Tested in both dextrose 5% in water and sodium chloride 0.9%.*
[d]*Tested in dextrose 5% in water with human albumin 2 mg/ml.*
[e]*Lyophilized formulation tested.*
[f]*Refer to Appendix I for the composition of parenteral nutrition solutions. TNA indicates a 3-in-1 admixture, and TPN indicates a 2-in-1 admixture.*

Additional Compatibility Information

The manufacturer recommends not physically combining imipenem–cilastatin with other anti-infectives such as aminoglycosides. However, the drugs may be administered from separate containers through the same tubing (2; 4).

Tobramycin— The potential for inactivation of tobramycin sulfate by the carbapenem antibiotic imipenem–cilastatin sodium was investigated by Ariano et al. Tobramycin sulfate 10 μg/ml was incubated at 37 °C for five days with imipenem–cilastatin sodium at concentrations ranging from 10 to 40 μg/ml in human serum. Degradation rates of tobramycin sulfate determined by fluorescence polarization immunoassay were not enhanced by the presence of imipenem–cilastatin sodium (2013).

Infusion Solutions— The manufacturer recommends the following infusion solutions for the dilution of imipenem–cilastatin (2):

> Dextrose 5% with potassium chloride 0.15%
> Dextrose 5% in sodium chloride 0.225, 0.45, and 0.9%
> Dextrose 5 and 10% in water
> Mannitol 5 and 10% in water
> Sodium chloride 0.9%

Imipenem–cilastatin is stated to be stable in these infusion solutions for four hours at room temperature or 24 hours when refrigerated at 5 °C (4).

The utility time, or time to 10% decomposition (t_{90}), for imipenem–cilastatin in various infusion solutions has been determined (1141). The results are presented in Table 1.

Table 1. Utility Time (t_{90}) of Imipenem–Cilastatin in Infusion Solutions (1141)

Infusion Solution	Time (hr) to 10% Decomposition			
	25 °C		4 °C	
	250 mg/100 ml	500 mg/100 ml	250 mg/100 ml	500 mg/100 ml
Dextrose 5% with potassium chloride 0.15%	6.3	4.2	51.4	35.4
Dextrose 5% in Ringer's injection, lactated	4.1	2.5	30.9	24.7
Dextrose 5% with sodium bicarbonate 0.02%	5.5	5.4	37.1	34.6
Dextrose 5% in sodium chloride 0.225%	7.3	5.4	52.9	36.7
Dextrose 5% in sodium chloride 0.45%	7.8	5.8	53.0	37.7
Dextrose 5% in sodium chloride 0.9%	9.0	5.5	46.6	39.7
Dextrose 5% in water	6.6	4.7	37.0	36.4
Dextrose 10% in water	5.9	4.3	39.0	31.3
Mannitol 2.5% in water	10.1	6.3	65.0	43.6
Mannitol 5% in water	6.4	5.9	54.9	44.7
Mannitol 10% in water	5.9	3.9	43.6	41.7
Normosol M in dextrose 5%	5.2	4.6	26.8	33.4
Ringer's injection, lactated	6.8	5.4	47.4	41.9
Sodium bicarbonate 5%	0.5	0.4	2.6	2.9
Sodium chloride 0.9%	15.0	11.1	103.0	67.3
Sodium lactate ⅙ M	2.2	1.9	33.6	19.3

IMMUNE GLOBULIN INTRAVENOUS
AHFS 80:04

Gamimune N   **Bayer**
Sandoglobulin   **Novartis**

Products— Immune globulin intravenous 5% (Bayer) is available in 10-, 50-, 100-, and 250-ml sizes. Each milliliter of sterile solution contains approximately 4.5 to 5.5% protein stabilized with 9 to 11% maltose. It also is available in 10-, 50-, 100-, and 200-ml sizes as a 10% solution. Each milliliter of sterile solution contains approximately 9 to 11% protein in 0.16 to 0.24 M glycine. A minimum of 98% of the protein is gamma globulin (immunoglobulin G, IgG) (2; 4).

Immune globulin intravenous (Novartis) is available as a lyophilized product in vials containing 1, 3, 6, or 12 g with 1.67 g of sucrose per gram of protein along with small amounts of sodium chloride. The vials may be reconstituted with dextrose 5% in water, sodium chloride 0.9% injection, or sterile water for injection, using a syringe, in the following amounts to yield a 3 to 12% (30 to 120 mg/ml) solution (2; 4):

Vial Size	3%	6%	9%	12%
1 g	33 ml	16.5 ml	11 ml	8.3 ml
3 g	100 ml	50 ml	33 ml	25 ml
6 g	200 ml	100 ml	66 ml	50 ml
12 g	a	200 ml	132 ml	100 ml

aContainer size precludes this concentration.

Do not shake the product. Rotate or swirl the vial to dissolve particles. Foaming results from shaking and should be avoided (2) because it may impede dissolution (1499).

pH— Gamimune N: 4 to 4.5. Sandoglobulin: 6.4 to 6.8 (2; 4).

Osmotic Values— Gamimune N 5% has an osmolality of 309 mOsm/kg (2; 4). The 10% product has an osmolality of 274 mOsm/kg (2).
Sandoglobulin in various concentrations has the following osmolarities (mOsm/L) (2):

Diluent	Sandoglobulin Concentration			
	3%	6%	9%	12%
Dextrose 5% in water	444	636	828	1020
Sodium chloride 0.9%	498	690	882	1074
Sterile water for injection	192	384	576	768

Administration— Immune globulin intravenous is administered initially by slow intravenous infusion; the rate is gradually increased after 15 to 30 minutes according to patient tolerance (2; 4).

Stability— Gamimune N should be stored under refrigeration at 2 to 8 °C and protected from freezing (2; 4).
Sandoglobulin should be stored at a room temperature not exceeding 30 °C, but it should not be frozen. The reconstituted solution should be used only if it is clear (2; 4). Administration may be initiated within 24 hours of reconstitution if the solution is stored under refrigeration and prepared using aseptic technique in a laminar airflow hood (2).

Compatibility Information

Solution Compatibility

Immune globulin intravenous

Solution	Mfr	Mfr	Conc/L	Remarks	Ref	C/I
Dextrose 5% in water	a	HY	2.5%	Visually compatible with no alteration of IgG concentration or functional activity by bioassay	1885	C
Dextrose 15% in water	a	HY	2.5%	Visually compatible with no alteration of IgG concentration or functional activity by bioassay	1885	C
Dextrose 5% in sodium chloride 0.225%	a	HY	2.5%	Visually compatible with no alteration of IgG concentration or functional activity by bioassay	1885	C
TPN #194 and #195[b]	a	HY	2.5%	Visually compatible with no alteration of IgG concentration or functional activity by bioassay	1885	C

[a]Tested in PVC containers.
[b]Refer to Appendix I for the composition of parenteral nutrition solutions. TPN indicates a 2-in-1 admixture.

Y-Site Injection Compatibility (1:1 Mixture)

Immune globulin intravenous

Drug	Mfr	Conc	Mfr	Conc	Remarks	Ref	C/I
Fluconazole	RR	2 mg/ml	CU	50 mg/ml	Physically compatible for 24 hr at 25 °C under fluorescent light	1407	C
Sargramostim	IMM	6[a] and 15 μg/ml[b]	CU	50 mg/ml	Visually compatible for 2 hr	1618	C

[a]With human albumin 0.1%.
[b]Tested in sodium chloride 0.9%.

Additional Compatibility Information

The manufacturers recommend that other medications not be mixed with immune globulin intravenous and that it be given by a separate infusion line (2).

Gamimune N may be diluted, when necessary, with dextrose 5% in water (2).

Alpha Therapeutic recommends that Venoglobulin-I not be mixed in bacteriostatic water for injection, dextrose injections, and other injections with an acidic pH because of instability (4).

Reconstitution of Sandoglobulin with dextrose 5% in water has resulted in extended dissolution times of 75 and 135 minutes for the 3 and 6% solutions, respectively. With the usual sodium chloride 0.9% diluent, dissolution occurs over a few minutes; exceptional cases take up to 20 minutes (1498).

INDOMETHACIN SODIUM TRIHYDRATE
AHFS 28:08.04

Indocin I.V.   **Merck**

Products— Indomethacin sodium trihydrate (Merck) is supplied as a lyophilized product in vials containing the equivalent of 1 mg of indomethacin. Reconstitute with 1 or 2 ml of preservative-free sterile water for injection or sodium chloride 0.9% to yield a 1- or 0.5-mg/ml solution, respectively (2).

pH— From 6 to 7.5 (4).

Administration— Indomethacin sodium trihydrate is usually administered by intravenous injection over five to 10 seconds. Dilution after reconstitution is not recommended. Extravasation should be avoided (2; 4).

Stability— Indomethacin sodium trihydrate is supplied as a white to yellow powder. Color variations have no relationship to indomethacin content. The vials should be stored at room temperature and protected from light (2).

The manufacturer recommends discarding any unused solution because of the absence of an antibacterial preservative (2). However, at 1 mg/ml in sodium chloride 0.9%, the drug is stated to be chemically stable for 16 days at room temperature (4).

Solutions of indomethacin sodium trihydrate (Abbott and Fujisawa) diluted in sodium chloride 0.9% to a concentration of 0.1 mg/ml were evaluated for visual and chemical stability stored in the original vials. Little or no loss was found by HPLC analysis after storage for 10 days at 25 °C (2105).

Walker et al. reported on the stability of indomethacin sodium trihydrate (Merck Sharp & Dohme) 0.5 mg/ml reconstituted with sterile water for injection in the original vials. The reconstituted solutions were stored at room temperature (about 23 °C) exposed to fluorescent light for 12 hours daily and under refrigeration (about 4 °C) in the dark. Stability-indicating HPLC analysis found little or no loss of indomethacin in the refrigerated solutions after 14 days of storage. The solutions stored at room temperature exhibited 9% loss in 10 days. The solutions at both temperatures remained visually clear and colorless throughout the study (2228).

Syringes— Walker et al. also evaluated the stability of indomethacin

sodium trihydrate 0.5 mg/ml reconstituted with sterile water for injection and repackaged into 1-ml polypropylene syringes (Sherwood). The syringes were stored at room temperature (about 23 °C) exposed to fluorescent light for 12 hours daily and under refrigeration (about 4 °C) in the dark. Stability-indicating HPLC analysis found little or no loss of indomethacin in samples stored at either temperature after 14 days of storage. The solutions stored at both temperatures remained visually clear and colorless throughout the study (2228).

pH Effects— Reconstitution of indomethacin sodium trihydrate with solutions having pH values below 6 may result in precipitation of free indomethacin (2; 4).

Compatibility Information

Y-Site Injection Compatibility (1:1 Mixture)

Indomethacin sodium trihydrate

Drug	Mfr	Conc	Mfr	Conc	Remarks	Ref	C/I
Amino acid injection (TrophAmine)	MG	1 and 2%[a]	MSD	1 mg/ml[b]	Haze forms in 2 hr and white precipitate forms in 4 hr	1527	I
	MG	1 and 2%[c]	MSD	1 mg/ml[b]	Haze forms in 30 min and white precipitate forms in 1 hr	1527	I
Calcium gluconate	AMR	100 mg/ml	MSD	1 mg/ml[b]	Fine yellow precipitate forms within 1 hr	1527	I
Cimetidine HCl	SKB	6 mg/ml[d]	MSD	1 mg/ml[b]	Haze and fine precipitate form immediately	1527	I
Dextrose injection	BA	2.5%	MSD	1 mg/ml[b]	Visually compatible for 24 hr at 28 °C	1527	C
	BA	5%	MSD	1 mg/ml[b]	Visually compatible for 24 hr at 28 °C	1527	C
	BA	7.5%	MSD	1 mg/ml[b]	Haze forms in 2 hr and precipitate forms in 4 hr	1527	I
	BA	10%	MSD	1 mg/ml[b]	Haze forms in 2 hr and precipitate forms in 4 hr	1527	I
Dobutamine HCl	LI	1.2 mg/ml[d]	MSD	1 mg/ml[b]	Haze and fine precipitate form immediately	1527	I
Dopamine HCl	AB	1.2 mg/ml[d]	MSD	1 mg/ml[b]	Haze and fine precipitate form immediately	1527	I
Furosemide	AB	10 mg/ml	MSD	1 mg/ml[b]	Visually compatible for 24 hr at 28 °C	1527	C
Gentamicin sulfate		1 mg/ml[d]	MSD	0.5 and 1 mg/ml[d]	White turbidity forms immediately and becomes white flakes in 1 hr	1550	I
Insulin, regular	NOV	1 unit/ml[b]	MSD	1 mg/ml[b]	Visually compatible for 24 hr at 28 °C	1527	C
Potassium chloride	AB	0.2 mEq/ml[d]	MSD	1 mg/ml[b]	Visually compatible for 24 hr at 28 °C	1527	C
Sodium bicarbonate	AB	0.5 mEq/ml[d]	MSD	1 mg/ml[b]	Visually compatible for 24 hr at 28 °C	1527	C
Sodium nitroprusside	AB	0.2 mg/ml[d]	MSD	1 mg/ml[b]	Visually compatible for 24 hr at 28 °C	1527	C
Tobramycin sulfate		1 mg/ml[d]	MSD	0.5 and 1 mg/ml[d]	White turbidity forms immediately and becomes white flakes in 1 hr	1550	I
Tolazoline HCl		0.1 mg/ml[d]	MSD	1 mg/ml	White precipitate forms within 30 min	1363	I

[a]Tested TrophAmine in dextrose 10% in water.
[b]Tested in sodium chloride 0.9%.
[c]Tested TrophAmine in sterile water for injection.
[d]Tested in dextrose 5% in water.

INSULIN
AHFS 68:20.08

Humulin R	**Lilly**
Regular Iletin I	**Lilly**
Novolin R	**Novo Nordisk**
Velosulin BR	**Novo Nordisk**

Products— Regular insulin is available from several manufacturers in 10-ml vials at a concentration of 100 units/ml. The insulin may be derived from beef and/or pork sources or may be human insulin produced using recombinant DNA technology. Regular concentrated insulin (Lilly) also is available in 20-ml vials containing 500 units/ml. Glycerin 1.4 to 1.8% and phenol or cresol 0.1 to 0.25% may also be present (2; 4).

Several modified forms of insulin (Isophane, Lente, etc.) are available, each having a characteristic onset of action, time to peak effect, and duration of action (4).

pH— All regular insulin products have a neutral pH of approximately 7 to 7.8 (4; 261). Prior to 1973, the older acidic form having a pH of 2.5 to 3.5 was available (4; 263).

Administration— Regular insulin is usually administered by subcutaneous injection into the thighs, arms, buttocks, or abdomen, with sites rotated. Syringes calibrated for the particular concentration of insulin to be given must be used. Regular insulin may also be administered intramuscularly or by intravenous infusion, usually diluted in sodium chloride 0.9%. Regular insulin is the only form of insulin that can be given intravenously (4).

Stability— Regular insulin should be stored under refrigeration and protected from freezing (2; 4). Freezing of insulin products may alter the protein structure, decreasing potency (559). In one study of several insulin products, one cycle of freezing for 45 hours followed by slow thawing at 21 °C or rapid thawing in a water bath at 37 °C did not result in a loss of bioactivity. However, microscopic examination revealed particle aggregation, and some crystal damage had occurred (680).

The currently available regular insulin formulations having a neutral pH are more stable than the older acidic forms used to be (413; 907). At 25 °C, regular insulin has been found to be stable for 24 to 30 months (414), although Lilly has recommended a maximum of 30 days (1433). One study found approximately 5% loss of biological potency after about 36 months at 25 °C. At 37 °C, a 5% loss occurred in about five months (907).

As with other protein and peptide products, insulin aggregation with possible reduced bioactivity can be a problem. Aggregates have been found to form in a variety of infusion devices and under various storage conditions, including static storage and continuous rotational or reciprocating motion. (1948; 1995–1998). Aggregation may occur at air-water interfaces. Such interfaces have been generated by turbulence, such as shaking and repeatedly passing insulin through a syringe and needle. With sufficient vigor, both actions can turn the insulin turbid from insoluble aggregates (1948). In addition, contact with silicone rubber appears to promote insulin aggregation (1995).

Gregory et al. evaluated factors that increase the formation rate of insulin transformation products (such as deamidated insulin, covalent dimers, and higher oligamers) in beef and human insulin products during six months of storage. HPLC analysis showed a low rate of transformation product appearance at 4 °C. Higher temperatures, as might occur when insulin is carried in a shirt pocket or car glove compartment, accelerated this production (especially for human insulin) and also fibril formation. Exposure to light increased the dimer and higher oligamer content. According to these authors, insulin should not be exposed to direct sunlight or subjected to vibration or extremes of temperature (1663).

Regular insulin, containing 100 units/ml, is clear and colorless or almost colorless. The concentrated injection containing 500 units/ml may be straw colored. Discoloration, turbidity, or unusual viscosity indicates deterioration or contamination (4).

It has been stated that neutral regular insulin (and also NPH and Lente insulin) can be stored for five to seven days under refrigeration in either glass or plastic syringes. Mixtures of these insulins can also be stored similarly (679).

In a study by Simmons and Allwood, insulin soluble, BP, 1.6 units/2 ml diluted in sodium chloride 0.9% was stored for 18 hours at room temperature in the following plastic syringes: Brunswick (Sherwood Medical), Plastipak (Becton-Dickinson), and Sabre (Gillette U.K.). The first two syringes have polypropylene barrels; the Sabre has a combination polypropylene–polystyrene barrel. No significant loss of insulin occurred due to sorption. Significant (but unspecified) losses did occur when the concentration was reduced to 0.2 unit/ml, but the make of syringe did not influence this adsorption (784).

Zell and Paone, using a radioimmunoassay, found no apparent degradation or binding for at least 14 days when insulin, USP (Lilly), 100 units/ml was stored under refrigeration in 1-ml polypropylene syringes (Becton-Dickinson) (805).

Adams et al. reported that the soluble insulins Velosulin (Nordisk), Actrapid and Human Actrapid (Novo), Humulin S (Lilly), Neusulin (Wellcome), and Quicksol (Boots) in 1-ml 100-unit Plastipak syringes (Becton-Dickinson) exhibited no loss of potency by HPLC in 29 days when stored at 4 and 20 °C (1275).

Infusion Pumps— Insulin solutions may form highly insoluble polymers. In areas having high shear rates such as the tubing, cannula, and needle, aggregation can lead to blockage. In low shear areas such as the insulin reservoir of implantable pumps, gentle agitation can lead to the formation of a cross-linked gel (1112).

Sorption— The adsorption of insulin to the surfaces of intravenous infusion solution containers, glass and plastic (including PVC, ethylene vinyl acetate, polyethylene, and other polyolefins), tubing, and filters has been demonstrated. Estimates of the potency loss range up to about 80% for the entire infusion apparatus, although varying results using differing test methods, equipment, and procedures have been reported. Estimates of adsorption of around 20 to 30% are common. The percent adsorbed is inversely proportional to the concentration of insulin. Other important factors are the amount of container surface area and the fill volume of the solution. The amount of insulin adsorbed varies directly with the available surface area and indirectly with the ratio of fluid volume to container capacity. The container material is a factor, with glass possibly adsorbing insulin more extensively than some plastics. Other factors influencing the extent of insulin adsorption include the type of solution, type and length of administration set, temperature, previous exposure of tubing to insulin, and presence of albumin, whole blood, electrolytes, and other drugs (266–269; 420; 422–426; 428; 533; 681–690; 854; 908–913; 1111; 1112; 1274; 1408; 1497; 1664; 1665; 2079).

The adsorption of insulin to container surfaces is an instantaneous process (267; 425; 911–913). However, the effect of adsorption on the deliverable amount of insulin appears to vary with time. Several investigators reported a dramatic initial drop in delivered insulin followed by a return to higher (although variable) levels. The bulk of the insulin adsorption apparently occurs in the first 30 to 60 minutes. Although flow rate does not influence total insulin binding, the plateau phase of delivered insulin may be reached more quickly at faster infusion rates (422; 424–426; 428; 687–689; 854).

The addition of human serum albumin to infusion solutions helps to reduce the adsorption of insulin. The degree to which human serum albumin prevents adsorption is uncertain. Reported losses of insulin in albumin-containing solutions have varied from about zero to approximately 30%. However, most work indicates a substantial reduction in insulin adsorption (266–269; 418; 428; 683–685; 908; 909). Other additives such as vitamins, electrolytes, and drugs may also have a similar effect (425; 909; 914).

Other recommended approaches to avoiding or minimizing adsorption include adding a small amount of the patient's blood to the insulin solution (689–691) and storing or flushing the administration apparatus with the insulin solution to saturate the set prior to administration (428; 1111). Addition of extra insulin to compensate for the losses has also been suggested (1112). As an alternative, administration of insulin using a syringe pump with a short cannula has been recommended. This procedure will reduce the surface area in relation to the amount of insulin present (1033).

The clinical significance of this adsorption is uncertain. Some clinical studies indicated no relevant effect on the success of therapy (415; 427; 685). Some investigators felt that the importance of insulin adsorption to the surfaces of the infusion container and tubing may be a moot point since the dosage is individualized on the basis of blood and urine glucose determinations. Simply adding more insulin may saturate binding sites and yield the desired response (270; 271; 854; 909).

Still others indicated that the adsorption may indeed be relevant for solutions with an insulin content of less than 100 or 200 units/L (424; 426; 428; 908).

If the apparent dose of intravenous insulin is used as the basis for determining the subsequent dose upon discontinuing the intravenous one, then a potential for dosing error exists. The actual amount of insulin being administered could be substantially less than the apparent amount (533).

Whether one attempts to prevent insulin adsorption or not, it does not appear to be possible to add an amount of insulin to an infusion solution and know precisely what portion of that amount will actually be given to the patient. Monitoring the patient's response to therapy and making the appropriate adjustments on the basis of that response are, therefore, of prime importance (690; 854; 1664).

Filtration— A filter material specially treated with a proprietary agent was evaluated for a reduction in insulin binding. Insulin, regular (Lilly), 40 units/L in dextrose 5% in water and sodium chloride 0.9% was run through an administration set with a treated 0.22-μm cellulose ester inline filter at a rate of 2 ml/min. Cumulative insulin losses from the first 150 ml of solution was about 12% from dextrose 5% in water and 4% from sodium chloride 0.9%, compared to much higher losses previously reported for untreated cellulose ester filter material. Furthermore, equilibrium binding studies showed a reduction to 5% of the binding to untreated filter material from either solution (904). All Abbott Ivex integral filter and extension sets currently use this treated filter material (1074).

Compatibility Information

Solution Compatibility

Insulin, regular

Solution	Mfr	Mfr	Conc/L	Remarks	Ref	C/I
Amino acids 4.25%, dextrose 25%	MG	LI	100 units	No increase in particulate matter in 24 hr at 5 °C	349	C
Sodium chloride 0.9%	BA[a]	LI[b]	1000 units	10% insulin loss by HPLC in 1 hr in 50-ml bag and in 4 hr in 250-ml bag	2079	I
TPN #38 to #45 and #47[c]		LI	10 to 50 units	Physically compatible for 24 hr at 22 °C	313	C
TPN #46[c]		LI	10 to 30 units	Physically compatible for 24 hr at 22 °C	313	C
		LI	40 and 50 units	White crystalline precipitate forms in 24 hr at 22 °C	313	I

[a]*Tested in PVC containers.*
[b]*Regular human insulin.*
[c]*Refer to Appendix I for the composition of parenteral nutrition solutions. TPN indicates a 2-in-1 admixture.*

Additive Compatibility

Insulin, regular

Drug	Mfr	Conc/L	Mfr	Conc/L	Test Soln	Remarks	Ref	C/I
Aminophylline	SE	1 g	LI[a]	20 units	D5W	pH outside stability range for insulin	41	I

Additive Compatibility (Cont.)

Insulin, regular

Drug	Mfr	Conc/L	Mfr	Conc/L	Test Soln	Remarks	Ref	C/I
Amobarbital sodium		a				Physically incompatible	9	I
Bretylium tosylate	ACC	1 g	SQ	1000 units	D5W, NS	Physically compatible for 48 hr at 25 °C	756	C
Chlorothiazide sodium	MSD	a				Physically incompatible	9	I
Cimetidine HCl	SKF	1.2 and 5 g	LI	100 units	D5W, NS	Physically compatible and cimetidine chemically stable for 24 hr at room temperature. Insulin not tested	551	C
Cytarabine	UP	100 and 500 mg		40 units	D5W	Fine precipitate forms	174	I
Dobutamine HCl	LI	1 g	LI	1000 units	D5W, NS	Slightly pink in 24 hr at 25 °C	789	I
	LI	1 g	LI	50,000 units	D5W, NS	White precipitate forms rapidly	812	I
Lidocaine HCl	AST	2 g	SQ	1000 units	D5W, LR, NS	Physically compatible for 24 hr at 25 °C	775	C
Meropenem	ZEN	1 and 20 g	LI	1000 units	NS	Visually compatible for 4 hr at room temperature	1994	C
Pentobarbital sodium		a				Physically incompatible	9	I
Phenobarbital sodium	WI	a				Physically incompatible	9	I
Phenytoin sodium	PD	a				Physically incompatible	9	I
Ranitidine HCl	GL	50 mg and 2 g		100 units	NS	Physically compatible and ranitidine chemically stable by HPLC for 24 hr at 25 °C. Insulin not tested	1515	C
	GL	600 mg	LI	1000 units[c]	NS[b]	Visually compatible with little or no loss by HPLC of ranitidine in 24 hr at ambient temperature but insulin losses of 9% in 4 hr and 14% in 24 hr, presumably due to sorption	2079	I
Thiopental sodium	AB	a				Physically incompatible	9	I
Verapamil HCl	KN	80 mg	SQ	200 units	D5W, NS	Physically compatible for 48 hr	739	C

[a]Test performed prior to availability of neutral regular insulin.
[b]Tested in PVC containers.
[c]Regular human insulin.

Drugs in Syringe Compatibility

Insulin, regular

Drug (in syringe)	Mfr	Amt	Mfr	Amt	Remarks	Ref	C/I
Metoclopramide HCl	RB	10 mg/ 2 ml	LI	10 units/ 2 ml[a]	Physically compatible for 24 hr at room temperature	924	C
	RB	10 mg/ 2 ml	LI	20 units/ 4 ml[a]	Physically compatible for 24 hr at room temperature	924	C
	RB	10 mg/ 2 ml	LI	10 units/ 2 ml	Physically compatible for 24 hr at 25 °C	1167	C
	RB	10 mg/ 2 ml	LI	20 units/ 4 ml	Physically compatible for 24 hr at 25 °C	1167	C

Drugs in Syringe Compatibility (Cont.)

Insulin, regular

Drug (in syringe)	Mfr	Amt	Mfr	Amt	Remarks	Ref	C/I
	RB	160 mg/ 32 ml	LI	80 units/ 16 ml	Physically compatible for 24 hr at 25 °C	1167	C

[a]Brought to volume with distilled water.

Y-Site Injection Compatibility (1:1 Mixture)

Insulin, regular

Drug	Mfr	Conc	Mfr	Conc	Remarks	Ref	C/I
Amiodarone HCl	WY	4.8 mg/ml[a]	LI	1 unit/ml[a]	Visually compatible for 24 hr at 23 °C	1877	C
Ampicillin sodium	WY	20 mg/ml[b]	LI	0.2 unit/ml[b]	Physically compatible for 2 hr at 25 °C	1395	C
Ampicillin sodium–sulbactam sodium	RR	20 + 10 mg/ ml[b]	LI	0.2 unit/ml[b]	Physically compatible for 2 hr at 25 °C	1395	C
Aztreonam	SQ	20 mg/ml	LI	0.2 unit/ml[b]	Physically compatible for 2 hr at 25 °C	1395	C
Cefazolin sodium	LI	20 mg/ml[a]	LI	0.2 unit/ml[b]	Physically compatible for 2 hr at 25 °C	1395	C
Cefotetan disodium	STU	20 and 40 mg/ml[a]	LI	0.2 unit/ml[b]	Physically compatible for 2 hr at 25 °C	1395	C
Clarithromycin	AB	4 mg/ml[a]	NOV[l]	4 units/ml[a]	Visually compatible for 72 hr at both 30 and 17 °C	2174	C
Digoxin	ES	0.005 mg/ ml[b]	LI[c]	1 unit/ml[b]	Physically compatible for 3 hr	1316	C
	ES	0.005 mg/ ml[b]	LI[d]	1 unit/ml[b]	Physically compatible for 3 hr	1316	C
	ES	0.005 mg/ ml[a]	LI[c]	1 unit/ml[a]	Slight haze in 1 hr	1316	I
	ES	0.005 mg/ ml[a]	LI[d]	1 unit/ml[a]	Slight haze in 1 hr	1316	I
Diltiazem HCl	MMD	1[b] and 5 mg/ ml	NOV	100 units/ml	Precipitate forms and persists	1807	I
	MMD	5 mg/ml	NOV	0.4 unit/ml	Visually compatible	1807	C
Dobutamine HCl	LI	4 mg/ml[e]	LI[c]	1 unit/ml[e]	Physically compatible for 3 hr	1316	C
	LI	4 mg/ml[e]	LI[d]	1 unit/ml[e]	Physically compatible for 3 hr	1316	C
Dopamine HCl	DU	3.2 mg/ml[a]	LI	1 unit/ml[a]	White precipitate forms immediately, dissolves quickly, and reforms in 24 hr at 23 °C	1877	I
Esmolol HCl	DU	40 mg/ml[a]	LI	1 unit/ml[a]	Visually compatible for 24 hr at 23 °C	1877	C
Famotidine	MSD	0.2 mg/ml[a]	LI	0.03 unit/ml[a]	Physically compatible for 4 hr at 25 °C	1188	C
Gentamicin sulfate	TR	1.2 mg/ml[b]	LI	0.2 unit/ml[b]	Physically compatible for 2 hr at 25 °C	1395	C
Heparin sodium	ES	60 units/ml[a]	LI	0.2 unit/ml[b]	Physically compatible for 2 hr at 25 °C	1395	C
Heparin sodium with hydrocortisone sodium succinate	RI UP	1000 units + 100 mg/L[f]	LI	40 units/ml	Physically compatible for at least 4 hr at room temperature by visual and microscopic examination	322	C
Imipenem–cilastatin sodium	MSD	4 and 5 mg/ ml[b]	LI	0.2 unit/ml[b]	Physically compatible for 2 hr at 25 °C	1395	C
Indomethacin sodium trihydrate	MSD	1 mg/ml[b]	NOV	1 unit/ml[b]	Visually compatible for 24 hr at 28 °C	1527	C
Labetalol HCl	GL	5 mg/ml	LI	1 unit/ml[a]	Visually compatible for 4 hr. White precipitate forms in 24 hr 23 °C	1877	?

Y-Site Injection Compatibility (1:1 Mixture) (Cont.)

Insulin, regular

Drug	Mfr	Conc	Mfr	Conc	Remarks	Ref	C/I
Magnesium sulfate	LY	40 mg/ml[g]	LI	0.2 unit/ml[b]	Physically compatible for 2 hr at 25 °C	1395	**C**
Meperidine HCl	WY	10 mg/ml[b]	LI	0.2 unit/ml[b]	Physically compatible for 1 hr at 25 °C	1338	**C**
	AST	50 mg/ml[a]	LI	0.2 unit/ml[b]	Physically compatible for 2 hr at 25 °C	1395	**C**
Meropenem	ZEN	1 and 50 mg/ml[b]	LI	0.2 unit/ml[a]	Visually compatible for 4 hr at room temperature	1994	**C**
Midazolam HCl	RC	1 mg/ml[a]	LI	1 unit/ml[a]	Visually compatible for 24 hr at 23 °C	1877	**C**
Milrinone lactate	SW	0.4 mg/ml[a]	NOV[l]	1 unit/ml[b]	Visually compatible with little or no loss of either drug by HPLC in 4 hr at 23 °C	2214	**C**
Morphine sulfate	ES	1 mg/ml[b]	LI	0.2 unit/ml[b]	Physically compatible for 1 hr at 25 °C	1338	**C**
	ES	5 mg/ml[a]	LI	0.2 unit/ml[b]	Physically compatible for 2 hr at 25 °C	1395	**C**
	SX	1 mg/ml[a]	LI	1 unit/ml[a]	Visually compatible for 24 hr at 23 °C	1877	**C**
Nafcillin sodium	BA	20 and 40 mg/ml[a]	LI	0.2 unit/ml[b]	Immediate precipitation	1395	**I**
Nitroglycerin	OM	0.2 mg/ml[a]	LI	1 unit/ml[a]	Visually compatible for 24 hr at 23 °C	1877	**C**
Norepinephrine bitartrate	STR	0.064 mg/ml[a]	LI	1 unit/ml[a]	White precipitate forms immediately	1877	**I**
Oxytocin	PD	0.02 unit/ml[i]	LI	0.2 unit/ml[b]	Physically compatible for 2 hr at 25 °C	1395	**C**
Pentobarbital sodium	WY	2 mg/ml[e]	LI[c]	1 unit/ml[e]	Physically compatible for 3 hr	1316	**C**
	WY	2 mg/ml[e]	LI[d]	1 unit/ml[e]	Physically compatible for 3 hr	1316	**C**
Potassium chloride		40 mEq/L[f]	LI	40 units/ml	Physically compatible for at least 4 hr at room temperature by visual and microscopic examination	322	**C**
Propofol	ZEN	10 mg/ml	NOV	1 unit/ml[a]	Physically compatible for 1 hr at 23 °C with no increase in particle content	2066	**C**
Ranitidine HCl	GL	1 mg/ml[b]	LI[c]	1 unit/ml[b]	Visually compatible with little or no loss by HPLC of ranitidine in 4 hr at ambient temperature but insulin losses of 10% in 1 hr and 22% in 4 hr, presumably due to sorption	2079	**I**
Ritodrine HCl	AST	0.3 mg/ml[a]	LI	0.2 unit/ml[b]	Physically compatible for 2 hr at 25 °C	1395	**C**
Sodium bicarbonate	AB	1 mEq/ml[e]	LI[c]	1 unit/ml[e]	Physically compatible for 3 hr	1316	**C**
	AB	1 mEq/ml[e]	LI[d]	1 unit/ml[e]	Physically compatible for 3 hr	1316	**C**
Sodium nitroprusside	RC	0.2 mg/ml[a]	LI	1 unit/ml[a]	Visually compatible for 24 hr at 23 °C	1877	**C**
Tacrolimus	FUJ	1 mg/ml[b]	LI	0.1 unit/ml[a]	Visually compatible for 24 hr at 25 °C	1630	**C**
Terbutaline sulfate	CI	0.02 mg/ml[a]	LI	0.2 unit/ml[b]	Physically compatible for 2 hr at 25 °C	1395	**C**
Ticarcillin disodium	BE	30 mg/ml[b]	LI	0.2 unit/ml[b]	Physically compatible for 2 hr at 25 °C	1395	**C**
Ticarcillin disodium–clavulanate potassium	BE	31 mg/ml[b]	LI	0.2 unit/ml[b]	Physically compatible for 2 hr at 25 °C	1395	**C**
Tobramycin sulfate	LI	1.6 and 2 mg/ml[a]	LI	0.2 unit/ml[b]	Physically compatible for 2 hr at 25 °C	1395	**C**
TNA #218 to #226[j]			NOV	1 unit/ml[a]	Visually compatible with no precipitate or emulsion damage apparent in 4 hr at 23 °C	2215	**C**
TPN #189[j]			NOV	2 units/ml[k]	Visually compatible for 24 hr at 22 °C	1767	**C**

Y-Site Injection Compatibility (1:1 Mixture) (Cont.)

Insulin, regular

Drug	Mfr	Conc	Mfr	Conc	Remarks	Ref	C/I
TPN #212 to #215[j]			NOV	1 unit/ml[b]	Physically compatible with no change in measured turbidity or increase in particle content in 4 hr at 23 °C	2109	C
Vancomycin HCl	LI	4 mg/ml[a]	LI	0.2 unit/ml[b]	Physically compatible for 2 hr at 25 °C	1395	C
Vitamin B complex with C	RC	2 ml/L[f]	LI	40 units/ml	Physically compatible for at least 4 hr at room temperature by visual and microscopic examination	322	C

[a]*Tested in dextrose 5% in water.*
[b]*Tested in sodium chloride 0.9%.*
[c]*Humulin R.*
[d]*Beef pork.*
[e]*Tested in both dextrose 5% in water and sodium chloride 0.9%.*
[f]*Tested in dextrose 5% in water, sodium chloride 0.9%, and Ringer's injection, lactated.*
[g]*Tested in Ringer's injection, lactated.*
[h]*Tested in sterile water for injection.*
[i]*Tested in dextrose 5% in Ringer's injection, lactated.*
[j]*Refer to Appendix I for the composition of parenteral nutrition solutions. TNA indicates a 3-in-1 admixture, and TPN indicates a 2-in-1 admixture.*
[k]*Tested in Haemaccel (Behring).*
[l]*Regular human insulin.*

Additional Compatibility Information

It has been stated that neutral regular insulin may be combined with modified insulin in any proportions (263; 264). However, losses of soluble insulins when mixed with zinc and isophane insulins were reported by Adams et al. These losses generally ranged from about 20 to 50% but were as high as 99%, depending on the ratio and sources of the two insulins in the mixture. The reaction occurred within the first 90 to 120 seconds after mixing, with no further losses occurring after this time. The authors indicated that this phenomenon could explain clinical reports of failure to control postprandial blood sugar levels (1275).

Nolte et al. reported on the loss of solubility when short-acting insulins were mixed in ratios of 1:1, 1:2, 1:3, and 1:5 with long-acting insulins. Iletin II Regular (Lilly) was mixed with Iletin II Lente, NPH, or Ultralente (Lilly). Actrapid (Novo) was mixed with Monotard (Novo). Velosulin (Nordisk) was mixed with Insulatard (Nordisk). The mixtures were centrifuged after storage times of approximately 20 minutes and 75 seconds. The level of soluble short-acting insulin in the supernatant was determined by radioimmunoassay. In a 1:1 ratio, no significant loss of solubility occurred with the Iletin II Lente combination within 20 minutes and with the Actrapid–Monotard combination in 75 seconds. All other combinations, ratios, and time periods had losses ranging from 10 to 75%. The worst losses were experienced with the highest ratios of long-acting insulins and with the longer time period. The authors noted that the method used to prolong insulin action (precipitation) might affect the solubility of the short-acting insulin when admixed (1156).

Muhlhauser et al. noted the loss of initial hypoglycemic effect when Actrapid HM (Novo) was mixed with Ultratard HM (Novo), an ultralente insulin, for five minutes before injection. The authors recommended not mixing the two types of insulin to preserve the rapid hypoglycemic effect of regular insulin (73).

Methylprednisolone sodium succinate (Upjohn) has been stated to be incompatible with insulin (329).

Parenteral Nutrition Solutions— Regular insulin is not inactivated in amino acid injection (McGaw), but a physical separation may occur if it is not mixed thoroughly; occasional shaking prevents a bolus of insulin from being administered (189).

Regular insulin (Lilly) 20 to 100 units/L was tested for compatibility in parenteral nutrition solutions composed of protein hydrolysate 7% 590 ml/dextrose 50% 410 ml (Cutter) with calcium, magnesium, phosphate, phytonadione, cyanocobalamin, folic acid, and multivitamin infusion (USV) or Solu B Forte present. The parenteral nutrition solutions were physically compatible with little pH alteration in 24 hours at room temperature (464).

Octreotide— Radioimmunoassays of insulin levels in a 3-L bag of parenteral nutrition solution showed a marked reduction when octreotide 150 μg was added to the container. Sample parenteral nutrition solutions, with and without octreotide, were prepared with regular insulin 15 units/3-L bag. Subsequent analysis found an insulin level of 3.5 units/L in the plain parenteral nutrition solution, an amount consistent with the losses occurring due to surface adsorption. (See Stability above.) However, in the parenteral nutrition solution containing octreotide, the insulin level was only 0.6 unit/L. The reason for this potential incompatibility is not known (1377).

Other Information

Mixing Insulin Admixtures— Care is required when adding insulin to infusion solutions, especially in flexible containers. Adding insulin to a polygeline (plasma expander) carrier solution hanging in the use position resulted in stratification, with the insulin floating to the top. Little insulin was delivered initially, and 87% of the insulin appeared in the last 28% of the solution. Repeated inversion and agitation of the container to effect thorough mixture eliminates this stratification, yielding an even distribution and a constant delivery concentration (85).

Reuse of Disposable Insulin Syringes—— Reuse of disposable insulin syringes has been suggested to reduce cost to patients. However, disposable insulin syringes are usually siliconized. Reuse of disposable plastic insulin syringes (Plastipak Microfine II, Becton-Dickinson) has resulted in contamination of vials of insulin with silicone oil, causing a white precipitate and impairment of biological effects. In a test of insulin from several sources, repeated drawing of the insulin into the disposable syringes and then expulsion of it back into the vials introduced substantial amounts of silicone oil; a white precipitate formed within 12 hours at 8 °C (1110).

INTERFERON ALFA-2B
AHFS 10:00

Intron A   **Schering**

Products—— Interferon alfa-2b (Schering) is available as a dry powder in vials containing 3, 5, 10, 18, 25, and 50 million International Units (I.U.) packaged with bacteriostatic water for injection containing benzyl alcohol 0.9% diluent. See Table 1. Only the 10-million I.U. vial is recommended for intralesional use. The 50-million I.U. vials are used in malignant melanoma and AIDS-related Kaposi's sarcoma only (2).

For intramuscular, subcutaneous, or intralesional use, reconstitute the appropriate-size vial contents with the bacteriostatic water for injection diluent using the requisite volume noted in Table 1. Direct the stream at the vial wall and not at the powder in the bottom of the vial. Swirl gently to dissolve the powder; do not shake (2).

In addition to interferon alfa-2b, the reconstituted solutions also contain in each milliliter glycine 20 mg, sodium phosphate dibasic 2.3 mg, sodium phosphate monobasic 0.55 mg, and human albumin 1 mg (2).

For intravenous infusion, reconstitute the appropriate-size vial contents with the diluent provided. Swirl gently to dissolve the powder; do not shake. Withdraw the appropriate dose and add it to 100 ml of sodium chloride 0.9%, ensuring that the final concentration is not less than 10 million I.U./100 ml (2).

Interferon alfa-2b is also available for intramuscular or subcutaneous use as solutions in vials of 3 million I.U./0.5 ml, 5 million I.U./0.5 ml, and 10 million I.U./1 ml. Multidose vials are available labeled as 18 million I.U., which contain 22.8 million I.U./3.8 ml (6 million I.U./ml), and 25 million I.U., which contain 32 million I.U./3.2 ml (10 million I.U./ml). Multidose injection "pens" are also available containing 3, 5, and 10 million I.U. per 0.2 ml injection with a total of 1.5 ml per pen for subcutaneous injection (2).

In addition to intramuscular and subcutaneous use, the 5-, 10-, and 25-million I.U. vials are also for intralesional use. However, the solution products are not recommended for intravenous administration. Vial size to be used and appropriate concentration are dependent on the intended use of the product. Each milliliter of solution also contains sodium chloride 7.5 mg, sodium phosphate dibasic 1.8 mg, sodium phosphate monobasic 1.3 mg, edetate disodium 0.1 mg, polysorbate 80 0.1 mg, and meta-cresol 1.5 mg (2).

pH—— The reconstituted powder for injection has a pH in the range of 6.9 to 7.5 (4).

Tonicity—— Reconstitution of the 10-million I.U. vial with 1 ml of water for injection results in an isotonic solution (1369).

Specific Activity—— Approximately 2×10^8 I.U./mg of protein (2).

Administration—— The administration of interferon alfa-2b is dependent on the intended use and specific dosage form. The dry powder products, reconstituted as directed, may be administered by intramuscular and subcutaneous injection or intravenous infusion. The contents of the 10-million I.U. vial, reconstituted as directed, may also be given intralesionally. For intravenous infusions, interferon alfa-2b may be diluted further to a concentration of not less than 10 million I.U./100 ml of sodium chloride 0.9% for intravenous infusion over 20 minutes (2).

The solution products are administered by intramuscular or subcutaneous injection. The 5-million I.U. and 10-million I.U. vials and the 25-million I.U. multidose vials may also be used for intralesional injection. The solution products are not for use in malignant melanoma or AIDS-related Kaposi's sarcoma (2).

Stability—— Interferon alfa-2b dry powder in vials is a white to cream color (2). It is not photosensitive (1369). The reconstituted solution is clear and colorless to light yellow. Intact vials should be stored under refrigeration at 2 to 8 °C but are stable up to seven days at 45 °C (4) or 28 days at room temperature (1369). The reconstituted solution should be stored under refrigeration. In concentrations between 3 and 50 million I.U./ml, reconstituted solutions are stable for up to one month under refrigeration and up to two days at ambient temperatures up to 40 °C (2).

Interferon alfa-2b solution in vials is colorless. Intact vials of solution should be stored under refrigeration at 2 to 8 °C. The solution products are stable for up to seven days at 35 °C and up to 14 days at 30 °C. Interferon alfa-2b in multidose pens is stable for up to two days at 30 °C (2).

Interferon alfa-2b (Schering) containing albumin in the formulation reconstituted with the accompanying diluent and diluted further to 2 million I.U./ml with sterile water for injection was stored at 4 °C for 21 days in polypropylene centrifuge tubes. Biological ac-

Table 1. Reconstitution of Interferon Alfa-2b Powder for Injection Vials (2).

Vial Size (million I.U.)	Diluent Volume (ml)	Concentration (I.U./ml)
3	1	3
5	1	5
10	2	5
10	1	10 (for intralesional use only)
18	1	18
25	5	5
50	1	50 (for malignant melanoma and AIDS-related Kaposi's sarcoma only)

tivity was retained throughout the study period determined by a cell proliferation inhibition bioassay (2022).

In another study, the retention of bioactivity by albumin-free interferon alfa-2b 6 million units/ml stability was compared to samples of that product to which albumin 1 mg/ml was added and also to the reconstituted product containing albumin in the formulation. The solutions were packaged as 0.5 ml in polypropylene syringes and stored at 4 °C for 42 days. In addition, the albumin-free product was diluted to 2 million units/ml with sterile water for injection and stored in a 60-ml polypropylene syringe under the same conditions. No substantial loss of biological activity was found in any of the samples tested by a cell proliferation inhibition bioassay and by a separate interferon-mediated gene induction bioassay (2188).

pH Effects— Reconstituted interferon alfa-2b is stable over a pH range of 6.5 to 8 (4), with greatest stability between pH 6.9 and 7.5 (1369).

Freezing Solutions— Reconstituted interferon alfa-2b 10 million I.U./ ml packaged in plastic syringes is stated to be stable for up to four weeks when frozen at −10 °C or colder (4). Solutions frozen at −20 °C are stated to be stable for 56 days including four freeze-thaw cycles. Frozen solutions stored at −80 °C are stable for one year (1369).

Sorption— Like other interferons, interferon alfa-2b can bind to surfaces, including glass and plastics. Consequently, human albumin is incorporated into the formulation to minimize adsorption and permit the use of glass or plastic syringes for administration without substantial loss (4).

Compatibility Information

Solutions— Sodium chloride 0.9% is recommended for preparation of intravenous infusion admixtures (2).

Interferon alfa-2b is stated to be compatible with sodium chloride 0.9%, Ringer's injection, and Ringer's injection, lactated. It is stated to be incompatible with dextrose solutions (1369).

IODIPAMIDE MEGLUMINE
AHFS 36:68

Cholografin Meglumine　　　　　　　　　　　　　**Bracco**

Products— Iodipamide meglumine (Bracco) is available in 20-ml vials containing an aqueous solution composed of 52% iodipamide meglumine (5.2 g bound iodine/20 ml) with 0.32% sodium citrate buffer and 0.04% edetate disodium (4; 154).

pH— From 6.5 to 7.7 (4).

Sodium Content— The 52% solution contains approximately 18.2 mg of sodium per 20 ml (1-7/98).

Administration— Iodipamide meglumine is administered slowly intravenously only. After warming to body temperature, the 52% injection is injected over 10 minutes (1-7/98; 4).

Stability— The solutions may vary from colorless to pale yellow or light amber. Darker solutions should not be used. Crystallization may occur in the 52% solution. To redissolve it, place the vial in hot water and shake gently for several minutes. If cloudiness does not disappear, the solution should not be used (1-7/98; 4).

Plastic syringes have been stated to be unsuitable for accommodating radiopaque solutions for any length of time. The plastic is attacked, and the plunger tends to freeze on prolonged storage (40). However, when iodipamide meglumine (Squibb) 52% was stored in polystyrene syringes (Pharmaseal) at 25 and 37 °C, no apparent changes were noted visually or spectrophotometrically over five days (530).

Iodipamide meglumine solutions should be protected from light and excessive heat (1-7/98).

Compatibility Information

Additive Compatibility

Iodipamide meglumine

Drug	Mfr	Conc/L	Mfr	Conc/L	Test Soln	Remarks	Ref	C/I
Diphenhydramine HCl	PD	20 to 200 mg	SQ	a	NS	Dense putty-like white precipitate forms immediately	309	**I**

aAmount and percent unspecified.

Drugs in Syringe Compatibility

Iodipamide meglumine 52%

Drug (in syringe)	Mfr	Amt	Mfr	Amt	Remarks	Ref	C/I
Chlorpheniramine maleate	SC	1 ml[a]	SQ	40 to 5 ml	Forms a precipitate initially but clears within 1 hr and remains clear for 48 hr	530	I
	SC	1 ml[a]	SQ	2 and 1 ml	Forms a precipitate initially but clears within 1 hr. Precipitate reforms within 48 hr	530	I
Dimenhydrinate	SE	50 mg/ 1 ml	SQ	40 ml	Forms a precipitate initially but clears within 1 hr and remains clear for 48 hr	530	I
	SE	50 mg/ 1 ml	SQ	20 to 1 ml	Forms a precipitate initially but clears within 1 hr. Precipitate reforms on standing	530	I
Diphenhydramine HCl	PD	5 mg/ 0.1 ml to 50 mg/ 1 ml	SQ	b	Dense putty-like white precipitate forms immediately	309	I
	PD	1 ml[a]	SQ	40 to 1 ml	Forms a precipitate initially but clears within 1 hr and remains clear for 48 hr	530	I
Hyaluronidase	WY	150 units/ 1 ml	SQ	40 to 2 ml	Physically compatible for 48 hr	530	C
	WY	150 units/ 1 ml	SQ	1 ml	Physically compatible for at least 1 hr but a precipitate forms within 48 hr	530	I
Promethazine HCl	WY	1 ml[a]	SQ	40 and 20 ml	Forms a precipitate initially but clears within 1 hr and remains clear for 48 hr	530	I
	WY	1 ml[a]	SQ	10 to 1 ml	Immediate precipitation	530	I

[a]*Concentration unspecified.*
[b]*Amount and concentration unspecified.*

Additional Compatibility Information

Antihistamines—— Iodipamide meglumine (Squibb) was found to be physically incompatible with chlorpheniramine maleate (Schering), diphenhydramine HCl (Parke-Davis), and promethazine HCl (Wyeth) (40).

The manufacturer recommends that antihistamines be administered separately and not be mixed with iodipamide meglumine (1-7/98).

Gentamicin—— Administration of iodipamide meglumine (Squibb) via a Y-injection site of an administration set through which gentamicin sulfate had been previously administered resulted in the immediate formation of a white precipitate downstream to the Y-site (324).

IOHEXOL
AHFS 36:68

Omnipaque   **Nycomed**

Products—— Iohexol (Nycomed) is available in concentrations ranging from 30.2% (140 mg/ml organically bound iodine) to 75.5% (350 mg/ml organically bound iodine) in numerous vial and bottle sizes from 10 to 250 ml; not all concentrations are available in all sizes. Also present in each milliliter are tromethamine 1.21 mg, edetate calcium disodium 0.1 mg, and hydrochloric acid or sodium hydroxide to adjust the pH (1-7/96). Table 1 presents the characteristics of iohexol products.

Table 1. Iohexol Product Characteristics (1-7/96)

Iohexol Concentration (%)	Iodine Concentration (mg/ml)	Osmolality (mOsm/kg)	Specific Gravity (37 °C)
30.2	140	322	1.164
38.8	180	408	1.209
45.3	210	460	1.244
51.8	240	520	1.280
64.7	300	672	1.349
75.5	350	844	1.406

pH—— From 6.8 to 7.7 (1-7/96).

Administration— Iohexol may be administered intravenously, intra-arterially, intrathecally slowly over one to two minutes, intra-articularly, or directly into selected areas for visualization. Solutions should be warmed to body temperature prior to administration (1-7/96).

Stability— Iohexol is colorless to pale yellow. Intact vials should be stored at controlled room temperature and protected from direct ex-posure to sunlight and freezing. The product should not be used if particulate matter is present. If a plastic syringe is to be used, io-hexol should be injected immediately after being drawn into it. Do not remove the iohexol containers from the moisture- and light-protective foil overwrap until immediately before use (1-7/96).

Compatibility Information

Drugs in Syringe Compatibility

				Iohexol			
Drug (in syringe)	Mfr	Amt	Mfr	Amt	Remarks	Ref	C/I
Ampicillin sodium	BR	30 mg/ 1 ml	WI	64.7%, 5 ml	Physically compatible for at least 2 hr	1438	C
Bupivacaine HCl	AST	0.25%, 4 ml		1 ml[a]	Visually compatible with no bupivacaine loss by HPLC in 24 hr at room temperature. Iohexol not tested	1611	C
	AST	0.125%[b], 4 ml		1 ml[a]	Visually compatible with no bupivacaine loss by HPLC in 24 hr at room temperature. Iohexol not tested	1611	C
Chloramphenicol sodium succinate	PD	33 mg/ 1 ml	WI	64.7%, 5 ml	Physically compatible for at least 2 hr	1438	C
Cimetidine HCl	SKF	150 mg/ 1 ml	WI	64.7%, 5 ml	Physically compatible for at least 2 hr	1438	C
Diphenhydramine HCl	PD	12.5 mg/ 0.25 ml	WI	64.7%, 5 ml	Physically compatible for at least 2 hr	1438	C
Epinephrine HCl	PD	1 mg/ 1 ml	WI	64.7%, 5 ml	Physically compatible for at least 2 hr	1438	C
Gentamicin sulfate	SC	0.8 mg/ 1 ml	WI	64.7%, 5 ml	Physically compatible for at least 2 hr	1438	C
Heparin sodium	OR	5000 units/ 0.5 ml	WI	64.7%, 5 ml	Physically compatible for at least 2 hr	1438	C
Hydrocortisone sodium succinate	UP	10 mg/ 1 ml	WI	64.7%, 5 ml	Physically compatible for at least 2 hr	1438	C
Methylprednisolone sodium succinate	UP	10 mg/ 1 ml	WI	64.7%, 5 ml	Physically compatible for at least 2 hr	1438	C
Papaverine HCl	LI	30 mg/ 1 ml	WI	64.7%, 5 ml	Physically compatible for at least 2 hr	1438	C
Protamine sulfate	LI	10 mg/ 1 ml	WI	64.7%, 5 ml	Physically compatible for at least 2 hr	1438	C

[a]Concentration unspecified.
[b]Diluted 1:1 in sodium chloride 0.9%.

Additional Compatibility Information

The manufacturer recommends not mixing iohexol products with any other pharmaceutical (1-7/96).

IOPAMIDOL
AHFS 36:68

Isovue **Bracco Diagnostics**

Products— Isovue products (Bracco Diagnostics) are available in concentrations ranging from 41% (200 mg/ml organically bound iodine) to 76% (370 mg/ml organically bound iodine) in numerous vial and bottle sizes from 20 to 200 ml; not all concentrations are available in all sizes. Also present in each milliliter are tromethamine 1 mg, edetate calcium disodium, with hydrochloric acid and/or sodium hydroxide to adjust the pH (1-8/98). Table 1 presents the characteristics of iopamidol products.

pH— From 6.5 to 7.5 (1-8/98).

Administration— Iopamidol may be administered intravenously or intra-arterially. Solutions should be warmed to body temperature prior to administration (1-8/98).

Table 1. Iopamidol Product Characteristics (1-8/98)

Iopamidol Concentration (%)	Iodine Concentration (mg/ml)	Osmolality (mOsm/kg)	Specific Gravity (37 °C)
41	200	413	1.227
51	250	524	1.281
61	300	616	1.339
76	370	796	1.405

Stability— Iopamidol injection is colorless to pale yellow. Intact vials should be stored at controlled room temperature and protected from light. If crystals form, they should be dissolved by warming of the vial in hot (60 to 100 °C) water for about five minutes and gentle shaking. The vials should cool to body temperature before use. If crystals fail to dissolve, the vials should be discarded (1-8/98).

Compatibility Information

Drugs in Syringe Compatibility

Iopamidol

Drug (in syringe)	Mfr	Amt	Mfr	Amt	Remarks	Ref	C/I
Ampicillin sodium	BR	30 mg/ 1 ml	SQ	61%, 5 ml	Physically compatible for at least 2 hr	1438	C
Chloramphenicol sodium succinate	PD	33 mg/ 1 ml	SQ	61%, 5 ml	Physically compatible for at least 2 hr	1438	C
Cimetidine HCl	SKF	150 mg/ 1 ml	SQ	61%, 5 ml	Physically compatible for at least 2 hr	1438	C
Diphenhydramine HCl	PD	12.5 mg/ 0.25 ml	SQ	61%, 5 ml	Physically compatible for at least 2 hr	1438	C
Epinephrine HCl	PD	1 mg/ 1 ml	SQ	61%, 5 ml	Physically compatible for at least 2 hr	1438	C
Gentamicin sulfate	SC	0.8 mg/ 1 ml	SQ	61%, 5 ml	Physically compatible for at least 2 hr	1438	C
Heparin sodium	OR	5000 units/ 0.5 ml	SQ	61%, 5 ml	Physically compatible for at least 2 hr	1438	C
Hydrocortisone sodium succinate	UP	10 mg/ 1 ml	SQ	61%, 5 ml	Physically compatible for at least 2 hr	1438	C
Methylprednisolone sodium succinate	UP	10 mg/ 1 ml	SQ	61%, 5 ml	Physically compatible for at least 2 hr	1438	C
Papaverine HCl	LI	30 mg/ 1 ml	SQ	61%, 5 ml	Physically compatible for at least 2 hr	1438	C
Protamine sulfate	LI	10 mg/ 1 ml	SQ	61%, 5 ml	Physically compatible for at least 2 hr	1438	C

Additional Compatibility Information

The manufacturer recommends not mixing iopamidol products with any other pharmaceutical (1-8/98).

IOTHALAMATE MEGLUMINE
AHFS 36:68

Conray   **Mallinckrodt**

Products— Iothalamate meglumine is available in concentrations ranging from 17.2 to 60%. It is also available in combination with other radiopaque contrast agents. The formulations may also contain edetate and phosphate buffers. Some examples of single-agent products are listed in Table 1 (4; 154).

Table 1. Some Representative Iothalamate Meglumine Products

Iothalamate Meglumine Content (%)	Bound Iodine (mg/ml)	Representative Trade Names
Urogenital solutions (not for intravascular use)		
17.2	81	Cysto-Conray II
43	202	Cysto-Conray
Parenteral solutions		
30	141	Conray 30
43	202	Conray 43
60	282	Conray

pH— From 6.5 to 7.7 (4).

Osmolarity— The injections have osmolarities from 750 to 1500 mOsm/L (4).

Administration— Iothalamate meglumine solutions may be administered intravenously, intra-arterially, by injection into pancreatic and biliary ducts, and by bladder, ureter, or renal pelvis instillation. Solutions should be warmed to body temperature before administration (4).

Stability— Iothalamate meglumine solutions are colorless to pale yellow. They should be stored below 30 °C. Crystallization does not occur at room temperature, but exposure to cold temperatures may result in crystallization. Should crystallization occur, the solution should be brought to room temperature, with shaking of the container if necessary to redissolve the crystals. The speed of dissolution may be increased by heating the vials in warm air (1-1/98).

Iothalamate meglumine is sensitive to light and should be protected from strong daylight and direct exposure to sunlight (4).

Iothalamate meglumine is also sensitive to low pH values. At pH values reported as about 2.4 to 2.7 (479) and below 3 (4), turbidity or frank precipitation may appear in the 60% product (479).

Iothalamate meglumine 60% (Conray) was stored in polystyrene syringes (Pharmaseal) at 25 and 37 °C. No apparent changes were noted visually or spectrophotometrically over five days (530).

Compatibility Information

Drugs in Syringe Compatibility

Iothalamate meglumine 60%

Drug (in syringe)	Mfr	Amt	Mfr	Amt	Remarks	Ref	C/I
Ampicillin sodium	BR	30 mg/ 1 ml	MA	60%, 5 ml	Physically compatible for at least 2 hr	1438	C
Chloramphenicol sodium succinate	PD	33 mg/ 1 ml	MA	60%, 5 ml	Physically compatible for at least 2 hr	1438	C
Chlorpheniramine maleate	SC	1 ml[a]	MA	40 to 1 ml	Physically compatible for 48 hr	530	C
Cimetidine HCl	SKF	150 mg/ 1 ml	MA	60%, 5 ml	Physically compatible for at least 2 hr	1438	C
Dimenhydrinate	SE	50 mg/ 1 ml	MA	40 to 1 ml	Physically compatible for 48 hr	530	C
Diphenhydramine HCl	PD	1 ml[a]	MA	40 to 1 ml	Physically compatible for 48 hr	530	C
	PD	50 mg/ 1 ml	MA	5 ml[a]	No precipitate observed	309	C
	PD	12.5 mg/ 0.25 ml	MA	60%, 5 ml	Physically compatible for at least 2 hr	1438	C
Epinephrine HCl	PD	1 mg/ 1 ml	MA	60%, 5 ml	Physically compatible for at least 2 hr	1438	C
Gentamicin sulfate	SC	0.8 mg/ 1 ml	MA	60%, 5 ml	Physically compatible for at least 2 hr	1438	C
Heparin sodium	OR	5000 units/ 0.5 ml	MA	60%, 5 ml	Physically compatible for at least 2 hr	1438	C

Drugs in Syringe Compatibility (Cont.)

Iothalamate meglumine 60%

Drug (in syringe)	Mfr	Amt	Mfr	Amt	Remarks	Ref	C/I
Hyaluronidase	WY	150 units/ 1 ml	MA	40 to 1 ml	Physically compatible for 48 hr	530	**C**
Hydrocortisone sodium succinate	UP	10 mg/ 1 ml	MA	60%, 5 ml	Physically compatible for at least 2 hr	1438	**C**
Methylprednisolone sodium succinate	UP	10 mg/ 1 ml	MA	60%, 5 ml	Physically compatible for at least 2 hr	1438	**C**
Papaverine HCl	LI	30 mg/ 1 ml	MA	60%, 5 ml	Physically compatible for at least 2 hr	1438	**C**
Promethazine HCl	WY	1 ml[a]	MA	40 to 1 ml	Immediate precipitation	530	**I**
Protamine sulfate	LI	10 mg/ 1 ml	MA	60%, 5 ml	Physically compatible for at least 2 hr	1438	**C**

[a]*Concentration unspecified.*

IOTHALAMATE SODIUM
AHFS 36:68

Conray 400   **Mallinckrodt**
Conray 325   **Mallinckrodt**

Products— Iothalamate sodium is available in concentrations of 54.3 and 66.8%. It is also available in combination with other radiopaque contrast agents. The formulations may also contain edetate and phosphate buffers. Some examples of single-agent products are listed in Table 1 (4; 154).

pH— From 6.5 to 7.7 (4).

Table 1. Some Representative Iothalamate Sodium Products

Iothalamate Sodium Content (%)	Bound Iodine (mg/ml)	Representative Trade Names
54.3	325	Conray 325
66.8	400	Conray-400

Osmolarity— The injections have osmolarities of (54.3%) 1700 mOsm/L and (66.8%) 2300 mOsm/L (1-1/98; 4).

Sodium Content— Iothalamate sodium contains approximately 1.57 mEq of sodium per gram of drug (4).

Administration— Iothalamate sodium solutions may be administered intravenously, intra-arterially, or by injection through a catheter into the chambers of the heart or associated large blood vessels. Solutions should be warmed to body temperature before administration (4).

Stability— Iothalamate sodium solutions are colorless to pale yellow. Solutions should be protected from strong daylight and direct exposure to the sun and should be stored below 30 °C. Crystallization does not occur at room temperature, but exposure to cold temperatures may result in it. Should crystallization occur, the solution should be warmed to room temperature, with shaking of the container if necessary to redissolve the crystals (1-1/98; 4). The speed of crystal dissolution may be increased by heating with circulating warm air. Submersion of prefilled syringes in water is not recommended. The prefilled plastic syringes should not be re-autoclaved because of possible damage (1-1/98).

Iothalamate sodium 80% (Angio-Conray) was stored in polystyrene syringes (Pharmaseal) at 25 and 37 °C. No apparent changes were noted visually or spectrophotometrically over five days (550).

Compatibility Information

Drugs in Syringe Compatibility

Iothalamate sodium

Drug (in syringe)	Mfr	Amt	Mfr	Amt	Remarks	Ref	C/I
Chlorpheniramine maleate	SC	1 ml[b]	MA	80%[a], 40 to 1 ml	Physically compatible for 48 hr	530	C
Dimenhydrinate	SE	50 mg/ 1 ml	MA	80%[a], 40 to 1 ml	Physically compatible for 48 hr	530	C
Diphenhydramine HCl	PD	1 ml[b]	MA	80%[a], 40 to 1 ml	Physically compatible for 48 hr	530	C
Hyaluronidase	WY	150 units/ 1 ml	MA	80%[a], 40 to 1 ml	Physically compatible for 48 hr	530	C
Papaverine HCl	LI	30 mg/ 1 ml	MA	60%, 3 ml	Physically compatible	1437	C
Promethazine HCl	WY	1 ml[b]	MA	80%[a], 40 to 1 ml	Immediate precipitation	530	I

[a]*This concentration is no longer available.*
[b]*Concentration unspecified.*

IOXAGLATE MEGLUMINE AND IOXAGLATE SODIUM
AHFS 36:68

Hexabrix **Mallinckrodt**

Products— Ioxaglate meglumine 39.3% and ioxaglate sodium 19.6% (Mallinckrodt) is available in containers ranging in size from 20 to 200 ml. Each milliliter contains ioxaglate meglumine 393 mg, ioxaglate sodium 196 mg, and edetate calcium disodium 0.1 mg as a stabilizer. The product provides 32% organically bound iodine (1-1/98).

pH— From 6 to 7.6 (1-1/98).

Osmolality— The osmolality of the product is approximately 600 mOsm/kg (1-1/98).

Sodium Content— Each milliliter provides 0.15 mEq (3.48 mg) of sodium (1-1/98).

Administration— The product may be administered intravenously, intra-arterially, or intra-articularly. It also may be injected or instilled directly into selected areas to be visualized. The solutions should be warmed to body temperature before administration (1-1/98).

Stability— The product should be stored below 30 °C and protected from freezing and direct exposure to sun or strong daylight. The solution is colorless to pale yellow. Crystallization does not occur at normal room temperatures. If the product is frozen or crystallization occurs, bring it to room temperature and shake vigorously to dissolve all crystals. Warming with circulating warm air is recommended to speed dissolution. Submersion of syringes in water is not recommended (1-1/98).

Compatibility Information

Drugs in Syringe Compatibility

Ioxaglate meglumine 39.3% + Ioxaglate sodium 19.6%

Drug (in syringe)	Mfr	Amt	Mfr	Amt	Remarks	Ref	C/I
Ampicillin sodium	BR	30 mg/ 1 ml	MA	5 ml	Physically compatible for at least 2 hr	1438	C
Chloramphenicol sodium succinate	PD	33 mg/ 1 ml	MA	5 ml	Physically compatible for at least 2 hr	1438	C

Drugs in Syringe Compatibility (Cont.)

Ioxaglate meglumine 39.3% + Ioxaglate sodium 19.6%

Drug (in syringe)	Mfr	Amt	Mfr	Amt	Remarks	Ref	C/I
Cimetidine HCl	SKF	150 mg/ 1 ml	MA	5 ml	Precipitate forms immediately and persists for at least 2 hr	1438	I
Diphenhydramine HCl	PD	12.5 mg/ 0.25 ml	MA	5 ml	Precipitate forms immediately and persists for at least 2 hr	1438	I
Epinephrine HCl	PD	1 mg/ 1 ml	MA	5 ml	Physically compatible for at least 2 hr	1438	C
Gentamicin sulfate	SC	0.8 mg/ 1 ml	MA	5 ml	Transient precipitate clears within 5 min	1438	?
Heparin sodium	OR	5000 units/ 0.5 ml	MA	5 ml	Physically compatible for at least 2 hr	1438	C
Hydrocortisone sodium succinate	UP	10 mg/ 1 ml	MA	5 ml	Physically compatible for at least 2 hr	1438	C
Methylprednisolone sodium succinate	UP	10 mg/ 1 ml	MA	5 ml	Physically compatible for at least 2 hr	1438	C
Papaverine HCl	ME	32 mg/ 1 ml	MA	5 ml	Precipitate forms immediately and persists for at least 2 hr	1438	I
	LI	30 mg/ 1 ml	MA	3 and 5 ml	White amorphous precipitate forms immediately and persists for 24 hr. If shaken, it dissolves in 20 to 30 min	1437	I
	LI	30 mg/2 to 6 ml[a]	MA	5 ml	Precipitate forms	1437	I
	LI	30 mg/ 11 and 16 ml[a]	MA	5 ml	Precipitate forms and then dissolves	1437	?
	LI	30 mg/ 21 ml[a]	MA	5 ml	Physically compatible	1437	C
	LI	30 mg/ 11 ml[a]	MA	15 and 30 ml	Physically compatible	1437	C
	LI	60 mg/ 12 and 17 ml[a]	MA	5 ml	Precipitate forms	1437	I
	LI	60 mg/ 22 ml[a]	MA	5 ml	Precipitate forms and then dissolves	1437	?
Protamine sulfate	LI	10 mg/ 1 ml	MA	5 ml	Precipitate forms immediately and persists for at least 2 hr	1438	I

[a]*Diluted in sodium chloride 0.9%.*

IRINOTECAN HCL
AHFS 10:00

Camptosar　　　　　　　**Pharmacia & Upjohn**

Products— Irinotecan HCl (Pharmacia & Upjohn) is available in 2- and 5-ml single-use vials containing 40 and 100 mg of drug, respectively, on the basis of the trihydrate. Each milliliter of solution contains irinotecan HCl trihydrate 20 mg, sorbitol 45 mg, lactic acid 0.9 mg, and hydrochloric acid or sodium hydroxide to adjust the pH. The product must be diluted prior to use (2).

pH— From 3 to 3.8 (2).

Administration— Irinotecan HCl is administered by intravenous infusion over 90 minutes after dilution to a final concentration in the range of 0.12 to 1.1 mg/ml in dextrose 5% in water or sodium chloride 0.9%. In most clinical trials, the doses were given in

500 ml of dextrose 5% in water (2). Use of concentrations up to 2.8 mg/ml and in volumes down to 250 ml has also been cited (4).

Stability— Irinotecan HCl injection is supplied as a clear pale yellow solution. Intact vials should be stored at controlled room temperature and protected from light. Freezing of irinotecan HCl solutions may result in precipitation and should be avoided (2).

Photodegradation— Irinotecan HCl is subject to photodegradation, including the formation of a precipitate (1997; 1998; 2137). Exposure to ultraviolet light for three days produced a darkening in the solution color and the formation of a yellow precipitate composed of several decomposition products (1997). Photodegradation of irinotecan HCl occurs under any pH condition but is accelerated in neutral and alkaline solutions compared with acidic solutions. At pH 10,

photodegradation is very rapid; at pH 3 it is much slower. At pH 7, irinotecan 0.34 mg/ml lost 32% in six hours exposed to a daylight lamp and 19% exposed to a white fluorescent light. In infusion solutions having neutral pH, irinotecan HCl exposed to lighting (such as that of a medical facility) may have rapid decomposition. Protection from light exposure has been recommended to maintain product quality during administration (1998). The structural changes exhibited by the decomposition products would indicate that they are unlikely to be active antineoplastic compounds (2137).

pH Effects— Irinotecan in solution at acidic pH is stable, but raising the pH to more than 6.5 has resulted in 10% loss in as little as three hours (1881).

Compatibility Information

Y-Site Injection Compatibility (1:1 Mixture)

Drug	Mfr	Conc	Mfr	Conc	Remarks	Ref	C/I
Gemcitabine HCl	PHU	5 mg/ml[b]	LI	10 mg/ml[b]	Subvisual haze with green discoloration forms immediately	2226	**I**

[b]Tested in sodium chloride 0.9%.

Additional Compatibility Information

Infusion Solutions— Dextrose 5% in water and sodium chloride 0.9% are recommended for administration of irinotecan HCl. Admixtures of the drug in dextrose 5% in water and sodium chloride 0.9% at concentrations between 0.12 and 1.1 mg/ml are stated to be physically and chemically stable for up to 24 hours at room temperatures around 25 °C exposed to ambient fluorescent light. Under refrigeration and protected from light, admixtures in dextrose 5% in water are stable for 48 hours. However, refrigerated storage of iri-

notecan HCl in sodium chloride 0.9% is not recommended because of occasional visible precipitation. The manufacturer recommends use of the drug admixtures within six hours at room temperature and 24 hours under refrigeration because of concern for possible microbiological contamination during preparation (2).

Methylprednisolone— Adding methylprednisolone sodium succinate to irinotecan was found to result in an admixture having a pH greater than 6.5. Approximately 10% irinotecan loss occurs within three hours at this pH (1881).

IRON DEXTRAN
AHFS 20:04.04

INFeD   **Schein**
Dexferrum   **American Regent**

Products— Iron dextran is available in 2-ml vials for intravenous or intramuscular use. It is composed of a dark brown, slightly viscous liquid complex of ferric hydroxide and dextran in sodium chloride 0.9%, providing 50 mg of elemental iron per milliliter (2).

pH— From 5.2 to 6.5 (2).

Osmolality— Iron dextran injection has an osmolality exceeding 2000 mOsm/kg (1689).

Administration— Iron dextran may be administered by slow intravenous injection at a rate of no more than 1 ml/min or by deep intramuscular injection into the upper outer quadrant of the buttock.

Subsequent injections should be made into alternate buttocks. Staining of the skin can be minimized by using a separate needle to withdraw the drug from the container and by displacing the skin laterally prior to injection (2; 4). Iron dextran also has been administered by intravenous infusion over one to six hours after dilution in sodium chloride 0.9% (4). A test dose of 25 mg should be given over five minutes, with the remainder given after one hour has elapsed if no hypersensitivity reaction occurs (2; 4).

Stability— The commercial injection should be stored at controlled room temperature (2; 4). High temperatures, such as during autoclaving, precipitate the iron dextran complex (692).

A stable dilute solution of iron dextran for use in parenteral nutrition has been prepared. A 0.5-mg/ml diluted solution was prepared by diluting 5 ml of iron dextran to 200 ml with sterile water for injection, adding benzyl alcohol 4.5 ml, and adding more sterile water for injection to a final volume of 500 ml. The diluted solution was sterilized by filtration through a 0.22-µm filter. The dilution was stable for at least three months when stored under refrigeration (692).

Filtration— Iron dextran is reported to be adsorbed to sterilizing membrane filters composed of cellulose nitrate and acetate combined (such as the Millex G.S. and Gelman Acrodisc). The initial concern resulted from a reddish brown stain on the filters. In subsequent studies, an iron dextran solution containing 5 µg/ml in water was estimated to lose 93% of the iron from the first milliliter passed through the filter. As more solution was passed through the filter, a decreasing proportion of the iron was adsorbed, indicating that the filter was approaching saturation. The extent of iron adsorption increased in the presence of electrolytes and trace elements. The authors concluded that adsorption can be significant, especially when small amounts of iron dextran are involved (918).

Compatibility Information

Solution Compatibility

Iron dextran

Solution	Mfr	Mfr	Conc/L	Remarks	Ref	C/I
TNA #122[a]		FI	50 mg	Lipid oiling out in 18 to 19 hr with formation of yellow-brown layer on admixture surface	1383	I
TNA #159 to #166[a]		FI	2 mg	Physically compatible with no change visually, microscopically, or in particle size distribution in 48 hr at 4 and 25 °C	1648	C
TPN #31 to #33[a]		FI	100 mg	Physically compatible with minimal changes to iron dextran and amino acids for 18 hr at room temperature	692	C
TPN #207 and #208[a]		SCN	10 mg	Rust-colored precipitate forms in 12 hr at 19 °C protected from sunlight	2103	I
TPN #209[a]		SCN	10 mg	Rust-colored precipitate forms in 18 to 24 hr at 19 °C protected from sunlight	2103	I
TPN #210[a]		SCN	10 mg	Visually compatible for 48 hr at 19 °C protected from sunlight. Trace iron precipitation found by filtration and analysis after 48 hr	2103	?
TPN #211[a]		SCN	10 mg	Visually compatible for 48 hr at 19 °C protected from sunlight. No iron precipitation found by filtration and analysis after 48 hr	2103	C

[a]*Refer to Appendix I for the composition of parenteral nutrition solutions. TNA indicates a 3-in-1 admixture, and TPN indicates a 2-in-1 admixture.*

Additive Compatibility

Iron dextran

Drug	Mfr	Conc/L	Mfr	Conc/L	Test Soln	Remarks	Ref	C/I
Netilmicin sulfate	SC	3 g	MRN	8 ml	D5S	Physically compatible and netilmicin chemically stable for 7 days at 4 and 25 °C. Iron dextran not tested	558	C

Additional Compatibility Information

Sodium chloride 0.9% has been suggested as a diluent for infusion of iron dextran (75; 76; 429; 919–921). Dilution in dextrose 5% in water results in a greater incidence of pain and phlebitis (75).

Cyanocobalamin is stated to be stable in the presence of iron dextran (52).

The manufacturer recommends not mixing iron dextran injection with other medications or adding it to parenteral nutrition solutions (2).

Mayhew and Quick evaluated the effect of amino acid concentration on precipitation of iron from iron dextran (INFeD, Schein) 10 mg/L in neonatal parenteral nutrition mixtures (TPN #207 to #211) formulated with TrophAmine (McGaw). Rust-colored precipitate formed in the neonatal formulations having amino acid concentrations of 1.5% or less. The precipitate formed more rapidly and in greater amounts at lower amino acid concentrations. Parenteral nutrition admixtures with amino acid concentrations of 2 and 2.5% were visually compatible for 48 hr at 19 °C, but trace precipitation was found on filtration and analysis of the 2% admixture. Extrapolation of the information to other iron dextran products may not be appropriate because of possible product differences (2103).

Iron dextran (Fisons) 2 mg/L was physically compatible with several fat-containing parenteral nutrition solutions (TNA #159 to #166, Appendix I) for 48 hours at 4 and 25 °C. The order of mixing and deliberate agitation had no effect on physical compatibility and particle size distribution (1648).

The influence of six factors on the stability of fat emulsion in 45 different 3-in-1 parenteral nutrition mixtures was evaluated. The factors were amino acid concentration (2.5 to 7%); dextrose (5 to 20%); fat emulsion, intravenous (2 to 5%); monovalent cations (0 to 150 mEq/L); divalent cations (4 to 20 mEq/L); and trivalent cations from iron dextran (0 to 10 mg elemental iron/L). Although many formulations were unstable, visual examination could identify instability in only 65% of the samples. Electronic evaluation of particle size identified the remaining unstable mixtures. Furthermore, only the concentration of trivalent ferric ions significantly and consistently affected the emulsion stability during the 30-hour test period. Of the parenteral nutrition mixtures containing iron dextran, 16% were unstable, exhibiting emulsion cracking. The authors suggested that iron dextran should not be incorporated into 3-in-1 mixtures (1814).

ISOPROTERENOL HCL (ISOPRENALINE HCL) AHFS 12:12

Abbott

Products— Isoproterenol HCl (Abbott) is available as a 1:50,000 solution in 10-ml (0.2 mg) unit-of-use syringes. It is also available as a 1:5000 concentrated solution in 5-ml (1 mg) and 10-ml (2 mg) Universal Additive Syringes intended for dilution in an intravenous infusion solution (1-2/97). The drug is also available in a concentration of 0.2 mg/ml in 1- and 5-ml ampuls (29; 154).

Each milliliter of isoproterenol HCl solutions (Abbott) contains (1-2/97):

	1:50,000 injection	1:5000 injection
Isoproterenol HCl	0.02 mg	0.2 mg
Sodium chloride	4.7 mg	4.25 mg
Sodium metabisulfite	0.9 mg	0.5 mg
Citric acid, anhydrous	2 mg	2 mg
Sodium citrate dihydrate	0.4 mg	1.6 mg

(Additional citric acid and/or sodium citrate may have been added to adjust pH.)

pH— The 0.02-mg/ml concentration has a pH in the range of 2.5 to 3.5. The 0.2-mg/ml concentration has a pH in the range of 3.5 to 4.5 (1-2/97).

Osmolality— The osmolality of isoproterenol HCl (Breon) 0.2 mg/ml was determined to be 277 mOsm/kg by freezing-point depression and 293 mOsm/kg by vapor pressure (1071).

Administration— Isoproterenol HCl may be administered by intravenous infusion; by direct intravenous, intramuscular, or subcutaneous injection; and, in extreme emergencies, by intracardiac injection. For direct intravenous injection, 1 ml of the 1:5000 injection should be diluted to 10 ml with sodium chloride 0.9% or dextrose 5% in water to provide a 20-μg/ml solution. Intravenous infusions are prepared by adding 1 to 10 ml of the 1:5000 injection to 500 ml of compatible diluent (1-2/97; 4).

Stability— Isoproterenol HCl injection in intact containers should be stored in a cool place between 2 and 15 °C and protected from light. Ampuls should be kept in opaque containers until used. The drug should not be used if a color or precipitate is present. Exposure to air, light, or increased temperature may cause a pink to brownish pink color to develop (1-2/97; 4; 975). Isoproterenol HCl 5 mg/L was stable at pH 3.7 to 5.7 in dextrose 5% in water at 25 °C for more than 24 hours (59). At pH values above 6, it displayed significant decomposition (48; 59; 430). The pH of a solution is the primary determinant of catecholamine stability in intravenous admixtures (527).

Isoproterenol HCl (Winthrop) 4 mg/L in dextrose 5% in water in PVC bags retained biological activity after 30 months of storage at room temperature. However, spectrophotometric analysis of the PVC stored solutions was not possible because of interference by substances leached from the plastic (430).

Filtration— Isoproterenol HCl (Winthrop) 2 mg/L in dextrose 5% in water, sodium chloride 0.9%, and Ringer's injection, lactated, filtered over 12 hours through a 5-μm stainless steel depth filter (Argyle Filter Connector), a 0.22-μm cellulose ester membrane filter (Ivex-2 Filter Set), and a 0.22-μm polycarbonate membrane filter (In-Sure Filter Set), showed no significant reduction in potency due to binding to the filters (320).

In another study, isoproterenol HCl (Winthrop) 4 mg/L in dextrose 5% in water and sodium chloride 0.9% did not display significant sorption to a 0.45-μm cellulose membrane filter (Abbott S-A-I-F) during an eight-hour simulated infusion (567).

Compatibility Information

Solution Compatibility

Isoproterenol[a]

Solution	Mfr	Mfr	Conc/L	Remarks	Ref	C/I
Amino acids 4.25%, dextrose 25%	MG	WI	2 mg (H)	No increase in particulate matter in 24 hr at 5 °C	349	C

Solution Compatibility (Cont.)

Isoproterenol[a]

Solution	Mfr	Mfr	Conc/L	Remarks	Ref	C/I
Dextran 6% in dextrose 5%	AB	AB	0.02 mg (S)	Physically compatible	3	**C**
Dextran 6% in sodium chloride 0.9%	AB	AB	0.02 mg (S)	Physically compatible	3	**C**
Dextrose–Ringer's injection combinations	AB	AB	0.02 mg (S)	Physically compatible	3	**C**
Dextrose–Ringer's injection, lactated, combinations	AB	AB	0.02 mg (S)	Physically compatible	3	**C**
Dextrose 5% in Ringer's injection, lactated	TR[b]	WI	2 mg (H)	Potency retained for 24 hr at 5 °C	282	**C**
Dextrose–saline combinations	AB	AB	0.02 mg (S)	Physically compatible	3	**C**
Dextrose 5% in sodium chloride 0.9%	TR[b]	WI	2 mg (H)	Potency retained for 24 hr at 5 °C	282	**C**
Dextrose 2½% in water	AB	AB	0.02 mg (S)	Physically compatible	3	**C**
Dextrose 5% in water	AB	AB	0.02 mg (S)	Physically compatible	3	**C**
	TR[b]	WI	2 mg (H)	Potency retained for 24 hr at 5 °C	282	**C**
	AB	BN	2 mg (H)	Physically compatible and chemically stable. 10% decomposition is calculated to occur in 24 hr in the light and 250 hr in the dark at 25 °C	527	**C**
Dextrose 10% in water	AB	AB	0.02 mg (S)	Physically compatible	3	**C**
Fructose 10% in sodium chloride 0.9%	AB	AB	0.02 mg (S)	Physically compatible	3	**C**
Fructose 10% in water	AB	AB	0.02 mg (S)	Physically compatible	3	**C**
Invert sugar 5 and 10% in sodium chloride 0.9%	AB	AB	0.02 mg (S)	Physically compatible	3	**C**
Invert sugar 5 and 10% in water	AB	AB	0.02 mg (S)	Physically compatible	3	**C**
Ionosol products	AB	AB	0.02 mg (S)	Physically compatible	3	**C**
Ringer's injection	AB	AB	0.02 mg (S)	Physically compatible	3	**C**
Ringer's injection, lactated	AB	AB	0.02 mg (S)	Physically compatible	3	**C**
	TR[b]	WI	2 mg (H)	Potency retained for 24 hr at 5 °C	282	**C**
Sodium bicarbonate 5%		WI	5 mg (H)	Isoproterenol decomposition	48	**I**
Sodium chloride 0.45%	AB	AB	0.02 mg (S)	Physically compatible	3	**C**
Sodium chloride 0.9%	AB	AB	0.02 mg (S)	Physically compatible	3	**C**

Solution Compatibility (Cont.)

Solution Compatibility (Cont.)

Isoproterenol[a]

Solution	Mfr	Mfr	Conc/L	Remarks	Ref	C/I
	TR[b]	WI	2 mg (H)	Potency retained for 24 hr at 5 °C	282	C
Sodium lactate ⅙ M	AB	AB	0.02 mg (S)	Physically compatible	3	C

[a]Combinations with designation "(H)" in the Conc/L column were tested as the hydrochloride salt; "(S)" indicates the sulfate salt of isoproterenol.
[b]Tested in both glass and PVC containers.

Additive Compatibility

Isoproterenol HCl

Drug	Mfr	Conc/L	Mfr	Conc/L	Test Soln	Remarks	Ref	C/I
Aminophylline	SE	500 mg	BN	2 mg	D5W	10% isoproterenol decomposition in 2.2 to 2.5 hr in the light and dark at 25 °C	527	I
Atracurium besylate	BW	500 mg		4 mg	D5W	Physically compatible and atracurium chemically stable for 24 hr at 5 and 30 °C	1694	C
Calcium chloride	UP	1 g	WI	4 mg		Physically compatible	59	C
Cibenzoline succinate		2 g	WB	4 mg	D5W, NS	Physically compatible for 24 hr at 25 °C by visual and microscopic examination	1182	C
Cimetidine HCl	SKF	3 g	WI	20 mg	D5W	Physically compatible and cimetidine chemically stable for 24 hr at room temperature. Isoproterenol not tested	551	C
Dobutamine HCl	LI	1 g	ES	2 mg	D5W, NS	Physically compatible for 24 hr at 21 °C	812	C
Floxacillin sodium	BE	20 g	PX	4 mg	D5W	Physically compatible for 24 hr at 15 and 30 °C. Haze forms in 48 hr and precipitate forms in 72 hr	1479	C
Furosemide	HO	1 g	PX	4 mg	D5W	Immediate precipitation	1479	I
Heparin sodium		32,000 units		2 mg	NS	Physically compatible and heparin activity retained for 24 hr	57	C
	AB	20,000 units	WI	4 mg		Physically compatible	59	C
Magnesium sulfate		1 g	WI	4 mg		Physically compatible	59	C
Multivitamins	USV	10 ml	WI	4 mg		Physically compatible	59	C
Netilmicin sulfate	SC	3 g	WI	400 mg	D5S	Physically compatible and netilmicin chemically stable for 7 days at 4 and 25 °C. Isoproterenol not tested	558	C
Potassium chloride	AB	40 mEq	WI	4 mg		Physically compatible	59	C
Ranitidine HCl	GL	50 mg and 2 g		20 mg	D5W	Physically compatible and ranitidine chemically stable by HPLC for 24 hr at 25 °C. Isoproterenol not tested	1515	C
Sodium bicarbonate	AB	2.4 mEq[a]	BN	1 mg	D5W	Isoproterenol inactivated	772	I
Succinylcholine chloride	AB	2 g	WI	4 mg		Physically compatible	59	C
Verapamil HCl	KN	80 mg	BN	10 mg	D5W, NS	Physically compatible for 24 hr	764	C
Vitamin B complex with C	AB	10 ml	WI	4 mg		Physically compatible	59	C
	UP	10 ml	WI	4 mg		Physically compatible	59	C

[a]One vial of Neut added to a liter of admixture.

Drugs in Syringe Compatibility

Isoproterenol[a]

Drug (in syringe)	Mfr	Amt	Mfr	Amt	Remarks	Ref	C/I
Ranitidine HCl	GL	50 mg/ 5 ml	BI	0.2 mg	Physically compatible for 4 hr at ambient temperature under fluorescent light	1151	C

[a]*Tested as the sulfate salt of isoproterenol.*

Y-Site Injection Compatibility (1:1 Mixture)

Isoproterenol HCl

Drug	Mfr	Conc	Mfr	Conc	Remarks	Ref	C/I
Amiodarone HCl	LZ	4 mg/ml[c]	ES	0.004 mg/ml[c]	Physically compatible for 24 hr at 21 °C	1032	C
Amrinone lactate	WB	3 mg/ml[b]	BR	0.004 mg/ml[a]	Physically compatible for at least 4 hr at 25 °C under fluorescent light	992	C
Atracurium besylate	BW	0.5 mg/ml[a]	ES	4 μg/ml[a]	Physically compatible for 24 hr at 28 °C	1337	C
Bretylium tosylate	LY	4 mg/ml[c]	ES	0.032 mg/ml[c]	Physically compatible for 3 hr	1316	C
Cisatracurium besylate	GW	0.1, 2, 5 mg/ml[a]	AB	0.02 mg/ml[a]	Physically compatible with no change in measured turbidity or increase in particle content in 4 hr at 23 °C	2074	C
Famotidine	MSD	0.2 mg/ml[a]	ES	0.004 mg/ml[a]	Physically compatible for 4 hr at 25 °C	1188	C
Heparin sodium	UP	1000 units/ L[d]	WI	0.2 mg/ml	Physically compatible for at least 4 hr at room temperature by visual and microscopic examination	534	C
Hydrocortisone sodium succinate	UP	10 mg/L[d]	WI	0.2 mg/ml	Physically compatible for at least 4 hr at room temperature by visual and microscopic examination	534	C
Milrinone lactate	SW	0.4 mg/ml[a]	ES	8 μg/ml[a]	Visually compatible with little or no loss of either drug by HPLC in 4 hr at 23 °C	2214	C
Pancuronium bromide	ES	0.05 mg/ml[a]	ES	4 μg/ml[a]	Physically compatible for 24 hr at 28 °C	1337	C
Potassium chloride	AB	40 mEq/L[d]	WI	0.2 mg/ml	Physically compatible for at least 4 hr at room temperature by visual and microscopic examination	534	C
Propofol	ZEN	10 mg/ml	AB	0.004 mg/ml[a]	Physically compatible for 1 hr at 23 °C with no increase in particle content	2066	C
Remifentanil HCl	GW	0.025 and 0.25 mg/ml[b]	SW	0.02 mg/ml[a]	Physically compatible with no change in measured turbidity or increase in particle content in 4 hr at 23 °C	2075	C
Tacrolimus	FUJ	1 mg/ml[b]	ES	0.04 mg/ml[a]	Visually compatible for 24 hr at 25 °C	1630	C
TNA #73[e]			BR	0.2 mg/ 50 ml[c]	Physically compatible for 4 hr by visual observation	1009	C
Vecuronium bromide	OR	0.1 mg/ml[a]	ES	4 μg/ml[a]	Physically compatible for 24 hr at 28 °C	1337	C
Vitamin B complex with C	RC	2 ml/L[d]	WI	0.2 mg/ml	Physically compatible for at least 4 hr at room temperature by visual and microscopic examination	534	C

[a]*Tested in dextrose 5% in water.*

[b]*Tested in sodium chloride 0.9%.*

[c]*Tested in both dextrose 5% in water and sodium chloride 0.9%.*

[d]*Tested in dextrose 5% in Ringer's injection, dextrose 5% in Ringer's injection, lactated, dextrose 5% in water, Ringer's injection, lactated, and sodium chloride 0.9%.*

[e]*Refer to Appendix I for the composition of parenteral nutrition solutions. TNA indicates a 3-in-1 admixture.*

Additional Compatibility Information

Infusion Solutions— Dilution of isoproterenol HCl with sodium chloride 0.9% or dextrose 5% in water has been recommended (1-2/97; 4). Isoproterenol HCl (Winthrop) at 4 mg/L is stated to be physically compatible with all Abbott infusion solutions (59).

pH Effects— Isoproterenol HCl (Winthrop) at 5 mg/L displayed significant decomposition at a pH above approximately 6 (48; 59). Caution should be used when attempting to mix this drug in a solution with a final pH above this value. Drugs that may raise the pH above 6 include sodium bicarbonate, barbiturates, alkaline-buffered antibiotics (59), lidocaine HCl (24), and aminophylline (6). If these drugs are mixed, they should be administered immediately after preparation (59), or separate administration should be considered (24).

Visual inspection for color changes related to decomposition may be inadequate to assess the compatibility of admixtures. In one evaluation with aminophylline stored at 25 °C, a color change was not noted until 24 hours had elapsed. However, no intact isoproterenol HCl was present in the admixture at 24 hours (527).

KANAMYCIN SULFATE
AHFS 8:12.02

Kantrex   Apothecon

Products— Kanamycin sulfate is available in 3-ml vials containing 1 g, 2-ml vials containing 500 mg, and a pediatric injection in 2-ml vials containing 75 mg of kanamycin as the sulfate. The products also contain sodium bisulfite as an antioxidant (4; 154).

pH— Adjusted by the manufacturer to pH 4.5 with sulfuric acid (4).

Osmolality— The osmolality of kanamycin sulfate (Beecham) 250 mg/ml was determined to be 858 mOsm/kg by freezing-point depression and 952 mOsm/kg by vapor pressure (1071).

Administration— Kanamycin sulfate may be administered by deep intramuscular injection into the upper outer quadrant of the gluteal muscle or by intermittent intravenous infusion over 30 to 60 minutes in dextrose 5% in water or sodium chloride 0.9%. The drug also is administered by intraperitoneal instillation and irrigation (4).

Stability— Kanamycin sulfate injection is a clear colorless solution. Although some vials may darken during storage, the manufacturer states that this darkening does not indicate a loss of potency. Kanamycin sulfate injection should be stored at room temperature and protected from temperatures above 40 °C and from freezing (4).

Sorption— Kanamycin sulfate (Bristol) 15 mg/L in sodium chloride 0.9% (Travenol) in PVC bags did not exhibit significant sorption to the plastic during one week of storage at room temperature (15 to 20 °C) (536).

In another study, kanamycin sulfate (Bristol) 15 mg/L in sodium chloride 0.9% did not exhibit any loss due to sorption during a seven-hour simulated infusion through an infusion set (Travenol) consisting of a cellulose propionate burette chamber and 170 cm of PVC tubing (606).

The drug also was tested as a simulated infusion over at least one hour by a syringe pump system. A glass syringe on a syringe pump was fitted with 20 cm of polyethylene tubing or 50 cm of Silastic tubing. No loss of drug due to sorption was observed with either tubing (606).

A 25-ml aliquot of kanamycin sulfate (Bristol) 15 mg/L in sodium chloride 0.9% was stored in all-plastic syringes composed of polypropylene barrels and polyethylene plungers for 24 hours at room temperature in the dark. No loss due to sorption occurred (606).

Compatibility Information

Solution Compatibility

Kanamycin sulfate

Solution	Mfr	Mfr	Conc/L	Remarks	Ref	C/I
Amino acids 4.25%, dextrose 25%	MG	BR	500 mg	No increase in particulate matter in 24 hr at 5 °C	349	C
Dextrose 5% in sodium chloride 0.9%	MG	BR	250 mg	Potency retained for 24 hr at 4 and 25 °C	105	C
Dextrose 5% in water	MG	BR	250 mg	Potency retained for 24 hr at 4 and 25 °C	105	C
Dextrose 10% in water	MG	BR	250 mg	Potency retained for 24 hr at 4 and 25 °C	105	C
Isolyte M with dextrose 5%	MG	BR	250 mg	Potency retained for 24 hr at 4 and 25 °C	105	C
Isolyte P with dextrose 5%	MG	BR	250 mg	Potency retained for 24 hr at 4 and 25 °C	105	C
Ringer's injection, lactated	MG	BR	250 mg	Potency retained for 24 hr at 4 and 25 °C	105	C
Sodium chloride 0.9%	MG	BR	250 mg	Potency retained for 24 hr at 4 and 25 °C	105	C

Solution Compatibility (Cont.)

Kanamycin sulfate

Solution	Mfr	Mfr	Conc/L	Remarks	Ref	C/I
TPN #1, #3, #6, #9[a]		BR	500 mg	Physically incompatible with a precipitate forming in 8 to 12 hr at 22 °C	313	**I**
TPN #2, #4, #5, #7, #8[a]		BR	500 mg	Physically compatible for 24 hr at 22 °C	313	**C**
TPN #1[a]		BR	400 mg	Antibiotic potency retained for at least 12 hr at 22 °C	313	**C**
TPN #10[a]		BR	500 mg	Physically compatible for 24 hr and antibiotic potency retained for at least 12 hr at 22 °C	313	**C**
TPN #21[a]		BR	250 mg	Antibiotic potency retained for 24 hr at 4 °C	87	**C**
		BR	250 mg	11 to 13% kanamycin decomposition in 24 hr at 25 °C	87	**I**

[a]Refer to Appendix I for the composition of parenteral nutrition solutions. TPN indicates a 2-in-1 admixture.

Additive Compatibility

Kanamycin sulfate

Drug	Mfr	Conc/L	Mfr	Conc/L	Test Soln	Remarks	Ref	C/I
Amphotericin B		200 mg	BPC	4 g	D5W	Haze develops over 3 hr	26	**I**
Ascorbic acid injection	UP	500 mg	BR	4 g	D5W	Physically compatible	15	**C**
Cefoxitin sodium	MSD	5 g	BR	5 g	D5S	9% cefoxitin decomposition at 25 °C and 1% at 5 °C in 48 hr. 6% kanamycin decomposition at 25 °C and none at 5 °C in 48 hr	308	**C**
Chloramphenicol sodium succinate	PD	10 g	BR	4 g	D5W	Physically compatible	15	**C**
	PD	10 g	BR	4 g		Physically compatible	21	**C**
Chlorpheniramine maleate	SC	100 mg	BR	4 g	D5W	Physically incompatible	15	**I**
Clindamycin phosphate	UP	2.4 g		1 g	D5W	Physically compatible and clindamycin potency retained for 24 hr at room temperature	104	**C**
	UP	1.2 g		0.5 g	D5W	Physically compatible and clindamycin potency retained for 24 hr at room temperature	104	**C**
Colistimethate sodium	WC	500 mg	BR	4 g	D5W	Physically incompatible	15	**I**
Dopamine HCl	AS	800 mg	BR	2 g	D5W	Kanamycin and dopamine potency retained for 24 hr at 23 to 25 °C	78	**C**
Furosemide	HO	160 mg	BE	2 g	D5W, NS	Transient cloudiness during admixture. Then physically compatible for 24 hr at 21 °C	876	**C**
Heparin sodium		12,000 units	BR	250 mg	D5S, D5W, D10W, IM, IP, LR, NS	Immediate precipitation	87	**I**
	UP	4000 units	BR	4 g	D5W	Physically incompatible	15	**I**
	BP	20,000 units	BPC	4 g	D5W, NS	Immediate precipitation	26	**I**

Additive Compatibility (Cont.)

Kanamycin sulfate

Drug	Mfr	Conc/L	Mfr	Conc/L	Test Soln	Remarks	Ref	C/I
	AB	20,000 units	BR	500 mg		Precipitate forms within 1 hr	21	I
	OR	20,000 units	TE	2 g	NS	Precipitate forms	113	I
Hydrocortisone sodium succinate	UP	500 mg	BR	4 g	D5W	Physically incompatible	15	I
		1.8 g	BR	250 mg	D5S, D5W, D10W, IM, IP, NS	Kanamycin potency retained for 24 hr at 4 and 25 °C	87	C
Methohexital sodium	BR	2 g	BPC	4 g	D5W, NS	Immediate precipitation	26	I
Penicillin G potassium	SQ	20 million units	BR	4 g	D5W	Physically compatible	15	C
	SQ	5 million units	BR	4 g	D	Physically compatible	47	C
Penicillin G sodium	UP	20 million units	BR	4 g	D5W	Physically compatible	15	C
Polymyxin B sulfate	BW	200 mg	BR	4 g	D5W	Physically compatible	15	C
Sodium bicarbonate	AB	80 mEq	BR	4 g	D5W	Physically compatible	15	C
Vitamin B complex with C	AB	5 ml	BR	4 g	D5W	Physically compatible	15	C

Drugs in Syringe Compatibility

Kanamycin sulfate

Drug (in syringe)	Mfr	Amt	Mfr	Amt	Remarks	Ref	C/I
Ampicillin sodium	AY	500 mg		1 g/4 ml	Physically incompatible within 1 hr at room temperature	99	I
	AY	500 mg		1 g/2 ml	Precipitate forms in 1 hr at room temperature	300	I
Heparin sodium	AB	20,000 units/ 1 ml	BR	500 mg	Physically incompatible	21	I
Penicillin G sodium		1 million units		1 g/4 ml	No precipitate or color change within 1 hr at room temperature	99	C

Y-Site Injection Compatibility (1:1 Mixture)

Kanamycin sulfate

Drug	Mfr	Conc	Mfr	Conc	Remarks	Ref	C/I
Cyclophosphamide	MJ	20 mg/ml[a]	BR	2.5 mg/ml[a]	Physically compatible for 4 hr at 25 °C	1194	C
Furosemide	HO	10 mg/ml	BE	2 mg/ml[b]	Physically compatible for 24 hr at 21 °C	876	C
Heparin sodium with hydrocortisone sodium succinate	RI	1000 units + 100 mg/L[c]	BR	250 mg/ml	Physically compatible for at least 4 hr at room temperature by visual and microscopic examination	322	C

Y-Site Injection Compatibility (1:1 Mixture) (Cont.)

Kanamycin sulfate

Drug	Mfr	Conc	Mfr	Conc	Remarks	Ref	C/I
Hydromorphone HCl	WY	0.2 mg/ml[a]	BR	2.5 mg/ml[a]	Physically compatible for at least 4 hr at 25 °C under fluorescent light	987	C
Magnesium sulfate	IX	16.7, 33.3, 66.7, 100 mg/ml[a]	BR	2.5 mg/ml[a]	Physically compatible for at least 4 hr at 32 °C	813	C
Meperidine HCl	WY	10 mg/ml[a]	BR	2.5 mg/ml[a]	Physically compatible for at least 4 hr at 25 °C under fluorescent light	987	C
Morphine sulfate	WI	1 mg/ml[a]	BR	2.5 mg/ml[a]	Physically compatible for at least 4 hr at 25 °C under fluorescent light	987	C
Perphenazine	SC	0.02 mg/ml[a]	BR	2.5 mg/ml[a]	Physically compatible for 4 hr at 25 °C	1155	C
Potassium chloride		40 mEq/L[c]	BR	250 mg/ml	Physically compatible for at least 4 hr at room temperature by visual and microscopic examination	322	C
TNA #73[d]		32.5 ml[e]	BR	500 mg/50 ml[a]	Physically compatible by visual observation for 4 hr at 25 °C	1008	C
Vitamin B complex with C	RC	2 ml/L[c]	BR	250 mg/ml	Physically compatible for at least 4 hr at room temperature by visual and microscopic examination	322	C

[a]Tested in dextrose 5% in water.
[b]Tested in both dextrose 5% in water and sodium chloride 0.9%.
[c]Tested in dextrose 5% in water, sodium chloride 0.9%, and Ringer's injection, lactated.
[d]Refer to Appendix I for the composition of parenteral nutrition solutions. TNA indicates a 3-in-1 admixture.
[e]A 32.5-ml sample of parenteral nutrition solution mixed with 50 ml of antibiotic.

Additional Compatibility Information

Solutions— Kanamycin sulfate is stated to be stable for 24 hours at room temperature in most intravenous infusion solutions, including dextrose 5% in water and sodium chloride 0.9% (4).

Additives— It is recommended that other drugs not be physically combined with kanamycin sulfate (4).

In vitro testing of thiamine HCl, riboflavin-5′-phosphate, pyridoxine HCl, niacinamide, and ascorbic acid individually at concentrations of 0.1% with kanamycin sulfate 0.025% in sterile distilled water showed a significant reduction in antibiotic activity in one hour at 25 °C (314).

Kanamycin sulfate is stated to be physically incompatible with lincomycin HCl (154) and cefotetan disodium (4). Kanamycin sulfate also appears to be incompatible with cefazolin sodium (278).

Cefotaxime sodium (Hoechst-Roussel) should not be mixed with aminoglycosides in the same solution, but they may be administered to the same patient separately (792).

Although piperacillin sodium and aminoglycosides act synergistically and have been used successfully clinically when recommended doses of each drug were administered, mixing piperacillin sodium directly in a syringe or infusion bottle with an aminoglycoside can result in substantial inactivation of the aminoglycoside (740).

The comparative inactivation of five aminoglycosides by seven β-lactam antibiotics in human serum at 37 °C was reported by Riff and Thomason. Amikacin, followed by netilmicin, had the lowest degree of inactivation; tobramycin sustained the most pronounced losses. Gentamicin and kanamycin were intermediate in the extent of losses. The six penicillins that were tested all produced aminoglycoside inactivation; the greatest extent of inactivation was caused by carbenicillin followed by ticarcillin, penicillin G, oxacillin, methicillin, and ampicillin, in approximate descending order. Cephalothin produced minimal inactivation (5 to 10% in 24 hours). The rate of inactivation could be reduced by storage at 4 °C and further reduced by storage at −20 °C. The authors suggested processing blood samples rapidly to avoid inaccurate serum determinations. Storage of specimens at low temperature until analysis may be helpful (1052).

Concentrated Solutions— The following incompatibility determinations were performed with concentrated solutions. The drugs in dry form were constituted according to the manufacturers' recommendations. One milliliter of kanamycin sulfate (Bristol) was added to 5 ml of sterile distilled water along with 1 ml of each of the following drugs. Particulate matter was noted within two hours (28):

Heparin sodium
Hydrocortisone sodium succinate (Upjohn)
Phenobarbital sodium (Winthrop)
Phenytoin sodium (Parke-Davis)

KETAMINE HCL
AHFS 28:04

Ketalar

Abbott

Monarch

Products— Ketamine HCl is available in concentrations equivalent to 10, 50, or 100 mg/ml of ketamine base. The injections also contain 0.1 mg/ml of benzethonium chloride. The 10-mg/ml concentration is made isotonic with sodium chloride and is available in 20-ml vials. The 50-mg/ml concentration is available in 10-ml vials, and the 100-mg/ml concentration is available in 5-ml vials (1-2/95; 1-3/98).

The 100-mg/ml concentration must be diluted before intravenous use. Dilution of the dose with an equal volume of sterile water for injection, dextrose 5% in water, or sodium chloride 0.9% is recommended (1-3/98).

pH— From 3.5 to 5.5 (1-3/98).

Osmolality— The osmolalities of ketamine HCl products were determined to be 300 mOsm/kg for the 10-mg/ml concentration and 387 mOsm/kg for the 50-mg/ml concentration (1233).

Administration— Ketamine HCl may be administered intramuscularly or by slow intravenous injection over at least 60 seconds. The 100-mg/ml preparation should not be given undiluted. See Products section above. For intravenous infusion, a 1- or 2-mg/ml solution may be prepared by adding 500 mg of ketamine to 500 ml or to 250 ml, respectively, of dextrose 5% in water or sodium chloride 0.9% (1-3/98).

Stability— Intact vials of ketamine HCl should be stored at controlled room temperature and protected from light. Ketamine HCl injection is a colorless to slightly yellow solution. Although the drug may darken upon prolonged exposure to light, this darkening does not affect potency. Do not use the product if a precipitate is present (1-3/98).

Compatibility Information

Drugs in Syringe Compatibility

Ketamine HCl

Drug (in syringe)	Mfr	Amt	Mfr	Amt	Remarks	Ref	C/I
Bupivacaine HCl with fentanyl citrate	SW JN	1.5 mg/ml 0.01 mg/ml	PD	2 mg/ml	Diluted to 5 ml with NS. Visually compatible with no new GC/MS peaks appearing in 1 hr at room temperature	1956	C
Clonidine HCl with tetracaine HCl	BI SW	0.03 mg/ml 2 mg/ml	PD	2 mg/ml	Diluted to 5 ml with NS. Visually compatible with no new GC/MS peaks appearing in 1 hr at room temperature	1956	C
Doxapram HCl	RB	400 mg/20 ml	PD	200 mg/20 ml	Physically compatible with no doxapram loss in 9 hr but 12% loss in 24 hr	1177	I
Lidocaine HCl with morphine sulfate	AST ES	2 mg/ml 0.2 mg/ml	PD	2 mg/ml	Diluted to 5 ml with NS. Visually compatible with no new GC/MS peaks appearing in 1 hr at room temperature	1956	C
Meperidine HCl	DB	12 mg/ml	PD	2 mg/ml	Diluted to 50 ml with NS. Visually compatible for 48 hr at 25 °C	2059	C
Morphine tartrate		240 mg		100 mg	Brought to 9 ml with NS. Visually compatible for 8 days refrigerated and at room temperature protected from light	1899	C

Y-Site Injection Compatibility (1:1 Mixture)

Ketamine HCl

Drug	Mfr	Conc	Mfr	Conc	Remarks	Ref	C/I
Propofol	ZEN	10 mg/ml	PD	10 mg/ml	Physically compatible for 1 hr at 23 °C with no increase in particle content	2066	C

Additional Compatibility Information

Dextrose 5% in water and sodium chloride 0.9% have been recommended as diluents for ketamine HCl (1-3/98).

Ketamine HCl is incompatible with barbiturates because of precipitate formation. Consequently, they should not be combined in the same syringe. Diazepam must be given separately from ketamine HCl and not be mixed in the same syringe or infusion container (1-3/98).

KETOROLAC TROMETHAMINE
AHFS 28:08.04

Toradol   **Roche**

Products— Ketorolac tromethamine (Roche) is available as a 15-mg/ml solution in 1-ml Tubex cartridge-needle units and vials and also as a 30-mg/ml solution in 1- and 2-ml Tubex cartridge-needle units or vials. The 15- and 30-mg/ml concentrations are also available in 1-ml Tubex needle-less cartridges. Each milliliter of the two concentrations contains (2):

Ketorolac tromethamine	15 mg	30 mg
Ethanol	10% (w/v)	10% (w/v)
Sodium chloride	6.68 mg	4.35 mg
Water for injection	qs	qs

The product also contains sodium hydroxide or hydrochloric acid to adjust the pH (2).

pH— From 6.9 to 7.9 (4).

Tonicity— Both ketorolac tromethamine concentrations are isotonic (4).

Administration— Ketorolac tromethamine is administered slowly by deep intramuscular injection or by intravenous injection over no less than 15 seconds (2; 4). The 60 mg/2 ml injection is for intramuscular use only (2).

Stability— Ketorolac tromethamine injection should be stored at controlled room temperature and protected from light. The injection is clear and has a slight yellow color (2; 4). Prolonged exposure to light may result in discoloration of the solution and precipitation. Precipitation may also occur in solutions having a relatively low pH (4).

Sorption— Ketorolac tromethamine (Syntex) 30 mg/50 ml in dextrose 5% in sodium chloride 0.9%, dextrose 5% in water, Plasma-Lyte A (pH 7.4), Ringer's injection, Ringer's injection, lactated, and sodium chloride 0.9% and 30 mg/500 ml in Plasma-Lyte A (pH 7.4) and Ringer's injection did not exhibit sorption to PVC containers over 48 hours or to administration set tubing in static contact or in simulated infusion (1646).

Compatibility Information

Solution Compatibility

Ketorolac tromethamine

Solution	Mfr	Mfr	Conc/L	Remarks	Ref	C/I
Dextrose 5% in sodium chloride 0.9%	TR[a]	SY	600 mg	Physically compatible by visual examination and particle assessment. No ketorolac loss by HPLC in 48 hr at room temperature	1646	C
Dextrose 5% in water	TR[b]	SY	600 mg	Physically compatible by visual examination and particle assessment. No ketorolac loss by HPLC in 48 hr at room temperature	1646	C
	BA[a]	RC	600 mg	Visually compatible with little or no loss by HPLC in 7 days and 14% loss in 14 days at 25 °C. Less than 2% loss in 50 days at 5 °C	2095	C
Plasma-Lyte A, pH 7.4	TR[a]	SY	600 mg	Physically compatible by visual examination and particle assessment. No ketorolac loss by HPLC in 48 hr at room temperature	1646	C
	TR[b]	SY	60 mg	Physically compatible by visual examination and particle assessment. Little or no ketorolac loss by HPLC in 48 hr at room temperature	1646	C
Ringer's injection	TR[a]	SY	600 mg	Physically compatible by visual examination and particle assessment. No ketorolac loss by HPLC in 48 hr at room temperature	1646	C
	TR[b]	SY	60 mg	Physically compatible by visual examination and particle assessment. Little or no ketorolac loss by HPLC in 48 hr at room temperature	1646	C
Ringer's injection, lactated	TR[a]	SY	600 mg	Physically compatible by visual examination and particle assessment. No ketorolac loss by HPLC in 48 hr at room temperature	1646	C
Sodium chloride 0.9%	TR[b]	SY	600 mg	Physically compatible by visual examination and particle assessment. No ketorolac loss by HPLC in 48 hr at room temperature	1646	C

Solution Compatibility (Cont.)

Ketorolac tromethamine

Solution	Mfr	Mfr	Conc/L	Remarks	Ref	C/I
	BA[a]	RC	600 mg	Visually compatible with no loss by HPLC in 35 days at 25 °C and in 50 days at 25 °C	2095	C

[a]Tested in PVC containers.
[b]Tested in both glass and PVC containers.

Drugs in Syringe Compatibility

Ketorolac tromethamine

Drug (in syringe)	Mfr	Amt	Mfr	Amt	Remarks	Ref	C/I
Diazepam	ES	15 mg/ 3 ml	SY	180 mg/ 6 ml	Visually compatible for 4 hr at 24 °C under ambient light. Spectrophotometric absorbance increases immediately and persists for 30 min but dissipates by 1 hr	1703	?
Haloperidol lactate	SO	5 mg/ 1 ml	SY	30 mg/ 1 ml	White crystalline precipitate forms immediately	1786	I
Hydromorphone HCl	KN	10 mg/ 1 ml	SY	30 mg/ 1 ml	Cloudiness forms immediately but clears with swirling	1785	?
	KN	1 mg/ 1 ml[a]	SY	30 mg/ 1 ml	Visually compatible for 24 hr at 25 °C	1785	C
	KN	1[a] and 10 mg/ 1 ml	SY	15 mg/ 1 ml[a]	Visually compatible for 24 hr at 25 °C	1785	C
Hydroxyzine HCl	SO	150 mg/ 3 ml	SY	180 mg/ 6 ml	Heavy white precipitate forms immediately, separating into two layers over time	1703	I
Nalbuphine HCl	DU	30 mg/ 3 ml	SY	180 mg/ 6 ml	Solid white precipitate forms immediately and settles to bottom	1703	I
Prochlorperazine edisylate	STS	15 mg/ 3 ml	SY	180 mg/ 6 ml	Heavy white precipitate forms immediately, separating into two layers over time	1703	I
Promethazine HCl	ES	75 mg/ 3 ml	SY	180 mg/ 6 ml	Heavy white precipitate forms immediately, separating into two layers over time	1703	I
Sufentanil citrate	JN	50 μg/ml	SY	30 mg/ ml	Physically compatible with no subvisual haze or particle formation in 24 hr at 23 °C	1711	C
Thiethylperazine maleate	ROX	5 mg/ 1 ml	SY	30 mg/ 1 ml	White crystalline precipitate forms immediately	1785	I

[a]Dilutions prepared with sterile water for injection.

Y-Site Injection Compatibility (1:1 Mixture)

Ketorolac tromethamine

Drug	Mfr	Conc	Mfr	Conc	Remarks	Ref	C/I
Cisatracurium besylate	GW	0.1, 2, 5 mg/ml[a]	RC	15 mg/ml[a]	Physically compatible with no change in measured turbidity or increase in particle content in 4 hr at 23 °C	2074	C
Remifentanil HCl	GW	0.025 and 0.25 mg/ml[b]	RC	15 mg/ml[a]	Physically compatible with no change in measured turbidity or increase in particle content in 4 hr at 23 °C	2075	C

Y-Site Injection Compatibility (1:1 Mixture) (Cont.)

Ketorolac tromethamine

Drug	Mfr	Conc	Mfr	Conc	Remarks	Ref	C/I
Sufentanil citrate	JN	12.5 μg/ml[a]	SY	1 mg/ml[a]	Physically compatible with no subvisual haze or particle formation in 24 hr at 23 °C	1711	C

[a]Tested in dextrose 5% in water.
[b]Tested in sodium chloride 0.9%.

Additional Compatibility Information

Additives— Ketorolac tromethamine should not be admixed with drugs that result in a relatively low pH such as hydroxyzine HCl, meperidine HCl, morphine sulfate, and promethazine HCl because ketorolac may precipitate (2; 4).

LABETALOL HCL
AHFS 24:08

Normodyne   **Schering**
Trandate   **Glaxo Wellcome**

Products— Labetalol HCl (Schering) is available in 20- and 40-ml multiple-dose vials and 4- and 8-ml disposable syringes. Each milliliter of solution contains (2):

Labetalol HCl	5 mg
Dextrose, anhydrous	45 mg
Edetate disodium	0.1 mg
Methylparaben	0.8 mg
Propylparaben	0.1 mg

The product also contains citric acid monohydrate and sodium hydroxide, as necessary, to adjust the pH (2).

pH— From 3 to 4 (2).

Osmolality— Labetalol HCl 5 mg/ml has an osmolality of 287 mOsm/kg (1689).

Administration— Labetalol HCl is administered slowly, over two minutes, by direct intravenous injection, or by continuous intravenous infusion at an initial rate of 2 mg/min with subsequent adjustments based on blood pressure response. For continuous infusion, concentrations of 1 mg/ml or 2 mg/3 ml can be made by adding 200 mg (40 ml) to 160 or 250 ml of compatible infusion solution (2; 4).

Stability— Labetalol HCl may be stored at room temperature or under refrigeration and should be protected from light and freezing. The solution is clear and colorless to slightly yellow (2). The drug has optimal stability at pH 3 to 4. Addition to an alkaline admixture, such as sodium bicarbonate 5% with a pH of 7.6 to 8, has resulted in a precipitate (757).

Compatibility Information

Solution Compatibility

Labetalol HCl

Solution	Mfr	Mfr	Conc/L	Remarks	Ref	C/I
Dextrose 5% in Ringer's injection	TR	SC	1.25 and 3.75 g	Physically compatible and chemically stable for 72 hr at 4 and 25 °C	757	C
Dextrose 5% in Ringer's injection, lactated	TR	SC	1.25 and 3.75 g	Physically compatible and chemically stable for 72 hr at 4 and 25 °C	757	C
Dextrose 2½% in sodium chloride 0.45%	TR	SC	1.25 and 3.75 g	Physically compatible and chemically stable for 72 hr at 4 and 25 °C	757	C
Dextrose 5% in sodium chloride 0.2%	TR	SC	1.25 and 3.75 g	Physically compatible and chemically stable for 72 hr at 4 and 25 °C	757	C

Solution Compatibility (Cont.)

Labetalol HCl

Solution	Mfr	Mfr	Conc/L	Remarks	Ref	C/I
Dextrose 5% in sodium chloride 0.33%	TR	SC	1.25 and 3.75 g	Physically compatible and chemically stable for 72 hr at 4 and 25 °C	757	**C**
Dextrose 5% in sodium chloride 0.9%	TR	SC	1.25 and 3.75 g	Physically compatible and chemically stable for 72 hr at 4 and 25 °C	757	**C**
Dextrose 5% in water	TR	SC	1.25 and 3.75 g	Physically compatible and chemically stable for 72 hr at 4 and 25 °C	757	**C**
Polysal in dextrose 5%	CU	SC	1.25 and 3.75 g	Physically compatible and chemically stable for 72 hr at 4 and 25 °C	757	**C**
Ringer's injection	TR	SC	1.25 and 3.75 g	Physically compatible and chemically stable for 72 hr at 4 and 25 °C	757	**C**
Ringer's injection, lactated	TR	SC	1.25 and 3.75 g	Physically compatible and chemically stable for 72 hr at 4 and 25 °C	757	**C**
Sodium bicarbonate 5%	TR	SC	1.25, 2.5, 3.75 g	White precipitate forms within 6 hr after mixing at 4 and 25 °C	757	**I**

Y-Site Injection Compatibility (1:1 Mixture)

Labetalol HCl

Drug	Mfr	Conc	Mfr	Conc	Remarks	Ref	C/I
Amikacin sulfate	BR	5 mg/ml[a]	SC	1 mg/ml[a]	Physically compatible for 24 hr at 18 °C	1171	**C**
Aminophylline	ES	1 mg/ml[a]	SC	1 mg/ml[a]	Physically compatible for 24 hr at 18 °C	1171	**C**
Amiodarone HCl	WY	4.8 mg/ml[a]	GL	5 mg/ml	Visually compatible for 24 hr at 23 °C	1877	**C**
Amphotericin B cholesteryl sulfate complex	SEQ	0.83 mg/ml[a]	AH	5 mg/ml	Gross precipitate forms	2117	**I**
Ampicillin sodium	WY	10 mg/ml[b]	SC	1 mg/ml[a]	Physically compatible for 24 hr at 18 °C	1171	**C**
Butorphanol tartrate	BR	0.04 mg/ml[a]	SC	1 mg/ml[a]	Physically compatible for 24 hr at 18 °C	1171	**C**
Calcium gluconate	AMR	0.23 mEq/ml[a]	SC	1 mg/ml[a]	Physically compatible for 24 hr at 18 °C	1171	**C**
Cefazolin sodium	LI	10 mg/ml[a]	SC	1 mg/ml[a]	Physically compatible for 24 hr at 18 °C	1171	**C**
Cefoperazone sodium	RR	10 mg/ml[a]	SC	1 mg/ml[a]	Cloudiness and fine precipitate form immediately	1171	**I**
Ceftazidime	GL[e]	10 mg/ml[a]	SC	1 mg/ml[a]	Physically compatible for 24 hr at 18 °C	1171	**C**
Ceftizoxime sodium	SKF	10 mg/ml[a]	SC	1 mg/ml[a]	Physically compatible for 24 hr at 18 °C	1171	**C**
Ceftriaxone sodium	RC	20[a,b] and 100[c] mg/ml	GL	2.5[c] and 5 mg/ml	Fluffy white precipitate formed immediately	1964	**I**
Chloramphenicol sodium succinate	PD	10 mg/ml[a]	SC	1 mg/ml[a]	Physically compatible for 24 hr at 18 °C	1171	**C**
Cimetidine HCl	SKF	3 mg/ml[a]	SC	1 mg/ml[a]	Physically compatible for 24 hr at 18 °C	1171	**C**
Clindamycin phosphate	UP	9 mg/ml[a]	SC	1 mg/ml[a]	Physically compatible for 24 hr at 18 °C	1171	**C**
Diltiazem HCl	MMD	1 mg/ml[a]	AH	2 mg/ml[a]	Visually compatible for 4 hr at 27 °C	2062	**C**
Dobutamine HCl	LI	2.5 mg/ml[a]	GL	1 mg/ml[a]	Visually compatible with little or no loss of either drug by HPLC in 4 hr at room temperature	1762	**C**
	LI	4 mg/ml[a]	GL	5 mg/ml	Visually compatible for 24 hr at 23 °C	1877	**C**
	LI	4 mg/ml[a]	AH	2 mg/ml[a]	Visually compatible for 4 hr at 27 °C	2062	**C**

Y-Site Injection Compatibility (1:1 Mixture) (Cont.)

Labetalol HCl

Drug	Mfr	Conc	Mfr	Conc	Remarks	Ref	C/I
Dopamine HCl	IMS	1.6 mg/ml[a]	SC	1 mg/ml[a]	Physically compatible for 24 hr at 18 °C	1171	**C**
	ES	1.6 mg/ml[a]	GL	1 mg/ml[a]	Visually compatible with little or no loss of either drug by HPLC in 4 hr at room temperature	1762	**C**
	AB	3.2 mg/ml[a]	AH	2 mg/ml[a]	Visually compatible for 4 hr at 27 °C	2062	**C**
Enalaprilat	MSD	0.05 mg/ml[b]	GL	1 mg/ml[a]	Physically compatible for 24 hr at room temperature under fluorescent light	1355	**C**
Epinephrine HCl	AB	0.02 mg/ml[a]	AH	2 mg/ml[a]	Visually compatible for 4 hr at 27 °C	2062	**C**
Erythromycin lactobionate	AB	5 mg/ml[a]	SC	1 mg/ml[a]	Physically compatible for 24 hr at 18 °C	1171	**C**
Esmolol HCl	DU	40 mg/ml[a]	GL	5 mg/ml	Visually compatible for 24 hr at 23 °C	1877	**C**
Famotidine	MSD	0.2 mg/ml[a]	SC	1 mg/ml[a]	Physically compatible for 4 hr at 25 °C	1188	**C**
Fentanyl citrate	JN	10 mg/ml[a]	SC	1 mg/ml[a]	Physically compatible for 24 hr at 18 °C	1171	**C**
	ES	0.05 mg/ml	AH	2 mg/ml[a]	Visually compatible for 4 hr at 27 °C	2062	**C**
Furosemide	AB	10 mg/ml	SC	2.5 mg/ml[a]	White turbidity forms immediately; flocculent precipitate forms in 4 hr	1704	**I**
	AB	0.5 mg/ml[a]	SC	2.5 mg/ml[a]	Physically compatible with no change in measured turbidity or increase in particle content in 4 hr at 22 °C	1704	**C**
	AB	0.5[a] and 10 mg/ml	SC	0.25 mg/ml[a]	Physically compatible with no change in measured turbidity or increase in particle content in 4 hr at 22 °C	1704	**C**
	ES	10 mg/ml[d]	SC	1.6 mg/ml[d]	White precipitate forms immediately	1714	**I**
	AMR	10 mg/ml	AH	2 mg/ml[a]	Precipitate forms immediately	2062	**I**
Gentamicin sulfate	ES	0.8 mg/ml[a]	SC	1 mg/ml[a]	Physically compatible for 24 hr at 18 °C	1171	**C**
Heparin sodium	IX	40 units/ml[a]	SC	1 mg/ml[a]	Physically compatible for 24 hr at 18 °C	1171	**C**
	OR	100 units/ml[a]	GL	5 mg/ml	Cloudiness with particles forms immediately	1877	**I**
	ES	100 units/ml[a]	AH	2 mg/ml[a]	Visually compatible for 4 hr at 27 °C	2062	**C**
Hydromorphone HCl	KN	1 mg/ml	AH	2 mg/ml[a]	Visually compatible for 4 hr at 27 °C	2062	**C**
Insulin, regular	LI	1 unit/ml[a]	GL	5 mg/ml	Visually compatible for 4 hr. White precipitate forms in 24 hr at 23 °C	1877	**?**
Lidocaine HCl	AST	20 mg/ml[a]	SC	1 mg/ml[a]	Physically compatible for 24 hr at 18 °C	1171	**C**
Lorazepam	WY	0.5 mg/ml[a]	AH	2 mg/ml[a]	Visually compatible for 4 hr at 27 °C	2062	**C**
Magnesium sulfate	LY	10 mg/ml[a]	SC	1 mg/ml[a]	Physically compatible for 24 hr at 18 °C	1171	**C**
Meperidine HCl	AB	10 mg/ml	GL	5 mg/ml	Physically compatible for 4 hr at 25 °C	1397	**C**
Metronidazole	SE	5 mg/ml	SC	1 mg/ml[a]	Physically compatible for 24 hr at 18 °C	1171	**C**
Midazolam HCl	RC	1 mg/ml[a]	GL	5 mg/ml	Visually compatible for 24 hr at 23 °C	1877	**C**
	RC	2 mg/ml[a]	AH	2 mg/ml[a]	Visually compatible for 4 hr at 27 °C	2062	**C**
Milrinone lactate	SW	0.2 mg/ml[a]	AH	2 mg/ml[a]	Visually compatible for 4 hr at 27 °C	2062	**C**
Morphine sulfate	WY	1 mg/ml[a]	SC	1 mg/ml[a]	Physically compatible for 24 hr at 18 °C	1171	**C**
	AB	1 mg/ml	GL	5 mg/ml	Physically compatible for 4 hr at 25 °C	1397	**C**
	ES	0.5 mg/ml[a]	GL	1 mg/ml[a]	Visually compatible with little or no loss of either drug by HPLC in 4 hr at room temperature	1762	**C**
	SCN	2 mg/ml[a]	AH	2 mg/ml[a]	Visually compatible for 4 hr at 27 °C	2062	**C**
Nafcillin sodium	BR	10 mg/ml[a]	SC	1 mg/ml[a]	Cloudiness and fine precipitate form immediately	1171	**I**

Y-Site Injection Compatibility (1:1 Mixture) (Cont.)

			Labetalol HCl				
Drug	*Mfr*	*Conc*	*Mfr*	*Conc*	*Remarks*	*Ref*	*C/I*
Nicardipine HCl	WY	1 mg/ml[a]	AH	2 mg/ml[a]	Visually compatible for 4 hr at 27 °C	2062	**C**
Nitroglycerin	DU	0.2 mg/ml[a]	GL	1 mg/ml[a]	Visually compatible with no labetalol loss and 6% nitroglycerin loss by HPLC in 4 hr at room temperature	1762	**C**
	OM	0.2 mg/ml[a]	GL	5 mg/ml	Visually compatible for 24 hr at 23 °C	1877	**C**
	AB	0.4 mg/ml[a]	AH	2 mg/ml[a]	Visually compatible for 4 hr at 27 °C	2062	**C**
Norepinephrine bitartrate	STR	0.064 mg/ml[a]	GL	5 mg/ml	Visually compatible for 24 hr at 23 °C	1877	**C**
	AB	0.128 mg/ml[a]	AH	2 mg/ml[a]	Visually compatible for 4 hr at 27 °C	2062	**C**
Oxacillin sodium	BR	10 mg/ml[a]	SC	1 mg/ml[a]	Physically compatible for 24 hr at 18 °C	1171	**C**
Penicillin G potassium	PF	50,000 units/ml[a]	SC	1 mg/ml[a]	Physically compatible for 24 hr at 18 °C	1171	**C**
Piperacillin sodium	LE	10 mg/ml[a]	SC	1 mg/ml[a]	Physically compatible for 24 hr at 18 °C	1171	**C**
Potassium chloride	IX	0.4 mEq/ml[a]	SC	1 mg/ml[a]	Physically compatible for 24 hr at 18 °C	1171	**C**
Potassium phosphates	LY	0.44 mEq/ml[a]	SC	1 mg/ml[a]	Physically compatible for 24 hr at 18 °C	1171	**C**
Propofol	ZEN	10 mg/ml	AH	5 mg/ml	Physically compatible for 1 hr at 23 °C with no increase in particle content	2066	**C**
Ranitidine HCl	GL	0.5 mg/ml[a]	SC	1 mg/ml[a]	Physically compatible for 24 hr at 18 °C	1171	**C**
	GL	0.6 mg/ml[a]	GL	1 mg/ml[a]	Visually compatible with 5% labetalol loss and little or no ranitidine loss by HPLC in 4 hr at room temperature	1762	**C**
	GL	1 mg/ml[a]	AH	2 mg/ml[a]	Visually compatible for 4 hr at 27 °C	2062	**C**
Sodium acetate	LY	0.4 mEq/ml[a]	SC	1 mg/ml[a]	Physically compatible for 24 hr at 18 °C	1171	**C**
Sodium nitroprusside	RC	0.2 mg/ml[a]	GL	5 mg/ml	Visually compatible for 24 hr at 23 °C	1877	**C**
Thiopental sodium	AB	25 mg/ml[c]	AH	2 mg/ml[a]	Precipitate forms immediately	2062	**I**
Tobramycin sulfate	LI	0.8 mg/ml[a]	SC	1 mg/ml[a]	Physically compatible for 24 hr at 18 °C	1171	**C**
Trimethoprim–sulfamethoxazole	BW	0.8 + 4 mg/ml[a]	SC	1 mg/ml[a]	Physically compatible for 24 hr at 18 °C	1171	**C**
Vancomycin HCl	LE	5 mg/ml[a]	SC	1 mg/ml[a]	Physically compatible for 24 hr at 18 °C	1171	**C**
Vecuronium bromide	OR	1 mg/ml	AH	2 mg/ml[a]	Visually compatible for 4 hr at 27 °C	2062	**C**
Warfarin sodium	DU	2 mg/ml[c]	SCH	0.8 mg/ml[a]	Haze forms immediately	2010	**I**
	DME	2 mg/ml[c]	SC	0.8 mg/ml[a]	Haze forms immediately	2078	**I**

[a]*Tested in dextrose 5% in water.*
[b]*Tested in sodium chloride 0.9%.*
[c]*Tested in sterile water for injection.*
[d]*Furosemide 0.5 ml injected in the Y-site port of a running infusion of labetalol HCl in dextrose 5% in water.*
[e]*Sodium carbonate–containing formulation tested.*

Additional Compatibility Information

In addition to the solutions noted in the compatibility table, the manufacturer states that labetalol is physically compatible and chemically stable in sodium chloride 0.9% for 24 hours at room temperature or under refrigeration (2).

Sodium Bicarbonate— The precipitate observed when labetalol HCl is admixed with sodium bicarbonate 5% (757) is believed to be labetalol free base. At the alkaline pH of the sodium bicarbonate solution (pH 7.6 to 8), the amine is no longer protonated but is partially or completely the free base. The free base is unionized and less soluble, precipitating in the aqueous medium (927).

LEUCOVORIN CALCIUM
AHFS 92:00

Wellcovorin

Immunex
Glaxo Wellcome

Products— Leucovorin calcium is available in lyophilized form in vials containing leucovorin 50, 100, and 350 mg as the calcium salt with sodium chloride 40, 80, and 140 mg, respectively, and sodium hydroxide or hydrochloric acid to adjust the pH. Reconstitution with 5 ml of bacteriostatic water for injection containing benzyl alcohol or sterile water for injection for the 50-mg vial or with 10 ml for the 100-mg vial results in a solution containing 10 mg/ml leucovorin. Reconstitute the 350-mg vial with 17 ml of sterile water for injection or bacteriostatic water for injection containing benzyl alcohol to yield a concentration of 20 mg/ml (2; 4).

pH— The vials have a pH of approximately 8.1 (2).

Osmolality— Leucovorin calcium 10 mg/ml in sterile water for injection has an osmolality of 274 mOsm/kg (1689).

Administration— Leucovorin calcium is administered by intramuscular or intravenous injection or infusion at a rate not exceeding 160 mg/min. When doses greater than 10 mg/m^2 are required, diluents containing benzyl alcohol should not be used for reconstitution (2; 4).

Stability— Leucovorin calcium injection should be stored at room temperature and protected from light (2; 4).

The reconstituted solution of leucovorin calcium is stated to be chemically stable for seven days. However, when constituted with diluents that contain no preservatives, immediate use is recommended (2).

Leucovorin calcium (Lederle) 10 mg/ml in sterile water for injection was determined by UV spectroscopy to be stable for seven days at 4 and 25 °C when protected from light (1669).

pH Effects— Leucovorin calcium in aqueous solution exhibits good stability at pH 6.5 to 10. The pH of maximum stability was determined to be 7.1 to 7.4. Below pH 6, increased decomposition rates were observed (1276).

Compatibility Information

Solution Compatibility

Leucovorin calcium

Solution	Mfr	Mfr	Conc/L	Remarks	Ref	C/I
Dextrose 10% in sodium chloride 0.9%		LE	50 mg	Less than 10% decomposition in 24 hr at room temperature protected from light	488	**C**
Dextrose 5% in water	TR[a]	LE	910 mg	Less than 10% decomposition in 24 hr at room temperature	519	**C**
	[a]	LE	0.1, 0.5, 1, 1.5 g	Little or no loss by HPLC in 4 days at 4 and 23 °C protected from light	1596	**C**
	MG[b]		910 mg	Less than 10% loss by HPLC in 24 hr at room temperature exposed to light	1658	**C**
Dextrose 10% in water		LE	50 mg	Less than 10% decomposition in 24 hr at room temperature protected from light	488	**C**
Ringer's injection		LE	50 mg	Less than 10% decomposition in 24 hr at room temperature protected from light	488	**C**
Ringer's injection, lactated		LE	50 mg	Less than 10% decomposition in 24 hr at room temperature protected from light	488	**C**
Sodium chloride 0.9%	[a]	LE	1 and 1.5 g	Little or no loss by HPLC in 4 days at 4 and 23 °C protected from light	1596	**C**
	[c]	LE	0.5 g	Little or no loss by HPLC in 4 days at 4 and 23 °C protected from light	1596	**C**
	[c]	LE	0.1 g	Approximately 9% loss by HPLC in 4 days at 4 and 23 °C protected from light	1596	**C**
	[d]	LE	0.1 and 0.5 g	Variable losses, up to 24%, by HPLC in 4 days at 4 and 23 °C protected from light	1596	**I**
	[b]	LE	1 g	Chemically stable by UV spectroscopy for 7 days at 4 and 25 °C protected from light	1669	**C**

[a]*Tested in both glass and PVC containers.*
[b]*Tested in both glass and polyolefin containers.*
[c]*Tested in glass containers.*
[d]*Tested in PVC containers.*

Additive Compatibility

Leucovorin calcium

Drug	Mfr	Conc/L	Mfr	Conc/L	Test Soln	Remarks	Ref	C/I
Cisplatin		200 mg		140 mg	NS	Both drugs stable for 15 days at room temperature protected from light	1379	C
Cisplatin with floxuridine		200 mg 700 mg		140 mg	NS	All drugs stable for 7 days at room temperature	1379	C
Floxuridine	QU	1 g	QU	30 mg	NS	Physically compatible and chemically stable for 48 hr at 4 and 20 °C. No floxuridine loss and 10% leucovorin loss in 48 hr at 40 °C	1317	C
	QU	2 g	QU	240 mg	NS	Physically compatible and chemically stable for 48 hr at 4 and 20 °C. No floxuridine loss and 7% leucovorin loss in 48 hr at 40 °C	1317	C
	QU	4 g	QU	960 mg	NS	Physically compatible and chemically stable for 48 hr at 4, 20 and 40 °C	1317	C
		10 g		200 mg	NS	Both drugs stable for 15 days at room temperature protected from light	1387	C
Fluorouracil	AD	16.7 to 46.2 g	LE	1.5 to 13.3 g	a	Subvisual particulate matter forms in all combinations in variable periods from 1 to 4 days at 4, 23, and 32 °C	1816	I

[a]Tested with both drugs undiluted and diluted by 25% with dextrose 5% in water.

Drugs in Syringe Compatibility

Leucovorin calcium

Drug (in syringe)	Mfr	Amt	Mfr	Amt	Remarks	Ref	C/I
Bleomycin sulfate		1.5 units/ 0.5 ml		5 mg/ 0.5 ml	Physically compatible for 5 min at room temperature followed by 8 min of centrifugation	980	C
Cisplatin		0.5 mg/ 0.5 ml		5 mg/ 0.5 ml	Physically compatible for 5 min at room temperature followed by 8 min of centrifugation	980	C
Cyclophosphamide		10 mg/ 0.5 ml		5 mg/ 0.5 ml	Physically compatible for 5 min at room temperature followed by 8 min of centrifugation	980	C
Doxorubicin HCl		1 mg/ 0.5 ml		5 mg/ 0.5 ml	Physically compatible for 5 min at room temperature followed by 8 min of centrifugation	980	C
Droperidol		1.25 mg/ 0.5 ml		5 mg/ 0.5 ml	Immediate precipitation	980	I
Fluorouracil		25 mg/ 0.5 ml		5 mg/ 0.5 ml	Physically compatible for 5 min at room temperature followed by 8 min of centrifugation	980	C
Furosemide		5 mg/ 0.5 ml		5 mg/ 0.5 ml	Physically compatible for 5 min at room temperature followed by 8 min of centrifugation	980	C
Heparin sodium		500 units/ 0.5 ml		5 mg/ 0.5 ml	Physically compatible for 5 min at room temperature followed by 8 min of centrifugation	980	C

Drugs in Syringe Compatibility (Cont.)

Leucovorin calcium

Drug (in syringe)	Mfr	Amt	Mfr	Amt	Remarks	Ref	C/I
Methotrexate sodium		12.5 mg/ 0.5 ml		5 mg/ 0.5 ml	Physically compatible for 5 min at room temperature followed by 8 min of centrifugation	980	C
Metoclopramide HCl		2.5 mg/ 0.5 ml		5 mg/ 0.5 ml	Physically compatible for 5 min at room temperature followed by 8 min of centrifugation	980	C
Mitomycin		0.25 mg/ 0.5 ml		5 mg/ 0.5 ml	Physically compatible for 5 min at room temperature followed by 8 min of centrifugation	980	C
Vinblastine sulfate		0.5 mg/ 0.5 ml		5 mg/ 0.5 ml	Physically compatible for 5 min at room temperature followed by 8 min of centrifugation	980	C
Vincristine sulfate		0.5 mg/ 0.5 ml		5 mg/ 0.5 ml	Physically compatible for 5 min at room temperature followed by 8 min of centrifugation	980	C

Y-Site Injection Compatibility (1:1 Mixture)

Leucovorin calcium

Drug	Mfr	Conc	Mfr	Conc	Remarks	Ref	C/I
Amifostine	USB	10 mg/ml[a]	LE	2 mg/ml[a]	Physically compatible with no change in measured turbidity or increase in particle content in 4 hr at 23 °C	1845	C
Amphotericin B cholesteryl sulfate complex	SEQ	0.83 mg/ml[a]	IMM	2 mg/ml[a]	Gross precipitate forms	2117	I
Aztreonam	SQ	40 mg/ml[a]	LE	2 mg/ml[a]	Physically compatible with no subvisual haze or particle formation in 4 hr at 23 °C	1758	C
Bleomycin sulfate		3 units/ml		10 mg/ml	Drugs injected sequentially into Y-site with no flush between. No visually apparent precipitate	980	C
Cefepime HCl	BR	20 mg/ml[a]	LE	2 mg/ml[a]	Physically compatible with no change in measured turbidity or increase in particle content in 4 hr at 22 °C	1689	C
Cisplatin		1 mg/ml		10 mg/ml	Drugs injected sequentially into Y-site with no flush between. No visually apparent precipitate	980	C
Cladribine	ORT	0.015[b] and 0.5[c] mg/ml	IMM	2 mg/ml[b]	Physically compatible with no change in measured turbidity or increase in particle content in 4 hr at 23 °C	1969	C
Cyclophosphamide		20 mg/ml		10 mg/ml	Drugs injected sequentially into Y-site with no flush between. No visually apparent precipitate	980	C
Docetaxel	RPR	0.9 mg/ml[a]	ES	2 mg/ml[a]	Physically compatible with no change in measured turbidity or increase in particle content in 4 hr at 23 °C	2224	C
Doxorubicin HCl		2 mg/ml		10 mg/ml	Drugs injected sequentially into Y-site with no flush between. No visually apparent precipitate	980	C

Y-Site Injection Compatibility (1:1 Mixture) (Cont.)

Leucovorin calcium

Drug	Mfr	Conc	Mfr	Conc	Remarks	Ref	C/I
Doxorubicin HCl liposome injection	SEQ	0.4 mg/ml[a]	IMM	2 mg/ml[a]	Physically compatible with little or no change in measured turbidity and no increase in particle content in 4 hr at 23 °C	2087	C
Droperidol		2.5 mg/ml		10 mg/ml	Drugs injected sequentially into Y-site with no flush between. Immediate precipitation	980	I
Etoposide phosphate	BR	5 mg/ml[a]	IMM	2 mg/ml[a]	Physically compatible with no change in measured turbidity or increase in particle content in 4 hr at 23 °C	2218	C
Filgrastim	AMG	30 μg/ml[a]	LE	2 mg/ml[a]	Physically compatible with no change in measured turbidity or increase in particle content in 4 hr at 22 °C	1687	C
Fluconazole	RR	2 mg/ml	LE	10 mg/ml	Physically compatible for 24 hr at 25 °C	1407	C
Fluorouracil		50 mg/ml		10 mg/ml	Drugs injected sequentially into Y-site with no flush between. No visually apparent precipitate	980	C
Foscarnet sodium	AST	24 mg/ml	QU	10 mg/ml	Cloudy yellow solution	1335	I
Furosemide		10 mg/ml		10 mg/ml	Drugs injected sequentially into Y-site with no flush between. No visually apparent precipitate	980	C
Gemcitabine HCl	LI	10 mg/ml[b]	IMM	2 mg/ml[b]	Physically compatible with no change in measured turbidity or increase in particle content in 4 hr at 23 °C	2226	C
Granisetron HCl	SKB	0.05 mg/ml[a]	IMM	2 mg/ml[a]	Physically compatible with no change in measured turbidity or increase in particle content in 4 hr at 23 °C	2000	C
Heparin sodium		1000 units/ml		10 mg/ml	Drugs injected sequentially into Y-site with no flush between. No visually apparent precipitate	980	C
Methotrexate sodium		25 mg/ml		10 mg/ml	Drugs injected sequentially into Y-site with no flush between. No visually apparent precipitate	980	C
		30 mg/ml	LE	10 mg/ml	Visually compatible for 4 hr at room temperature	1788	C
Metoclopramide HCl		5 mg/ml		10 mg/ml	Drugs injected sequentially into Y-site with no flush between. No visually apparent precipitate	980	C
Mitomycin		0.5 mg/ml		10 mg/ml	Drugs injected sequentially into Y-site with no flush between. No visually apparent precipitate	980	C
Piperacillin sodium–tazobactam sodium	LE	40 + 5 mg/ml[a]	LE	2 mg/ml[a]	Physically compatible with no change in measured turbidity or increase in particle content in 4 hr at 22 °C	1688	C
Sodium bicarbonate		1.4%	LE	10 mg/ml	Yellow precipitate forms in 0.5 hr at room temperature	1788	I
Tacrolimus	FUJ	1 mg/ml[b]	ES	10 mg/ml[a]	Visually compatible for 24 hr at 25 °C	1630	C

Y-Site Injection Compatibility (1:1 Mixture) (Cont.)

Leucovorin calcium

Drug	Mfr	Conc	Mfr	Conc	Remarks	Ref	C/I
Teniposide	BR	0.1 mg/ml[a]	LE	2 mg/ml[a]	Physically compatible with no subvisual haze or particle formation in 4 hr at 23 °C	1725	C
Thiotepa	IMM[d]	1 mg/ml[a]	LE	2 mg/ml[a]	Physically compatible with no change in measured turbidity or increase in particle content in 4 hr at 23 °C	1861	C
TNA #218 to #226[e]			IMM	2 mg/ml[a]	Visually compatible with no precipitate or emulsion damage apparent in 4 hr at 23 °C	2215	C
TPN #212 to #215[e]			IMM	2 mg/ml[a]	Physically compatible with no change in measured turbidity or increase in particle content in 4 hr at 23 °C	2109	C
Vinblastine sulfate		1 mg/ml		10 mg/ml	Drugs injected sequentially into Y-site with no flush between. No visually apparent precipitate	980	C
Vincristine sulfate		1 mg/ml		10 mg/ml	Drugs injected sequentially into Y-site with no flush between. No visually apparent precipitate	980	C

[a]*Tested in dextrose 5% in water.*
[b]*Tested in sodium chloride 0.9%.*
[c]*Tested in bacteriostatic sodium chloride 0.9% preserved with benzyl alcohol 0.9%.*
[d]*Lyophilized formulation tested.*
[e]*Refer to Appendix I for the composition of parenteral nutrition solutions. TNA indicates a 3-in-1 admixture, and TPN indicates a 2-in-1 admixture.*

Additional Compatibility Information

Fluorouracil— Several articles reported the chemical stability and physical compatibility of fluorouracil with leucovorin calcium (980; 1387; 1817). However, more recent work found substantial amounts of subvisual particles in this drug combination over numerous concentrations when stored at 4, 23, and 32 °C. Particulate formation sometimes clogged filters and disrupted multiple-day treatment. Particulate formation began in about 24 hours in most samples, and particles were found in all samples within seven days. Fluorouracil and leucovorin calcium in the same container can no longer be considered a compatible combination (1816).

Floxuridine— Leucovorin calcium (Quad) and floxuridine (Quad) in concentrations ranging from 30 mg and 1 g, respectively, to 960 mg and 4 g, respectively, per liter of sodium chloride 0.9% were evaluated for stability under a sequence of temperatures to simulate use conditions as intraperitoneal chemotherapy solutions. The admixtures were stored for 48 hours at 4 °C, followed by 12 hours at 20 °C, and finally followed by 12 hours at 40 °C (near-physiologic temperature). No floxuridine loss and about a 3 to 6% leucovorin calcium loss occurred during the study period (1317).

LEVOFLOXACIN
AHFS 8:22

Levaquin   **Ortho-McNeil**

Products— Levofloxacin (Ortho-McNeil) is available as a 25-mg/ml preservative-free aqueous solution in 20-ml (500-mg) single-use vials. This concentration must be diluted to a 5-mg/ml concentration for administration. Adding 250 mg (10 ml) to 40 ml of diluent or 500 mg (20 ml) to 80 ml of diluent will result in a 5-mg/ml concentration (2).

The drug is also available as premixed infusion solutions of 5 mg/ml in dextrose 5% in water in 50-ml (250-mg) and 100-ml (500-mg) flexible plastic bags. The solutions in plastic bags are ready to use and require no dilution. Sodium hydroxide and hydrochloric acid may have been added during manufacture to adjust the pH (2).

pH— From 3.8 to 5.8 (2).

The pH of a 5-mg/ml concentration in dextrose or sodium chloride solutions is about 4.6 to 4.7. In solutions with a greater buffering capacity, pH values are higher. A 5-mg/ml concentration had a pH of 4.9 in dextrose 5% in Ringer's injection, lactated, a pH of

5.0 in Plasma-Lyte 56/5% dextrose, and a pH of 5.5 in sodium lactate ⅙ M (2).

Tonicity— The premixed infusion solutions are nearly isotonic (2).

Administration— Levofloxacin is administered only at a concentration of 5-mg/ml by slow intravenous infusion over 60 minutes. No other route is recommended. Rapid infusion or bolus administration must not be used because of the potential for hypotension. The 25-mg/ml concentrate must be diluted to 5 mg/ml with a compatible diluent for administration (2).

Stability— Intact vials should be stored at controlled room temperature and protected from light. The premixed infusion solutions should be stored at or below 25 °C and protected from light, freezing, and excessive heat. A brief exposure to temperatures up to 40 °C does not adversely affect potency (2). The injection and infusion admixtures are clear and yellow to greenish yellow in appearance. This color does not adversely affect the product (2; 1986).

Levofloxacin diluted in a compatible diluent to 5 mg/ml is stated to be stable for 72 hours stored at or below 25 °C and for 14 days stored at 5 °C (2).

pH Effects— Levofloxacin has a solubility of about 100 mg/ml at pH values ranging from 0.6 to 5.8. The solubility increases as pH increases up to 6.7, with a maximum solubility of 272 mg/ml. Above pH 6.7, solubility decreases to a minimum of 50 mg/ml at pH 6.9 (2).

Freezing Solutions— Levofloxacin 5 mg/ml diluted in a compatible diluent in glass bottles or plastic infusion containers is stable for six months frozen at −20 °C. Frozen solutions should be thawed at room temperature or in the refrigerator. Accelerated thawing using microwaves or hot water immersion is not recommended. Thawed solutions should not be refrozen (2).

Levofloxacin (OMJ Pharmaceuticals) 0.5 and 5 g/L in mannitol 20% and 0.5 g/L in sodium bicarbonate 5% formed a precipitate during frozen storage at −20 °C for 13 weeks. In several other infusion solutions at 0.5 and 5 g/L, no precipitate formed and little or no loss of levofloxacin by HPLC analysis occurred during 26 weeks of storage at −20 °C (1986). See Solution Compatibility below.

Compatibility Information

Solution Compatibility

Levofloxacin

Solution	Mfr	Mfr	Conc/L	Remarks	Ref	C/I
Dextrose 5% in Ringer's injection, lactated	BA[a]	OMJ	0.5 and 5 g	Physically compatible with no loss by HPLC in 3 days at 25 °C, 14 days at 5 °C, and 26 weeks at −20 °C, all protected from light	1986	C
Dextrose 5% in sodium chloride 0.9%	BA[a]	OMJ	0.5 and 5 g	Physically compatible with no loss by HPLC in 3 days at 25 °C, 14 days at 5 °C, and 26 weeks at −20 °C, all protected from light	1986	C
Dextrose 5% in sodium chloride 0.45% with potassium chloride 0.15%	BA[a]	OMJ	0.5 and 5 g	Physically compatible with little or no loss by HPLC in 3 days at 25 °C, 14 days at 5 °C, and 26 weeks at −20 °C, all protected from light	1986	C
Dextrose 5% in water	BA[a]	OMJ	0.5 and 5 g	Physically compatible with no loss by HPLC in 3 days at 25 °C, 14 days at 5 °C, and 26 weeks at −20 °C, all protected from light	1986	C
Mannitol 20%	BA[a]	OMJ	0.5 g	Precipitate forms within a few hours	1986	I
	BA[a]	OMJ	5 g	Physically compatible with 4% or less loss by HPLC in 3 days at 25 °C and 14 days at 5 °C protected from light	1986	C
	BA[a]	OMJ	5 g	Precipitate forms within 13 weeks at −20 °C	1986	I
Plasma-Lyte 56 and dextrose 5%	BA[a]	OMJ	0.5 and 5 g	Physically compatible with no loss by HPLC in 3 days at 25 °C, 14 days at 5 °C, and 26 weeks at −20 °C, all protected from light	1986	C
Sodium bicarbonate 5%	BA[a]	OMJ	0.5 g	Physically compatible with no loss by HPLC in 3 days at 25 °C and 14 days at 5 °C, protected from light	1986	C
	BA[a]	OMJ	0.5 g	Precipitate forms within 13 weeks at −20 °C	1986	I
	BA[a]	OMJ	5 g	Physically compatible with no loss by HPLC in 3 days at 25 °C, 14 days at 5 °C, and 26 weeks at −20 °C, all protected from light	1986	C

Solution Compatibility (Cont.)

Levofloxacin

Solution	Mfr	Mfr	Conc/L	Remarks	Ref	C/I
Sodium chloride 0.9%	BA[a]	OMJ	0.5 and 5 g	Physically compatible with no loss by HPLC in 3 days at 25 °C, 14 days at 5 °C, and 26 weeks at −20 °C, all protected from light	1986	C
Sodium lactate ⅙ M	BA[a]	OMJ	0.5 and 5 g	Physically compatible with 4% or less loss by HPLC in 3 days at 25 °C, 14 days at 5 °C, and 26 weeks at −20 °C, all protected from light	1986	C

[a]*Tested in PVC containers.*

Additional Compatibility Information

The manufacturer recommends that no other drugs be added to levofloxacin or infused simultaneously through the same line (2).

Solutions—— The manufacturer recommends the following infusion solutions for dilution of levofloxacin to a 5-mg/ml concentration (2):

Dextrose in Ringer's injection, lactated
Dextrose 5% in sodium chloride 0.9%
Dextrose 5% in sodium chloride 0.45% and potassium chloride 0.15%
Dextrose 5% in water
Plasma-Lyte 56/5% dextrose
Sodium chloride 0.9%
Sodium lactate ⅙ M

Metal Ions—— Levofloxacin may form stable coordination compounds with metal ions. The chelation potential is greatest with Al^{3+} and declines from Cu^{2+} to Zn^{2+} to Mg^{2+} to Ca^{2+} (2).

LEVORPHANOL TARTRATE
AHFS 28:08.08

Levo-Dromoran   **ICN**

Products—— Levorphanol tartrate (ICN) is available in 1-ml ampuls and 10-ml multiple-dose vials. Each milliliter of solution contains (2):

Component	Ampul	Vial
Levorphanol tartrate	2 mg	2 mg
Methylparaben	1.8 mg	
Propylparaben	0.2 mg	
Phenol		4.5 mg
Sodium hydroxide	to adjust pH	to adjust pH
Water for injection	qs 1 ml	qs 1 ml

pH—— The pH is adjusted to approximately 4.3 (2).

Administration—— Levorphanol tartrate may be administered by subcutaneous or slow intravenous injection or infusion (2; 4).

Stability—— The product should be stored at room temperature. Freezing should be avoided (4).

Compatibility Information

Additive Compatibility

Levorphanol tartrate

Drug	Mfr	Conc/L	Mfr	Conc/L	Test Soln	Remarks	Ref	C/I
Aminophylline		RC				Physically incompatible	9	I
Ammonium chloride		RC				Physically incompatible	9	I
Amobarbital sodium		RC				Physically incompatible	9	I
Chlorothiazide sodium	MSD	RC				Physically incompatible	9	I

Additive Compatibility (Cont.)

Levorphanol tartrate

Drug	Mfr	Conc/L	Mfr	Conc/L	Test Soln	Remarks	Ref	C/I
Heparin sodium		RC				Physically incompatible	9	I
Pentobarbital sodium		RC				Physically incompatible	9	I
Phenobarbital sodium	WI	RC				Physically incompatible	9	I
Phenytoin sodium	PD	RC				Physically incompatible	9	I
Sodium bicarbonate		RC				Physically incompatible	9	I
Thiopental sodium	AB	RC				Physically incompatible	9	I

Drugs in Syringe Compatibility

Levorphanol tartrate

Drug (in syringe)	Mfr	Amt	Mfr	Amt	Remarks	Ref	C/I
Glycopyrrolate	RB	0.2 mg/ 1 ml	RC	2 mg/ 1 ml	Physically compatible and pH in stability range for glycopyrrolate for 48 hr at 25 °C	331	C
	RB	0.2 mg/ 1 ml	RC	4 mg/ 2 ml	Physically compatible and pH in stability range for glycopyrrolate for 48 hr at 25 °C	331	C
	RB	0.4 mg/ 2 ml	RC	2 mg/ 1 ml	Physically compatible and pH in stability range for glycopyrrolate for 48 hr at 25 °C	331	C

Y-Site Injection Compatibility (1:1 Mixture)

Levorphanol tartrate

Drug	Mfr	Conc	Mfr	Conc	Remarks	Ref	C/I
Propofol	ZEN	10 mg/ml	RC	0.5 mg/ml[a]	Physically compatible for 1 hr at 23 °C with no increase in particle content	2066	C
TNA #218 to #226[b]			RC	0.5 mg/ml[a]	Damage to emulsion integrity occurs immediately with free oil formation possible	2215	I
TPN #212 to #215[b]			RC	0.5 mg/ml[a]	Physically compatible with no change in measured turbidity or increase in particle content in 4 hr at 23 °C	2109	C

[a]*Tested in dextrose 5% in water.*
[b]*Refer to Appendix I for the composition of parenteral nutrition solutions. TNA indicates a 3-in-1 admixture, and TPN indicates a 2-in-1 admixture.*

LIDOCAINE HCL
(LIGNOCAINE HCL)
AHFS 24:04

Xylocaine HCl I.V.　　　　　　　　**Astra**

Products— Lidocaine HCl for direct intravenous use is available in concentrations of 10 and 20 mg/ml in ampuls and vials from 5 to 50 ml and in 5-ml prefilled syringes. The drug is also available as 40-, 100-, and 200-mg/ml concentrates for intravenous admixture preparation. Multiple-dose vials and automatic injection devices may also have methylparaben and EDTA or sulfites (4; 154).

The pH of these solutions is adjusted with sodium hydroxide and/or hydrochloric acid (4).

Lidocaine HCl is also available premixed in dextrose 5% in water in concentrations of 0.2, 0.4, and 0.8% (2, 4, and 8 mg/ml, respectively). The solutions come in container sizes ranging from 250 to 1000 ml (4).

pH— The pH of the injection is about 6.5 but may range from 5 to 7

(2; 4). The premixed infusion solutions in dextrose 5% in water have a pH of 3 to 7 (4; 17).

Osmolality— The osmolalities of lidocaine HCl products were determined to be 296 mOsm/kg for the 10-mg/ml concentration and 352 mOsm/kg for the 20-mg/ml concentration (1233).

The commercially available lidocaine HCl 0.2, 0.4, and 0.8% premixed solutions have osmolarities of approximately 266, 281, and 308 mOsm/L, respectively (4).

Administration— Lidocaine HCl is administered by direct intravenous injection and continuous intravenous infusion (4; 8; 338). It may also be administered by intramuscular injection (4; 118–120). Products containing 40, 100, or 200 mg/ml should not be administered by direct intravenous injection without prior dilution. Usually 1 or 2 g of lidocaine HCl is added to 1 L of dextrose 5% in water to form a 1- or 2-mg/ml (0.1 or 0.2%) solution, respectively. Concentrations up to 8 mg/ml have been recommended in fluid-restricted patients. Lidocaine HCl products containing preservatives should not be given intravenously. Products containing epinephrine should not be used to treat arrhythmias (4).

Stability— Lidocaine HCl injection and premixed infusion solutions should be stored at controlled room temperature and protected from excessive heat and freezing (4). Aqueous solutions are reported to be stable to heat, acids, and alkalies (24). Although lidocaine HCl is stable across a broad pH range, its pH of maximum stability was determined to be 3 to 6 (1277). Lidocaine HCl (Astra) 20 mg/ml retained potency for three months at room temperature when 2 ml of solution was packaged in Tubex cartridges (13).

pH Effects— Bonhomme et al. studied the stability of lidocaine HCl 2%, with and without epinephrine HCl, after alkalinization with sodium bicarbonate. Lidocaine HCl alone was alkalinized to pH 7.2, while the lidocaine–epinephrine combination was adjusted to pH 6.5 and also 7.05. The combinations were compatible, and no loss of lidocaine or epinephrine occurred over six hours (1401).

Elastomeric Reservoir Pumps— Lidocaine HCl (Lyphomed) 4 mg/ml in both dextrose 5% in water and sodium chloride 0.9% was evaluated for binding potential to natural rubber elastomeric reservoirs (Baxter). Less than 1% loss was found after storage for two weeks at 35 °C with gentle agitation (2014).

Sorption— Lidocaine HCl (Astra) 200 mg/L did not display significant sorption to a PVC plastic test strip in 24 hours (12).

Similarly, lidocaine HCl (Sigma) 200 mg/L in sodium chloride 0.9% (Travenol) in PVC bags did not exhibit significant sorption to the plastic during one week of storage at room temperature (15 to 20 °C) (536).

In another study, lidocaine HCl (Sigma) 200 mg/L in sodium chloride 0.9% did not exhibit any loss due to sorption during a seven-hour simulated infusion through an infusion set (Travenol) consisting of a cellulose propionate burette chamber and 170 cm of PVC tubing (606).

The drug was also tested as a simulated infusion over at least one hour by a syringe pump system. A glass syringe on a syringe pump was fitted with 20 cm of polyethylene tubing or 50 cm of Silastic tubing. No loss of drug due to sorption was observed with either tubing (606).

In addition, a 25-ml aliquot of lidocaine HCl (Sigma) 200 mg/L in sodium chloride 0.9% was stored in all-plastic syringes composed of polypropylene barrels and polyethylene plungers for 24 hours at room temperature in the dark. No loss due to sorption occurred (606).

However, in a slightly alkaline (pH 8) cardioplegic solution, the percentage of unionized lidocaine base increased to 58%. This amount compares to less than 3% in dextrose 5% in water and sodium chloride 0.9% at around pH 6. This unionized form is highly lipid soluble and may interact with PVC bags. Storage of the cardioplegic solutions in 500- and 250-ml PVC bags at 22 °C resulted in a 12 to 19% lidocaine loss in two days and a 65 to 75% loss in 21 days. Degradation was not likely because storage of the same solution in glass bottles did not result in any lidocaine loss after 21 days at 22 °C. Refrigeration of the PVC bags at 4 °C slowed the lidocaine loss to 9% or less in 21 days (776).

Filtration— Lidocaine HCl (Astra) 200 mg/L in dextrose 5% in water and sodium chloride 0.9% did not display significant sorption to a 0.45-μm cellulose membrane filter (Abbott S-A-I-F) during an eight-hour simulated infusion (567).

Compatibility Information

Solution Compatibility

Lidocaine HCl

Solution	Mfr	Mfr	Conc/L	Remarks	Ref	C/I
Amino acids 4.25%, dextrose 25%	MG	AST	1 g	No increase in particulate matter in 24 hr at 5 °C	349	C
Dextrose 5% in Ringer's injection, lactated	TR[a]	AST	1 g	Potency retained for 24 hr at 5 °C	282	C
	TR[a]	AST	2 g	Physically compatible with little or no lidocaine loss in 14 days at 25 °C	775	C
Dextrose 5% in sodium chloride 0.45%	CU, AB[a]	AST	2 g	Physically compatible with little or no lidocaine loss in 14 days at 25 °C	775	C
Dextrose 5% in sodium chloride 0.9%	TR[a]	AST	1 g	Potency retained for 24 hr at 5 °C	282	C
Dextrose 5% in water	TR[a]	AST	2 g	Physically compatible with no lidocaine loss in 14 days at 25 °C	775	C
	AB[b]	ES	518 mg	No lidocaine loss over 21 days at 20 to 24 °C	776	C

Solution Compatibility (Cont.)

Lidocaine HCl

Solution	Mfr	Mfr	Conc/L	Remarks	Ref	C/I
	TR[a]	AST	1 g	Potency retained for 24 hr at 5 °C	282	C
	TR[a]	ES	4 g	Chemically stable for 120 days at 4 and 30 °C	543	C
	TR[b]	AST	1 and 8 g	Visually compatible with no lidocaine loss by HPLC in 48 hr at room temperature	1802	C
Ringer's injection, lactated	TR[a]	AST	1 g	Potency retained for 24 hr at 5 °C	282	C
	TR[a]	AST	2 g	Physically compatible with no lidocaine loss in 14 days at 25 °C	775	C
Sodium chloride 0.45%	AB[a]	AST	2 g	Physically compatible with no lidocaine loss in 14 days at 25 °C	775	C
Sodium chloride 0.9%	TR[a]	AST	2 g	Physically compatible with no lidocaine loss in 14 days at 25 °C	775	C
	AB[b]	ES	518 mg	No lidocaine loss over 21 days at 20 to 24 °C	776	C
	BA	AST		Potency retained for 24 hr	45	C
	TR[a]	AST	1 g	Potency retained for 24 hr at 5 °C	282	C
	TR[b]	AST	1 g	Potency retained for 24 hr	45	C
	TR[b]	AST	1 and 8 g	Visually compatible with little or no lidocaine loss by HPLC in 48 hr at room temperature	1802	C

[a]Tested in both glass and PVC containers.
[b]Tested in PVC containers.

Additive Compatibility

Lidocaine HCl

Drug	Mfr	Conc/L	Mfr	Conc/L	Test Soln	Remarks	Ref	C/I
Alteplase	GEN	0.5 g	AST	4 g	D5W	Visually compatible with no alteplase clot-lysis activity loss in 24 hr at 25 °C	1856	C
	GEN	0.5 g	AST	4 g	NS	Visually compatible with 7% alteplase clot-lysis activity loss in 24 hr at 25 °C	1856	C
Aminophylline	SE	500 mg	AST	2 g		Physically compatible	24	C
	AQ	1 g	AST	2 g	D5W, LR, NS	Physically compatible for 24 hr at 25 °C	775	C
Amiodarone HCl	LZ	1.8 g	AB	4 g	D5W, NS[a,d]	Physically compatible with 9% or less amiodarone loss in 24 hr at 24 °C under fluorescent light	1031	C
Atracurium besylate	BW	500 mg		2 g	D5W	Physically compatible and atracurium chemically stable for 24 hr at 5 and 30 °C	1694	C
Bretylium tosylate	ACC	10 g	AST	1 g	D5S[b]	Physically compatible and both drugs chemically stable for 48 hr at room temperature and 7 days at 4 °C	522	C
	AS	1 g	AST	2 g	D5W, LR, NS	Physically compatible for 24 hr at 25 °C	775	C
	ACC	1 g	AST	2 g	D5W, NS	Physically compatible for 48 hr at 25 °C	756	C
Calcium chloride	UP	1 g	AST	2 g		Physically compatible	24	C
Calcium gluconate	ES	2 g	AST	2 g	D5W, LR, NS	Physically compatible for 24 hr at 25 °C	775	C
Chloramphenicol sodium succinate	PD	1 g	AST	2 g		Physically compatible	24	C
Chlorothiazide sodium	MSD	500 mg	AST	2 g		Physically compatible	24	C

Additive Compatibility (Cont.)

Lidocaine HCl

Drug	Mfr	Conc/L	Mfr	Conc/L	Test Soln	Remarks	Ref	C/I
Cibenzoline succinate		2 g	AB	8 g	D5W, NS	Physically compatible for 24 hr at 25 °C by visual and microscopic examination	1182	C
Cimetidine HCl	SKF	3 g	AST	2.5 g	D5W	Physically compatible and cimetidine chemically stable for 24 hr at room temperature. Lidocaine not tested	551	C
Dexamethasone sodium phosphate	MSD	4 mg	AST	2 g		Physically compatible	24	C
Digoxin	ES	1 mg	AST	2 g	D5W, LR, NS	Physically compatible for 24 hr at 25 °C	775	C
Diphenhydramine HCl	PD	50 mg	AST	2 g		Physically compatible	24	C
Dobutamine HCl	LI	1 g	ES	4 g	D5W, NS	Physically compatible with no color change in 24 hr at 25 °C	789	C
	LI	1 g	AST	4 and 10 g	D5W, NS	Physically compatible for 24 hr at 21 °C	812	C
Dopamine HCl	ACC	800 mg	AST	2 g	D5W, LR, NS	Physically compatible for 24 hr at 25 °C	775	C
	AS	800 mg	AST	4 g	D5W	No dopamine or lidocaine decomposition in 24 hr at 25 °C	312	C
	AS	800 mg	AST	4 g	D5W[a]	No dopamine or lidocaine decomposition in 24 hr at 25 °C	312	C
Ephedrine sulfate		50 mg	AST	2 g		Physically compatible	24	C
Erythromycin lactobionate	AB	1 g	AST	2 g		Physically compatible	24	C
Floxacillin sodium	BE	20 g	ANT	2 g	NS	Physically compatible for 72 hr at 15 and 30 °C	1479	C
Flumazenil	RC	20 mg	AB	4 g	D5W[a]	Visually compatible with 4% flumazenil loss by HPLC in 24 hr at 23 °C under fluorescent light. Lidocaine not tested	1710	C
Furosemide	HO	1 g	ANT	2 g	NS	Physically compatible for 72 hr at 15 and 30 °C	1479	C
Heparin sodium		32,000 units		4 g	NS	Physically compatible and heparin activity retained for 24 hr	57	C
	AB	20,000 units	AST	2 g		Physically compatible	24	C
Hydrocortisone sodium succinate	UP	250 mg	AST	2 g		Physically compatible	24	C
Hydroxyzine HCl	PF	100 mg	AST	2 g		Physically compatible	24	C
Insulin, regular	SQ	1000 units	AST	2 g	D5W, LR, NS	Physically compatible for 24 hr at 25 °C	775	C
Mephentermine sulfate	WY	1 g	AST	2 g		Physically compatible	24	C
Metaraminol bitartrate	MSD	100 mg	AST	2 g		Physically compatible	24	C
Methohexital sodium	BP	2 g	BP	2 g	D5W	Immediate precipitation	26	I
Nafcillin sodium	AP	20 g	AST	0.6 g	D5W[a], NS[d]	Visually compatible with little or no nafcillin loss by HPLC in 48 hr at 23 °C. Lidocaine not tested	1806	C
Nitroglycerin	ACC	400 mg	IMS	4 g	D5W, NS[e]	Physically compatible with no nitroglycerin loss in 48 hr at 23 °C. Lidocaine not tested	929	C

Additive Compatibility (Cont.)

Lidocaine HCl

Drug	Mfr	Conc/L	Mfr	Conc/L	Test Soln	Remarks	Ref	C/I
Penicillin G potassium	SQ	1 million units	AST	2 g		Physically compatible	24	**C**
Pentobarbital sodium	AB	500 mg	AST	2 g		Physically compatible	24	**C**
Phenylephrine HCl	WI	20 mg	AST	2 g		Physically compatible	24	**C**
Phenytoin sodium	ES	1 g	AST	2 g	D5W, LR, NS	Immediate formation of a white cloudy precipitate	775	**I**
Potassium chloride	AB	40 mEq	AST	2 g		Physically compatible	24	**C**
Procainamide HCl	SQ	1 g	AST	2 g	D5W, LR, NS	Physically compatible for 24 hr at 25 °C	775	**C**
Prochlorperazine edisylate	SKF	10 mg	AST	2 g		Physically compatible	24	**C**
Promazine HCl	WY	100 mg	AST	2 g		Physically compatible	24	**C**
Propafenone HCl	KN	0.54 g	AST	4.5 g[c]	D5W	Visually compatible with little or no propafenone loss by HPLC in 24 hr at 22 °C exposed to fluorescent light. Lidocaine not tested	412	**C**
Ranitidine HCl	GL	50 mg and 2 g	AST	1 and 8 g	D5W, NS[a]	Physically compatible with 3% or less ranitidine loss in 24 hr at room temperature under fluorescent light. Lidocaine not tested	1361	**C**
	GL	50 mg and 2 g		2.5 g	D5W	Physically compatible and ranitidine chemically stable by HPLC for 24 hr at 25 °C. Lidocaine not tested	1515	**C**
	GL	50 mg and 2 g	AST	1 and 8 g	D5W, NS[a]	Visually compatible with little or no loss of either drug by HPLC in 48 hr at room temperature	1802	**C**
Sodium bicarbonate	AB	40 mEq	AST	2 g		Physically compatible	24	**C**
	AB	2.4 mEq[f]		1 g	D5W	Physically compatible for 24 hr	772	**C**
Sodium lactate	AB	50 mEq	AST	2 g		Physically compatible	24	**C**
Theophylline		2 g		380 mg	D5W	Visually compatible with little or no loss of either drug in 48 hr	1909	**C**
Verapamil HCl	KN	80 mg	IMS	2 g	D5W, NS	Physically compatible for 48 hr	739	**C**
Vitamin B complex with C	AB	10 ml	AST	2 g		Physically compatible	24	**C**

[a]Tested in PVC containers.
[b]Tested in both glass and PVC containers.
[c]Approximate concentration.
[d]Tested in polyolefin containers.
[e]Tested in glass containers.
[f]One vial of Neut added to a liter of admixture.

Drugs in Syringe Compatibility

Lidocaine HCl

Drug (in syringe)	Mfr	Amt	Mfr	Amt	Remarks	Ref	C/I
Ampicillin sodium	BE	500 mg		0.5 and 2.5%/ 1.5 ml	Physically compatible	89	**C**

Drugs in Syringe Compatibility (Cont.)

Lidocaine HCl

Drug (in syringe)	Mfr	Amt	Mfr	Amt	Remarks	Ref	C/I
	BE	250 mg		0.5 and 2.5%/ 1.5 ml	Occasional turbidity	89	**I**
Cefazolin sodium	SKF	1 g	AST	0.5%/ 3 ml	Precipitate forms within 3 to 4 hr at 4 °C	532	**I**
Ceftriaxone sodium	RC	450 mg/ ml	LY	1%	5% or less ceftriaxone loss by HPLC in 8 weeks at −15 °C but solution failed the particulate matter test	1824	**I**
	RC	250 and 450 mg/ ml	DW	1%	10% ceftriaxone loss in 3 days at 20 °C, 7 to 8% loss in 35 days at 4 °C, and 4 to 6% loss in 168 days at −20 °C. Lidocaine not tested	1991	**C**
Clonidine HCl with fentanyl citrate	BI JN	0.03 mg/ ml 0.01 mg/ ml	AST	2 mg/ml	Diluted to 5 ml with NS. Visually compatible with no new GC/MS peaks appearing in 1 hr at room temperature	1956	**C**
Glycopyrrolate	RB	0.2 mg/ 1 ml	ES	10 mg/ 1 ml	Physically compatible and pH in stability range for glycopyrrolate for 48 hr at 25 °C	331	**C**
	RB	0.2 mg/ 1 ml	ES	20 mg/ 2 ml	Physically compatible and pH in stability range for glycopyrrolate for 48 hr at 25 °C	331	**C**
	RB	0.4 mg/ 2 ml	ES	10 mg/ 1 ml	Physically compatible and pH in stability range for glycopyrrolate for 48 hr at 25 °C	331	**C**
	RB	0.2 mg/ 1 ml	ES	20 mg/ 1 ml	Physically compatible and pH in stability range for glycopyrrolate for 48 hr at 25 °C	331	**C**
	RB	0.2 mg/ 1 ml	ES	40 mg/ 2 ml	Physically compatible and pH in stability range for glycopyrrolate for 48 hr at 25 °C	331	**C**
	RB	0.4 mg/ 2 ml	ES	20 mg/ 1 ml	Physically compatible and pH in stability range for glycopyrrolate for 48 hr at 25 °C	331	**C**
Heparin sodium		2500 units/ 1 ml	AST	100 mg/ 5 ml	Physically compatible for at least 5 min	1053	**C**
Hydroxyzine HCl	PF	50 mg/ 2 ml	AST	2%/2 ml	Physically compatible	771	**C**
	PF	100 mg/ 2 ml	AST	2%/2 ml	Physically compatible	771	**C**
Ketamine HCl with morphine sulfate	PD ES	2 mg/ml 0.2 mg/ ml	AST	2 mg/ml	Diluted to 5 ml with NS. Visually compatible with no new GC/MS peaks appearing in 1 hr at room temperature	1956	**C**
Metoclopramide HCl	RB	10 mg/ 2 ml	ES	50 mg/ 5 ml	Physically compatible for 48 hr at room temperature	924	**C**
	RB	10 mg/ 2 ml	ES	100 mg/ 10 ml	Physically compatible for 48 hr at room temperature	924	**C**
	RB	10 mg/ 2 ml	ES	50 mg/ 5 ml	Physically compatible for 48 hr at 25 °C	1167	**C**
	RB	10 mg/ 2 ml	ES	100 mg/ 10 ml	Physically compatible for 48 hr at 25 °C	1167	**C**
	RB	160 mg/ 32 ml	ES	50 mg/ 5 ml	Physically compatible for 48 hr at 25 °C	1167	**C**
	RB	160 mg/ 32 ml	ES	100 mg/ 10 ml	Physically compatible for 48 hr at 25 °C	1167	**C**

Drugs in Syringe Compatibility (Cont.)

Lidocaine HCl

Drug (in syringe)	Mfr	Amt	Mfr	Amt	Remarks	Ref	C/I
Milrinone lactate	WI	5.25 mg/ 5.25 ml	AB	100 mg/ 10 ml	Physically compatible with no loss of either drug in 20 min at 23 °C under fluorescent light	1410	C
Moxalactam disodium	LI	1 g		0.5 and 1%/3 ml	Physically compatible with 7% moxalactam decomposition in 24 hr at 25 °C and 4% in 96 hr at 5 °C	693	C
Nalbuphine HCl	DU	10 mg/ 1 ml		40 mg	Physically compatible for 48 hr	128	C
	DU	20 mg/ 1 ml		40 mg	Physically compatible for 48 hr	128	C
Sodium bicarbonate	AB	3 mEq/ 3 ml	ES	2%[a], 30 ml	11% lidocaine loss in 1 week and 22% loss in 2 weeks at 25 °C by GC. 28% epinephrine loss by HPLC in 1 week at 25 °C	1712	I
	AB	3 mEq/ 3 ml	ES	2%[a], 30 ml	6% lidocaine loss by GC in 4 weeks at 4 °C. 2% epinephrine loss in 1 week and 12% loss in 3 weeks at 4 °C by HPLC	1712	C
	LY	0.1 mEq/ml	AST	1%[a], 30 ml	25% epinephrine loss by HPLC in 1 week at room temperature. Lidocaine not tested	1713	I
		0.088 mEq/ml		0.9%	11% lidocaine loss by fluorescence polarization immunoassay in 7 days at room temperature	1723	C
	AST	8.4%, 2 ml	AST	1 and 1.5%[b], 20 ml	Visually compatible for up to 5 hr at room temperature	1724	C
	AST	8.4%, 2 ml	AST	2%[b], 20 ml	Haze forms but clarifies with gentle agitation	1724	?
	AB	4%, 4 ml	AST	1 and 1.5%[b], 20 ml	Visually compatible for up to 5 hr at room temperature	1724	C
	AB	4%, 4 ml	AST	2%[b], 20 ml	Haze forms but clarifies with gentle agitation	1724	?
		1.4 and 8.4%, 1.5 ml	BEL	2%[c], 20 ml	8% epinephrine loss by HPLC in 7 days at room temperature. Lidocaine not tested	1743	C

[a]*Tested with epinephrine HCl 1:100,000 added.*
[b]*Tested with epinephrine HCl 1:200,000 added.*
[c]*Tested with epinephrine HCl 1:80,000 added.*

Y-Site Injection Compatibility (1:1 Mixture)

Lidocaine HCl

Drug	Mfr	Conc	Mfr	Conc	Remarks	Ref	C/I
Alteplase	GEN	1 mg/ml	AB	8 mg/ml[a]	Physically compatible for 12 days by spectrophotometric and visual examination	1340	C
Amiodarone HCl	LZ	4 mg/ml[c]	AST	8 mg/ml[c]	Physically compatible for 24 hr at 21 °C	1032	C
Amphotericin B cholesteryl sulfate complex	SEQ	0.83 mg/ml[a]	AST	10 mg/ml	Gross precipitate forms	2117	I
Amrinone lactate	WB	3 mg/ml[b]	ES	1 mg/ml[a]	Physically compatible for at least 4 hr at 25 °C under fluorescent light	992	C
Cefazolin sodium	LI	40 mg/ml[c]	AB	8 mg/ml[c]	Physically compatible for 3 hr	1316	C

Y-Site Injection Compatibility (1:1 Mixture) (Cont.)

Lidocaine HCl

Drug	Mfr	Conc	Mfr	Conc	Remarks	Ref	C/I
Ciprofloxacin	MI	2 mg/ml[c]	AB	4[a] and 20 mg/ml	Visually compatible for 24 hr at 24 °C	1655	**C**
Cisatracurium besylate	GW	0.1, 2, 5 mg/ml[a]	AST	8 mg/ml[a]	Physically compatible with no change in measured turbidity or increase in particle content in 4 hr at 23 °C	2074	**C**
Clarithromycin	AB	4 mg/ml[a]	ANT	4 mg/ml[a]	Visually compatible for 72 hr at both 30 and 17 °C	2174	**C**
Diltiazem HCl	MMD	1 mg/ml[a]	AST	8 mg/ml[a]	Visually compatible for 24 hr at 25 °C	1530	**C**
	MMD	1[b] and 5 mg/ml	AB	10 mg/ml[b]	Visually compatible	1807	**C**
	MMD	5 mg/ml	AB, SCN	4 and 8 mg/ml[a]	Visually compatible	1807	**C**
Dobutamine HCl	LI	4 mg/ml[c]	AB	8 mg/ml[c]	Physically compatible for 3 hr	1316	**C**
Dobutamine HCl with dopamine HCl	LI DCC	4 mg/ml[c] 3.2 mg/ml[c]	AB	8 mg/ml[c]	Physically compatible for 3 hr	1316	**C**
Dobutamine HCl with nitroglycerin	LI LY	4 mg/ml[c] 0.4 mg/ml[c]	AB	8 mg/ml[c]	Physically compatible for 3 hr	1316	**C**
Dobutamine HCl with sodium nitroprusside	LI ES	4 mg/ml[c] 0.4 mg/ml[c]	AB	8 mg/ml[c]	Physically compatible for 3 hr	1316	**C**
Dopamine HCl	DCC	3.2 mg/ml[c]	AB	8 mg/ml[c]	Physically compatible for 3 hr	1316	**C**
Dopamine HCl with dobutamine HCl	DCC LI	3.2 mg/ml[c] 4 mg/ml[c]	AB	8 mg/ml[c]	Physically compatible for 3 hr	1316	**C**
Dopamine HCl with nitroglycerin	DCC LY	3.2 mg/ml[c] 0.4 mg/ml[c]	AB	8 mg/ml[c]	Physically compatible for 3 hr	1316	**C**
Dopamine HCl with sodium nitroprusside	DCC ES	3.2 mg/ml[c] 0.4 mg/ml[c]	AB	8 mg/ml[c]	Physically compatible for 3 hr	1316	**C**
Enalaprilat	MSD	0.05 mg/ml[b]	AST	4 mg/ml[a]	Physically compatible for 24 hr at room temperature under fluorescent light	1355	**C**
Etomidate	AB	2 mg/ml	AST	20 mg/ml	Visually compatible for up to 7 days at 25 °C	1801	**C**
Famotidine	MSD	0.2 mg/ml[a]	TR	4 mg/ml[a]	Physically compatible for 4 hr at 25 °C	1188	**C**
	MSD	0.2 mg/ml[a]	LY	1 mg/ml[a]	Physically compatible for 14 hr	1196	**C**
Haloperidol lactate	MN	0.5[a] and 5 mg/ml	AB	4 mg/ml[a]	Visually compatible for 24 hr at 21 °C	1523	**C**
Heparin sodium	TR	50 units/ml	TR	4 mg/ml	Visually compatible for 6 hr at 25 °C	1793	**C**
Heparin sodium with hydrocortisone sodium succinate	RI UP	1000 units + 100 mg/L[d]	AST	20 mg/ml	Physically compatible for at least 4 hr at room temperature by visual and microscopic examination	322	**C**
Labetalol HCl	SC	1 mg/ml[a]	AST	20 mg/ml[a]	Physically compatible for 24 hr at 18 °C	1171	**C**
Meperidine HCl	AB	10 mg/ml	AB	1 mg/ml[a]	Physically compatible for 4 hr at 25 °C	1397	**C**
Morphine sulfate	AB	1 mg/ml	AB	1 mg/ml[a]	Physically compatible for 4 hr at 25 °C	1397	**C**
Nitroglycerin	LY	0.4 mg/ml[c]	AB	8 mg/ml[c]	Physically compatible for 3 hr	1316	**C**
Nitroglycerin with dobutamine HCl	LY LI	0.4 mg/ml[c] 4 mg/ml[c]	AB	8 mg/ml[c]	Physically compatible for 3 hr	1316	**C**
Nitroglycerin with dopamine HCl	LY DCC	0.4 mg/ml[c] 3.2 mg/ml[c]	AB	8 mg/ml[c]	Physically compatible for 3 hr	1316	**C**

Y-Site Injection Compatibility (1:1 Mixture) (Cont.)

Lidocaine HCl

Drug	Mfr	Conc	Mfr	Conc	Remarks	Ref	C/I
Nitroglycerin with sodium nitroprusside	LY ES	0.4 mg/ml[c] 0.4 mg/ml[c]	AB	8 mg/ml[c]	Physically compatible for 3 hr	1316	C
Potassium chloride		40 mEq/L[d]	AST	20 mg/ml	Physically compatible for at least 4 hr at room temperature by visual and microscopic examination	322	C
Propofol	ZEN	10 mg/ml	AST	10 mg/ml	Physically compatible for 1 hr at 23 °C with no increase in particle content	2066	C
Remifentanil HCl	GW	0.025 and 0.25 mg/ml[b]	AST	8 mg/ml[a]	Physically compatible with no change in measured turbidity or increase in particle content in 4 hr at 23 °C	2075	C
Sodium nitroprusside	ES	0.4 mg/ml[c]	AB	8 mg/ml[c]	Physically compatible for 3 hr	1316	C
Sodium nitroprusside with dobutamine HCl	ES LI	0.4 mg/ml[c] 4 mg/ml[c]	AB	8 mg/ml[c]	Physically compatible for 3 hr	1316	C
Sodium nitroprusside with dopamine HCl	ES DCC	0.4 mg/ml[c] 3.2 mg/ml[c]	AB	8 mg/ml[c]	Physically compatible for 3 hr	1316	C
Sodium nitroprusside with nitroglycerin	ES LY	0.4 mg/ml[c] 0.4 mg/ml[c]	AB	8 mg/ml[c]	Physically compatible for 3 hr	1316	C
Streptokinase	HO	30,000 units/ml[a]	AB	8 mg/ml[a]	Physically compatible for at least 3 days by visual examination	1340	C
Theophylline	TR	4 mg/ml	TR	4 mg/ml	Visually compatible for 6 hr at 25 °C	1793	C
Thiopental sodium	AB	25 mg/ml	AST	20 mg/ml	White cloudiness forms immediately but clears within 24 hr at 25 °C	1801	I
TNA #73[e]			ES	200 mg/ 50 ml[c]	Physically compatible for 4 hr by visual observation	1009	C
Vitamin B complex with C	RC	2 ml/L[d]	AST	20 mg/ml	Physically compatible for at least 4 hr at room temperature by visual and microscopic examination	322	C
Warfarin sodium	DU	2 mg/ml[f]	AST	2 mg/ml[a]	Visually compatible with no warfarin loss by HPLC in 30 min	2010	C
	DME	2 mg/ml[f]	AST	2 mg/ml[a]	Visually compatible for 24 hr at 24 °C	2078	C

[a]*Tested in dextrose 5% in water.*
[b]*Tested in sodium chloride 0.9%.*
[c]*Tested in both dextrose 5% in water and sodium chloride 0.9%.*
[d]*Tested in dextrose 5% in water, sodium chloride 0.9%, and Ringer's injection, lactated.*
[e]*Refer to Appendix I for the composition of parenteral nutrition solutions. TNA indicates a 3-in-1 admixture.*
[f]*Tested in sterile water for injection.*

Additional Compatibility Information

Infusion Solutions— At a concentration in the range of 1 to 4 mg/ml in dextrose 5% in water, lidocaine HCl appears to be stable for at least 24 hours at room temperature (4). At a concentration of 2 g/L, lidocaine HCl is physically compatible with most Abbott infusion solutions (24).

Miscellaneous Additives— Dacarbazine is stated to be physically incompatible when mixed with lidocaine HCl 1 or 2% (524). Also, local anesthetics such as lidocaine HCl cause precipitation of amphotericin B (107). Lidocaine HCl is stated to be physically compatible with alteplase when administered by Y-site injection into a running alteplase solution (4).

Cefazolin— Cefazolin sodium (SKF) constituted with 0.5% lidocaine HCl (Astra) to a concentration of 1 g/3 ml and frozen at −20 °C in glass syringes (Hy-Pod) did not yield a clear solution on thawing. The solution was unsuitable for injection (532).

Dobutamine, Dopamine, Nitroglycerin, and Nitroprusside— Dobutamine HCl (Lilly) 4 mg/ml, dopamine HCl (Dupont Critical Care) 3.2 mg/ml, lidocaine HCl (Abbott) 8 mg/ml, nitroglycerin (Lyphomed) 0.4 mg/ml, and sodium nitroprusside (Elkins-Sinn) 0.4 mg/ml, prepared in dextrose 5% in water and sodium chloride 0.9%, were combined in equal quantities in all possible combinations of two, three, four, and five drugs and then evaluated for physical compatibility. No physical incompatibility was observed in any combination within the three-hour study period (1316).

Sympathomimetic Amines— Lidocaine HCl mixed with certain acid-stable drugs may present a problem. In combination with epinephrine HCl, norepinephrine bitartrate, and isoproterenol HCl, lidocaine HCl is stable, but its buffering action may raise the pH of intravenous admixtures above 5.5, the maximum pH for stability of the other drugs. The final pH is usually about 6. These drugs begin to deteriorate within several hours. Therefore, admixtures should be used promptly after preparation, or the separate administration of the sympathomimetic amines should be considered. Note: This does not apply to commercial lidocaine–epinephrine combinations, which have the pH adjusted to retain the maximum epinephrine potency (24).

Phenylephrine— Lidocaine HCl 2% in combination with phenylephrine HCl 0.25% was stable for at least 66 days at 25 °C. No loss of either drug was found by HPLC analysis, and little change in pH occurred during the test period (1278).

Multiple Drugs— A seven-drug combination consisting of bupivacaine HCl (Sanofi Winthrop) 1.5 mg/1 ml, clonidine HCl (Boehringer Ingelheim) 0.03 mg/1 ml, fentanyl citrate (Janssen) 0.01 mg/1 ml, ketamine (Parke-Davis) 2 mg/ml, lidocaine HCl (Astra) 2 mg/ml, morphine sulfate (Elkins-Sinn) 0.2 mg/ml, and tetracaine HCl (Sanofi Winthrop) 2 mg/ml mixed together in equal quantities was found to be visually compatible with no new GC/MS peaks appearing in one hour at room temperature (1956).

Cardioplegic Solution— The stability of lidocaine was assessed in a cardioplegic solution of the following composition:

Component	Final Concentration per Liter
Lidocaine (as HCl)	448 mg
Potassium chloride	20 mEq
Sodium bicarbonate	25 mEq
Dextrose	17 g
Sodium chloride	8.3 g

Because insulin is not added to the cardioplegic solution until just before use, it was not included in this study. The cardioplegic solution was stored in glass and PVC containers at 22 and 4 °C for 21 days. No loss of lidocaine occurred in glass containers during this period. However, storage in PVC bags at 22 °C resulted in a 12 to 19% loss in two days and a 65 to 75% loss in 21 days, believed to be due to sorption to the plastic. Refrigeration at 4 °C slowed the loss in PVC bags to 9% or less in 21 days. Concentrations of the other components did not change during the study (776).

LINCOMYCIN HCL
AHFS 8:12.28

Lincocin Hydrochloride　　　　　　**Pharmacia & Upjohn**

Products— Lincomycin HCl (Pharmacia & Upjohn) is available in 2- and 10-ml vials. Each milliliter contains lincomycin HCl equivalent to lincomycin base 300 mg and benzyl alcohol 9.45 mg in water for injection (1-6/99; 4).

pH— From 3 to 5.5 (4).

Administration— Lincomycin HCl may be administered by deep intramuscular injection, slow intravenous infusion, or subconjunctival injection (1-6/99; 4).

Stability— Lincomycin HCl injection should be stored at controlled room temperature and protected from freezing (1-6/99; 4).

Compatibility Information

Solution Compatibility

Lincomycin HCl

Solution	Mfr	Mfr	Conc/L	Remarks	Ref	C/I
Dextrose 5% in sodium chloride 0.9%		UP	1.2 g	Potency retained for 24 hr	109	C
Dextrose 5% in water		UP	1.2 g	Potency retained for 24 hr	109	C
Dextrose 10% in water		UP	1.2 g	Potency retained for 24 hr	109	C
Sodium chloride 0.9%		UP	1.2 g	Potency retained for 24 hr	109	C

Additive Compatibility

Lincomycin HCl

Drug	Mfr	Conc/L	Mfr	Conc/L	Test Soln	Remarks	Ref	C/I
Amikacin sulfate	BR	5 g	UP	10 g	D5LR, D5R, D5S, D5W, D10W, IS10, LR, NS, R, SL	Physically compatible and potency of both retained for 24 hr at 25 °C	294	C
Cimetidine HCl	SKF	3 g	UP	6 g	D5W	Physically compatible and cimetidine chemically stable for 24 hr at room temperature. Lincomycin not tested	551	C
Cytarabine	UP	500 mg		1, 1.5, 2, 2.4, 3 g		Physically compatible for 48 hr	174	C
Heparin sodium	AB	20,000 units	UP	600 mg		Physically compatible	21	C
Penicillin G potassium	SQ	20 million units	UP	6 g	D5W	Physically compatible	15	C
	SQ	5 million units	UP	600 mg	D	Physically compatible	47	C
			UP			Physically incompatible	9	I
Penicillin G sodium	UP	20 million units	UP	6 g	D5W	Physically compatible	15	C
			UP			Physically incompatible	9	I
Phenytoin sodium	PD		UP			Physically incompatible	9	I
Ranitidine HCl	GL	50 mg and 2 g		2.4 g	D5W	Physically compatible and ranitidine chemically stable by HPLC for 24 hr at 25 °C. Lincomycin not tested	1515	C

Drugs in Syringe Compatibility

Lincomycin HCl

Drug (in syringe)	Mfr	Amt	Mfr	Amt	Remarks	Ref	C/I
Ampicillin sodium	AY	500 mg	UP	600 mg/ 2 ml	Physically incompatible within 1 hr at room temperature	99	I
	AY	500 mg	UP	600 mg/ 2 ml	Precipitate forms within 1 hr at room temperature	300	I
Doxapram HCl	RB	400 mg/ 20 ml		300 mg/ 1 ml	Physically compatible with no doxapram loss in 24 hr	1177	C
Heparin sodium	AB	20,000 units/ 1 ml	UP	600 mg/ 2 ml	Physically compatible for at least 30 min	21	C
Penicillin G sodium		1 million units	UP	600 mg/ 2 ml	No precipitate or color change within 1 hr at room temperature	99	C

Additional Compatibility Information

Lincomycin HCl is stated to be physically compatible for 24 hours at room temperature with the following infusion solutions and drugs in infusion solutions (1-6/99; 154):

Infusion Solutions

Dextran 6% in sodium chloride 0.9%
Dextrose 5% in sodium chloride 0.9%
Dextrose 10% in sodium chloride 0.9%
Dextrose 5% in water
Dextrose 10% in water
Invert sugar 10% in Electrolyte #1
Ringer's injection
Sodium lactate ⅙ M

Drugs in Infusion Solutions

Ampicillin sodium
Chloramphenicol sodium succinate
Polymyxin B sulfate
Vitamin B complex
Vitamin B complex with C

Lincomycin HCl is stated to be physically incompatible with kanamycin sulfate and to be physically compatible for only four hours with colistimethate sodium and penicillin G sodium (1-6/99; 154).

In vitro testing of riboflavin-5'-phosphate at a concentration of 0.1% with lincomycin HCl 0.025% in sterile distilled water showed significant reduction in antibiotic activity in one hour at 25 °C (314).

LORAZEPAM
AHFS 28:24.08

Ativan   **Wyeth-Ayerst**

Products— Lorazepam (Wyeth-Ayerst) is available in 2- and 4-mg/ml concentrations in 1- and 10-ml vials. The 2-mg/ml concentration is also available in 0.5- and 1-ml Tubex disposable cartridge units, and the 4-mg/ml concentration is available in 1-ml Tubex units. Each milliliter also contains 0.18 ml of polyethylene glycol 400 and 2% benzyl alcohol in propylene glycol (2).

For intramuscular use, lorazepam (Wyeth-Ayerst) may be injected as is. For intravenous use, however, lorazepam *must* be diluted immediately prior to injection with an equal volume of compatible diluent. To dilute the dose in a Tubex or when aspirated from a vial into a syringe, first eliminate all air and then aspirate the proper volume of diluent. Pull the plunger back slightly to provide some mixing space and gently invert the Tubex or syringe repeatedly to mix the contents thoroughly. To avoid air entrapment, do not shake vigorously (2).

Administration— Lorazepam may be administered by deep intramuscular injection or by intravenous injection when diluted immediately before use with an equal volume of compatible diluent. Intravenous injection is made directly into a vein or into the tubing of a running intravenous infusion at a rate not exceeding 2 mg/min (2; 4).

Stability— Intact vials of lorazepam should be refrigerated and protected from light and freezing (2; 4). The manufacturer has stated that the product may be stored for up to two weeks at room temperature (1181). However, in response to an inquiry, the manufacturer acknowledged that both physical and chemical stability are acceptable for up to 60 days at room temperature (1674). As with other parenteral products, lorazepam should be inspected visually for particulate matter and discoloration before use (2).

Lorazepam solutions should not be used if they are discolored or contain a precipitate (4).

The choice of commercial lorazepam concentration to use in the preparation of dilutions is a critical factor in the physical stability of the dilutions. Both the 2- and 4-mg/ml concentrations utilize the same concentrations of solubilizing solvents. On admixture, the solvents that keep the aqueous insoluble lorazepam in solution are diluted twice as much using the 4-mg/ml concentration than if the 2-mg/ml were used, resulting in different precipitation potentials for the same concentration of lorazepam. Care should be taken to ensure that the compounding procedure that is to be used for lorazepam admixtures has been demonstrated to result in solutions in which the lorazepam remains soluble.

Lorazepam concentrations up to 0.08 mg/ml have been reported to be physically stable, while occasional precipitate formation in admixtures of lorazepam 0.1 to 0.2 mg/ml has been reported. The precipitate has been observed in both containers and in administration set tubing (1943; 1979; 1980). In one case, a visible precipitate formed in a lorazepam 0.5-mg/ml admixture in sodium chloride 0.9% in a glass bottle (1945). However, a 0.5-mg/ml concentration may remain in solution longer if prepared from the 2-mg/ml concentration, yielding a higher concentration of organic solvents in the final admixture (1981; 2207). Concentrations of 1 and 2 mg/ml have been reported to be physically stable for up to 24 hours as well as concentrations below 0.08 mg/ml (1980; 2208). Concentrations in the middle range of 0.08 to 1 mg/ml may be problematic (1980). In one report, use of lorazepam 2 mg/ml to prepare lorazepam 1-mg/ml admixtures in dextrose 5% in water or sodium chloride 0.9% was acceptable but use of the lorazepam 4-mg/ml concentration to prepare the same solutions resulted in almost immediate precipitation (2207). Also see Solubility in Solutions under Additional Compatibility Information below.

Freezing— Although freezing is not recommended by the manufacturer (2), lorazepam (Wyeth-Ayerst) 0.1 mg/ml in dextrose 5% in water (McGaw) in polyolefin bags exhibited no loss when frozen at −20 °C for seven days (1683).

Bacteriostatic Water— Dilution of lorazepam (Wyeth) to 1 mg/ml with bacteriostatic water for injection (bacteriostat not noted), packaged in glass vials, resulted in lorazepam losses. HPLC analysis showed losses of about 10% at 4 °C and 12% at 22 °C in seven days. Drug crystals precipitated from solutions in varying periods after the first week of storage (1840).

Syringes— Lorazepam (Wyeth) 2 mg/ml was packaged as 3 ml in 10-ml polypropylene infusion pump syringes (Pharmacia Deltec). About 12 to 14% loss by HPLC analysis occurred in three days and 25% loss in 10 days at 5 and 30 °C. The authors recommended not storing lorazepam in the syringes for these time periods (1967).

Lorazepam (Wyeth) 1 mg/ml, prepared from the 2-mg/ml commercial concentration, diluted in dextrose 5% in water or in sodium chloride 0.9% was filled as 40 ml in 60-ml polypropylene syringes (Becton-Dickinson). The filled syringes were stored at 22 °C for 28 hours. Visual inspection found the solutions remained physically stable, and HPLC analysis found less than 3% drug loss in this time period (2208).

Sorption— Lorazepam (Wyeth-Ayerst) 0.1 mg/ml underwent substantial sorption to PVC containers of infusion solutions. In 50-ml bags of dextrose 5% in water or sodium chloride 0.9%, losses of 11 to 13% in eight hours and of 27 to 29% in 24 hr occurred at 37 °C. At 24 °C, approximately 17% was lost in 24 hr and 30% was lost in 72 hours. At 4 °C, 8 to 9% losses occurred in seven days. In Ringer's injection, lactated, losses due to sorption averaged about 50% more than with the other two infusion solutions. The use of PVC administration sets can be expected to contribute to sorption losses as well, while the use of polyolefin containers reduces losses dramatically. See Compatibility Table (1684).

Lorazepam (Wyeth) 2- and 4-mg/ml concentrations were diluted 1:1 using dextrose 5% in water, sodium chloride 0.9%, and water for injection. A 2-ml sample of each dilution was injected into the Y-sites of administration sets from five different manufacturers through which dextrose 5% in water, sodium chloride 0.9%, Ringer's injection, or Ringer's injection, lactated, was flowing at rates of 30 and 125 ml/hr. No differences were found among the various infusion sets, infusion solutions, or flow rates. All effluent solutions were visually acceptable and had no loss of lorazepam (786).

In another study, lorazepam (Wyeth) 2 mg/50 ml in dextrose 5% in water was delivered at rates of 600, 200, and 100 ml/hr using an infusion controller fitted with 180 or 350 cm of PVC tubing. Lorazepam loss due to sorption was greater with the longer tubing and at slower rates. Losses ranged from a high of 5% (350 cm, 100 ml/hr) to a low of 0.7% (180 cm, 600 ml/hr) (787).

In static sorption studies, lorazepam (Wyeth) 2 mg/50 ml in dextrose 5% in water was filled into PVC containers in the following amounts: 50 ml into 50-ml bags, 100 ml into 50-ml bags, and 100 ml into 250-ml bags. The bags were stored at 23 °C. A rapid initial loss of lorazepam occurred (about 3.9 to 5.8% in the first hour) followed by a slower, approximately constant loss after eight hours. Cumulative losses of 6 to 8% occurred in about five hours in the smaller bags with smaller bag surface area to volume ratios. The solution in the larger bags exhibited over a 10% loss in two hours (787).

Martens et al. found less than a 3% lorazepam loss from a 40-µg/ml solution in 500-ml PVC containers of sodium chloride 0.9% in 24 hours at 21 °C in the dark. In glass and polyethylene-lined laminated containers, virtually no loss was observed (1392).

Lorazepam (Wyeth) at a high concentration of 1 mg/ml admixed in dextrose 5% in water in PVC containers (Baxter) was stored for 24 hours at 25 °C. HPLC analysis found about 6% loss due to sorption, primarily during the first six hours with little additional loss occurring. This was substantially less loss than if the same solution was evaluated with a spectrophotometric method. The authors attributed the difference to interference of the benzyl alcohol preservative with the spectrophotometric analysis (2203).

Plasticizer Leaching— Lorazepam (Wyeth-Ayerst) 0.1 mg/ml in dextrose 5% in water did not leach diethylhexyl phthalate (DEHP) plasticizer from 50-ml PVC bags in 24 hours at 24 °C (1683).

Compatibility Information

Solution Compatibility

Lorazepam

Solution	Mfr	Mfr	Conc/L	Remarks	Ref	C/I
Dextrose 5% in water	BA[a]	WY	0.1 g	Losses due to sorption of 11% in 8 hr and 27% in 24 hr at 37 °C, 8% in 8 hr and 17% in 24 hr at 24 °C, and 3% in 24 hr and 8% in 7 days at 4 °C	1684	I
	MG[b]	WY	0.1 g	3% loss in 24 hr and 9% in 72 hr at 37 °C, little or no loss in 24 hr and 5% in 7 days at 24 °C, and no loss in 7 days at 4 °C	1684	C
	AB[c]	WY	0.16, 0.24, 0.5 g	About 10 to 20% loss due to sorption throughout 24-hr delivery at 24 °C under fluorescent light	1858	I
	BA[a]	WY	0.08 g	10 to 17% loss due to sorption in 4 hr at 4 °C. 17% loss in 1 hr, increasing to over 30% in 24 hr at 21 °C	1873	I
	BA[a]	WY	0.5 g	About 14% loss due to sorption in 4 hr at 21 °C	1873	I

Solution Compatibility (Cont.)

Lorazepam

Solution	Mfr	Mfr	Conc/L	Remarks	Ref	C/I
	BA[a]	WY	1 g	Approximately 6% loss by HPLC due to sorption in 6 hr with no further loss in 24 hr at 25 °C	2203	C
	AB[e]	WY	1 g	Prepared with 4-mg/ml lorazepam. White precipitate forms in 8 hours at 22 °C	2208	I
	AB[e]	WY	1 g	Prepared with 2-mg/ml lorazepam. Visually compatible with little or no lorazepam loss by HPLC in 28 hr at 22 °C under fluorescent light	2208	C
	AB[e]	WY	2 g	Prepared with 4-mg/ml lorazepam. Visually compatible with little or no lorazepam loss by HPLC in 28 hr at 22 °C under fluorescent light	2208	C
Ringer's injection, lactated	BA[a]	WY	0.1 g	Losses due to sorption of 25% in 8 hr at 37 °C, 14% in 8 hr at 24 °C, and 5% in 24 hr and 9% in 72 hr at 4 °C	1684	I
	MG[b]	WY	0.1 g	2% loss in 24 hr and 7% in 72 hr at 37 °C, little or no loss in 24 hr and 4% in 7 days at 24 °C, and no loss in 7 days at 4 °C	1684	C
Sodium chloride 0.9%	[d]		40 mg	Physically compatible with less than 3% loss in 24 hr at 21 °C in the dark	1392	C
	BA[a]	WY	0.1 g	Losses due to sorption of 13% in 8 hr and 29% in 24 hr at 37 °C, 8% in 8 hr and 17% in 24 hr at 24 °C, and 3% in 24 hr and 8% in 7 days at 4 °C	1684	I
	MG[b]	WY	0.1 g	2% loss in 24 hr and 7% in 72 hr at 37 °C, little or no loss in 24 hr and 4% in 7 days at 24 °C, and no loss in 7 days at 4 °C	1684	C
	AB[c]	WY	0.16, 0.24, 0.5 g	About 10 to 20% loss due to sorption throughout 24-hr delivery at 24 °C under fluorescent light	1858	I
	BA[a]	WY	0.08 g	8 to 10% loss due to sorption in 4 hr at 4 °C. 17 to 23% loss in 1 hr, increasing to 25 to 30% loss in 4 hr at 21 °C	1873	I
	BA[a]	WY	0.5 g	17% or more loss due to sorption in 4 hr at 21 °C	1873	I

[a]Tested in PVC containers.
[b]Tested in polyolefin containers.
[c]Tested in PVC containers and delivered through PVC administration sets.
[d]Tested in PVC, glass, and polyethylene-lined laminated containers.
[e]Tested in glass containers.

Additive Compatibility

Lorazepam

Drug	Mfr	Conc/L	Mfr	Conc/L	Test Soln	Remarks	Ref	C/I
Dexamethasone sodium phosphate with diphenhydramine HCl and metoclopramide HCl	AMR ES DU	400 mg 2 g 4 g	WY	40 mg	NS[a]	Rapid lorazepam losses of 8, 10, and 15% at 3, 23, and 30 °C, respectively, in 24 hr by HPLC. Other drugs stable for 14 days by HPLC at all three storage temperatures	1733	I

[a]Tested in Pharmacia-Deltec PVC pump reservoirs.

Drugs in Syringe Compatibility

Drug (in syringe)	Mfr	Amt	Mfr	Amt	Remarks	Ref	C/I
		Lorazepam					
Cimetidine HCl	SKF	300 mg/ 2 ml	WY	2 mg/ 1 ml	Physically compatible for 4 hr at 25 °C	25	C
Hydromorphone HCl	KN	1, 10, 40 mg/ 1 ml	WY	4 mg/ 1 ml	Visually compatible with 10% lorazepam loss by HPLC in 6 days at 4 °C, 4 days at 23 °C, and 24 hr at 37 °C. Little or no hydromorphone loss in 7 days at all three temperatures	1776	C
Ranitidine HCl	GL	50 mg/ 2 ml	WY	4 mg/ 1 ml	Lorazepam viscosity caused poor mixing and layering, which disappeared following vortex mixing	978	?
Sufentanil citrate	JN	50 µg/ml	WY	2 mg/ml	Turbidity increases within 0.5 hr and continues to increase over 24 hr at 23 °C	1711	I

Y-Site Injection Compatibility (1:1 Mixture)

Drug	Mfr	Conc	Mfr	Conc	Remarks	Ref	C/I
		Lorazepam					
Acyclovir sodium	BW	5 mg/ml[a]	WY	0.04 mg/ml[a]	Physically compatible for 4 hr at 25 °C	1157	C
Albumin		200 mg/ml	WY	0.33 mg/ml[b]	Visually compatible for 24 hr at 22 °C	1855	C
Aldesleukin	CHI	33,800 I.U./ ml[a]	WY	2 mg/ml	Globules form immediately	1857	I
Allopurinol sodium	BW	3 mg/ml[b]	WY	0.1 mg/ml[b]	Physically compatible with no change in measured turbidity or increase in particle content in 4 hr at 22 °C	1686	C
Amifostine	USB	10 mg/ml[a]	WY	0.1 mg/ml[a]	Physically compatible with no change in measured turbidity or increase in particle content in 4 hr at 23 °C	1845	C
Amikacin sulfate	BMS	5 mg/ml	WY	0.33 mg/ml[b]	Visually compatible for 24 hr at 22 °C	1855	C
Amoxicillin sodium	SKB	50 mg/ml	WY	0.33 mg/ml[b]	Visually compatible for 24 hr at 22 °C	1855	C
Amoxicillin sodium–clavulanate potassium	SKB	20 + 2 mg/ ml	WY	0.33 mg/ml[b]	Visually compatible for 24 hr at 22 °C	1855	C
Amphotericin B cholesteryl sulfate complex	SEQ	0.83 mg/ml[a]	WY	0.1 mg/ml[a]	Physically compatible with little or no change in measured turbidity or increase in particle content in 4 hr at 23 °C under fluorescent light	2117	C
Amsacrine	NCI	1 mg/ml[a]	WY	0.1 mg/ml[a]	Physically compatible for 4 hr at room temperature under fluorescent light	1381	C
Atracurium besylate	BW	0.5 mg/ml[a]	WY	0.5 mg/ml[a]	Physically compatible for 24 hr at 28 °C	1337	C
Aztreonam	SQ	40 mg/ml[a]	WY	0.1 mg/ml[a]	Haze forms within 1 hr	1758	I
Bumetanide	LEO	0.5 mg/ml	WY	0.33 mg/ml[b]	Visually compatible for 24 hr at 22 °C	1855	C
Cefepime HCl	BR	20 mg/ml[a]	WY	0.1 mg/ml[a]	Physically compatible with no change in measured turbidity or increase in particle content in 4 hr at 22 °C	1689	C
Cefotaxime sodium	RS	10 mg/ml	WY	0.33 mg/ml[b]	Visually compatible for 24 hr at 22 °C	1855	C
Ciprofloxacin	BAY	2 mg/ml	WY	0.33 mg/ml[b]	Visually compatible for 24 hr at 22 °C	1855	C

Y-Site Injection Compatibility (1:1 Mixture) (Cont.)

			Lorazepam				
Drug	*Mfr*	*Conc*	*Mfr*	*Conc*	*Remarks*	*Ref*	*C/I*
Cisatracurium besylate	GW	0.1, 2, 5 mg/ml[a]	WY	0.5 mg/ml[a]	Physically compatible with no change in measured turbidity or increase in particle content in 4 hr at 23 °C	2074	**C**
Cisplatin	BR	1 mg/ml	WY	0.1 mg/ml[a]	Visually compatible for 4 hr at room temperature under fluorescent light	1685	**C**
Cladribine	WY	0.1 mg/ml[b]	ORT	0.015[b] and 0.5[d] mg/ml	Physically compatible with no change in measured turbidity or increase in particle content in 4 hr at 23 °C	1969	**C**
Clonidine HCl	BI	0.015 mg/ml	WY	0.33 mg/ml[b]	Visually compatible for 24 hr at 22 °C	1855	**C**
Cyclophosphamide	MJ	10 mg/ml	WY	0.1 mg/ml[a]	Visually compatible for 4 hr at room temperature under fluorescent light	1685	**C**
Cytarabine	UP	50 mg/ml	WY	0.1 mg/ml[a]	Visually compatible for 4 hr at room temperature under fluorescent light	1685	**C**
Dexamethasone sodium phosphate		4 mg/ml	WY	0.33 mg/ml[b]	Visually compatible for 24 hr at 22 °C	1855	**C**
Diltiazem HCl	MMD	5 mg/ml	WY	4 mg/ml	Visually compatible	1807	**C**
	MMD	1 mg/ml[b]	WY	2 mg/ml[b]	Visually compatible	1807	**C**
	MMD	1 mg/ml[a]	WY	0.5 mg/ml[a]	Visually compatible for 4 hr at 27 °C	2062	**C**
Dobutamine HCl	LI	4 mg/ml[a]	WY	0.5 mg/ml[a]	Visually compatible for 4 hr at 27 °C	2062	**C**
Docetaxel	RPR	0.9 mg/ml[a]	WY	0.5 mg/ml[a]	Physically compatible with no change in measured turbidity or increase in particle content in 4 hr at 23 °C	2224	**C**
Dopamine HCl	AB	3.2 mg/ml[a]	WY	0.5 mg/ml[a]	Visually compatible for 4 hr at 27 °C	2062	**C**
Doxorubicin HCl	AD	0.2 mg/ml[a]	WY	0.1 mg/ml[a]	Visually compatible for 4 hr at room temperature under fluorescent light	1685	**C**
Doxorubicin HCl liposome injection	SEQ	0.4 mg/ml[a]	WY	0.1 mg/ml[a]	Physically compatible with little or no change in measured turbidity and no increase in particle content in 4 hr at 23 °C	2087	**C**
Epinephrine HCl	AB	0.02 mg/ml[a]	WY	0.5 mg/ml[a]	Visually compatible for 4 hr at 27 °C	2062	**C**
Erythromycin lactobionate	AB	5 mg/ml	WY	0.33 mg/ml[b]	Visually compatible for 24 hr at 22 °C	1855	**C**
Etomidate	AB	2 mg/ml	WY	2 mg/ml	Visually compatible for up to 7 days at 25 °C	1801	**C**
Etoposide phosphate	BR	5 mg/ml[a]	WY	0.5 mg/ml[a]	Physically compatible with no change in measured turbidity or increase in particle content in 4 hr at 23 °C	2218	**C**
Famotidine	ME	2 mg/ml[b]		0.1 mg/ml[a]	Visually compatible for 4 hr at 22 °C	1936	**C**
Fentanyl citrate		0.05 mg/ml	WY	0.33 mg/ml[b]	Visually compatible for 24 hr at 22 °C	1855	**C**
	ES	0.05 mg/ml	WY	0.5 mg/ml[a]	Visually compatible for 4 hr at 27 °C	2062	**C**
Filgrastim	AMG	30 μg/ml[a]	WY	0.1 mg/ml[a]	Physically compatible with no change in measured turbidity or increase in particle content in 4 hr at 22 °C	1687	**C**
Floxacillin sodium	SKB	50 mg/ml	WY	0.33 mg/ml[b]	White opalescence forms in 4 hr	1855	**I**
Fluconazole	PF	2 mg/ml	WY	0.33 mg/ml[b]	Visually compatible for 24 hr at 22 °C	1855	**C**
Fludarabine phosphate	BX	1 mg/ml[a]	WY	0.1 mg/ml[a]	Physically compatible for 4 hr at room temperature under fluorescent light	1439	**C**

Y-Site Injection Compatibility (1:1 Mixture) (Cont.)

		Lorazepam					
Drug	*Mfr*	*Conc*	*Mfr*	*Conc*	*Remarks*	*Ref*	*C/I*
Foscarnet sodium	AST	24 mg/ml	WY	4 mg/ml	Gas production	1335	**I**
	AST	24 mg/ml	WY	0.08 mg/ml[a]	Physically compatible for 24 hr at 25 °C under fluorescent light by visual and microscopic examination	1393	**C**
Fosphenytoin sodium	PD	1 mgPE/ml[b,h]	WY	2 mg/ml	Samples remained clear with no loss of either drug by HPLC in 8 hr	2223	**C**
Furosemide	CNF	10 mg/ml	WY	0.33 mg/ml[b]	Visually compatible for 24 hr at 22 °C	1855	**C**
	AMR	10 mg/ml	WY	0.5 mg/ml[a]	Visually compatible for 4 hr at 27 °C	2062	**C**
Gemcitabine HCl	LI	10 mg/ml[b]	WY	0.5 mg/ml[a]	Physically compatible with no change in measured turbidity or increase in particle content in 4 hr at 23 °C	2226	**C**
Gentamicin sulfate	CNF	3 mg/ml	WY	0.33 mg/ml[b]	Visually compatible for 24 hr at 22 °C	1855	**C**
Granisetron HCl	SKB	1 mg/ml	WY	0.1 mg/ml[b]	Physically compatible with little or no loss of either drug by HPLC in 4 hr at 22 °C	1883	**C**
	SKB	0.05 mg/ml[a]	WY	0.1 mg/ml[a]	Physically compatible with no change in measured turbidity or increase in particle content in 4 hr at 23 °C	2000	**C**
Haloperidol lactate	MN	5 mg/ml	WY	2 mg/ml	Physically compatible and chemically stable for 16 hr at room temperature	1838	**C**
	JN	0.5 and 5 mg/ml	WY	0.33 mg/ml[b]	Visually compatible for 24 hr at 22 °C	1855	**C**
Heparin sodium		417 units/ml	WY	0.33 mg/ml[b]	Visually compatible for 24 hr at 22 °C	1855	**C**
	ES	100 units/ml[a]	WY	0.5 mg/ml[a]	Visually compatible for 4 hr at 27 °C	2062	**C**
Hydrocortisone sodium succinate	UP	50 mg/ml	WY	0.33 mg/ml[b]	Visually compatible for 24 hr at 22 °C	1855	**C**
Hydromorphone HCl	KN	1 mg/ml	WY	0.5 mg/ml[a]	Visually compatible for 4 hr at 27 °C	2062	**C**
Idarubicin HCl	AD	1 mg/ml[b]	WY	2 mg/ml	Color changes immediately	1525	**I**
Imipenem–cilastatin sodium	MSD	5 mg/ml	WY	0.33 mg/ml[b]	Yellow precipitate forms in 24 hr	1855	**I**
Ketanserin tartrate	JN	1 mg/ml	WY	0.33 mg/ml[b]	Visually compatible for 24 hr at 22 °C	1855	**C**
Labetalol HCl	AH	2 mg/ml[a]	WY	0.5 mg/ml[a]	Visually compatible for 4 hr at 27 °C	2062	**C**
Melphalan HCl	BW	0.1 mg/ml[b]	WY	0.1 mg/ml[b]	Physically compatible with no change in measured turbidity or increase in particle content in 3 hr at 22 °C	1557	**C**
Methotrexate sodium	AD	15 mg/ml[e]	WY	0.1 mg/ml[a]	Visually compatible for 4 hr at room temperature under fluorescent light	1685	**C**
Metronidazole	BRN	5 mg/ml	WY	0.33 mg/ml[b]	Visually compatible for 24 hr at 22 °C	1855	**C**
Midazolam HCl	RC	2 mg/ml[a]	WY	0.5 mg/ml[a]	Visually compatible for 4 hr at 27 °C	2062	**C**
Milrinone lactate	SW	0.2 mg/ml[a]	WY	0.5 mg/ml[a]	Visually compatible for 4 hr at 27 °C	2062	**C**
	SW	0.4 mg/ml[a]	WY	0.2 mg/ml[a]	Visually compatible with little or no loss of either drug by HPLC in 4 hr at 23 °C	2214	**C**
Morphine HCl	CNF	1 mg/ml	WY	0.33 mg/ml[b]	Visually compatible for 24 hr at 22 °C	1855	**C**
Morphine sulfate	SCN	2 mg/ml[a]	WY	0.5 mg/ml[a]	Visually compatible for 4 hr at 27 °C	2062	**C**
Nicardipine HCl	WY	1 mg/ml[a]	WY	0.5 mg/ml[a]	Visually compatible for 4 hr at 27 °C	2062	**C**
Nitroglycerin	AB	0.4 mg/ml[a]	WY	0.5 mg/ml[a]	Visually compatible for 4 hr at 27 °C	2062	**C**

Y-Site Injection Compatibility (1:1 Mixture) (Cont.)

		Lorazepam					
Drug	*Mfr*	*Conc*	*Mfr*	*Conc*	*Remarks*	*Ref*	*C/I*
Norepinephrine bitartrate	AB	0.128 mg/ml[a]	WY	0.5 mg/ml[a]	Visually compatible for 4 hr at 27 °C	2062	**C**
Omeprazole sodium	AST	4 mg/ml	WY	0.33 mg/ml[b]	Yellow discoloration forms	1855	**I**
Ondansetron HCl	GL	1 mg/ml[b]	WY	0.1 mg/ml[a]	Light haze forms immediately	1365	**I**
Paclitaxel	NCI	1.2 mg/ml[a]		0.1 mg/ml[a]	Physically compatible with no change in measured turbidity in 4 hr at 22 °C	1528	**C**
Pancuronium bromide	ES	0.05 mg/ml[a]	WY	0.5 mg/ml[a]	Physically compatible for 24 hr at 28 °C	1337	**C**
Piperacillin sodium	LE	150 mg/ml	WY	0.33 mg/ml[b]	Visually compatible for 24 hr at 22 °C	1855	**C**
Piperacillin sodium–tazobactam sodium	LE	40 + 5 mg/ml[a]	WY	0.1 mg/ml[a]	Physically compatible with no change in measured turbidity or increase in particle content in 4 hr at 22 °C	1688	**C**
Potassium chloride	BRN	1 mEq/ml	WY	0.33 mg/ml[b]	Visually compatible for 24 hr at 22 °C	1855	**C**
Propofol	ZEN	10 mg/ml	WY	0.1 mg/ml[a]	Physically compatible for 1 hr at 23 °C with no increase in particle content	2066	**C**
Ranitidine HCl	GL	0.5 mg/ml	WY	0.33 mg/ml[b]	Visually compatible for 24 hr at 22 °C	1855	**C**
	GL	1 mg/ml[a]	WY	0.5 mg/ml[a]	Visually compatible for 4 hr at 27 °C	2062	**C**
Remifentanil HCl	GW	0.025 and 0.25 mg/ml[b]	WY	0.5 mg/ml[a]	Physically compatible with no change in measured turbidity or increase in particle content in 4 hr at 23 °C	2075	**C**
Sargramostim	IMM	10 μg/ml[b]	WY	0.1 mg/ml[b]	Slightly bluish haze, visible with high intensity light, forms in 1 hr	1436	**I**
Sufentanil citrate	JN	12.5 μg/ml[a]	WY	0.1 mg/ml[a]	Large increase in turbidity occurs immediately and persists for 24 hr at 23 °C	1711	**I**
Tacrolimus	FUJ	1 mg/ml[b]	WY	1 mg/ml[a]	Visually compatible for 24 hr at 25 °C	1630	**C**
Teniposide	BR	0.1 mg/ml[a]	WY	0.1 mg/ml[a]	Physically compatible with no subvisual haze or particle formation in 4 hr at 23 °C	1725	**C**
Thiopental sodium	AB	25 mg/ml	WY	2 mg/ml	Yellow discoloration forms	1801	**I**
	AB	25 mg/ml[c]	WY	0.5 mg/ml[a]	Visually compatible for 4 hr at 27 °C	2062	**C**
Thiotepa	IMM[f]	1 mg/ml[a]	WY	0.1 mg/ml[a]	Physically compatible with no change in measured turbidity or increase in particle content in 4 hr at 23 °C	1861	**C**
TNA #218 to #226[g]			WY	0.1 mg/ml[a]	Damage to emulsion integrity occurs in 1 hr	2215	**I**
TPN #212 to #215[g]			WY	0.1 mg/ml[a]	Physically compatible with no change in measured turbidity or increase in particle content in 4 hr at 23 °C	2109	**C**
Trimethoprim–sulfamethoxazole	RC	0.8 + 4 mg/ml	WY	0.33 mg/ml[b]	Visually compatible for 24 hr at 22 °C	1855	**C**
Vancomycin HCl	LI	5 mg/ml	WY	0.33 mg/ml[b]	Visually compatible for 24 hr at 22 °C	1855	**C**
Vecuronium bromide	OR	0.1 mg/ml[a]	WY	0.5 mg/ml[a]	Physically compatible for 24 hr at 28 °C	1337	**C**
	OR	4 mg/ml	WY	0.33 mg/ml[b]	Visually compatible for 24 hr at 22 °C	1855	**C**
	OR	1 mg/ml	WY	0.5 mg/ml[a]	Visually compatible for 4 hr at 27 °C	2062	**C**
Vinorelbine tartrate	BW	1 mg/ml[b]	WY	0.1 mg/ml[b]	Physically compatible with no change in measured turbidity or increase in particle content in 4 hr at 22 °C	1558	**C**

Y-Site Injection Compatibility (1:1 Mixture) (Cont.)

Lorazepam

Drug	Mfr	Conc	Mfr	Conc	Remarks	Ref	C/I
Zidovudine	BW	4 mg/ml[a]	WY	80 μg/ml[a]	Physically compatible for 4 hr at 25 °C under fluorescent light by visual and microscopic examination	1193	C

[a]*Tested in dextrose 5% in water.*
[b]*Tested in sodium chloride 0.9%.*
[c]*Tested in sterile water for injection.*
[d]*Tested in bacteriostatic sodium chloride 0.9% preserved with benzyl alcohol 0.9%.*
[e]*Tested in dextrose 5% in water with sodium bicarbonate 0.05 mEq/ml.*
[f]*Lyophilized formulation tested.*
[g]*Refer to Appendix I for the composition of parenteral nutrition solutions. TNA indicates a 3-in-1 admixture, and TPN indicates a 2-in-1 admixture.*
[h]*Concentration expressed in milligrams of phenytoin sodium equivalents (PE) per milliliter.*

Additional Compatibility Information

Solutions—— For dilution of intravenous doses, lorazepam (Wyeth) is stated to be compatible with dextrose 5% in water, sodium chloride 0.9%, and sterile water for injection (2).

Solubility in Solutions—— Lorazepam solubility in common infusion solutions has been reported (Table 1). Its solubility in sodium chloride 0.9% is approximately half that found in the other tested solutions. This result was attributed to the pH of the sodium chloride 0.9% (pH 6.3) being essentially the same as the isoelectric point of lorazepam (pH 6.4), where aqueous solubility would be the lowest. Dextrose 5% in water was the best diluent for lorazepam (787).

Table 1. Lorazepam Equilibrium Solubility (787)

Solution	Lorazepam Solubility (mg/ml)	Solution pH
Deionized water	0.054	7.09
Dextrose 5% in water	0.062	4.41
Ringer's injection, lactated	0.055	7.21
Sodium chloride 0.9%	0.027	6.30

Buprenorphine—— Lorazepam is stated to be incompatible with buprenorphine HCl (4).

MAGNESIUM SULFATE
AHFS 28:12.92

American Pharmaceutical Partners

Products—— Magnesium sulfate is available from various manufacturers in concentrations of 50, 20, 12.5, 10, 8, 4, 2, and 1% in a variety of container sizes (4; 154). The 50% solution provides 500 mg/ml of magnesium sulfate (magnesium 4.06 mEq/ml). The 12.5% solution contains 125 mg/ml of magnesium sulfate (magnesium 1 mEq/ml). Magnesium sulfate 10% contains 100 mg/ml of magnesium sulfate (magnesium 0.8 mEq/ml). The pH of these concentrations may have been adjusted with sodium hydroxide and/or sulfuric acid (1-8/98; 4; 154).

Magnesium sulfate is also available as 4 and 8% (40 and 80 mg/ml, respectively) solutions in water for injection and 1 and 2% (10 and 20 mg/ml, respectively) solutions in dextrose 5% in water (4).

pH— Magnesium sulfate injection has a pH adjusted to 5.5 to 7.0 when diluted to a 5% concentration (1-8/98). The premixed infusion solutions have pH values in the range of 3.5 to 6.5 (17).

Osmotic Values— The osmolality of magnesium sulfate 50% (Invenex) was determined to be 2620 mOsm/kg by freezing-point depression and 2875 mOsm/kg by vapor pressure (1071).

The 50% solution has a calculated osmolarity of 4060 mOsm/L (1-8/98).

Administration—— Magnesium sulfate may be administered by intramuscular or direct intravenous injection and by continuous or intermittent intravenous infusion. For intravenous injection, a concentration of 20% or less should be used; the rate of injection should not exceed 1.5 ml of a 10% solution (or equivalent) per minute. For intramuscular injection, a 25 or 50% concentration is satisfactory for adults, but dilution to 20% is necessary for infants and children (1-8/98; 4; 431).

Stability—— Magnesium sulfate injection and magnesium sulfate in dextrose 5% in water should be stored at room temperature and protected from temperatures above 40 °C and from freezing (4). Refrigeration of intact ampuls may result in precipitation or crystallization (593).

At a concentration of 40 g/L in dextrose 5% in water in polyolefin bottles (McGaw), magnesium sulfate (Abbott) was found to be stable for at least 60 days at 0 °C (922).

Compatibility Information

Solution Compatibility

Magnesium sulfate

Solution	Mfr	Mfr	Conc/L	Remarks	Ref	C/I
Dextrose 5% in water	MG	AB	40 g	Physically compatible and chemically stable for 60 days at 0 °C	922	C
Fat emulsion 10%, intravenous	CU		13.6 mEq[a]	Immediate flocculation with visually apparent layer within 2 hr at room temperature	656	I
Ringer's injection, lactated	BA[b,c]	AMR	37 g	Visually compatible with no consistent change in elemental composition over 3 months stored at room temperature	2184	C
Sodium chloride 0.9%	BA[b,c]	AMR	37 g	Visually compatible with no consistent change in elemental composition over 3 months stored at room temperature	2184	C

[a]Tested as magnesium chloride.
[b]Tested in PVC containers.
[c]Tested in glass containers.

Additive Compatibility

Magnesium sulfate

Drug	Mfr	Conc/L	Mfr	Conc/L	Test Soln	Remarks	Ref	C/I
Amphotericin B	SQ	40 and 80 mg	IMS	2 and 4 g	D5W	Physically incompatible in 3 hr at 24 °C with decreased clarity and development of supernatant. Total loss of amphotericin B in supernatant by HPLC	1578	I
Calcium gluconate	PR	10, 20, 30, 40 mEq	LI	1, 2, 3, 4 mEq	AA 4%, D 25%	Physically compatible for 24 hr at 22 °C	313	C
	PR	4 to 100 mEq	LI	4 to 100 mEq	PH 4%, D 20%	Physically compatible for 24 hr at room temperature	464	C
Chloramphenicol sodium succinate	PD	10 g	LI	16 mEq	D5W	Physically compatible	15	C
Cisplatin	BR	50 and 200 mg		1 and 2 g	D5½S[a]	Compatible for 48 hr at 25 °C and 96 hr at 4 °C followed by 48 hr at 25 °C	1088	C
Cyclosporine	SZ	2 g	LY	30 g	D5W	Transient turbidity appears upon preparation but dissipates in 30 sec and remains clear for 36 hr at 24 °C. 5% cyclosporine loss in 6 hr and 10% loss in 12 hr by HPLC at 24 °C under fluorescent light	1629	I
Dobutamine HCl	LI	167 mg	ES	83 g	NS	Physically compatible for 20 hr. Haze forms at 24 hr	552	I
	LI	1 g	TO	2 g	D5W, NS	Slightly pink in 24 hr at 25 °C	789	I
Heparin sodium		50,000 units		130 mEq	NS[b]	Visually compatible with heparin activity retained for 14 days at 24 °C under fluorescent light	1908	C
Hydrocortisone sodium succinate	UP	100 mg	ES	750 mg	AA 3.5%, D 25%	Physically compatible	302	C
Isoproterenol HCl	WI	4 mg		1 g		Physically compatible	59	C

Additive Compatibility (Cont.)

Magnesium sulfate

Drug	Mfr	Conc/L	Mfr	Conc/L	Test Soln	Remarks	Ref	C/I
Meropenem	ZEN	1 and 20 g	AST	1 g	NS	Visually compatible for 4 hr at room temperature	1994	C
Methyldopate HCl	MSD	1 g		1 g	D, D–S, S	Physically compatible	23	C
Norepinephrine bitartrate	WI	8 mg		1 g	D, D–S, S	Physically compatible	77	C
Penicillin G potassium	PF	500 mg		1 g	W	5% penicillin loss in 1 day and 13% loss in 2 days at 24 °C	999	C
	PF	500 mg		2 to 8 g	W	7 to 8% penicillin loss in 1 day and 20 to 25% loss in 2 days at 24 °C	999	C
Polymyxin B sulfate	BW	200 mg	LI	16 mEq	D5W	Physically incompatible	15	I
Potassium phosphate	MG	10, 20, 30, 40 mEq	LI	1, 2, 3, 4 mEq	AA 4%, D 25%	Physically compatible for 24 hr at 22 °C	313	C
	MG	4 to 100 mEq	LI	4 to 100 mEq	PH 4%, D 20%	Physically compatible for 24 hr at room temperature	464	C
Procaine HCl						Physically incompatible	9	I
	WI	1 g	LI	16 mEq	D5W	Physically incompatible	15	I
Sodium bicarbonate						Physically incompatible	9	I
	AB	80 mEq	LI	16 mEq	D5W	Physically incompatible	15	I
Verapamil HCl	KN	80 mg	IX	10 g	D5W, NS	Physically compatible for 24 hr	764	C

[a]Tested in PVC containers.
[b]Tested in glass bottles.

Drugs in Syringe Compatibility

Magnesium sulfate

Drug (in syringe)	Mfr	Amt	Mfr	Amt	Remarks	Ref	C/I
Metoclopramide HCl	RB	10 mg/ 2 ml	ES	500 mg/ 1 ml	Physically compatible for 48 hr at room temperature	924	C
	RB	10 mg/ 2 ml	ES	1 g/2 ml	Physically compatible for 48 hr at room temperature	924	C
	RB	10 mg/ 2 ml	ES	500 mg/ 1 ml	Physically compatible for 48 hr at 25 °C	1167	C
	RB	10 mg/ 2 ml	ES	1 g/2 ml	Physically compatible for 48 hr at 25 °C	1167	C
	RB	160 mg/ 32 ml	ES	1 g/2 ml	Physically compatible for 48 hr at 25 °C	1167	C

Y-Site Injection Compatibility (1:1 Mixture)

Magnesium sulfate

Drug	Mfr	Conc	Mfr	Conc	Remarks	Ref	C/I
Acyclovir sodium	BW	5 mg/ml[a]	LY	20 mg/ml[a]	Physically compatible for 4 hr at 25 °C	1157	C
Aldesleukin	CHI	33,800 I.U./ ml[a]	LY	20 mg/ml[a]	Visually compatible with little or no loss of aldesleukin activity by bioassay	1857	C
Amifostine	USB	10 mg/ml[a]	AST	100 mg/ml[a]	Physically compatible with no change in measured turbidity or increase in particle content in 4 hr at 23 °C	1845	C

Y-Site Injection Compatibility (1:1 Mixture) (Cont.)

Magnesium sulfate

Drug	Mfr	Conc	Mfr	Conc	Remarks	Ref	C/I
Amikacin sulfate	BR	5 mg/ml[a]	IX	16.7, 33.3, 66.7, 100 mg/ml[a]	Physically compatible for at least 4 hr at 32 °C	813	C
Amphotericin B cholesteryl sulfate complex	SEQ	0.83 mg/ml[a]	AST	100 mg/ml[a]	Gross precipitate forms	2117	I
Ampicillin sodium	WY	20 mg/ml[b]	IX	16.7, 33.3, 66.7, 100 mg/ml[a]	Physically compatible for at least 4 hr at 32 °C	813	C
Aztreonam	SQ	40 mg/ml[a]	AST	100 mg/ml[a]	Physically compatible with no subvisual haze or particle formation in 4 hr at 23 °C	1758	C
Cefamandole nafate	LI	20 mg/ml[a]	IX	16.7, 33.3, 66.7, 100 mg/ml[a]	Physically compatible for at least 4 hr at 32 °C	813	C
Cefazolin sodium	LI	20 mg/ml[a]	IX	16.7, 33.3, 66.7, 100 mg/ml[a]	Physically compatible for at least 4 hr at 32 °C	813	C
Cefepime HCl	BR	20 mg/ml[a]	AST	100 mg/ml[a]	Haze forms immediately	1689	I
Cefoperazone sodium	RR	20 mg/ml[a]	IX	16.7, 33.3, 66.7, 100 mg/ml[a]	Physically compatible for at least 4 hr at 32 °C	813	C
Cefotaxime sodium	HO	20 mg/ml[a]	IX	16.7, 33.3, 66.7, 100 mg/ml[a]	Physically compatible for at least 4 hr at 32 °C	813	C
Cefoxitin sodium	MSD	20 mg/ml[a]	IX	16.7, 33.3, 66.7, 100 mg/ml[a]	Physically compatible for at least 4 hr at 32 °C	813	C
Chloramphenicol sodium succinate	PD	20 mg/ml[a]	IX	16.7, 33.3, 66.7, 100 mg/ml[a]	Physically compatible for at least 4 hr at 32 °C	813	C
Ciprofloxacin	MI	2 mg/ml[a]	LY	50%	Visually compatible for 2 hr at 25 °C	1628	C
	MI	2 mg/ml[d]	AB	4 mEq/ml	Precipitate forms in 4 hr in D5W and after 4 hr in NS at 24 °C	1655	I
Cisatracurium besylate	GW	0.1, 2, 5 mg/ml[a]	AB	100 mg/ml[a]	Physically compatible with no change in measured turbidity or increase in particle content in 4 hr at 23 °C	2074	C
Clindamycin phosphate	UP	12 mg/ml[a]	IX	16.7, 33.3, 66.7, 100 mg/ml[a]	Physically compatible for at least 4 hr at 32 °C	813	C
Dobutamine HCl	LI	4 mg/ml[d]	LY	40 mg/ml[d]	Physically compatible for 3 hr	1316	C
Docetaxel	RPR	0.9 mg/ml[a]	AST	100 mg/ml[a]	Physically compatible with no change in measured turbidity or increase in particle content in 4 hr at 23 °C	2224	C
Doxorubicin HCl liposome injection	SEQ	0.4 mg/ml[a]	AST	100 mg/ml[a]	Physically compatible with little or no change in measured turbidity and no increase in particle content in 4 hr at 23 °C	2087	C

Y-Site Injection Compatibility (1:1 Mixture) (Cont.)

Drug	Mfr	Conc	Mfr	Conc	Remarks	Ref	C/I
				Magnesium sulfate			
Doxycycline hyclate	PF	1 mg/ml[a]	IX	16.7, 33.3, 66.7, 100 mg/ml[a]	Physically compatible for at least 4 hr at 32 °C	813	**C**
Enalaprilat	MSD	0.05 mg/ml[b]	LY	10 mEq/ml[a]	Physically compatible for 24 hr at room temperature under fluorescent light	1355	**C**
Erythromycin lactobionate	AB	5 mg/ml[a]	IX	16.7, 33.3, 66.7, 100 mg/ml[a]	Physically compatible for at least 4 hr at 32 °C	813	**C**
Esmolol HCl	DCC	10 mg/ml[a]	LY	10 mg/ml[a]	Physically compatible for 24 hr at 22 °C	1169	**C**
Etoposide phosphate	BR	5 mg/ml[a]	AST	100 mg/ml[a]	Physically compatible with no change in measured turbidity or increase in particle content in 4 hr at 23 °C	2218	**C**
Famotidine	MSD ME	0.2 mg/ml[a] 2 mg/ml[b]	SO	100 mg/ml[b] 100 mg/ml[a]	Physically compatible for 14 hr Visually compatible for 4 hr at 22 °C	1196 1936	**C** **C**
Fludarabine phosphate	BX	1 mg/ml[a]	SO	100 mg/ml[a]	Physically compatible for 4 hr at room temperature under fluorescent light	1439	**C**
Gentamicin sulfate	SC	0.8 mg/ml[a]	IX	16.7, 33.3, 66.7, 100 mg/ml[a]	Physically compatible for at least 4 hr at 32 °C	813	**C**
Granisetron HCl	SKB	1 mg/ml	AB	16 mg/ml[b]	Physically compatible with little or no loss of granisetron by HPLC in 4 hr at 22 °C	1883	**C**
	SKB	0.05 mg/ml[a]	AB	100 mg/ml[a]	Physically compatible with no change in measured turbidity or increase in particle content in 4 hr at 23 °C	2000	**C**
Heparin sodium	UP	1000 units/L[e]	AB	500 mg/ml	Physically compatible for at least 4 hr at room temperature by visual and microscopic examination	534	**C**
Hydrocortisone sodium succinate	UP	10 mg/L[e]	AB	500 mg/ml	Physically compatible for at least 4 hr at room temperature by visual and microscopic examination	534	**C**
Hydromorphone HCl	KN	2 mg/ml[a]	LY	16.7, 33.3, 50, 100 mg/ml[a]	Visually compatible for 4 hr at 25 °C under fluorescent light	1549	**C**
Idarubicin HCl	AD	1 mg/ml[b]	SO	2 mg/ml[b]	Visually compatible for 24 hr at 25 °C	1525	**C**
Insulin, regular	LI	0.2 unit/ml[b]	LY	40 mg/ml[f]	Physically compatible for 2 hr at 25 °C	1395	**C**
Kanamycin sulfate	BR	2.5 mg/ml[a]	IX	16.7, 33.3, 66.7, 100 mg/ml[a]	Physically compatible for at least 4 hr at 32 °C	813	**C**
Labetalol HCl	SC	1 mg/ml[a]	LY	10 mg/ml[a]	Physically compatible for 24 hr at 18 °C	1171	**C**
Meperidine HCl	WI	10 mg/ml[a]	LY	16.7, 33.3, 50, 100 mg/ml[a]	Visually compatible for 4 hr at 25 °C under fluorescent light	1549	**C**
Metronidazole	SE	5 mg/ml	IX	16.7, 33.3, 66.7, 100 mg/ml[a]	Physically compatible for at least 4 hr at 32 °C	813	**C**
Milrinone lactate	SW	0.4 mg/ml[a]	SO	40 mg/ml[a]	Visually compatible with no loss of milrinone by HPLC in 4 hr at 23 °C	2214	**C**

Y-Site Injection Compatibility (1:1 Mixture) (Cont.)

Magnesium sulfate

Drug	Mfr	Conc	Mfr	Conc	Remarks	Ref	C/I
Minocycline HCl	LE	0.2 mg/ml[a]	IX	16.7, 33.3, 66.7, 100 mg/ml[a]	Physically compatible for at least 4 hr at 32 °C	813	**C**
Morphine sulfate	ES	1 mg/ml[a]	LY	16.7, 33.3, 50, 100 mg/ml[a]	Visually compatible for 4 hr at 25 °C under fluorescent light	1549	**C**
	g	2 mg/ml[b]	AB	2, 4, 8 mg/ml[b]	Visually compatible for 8 hr at room temperature	1719	**C**
Nafcillin sodium	WY	20 mg/ml[a]	IX	16.7, 33.3, 66.7, 100 mg/ml[a]	Physically compatible for at least 4 hr at 32 °C	813	**C**
Ondansetron HCl	GL	1 mg/ml[b]	SO	100 mg/ml[a]	Physically compatible for 4 hr at 22 °C	1365	**C**
Oxacillin sodium	BE	20 mg/ml[a]	IX	16.7, 33.3, 66.7, 100 mg/ml[a]	Physically compatible for at least 4 hr at 32 °C	813	**C**
Paclitaxel	NCI	1.2 mg/ml[a]	AST	100 mg/ml[a]	Physically compatible with no change in measured turbidity in 4 hr at 22 °C	1556	**C**
Penicillin G potassium	SQ	100,000 units/ml[a]	IX	16.7, 33.3, 66.7, 100 mg/ml[a]	Physically compatible for at least 4 hr at 32 °C	813	**C**
Piperacillin sodium	LE	60 mg/ml[a]	IX	16.7, 33.3, 66.7, 100 mg/ml[a]	Physically compatible for at least 4 hr at 32 °C	813	**C**
Piperacillin sodium–tazobactam sodium	LE	40 + 5 mg/ml[a]	AST	100 mg/ml[a]	Physically compatible with no change in measured turbidity or increase in particle content in 4 hr at 22 °C	1688	**C**
Potassium chloride	AB	40 mEq/L[e]	AB	500 mg/ml	Physically compatible for at least 4 hr at room temperature by visual and microscopic examination	534	**C**
Propofol	ZEN	10 mg/ml	AST	100 mg/ml[a]	Physically compatible for 1 hr at 23 °C with no increase in particle content	2066	**C**
Remifentanil HCl	GW	0.025 and 0.25 mg/ml[b]	AB	100 mg/ml[a]	Physically compatible with no change in measured turbidity or increase in particle content in 4 hr at 23 °C	2075	**C**
Sargramostim	IMM	10 µg/ml[b]	LY	100 mg/ml[b]	Physically compatible for 4 hr at 22 °C	1436	**C**
Thiotepa	IMM[h]	1 mg/ml[a]	AST	100 mg/ml[a]	Physically compatible with no change in measured turbidity or increase in particle content in 4 hr at 23 °C	1861	**C**
Ticarcillin disodium	BE	60 mg/ml[a]	IX	16.7, 33.3, 66.7, 100 mg/ml[a]	Physically compatible for at least 4 hr at 32 °C	813	**C**
TNA #218 to #226[i]			AB	100 mg/ml[a]	Visually compatible with no precipitate or emulsion damage apparent in 4 hr at 23 °C	2215	**C**
Tobramycin sulfate	DI	0.8 mg/ml[a]	IX	16.7, 33.3, 66.7, 100 mg/ml[a]	Physically compatible for at least 4 hr at 32 °C	813	**C**

Y-Site Injection Compatibility (1:1 Mixture) (Cont.)

Magnesium sulfate

Drug	Mfr	Conc	Mfr	Conc	Remarks	Ref	C/I
TPN #212 to #215[i]			AB	100 mg/ml[a]	Physically compatible with no change in measured turbidity or increase in particle content in 4 hr at 23 °C	2109	**C**
Trimethoprim–sulfamethoxazole	RC	0.8 + 4 mg/ml[a]	IX	16.7, 33.3, 66.7, 100 mg/ml[a]	Physically compatible for at least 4 hr at 32 °C	813	**C**
Vancomycin HCl	LI	5 mg/ml[a]	IX	16.7, 33.3, 66.7, 100 mg/ml[a]	Physically compatible for at least 4 hr at 32 °C	813	**C**
Vitamin B complex with C	RC	2 ml/L[e]	AB	500 mg/ml	Physically compatible for at least 4 hr at room temperature by visual and microscopic examination	534	**C**

[a]*Tested in dextrose 5% in water.*
[b]*Tested in sodium chloride 0.9%.*
[c]*Tested in sterile water for injection.*
[d]*Tested in both dextrose 5% in water and sodium chloride 0.9%.*
[e]*Tested in dextrose 5% in Ringer's injection, dextrose 5% in Ringer's injection, lactated, dextrose 5% in water, Ringer's injection, lactated, and sodium chloride 0.9%.*
[f]*Tested in Ringer's injection, lactated.*
[g]*Extemporaneously prepared product.*
[h]*Lyophilized formulation tested.*
[i]*Refer to Appendix I for the composition of parenteral nutrition solutions. TNA indicates a 3-in-1 admixture, and TPN indicates a 2-in-1 admixture.*

Additional Compatibility Information

Additives— Magnesium sulfate is stated to be incompatible with soluble phosphates and with alkali hydroxides and carbonates (4).

Clindamycin phosphate (Upjohn) has been reported to be physically incompatible with magnesium sulfate (2p2462).

The activity of tobramycin sulfate apparently is inhibited by magnesium ions (145).

Hydrocortisone— A white flocculent precipitate was observed when hydrocortisone sodium succinate (Upjohn) 100 mg in 2 ml was drawn into a syringe previously used to add magnesium sulfate 50% (Elkins-Sinn) 1.5 ml to a parenteral nutrition solution. Hydrocortisone sodium succinate (Upjohn) contains phosphate buffers, and it was postulated that insoluble magnesium phosphate was formed. This finding indicates that magnesium sulfate and hydrocortisone sodium succinate should not be admixed as the concentrated solutions but rather should be added separately to large volume parenteral solutions with thorough mixing after each addition (302).

MANNITOL
AHFS 36:40 and 40:28

American Pharmaceutical Partners
Baxter

Osmitrol

Products— Mannitol is available from several manufacturers in concentrations ranging from 5 to 25% (4; 29):

Concentration	Osmolarity	Available Sizes
5%	275 mOsm/L	1000 ml
10%	550 mOsm/L	500 and 1000 ml
15%	825 mOsm/L	500 ml
20%	1100 mOsm/L	250 and 500 ml
25%	1375 mOsm/L	50 ml

pH— From 4.5 to 7 (4).

Administration— Mannitol is administered by intravenous infusion. An administration set with a filter should be used for infusion solutions containing mannitol 20% or more. The dosage, concentration, and administration rate are dependent on the patient's condition and response (4).

Stability— Mannitol solutions should be stored at room temperature and protected from freezing (4). The solutions are chemically stable. Mannitol 25% (Invenex) was chemically and physically stable after five autoclavings at 250 °F for 15 minutes. In addition, no extracts or visible particles from the rubber closures were found (83).

Crystallization— In concentrations of 15% or greater, mannitol may crystallize when exposed to low temperatures (4; 593). Do not use a mannitol solution containing crystals. If such crystallization occurs, the recommended procedure for resolubilization is to heat the mannitol in hot water at 60 to 80 °C with vigorous shaking periodically. The solution should cool to body temperature before use (1-9/98; 4).

The use of a microwave oven to resolubilize crystallized mannitol in glass ampuls has been suggested. Exposure to microwave radiation followed by shaking satisfactorily resolubilized the crystals in a shorter total time than the water bath and autoclave methods and resulted in no chemical decomposition (694).

Unfortunately, the use of microwave radiation to solubilize mannitol crystals is a highly risky undertaking. Explosions of mannitol ampuls during microwave exposure have been reported (695; 697). Such explosions could injure someone as well as ruin the microwave oven. The explosion results from pressure building during the heating of the solution that occurs from the microwave exposure (696; 697).

One inventive pharmacist redissolved mannitol crystals using a coffeemaker (1114).

As an alternative to resolubilizing techniques, the use of warming chambers to maintain the solutions in a crystal-free condition has been recommended (698–700). Various chambers have been described including a wooden cabinet (698), a metal kettle (699), and even a bun warmer (700). Storage temperatures of 35 and 50 °C have been utilized (698; 699).

A related but differing effect is seen when supersaturated solutions of mannitol are placed in PVC bags. Within a few minutes, a heavy white flocculent precipitate forms. The needle-like crystals in mannitol solutions result from slow undisturbed growth. The white flocculent mannitol precipitate results from contact with the PVC surfaces, which act as nuclei for rapid rate crystallization of small crystals. Attempts to resolubilize the white flocculent precipitate with the aid of heat are not fruitful because crystallization may recur in a short time (432).

Compatibility Information

Additive Compatibility

			Mannitol				
Drug	Mfr	Conc	Mfr	Conc	Remarks	Ref	C/I
Amikacin sulfate	BR	250 mg and 5 g		20%	Physically compatible and chemically stable for 24 hr at 25 °C	292	C
Bretylium tosylate	ACC	10 g	MG	20%	Physically compatible and chemically stable for 48 hr at room temperature. Mannitol crystallized when stored in refrigerator	541	C
Cefamandole nafate	LI	20 g	TR	15%	9% cefamandole decomposition in 72 hr at 25 °C and 2% in 7 days at 5 °C	376	C
		2 g		10 and 20%	Physically compatible and chemically stable for 24 hr at 25 °C	596	C
	LI	20 g	TR	15%	Physically compatible with 9% cefamandole loss in 72 hr at 25 °C and 5% loss in 10 days at 5 °C	788	C
Cefoxitin sodium	MSD	1, 2, 10, 20 g		10%	4 to 5% cefoxitin decomposition in 24 hr and 10 to 11% in 48 hr at 25 °C. 2 to 5% cefoxitin decomposition in 7 days at 5 °C	308	C
Cimetidine HCl	SKF	1.2 and 5 g	TR	10%	Physically compatible and chemically stable for 1 week at room temperature	549	C
Cisplatin	BR	50 and 200 mg		18.75 g	In D5½S.[a] Compatible for 48 hr at 25 °C and 96 hr at 4 °C followed by 48 hr at 25 °C	1088	C
Dopamine HCl	AS	800 mg		20%	5% dopamine decomposition in 48 hr at 25 °C	79	C
Etoposide with cisplatin and potassium chloride	BR BR LY	400 mg 200 mg 20 mEq	LY	1.875%	In NS.[b] Physically compatible and etoposide and cisplatin chemically stable for 8 hr at 22 °C. Precipitate forms within 24 hr	1329	I
Etoposide with cisplatin and potassium chloride	BR BR LY	400 mg 200 mg 20 mEq	LY	1.875%	In D5½S.[b] Physically compatible and etoposide and cisplatin chemically stable for 8 hr at 22 °C. Precipitate forms within 48 hr	1329	C

Additive Compatibility (Cont.)

		Mannitol					
Drug	*Mfr*	*Conc*	*Mfr*	*Conc*	*Remarks*	*Ref*	*C/I*
Fosphenytoin sodium	PD	2, 8, 20 mgPE/ml[g]	BA[a]	20%	Visually compatible with little or no loss of fosphenytoin by HPLC in 7 days at 25 °C under fluorescent light	2083	**C**
Furosemide	AB	200, 400, 800 mg	BA[a]	20%	Visually compatible for 72 hr at 22 °C	1803	**C**
Gentamicin sulfate		120 mg		20%	Physically compatible and gentamicin stable by microbiological assay for 24 hr at 25 °C	897	**C**
Imipenem–cilastatin	MSD	2.5 g	AB[c]	2.5%	9% imipenem loss in 9 hr at 25 °C. 7% imipenem loss in 48 hr and 11% in 72 hr at 4 °C	1141	**I**[d]
	MSD	5 g	AB[c]	2.5%	6% imipenem loss in 3 hr and 12% in 6 hr at 25 °C. 7% imipenem loss in 24 hr and 10% in 48 hr at 4 °C	1141	**I**[d]
	MSD	2.5 g	AB[c]	5%	6% imipenem loss in 3 hr and 10% in 6 hr at 25 °C. 9% imipenem loss in 48 hr and 13% in 72 hr at 4 °C	1141	**I**[d]
	MSD	5 g	AB[c]	5%	7% imipenem loss in 3 hr and 12% in 6 hr at 25 °C. 12% imipenem loss in 48 hr at 4 °C	1141	**I**[d]
	MSD	2.5 g	AB[c]	10%	6% imipenem loss in 3 hr and 10% in 6 hr at 25 °C. 7% imipenem loss in 24 hr and 12% in 48 hr at 4 °C	1141	**I**[d]
	MSD	5 g	AB[c]	10%	12% imipenem loss in 3 hr at 25 °C. 13% imipenem loss in 48 hr at 4 °C	1141	**I**[d]
Meropenem	ZEN	1 g	BA[a]	2.5%	7 to 8% meropenem loss by HPLC in 8 hr at 24 °C and in 24 hr at 4 °C	2089	**I**[d]
	ZEN	20 g	BA[a]	2.5%	7 to 9% meropenem loss by HPLC in 4 hr at 24 °C and 6% loss in 20 hr at 4 °C	2089	**I**[d]
	ZEN	1 g	BA[a]	10%	10 to 11% meropenem loss by HPLC in 4 hr at 24 °C and in 20 hr at 4 °C	2089	**I**[d]
	ZEN	20 g	BA[a]	10%	10% meropenem loss by HPLC in 3 hr at 24 °C and in 20 hr at 4 °C	2089	**I**[d]
Metoclopramide HCl	RB	40 and 100 mg	AB	20%	Physically compatible for 48 hr at room temperature	924	**C**
	RB	40 and 100 mg	AB	20%	Physically compatible for 48 hr at 25 °C	1167	**C**
	RB	640 mg and 1.6 g	AB	20%	Physically compatible for 48 hr at 25 °C	1167	**C**
Netilmicin sulfate	SC	3 g	TR	10 and 20%	Physically compatible and chemically stable for 7 days at 4 and 25 °C	558	**C**
Nizatidine	LI	0.75, 1.5, 3 g	MG	20%[c]	Visually compatible and nizatidine potency by HPLC retained for 7 days at 4 and 25 °C	1533	**C**
Ofloxacin	ORT	0.4 and 4 g	BA[a]	20%	Physically compatible with little or no ofloxacin loss by HPLC in 3 days at 24 °C	1636	**C**
	ORT	0.4 and 4 g	BA[a]	20%	White mannitol crystals form upon refrigeration at 5 °C and freezing at −20 °C but disappear with warming	1636	**C**

Additive Compatibility (Cont.)

Mannitol

Drug	Mfr	Conc	Mfr	Conc	Remarks	Ref	C/I
Ondansetron HCl	GL	16 mg	BP[a]	10%	Physically compatible and chemically stable for 7 days at room temperature exposed to light and at 4 °C	1366	C
Sodium bicarbonate	AB	44.6 mEq[e]	AMR	25 g[e]	Visually compatible for 24 hr at 24 °C	1853; 1973	C
Tobramycin sulfate	LI	200 mg and 1 g		20%	Physically compatible and chemically stable for 48 hr at 25 °C	147	C
Verapamil HCl	KN	80 mg[f]	IX	25 g[f]	Physically compatible for 24 hr	764	C

[a]*Tested in PVC containers.*
[b]*Tested in both PVC and glass containers.*
[c]*Tested in glass containers.*
[d]*Incompatible by conventional standards but may be used in shorter periods of time.*
[e]*Tested in dextrose 5% in Ringer's injection, lactated, dextrose 5% in sodium chloride 0.225%, dextrose 5% in sodium chloride 0.45%, dextrose 5% in sodium chloride 0.9%, dextrose 10% in water, sodium chloride 0.45%, and sodium chloride 0.9% in polyolefin containers.*
[f]*Tested in both dextrose 5% in water and sodium chloride 0.9%.*
[g]*Concentration expressed in milligrams of phenytoin sodium equivalents (PE) per milliliter.*

Y-Site Injection Compatibility (1:1 Mixture)

Mannitol

Drug	Mfr	Conc	Mfr	Conc	Remarks	Ref	C/I
Allopurinol sodium	BW	3 mg/ml[b]	BA	15%	Physically compatible with no change in measured turbidity or increase in particle content in 4 hr at 22 °C	1686	C
Amifostine	USB	10 mg/ml[a]	BA	15%	Physically compatible with no change in measured turbidity or increase in particle content in 4 hr at 23 °C	1845	C
Amphotericin B cholesteryl sulfate complex	SEQ	0.83 mg/ml[a]	BA	15%	Physically compatible with little or no change in measured turbidity or increase in particle content in 4 hr at 23 °C under fluorescent light	2117	C
Aztreonam	SQ	40 mg/ml[a]	BA	15%	Physically compatible with no subvisual haze or particle formation in 4 hr at 23 °C	1758	C
Cefepime HCl	BR	20 mg/ml[a]	BA	15%	Slight haze with particles forms immediately	1689	I
Cisatracurium besylate	GW	0.1, 2, 5 mg/ml[a]	BA	15%	Physically compatible with no change in measured turbidity or increase in particle content in 4 hr at 23 °C	2074	C
Cladribine	ORT	0.015[b] and 0.5[c] mg/ml	BA	15%	Physically compatible with no change in measured turbidity or increase in particle content in 4 hr at 23 °C	1969	C
Docetaxel	RPR	0.9 mg/ml[a]	BA	15%	Physically compatible with no change in measured turbidity or increase in particle content in 4 hr at 23 °C	2224	C
Doxorubicin HCl liposome injection	SEQ	0.4 mg/ml[a]	BA	15%	Partial loss of measured natural turbidity	2087	I
Etoposide phosphate	BR	5 mg/ml[a]	BA	15%	Physically compatible with no change in measured turbidity or increase in particle content in 4 hr at 23 °C	2218	C

Y-Site Injection Compatibility (1:1 Mixture) (Cont.)

Mannitol

Drug	Mfr	Conc	Mfr	Conc	Remarks	Ref	C/I
Filgrastim	AMG	30 μg/ml[a]	BA	15%	Filaments form immediately	1687	**I**
Fludarabine phosphate	BX	1 mg/ml[a]	BA	15%	Physically compatible for 4 hr at room temperature under fluorescent light	1439	**C**
Fluorouracil	SO	1 and 2 mg/ml[d]		20%	Physically compatible both visually and microscopically and fluorouracil chemically stable by HPLC for 24 hr. Mannitol not tested	1526	**C**
Gemcitabine HCl	LI	10 mg/ml[b]	BA	15%	Physically compatible with no change in measured turbidity or increase in particle content in 4 hr at 23 °C	2226	**C**
Idarubicin HCl	AD	1 mg/ml[b]	AB	12.5 mg/ml[b]	Visually compatible for 24 hr at 25 °C	1525	**C**
Melphalan HCl	BW	0.1 mg/ml[b]	BA	15%	Physically compatible with no change in measured turbidity or increase in particle content in 3 hr at 22 °C	1557	**C**
Ondansetron HCl	GL	1 mg/ml[b]	BA	15%	Physically compatible for 4 hr at 22 °C	1365	**C**
Paclitaxel	NCI	1.2 mg/ml[a]	BA	15%	Physically compatible with no change in measured turbidity in 4 hr at 22 °C	1556	**C**
Piperacillin sodium–tazobactam sodium	LE	40 + 5 mg/ml[a]	BA	15%	Physically compatible with no change in measured turbidity or increase in particle content in 4 hr at 22 °C	1688	**C**
Propofol	ZEN	10 mg/ml	BA	15%	Physically compatible for 1 hr at 23 °C with no increase in particle content	2066	**C**
Remifentanil HCl	GW	0.025 and 0.25 mg/ml[b]	BA	15%	Physically compatible with no change in measured turbidity or increase in particle content in 4 hr at 23 °C	2075	**C**
Sargramostim	IMM	10 μg/ml[b]	BA	15%	Physically compatible for 4 hr at 22 °C	1436	**C**
Teniposide	BR	0.1 mg/ml[a]	BA	15%	Physically compatible with no subvisual haze or particle formation in 4 hr at 23 °C	1725	**C**
Thiotepa	IMM[e]	1 mg/ml[b]	BA	15%	Physically compatible with no change in measured turbidity or increase in particle content in 4 hr at 23 °C	1861	**C**
TNA #218 to #226[f]			BA	15%	Visually compatible with no precipitate or emulsion damage apparent in 4 hr at 23 °C	2215	**C**
TPN #212 to #215[f]			BA	15%	Physically compatible with no change in measured turbidity or increase in particle content in 4 hr at 23 °C	2109	**C**
Vinorelbine tartrate	BW	1 mg/ml[b]	BA	15%	Physically compatible with no change in measured turbidity or increase in particle content in 4 hr at 22 °C	1558	**C**

[a]Tested in dextrose 5% in water.
[b]Tested in sodium chloride 0.9%.
[c]Tested in bacteriostatic sodium chloride 0.9% preserved with benzyl alcohol 0.9%.
[d]Tested in dextrose 5% in sodium chloride 0.45%, dextrose 5% in water, and sodium chloride 0.9%.
[e]Lyophilized formulation tested.
[f]Refer to Appendix I for the composition of parenteral nutrition solutions. TNA indicates a 3-in-1 admixture, and TPN indicates a 2-in-1 admixture.

Additional Compatibility Information

Miscellaneous— The addition of potassium chloride or sodium chloride to mannitol 20 or 25% solutions may cause precipitation of the mannitol (4; 38). Also, the addition of cephapirin sodium (Bristol) 2 or 30 g/L to mannitol 20% results in a haze after eight hours at 25 °C (111).

Mannitol should not be mixed with blood (4).

It has been stated that mannitol is incompatible in strongly acidic and alkaline solutions (18).

When mannitol 25 g was added to amphotericin B in dextrose 5% in water, serum amphotericin B levels were satisfactory during therapy (84).

Although short-term combinations of cisplatin and mannitol are feasible and convenient and they reduce renal toxicity of the cisplatin, advanced premixing of the two agents should be avoided because of complex formation (524).

MECHLORETHAMINE HCL (MUSTINE HCL) AHFS 10:00

Mustargen   **Merck**

Products— Mechlorethamine HCl (Merck) is available in vials containing 10 mg of drug and sodium chloride qs 100 mg. While taking appropriate protective measures, including wearing protective gloves, reconstitute the vial with 10 ml of water for injection or sodium chloride 0.9%. With the needle in the rubber stopper, shake the vial several times to dissolve the drug. The resultant solution contains mechlorethamine HCl 1 mg/ml (2).

pH— The reconstituted solution has a pH of 3 to 5 (2; 4).

Osmolality— Mechlorethamine HCl 1 mg/ml in sterile water for injection has an osmolality of 300 mOsm/kg (1689).

Administration— Mechlorethamine HCl is administered intravenously or into body cavities (2; 4). The drug is extremely irritating to tissues and should not be given intramuscularly or subcutaneously (4). For intravenous use, the drug may be injected over a few minutes directly into the vein or into the tubing of a running infusion solution (2; 4). The drug is a powerful vesicant, and extravasation should be avoided (2; 4; 377). For intracavitary administration, the drug may be diluted up to 100 ml with sodium chloride 0.9% (2; 4).

Stability— In dry form, the drug is a light yellow-brown and is stable at temperatures up to 40 °C (4). Solutions of mechlorethamine HCl decompose on standing and should be prepared immediately before use. Mechlorethamine HCl is even less stable in neutral or alkaline solutions than in the acidic reconstituted solution. Do not use if the solution is discolored or if water droplets form within the vial before reconstitution. Discard unused portions after neutralization (2; 4). (See Other Information section.)

Using HPLC, Kirk determined the stability of mechlorethamine HCl (Boots) 1 mg/ml when reconstituted with water for injection or sodium chloride 0.9% in vials and plastic syringes. About an 8 to 10% loss occurred in samples over six hours at 22 °C; losses of 4 to 6% occurred in six hours in samples stored at 4 °C (1279).

Freezing Solutions— Using HPLC, Kirk also determined the stability of mechlorethamine HCl (Boots) 1 mg/ml in water for injection and sodium chloride 0.9% frozen at −20 °C. In water for injection, about a 7% loss occurred after 12 weeks; about a 15% loss occurred in eight weeks with sodium chloride 0.9% as the diluent. At a concentration of 10 mg/500 ml in sodium chloride 0.9% in PVC bags, about a 10% loss occurred in eight weeks frozen at −20 °C (1279).

Sorption— Mechlorethamine HCl apparently does not undergo sorption to PVC infusion containers. During stability studies, mechlorethamine HCl losses were similar for both PVC and glass containers (1279).

Compatibility Information

Solution Compatibility

Mechlorethamine HCl

Solution	Mfr	Mfr	Conc/L	Remarks	Ref	C/I
Dextrose 5% in water	a	BT	20 mg	10% loss in about 5 hr at 22 °C. 4% loss in 6 hr at 4 °C	1279	I
Sodium chloride 0.9%	a	BT	20 mg	10% loss in about 3 hr at 22 °C. 10% loss in 4 hr at 4 °C	1279	I

*a*Tested in PVC containers.

Additive Compatibility

Mechlorethamine HCl

Drug	Mfr	Conc/L	Mfr	Conc/L	Test Soln	Remarks	Ref	C/I
Methohexital sodium	BP	2 g	BP	40 mg	D5W, NS	Haze develops within 3 hr	26	I

Y-Site Injection Compatibility (1:1 Mixture)

Mechlorethamine HCl

Drug	Mfr	Conc	Mfr	Conc	Remarks	Ref	C/I
Allopurinol sodium	BW	3 mg/ml[a]	MSD	1 mg/ml	Haze and small particles form immediately and become numerous large particles in 4 hr	1686	I
Amifostine	USB	10 mg/ml[b]	MSD	1 mg/ml	Physically compatible with no change in measured turbidity or increase in particle content in 4 hr at 23 °C	1845	C
Aztreonam	SQ	40 mg/ml[b]	MSD	1 mg/ml	Physically compatible with no subvisual haze or particle formation in 4 hr at 23 °C	1758	C
Cefepime HCl	BR	20 mg/ml[b]	MSD	1 mg/ml[b]	Slight haze with particles forms immediately	1689	I
Filgrastim	AMG	30 μg/ml[b]	MSD	1 mg/ml[b]	Physically compatible with no change in measured turbidity or increase in particle content in 4 hr at 22 °C	1687	C
Fludarabine phosphate	BX	1 mg/ml[b]	MSD	1 mg/ml	Physically compatible for 4 hr at room temperature under fluorescent light	1439	C
Granisetron HCl	SKB	1 mg/ml	MSD	0.5 mg/ml[a]	Physically compatible with little or no loss of either drug by HPLC in 4 hr at 22 °C	1883	C
Melphalan HCl	BW	0.1 mg/ml[a]	MSD	1 mg/ml	Physically compatible with no change in measured turbidity or increase in particle content in 3 hr at 22 °C	1557	C
Ondansetron HCl	GL	1 mg/ml[a]	MSD	1 mg/ml	Physically compatible for 4 hr at 22 °C	1365	C
Sargramostim	IMM	10 μg/ml[a]	MSD	1 mg/ml	Physically compatible for 4 hr at 22 °C	1436	C
Teniposide	BR	0.1 mg/ml[b]	MSD	1 mg/ml	Physically compatible with no subvisual haze or particle formation in 4 hr at 23 °C	1725	C
Vinorelbine tartrate	BW	1 mg/ml[a]	MSD	1 mg/ml	Physically compatible with no change in measured turbidity or increase in particle content in 4 hr at 22 °C	1558	C

[a]Tested in sodium chloride 0.9%.
[b]Tested in dextrose 5% in water.

Additional Compatibility Information

Solutions— Because of the rapid decomposition of mechlorethamine HCl in solution, administration in intravenous infusion solutions is not recommended (4). One report indicated a 7% loss of mechlorethamine in one hour at room temperature when diluted to 0.1 mg/ml in sodium chloride 0.9% (923). Injecting the drug into the tubing of a running intravenous infusion rather than adding it to the entire volume of the solution minimizes the extent of chemical decomposition (2).

For intracavitary administration, up to 100 ml of sodium chloride 0.9% has been used for dilution of mechlorethamine (2; 4).

Aluminum— Ogawa et al. reported that immersion of a needle with an aluminum component in mechlorethamine (MSD) 1 mg/ml resulted in no visually apparent reaction after seven days at 24 °C (988).

Other Information

Neutralization— Spillage of the drug on gloves, etc., can be neutralized by soaking in an aqueous solution containing equal amounts of sodium thiosulfate 5% and sodium bicarbonate 5% for 45 minutes. Unused injection solution also may be neutralized by mixing with an equal volume of the sodium thiosulfate–sodium bicarbonate solution for 45 minutes (2; 1200).

MELPHALAN HCL
AHFS 10:00

Alkeran   **Glaxo Wellcome**

Products— Melphalan HCl (Glaxo Wellcome) is available as a lyophilized powder in vials containing 50 mg with povidone 20 mg. It is packaged with a vial of special diluent containing sodium citrate 0.2 g, propylene glycol 6 ml, ethanol (96%) 0.52 ml, and sterile water for injection qs to 10 ml. While taking appropriate protective measures, including wearing protective gloves, reconstitute with 10 ml of special diluent and shake vigorously to yield a 5-mg/ml melphalan concentration (2).

pH— The reconstituted solution has a pH of about 7 (4).

Administration— Melphalan is administered intravenously. Immediately after reconstitution, the drug should be diluted in sodium chloride 0.9% to a concentration not greater than 0.45 mg/ml. It should be infused over 15 to 20 minutes (2; 4). Melphalan has also been administered intra-arterially and intraperitoneally (4).

Stability— Intact vials should be stored at controlled room temperature and protected from light. The reconstituted solution is stable for no more than 90 minutes at room temperature (4). Refrigeration of the reconstituted solution results in precipitation (2; 4).

Because of rapid decomposition, the manufacturer recommends that drug administration be completed within 60 minutes of initial reconstitution. Degradation products are detected within 30 minutes (2); a 10% loss of initial potency occurs within approximately three hours at 30 °C (234). After dilution in sodium chloride 0.9%, nearly 1% of melphalan HCl is hydrolyzed every 10 minutes (2).

Melphalan HCl, reconstituted according to the manufacturer's instructions, was cultured with human lymphoblasts to determine whether its cytotoxic activity was retained. The solution retained cytotoxicity for 24 hours at 4 °C and room temperature (1575).

Melphalan is stated to be compatible with various medical plastic items, including containers, administration sets, and syringes (1396).

pH Effects— Melphalan is most stable over a pH range of 3 to 7; decomposition increases at pH 9 (971).

Filtration— Melphalan HCl 20 µg/ml in 1 ml of sodium chloride 0.9% was filtered through the following filters; minimal adsorption occurred in all cases (970):

Filter	Delivered Concentration (% of initial)
Cellulose acetate 0.2 µm (Minisart-N, Sartorius)	99
Polysulfone 0.45 µm (Acrodisc, Gelman)	98
Polytetrafluoroethylene 0.45 µm (Acrodisc-CR, Gelman)	96

Freezing Solutions— Melphalan HCl 20 µg/ml in sodium chloride 0.9% did not undergo significant decomposition after storage at −20 °C for six or seven months. Test samples exhibited about a 2 to 4% loss over this period. Repeated freeze–thaw cycles also had little effect on melphalan concentration. After four such cycles, the loss was less than 2% (970).

Melphalan HCl (Wellcome) 0.2 mg/ml in sodium chloride 0.9% in PVC containers was frozen at −20 °C for 72 hours. The thawed solutions were visually clear, and no loss was found by HPLC analysis (1841).

Compatibility Information

Solution Compatibility

Melphalan HCl

Solution	Mfr	Mfr	Conc/L	Remarks	Ref	C/I
Dextrose 5% in water		BW	40 and 400 mg	10% loss in 90 min at 20 °C and 36 min at 25 °C	971	I
Ringer's injection, lactated		BW	40 and 400 mg	10% loss in 2.9 hr at 20 °C and 90 min at 25 °C	971	I
Sodium chloride 0.9%		BW	40 and 400 mg	10% loss in 4.5 hr at 20 °C and 2.4 hr at 25 °C	971	I[a]
		BW	100 and 450 mg	10% loss in 45 min at 30 °C	234	I
		BW	100 mg	10% loss in 3 hr at 20 °C	234	I[a]

Solution Compatibility (Cont.)

Melphalan HCl

Solution	Mfr	Mfr	Conc/L	Remarks	Ref	C/I
[b]		WEL	200 mg	Visually compatible with losses by HPLC of 6% in 3 hr and 17% in 6 hr at room temperature and 6% in 6 hr and 13% in 24 hr at 4 °C	1841	I[a]

[a]Incompatible by conventional standards. May be used in shorter time periods.
[b]Tested in PVC containers.

Y-Site Injection Compatibility (1:1 Mixture)

Melphalan HCl

Drug	Mfr	Conc	Mfr	Conc	Remarks	Ref	C/I
Acyclovir sodium	BW	7 mg/ml[b]	BW	0.1 mg/ml[b]	Physically compatible with no change in measured turbidity or increase in particle content in 3 hr at 22 °C	1557	C
Amikacin sulfate	BR	5 mg/ml[b]	BW	0.1 mg/ml[b]	Physically compatible with no change in measured turbidity or increase in particle content in 3 hr at 22 °C	1557	C
Aminophylline	AB	2.5 mg/ml[b]	BW	0.1 mg/ml[b]	Physically compatible with no change in measured turbidity or increase in particle content in 3 hr at 22 °C	1557	C
Amphotericin B	SQ	0.6 mg/ml[a]	BW	0.1 mg/ml[b]	Immediate two- to fourfold increase in measured turbidity due to sodium chloride	1557	I
	SQ	0.6 mg/ml[a]	BW	0.1 mg/ml[a]	Physically compatible but rapid melphalan loss in D5W precludes use	1557	I
Ampicillin sodium	WY	20 mg/ml[b]	BW	0.1 mg/ml[b]	Physically compatible with no change in measured turbidity or increase in particle content in 3 hr at 22 °C	1557	C
Aztreonam	SQ	40 mg/ml[b]	BW	0.1 mg/ml[b]	Physically compatible with no change in measured turbidity or increase in particle content in 3 hr at 22 °C	1557	C
Bleomycin sulfate	BR	1 unit/ml[b]	BW	0.1 mg/ml[b]	Physically compatible with no change in measured turbidity or increase in particle content in 3 hr at 22 °C	1557	C
Bumetanide	RC	0.04 mg/ml[b]	BW	0.1 mg/ml[b]	Physically compatible with no change in measured turbidity or increase in particle content in 3 hr at 22 °C	1557	C
Buprenorphine HCl	RKC	0.04 mg/ml[b]	BW	0.1 mg/ml[b]	Physically compatible with no change in measured turbidity or increase in particle content in 3 hr at 22 °C	1557	C
Butorphanol tartrate	BR	0.04 mg/ml[b]	BW	0.1 mg/ml[b]	Physically compatible with no change in measured turbidity or increase in particle content in 3 hr at 22 °C	1557	C
Calcium gluconate	AST	40 mg/ml[b]	BW	0.1 mg/ml[b]	Physically compatible with no change in measured turbidity or increase in particle content in 3 hr at 22 °C	1557	C
Carboplatin	BR	5 mg/ml[b]	BW	0.1 mg/ml[b]	Physically compatible with no change in measured turbidity or increase in particle content in 3 hr at 22 °C	1557	C

Y-Site Injection Compatibility (1:1 Mixture) (Cont.)

Melphalan HCl

Drug	Mfr	Conc	Mfr	Conc	Remarks	Ref	C/I
Carmustine	BR	1.5 mg/ml[b]	BW	0.1 mg/ml[b]	Physically compatible with no change in measured turbidity or increase in particle content in 3 hr at 22 °C	1557	C
Cefazolin sodium	GEM	20 mg/ml[b]	BW	0.1 mg/ml[b]	Physically compatible with no change in measured turbidity or increase in particle content in 3 hr at 22 °C	1557	C
Cefepime HCl	BR	20 mg/ml[a]	BW	0.1 mg/ml[a]	Physically compatible with no change in measured turbidity or increase in particle content in 4 hr at 22 °C	1689	C
Cefoperazone sodium	RR	40 mg/ml[b]	BW	0.1 mg/ml[b]	Physically compatible with no change in measured turbidity or increase in particle content in 3 hr at 22 °C	1557	C
Cefotaxime sodium	HO	20 mg/ml[b]	BW	0.1 mg/ml[b]	Physically compatible with no change in measured turbidity or increase in particle content in 3 hr at 22 °C	1557	C
Cefotetan disodium	STU	20 mg/ml[b]	BW	0.1 mg/ml[b]	Physically compatible with no change in measured turbidity or increase in particle content in 3 hr at 22 °C	1557	C
Ceftazidime	LI[c]	40 mg/ml[b]	BW	0.1 mg/ml[b]	Physically compatible with no change in measured turbidity or increase in particle content in 3 hr at 22 °C	1557	C
Ceftizoxime sodium	FUJ	20 mg/ml[b]	BW	0.1 mg/ml[b]	Physically compatible with no change in measured turbidity or increase in particle content in 3 hr at 22 °C	1557	C
Ceftriaxone sodium	RC	20 mg/ml[b]	BW	0.1 mg/ml[b]	Physically compatible with no change in measured turbidity or increase in particle content in 3 hr at 22 °C	1557	C
Cefuroxime sodium	GL	20 mg/ml[b]	BW	0.1 mg/ml[b]	Physically compatible with no change in measured turbidity or increase in particle content in 3 hr at 22 °C	1557	C
Chlorpromazine HCl	ES	2 mg/ml[b]	BW	0.1 mg/ml[b]	Large increase in measured turbidity occurs within 1 hr and grows over 4 hr	1557	I
Cimetidine HCl	SKB	12 mg/ml[b]	BW	0.1 mg/ml[b]	Physically compatible with no change in measured turbidity or increase in particle content in 3 hr at 22 °C	1557	C
Cisplatin	BR	1 mg/ml	BW	0.1 mg/ml[b]	Physically compatible with no change in measured turbidity or increase in particle content in 3 hr at 22 °C	1557	C
Clindamycin phosphate	AB	10 mg/ml[b]	BW	0.1 mg/ml[b]	Physically compatible with no change in measured turbidity or increase in particle content in 3 hr at 22 °C	1557	C
Cyclophosphamide	BR	10 mg/ml[b]	BW	0.1 mg/ml[b]	Physically compatible with no change in measured turbidity or increase in particle content in 3 hr at 22 °C	1557	C
Cytarabine	UP	50 mg/ml	BW	0.1 mg/ml[b]	Physically compatible with no change in measured turbidity or increase in particle content in 3 hr at 22 °C	1557	C

Y-Site Injection Compatibility (1:1 Mixture) (Cont.)

Melphalan HCl

Drug	Mfr	Conc	Mfr	Conc	Remarks	Ref	C/I
Dacarbazine	MI	4 mg/ml[b]	BW	0.1 mg/ml[b]	Physically compatible with no change in measured turbidity or increase in particle content in 3 hr at 22 °C	1557	**C**
Dactinomycin	MSD	0.01 mg/ml[b]	BW	0.1 mg/ml[b]	Physically compatible with no change in measured turbidity or increase in particle content in 3 hr at 22 °C	1557	**C**
Daunorubicin HCl	WY	1 mg/ml[b]	BW	0.1 mg/ml[b]	Physically compatible with little change in measured turbidity or increase in particle content in 3 hr at 22 °C	1557	**C**
Dexamethasone sodium phosphate	LY	1 mg/ml[b]	BW	0.1 mg/ml[b]	Physically compatible with no change in measured turbidity or increase in particle content in 3 hr at 22 °C	1557	**C**
Diphenhydramine HCl	WY	2 mg/ml[b]	BW	0.1 mg/ml[b]	Physically compatible with no change in measured turbidity or increase in particle content in 3 hr at 22 °C	1557	**C**
Doxorubicin HCl	AD	2 mg/ml	BW	0.1 mg/ml[b]	Physically compatible with no change in measured turbidity or increase in particle content in 3 hr at 22 °C	1557	**C**
Doxycycline hyclate	LY	1 mg/ml[b]	BW	0.1 mg/ml[b]	Physically compatible with no change in measured turbidity or increase in particle content in 3 hr at 22 °C	1557	**C**
Droperidol	JN	0.4 mg/ml[b]	BW	0.1 mg/ml[b]	Physically compatible with no change in measured turbidity or increase in particle content in 3 hr at 22 °C	1557	**C**
Enalaprilat	MSD	0.1 mg/ml[b]	BW	0.1 mg/ml[b]	Physically compatible with no change in measured turbidity or increase in particle content in 3 hr at 22 °C	1557	**C**
Etoposide	BR	0.4 mg/ml[b]	BW	0.1 mg/ml[b]	Physically compatible with no change in measured turbidity or increase in particle content in 3 hr at 22 °C	1557	**C**
Famotidine	MSD	2 mg/ml[b]	BW	0.1 mg/ml[b]	Physically compatible with no change in measured turbidity or increase in particle content in 3 hr at 22 °C	1557	**C**
Floxuridine	RC	3 mg/ml[b]	BW	0.1 mg/ml[b]	Physically compatible with no change in measured turbidity or increase in particle content in 3 hr at 22 °C	1557	**C**
Fluconazole	RR	2 mg/ml	BW	0.1 mg/ml[b]	Physically compatible with no change in measured turbidity or increase in particle content in 3 hr at 22 °C	1557	**C**
Fludarabine phosphate	BX	1 mg/ml[b]	BW	0.1 mg/ml[b]	Physically compatible with no change in measured turbidity or increase in particle content in 3 hr at 22 °C	1557	**C**
Fluorouracil	LY	16 mg/ml[b]	BW	0.1 mg/ml[b]	Physically compatible with no change in measured turbidity or increase in particle content in 3 hr at 22 °C	1557	**C**
Furosemide	AB	3 mg/ml[b]	BW	0.1 mg/ml[b]	Physically compatible with no change in measured turbidity or increase in particle content in 3 hr at 22 °C	1557	**C**

Y-Site Injection Compatibility (1:1 Mixture) (Cont.)

Melphalan HCl

Drug	Mfr	Conc	Mfr	Conc	Remarks	Ref	C/I
Ganciclovir sodium	SY	20 mg/ml[b]	BW	0.1 mg/ml[b]	Physically compatible with no change in measured turbidity or increase in particle content in 3 hr at 22 °C	1557	C
Gentamicin sulfate	LY	5 mg/ml[b]	BW	0.1 mg/ml[b]	Physically compatible with no change in measured turbidity or increase in particle content in 3 hr at 22 °C	1557	C
Granisetron HCl	SKB	0.05 mg/ml[a]	BW	0.1 mg/ml[b]	Physically compatible with no change in measured turbidity or increase in particle content in 4 hr at 23 °C	2000	C
Haloperidol lactate	MN	0.2 mg/ml[b]	BW	0.1 mg/ml[b]	Physically compatible with no change in measured turbidity or increase in particle content in 3 hr at 22 °C	1557	C
Heparin sodium	WY	100 units/ml[b]	BW	0.1 mg/ml[b]	Physically compatible with no change in measured turbidity or increase in particle content in 3 hr at 22 °C	1557	C
Hydrocortisone sodium phosphate	MSD	1 mg/ml[b]	BW	0.1 mg/ml[b]	Physically compatible with no change in measured turbidity or increase in particle content in 3 hr at 22 °C	1557	C
Hydrocortisone sodium succinate	UP	1 mg/ml[b]	BW	0.1 mg/ml[b]	Physically compatible with no change in measured turbidity or increase in particle content in 3 hr at 22 °C	1557	C
Hydromorphone HCl	KN	0.5 mg/ml[b]	BW	0.1 mg/ml[b]	Physically compatible with no change in measured turbidity or increase in particle content in 3 hr at 22 °C	1557	C
Hydroxyzine HCl	WI	4 mg/ml[b]	BW	0.1 mg/ml[b]	Physically compatible with no change in measured turbidity or increase in particle content in 3 hr at 22 °C	1557	C
Idarubicin HCl	AD	0.5 mg/ml[b]	BW	0.1 mg/ml[b]	Increase in measured turbidity no greater than dilution of idarubicin with sodium chloride 0.9%. No increase in particle content in 4 hr at 22 °C	1557; 1675	C
Ifosfamide	BR	25 mg/ml[b]	BW	0.1 mg/ml[b]	Physically compatible with no change in measured turbidity or increase in particle content in 3 hr at 22 °C	1557	C
Imipenem–cilastatin sodium	MSD	10 mg/ml[b]	BW	0.1 mg/ml[b]	Physically compatible with no change in measured turbidity or increase in particle content in 3 hr at 22 °C	1557	C
Lorazepam	WY	0.1 mg/ml[b]	BW	0.1 mg/ml[b]	Physically compatible with no change in measured turbidity or increase in particle content in 3 hr at 22 °C	1557	C
Mannitol	BA	15%	BW	0.1 mg/ml[b]	Physically compatible with no change in measured turbidity or increase in particle content in 3 hr at 22 °C	1557	C
Mechlorethamine HCl	MSD	1 mg/ml	BW	0.1 mg/ml[b]	Physically compatible with no change in measured turbidity or increase in particle content in 3 hr at 22 °C	1557	C
Meperidine HCl	WY	4 mg/ml[b]	BW	0.1 mg/ml[b]	Physically compatible with no change in measured turbidity or increase in particle content in 3 hr at 22 °C	1557	C

Y-Site Injection Compatibility (1:1 Mixture) (Cont.)

Melphalan HCl

Drug	Mfr	Conc	Mfr	Conc	Remarks	Ref	C/I
Mesna	BR	10 mg/ml[b]	BW	0.1 mg/ml[b]	Physically compatible with no change in measured turbidity or increase in particle content in 3 hr at 22 °C	1557	**C**
Methotrexate sodium	LE	15 mg/ml[b]	BW	0.1 mg/ml[b]	Physically compatible with no change in measured turbidity or increase in particle content in 3 hr at 22 °C	1557	**C**
Methylprednisolone sodium succinate	AB	5 mg/ml[b]	BW	0.1 mg/ml[b]	Physically compatible with no change in measured turbidity or increase in particle content in 3 hr at 22 °C	1557	**C**
Metoclopramide HCl	RB	5 mg/ml	BW	0.1 mg/ml[b]	Physically compatible with no change in measured turbidity or increase in particle content in 3 hr at 22 °C	1557	**C**
Metronidazole	AB	5 mg/ml	BW	0.1 mg/ml[b]	Physically compatible with no change in measured turbidity or increase in particle content in 3 hr at 22 °C	1557	**C**
Minocycline HCl	LE	0.2 mg/ml[b]	BW	0.1 mg/ml[b]	Physically compatible with no change in measured turbidity or increase in particle content in 3 hr at 22 °C	1557	**C**
Mitomycin	BR	0.5 mg/ml	BW	0.1 mg/ml[b]	Physically compatible with no change in measured turbidity or increase in particle content in 3 hr at 22 °C	1557	**C**
Mitoxantrone HCl	LE	0.5 mg/ml[b]	BW	0.1 mg/ml[b]	Physically compatible with no change in measured turbidity or increase in particle content in 3 hr at 22 °C	1557	**C**
Morphine sulfate	WI	1 mg/ml[b]	BW	0.1 mg/ml[b]	Physically compatible with no change in measured turbidity or increase in particle content in 3 hr at 22 °C	1557	**C**
Nalbuphine HCl	AST	10 mg/ml	BW	0.1 mg/ml[b]	Physically compatible with no change in measured turbidity or increase in particle content in 3 hr at 22 °C	1557	**C**
Netilmicin sulfate	SC	5 mg/ml[b]	BW	0.1 mg/ml[b]	Physically compatible with no change in measured turbidity or increase in particle content in 3 hr at 22 °C	1557	**C**
Ondansetron HCl	GL	1 mg/ml[b]	BW	0.1 mg/ml[b]	Physically compatible with no change in measured turbidity or increase in particle content in 3 hr at 22 °C	1557	**C**
Pentostatin	PD	0.4 mg/ml[b]	BW	0.1 mg/ml[b]	Physically compatible with no change in measured turbidity or increase in particle content in 3 hr at 22 °C	1557	**C**
Piperacillin sodium	LE	40 mg/ml[b]	BW	0.1 mg/ml[b]	Physically compatible with no change in measured turbidity or increase in particle content in 3 hr at 22 °C	1557	**C**
Plicamycin	MI	0.01 mg/ml[b]	BW	0.1 mg/ml[b]	Physically compatible with no change in measured turbidity or increase in particle content in 3 hr at 22 °C	1557	**C**
Potassium chloride	AB	0.1 mEq/ml[b]	BW	0.1 mg/ml[b]	Physically compatible with no change in measured turbidity or increase in particle content in 3 hr at 22 °C	1557	**C**

Y-Site Injection Compatibility (1:1 Mixture) (Cont.)

Melphalan HCl

Drug	Mfr	Conc	Mfr	Conc	Remarks	Ref	C/I
Prochlorperazine edisylate	SKB	0.5 mg/ml[b]	BW	0.1 mg/ml[b]	Physically compatible with no change in measured turbidity or increase in particle content in 3 hr at 22 °C	1557	**C**
Promethazine HCl	WY	2 mg/ml[b]	BW	0.1 mg/ml[b]	Physically compatible with no change in measured turbidity or increase in particle content in 3 hr at 22 °C	1557	**C**
Ranitidine HCl	GL	2 mg/ml[b]	BW	0.1 mg/ml[b]	Physically compatible with no change in measured turbidity or increase in particle content in 3 hr at 22 °C	1557	**C**
Sodium bicarbonate	AB	1 mEq/ml	BW	0.1 mg/ml[b]	Physically compatible with no change in measured turbidity or increase in particle content in 3 hr at 22 °C	1557	**C**
Streptozocin	UP	40 mg/ml[b]	BW	0.1 mg/ml[b]	Physically compatible with no change in measured turbidity or increase in particle content in 3 hr at 22 °C	1557	**C**
Teniposide	BR	0.1 mg/ml[a]	BW	0.1 mg/ml[a]	Physically compatible with no subvisual haze or particle formation in 4 hr at 23 °C	1725	**C**
Thiotepa	LE	10 mg/ml[b]	BW	0.1 mg/ml[b]	Physically compatible with no change in measured turbidity or increase in particle content in 3 hr at 22 °C	1557	**C**
Ticarcillin disodium	BE	30 mg/ml[b]	BW	0.1 mg/ml[b]	Physically compatible with no change in measured turbidity or increase in particle content in 3 hr at 22 °C	1557	**C**
Ticarcillin disodium–clavulanate potassium	SKB	31 mg/ml[b]	BW	0.1 mg/ml[b]	Physically compatible with no change in measured turbidity or increase in particle content in 3 hr at 22 °C	1557	**C**
Tobramycin sulfate	LI	5 mg/ml[b]	BW	0.1 mg/ml[b]	Physically compatible with no change in measured turbidity or increase in particle content in 3 hr at 22 °C	1557	**C**
Trimethoprim–sulfamethoxazole	ES	0.8 + 4 mg/ml[b]	BW	0.1 mg/ml[b]	Physically compatible with no change in measured turbidity or increase in particle content in 3 hr at 22 °C	1557	**C**
Vancomycin HCl	LY	10 mg/ml[b]	BW	0.1 mg/ml[b]	Physically compatible with no change in measured turbidity or increase in particle content in 3 hr at 22 °C	1557	**C**
Vinblastine sulfate	LI	0.12 mg/ml[b]	BW	0.1 mg/ml[b]	Physically compatible with no change in measured turbidity or increase in particle content in 3 hr at 22 °C	1557	**C**
Vincristine sulfate	LI	0.05 mg/ml[b]	BW	0.1 mg/ml[b]	Physically compatible with no change in measured turbidity or increase in particle content in 3 hr at 22 °C	1557	**C**
Vinorelbine tartrate	BW	1 mg/ml[b]	BW	0.1 mg/ml[b]	Physically compatible with no change in measured turbidity or increase in particle content in 4 hr at 22 °C	1558	**C**

Y-Site Injection Compatibility (1:1 Mixture) (Cont.)

Melphalan HCl

Drug	Mfr	Conc	Mfr	Conc	Remarks	Ref	C/I
Zidovudine	BW	4 mg/ml[b]	BW	0.1 mg/ml[b]	Physically compatible with no change in measured turbidity or increase in particle content in 3 hr at 22 °C	1557	C

[a]Tested in dextrose 5% in water.
[b]Tested in sodium chloride 0.9%.
[c]Sodium carbonate–containing formulation tested.

MEPERIDINE HCL
(PETHIDINE HCL)
AHFS 28:08.08

Demerol Hydrochloride   **Abbott**

Products— Meperidine HCl is available in concentrations of 10, 25, 50, 75, and 100 mg/ml in a variety of packaging sizes and configurations, including ampuls, vials, and disposable cartridge units (29).

In addition to meperidine HCl, each milliliter of drug solution in disposable cartridge units (Wyeth) contains sodium acetate buffer. Each milliliter of drug solution in multiple-dose vials (Wyeth) contains sodium acetate buffer, not more than 1.5 mg of sodium metabisulfite, and 5 mg of phenol as a preservative (1-3/22/95). Other products may be preservative free in single-dose containers or incorporate 0.1% metacresol as a preservative in multiple-dose containers (4).

pH— The pH is adjusted to 3.5 to 6 (4).

Osmolality— The osmolality of meperidine HCl 50 mg/ml was determined to be 302 mOsm/kg (1233).

Administration— Meperidine HCl is administered by intramuscular injection into a large muscle mass. It may also be given subcutaneously or slowly by intravenous injection or infusion in a diluted solution. A 10-mg/ml concentration has been recommended for slow intravenous injection. The 10-mg/ml commercial injection does not require further dilution and is for use with a compatible infusion device. Intravenous infusion of a 1-mg/ml concentration has been used to supplement anesthesia (4).

Stability— Meperidine HCl should be stored at temperatures between 15 and 25 °C and protected from light and freezing (4).

Syringes— Meperidine HCl (Wyeth) 5 and 10 mg/ml in dextrose 5% in water and sodium chloride 0.9% was packaged in 30-ml Plastipak (Becton-Dickinson) syringes capped with Monoject (Sherwood) tip caps. Syringes were stored at 23 °C exposed to light and protected from light, 4 °C protected from light, and frozen at −20 °C protected from light for 12 weeks. HPLC analysis found that both concentrations at all storage conditions were stable for at least 12 weeks (1894).

Preservative-free meperidine HCl (Abbott) was diluted to concentrations of 0.25, 1, 10, 20, and 30 mg/ml with dextrose 5% in water and with sodium chloride 0.9%. The solutions were packaged in 60-ml polypropylene syringes (Becton-Dickinson), sealed with Luer lock caps, and stored at 22 and 4 °C for 28 days protected from light. The solutions were visually colorless and free of precipitation over the course of the study. Stability-indicating HPLC analysis found little or no loss of meperidine HCl in either solution at either temperature in 28 days (2200).

Sorption— Meperidine HCl (David Bull Laboratories) 71 mg/L in sodium chloride 0.9% (Travenol) in PVC bags did not exhibit significant sorption to the plastic during one week of storage at room temperature (15 to 20 °C) (536).

In another study, meperidine HCl (David Bull Laboratories) 71 mg/L in sodium chloride 0.9% did not exhibit any loss due to sorption during a seven-hour simulated infusion through an infusion set (Travenol) consisting of a cellulose propionate burette chamber and 170 cm of PVC tubing (606).

The drug was also tested as a simulated infusion over at least one hour by a syringe pump system. A glass syringe on a syringe pump was fitted with 20 cm of polyethylene tubing or 50 cm of Silastic tubing. No loss of drug due to sorption was observed with either tubing (606).

A 25-ml aliquot of meperidine HCl (David Bull Laboratories) 71 mg/L in sodium chloride 0.9% was stored in all-plastic syringes composed of polypropylene barrels and polyethylene plungers for 24 hours at room temperature in the dark. No loss due to sorption occurred (606).

Compatibility Information

Solution Compatibility

Meperidine HCl

Solution	Mfr	Mfr	Conc/L	Remarks	Ref	C/I
Dextran 6% in dextrose 5%	AB	WI	100 mg	Physically compatible	3	C
Dextran 6% in sodium chloride 0.9%	AB	WI	100 mg	Physically compatible	3	C
Dextrose–Ringer's injection combinations	AB	WI	100 mg	Physically compatible	3	C
Dextrose–Ringer's injection, lactated, combinations	AB	WI	100 mg	Physically compatible	3	C
Dextrose–saline combinations	AB	WI	100 mg	Physically compatible	3	C
Dextrose 2½% in water	AB	WI	100 mg	Physically compatible	3	C
Dextrose 5% in water	AB	WI	100 mg	Physically compatible	3	C
	TR[a]	WI	1.2 g	Physically compatible with no meperidine loss in 36 hr at 22 °C	1000	C
Dextrose 10% in water	AB	WI	100 mg	Physically compatible	3	C
Fructose 10% in sodium chloride 0.9%	AB	WI	100 mg	Physically compatible	3	C
Fructose 10% in water	AB	WI	100 mg	Physically compatible	3	C
Invert sugar 5 and 10% in sodium chloride 0.9%	AB	WI	100 mg	Physically compatible	3	C
Invert sugar 5 and 10% in water	AB	WI	100 mg	Physically compatible	3	C
Ionosol products	AB	WI	100 mg	Physically compatible	3	C
Ringer's injection	AB	WI	100 mg	Physically compatible	3	C
Ringer's injection, lactated	AB	WI	100 mg	Physically compatible	3	C
Sodium chloride 0.45%	AB	WI	100 mg	Physically compatible	3	C
Sodium chloride 0.9%	AB	WI	100 mg	Physically compatible	3	C
	FRE[a]		2.5 g	Visually compatible with little or no loss by GC in 24 days at room temperature	1791	C
Sodium lactate ⅙ M	AB	WI	100 mg	Physically compatible	3	C
TPN #71[b]	[a]	WI	100 mg	Physically compatible with no meperidine loss in 36 hr at 22 °C	1000	C

[a]Tested in PVC bags.
[b]Refer to Appendix I for the composition of parenteral nutrition solutions. TPN indicates a 2-in-1 admixture.

Additive Compatibility

Meperidine HCl

Drug	Mfr	Conc/L	Mfr	Conc/L	Test Soln	Remarks	Ref	C/I
Aminophylline			WI			Physically incompatible	9	I
Amobarbital sodium			WI			Physically incompatible	9	I
Cefazolin sodium	FUJ	10 g		0.5 g	D5W	Visually compatible with about 5% loss by HPLC of each drug in 5 days at 25 °C. 5% cefazolin loss and 7% meperidine loss in 20 days at 4 °C.	1966	C
Dobutamine HCl	LI	1 g	ES	50 g	D5W, NS	Physically compatible for 24 hr at 21 °C	812	C
Floxacillin sodium	BE	20 g	RC	5 g	W	Haze forms immediately and precipitate forms in 5 to 24 hr	1479	I
Furosemide	HO	1 g	RC	5 g	W	Fine precipitate forms immediately	1479	I

Additive Compatibility (Cont.)

Meperidine HCl

Drug	Mfr	Conc/L	Mfr	Conc/L	Test Soln	Remarks	Ref	C/I
Heparin sodium			WI			Physically incompatible	9	I
Morphine sulfate			WI			Physically incompatible	9	I
Ondansetron HCl	GL	100 mg and 1 g	WY	4 g	NS[a]	Physically compatible with no change in measured turbidity or increase in particle content and no loss of either drug by HPLC in 31 days at 4 and 22 °C and in 7 days at 32 °C	1862	C
Phenobarbital sodium	WI		WI			Physically incompatible	9	I
Phenytoin sodium	PD		WI			Physically incompatible	9	I
Scopolamine HBr		0.43 mg	WI	100 mg		Physically compatible	3	C
Sodium bicarbonate			WI			Physically incompatible	9	I
	AB	2.4 mEq[b]	WI	100 mg	D5W	Physically compatible for 24 hr	772	C
Succinylcholine chloride	AB	2 g	WI	100 mg		Physically compatible	3	C
Thiopental sodium			WI			Physically incompatible	9	I
Triflupromazine HCl	SQ					Physically compatible	40	C
Verapamil HCl	KN	80 mg	WI	150 mg	D5W, NS	Physically compatible for 24 hr	764	C

[a]Tested in PVC containers.
[b]One vial of Neut added to a liter of admixture.

Drugs in Syringe Compatibility

Meperidine HCl

Drug (in syringe)	Mfr	Amt	Mfr	Amt	Remarks	Ref	C/I
Atropine sulfate		0.6 mg/ 1.5 ml	WY	100 mg/ 1 ml	Physically compatible for at least 15 min	14	C
	ST	0.4 mg/ 1 ml	WI	50 mg/ 1 ml	Physically compatible for at least 15 min	326	C
Atropine sulfate with hydroxyzine HCl[a]	ES PF	0.4 mg 50 mg	WI	50 mg/ 2.5 ml	No alteration of UV spectra in 10 days at 3 and 25 °C	301	C
Atropine sulfate with promethazine HCl	WY	0.6 mg/ 1.5 ml 50 mg/ 2 ml	WY	100 mg/ 1 ml	Physically compatible	14	C
Atropine sulfate with promethazine HCl	LI WY	0.4 mg/ 1 ml 25 mg/ 1 ml	WI	50 mg/ 1 ml	No loss of any drug in 24 hr at 25 °C. Slight haze, not present at 6 hr, developed by 24 hr	991	C
Butorphanol tartrate	BR	4 mg/ 2 ml	WI	50 mg/ 1 ml	Physically compatible both macroscopically and microscopically for 30 min at room temperature	566	C
Chlorpromazine HCl	SKF	50 mg/ 2 ml	WY	100 mg/ 1 ml	Physically compatible for at least 15 min	14	C
	PO	50 mg/ 2 ml	WI	50 mg/ 1 ml	Physically compatible for at least 15 min	326	C

Drugs in Syringe Compatibility (Cont.)

Meperidine HCl

Drug (in syringe)	Mfr	Amt	Mfr	Amt	Remarks	Ref	C/I
Cimetidine HCl	SKF	300 mg/ 2 ml	WI	100 mg/ 2 ml	Physically compatible for 4 hr at 25 °C	25	C
Dimenhydrinate	HR	50 mg/ 1 ml	WI	50 mg/ 1 ml	Physically compatible for at least 15 min	326	C
Diphenhydramine HCl	PD	50 mg/ 1 ml	WY	100 mg/ 1 ml	Physically compatible for at least 15 min	14	C
	PD	50 mg/ 1 ml	WI	50 mg/ 1 ml	Physically compatible for at least 15 min	326	C
Droperidol	MN	2.5 mg/ 1 ml	WI	50 mg/ 1 ml	Physically compatible for at least 15 min	326	C
Fentanyl citrate	MN	0.05 mg/ 1 ml	WI	50 mg/ 1 ml	Physically compatible for at least 15 min	326	C
Glycopyrrolate	RB	0.2 mg/ 1 ml	WI	50 mg/ 1 ml	Physically compatible and pH in stability range for glycopyrrolate for 48 hr at 25 °C	331	C
	RB	0.2 mg/ 1 ml	WI	100 mg/ 2 ml	Physically compatible and pH in stability range for glycopyrrolate for 48 hr at 25 °C	331	C
	RB	0.4 mg/ 2 ml	WI	50 mg/ 1 ml	Physically compatible and pH in stability range for glycopyrrolate for 48 hr at 25 °C	331	C
Heparin sodium		2500 units/ 1 ml	HO	100 mg/ 2 ml	Turbidity or precipitate forms within 5 min	1053	I
Hydroxyzine HCl	PF	100 mg/ 4 ml	WY	100 mg/ 1 ml	Physically compatible for at least 15 min	14	C
	PF	50 mg/ 1 ml	WI	50 mg/ 1 ml	Physically compatible for at least 15 min	326	C
	PF	50 mg/ 1 ml	WI	100 mg/ 2 ml	Physically compatible	771	C
	PF	100 mg/ 2 ml	WI	50 mg/ 1 ml	Physically compatible	771	C
Hydroxyzine HCl with atropine sulfate[a]	PF ES	50 mg 0.4 mg	WI	50 mg/ 2.5 ml	No alteration of UV spectra in 10 days at 3 and 25 °C	301	C
Ketamine HCl	PD	2 mg/ml	DB	12 mg/ ml	Diluted to 50 ml with NS. Visually compatible for 48 hr at 25 °C	2059	C
Metoclopramide HCl	NO	10 mg/ 2 ml	WI	50 mg/ 1 ml	Physically compatible both macroscopically and microscopically for 15 min at room temperature	565	C
Midazolam HCl	RC	5 mg/ 1 ml	WB	100 mg/ 1 ml	Physically compatible for 4 hr at 25 °C under fluorescent light	1145	C
Morphine sulfate	ST	15 mg/ 1 ml	WI	50 mg/ 1 ml	Physically incompatible within 15 min	326	I
Ondansetron HCl	GW	1.33 mg/ ml[b]	ES	8.33 mg/ ml[b]	Physically compatible with no measured increase in particulates and little or no loss of either drug by HPLC in 24 hr at 4 or 23 °C	2199	C
Pentazocine lactate	WI	30 mg/ 1 ml	WI	50 mg/ 1 ml	Physically compatible for at least 15 min	326	C
Pentazocine lactate with perphenazine		15 mg 5 mg		150 mg	Physically compatible for at least 15 min	815	C

Drugs in Syringe Compatibility (Cont.)

Meperidine HCl

Drug (in syringe)	Mfr	Amt	Mfr	Amt	Remarks	Ref	C/I
Pentobarbital sodium	WY	100 mg/ 2 ml	WY	100 mg/ 1 ml	Precipitate forms within 15 min	14	I
	AB	500 mg/ 10 ml	WI	100 mg/ 2 ml	Physically incompatible	55	I
	AB	50 mg/ 1 ml	WI	50 mg/ 1 ml	Physically incompatible within 15 min	326	I
Perphenazine	SC	5 mg/ 1 ml	WI	50 mg/ 1 ml	Physically compatible both macroscopically and microscopically for 30 min at room temperature	566	C
Perphenazine with pentazocine lactate		5 mg 15 mg[b]		150 mg	Physically compatible for at least 15 min	815	C
Prochlorperazine edisylate	SKF		WY	100 mg/ 1 ml	Physically compatible for at least 15 min	14	C
	PO	5 mg/ 1 ml	WI	50 mg/ 1 ml	Physically compatible for at least 15 min	326	C
Promazine HCl	WY	50 mg/ 1 ml	WI	50 mg/ 1 ml	Physically compatible for at least 15 min	326	C
Promethazine HCl	WY	50 mg/ 2 ml	WY	100 mg/ 1 ml	Physically compatible for at least 15 min	14	C
	PO	50 mg/ 2 ml	WI	50 mg/ 1 ml	Physically compatible for at least 15 min	326	C
Promethazine HCl with atropine sulfate	WY	50 mg/ 2 ml 0.6 mg/ 1.5 ml	WY	100 mg/ 1 ml	Physically compatible	14	C
Promethazine HCl with atropine sulfate	WY LI	25 mg/ 1 ml 0.4 mg/ 1 ml	WI	50 mg/ 1 ml	No loss of any drug in 24 hr at 25 °C. Slight haze, not present at 6 hr, developed by 24 hr	991	C
Ranitidine HCl	GL	50 mg/ 2 ml	WI	100 mg/ 1 ml	Physically compatible for 1 hr at 25 °C both macroscopically and microscopically	978	C
Scopolamine HBr		0.6 mg/ 1.5 ml	WY	100 mg/ 1 ml	Physically compatible for at least 15 min	14	C
	ST	0.4 mg/ 1 ml	WI	50 mg/ 1 ml	Physically compatible for at least 15 min	326	C

[a]Tested in both glass and plastic syringes.
[b]Tested in sodium chloride 0.9%.

Y-Site Injection Compatibility (1:1 Mixture)

Meperidine HCl

Drug	Mfr	Conc	Mfr	Conc	Remarks	Ref	C/I
Acyclovir sodium	BW	5 mg/ml[a]	WB	1 mg/ml[a]	Physically compatible for 4 hr at 25 °C	1157	C
	BW	5 mg/ml[a]	AB	10 mg/ml	White crystalline precipitate forms within 1 hr at 25 °C under fluorescent light	1397	I
	BW	5 mg/ml[a,b]	WY	100 mg/ml	Visually compatible for 24 hr at room temperature in test tubes. No precipitate found on filter from Y-site delivery	2063	C

Y-Site Injection Compatibility (1:1 Mixture) (Cont.)

Meperidine HCl

Drug	Mfr	Conc	Mfr	Conc	Remarks	Ref	C/I
Allopurinol sodium	BW	3 mg/ml[b]	WY	4 mg/ml[b]	Tiny particles form immediately and increase in number over 4 hr	1686	I
Amifostine	USB	10 mg/ml[a]	WY	4 mg/ml[a]	Physically compatible with no change in measured turbidity or increase in particle content in 4 hr at 23 °C	1845	C
Amikacin sulfate	BR	5 mg/ml[a]	WY	10 mg/ml[a]	Physically compatible for at least 4 hr at 25 °C under fluorescent light	987	C
Amphotericin B cholesteryl sulfate complex	SEQ	0.83 mg/ml[a]	AST	4 mg/ml[a]	Increased turbidity forms immediately	2117	I
Ampicillin sodium	BR	20 mg/ml[b]	WY	10 mg/ml[a]	Physically compatible for at least 4 hr at 25 °C under fluorescent light	987	C
Ampicillin sodium–sulbactam sodium	RR	20 + 10 mg/ml[b]	WY	10 mg/ml[b]	Physically compatible for 1 hr at 25 °C	1338	C
Atenolol	ICI	0.5 mg/ml	AB	10 mg/ml	Physically compatible for 4 hr at 25 °C	1397	C
Aztreonam	SQ	20 mg/ml[a]	AB	10 mg/ml	Physically compatible for 4 hr at 25 °C	1397	C
	SQ	40 mg/ml[a]	WY	4 mg/ml[a]	Physically compatible with no subvisual haze or particle formation in 4 hr at 23 °C	1758	C
Bumetanide	RC	0.25 mg/ml	AB	10 mg/ml	Physically compatible for 4 hr at 25 °C	1397	C
Cefamandole nafate	LI	20 mg/ml[a]	WY	10 mg/ml[a]	Physically compatible for at least 4 hr at 25 °C under fluorescent light	987	C
	LI	40 mg/ml[a]	WY	10 mg/ml[b]	Physically compatible for 1 hr at 25 °C	1338	C
Cefazolin sodium	SKF	20 mg/ml[a]	WY	10 mg/ml[a]	Physically compatible for at least 4 hr at 25 °C under fluorescent light	987	C
Cefepime HCl	BR	20 mg/ml[a]	WY	4 mg/ml[a]	Haze forms immediately with numerous particles in 1 hr	1689	I
Cefoperazone sodium	RR	20 mg/ml[a]	WY	10 mg/ml[a]	Immediate precipitation	987	I
Cefotaxime sodium	HO	20 mg/ml[a]	WY	10 mg/ml[a]	Physically compatible for at least 4 hr at 25 °C under fluorescent light	987	C
Cefotetan disodium	STU	20 and 40 mg/ml[a]	WY	10 mg/ml[b]	Physically compatible for 1 hr at 25 °C	1338	C
Cefoxitin sodium	MSD	20 mg/ml[a]	WY	10 mg/ml[a]	Physically compatible for at least 4 hr at 25 °C under fluorescent light	987	C
Ceftazidime	LI[c]	20 and 40 mg/ml[a]	AB	10 mg/ml	Physically compatible for 4 hr at 25 °C	1397	C
Ceftizoxime sodium	SKF	20 mg/ml[a]	WY	10 mg/ml[a]	Physically compatible for at least 4 hr at 25 °C under fluorescent light	987	C
Ceftriaxone sodium	RC	20 and 40 mg/ml[a]	AB	10 mg/ml	Physically compatible for 4 hr at 25 °C	1397	C
Cefuroxime sodium	GL	30 mg/ml[a]	WY	10 mg/ml[a]	Physically compatible for at least 4 hr at 25 °C under fluorescent light	987	C
Chloramphenicol sodium succinate	LY	20 mg/ml[a]	WY	10 mg/ml[a]	Physically compatible for at least 4 hr at 25 °C under fluorescent light	987	C
Cisatracurium besylate	GW	0.1, 2, 5 mg/ml[a]	AST	4 mg/ml[a]	Physically compatible with no change in measured turbidity or increase in particle content in 4 hr at 23 °C	2074	C

Y-Site Injection Compatibility (1:1 Mixture) (Cont.)

Meperidine HCl

Drug	Mfr	Conc	Mfr	Conc	Remarks	Ref	C/I
Cladribine	ORT	0.015[b] and 0.5[e] mg/ml	WY	4 mg/ml[b]	Physically compatible with no change in measured turbidity or increase in particle content in 4 hr at 23 °C	1969	C
Clindamycin phosphate	UP	12 mg/ml[a]	WY	10 mg/ml[a]	Physically compatible for at least 4 hr at 25 °C under fluorescent light	987	C
Dexamethasone sodium phosphate	LY	0.2 mg/ml[a]	AB	10 mg/ml	Physically compatible for 4 hr at 25 °C	1397	C
Diltiazem HCl	MMD	1[b] and 5 mg/ml	WY	100 mg/ml	Visually compatible	1807	C
	MMD	5 mg/ml	WY	10 mg/ml[b]	Visually compatible	1807	C
Diphenhydramine HCl	ES	1[a] and 50 mg/ml	AB	10 mg/ml	Physically compatible for 4 hr at 25 °C	1397	C
Dobutamine HCl	LI	1 mg/ml	AB	10 mg/ml	Physically compatible for 4 hr at 25 °C	1397	C
Docetaxel	RPR	0.9 mg/ml[a]	AST	4 mg/ml[a]	Physically compatible with no change in measured turbidity or increase in particle content in 4 hr at 23 °C	2224	C
Dopamine HCl	AB	1.6 mg/ml	AB	10 mg/ml	Physically compatible for 4 hr at 25 °C	1397	C
Doxorubicin HCl liposome injection	SEQ	0.4 mg/ml[a]	AST	4 mg/ml[a]	Increase in measured turbidity	2087	I
Doxycycline hyclate	ES	1 mg/ml[a]	WY	10 mg/ml[a]	Physically compatible for at least 4 hr at 25 °C under fluorescent light	987	C
Droperidol	AMR	2.5 mg/ml[a]	AB	10 mg/ml	Physically compatible for 4 hr at 25 °C	1397	C
Erythromycin lactobionate	AB	5 mg/ml[a]	WY	10 mg/ml[a]	Physically compatible for at least 4 hr at 25 °C under fluorescent light	987	C
Etoposide phosphate	BR	5 mg/ml[a]	AST	4 mg/ml[a]	Physically compatible with no change in measured turbidity or increase in particle content in 4 hr at 23 °C	2218	C
Famotidine	MSD	0.2 mg/ml[a]	AB	10 mg/ml	Physically compatible for 4 hr at 25 °C	1397	C
	ME	2 mg/ml[b]		4 mg/ml[a]	Visually compatible for 4 hr at 22 °C	1936	C
Filgrastim	AMG	3 μg/ml[a]	WY	4 mg/ml[a]	Physically compatible with no change in measured turbidity or increase in particle content in 4 hr at 22 °C	1687	C
Fluconazole	RR	2 mg/ml	AB	10 mg/ml	Physically compatible for 4 hr at 25 °C	1397	C
Fludarabine phosphate	BX	1 mg/ml[a]	WI	4 mg/ml[a]	Physically compatible for 4 hr at room temperature under fluorescent light	1439	C
Furosemide	ES	0.8 mg/ml[a]	AB	10 mg/ml	Physically compatible for 4 hr at 25 °C	1397	C
	ES	2.4 mg/ml[a]	AB	10 mg/ml	White cloudiness forms immediately	1397	I
	ES	10 mg/ml	AB	10 mg/ml	White flocculent precipitate forms immediately	1397	I
Gemcitabine HCl	LI	10 mg/ml[b]	AST	4 mg/ml[b]	Physically compatible with no change in measured turbidity or increase in particle content in 4 hr at 23 °C	2226	C
Gentamicin sulfate	TR	0.8 mg/ml[a]	WY	10 mg/ml[a]	Physically compatible for at least 4 hr at 25 °C under fluorescent light	987	C
	ES	1.2 and 2 mg/ml[b]	WY	10 mg/ml[b]	Physically compatible for 1 hr at 25 °C	1338	C

Y-Site Injection Compatibility (1:1 Mixture) (Cont.)

Meperidine HCl

Drug	Mfr	Conc	Mfr	Conc	Remarks	Ref	C/I
Granisetron HCl	SKB	0.05 mg/ml[a]	WY	4 mg/ml[a]	Physically compatible with no change in measured turbidity or increase in particle content in 4 hr at 23 °C	2000	C
Heparin sodium		50 units/ml/min[b]	HO	100 mg/2 ml[f]	Clear solution	1053	C
	ES	60 units/ml[a]	WY	10 mg/ml[b]	Physically compatible for 1 hr at 25 °C	1338	C
Hydrocortisone sodium succinate	AB	2 mg/ml[a]	AB	10 mg/ml	Physically compatible for 4 hr at 25 °C	1397	C
Idarubicin HCl	AD	1 mg/ml[b]	WY	1[a] and 50 mg/ml	Color changes immediately	1525	I
Imipenem–cilastatin sodium	MSD	5 mg/ml[a]	AB	10 mg/ml	Yellow discoloration forms within 2 hr at 25 °C under fluorescent light	1397	I
Insulin, regular	LI	0.2 unit/ml[b]	WY	10 mg/ml[b]	Physically compatible for 1 hr at 25 °C	1338	C
	LI	0.2 unit/ml[b]	AST	50 mg/ml[a]	Physically compatible for 2 hr at 25 °C	1395	C
Kanamycin sulfate	BR	2.5 mg/ml[a]	WY	10 mg/ml[a]	Physically compatible for at least 4 hr at 25 °C under fluorescent light	987	C
Labetalol HCl	GL	5 mg/ml	AB	10 mg/ml	Physically compatible for 4 hr at 25 °C	1397	C
Lidocaine HCl	AB	1 mg/ml[a]	AB	10 mg/ml	Physically compatible for 4 hr at 25 °C	1397	C
Magnesium sulfate	LY	16.7, 33.3, 50, 100 mg/ml[a]	WI	10 mg/ml[a]	Visually compatible for 4 hr at 25 °C under fluorescent light	1549	C
Melphalan HCl	BW	0.1 mg/ml[b]	WY	4 mg/ml[b]	Physically compatible with no change in measured turbidity or increase in particle content in 3 hr at 22 °C	1557	C
Methyldopate HCl	AMR	2.5 mg/ml[a]	AB	10 mg/ml	Physically compatible for 4 hr at 25 °C	1397	C
Methylprednisolone sodium succinate	UP	2.5 mg/ml[a]	AB	10 mg/ml	Physically compatible for 4 hr at 25 °C	1397	C
Metoclopramide HCl	SN	0.2 mg/ml[a]	AB	10 mg/ml	Physically compatible for 4 hr at 25 °C	1397	C
Metoprolol tartrate	CI	1 mg/ml	AB	10 mg/ml	Physically compatible for 4 hr at 25 °C	1397	C
Metronidazole	SE	5 mg/ml	WY	10 mg/ml[a]	Physically compatible for at least 4 hr at 25 °C under fluorescent light	987	C
Minocycline HCl	LE	0.2 mg/ml[a]	WY	10 mg/ml[a]	Color change from pale yellow to light green within 1 hr at 25 °C	987	I
Nafcillin sodium	WY	20 mg/ml[a]	WY	10 mg/ml[a]	Cloudy haze cleared on mixing and remained clear for 4 hr at 25 °C	987	C
	WY	20 and 30 mg/ml[a]	WY	10 mg/ml[b]	Cloudy solution formed immediately and persisted for at least 1 hr at 25 °C	1338	I
Ondansetron HCl	GL	1 mg/ml[b]	WI	4 mg/ml[a]	Physically compatible for 4 hr at 22 °C	1365	C
Oxacillin sodium	BE	20 mg/ml[a]	WY	10 mg/ml[a]	Physically compatible for at least 4 hr at 25 °C under fluorescent light	987	C
Oxytocin	PD	0.02 mg/ml[h]	WY	10 mg/ml[b]	Physically compatible for 1 hr at 25 °C	1338	C
Paclitaxel	NCI	1.2 mg/ml[a]	WY	4 mg/ml[a]	Physically compatible with no change in measured turbidity in 4 hr at 22 °C	1556	C
Penicillin G potassium	PF	100,000 units/ml[a]	WY	10 mg/ml[a]	Physically compatible for at least 4 hr at 25 °C under fluorescent light	987	C

Y-Site Injection Compatibility (1:1 Mixture) (Cont.)

Meperidine HCl

Drug	Mfr	Conc	Mfr	Conc	Remarks	Ref	C/I
Piperacillin sodium	LE	60 mg/ml[a]	WY	10 mg/ml[a]	Physically compatible for at least 4 hr at 25 °C under fluorescent light	987	**C**
Piperacillin sodium–tazobactam sodium	LE	40 + 5 mg/ml[a]	WY	4 mg/ml[a]	Physically compatible with no change in measured turbidity or increase in particle content in 4 hr at 22 °C	1688	**C**
Potassium chloride	AB	0.4 mEq/ml[a]	AB	10 mg/ml	Physically compatible for 4 hr at 25 °C	1397	**C**
Propofol	ZEN	10 mg/ml	WY	4 mg/ml[a]	Physically compatible for 1 hr at 23 °C with no increase in particle content	2066	**C**
Propranolol HCl	WY	1 mg/ml	AB	10 mg/ml	Physically compatible for 4 hr at 25 °C	1397	**C**
Ranitidine HCl	GL	0.5 mg/ml[i]	WY	10 mg/ml[b]	Physically compatible for 1 hr at 25 °C	1338	**C**
Remifentanil HCl	GW	0.025 and 0.25 mg/ml[b]	AST	4 mg/ml[a]	Physically compatible with no change in measured turbidity or increase in particle content in 4 hr at 23 °C	2075	**C**
Sargramostim	IMM	10 μg/ml[b]	WI	4 mg/ml[b]	Physically compatible for 4 hr at 22 °C	1436	**C**
Teniposide	BR	0.1 mg/ml[a]	WY	4 mg/ml[a]	Physically compatible with no subvisual haze or particle formation in 4 hr at 23 °C	1725	**C**
Thiotepa	IMM[j]	1 mg/ml[a]	WY	4 mg/ml[a]	Physically compatible with no change in measured turbidity or increase in particle content in 4 hr at 23 °C	1861	**C**
Ticarcillin disodium	BE	60 mg/ml[a]	WY	10 mg/ml[a]	Physically compatible for at least 4 hr at 25 °C under fluorescent light	987	**C**
Ticarcillin disodium–clavulanate potassium	BE	31 mg/ml[b]	WY	10 mg/ml[b]	Physically compatible for 1 hr at 25 °C	1338	**C**
TNA #218 to #226[g]			AST	4 mg/ml[a]	Visually compatible with no precipitate or emulsion damage apparent in 4 hr at 23 °C	221?	**C**
Tobramycin sulfate	DI	0.8 mg/ml[a]	WY	10 mg/ml[a]	Physically compatible for at least 4 hr at 25 °C under fluorescent light	987	**C**
	LI	1.6, 2, 2.4 mg/ml[a]	WY	10 mg/ml[b]	Physically compatible for 1 hr at 25 °C	1338	**C**
TPN #131 and #132[g]			AB	10 mg/ml	Physically compatible for 4 hr at 25 °C	1397	**C**
TPN #189[g]			DB	50 mg/ml	Visually compatible for 24 hr at 22 °C	1767	**C**
TPN #212 to #215[g]			AST	4 mg/ml[a]	Physically compatible with no change in measured turbidity or increase in particle content in 4 hr at 23 °C	2109	**C**
Trimethoprim–sulfamethoxazole	BW	0.8 + 4 mg/ml[a]	WY	10 mg/ml[a]	Physically compatible for at least 4 hr at 25 °C under fluorescent light	987	**C**
Vancomycin HCl	LI	5 mg/ml[a]	WY	10 mg/ml[a]	Physically compatible for at least 4 hr at 25 °C under fluorescent light	987	**C**
Verapamil HCl	DU	2.5 mg/ml	AB	10 mg/ml	Physically compatible for 4 hr at 25 °C	1397	**C**

Y-Site Injection Compatibility (1:1 Mixture) (Cont.)

Meperidine HCl

Drug	Mfr	Conc	Mfr	Conc	Remarks	Ref	C/I
Vinorelbine tartrate	BW	1 mg/ml[b]	WY	4 mg/ml[b]	Physically compatible with no change in measured turbidity or increase in particle content in 4 hr at 22 °C	1558	C

[a]Tested in dextrose 5% in water.
[b]Tested in sodium chloride 0.9%.
[c]Sodium carbonate–containing formulation tested.
[d]Tested in sterile water for injection.
[e]Tested in bacteriostatic sodium chloride 0.9% preserved with benzyl alcohol 0.9%.
[f]Given over three minutes via a Y-site into a running infusion solution.
[g]Refer to Appendix I for the composition of parenteral nutrition solutions. TNA indicates a 3-in-1 admixture, and TPN indicates a 2-in-1 admixture.
[h]Tested in dextrose 5% in Ringer's injection, lactated.
[i]Tested in sodium chloride 0.45%.
[j]Lyophilized formulation tested.

Additional Compatibility Information

Promethazine and Scopolamine— Promethazine HCl (Wyeth) 50 mg/2 ml, meperidine HCl (Wyeth) 100 mg/ml, and scopolamine hydrobromide 0.6 mg/1.5 ml have been reported to be conditionally compatible when packaged in syringes. The mixture is physically compatible when the order of mixing is as stated above (14).

Chlorpromazine and Hydroxyzine— Chlorpromazine HCl (Elkins-Sinn) 6.25 mg/ml, hydroxyzine HCl (Pfizer) 12.5 mg/ml, and meperidine HCl (Winthrop) 25 mg/ml, in both glass and plastic syringes, have been reported to be physically compatible and chemically stable for at least one year at 4 and 25 °C when protected from light. Significant discoloration, ranging from yellow to brownish yellow, occurred on storage at 44 °C (989).

Chlorpromazine and Promethazine— Chlorpromazine HCl (Elkins-Sinn), meperidine HCl (Winthrop), and promethazine HCl (Elkins-Sinn), combined as an extemporaneous mixture for preoperative sedation, developed a brownish-yellow color after two weeks of storage with protection from light. The discoloration was attributed to the metacresol preservative content of Winthrop's meperidine HCl. Use of Wyeth's meperidine HCl instead, which contains a different preservative, resulted in a solution that remained clear and colorless for at least three months when protected from light (1148).

Heparin— If meperidine HCl is injected into a heparinized scalp vein infusion set, a precipitate will form. It has been suggested that these heparinized sets be flushed with sodium chloride 0.9% before and after drug administration. Heparin lock flush solution may then be reinjected into the device (4; 97).

MEPERIDINE HCL AND PROMETHAZINE HCL
AHFS 4:00, 28:08.08, and 28:24.92

Mepergan   **Wyeth-Ayerst**

Products— Mepergan is available in 10-ml vials and 2-ml Tubex cartridges. Each milliliter contains meperidine HCl 25 mg and promethazine HCl 25 mg with edetate disodium 0.1 mg, calcium chloride 0.04 mg, sodium metabisulfite 0.25 mg, phenol 5 mg, not more than 0.75 mg sodium formaldehyde sulfoxylate, and sodium acetate buffer (2).

Administration— Mepergan may be administered intravenously but is usually given by deep intramuscular injection. When given intravenously, the rate of administration should not exceed 1 ml/min, preferably through the tubing of a running intravenous solution. Subcutaneous administration is contraindicated because of possible tissue necrosis (2).

Stability— Mepergan in intact containers should be stored at room temperature and protected from light (2).

Compatibility Information

Drugs in Syringe Compatibility

Meperidine HCl and Promethazine HCl

Drug (in syringe)	Mfr	Amt	Mfr	Amt	Remarks	Ref	C/I
Glycopyrrolate	RB	0.2 mg/ 1 ml	WY	25 mg + 25 mg/ 1 ml	Physically compatible and pH in stability range for glycopyrrolate for 48 hr at 25 °C	331	C
	RB	0.2 mg/ 1 ml	WY	50 mg + 50 mg/ 2 ml	Physically compatible and pH in stability range for glycopyrrolate for 48 hr at 25 °C	331	C
	RB	0.4 mg/ 2 ml	WY	25 mg + 25 mg/ 1 ml	Physically compatible and pH in stability range for glycopyrrolate for 48 hr at 25 °C	331	C

Additional Compatibility Information

Mepergan may be combined in the same syringe with 0.3 to 0.4 mg of atropine sulfate or 0.25 to 0.4 mg of scopolamine hydrobromide (2).

Mepergan is incompatible with barbiturates. Consequently, they should not be mixed in the same syringe (2).

Also see the monographs on meperidine HCl and promethazine HCl.

MEPHENTERMINE SULFATE
AHFS 12:12

Wyamine Sulfate   **Wyeth-Ayerst**

Products— Mephentermine sulfate (Wyeth-Ayerst) is available at a concentration of 15 mg/ml in 10-ml vials and 2-ml ampuls. It is also available at a concentration of 30 mg/ml in 10-ml vials. Also present in each milliliter are sodium acetate buffer, methylparaben 1.8 mg, and propylparaben 0.2 mg (1-5/10/95).

pH— From 4 to 6.5 (1-5/10/95).

Administration— Mephentermine sulfate may be administered by intramuscular or intravenous injection (1-5/10/95; 4). It may also be administered by intravenous infusion, usually as a solution containing about 1 to 1.2 mg/ml of drug. The flow rate and duration of therapy should be individualized to the response of the patient (1-5/10/95), but mephentermine sulfate is usually infused at 1 to 5 mg/min (4).

Stability— Intact containers of mephentermine sulfate injection should be stored at controlled room temperature (4). Mephentermine sulfate is stable at pH 3.5 to 7.5 (48).

Compatibility Information

Solution Compatibility

Mephentermine sulfate

Solution	Mfr	Mfr	Conc/L	Remarks	Ref	C/I
Dextrose 5% in water		WY	1 g	Potency retained for 24 hr at 25 °C	48	C
Sodium bicarbonate 5%		WY	1 g	Potency retained for 48 hr at 25 °C	48	C

Additive Compatibility

Mephentermine sulfate

Drug	Mfr	Conc/L	Mfr	Conc/L	Test Soln	Remarks	Ref	C/I
Aminophylline		625 mg		750 mg	D5W	Physically compatible and chemically stable for 24 hr at 3 and 30 °C	520	C

Additive Compatibility (Cont.)

Mephentermine sulfate

Drug	Mfr	Conc/L	Mfr	Conc/L	Test Soln	Remarks	Ref	C/I
Epinephrine HCl	PD		WY			Physically incompatible	10	I
Hydralazine HCl	BP	80 mg	BP	120 mg	D5W	Yellow color produced	26	I
Hydrocortisone sodium succinate		250 mg		750 mg	D5W	Physically compatible and chemically stable for 24 hr at 3 and 30 °C	520	C
Lidocaine HCl	AST	2 g	WY	1 g		Physically compatible	24	C

Additional Compatibility Information

Mephentermine sulfate appears to be compatible with most intravenous infusion solutions (4). Dextrose 5% in water (1-5/10/95) and sodium chloride 0.9% (4) have been recommended for the preparation of mephentermine sulfate infusions.

Mephentermine sulfate (Wyeth) has been stated to be incompatible with oxidizing agents because of color formation (10).

MEPIVACAINE HCL
AHFS 72:00

Carbocaine   **Abbott**

Products— Mepivacaine HCl is available in concentrations of 1, 1.5, 2, and 3%. Methylparaben is incorporated into multiple-dose containers, but single-dose containers may be preservative free. The pH may have been adjusted with sodium hydroxide and/or hydrochloric acid. A 2% product with levonordefrin is also available (4; 29).

pH— From 4.5 to 6.8 (4).

Administration— Mepivacaine HCl may be administered by infiltration and by peripheral or sympathetic nerve block. Mepivacaine HCl *without* preservatives may be administered by epidural block, including caudal anesthesia; forms containing preservatives should not be administered by this route. Mepivacaine HCl 2% with levonordefrin is used in dental infiltration and nerve block procedures (4).

Stability— Mepivacaine HCl in intact containers should be stored at room temperature and protected from temperatures above 40 °C and from freezing. Mepivacaine HCl is resistant to hydrolysis and may be autoclaved repeatedly. However, mepivacaine HCl in dental cartridges and mepivacaine HCl 2% with levonordefrin should not be subjected to autoclaving because of breakdown of the dental cartridge closures and instability of the levonordefrin, respectively (4).

Syringes— The stability of mepivacaine (salt form unspecified) 10 mg/ml repackaged in polypropylene syringes was evaluated by spectrophotometric and potentiometric methods. Little or no change in concentration was found after four weeks of storage at room temperature not exposed to direct light (2164).

MEROPENEM
AHFS 8:12.07

Merrem   **AstraZeneca**

Products— Meropenem is available in dosage forms containing 500 mg and 1 g of drug along with sodium carbonate (2).

Reconstitute the 500-mg vials with 10 ml and the 1-g vials with 20 ml of sterile water for injection, shake the vial, and allow it to stand until the solution is clear. Each milliliter of the resultant solution contains 50 mg of meropenem (2).

Meropenem is also available in ADD-Vantage vials of 500 mg and 1 g. These vials are to be reconstituted only with sodium chloride 0.45%, sodium chloride 0.9%, and dextrose 5% in water in 50-, 100-, or 250-ml ADD-Vantage flexible diluent containers (2).

Meropenem is provided in 100-ml infusion vials containing 500 mg and 1 g of drug. The contents may be reconstituted directly with 100 ml of compatible diluent (2).

pH— The reconstituted solution has a pH from 7.3 to 8.3 (2).

Sodium Content— Each gram of meropenem provides 3.92 mEq (90.2 mg) of sodium from the sodium carbonate present in the formulation (2).

Administration— Meropenem is administered by direct intravenous injection of 5 to 20 ml over three to five minutes or by intravenous infusion diluted in a compatible infusion solution over 15 to 30 minutes (2).

Stability— Intact vials should be stored at controlled room temperature between 20 and 25 °C. The drug is a white to pale yellow powder that yields a colorless to yellow solution on reconstitution (2).

The manufacturer indicates that reconstituted solutions in vials of meropenem up to 50 mg/ml in sterile water for injection are stable for two hours at room temperature and up to 12 hours under refrigeration. The infusion vials diluted in sodium chloride 0.9% to a meropenem concentration of 2.5 to 50 mg/ml are stated to be stable for two hours at room temperature and 18 hours under refrigeration; in dextrose 5% in water at these concentrations, stability is only one hour at room temperature and eight hours under refrigeration (2).

Solutions of meropenem 2.5 to 20 mg/ml in sodium chloride 0.9% in the Minibag Plus (Baxter) are stable for up to four hours at room temperature and up to 24 hours under refrigeration. In dextrose 5% in water in the same concentration range, the drug is stable for only one hour at room temperature and up to six hours under refrigeration (2).

Meropenem in ADD-Vantage containers reconstituted to a concentration in the range of 5 to 20 mg/ml in sodium chloride 0.45% or 1 to 20 mg/ml in sodium chloride 0.9% is stable for six or four hours, respectively, at room temperature and up to 24 hours under refrigeration. In dextrose 5% in water at a concentration in the range of 1 to 20 mg/ml, the drug is stable for only one hour at room temperature and up to eight hours under refrigeration (2).

In addition, the manufacturer notes that meropenem 1 to 20 mg/ml in sterile water for injection or sodium chloride 0.9% is stable for up to four hours and in dextrose 5% in water for up to two hours at room temperature in plastic syringes, plastic administration set tubing, drip chambers, and volume control devices (2).

The manufacturer recommends that solutions of meropenem not be frozen (2).

Also see Infusion Solutions under Additional Compatibility Information below.

Elastomeric Infusion Devices— Meropenem (Zeneca) 5 and 10 mg/ml in sodium chloride 0.9% protected from light was evaluated for stability in Intermate SV 200 ml/hr (Baxter) infusion devices having polyisoprene elastomeric reservoirs. By visual inspection, the lower concentration was a faint yellow solution and remained unchanged in color while the higher concentration exhibited an increased yellow coloring on storage. Based on HPLC analysis of the solutions, the calculated time to 10% loss at room temperature (about 24 °C) was 34 hours for the 5-mg/ml concentration and 20 hours for the 10-mg/ml concentration. Under refrigeration, both concentrations had a calculated time to 10% loss of 120 hours. Solutions refrigerated for 96 hours maintained adequate meropenem concentrations for an additional six hours at room temperature but became unacceptable on longer room-temperature storage. The stability characteristics of the meropenem solutions in Intermate SV units was very similar to the solution controls in glass containers (2152).

Compatibility Information

Solution Compatibility

Meropenem

Solution	Mfr	Mfr	Conc/L	Remarks	Ref	C/I
Dextrose 5% with potassium chloride 0.15%	BA[a]	ZEN	1 g	10 to 11% loss by HPLC in 4 hr at 24 °C and in 18 hr at 4 °C	2089	I[c]
	BA[a]	ZEN	20 g	8 to 10% loss by HPLC in 3 hr at 24 °C and in 18 hr at 4 °C	2089	I[c]
Dextrose 5% in Ringer's injection, lactated	BA[a]	ZEN	1 g	11% loss by HPLC in 8 hr at 24 °C and 4 to 5% loss in 8 hr at 4 °C	2089	I[c]
	BA[a]	ZEN	20 g	15% loss by HPLC in 4 hr at 24 °C and 10% loss in 18 hr at 4 °C	2089	I[c]
Dextrose 5% with sodium bicarbonate 0.02%	BA[a]	ZEN	1 g	11% loss by HPLC in 4 hr at 24 °C and 9% in 18 hr at 4 °C	2089	I[c]
	BA[a]	ZEN	20 g	10 to 12% loss by HPLC in 3 hr at 24 °C and 10% loss in 20 hr at 4 °C	2089	I[c]
Dextrose 2.5% in sodium chloride 0.45%	BA[a]	ZEN	1 g	10% loss by HPLC in 6 hr at 24 °C and 7% loss in 24 hr at 4 °C	2089	I[c]
	BA[a]	ZEN	20 g	8% loss by HPLC in 4 hr at 24 °C and 7% loss in 24 hr at 4 °C	2089	I[c]
Dextrose 5% in sodium chloride 0.2%	BA[a]	ZEN	1 g	10 to 11% loss by HPLC in 4 hr at 24 °C and in 16 hr at 4 °C	2089	I[c]
	BA[a]	ZEN	20 g	Up to 10% loss by HPLC in 3 hr at 24 °C and 9% loss in 18 hr at 4 °C	2089	I[c]
Dextrose 5% in sodium chloride 0.9%	BA[a]	ZEN	1 g	11 to 13% loss by HPLC in 4 hr at 24 °C and in 14 hr at 4 °C	2089	I[c]

Solution Compatibility (Cont.)

Solution	Mfr	Mfr	Conc/L	Remarks	Ref	C/I
	BA[a]	ZEN	20 g	9 to 11% loss by HPLC in 3 hr at 24 °C and in 14 hr at 4 °C	2089	I[c]
Dextrose 5% in water	BA[a]	ZEN	1 g	9% loss by HPLC in 4 hr at 24 °C and in 14 hr at 4 °C	2089	I[c]
	BA[b]	ZEN	2.5 g	6 to 7% loss by HPLC in 4 hr at 24 °C and 8 to 10% in 24 hr at 4 °C	2089	I[c]
	BA[a]	ZEN	20 g	11 to 12% loss by HPLC in 4 hr at 24 °C and in 18 hr at 4 °C	2089	I[c]
	BA[b]	ZEN	50 g	9 to 10% loss by HPLC in 3 hr at 24 °C and in 24 hr at 4 °C	2089	I[c]
Dextrose 10% in water	BA[a]	ZEN	1 g	10 to 12% loss by HPLC in 3 hr at 24 °C and in 8 hr at 4 °C	2089	I[c]
	BA[a]	ZEN	20 g	9 to 10% loss by HPLC in 2 hr at 24 °C and in 8 hr at 4 °C	2089	I[c]
Mannitol 2.5%	BA[a]	ZEN	1 g	7 to 8% loss by HPLC in 8 hr at 24 °C and in 24 hr at 4 °C	2089	I[c]
	BA[a]	ZEN	20 g	7 to 9% loss by HPLC in 4 hr at 24 °C and 6% loss in 20 hr at 4 °C	2089	I[c]
Mannitol 10%	BA[a]	ZEN	1 g	10 to 11% loss by HPLC in 4 hr at 24 °C and in 20 hr at 4 °C	2089	I[c]
	BA[a]	ZEN	20 g	10% loss by HPLC in 3 hr at 24 °C and in 20 hr at 4 °C	2089	I[c]
Normosol M with dextrose 5%	AB[a]	ZEN	1 g	5% loss by HPLC in 8 hr at 24 °C and 4% loss in 48 hr at 4 °C	2089	I[c]
	AB[a]	ZEN	20 g	7 to 8% loss by HPLC in 8 hr at 24 °C and 7 to 8% loss in 24 hr at 4°C	2089	I[c]
Ringer's injection	BA[a]	ZEN	1 g	6% loss by HPLC in 10 hr at 24 °C and 4 to 5% loss in 48 hr at 4 °C	2089	I[c]
	BA[a]	ZEN	20 g	7% loss by HPLC in 8 hr at 24 °C and 7% loss in 48 hr at 4 °C	2089	I[c]
Ringer's injection, lactated	BA[a]	ZEN	1 g	10 to 12% loss by HPLC in 10 hr at 24 °C and 6 to 7% loss in 48 hr at 4 °C	2089	I[c]
	BA[a]	ZEN	20 g	9% loss by HPLC in 8 hr at 24 °C and 7% loss in 48 hr at 4 °C	2089	I[c]
Sodium bicarbonate 5%	BA[a]	ZEN	1 g	10% loss by HPLC in 4 hr at 24 °C and in 18 hr at 4 °C	2089	I[c]
	BA[a]	ZEN	20 g	9 to 10% loss by HPLC in 3 hr at 24 °C and in 18 hr at 4 °C	2089	I[c]
Sodium chloride 0.45%	AB[d]	ZEN	5 g	9 to 10% loss by HPLC in 22 hr at 24 °C and 3% loss in 48 hr at 4 °C	2089	I[c]
	AB[d]	ZEN	20 g	6 to 8% loss by HPLC in 10 hr at 24 °C and 5 to 6% loss in 48 hr at 4 °C	2089	I[c]
Sodium chloride 0.9%	BA[a]	ZEN	1 g	8 to 10% loss by HPLC in 20 hr at 24 °C and 3 to 4% loss in 48 hr at 4 °C	2089	I[c]
	BA[b]	ZEN	2.5 g	6 to 7% loss by HPLC in 24 hr at 24 °C and 2% loss in 48 hr at 4 °C	2089	C
	BA[a]	ZEN	20 g	8% loss by HPLC in 10 hr at 24 °C and 5 to 7% loss in 48 hr at 4 °C	2089	I[c]
	BA[b]	ZEN	50 g	9 to 10% loss by HPLC in 8 hr at 24 °C and in 48 hr at 4 °C	2089	I[c]

Solution Compatibility (Cont.)

				Meropenem		
Solution	Mfr	Mfr	Conc/L	Remarks	Ref	C/I
Sodium lactate ⅙ M	BA[a]	ZEN	1 g	7% loss by HPLC in 8 hr at 24 °C and 6 to 7% loss in 48 hr at 4 °C	2089	I[c]
	BA[a]	ZEN	20 g	9% loss by HPLC in 8 hr at 24 °C and 4 to 5% loss in 24 hr at 4 °C	2089	I[c]

[a]Tested in PVC containers.
[b]Tested in glass containers.
[c]Incompatible by conventional standards but recommended for dilution of meropenem with use in shorter periods of time.
[d]Tested in Abbott ADD-Vantage system.

Additive Compatibility

				Meropenem				
Drug	Mfr	Conc/L	Mfr	Conc/L	Test Soln	Remarks	Ref	C/I
Acyclovir sodium	BW	5 g	ZEN	1 g	NS	Visually compatible for 4 hr at room temperature	1994	C
	BW	5 g	ZEN	20 g	NS	Immediate precipitation	1994	I
Aminophylline	AMR	1 g	ZEN	1 and 20 g	NS	Visually compatible for 4 hr at room temperature	1994	C
Amphotericin B	SQ	200 mg	ZEN	1 and 20 g	NS	Precipitate forms	2068	I
Atropine sulfate	ES	40 mg	ZEN	1 and 20 g	NS	Visually compatible for 4 hr at room temperature	1994	C
Cimetidine HCl	SKB	3 g	ZEN	1 and 20 g	NS	Visually compatible for 4 hr at room temperature	1994	C
Dexamethasone sodium phosphate	MSD	4 g	ZEN	1 and 20 g	NS	Visually compatible for 4 hr at room temperature	1994	C
Dobutamine HCl	LI	1 g	ZEN	1 and 20 g	NS	Visually compatible for 4 hr at room temperature	1994	C
Dopamine HCl	DU	800 mg	ZEN	1 and 20 g	NS	Visually compatible for 4 hr at room temperature	1994	C
Doxycycline hyclate	RR	200 mg	ZEN	1 g	NS	Visually compatible for 4 hr at room temperature	1994	C
	RR	200 mg	ZEN	20 g	NS	Brown discoloration forms in 1 hr at room temperature	1994	I
Enalaprilat	MSD	50 mg	ZEN	1 and 20 g	NS	Visually compatible for 4 hr at room temperature	1994	C
Fluconazole	RR	2 g	ZEN	1 and 20 g	NS	Visually compatible for 4 hr at room temperature	1994	C
Furosemide	HO	1 g	ZEN	1 and 20 g	NS	Visually compatible for 4 hr at room temperature	1994	C
Gentamicin sulfate	SCH	800 mg	ZEN	1 and 20 g	NS	Visually compatible for 4 hr at room temperature	1994	C
Heparin sodium	ES	20,000 units	ZEN	1 and 20 g	NS	Visually compatible for 4 hr at room temperature	1994	C
Insulin, regular	LI	1000 units	ZEN	1 and 20 g	NS	Visually compatible for 4 hr at room temperature	1994	C
Magnesium sulfate	AST	1 g	ZEN	1 and 20 g	NS	Visually compatible for 4 hr at room temperature	1994	C

Additive Compatibility (Cont.)

Meropenem

Drug	Mfr	Conc/L	Mfr	Conc/L	Test Soln	Remarks	Ref	C/I
Metoclopramide HCl	RB	100 mg	ZEN	1 and 20 g	NS	Visually compatible for 4 hr at room temperature	1994	C
Metronidazole HCl	SE	5 g	ZEN	1 and 20 g	NS	Discoloration forms	2068	I
Morphine sulfate	ES	1 g	ZEN	1 and 20 g	NS	Visually compatible for 4 hr at room temperature	1994	C
Multivitamins	AST	50 ml	ZEN	1 and 20 g	NS	Color darkened in 4 hr at room temperature	1994	I
Norepinephrine bitartrate	WI	8 g	ZEN	1 and 20 g	NS	Visually compatible for 4 hr at room temperature	1994	C
Ondansetron HCl	GL	1 g	ZEN	1 g	NS	Visually compatible for 4 hr at room temperature	1994	C
	GL	1 g	ZEN	20 g	NS	White precipitate forms immediately	1994	I
Phenobarbital sodium	ES	200 mg	ZEN	1 and 20 g	NS	Visually compatible for 4 hr at room temperature	1994	C
Ranitidine HCl	GL	100 mg	ZEN	1 and 20 g	NS	Visually compatible for 4 hr at room temperature	1994	C
Vancomycin HCl	LI	1 g	ZEN	1 and 20 g	NS	Visually compatible for 4 hr at room temperature	1994	C
Zidovudine	BW	4 g	ZEN	1 g	NS	Visually compatible for 4 hr at room temperature	1994	C
	BW	4 g	ZEN	20 g	NS	Dark yellow discoloration forms in 4 hr at room temperature	1994	I

Y-Site Injection Compatibility (1:1 Mixture)

Meropenem

Drug	Mfr	Conc	Mfr	Conc	Remarks	Ref	C/I
Acyclovir sodium	BW	5 mg/ml[c]	ZEN	1 mg/ml[b]	Visually compatible for 4 hr at room temperature	1994	C
	BW	5 mg/ml[c]	ZEN	50 mg/ml[c]	Precipitate forms	2068	I
Aminophylline	AMR	25 mg/ml	ZEN	1 and 50 mg/ml[b]	Visually compatible for 4 hr at room temperature	1994	C
Amphotericin B	SQ	5 mg/ml	ZEN	1 and 50 mg/ml[b]	Precipitate forms	2068	I
Atenolol	ICI	0.5 mg/ml	ZEN	1 and 50 mg/ml[b]	Visually compatible for 4 hr at room temperature	1994	C
Atropine sulfate	ES	0.4 mg/ml[c]	ZEN	1 and 50 mg/ml[b]	Visually compatible for 4 hr at room temperature	1994	C
Calcium gluconate	AMR	4 mg/ml[c]	ZEN	1 mg/ml[b]	Visually compatible for 4 hr at room temperature	1994	C
	AMR	4 mg/ml[c]	ZEN	50 mg/ml[b]	Yellow discoloration forms in 4 hr at room temperature	1994	I
Cimetidine HCl	SKB	150 mg/ml	ZEN	1 and 50 mg/ml[b]	Visually compatible for 4 hr at room temperature	1994	C
Dexamethasone sodium phosphate	MSD	10 mg/ml[c]	ZEN	1 and 50 mg/ml[b]	Visually compatible for 4 hr at room temperature	1994	C

Y-Site Injection Compatibility (1:1 Mixture) (Cont.)

		Meropenem					
Drug	*Mfr*	*Conc*	*Mfr*	*Conc*	*Remarks*	*Ref*	*C/I*
Diazepam	RC	5 mg/ml	ZEN	1 and 50 mg/ml[b]	White precipitate forms immediately	1994	I
Digoxin	BW	0.25 mg/ml	ZEN	1 and 50 mg/ml[b]	Visually compatible for 4 hr at room temperature	1994	C
Diphenhydramine HCl	PD	50 mg/ml	ZEN	1 and 50 mg/ml[b]	Visually compatible for 4 hr at room temperature	1994	C
Docetaxel	RPR	0.9 mg/ml[a]	ZEN	20 mg/ml[b]	Physically compatible with no change in measured turbidity or increase in particle content in 4 hr at 23 °C	2224	C
Doxycycline hyclate	RR	1 mg/ml[c]	ZEN	1 mg/ml[b]	Visually compatible for 4 hr at room temperature	1994	C
	RR	1 mg/ml[c]	ZEN	50 mg/ml[b]	Amber discoloration forms within 30 min	1994	I
Enalaprilat	MSD	0.05 mg/ml[c]	ZEN	1 and 50 mg/ml[b]	Visually compatible for 4 hr at room temperature	1994	C
Fluconazole	RR	2 mg/ml	ZEN	1 and 50 mg/ml[b]	Visually compatible for 4 hr at room temperature	1994	C
Furosemide	HO	10 mg/ml	ZEN	1 and 50 mg/ml[b]	Visually compatible for 4 hr at room temperature	1994	C
Gentamicin sulfate	SCH	4 mg/ml[c]	ZEN	1 and 50 mg/ml[b]	Visually compatible for 4 hr at room temperature	1994	C
Heparin sodium	ES	1 unit/ml[c]	ZEN	1 and 50 mg/ml[b]	Visually compatible for 4 hr at room temperature	1994	C
Insulin, regular	LI	0.2 unit/ml[c]	ZEN	1 and 50 mg/ml[b]	Visually compatible for 4 hr at room temperature	1994	C
Metoclopramide HCl	RB	5 mg/ml	ZEN	1 and 50 mg/ml[b]	Visually compatible for 4 hr at room temperature	1994	C
Metronidazole HCl	SE	5 mg/ml[c]	ZEN	1 and 50 mg/ml[b]	Discoloration forms	2068	I
Morphine sulfate	ES	1 mg/ml[c]	ZEN	1 and 50 mg/ml[b]	Visually compatible for 4 hr at room temperature	1994	C
Norepinephrine bitartrate	WI	1 mg/ml[c]	ZEN	1 and 50 mg/ml[b]	Visually compatible for 4 hr at room temperature	1994	C
Ondansetron HCl	GL	1 mg/ml[c]	ZEN	1 mg/ml[b]	Visually compatible for 4 hr at room temperature	1994	C
	GL	1 mg/ml[c]	ZEN	50 mg/ml[b]	White precipitate forms immediately	1994	I
Phenobarbital sodium	ES	0.32 mg/ml[c]	ZEN	1 and 50 mg/ml[b]	Visually compatible for 4 hr at room temperature	1994	C
TNA #218 to #226[d]			ZEN	20 mg/ml[a]	Visually compatible with no precipitate or emulsion damage apparent in 4 hr at 23 °C	2215	C
Vancomycin HCl	LI	5 mg/ml[c]	ZEN	1 and 50 mg/ml[b]	Visually compatible for 4 hr at room temperature	1994	C
Zidovudine	BW	4 mg/ml[c]	ZEN	1 mg/ml[b]	Visually compatible for 4 hr at room temperature	1994	C

Y-Site Injection Compatibility (1:1 Mixture) (Cont.)

Meropenem

Drug	Mfr	Conc	Mfr	Conc	Remarks	Ref	C/I
	BW	4 mg/ml[c]	ZEN	50 mg/ml[b]	Yellow discoloration forms in 4 hr at room temperature	1994	I

[a]*Tested in dextrose 5% in water.*
[b]*Tested in sodium chloride 0.9%.*
[c]*Tested in sterile water for injection.*
[d]*Refer to Appendix I for the composition of parenteral nutrition solutions. TNA indicates a 3-in-1 admixture.*

Additional Compatibility Information

Infusion Solutions— Meropenem 1 to 20 mg/ml as infusion admixtures is stable for the time periods indicated in the following infusion solutions (2):

	Time (hr)	
Infusion Solution	Stored at 15–25 °C	Stored at 4 °C
Dextrose 2.5% in sodium chloride 0.45%	3	12
Dextrose 5% and potassium chloride 0.15%	1	6
Dextrose 5% in Ringer's injection, lactated	1	4
Dextrose 5% in sodium chloride 0.2%	1	4
Dextrose 5% in sodium chloride 0.9%	1	2
Dextrose 5% in water	1	4
Dextrose 5% in water with sodium bicarbonate 0.02%	1	6
Dextrose 10% in water	1	2
Mannitol 2.5%	2	16
Normosol M with dextrose 5%	1	8
Ringer's injection	4	24
Ringer's injection, lactated	4	12
Sodium bicarbonate 5%	1	4
Sodium chloride 0.9%	4	24
Sodium lactate ⅙ M	2	24

MESNA
AHFS 92:00

Mesnex   **Bristol-Myers Squibb**

Products— Mesna (Bristol-Myers Squibb) is available as a 100-mg/ml solution in 2-ml ampuls and 10-ml multidose vials. Each milliliter of solution also contains edetate disodium 0.25 mg and sodium hydroxide to adjust the pH. In addition, the multidose vials contain benzyl alcohol 10.4 mg/ml (2).

pH— From 6.5 to 8.5 (2).

Osmolality— Mesna 100 mg/ml has an osmolality of 1563 mOsm/kg (1689).

Administration— Mesna may be administered by intravenous injection or infusion (2; 4). Infusion is usually performed over 15 to 30 minutes, but continuous infusion has also been utilized (4). Dilution to a concentration of 20 mg/ml in a compatible solution is recommended for intravenous infusion (2; 4).

Stability— Intact ampuls of mesna should be stored at room temperature. The solution is clear and colorless (2) and is not light sensitive (72). When exposed to oxygen, mesna oxidizes to the disulfide form, dimesna. Unused mesna injection in opened ampuls should be discarded after dose preparation. However, the multidose vials may be stored and used for up to eight days after initial entry (2).

Syringes— The short-term use of plastic syringes for preparing mesna infusions appears to be satisfactory. However, extended storage of mesna in a plastic syringe with a luer tip resulted in the formation of dark or thread-like particles and a change in viscosity after 12 hours at room temperature. Similar behavior also occurred in a glass syringe (72).

Mesna (Asta Pharma) 100 mg/ml was packaged as 10 ml in 20-ml polypropylene syringes (Becton-Dickinson). Samples having the air expelled from the syringes were stored at 5, 24, and 35 °C, and samples with air drawn into the syringes were stored at 24 °C. After nine days of storage, little or no change in the mesna concentration was determined by colorimetric analysis for thiols and disulfides in all samples with no air present. The maximum loss was less than 4% found in the samples stored at 35 °C. However, the syringes containing air exhibited 10% loss in eight days at 24 °C. Minimizing the exposure of mesna to air during storage was recommended to slow the formation of dimesna (2181).

Compatibility Information

Solution Compatibility

Mesna

Solution	Mfr	Mfr	Conc/L	Remarks	Ref	C/I
Dextrose 5% in sodium chloride 0.45%		AW	1 g	4% loss in 72 hr at room temperature	72	**C**
		AW	20 g	5% loss in 48 hr at room temperature	72	**C**
Dextrose 5% in water		AW	1 g	5% loss in 24 hr and 13% in 48 hr at room temperature	72	**C**
		AW	20 g	5% loss in 48 hr at room temperature	72	**C**
Ringer's injection, lactated		AW	1 g	4% loss in 24 hr and 11% in 48 hr at room temperature	72	**C**
Sodium chloride 0.9%		AW	1 g	10% loss in 48 hr at room temperature	72	**C**

Additive Compatibility

Mesna

Drug	Mfr	Conc/L	Mfr	Conc/L	Test Soln	Remarks	Ref	C/I
Carboplatin		1 g		1 g	W	More than 10% carboplatin loss within 24 hr at room temperature	1379	**I**
Cisplatin		67 mg		3.33 g	NS	Cisplatin not detected after 1 hr	1291	**I**
		67 mg		110 mg	NS	Cisplatin weakly detected after 1 hr	1291	**I**
Hydroxyzine HCl	LY	500 mg	AW	3 g	D5W[a]	Physically compatible for 48 hr	1190	**C**
Ifosfamide	MJ	3.3 g	AW	3.3 g	D5W, LR	Physically compatible with no ifosfamide loss and about 5% mesna loss in 24 hr at 21 °C exposed to light	72	**C**
	MJ	5 g	AW	5 g	D5W, LR	Physically compatible with no ifosfamide loss and about 5% mesna loss in 24 hr at 21 °C exposed to light	72	**C**
		50 g		40 g	NS	Both drugs stable for 14 days at room temperature	1380	**C**
	BI	83.3 g	BI	79 g	NS	Little or no ifosfamide loss in 9 days at room temperature and 7% loss in 9 days at 37 °C. Mesna not tested	1494	**C**
		2.6 g		1.6 g	D5S[b]	No increase in decomposition products in 8 hr at room temperature	1495	**C**
	BR	600 mg	BR	600 mg	D5½S, D5W, LR, NS[c]	Chemically stable for at least 24 hr at room temperature	1496	**C**
Ifosfamide with epirubicin HCl		50 g 500 mg		80 g	NS	More than 50% epirubicin loss in 7 days at room temperature	1380	**I**

[a]Tested in glass containers.
[b]Tested in polyethylene containers.
[c]Tested in PVC containers.

Drugs in Syringe Compatibility

Mesna

Drug (in syringe)	Mfr	Amt	Mfr	Amt	Remarks	Ref	C/I
Ifosfamide		500 mg/ 10 ml		400 mg/ 10 ml	3% ifosfamide loss in 7 days and 12% in 4 weeks at 4 °C and room temperature. No mesna loss	1290	**C**

Drugs in Syringe Compatibility (Cont.)

Drug (in syringe)	Mfr	Amt	Mfr	Amt	Remarks	Ref	C/I
		50 mg/ml[a]		40 mg/ml[a]	Little or no loss of either drug by HPLC in 28 days at 4 and 20 °C	1564	C
Ifosfamide with epirubicin HCl		50 mg/ml[a] 1 mg/ml[a]		40 mg/ml[a]	50% epirubicin loss by HPLC in 7 days at 4 and 20 °C. No loss of other drugs in 7 days	1564	I

[a] Diluted with sodium chloride 0.9%.

Y-Site Injection Compatibility (1:1 Mixture)

Mesna

Drug	Mfr	Conc	Mfr	Conc	Remarks	Ref	C/I
Allopurinol sodium	BW	3 mg/ml[b]	MJ	10 mg/ml[b]	Physically compatible with no change in measured turbidity or increase in particle content in 4 hr at 22 °C	1686	C
Amifostine	USB	10 mg/ml[a]	MJ	10 mg/ml[a]	Physically compatible with no change in measured turbidity or increase in particle content in 4 hr at 23 °C	1845	C
Amphotericin B cholesteryl sulfate complex	SEQ	0.83 mg/ml[a]	MJ	10 mg/ml[a]	Microprecipitate forms immediately	2117	I
Aztreonam	SQ	40 mg/ml[a]	MJ	10 mg/ml[a]	Physically compatible with no subvisual haze or particle formation in 4 hr at 23 °C	1758	C
Cefepime HCl	BR	20 mg/ml[a]	MJ	10 mg/ml[a]	Physically compatible with no change in measured turbidity or increase in particle content in 4 hr at 22 °C	1689	C
Cladribine	ORT	0.015[b] and 0.5[c] mg/ml	MJ	10 mg/ml[b]	Physically compatible with no change in measured turbidity or increase in particle content in 4 hr at 23 °C	1969	C
Docetaxel	RPR	0.9 mg/ml[a]	MJ	10 mg/ml[a]	Physically compatible with no change in measured turbidity or increase in particle content in 4 hr at 23 °C	2224	C
Doxorubicin HCl liposome injection	SEQ	0.4 mg/ml[a]	MJ	10 mg/ml[a]	Physically compatible with little or no change in measured turbidity and no increase in particle content in 4 hr at 23 °C	2087	C
Etoposide phosphate	BR	5 mg/ml[a]	MJ	10 mg/ml[a]	Physically compatible with no change in measured turbidity or increase in particle content in 4 hr at 23 °C	2218	C
Filgrastim	AMG	30 μg/ml[a]	MJ	10 mg/ml[a]	Physically compatible with no change in measured turbidity or increase in particle content in 4 hr at 22 °C	1687	C
Fludarabine phosphate	BR	1 mg/ml[a]	BR	10 mg/ml[a]	Physically compatible for 4 hr at room temperature under fluorescent light	1439	C
Gemcitabine HCl	LI	10 mg/ml[b]	MJ	10 mg/ml[b]	Physically compatible with no change in measured turbidity or increase in particle content in 4 hr at 23 °C	2226	C
Granisetron HCl	SKB	1 mg/ml	MJ	4 mg/ml[b]	Physically compatible with little or no loss of either drug by HPLC in 4 hr at 22 °C	1883	C

Y-Site Injection Compatibility (1:1 Mixture) (Cont.)

Drug	Mfr	Conc	Mfr	Conc	Remarks	Ref	C/I
			Mesna				
Melphalan HCl	BW	0.1 mg/ml[b]	BR	10 mg/ml[b]	Physically compatible with no change in measured turbidity or increase in particle content in 3 hr at 22 °C	1557	C
Methotrexate sodium		30 mg/ml		1.8 mg/ml[a]	Visually compatible for 4 hr at room temperature	1788	C
Ondansetron HCl	GL	1 mg/ml[b]	BR	10 mg/ml[a]	Physically compatible for 4 hr at 22 °C	1365	C
Paclitaxel	NCI	1.2 mg/ml[a]	MJ	10 mg/ml[a]	Physically compatible with no change in measured turbidity in 4 hr at 22 °C	1556	C
Piperacillin sodium–tazobactam sodium	LE	40 + 5 mg/ml[a]	MJ	10 mg/ml[a]	Physically compatible with no change in measured turbidity or increase in particle content in 4 hr at 22 °C	1688	C
Sargramostim	IMM	10 μg/ml[b]	MJ	10 mg/ml[b]	Physically compatible for 4 hr at 22 °C	1436	C
Sodium bicarbonate		1.4%		1.8 mg/ml[a]	Visually compatible for 4 hr at room temperature	1788	C
Teniposide	BR	0.1 mg/ml[a]	MJ	10 mg/ml[a]	Physically compatible with no subvisual haze or particle formation in 4 hr at 23 °C	1725	C
Thiotepa	IMM[d]	1 mg/ml[a]	MJ	10 mg/ml[a]	Physically compatible with no change in measured turbidity or increase in particle content in 4 hr at 23 °C	1861	C
TNA #218 to #226[e]			MJ	10 mg/ml[a]	Visually compatible with no precipitate or emulsion damage apparent in 4 hr at 23 °C	2215	C
TPN #212 to #215[e]			MJ	10 mg/ml[a]	Physically compatible with no change in measured turbidity or increase in particle content in 4 hr at 23 °C	2109	C
Vinorelbine tartrate	BW	1 mg/ml[b]	MJ	10 mg/ml[b]	Physically compatible with no change in measured turbidity or increase in particle content in 4 hr at 22 °C under fluorescent light	1558	C

[a]Tested in dextrose 5% in water.
[b]Tested in sodium chloride 0.9%.
[c]Tested in bacteriostatic sodium chloride 0.9% preserved with benzyl alcohol 0.9%.
[d]Lyophilized formulation tested.
[e]Refer to Appendix I for the composition of parenteral nutrition solutions. TNA indicates a 3-in-1 admixture, and TPN indicates a 2-in-1 admixture.

Additional Compatibility Information

Solutions— The manufacturer states that mesna is chemically and physically stable for 24 hours at 25 °C diluted to 20 mg/ml in the following infusion solutions (2):

Dextrose 5% in sodium chloride 0.2%
Dextrose 5% in sodium chloride 0.33%
Dextrose 5% in sodium chloride 0.45%
Dextrose 5% in water
Ringer's injection, lactated
Sodium chloride 0.9%

Other information indicates that admixtures may be stable for a longer time (72). (See the Solution Compatibility table.)

Cyclophosphamide and Ifosfamide— Mesna is stated to be stable for 24 hours in dextrose 5% in water or Ringer's injection, lactated, when admixed with cyclophosphamide or ifosfamide (4; 1292).

METARAMINOL BITARTRATE
AHFS 12:12

Aramine   **Merck**

Products— Metaraminol bitartrate (Merck) is available in 10-ml vials containing, in each milliliter, metaraminol bitartrate equivalent to metaraminol 10 mg, sodium chloride 4.4 mg, methylparaben 0.15%, propylparaben 0.02%, and sodium bisulfite 0.2% in water for injection (2).

pH— From 3.2 to 4.5 (4).

Osmolality— Metaraminol bitartrate 10 mg/ml has an osmolality of 290 mOsm/kg (1689).

Administration— Metaraminol bitartrate may be administered by intramuscular or subcutaneous injection and by direct intravenous injection in severe shock. The drug may also be given by intravenous infusion, usually in 500 ml of dextrose 5% in water or sodium chloride 0.9%, although the volume may be varied depending on the rate of administration and the patient's fluid needs (2; 4; 8; 19). Some clinicians recommend avoiding subcutaneous injection because of the possibility of local tissue injury (4).

Stability— Metaraminol bitartrate injection is a clear, colorless solution. Intact containers should be stored at controlled room temperature and protected from light. Temperatures above 40 °C and below −20 °C should be avoided (2; 4). Although the drug is sensitive to excessive heat (7), the manufacturer states that the vial can be sterilized by autoclaving as well as by immersion in a sterilizing solution (2).

pH Effects— Metaraminol bitartrate appears to be stable over a wide pH range. A stability profile of 100 mg/L in dextrose 5% in water at pH 3.6 to 7.6 did not show any significant loss in potency during 24 hours (7). Another study showed that metaraminol bitartrate 10, 20, and 30 mg/L in various buffer solutions ranging from pH 2.1 to 9.9 was stable for 48 hours (43).

Sorption— Metaraminol bitartrate 68 mg/L in sodium chloride 0.9% (Travenol) in PVC bags did not exhibit significant sorption to the plastic during one week of storage at room temperature (15 to 20 °C) (536).

In another study, metaraminol bitartrate 68 mg/L in sodium chloride 0.9% did not exhibit any loss due to sorption during a seven-hour simulated infusion through an infusion set (Travenol) consisting of a cellulose propionate burette chamber and 170 cm of PVC tubing (606).

The drug was also tested as a simulated infusion over at least one hour by a syringe pump system. A glass syringe on a syringe pump was fitted with 20 cm of polyethylene tubing or 50 cm of Silastic tubing. No loss of drug due to sorption was observed with either tubing (606).

A 25-ml aliquot of metaraminol bitartrate 68 mg/L in sodium chloride 0.9% stored in all-plastic syringes composed of polypropylene barrels and polyethylene plungers for 24 hours at room temperature in the dark did not exhibit any loss due to sorption (606).

Compatibility Information

Solution Compatibility

Metaraminol bitartrate

Solution	Mfr	Mfr	Conc/L	Remarks	Ref	C/I
Alcohol 5%, dextrose 5%	BA	MSD	1 g	Physically compatible for 24 hr	315	C
Amino acids 4.25%, dextrose 25%	MG	MSD	100 mg	No increase in particulate matter in 24 hr at 5 °C	349	C
Dextran 40,000	PH	MSD		Compatible	44	C
Dextran 6% in sodium chloride 0.9%	AB	MSD	100 mg	Potency retained for 24 hr	7	C
Dextrose 5% in Ringer's injection, lactated	TR[a]	MSD	100 mg	Potency retained for 24 hr at 5 °C	282	C
	BA	MSD	1 g	Physically compatible for 24 hr	315	C
Dextrose 5% in sodium chloride 0.9%	AB	MSD	100 mg	Potency retained for 24 hr	7	C
	AB	MSD	100 mg	Potency retained for 48 hr	46	C
		MSD	100, 200, 300 mg	Potency retained for 48 hr	43	C
	TR[a]	MSD	100 mg	Potency retained for 24 hr at 5 °C	282	C
	BA	MSD	1 g	Physically compatible for 24 hr	315	C
Dextrose 5% in water	AB	MSD	100 mg	Potency retained for 24 hr	7	C
	AB	MSD	100 mg	Potency retained for 48 hr	46	C
	TR[a]	MSD	100 mg	Potency retained for 24 hr	282	C
	BA	MSD	1 g	Physically compatible for 24 hr	315	C
Dextrose 10% in water	BA	MSD	1 g	Physically compatible for 24 hr	315	C
Dextrose 20% in water	BA	MSD	1 g	Physically compatible for 24 hr	315	C
Fructose 10% in water	BA	MSD	1 g	Physically compatible for 24 hr	315	C

Solution Compatibility (Cont.)

Metaraminol bitartrate

Solution	Mfr	Mfr	Conc/L	Remarks	Ref	C/I
Invert sugar 10% in Electrolyte #1	BA	MSD	1 g	Physically compatible for 24 hr	315	C
Invert sugar 10% in Electrolyte #2	BA	MSD	1 g	Physically compatible for 24 hr	315	C
Multielectrolyte solution	AB	MSD	100 mg	Potency retained for 48 hr	46	C
Normosol M in dextrose 5%	AB	MSD	100 mg	Potency retained for 24 hr	7	C
Normosol R	AB	MSD	100 mg	Potency retained for 24 hr	7	C
Normosol R, pH 7.4	AB	MSD	100 mg	Potency retained for 24 hr	7	C
Polysal M with dextrose 5%	CU	MSD	1 g	Physically compatible for 24 hr	315	C
Ringer's injection	AB	MSD	100 mg	Potency retained for 24 hr	7	C
Ringer's injection, lactated	AB	MSD	100 mg	Potency retained for 24 hr	7	C
	TR[a]	MSD	100 mg	Potency retained for 24 hr at 5 °C	282	C
	BA	MSD	1 g	Physically compatible for 24 hr	315	C
	AB	MSD	100 mg	Physically incompatible	15	I
Sodium bicarbonate 5%	AB	MSD	100 mg	Potency retained for 24 hr	7	C
Sodium chloride 0.9%	AB	MSD	100 mg	Potency retained for 24 hr	7	C
	AB	MSD	100 mg	Potency retained for 48 hr	46	C
	BA	MSD		Potency retained for 24 hr	45	C
	TR[a]	MSD	100 mg	Potency retained for 24 hr at 5 °C	282	C
	TR[b]	MSD		Potency retained for 24 hr	45	C
	BA	MSD	1 g	Physically compatible for 24 hr	315	C
Sodium lactate ⅙ M	BA	MSD	1 g	Physically compatible for 24 hr	315	C

[a]Tested in both glass and PVC containers.
[b]Tested in PVC containers.

Additive Compatibility

Metaraminol bitartrate

Drug	Mfr	Conc/L	Mfr	Conc/L	Test Soln	Remarks	Ref	C/I
Amikacin sulfate	BR	5 g	BR	200 mg	D5LR, D5R, D5S, D5W, D10W, IS10, LR, NS, R, SL	Physically compatible and potency of both retained for 24 hr at 25 °C	294	C
Amphotericin B		200 mg	BP	200 mg	D5W	Haze develops over 3 hr	26	I
Chloramphenicol sodium succinate	PD	1 g	MSD	100 mg		Physically compatible	7	C
	PD	1 g	MSD	200 mg		Physically compatible	6	C
Cibenzoline succinate		2 g	MSD	1 g	D5W, NS	Physically compatible for 24 hr at 25 °C by visual and microscopic examination	1182	C
Cimetidine HCl	SKF	3 g	MSD	1 g	D5W	Physically compatible and cimetidine chemically stable for 24 hr at room temperature. Metaraminol not tested	551	C
Cyanocobalamin	AB	1000 μg	MSD	100 mg		Physically compatible	7	C
Dexamethasone sodium phosphate	MSD	20 mg	MSD	100 mg	D5W, NS	Altered UV spectrum for dexamethasone within 1 hr at room temperature	42	I

Additive Compatibility (Cont.)

Metaraminol bitartrate

Drug	Mfr	Conc/L	Mfr	Conc/L	Test Soln	Remarks	Ref	C/I
	MSD	100 mg	MSD	500 mg	D5W	Altered UV spectrum for dexamethasone within 1 hr at room temperature	42	I
Dobutamine HCl	LI	1 g	MSD	100 mg	D5W, NS	Physically compatible for 24 hr at 21 °C	812	C
Ephedrine sulfate	AB	50 mg	MSD	100 mg		Physically compatible	7	C
Epinephrine HCl	PD	4 mg	MSD	100 mg		Physically compatible	7	C
Erythromycin lactobionate	AB	750 mg	MSD	100 mg	D5W	92% erythromycin decomposition in 24 hr at 25 °C	20	I
	AB	1 g	MSD	100 mg	D5W	44% erythromycin decomposition in 6 hr at 25 °C	48	I
Fibrinogen	CU	2 g	MSD	200 mg	D5W	Physically incompatible	11	I
Hydrocortisone sodium phosphate	MSD	250 mg	MSD	500 mg	D5W, NS	UV spectra of both not altered in 8 hr at room temperature	42	C
Hydrocortisone sodium succinate	UP	100 mg	MSD	100 mg	D5S	Potency of both retained for 24 hr	43	C
			MSD			Physically incompatible	9	I
	UP	250 mg	MSD	100 mg		Precipitate forms within 1 hr	7	I
	UP	200 and 300 mg	MSD	100, 200, 300 mg	D5S	Precipitate forms and chemical decomposition of hydrocortisone	43	I
		250 mg	MSD	500 mg	D5W, NS	Precipitate forms within 1 hr	42	I
Lidocaine HCl	AST	2 g	MSD	100 mg		Physically compatible	24	C
Methylprednisolone sodium succinate	UP	125 mg	MSD	400 mg	D5W, NS	Precipitate forms within 4 hr	42	I
Oxytocin	PD	5 units	MSD	100 mg		Physically compatible	7	C
Penicillin G potassium	SQ	1 million units	MSD	100 mg	D5W	59% penicillin decomposition in 24 hr at 25 °C	47	I
	[a]	900,000 units	MSD	100 mg	D5W	17% penicillin decomposition in 6 hr at 25 °C	48	I
Phenytoin sodium	PD		MSD			Physically incompatible	9	I
Potassium chloride	AB	40 mEq	MSD	100 mg		Physically compatible	7	C
Promazine HCl	WY	100 mg	MSD	100 mg		Physically compatible	7	C
Sodium bicarbonate	AB	3.75 g	MSD	100 mg		Physically compatible	7	C
	AB	4.8 mEq[b]	MSD	100 mg	D5W	Physically compatible for 24 hr	772	C
Thiopental sodium	AB	2.5 g	MSD	200 mg	D5W	Precipitate forms within 1 hr	21	I
	AB	2.5 g	MSD	100 mg		Precipitate forms within 1 hr	7	I
	AB	2.5 g	MSD	200 mg	D5W	Physically incompatible	11	I
Verapamil HCl	KN	80 mg	MSD	20 mg	D5W, NS	Physically compatible for 24 hr	764	C

[a]A buffered preparation was specified.
[b]Two vials of Neut added to a liter of admixture.

Y-Site Injection Compatibility (1:1 Mixture)

Metaraminol bitartrate

Drug	Mfr	Conc	Mfr	Conc	Remarks	Ref	C/I
Amiodarone HCl	LZ	4 mg/ml[a]	MSD	0.2 mg/ml[a]	Physically compatible for 24 hr at 21 °C	1032	C
Amrinone lactate	WB	3 mg/ml[b]	MSD	0.2 mg/ml[c]	Physically compatible for at least 4 hr at 25 °C under fluorescent light	992	C

Y-Site Injection Compatibility (1:1 Mixture) (Cont.)

Metaraminol bitartrate

Drug	Mfr	Conc	Mfr	Conc	Remarks	Ref	C/I
Warfarin sodium	DU	0.1[a] and 2 mg/ml[d]	MSD	0.2 mg/ml[a]	Physically compatible with no change in measured turbidity or increase in particle content in 24 hr at 23 °C	2011	C

[a]*Tested in both dextrose 5% in water and sodium chloride 0.9%.*
[b]*Tested in sodium chloride 0.9%.*
[c]*Tested in dextrose 5% in water.*
[d]*Tested in sterile water for injection.*

Additional Compatibility Information

Solutions—— At a concentration of 100 mg/L, metaraminol bitartrate is physically compatible with all Abbott infusion solutions (7). The manufacturer indicates that metaraminol bitartrate (MSD) is physically compatible and chemically stable at a concentration of 100 mg/L in the following infusion solutions (2; 4):

Dextran 6% in sodium chloride 0.9%
Dextrose 5% in sodium chloride 0.9%
Dextrose 5% in water
Normosol M in dextrose 5% in water
Normosol R
Normosol R, pH 7.4
Ringer's injection
Ringer's injection, lactated
Sodium bicarbonate 5%
Sodium chloride 0.9%

Use of the infusions within 24 hours is recommended because no preservatives are present in the solutions (2).

Acid-Sensitive Drugs—— Physical incompatibilities with metaraminol bitartrate may involve precipitation of drugs with poor solubility in an acidic medium. The incompatibilities occur to varying extents, depending on the concentration of the various additives and metaraminol bitartrate in the infusion solution. Examples include sodium salts of barbituric acid and sulfonamides. In addition, the rate of decomposition of acid-sensitive drugs such as penicillin G, erythromycin lactobionate, and nafcillin sodium may be increased (6; 7; 20; 27). Metaraminol bitartrate should not be mixed with acid-labile drugs (7).

Ranitidine—— Metaraminol bitartrate is stated to be incompatible with ranitidine HCl (1515).

Concentrated Solutions—— The following incompatibility determinations were performed in concentrated solutions. The drugs in dry form were constituted according to the manufacturers' recommendations. One milliliter of metaraminol bitartrate was added to 5 ml of sterile distilled water along with 1 ml of each of the following drugs. Particulate matter was noted within two hours (28):

Penicillin G potassium
Phenytoin sodium (Parke-Davis)

METHADONE HCL
AHFS 28:08.08

Dolophine Hydrochloride　　　　　　　　　**Roxane**

Products—— Methadone HCl (Roxane) is available 20-ml multidose vials. Each milliliter of solution contains methadone HCl 10 mg and sodium chloride 0.9% with sodium hydroxide and/or hydrochloric acid to adjust the pH. In addition, the 20-ml vials contain chlorobutanol 0.5% (1-5/26/95).

pH—— From 3 to 6.5 (4).

Administration—— Methadone HCl may be administered by subcutaneous or intramuscular injection (4).

Stability—— Methadone HCl in intact vials should be stored at controlled room temperature and protected from light (1-5/26/95).

Compatibility Information

Solution Compatibility

Methadone HCl

Solution	Mfr	Mfr	Conc/L	Remarks	Ref	C/I
Sodium chloride 0.9%	TR[a]	LI	1, 2, 5 g	Little or no loss by HPLC in 28 days at room temperature exposed to light	1500	C

[a]*Tested in PVC containers.*

METHOHEXITAL SODIUM
AHFS 28:24.04

Brevital Sodium   **Jones Pharma, Inc.**

Products— Methohexital sodium (Jones Pharma, Inc.) is available in 50-ml vials (with or without accompanying vials of sterile water for injection) containing methohexital sodium 500 mg with anhydrous sodium carbonate 30 mg, in vials containing methohexital sodium 2.5 g with sodium carbonate 150 mg, and in vials containing methohexital sodium 5 g with sodium carbonate 300 mg (1-5/7/96).

To prepare a 1% (10 mg/ml) solution of methohexital sodium, reconstitute with sterile water for injection, preferably, or dextrose 5% in water or sodium chloride 0.9% in the following amounts. Do not use diluents containing bacteriostats (1-5/7/96).

Size	Reconstitution Volume	Final Volume of Diluent
500 mg in 50-ml vial		50 ml
2.5 g in vial	15 ml	250 ml
5 g in vial	30 ml	500 ml

The initial dilution of the 2.5- and 5-g vials results in a yellow solution. When further diluted, the solution must be clear and colorless or it should not be used (1-5/7/96; 4).

To prepare a 0.2% (2 mg/ml) solution of methohexital sodium, add 500 mg to 250 ml of dextrose 5% in water or sodium chloride 0.9%. Sterile water for injection should not be used for this concentration to avoid extreme hypotonicity (1-5/7/96).

pH— A 0.2% solution in dextrose 5% in water has a pH of 9.5 to 10.5; a 1% solution in sterile water for injection has a pH of 10 to 11 (4).

Sodium Content— Methohexital sodium contains 4.652 mEq of sodium per gram of drug; the sodium carbonate provides 1.132 mEq while the balance comes from the drug itself (869).

Administration— Methohexital sodium is administered intravenously, by injection or continuous infusion, in concentrations no higher than 1%. Intra-arterial injection and extravasation should be avoided (4).

Stability— Intact vials should be stored at controlled room temperature (1-5/7/96; 4). Solutions of methohexital sodium in sterile water for injection are stable at 25 °C or below for at least six weeks. In dextrose 5% in water or sodium chloride 0.9%, it is stable for about 24 hours (4).

Methohexital sodium is alkaline in solution and is incompatible with acidic solutions and phenol-containing solutions (4).

Sorption— Methohexital sodium (Lilly) 32 mg/L displayed 7.9% sorption to a PVC plastic test strip in 24 hours (12). However, another test did not confirm this finding. No significant loss in PVC containers and no difference between glass and PVC containers were found (282).

Compatibility Information

Solution Compatibility

Methohexital sodium

Solution	Mfr	Mfr	Conc/L	Remarks	Ref	C/I
Dextrose 5% in Ringer's injection, lactated	TR[a]	LI	2 g	Potency retained for 24 hr at 5 °C	282	C
Dextrose 5% in sodium chloride 0.9%	TR[a]	LI	2 g	Potency retained for 24 hr at 5 °C	282	C
Dextrose 5% in water	TR[a]	LI	2 g	Potency retained for 24 hr at 5 °C	282	C
Ringer's injection, lactated	TR[a]	LI	2 g	Potency retained for 24 hr at 5 °C	282	C
Sodium chloride 0.9%	TR[a]	LI	2 g	Potency retained for 24 hr at 5 °C	282	C

[a]*Tested in both glass and PVC containers.*

Additive Compatibility

Methohexital sodium

Drug	Mfr	Conc/L	Mfr	Conc/L	Test Soln	Remarks	Ref	C/I
Chlorpromazine HCl	BP	200 mg	BP	2 g	D5W, NS	Immediate precipitation	26	I
Hydralazine HCl	BP	80 mg	BP	2 g	D5W, NS	Yellow color and precipitate forms within 3 hr	26	I
Kanamycin sulfate	BPC	4 g	BP	2 g	D5W, NS	Immediate precipitation	26	I
Lidocaine HCl	BP	2 g	BP	2 g	D5W	Immediate precipitation	26	I
Mechlorethamine HCl	BP	40 mg	BP	2 g	D5W, NS	Haze develops over 3 hr	26	I
Methyldopate HCl		1 g	BP	2 g	D5W	Haze develops over 3 hr	26	I
		1 g	BP	2 g	NS	Crystals produced	26	I
Prochlorperazine mesylate	BP	100 mg	BP	2 g	D5W	Haze develops over 3 hr	26	I
Promazine HCl	BP	200 mg	BP	2 g	D5W, NS	Immediate precipitation	26	I
Promethazine HCl	BP	100 mg	BP	2 g	D5W, NS	Immediate precipitation	26	I
Streptomycin sulfate	BP	4 g	BP	2 g	NS	Crystals produced	26	I

Drugs in Syringe Compatibility

Methohexital sodium

Drug (in syringe)	Mfr	Amt	Mfr	Amt	Remarks	Ref	C/I
Glycopyrrolate	RB	0.2 mg/ 1 ml	LI	10 mg/ 1 ml	Immediate precipitation	331	I
	RB	0.2 mg/ 1 ml	LI	20 mg/ 2 ml	Immediate precipitation	331	I
	RB	0.4 mg/ 2 ml	LI	10 mg/ 1 ml	Immediate precipitation	331	I

Additional Compatibility Information

Solutions— Although the manufacturer does not recommend the use of Ringer's injection, lactated, as a diluent, methohexital sodium has been determined to be compatible in dextrose 5% in Ringer's injection, lactated, as well as Ringer's injection, lactated. (See the table above.) However, the potential for incompatibility does exist between the sodium carbonate in the drug formulation and the calcium ions of the infusion solutions (282).

Acidic Drugs— Drugs such as methohexital sodium that exhibit poor solubility in an acidic medium may precipitate in solutions containing acidic drugs (22). Metaraminol bitartrate is acidic and may cause precipitation, depending on the concentration of the additives (7). In addition, the acidic methyldopate HCl imparts some buffer capacity to admixtures and may pose solubility problems with barbiturate salts (23).

Since solubility is maintained only at relatively high pH, mixing methohexital sodium with acidic solutions is not recommended (4). Mixed with methohexital sodium, a haze or precipitate forms in 15 minutes with atropine sulfate and tubocurarine chloride, in 30 minutes with metocurine iodide and succinylcholine chloride, and in 60 minutes with scopolamine HBr (1-5/7/96).

When barbiturates are mixed with succinylcholine chloride, either free barbiturate precipitates or the succinylcholine chloride is hydrolyzed, depending on the final pH of the admixture (4; 21). Similarly, atracurium besylate may be inactivated by alkaline solutions, such as barbiturates, and a free acid of the admixed drug may precipitate, depending on the resultant pH of the admixture (4).

Alkaline-Sensitive Drugs— Methohexital sodium may raise the pH of admixture solutions to the alkaline range and, therefore, should not be mixed with drugs that are alkali labile such as penicillin G (47). Significant decomposition of isoproterenol HCl and norepinephrine bitartrate may also occur. If either of these two drugs is mixed with methohexital sodium, the admixture should be used immediately after preparation (59; 77). Thiamine HCl is also stated to be unstable in the alkaline solutions of barbiturates (4).

Other Drugs— Other drugs stated to be incompatible with barbiturate salts include clindamycin phosphate (106), pentazocine lactate, propiomazine HCl, fentanyl citrate (4), cimetidine HCl (360), and droperidol (4).

A visible precipitate may form if pancuronium bromide is mixed with barbiturates (4). However, a visible precipitate was not produced when pancuronium bromide was mixed in a syringe with thiopental or methohexital (134).

In addition, methohexital sodium is stated to be incompatible with silicone and, as a consequence, should not contact rubber stoppers or parts of disposable syringes that have been treated with silicone (4).

METHOTREXATE SODIUM
AHFS 10:00

Immunex

Products— Methotrexate sodium is available in liquid and lyophilized dosage forms.

The liquid dosage forms from Immunex are supplied both in preserved and preservative-free formulations. The compositions of the various products are as follows (2):

Component	50 and 250 mg	50, 100, 200, 250 mg
Methotrexate (as sodium salt)	25 mg/ml	25 mg/ml
Benzyl alcohol	0.9% w/v	
Sodium chloride	0.26% w/v	0.49% w/v
Water for injection	qs	qs
Vial sizes	2 and 10 ml	2, 4, 8, 10 ml

The pH is adjusted with sodium hydroxide and, if necessary, hydrochloric acid (2).

The single-use lyophilized dosage forms of methotrexate (as the sodium salt) available from Immunex include 20-mg and 1-g vials. The pH is adjusted with sodium hydroxide. Immunex recommends reconstitution of the 20-mg vial to a concentration no greater than 25 mg/ml with a sterile, preservative-free medium such as dextrose 5% in water or sodium chloride 0.9%. The 1-g vial requires 19.4 ml of sterile, preservative-free diluent for reconstitution to yield a 50-mg/ml concentration (2).

pH— The pH of the commercially available dosage forms of methotrexate sodium is adjusted to approximately 8.5 (2; 4).

Tonicity— The liquid dosage forms of methotrexate sodium are isotonic solutions (4).

Sodium Content— The sodium content of some methotrexate sodium dosage forms is listed here (2):

Preservative-Free Liquid Forms	Approximate Sodium Content (mEq)
50 mg (25 mg/ml; 2 ml)	0.43
100 mg (25 mg/ml; 4 ml)	0.86
200 mg (25 mg/ml; 8 ml)	1.72
250 mg (25 mg/ml; 10 ml)	2.15
Lyophilized Forms	
20 mg	0.14
1 g	7.00

Administration— Methotrexate sodium may be administered by intramuscular, intra-arterial, or intrathecal injection, by direct intravenous injection, or by continuous or intermittent intravenous infusion (2; 4; 8; 338). For intrathecal injection, a preservative-free form is diluted to a 1-mg/ml concentration in sodium chloride 0.9%, Elliott's B solution, or the patient's own spinal fluid (2; 4; 435; 830). For high-dose regimens, it is recommended that preservative-free forms of methotrexate sodium be used (2; 241; 242); high doses of methotrexate sodium require leucovorin rescue (2).

Stability— Storage of the lyophilized powder and injection at controlled room temperature with protection from light is recommended (2; 4).

For intrathecal injection, the preservative-free dosage forms should be diluted immediately prior to use (2; 4). Immunex also recommends reconstitution of the lyophilized vials immediately prior to use (2). However, other information indicates that the reconstituted solution is stable for at least one week at room temperature (234).

Methotrexate is most stable between pH 6 and 8. Drugs producing extremes of pH should not be added to methotrexate (1072; 1369; 1379).

Methotrexate sodium, reconstituted according to the manufacturer's instructions, was cultured with human lymphoblasts to determine whether its cytotoxic activity was retained. The solution retained cytotoxicity for 24 hours at 4 °C and room temperature (1575).

Repackaging in Syringes— Wright and Newton found that methotrexate (Lederle) 50 mg/ml was stable for up to eight months when stored in Monoject (Sherwood) or Plastipak (Becton-Dickinson) plastic syringes at 25 °C. Because of possible alteration in water vapor permeability, use of Sabre (Gillette) and Sterisceal (Needle Industries) plastic syringes is limited to 70 days at 25 °C (1280).

Methotrexate sodium (Lederle) 2.5 mg/ml was repackaged into 10-ml plastic syringes (Becton-Dickinson) and stored at 4 and 25 °C for seven days. No loss of methotrexate was found by HPLC analysis. Furthermore, no contaminants from the syringes were observed (1913).

Freezing Solutions— Karlsen et al. found that methotrexate sodium (Lederle) 50 mg/100 ml in PVC bags of dextrose 5% in water (Travenol) could be frozen at −20 °C for at least 30 days and thawed by microwave radiation for two minutes with no significant change in concentration. Even after five repetitions of the freeze–thaw treatment, the methotrexate concentration showed no significant change (818).

Dyvik et al. evaluated the stability of methotrexate 5 mg, 50 mg, and 1 g in 50 ml of sodium chloride 0.9% in PVC bags frozen at −20 °C for up to 12 weeks and thawed in a microwave oven. No loss of methotrexate was found in any of the concentrations (1281).

Intrathecal Injections— In a study of solutions for intrathecal injection, the investigational form of preservative-free methotrexate sodium (Ben Venue) was reconstituted to a concentration of 2.5 mg/ml with Elliott's B solution (305 mOsm/kg, pH 7.2), sodium chloride 0.9% injection (303 mOsm/kg, pH 7.6), or Ringer's injection, lactated (270 mOsm/kg, pH 7.6). In all three solutions, methotrexate exhibited no change in concentration by UV spectroscopy over seven days under fluorescent light at 30 °C (327).

In another study, the stability and compatibility of cytarabine (Upjohn), methotrexate (National Cancer Institute), and hydrocortisone (Upjohn), mixed together in intrathecal injections, were evaluated. Two combinations were tested: (1) cytarabine 50 mg, methotrexate 12 mg (as the sodium salt), and hydrocortisone 25 mg (as the sodium succinate salt); and (2) cytarabine 30 mg, methotrexate 12 mg (as the sodium salt), and hydrocortisone 15 mg (as the sodium succinate salt). Each drug combination was added to 12 ml of Elliott's B solution (National Cancer Institute), sodium chloride 0.9% (Abbott), dextrose 5% in water (Abbott), and Ringer's injection, lactated (Abbott), and stored for 24 hours at 25 °C. Cytarabine and methotrexate were both chemically stable, with no drug loss after the full 24 hours in all solutions. Hydrocortisone was also stable in the sodium chloride 0.9%, dextrose 5% in water, and Ringer's injection, lactated, with about a 2% drug loss. However, in Elliott's B solution, hydrocortisone was significantly less stable, with a 6% loss in the 25-mg concentration over 24 hours. The 15-mg concentration was worse, with a 5% loss in 10 hours and a 13% loss in 24 hours. The higher pH of Elliott's B solution and the lower concentration of hydrocortisone may have been factors in this increased decomposition. All mixtures were physically compatible during this study, but a precipitate formed after several days of storage (819).

Methotrexate sodium (Lederle) 2 mg/ml diluted in Elliott's B solution (Orphan Medical) was packaged as 20 ml in 30-ml glass vials and 20-ml plastic syringes (Becton-Dickinson) with Red Cap (Burron) Luer-Lok syringe tip caps. The solution was physically compatible with no increase in measured turbidity or particulates and was chemically stable, exhibiting little or no loss by HPLC analysis during storage for 48 hours at 4 and 23 °C (1976).

Bacterially contaminated intrathecal solutions can pose very grave risks. Consequently, intrathecal solutions should be administered as soon as possible after preparation (328).

Effects of Light— Photolability, although unrecognized for many years, is a stability problem that is increased by dilution and mixture with sodium bicarbonate (1202).

In dilute solutions of 0.1 mg/ml, methotrexate is reported to undergo photodegradation on exposure to light. Decomposition of 5 to 8% in 10 days and 11 to 17% in 20 days was reported. This effect was not observed in the more concentrated solutions of the commercial preparation (25 mg/ml) (433) or in admixtures of methotrexate during short-term light exposure. Dyvik et al. found no

significant loss of methotrexate due to light exposure for four hours in solutions composed of 5 mg, 50 mg, or 1 g of methotrexate in 50 ml of sodium chloride 0.9% in PVC containers (1281).

McElnay et al. found little methotrexate loss from a 1-mg/ml solution in sodium chloride 0.9% in three burette drip chambers made of cellulose propionate (Avon A200 standard and A2000 Amberset) and methacrylate butadiene styrene (Avon A2001 Sureset) when exposed to normal mixed daylight and fluorescent lighting conditions for 24 hours. However, in 48 hours about 10 and 12% losses were observed in the A200 and A2001, respectively. With exposure to direct sunlight, an 11% loss occurred in the A200 in seven hours. No loss occurred when the Amberset or Sureset was wrapped in foil and exposed to either light condition for 48 hours (1378).

Exposure of the methotrexate 1-mg/ml solution in PVC and polybutadiene tubing to mixed daylight and fluorescent light produced significant losses after eight to 12 hours. Use of the Amberset PVC tubing or of foil wrapping for the polybutadiene tubing to protect static solutions from light reduced losses to 12 to 16% in 48 hours (1378).

Methotrexate sodium (R. Bellon), reconstituted to a concentration of 1 mg/ml with sodium chloride 0.9%, was evaluated for stability in translucent containers (Perfupack, Baxter) and five opaque containers [green PVC Opafuseur (Bruneau), white EVA Perfu-opaque (Baxter), orange PVC PF170 (Cair), white PVC V86 (Codan), and white EVA Perfecran (Fandre)] when exposed to sunlight for 28 days. Photodegradation was found by HPLC analysis after storage in the translucent Perfupack. Losses ranged from 18.5 to 27% after 24 hours of exposure to sunlight; losses dropped to about 5% in 24 hours at a methotrexate sodium concentration of 5 mg/ml. At 1 mg/ml, losses of 4% or less occurred in 24 hours in the opaque containers (1750).

Sorption— Methotrexate sodium 22.5 mg/100 ml and 12 g/500 ml in both dextrose 5% in water and sodium chloride 0.9% in PVC containers (Macroflex, Macopharma) exhibited no loss due to sorption during 30 days of storage at 4 °C protected from light. Simulated infusion of methotrexate sodium 2.25 g/500 ml in dextrose 5% in water and sodium chloride 0.9% over 24 hours through opaque PVC infusion sets (Perfecran, Fandre) also showed no loss of drug due to sorption to the PVC tubing (1867).

Filtration— Methotrexate sodium (David Bull Laboratories) 50 mg/100 ml in sodium chloride 0.9% in a burette was filtered through a nylon 0.2-μm filter (Pall, ELD96LL). Little or no drug loss due to sorption was found spectrophotometrically (1568).

Compatibility Information

Solution Compatibility

Methotrexate sodium

Solution	Mfr	Mfr	Conc/L	Remarks	Ref	C/I
Amino acids 4.25%, dextrose 25%	MG	LE	50 mg	No increase in particulate matter in 24 hr at 5 °C	349	C
Dextrose 5% in water	TR[a]	LE	960 mg	Less than 10% decrease in 24 hr at room temperature	519	C
	b		225 mg and 24 g	Visually compatible with no loss by HPLC in 30 days at 4 °C protected from light	1867	C

Solution Compatibility (Cont.)

Methotrexate sodium

Solution	Mfr	Mfr	Conc/L	Remarks	Ref	C/I
Sodium bicarbonate 0.05 M			2 g	No photodegradation products in 12 hr exposed to room light	433	C
Sodium chloride 0.9%	a	FA	1.25 and 12.5 g	Visually compatible with little or no loss by HPLC in 105 days at 4 °C followed by 7 days at 25 °C in the dark	1567	C
	b		225 mg and 24 g	Visually compatible with no loss by HPLC in 30 days at 4 °C protected from light	1867	C

[a]Tested in both glass and PVC containers.
[b]Tested in PVC containers.

Additive Compatibility

Methotrexate sodium

Drug	Mfr	Conc/L	Mfr	Conc/L	Test Soln	Remarks	Ref	C/I
Bleomycin sulfate	BR	20 and 30 units	LE	250 and 500 mg	NS	About 60% loss of bleomycin activity in 1 week at 4 °C	763	I
Cyclophosphamide		1.67 g		25 mg	NS	6.6% cyclophosphamide loss in 14 days at room temperature	1379; 1389	C
Cyclophosphamide with fluorouracil		1.67 g 8.3 g		25 mg	NS	9.3% cyclophosphamide loss in 7 days at room temperature. No loss of other drugs observed	1389	C
Cytarabine	UP	400 mg	LE	200 mg	D5W	Physically compatible. Very little change in UV spectra in 8 hr at room temperature	207	C
Fluorouracil		10 g		30 mg	NS	Both drugs stable for 15 days at room temperature	1379	C
Hydroxyzine HCl	LY	500 mg	BV	1 and 3 g	D5W[a]	Physically compatible for 48 hr	1198	C
Mercaptopurine sodium	BW	1 g	LE	100 mg	D5W	Physically compatible	15	C
Ondansetron HCl	GL	30 and 300 mg	LE	500 mg	D5W[b]	Physically compatible with little or no loss of either drug by HPLC in 48 hr at 23 °C	1876	C
	GL	30 and 300 mg	LE	6 g	D5W[b]	Physically compatible with little or no loss of either drug by HPLC in 48 hr at 23 °C	1876	C
Sodium bicarbonate		50 mEq	LE	750 mg	D5W	1.4% methotrexate decomposition in 72 hr and 6% in 1 week at 5 °C protected from light. At 23 °C exposed to light, 6% methotrexate decomposition in 72 hr and 15% in 1 week	465	C
Vincristine sulfate	LI	10 mg	LE	100 mg	D5W	Physically compatible	15	C
	LI	4 mg	LE	8 mg	D5W	Physically compatible. No change in UV spectra in 8 hr at room temperature	207	C

[a]Tested in glass containers.
[b]Tested in PVC containers.

Drugs in Syringe Compatibility

Methotrexate sodium

Drug (in syringe)	Mfr	Amt	Mfr	Amt	Remarks	Ref	C/I
Bleomycin sulfate		1.5 units/ 0.5 ml		12.5 mg/ 0.5 ml	Physically compatible for 5 min at room temperature followed by 8 min of centrifugation	980	C
Cisplatin		0.5 mg/ 0.5 ml		12.5 mg/ 0.5 ml	Physically compatible for 5 min at room temperature followed by 8 min of centrifugation	980	C
Cyclophosphamide		10 mg/ 0.5 ml		12.5 mg/ 0.5 ml	Physically compatible for 5 min at room temperature followed by 8 min of centrifugation	980	C
Doxapram HCl	RB	400 mg/ 20 ml		50 mg/ 20 ml	Physically compatible with 4% doxapram loss in 24 hr	1177	C
Doxorubicin HCl		1 mg/ 0.5 ml		12.5 mg/ 0.5 ml	Physically compatible for 5 min at room temperature followed by 8 min of centrifugation	980	C
Droperidol		1.25 mg/ 0.5 ml		12.5 mg/ 0.5 ml	Immediate precipitation	980	I
Fluorouracil		25 mg/ 0.5 ml		12.5 mg/ 0.5 ml	Physically compatible for 5 min at room temperature followed by 8 min of centrifugation	980	C
Furosemide		5 mg/ 0.5 ml		12.5 mg/ 0.5 ml	Physically compatible for 5 min at room temperature followed by 8 min of centrifugation	980	C
Heparin sodium		500 units/ 0.5 ml		12.5 mg/ 0.5 ml	Physically compatible for 5 min at room temperature followed by 8 min of centrifugation	980	C
Leucovorin calcium		5 mg/ 0.5 ml		12.5 mg/ 0.5 ml	Physically compatible for 5 min at room temperature followed by 8 min of centrifugation	980	C
Metoclopramide HCl	RB	10 mg/ 2 ml	LE	50 mg/ 2 ml	Incompatible. If mixed, use immediately	924	I
		2.5 mg/ 0.5 ml		12.5 mg/ 0.5 ml	Physically compatible for 5 min at room temperature followed by 8 min of centrifugation	980	C
	RB	10 mg/ 2 ml	LE	50 mg/ 2 ml	Incompatible. If mixed, use immediately	1167	I
	RB	160 mg/ 32 ml	LE	200 mg/ 8 ml	Incompatible. If mixed, use immediately	1167	I
Mitomycin		0.25 mg/ 0.5 ml		12.5 mg/ 0.5 ml	Physically compatible for 5 min at room temperature followed by 8 min of centrifugation	980	C
Vinblastine sulfate		0.5 mg/ 0.5 ml		12.5 mg/ 0.5 ml	Physically compatible for 5 min at room temperature followed by 8 min of centrifugation	980	C
Vincristine sulfate		0.5 mg/ 0.5 ml		12.5 mg/ 0.5 ml	Physically compatible for 5 min at room temperature followed by 8 min of centrifugation	980	C

Y-Site Injection Compatibility (1:1 Mixture)

Methotrexate sodium

Drug	Mfr	Conc	Mfr	Conc	Remarks	Ref	C/I
Allopurinol sodium	BW	3 mg/ml[b]	LE	15 mg/ml[b]	Physically compatible with no change in measured turbidity or increase in particle content in 4 hr at 22 °C	1686	**C**
Amifostine	USB	10 mg/ml[a]	LE	15 mg/ml[a]	Physically compatible with no change in measured turbidity or increase in particle content in 4 hr at 23 °C	1845	**C**
Amphotericin B cholesteryl sulfate complex	SEQ	0.83 mg/ml[a]	IMM	15 mg/ml[a]	Physically compatible with little or no change in measured turbidity or increase in particle content in 4 hr at 23 °C under fluorescent light	2117	**C**
Asparaginase	BEL	120 I.U./ml[a]		30 mg/ml	Visually compatible for 4 hr at room temperature	1788	**C**
Aztreonam	SQ	40 mg/ml[a]	LE	15 mg/ml[a]	Physically compatible with no subvisual haze or particle formation in 4 hr at 23 °C	1758	**C**
Bleomycin sulfate		3 units/ml		25 mg/ml	Drugs injected sequentially into Y-site with no flush between. No visually apparent precipitate	980	**C**
Cefepime HCl	BR	20 mg/ml[a]	LE	15 mg/ml[a]	Physically compatible with no change in measured turbidity or increase in particle content in 4 hr at 22 °C	1689	**C**
Ceftriaxone sodium	RC	100 mg/ml		30 mg/ml	Visually compatible for 4 hr at room temperature	1788	**C**
Chlorpromazine HCl	SKF	2 mg/ml[a]	AD	15 mg/ml[c]	Turbidity and yellow precipitate form immediately	1685	**I**
Cimetidine HCl	SKF	12 mg/ml[a]	AD	15 mg/ml[c]	Visually compatible for 4 hr at room temperature under fluorescent light	1685	**C**
Cisplatin		1 mg/ml		25 mg/ml	Drugs injected sequentially into Y-site with no flush between. No visually apparent precipitate	980	**C**
Cyclophosphamide		20 mg/ml		25 mg/ml	Drugs injected sequentially into Y-site with no flush between. No visually apparent precipitate	980	**C**
		20 mg/ml[a]		30 mg/ml	Visually compatible for 4 hr at room temperature	1788	**C**
Cytarabine	UP	0.6 mg/ml[a]		30 mg/ml	Visually compatible for 4 hr at room temperature	1788	**C**
Daunorubicin HCl	BEL	0.52 mg/ml[a]		30 mg/ml	Visually compatible for 4 hr at room temperature	1788	**C**
Dexamethasone sodium phosphate	QU	1 mg/ml[a]	AD	15 mg/ml[c]	Visually compatible for 4 hr at room temperature under fluorescent light	1685	**C**
	MSD	4 mg/ml		30 mg/ml	Visually compatible for 2 hr at room temperature. Dark yellow precipitate forms in 4 hr	1788	**I**
Dexchlorpheniramine maleate		5 mg/ml		30 mg/ml	Visually compatible for 4 hr at room temperature	1788	**C**
Diphenhydramine HCl	PD	2 mg/ml[a]	AD	15 mg/ml[c]	Visually compatible for 4 hr at room temperature under fluorescent light	1685	**C**

Y-Site Injection Compatibility (1:1 Mixture) (Cont.)

			Methotrexate sodium				
Drug	Mfr	Conc	Mfr	Conc	Remarks	Ref	C/I
Doxorubicin HCl		2 mg/ml		25 mg/ml	Drugs injected sequentially into Y-site with no flush between. No visually apparent precipitate	980	C
	FA	0.4 mg/ml[a]		30 mg/ml	Visually compatible for 4 hr at room temperature	1788	C
Doxorubicin HCl liposome injection	SEQ	0.4 mg/ml[a]	IMM	15 mg/ml[a]	Physically compatible with little or no change in measured turbidity and no increase in particle content in 4 hr at 23 °C	2087	C
Droperidol		2.5 mg/ml		25 mg/ml	Precipitate forms	977	I
		2.5 mg/ml		25 mg/ml	Drugs injected sequentially into Y-site with no flush between. Immediate precipitation	980	I
	JA	20 µg/ml[a]	AD	15 mg/ml[c]	Visually compatible for 4 hr at room temperature under fluorescent light	1685	C
Etoposide	BR	0.6 mg/ml[b]		30 mg/ml	Visually compatible for 4 hr at room temperature	1788	C
Etoposide phosphate	BR	5 mg/ml[a]	IMM	15 mg/ml[a]	Physically compatible with no change in measured turbidity or increase in particle content in 4 hr at 23 °C	2218	C
Famotidine	MSD	2 mg/ml[a]	AD	15 mg/ml[c]	Visually compatible for 4 hr at room temperature under fluorescent light	1685	C
Filgrastim	AMG	30 µg/ml[a]	LE	15 mg/ml[a]	Physically compatible with no change in measured turbidity or increase in particle content in 4 hr at 22 °C	1687	C
Fludarabine phosphate	BX	1 mg/ml[a]	CET	15 mg/ml[a]	Physically compatible for 4 hr at room temperature under fluorescent light	1439	C
Fluorouracil		50 mg/ml		25 mg/ml	Drugs injected sequentially into Y-site with no flush between. No visually apparent precipitate	980	C
Furosemide		10 mg/ml		25 mg/ml	Drugs injected sequentially into Y-site with no flush between. No visually apparent precipitate	980	C
	ES	3 mg/ml[a]	AD	15 mg/ml[c]	Visually compatible for 4 hr at room temperature under fluorescent light	1685	C
Ganciclovir sodium	SY	20 mg/ml[a]	AD	15 mg/ml[c]	Visually compatible for 4 hr at room temperature under fluorescent light	1685	C
Gemcitabine HCl	LI	10 mg/ml[b]	IMM	15 mg/ml[b]	Gross precipitate forms immediately, redissolves, but reprecipitates within 15 to 20 min	2226	I
Granisetron HCl	SKB	1 mg/ml	CET	12.5 mg/ml[b]	Physically compatible with little or no loss of either drug by HPLC in 4 hr at 22 °C	1883	C
Heparin[d]	CH	500 units/ml[b]		30 mg/ml	Visually compatible for 4 hr at room temperature	1788	C
Heparin sodium		1000 units/ml		25 mg/ml	Drugs injected sequentially into Y-site with no flush between. No visually apparent precipitate	980	C
	SO	40 units/ml[a]	AD	15 mg/ml[c]	Visually compatible for 4 hr at room temperature under fluorescent light	1685	C

Y-Site Injection Compatibility (1:1 Mixture) (Cont.)

Methotrexate sodium

Drug	Mfr	Conc	Mfr	Conc	Remarks	Ref	C/I
Hydromorphone HCl	ES	0.04 mg/ml[a]	AD	15 mg/ml[c]	Visually compatible for 4 hr at room temperature under fluorescent light	1685	**C**
Idarubicin HCl	AD	1 mg/ml[b]	LE	25 mg/ml	Color changes immediately	1525	**I**
Ifosfamide		36 mg/ml[a]		30 mg/ml	Visually compatible for 2 hr at room temperature. Dark yellow precipitate forms in 4 hr	1788	**I**
Imipenem–cilastatin sodium	MSD	5 mg/ml		30 mg/ml	Visually compatible for 4 hr at room temperature	1788	**C**
Leucovorin calcium		10 mg/ml		25 mg/ml	Drugs injected sequentially into Y-site with no flush between. No visually apparent precipitate	980	**C**
	LE	10 mg/ml		30 mg/ml	Visually compatible for 4 hr at room temperature	1788	**C**
Lorazepam	WY	0.1 mg/ml[a]	AD	15 mg/ml[c]	Visually compatible for 4 hr at room temperature under fluorescent light	1685	**C**
Melphalan HCl	BW	0.1 mg/ml[b]	LE	15 mg/ml[b]	Physically compatible with no change in measured turbidity or increase in particle content in 3 hr at 22 °C	1557	**C**
Mesna		1.8 mg/ml[a]		30 mg/ml	Visually compatible for 4 hr at room temperature	1788	**C**
Methylprednisolone sodium succinate	UP	0.5 mg/ml[a]	AD	15 mg/ml[c]	Visually compatible for 4 hr at room temperature under fluorescent light	1685	**C**
Metoclopramide HCl		5 mg/ml		25 mg/ml	Drugs injected sequentially into Y-site with no flush between. No visually apparent precipitate	980	**C**
	RB	2.5 mg/ml[a]	AD	15 mg/ml[c]	Visually compatible for 4 hr at room temperature under fluorescent light	1685	**C**
Midazolam HCl	RC	5 mg/ml		30 mg/ml	Yellow precipitate forms immediately	1788	**I**
Mitomycin		0.5 mg/ml		25 mg/ml	Drugs injected sequentially into Y-site with no flush between. No visually apparent precipitate	980	**C**
Morphine sulfate	ES	0.12 mg/ml[a]	AD	15 mg/ml[c]	Visually compatible for 4 hr at room temperature under fluorescent light	1685	**C**
Nalbuphine HCl	DU	10 mg/ml		30 mg/ml	Heavy yellow precipitate forms immediately	1788	**I**
Ondansetron HCl	GL	1 mg/ml[b]	CET	15 mg/ml[a]	Physically compatible for 4 hr at 22 °C	1365	**C**
	GL	2 mg/ml		30 mg/ml	Visually compatible for 4 hr at room temperature	1788	**C**
Oxacillin sodium	BR	250 mg/ml		30 mg/ml	Visually compatible for 4 hr at room temperature	1788	**C**
Paclitaxel	NCI	1.2 mg/ml[a]		15 mg/ml[a]	Physically compatible with no change in measured turbidity in 4 hr at 22 °C	1528	**C**
Piperacillin sodium–tazobactam sodium	LE	40 + 5 mg/ml[a]	LE	15 mg/ml[a]	Physically compatible with no change in measured turbidity or increase in particle content in 4 hr at 22 °C	1688	**C**
Prochlorperazine edisylate	SKF	0.5 mg/ml[a]	AD	15 mg/ml[c]	Visually compatible for 4 hr at room temperature under fluorescent light	1685	**C**
Promethazine HCl	WY	2 mg/ml[a]	AD	15 mg/ml[c]	Turbidity forms in 30 min	1685	**I**

Y-Site Injection Compatibility (1:1 Mixture) (Cont.)

Methotrexate sodium

Drug	Mfr	Conc	Mfr	Conc	Remarks	Ref	C/I
Propofol	ZEN	10 mg/ml	LE	15 mg/ml[a]	Small amount of white precipitate forms in 1 hr	2066	**I**
Ranitidine HCl	GL	1 mg/ml[a]	AD	15 mg/ml[c]	Visually compatible for 4 hr at room temperature under fluorescent light	1685	**C**
Sargramostim	IMM	10 μg/ml[b]	CET	15 mg/ml[b]	Physically compatible for 4 hr at 22 °C	1436	**C**
Teniposide	BR	0.1 mg/ml[a]	LE	15 mg/ml[a]	Physically compatible with no subvisual haze or particle formation in 4 hr at 23 °C	1725	**C**
Thiotepa	IMM[e]	1 mg/ml[a]	LE	15 mg/ml[a]	Physically compatible with no change in measured turbidity or increase in particle content in 4 hr at 23 °C	1861	**C**
TNA #218 to #226[h]			IMM	15 mg/ml[a]	Visually compatible with no precipitate or emulsion damage apparent in 4 hr at 23 °C	2215	**C**
TPN #212 to #215[h]			LE	15 mg/ml[a]	Substantial loss of natural subvisual turbidity with a hazy subvisual precipitate in 0 to 1 hr	2109	**I**
Vancomycin HCl	AB	510 mg[f]	LE	[g]	Physically compatible during 1-hr simultaneous infusion	1405	**C**
		5 mg/ml[a]		30 mg/ml	Visually compatible for 2 hr at room temperature. Dark yellow precipitate forms in 4 hr	1788	**I**
Vinblastine sulfate		1 mg/ml		25 mg/ml	Drugs injected sequentially into Y-site with no flush between. No visually apparent precipitate	980	**C**
Vincristine sulfate		1 mg/ml		25 mg/ml	Drugs injected sequentially into Y-site with no flush between. No visually apparent precipitate	980	**C**
	LI	0.1 mg/ml		30 mg/ml	Visually compatible for 4 hr at room temperature	1788	**C**
Vindesine sulfate	LI	0.1 mg/ml		30 mg/ml	Visually compatible for 4 hr at room temperature	1788	**C**
Vinorelbine tartrate	BW	1 mg/ml[b]	LE	15 mg/ml[b]	Physically compatible with no change in measured turbidity or increase in particle content in 4 hr at 22 °C	1558	**C**

[a]*Tested in dextrose 5% in water.*
[b]*Tested in sodium chloride 0.9%.*
[c]*Tested in dextrose 5% in water with sodium bicarbonate 0.05 mEq/ml.*
[d]*Salt form unspecified.*
[e]*Lyophilized formulation tested.*
[f]*Infused over one hour simultaneously with methotrexate.*
[g]*Diluted in dextrose 5% in water; concentration not cited.*
[h]*Refer to Appendix I for the composition of parenteral nutrition solutions. TNA indicates a 3-in-1 admixture, and TPN indicates a 2-in-1 admixture.*

Additional Compatibility Information

Solutions—— Methotrexate sodium is stated to be stable in dextrose 5% in water, sodium chloride 0.9%, or dextrose 5% in sodium chloride 0.9% for at least one week at room temperature (234).

Methotrexate sodium 0.03 mg/ml in dextrose 5% in water ex-

hibited less than a 10% loss in seven days at room temperature when protected from light (1379).

Dacarbazine—— No alteration in the ultraviolet/visible spectra was observed when dacarbazine was combined in solution with methotrexate sodium (492).

Fluorouracil—— The reported incompatibility of fluorouracil (Roche) 250 mg/L with methotrexate sodium (Lederle) 200 mg/L in dextrose 5% in water (207) has been questioned on the grounds that the observed alteration in UV spectra for both drugs might be an artifact of the experiment, merely being a result of methotrexate's altered UV spectra at varying pH values. It was observed that the altered methotrexate spectrum could contribute to an altered spectrum for fluorouracil (318).

In reply, King noted that the pH of fluorouracil, rather than the drug itself, might be responsible for changes in methotrexate's UV spectrum. However, using a buffered aqueous solution to simulate the admixture with a pH of approximately 8 and decreasing the pH with 0.2 M HCl back to the range of methotrexate sodium in dextrose 5% in water (pH 6.5) failed to return the UV spectrum to that of the pH 6.5 solution; in fact, the UV spectrum was not signifi-

cantly different than the pH 8 scan. King concluded that irreversible changes were occurring, which make the compatibility of the admixture suspect (319).

However, it should be noted that the commercial methotrexate sodium (Lederle) used in the studies is formulated in solution at a pH of approximately 8.5, not significantly different than that of the admixture suspected of incompatibility, and yet is stable until expiration, a period of at least two years (4).

Aluminum— Ogawa et al. reported that immersion of a needle with an aluminum component in methotrexate sodium (Lederle) 25 mg/ml resulted in the formation of orange crystals on the aluminum surface after 36 hours at 24 °C with protection from light (988).

METHOXAMINE HCL
AHFS 12:12

Vasoxyl   **Glaxo Wellcome**

Products— Methoxamine HCl (Glaxo Wellcome) is available in 1-ml ampuls. Each milliliter of aqueous solution contains methoxamine HCl 20 mg with citric acid anhydrous 0.3%, sodium citrate 0.3%, potassium metabisulfite 0.1%, and sodium chloride for isotonicity (2).

pH— From 3 to 5 (4).

Administration— Methoxamine HCl is administered intramuscularly or, in emergencies, intravenously by direct injection (2; 4). Alternatively, 35 to 40 mg of methoxamine HCl diluted in 250 ml of dextrose 5% in water may be infused slowly intravenously (4).

Stability— Methoxamine HCl in intact containers should be stored at controlled room temperature. The drug is stated to be sensitive to light and should be stored protected from light (2; 4).

Compatibility Information

Y-Site Injection Compatibility (1:1 Mixture)

Methoxamine HCl

Drug	Mfr	Conc	Mfr	Conc	Remarks	Ref	C/I
Heparin sodium	UP	1000 units/L[a]	BW	10 mg/ml	Physically compatible for at least 4 hr at room temperature by visual and microscopic examination	534	C
Hydrocortisone sodium succinate	UP	10 mg/L[a]	BW	10 mg/ml	Physically compatible for at least 4 hr at room temperature by visual and microscopic examination	534	C
Potassium chloride	AB	40 mEq/L[a]	BW	10 mg/ml	Physically compatible for at least 4 hr at room temperature by visual and microscopic examination	534	C
Vitamin B complex with C	RC	2 ml/L[a]	BW	10 mg/ml	Physically compatible for at least 4 hr at room temperature by visual and microscopic examination	534	C

[a]*Tested in dextrose 5% in Ringer's injection, dextrose 5% in Ringer's injection, lactated, dextrose 5% in water, Ringer's injection, lactated, and sodium chloride 0.9%.*

METHYLDOPATE HCL
AHFS 24:08

Aldomet Ester Hydrochloride   **American Regent**

Products— Methyldopate HCl (American Regent) is available in 5-ml vials containing 250 mg of drug. Each milliliter of solution contains (2):

Methyldopate HCl	50 mg
Citric acid, anhydrous	5 mg
Sodium bisulfite	3.2 mg
Monothioglycerol	2 mg
Methylparaben	1.5 mg
Disodium edetate	0.5 mg
Propylparaben	0.2 mg
Sodium hydroxide	to adjust pH
Water for injection	qs 1 ml

pH— From 3 to 4.2 (4).

Osmolality— Methyldopate HCl 50 mg/ml has an osmolality of 481 mOsm/kg (1689).

Administration— Methyldopate HCl is administered by intravenous infusion (2; 4; 8; 19). It is recommended that the desired dose be added to 100 ml of dextrose 5% in water. Alternatively, the dose may be administered at a concentration of 100 mg/10 ml in dextrose 5% in water. The dose should be infused slowly over 30 to 60 minutes (2; 4).

Stability— Intact vials should be stored at controlled room temperature and protected from freezing (2; 4). In aqueous solutions, the drug is most stable at acid to neutral pH. Oxidation of the catechol ring is the most important degradation process. The rate of such oxidation increases with increasing oxygen supply, increasing pH, and decreasing drug concentration (1072). Oxidizing agents decompose the drug (4); such oxidation is facilitated in alkaline solutions, yielding inactive dark-colored compounds (436). In dextrose 5% in water over a pH range of 3.5 to 7.8, no loss of potency occurred over 24 hours (23). However, at pH 7.8, more than a 5% potency loss occurred after the 24-hour study period (437).

Compatibility Information

Solution Compatibility

Methyldopate HCl

Solution	Mfr	Mfr	Conc/L	Remarks	Ref	C/I
Amino acids 4.25%, dextrose 25%	MG	MSD	500 mg	No increase in particulate matter in 24 hr at 5 °C	349	C
Dextran 6% in sodium chloride 0.9%	AB	MSD	1 g	Potency retained for 24 hr	23	C
Dextrose 5% in sodium chloride 0.9%	AB	MSD	1 g	Potency retained for 24 hr	23	C
Dextrose 5% in water	AB	MSD	1 g	Potency retained for 24 hr	23	C
	AB	MSD	1 g	Physically compatible and chemically stable. 10% decomposition is calculated to occur in 125 hr at 25 °C	527	C
Normosol M in dextrose 5% in water	AB	MSD	1 g	Potency retained for 24 hr	23	C
Normosol R	AB	MSD	1 g	Potency retained for 24 hr	23	C
Ringer's injection	AB	MSD	1 g	Potency retained for 24 hr	23	C
Sodium bicarbonate 5%	AB	MSD	1 g	Potency retained for 24 hr	23	C
Sodium chloride 0.9%	AB	MSD	1 g	Potency retained for 24 hr	23	C

Additive Compatibility

Methyldopate HCl

Drug	Mfr	Conc/L	Mfr	Conc/L	Test Soln	Remarks	Ref	C/I
Aminophylline	SE	500 mg	MSD	1 g	D, D–S, S	Physically compatible	23	C
	SE	500 mg	MSD	1 g	D5W	Physically compatible. 10% methyldopate decomposition in 90 hr at 25 °C	527	C
Amphotericin B		200 mg		1 g	D5W	Haze develops over 3 hr	26	I
Ascorbic acid injection	AB	1 g	MSD	1 g	D, D–S, S	Physically compatible	23	C
Chloramphenicol sodium succinate	PD	1 g	MSD	1 g	D, D–S, S	Physically compatible	23	C
Diphenhydramine HCl	PD	50 mg	MSD	1 g	D, D–S, S	Physically compatible	23	C

Additive Compatibility (Cont.)

Methyldopate HCl

Drug	Mfr	Conc/L	Mfr	Conc/L	Test Soln	Remarks	Ref	C/I
Heparin sodium	AB	20,000 units	MSD	1 g	D, D–S, S	Physically compatible	23	C
Magnesium sulfate		1 g	MSD	1 g	D, D–S, S	Physically compatible	23	C
Methohexital sodium	BP	2 g		1 g	D5W	Haze develops over 3 hr	26	I
	BP	2 g		1 g	NS	Crystals produced	26	I
Multivitamins	USV	10 ml	MSD	1 g	D, D–S, S	Physically compatible	23	C
Netilmicin sulfate	SC	3 g	MSD	1 g	D5S	Physically compatible and netilmicin chemically stable for 7 days at 4 and 25 °C. Methyldopate not tested	558	C
Potassium chloride		40 mEq	MSD	1 g	D, D–S, S	Physically compatible	23	C
Promazine HCl	WY	100 mg	MSD	1 g	D, D–S, S	Physically compatible	23	C
Sodium bicarbonate		50 mEq	MSD	1 g	D, D–S, S	Physically compatible	23	C
Succinylcholine chloride	AB	2 g	MSD	1 g	D, D–S, S	Physically compatible	23	C
Verapamil HCl	KN	80 mg	MSD	500 mg	D5W, NS	Physically compatible for 24 hr	764	C
Vitamin B complex with C	AB	10 ml	MSD	1 g	D, D–S, S	Physically compatible	23	C
	UP	10 ml	MSD	1 g	D, D–S, S	Physically compatible	23	C

Y-Site Injection Compatibility (1:1 Mixture)

Methyldopate HCl

Drug	Mfr	Conc	Mfr	Conc	Remarks	Ref	C/I
Esmolol HCl	DCC	10 mg/ml[a]	MSD	5 mg/ml[a]	Physically compatible for 24 hr at 22 °C under fluorescent light	1169	C
Heparin sodium	TR	50 units/ml	ES	5 mg/ml[a]	Visually compatible for 6 hr at 25 °C	1793	C
Meperidine HCl	AB	10 mg/ml	AMR	2.5 mg/ml[a]	Physically compatible for 4 hr at 25 °C under fluorescent light	1397	C
Morphine sulfate	AB	1 mg/ml	AMR	2.5 mg/ml[a]	Physically compatible for 4 hr at 25 °C under fluorescent light	1397	C
Theophylline	TR	4 mg/ml	ES	5 mg/ml[a]	Visually compatible for 6 hr at 25 °C	1793	C
TNA #73[b]			MSD	250 mg/ 50 ml[a]	Cracked the lipid emulsion	1009	I
			MSD	250 mg/ 50 ml[c]	Physically compatible for 4 hr by visual observation	1009	C

[a]*Tested in dextrose 5% in water.*
[b]*Refer to Appendix I for the composition of parenteral nutrition solutions. TNA indicates a 3-in-1 admixture.*
[c]*Tested in sodium chloride 0.9%.*

Additional Compatibility Information

Solutions— Dextrose 5% in water has been recommended as the diluent for infusion (2). Methyldopate HCl (MSD) 1 g/L is, however, physically compatible with all Abbott infusion solutions (23). The drug is stable in most intravenous fluids at pH 3.5 to 6 for 24 hours (4).

Acid-Sensitive Drugs— The pH of infusion solutions containing methyldopate HCl tends to be 7 or less, even when alkaline intravenous infusion solutions are used (4). It has been suggested that drugs poorly soluble in acidic media, such as barbiturate salts and sulfonamides, be mixed cautiously with methyldopate HCl since its acidity imparts some buffer capacity to intravenous admixtures. Furthermore, it should not be used with drugs known to be acid labile (23). The oxidation of methyldopate HCl in solution is catalyzed by the presence of iron (436; 437).

Metal Ions— Oxidative degradation of methyldopate HCl is catalyzed by manganese, cupric, cobalt, nickel, and ferric ions (1072).

METHYLERGONOVINE MALEATE
AHFS 76:00

Methergine   **Sandoz**

Products— Methylergonovine maleate (Sandoz) is available in 1-ml ampuls. Each milliliter of solution contains (1-10/96):

Methylergonovine maleate	0.2 mg
Tartaric acid	0.25 mg
Sodium chloride	3 mg
Water for injection	qs 1 ml

pH— From 2.7 to 3.5 (4).

Administration— Methylergonovine maleate may be administered intramuscularly or, in severe or life-threatening situations, intravenously slowly over no less than one minute (1-10/96; 4). Dilution of the dose to 5 ml with sodium chloride 0.9% has also been recommended for intravenous injection (4).

Stability— Methylergonovine maleate injection is a clear, colorless solution. If the product becomes discolored, it should not be used (1-10/96; 4). The drug darkens with age and exposure to light (4). The manufacturer recommends storage of intact ampuls below 25 °C and protection from light (1-10/96).

Compatibility Information

Y-Site Injection Compatibility (1:1 Mixture)

Methylergonovine maleate

Drug	Mfr	Conc	Mfr	Conc	Remarks	Ref	C/I
Heparin sodium	UP	1000 units/L[a]	SZ	0.2 mg/ml	Physically compatible for at least 4 hr at room temperature by visual and microscopic examination	534	C
Hydrocortisone sodium succinate	UP	10 mg/L[a]	SZ	0.2 mg/ml	Physically compatible for at least 4 hr at room temperature by visual and microscopic examination	534	C
Potassium chloride	AB	40 mEq/L[a]	SZ	0.2 mg/ml	Physically compatible for at least 4 hr at room temperature by visual and microscopic examination	534	C
Vitamin B complex with C	RC	2 ml/L[a]	SZ	0.2 mg/ml	Physically compatible for at least 4 hr at room temperature by visual and microscopic examination	534	C

[a]*Tested in dextrose 5% in Ringer's injection, dextrose 5% in Ringer's injection, lactated, dextrose 5% in water, Ringer's injection, lactated, and sodium chloride 0.9%.*

Additional Compatibility Information

Sodium chloride 0.9% has been recommended as a diluent for methylergonovine maleate (4).

METHYLPREDNISOLONE SODIUM SUCCINATE
AHFS 68:04

Solu-Medrol   **Pharmacia & Upjohn**

Products— Methylprednisolone sodium succinate (Pharmacia & Upjohn) is available in 40-mg (1 ml), 125-mg (2 ml), 500-mg (4 ml), and 1-g (8 ml) "Act-O-Vial" containers and 500-mg (8 ml), 1-g (16 ml), and 2-g (30.6 ml) vials with and without diluent (2). Use only the special diluent or bacteriostatic water for injection with benzyl alcohol to reconstitute the vials. When reconstituted as directed, each milliliter of solution contains (2):

Component	40 mg	125 mg, 500 mg, 1 g (16 ml)	1 g (8 ml)	2 g
Methylprednisolone equivalent (as sodium succinate)	40 mg	62.5 mg	125 mg	65.3 mg
Monobasic sodium phosphate anhydrous	1.6 mg	0.8 mg	1.6 mg	0.8 mg
Dibasic sodium phosphate dried	17.46 mg	8.7 mg	17.4 mg	9.1 mg
Benzyl alcohol	8.8 mg	8.8 mg	8.4 mg	8.9 mg
Lactose hydrous	25 mg			

pH— The pH is adjusted to 7 to 8 with sodium hydroxide when necessary (2; 4).

Osmotic Values— The osmolarities of the 40-, 62.5-, 125-, and 65.3-mg/ml concentrations are 500, 400, 440, and 420 mOsm/L, respectively (2).

The osmolality of methylprednisolone sodium succinate was calculated for the following dilutions (1054):

	Osmolality (mOsm/kg)	
Diluent	50 ml	100 ml
500 mg		
Dextrose 5% in water	291	275
Sodium chloride 0.9%	317	301
1 g		
Dextrose 5% in water	318	292
Sodium chloride 0.9%	345	319

Sodium Content— Each gram of methylprednisolone sodium succinate contains 2.01 mEq of sodium (846).

Administration— Methylprednisolone sodium succinate may be administered by intramuscular and direct intravenous injection and by intermittent or continuous intravenous infusion (2; 4; 8; 338). Direct intravenous injection should be performed over at least one minute (4) or over several minutes (2). High-dose therapy is given intravenously over at least 30 minutes (2).

Stability— Intact vials should be stored between 20 and 25 °C and protected from light. Reconstituted solutions also should be stored between 20 and 25 °C and should used within 48 hours (2).

The drug is subject to both ester hydrolysis and acyl migration. Degradation products include free methylprednisolone, succinate, and methylprednisolone-17-succinate (1072). The solution should not be used unless it is clear and free of particulate matter (4).

Methylprednisolone sodium succinate (Upjohn) diluted to a concentration of 4 mg/ml with sterile water for injection and packaged in glass vials was evaluated for stability by HPLC analysis. The samples stored at 22 °C lost 10% in 24 hours while those stored at 4 °C lost 6% in seven days and 17% in 14 days (1938).

pH Effects— The minimum rate of hydrolysis occurs at pH 3.5. Between pH 3.4 and 7.4, acyl migration is the dominant effect (1501).

Freezing Solutions— Reconstituted methylprednisolone sodium succinate (Upjohn) 125 mg/2 ml, when stored frozen, exhibited no loss of potency over four weeks (69).

When stored frozen at −20 °C, methylprednisolone sodium succinate (Upjohn) 500 mg/108 ml in sodium chloride 0.9% in PVC bags exhibited no loss by HPLC assay after 12 months followed by microwave thawing. Furthermore, the solution was physically compatible, with no increase in subvisual particles (1612).

Compatibility Information

Solution Compatibility

Methylprednisolone sodium succinate

Solution	Mfr	Mfr	Conc/L	Remarks	Ref	C/I
Amino acids 4.25%, dextrose 25%	MG	UP	250 mg	No increase in particulate matter in 24 hr at 5 °C	349	**C**
Dextrose 5% in sodium chloride 0.45%		UP	5 to 10 g	Physically incompatible	329	**I**
Dextrose 5% in sodium chloride 0.9%		UP	80 mg	Physically compatible for 24 hr	329	**C**
		UP	500 mg to 10 g	Physically incompatible	329	**I**
Dextrose 5% in water	MG	UP	1.25, 2.5, 5 g	Physically compatible for 24 hr at room temperature. Approximately 2 to 3% increase in free methylprednisolone in 24 hr	702	**C**
	MG	UP	10 g	Physically compatible for 12 to 24 hr at room temperature with haze developing. Approximately 2 to 3% increase in free methylprednisolone in 24 hr	702	**I**
	MG	UP	20 g	Haze forms after 6 hr at room temperature. Approximately 2 to 3% increase in free methylprednisolone in 24 hr	702	**I**

Solution Compatibility (Cont.)

Methylprednisolone sodium succinate

Solution	Mfr	Mfr	Conc/L	Remarks	Ref	C/I
	MG	UP	30 g	Haze forms after 12 hr at room temperature. Approximately 2 to 3% increase in free methylprednisolone in 24 hr	702	**I**
	MG	UP	40 and 60 g	Physically compatible for 24 hr at room temperature. Approximately 2 to 3% increase in free methylprednisolone in 24 hr	702	**C**
	AB	AB	500 mg to 1 g	Physically compatible and chemically stable for 24 hr at 25 °C	758	**C**
	AB	AB	1.25 g	Physically compatible for 12 hr at 25 °C. Turbidity due to free methylprednisolone may develop after 12 hr	758	**I**
	AB	AB	2 to 20 g	Physically compatible for 8 hr at 25 °C. Turbidity due to free methylprednisolone may develop after 8 hr	758	**I**
	AB	AB	30 g	Physically compatible and chemically stable for 24 hr at 25 °C	758	**C**
	TR[a]	UP	400 mg and 1.25 g	Physically compatible with 6 to 8% methylprednisolone 21-succinate ester loss in 24 hr at 24 °C	1418	**C**
	TR[a]	UP	40 mg and 2 g	Visually compatible with 4% or less loss by HPLC in 48 hr at room temperature	1802	**C**
Ringer's injection, lactated		UP	80 mg	Physically compatible for 24 hr	329	**C**
		UP	500 mg to 10 g	Physically incompatible	329	**I**
Sodium chloride 0.9%	MG	UP	1.25 g	Physically compatible for 24 hr at room temperature. Approximately 2 to 3% increase in free methylprednisolone	702	**C**
	MG	UP	2.5 g	Physically compatible for 12 to 24 hr at room temperature. Approximately 2 to 3% increase in free methylprednisolone in 24 hr	702	**I**
	MG	UP	5 g	Haze forms after 8 to 12 hr at room temperature. Approximately 2 to 3% increase in free methylprednisolone in 24 hr	702	**I**
	MG	UP	10 g	Haze forms within 6 hr at room temperature. Approximately 2 to 3% increase in free methylprednisolone in 24 hr	702	**I**
	MG	UP	20 g	Haze forms after 12 hr at room temperature. Approximately 2 to 3% increase in free methylprednisolone in 24 hr	702	**I**
	MG	UP	30 to 60 g	Physically compatible for 24 hr at room temperature. Approximately 2 to 3% increase in free methylprednisolone in 24 hr	702	**C**
	AB	AB	500 mg to 30 g	Physically compatible and chemically stable for 24 hr at 25 °C	758	**C**
	TR[a]	UP	40 mg	Visually compatible with 6% loss by HPLC in 48 hr at room temperature	1802	**C**
	TR[a]	UP	2 g	Visually compatible with 9% loss by HPLC in 24 hr and 12% loss in 48 hr at room temperature	1802	**C**

[a]Tested in PVC containers.

Additive Compatibility

Methylprednisolone sodium succinate

Drug	Mfr	Conc/L	Mfr	Conc/L	Test Soln	Remarks	Ref	C/I
Aminophylline		500 mg	UP	40 to 250 mg	D5W, NS	Clear solution for 24 hr	329	C
		1 g	UP	80 mg	D5W	Clear solution for 24 hr	329	C
	SE	500 mg	UP	125 mg		Precipitate forms after 6 hr but within 24 hr	6	I
		1 g	UP	250 mg to 1 g	D5W	Precipitate forms	329	I
	SE	1 g	UP	500 mg and 2 g	D5W	Physically compatible with no aminophylline or methylprednisolone alcohol loss in 3 hr at room temperature. 7 to 10% ester hydrolysis termed not clinically important	1022	C
	SE	1 g	UP	500 mg and 2 g	NS	Physically compatible with no aminophylline or methylprednisolone alcohol loss in 3 hr at room temperature. 12 to 18% ester hydrolysis termed not clinically important	1022	C
Calcium gluconate		1 g	UP	40 mg	D5S	Physically incompatible	329	I
Chloramphenicol sodium succinate	PD	1 g	UP	40 mg	D5W	Clear solution for 20 hr	329	C
	PD	2 g	UP	80 mg	D5W	Clear solution for 20 hr	329	C
Cimetidine HCl	SKF	3 g	UP	400 mg	D5W	Physically compatible and cimetidine chemically stable for 24 hr at room temperature. Methylprednisolone not tested	551	C
	SKF	3 g	UP	400 mg	D5W[a]	Physically compatible with no cimetidine loss and 3% methylprednisolone 21-succinate ester loss in 24 hr at 24 °C	1418	C
	SKF	3 g	UP	1.25 g	D5W[a]	Physically compatible with no cimetidine loss and 8% methylprednisolone 21-succinate ester loss in 24 hr at 24 °C	1418	C
Clindamycin phosphate	UP	1.2 g	UP	500 mg	D5W, W	Clindamycin stable for 24 hr	101	C
Cytarabine	UP	360 mg	UP	250 mg	D5S, D10S, NS	Clear solution for 24 hr	329	C
	UP	360 mg	UP	250 mg	R, SL	Physically incompatible	329	I
Dopamine HCl	AS	800 mg	UP	500 mg	D5W	Clear solution for 24 hr	329	C
	AS	800 mg	UP	500 mg	D5W	No dopamine decomposition in 18 hr at 25 °C	312	C
Glycopyrrolate	RB	1.33 mg	UP	250 mg	D5½S	Physically incompatible	329	I
Granisetron HCl	BE	56 mg	DAK	2.26 g	D5W, NS[a]	Visually compatible with little or no loss of either drug by HPLC in 72 hr at room temperature	1884	C
Heparin sodium		5000 units	UP	125 mg	D5S, D5W, R, LR	Clear solution for 24 hr	329	C
		10,000 units	UP	40 mg	D5S	Clear solution for 24 hr	329	C
		40,000 units	UP	25 g	NS	Clear solution for 24 hr	329	C
Metaraminol bitartrate	MSD	400 mg	UP	125 mg	D5W, NS	Precipitate forms within 4 hr	42	I
Nafcillin sodium	WY	500 mg	UP	125 mg	D5W	Precipitate forms	329	I

Additive Compatibility (Cont.)

Methylprednisolone sodium succinate

Drug	Mfr	Conc/L	Mfr	Conc/L	Test Soln	Remarks	Ref	C/I
Norepinephrine bitartrate	WI	8 mg	UP	40 mg	D5S	Physically compatible	329	C
Penicillin G potassium		2 to 10 million units	UP	80 mg	D5S, D5W, LR	Clear solution for 24 hr	329	C
Penicillin G sodium		5 million units	UP	125 mg	D5W, LR	Precipitate forms	329	I
Ranitidine HCl	GL	50 mg	UP	40 mg	D5W[a]	Visually compatible with 7% ranitidine loss and no methylprednisolone loss by HPLC in 48 hr at room temperature	1802	C
	GL	50 mg	UP	2 g	D5W[a]	Visually compatible with 6% ranitidine loss and 10% methylprednisolone loss by HPLC in 48 hr at room temperature	1802	C
	GL	2 g	UP	40 mg and 2 g	D5W[a]	Visually compatible with no loss of either drug by HPLC in 48 hr at room temperature	1802	C
	GL	50 mg and 2 g	UP	40 mg and 2 g	NS[a]	Visually compatible with no ranitidine loss and about 10% methylprednisolone loss by HPLC in 48 hr at room temperature	1802	C
Theophylline	AB	4 g	UP	500 mg and 2 g	D5W[b]	Physically compatible with little or no theophylline or methylprednisolone alcohol loss in 24 hr at room temperature. 8% ester hydrolysis termed not clinically important	1150	C
	AB	400 mg	UP	500 mg and 2 g	D5W[b]	Physically compatible with little or no theophylline or methylprednisolone alcohol loss in 24 hr at room temperature. 11% ester hydrolysis termed not clinically important	1150	C
Verapamil HCl	KN	80 mg	UP	250 mg	D5W, NS	Physically compatible for 24 hr	764	C

[a]Tested in PVC containers.
[b]Premixed theophylline infusion.

Drugs in Syringe Compatibility

Methylprednisolone sodium succinate

Drug (in syringe)	Mfr	Amt	Mfr	Amt	Remarks	Ref	C/I
Diatrizoate meglumine 52%, diatrizoate sodium 8%	MA	5 ml	UP	10 mg/ 1 ml	Physically compatible for at least 2 hr	1438	C
Diatrizoate sodium 60%	WI	5 ml	UP	10 mg/ 1 ml	Physically compatible for at least 2 hr	1438	C
Doxapram HCl	RB	400 mg/ 20 ml	UP	40 mg/ 2 ml	Immediate turbidity and precipitation	1177	I
Granisetron HCl	BE	0.15 mg/ ml[a]	DAK	6 mg/ml[a]	Visually compatible with little or no loss of either drug by HPLC in 72 hr at room temperature	1884	C
Iohexol	WI	64.7%, 5 ml	UP	10 mg/ 1 ml	Physically compatible for at least 2 hr	1438	C

Drugs in Syringe Compatibility (Cont.)

Methylprednisolone sodium succinate

Drug (in syringe)	Mfr	Amt	Mfr	Amt	Remarks	Ref	C/I
Iopamidol	SQ	61%, 5 ml	UP	10 mg/ 1 ml	Physically compatible for at least 2 hr	1438	C
Iothalamate meglumine 60%	MA	5 ml	UP	10 mg/ 1 ml	Physically compatible for at least 2 hr	1438	C
Ioxaglate meglumine 39.3%, ioxaglate sodium 19.6%	MA	5 ml	UP	10 mg/ 1 ml	Physically compatible for at least 2 hr	1438	C
Metoclopramide HCl	RB	10 mg/ 2 ml	ES	62.5 mg/ 1 ml	Physically compatible for 24 hr at room temperature	924	C
	RB	10 mg/ 2 ml	ES	250 mg/ 4 ml	Physically compatible for 24 hr at room temperature	924	C
	RB	10 mg/ 2 ml	ES	62.5 mg/ 1 ml	Physically compatible for 24 hr at 25 °C	1167	C
	RB	10 mg/ 2 ml	ES	250 mg/ 4 ml	Physically compatible for 24 hr at 25 °C	1167	C
	RB	160 mg/ 32 ml	ES	250 mg/ 4 ml	Physically compatible for 24 hr at 25 °C	1167	C

[a]Granisetron HCl in sodium chloride 0.9% and dextrose 5% in water. Diluted further with 17 ml of water.

Y-Site Injection Compatibility (1:1 Mixture)

Methylprednisolone sodium succinate

Drug	Mfr	Conc	Mfr	Conc	Remarks	Ref	C/I
Acyclovir sodium	BW	5 mg/ml[a]	LY	0.8 mg/ml[a]	Physically compatible for 4 hr at 25 °C	1157	C
Allopurinol sodium	BW	3 mg/ml[b]	AB	5 mg/ml[b]	Haze forms in 1 hr with white precipitate in 24 hr	1686	I
Amifostine	USB	10 mg/ml[a]	AB	5 mg/ml[a]	Physically compatible with no change in measured turbidity or increase in particle content in 4 hr at 23 °C	1845	C
Amphotericin B cholesteryl sulfate complex	SEQ	0.83 mg/ml[a]	PHU	5 mg/ml[a]	Physically compatible with little or no change in measured turbidity or increase in particle content in 4 hr at 23 °C under fluorescent light	2117	C
Amrinone lactate	WB	3 mg/ml[b]	ES	1 mg/ml[a]	Physically compatible for at least 4 hr at 25 °C under fluorescent light	992	C
Amsacrine	NCI	1 mg/ml[a]	UP	5 mg/ml[a]	Immediate orange turbidity and precipitate in 4 hr	1381	I
Aztreonam	SQ	40 mg/ml[a]	AB	5 mg/ml[a]	Physically compatible with no subvisual haze or particle formation in 4 hr at 23 °C	1758	C
Cefepime HCl	BR	20 mg/ml[a]	AB	5 mg/ml[a]	Physically compatible with no change in measured turbidity or increase in particle content in 4 hr at 22 °C	1689	C
Ciprofloxacin	MI	2 mg/ml[c]	UP	62.5 mg/ml	Transient white cloudiness rapidly dissipates. White crystals form in 2 hr at 24 °C	1655	I
Cisatracurium besylate	GW	0.1 mg/ml[a]	AB	5 mg/ml[a]	Physically compatible with no change in measured turbidity or increase in particle content in 4 hr at 23 °C	2074	C
	GW	2 mg/ml[a]	AB	5 mg/ml[a]	Subvisual haze forms immediately	2074	I

Y-Site Injection Compatibility (1:1 Mixture) (Cont.)

Methylprednisolone sodium succinate

Drug	Mfr	Conc	Mfr	Conc	Remarks	Ref	C/I
	GW	5 mg/ml[a]	AB	5 mg/ml[a]	Haze forms immediately	2074	I
Cisplatin	BR	1 mg/ml	UP	0.5 mg/ml[a]	Visually compatible for 4 hr at room temperature under fluorescent light	1685	C
Cladribine	ORT	0.015[b] and 0.5[d] mg/ml	AB	5 mg/ml[b]	Physically compatible with no change in measured turbidity or increase in particle content in 4 hr at 23 °C	1969	C
Cyclophosphamide	MJ	10 mg/ml	UP	0.5 mg/ml[a]	Visually compatible for 4 hr at room temperature under fluorescent light	1685	C
Cytarabine	UP	50 mg/ml	UP	0.5 mg/ml[a]	Visually compatible for 4 hr at room temperature under fluorescent light	1685	C
	UP	16 mg/ml[b]	UP	5 mg/ml[a]	Visually compatible for 24 hr at room temperature in test tubes. No precipitate found on filter from Y-site delivery	2063	C
Diltiazem HCl	MMD	5 mg/ml	UP	2.5 mg/ml[a]	Cloudiness forms	1807	I
	MMD	5 mg/ml	UP	20 mg/ml[b]	Precipitate forms	1807	I
	MMD	5 mg/ml	UP	62.5 mg/ml	Cloudiness forms but clears with swirling	1807	?
	MMD	1 mg/ml[b]	UP	2.5[a], 20[b], 62.5 mg/ml	Visually compatible	1807	C
Docetaxel	RPR	0.9 mg/ml[a]	PHU	5 mg/ml[a]	Partial loss of measured natural turbidity occurs immediately	2224	I
Dopamine HCl	AB	0.8 mg/ml[a]	UP	5 mg/ml[a]	Visually compatible for 24 hr at room temperature in test tubes. No precipitate found on filter from Y-site delivery	2063	C
Doxorubicin HCl	AD	0.2 mg/ml[a]	UP	0.5 mg/ml[a]	Visually compatible for 4 hr at room temperature under fluorescent light	1685	C
Doxorubicin HCl liposome injection	SEQ	0.4 mg/ml[a]	UP	5 mg/ml[a]	Physically compatible with little or no change in measured turbidity and no increase in particle content in 4 hr at 23 °C	2087	C
Enalaprilat	MSD	0.05 mg/ml[b]	UP	0.8 mg/ml[a]	Physically compatible for 24 hr at room temperature under fluorescent light	1355	C
Etoposide phosphate	BR	5 mg/ml[a]	AB	5 mg/ml[a]	Haze with small subvisual particles forms immediately. Particle content increases fivefold over 4 hr at 23 °C	2218	I
Famotidine	MSD	0.2 mg/ml[a]	AB	1 mg/ml[a]	Physically compatible for 4 hr at 25 °C	1188	C
	MSD	0.2 mg/ml[a]	QU	40 mg/ml	Physically compatible for 14 hr	1196	C
	ME	2 mg/ml[b]		5 mg/ml[a]	Visually compatible for 4 hr at 22 °C	1936	C
Filgrastim	AMG	30 µg/ml[a]	AB	5 mg/ml[a]	Haze, particles, and filaments form immediately	1687	I
Fludarabine phosphate	BX	1 mg/ml[a]	UP	5 mg/ml[a]	Physically compatible for 4 hr at room temperature under fluorescent light	1439	C
Gemcitabine HCl	LI	10 mg/ml[b]	AB	5 mg/ml[b]	Gross precipitation occurs immediately	2226	I
Granisetron HCl	SKB	0.05 mg/ml[a]	WY	5 mg/ml[a]	Physically compatible with no change in measured turbidity or increase in particle content in 4 hr at 23 °C	2000	C
Heparin sodium	TR	50 units/ml	UP	2.5 mg/ml[a]	Visually compatible for 6 hr at 25 °C	1793	C
	ES	100 units/ml[c]	UP	5 mg/ml[a]	Visually compatible for 24 hr at room temperature in test tubes. No precipitate found on filter from Y-site delivery	2063	C

Y-Site Injection Compatibility (1:1 Mixture) (Cont.)

		Methylprednisolone sodium succinate					
Drug	*Mfr*	*Conc*	*Mfr*	*Conc*	*Remarks*	*Ref*	*C/I*
Heparin sodium with hydrocortisone sodium succinate	RI UP	1000 units + 100 mg/L[a]	UP	40 mg/ml	Physically compatible for at least 4 hr at room temperature by visual and microscopic examination	332	C
Heparin sodium with hydrocortisone sodium succinate	RI UP	1000 units + 100 mg/L[e]	UP	40 mg/ml	Physically compatible initially but haziness noted in 4 hr at room temperature	322	I
Melphalan HCl	BW	0.1 mg/ml[b]	AB	5 mg/ml[b]	Physically compatible with no change in measured turbidity or increase in particle content in 3 hr at 22 °C	1557	C
Meperidine HCl	AB	10 mg/ml	UP	2.5 mg/ml[a]	Physically compatible for 4 hr at 25 °C	1397	C
Methotrexate sodium	AD	15 mg/ml[f]	UP	0.5 mg/ml[a]	Visually compatible for 4 hr at room temperature under fluorescent light	1685	C
		30 mg/ml	UP	20 mg/ml	Visually compatible for 4 hr at room temperature	1788	C
Metronidazole	MG	5 mg/ml	UP	5 mg/ml[a]	Visually compatible for 24 hr at room temperature in test tubes. No precipitate found on filter from Y-site delivery	2063	C
Midazolam HCl	RC	1 mg/ml[a]	UP	40 mg/ml	Visually compatible for 24 hr at 23 °C	1847	C
Morphine sulfate	AB	1 mg/ml	UP	2.5 mg/ml[a]	Physically compatible for 4 hr at 25 °C	1397	C
Ondansetron HCl	GL	1 mg/ml[b]	UP	5 mg/ml[a]	Light haze develops in 30 min	1365	I
Paclitaxel	NCI	1.2 mg/ml[a]	UP	5 mg/ml[a]	Normal inherent haze from paclitaxel decreases immediately	1556	I
Piperacillin sodium–tazobactam sodium	LE	40 + 5 mg/ml[a]	AB	5 mg/ml[a]	Physically compatible with no change in measured turbidity or increase in particle content in 4 hr at 22 °C	1688	C
Potassium chloride		40 mEq/L[a]	UP	40 mg/ml	Physically compatible for at least 4 hr at room temperature by visual and microscopic examination	322	C
		40 mEq/L[b]	UP	40 mg/ml	Physically compatible initially but haziness noted in 4 hr at room temperature	322	I
		40 mEq/L[g]	UP	40 mg/ml	Immediate haze formation	322	I
Propofol	ZEN	10 mg/ml	AB	5 mg/ml[a]	Small amount of white precipitate forms immediately	2066	I
Remifentanil HCl	GW	0.025 and 0.25 mg/ml[b]	AB	5 mg/ml[a]	Physically compatible with no change in measured turbidity or increase in particle content in 4 hr at 23 °C	2075	C
Sargramostim	IMM	10 μg/ml[b]	UP	5 mg/ml[b]	Small amount of particles and filaments form in 4 hr	1436	I
Sodium bicarbonate		1.4%	UP	20 mg/ml	Visually compatible for 4 hr at room temperature	1788	C
Tacrolimus	FUJ	1 mg/ml[b]	UP	0.8 mg/ml[a]	Visually compatible for 24 hr at 25 °C	1630	C
Teniposide	BR	0.1 mg/ml[a]	AB	5 mg/ml[a]	Physically compatible with no subvisual haze or particle formation in 4 hr at 23 °C	1725	C
Theophylline	TR	4 mg/ml	UP	2.5 mg/ml[a]	Visually compatible for 6 hr at 25 °C	1793	C
Thiotepa	IMM[h]	1 mg/ml[a]	AB	5 mg/ml[a]	Physically compatible with no change in measured turbidity or increase in particle content in 4 hr at 23 °C	1861	C

Y-Site Injection Compatibility (1:1 Mixture) (Cont.)

Methylprednisolone sodium succinate

Drug	Mfr	Conc	Mfr	Conc	Remarks	Ref	C/I
TNA #218 to #226[i]			AB	5 mg/ml[a]	Visually compatible with no precipitate or emulsion damage apparent in 4 hr at 23 °C	2215	**C**
TPN #212 to #215[i]			AB	5 mg/ml[a]	Physically compatible with no change in measured turbidity or increase in particle content in 4 hr at 23 °C	2109	**C**
Vinorelbine tartrate	BW	1 mg/ml[b]	AB	5 mg/ml[b]	Heavy white precipitate forms immediately	1558	**I**
Vitamin B complex with C	RC	2 ml/L[c]	UP	40 mg/ml	Physically compatible for at least 4 hr at room temperature by visual and microscopic examination	322	**C**
	RC	2 ml/L[g]	UP	40 mg/ml	Physically compatible initially but haziness noted in 4 hr at room temperature	322	**I**

[a]*Tested in dextrose 5% in water.*
[b]*Tested in sodium chloride 0.9%.*
[c]*Tested in both dextrose 5% in water and sodium chloride 0.9%.*
[d]*Tested in bacteriostatic sodium chloride 0.9% preserved with benzyl alcohol 0.9%.*
[e]*Tested in both Ringer's injection, lactated, and sodium chloride 0.9%.*
[f]*Tested in dextrose 5% in water with sodium bicarbonate 0.05 mEq/ml.*
[g]*Tested in Ringer's injection, lactated.*
[h]*Lyophilized formulation tested.*
[i]*Refer to Appendix I for the composition of parenteral nutrition solutions. TNA indicates a 3-in-1 admixture, and TPN indicates a 2-in-1 admixture.*

Additional Compatibility Information

Solutions— Dextrose 5% in water, sodium chloride 0.9%, and dextrose 5% in sodium chloride 0.9% have been recommended as diluents for intravenous infusions (2; 4).

The haze formation in solutions of methylprednisolone sodium succinate in intravenous fluids is caused by hydrolysis of the ester to free methylprednisolone. The time it takes for this haze to appear in solutions is quite variable, however, even among solutions of the same concentration (702).

In a study of the turbidity produced by methylprednisolone sodium succinate (Abbott) 500 mg to 30 g/L, turbidity was substantially higher in dextrose 5% in water than in sodium chloride 0.9% (758). Another important factor was the concentration of methylprednisolone sodium succinate. Turbidity was generally higher at intermediate concentrations (2 to 15 g/L) than at low (300 mg/L) or high (20 g/L) concentrations (758).

These differences in the development of turbidity cannot be explained by simple increased ester hydrolysis due to differing pH values and drug concentrations. Rather, the solubility of free methylprednisolone in various concentrations of methylprednisolone sodium succinate has been suggested as the primary factor. The solubility of free methylprednisolone is increased as the concentration of the sodium succinate ester increases. The increased solubi-lization is believed to overshadow increased formation of free methylprednisolone in concentrations over 10 g/L, preventing or minimizing precipitation and turbidity. Differences in turbidity between the drug in dextrose 5% in water and sodium chloride 0.9% are believed to result primarily from the electrolyte content of sodium chloride 0.9% and, to a much lesser extent, the slightly higher pH of the dextrose admixtures. These differences are presumed to affect the solubilizing capacity and reactivity of the ester (758).

Other Drugs— Amphotericin B in infusions appears to be compatible with limited amounts of methylprednisolone sodium succinate (4). However, insulin has been stated to be incompatible with methylprednisolone sodium succinate (Upjohn) (329).

Irinotecan admixed with methylprednisolone sodium succinate resulted in an admixture having a pH greater than 6.5. Approximately 10% irinotecan loss occurs within three hours at this pH (1881).

The compatibility of methylprednisolone sodium succinate (Upjohn) with several drugs added to auxiliary medication infusion units has been studied. Primary admixtures were prepared by adding various drugs to dextrose 5% in water, dextrose 5% in sodium chloride 0.9%, and Ringer's injection, lactated. Up to 100 ml of the primary admixture was added along with methylprednisolone sodium succinate (Upjohn) to the auxiliary medication infusion unit with the following results (329):

Methylprednisolone Sodium Succinate	Primary Solution	Result
Aminophylline 500 mg/L		
500 mg	D5S, D5W qs 100 ml	Clear solution for 24 hr
500 mg	LR qs 100 ml	Clear solution for 24 hr
500 mg	Added to 100 ml LR	Clear solution for 1 hr
1000 mg	D5W qs 100 ml	Yellow solution, clear for 24 hr
1000 mg	D5S qs 100 ml	Yellow solution, clear for 6 hr
1000 mg	Added to 100 ml D5S	Yellow solution, clear for 24 hr
1000 mg	LR qs 100 ml or added to 100 ml LR	Yellow solution, clear for 4 hr
2000 mg	D5S, D5W, LR qs 100 ml	Yellow solution, clear for 24 hr
Heparin Sodium 10,000 units/L		
500 mg	D5S, D5W qs 100 ml	Clear solution for 24 hr
500 mg	LR qs 100 ml or added to 100 ml LR	Clear solution for 6 hr
1000 mg	D5S, D5W qs 100 ml	Clear solution for 6 hr
1000 mg	Added to 100 ml D5W	Clear solution for 24 hr
1000 mg	LR qs 100 ml or added to 100 ml LR	Clear solution for 4 to 6 hr
2000 mg	D5W qs 100 ml	Clear solution for 6 hr
2000 mg	D5S, LR qs 100 ml	Clear solution for 24 hr
Potassium Chloride 40 mEq/L		
500 mg	D5S, D5W, LR qs 100 ml	Clear solution for 24 hr
1000 mg	D5W qs 100 ml	Clear solution for 24 hr
1000 mg	D5S, LR qs 100 ml or added to 100 ml D5S, LR	Clear solution for 6 hr
2000 mg	D5S, D5W, LR qs 100 ml	Clear solution for 24 hr
Sodium Bicarbonate 44.6 mEq/L		
500 mg	D5S, D5W qs 100 ml	Clear solution for 24 hr
500 mg	LR qs 100 ml or added to 100 ml LR	Clear solution for 1 hr
1000 mg	D5W qs 100 ml	Clear solution for 24 hr
1000 mg	D5S qs 100 ml or added to 100 ml D5S	Clear solution for 24 hr
1000 mg	LR qs 100 ml	Clear solution for 1 hr
1000 mg	Added to 100 ml LR	Clear solution for 4 hr
2000 mg	D5S, D5W qs 100 ml	Clear solution for 24 hr
2000 mg	LR qs 100 ml	Clear solution for 30 min
2000 mg	Added to 100 ml LR	Clear solution for 4 hr
Ticarcillin Disodium 6 g/L		
500 mg	D5S, D5W qs 100 ml	Clear solution for 24 hr
500 mg	LR qs 100 ml	Clear solution for 6 hr
500 mg	Added to 100 ml LR	Clear solution for 24 hr
1000 mg	D5W qs 100 ml	Clear solution for 24 hr
1000 mg	D5S qs 100 ml or added to 100 ml D5S	Clear solution for 6 hr
1000 mg	LR qs 100 ml	Clear solution for 1 hr
1000 mg	Added to 100 ml LR	Clear solution for 6 hr

METOCLOPRAMIDE HCL
AHFS 56:40

Reglan   **Robins**

Products— Metoclopramide HCl (Robins) is available in 2-ml ampuls and 2-, 10-, and 30-ml vials. Each milliliter of solution contains metoclopramide (as the hydrochloride) 5 mg with sodium chloride 8.5 mg in water for injection. The pH may be adjusted with hydrochloric acid and/or sodium hydroxide, if necessary (2).

pH— From 4.5 to 6.5 (2). Metoclopramide HCl (Delta West) 1.25, 2.22, and 3.75 mg/ml in sodium chloride 0.9% for continuous sub-cutaneous infusion had pH values of 4.4, 4.1, and 4.0, respectively (2161).

Osmolality— The osmolality of metoclopramide HCl 5 mg/ml was determined to be 280 mOsm/kg (1233). Metoclopramide HCl (Delta West) 1.25, 2.22, and 3.75 mg/ml in sodium chloride 0.9% for continuous subcutaneous infusion had osmolalities of 285, 286, and 294 mOsm/kg, respectively (2161).

Administration— Metoclopramide HCl is administered by intramuscular injection, by direct intravenous injection undiluted slowly over one or two minutes for 10 mg doses of drug, or by intermittent intravenous infusion over 15 minutes diluted in 50 ml of compatible diluent for larger doses (2; 4).

Stability— Metoclopramide HCl injection is a clear, colorless solution; it should be stored at controlled room temperature and protected from freezing. The drug is stable over a pH range of 2 to 9. Metoclopramide HCl is photosensitive; protection from light for the product during storage has been recommended (4). However, the manufacturer no longer recommends light protection for dilutions under normal lighting conditions, stating that they may be stored up to 24 hours (2).

Freezing Solutions— Metoclopramide HCl diluted in sodium chloride 0.9% in PVC bags is stable for up to four weeks when frozen at −20 °C. However, under the same storage conditions, dilutions in dextrose 5% in water lose up to 40% of their potency (4).

Metoclopramide HCl (Robins) 10 and 160 mg in 50 ml of sodium chloride 0.9% and dextrose 5% in water in PVC containers was stored frozen at −20 °C. The bags were subsequently thawed for 24 hours at room temperature. In sodium chloride 0.9%, no metoclopramide loss occurred in four weeks. However, in dextrose 5% in water, the lower concentration lost 9% in two weeks and 14% in four weeks. At 160 mg/50 ml in dextrose 5% in water, 11% was lost in one week and 37% in four weeks. The mechanism of this degradation is not fully understood but may be the result of reaction with dextrose breakdown products or impurities (1167).

Undiluted metoclopramide HCl (Robins) 5 mg/ml packaged as 3 ml in plastic infusion-pump syringes (MiniMed) fitted with Luer-Lok tip caps (Burron) exhibited microprecipitation that did not redissolve upon warming to room temperature when stored frozen at −20 °C for as little as one day. The precipitate was not visible with the unaided eye. Freezing is not an acceptable storage method for undiluted metoclopramide HCl injection (2001).

Light Exposure— Metoclopramide HCl (Robins) 10 and 160 mg/50 ml of dextrose 5% in water, dextrose 5% in sodium chloride 0.45%, and sodium chloride 0.9% was stored exposed to normal room light and to extreme high intensity light. Little or no drug loss occurred in any solution at either concentration exposed to normal room light for 24 hours. The accelerated study under high intensity light showed little or no loss of either concentration in sodium chloride 0.9% or of the high concentration in the dextrose-containing solutions in 24 hours. However, the 10-mg/50 ml concentration in the dextrose-containing solutions exhibited a 1 to 4% loss in four hours and an 11 to 14% loss in 24 hours under the high intensity light (1167).

Syringes— Undiluted metoclopramide HCl (Robins) 5 mg/ml packaged as 3 ml in plastic infusion-pump syringes (MiniMed) fitted with Luer-Lok tip caps (Burron) was evaluated for physical stability, including subvisual particulates, and chemical stability by HPLC analysis. Stored for seven days at 32 °C to simulate wearing a portable infusion pump close to the body, metoclopramide HCl was physically stable and little or no loss occurred. At 23 °C, metoclopramide HCl was physically and chemically stable for up to 60 days with little or no loss occurring. However, large quantities of subvisual particulates formed after that time, making the drug unsuitable for use. Stored under refrigeration at 4 °C, metoclopramide HCl remained both physically and chemically stable for up to 90 days (2001).

Metoclopramide HCl (Solopak) 2.5 mg/ml in sodium chloride 0.9% packaged in polypropylene syringes (Sherwood) was physically stable and exhibited not more than 5% loss by stability-indicating HPLC analysis in 24 hours stored at 4 and 23 °C (2199).

Compatibility Information

Solution Compatibility

Metoclopramide HCl

Solution	Mfr	Mfr	Conc/L	Remarks	Ref	C/I
Amino acids 2.75%, dextrose 25%, electrolytes	TR	RB	5 and 20 mg	Metoclopramide chemically stable for 72 hr at room temperature	854	C
Dextrose 5% in sodium chloride 0.45%	TR[a]	RB	200 mg	Physically compatible with 2% loss in 24 hr at 25 °C exposed to normal room light	1167	C
	TR[a]	RB	3.2 g	Physically compatible with 4 to 5% loss in 24 hr at 25 °C exposed to normal room light	1167	C
Dextrose 5% in water	TR[a]	RB	200 mg	Physically compatible with no loss in 24 hr at 25 °C exposed to normal room light	1167	C
	TR[a]	RB	200 mg	9% loss after 2 weeks and 14% loss after 4 weeks frozen at −20 °C followed by 24 hr at room temperature	1167	C
	TR[a]	RB	3.2 g	Physically compatible with 5% loss in 24 hr at 25 °C exposed to normal room light	1167	C
	TR[a]	RB	3.2 g	11% loss after 1 week and 37% loss after 4 weeks frozen at −20 °C followed by 24 hr at room temperature	1167	I
Mannitol 20%	AB	RB	40 and 100 mg	Physically compatible for 48 hr at room temperature	924	C
	AB	RB	40 and 100 mg	Physically compatible for 48 hr at 25 °C	1167	C

Solution Compatibility (Cont.)

Metoclopramide HCl

Solution	Mfr	Mfr	Conc/L	Remarks	Ref	C/I
	AB	RB	640 mg and 1.6 g	Physically compatible for 48 hr at 25 °C	1167	C
Sodium chloride 0.9%	TR[a]	RB	200 mg and 3.2 g	No loss after 4 weeks frozen at −20 °C followed by 24 hr at room temperature	1167	C
	TR[a]	RB	200 mg and 3.2 g	Physically compatible with no loss in 24 hr at 25 °C exposed to normal room light	1167	C
TPN #89[b]		RB	5 mg	Physically compatible with no metoclopramide loss in 24 hr and 10% loss in 48 hr at 25 °C	1167	C
		RB	20 mg	Physically compatible with no metoclopramide loss in 72 hr at 25 °C	1167	C
TPN #90[b]		RB	5 mg	Physically compatible with no metoclopramide loss in 72 hr at 25 °C	1167	C
		RB	20 mg	Physically compatible with 3% metoclopramide loss in 72 hr at 25 °C	1167	C

[a]Tested in PVC containers.
[b]Refer to Appendix I for the composition of parenteral nutrition solutions. TPN indicates a 2-in-1 admixture.

Additive Compatibility

Metoclopramide HCl

Drug	Mfr	Conc/L	Mfr	Conc/L	Test Soln	Remarks	Ref	C/I
Cimetidine HCl	SKF	3 g	RB	100 mg	NS	Physically compatible for 48 hr at room temperature, but bioavailability of cimetidine may be reduced	924	?
	SKF	3 g	RB	100 mg and 1.6 g		Physically compatible for 48 hr at 25 °C	1167	C
Clindamycin phosphate	UP	6 g	RB	100 and 200 mg	NS	Physically compatible for 24 hr at room temperature	924	C
	UP	6 g	RB	100 and 200 mg		Physically compatible for 24 hr at 25 °C	1167	C
	UP	3.5 g	RB	1.9 g		Physically compatible for 24 hr at 25 °C	1167	C
	UP	4.4 g	RB	1.2 g		Physically compatible for 24 hr at 25 °C	1167	C
Dexamethasone sodium phosphate with lorazepam and diphenhydramine HCl	AMR WY ES	400 mg 40 mg 2 g	DU	4 g	NS[a]	Rapid lorazepam losses of 8, 10, and 15% at 3, 23, and 30 °C, respectively, in 24 hr by HPLC. Other drugs stable for 14 days by HPLC at all three storage temperatures	1733	I
Erythromycin lactobionate	AB	4 g	RB	400 mg	NS	Incompatible. If mixed, use immediately	924	I
	AB	4.1 g	RB	416 mg		Incompatible. If mixed, use immediately	1167	I
	AB	5 g	RB	100 mg	NS	Incompatible. If mixed, use immediately	924	I
	AB	5 g	RB	100 mg		Incompatible. If mixed, use immediately	1167	I
	AB	3.5 g	RB	1.1 g		Incompatible. If mixed, use immediately	1167	I
Floxacillin sodium	BE	20 g	ANT	1 g	NS	Immediate white precipitation	1479	I

Additive Compatibility (Cont.)

<table>
<tr><td colspan="9" align="center">Metoclopramide HCl</td></tr>
<tr>
<th>Drug</th>
<th>Mfr</th>
<th>Conc/L</th>
<th>Mfr</th>
<th>Conc/L</th>
<th>Test Soln</th>
<th>Remarks</th>
<th>Ref</th>
<th>C/I</th>
</tr>
<tr>
<td>Fluorouracil</td>
<td>RC</td>
<td>2.5 g</td>
<td>FUJ</td>
<td>100 mg</td>
<td>D5W</td>
<td>10% metoclopramide loss in 6 hr and 27% loss in 24 hr at 25 °C. 5% meto-clopramide loss in 120 hr at 4 °C. 5 and 7% fluorouracil losses in 120 hr at 4 and 25 °C, respectively</td>
<td>1780</td>
<td>I</td>
</tr>
<tr>
<td>Furosemide</td>
<td>HO</td>
<td>1 g</td>
<td>ANT</td>
<td>1 g</td>
<td>NS</td>
<td>Immediate precipitation</td>
<td>1479</td>
<td>I</td>
</tr>
<tr>
<td>Meropenem</td>
<td>ZEN</td>
<td>1 and 20 g</td>
<td>RB</td>
<td>100 mg</td>
<td>NS</td>
<td>Visually compatible for 4 hr at room temperature</td>
<td>1994</td>
<td>C</td>
</tr>
<tr>
<td>Morphine sulfate</td>
<td>EV</td>
<td>1 g</td>
<td>SKB</td>
<td>500 mg</td>
<td>NS[b]</td>
<td>Visually compatible with little or no loss of either drug by HPLC in 35 days at 22 °C and 182 days at 4 °C followed by 7 days at 32 °C</td>
<td>1938</td>
<td>C</td>
</tr>
<tr>
<td></td>
<td>EV</td>
<td>1 g</td>
<td>SKB</td>
<td>500 mg</td>
<td>NS[c]</td>
<td>Visually compatible with 8% metoclopra-mide loss by HPLC in 14 days at 22 °C and 98 days at 4 °C. No morphine loss occurs</td>
<td>1938</td>
<td>C</td>
</tr>
<tr>
<td>Multivitamins (M.V.I.)</td>
<td>USV</td>
<td>20 ml</td>
<td>RB</td>
<td>20 and 320 mg</td>
<td>NS</td>
<td>Physically compatible for 48 hr at room temperature</td>
<td>924</td>
<td>C</td>
</tr>
<tr>
<td>(M.V.I.)</td>
<td>USV</td>
<td>20 ml</td>
<td>RB</td>
<td>20 and 320 mg</td>
<td></td>
<td>Physically compatible for 48 hr at 25 °C</td>
<td>1167</td>
<td>C</td>
</tr>
<tr>
<td>(M.V.I.-12)</td>
<td>USV</td>
<td>20 ml</td>
<td>RB</td>
<td>20 and 320 mg</td>
<td>NS</td>
<td>Physically compatible for 48 hr at room temperature</td>
<td>924</td>
<td>C</td>
</tr>
<tr>
<td>(M.V.I.-12)</td>
<td>USV</td>
<td>20 ml</td>
<td>RB</td>
<td>20 and 320 mg</td>
<td></td>
<td>Physically compatible for 48 hr at 25 °C</td>
<td>1167</td>
<td>C</td>
</tr>
<tr>
<td>Potassium acetate</td>
<td>IX</td>
<td>20 mEq</td>
<td>RB</td>
<td>10 and 160 mg</td>
<td>NS</td>
<td>Physically compatible for 48 hr at room temperature</td>
<td>924</td>
<td>C</td>
</tr>
<tr>
<td></td>
<td>IX</td>
<td>20 mEq</td>
<td>RB</td>
<td>10 and 160 mg</td>
<td></td>
<td>Physically compatible for 48 hr at 25 °C</td>
<td>1167</td>
<td>C</td>
</tr>
<tr>
<td>Potassium chloride</td>
<td>ES</td>
<td>30 mEq</td>
<td>RB</td>
<td>10 and 160 mg</td>
<td>NS</td>
<td>Physically compatible for 48 hr at room temperature</td>
<td>924</td>
<td>C</td>
</tr>
<tr>
<td></td>
<td>ES</td>
<td>30 mEq</td>
<td>RB</td>
<td>10 and 160 mg</td>
<td></td>
<td>Physically compatible for 48 hr at 25 °C</td>
<td>1167</td>
<td>C</td>
</tr>
<tr>
<td>Potassium phosphates</td>
<td>IX</td>
<td>15 mM</td>
<td>RB</td>
<td>10 and 160 mg</td>
<td>NS</td>
<td>Physically compatible for 48 hr at room temperature</td>
<td>924</td>
<td>C</td>
</tr>
<tr>
<td></td>
<td>IX</td>
<td>15 mM</td>
<td>RB</td>
<td>10 and 160 mg</td>
<td></td>
<td>Physically compatible for 48 hr at 25 °C</td>
<td>1167</td>
<td>C</td>
</tr>
<tr>
<td>Verapamil HCl</td>
<td>KN</td>
<td>80 mg</td>
<td>RB</td>
<td>20 mg</td>
<td>D5W, NS</td>
<td>Physically compatible for 24 hr</td>
<td>764</td>
<td>C</td>
</tr>
</table>

[a]Tested in Pharmacia-Deltec PVC pump reservoirs.
[b]Tested in PVC containers.
[c]Tested in PCA Infusors (Baxter).

Drugs in Syringe Compatibility

<table>
<tr><td colspan="8" align="center">Metoclopramide HCl</td></tr>
<tr>
<th>Drug (in syringe)</th>
<th>Mfr</th>
<th>Amt</th>
<th>Mfr</th>
<th>Amt</th>
<th>Remarks</th>
<th>Ref</th>
<th>C/I</th>
</tr>
<tr>
<td>Aminophylline</td>
<td>ES</td>
<td>80 mg/ 3.2 ml</td>
<td>RB</td>
<td>10 mg/ 2 ml</td>
<td>Physically compatible for 24 hr at room temperature</td>
<td>924</td>
<td>C</td>
</tr>
<tr>
<td></td>
<td>ES</td>
<td>500 mg/ 20 ml</td>
<td>RB</td>
<td>10 mg/ 2 ml</td>
<td>Physically compatible for 24 hr at room temperature</td>
<td>924</td>
<td>C</td>
</tr>
</table>

Drugs in Syringe Compatibility (Cont.)

Metoclopramide HCl

Drug (in syringe)	Mfr	Amt	Mfr	Amt	Remarks	Ref	C/I
	ES	500 mg/ 20 ml	RB	160 mg/ 32 ml	Physically compatible for 24 hr at 25 °C	1167	**C**
	ES	80 mg/ 3.2 ml	RB	10 mg/ 2 ml	Physically compatible for 24 hr at 25 °C	1167	**C**
	ES	500 mg/ 20 ml	RB	10 mg/ 2 ml	Physically compatible for 24 hr at 25 °C	1167	**C**
Ampicillin sodium	BR	250 mg/ 2.5 ml	RB	10 mg/ 2 ml	Incompatible. If mixed, use immediately	1167	**I**
	BR	1 g/ 10 ml	RB	10 mg/ 2 ml	Incompatible. If mixed, use immediately	1167	**I**
	BR	1 g/ 10 ml	RB	160 mg/ 32 ml	Incompatible. If mixed, use immediately	1167	**I**
Ascorbic acid injection	AB	250 mg/ 0.5 ml	RB	10 mg/ 2 ml	Physically compatible for 48 hr at room temperature	924	**C**
	AB	250 mg/ 0.5 ml	RB	160 mg/ 32 ml	Physically compatible for 48 hr at 25 °C	1167	**C**
	AB	250 mg/ 0.5 ml	RB	10 mg/ 2 ml	Physically compatible for 48 hr at 25 °C	1167	**C**
Atropine sulfate	GL	0.4 mg/ 1 ml	NO	10 mg/ 2 ml	Physically compatible both macroscopically and microscopically for 15 min at room temperature	565	**C**
Benztropine mesylate	MSD	2 mg/ 2 ml	RB	10 mg/ 2 ml	Physically compatible for 48 hr at room temperature	924	**C**
	MSD	2 mg/ 2 ml	RB	160 mg/ 32 ml	Physically compatible for 48 hr at 25 °C	1167	**C**
	MSD	2 mg/ 2 ml	RB	10 mg/ 2 ml	Physically compatible for 48 hr at 25 °C	1167	**C**
Bleomycin sulfate		1.5 units/ 0.5 ml		2.5 mg/ 0.5 ml	Physically compatible for 5 min at room temperature followed by 8 min of centrifugation	980	**C**
Butorphanol tartrate	BR	4 mg/ 2 ml	NO	10 mg/ 2 ml	Physically compatible for 30 min at room temperature both macroscopically and microscopically	566	**C**
Calcium gluconate	ES	1 g/ 10 ml	RB	10 mg/ 2 ml	Possible precipitate formation	924	**I**
	ES	1 g/ 10 ml	RB	10 mg/ 2 ml	Incompatible. If mixed, use immediately	1167	**I**
	ES	1 g/ 10 ml	RB	160 mg/ 32 ml	Incompatible. If mixed, use immediately	1167	**I**
Chloramphenicol sodium succinate	PD	250 mg/ 2.5 ml	RB	10 mg/ 2 ml	Incompatible. Do not mix	924	**I**
	PD	2 g/ 20 ml	RB	10 mg/ 2 ml	Incompatible. Do not mix	924	**I**
	PD	250 mg/ 2.5 ml	RB	10 mg/ 2 ml	White precipitate forms within 1 hr at 25 °C	1167	**I**
	PD	2 g/ 20 ml	RB	10 mg/ 2 ml	White precipitate forms within 1 hr at 25 °C	1167	**I**
	PD	2 g/ 20 ml	RB	160 mg/ 32 ml	White precipitate forms within 1 hr at 25 °C	1167	**I**
Chlorpromazine HCl	MB	25 mg/ 1 ml	NO	10 mg/ 2 ml	Physically compatible both macroscopically and microscopically for 15 min at room temperature	565	**C**

Drugs in Syringe Compatibility (Cont.)

Metoclopramide HCl

Drug (in syringe)	Mfr	Amt	Mfr	Amt	Remarks	Ref	C/I
Cisplatin		0.5 mg/ 0.5 ml		2.5 mg/ 0.5 ml	Physically compatible for 5 min at room temperature followed by 8 min of centrifugation	980	**C**
Cyclophosphamide	MJ	40 mg/ 2 ml	RB	10 mg/ 2 ml	Physically compatible for 24 hr at room temperature	924	**C**
		10 mg/ 0.5 ml		2.5 mg/ 0.5 ml	Physically compatible for 5 min at room temperature followed by 8 min of centrifugation	980	**C**
	MJ	1 g/ 50 ml	RB	10 mg/ 2 ml	Physically compatible for 24 hr at 25 °C	1167	**C**
	MJ	1 g/ 50 ml	RB	160 mg/ 32 ml	Physically compatible for 24 hr at 25 °C	1167	**C**
	MJ	40 mg/ 2 ml	RB	10 mg/ 2 ml	Physically compatible for 24 hr at 25 °C	1167	**C**
Cytarabine	UP	50 mg/ 1 ml	RB	10 mg/ 2 ml	Physically compatible for 48 hr at room temperature	924	**C**
	UP	500 mg/ 10 ml	RB	160 mg/ 32 ml	Physically compatible for 48 hr at 25 °C	1167	**C**
	UP	50 mg/ 1 ml	RB	10 mg/ 2 ml	Physically compatible for 48 hr at 25 °C	1167	**C**
Dexamethasone sodium phosphate	ES, MSD	8 mg/ 2 ml	RB	10 mg/ 2 ml	Physically compatible for 48 hr at room temperature	924	**C**
	ES, MSD	8 mg/ 2 ml	RB	160 mg/ 32 ml	Physically compatible for 48 hr at 25 °C	1167	**C**
	ES, MSD	8 mg/ 2 ml	RB	10 mg/ 2 ml	Physically compatible for 48 hr at 25 °C	1167	**C**
Diamorphine HCl	MB	10, 25, 50 mg/ 1 ml	BK	5 mg/ 1 ml	Physically compatible and diamorphine potency retained for 24 hr at room temperature	1454	**C**
	EV	50 and 150 mg/ 1 ml	LA	5 mg/ 1 ml	Slight discoloration with 8% metoclopramide loss and 9% diamorphine loss in 7 days at room temperature	1455	**C**
Dimenhydrinate	HR	50 mg/ 1 ml	NO	10 mg/ 2 ml	Physically compatible both macroscopically and microscopically for 15 min at room temperature	565	**C**
Diphenhydramine HCl	PD	50 mg/ 1 ml	NO	10 mg/ 2 ml	Physically compatible both macroscopically and microscopically for 15 min at room temperature	565	**C**
	PD	50 mg/ 5 ml	RB	10 mg/ 2 ml	Physically compatible for 48 hr at room temperature	924	**C**
	PD	250 mg/ 25 ml	RB	10 mg/ 2 ml	Physically compatible for 48 hr at room temperature	924	**C**
	PD	40 mg/ 4 ml	RB	160 mg/ 32 ml	Physically compatible for 48 hr at 25 °C	1167	**C**
	PD	200 mg/ 20 ml	RB	160 mg/ 32 ml	Physically compatible for 48 hr at 25 °C	1167	**C**
	PD	50 mg/ 5 ml	RB	10 mg/ 2 ml	Physically compatible for 48 hr at 25 °C	1167	**C**
	PD	250 mg/ 25 ml	RB	10 mg/ 2 ml	Physically compatible for 48 hr at 25 °C	1167	**C**
Doxorubicin HCl	AD	40 mg/ 20 ml	RB	10 mg/ 2 ml	Physically compatible for 48 hr at room temperature	924	**C**

Drugs in Syringe Compatibility (Cont.)

Metoclopramide HCl

Drug (in syringe)	Mfr	Amt	Mfr	Amt	Remarks	Ref	C/I
		1 mg/ 0.5 ml		2.5 mg/ 0.5 ml	Physically compatible for 5 min at room temperature followed by 8 min of centrifugation	980	**C**
	AD	90 mg/ 45 ml	RB	160 mg/ 32 ml	Physically compatible for 48 hr at 25 °C	1167	**C**
	AD	40 mg/ 20 ml	RB	10 mg/ 2 ml	Physically compatible for 48 hr at 25 °C	1167	**C**
Droperidol	MN	2.5 mg/ 1 ml	NO	10 mg/ 2 ml	Physically compatible both macroscopically and microscopically for 15 min at room temperature	565	**C**
		1.25 mg/ 0.5 ml		2.5 mg/ 0.5 ml	Physically compatible for 5 min at room temperature followed by 8 min of centrifugation	980	**C**
Fentanyl citrate	MN	0.05 mg/ 1 ml	NO	10 mg/ 2 ml	Physically compatible both macroscopically and microscopically for 15 min at room temperature	565	**C**
Fluorouracil		25 mg/ 0.5 ml		2.5 mg/ 0.5 ml	Physically compatible for 5 min at room temperature followed by 8 min of centrifugation	980	**C**
Furosemide		5 mg/ 0.5 ml		2.5 mg/ 0.5 ml	Immediate precipitation	980	**I**
Heparin sodium	ES	2000 units/ 2 ml	RB	10 mg/ 2 ml	Physically compatible for 48 hr at room temperature	924	**C**
	ES	4000 units/ 4 ml	RB	10 mg/ 2 ml	Physically compatible for 48 hr at room temperature	924	**C**
		500 units/ 0.5 ml		2.5 mg/ 0.5 ml	Physically compatible for 5 min at room temperature followed by 8 min of centrifugation	980	**C**
		2500 units/ 1 ml		10 mg/ 2 ml	Physically compatible for at least 5 min	1053	**C**
	ES	16,000 units/ 16 ml	RB	160 mg/ 32 ml	Physically compatible for 48 hr at 25 °C	1167	**C**
	ES	2000 units/ 2 ml	RB	10 mg/ 2 ml	Physically compatible for 48 hr at 25 °C	1167	**C**
	ES	4000 units/ 4 ml	RB	10 mg/ 2 ml	Physically compatible for 48 hr at 25 °C	1167	**C**
Hydrocortisone sodium phosphate	MSD	10 mg/ 2 ml	RB	10 mg/ 2 ml	Physically compatible for 48 hr at 25 °C	1167	**C**
	MSD	20 mg/ 4 ml	RB	10 mg/ 2 ml	Physically compatible for 48 hr at 25 °C	1167	**C**
	MSD	80 mg/ 16 ml	RB	160 mg/ 32 ml	Physically compatible for 48 hr at 25 °C	1167	**C**
Hydrocortisone sodium succinate	MSD	10 mg/ 2 ml[a]	RB	10 mg/ 2 ml	Physically compatible for 48 hr at room temperature	924	**C**
	MSD	20 mg/ 4 ml[a]	RB	10 mg/ 2 ml	Physically compatible for 48 hr at room temperature	924	**C**

Drugs in Syringe Compatibility (Cont.)

Metoclopramide HCl

Drug (in syringe)	Mfr	Amt	Mfr	Amt	Remarks	Ref	C/I
Hydroxyzine HCl	PF	50 mg/ 1 ml	NO	10 mg/ 2 ml	Physically compatible both macroscopically and microscopically for 15 min at room temperature	565	C
Insulin, regular	LI	10 units/ 2 ml[a]	RB	10 mg/ 2 ml	Physically compatible for 24 hr at room temperature	924	C
	LI	20 units/ 4 ml[a]	RB	10 mg/ 2 ml	Physically compatible for 24 hr at room temperature	924	C
	LI	80 units/ 16 ml	RB	160 mg/ 32 ml	Physically compatible for 24 hr at 25 °C	1167	C
	LI	10 units/ 2 ml	RB	10 mg/ 2 ml	Physically compatible for 24 hr at 25 °C	1167	C
	LI	20 units/ 4 ml	RB	10 mg/ 2 ml	Physically compatible for 24 hr at 25 °C	1167	C
Leucovorin calcium		5 mg/ 0.5 ml		2.5 mg/ 0.5 ml	Physically compatible for 5 min at room temperature followed by 8 min of centrifugation	980	C
Lidocaine HCl	ES	50 mg/ 5 ml	RB	10 mg/ 2 ml	Physically compatible for 48 hr at room temperature	924	C
	ES	100 mg/ 10 ml	RB	10 mg/ 2 ml	Physically compatible for 48 hr at room temperature	924	C
	ES	50 mg/ 5 ml	RB	160 mg/ 32 ml	Physically compatible for 48 hr at 25 °C	1167	C
	ES	100 mg/ 10 ml	RB	160 mg/ 32 ml	Physically compatible for 48 hr at 25 °C	1167	C
	ES	50 mg/ 5 ml	RB	10 mg/ 2 ml	Physically compatible for 48 hr at 25 °C	1167	C
	ES	100 mg/ 10 ml	RB	10 mg/ 2 ml	Physically compatible for 48 hr at 25 °C	1167	C
Magnesium sulfate	ES	500 mg/ 1 ml	RB	10 mg/ 2 ml	Physically compatible for 48 hr at room temperature	924	C
	ES	1 g/2 ml	RB	10 mg/ 2 ml	Physically compatible for 48 hr at room temperature	924	C
	ES	1 g/2 ml	RB	160 mg/ 32 ml	Physically compatible for 48 hr at 25 °C	1167	C
	ES	500 mg/ 1 ml	RB	10 mg/ 2 ml	Physically compatible for 48 hr at 25 °C	1167	C
	ES	1 g/2 ml	RB	10 mg/ 2 ml	Physically compatible for 48 hr at 25 °C	1167	C
Meperidine HCl	WI	50 mg/ 1 ml	NO	10 mg/ 2 ml	Physically compatible both macroscopically and microscopically for 15 min at room temperature	565	C
Methotrexate sodium	LE	50 mg/ 2 ml	RB	10 mg/ 2 ml	Incompatible. If mixed, use immediately	924	I
		12.5 mg/ 0.5 ml		2.5 mg/ 0.5 ml	Physically compatible for 5 min at room temperature followed by 8 min of centrifugation	980	C
	LE	200 mg/ 8 ml	RB	160 mg/ 32 ml	Incompatible. If mixed, use immediately	1167	I
	LE	50 mg/ 2 ml	RB	10 mg/ 2 ml	Incompatible. If mixed, use immediately	1167	I
Methotrimeprazine	RP	10 mg/ 2 ml	NO	10 mg/ 2 ml	Physically compatible both microscopically and macroscopically for 15 min at room temperature	565	C

Drugs in Syringe Compatibility (Cont.)

Metoclopramide HCl

Drug (in syringe)	Mfr	Amt	Mfr	Amt	Remarks	Ref	C/I
Methylprednisolone sodium succinate	ES	62.5 mg/ 1 ml	RB	10 mg/ 2 ml	Physically compatible for 24 hr at room temperature	924	C
	ES	250 mg/ 4 ml	RB	10 mg/ 2 ml	Physically compatible for 24 hr at room temperature	924	C
	ES	250 mg/ 4 ml	RB	160 mg/ 32 ml	Physically compatible for 24 hr at 25 °C	1167	C
	ES	62.5 mg/ 1 ml	RB	10 mg/ 2 ml	Physically compatible for 24 hr at 25 °C	1167	C
	ES	250 mg/ 4 ml	RB	10 mg/ 2 ml	Physically compatible for 24 hr at 25 °C	1167	C
Midazolam HCl	RC	5 mg/ 1 ml	RB	10 mg/ 2 ml	Physically compatible for 4 hr at 25 °C under fluorescent light	1145	C
Mitomycin		0.25 mg/ 0.5 ml		2.5 mg/ 0.5 ml	Physically compatible for 5 min at room temperature followed by 8 min of centrifugation	980	C
Morphine sulfate	AH	10 mg/ 1 ml	NO	10 mg/ 2 ml	Physically compatible both macroscopically and microscopically for 15 min at room temperature	565	C
	EV	1 mg/ml	SKB	0.5 mg/ ml	Diluted with NS. 5% or less loss of both drugs by HPLC in 35 days at 22 °C and 182 days at 4 °C followed by 7 days at 32 °C	1938	C
Morphine tartrate	DB	[b]	DB	10 mg/ 2 ml	Visually compatible with about 5% morphine loss by HPLC in 48 hr at room temperature protected from light. Metoclopramide not tested	1599	C
Ondansetron HCl	GW	1 mg/ml[c]	SO	2.5 mg/ ml[c]	Physically compatible with no measured increase in particulates and less than 6% loss of ondansetron and less than 5% loss of metoclopramide by HPLC in 24 hr at 4 or 23 °C	2199	C
Penicillin G potassium	SQ	250,000 units/ 1 ml	RB	10 mg/ 2 ml	Incompatible. If mixed, use immediately	924; 1167	I
	SQ	1 million units/ 4 ml	RB	10 mg/ 2 ml	Incompatible. If mixed, use immediately	924; 1167	I
	SQ	1 million units/ 4 ml	RB	160 mg/ 32 ml	Incompatible. If mixed, use immediately	1167	I
Pentazocine lactate	WI	30 mg/ 1 ml	NO	10 mg/ 2 ml	Physically compatible both macroscopically and microscopically for 15 min at room temperature	565	C
Perphenazine	SC	5 mg/ 1 ml	NO	10 mg/ 2 ml	Physically compatible both macroscopically and microscopically for 15 min at room temperature	565; 566	C
Prochlorperazine edisylate	MB	10 mg/ 2 ml	NO	10 mg/ 2 ml	Physically compatible both macroscopically and microscopically for 15 min at room temperature	565	C

Drugs in Syringe Compatibility (Cont.)

Metoclopramide HCl

Drug (in syringe)	Mfr	Amt	Mfr	Amt	Remarks	Ref	C/I
Promazine HCl	MY	50 mg/ 1 ml	NO	10 mg/ 2 ml	Physically compatible both macroscopically and microscopically for 15 min at room temperature	565	C
Promethazine HCl	WY	25 mg/ 1 ml	NO	10 mg/ 2 ml	Physically compatible both macroscopically and microscopically for 15 min at room temperature	565	C
Ranitidine HCl	GL	50 mg/ 2 ml	RB	10 mg/ 1 ml	Physically compatible for 1 hr at 25 °C both macroscopically and microscopically	978	C
Scopolamine HBr	ST	0.4 mg/ 1 ml	NO	10 mg/ 2 ml	Physically compatible both macroscopically and microscopically for 15 min at room temperature	565	C
Sodium bicarbonate	AB	100 mEq/ 100 ml	RB	10 mg/ 2 ml	Incompatible. Do not mix	924	I
	AB	100 mEq/ 100 ml	RB	10 mg/ 2 ml	Gas evolves	1167	I
	AB	100 mEq/ 100 ml	RB	160 mg/ 32 ml	Gas evolves	1167	I
Sufentanil citrate	JN	50 µg/ml	RB	5 mg/ml	Physically compatible with no subvisual haze or particle formation in 24 hr at 23 °C	1711	C
Vinblastine sulfate		0.5 mg/ 0.5 ml		2.5 mg/ 0.5 ml	Physically compatible for 5 min at room temperature followed by 8 min of centrifugation	980	C
Vincristine sulfate		0.5 mg/ 0.5 ml		2.5 mg/ 0.5 ml	Physically compatible for 5 min at room temperature followed by 8 min of centrifugation	980	C
Vitamin B complex with C	RC	2 ml	RB	10 mg/ 2 ml	Physically compatible for 48 hr at room temperature	924	C
	RC	2 ml	RB	160 mg/ 32 ml	Physically compatible for 48 hr at 25 °C	1167	C
	RC	2 ml	RB	10 mg/ 2 ml	Physically compatible for 48 hr at 25 °C	1167	C

[a]Brought to volume with distilled water.
[b]Amount unspecified.
[c]Tested in sodium chloride 0.9%.

Y-Site Injection Compatibility (1:1 Mixture)

Metoclopramide HCl

Drug	Mfr	Conc	Mfr	Conc	Remarks	Ref	C/I
Acyclovir sodium	BW	5 mg/ml[a]	ES	0.2 mg/ml[a]	Physically compatible for 4 hr at 25 °C	1157	C
Aldesleukin	CHI	33,800 I.U./ ml[a]	DU	5 mg/ml	Visually compatible with little or no loss of aldesleukin activity by bioassay	1857	C
Allopurinol sodium	BW	3 mg/ml[b]	DU	5 mg/ml	Heavy white precipitate forms immediately	1686	I
Amifostine	USB	10 mg/ml[a]	ES	5 mg/ml	Physically compatible with no change in measured turbidity or increase in particle content in 4 hr at 23 °C	1845	C
Amphotericin B cholesteryl sulfate complex	SEQ	0.83 mg/ml[a]	FAU	5 mg/ml	Gross precipitate forms	2117	I

Y-Site Injection Compatibility (1:1 Mixture) (Cont.)

Metoclopramide HCl

Drug	Mfr	Conc	Mfr	Conc	Remarks	Ref	C/I
Amsacrine	NCI	1 mg/ml[a]	RB	2.5 mg/ml[a]	Yellow-orange turbidity develops in 15 min, becoming heavy flocculent orange precipitate in 1 hr	1381	I
Aztreonam	SQ	40 mg/ml[a]	ES	5 mg/ml	Physically compatible with no subvisual haze or particle formation in 4 hr at 23 °C	1758	C
Bleomycin sulfate		3 units/ml		5 mg/ml	Drugs injected sequentially into Y-site with no flush between. No visually apparent precipitate	980	C
Cefepime HCl	BR	20 mg/ml[a]	RB	5 mg/ml	Haze forms immediately	1689	I
Ciprofloxacin	MI	2 mg/ml[c]	DU	5 mg/ml	Visually compatible for 24 hr at 24 °C	1655	C
	BAY	2 mg/ml[b]		5 mg/ml	Visually compatible with no ciprofloxacin loss by HPLC in 15 min. Metoclopramide not tested.	1934	C
Cisatracurium besylate	GW	0.1, 2, 5 mg/ml[a]	AB	5 mg/ml	Physically compatible with no change in measured turbidity or increase in particle content in 4 hr at 23 °C	2074	C
Cisplatin		1 mg/ml		5 mg/ml	Drugs injected sequentially into Y-site with no flush between. No visually apparent precipitate	980	C
	BR	1 mg/ml	RB	2.5 mg/ml[a]	Visually compatible for 4 hr at room temperature under fluorescent light	1685	C
Cladribine	ORT	0.015[b] and 0.5[d] mg/ml	RB	5 mg/ml	Physically compatible with no change in measured turbidity or increase in particle content in 4 hr at 23 °C	1969	C
Clarithromycin	AB	4 mg/ml[a]	ANT	5 mg/ml	Visually compatible for 72 hr at both 30 and 17 °C	2174	C
Cyclophosphamide		20 mg/ml		5 mg/ml	Drugs injected sequentially into Y-site with no flush between. No visually apparent precipitate	980	C
	MJ	10 mg/ml	RB	2.5 mg/ml[a]	Visually compatible for 4 hr at room temperature under fluorescent light	1685	C
Cytarabine	UP	50 mg/ml	RB	2.5 mg/ml[a]	Visually compatible for 4 hr at room temperature under fluorescent light	1685	C
Diltiazem HCl	MMD	1[b] and 5 mg/ml	RB	5 mg/ml	Visually compatible	1807	C
	MMD	5 mg/ml	RB	0.2 mg/ml[b]	Visually compatible	1807	C
Docetaxel	RPR	0.9 mg/ml[a]	AB	5 mg/ml	Physically compatible with no change in measured turbidity or increase in particle content in 4 hr at 23 °C	2224	C
Doxorubicin HCl		2 mg/ml		5 mg/ml	Drugs injected sequentially into Y-site with no flush between. No visually apparent precipitate	980	C
	AD	0.2 mg/ml[a]	RB	2.5 mg/ml[a]	Visually compatible for 4 hr at room temperature under fluorescent light	1685	C
Doxorubicin HCl liposome injection	SEQ	0.4 mg/ml[a]	GNS	5 mg/ml	Increase in measured turbidity	2087	I

Y-Site Injection Compatibility (1:1 Mixture) (Cont.)

Metoclopramide HCl

Drug	Mfr	Conc	Mfr	Conc	Remarks	Ref	C/I
Droperidol		2.5 mg/ml		5 mg/ml	Drugs injected sequentially into Y-site with no flush between. No visually apparent precipitate	980	C
Etoposide phosphate	BR	5 mg/ml[a]	FAU	5 mg/ml	Physically compatible with no change in measured turbidity or increase in particle content in 4 hr at 23 °C	2218	C
Famotidine	MSD ME	0.2 mg/ml[a] 2 mg/ml[b]	RB	5 mg/ml 5 mg/ml	Physically compatible for 14 hr Visually compatible for 4 hr at 22 °C	1196 1936	C C
Filgrastim	AMG	30 μg/ml[a]	ES	5 mg/ml	Physically compatible with no change in measured turbidity or increase in particle content in 4 hr at 22 °C	1687	C
Fluconazole	RR	2 mg/ml	RB	5 mg/ml	Physically compatible for 24 hr at 25 °C	1407	C
Fludarabine phosphate	BX	1 mg/ml[a]	DU	5 mg/ml	Physically compatible for 4 hr at room temperature under fluorescent light	1439	C
Fluorouracil		50 mg/ml		5 mg/ml	Drugs injected sequentially into Y-site with no flush between. No visually apparent precipitate	980	C
Foscarnet sodium	AST	24 mg/ml	RB	4 mg/ml	Physically compatible for 24 hr at room temperature under fluorescent light	1335	C
	AST	24 mg/ml	RB	2 mg/ml[c]	Physically compatible for 24 hr at 25 °C under fluorescent light by visual and microscopic examination	1393	C
Furosemide		10 mg/ml		5 mg/ml	Drugs injected sequentially into Y-site with no flush between. Immediate precipitation	980	I
Gemcitabine HCl	LI	10 mg/ml[b]	FAU	5 mg/ml	Physically compatible with no change in measured turbidity or increase in particle content in 4 hr at 23 °C	2226	C
Granisetron HCl	SKB	0.05 mg/ml[a]	AB	5 mg/ml	Physically compatible with no change in measured turbidity or increase in particle content in 4 hr at 23 °C	2000	C
Heparin sodium		1000 units/ml		5 mg/ml	Drugs injected sequentially into Y-site with no flush between. No visually apparent precipitate	980	C
Idarubicin HCl	AD	1 mg/ml[b]	SO	5 mg/ml	Visually compatible for 24 hr at 25 °C	1525	C
Leucovorin calcium		10 mg/ml		5 mg/ml	Drugs injected sequentially into Y-site with no flush between. No visually apparent precipitate	980	C
Melphalan HCl	BW	0.1 mg/ml[b]	RB	5 mg/ml	Physically compatible with no change in measured turbidity or increase in particle content in 3 hr at 22 °C	1557	C
Meperidine HCl	AB	10 mg/ml	SN	0.2 mg/ml[a]	Physically compatible for 4 hr at 25 °C	1397	C
Meropenem	ZEN	1 and 50 mg/ml[b]	RB	5 mg/ml	Visually compatible for 4 hr at room temperature	1994	C
Methotrexate sodium		25 mg/ml		5 mg/ml	Drugs injected sequentially into Y-site with no flush between. No visually apparent precipitate	980	C
	AD	15 mg/ml[e]	RB	2.5 mg/ml[a]	Visually compatible for 4 hr at room temperature under fluorescent light	1685	C

Y-Site Injection Compatibility (1:1 Mixture) (Cont.)

Metoclopramide HCl

Drug	Mfr	Conc	Mfr	Conc	Remarks	Ref	C/I
Mitomycin		0.5 mg/ml		5 mg/ml	Drugs injected sequentially into Y-site with no flush between. No visually apparent precipitate	980	C
Morphine sulfate	AB	1 mg/ml	SN	0.2 mg/ml[a]	Physically compatible for 4 hr at 25 °C	1397	C
Ondansetron HCl	GL	1 mg/ml[b]	DU	5 mg/ml	Physically compatible for 4 hr at 22 °C	1365	C
Paclitaxel	NCI	1.2 mg/ml[a]		5 mg/ml	Physically compatible with no change in measured turbidity in 4 hr at 22 °C	1528	C
Piperacillin sodium–tazobactam sodium	LE	40 + 5 mg/ml[a]	RB	5 mg/ml	Physically compatible with no change in measured turbidity or increase in particle content in 4 hr at 22 °C	1688	C
Propofol	ZEN	10 mg/ml	RB	5 mg/ml	Emulsion broke and oiled out	1916	I
Remifentanil HCl	GW	0.025 and 0.25 mg/ml[b]	AB	5 mg/ml	Physically compatible with no change in measured turbidity or increase in particle content in 4 hr at 23 °C	2075	C
Sargramostim	IMM	10 μg/ml[b]	DU	5 mg/ml	Physically compatible for 4 hr at 22 °C	1436	C
Sufentanil citrate	JN	12.5 μg/ml[a]	RB	5 mg/ml	Physically compatible with no subvisual haze or particle formation in 24 hr at 23 °C	1711	C
Tacrolimus	FUJ	1 mg/ml[b]	DU	0.2 mg/ml[a]	Visually compatible for 24 hr at 25 °C	1630	C
Teniposide	BR	0.1 mg/ml[a]	ES	5 mg/ml	Physically compatible with no subvisual haze or particle formation in 4 hr at 23 °C	1725	C
Thiotepa	IMM[f]	1 mg/ml[a]	RB	5 mg/ml	Physically compatible with no change in measured turbidity or increase in particle content in 4 hr at 23 °C	1861	C
TNA #218 to #226[g]			AB	5 mg/ml	Visually compatible with no precipitate or emulsion damage apparent in 4 hr at 23 °C	2215	C
TPN #212 to #215[g]			AB	5 mg/ml	Substantial loss of natural subvisual turbidity occurs immediately	2109	I
Vinblastine sulfate		1 mg/ml		5 mg/ml	Drugs injected sequentially into Y-site with no flush between. No visually apparent precipitate	980	C
Vincristine sulfate		1 mg/ml		5 mg/ml	Drugs injected sequentially into Y-site with no flush between. No visually apparent precipitate	980	C
Vinorelbine tartrate	BW	1 mg/ml[b]	RB	5 mg/ml	Physically compatible with no change in measured turbidity or increase in particle content in 4 hr at 22 °C	1558	C
Zidovudine	BW	4 mg/ml[a]	RB	2 mg/ml[a]	Physically compatible for 4 hr at 25 °C under fluorescent light by visual and microscopic examination	1193	C

[a]*Tested in dextrose 5% in water.*
[b]*Tested in sodium chloride 0.9%.*
[c]*Tested in both dextrose 5% in water and sodium chloride 0.9%.*
[d]*Tested in bacteriostatic sodium chloride 0.9% preserved with benzyl alcohol 0.9%.*
[e]*Tested in dextrose 5% in water with sodium bicarbonate 0.05 mEq/ml.*
[f]*Lyophilized formulation tested.*
[g]*Refer to Appendix I for the composition of parenteral nutrition solutions. TNA indicates a 3-in-1 admixture, and TPN indicates a 2-in-1 admixture.*

Additional Compatibility Information

Solutions— Metoclopramide HCl has been stated to be compatible for up to 48 hours at room temperature, protected from light, in the following infusion solutions (2; 4):

Dextrose 5% in sodium chloride 0.45%
Dextrose 5% in water
Ringer's injection
Ringer's injection, lactated
Sodium chloride 0.9%

The manufacturer indicates dilutions may be stored under normal light conditions, without light protection, for up to 24 hours (2).

Cisplatin— The sodium metabisulfite antioxidant present in the former metoclopramide HCl formulation reacted rapidly and extensively with cisplatin, displacing the chloride ligands. At clinically relevant concentrations, a 10% cisplatin loss occurred in less than five minutes. Total cisplatin loss occurred in about 30 minutes (1175). The current Reglan and Maxolon formulations contain no sulfites (2; 4; 1247).

Diamorphine HCl— Metoclopramide HCl is stated to be stable and compatible with diamorphine HCl (1442).

METOPROLOL TARTRATE
AHFS 24:04

Lopressor   **Novartis**

Products— Metoprolol tartrate (Novartis) is available in 5-ml ampuls. Each milliliter of solution contains 1 mg of metoprolol tartrate and 9 mg of sodium chloride (2).

pH— Approximately 7.5 (175).

Administration— Metoprolol tartrate is administered intravenously (2; 4).

Stability— Metoprolol tartrate injection should be stored at controlled room temperature and protected from light and freezing (2; 4).

Compatibility Information

Solution Compatibility

Metoprolol tartrate

Solution	Mfr	Mfr	Conc/L	Remarks	Ref	C/I
Dextrose 5% in water	BA[a]	CI	300 mg	Visually compatible with little or no metoprolol loss by HPLC in 36 hr at 24 °C under fluorescent light	1679	C
Sodium chloride 0.9%	BA[a]	CI	300 mg	Visually compatible with little or no metoprolol loss by HPLC in 36 hr at 24 °C under fluorescent light	1679	C

[a]Tested in PVC containers.

Y-Site Injection Compatibility (1:1 Mixture)

Metoprolol tartrate

Drug	Mfr	Conc	Mfr	Conc	Remarks	Ref	C/I
Alteplase	GEN	1 mg/ml	CI	1 mg/ml	Visually compatible with no alteplase clot-lysis activity loss in 24 hr at 25 °C	1856	C
Amphotericin B cholesteryl sulfate complex	SEQ	0.83 mg/ml[a]	GEN	1 mg/ml	Gross precipitate forms	2117	I
Meperidine HCl	AB	10 mg/ml	CI	1 mg/ml	Physically compatible for 4 hr at 25 °C	1397	C
Morphine sulfate	AB	1 mg/ml	CI	1 mg/ml	Physically compatible for 4 hr at 25 °C	1397	C

[a]Tested in dextrose 5% in water.

METRONIDAZOLE
AHFS 8:40

Flagyl I.V. RTU

Abbott
SCS Pharmaceuticals

Products—— Metronidazole (SCS Pharmaceuticals) is available as a ready-to-use solution in 100-ml single-dose PVC plastic bags. No dilution or buffering is required. Each bag contains (2):

Metronidazole	500 mg
Sodium phosphate	47.6 mg
Citric acid	22.9 mg
Sodium chloride	790 mg
Water for injection	qs 100 ml

pH—— Metronidazole ready-to-use has a pH of 5 to 7 (2).

Osmolarity—— Metronidazole ready-to-use has an osmolarity of 310 mOsm/L (2).

Sodium Content—— Metronidazole ready-to-use contains 14 mEq of sodium from the excipients per 500 mg of metronidazole (2; 4).

Administration—— Metronidazole ready-to-use is administered by continuous intravenous infusion or by intermittent intravenous infusion over one hour. Metronidazole ready-to-use may be administered without dilution or buffering.

Stability—— Metronidazole ready-to-use is a clear, colorless solution which should be stored between 15 and 30 °C and protected from light (2; 4). It should not be stored under refrigeration (2). Refrigeration may result in crystal formation. However, the crystals redissolve on warming to room temperature (1115).

Prolonged exposure to light will cause a darkening of the product (4). However, most manufacturers indicate that short-term exposure to normal room light does not adversely affect metronidazole stability. Direct sunlight should be avoided (1115).

Sorption—— Metronidazole (May & Baker) 30 mg/L in sodium chloride 0.9% (Travenol) in PVC bags did not exhibit significant sorption to the plastic during one week of storage at room temperature (15 to 20 °C) (536).

In another study, metronidazole (May & Baker) 30 mg/L in sodium chloride 0.9% did not exhibit any loss due to sorption during a seven-hour simulated infusion through an infusion set (Travenol) consisting of a cellulose propionate burette chamber and 170 cm of PVC tubing (606).

The drug was also tested as a simulated infusion over at least one hour by a syringe pump system. A glass syringe on a syringe pump was fitted with 20 cm of polyethylene tubing or 50 cm of Silastic tubing. No loss of drug due to sorption was observed with either tubing (606).

A 25-ml aliquot of metronidazole (May & Baker) 30 mg/L in sodium chloride 0.9% was stored in all-plastic syringes composed of polypropylene barrels and polyethylene plungers for 24 hours at room temperature in the dark. No loss due to sorption occurred (606).

Filtration—— Metronidazole (Specia) 5 mg/ml in dextrose 5% in water and sodium chloride 0.9% was filtered through a 0.22-μm cellulose ester membrane filter (Ivex-HP, Millipore) over six hours. No significant drug loss due to binding to the filter was noted (1034).

Compatibility Information

Additive Compatibility

Metronidazole

Drug	Mfr	Conc/L	Mfr	Conc/L	Test Soln	Remarks	Ref	C/I
Amikacin sulfate	BR	5 g	RP	5 g[a]		Physically compatible with little or no pH change for at least 12 hr at 23 °C	807	**C**
Amoxicillin sodium–clavulanate potassium	BE	20 + 2 g	BAY	5 g		Physically compatible with 8% clavulanate loss in 2 hr and 25% loss in 6 hr at 21 °C by HPLC. 7 to 8% amoxicillin and no metronidazole loss in 6 hr at 21 °C.	1920	**I**
Ampicillin sodium	AY	20 g	RP	5 g[a]		Physically compatible for at least 24 hr at 23 °C, but pH changed significantly	807	**?**
	BR	20 g	SE	5 g		9% ampicillin loss in 22 hr at 25 °C and 12 days at 5 °C. No metronidazole loss	993	**C**
Aztreonam	SQ	10 and 20 g	MG	5 g		Pink color develops in 12 hr, becoming cherry red in 48 hr at 25 °C. Pink color develops in 3 days at 4 °C. No loss of either drug detected	1023	**I**
Cefamandole nafate	LI	20 g	RP	5 g[a]		Physically compatible with little or no pH change for at least 72 hr at 4 °C	807	**C**
	LI	20 g	RP	5 g[a]		Physically compatible for at least 24 hr at 23 °C, but pH changed significantly	807	**?**

Additive Compatibility (Cont.)

Metronidazole

Drug	Mfr	Conc/L	Mfr	Conc/L	Test Soln	Remarks	Ref	C/I
	LI	20 g	SE	5 g		10% metronidazole loss in 2 hr at 25 °C and 6 hr at 5 °C with no further loss occurring in up to 3 days. No cefamandole loss	979	I
	LI	800 mg	SE	200 mg	W	No immediate loss of potency of either drug	979	C
	LI	16.7 g	BAY	4.2 g	b	Visually compatible with little cefamandole loss and 8% or less metronidazole loss in 4 hr at room temperature by HPLC	1888	C
Cefazolin sodium	LI	10 g	RP	5 g[a]		Physically compatible with little or no pH change for at least 24 hr at 23 °C and 72 hr at 4 °C	807	C
	LI	10 g	SE	5 g		5% cefazolin loss and no metronidazole loss in 7 days at 25 °C. No loss of either drug in 12 days at 5 °C	993	C
	LI	10 g	AB	5 g		Visually compatible with no loss of either drug by HPLC in 72 hr at 8 °C	1649	C
Cefepime HCl	BR	40 g	AB, ES, SE	5 g		7% cefepime loss by HPLC in 24 hr at room temperature exposed to light and 8% loss in 5 days at 5 °C. Little or no metronidazole loss by HPLC. However, orange color develops in 18 hr at room temperature and 24 hr at 5 °C	1682	?
	BR	4 g	AB, ES, SE	5 g		6% cefepime loss by HPLC in 24 hr at room temperature exposed to light and 3% loss in 5 days at 5 °C. Little or no metronidazole loss by HPLC. However, orange color develops in 18 hr at room temperature and 24 hr at 5 °C	1682	?
Cefotaxime sodium	RS	20 g	RP	5 g[a]		Physically compatible with little or no pH change for at least 24 hr at 4 °C	807	C
	HO	10 g	AB	5 g		Potency of both drugs by HPLC retained for 72 hr at 8 °C	1547	C
	HO	10 g	AB	5 g		Visually compatible with 10% cefotaxime loss by HPLC in 19 hr at 28 °C and 8% loss in 96 hr at 5 °C. No metronidazole loss in 96 hr at 5 or 28 °C	1754	C
Cefotiam HCl	TAK	20 g		5 g		Visually compatible with no little or no loss of either drug by HPLC in 4 hr at room temperature	1737	C
Cefoxitin sodium	FC	30 g	RP	5 g[a]		Physically compatible with little or no pH change for at least 24 hr at 4 °C	807	C
	FC	30 g	RP	5 g[a]		Physically compatible, but pH changed significantly in 6 to 12 hr at 23 °C	807	?
	MSD	30 g	SE	5 g		9% cefoxitin loss in 48 hr at 25 °C and 3% in 12 days at 5 °C. No metronidazole loss	993	C
Ceftazidime	GL[e]	20 g		5 g		No loss of either drug in 4 hr	1345	C
	LI[e]	10 g	AB	5 g		Visually compatible with little or no loss of either drug by HPLC in 72 hr at 8 °C	1849	C

Additive Compatibility (Cont.)

Metronidazole

Drug	Mfr	Conc/L	Mfr	Conc/L	Test Soln	Remarks	Ref	C/I
Ceftizoxime sodium	FUJ	10 g	AB	5 g		Visually compatible with little or no loss of either drug by HPLC in 72 hr at 8 °C	1849	C
	SKB	10 g	AB	5 g		Visually compatible with 8 to 9% loss of both drugs by HPLC in 14 days at 4 °C followed by 48 hr at 25 °C. 3 to 4% loss of both drugs in 3 days and 10 to 13% in 5 days at 25 °C	1879	C
Ceftriaxone sodium	RC	10 g	AB	5 g		Visually compatible with little or no loss of either drug by HPLC in 72 hr at 8 °C	1849	C
	RC	10 g	BA	5 g		Visually compatible with no metronidazole loss by HPLC and with 6% ceftriaxone loss in 3 days and 8% in 4 days at 25 °C	2101	C
Cefuroxime sodium	GL	7.5 g		5 g		Physically compatible with no loss of either drug in 1 hr	1036	C
	GL	15 g		5 g		No loss of either drug in 4 hr at 24 °C	1376	C
	GL	7.5 g		5 g		10% cefuroxime loss by HPLC in 16 days at 4 °C and 35 hr at 25 °C. No metronidazole loss by HPLC in 15 days at 4 and 25 °C	1565	C
	GL	7.5 and 15 g	IVX	5 g		Physically compatible with no visible precipitation or increase in measured particulates. No loss of metronidazole and about 6% cefuroxime loss in 49 days at 5 °C	2192	C
Chloramphenicol sodium succinate	PD	10 g	RP	5 g[a]		Physically compatible with little or no pH change for at least 72 hr at 23 °C	807	C
Ciprofloxacin		2 g		5 g		No loss of either drug in 4 hr at 24 °C	1346	C
	MI	1.6 g	SE	4.2 g		Visually compatible and potency of both drugs by HPLC retained for 48 hr at 25 °C under fluorescent light and 4 °C in the dark	1541	C
Clindamycin phosphate	UP	10 g	RP	5 g[a]		Physically compatible with little or no pH change for at least 24 hr at 23 °C	807	C
Floxacillin sodium	BE	10 g		5 g		Physically compatible for 48 hr. Potency of both drugs retained when assayed after 1 hr at room temperature	1036	C
Fluconazole	PF	1 g	AB	2.5 g		Visually compatible with no fluconazole loss by HPLC in 72 hr at 25 °C under fluorescent light. Metronidazole not tested	1677	C
Gentamicin sulfate	RS	800 mg	RP	5 g[a]		Physically compatible with little or no pH change for at least 72 hr at 23 °C	807	C
	EX	800 mg[d]		5 g		Physically compatible with no loss of either drug in 1 hr	1036	C
	SC	800 mg and 1.2 g	SE	5 g		Physically compatible with no loss of either drug in 2 days at 18 °C. At 4 °C, no metronidazole loss but up to 10% gentamicin loss in 7 days	1242	C

Additive Compatibility (Cont.)

Metronidazole

Drug	Mfr	Conc/L	Mfr	Conc/L	Test Soln	Remarks	Ref	C/I
		800 mg	RP	5 g		Visually compatible with no loss of metronidazole by HPLC in 15 days at 5 and 25 °C. 10% gentamicin loss by immunoassay in 63 hr at 25 °C and 10.6 days at 5 °C	1931	C
Hydrocortisone sodium succinate	UP	10 g	RP	5 g[a]		Physically compatible for at least 72 hr at 23 °C, but pH changed significantly	807	?
	ES	10 g	SE	5 g		No loss of either drug for 7 days at 25 °C and 12 days at 5 °C	993	C
Netilmicin sulfate	SC	1.4 g	RP	5 g[a]		Physically compatible with little or no pH change for at least 24 hr at 23 °C and 72 hr at 4 °C	807	C
	EX	1 g		5 g		Physically compatible with no loss of either drug in 1 hr	1036	C
Penicillin G potassium	AY	12 million units	RP	5 g[a]		Physically compatible for at least 72 hr at 23 °C, but pH changed significantly	807	?
	PF	200 million units	SE	5 g		5% penicillin loss in 22 hr and 8% in 72 hr at 25 °C. 2% penicillin loss in 12 days at 5 °C. No metronidazole loss	993	C
Tobramycin sulfate	LI	800 mg	RP	5 g[a]		Physically compatible with little or no pH change for at least 72 hr at 23 °C	807	C
	LI	1 g	RP	5 g		Visually compatible with no loss of metronidazole by HPLC in 15 days at 5 and 25 °C. 10% tobramycin loss by immunoassay in 73 hr at 25 °C and 12.1 days at 5 °C	1931	C

[a]Minibags (100 ml) containing metronidazole 500 mg with disodium phosphate 150 mg, citric acid 44 mg, and sodium chloride 740 mg. This product differs from the SCS Pharmaceuticals product.
[b]Cefamandole reconstituted with water and added to metronidazole infusion.
[c]Sodium carbonate-containing formulation tested.
[d]Tested in both dextrose 5% in water and sodium chloride 0.9%.

Y-Site Injection Compatibility (1:1 Mixture)

Metronidazole

Drug	Mfr	Conc	Mfr	Conc	Remarks	Ref	C/I
Acyclovir sodium	BW	5 mg/ml[a]	SE	5 mg/ml	Physically compatible for 4 hr at 25 °C	1157	C
Allopurinol sodium	BW	3 mg/ml[b]	BA	5 mg/ml	Physically compatible with no change in measured turbidity or increase in particle content in 4 hr at 22 °C	1686	C
Amifostine	USB	10 mg/ml[a]	BA	5 mg/ml	Physically compatible with no change in measured turbidity or increase in particle content in 4 hr at 23 °C	1845	C
Amphotericin B cholesteryl sulfate complex	SEQ	0.83 mg/ml[a]	AB	5 mg/ml	Gross precipitate forms	2117	I
Aztreonam	SQ	40 mg/ml[a]	BA	5 mg/ml	Color changes from colorless to orange in 4 hr	1758	I

Y-Site Injection Compatibility (1:1 Mixture) (Cont.)

Metronidazole

Drug	Mfr	Conc	Mfr	Conc	Remarks	Ref	C/I
Cefepime HCl	BR	20 mg/ml[a]	BA	5 mg/ml	Physically compatible with no change in measured turbidity or increase in particle content in 4 hr at 22 °C	1689	C
Cisatracurium besylate	GW	0.1, 2, and 5 mg/ml[a]	AB	5 mg/ml	Physically compatible with no change in measured turbidity or increase in particle content in 4 hr at 23 °C	2074	C
Clarithromycin	AB	4 mg/ml[a]	PRK	5 mg/ml	Visually compatible for 72 hr at both 30 and 17 °C	2174	C
Cyclophosphamide	MJ	20 mg/ml[a]	SE	5 mg/ml	Physically compatible for 4 hr at 25 °C	1194	C
Diltiazem HCl	MMD	5 mg/ml	SE	5 mg/ml	Visually compatible	1807	C
Docetaxel	RPR	0.9 mg/ml[a]	BA	5 mg/ml	Physically compatible with no change in measured turbidity or increase in particle content in 4 hr at 23 °C	2224	C
Dopamine HCl	AB	0.8 mg/ml[a]	MG	5 mg/ml	Visually compatible for 24 hr at room temperature in test tubes. No precipitate found on filter from Y-site delivery	2063	C
Doxorubicin HCl liposome injection	SEQ	0.4 mg/ml[a]	AB	5 mg/ml	Physically compatible with little or no change in measured turbidity and no increase in particle content in 4 hr at 23 °C	2087	C
Enalaprilat	MSD	0.05 mg/ml[b]	SE	5 mg/ml	Physically compatible for 24 hr at room temperature under fluorescent light	1355	C
Esmolol HCl	DCC	10 mg/ml[a]	SE	5 mg/ml	Physically compatible for 24 hr at 22 °C	1169	C
Etoposide phosphate	BR	5 mg/ml[a]	AB	5 mg/ml	Physically compatible with no change in measured turbidity or increase in particle content in 4 hr at 23 °C	2218	C
Filgrastim	AMG	30 μg/ml[a]	BA	5 mg/ml	Particles form immediately with filaments in 1 hr	1687	I
Fluconazole	RR	2 mg/ml	AB	5 mg/ml	Physically compatible for 24 hr at 25 °C	1407	C
Foscarnet sodium	AST	24 mg/ml	AB	5 mg/ml	Physically compatible for 24 hr at room temperature under fluorescent light	1335	C
	AST	24 mg/ml	SE	5 mg/ml	Physically compatible for 24 hr at 25 °C under fluorescent light by visual and microscopic examination	1393	C
Gemcitabine HCl	LI	10 mg/ml[b]	AB	5 mg/ml	Physically compatible with no change in measured turbidity or increase in particle content in 4 hr at 23 °C	2226	C
Granisetron HCl	SKB	0.05 mg/ml[a]	BA	5 mg/ml	Physically compatible with no change in measured turbidity or increase in particle content in 4 hr at 23 °C	2000	C
Heparin sodium	TR	50 units/ml	MG	5 mg/ml	Visually compatible for 6 hr at 25 °C	1793	C
Hydromorphone HCl	WY	0.2 mg/ml[a]	SE	5 mg/ml	Physically compatible for at least 4 hr at 25 °C under fluorescent light	987	C
Labetalol HCl	SC	1 mg/ml[a]	SE	5 mg/ml	Physically compatible for 24 hr at 18 °C	1171	C
Lorazepam	WY	0.33 mg/ml[b]	BRN	5 mg/ml	Visually compatible for 24 hr at 22 °C	1855	C

Y-Site Injection Compatibility (1:1 Mixture) (Cont.)

		Metronidazole					
Drug	*Mfr*	*Conc*	*Mfr*	*Conc*	*Remarks*	*Ref*	*C/I*
Magnesium sulfate	IX	16.7, 33.3, 66.7, 100 mg/ml[a]	SE	5 mg/ml	Physically compatible for at least 4 hr at 32 °C	813	**C**
Melphalan HCl	BW	0.1 mg/ml[b]	AB	5 mg/ml	Physically compatible with no change in measured turbidity or increase in particle content in 3 hr at 22 °C	1557	**C**
Meperidine HCl	WY	10 mg/ml[a]	SE	5 mg/ml	Physically compatible for at least 4 hr at 25 °C under fluorescent light	987	**C**
Methylprednisolone sodium succinate	UP	5 mg/ml[a]	MG	5 mg/ml	Visually compatible for 24 hr at room temperature in test tubes. No precipitate found on filter from Y-site delivery	2063	**C**
Midazolam HCl	RC	1 mg/ml[a]	BA	5 mg/ml	Visually compatible for 24 hr at 23 °C	1847	**C**
	RC	5 mg/ml	BRN	5 mg/ml	Visually compatible for 24 hr at 22 °C	1855	**C**
Morphine sulfate	WI	1 mg/ml[a]	SE	5 mg/ml	Physically compatible for at least 4 hr at 25 °C under fluorescent light	987	**C**
Perphenazine	SC	0.02 mg/ml[a]	SE	5 mg/ml	Physically compatible for 4 hr at 25 °C	1155	**C**
Piperacillin sodium–tazobactam sodium	LE	40 + 5 mg/ml[a]	BA	5 mg/ml	Physically compatible with no change in measured turbidity or increase in particle content in 4 hr at 22 °C	1688	**C**
Remifentanil HCl	GW	0.025 and 0.25 mg/ml[b]	AB	5 mg/ml	Physically compatible with no change in measured turbidity or increase in particle content in 4 hr at 23 °C	2075	**C**
Sargramostim	IMM	10 μg/ml[b]	MG	5 mg/ml	Physically compatible for 4 hr at 22 °C	1436	**C**
Tacrolimus	FUJ	1 mg/ml[b]	AB	5 mg/ml	Visually compatible for 24 hr at 25 °C	1630	**C**
Teniposide	BR	0.1 mg/ml[a]	BA	5 mg/ml	Physically compatible with no subvisual haze or particle formation in 4 hr at 23 °C	1725	**C**
Theophylline	MG	5 mg/ml	TR	4 mg/ml	Visually compatible for 6 hr at 25 °C	1793	**C**
Thiotepa	IMM[c]	1 mg/ml[a]	BA	5 mg/ml	Physically compatible with no change in measured turbidity or increase in particle content in 4 hr at 23 °C	1861	**C**
TNA #218 to #226[d]			AB	5 mg/ml	Visually compatible with no precipitate or emulsion damage apparent in 4 hr at 23 °C	2215	**C**
TPN #189[d]			DB	5 mg/ml	Visually compatible for 24 hr at 22 °C	1767	**C**
TPN #203 and #204[d]			AB	5 mg/ml	Visually compatible for 2 hr at 23 °C	1974	**C**
TPN #212 to #215[d]			SCS	5 mg/ml	Physically compatible with no change in measured turbidity or increase in particle content in 4 hr at 23 °C	2109	**C**
Vinorelbine tartrate	BW	1 mg/ml[b]	BA	5 mg/ml	Physically compatible with no change in measured turbidity or increase in particle content in 4 hr at 22 °C	1558	**C**

[a]*Tested in dextrose 5% in water.*
[b]*Tested in sodium chloride 0.9%.*
[c]*Lyophilized formulation tested.*
[d]*Refer to Appendix I for the composition of parenteral nutrition solutions. TNA indicates a 3-in-1 admixture, and TPN indicates a 2-in-1 admixture.*
[e]*Sodium carbonate–containing formulation tested.*

Additional Compatibility Information

It is recommended that no other drug be added to infusions of metronidazole ready-to-use. Furthermore, if administration of metronidazole is to be made through the tubing of an ongoing primary infusion, the primary infusion should be stopped, if possible, during metronidazole administration (2; 4).

However, ceftazidime (Ceptaz) is stated to be stable for 24 hours at room temperature or for seven days under refrigeration with metronidazole 5 mg/ml (4).

Reaction with Aluminum— The discoloration interaction that occurs between reconstituted metronidazole HCl and aluminum in needle hubs does not occur as readily with the ready-to-use metronidazole solution. Discoloration is not apparent when administration is completed within one hour. However, the solution may discolor and a precipitate may form after contact with aluminum for six or more hours (4; 707; 1116; 1117). Also see metronidazole HCl monograph.

METRONIDAZOLE HCL
AHFS 8:40

Flagyl I.V.   **SCS Pharmaceuticals**

Products— Metronidazole HCl (SCS Pharmaceuticals) is available in single-dose lyophilized vials containing metronidazole 500 mg as the hydrochloride and mannitol 415 mg. The correct order of mixing must be followed in preparing the dose for administration (2).

To prepare the solution, add 4.4 ml of one of the following diluents to the vial and mix thoroughly:

Sterile water for injection
Bacteriostatic water for injection
Sodium chloride 0.9%
Bacteriostatic sodium chloride 0.9%

The resulting solution volume of 5 ml will contain 100 mg/ml of metronidazole as the hydrochloride. Further dilute this reconstituted solution to a concentration not more than 8 mg/ml in one of the following infusion solutions:

Dextrose 5% in water
Ringer's injection, lactated
Sodium chloride 0.9%

Addition of 500 mg of metronidazole as the hydrochloride to 100 ml of infusion solution will result in a 5-mg/ml solution. Concentrations exceeding 8 mg/ml may result in precipitation. Use only needles with plastic hubs for this dilution. Do not allow the reconstituted solution to contact aluminum (2; 4).

The diluted solution has an acidic pH and must be neutralized before administration. Approximately 5 mEq of sodium bicarbonate should be added to the diluted solution for each 500 mg of metronidazole and mixed thoroughly. Carbon dioxide gas will be generated, and it may be necessary to relieve the pressure in the container (2; 4).

pH— After reconstitution, metronidazole HCl has a pH of 0.5 to 2. On further dilution and subsequent neutralization, the pH is approximately 6 to 7 (2; 4).

Administration— Metronidazole HCl is administered by continuous intravenous infusion or by intermittent intravenous infusion over one hour. Metronidazole HCl must be diluted to 8 mg/ml or less and neutralized prior to administration. Because of the very low pH of the reconstituted solution, it cannot be given by direct intravenous injection (2; 4).

Stability— Metronidazole HCl should be stored below 30 °C and protected from light (2; 4). Prolonged exposure to light will cause darkening of the product (4). However, most manufacturers indicate that short-term exposure to normal room light does not adversely affect metronidazole stability. Direct sunlight should be avoided (1115).

Initial reconstitution results in a pale yellow to yellow-green solution, which is chemically stable for 96 hours when stored below 30 °C in normal room light. Once further diluted in infusion solutions and neutralized, the solutions should be stored at room temperature and used within 24 hours. Do not refrigerate the neutralized diluted solution because precipitation may occur (2; 4).

Do not attempt to neutralize the reconstituted metronidazole HCl solution prior to dilution in intravenous solutions. Direct addition of sodium bicarbonate to the reconstituted solution will result in immediate precipitation along with the formation of carbon dioxide gas (706).

Compatibility Information

Solution Compatibility

Metronidazole HCl

Solution	Mfr	Mfr	Conc/L	Remarks	Ref	C/I
Amino acids 10%	AB	SE	5 g[a]	Initial yellow color becomes dark yellow in 24 hr	765	I

[a]*Reconstituted metronidazole HCl neutralized with sodium bicarbonate 50 mEq/L was tested.*

Additive Compatibility

Metronidazole HCl

Drug	Mfr	Conc/L	Mfr	Conc/L	Test Soln	Remarks	Ref	C/I
Amikacin sulfate	BR	2.25 g	SE	5 g[a]	D5W, NS	Physically compatible for 48 hr	765	**C**
Aminophylline	SE	2 g	SE	5 g[a]	D5W, NS	Physically compatible for 48 hr	765	**C**
Ampicillin sodium	BR	2 g	SE	5 g[a]	D5W, NS	Physically compatible for 48 hr but ampicillin instability may be determining factor	765	**?**
Cefamandole nafate	LI	2 g	SE	5 g[a]	D5W, NS	Physically compatible for 48 hr. Gradual darkening attributed to normal cephalosporin color change with time	765	**C**
Cefazolin sodium	SKF	5 g	SE	5 g[a]	D5W, NS	Physically compatible for 48 hr. Gradual darkening attributed to normal cephalosporin color change with time	765	**C**
Cefepime HCl	BR	40 g	SE	5 g[a]	D5W, NS	7% cefepime loss by HPLC in 24 hr at room temperature exposed to light and 8% loss in 5 days at 5 °C. Little or no metronidazole loss by HPLC. However, orange color develops in 18 hr at room temperature and 24 hr at 5 °C	1682	**?**
	BR	4 g	SE	8 g[a]	D5W, NS	6% cefepime loss by HPLC in 24 hr at room temperature exposed to light and 3% loss in 5 days at 5 °C. Little or no metronidazole loss by HPLC. However, orange color develops in 18 hr at room temperature and 24 hr at 5 °C. Precipitate forms in 48 hr at 5 °C	1682	**?**
Cefotaxime sodium	HO	10 g	SE	5 g[a]	NS	Visually compatible with 10% cefotaxime loss by HPLC in 24 hr at 28 °C and no loss in 96 hr at 5 °C. No metronidazole loss in 96 hr at 5 or 28 °C	1754	**C**
Cefoxitin sodium	MSD	2 g	SE	5 g[a]	D5W, NS	Physically compatible for 48 hr	765	**C**
Ceftriaxone sodium	RC	20 g	SCS	15 g	D5W, NS	Metronidazole begins to precipitate immediately and increases with time stored at 4 and 24 °C. 22 to 50% of the metronidazole precipitates in 4 hr	2091	**I**
	RC	10 g	SCS	7.5 g	D5W, NS	Visually compatible with little or no loss of either drug by HPLC at 24 °C in 72 hr	2091	**C**
	RC	10 g	SCS	7.5 g	D5W, NS	Visually compatible with little or no loss of either drug by HPLC at 4 °C through 24 hr. Slight precipitation occurred in 48 hr	2091	**C**
Chloramphenicol sodium succinate	PD	2 g	SE	5 g[a]	D5W, NS	Physically compatible for 48 hr	765	**C**
Clindamycin phosphate	UP	2.4 g	SE	5 g[a]	D5W, NS	Physically compatible for 48 hr	765	**C**
Disopyramide phosphate	SE	720 mg	SE	5 g[a]	D5W, NS	Physically compatible for 48 hr	765	**C**
Dopamine HCl	ACC	1 g	SE	5 g[a]	D5W, NS	Becomes markedly discolored, turning yellow then brown	765	**I**
Gentamicin sulfate	SC	320 mg	SE	5 g[a]	D5W, NS	Physically compatible for 48 hr	765	**C**
Heparin sodium	UP	30,000 units	SE	5 g[a]	D5W, NS	Physically compatible for 48 hr	765	**C**

Additive Compatibility (Cont.)

Metronidazole HCl

Drug	Mfr	Conc/L	Mfr	Conc/L	Test Soln	Remarks	Ref	C/I
Hydrocortisone sodium succinate	UP	1 g	SE	5 g[a]	D5W, NS	Physically compatible for 48 hr	765	C
Meropenem	ZEN	1 and 20 g	SE	5 g	NS	Discoloration forms	2068	I
Multielectrolyte concentrate	MG	200 ml	SE	5 g[a]	D5W, NS	Physically compatible for 48 hr	765	C
Multivitamins	USV	20 ml	SE	5 g[a]	D5W, NS	Physically compatible for 48 hr	765	C
Penicillin G potassium	SQ	5 million units	SE	5 g[a]	D5W, NS	Physically compatible for 48 hr	765	C
Tobramycin sulfate	LI	700 mg	SE	5 g[a]	D5W, NS	Physically compatible for 48 hr	765	C

[a]*Reconstituted metronidazole HCl neutralized with sodium bicarbonate 50 mEq/L*

Y-Site Injection Compatibility (1:1 Mixture)

Metronidazole HCl

Drug	Mfr	Conc	Mfr	Conc	Remarks	Ref	C/I
Amiodarone HCl	LZ	4 mg/ml[a,b]	LY	5 mg/ml[a,b]	Physically compatible for 4 hr at room temperature	1444	C
Diltiazem HCl	MMD	5 mg/ml	SE	8 mg/ml[b]	Visually compatible	1807	C
Meropenem	ZEN	1 and 50 mg/ml[b]	SE	5 mg/ml[c]	Discoloration forms	2068	I
Warfarin sodium	DME	2 mg/ml[c]	SCS	5 mg/ml[b]	Slight haze forms in 24 hr at 24 °C	2078	I

[a]*Tested in dextrose 5% in water.*
[b]*Tested in sodium chloride 0.9%.*
[c]*Tested in sterile water for injection.*

Additional Compatibility Information

It is recommended that no other drug be added to infusions of metronidazole HCl. Furthermore, if administration of metronidazole HCl is to be made through the tubing of an ongoing primary infusion, the primary infusion should be stopped, if possible, during the metronidazole administration (2; 4).

Reaction with Aluminum— Because of the low pH of the initial reconstituted solution of metronidazole HCl, an interaction with aluminum results on contact. Solutions develop a discoloration variously described as bright orange, rust, and reddish brown. Although this interaction is stated not to affect the potency of the solution, aluminum hub needles should not be used in handling this initial solution. Plastic hub needles are recommended. This discoloration interaction does not occur as readily with the diluted and neutralized infusion solution or with metronidazole ready-to-use. It is not apparent when administration is completed within one hour. However, the solution may discolor and a precipitate may form after contact with aluminum for six or more hours (4; 707; 1116; 1117). Also see the Metronidazole monograph.

MIDAZOLAM HCL
AHFS 28:24.08

Versed   **Roche**

Products— Midazolam HCl (Roche) is available at a concentration equivalent to midazolam 5 mg/ml in vials containing 1, 2, 5, or 10 ml and in 2-ml disposable syringes. It also is available at a concentration equivalent to midazolam 1 mg/ml in vials containing 2, 5, or 10 ml. Each milliliter also contains sodium chloride 0.8%, disodium edetate 0.01%, and benzyl alcohol 1%, with hydrochloric acid and, if necessary, sodium hydroxide to adjust the pH (2; 4).

pH— The pH of the commercial injection has been adjusted to approximately 3 (2; 4). Midazolam (Roche) 0.625, 1.25, and 1.67

mg/ml in sodium chloride 0.9% had pH values of 3.6, 3.4, and 3.4, respectively (2161).

Osmolality— The 5-mg/ml concentration has an osmolality of 385 mOsm/kg (4). Midazolam (Roche) 0.625, 1.25, and 1.67 mg/ml in sodium chloride 0.9% had osmolalities of 274, 262, and 259 mOsm/kg, respectively (2161).

Sodium Content— Each milliliter of the available products contains about 0.14 mEq of sodium (4).

Administration— Midazolam HCl is administered by intramuscular injection deep into a large muscle mass or by slow intravenous injection in incremental doses (2; 4) or intravenous infusion (4). Use of the 1-mg/ml concentration is recommended to facilitate slower injection and dosage titration. Both concentrations may be diluted with sodium chloride 0.9% or dextrose 5% in water to facilitate slow administration (2; 4).

Stability— Midazolam HCl (Roche) is a colorless to light yellow solution. If stored at room temperature and protected from light, it has an expiration date of two years from manufacture. Admixtures of midazolam HCl in compatible infusion solutions do not require protection from light for short-term storage and administration (4). However, exposure of the commercial injection (Roche) to sunlight for four months resulted in the yellowing of the solution in one month and the loss of about 8% by HPLC in four months (1944).

pH Effects— Midazolam HCl is stable at pH 3 to 3.6 (4). It is highly water soluble at pH 4 or less; at higher pH values, increased lipid solubility occurs (1145). The rate of photodecomposition increases with increasing pH from 1.3 to 6.4 (1944).

Exposure to Light— Midazolam HCl (Roche) 1 mg/ml in PVC bags of sodium chloride 0.9% (Baxter) with benzyl alcohol added to a concentration of 1% was stored for 10 days at 23 °C both protected from and exposed to bright fluorescent light. No difference in midazolam content and no increase in photodecomposition products were found by HPLC analysis (1859). Consequently, protection of midazolam solutions from light exposure is not necessary (4).

Syringes— Midazolam HCl (Roche) 2 mg/ml in sodium chloride 0.9% was packaged as 3 ml in 10-ml polypropylene infusion pump syringes (Pharmacia Deltec). Little or no loss by HPLC analysis occurred during 10 days of storage at 5 and 30 °C (1967).

Midazolam HCl (Roche) 3 mg/ml in sodium chloride 0.9% exhibited no visual changes and had losses by HPLC analysis of 6.5% at 20 °C and 8.7% at 32 °C in polypropylene syringes (Terumo) and of 8.9% at 32 °C in glass vials after 13 days (1595).

The stability of midazolam (salt form unspecified) 1 mg/ml repackaged in polypropylene syringes was evaluated by spectrophotometric and potentiometric methods. Little or no change in concentration was found after four weeks of storage at room temperature not exposed to direct light (2164).

Midazolam HCl (Roche) 5 mg/ml was packaged as 10 ml in 12-ml polypropylene syringes (Sherwood). No loss by HPLC analysis occurred in 36 days when stored at 25 °C protected from light (2088).

Freezing Solutions— The injection was physically stable when frozen for three days followed by room temperature thawing (4).

Sorption— Midazolam (Roche) 40 μg/ml in sodium chloride 0.9% exhibited no loss due to sorption in 24 hours at 21 °C when protected from light in PVC, glass, and polyethylene-lined laminated containers (1392).

Midazolam (Roche) 0.03 mg/ml in sodium chloride 0.9% or dextrose 5% in water was determined by UV spectroscopy to exhibit no loss due to sorption to PVC containers over 72 hours at 20 °C. However, adjustment of the natural pH of 4.3 to 4.8 in the infusion solutions to pH 7 with phosphate buffer resulted in extensive losses. Losses were 8% in one hour, 20% in six hours, and 46% in 24 hours (1798).

Midazolam (Roche) 1 mg/ml in PVC bags of sodium chloride 0.9% (Baxter) with benzyl alcohol added to a concentration of 1% exhibited little or no loss of drug due to sorption during 10 days of storage at 23 °C. Midazolam losses of about 5% were determined by HPLC analysis (1859).

Compatibility Information

Solution Compatibility

Midazolam HCl

Solution	Mfr	Mfr	Conc/L	Remarks	Ref	C/I
Dextrose 5% in water with potassium chloride 0.15%	BA[a]	RC	0.1 and 0.5 g	13% midazolam loss by HPLC in 24 hr at ambient temperature. 10% loss calculated in 20 hr	1868	I
	BA[a]	RC	1 g	7% midazolam loss by HPLC in 24 hr at ambient temperature. 10% loss calculated in 35 hr	1868	C
Dextrose 5% in sodium chloride 0.9%	GRI	RC	0.1 and 0.5 g	8 to 10% midazolam loss by HPLC in 24 hr at ambient temperature	1868	C
	GRI	RC	1 g	4% midazolam loss by HPLC in 24 hr at ambient temperature. 10% loss calculated in 54 hr	1868	C
Dextrose 5% in water	MG[b]	RC	0.5 g	Visually compatible with no midazolam loss by HPLC in 30 days at 23 °C in the dark or at 4 °C	1717	C
	[c]	RC	30 mg	No loss by UV spectroscopy in 72 hr at 20 °C	1798	C
	AB	RC	0.1 and 0.5 g	Visually compatible with no midazolam loss by HPLC in 3 hr at 24 °C	1852	C

Solution Compatibility (Cont.)

Midazolam HCl

Solution	Mfr	Mfr	Conc/L	Remarks	Ref	C/I
	GRI	RC	0.1, 0.5, 1 g	3 to 5% midazolam loss by HPLC in 24 hr at ambient temperature. 10% loss calculated in 63 to 112 hr (0.1 to 1 g/L)	1868	**C**
	BA[g]	RC	500 mg	Visually compatible with no loss by HPLC in 36 days at 4, 25, and 40 °C protected from light	2088	**C**
Ringer's injection, lactated	GRI	RC	0.1 g	10% midazolam loss calculated in 2 hr at ambient temperature	1868	**I**
	GRI	RC	0.5 g	10% midazolam loss calculated in 6 hr at ambient temperature	1868	**I**
	GRI	RC	1 g	10% midazolam loss calculated in 10 hr at ambient temperature	1868	**I**
Sodium chloride 0.9%	[d]	RC	40 mg	Physically compatible with no midazolam loss in 24 hr at 21 °C in the dark	1392	**C**
	MG[b]	RC	0.5 g	Visually compatible with no midazolam loss by HPLC in 30 days at 23 °C in the dark or at 4 °C	1717	**C**
	[c]	RC	30 mg	No loss by UV spectroscopy in 72 hr at 20 °C	1798	**C**
	BA[a]	RC	1 g[e]	Visually compatible with 5% or less midazolam loss by HPLC in 10 days at 23 °C both protected from and exposed to fluorescent light	1859	**C**
	BA[a]	RC	1 g	Visually compatible with 4 to 6% midazolam loss by HPLC in 49 days at 4 and 20 °C exposed to fluorescent light and at 20 °C protected from light	1863	**C**
	GRI	RC	0.1, 0.5, 1 g	8 to 10% midazolam loss by HPLC in 24 hr at ambient temperature	1868	**C**
	BA[g]	RC	500 mg	Visually compatible with no loss by HPLC in 36 days at 4, 25, and 40 °C protected from light	2088	**C**
TPN #174 to #176[f]		RC	600 mg to 1 g	Immediate precipitation	1624	**I**
		RC	100 and 500 mg	Visually compatible with little or no midazolam loss by HPLC and less than 10% loss of any amino acid by HPLC in 5 hr at 22 °C under fluorescent light	1624	**C**

[a]Tested in PVC containers.
[b]Tested in polyolefin containers.
[c]Tested in both glass and PVC containers.
[d]Tested in PVC, glass, and polyethylene-lined laminated containers.
[e]Also contained benzyl alcohol 1%.
[f]Refer to Appendix I for the composition of parenteral nutrition solutions. TPN indicates a 2-in-1 admixture.
[g]Tested in glass bottles.

Additive Compatibility

Midazolam HCl

Drug	Mfr	Conc/L	Mfr	Conc/L	Test Soln	Remarks	Ref	C/I
Hydromorphone HCl	KN	0.5 to 45 g	RC	0.1 to 4.5 g	D5W, NS	Visually compatible for 24 hr at room temperature	2086	**C**
	KN	2 and 20 g	RC	100 mg	D5W, NS	Visually compatible with less than 7% hydromorphone loss and less than 3% midazolam loss by HPLC in 23 days at 4 and 23 °C	2086	**C**

Additive Compatibility (Cont.)

Midazolam HCl

Drug	Mfr	Conc/L	Mfr	Conc/L	Test Soln	Remarks	Ref	C/I
	KN	2 and 20 g	RC	500 mg	D5W, NS	Visually compatible with less than 6% hydromorphone loss and less than 7% midazolam loss by HPLC in 23 days at 4 and 23 °C	2086	C

Drugs in Syringe Compatibility

Midazolam HCl

Drug (in syringe)	Mfr	Amt	Mfr	Amt	Remarks	Ref	C/I
Alfentanil HCl	JN	0.5 mg/ml[a]	RC	0.2 mg/ml[a]	Visually compatible with 8% midazolam and 2% alfentanil loss in 3 weeks at 20 °C exposed to light. No alfentanil loss and 7% midazolam loss in 4 weeks at 6 °C in the dark	2133	C
Atracurium besylate	BW	10 mg/1 ml		5 mg/1 ml	Physically compatible and atracurium chemically stable for 24 hr at 5 and 25 °C	1694	C
Atropine sulfate	IX	0.4 mg/1 ml	RC	5 mg/1 ml	Physically compatible for 4 hr at 25 °C under fluorescent light	1145	C
Buprenorphine HCl	NE	0.3 mg/1 ml	RC	5 mg/1 ml	Physically compatible for 4 hr at 25 °C under fluorescent light	1145	C
Butorphanol tartrate	BR	2 mg/1 ml	RC	5 mg/1 ml	Physically compatible for 4 hr at 25 °C under fluorescent light	1145	C
Chlorpromazine HCl	SKF	50 mg/2 ml	RC	5 mg/1 ml	Physically compatible for 4 hr at 25 °C under fluorescent light	1145	C
Cimetidine HCl	SKF	300 mg/2 ml	RC	5 mg/1 ml	Physically compatible for 4 hr at 25 °C under fluorescent light	1145	C
Diamorphine HCl	EV	10 mg	RC	10[b] and 75[c] mg	Visually compatible with 10% diamorphine loss and no midazolam loss by HPLC in 15.9 days at 22 °C	1792	C
	EV	500 mg	RC	10[b] and 75[c] mg	Visually compatible with 10% diamorphine loss and no midazolam loss in 22.2 days at 22 °C	1792	C
Dimenhydrinate	SE	50 mg/1 ml	RC	5 mg/1 ml	White precipitate forms immediately	1145	I
Diphenhydramine HCl	ES	50 mg/1 ml	RC	5 mg/1 ml	Physically compatible for 4 hr at 25 °C under fluorescent light	1145	C
Droperidol	JN	2.5 mg/1 ml	RC	5 mg/1 ml	Physically compatible for 4 hr at 25 °C under fluorescent light	1145	C
Fentanyl citrate	ES	0.1 mg/2 ml	RC	5 mg/1 ml	Physically compatible for 4 hr at 25 °C under fluorescent light	1145	C
	DB	12.5 µg/ml[a]	RC	0.625 and 0.938 mg/ml[a]	Visually compatible with little fentanyl loss and 7 to 9% midazolam loss by HPLC in 7 days at 5 and 22 °C, respectively	2202	C
	DB	37.5 µg/ml[a]	RC	0.625 mg/ml[a]	Visually compatible with no fentanyl loss and 5 to 8% midazolam loss by HPLC in 7 days at 5 and 22 °C, respectively	2202	C

Drugs in Syringe Compatibility (Cont.)

Midazolam HCl

Drug (in syringe)	Mfr	Amt	Mfr	Amt	Remarks	Ref	C/I
	DB	37.5 μg/ml[a]	RC	0.938 mg/ml[a]	Visually compatible with little fentanyl loss and 7 to 9% midazolam loss by HPLC in 7 days at 5 and 22 °C, respectively	2202	C
	DB	33.3 μg/ml[a]	RC	0.278 and 0.833 mg/ml[a]	Visually compatible with no fentanyl loss and not more than 5 to 7% midazolam loss by HPLC in 7 days at 5 and 22 °C, respectively	2202	C
Glycopyrrolate	RB	0.2 mg/1 ml	RC	5 mg/1 ml	Physically compatible for 4 hr at 25 °C under fluorescent light	1145	C
Hydromorphone HCl	WB	2 mg/0.5 ml	RC	5 mg/1 ml	Physically compatible for 4 hr at 25 °C under fluorescent light	1145	C
Hydroxyzine HCl	ES	100 mg/2 ml	RC	5 mg/1 ml	Physically compatible for 4 hr at 25 °C under fluorescent light	1145	C
Meperidine HCl	WB	100 mg/1 ml	RC	5 mg/1 ml	Physically compatible for 4 hr at 25 °C under fluorescent light	1145	C
Metoclopramide HCl	RB	10 mg/2 ml	RC	5 mg/1 ml	Physically compatible for 4 hr at 25 °C under fluorescent light	1145	C
Morphine sulfate	WB	10 mg/1 ml	RC	5 mg/1 ml	Physically compatible for 4 hr at 25 °C under fluorescent light	1145	C
		5 and 10 mg/1 ml[d]	RC	5 mg/1 ml	Visually compatible with 9% or less morphine loss and 8% or less midazolam loss by HPLC in 14 days at 22 °C protected from light. Subvisual microprecipitate may form, requiring filtration	1901	C
		5 and 10 mg/1 ml[e]	RC	5 mg/1 ml	Visually compatible with 8% or less morphine loss and 3% or less midazolam loss by HPLC in 14 days at 22 °C protected from light. Subvisual microprecipitate may form, requiring filtration	1901	C
Morphine tartrate	DB	24 mg/ml	RC	3 mg/ml[a]	Visually compatible with 4.4% midazolam loss by HPLC in 13 days at 32 °C. Morphine not tested	1595	C
Nalbuphine HCl	DU	10 mg/1 ml	RC	5 mg/1 ml	Physically compatible for 4 hr at 25 °C under fluorescent light	1145	C
Ondansetron HCl	GW	1.33 mg/ml[a]	RC	1.66 mg/ml[a]	Physically compatible with no measured increase in particulates and less than 4% loss of ondansetron and less than 7% loss of midazolam by HPLC in 24 hr at 4 or 23 °C	2199	C
Pentobarbital sodium	WY	100 mg/2 ml	RC	5 mg/1 ml	White precipitate forms immediately	1145	I
Perphenazine	SC	5 mg/1 ml	RC	5 mg/1 ml	White precipitate forms immediately	1145	I
Prochlorperazine edisylate	SKF	10 mg/2 ml	RC	5 mg/1 ml	White precipitate forms immediately	1145	I
Promazine HCl	WY	50 mg/1 ml	RC	5 mg/1 ml	Physically compatible for 4 hr at 25 °C under fluorescent light	1145	C
Promethazine HCl	WY	25 mg/1 ml	RC	5 mg/1 ml	Physically compatible for 4 hr at 25 °C under fluorescent light	1145	C

Drugs in Syringe Compatibility (Cont.)

Midazolam HCl

Drug (in syringe)	Mfr	Amt	Mfr	Amt	Remarks	Ref	C/I
Ranitidine HCl	GL	50 mg/ 2 ml	RC	5 mg/ 1 ml	White precipitate forms immediately	1145	I
Scopolamine HBr	BW	0.43 mg/ 0.5 ml	RC	5 mg/ 1 ml	Physically compatible for 4 hr at 25 °C under fluorescent light	1145	C
Sufentanil citrate	JN	50 μg/ml	RC	5 mg/ml	Physically compatible with no subvisual haze or particle formation in 24 hr at 23 °C	1711	C
Thiethylperazine malate	BI	10 mg/ 2 ml	RC	5 mg/ 1 ml	Physically compatible for 4 hr at 25 °C under fluorescent light	1145	C
Trimethobenzamide HCl	BE	200 mg/ 2 ml	RC	5 mg/ 1 ml	Physically compatible for 4 hr at 25 °C under fluorescent light	1145	C

[a]Diluted with sodium chloride 0.9%.
[b]Diluted with sterile water to 15 ml.
[c]Diamorphine HCl constituted with midazolam injection.
[d]Morphine sulfate powder dissolved in dextrose 5% in water.
[e]Morphine sulfate powder dissolved in water and sodium chloride 0.9%.

Y-Site Injection Compatibility (1:1 Mixture)

Midazolam HCl

Drug	Mfr	Conc	Mfr	Conc	Remarks	Ref	C/I
Albumin		200 mg/ml	RC	5 mg/ml	White precipitate forms immediately	1855	I
Amikacin sulfate	BMS	5 mg/ml	RC	5 mg/ml	Visually compatible for 24 hr at 22 °C	1855	C
Amiodarone HCl	WY	4.8 mg/ml[a]	RC	1 mg/ml[a]	Visually compatible for 24 hr at 23 °C	1877	C
Amoxicillin sodium	SKB	50 mg/ml	RC	5 mg/ml	White precipitate forms immediately	1855	I
Amoxicillin sodium–clavulanate potassium	SKB	20 + 2 mg/ ml	RC	5 mg/ml	White precipitate forms immediately	1855	I
Amphotericin B cholesteryl sulfate complex	SEQ	0.83 mg/ml[a]	RC	2 mg/ml[a]	Gross precipitate forms	2117	I
Ampicillin sodium	WY	20 mg/ml[b]	RC	1 mg/ml[a]	Haze forms immediately	1847	I
Atracurium besylate	BW	0.5 mg/ml[a]	RC	0.05 mg/ml[a]	Physically compatible for 24 hr at 28 °C	1337	C
	GW	1 and 5 mg/ ml[a]	RC	0.1 mg/ml[a]	Visually compatible with no loss of either drug by HPLC in 3 hr at 25 °C under fluorescent light	2112	C
	GW	5 mg/ml[a]	RC	0.5 mg/ml[a]	Visually compatible with no loss of either drug by HPLC in 3 hr at 25 °C under fluorescent light	2112	C
	GW	1 mg/ml[a]	RC	0.5 mg/ml[a]	Visually compatible with no loss of midazolam and 4% loss of atracurium by HPLC in 3 hr at 25 °C under fluorescent light	2112	C
Bumetanide	LEO	0.5 mg/ml	RC	5 mg/ml	White precipitate forms immediately	1855	I
Butorphanol tartrate	BR	[f]	RC	[f]	Crystalline precipitate identified by HPLC as midazolam formed in infusion line several hours after administration was completed	2144	I
Calcium gluconate	FUJ	100 mg/ml	RC	1 mg/ml[a]	Visually compatible for 24 hr at 23 °C	1847	C
Cefazolin sodium	MAR	20 mg/ml[a]	RC	1 mg/ml[a]	Visually compatible for 24 hr at 23 °C	1847	C
Cefotaxime sodium	HO	20 mg/ml[a]	RC	1 mg/ml[a]	Visually compatible for 24 hr at 23 °C	1847	C
	RS	10 mg/ml	RC	5 mg/ml	Visually compatible for 24 hr at 22 °C	1855	C

Y-Site Injection Compatibility (1:1 Mixture) (Cont.)

Midazolam HCl

Drug	Mfr	Conc	Mfr	Conc	Remarks	Ref	C/I
Ceftazidime	LI[d]	20 mg/ml[a]	RC	1 mg/ml[a]	Haze forms in 1 hr	1847	**I**
Cefuroxime sodium	LI	15 mg/ml[a]	RC	1 mg/ml[a]	Particles form in 8 hr	1847	**I**
Cimetidine HCl	SKB	15 mg/ml[a]	RC	1 mg/ml[a]	Visually compatible for 24 hr at 23 °C	1847	**C**
Ciprofloxacin	BAY	2 mg/ml	RC	5 mg/ml	Visually compatible for 24 hr at 22 °C	1855	**C**
Cisatracurium besylate	GW	0.1, 2, 5 mg/ml[a]	RC	1 mg/ml[a]	Physically compatible with no change in measured turbidity or increase in particle content in 4 hr at 23 °C	2074	**C**
Clindamycin phosphate	UP	9 mg/ml[a]	RC	1 mg/ml[a]	Visually compatible for 24 hr at 23 °C	1847	**C**
Clonidine HCl	BI	0.015 mg/ml	RC	5 mg/ml	Orange discoloration forms in 24 hr at 22 °C	1855	**I**
Dexamethasone sodium phosphate	ES	4 mg/ml	RC	1 mg/ml[a]	Haze forms immediately. Precipitate forms in 8 hr	1847	**I**
		4 mg/ml	RC	5 mg/ml	White precipitate forms immediately	1855	**I**
Digoxin	BW	0.1 mg/ml	RC	1 mg/ml[a]	Visually compatible for 24 hr at 23 °C	1847	**C**
Diltiazem HCl	MMD	1 mg/ml[a]	RC	2 mg/ml[a]	Visually compatible for 4 hr at 27 °C	2062	**C**
Dobutamine HCl	GNS	2 mg/ml[a]	RC	1 mg/ml[a]	Particles form in 8 hr	1847	**I**
	LI	4 mg/ml[a]	RC	1 mg/ml[a]	Visually compatible for 24 hr at 23 °C	1877	**C**
	LI	4 mg/ml[a]	RC	2 mg/ml[a]	Visually compatible for 4 hr at 27 °C	2062	**C**
Dopamine HCl	AB	1.6 mg/ml[a]	RC	1 mg/ml[a]	Visually compatible for 24 hr at 23 °C	1847	**C**
	DU	3.2 mg/ml[a]	RC	1 mg/ml[a]	Visually compatible for 24 hr at 23 °C	1877	**C**
	AB	3.2 mg/ml[a]	RC	2 mg/ml[a]	Visually compatible for 4 hr at 27 °C	2062	**C**
Epinephrine HCl	AB	0.02 mg/ml[a]	RC	2 mg/ml[a]	Visually compatible for 4 hr at 27 °C	2062	**C**
Erythromycin lactobionate	AB	5 mg/ml	RC	5 mg/ml	Visually compatible for 24 hr at 22 °C	1855	**C**
Esmolol HCl	DU	40 mg/ml[a]	RC	1 mg/ml[a]	Visually compatible for 24 hr at 23 °C	1877	**C**
Etomidate	AB	2 mg/ml	RC	5 mg/ml	Visually compatible for up to 7 days at 25 °C	1801	**C**
Famotidine	MSD	0.2 mg/ml[a]	RC	0.15 mg/ml[a]	Physically compatible for 4 hr at 25 °C	1188	**C**
	ME	2 mg/ml[b]	RC	1.5 mg/ml[a]	Visually compatible for 4 hr at 22 °C	1936	**C**
Fentanyl citrate	JN	40 μg/ml[a]	RC	0.1 and 0.5 mg/ml[a]	Visually compatible with little or no loss of either drug by HPLC in 3 hr at 24 °C	1813	**C**
	JN	20 μg/ml[a]	RC	0.1 and 0.5 mg/ml[a]	Visually compatible with little or no midazolam loss and 3 to 4% fentanyl loss by HPLC in 3 hr at 24 °C	1813	**C**
	ES	0.05 mg/ml	RC	1 mg/ml[a]	Visually compatible for 24 hr at 23 °C	1847	**C**
	JN	0.02 mg/ml[a]	RC	0.1 and 0.5 mg/ml[a]	Visually compatible with no midazolam loss and 3 to 4% fentanyl loss by HPLC in 3 hr at 24 °C	1852	**C**
	JN	0.04 mg/ml[a]	RC	0.1 and 0.5 mg/ml[a]	Visually compatible with no loss of either drug by HPLC in 3 hr at 24 °C	1852	**C**
		0.05 mg/ml	RC	5 mg/ml	Visually compatible for 24 hr at 22 °C	1855	**C**
	ES	0.05 mg/ml	RC	2 mg/ml[a]	Visually compatible for 4 hr at 27 °C	2062	**C**
Floxacillin sodium	SKB	50 mg/ml	RC	5 mg/ml	White precipitate forms immediately	1855	**I**
Fluconazole	RR	2 mg/ml	RC	5 mg/ml	Physically compatible for 24 hr at 25 °C	1407	**C**
	PF	2 mg/ml	RC	5 mg/ml	Visually compatible for 24 hr at 22 °C	1855	**C**
Foscarnet sodium	AST	24 mg/ml	RC	5 mg/ml	Gas production	1335	**I**

Y-Site Injection Compatibility (1:1 Mixture) (Cont.)

Midazolam HCl

Drug	Mfr	Conc	Mfr	Conc	Remarks	Ref	C/I
Fosphenytoin sodium	PD	1 mgPE/ml[b,g]	RC	2 mg/ml[b]	Midazolam base precipitates immediately	2223	I
Furosemide	AST	10 mg/ml[a]	RC	1 mg/ml[a]	Haze forms immediately. Precipitate forms in 2 hr	1847	I
	CNF	10 mg/ml	RC	5 mg/ml	White precipitate forms immediately	1855	I
	AMR	10 mg/ml	RC	2 mg/ml[a]	Precipitate forms immediately	2062	I
Gentamicin sulfate	ES	10 mg/ml	RC	1 mg/ml[a]	Visually compatible for 24 hr at 23 °C	1847	C
	CNF	3 mg/ml	RC	5 mg/ml	Visually compatible for 24 hr at 22 °C	1855	C
Haloperidol lactate	JN	0.5 and 5 mg/ml	RC	5 mg/ml	Visually compatible for 24 hr at 22 °C	1855	C
Heparin sodium		417 units/ml	RC	5 mg/ml	Visually compatible for 24 hr at 22 °C	1855	C
	ES	100 units/ml[a]	RC	2 mg/ml[a]	Visually compatible for 4 hr at 27 °C	2062	C
Hydrocortisone sodium succinate	UP	50 mg/ml	RC	5 mg/ml	White precipitate forms immediately	1855	I
Hydromorphone HCl	KN	1 mg/ml	RC	2 mg/ml[a]	Visually compatible for 4 hr at 27 °C	2062	C
Imipenem–cilastatin sodium	MSD	5 mg/ml	RC	5 mg/ml	Haze forms in 24 hr	1855	I
Insulin, regular	LI	1 unit/ml[a]	RC	1 mg/ml[a]	Visually compatible for 24 hr at 23 °C	1877	C
Ketanserin tartrate	JN	1 mg/ml	RC	5 mg/ml	Visually compatible for 24 hr at 22 °C	1855	C
Labetalol HCl	GL	5 mg/ml	RC	1 mg/ml[a]	Visually compatible for 24 hr at 23 °C	1877	C
	AH	2 mg/ml[a]	RC	2 mg/ml[a]	Visually compatible for 4 hr at 27 °C	2062	C
Lorazepam	WY	0.5 mg/ml[a]	RC	2 mg/ml[a]	Visually compatible for 4 hr at 27 °C	2062	C
Methotrexate sodium		30 mg/ml	RC	5 mg/ml	Yellow precipitate forms immediately	1788	I
Methylprednisolone sodium succinate	UP	40 mg/ml	RC	1 mg/ml[a]	Visually compatible for 24 hr at 23 °C	1847	C
Metronidazole	BA	5 mg/ml	RC	1 mg/ml[a]	Visually compatible for 24 hr at 23 °C	1847	C
	BRN	5 mg/ml	RC	5 mg/ml	Visually compatible for 24 hr at 22 °C	1855	C
Milrinone lactate	SW	0.2 mg/ml[a]	RC	2 mg/ml[a]	Visually compatible for 4 hr at 27 °C	2062	C
	SW	0.4 mg/ml[a]	RC	1 mg/ml	Visually compatible with little or no loss of either drug by HPLC in 4 hr at 23 °C	2214	C
Morphine HCl	CNF	1 mg/ml	RC	5 mg/ml	Visually compatible for 24 hr at 22 °C	1855	C
Morphine sulfate	ES	0.25 mg/ml[a]	RC	0.1 and 0.5 mg/ml[a]	Visually compatible with no loss of either drug by HPLC in 3 hr at 24 °C	1789	C
	ES	1 mg/ml[a]	RC	0.1 and 0.5 mg/ml[a]	Visually compatible with no loss of either drug by HPLC in 3 hr at 24 °C	1789	C
	SX	1 mg/ml[a]	RC	1 mg/ml[a]	Visually compatible for 24 hr at 23 °C	1877	C
	SCN	2 mg/ml[a]	RC	2 mg/ml[a]	Visually compatible for 4 hr at 27 °C	2062	C
Nafcillin sodium	WY	20 mg/ml[a]	RC	1 mg/ml[a]	Haze forms immediately. Particles form in 4 hr	1847	I
Nicardipine HCl	WY	1 mg/ml[a]	RC	2 mg/ml[a]	Visually compatible for 4 hr at 27 °C	2062	C
Nitroglycerin	SO	0.2 mg/ml[a]	RC	1 mg/ml[a]	Visually compatible for 24 hr at 23 °C	1847	C
	OM	0.2 mg/ml[a]	RC	1 mg/ml[a]	Visually compatible for 24 hr at 23 °C	1877	C
	AB	0.4 mg/ml[a]	RC	2 mg/ml[a]	Visually compatible for 4 hr at 27 °C	2062	C
Norepinephrine bitartrate	STR	0.064 mg/ml[a]	RC	1 mg/ml[a]	Visually compatible for 24 hr at 23 °C	1877	C
	AB	0.128 mg/ml[a]	RC	2 mg/ml[a]	Visually compatible for 4 hr at 27 °C	2062	C

Y-Site Injection Compatibility (1:1 Mixture) (Cont.)

Midazolam HCl

Drug	Mfr	Conc	Mfr	Conc	Remarks	Ref	C/I
Omeprazole sodium	AST	4 mg/ml	RC	5 mg/ml	Brown discoloration forms, followed by a brown precipitate	1855	**I**
Pancuronium bromide	ES	0.05 mg/ml[a]	RC	0.05 mg/ml[a]	Physically compatible for 24 hr at 28 °C	1337	**C**
Piperacillin sodium	LE	150 mg/ml	RC	5 mg/ml	Visually compatible for 24 hr 22 °C	1855	**C**
Potassium chloride	BRN	1 mEq/ml	RC	5 mg/ml	Visually compatible for 24 hr at 22 °C	1855	**C**
Propofol	STU	2 mg/ml	RC	5 mg/ml	Oil droplets form within 7 days at 25 °C. No visible change in 24 hr	1801	**?**
	ZEN	10 mg/ml	RC	2 mg/ml[a]	Physically compatible for 1 hr at 23 °C with no increase in particle content	2066	**C**
Ranitidine HCl	GL	0.5 mg/ml	RC	5 mg/ml	Visually compatible for 24 hr at 22 °C	1855	**C**
	GL	1 mg/ml[a]	RC	2 mg/ml[a]	Visually compatible for 4 hr at 27 °C	2062	**C**
Remifentanil HCl	GW	0.025 and 0.25 mg/ml[b]	RC	1 mg/ml[a]	Physically compatible with no change in measured turbidity or increase in particle content in 4 hr at 23 °C	2075	**C**
Sodium bicarbonate		1.4%	RC	5 mg/ml	White precipitate forms immediately	1788	**I**
	IMS	1 mEq/ml	RC	1 mg/ml[a]	Haze forms immediately. Precipitate forms in 2 hr	1847	**I**
Sodium nitroprusside	ES	0.2 mg/ml[a]	RC	1 mg/ml[a]	Visually compatible for 24 hr at 23 °C	1847	**C**
	RC	0.2 mg/ml[a]	RC	1 mg/ml[a]	Visually compatible for 24 hr at 23 °C	1877	**C**
Sufentanil citrate	JN	12.5 μg/ml[a]	RC	0.2 mg/ml[a]	Physically compatible with no subvisual haze or particle formation in 24 hr at 23 °C	1711	**C**
Theophylline	BA	1.6 mg/ml[a]	RC	1 mg/ml[a]	Visually compatible for 24 hr at 23 °C	1847	**C**
Thiopental sodium	AB	25 mg/ml	RC	5 mg/ml	White precipitate forms immediately	1801	**I**
	AB	25 mg/ml[b]	RC	2 mg/ml[a]	Precipitate forms immediately	2062	**I**
TNA #218 to #226[e]			RC	2 mg/ml[a]	Damage to emulsion integrity occurs immediately with free oil formation possible	2215	**I**
Tobramycin sulfate	LI	10 mg/ml	RC	1 mg/ml[a]	Visually compatible for 24 hr at 23 °C	1847	**C**
TPN #189[e]			RC	5 mg/ml	White haze and light, white precipitate form immediately. Crystals form in 24 hr	1767	**I**
TPN #212 to #215[e]			RC	2 mg/ml[a]	White cloudiness forms rapidly	2109	**I**
Trimethoprim–sulfamethoxazole	RC	0.8 + 4 mg/ml	RC	5 mg/ml	White precipitate forms immediately	1855	**I**
Vancomycin HCl	LI	5 mg/ml[a]	RC	1 mg/ml[a]	Visually compatible for 24 hr at 23 °C	1847	**C**
	LI	5 mg/ml	RC	5 mg/ml	Visually compatible for 24 hr at 22 °C	1855	**C**
Vecuronium bromide	OR	0.1 mg/ml[a]	RC	0.05 mg/ml[a]	Physically compatible for 24 hr at 28 °C	1337	**C**
	OR	4 mg/ml	RC	5 mg/ml	Visually compatible for 24 hr at 22 °C	1855	**C**
	OR	1 mg/ml	RC	2 mg/ml[a]	Visually compatible for 4 hr at 27 °C	2062	**C**

[a]Tested in dextrose 5% in water.
[b]Tested in sodium chloride 0.9%.
[c]Tested in sterile water for injection.
[d]Sodium carbonate-containing formulation tested.
[e]Refer to Appendix I for the composition of parenteral nutrition solutions. TNA indicates a 3-in-1 admixture, and TPN indicates a 2-in-1 admixture.
[f]Concentration unspecified.
[g]Concentration expressed in milligrams of phenytoin sodium equivalents (PE) per milliliter.

Solutions— Midazolam HCl 0.5 mg/ml or less is physically compatible and chemically stable at 25 °C for 24 hours in dextrose 5% in water and sodium chloride 0.9% and for four hours in Ringer's injection, lactated, in both glass and PVC containers (4).

MILRINONE LACTATE
AHFS 24:04

Primacor   **Sanofi**

Products— Milrinone lactate (Sanofi) is available as a solution containing the equivalent of milrinone 1 mg/ml in 10-, 20-, and 50-ml single-dose vials and 5-ml cartridge units with and without needles. Each milliliter also contains dextrose, anhydrous, 47 mg in water for injection. Lactic acid or sodium hydroxide may have been used to adjust the pH. The total lactic acid concentration may vary between 0.95 and 1.29 mg/ml (2).

Milrinone lactate is also available as a ready-to-use solution in 100- and 200-ml flexible PVC plastic containers at a concentration equivalent to milrinone 0.2 mg/ml (200 μg/ml). The solution has a nominal lactic acid concentration of 0.282 mg/ml and also contains dextrose, anhydrous 49.4 mg/ml. The 1-mg/ml concentration must be diluted for use (2).

pH— From 3.2 to 4 (2).

Administration— Milrinone lactate is administered intravenously. For maintenance administration by continuous intravenous infusion, milrinone lactate in vials is diluted in a compatible diluent, usually to 200 μg/ml. The premixed 200-μg/ml infusion in flexible plastic containers need not be diluted for use (2).

Stability— Milrinone lactate solutions are colorless to pale yellow. The 1-mg/ml concentration should be stored at controlled room temperature and protected from freezing. The 0.2-mg/ml concentration in PVC containers should be stored at room temperature of 25 °C and should be protected from freezing and exposure to excessive heat. Brief exposure to temperatures up to 40 °C does not adversely affect the product (2).

Milrinone lactate (Sterling Winthrop) 0.2 mg/ml in sodium chloride 0.45 or 0.9% or dextrose 5% in water was stored in glass (Abbott), Accumed (McGaw), or PVC (Travenol) containers for 72 hours at room temperature in normal light. The milrinone concentration remained constant at about 100% of the initial amount over the study period by HPLC analysis. In addition, the solutions remained physically compatible and the pH remained constant (1468).

Sorption— Milrinone lactate (Sterling Winthrop) 0.2 mg/ml in sodium chloride 0.45 or 0.9% or dextrose 5% in water did not exhibit any loss due to sorption to glass, PVC, or Accumed containers during storage for 72 hours at room temperature (1468).

Compatibility Information

Solution Compatibility

Milrinone lactate

Solution	Mfr	Mfr	Conc/L	Remarks	Ref	C/I
Dextrose 5% in water	c	WI	200 mg	Physically compatible and potency retained for 72 hr at room temperature under normal light or in the dark	1468	C
	a	SW	0.2 g	Visually compatible with little or no loss by HPLC after 14 days at 23 °C in normal room light and at 4 °C	2106	C
	BA[a]	SW	0.4, 0.6, 0.8 g	Visually compatible with little or no loss by HPLC after 14 days at 23 °C and at 4 °C	2107	C
	BA[a]	SW	0.4 g	Visually compatible with no loss by HPLC after 7 days at 23 °C under fluorescent light	2214	C
Ringer's injection, lactated	BA[a]	SW	0.4 g	Visually compatible with 3% loss by HPLC after 7 days at 23 °C under fluorescent light	2214	C
Sodium chloride 0.45%	c	WI	200 mg	Physically compatible and potency retained for 72 hr at room temperature under normal light or in the dark	1468	C
	BA[a]	SW	0.4 g	Visually compatible with no loss by HPLC after 7 days at 23 °C under fluorescent light	2214	C

Solution Compatibility (Cont.)

Milrinone lactate

Solution	Mfr	Mfr	Conc/L	Remarks	Ref	C/I
Sodium chloride 0.9%	c	WI	200 mg	Physically compatible and potency retained for 72 hr at room temperature under normal light or in the dark	1468	**C**
	a	SW	0.2 g	Visually compatible with little or no loss by HPLC after 14 days at 23 °C in normal room light and at 4 °C	2106	**C**
	MG[b]	SW	0.4, 0.6, 0.8 g	Visually compatible with little or no loss by HPLC after 14 days at 23 and 4 °C	2107	**C**
	BA[a]	SW	0.4 g	Visually compatible with no loss by HPLC after 7 days at 23 °C under fluorescent light	2214	**C**

[a]Tested in PVC containers.
[b]Tested in polyolefin containers.
[c]Tested in glass (Abbott), Accumed (McGaw), and PVC (Travenol) containers.

Additive Compatibility

Milrinone lactate

Drug	Mfr	Conc/L	Mfr	Conc/L	Test Soln	Remarks	Ref	C/I
Procainamide HCl	SQ	2 and 4 g	WI	200 mg	D5W	2 to 3% procainamide loss in 1 hr and 10 to 11% loss in 4 hr at 23 °C. No milrinone loss	1191	**I**
Quinidine gluconate	LI	16 g	WI	200 mg	D5W	Physically compatible with no loss of either drug in 4 hr at 23 °C	1191	**C**

Drugs in Syringe Compatibility

Milrinone lactate

Drug (in syringe)	Mfr	Amt	Mfr	Amt	Remarks	Ref	C/I
Atropine sulfate	IX	2 mg/ 2 ml	WI	5.25 mg/ 5.25 ml	Physically compatible with no loss of either drug in 20 min at 23 °C under fluorescent light	1410	**C**
Calcium chloride	AB	3 g/ 30 ml	WI	5.25 mg/ 5.25 ml	Physically compatible with no milrinone loss in 20 min at 23 °C under fluorescent light	1410	**C**
Digoxin	BW	0.5 mg/ 2 ml	WI	3.5 mg/ 3.5 ml	Brought to 10-ml total volume with D5W. Physically compatible with no loss of either drug in 4 hr at 23 °C	1191	**C**
Epinephrine HCl	AB	0.5 mg/ 0.5 ml	WI	5.25 mg/ 5.25 ml	Physically compatible with no loss of either drug in 20 min at 23 °C under fluorescent light	1410	**C**
Furosemide	LY	40 mg/ 4 ml	WI	3.5 mg/ 3.5 ml	Brought to 10-ml total volume with D5W. Immediate precipitation	1191	**I**
Lidocaine HCl	AB	100 mg/ 10 ml	WI	5.25 mg/ 5.25 ml	Physically compatible with no loss of either drug in 20 min at 23 °C under fluorescent light	1410	**C**
Morphine sulfate	WI	40 mg/ 5 ml	WI	5.25 mg/ 5.25 ml	Physically compatible with no loss of either drug in 20 min at 23 °C under fluorescent light	1410	**C**

Drugs in Syringe Compatibility (Cont.)

Drug (in syringe)	Mfr	Amt	Mfr	Amt	Remarks	Ref	C/I
				Milrinone lactate			
Propranolol HCl	AY	3 mg/ 3 ml	WI	3.5 mg/ 3.5 ml	Brought to 10-ml total volume with D5W. Physically compatible with no loss of either drug in 4 hr at 23 °C	1191	C
Sodium bicarbonate	AB	3.75 g/ 50 ml	WI	5.25 mg/ 5.25 ml	Physically compatible with no milrinone loss in 20 min at 23 °C under fluorescent light	1410	C
Verapamil HCl	KN	10 mg/ 4 ml	WI	3.5 mg/ 3.5 ml	Brought to 10-ml total volume with D5W. Physically compatible with no loss of either drug in 4 hr at 23 °C	1191	C

Y-Site Injection Compatibility (1:1 Mixture)

Drug	Mfr	Conc	Mfr	Conc	Remarks	Ref	C/I
				Milrinone lactate			
Atracurium besylate	BW	1 mg/ml[a]	SW	0.4 mg/ml[a]	Visually compatible with little or no loss of either drug by HPLC in 4 hr at 23 °C	2214	C
Bumetanide	RC	0.25 mg/ml	SW	0.4 mg/ml[a]	Visually compatible with little or no loss of either drug by HPLC in 4 hr at 23 °C	2214	C
Calcium gluconate	LY	0.465 mEq/ml	SW	0.4 mg/ml[a]	Visually compatible with no loss of milrinone by HPLC in 4 hr at 23 °C	2214	C
Cimetidine HCl	SKB	6 mg/ml[a]	SW	0.4 mg/ml[a]	Visually compatible with little or no loss of either drug by HPLC in 4 hr at 23 °C	2214	C
Digoxin	BW	0.25 mg/ml	WI	200 μg/ml[a]	Physically compatible with no loss of either drug in 4 hr at 23 °C	1191	C
Diltiazem HCl	MMD	1 mg/ml[a]	SW	0.2 mg/ml[a]	Visually compatible for 4 hr at 27 °C	2062	C
	MMD	1 mg/ml[a]	SW	0.4 mg/ml[a]	Visually compatible with little or no loss of either drug by HPLC in 4 hr at 23 °C	2214	C
Dobutamine HCl	LI	4 mg/ml[a]	SW	0.2 mg/ml[a]	Visually compatible for 4 hr at 27 °C	2062	C
	GEN	8 mg/ml[a]	SW	0.4 mg/ml[a]	Visually compatible with little or no loss of either drug by HPLC in 4 hr at 23 °C	2214	C
Dopamine HCl	AB	3.2 mg/ml[a]	SW	0.2 mg/ml[a]	Visually compatible for 4 hr at 27 °C	2062	C
	SO	6.4 mg/ml[a]	SW	0.4 mg/ml[a]	Visually compatible with little or no loss of either drug by HPLC in 4 hr at 23 °C	2214	C
Epinephrine HCl	AB	0.02 mg/ml[a]	SW	0.2 mg/ml[a]	Visually compatible for 4 hr at 27 °C	2062	C
	AB	0.064 mg/ ml[a]	SW	0.4 mg/ml[a]	Visually compatible with little or no loss of either drug by HPLC in 4 hr at 23 °C	2214	C
Fentanyl citrate	ES	0.05 mg/ml	SW	0.2 mg/ml[a]	Visually compatible for 4 hr at 27 °C	2062	C
	ES	50 μg/ml	SW	0.4 mg/ml[a]	Visually compatible with little or no loss of either drug by HPLC in 4 hr at 23 °C	2214	C
Furosemide	LY	10 mg/ml	WI	200 μg/ml[a]	Immediate precipitation	1191	I
	AMR	10 mg/ml	SW	0.2 mg/ml[a]	Precipitate forms in 4 hr at 27 °C	2062	I
Heparin sodium	ES	100 units/ml[a]	SW	0.2 mg/ml[a]	Visually compatible for 4 hr at 27 °C	2062	C

Y-Site Injection Compatibility (1:1 Mixture) (Cont.)

Milrinone lactate

Drug	Mfr	Conc	Mfr	Conc	Remarks	Ref	C/I
	ES	100 units/ml[a]	SW	0.4 mg/ml[a]	Visually compatible with little or no loss of milrinone by HPLC and heparin by immunoassay in 4 hr at 23 °C	2214	C
Hydromorphone HCl	KN	1 mg/ml	SW	0.2 mg/ml[a]	Visually compatible for 4 hr at 27 °C	2062	C
Insulin, regular human	NOV	1 unit/ml[b]	SW	0.4 mg/ml[a]	Visually compatible with little or no loss of either drug by HPLC in 4 hr at 23 °C	2214	C
Isoproterenol HCl	ES	8 μg/ml[a]	SW	0.4 mg/ml[a]	Visually compatible with little or no loss of either drug by HPLC in 4 hr at 23 °C	2214	C
Labetalol HCl	AH	2 mg/ml[a]	SW	0.2 mg/ml[a]	Visually compatible for 4 hr at 27 °C	2062	C
Lorazepam	WY	0.5 mg/ml[a]	SW	0.2 mg/ml[a]	Visually compatible for 4 hr at 27 °C	2062	C
	WY	0.2 mg/ml[a]	SW	0.4 mg/ml[a]	Visually compatible with little or no loss of either drug by HPLC in 4 hr at 23 °C	2214	C
Magnesium sulfate	SO	40 mg/ml[a]	SW	0.4 mg/ml[a]	Visually compatible with no loss of milrinone by HPLC in 4 hr at 23 °C	2214	C
Midazolam HCl	RC	2 mg/ml[a]	SW	0.2 mg/ml[a]	Visually compatible for 4 hr at 27 °C	2062	C
	RC	1 mg/ml	SW	0.4 mg/ml[a]	Visually compatible with little or no loss of either drug by HPLC in 4 hr at 23 °C	2214	C
Morphine sulfate	SCN	2 mg/ml[a]	SW	0.2 mg/ml[a]	Visually compatible for 4 hr at 27 °C	2062	C
	AST	1 mg/ml[a]	SW	0.4 mg/ml[a]	Visually compatible with little or no loss of either drug by HPLC in 4 hr at 23 °C	2214	C
Nicardipine HCl	WY	1 mg/ml[a]	SW	0.2 mg/ml[a]	Visually compatible for 4 hr at 27 °C	2062	C
Nitroglycerin	AB	0.4 mg/ml[a]	SW	0.2 mg/ml[a]	Visually compatible for 4 hr at 27 °C	2062	C
	SO	0.8 mg/ml[a]	SW	0.4 mg/ml[a]	Visually compatible with little or no loss of either drug by HPLC in 4 hr at 23 °C	2214	C
Norepinephrine bitartrate	AB	0.128 mg/ml[a]	SW	0.2 mg/ml[a]	Visually compatible for 4 hr at 27 °C	2062	C
	SW	0.064 mg/ml[a]	SW	0.4 mg/ml[a]	Visually compatible with little or no loss of either drug by HPLC in 4 hr at 23 °C	2214	C
Pancuronium bromide	GEN	1 mg/ml	SW	0.4 mg/ml[a]	Visually compatible with little or no loss of either drug by HPLC in 4 hr at 23 °C	2214	C
Potassium chloride	AB	1 mEq/ml[a]	SW	0.4 mg/ml[a]	Visually compatible with no loss of milrinone by HPLC in 4 hr at 23 °C	2214	C
Procainamide HCl	SQ	2 and 4 mg/ml[a]	WI	350 μg/ml[a]	3 to 6% procainamide loss in 1 hr and 10 to 13% loss in 4 hr at 23 °C. No milrinone loss	1191	I
Propofol	ZEN	10 mg/ml	SW	0.4 mg/ml[a]	Little or no loss of either drug by HPLC in 4 hr at 23 °C	2214	C
Propranolol HCl	AY	1 mg/ml[a]	WI	200 μg/ml[a]	Physically compatible with no loss of either drug in 4 hr at 23 °C	1191	C
Quinidine gluconate	LI	16 mg/ml[a]	WI	350 μg/ml[a]	Physically compatible with no loss of either drug in 4 hr at 23 °C	1191	C

Y-Site Injection Compatibility (1:1 Mixture) (Cont.)

Milrinone lactate

Drug	Mfr	Conc	Mfr	Conc	Remarks	Ref	C/I
Ranitidine HCl	GL	1 mg/ml[a]	SW	0.2 mg/ml[a]	Visually compatible for 4 hr at 27 °C	2062	C
	GL	2 mg/ml[a]	SW	0.4 mg/ml[a]	Visually compatible with little or no loss of either drug by HPLC in 4 hr at 23 °C	2214	C
Rocuronium bromide	OR	2 mg/ml[a]	SW	0.4 mg/ml[a]	Visually compatible with little or no loss of either drug by HPLC in 4 hr at 23 °C	2214	C
Sodium bicarbonate	AB	1 mEq/ml	SW	0.4 mg/ml[a]	Visually compatible with 4% loss of milrinone by HPLC in 4 hr at 23 °C	2214	C
Sodium nitroprusside	AB	0.8 mg/ml[a]	SW	0.4 mg/ml[a]	Visually compatible with little or no loss of either drug by HPLC in 4 hr at 23 °C protected from light	2214	C
Theophylline	AB	1.6 mg/ml[a]	SW	0.4 mg/ml[a]	Visually compatible with little or no loss of milrinone by HPLC and theophylline by immunoassay in 4 hr at 23 °C	2214	C
Thiopental sodium	AB	25 mg/ml[c]	SW	0.2 mg/ml[a]	Visually compatible for 4 hr at 27 °C	2062	C
Torsemide	BM	10 mg/ml	SW	0.4 mg/ml[a]	Visually compatible with little or no loss of either drug by HPLC in 4 hr at 23 °C	2214	C
TPN #217[d]			SW	0.4 mg/ml[a]	Visually compatible with no loss of milrinone by HPLC in 4 hr at 23 °C	2214	C
Vecuronium bromide	OR	1 mg/ml	SW	0.2 mg/ml[a]	Visually compatible for 4 hr at 27 °C	2062	C
	OR	1 mg/ml[a]	SW	0.4 mg/ml[a]	Visually compatible with little or no loss of either drug by HPLC in 4 hr at 23 °C	2214	C

[a]*Tested in dextrose 5% in water.*
[b]*Tested in sodium chloride 0.9%.*
[c]*Tested in sterile water for injection.*
[d]*Refer to Appendix I for the composition of parenteral nutrition solutions. TPN indicates a 2-in-1 admixture.*

Additional Compatibility Information

Solutions— Dextrose 5% in water and sodium chloride 0.45 and 0.9% are recommended for milrinone lactate dilution for intravenous infusion (2).

Miscellaneous— Furosemide and bumetanide may precipitate if mixed with milrinone lactate infusions (1442).

MINOCYCLINE HCL
AHFS 8:12.24

Minocin   **Lederle**

Products— Minocycline HCl (Lederle) is available in vials containing 100 mg of drug in lyophilized form. The vials should be reconstituted with 5 ml of sterile water for injection to yield a 20-mg/ml solution (2; 4).

pH— From 2 to 2.8 (2; 4).

Osmolality— Minocycline HCl 20 mg/ml in sterile water for injection has an osmolality of 107 mOsm/kg (1689).

Administration— Minocycline HCl is administered by intravenous infusion. The reconstituted drug is further diluted to a concentration of 100 to 200 µg/ml in 500 to 1000 ml of a compatible infusion solution. Minocycline HCl is infused slowly, usually over a six-hour period (2; 4).

Stability— Minocycline HCl should be stored at controlled room temperature and protected from temperatures above 40 °C and from light (4). The reconstituted solution is stable for 24 hours at room temperature (2; 4).

Compatibility Information

Solution Compatibility

Minocycline HCl

Solution	Mfr	Mfr	Conc/L	Remarks	Ref	C/I
Dextrose 5% in water	BA[a]	LE	0.1 g	Physically compatible with approximately 8% minocycline loss at 24 °C and 2% loss at 4 °C in 7 days	1559	**C**
Sodium chloride 0.9%	BA[a]	LE	0.1 g	Physically compatible with approximately 8% minocycline loss at 24 °C and 2% loss at 4 °C in 7 days	1559	**C**

[a]*Tested in PVC containers.*

Additive Compatibility

Minocycline HCl

Drug	Mfr	Conc/L	Mfr	Conc/L	Test Soln	Remarks	Ref	C/I
Rifampin	MMD	0.1 g	LE	0.1 g	NS	Brownish color appears in 4 hr at 37 and 24 °C and 8 hr at 4 °C. 10% rifampin loss by HPLC in 3 days at 4 °C and 8 hr at 24 °C; 14% loss in 4 hr at 37 °C. Less than 2% minocycline loss by HPLC under these conditions	1559	**I**

Drugs in Syringe Compatibility

Minocycline HCl

Drug (in syringe)	Mfr	Amt	Mfr	Amt	Remarks	Ref	C/I
Doxapram HCl	RB	400 mg/ 20 ml		100 mg/ 5 ml	8% doxapram loss in 3 hr and 13% loss in 6 hr	1177	**I**

Y-Site Injection Compatibility (1:1 Mixture)

Minocycline HCl

Drug	Mfr	Conc	Mfr	Conc	Remarks	Ref	C/I
Allopurinol sodium	BW	3 mg/ml[b]	LE	0.2 mg/ml[b]	Greenish-yellow color forms in 4 hr	1686	**I**
Amifostine	USB	10 mg/ml[b]	LE	0.2 mg/ml[b]	Bright yellow discoloration forms immediately	1845	**I**
Aztreonam	SQ	40 mg/ml[a]	LE	0.2 mg/ml[a]	Physically compatible with no subvisual haze or particle formation in 4 hr at 23 °C	1758	**C**
Cisatracurium besylate	GW	0.1, 2, 5 mg/ml[a]	LE	0.2 mg/ml[a]	Physically compatible with no change in measured turbidity or increase in particle content in 4 hr at 23 °C	2074	**C**
Cyclophosphamide	MJ	20 mg/ml[a]	LE	0.2 mg/ml[a]	Physically compatible for 4 hr at 25 °C	1194	**C**
Docetaxel	RPR	0.9 mg/ml[a]	LE	0.2 mg/ml[a]	Physically compatible with no change in measured turbidity or increase in particle content in 4 hr at 23 °C	2224	**C**

Y-Site Injection Compatibility (1:1 Mixture) (Cont.)

Minocycline HCl

Drug	Mfr	Conc	Mfr	Conc	Remarks	Ref	C/I
Etoposide phosphate	BR	5 mg/ml[a]	LE	0.2 mg/ml[a]	Physically compatible with no change in measured turbidity or increase in particle content in 4 hr at 23 °C	2218	C
Filgrastim	AMG	30 µg/ml[a]	LE	0.2 mg/ml[a]	Physically compatible with no change in measured turbidity or increase in particle content in 4 hr at 22 °C	1687	C
Fludarabine phosphate	BX	1 mg/ml[a]	LE	0.2 mg/ml[a]	Physically compatible for 4 hr at room temperature under fluorescent light	1439	C
Gemcitabine HCl	LE	0.2 mg/ml[b]	LI	10 mg/ml[b]	Physically compatible with no change in measured turbidity or increase in particle content in 4 hr at 23 °C	2226	C
Granisetron HCl	SKB	0.05 mg/ml[a]	LE	0.2 mg/ml[a]	Physically compatible with no change in measured turbidity or increase in particle content in 4 hr at 23 °C	2000	C
Heparin sodium	UP	1000 units/L[c]	LE	50 mg/ml	Physically compatible for at least 4 hr at room temperature by visual and microscopic examination	534	C
Hydrocortisone sodium succinate	UP	10 mg/L[c]	LE	50 mg/ml	Physically compatible for at least 4 hr at room temperature by visual and microscopic examination	534	C
Hydromorphone HCl	WY	0.2 mg/ml[a]	LE	0.2 mg/ml[a]	Color changed from pale yellow to light green within 1 hr at 25 °C	987	I
Magnesium sulfate	IX	16.7, 33.3, 66.7, 100 mg/ml[a]	LE	0.2 mg/ml[a]	Physically compatible for at least 4 hr at 32 °C	813	C
Melphalan HCl	BW	0.1 mg/ml[b]	LE	0.2 mg/ml[b]	Physically compatible with no change in measured turbidity or increase in particle content in 3 hr at 22 °C	1557	C
Meperidine HCl	WY	10 mg/ml[a]	LE	0.2 mg/ml[a]	Color changed from pale yellow to light green within 1 hr at 25 °C	987	I
Morphine sulfate	WI	1 mg/ml[a]	LE	0.2 mg/ml[a]	Color changed from pale yellow to light green within 1 hr at 25 °C	987	I
Perphenazine	SC	0.02 mg/ml[a]	LE	0.2 mg/ml[a]	Physically compatible for 4 hr at 25 °C	1155	C
Piperacillin sodium–tazobactam sodium	LE	40 + 5 mg/ml[a]	LE	1 mg/ml[a]	Particles form immediately, becoming numerous in 4 hr	1688	I
Potassium chloride	AB	40 mEq/L[c]	LE	50 mg/ml	Physically compatible for at least 4 hr at room temperature by visual and microscopic examination	534	C
Propofol	ZEN	10 mg/ml	LE	0.2 mg/ml[a]	Small amount of white particles forms immediately	2066	I
Remifentanil HCl	GW	0.025 and 0.25 mg/ml[b]	LE	0.2 mg/ml[a]	Physically compatible with no change in measured turbidity or increase in particle content in 4 hr at 23 °C	2075	C
Sargramostim	IMM	10 µg/ml[b]	LE	0.2 mg/ml[b]	Physically compatible for 4 hr at 22 °C	1436	C
Teniposide	BR	0.1 mg/ml[a]	LE	0.2 mg/ml[a]	Physically compatible with no subvisual haze or particle formation in 4 hr at 23 °C	1725	C

Y-Site Injection Compatibility (1:1 Mixture) (Cont.)

Minocycline HCl

Drug	Mfr	Conc	Mfr	Conc	Remarks	Ref	C/I
Thiotepa	IMM[d]	1 mg/ml[a]	LE	0.2 mg/ml[a]	Yellow-green discoloration forms in 1 hr at 23 °C	1861	I
TNA #218 to #226[e]			LE	0.2 mg/ml[a]	Damage to emulsion integrity occurs immediately with free oil formation possible	2215	I
TPN #212 to #215[e]			LE	0.2 mg/ml[a]	Bright yellow discoloration forms immediately	2109	I
Vinorelbine tartrate	BW	1 mg/ml[b]	LE	0.2 mg/ml[b]	Physically compatible with no change in measured turbidity or increase in particle content in 4 hr at 22 °C	1558	C
Vitamin B complex with C	RC	2 ml/L[c]	LE	50 mg/ml	Physically compatible for at least 4 hr at room temperature by visual and microscopic examination	534	C

[a]*Tested in dextrose 5% in water.*
[b]*Tested in sodium chloride 0.9%.*
[c]*Tested in dextrose 5% in Ringer's injection, dextrose 5% in Ringer's injection, lactated, dextrose 5% in water, Ringer's injection, lactated, and sodium chloride 0.9%.*
[d]*Lyophilized formulation tested.*
[e]*Refer to Appendix I for the composition of parenteral nutrition solutions. TNA indicates a 3-in-1 admixture, and TPN indicates a 2-in-1 admixture.*

Additional Compatibility Information

Solutions— The manufacturer recommends further dilution of the reconstituted minocycline HCl solution in the following infusion solutions (2):

Dextrose 5% in sodium chloride 0.9%
Dextrose 5% in water
Ringer's injection
Ringer's injection, lactated
Sodium chloride 0.9%

Other calcium-containing solutions are not recommended because of possible precipitate formation (2; 4).

MITOMYCIN
AHFS 10:00

Mutamycin   **Bristol-Myers Squibb**

Products— Mitomycin (Bristol-Myers Squibb) is available in 5-mg vials with mannitol 10 mg, 20-mg vials with mannitol 40 mg, and 40-mg vials with mannitol 80 mg. Reconstitute the 5-mg vials with 10 ml, the 20-mg vials with 40 ml, and the 40-mg vials with 80 ml of sterile water for injection and shake to aid dissolution. The product should be allowed to stand at room temperature if dissolution does not take place immediately. The reconstituted solution contains 500 µg/ml of mitomycin (2; 4).

pH— From 6 to 8 (4).

Osmolality— Mitomycin (Bristol) 0.5 mg/ml in sterile water for injection has an osmolality of 9 mOsm/kg (2043).

Administration— Mitomycin is administered intravenously through a functioning intravenous catheter. Extravasation should be avoided because cellulitis, ulceration, and sloughing may occur. It has been recommended that mitomycin be administered through the tubing of a running infusion solution to avoid this problem (2; 4).

Stability— Intact vials of mitomycin should be stored at controlled room temperature. Temperatures exceeding 40 °C should be avoided. Reconstituted solutions are stable for two weeks when stored under refrigeration at 2 to 8 °C or for one week at room temperature (2; 4).

Mitomycin is very stable in solution at neutral pH but undergoes more rapid decomposition at acidic and basic pH (1119; 1203; 1204; 1866). The decomposition is complex and pH dependent, producing different decomposition products in acidic and basic solutions (1119; 1283; 1284). The pH of maximum stability is approximately pH 7 (1072; 1203; 1204; 1379). At pH 7, a 10% mitomycin loss occurs in seven days at room temperature (1072). At a concentration of 50 µg/ml in dextrose 5% in water buffered to pH 7.8 with a mixture of phosphates, mitomycin was stable for 15 days at room temperature and over 120 days when refrigerated (1118).

Mitomycin (Kyowa) 0.6 and 0.8 mg/ml in water for injection exhibited 10% loss in seven days at 21 °C in the dark. When stored at 4 °C in the dark, the 0.6-mg/ml concentration lost 7% in seven days. Although exhibiting no loss in 24 hours when stored at 4 °C in the dark, the 0.8-mg/ml concentration developed a fine, pink, needle-like precipitate in three days. At a higher concentration of 1 mg/ml in water for injection similar results were obtained. Refrigeration resulted in fine, pink, needle-like precipitate formation in 24 hours. The 1-mg/ml concentration stored at 21 °C exposed to fluorescent light exhibited 6% loss in 24 hours and developed the fine, pink, needle-like precipitate in four days. Stored at a higher temperature of 25 °C in the dark, losses of 6% in 24 hours and 10% in seven days were found with no precipitate forming (1503).

Heating mitomycin 0.6 mg/ml in sodium chloride 0.9% to 100 °C resulted in a 24% drug loss in 30 minutes and a 58% loss in one hour (1285).

The stability of mitomycin is not adversely affected by the presence or absence of normal fluorescent light (1503).

Mitomycin, reconstituted according to the manufacturer's instructions, was cultured with human lymphoblasts to determine whether its cytotoxic activity was retained. The solution retained cytotoxicity for 24 hours at 4 °C and room temperature (1575).

Syringes— Mitomycin (Bristol-Myers Squibb) reconstituted to a concentration of 0.5 mg/ml with sterile water was repackaged in 1-ml polypropylene tuberculin syringes (Sherwood). Syringes were stored at both 5 and 25 °C protected from light. Stability-indicating HPLC analysis found about 7% mitomycin loss in 11 days at 25 °C and about 8% loss in 42 days at 5 °C (2179).

Freezing Solutions— Mitomycin 0.6 mg/ml in sodium chloride 0.9% crystallized out of solution when frozen at −20 °C. The particles did not redissolve after thawing in a microwave oven. Freezing to −30 °C, below the eutectic temperature, resulted in no loss of mitomycin during four weeks of storage, microwave thawing, and refreezing at −30 °C for another four weeks (1285).

Sorption— Mitomycin (Kyowa) 20 to 50 mg in 50 ml of sterile water for injection or sodium chloride 0.9% in PVC containers exhibited no loss due to sorption (1503).

Filtration— Mitomycin 10 to 75 µg/ml exhibited little or no loss due to sorption to either cellulose nitrate/cellulose acetate ester (Millex OR) or Teflon (Millex FG) filters (1415; 1416).

Compatibility Information

Solution Compatibility

Mitomycin

Solution	Mfr	Mfr	Conc/L	Remarks	Ref	C/I
Dextrose 3.3% in sodium chloride 0.3%		BR	50 mg	10% mitomycin loss in 1.6 hr at 25 °C	1205	I
Dextrose 5% in water	TR[a]	BR	400 mg	10% mitomycin loss in 1 or 2 hr at room temperature	519	I
	TR[b]	CH	50 mg	Violet color appeared in 4 hr and intensified over 12 hr. 74% mitomycin loss in 12 hr at 28 °C under fluorescent light and 33% in 12 hr at 5 °C in the dark	1118	I
		BR	50 mg	10% mitomycin loss in 2.6 hr at 25 °C	1205	I
	MG[c]	BR	20 mg	10% mitomycin loss by HPLC in 3 hr at 25 °C	1866	I
	MG[c]	BR	40 mg	10% mitomycin loss by HPLC in 24 hr at 4 °C	1866	C
	TR[b]	BR	20 mg	10% mitomycin loss by HPLC in 7 hr at 25 °C	1866	I
	TR[b]	BR	40 mg	10% mitomycin loss by HPLC in 23 hr at 4 °C	1866	C
Ringer's injection, lactated		BR	50 mg	10% mitomycin loss in 43 hr at 25 °C	1205	C
	MG[c]	BR	20 mg	10% mitomycin loss by HPLC in 143 hr at 25 °C	1866	C
	MG[c]	BR	40 mg	10% mitomycin loss by HPLC in 480 hr at 4 °C	1866	C
	TR[b]	BR	20 mg	10% mitomycin loss by HPLC in 142 hr at 25 °C	1866	C
	TR[b]	BR	40 mg	10% mitomycin loss by HPLC in 370 hr at 4 °C	1866	C
Sodium chloride 0.3%	[b,d]	KY	400 mg	9% loss in 7 days at 4 °C in the dark	1503	C
Sodium chloride 0.5%	[a,d]	KY	600 mg	6 to 8% loss in 7 days at 4 °C in the dark	1503	C
Sodium chloride 0.9%	TR[a]	BR	400 mg	Less than 10% mitomycin loss in 24 hr at room temperature	519	C
	TR[b]	CH	50 mg	Violet color appeared in 4 hr and intensified over 12 hr. 10% mitomycin loss in 12 hr at 5 °C in the dark	1118	I
		BR	50 mg	10% mitomycin loss in 5 days at 25 °C	1205	C

Solution Compatibility (Cont.)

Mitomycin

Solution	Mfr	Mfr	Conc/L	Remarks	Ref	C/I
[a]	KY	600 mg		5% loss in 24 hr and 9% loss in 4 days at 4 °C in the dark	1503	C
	MG[c]	BR	40 mg	10% mitomycin loss by HPLC in 128 hr at 4 °C	1866	C
	TR[b]	BR	40 mg	10% mitomycin loss by HPLC in 126 hr at 4 °C	1866	C

[a]Tested in both glass and PVC containers.
[b]Tested in PVC containers.
[c]Tested in glass containers.
[d]Prepared from sodium chloride 0.9% and water for injection.

Additive Compatibility

Mitomycin

Drug	Mfr	Conc/L	Mfr	Conc/L	Test Soln	Remarks	Ref	C/I
Bleomycin sulfate	BR	20 and 30 units	BR	10 mg	NS	20% loss of bleomycin activity in 1 week at 4 °C	763	I
	BR	20 and 30 units	BR	50 mg	NS	52% loss of bleomycin activity in 1 week at 4 °C	763	I
Dexamethasone sodium phosphate	LY	5 g	BR	100 mg	NS[a]	Visually compatible with 10% mitomycin loss calculated in 68 hr and 10% dexamethasone loss calculated in 250 hr at 25 °C	1866	C
	LY	5 g	BR	100 mg	NS[b]	Visually compatible with 10% mitomycin loss calculated in 91 hr and 10% dexamethasone loss calculated in 154 hr at 25 °C	1866	C
	LY	5 g	BR	100 mg	NS[a]	Visually compatible with 10% mitomycin loss calculated in 211 hr and 10% dexamethasone loss calculated in 98 hr at 4 °C	1866	C
	LY	5 g	BR	100 mg	NS[b]	Visually compatible with 10% mitomycin loss calculated in 238 hr and 10% dexamethasone loss calculated in 355 hr at 25 °C	1866	C
Heparin sodium	ES	33,300 units	BR	167 mg	NS[a]	Visually compatible with 10% mitomycin loss calculated in 21 hr and no decrease in heparin bioactivity at 25 °C	1866	I
	ES	33,300 units	BR	167 mg	NS[b]	Visually compatible with 10% mitomycin loss calculated in 25 hr and no decrease in heparin bioactivity at 25 °C	1866	C
	ES	33,300 units	BR	500 mg	NS[a]	Visually compatible with 10% mitomycin loss calculated in 42 hr and no decrease in heparin bioactivity at 25 °C	1866	C
	ES	33,300 units	BR	500 mg	NS[b]	Visually compatible with 10% mitomycin loss calculated in 61 hr and no decrease in heparin bioactivity at 25 °C	1866	C
Hydrocortisone sodium succinate	AB	33.3 g	BR	1 g	W[a]	Visually compatible with 10% mitomycin loss calculated in 172 hr and 10% hydrocortisone loss calculated in 212 hr at 25 °C	1866	C

Additive Compatibility (Cont.)

Mitomycin

Drug	Mfr	Conc/L	Mfr	Conc/L	Test Soln	Remarks	Ref	C/I
	AB	33.3 g	BR	1 g	W[b]	Visually compatible with 10% mitomycin loss calculated in 206 hr and 10% hydrocortisone loss calculated in 218 hr at 25 °C	1866	**C**
	AB	33.3 g	BR	1 g	W[a]	Visually compatible with 10% mitomycin loss calculated in 1423 hr and 10% hydrocortisone loss calculated in 176 hr at 4 °C	1866	**C**
	AB	33.3 g	BR	1 g	W[b]	Visually compatible with 10% mitomycin loss calculated in 820 hr and 10% hydrocortisone loss calculated in 807 hr at 4 °C	1866	**C**

[a]*Tested in glass containers.*
[b]*Tested in PVC containers.*

Drugs in Syringe Compatibility

Mitomycin

Drug (in syringe)	Mfr	Amt	Mfr	Amt	Remarks	Ref	C/I
Bleomycin sulfate		1.5 units/ 0.5 ml		0.25 mg/ 0.5 ml	Physically compatible for 5 min at room temperature followed by 8 min of centrifugation	980	**C**
Cisplatin		0.5 mg/ 0.5 ml		0.25 mg/ 0.5 ml	Physically compatible for 5 min at room temperature followed by 8 min of centrifugation	980	**C**
Cyclophosphamide		10 mg/ 0.5 ml		0.25 mg/ 0.5 ml	Physically compatible for 5 min at room temperature followed by 8 min of centrifugation	980	**C**
Doxorubicin HCl		1 mg/ 0.5 ml		0.25 mg/ 0.5 ml	Physically compatible for 5 min at room temperature followed by 8 min of centrifugation	980	**C**
Droperidol		1.25 mg/ 0.5 ml		0.25 mg/ 0.5 ml	Physically compatible for 5 min at room temperature followed by 8 min of centrifugation	980	**C**
Fluorouracil		25 mg/ 0.5 ml		0.25 mg/ 0.5 ml	Physically compatible for 5 min at room temperature followed by 8 min of centrifugation	980	**C**
Furosemide		5 mg/ 0.5 ml		0.25 mg/ 0.5 ml	Physically compatible for 5 min at room temperature followed by 8 min of centrifugation	980	**C**
Heparin sodium		500 units/ 0.5 ml		0.25 mg/ 0.5 ml	Physically compatible for 5 min at room temperature followed by 8 min of centrifugation	980	**C**
Leucovorin calcium		5 mg/ 0.5 ml		0.25 mg/ 0.5 ml	Physically compatible for 5 min at room temperature followed by 8 min of centrifugation	980	**C**
Methotrexate sodium		12.5 mg/ 0.5 ml		0.25 mg/ 0.5 ml	Physically compatible for 5 min at room temperature followed by 8 min of centrifugation	980	**C**

Drugs in Syringe Compatibility (Cont.)

Drug (in syringe)	Mfr	Amt	Mfr	Amt	Remarks	Ref	C/I
		Mitomycin					
Metoclopramide HCl		2.5 mg/ 0.5 ml		0.25 mg/ 0.5 ml	Physically compatible for 5 min at room temperature followed by 8 min of centrifugation	980	C
Vinblastine sulfate		0.5 mg/ 0.5 ml		0.25 mg/ 0.5 ml	Physically compatible for 5 min at room temperature followed by 8 min of centrifugation	980	C
Vincristine sulfate		0.5 mg/ 0.5 ml		0.25 mg/ 0.5 ml	Physically compatible for 5 min at room temperature followed by 8 min of centrifugation	980	C

Y-Site Injection Compatibility (1:1 Mixture)

Drug	Mfr	Conc	Mfr	Conc	Remarks	Ref	C/I
		Mitomycin					
Amifostine	USB	10 mg/ml[a]	BR	0.5 mg/ml	Physically compatible with no change in measured turbidity or increase in particle content in 4 hr at 23 °C	1845	C
Aztreonam	SQ	40 mg/ml[a]	BMS	0.5 mg/ml	Color changes from pale blue to reddish purple in 4 hr	1758	I
Bleomycin sulfate		3 units/ml		0.5 mg/ml	Drugs injected sequentially into Y-site with no flush between. No visually apparent precipitate	980	C
Cefepime HCl	BR	20 mg/ml[a]	BR	0.5 mg/ml	Color changes to pinkish purple in 1 hr	1684	I
Cisplatin		1 mg/ml		0.5 mg/ml	Drugs injected sequentially into Y-site with no flush between. No visually apparent precipitate	980	C
Cyclophosphamide		20 mg/ml		0.5 mg/ml	Drugs injected sequentially into Y-site with no flush between. No visually apparent precipitate	980	C
Doxorubicin HCl		2 mg/ml		0.5 mg/ml	Drugs injected sequentially into Y-site with no flush between. No visually apparent precipitate	980	C
Droperidol		2.5 mg/ml		0.5 mg/ml	Drugs injected sequentially into Y-site with no flush between. No visually apparent precipitate	980	C
Etoposide phosphate	BR	5 mg/ml[a]	BR	0.5 mg/ml[a]	Color changed from light blue to reddish-purple in 4 hr at 23 °C	2218	I
Filgrastim	AMG	30 μg/ml[a]	BR	0.5 mg/ml	Color changes to reddish purple in 1 hr	1687	I
Fluorouracil		50 mg/ml		0.5 mg/ml	Drugs injected sequentially into Y-site with no flush between. No visually apparent precipitate	980	C
Furosemide		10 mg/ml		0.5 mg/ml	Drugs injected sequentially into Y-site with no flush between. No visually apparent precipitate	980	C
Gemcitabine HCl	LI	10 mg/ml[b]	BR	0.5 mg/ml[b]	Reddish-purple discoloration forms in 1 hr	2226	I

Y-Site Injection Compatibility (1:1 Mixture) (Cont.)

Drug		Mitomycin					
	Mfr	Conc	Mfr	Conc	Remarks	Ref	C/I
Granisetron HCl	SKB	0.05 mg/ml[a]	BMS	0.5 mg/ml	Physically compatible with no change in measured turbidity or increase in particle content in 4 hr at 23 °C	2000	C
Heparin sodium		1000 units/ml		0.5 mg/ml	Drugs injected sequentially into Y-site with no flush between. No visually apparent precipitate	980	C
Leucovorin calcium		10 mg/ml		0.5 mg/ml	Drugs injected sequentially into Y-site with no flush between. No visually apparent precipitate	980	C
Melphalan HCl	BW	0.1 mg/ml[b]	BR	0.5 mg/ml	Physically compatible with no change in measured turbidity or increase in particle content in 3 hr at 22 °C	1557	C
Methotrexate sodium		25 mg/ml		0.5 mg/ml	Drugs injected sequentially into Y-site with no flush between. No visually apparent precipitate	980	C
Metoclopramide HCl		5 mg/ml		0.5 mg/ml	Drugs injected sequentially into Y-site with no flush between. No visually apparent precipitate	980	C
Ondansetron HCl	GL	1 mg/ml[b]	BR	0.5 mg/ml	Physically compatible for 4 hr at 22 °C	1365	C
Piperacillin sodium–tazobactam sodium	LE	40 + 5 mg/ml[a]	BR	0.5 mg/ml	Blue color darkens in 4 hr, becoming reddish purple in 24 hr	1688	I
Sargramostim	IMM	10 μg/ml[b]	BR	0.5 mg/ml	Slight haze, visible with high intensity light, forms in 30 min	1436	I
Teniposide	BR	0.1 mg/ml[a]	BR	0.5 mg/ml	Physically compatible with no subvisual haze or particle formation in 4 hr at 23 °C	1725	C
Thiotepa	IMM[c]	1 mg/ml[a]	BMS	0.5 mg/ml	Physically compatible with no change in measured turbidity or increase in particle content in 4 hr at 23 °C	1861	C
Vinblastine sulfate		1 mg/ml		0.5 mg/ml	Drugs injected sequentially into Y-site with no flush between. No visually apparent precipitate	980	C
Vincristine sulfate		1 mg/ml		0.5 mg/ml	Drugs injected sequentially into Y-site with no flush between. No visually apparent precipitate	980	C
Vinorelbine tartrate	BW	1 mg/ml[b]	BR	0.5 mg/ml	Color changes from pale blue to reddish purple in 1 hr	1558	I

[a]Tested in dextrose 5% in water.
[b]Tested in sodium chloride 0.9%.
[c]Lyophilized formulation tested.

Additional Compatibility Information

The manufacturer indicates that mitomycin 20 to 40 μg/ml is stable at room temperature for three hours in dextrose 5% in water, 12 hours in sodium chloride 0.9%, and 24 hours in sodium lactate ⅙ M (2). Other reports indicated differing stability information (519; 1118; 1205; 1503). See both Stability and Solution Compatibility table.

Combining mitomycin 5 to 15 mg and heparin sodium 1000 to 10,000 units in 30 ml of sodium chloride 0.9% results in a solution that is stable for 48 hours at room temperature (2).

Other Information

Inactivation— In the event of spills or leaks, Bristol-Myers Squibb recommends the use of sodium hypochlorite 5% (household bleach) or potassium permanganate 1% to inactivate mitomycin (1200).

MITOXANTRONE HCL
AHFS 10:00

Novantrone   **Immunex**

Products— Mitoxantrone HCl (Immunex) is supplied as a concentrate for further dilution in 10-, 12.5-, and 15-ml multidose vials. Each milliliter of the dark blue aqueous solution contains mitoxantrone 2 mg (as the hydrochloride salt), sodium chloride 0.8%, sodium acetate 0.005%, and acetic acid 0.046% (2).

pH— From 3 to 4.5 (2).

Osmolality— Mitoxantrone HCl 2 mg/ml has an osmolality of 270 mOsm/kg (1689).

Sodium Content— Each milliliter of solution contains 0.14 mEq of sodium (2).

Administration— Mitoxantrone HCl is administered by slow intravenous infusion after dilution to at least 50 ml in dextrose 5% in water or sodium chloride 0.9%. Mitoxantrone HCl is usually administered over 15 to 30 minutes through the tubing of a freely running intravenous solution (2; 4) or by continuous intravenous infusion over 24 hours (4). It should not be given over less than three minutes (2; 4).

Stability— Intact vials of the dark blue concentrate should be stored at controlled room temperature and protected from freezing (2). Refrigeration of the concentrate may cause a precipitate, which redissolves upon warming to room temperature (72; 1369).

Mitoxantrone HCl is not photolabile. Exposure of the product to direct sunlight for one month caused no change in its appearance or potency (72; 1293).

The manufacturer indicates that mitoxantrone HCl concentrate remaining in partially used vials may be stored for up to seven days at 15 to 25 °C and up to 14 days under refrigeration but should not be stored frozen (4).

Mitoxantrone HCl was cultured with human lymphoblasts to determine whether its cytotoxic activity was retained. The solution retained cytotoxicity for 24 hours at 4 °C and room temperature (1575).

pH Effects— The pH range of maximum stability is 2 to 4.5. Mitoxantrone HCl was unstable when the pH was increased to 7.4 (1379).

Syringes— Mitoxantrone HCl 0.2 mg/ml in sodium chloride 0.9% in polypropylene syringes (Braun Omnifix) is reported to be stable for 28 days at 4 and 20 °C (1564) and for 24 hours at 37 °C (1369).

Mitoxantrone HCl (Lederle) 2 mg/ml in glass vials and drawn into 12-ml plastic syringes (Monoject) exhibited no visual changes and little or no loss by HPLC when stored for 42 days at 4 and 23 °C. Potential extractable materials from the syringes were not detectable during the study period (1593).

Micropumps— Mitoxantrone HCl (Lederle) 0.2 mg/ml in sterile water for injection was stable in Parker Micropump PVC reservoirs for 14 days at 4 and 37 °C, exhibiting no loss by HPLC (1696).

Sorption— Mitoxantrone HCl (Lederle) 1 mg/ml in sodium chloride 0.9% exhibited no loss by UV spectroscopy due to sorption to PVC and polyethylene administration lines during simulated infusion at 0.875 ml/hr for 2.5 hours via a syringe pump (1795).

Filtration— Although binding of mitoxantrone HCl to filters has been reported (1249; 1415; 1416), the manufacturer states that filtration of mitoxantrone HCl through a 0.22-μm filter (Millipore) results in no loss of potency (1293).

Mitoxantrone HCl (Lederle) 5 mg/100 ml in sodium chloride 0.9% in a burette was filtered through a nylon 0.2-μm filter (Pall, ELD96LL). No drug loss due to sorption was found spectrophotometrically (1568).

Mitoxantrone HCl (Lederle) 1 mg/ml in sodium chloride 0.9%, during simulated infusion at 0.875 ml/hr for 2.5 hours via a syringe pump, exhibited no loss by UV spectroscopy due to sorption to cellulose acetate (Minisart 45, Sartorius), polysulfone (Acrodisc 45, Gelman), and nylon (Posidyne ELD96, Pall) filters (1795).

Compatibility Information

Solution Compatibility

Mitoxantrone HCl

Solution	Mfr	Mfr	Conc/L	Remarks	Ref	C/I
Dextrose 5% in sodium chloride 0.9%	a	LE	20 to 500 mg	Physically compatible and at least 90% potency retained for 48 hr at room temperature	1293	**C**
Dextrose 5% in water	a	LE	20 to 500 mg	Physically compatible and at least 90% potency retained for 7 days at room temperature and under refrigeration	72; 1293	**C**
		LE	5 mg	Physically compatible and no decomposition in 48 hr	72	**C**
Sodium chloride 0.9%	a	LE	20 to 500 mg	Physically compatible and at least 90% potency retained for 7 days at room temperature and under refrigeration	72; 1293	**C**
	b	LE	20 to 500 mg	Physically compatible and at least 90% potency retained for 48 hr at room temperature	1293	**C**
		LE	5 mg	Physically compatible and no decomposition in 48 hr	72	**C**

aTested in PVC containers.
bTested in glass containers.

Additive Compatibility

<table>
<tr><td colspan="9" align="center">**Mitoxantrone HCl**</td></tr>
<tr>
<th>Drug</th>
<th>Mfr</th>
<th>Conc/L</th>
<th>Mfr</th>
<th>Conc/L</th>
<th>Test Soln</th>
<th>Remarks</th>
<th>Ref</th>
<th>C/I</th>
</tr>
<tr>
<td>Cyclophosphamide</td>
<td>AD</td>
<td>10 g</td>
<td>LE</td>
<td>500 mg</td>
<td>D5W</td>
<td>Visually compatible and mitoxantrone potency by HPLC retained for 24 hr at room temperature. Cyclophosphamide not tested</td>
<td>1531</td>
<td>C</td>
</tr>
<tr>
<td>Cytarabine</td>
<td>UP</td>
<td>500 mg</td>
<td>LE</td>
<td>500 mg</td>
<td>D5W</td>
<td>Visually compatible and mitoxantrone potency by HPLC retained for 24 hr at room temperature. Cytarabine not tested</td>
<td>1531</td>
<td>C</td>
</tr>
<tr>
<td>Fluorouracil</td>
<td></td>
<td>25 g</td>
<td>LE</td>
<td>500 mg</td>
<td>D5W</td>
<td>Visually compatible and mitoxantrone potency by HPLC retained for 24 hr at room temperature. Fluorouracil not tested</td>
<td>1531</td>
<td>C</td>
</tr>
<tr>
<td>Hydrocortisone sodium phosphate</td>
<td></td>
<td>100 mg to 2 g</td>
<td>LE</td>
<td>50 to 200 mg</td>
<td>NS[a]</td>
<td>Physically compatible and potency of both drugs retained for 24 hr at room temperature</td>
<td>1293</td>
<td>C</td>
</tr>
<tr>
<td></td>
<td></td>
<td>100 mg to 2 g</td>
<td>LE</td>
<td>50 to 200 mg</td>
<td>D5W[a]</td>
<td>Small blue particles form on inner surface of bag</td>
<td>1293</td>
<td>I</td>
</tr>
<tr>
<td></td>
<td></td>
<td>100 mg to 2 g</td>
<td>LE</td>
<td>50 to 200 mg</td>
<td>D5W[b]</td>
<td>Physically compatible</td>
<td>1293</td>
<td>C</td>
</tr>
<tr>
<td>Hydrocortisone sodium succinate</td>
<td></td>
<td>100 mg to 2 g</td>
<td>LE</td>
<td>50 to 200 mg</td>
<td>D5W, NS[a]</td>
<td>Physically compatible and potency of both drugs retained for 24 hr at room temperature</td>
<td>1293</td>
<td>C</td>
</tr>
<tr>
<td>Potassium chloride</td>
<td></td>
<td>50 mEq</td>
<td>LE</td>
<td>500 mg</td>
<td>D5W</td>
<td>Visually compatible and mitoxantrone potency by HPLC retained for 24 hr at room temperature. Potassium chloride not tested</td>
<td>1531</td>
<td>C</td>
</tr>
</table>

[a]*Tested in PVC containers.*
[b]*Tested in glass containers.*

Y-Site Injection Compatibility (1:1 Mixture)

<table>
<tr><td colspan="9" align="center">**Mitoxantrone HCl**</td></tr>
<tr>
<th>Drug</th>
<th>Mfr</th>
<th>Conc</th>
<th>Mfr</th>
<th>Conc</th>
<th>Remarks</th>
<th>Ref</th>
<th>C/I</th>
</tr>
<tr>
<td>Allopurinol sodium</td>
<td>BW</td>
<td>3 mg/ml[b]</td>
<td>LE</td>
<td>0.5 mg/ml[b]</td>
<td>Physically compatible with no change in measured turbidity or increase in particle content in 4 hr at 22 °C</td>
<td>1686</td>
<td>C</td>
</tr>
<tr>
<td>Amifostine</td>
<td>USB</td>
<td>10 mg/ml[a]</td>
<td>LE</td>
<td>0.5 mg/ml[a]</td>
<td>Physically compatible with no change in measured turbidity or increase in particle content in 4 hr at 23 °C</td>
<td>1845</td>
<td>C</td>
</tr>
<tr>
<td>Amphotericin B cholesteryl sulfate complex</td>
<td>SEQ</td>
<td>0.83 mg/ml[a]</td>
<td>IMM</td>
<td>0.5 mg/ml[a]</td>
<td>Gross precipitate forms</td>
<td>2117</td>
<td>I</td>
</tr>
<tr>
<td>Aztreonam</td>
<td>SQ</td>
<td>40 mg/ml[a]</td>
<td>LE</td>
<td>0.5 mg/ml[a]</td>
<td>Heavy precipitate forms in 1 hr</td>
<td>1758</td>
<td>I</td>
</tr>
<tr>
<td>Cefepime HCl</td>
<td>BR</td>
<td>20 mg/ml[a]</td>
<td>LE</td>
<td>0.5 mg/ml[a]</td>
<td>Haze forms immediately and becomes flocculent precipitate in 4 hr</td>
<td>1689</td>
<td>I</td>
</tr>
<tr>
<td>Cladribine</td>
<td>ORT</td>
<td>0.015[b] and 0.5[c] mg/ml</td>
<td>LE</td>
<td>0.5 mg/ml[b]</td>
<td>Physically compatible with no change in measured turbidity or increase in particle content in 4 hr at 23 °C</td>
<td>1969</td>
<td>C</td>
</tr>
<tr>
<td>Doxorubicin HCl liposome injection</td>
<td>SEQ</td>
<td>0.4 mg/ml[a]</td>
<td>IMM</td>
<td>0.5 mg/ml[a]</td>
<td>Partial loss of measured natural turbidity</td>
<td>2087</td>
<td>I</td>
</tr>
</table>

Y-Site Injection Compatibility (1:1 Mixture) (Cont.)

Mitoxantrone HCl

Drug	Mfr	Conc	Mfr	Conc	Remarks	Ref	C/I
Etoposide phosphate	BR	5 mg/ml[a]	IMM	0.5 mg/ml[a]	Physically compatible with no change in measured turbidity or increase in particle content in 4 hr at 23 °C	2218	C
Filgrastim	AMG	30 μg/ml[a]	LE	0.5 mg/ml[a]	Physically compatible with no change in measured turbidity or increase in particle content in 4 hr at 22 °C	1687	C
Fludarabine phosphate	BX	1 mg/ml[a]	LE	0.5 mg/ml[a]	Physically compatible for 4 hr at room temperature under fluorescent light	1439	C
Gemcitabine HCl	LI	10 mg/ml[b]	IMM	0.5 mg/ml[b]	Physically compatible with no change in measured turbidity or increase in particle content in 4 hr at 23 °C	2226	C
Granisetron HCl	SKB	0.05 mg/ml[a]	IMM	0.5 mg/ml[a]	Physically compatible with no change in measured turbidity or increase in particle content in 4 hr at 23 °C	2000	C
Melphalan HCl	BW	0.1 mg/ml[b]	LE	0.5 mg/ml[b]	Physically compatible with no change in measured turbidity or increase in particle content in 3 hr at 22 °C	1557	C
Ondansetron HCl	GL	1 mg/ml[b]	LE	0.5 mg/ml[a]	Physically compatible for 4 hr at 22 °C	1365	C
Paclitaxel	NCI	1.2 mg/ml[a]	LE	0.5 mg/ml[a]	Normal inherent haze from paclitaxel decreases immediately	1556	I
Piperacillin sodium–tazobactam sodium	LE	40 + 5 mg/ml[a]	LE	0.5 mg/ml[a]	Haze and particles form immediately. Large particles form in 4 hr	1688	I
Propofol	ZEN	10 mg/ml	IMM	0.5 mg/ml[a]	Small amount of particles forms immediately	2066	I
Sargramostim	IMM	10 μg/ml[b]	LE	0.5 mg/ml[b]	Physically compatible for 4 hr at 22 °C	1436	C
Teniposide	BR	0.1 mg/ml[a]	LE	0.5 mg/ml[a]	Physically compatible with no subvisual haze or particle formation in 4 hr at 23 °C	1725	C
Thiotepa	IMM[d]	1 mg/ml[a]	IMM	0.5 mg/ml[a]	Physically compatible with no change in measured turbidity or increase in particle content in 4 hr at 23 °C	1861	C
TNA #218 to #226[e]			IMM	0.5 mg/ml[a]	Visually compatible with no precipitate or emulsion damage apparent in 4 hr at 23 °C	2215	C
TPN #212 to #215[e]			IMM	0.5 mg/ml[a]	Substantial loss of natural subvisual turbidity occurs immediately	2109	I
Vinorelbine tartrate	BW	1 mg/ml[b]	LE	0.5 mg/ml[b]	Physically compatible with little change in measured turbidity or increase in particle content in 4 hr at 22 °C	1558	C

[a]*Tested in dextrose 5% in water.*
[b]*Tested in sodium chloride 0.9%.*
[c]*Tested in bacteriostatic sodium chloride 0.9% preserved with benzyl alcohol 0.9%.*
[d]*Lyophilized formulation tested.*
[e]*Refer to Appendix I for the composition of parenteral nutrition solutions. TNA indicates a 3-in-1 admixture, and TPN indicates a 2-in-1 admixture.*

Additional Compatibility Information

Solutions— The manufacturer recommends the use of dextrose 5% in sodium chloride 0.9%, dextrose 5% in water, or sodium chloride 0.9% for dilution of mitoxantrone HCl concentrate (2).

Heparin— The manufacturer does not recommend combining heparin with mitoxantrone HCl in the same admixture because of possible precipitate formation (2; 1293).

Other Information

Inactivation— The manufacturer recommends that mitoxantrone HCl spilled on equipment or surfaces be inactivated with an aqueous solution of calcium hypochlorite, 5.5 parts in 13 parts (by weight) of water for each one part of mitoxantrone HCl (2; 1293).

MIVACURIUM CHLORIDE
AHFS 12:20

Mivacron   **Abbott**

Products— Mivacurium chloride (Abbott) is available in 5- and 10-ml single-use vials and 20- and 50-ml multiple-use vials. Each milliliter contains mivacurium 2 mg (as the chloride) with hydrochloric acid, if necessary, to adjust the pH. The multiple-use vials also contain benzyl alcohol 0.9% (2).

A premixed mivacurium chloride infusion (Abbott) is available in dextrose 5% in water in 50- and 100-ml flexible plastic containers. Each milliliter contains mivacurium 0.5 mg (as the chloride) (2).

pH— From 3.5 to 5 (2).

Osmolarity— The premixed infusion has an osmolarity of 260 mOsm/L (2).

Administration— Mivacurium chloride is administered by rapid intravenous injection or by intravenous infusion (2; 4).

Stability— Mivacurium chloride solutions are clear and colorless. Both the injection and premixed infusion should be stored at 15 to 25 °C and protected from direct ultraviolet light, excessive heat, and freezing (2).

pH Effects— Mivacurium chloride is incompatible with alkaline solutions having a pH greater than 8.5 (2).

Compatibility Information

Y-Site Injection Compatibility (1:1 Mixture)

Mivacurium chloride

Drug	Mfr	Conc	Mfr	Conc	Remarks	Ref	C/I
Etomidate	AB	2 mg/ml	BW	2 mg/ml	Visually compatible for up to 7 days at 25 °C	1801	C
Thiopental sodium	AB	25 mg/ml	BW	2 mg/ml	Visually compatible for up to 7 days at 25 °C	1801	C

Additional Compatibility Information

Solutions— The manufacturer states that mivacurium chloride 0.5 mg/ml is physically and chemically stable for 24 hours at 5 to 25 °C in the following infusion solutions (2):

    Dextrose 5% in Ringer's injection, lactated
    Dextrose 5% in sodium chloride 0.9%
    Dextrose 5% in water
    Ringer's injection, lactated
    Sodium chloride 0.9%

Additives— The manufacturer recommends that, in general, no drugs should be admixed with mivacurium chloride. However, alfentanil HCl, droperidol, fentanyl citrate, midazolam HCl, and sufentanil citrate are compatible by Y-site administration with mivacurium chloride (2).

MORPHINE SULFATE
AHFS 28:08.08

Astramorph PF   **Astra**
Duramorph   **Elkins-Sinn**

Products— Morphine sulfate is available in a variety of concentrations and sizes ranging from 0.5 to 50 mg/ml. The Astramorph PF and Duramorph 0.5- and 1-mg/ml concentrations and the Infumorph 200 (10 mg/ml) and Infumorph 500 (25 mg/ml) formulations are preservative free. Other morphine sulfate products may contain various preservatives, antioxidants, and buffers, including chlorobutanol, phenol, sodium bisulfite, sodium phosphates, and sodium formaldehyde sulfoxylate (4; 154).

pH— From 2.5 to 6 for most products. Duramorph has a pH of 3.5 to 7, and Infumorph has a pH of about 4.5 (4). Morphine sulfate (David Bull) 7.5 mg/ml in sodium chloride 0.9% had a pH of 3.5 (2161).

Osmotic Values— The osmolality of morphine (as the hydrochloride) 10 mg/ml was determined to be 54 mOsm/kg (1233). Morphine sulfate (David Bull) 7.5 mg/ml in sodium chloride 0.9% had an osmolality of 236 mOsm/kg (2161).

Solubility— The maximum aqueous solubility of morphine sulfate at room temperature has been reported to be about 62.5 mg/ml (4). However, a lower practical morphine sulfate solubility was found during an evaluation of concentrations ranging from 10 to 50 mg/ml in water, dextrose 5% in water, and sodium chloride 0.9%. The maximum practical solubility in dextrose 5% in water was essentially the same as in water over the temperature range of 4 to 40 °C and was about 50 mg/ml at 22 °C. However, the solubility in sodium chloride 0.9% was markedly reduced about 40% to about 30 mg/ml at 22 °C. Under refrigeration, the maximum solubilities were reduced to 30 mg/ml in water and dextrose 5% in water and to 20 mg/ml in sodium chloride 0.9% (2162).

Administration— Morphine sulfate is usually administered subcutaneously but may be administered by intramuscular or slow intravenous injection and by slow continuous subcutaneous or intravenous infusion. For continuous intravenous infusion, a concentration of 0.1 to 1 mg/ml in dextrose 5% in water may be infused using an infusion control device, although more concentrated solutions also have been used. Duramorph, Infumorph, and Astramorph PF contain no preservatives and may be administered intrathecally or epidurally (2; 4).

High-concentration morphine sulfate is not recommended for subcutaneous, intramuscular, or intravenous injection of individual doses or for intrathecal or epidural administration. The products are intended for continuous intravenous infusion using a suitable microinfusion control device (4).

Stability— Morphine sulfate injections are clear, colorless solutions. Intact containers should be stored at controlled room temperature and protected from freezing and light. Morphine sulfate darkens upon prolonged exposure to light (4).

Morphine sulfate is relatively stable at acidic pH, especially below pH 4, but degradation increases greatly at neutral or basic pH. Degradation is often accompanied by a yellow to brown discoloration in the normally colorless solution (1072; 2170).

Undiluted morphine sulfate (Allen & Hanburys) 10 mg/ml, stored in 100-ml glass vials and PVC bags, exhibited no loss in 30 days at 23 °C (1394).

Morphine sulfate (Wyeth) 1 mg/ml in bacteriostatic sodium chloride 0.9% containing benzyl alcohol 0.9%, when stored in glass vials with protection from light, exhibited no loss by HPLC at 4 °C and a 4% loss at 22 °C after 91 days (1583).

Duafala et al. studied the stability of morphine sulfate 15 and 2 mg/ml diluted with sterile water for injection at 4 and 24 °C in 200-ml PVC bags (Baxter). Both concentrations were stable at both temperatures with little or no loss in 15 days (1504).

Morphine sulfate physical and chemical stability were evaluated at concentrations ranging from 10 to 50 mg/ml in water, dextrose 5% in water, and sodium chloride 0.9% for use in subcutaneous infusion. The solutions were stored in glass containers, polypropylene syringes, and PVC containers at 4, 22, and 40 °C for up to three months in the absence of light. At concentrations above 20 mg/ml, refrigerated storage resulted in the formation of visually apparent precipitation that was difficult to redissolve. Precipitation also occurred at concentrations above 30 mg/ml using sodium chloride 0.9% as the diluent. The solution color increased progressively from colorless to pale yellow initially to darker yellow and to brown in the 40 °C samples. HPLC analysis of morphine sulfate 30-mg/ml aqueous solutions found no substantial decomposition of morphine sulfate within three months at 22 °C, but the authors recommended that refrigerated storage be avoided because of the potential for precipitation. In addition, the solutions in PVC containers exhibited a gradual increase in drug concentration and osmolality possibly indicating a loss of water through the PVC. The morphine concentration increased to over 105% after storage of one month and one week at 22 and 40 °C, respectively. In addition, a white precipitate formed, possibly because of water evaporation. Storage in PVC containers for longer time periods was not recommended (2162).

Freezing Solutions— Morphine sulfate (Lilly) 1 and 2 mg/ml in dextrose 5% in water and sodium chloride 0.9% in PVC bags exhibited no loss during 14 weeks of frozen storage at −20 °C (1286).

Syringes— Prefilled into plastic syringes with syringe caps (Braun), morphine sulfate is stated to remain within acceptable limits of degradation for at least 69 days at room temperature (982).

In another study, less than a 3% loss of morphine sulfate occurred in 12 weeks when stored in plastic syringes at 22 °C and exposed to light. A smaller loss occurred when the morphine sulfate was stored at 3 °C with light protection (1287).

Duafala et al. studied the stability of morphine sulfate 15 and 2 mg/ml diluted with sterile water for injection at 4 and 24 °C in 3-ml disposable glass syringes (Hypod). Both concentrations were stable at both temperatures with little or no loss in 12 days (1504).

Morphine sulfate (Lilly) 1 and 5 mg/ml in dextrose 5% in water and sodium chloride 0.9% was packaged in 30-ml Plastipak (Becton-Dickinson) syringes capped with Monoject (Sherwood) tip caps. Syringes were stored at 23 °C exposed to light and protected from light, 4 °C protected from light, and frozen at −20 °C protected from light for 12 weeks. HPLC analysis found that both concentrations at all three temperatures were stable for at least six weeks when protected from light. However, the samples at 23 °C exposed to light were stable for a week, but some developed unacceptable losses after that (1894).

Grassby and Hutchings reported the stability of morphine sulfate 2 mg/ml in sodium chloride 0.9% packaged in 50-ml (Becton-Dickinson) and 30-ml (Becton-Dickinson and Sherwood) polypropylene syringes for use in patient-controlled analgesia and in stoppered glass vials. The morphine sulfate solution packaged in the syringes and glass vials was stored at room temperature in the dark for six weeks. Using HPLC analysis, the authors found little or no loss of morphine sulfate content in the 50-ml syringes and the glass vials in six weeks. About 5% loss occurred when packaged in both brands of 30-ml syringes. Addition of sodium metabisulfite 0.1% as an antioxidant substantially increased the rate of drug loss; up to 10% loss occurred in two weeks (2040).

The stability of morphine hydrochloride 1, 5, and 10 mg/ml in dextrose 5% in water and 0.9% sodium chloride packaged in 50-ml polypropylene syringes (B. Braun and Becton-Dickinson) was evaluated. HPLC analysis found little or no loss, with degradation products being less than 2% of the concentration when stored at 37 °C for two days (2169).

Morphine tartrate (David Bull) 80 mg/ml (undiluted) and 4 mg/ml diluted in sodium chloride 0.9% was packaged as 10 ml of solution in polypropylene syringes (Terumo) sealed with tip caps (Terumo). Samples were stored in the dark at 4 and 22 °C for 21 days. The refrigerated samples at both concentrations and the 4-mg/ml concentration at 22 °C underwent no visible changes and HPLC analysis found little or no loss. The 80-mg/ml samples stored at 22 °C developed a slight yellow discoloration within 21 days that was considered to be within the normal color range for this product. HPLC analysis found about 7% loss after 21 days (1461).

Ambulatory Infusion Pumps— Walker et al. reported the stability of morphine sulfate (Sabex) 50 and 25 mg/ml and 10 mg/ml diluted in dextrose 5% in water and sodium chloride 0.9%, with and without sodium metabisulfite preservative, in portable infusion pump cassettes (Pharmacia) stored at 4 and 23 °C. At all concentrations with or without preservatives at both temperatures, samples remained clear and colorless. Morphine sulfate losses of approximately 5 to 8% were found during 31 days of storage (1505).

Altman et al. evaluated the stability of morphine sulfate 0.5, 15, 30, and 60 mg/ml in sodium chloride 0.9% stored in Kalex (Cormed III) bags at 5 and 37 °C. The 60-mg/ml concentration exhibited precipitation in four to eight days when refrigerated. The maximum solubility of morphine sulfate at room temperature is 62.5 mg/ml; refrigeration reduced the solubility, causing precipitation. All other solutions were clear, with no evidence of precipitation. HPLC analysis showed no loss during 14 days of storage at either temperature. A small concentration increase in samples stored at 37 °C was attributed to water evaporation (1506).

Stiles et al. studied the stability of morphine sulfate 25, 15, 5 and 1 mg/ml (with the latter two concentrations prepared in sodium chloride 0.9%) in pump reservoirs (Pharmacia Deltec) stored at 5 and 25 °C for 30 days. After the initial storage period, the solutions were subsequently stored at 37 °C and pumped at a flow rate of 0.4 ml/hr to simulate patient use. No color change or precipitation occurred in any sample. No losses were detected by HPLC; in fact, increased concentrations were observed, especially at room temperature. The concentration increases were attributed to water evaporation during storage. The authors recommended a maximum storage of 30 days under refrigeration and 14 days at room temperature because of the evaporation (1507).

Morphine HCl (Merck) 20 mg/ml was filled into 50-ml ambulatory infusion pump cassette reservoirs (Pharmacia Deltec) and stored at room temperature and protected from light for 90 days. HPLC analysis found no loss of the drug. Instead, the drug concentration increased 13% during the observation period, possibly due to loss of water from the solutions (1850).

The stability of morphine HCl 20 mg/ml (undiluted) and 1 mg/ml diluted with dextrose 5% in water or sodium chloride 0.9% packaged in ambulatory infusion pump cassettes (B. Braun and Deltec)

was evaluated. HPLC analysis found no evidence of drug loss, with degradation products being less than 2% of the concentration when stored at 37 °C for 14 days. However, morphine concentration increases of up to 12% over the study period were observed in some samples presumably because of loss of water (2169).

Elastomeric Reservoir Pumps— Duafala et al. studied the stability of morphine sulfate 15 and 2 mg/ml diluted with sterile water for injection at 4 and 24 °C in Intermate 200 (Infusion Systems) and Infusor (Baxter) disposable elastomeric infusion devices. In the Intermate 200 with 100 ml of morphine sulfate solution, little or no loss occurred in 15 days at either 4 or 24 °C and even at 31 °C (simulating use next to a patient's skin or clothing). In the Infusor, with 50 ml, losses of 5% or more were observed in 12 days in some containers (1504).

Morphine sulfate 0.5 mg/ml in both dextrose 5% in water and sodium chloride 0.9% was evaluated for binding potential to natural rubber elastomeric reservoirs (Baxter). No loss was found after storage for two weeks at 35 °C with gentle agitation (2014).

Morphine HCl 2.5 and 5 mg/ml in 0.9% sodium chloride with and without the antioxidant sodium metabisulfite was filled into 60-ml Infusors (Baxter) and stored at room temperature exposed to or protected from light. HPLC analysis found 6% or less variation in the morphine concentration over a month. The formation of the decomposition product pseudomorphine was greatest without the metabisulfite in the samples exposed to light. Up to 1.5% formed in 30 days. No decomposition products formed if the metabisulfite was present (2176).

Implantable Infusion Pumps— Morphine sulfate 10 mg/ml was filled into a VIP 30 implantable infusion pump (Fresenius) and associated capillary tubing and stored at 37 °C. Samples were analyzed using an HPLC assay. No morphine loss and no contamination from components of pump materials occurred during eight weeks of storage (1903).

Baclofen (Ciba) 0.2 mg/ml with morphine sulfate (David Bull) 1 mg/ml in an implantable pump (Infusaid) was physically compatible and exhibited little or no loss of either drug within 30 days at 37 °C (1911).

In a follow-up study at higher concentrations, baclofen (Ciba) 1 mg/ml with morphine sulfate (David Bull) 15 mg/ml in an implantable pump (Infusaid) was physically compatible, with only a slight yellowing of the solution observed. HPLC analysis found no change in the baclofen concentration and 5% or less morphine loss after 30 days at 37 °C (2170).

Other Devices— Caute et al. evaluated the stability of two intrathecal solutions of morphine sulfate 10 mg/ml in sodium chloride 0.9% (isobaric) and 5 mg/ml in dextrose 7% in water (hyperbaric). The solutions were stored at 4 and 37 °C in glass ampuls and pump reservoirs composed of silicone rubber reinforced with polyester (Cordis Europa). No precipitation or discoloration and no loss of morphine sulfate or increase in degradation products occurred in the solutions in glass ampuls after two months at either temperature. However, in the pump reservoirs, the isobaric solution in sodium chloride 0.9% developed a yellow color. Furthermore, a decomposition product, pseudomorphine, was detectable in three days and increased to 1% in one month at 37 °C. This level was 20 times that of the pseudomorphine found in the hyperbaric dextrose 7% in water solution under the same conditions. The decomposition was attributed to dissolved oxygen, ethylene oxide sterilant, and silicone rubber (1508).

Sorption— Morphine HCl (British Drug Houses) 75 mg/L in sodium chloride 0.9% (Travenol) in PVC bags did not exhibit significant sorption to the plastic during one week of storage at room temperature (15 to 20 °C) (536).

In another study, morphine HCl (British Drug Houses) 75 mg/L in sodium chloride 0.9% did not exhibit any loss due to sorption during a seven-hour simulated infusion through an infusion set (Travenol) consisting of a cellulose propionate burette chamber and 170 cm of PVC tubing (606).

The drug was also tested as a simulated infusion over at least one hour by a syringe pump system. A glass syringe on a syringe pump was fitted with 20 cm of polyethylene tubing or 50 cm of Silastic tubing. No loss of drug due to sorption was observed with either tubing (606).

A 25-ml aliquot of morphine HCl (British Drug Houses) 75 mg/L in sodium chloride 0.9% was stored in all-plastic syringes composed of polypropylene barrels and polyethylene plungers for 24 hours at room temperature in the dark. No loss due to sorption occurred (606).

Filtration— Adsorption to cellulose acetate membrane filters was less than 3% for morphine sulfate 10 to 50 mg/ml in water, dextrose 5% in water, and sodium chloride 0.9% (2162).

Compatibility Information

Solution Compatibility

Morphine sulfate

Solution	Mfr	Mfr	Conc/L	Remarks	Ref	C/I
Dextran 6% in dextrose 5%	AB		16.2 mg	Physically compatible	3	C
Dextran 6% in sodium chloride 0.9%	AB		16.2 mg	Physically compatible	3	C
Dextrose–Ringer's injection combinations	AB		16.2 mg	Physically compatible	3	C
Dextrose–Ringer's injection, lactated, combinations	AB		16.2 mg	Physically compatible	3	C
Dextrose–saline combinations	AB		16.2 mg	Physically compatible	3	C
Dextrose 2½% in water	AB		16.2 mg	Physically compatible	3	C
Dextrose 5% in water	AB		16.2 mg	Physically compatible	3	C
	TR[a]	LI	1.2 g	Physically compatible and no morphine loss in 36 hr at 22 °C	1000	C
	TR[b]	AB, AH	40 and 400 mg	Physically compatible with little or no loss in 7 days at 23 and 4 °C	1349	C
	[a]	AH	5 g	No morphine loss in 30 days at 23 °C	1394	C
Dextrose 10% in water	AB		16.2 mg	Physically compatible	3	C
Fructose 10% in sodium chloride 0.9%	AB		16.2 mg	Physically compatible	3	C
Fructose 10% in water	AB		16.2 mg	Physically compatible	3	C
Invert sugar 5 and 10% in sodium chloride 0.9%	AB		16.2 mg	Physically compatible	3	C
Invert sugar 5 and 10% in water	AB		16.2 mg	Physically compatible	3	C
Ionosol products	AB		16.2 mg	Physically compatible	3	C
Ringer's injection	AB		16.2 mg	Physically compatible	3	C
Ringer's injection, lactated	AB		16.2 mg	Physically compatible	3	C
Sodium chloride 0.45%	AB		16.2 mg	Physically compatible	3	C
Sodium chloride 0.9%	AB		16.2 mg	Physically compatible	3	C
	TR[b]	AB, AH	40 and 400 mg	Physically compatible with little or no loss in 7 days at 23 and 4 °C	1349	C
	[a]	AH	5 g	No morphine loss in 30 days at 23 °C	1394	C
	GRI[a]		140 and 190 mg[c]	No change in concentration by UV in 28 days at 4 °C and room temperature	1910	C
	AB[a]	SCN	100 and 500 mg	Visually compatible with no loss by HPLC in 72 hr at 24 °C under fluorescent light	2058	C
Sodium lactate ⅙ M	AB		16.2 mg	Physically compatible	3	C

Solution Compatibility (Cont.)

Morphine sulfate

Solution	Mfr	Mfr	Conc/L	Remarks	Ref	C/I
TPN #71[d]	[a]	LI	100 mg	Physically compatible and no morphine loss in 36 hr at 22 °C	1000	C

[a]Tested in PVC containers.
[b]Tested in both glass and PVC containers.
[c]Tested as the HCl salt.
[d]Refer to Appendix I for the composition of parenteral nutrition solutions. TPN indicates a 2-in-1 admixture.

Additive Compatibility

Morphine sulfate

Drug	Mfr	Conc/L	Mfr	Conc/L	Test Soln	Remarks	Ref	C/I
Alteplase	GEN	0.5 g	WY	1 g	D5W, NS	Visually compatible with 5 to 8% alteplase clot-lysis activity loss in 24 hr at 25 °C	1856	C
Aminophylline						Physically incompatible	9	I
Amobarbital sodium						Physically incompatible	9	I
Atracurium besylate	BW	500 mg		1 g	D5W	Physically compatible and atracurium chemically stable for 24 hr at 5 and 30 °C	1694	C
Baclofen	CI	200 mg	DB	1 and 1.5 g	NS[d]	Physically compatible with little or no loss of either drug by HPLC in 30 days at 37 °C	1911	C
	CI	800 mg	DB	1 g	NS[d]	Physically compatible with little or no baclofen loss and less than 7% morphine loss by HPLC in 29 days at 37 °C	1911	C
	CI	800 mg	DB	1.5 g	NS[d]	Physically compatible with little or no loss of either drug by HPLC in 30 days at 37 °C	1911	C
	CI	1.5 g	DB	7.5 g	NS[d]	Physically compatible with little or no loss of either drug by HPLC in 30 days at 37 °C	2170	C
	CI	1 g	DB	15 g	NS[d]	Physically compatible with little or no loss of either drug by HPLC in 30 days at 37 °C	2170	C
	CI	200 mg	DB	21 g	NS[d]	Physically compatible with about 7% baclofen loss and little or no morphine loss by HPLC in 30 days at 37 °C	2170	C
Bupivacaine HCl		850 mg		140 and 190 mg[a]	NS[b]	No change in concentration by UV in 28 days at 4 °C and room temperature	1910	C
	AST	3 g		1 g	[a]	Little or no loss of either drug by HPLC in 30 days at 18 °C	1932	C
	AB	625 mg and 1.25 g	SCN	100 mg	NS[b]	Visually compatible with no loss of either drug by HPLC in 72 hr at 24 °C under fluorescent light	2058	C
	AB	625 mg and 1.25 g	SCN	500 mg	NS[b]	Visually compatible with no loss of either drug by HPLC in 72 hr at 24 °C under fluorescent light	2058	C
Chlorothiazide sodium	MSD					Physically incompatible	9	I
Dobutamine HCl	LI	1 g	ES	5 g	D5W, NS	Physically compatible for 24 hr at 21 °C	812	C
Floxacillin sodium	BE	20 g	EV	1 g	W	Haze forms in 24 hr and precipitate forms in 48 hr at 30 °C. No change at 15 °C	1479	I

Additive Compatibility (Cont.)

Morphine sulfate

Drug	Mfr	Conc/L	Mfr	Conc/L	Test Soln	Remarks	Ref	C/I
Fluconazole	PF	1 g	ES	0.25 g	D5W[b]	Fluconazole chemically stable by gas chromatography for at least 24 hr at 25 °C under fluorescent light. Morphine not tested	1676	C
Fluorouracil	AB	1 and 16 g	AST	1 g	D5W, NS[b]	Subvisual morphine precipitate forms immediately, becoming grossly visible within 24 hr. Morphine losses by HPLC of 60 to 80% occur within 1 day	1977	I
Furosemide	HO	1 g	EV	1 g	W	Physically compatible for 72 hr at 15 and 30 °C	1479	C
Heparin sodium						Physically incompatible	9	I
Meperidine HCl	WI					Physically incompatible	9	I
Meropenem	ZEN	1 and 20 g	ES	1 g	NS	Visually compatible for 4 hr at room temperature	1994	C
Metoclopramide HCl	SKB	500 mg	EV	1 g	NS[b]	Visually compatible with little or no loss of either drug by HPLC in 35 days at 22 °C and 182 days at 4 °C followed by 7 days at 32 °C	1938	C
	SKB	500 mg	EV	1 g	NS[c]	Visually compatible with 8% metoclopramide loss by HPLC in 14 days at 22 °C and 98 days at 4 °C. No morphine loss occurs	1938	C
Ondansetron HCl	GL	100 mg and 1 g	AST	1 g	NS[b]	Physically compatible with no ondansetron loss and 5% or less morphine loss by HPLC in 7 days at 32 °C or 31 days at 4 and 22 °C protected from light	1690	C
Phenobarbital sodium	WI					Physically incompatible	9	I
Phenytoin sodium	PD					Physically incompatible	9	I
Sodium bicarbonate						Physically incompatible	9	I
Succinylcholine chloride	AB	2 g		16.2 mg		Physically compatible	3	C
Thiopental sodium	AB					Physically incompatible	9	I
Verapamil HCl	KN	80 mg	KN	30 mg	D5W, NS	Physically compatible for 24 hr	764	C

[a]Tested as the HCl salt.
[b]Tested in PVC containers.
[c]Tested in PCA Infusors (Baxter).
[d]Tested in glass containers.

Drugs in Syringe Compatibility

Morphine sulfate

Drug (in syringe)	Mfr	Amt	Mfr	Amt	Remarks	Ref	C/I
Atropine sulfate		0.6 mg/ 1.5 ml	WY	15 mg/ 1 ml	Physically compatible for at least 15 min	14	C
	ST	0.4 mg/ 1 ml	ST	15 mg/ 1 ml	Physically compatible for at least 15 min	326	C
Bupivacaine HCl	AST	7.5 mg/ ml	MA	129 mg/ ml	Visually compatible for 30 days at 25 °C	1660	C

Drugs in Syringe Compatibility (Cont.)

Morphine sulfate

Drug (in syringe)	Mfr	Amt	Mfr	Amt	Remarks	Ref	C/I
	AST	3 mg/ml		1 mg/ml	Little or no loss of either drug by HPLC in 30 days at 18 °C	1932	C
Bupivacaine HCl with clonidine HCl	PD BI	2 mg/ml 0.03 mg/ml	SW	1.5 mg/ml	Diluted to 5 ml with NS. Visually compatible with no new GC/MS peaks appearing in 1 hr at room temperature	1956	C
Butorphanol tartrate	BR	4 mg/2 ml	AH	15 mg/1 ml	Physically compatible both macroscopically and microscopically for 30 min at room temperature	566	C
Chlorpromazine HCl	SKF	50 mg/2 ml	WY	15 mg/1 ml	Physically compatible for at least 15 min	14	C
	PO	50 mg/2 ml	ST	15 mg/1 ml	Physically compatible for at least 15 min	326	C
	DB	10 mg/2 ml	DB	a,b	Discoloration develops, although no morphine loss by HPLC in 48 hr at room temperature protected from light. Chlorpromazine not tested	1599	?
Cimetidine HCl	SKF	300 mg/2 ml	WI	10 mg/1 ml	Physically compatible for 4 hr at 25 °C	25	C
Dimenhydrinate	HR	50 mg/1 ml	ST	15 mg/1 ml	Physically compatible for at least 15 min	326	C
Diphenhydramine HCl	PD	50 mg/1 ml	WY	15 mg/1 ml	Physically compatible for at least 15 min	14	C
	PD	50 mg/1 ml	ST	15 mg/1 ml	Physically compatible for at least 15 min	326	C
Droperidol	MN	2.5 mg/1 ml	ST	15 mg/1 ml	Physically compatible for at least 15 min	326	C
Fentanyl citrate	MN	0.05 mg/1 ml	ST	15 mg/1 ml	Physically compatible for at least 15 min	326	C
Glycopyrrolate	RB	0.2 mg/1 ml	LI	15 mg/1 ml	Physically compatible and pH in stability range for glycopyrrolate for 48 hr at 25 °C	326	C
	RB	0.2 mg/1 ml	LI	30 mg/2 ml	Physically compatible and pH in stability range for glycopyrrolate for 48 hr at 25 °C	326	C
	RB	0.4 mg/2 ml	LI	15 mg/1 ml	Physically compatible and pH in stability range for glycopyrrolate for 48 hr at 25 °C	326	C
Haloperidol lactate	MN	5 mg/1 ml		5 and 10 mg/1 ml[c,d]	Cloudiness forms immediately, becoming a crystalline precipitate of haloperidol and parabens	1901	I
Heparin sodium	WY	100 and 200 units		1, 2, 5, 10 mg	Brought to 5 ml with sodium chloride 0.9%. Physically compatible with no morphine loss in 24 hr at 23 °C	985	C
	WY	100 and 200 units		1, 2, 5 mg	Brought to 5 ml with sterile water for injection. Physically compatible with no morphine loss in 24 hr at 23 °C	985	C
	WY	100 and 200 units		10 mg	Brought to 5 ml with sterile water for injection. Immediate haze with white precipitate and 5 to 7% loss of morphine potency	985	I
Hydroxyzine HCl	PF	100 mg/4 ml	WY	15 mg/1 ml	Physically compatible for at least 15 min	14	C
	PF	50 mg/1 ml	ST	15 mg/1 ml	Physically compatible for at least 15 min	326	C

Drugs in Syringe Compatibility (Cont.)

Drug (in syringe)	Morphine sulfate				Remarks	Ref	C/I
	Mfr	Amt	Mfr	Amt			
	PF	50 mg/ 1 ml		10 mg/ 0.7 ml	Physically compatible	771	C
	PF	100 mg/ 2 ml		5 mg/ 0.3 ml	Physically compatible	771	C
Ketamine HCl		100 mg		240 mg[a]	Brought to 9 ml with NS. Visually compatible for 8 days refrigerated and at room temperature protected from light	1899	C
Ketamine HCl with lidocaine HCl	PD AST	2 mg/ml 2 mg/ml	ES	0.2 mg/ ml	Diluted to 5 ml with NS. Visually compatible with no new GC/MS peaks appearing in 1 hr at room temperature	1956	C
Meperidine HCl	WI	50 mg/ 1 ml	ST	15 mg/ 1 ml	Physically incompatible within 15 min	326	I
Metoclopramide HCl	NO	10 mg/ 2 ml	AH	10 mg/ 1 ml	Physically compatible both macroscopically and microscopically for 15 min at room temperature	565	C
	DB	10 mg/ 2 ml	DB	a,b	Visually compatible with about 5% morphine loss by HPLC in 48 hr at room temperature protected from light. Metoclopramide not tested	1599	C
	SKB	0.5 mg/ ml	EV	1 mg/ml	Diluted with NS. 5% or less loss of both drugs by HPLC in 35 days at 22 °C and 182 days at 4 °C followed by 7 days at 32 °C	1939	C
Midazolam HCl	RC	5 mg/ 1 ml	WB	10 mg/ 1 ml	Physically compatible for 4 hr at 25 °C under fluorescent light	1145	C
	RC	3 mg/ml[e]	DB	24 mg/ ml[a]	Visually compatible with 4.4% midazolam loss by HPLC in 13 days at 32 °C. Morphine not tested	1595	C
	RC	5 mg/ 1 ml		5 and 10 mg/ 1 ml[c]	Visually compatible with 9% or less morphine loss and 8% or less midazolam loss by HPLC in 14 days at 22 °C protected from light. Subvisual microprecipitate may form, requiring filtration	1901	C
	RC	5 mg/ 1 ml		5 and 10 mg/ 1 ml[d]	Visually compatible with 8% or less morphine loss and 3% or less midazolam loss by HPLC in 14 days at 22 °C protected from light. Subvisual microprecipitate may form, requiring filtration	1901	C
Milrinone lactate	WI	5.25 mg/ 5.25 ml	WI	40 mg/ 5 ml	Physically compatible with no loss of either drug in 20 min at 23 °C under fluorescent light	1410	C
Ondansetron HCl	GW	1.33 mg/ ml[e]	ES	2.67 mg/ ml[e]	Physically compatible with no measured increase in particulates and less than 5% loss of ondansetron and less than 4% loss of morphine by HPLC in 24 hr at 4 or 23 °C	2199	C
Pentazocine lactate	WI	30 mg/ 1 ml	ST	15 mg/ 1 ml	Physically compatible for at least 15 min	326	C
Pentobarbital sodium	AB	500 mg/ 10 ml		16.2 mg/ 1 ml	Physically compatible	55	C
	WY	100 mg/ 2 ml	WY	15 mg/ 1 ml	Precipitate forms within 15 min	14	I

Drugs in Syringe Compatibility (Cont.)

Morphine sulfate

Drug (in syringe)	Mfr	Amt	Mfr	Amt	Remarks	Ref	C/I
	AB	50 mg/ 1 ml	ST	15 mg/ 1 ml	Physically incompatible within 15 min	326	I
Perphenazine	SC	5 mg/ 1 ml	AH	15 mg/ 1 ml	Physically compatible both macroscopically and microscopically for 30 min at room temperature	566	C
Prochlorperazine edisylate	SKF		WY	15 mg/ 1 ml	Physically compatible for at least 15 min	14	C
	PO	5 mg/ 1 ml	ST	15 mg/ 1 ml	Physically compatible for at least 15 min	326	C
	ES, SKF	10 mg/ 2 ml	WB	10 mg/ 1 ml	Immediate precipitation probably due to phenol in morphine formulation	1006	I
	SKF	5 mg/ 1 ml	WY	8, 10, 15 mg/ 1 ml	Physically compatible for 24 hr at 25 °C	1086	C
	DB	10 mg/ 2 ml	DB	a,b	Discoloration develops with 22% morphine loss by HPLC in 48 hr at room temperature protected from light. Prochlorperazine not tested	1599	I
Promazine HCl	WY	50 mg/ 1 ml	ST	15 mg/ 1 ml	Physically compatible for at least 15 min	326	C
Promethazine HCl	WY	50 mg/ 2 ml	WY	15 mg/ 1 ml	Physically compatible for at least 15 min	14	C
	PO	50 mg/ 2 ml	ST	15 mg/ 1 ml	Physically compatible for at least 15 min	326	C
	WY	12.5 mg	WY	8 mg	Cloudiness develops	98	I
Ranitidine HCl	GL	50 mg/ 2 ml	AH	10 mg/ 1 ml	Physically compatible for 1 hr at 25 °C both macroscopically and microscopically	978	C
Salbutamol	GL	2.5 mg/ 2.5 ml[f]	AB	5 mg/ 0.5 ml	Visually compatible for 1 hr both macroscopically and microscopically	1904	C
Scopolamine HBr		0.6 mg/ 1.5 ml	WY	15 mg/ 1 ml	Physically compatible for at least 15 min	14	C
	ST	0.4 mg/ 1 ml	ST	15 mg/ 1 ml	Physically compatible for at least 15 min	326	C
	BP	5 mg/ 5 ml	BP[g]	500 mg/ 5 ml	Little or no scopolamine loss by HPLC in 14 days at room temperature and 37 °C. Morphine not tested	1609	C
Thiopental sodium	AB	75 mg/ 3 ml	LI	16.2 mg/ 1 ml	Physically incompatible	21	I

[a]Present as the tartrate salt.
[b]Amount unspecified.
[c]Morphine sulfate powder dissolved in dextrose 5% in water.
[d]Morphine sulfate powder dissolved in water and sodium chloride 0.9%.
[e]Diluted in sodium chloride 0.9%.
[f]Both preserved (benzyl alcohol 0.9%; benzalkonium chloride 0.01%) and unpreserved sodium chloride 0.9% were used as a diluent.
[g]Tested as both sulfate and hydrochloride salts.

Y-Site Injection Compatibility (1:1 Mixture)

Morphine sulfate

Drug	Mfr	Conc	Mfr	Conc	Remarks	Ref	C/I
Acyclovir sodium	BW	5 mg/ml[a]	WB	0.08 mg/ml[a]	Physically compatible for 4 hr at 25 °C	1157	C

Y-Site Injection Compatibility (1:1 Mixture) (Cont.)

Morphine sulfate

Drug	Mfr	Conc	Mfr	Conc	Remarks	Ref	C/I
	BW	5 mg/ml[a]	AB	1 mg/ml	White crystalline precipitate forms within 2 hr at 25 °C under fluorescent light	1397	**I**
Allopurinol sodium	BW	3 mg/ml[b]	WI	1 mg/ml[b]	Physically compatible with no change in measured turbidity or increase in particle content in 4 hr at 22 °C	1686	**C**
Amifostine	USB	10 mg/ml[a]	AST	1 mg/ml[a]	Physically compatible with no change in measured turbidity or increase in particle content in 4 hr at 23 °C	1845	**C**
Amikacin sulfate	BR	5 mg/ml[a]	WI	1 mg/ml[a]	Physically compatible for at least 4 hr at 25 °C under fluorescent light	987	**C**
Aminophylline	ES	4 mg/ml[c]	WY	0.2 mg/ml[c]	Physically compatible for 3 hr	1316	**C**
Amiodarone HCl	WY	4.8 mg/ml[a]	SX	1 mg/ml[a]	Visually compatible for 24 hr at 23 °C	1877	**C**
Amphotericin B cholesteryl sulfate complex	SEQ	0.83 mg/ml[a]	ES	1 mg/ml[a]	Increased turbidity forms immediately	2117	**I**
Ampicillin sodium	BR	20 mg/ml[b]	WI	1 mg/ml[a]	Physically compatible for at least 4 hr at 25 °C under fluorescent light	987	**C**
Ampicillin sodium–sulbactam sodium	RR	20 + 10 mg/ml[b]	ES	1 mg/ml[b]	Physically compatible for 1 hr at 25 °C	1338	**C**
Amsacrine	NCI	1 mg/ml[a]	ES	1 mg/ml[a]	Physically compatible for 4 hr at room temperature under fluorescent light	1381	**C**
Atenolol	ICI	0.5 mg/ml	AB	1 mg/ml	Physically compatible for 4 hr at 25 °C	1397	**C**
Atracurium besylate	BW	0.5 mg/ml[a]	WY	1 mg/ml[a]	Physically compatible for 24 hr at 28 °C	1337	**C**
Aztreonam	SQ	20 mg/ml[a]	AB	1 mg/ml	Physically compatible for 4 hr at 25 °C	1397	**C**
	SQ	40 mg/ml[a]	AST	1 mg/ml[a]	Physically compatible with no subvisual haze or particle formation in 4 hr at 23 °C	1758	**C**
Bumetanide	RC	0.25 mg/ml	AB	1 mg/ml	Physically compatible for 4 hr at 25 °C	1397	**C**
Calcium chloride	AB	4 mg/ml[c]	WY	0.2 mg/ml[c]	Physically compatible for 3 hr	1316	**C**
Cefamandole nafate	LI	20 mg/ml[a]	WI	1 mg/ml[a]	Physically compatible for at least 4 hr at 25 °C under fluorescent light	987	**C**
	LI	40 mg/ml[a]	ES	1 mg/ml[b]	Physically compatible for 1 hr at 25 °C	1338	**C**
Cefazolin sodium	SKF	20 mg/ml[a]	WI	1 mg/ml[a]	Physically compatible for at least 4 hr at 25 °C under fluorescent light	987	**C**
Cefepime HCl	BR	20 mg/ml[a]	AST	1 mg/ml[a]	Haze forms immediately with numerous particles in 1 hr	1689	**I**
Cefoperazone sodium	RR	20 mg/ml[a]	WI	1 mg/ml[a]	Physically compatible for at least 4 hr at 25 °C under fluorescent light	987	**C**
Cefotaxime sodium	HO	20 mg/ml[a]	WI	1 mg/ml[a]	Physically compatible for at least 4 hr at 25 °C under fluorescent light	987	**C**
Cefotetan disodium	STU	20 and 40 mg/ml[a]	ES	1 mg/ml[b]	Physically compatible for 1 hr at 25 °C	1338	**C**
Cefoxitin sodium	MSD	20 mg/ml[a]	WI	1 mg/ml[a]	Physically compatible for at least 4 hr at 25 °C under fluorescent light	987	**C**
	MSD	40 mg/ml[a]	ES	1 mg/ml[b]	Physically compatible for 1 hr at 25 °C	1338	**C**
Ceftazidime	LI[l]	20 and 40 mg/ml[a]	AB	1 mg/ml	Physically compatible for 4 hr at 25 °C	1397	**C**

Y-Site Injection Compatibility (1:1 Mixture) (Cont.)

Morphine sulfate

Drug	Mfr	Conc	Mfr	Conc	Remarks	Ref	C/I
Ceftizoxime sodium	SKF	20 mg/ml[a]	WI	1 mg/ml[a]	Physically compatible for at least 4 hr at 25 °C under fluorescent light	987	C
Ceftriaxone sodium	RC	20 and 40 mg/ml[a]	AB	1 mg/ml	Physically compatible for 4 hr at 25 °C	1397	C
Cefuroxime sodium	GL	30 mg/ml[a]	WI	1 mg/ml[a]	Physically compatible for at least 4 hr at 25 °C under fluorescent light	987	C
Chloramphenicol sodium succinate	LY	20 mg/ml[a]	WI	1 mg/ml[a]	Physically compatible for at least 4 hr at 25 °C under fluorescent light	987	C
Cisatracurium besylate	GW	0.1, 2, 5 mg/ml[a]	AST	1 mg/ml[a]	Physically compatible with no change in measured turbidity or increase in particle content in 4 hr at 23 °C	2074	C
Cisplatin	BR	1 mg/ml	ES	0.12 mg/ml[a]	Visually compatible for 4 hr at room temperature under fluorescent light	1685	C
Cladribine	ORT	0.015[b] and 0.5[e] mg/ml	AST	1 mg/ml[b]	Physically compatible with no change in measured turbidity or increase in particle content in 4 hr at 23 °C	1969	C
Clindamycin phosphate	UP	12 mg/ml[a]	WI	1 mg/ml[a]	Physically compatible for at least 4 hr at 25 °C under fluorescent light	987	C
Cyclophosphamide	MJ	10 mg/ml	ES	0.12 mg/ml[a]	Visually compatible for 4 hr at room temperature under fluorescent light	1685	C
Cytarabine	UP	50 mg/ml	ES	0.12 mg/ml[a]	Visually compatible for 4 hr at room temperature under fluorescent light	1685	C
Dexamethasone sodium phosphate	LY	0.2 mg/ml[a]	AB	1 mg/ml	Physically compatible for 4 hr at 25 °C	1397	C
Digoxin	BW	0.25 mg/ml	AB	1 mg/ml	Physically compatible for 4 hr at 25 °C	1397	C
Diltiazem HCl	MMD	1[b] and 5 mg/ml	SCN	15 mg/ml	Visually compatible	1807	C
	MMD	5 mg/ml	SCN	0.4 mg/ml[b]	Visually compatible	1807	C
	MMD	1 mg/ml[a]	SCN	2 mg/ml[a]	Visually compatible for 4 hr at 27 °C	2062	C
Dobutamine HCl	LI	4 mg/ml[a]	SCN	2 mg/ml[a]	Visually compatible for 4 hr at 27 °C	2062	C
Docetaxel	RPR	0.9 mg/ml[a]	ES	1 mg/ml[a]	Physically compatible with no change in measured turbidity or increase in particle content	2224	C
Dopamine HCl	AB	1.6 mg/ml[a]	AB	1 mg/ml	Physically compatible for 4 hr at 25 °C	1397	C
	AB	3.2 mg/ml[a]	SCN	2 mg/ml[a]	Visually compatible for 4 hr at 27 °C	2062	C
Doxorubicin HCl	AD	0.2 mg/ml[a]	ES	0.12 mg/ml[a]	Visually compatible for 4 hr at room temperature under fluorescent light	1685	C
Doxorubicin HCl liposome injection	SEQ	0.4 mg/ml[a]	ES	1 mg/ml[a]	Partial loss of measured natural turbidity	2087	I
Doxycycline hyclate	ES	1 mg/ml[a]	WI	1 mg/ml[a]	Physically compatible for at least 4 hr at 25 °C under fluorescent light	987	C
Enalaprilat	MSD	0.05 mg/ml[b]	WY	0.2 mg/ml[a]	Physically compatible for 24 hr at room temperature under fluorescent light	1355	C
Epinephrine HCl	AB	0.02 mg/ml[a]	SCN	2 mg/ml[a]	Visually compatible for 4 hr at 27 °C	2062	C
Erythromycin lactobionate	AB	5 mg/ml[a]	WI	1 mg/ml[a]	Physically compatible for at least 4 hr at 25 °C under fluorescent light	987	C

Y-Site Injection Compatibility (1:1 Mixture) (Cont.)

Morphine sulfate

Drug	Mfr	Conc	Mfr	Conc	Remarks	Ref	C/I
Esmolol HCl	DCC	1 g/100 ml[f]	ES	15 mg/1 ml	Physically compatible when morphine is injected into Y-site of flowing admixture[g]	1168	C
	DCC	10 mg/ml[f]	ES	15 mg/ml	Physically compatible with no loss of either drug in 8 hr at ambient temperature exposed to light	1168	C
Etomidate	AB	2 mg/ml	ES	10 mg/ml	Visually compatible for up to 7 days at 25 °C	1801	C
Etoposide phosphate	BR	5 mg/ml[a]	ES	1 mg/ml[a]	Physically compatible with no change in measured turbidity or increase in particle content in 4 hr at 23 °C	2218	C
Famotidine	MSD	0.2 mg/ml[a]	ES	0.2 mg/ml[a]	Physically compatible for 4 hr at 25 °C	1188	C
	MSD	0.2 mg/ml[a]	AB	1 mg/ml	Physically compatible for 4 hr at 25 °C	1397	C
	ME	2 mg/ml[b]		1 mg/ml[a]	Visually compatible for 4 hr at 22 °C	1936	C
Fentanyl citrate	ES	0.05 mg/ml	SCN	2 mg/ml[a]	Visually compatible for 4 hr at 27 °C	2062	C
Filgrastim	AMG	30 μg/ml[a]	WY	1 mg/ml[a]	Physically compatible with no change in measured turbidity or increase in particle content in 4 hr at 22 °C	1687	C
Fluconazole	RR	2 mg/ml	IMS	25 mg/ml	Physically compatible for 24 hr at 25 °C	1407	C
	RR	2 mg/ml	AB	1 mg/ml	Physically compatible for 4 hr at 25 °C	1397	C
Fludarabine phosphate	BX	1 mg/ml[a]	WI	1 mg/ml[a]	Physically compatible for 4 hr at room temperature under fluorescent light	1439	C
Foscarnet sodium	AST	24 mg/ml	IMS	1 mg/ml	Physically compatible for 24 hr at room temperature under fluorescent light	1335	C
	AST	24 mg/ml	ES	1 mg/ml[c]	Physically compatible for 24 hr at 25 °C under fluorescent light by visual and microscopic examination	1393	C
	AST	24 mg/ml	ES	5[b] and 15 mg/ml	Visually compatible for 24 hr at 23 °C under fluorescent light	1529	C
Furosemide	ES	0.8[a], 2.4[a], 10 mg/ml	AB	1 mg/ml	White precipitate forms within 1 hr at 25 °C under fluorescent light	1397	I
	AMR	10 mg/ml	SCN	2 mg/ml[a]	Visually compatible for 4 hr at 27 °C	2062	C
Gemcitabine HCl	LI	10 mg/ml[b]	ES	1 mg/ml[b]	Physically compatible with no change in measured turbidity or increase in particle content in 4 hr at 23 °C	2226	C
Gentamicin sulfate	TR	0.8 mg/ml[a]	WI	1 mg/ml[a]	Physically compatible for at least 4 hr at 25 °C under fluorescent light	987	C
	ES	1.2 and 2 mg/ml[b]	ES	1 mg/ml[b]	Physically compatible for 1 hr at 25 °C	1338	C
Granisetron HCl	SKB	1 mg/ml	AST	1 mg/ml[b]	Physically compatible with little or no loss of either drug by HPLC in 4 hr at 22 °C	1883	C
	SKB	0.05 mg/ml[a]	AST	1 mg/ml[a]	Physically compatible with no change in measured turbidity or increase in particle content in 4 hr at 23 °C	2000	C
Heparin sodium	UP	1000 units/L[h]	WY	15 mg/ml	Physically compatible for at least 4 hr at room temperature by visual and microscopic examination	534	C
	ES	50 units/ml[c]	WY	0.2 mg/ml[c]	Physically compatible for 3 hr	1316	C
	ES	60 units/ml[a]	ES	1 mg/ml[b]	Physically compatible for 1 hr at 25 °C	1338	C

Y-Site Injection Compatibility (1:1 Mixture) (Cont.)

Morphine sulfate

Drug	Mfr	Conc	Mfr	Conc	Remarks	Ref	C/I
	ES	100 units/ml[a]	SCN	2 mg/ml[a]	Visually compatible for 4 hr at 27 °C	2062	C
Hydrocortisone sodium succinate	UP	10 mg/L[f]	WY	15 mg/ml	Physically compatible for at least 4 hr at room temperature by visual and microscopic examination	534	C
Hydromorphone HCl	KN	1 mg/ml	SCN	2 mg/ml[a]	Visually compatible for 4 hr at 27 °C	2062	C
IL-2	RC	4800 I.U./ml[b]	SCN	1 mg/ml	Visually compatible and IL-2 activity by bioassay retained. Morphine not tested	1552	C
Insulin, regular	LI	0.2 unit/ml[b]	ES	1 mg/ml[b]	Physically compatible for 1 hr at 25 °C	1338	C
	LI	0.2 unit/ml[b]	ES	5 mg/ml[b]	Physically compatible for 2 hr at 25 °C	1395	C
	LI	1 unit/ml[a]	SX	1 mg/ml[a]	Visually compatible for 24 hr at 23 °C	1877	C
Kanamycin sulfate	BR	2.5 mg/ml[a]	WI	1 mg/ml[a]	Physically compatible for at least 4 hr at 25 °C under fluorescent light	987	C
Labetalol HCl	SC	1 mg/ml[a]	WY	1 mg/ml[a]	Physically compatible for 24 hr at 18 °C	1171	C
	GL	5 mg/ml	AB	1 mg/ml	Physically compatible for 4 hr at 25 °C	1397	C
	GL	1 mg/ml[a]	ES	0.5 mg/ml[a]	Visually compatible with little or no loss of either drug by HPLC in 4 hr at room temperature	1762	C
	AH	2 mg/ml[a]	SCN	2 mg/ml[a]	Visually compatible for 4 hr at 27 °C	2062	C
Lidocaine HCl	AB	1 mg/ml[a]	AB	1 mg/ml	Physically compatible for 4 hr at 25 °C	1397	C
Lorazepam	WY	0.33 mg/ml[b]	CNF	1 mg/ml[i]	Visually compatible for 24 hr at 22 °C	1855	C
	WY	0.5 mg/ml[a]	SCN	2 mg/ml[a]	Visually compatible for 4 hr at 27 °C	2062	C
Magnesium sulfate	LY	16.7, 33.3, 50, 100 mg/ml[a]	ES	1 mg/ml[a]	Visually compatible for 4 hr at 25 °C under fluorescent light	1549	C
	AB	2, 4, 8 mg/ml[b]	[j]	2 mg/ml[b]	Visually compatible for 8 hr at room temperature	1719	C
Melphalan HCl	BW	0.1 mg/ml[b]	WI	1 mg/ml[b]	Physically compatible with no change in measured turbidity or increase in particle content in 3 hr at 22 °C	1557	C
Meropenem	ZEN	1 and 50 mg/ml[b]	ES	1 mg/ml[d]	Visually compatible for 4 hr at room temperature	1994	C
Methotrexate sodium	AD	15 mg/ml[k]	ES	0.12 mg/ml[a]	Visually compatible for 4 hr at room temperature under fluorescent light	1685	C
Methyldopa HCl	AMR	2.5 mg/ml[a]	AB	1 mg/ml	Physically compatible for 4 hr at 25 °C	1397	C
Methylprednisolone sodium succinate	UP	2.5 mg/ml[a]	AB	1 mg/ml	Physically compatible for 4 hr at 25 °C	1397	C
Metoclopramide HCl	SN	0.2 mg/ml[a]	AB	1 mg/ml	Physically compatible for 4 hr at 25 °C	1397	C
Metoprolol tartrate	CI	1 mg/ml	AB	1 mg/ml	Physically compatible for 4 hr at 25 °C	1397	C
Metronidazole	SE	5 mg/ml	WI	1 mg/ml[a]	Physically compatible for at least 4 hr at 25 °C under fluorescent light	987	C
Midazolam HCl	RC	0.1 and 0.5 mg/ml[a]	ES	0.25 mg/ml[a]	Visually compatible with no loss of either drug by HPLC in 3 hr at 24 °C	1789	C
	RC	0.1 and 0.5 mg/ml[a]	ES	1 mg/ml[a]	Visually compatible with no loss of either drug by HPLC in 3 hr at 24 °C	1789	C
	RC	5 mg/ml	CNF	1 mg/ml[i]	Visually compatible for 24 hr at 22 °C	1855	C
	RC	1 mg/ml[a]	SX	1 mg/ml[a]	Visually compatible for 24 hr at 23 °C	1877	C
	RC	2 mg/ml[a]	SCN	2 mg/ml[a]	Visually compatible for 4 hr at 27 °C	2062	C
Milrinone lactate	SW	0.2 mg/ml[a]	SCN	2 mg/ml[a]	Visually compatible for 4 hr at 27 °C	2062	C

Y-Site Injection Compatibility (1:1 Mixture) (Cont.)

					Morphine sulfate		
Drug	Mfr	Conc	Mfr	Conc	Remarks	Ref	C/I
	SW	0.4 mg/ml[a]	AST	1 mg/ml[a]	Visually compatible with little or no loss of either drug by HPLC in 4 hr at 23 °C	2214	C
Minocycline HCl	LE	0.2 mg/ml[a]	WI	1 mg/ml[a]	Color changed from pale yellow to light green in 1 hr	987	I
Nafcillin sodium	WY	20 mg/ml[a]	WI	1 mg/ml[a]	Physically compatible for at least 4 hr at 25 °C under fluorescent light	987	C
	WY	30 mg/ml[a]	ES	1 mg/ml[b]	Physically compatible for 1 hr at 25 °C	1338	C
Nicardipine HCl	WY	1 mg/ml[a]	SCN	2 mg/ml[a]	Visually compatible for 4 hr at 27 °C	2062	C
Nitroglycerin	AB	0.4 mg/ml[a]	SCN	2 mg/ml[a]	Visually compatible for 4 hr at 27 °C	2062	C
Norepinephrine bitartrate	STR	0.064 mg/ml[a]	SX	1 mg/ml[a]	Visually compatible for 24 hr at 23 °C	1877	C
	AB	0.128 mg/ml[a]	SCN	2 mg/ml[a]	Visually compatible for 4 hr at 27 °C	2062	C
Ondansetron HCl	GL	1 mg/ml[b]	WI	1 mg/ml[a]	Physically compatible for 4 hr at 22 °C	1365	C
Oxacillin sodium	BE	20 mg/ml[a]	WI	1 mg/ml[a]	Physically compatible for at least 4 hr at 25 °C under fluorescent light	987	C
Oxytocin	PD	0.02 mg/ml[m]	ES	1 mg/ml[b]	Physically compatible for 1 hr at 25 °C	1338	C
Paclitaxel	NCI	1.2 mg/ml[a]	WY	1 mg/ml[a]	Physically compatible with no change in measured turbidity in 4 hr at 22 °C	1556	C
Pancuronium bromide	ES	0.05 mg/ml[a]	WY	1 mg/ml[a]	Physically compatible for 24 hr at 28 °C	1337	C
Penicillin G potassium	PF	100,000 units/ml[a]	WI	1 mg/ml[a]	Physically compatible for at least 4 hr at 25 °C under fluorescent light	987	C
Piperacillin sodium	LE	60 mg/ml[a]	WI	1 mg/ml[a]	Physically compatible for at least 4 hr at 25 °C under fluorescent light	987	C
Piperacillin sodium–tazobactam sodium	LE	40 + 5 mg/ml[a]	WY	1 mg/ml[a]	Physically compatible with no change in measured turbidity or increase in particle content in 4 hr at 22 °C	1688	C
Potassium chloride	AB	40 mEq/L[f]	WY	15 mg/ml	Physically compatible for at least 4 hr at room temperature by visual and microscopic examination	534	C
Propofol	ZEN	10 mg/ml	AST	1 mg/ml[a]	Physically compatible for 1 hr at 23 °C with no increase in particle content	2066	C
Propranolol HCl	WY	1 mg/ml	AB	1 mg/ml	Physically compatible for 4 hr at 25 °C	1397	C
Ranitidine HCl	GL	0.5 mg/ml[n]	ES	1 mg/ml[b]	Physically compatible for 1 hr at 25 °C	1338	C
	GL	1 mg/ml[a]	SCN	2 mg/ml[a]	Visually compatible for 4 hr at 27 °C	2062	C
Remifentanil HCl	GW	0.025 and 0.25 mg/ml[b]	AST	1 mg/ml[a]	Physically compatible with no change in measured turbidity or increase in particle content in 4 hr at 23 °C	2075	C
Sargramostim	IMM	10 µg/ml[b]	WI	1 mg/ml[b]	Slight haze, visible with high intensity light, and small amount of particles formed in 1 hr in one of two samples	1436	I
Sodium bicarbonate	AB	1 mEq/ml[c]	WY	0.2 mg/ml[c]	Physically compatible for 3 hr	1316	C
Sodium nitroprusside	RC	0.2 mg/ml[a]	SX	1 mg/ml[a]	Visually compatible for 24 hr at 23 °C	1877	C

Y-Site Injection Compatibility (1:1 Mixture) (Cont.)

<table>
<tr><td colspan="5" align="center">Morphine sulfate</td><td></td><td></td></tr>
<tr><td>*Drug*</td><td>*Mfr*</td><td>*Conc*</td><td>*Mfr*</td><td>*Conc*</td><td>*Remarks*</td><td>*Ref*</td><td>*C/I*</td></tr>
<tr><td>Tacrolimus</td><td>FUJ</td><td>10 and 40 μg/ml[b]</td><td>SCN</td><td>1 mg/ml[b]</td><td>Visually compatible with no loss of either drug by HPLC in 4 hr at 24 °C under fluorescent light</td><td>2216</td><td>C</td></tr>
<tr><td></td><td>FUJ</td><td>10 and 40 μg/ml[b]</td><td>SCN</td><td>3 mg/ml[b]</td><td>Visually compatible with no loss of either drug by HPLC in 4 hr at 24 °C under fluorescent light</td><td>2216</td><td>C</td></tr>
<tr><td>Teniposide</td><td>BR</td><td>0.1 mg/ml[a]</td><td>AST</td><td>1 mg/ml[a]</td><td>Physically compatible with no subvisual haze or particle formation in 4 hr at 23 °C</td><td>1725</td><td>C</td></tr>
<tr><td>Thiopental sodium</td><td>AB</td><td>25 mg/ml</td><td>ES</td><td>10 mg/ml</td><td>White precipitate forms immediately</td><td>1801</td><td>I</td></tr>
<tr><td></td><td>AB</td><td>25 mg/ml[d]</td><td>SCN</td><td>2 mg/ml[a]</td><td>Visually compatible for 4 hr at 27 °C</td><td>2062</td><td>C</td></tr>
<tr><td>Thiotepa</td><td>IMM[o]</td><td>1 mg/ml[a]</td><td>AST</td><td>1 mg/ml[a]</td><td>Physically compatible with no change in measured turbidity or increase in particle content in 4 hr at 23 °C</td><td>1861</td><td>C</td></tr>
<tr><td>Ticarcillin disodium</td><td>BE</td><td>60 mg/ml[a]</td><td>WI</td><td>1 mg/ml[a]</td><td>Physically compatible for at least 4 hr at 25 °C under fluorescent light</td><td>987</td><td>C</td></tr>
<tr><td>Ticarcillin disodium–clavulanate potassium</td><td>BE</td><td>31 mg/ml[b]</td><td>ES</td><td>1 mg/ml[b]</td><td>Physically compatible for 1 hr at 25 °C</td><td>1338</td><td>C</td></tr>
<tr><td>TNA #218 to #226[p]</td><td></td><td></td><td>ES</td><td>1 mg/ml[a]</td><td>Visually compatible with no precipitate or emulsion damage apparent in 4 hr at 23 °C</td><td>2215</td><td>C</td></tr>
<tr><td>TNA #218 to #226[p]</td><td></td><td></td><td>ES</td><td>15 mg/ml</td><td>Damage to emulsion integrity occurs immediately with free oil formation possible</td><td>2215</td><td>I</td></tr>
<tr><td>Tobramycin sulfate</td><td>DI</td><td>0.8 mg/ml[a]</td><td>WI</td><td>1 mg/ml[a]</td><td>Physically compatible for at least 4 hr at 25 °C under fluorescent light</td><td>987</td><td>C</td></tr>
<tr><td></td><td>LI</td><td>1.6, 2, 2.4 mg/ml[a]</td><td>ES</td><td>1 mg/ml[b]</td><td>Physically compatible for 1 hr at 25 °C</td><td>1338</td><td>C</td></tr>
<tr><td>TPN #131 and #132[p]</td><td></td><td></td><td>AB</td><td>1 mg/ml</td><td>Physically compatible for 4 hr at 25 °C</td><td>1397</td><td>C</td></tr>
<tr><td>TPN #189[p]</td><td></td><td></td><td>DB</td><td>30 mg/ml</td><td>Visually compatible for 24 hr at 22 °C</td><td>1767</td><td>C</td></tr>
<tr><td>TPN #203 and #204[p]</td><td></td><td></td><td>ES</td><td>1 mg/ml</td><td>Visually compatible for 2 hr at 23 °C</td><td>1974</td><td>C</td></tr>
<tr><td>TPN #212 to #215[p]</td><td></td><td></td><td>AST</td><td>1 mg/ml[a]</td><td>Physically compatible with no change in measured turbidity or increase in particle content in 4 hr at 23 °C</td><td>2109</td><td>C</td></tr>
<tr><td>Trimethoprim–sulfamethoxazole</td><td>BW</td><td>0.8 + 4 mg/ml[a]</td><td>WI</td><td>1 mg/ml[a]</td><td>Physically compatible for at least 4 hr at 25 °C under fluorescent light</td><td>987</td><td>C</td></tr>
<tr><td>Vancomycin HCl</td><td>LI</td><td>5 mg/ml[a]</td><td>WI</td><td>1 mg/ml[a]</td><td>Physically compatible for at least 4 hr at 25 °C under fluorescent light</td><td>987</td><td>C</td></tr>
<tr><td>Vecuronium bromide</td><td>OR</td><td>0.1 mg/ml[a]</td><td>WY</td><td>1 mg/ml[a]</td><td>Physically compatible for 24 hr at 28 °C</td><td>1337</td><td>C</td></tr>
<tr><td></td><td>OR</td><td>1 mg/ml</td><td>SCN</td><td>2 mg/ml[a]</td><td>Visually compatible for 4 hr at 27 °C</td><td>2062</td><td>C</td></tr>
<tr><td>Vinorelbine tartrate</td><td>BW</td><td>1 mg/ml[b]</td><td>WI</td><td>1 mg/ml[b]</td><td>Physically compatible with no change in measured turbidity or increase in particle content in 4 hr at 22 °C</td><td>1558</td><td>C</td></tr>
<tr><td>Vitamin B complex with C</td><td>RC</td><td>2 ml/L[f]</td><td>WY</td><td>15 mg/ml</td><td>Physically compatible for at least 4 hr at room temperature by visual and microscopic examination</td><td>534</td><td>C</td></tr>
<tr><td>Warfarin sodium</td><td>DU</td><td>2 mg/ml[d]</td><td>ES</td><td>2 mg/ml[a]</td><td>Visually compatible with no warfarin loss by HPLC in 30 min</td><td>2010</td><td>C</td></tr>
</table>

Y-Site Injection Compatibility (1:1 Mixture) (Cont.)

Morphine sulfate

Drug	Mfr	Conc	Mfr	Conc	Remarks	Ref	C/I
	DME	2 mg/ml[d]	ES	2 mg/ml[a]	Visually compatible for 24 hr at 24 °C	2078	C
Zidovudine	BW	4 mg/ml[a]	ES	1 mg/ml[a]	Physically compatible for 4 hr at 25 °C under fluorescent light by visual and microscopic examination	1193	C

[a]*Tested in dextrose 5% in water.*
[b]*Tested in sodium chloride 0.9%.*
[c]*Tested in both dextrose 5% in water and sodium chloride 0.9%.*
[d]*Tested in sterile water for injection.*
[e]*Tested in bacteriostatic sodium chloride 0.9% preserved with benzyl alcohol 0.9%.*
[f]*Tested in dextrose 5% in sodium chloride 0.9%.*
[g]*Flowing at 1.6 ml/min.*
[h]*Tested in dextrose 5% in Ringer's injection, dextrose 5% in Ringer's injection, lactated, dextrose 5% in water, Ringer's injection, lactated, and sodium chloride 0.9%.*
[i]*Tested as the hydrochloride salt.*
[j]*Extemporaneously prepared product.*
[k]*Tested in dextrose 5% in water with sodium bicarbonate 0.05 mEq/ml.*
[l]*Sodium carbonate–containing formulation tested.*
[m]*Tested in dextrose 5% in Ringer's injection, lactated.*
[n]*Tested in sodium chloride 0.45%.*
[o]*Lyophilized formulation tested.*
[p]*Refer to Appendix I for the composition of parenteral nutrition solutions. TNA indicates a 3-in-1 admixture, and TPN indicates a 2-in-1 admixture.*

Additional Compatibility Information

Multiple Drugs— A seven-drug combination consisting of bupivacaine HCl (Sanofi Winthrop) 1.5 mg/1 ml, clonidine HCl (Boehringer Ingelheim) 0.03 mg/1 ml, fentanyl citrate (Janssen) 0.01 mg/1 ml, ketamine (Parke-Davis) 2 mg/1 ml, lidocaine HCl (Astra) 2 mg/1 ml, morphine sulfate (Elkins-Sinn) 0.2 mg/1 ml, and tetracaine HCl (Sanofi Winthrop) 2 mg/1 ml mixed together was found to be visually compatible with no new GC/MS peaks appearing in one hour at room temperature (1956).

Clonidine HCl (Boehringer) 30 μg/ml, bupivacaine HCl (Astra) 3 mg/ml, and morphine HCl (Merck) 6.66 mg/ml were combined in 50-ml ambulatory infusion pump cassette reservoirs (Pharmacia Deltec). The reservoirs were stored at room temperature and protected from light for 90 days. HPLC analysis found no loss of any of the drugs. Instead, drug concentrations increased 12 to 16% during the observation period, possibly due to loss of water from the solutions (1850).

Morphine tartrate (David Bull) 4 and 40 mg/ml was admixed with four other drugs and packaged in 10-ml polypropylene syringes with tip caps (Terumo). The formulas of the two admixtures to make 10 ml total volume are shown in Table 1. Samples were stored at 21 to 23 °C and 4 to 8 °C for two weeks. Most samples remained unchanged on visual inspection except Formulation 1 stored at room temperature that developed a slight straw color within 10 days.

Table 1. Formulas of Morphine Tartrate with Multiple Drug Admixtures Tested for Stability (2180)

Component	Formulation 1	Formulation 2
Morphine tartrate	400 mg	40 mg
Dexamethasone sodium phosphate	8 mg	8 mg
Droperidol HCl	2 mg	2 mg
Scopolamine butylbromide	20 mg	20 mg
Midazolam HCl	8 mg	5 mg
Sodium chloride 0.9%		qs to 10 ml

HPLC analysis found that the morphine tartrate and the other drug components except midazolam remained stable (less than 10% loss) throughout the 14-day study. Midazolam HCl was also stable for 14 days under refrigeration but was only stable through 12 days in Formulation 1 and five days in Formulation 2 stored at room temperature (2180).

Clonidine HCl— Clonidine HCl (Fujisawa) 100 μg/ml and morphine sulfate (Elkins-Sinn) 10 mg/ml were mixed in equal quantities, transferred to flint glass vials with rubber stoppers, and stored for 14 days at controlled room temperature protected from light. The solutions remained clear and colorless with no increase in particulate content. HPLC analysis found little or no change in concentration for either drug during the study period (2067).

MULTIVITAMINS
AHFS 88:28

M.V.I. Pediatric   **Astra**
M.V.I.-12   **Astra**

Products— Multivitamin products for parenteral administration are available in a variety of compositions and sizes from several manufacturers (154). The following products are representative formulations.

M.V.I.-12 consists of a two-chambered, single-dose 10-ml vial that must be mixed prior to use. To mix, remove the plastic cap, turn the plunger stopper 90 degrees, and press down to force the fluid in the upper chamber along with the center seal into the lower chamber. Gently mix the solution. The manufacturer states that the stopper must be "sterilized in the usual manner" before inserting a needle to withdraw the contents. After mixing, the solution contains (1-4/98):

Ascorbic acid	100 mg
Vitamin A (retinol)	1 mg
Vitamin D	
(ergocalciferol)	5 µg
Thiamine (as HCl)	3 mg
Riboflavin (as 5-	
phosphate sodium)	3.6 mg
Pyridoxine HCl	4 mg
Niacinamide	40 mg
Dexpanthenol	15 mg
Vitamin E	10 mg
(*dl*-alpha tocopheryl acetate)	
Biotin	60 µg
Folic acid	400 µg
Cyanocobalamin	
(vitamin B$_{12}$)	5 µg

M.V.I.-12 also contains propylene glycol 30%, gentisic acid ethanolamide 1%, polysorbate 80 0.8%, polysorbate 20 0.014%, butylated hydroxytoluene 0.001%, butylated hydroxyanisole 0.0003%, and citric acid, sodium citrate, and sodium hydroxide to adjust pH (1-4/98).

M.V.I. Pediatric is available as a lyophilized powder in vials containing a single dose. Each single dose contains (1-6/98):

Ascorbic acid	80 mg
Vitamin A (retinol)	0.7 mg
Vitamin D	
(ergocalciferol)	10 µg
Thiamine (as HCl)	1.2 mg
Riboflavin (as 5-	
phosphate sodium)	1.4 mg
Pyridoxine (as HCl)	1 mg
Niacinamide	17 mg
Dexpanthenol	5 mg
Vitamin E (*dl*-alpha	
tocopheryl acetate)	7 mg
Biotin	20 µg
Folic acid	140 µg
Cyanocobalamin	1 µg
Phytonadione	200 µg

M.V.I. Pediatric also contains, in each vial, mannitol 375 mg, polysorbate 80 50 mg, polysorbate 20 0.8 mg, butylated hydroxytoluene 58 µg, butylated hydroxyanisole 14 µg, and sodium hydroxide for pH adjustment (1-6/98).

Reconstitute the single-dose vial with 5 ml of sterile water for injection, dextrose 5% in water, or sodium chloride 0.9% and swirl gently. The solution is ready within three minutes. This solution must be further diluted for use; do not give it undiluted (1-6/98).

Osmolality— The osmolality of M.V.I.-12 was determined to be 4820 mOsm/kg by freezing-point depression and 4210 mOsm/kg by vapor pressure (1071).

Administration— Multivitamin infusion preparations are administered by intravenous infusion only. They should not be given by direct intravenous injection. M.V.I.-12 is diluted in not less than 500 ml but preferably 1000 ml of intravenous infusion solution for administration. M.V.I. Pediatric should be added to at least 100 ml of a compatible intravenous infusion solution for administration (1-4/98; 1-6/98).

Stability— M.V.I.-12 should be stored under refrigeration and protected from light. Do not store at room temperature. Since some of the vitamins, especially A, D, and riboflavin, are light sensitive, light protection is necessary (1-6/98).

M.V.I. Pediatric may be stored at controlled room temperature. After reconstitution, use of the product without delay is recommended. However, if this is not possible, the manufacturer permits use within a maximum of four hours from the initial penetration of the closure (1-6/98).

See Photodecomposition and Sorption under Additional Compatibility Information.

Compatibility Information

Solution Compatibility

Multivitamins

Solution	Mfr	Mfr	Conc/L	Remarks	Ref	C/I
Alcohol 5%, dextrose 5% in water	BA	USV	20 ml	Physically compatible for 24 hr	315	C
Amino acids 10%	TR	USV	1 vial	40% thiamine loss in 22 hr at 30 °C due to sulfite content	843	I

Solution Compatibility (Cont.)

Multivitamins

Solution	Mfr	Mfr	Conc/L	Remarks	Ref	C/I
Amino acids 8.5% (FreAmine III)	MG	RC	4 ml[a]	97% thiamine loss in 24 hr at 23 °C due to bisulfite content of solution. 63% loss in 24 hr at 7 °C	774	I
	MG	AB	[b]	96% thiamine loss in 24 hr at 23 °C due to bisulfite content of solution	774	I
	MG	USV	[c]	92% thiamine loss in 24 hr at 23 °C due to bisulfite content of solution	774	I
Amino acids 5.5% (Travasol)	TR	RC	4 ml[a]	About 70% thiamine loss in 24 hr at 23 °C due to bisulfite content of solution. 33% loss in 24 hr at 7 °C	774	I
Amino acids 4.25%, dextrose 25%	TR	USV	1 vial	No thiamine loss in 22 hr at 30 °C	843	C
Amino acids 2%, dextrose 12.5%		ROR	5 ml[d]	7% phytonadione loss in 4 hr and 27% loss in 24 hr by HPLC under ambient temperature and light	1815	I
Dextrose 5% in Ringer's injection, lactated	BA	USV	20 ml	Physically compatible for 24 hr	315	C
Dextrose 5% in sodium chloride 0.9%	BA	USV	20 ml	Physically compatible for 24 hr	315	C
Dextrose 5% in water	BA	USV	20 ml	Physically compatible for 24 hr	315	C
	TR[e]	RC	4 ml[a]	8% or less thiamine loss in 24 hr at 23 °C	774	C
Dextrose 10% in water	BA	USV	20 ml	Physically compatible for 24 hr	315	C
	TR[e]	RC	4 ml[a]	5% or less thiamine loss in 24 hr at 23 °C	774	C
	MG[f]	RC	4 ml[a]	11% or less thiamine loss in 24 hr at 23 °C	774	C
Dextrose 20% in water	BA	USV	20 ml	Physically compatible for 24 hr	315	C
Fat emulsion 10%, intravenous	VT	USV	4 ml	Physically compatible for 48 hr at 4 °C and room temperature	32	C
	KA	KA		Physically compatible for 24 hr at 26 °C with little loss of most vitamins by HPLC; up to 52% ascorbate loss	2050	C
Fructose 10% in water	BA	USV	20 ml	Physically compatible for 24 hr	315	C
Invert sugar 10% in Electrolyte #1	BA	USV	20 ml	Physically compatible for 24 hr	315	C
Invert sugar 10% in Electrolyte #2	BA	USV	20 ml	Physically compatible for 24 hr	315	C
Polysal M with dextrose 5%	CU	USV	20 ml	Physically compatible for 24 hr	315	C
Ringer's injection, lactated	BA	USV	20 ml	Physically compatible for 24 hr	315	C
	TR[e]	RC	4 ml[a]	5% or less thiamine loss in 24 hr at 23 °C	774	C
Sodium chloride 0.9%	BA	USV	20 ml	Physically compatible for 24 hr	315	C
	TR[e]	RC	4 ml[a]	Thiamine losses of 6 to 11% in 24 hr at 23 °C	774	C
Sodium lactate ⅙ M	BA	USV	20 ml	Physically compatible for 24 hr	315	C

[a] *Berocca Parenteral Nutrition.*
[b] *Multivitamin Additive.*
[c] *M.V.I.-12.*
[d] *M.V.I. Pediatric.*
[e] *Tested in both glass and PVC containers.*
[f] *Tested in polyolefin containers.*

Additive Compatibility

Multivitamins

Drug	Mfr	Conc/L	Mfr	Conc/L	Test Soln	Remarks	Ref	C/I
Cefoxitin sodium	MSD	10 g	USV	50 ml[a]	W	5% cefoxitin decomposition in 24 hr and 10% in 48 hr at 25 °C; 3% in 48 hr at 5 °C. TLC showed no other transformation products	308	**C**
Isoproterenol HCl	WI	4 mg	USV	10 ml		Physically compatible	59	**C**
Meropenem	ZEN	1 and 20 g	AST	50 ml	NS	Color darkened in 4 hr at room temperature	1994	**I**
Methyldopate HCl	MSD	1 g	USV	10 ml	D, D–S, S	Physically compatible	23	**C**
Metoclopramide HCl	RB	20 and 320 mg	USV	20 ml[b]	NS	Physically compatible for 48 hr at room temperature	924; 1167	**C**
	RB	20 and 320 mg	USV	20 ml[c]	NS	Physically compatible for 48 hr at room temperature	924; 1167	**C**
Metronidazole HCl with sodium bicarbonate	SE AB	5 g 50 mEq	USV	20 ml	D5W, NS	Physically compatible for 48 hr	765	**C**
Netilmicin sulfate	SC	3 g	USV	40 ml	D5S	Physically compatible and netilmicin chemically stable for 24 hr at 25 and 4 °C. 20% loss noted after 3 days. Multivitamins not tested	558	**C**
Norepinephrine bitartrate	WI	8 mg	USV	10 ml	D, D–S, S	Physically compatible	77	**C**
Sodium bicarbonate	AB	4.8 mEq[d]	USV	10 ml	D5W	Physically compatible for 24 hr	772	**C**
Verapamil HCl	KN	80 mg	USV	10 ml	D5W, NS	Physically compatible for 24 hr	764	**C**

[a]*Concentrate.*
[b]*M.V.I.*
[c]*M.V.I.-12.*
[d]*Two vials of Neut added to a liter of admixture.*

Y-Site Injection Compatibility (1:1 Mixture)

Multivitamins

Drug	Mfr	Conc	Mfr	Conc	Remarks	Ref	C/I
Acyclovir sodium	BW	5 mg/ml[a]	LY	0.01 ml/ml[a]	Physically compatible for 4 hr at 25 °C	1157	**C**
Ampicillin sodium	AY	1 g/50 ml[b]	USV	5 ml/L[a]	Physically compatible for 24 hr at room temperature	323	**C**
Cefazolin sodium	SKF	1 g/50 ml[a]	USV	5 ml/L[a]	Physically compatible for 24 hr at room temperature	323	**C**
Diltiazem HCl	MMD	5 mg/ml		[c]	Visually compatible	1807	**C**
Erythromycin lactobionate	AB	500 mg/ 250 ml[d]	USV	5 ml/L[a]	Physically compatible for 24 hr at room temperature	323	**C**
Fludarabine phosphate	BX	1 mg/ml[a]	RR	0.01 ml/ml[a]	Physically compatible for 4 hr at room temperature under fluorescent light	1439	**C**
Gentamicin sulfate	SC	80 mg/ 100 ml[a]	USV	5 ml/L[a]	Physically compatible for 24 hr at room temperature	323	**C**
Tacrolimus	FUJ	1 mg/ml[d]	LY	0.001 ml/ml[a]	Visually compatible for 24 hr at 25 °C	1630	**C**

Y-Site Injection Compatibility (1:1 Mixture) (Cont.)

Multivitamins

Drug	Mfr	Conc	Mfr	Conc	Remarks	Ref	C/I
TPN #189[e]			RR	[f]	Visually compatible for 24 hr at 22 °C	1767	C

[a]*Tested in dextrose 5% in water.*
[b]*Tested in both dextrose 5% in water and sodium chloride 0.9%.*
[c]*Concentration unspecified.*
[d]*Tested in sodium chloride 0.9%.*
[e]*Refer to Appendix I for the composition of parenteral nutrition solutions. TPN indicates a 2-in-1 admixture.*
[f]*M.V.I.-12.*

Additional Compatibility Information

Miscellaneous— Bleomycin sulfate is inactivated in vitro by ascorbic acid and riboflavin (4). In addition, some of the vitamins may react with vitamin K bisulfite. Folic acid has been reported to be unstable in the presence of calcium salts. A physical incompatibility may result from addition to moderately alkaline solutions such as a sodium bicarbonate solution and other alkaline drugs such as acetazolamide sodium, aminophylline, ampicillin sodium, and chlorothiazide sodium (1-4/98; 1-6/98).

Penicillin G— The times to 10% decomposition of combinations of penicillin G potassium buffered (Lilly, Pfizer, Squibb) with multivitamin infusion concentrate (USV) in dextrose 5% in water and sodium chloride 0.9% have been mathematically predicted on the basis of the final pH of the admixture (304):

Penicillin G Potassium	Multivitamin Infusion Concentrate	pH	Time to 10% Decomposition
1 million units/L	1 ml/L	5.1	6.51 hr
	5 ml/L	4.9	4.56 hr
3 million units/L	1 ml/L	5.4	13.54 hr
	5 ml/L	5.0	6.38 hr
5 million units/L	1 ml/L	5.7	22.01 hr
	5 ml/L	5.1	6.51 hr
10 million units/L	1 ml/L	5.9	over 24 hr
	5 ml/L	5.4	13.54 hr

Erythromycin— Erythromycin 5 mg/ml as the lactobionate in pH 8 buffer was combined with riboflavin in concentrations varying from 1 mg/ml to 20 μg/ml. On exposure to light for four hours, almost total decomposition of the erythromycin occurred, with only 4 to 12% remaining. Protection from light resulted in 12 to 25% decomposition. When no riboflavin was present, 10% or less decomposition of the erythromycin occurred. It was concluded that a photodynamic decomposition reaction was taking place (564).

Other Antibiotics— In vitro testing of thiamine HCl, riboflavin-5'-phosphate, pyridoxine HCl, niacinamide, and ascorbic acid individually at concentrations of 0.1% and the following antibiotics at 0.025% in sterile distilled water showed significant reduction in antibiotic activity in one hour at 25 °C (314):

Erythromycin (as estolate)
Kanamycin sulfate
Streptomycin sulfate

Riboflavin-5'-phosphate, but not the other vitamins, caused signif-icant reduction in antibiotic activity of the following (314):

Doxycycline HCl
Lincomycin HCl

Solutions— Dextrose and saline infusion solutions have been recommended as diluents for infusion of multivitamins (1-4/98).

Feroz et al. evaluated the stability of the vitamins in M.V.C. 9 + 3 (Lyphomed) in several infusion solutions. The contents of one package of two vials of M.V.C. 9 + 3 were added to 1000 ml of the following infusion solutions:

Amino acid injection (Abbott) 2.5%, dextrose 25% (in glass, PVC, and polyolefin containers)
Amino acid injection (McGaw) 4.25%, dextrose 25% (in glass, PVC, and polyolefin containers)
Dextrose 5% in sodium chloride 0.9% (in glass and PVC containers)
Dextrose 5% in water (in polyolefin containers)

The admixtures were stored for 24 hours at room temperature in the light and in the dark and at 4 °C. Under all three storage conditions, cyanocobalamin, biotin, folic acid, riboflavin, vitamin E, niacinamide, and dexpanthenol were stable in all solutions. Pyridoxine and vitamin D were moderately stable; vitamin A, ascorbic acid, and thiamine were unstable, with the higher temperature and light exposure adversely affecting their activity. However, all vitamins retained at least 90% of the labeled amounts for 24 hours when the admixtures were stored at 4 °C (926).

Parenteral Nutrition Solutions— Multivitamin infusion concentrate (USV) 5 and 10 ml/L was tested in parenteral nutrition solutions #38 through #42. (Refer to Appendix I for the composition of parenteral nutrition solutions.) The admixtures were physically compatible for 24 hours at 22 °C. However, the UV spectra for both the amino acids–dextrose and the vitamins altered markedly. Whether this result indicates an incompatibility is uncertain (313).

Additional tests were conducted with multivitamin infusion concentrate (USV) 10 ml/L in parenteral nutrition solutions #43 through #47. Once again, no physical incompatibility was observed in 24 hours at 22 °C. However, TLC changes were observed in similar solutions in 12 hours (313).

In a parenteral nutrition solution composed of amino acids, dextrose, electrolytes, trace elements, and multivitamins in PVC bags stored at 4 and 25 °C, vitamin A rapidly deteriorated to 10% of the initial concentration in eight hours at 25 °C when exposed to light. The decomposition was slowed by light protection and refrigeration, with a loss of about 25% in four days. Folic acid concentration dropped 40% initially on admixture and then remained relatively constant for 28 days of storage. About 35% of the ascorbic acid was lost in 39 hours at 25 °C when exposed to light. The loss was reduced substantially, to a negligible amount in four days, by refrigeration and light protection. Thiamine content dropped by about 50% initially but then remained unchanged over 120 hours of storage (1063).

The stability of ascorbic acid in parenteral nutrition solutions, with and without fat emulsion, was studied using HPLC analysis. Both with and without fat emulsion, the total vitamin C content (ascorbic acid plus dehydroascorbic acid) remained above 90% for 12 hours when the solutions were exposed to fluorescent light and for 24 hours when they were protected from light. When stored in a cool dark place, the solutions were stable for seven days (1227).

Photodecomposition— The effects of photoirradiation on a FreAmine II–dextrose 10% parenteral nutrition solution containing 1 ml/500 ml of multivitamins (USV) were evaluated. During simulated continuous administration to an infant at 0.156 ml/min, the amino acids were stable when the bottle, infusion tubing, and collection bottle were shielded with foil. Only 20 cm of tubing in the incubator was exposed to light. However, if the flow was stopped, marked reductions in methionine (40%), tryptophan (44%), and histidine (22%) occurred in the solution exposed to light for 24 hours. In a similar solution without vitamins, only the tryptophan concentration decreased. The difference was attributed to the presence of riboflavin, a photosensitizer. The authors recommended administering the multivitamins separately and shielding from light (833).

The stability of five B vitamins was studied over eight hours in representative parenteral nutrition solutions exposed to fluorescent light, indirect sunlight, or direct sunlight. One 5-ml vial of multivitamin concentrate (Lyphomed) and 1 mg of folic acid (Lederle) were added to a liter of parenteral nutrition solution composed of amino acids 4.25% and dextrose 25% (Travenol) with standard electrolytes and trace elements. The five B vitamins were stable for eight hours at room temperature when exposed to fluorescent light. In addition, folic acid and niacinamide were stable over eight hours in direct or indirect sunlight. Exposure to indirect sunlight appeared to have little or no effect on thiamine HCl and pyridoxine HCl in eight hours, but riboflavin-5-phosphate lost 47%. Direct sunlight caused a 26% loss of thiamine HCl and an 86% loss of pyridoxine HCl in eight hours. A four-hour exposure of riboflavin-5-phosphate to direct sunlight resulted in a 98% loss (842).

Samples from 24 1-L and four 2-L parenteral nutrition solutions, containing one vial each of multivitamin concentrate (USV), were evaluated for thiamine HCl content 48 to 72 hours after mixing. The parenteral nutrition solutions contained amino acids 2.75 to 5%, dextrose 15 to 25%, and electrolytes. Thiamine HCl was stable in all of the solutions tested in spite of approximately 0.05% sulfite content (843).

Kishi et al. reported on a parenteral nutrition solution in glass bottles exposed to sunlight. Vitamin A decomposed rapidly, losing more than 50% in three hours. The decomposition could be slowed by covering the bottle with a light-resistant vinyl bag, resulting in about a 25% loss in three hours (1040).

Kishi et al. also reported that vitamin E was stable in the parenteral nutrition solution in glass bottles exposed to sunlight, with no loss occurring during six hours of exposure (1040).

Allwood found that vitamin A was rapidly and significantly decomposed when exposed to daylight. The extent and rate of loss were dependent on the degree of exposure to daylight which, in turn, depended on various factors such as the direction of the radiation, time of day, and climatic conditions. Delivery of less than 10% of the expected amount was reported (1047). In controlled light experiments, the decomposition initially progressed exponentially.

Subsequently, the rate of decomposition slowed. This result was attributed to a protective effect of the degradation products on the remaining vitamin A. The presence of amino acids provided greater protection. Compared to degradation rates in dextrose 5% in water, decomposition was reduced by up to 50% in some amino acid mixtures (1048).

The stability of several water-soluble vitamins in dextrose 5% in water and sodium chloride 0.9% in PVC and ClearFlex containers was evaluated. HPLC analysis showed that thiamine, riboflavin, ascorbic acid, and folic acid were stable at 23 °C when protected from light, exhibiting 10% or less loss in 24 hours. When exposed to light, thiamine and folic acid were stable but ascorbic acid was reduced by approximately 50 to 65% and riboflavin was completely lost (1509).

The stability of phytonadione in a TPN solution containing amino acids 2%, dextrose 12.5%, "standard" electrolytes, and M.V.I. Pediatric over 24 hours while exposed to light was evaluated by HPLC analysis. Vitamin loss was about 7% in four hours and 27% in 24 hours. Some loss was attributed to the light sensitivity of the phytonadione (1815).

Billion-Rey et al. reported substantial loss by HPLC analysis of retinol all-*trans* palmitate and phytonadione from both TPN and TNA admixtures due to exposure to sunlight. In three hours of exposure to sunlight, essentially total loss of retinol and 50% loss of phytonadione had occurred. The presence or absence of lipids did not affect stability. In contrast, tocopherol concentrations remained essentially unchanged by exposure to sunlight through 12 hours. The container material used to store the nutrition admixtures affected the concentration of the vitamins as well. Losses were greatest (10 to 25%) in PVC containers and were slightly better in EVA and glass containers (2049).

Bisulfite Effects— A study of the stability of thiamine HCl in the multivitamin products Berocca Parenteral Nutrition (Roche), Multivitamin Additive (Abbott), and M.V.I-12 (USV) showed extensive decomposition when these products were admixed in infusion solutions containing sodium bisulfite. After 24 hours at 23 °C, thiamine losses ranged from 70% in Travasol 5.5% (pH 5.5) to 97% in FreAmine III 8.5% (pH 6.5). The extent of decomposition increased as the pH neared neutrality. The rate of decomposition could be slowed, but not eliminated, by refrigeration. When admixed in solutions not containing bisulfite, the thiamine was much more stable, showing losses of 0 to 11% in 24 hours at 23 °C. The authors noted that if bisulfite-containing solutions are necessary to administer the multivitamin preparations, the admixtures should be used immediately after preparation and patients on long-term therapy should be monitored for thiamine deficiency (774).

In another experiment, multivitamin concentrate (USV) was added to 500-ml glass bottles of amino acids 10% (Travenol) containing 0.1% sulfite and also to 1000-ml PVC bags containing amino acids 4.25%–dextrose 25% (Travenol) with about 0.05% sulfite. After 22 hours at 30 °C, a 40% loss of thiamine HCl occurred in the amino acids 10% solution, but no loss occurred in the PVC bags of parenteral nutrition solution. The authors concluded that the thiamine HCl content is retained in usual clinical parenteral nutrition solutions, probably because of the dilution of the sulfite and buffering of pH. However, direct addition to solutions with a high sulfite content (0.1%) may result in significant decomposition (843).

Sorption— Vitamin A (as the acetate) (Sigma) 7.5 mg/L displayed 66.7% sorption to a PVC plastic test strip in 24 hours. The presence of dextrose 5% and sodium chloride 0.9% increased the extent of the sorption (12).

In another report, vitamin A acetate displayed 78% sorption to 200-ml PVC containers after 24 hours at 25 °C with gentle shaking. The initial concentration was 3 mg/L. The sorption was increased by approximately 10% in sodium chloride 0.9% and by 20% in dextrose 5% in water (133).

However, Nedich noted that vitamin A delivery is also reduced in glass intravenous containers. At a concentration of 10,000 units/L in glass and PVC plastic containers protected from light with aluminum foil, 77 and 71%, respectively, of the vitamin A were delivered over a 10-hour period. Without light protection, 61% was delivered from glass and 49% from PVC plastic containers over a 10-hour period (290).

In another test using multivitamin infusion (USV), one ampul per liter of sodium chloride 0.9% in glass and PVC plastic containers not protected from light, 69.4 and 67.9% of the vitamin A were delivered from glass and PVC containers, respectively, over a 10-hour period. The amount of vitamin A was constant over the test period; it did not decrease with time (282).

Similar results were observed in a parenteral nutrition solution composed of protein hydrolysate 2%, dextrose 20%, electrolytes, and multivitamin infusion (USV) 10 ml in 1-L glass containers. Approximately 50 to 65% of the vitamin A content in the solution was lost in 24 hours and then it remained stable for three to seven days. When added to the cellulose propionate burette chambers of infusion sets, about 60% of the vitamin A was lost in six hours. Further, the effluent from the PVC tubing of the set was even worse. The concentration dropped from an initial 3 μg/ml to 1 μg/ml in two hours. Wrapping foil around the chambers to exclude light did not alter the vitamin A disappearance. About 50% of the lost vitamin A was recovered by hexane extraction of the administration sets (438).

The following vitamins did not reveal significant sorption to a PVC plastic test strip in 24 hours (12):

Ascorbic acid
Niacinamide
Pyridoxine HCl
Riboflavin
Thiamine HCl
Vitamin D
Vitamin E acetate

However, Gillis et al. evaluated the delivery of vitamins A, D, and E from a parenteral nutrition solution composed of 3% amino acid solution (Pharmacia) in dextrose 10% with electrolytes, trace elements, vitamin K, folate, and vitamin B_{12}. To this solution was added 6 ml of multivitamin infusion (USV). The solution was prepared in PVC bags (Travenol), and administration was simulated through a fluid chamber (Buretrol) and infusion tubing with a 0.5-μm filter at 10 ml/hr. During the first 60 to 90 minutes, minimal delivery of the vitamins occurred. This was followed by a rise and plateau in the delivered vitamins, which were attributed to an increasing saturation of adsorptive binding sites in the tubing. The total amounts delivered over 24 hours were 31% for vitamin A, 68% for vitamin D, and 64% for vitamin E. Sorption of the vitamins was found in the PVC bag, fluid chamber, and tubing. Decomposition was not a factor (836).

Riboflavin (Sigma) 5 mg/L in sodium chloride 0.9% (Travenol) in PVC bags wrapped in aluminum foil for light protection did not exhibit significant sorption to the plastic during one week of storage at room temperature (15 to 20 °C) (536).

In another study, riboflavin (Sigma) 5 mg/L in sodium chloride

0.9% did not exhibit any loss due to sorption during a seven-hour simulated infusion through an infusion set (Travenol) consisting of a cellulose propionate burette chamber and 170 cm of PVC tubing (606).

The riboflavin solution was also tested as a simulated infusion over at least one hour by a syringe pump system. A glass syringe on a syringe pump was fitted with 20 cm of polyethylene tubing or 50 cm of Silastic tubing. No loss of riboflavin due to sorption was observed with either tubing (606).

A 25-ml aliquot of riboflavin (Sigma) 5 mg/L in sodium chloride 0.9% was stored in all-plastic syringes composed of polypropylene barrels and polyethylene plungers for 24 hours at room temperature in the dark. No loss due to sorption occurred (606).

Howard et al. reported on a patient receiving 3000 I.U. of retinol daily in a parenteral nutrition solution; nevertheless, this patient experienced two episodes of night blindness. The pharmacy prepared the parenteral nutrition solution in 1-L PVC bags in weekly batches and stored them at 4 °C in the dark until use. A subsequent in vitro study showed losses of vitamin A of 23 and 77% in three- and 14-day periods, respectively, under these conditions. About 30% of the lost vitamin A could be extracted from the PVC bag (1038).

Shenai et al. reported on losses of vitamin A from multivitamin infusion (USV) in a neonatal parenteral nutrition solution. The solution was prepared in colorless glass bottles and run through an administration set with a burette (Travenol). The total loss of vitamin A was 75% in 24 hours, with about 16% as decomposition in the glass bottle. The decomposition was not noticeable during the first 12 hours, but then vitamin A levels fell rather precipitously to about one-third of the initial amount. The balance of the loss, averaging about 59%, occurred during transit through the administration set. Removal of the inline filter and treatment of the set with albumin had no effect on vitamin A delivery. The authors recommended a three- to fourfold increase in the amount of vitamin A to compensate for the losses (1039).

Riggle et al. noted a 50% loss of vitamin A from a bottle of parenteral nutrition solution prepared with multivitamin infusion (USV) after 5.5 hours of infusion. The amount delivered through an Ivex-2 filter set was only 6.3% of the added amount. Similar quantities were found after 20 hours of infusion. A reduced light exposure and use of ^{3}H-labeled vitamin A confirmed binding to the infusion bottles and tubing (704).

Subsequently, Riggle and Brandt incubated solutions containing multivitamin infusion (USV) spiked with ^{3}H-labeled retinol in intravenous tubing protected from light and agitated to simulate flow for five hours. About half of the vitamin A was lost in 30 minutes, and 88 to 96% was lost in five hours. Spectrophotometric assays correlated closely with the radioisotope assays. Hexane rinses and radioactivity determinations on the tubing accounted for the decrease in radioactivity (1049).

McGee et al. evaluated the stability of vitamin E (alpha-tocopherol acetate from M.V.I.-1000 or Soluzyme) and selenium (from Selepen) in amino acids (Abbott) and dextrose in PVC bags. Exposure to fluorescent light and room temperature (23 °C) for 24 hours and simulated infusion at 50 ml/hr for eight hours through a Medlon TPN administration set with a 0.22-μm filter did not affect the concentrations of vitamin E and selenium (1224).

Dahl et al. reported the stability of numerous vitamins in parenteral nutrition solutions composed of amino acids (Kabi-Vitrum), dextrose 30%, and fat emulsion 20% (Kabi-Vitrum) in a 2:1:1 ratio with electrolytes, trace elements, and both fat- and water-soluble vitamins. The admixtures were stored in darkness at 2 to 8 °C for

96 hours with no significant loss of retinyl palmitate, alpha-tocopherol, thiamine mononitrate, sodium riboflavin-5'-phosphate, pyridoxine HCl, nicotinamide, folic acid, biotin, sodium pantothenate, and cyanocobalamin. Sodium ascorbate and its biologically active degradation product, dehydroascorbic acid, totaled 59 and 42% of the nominal starting concentration at 24 and 96 hours, respectively. However, the actual initial concentration was only 66% of the nominal concentration (1225).

When the admixture was subjected to simulated infusion over 24 hours at 20 °C, either exposed to room light or light protected, or stored for six days in the dark under refrigeration and then subjected to the same simulated infusion, once again the retinyl palmitate, alpha-tocopherol, and sodium riboflavin-5'-phosphate did not undergo significant loss. However, sodium ascorbate and its degradation product, dehydroascorbic acid, had initial combined concentrations of 51 to 65% of the nominal initial concentration, with further declines during infusion. Light protection did not significantly alter the loss of total ascorbic acid (1225).

In another experiment, neonatal parenteral nutrition solutions containing multivitamin infusion prepared in bags were delivered at 10 ml/hr through Buretrol sets (Travenol). The bags and sets were protected from light. Spectrophotometric and radioisotope assays showed that about 26% of the vitamin A was lost before the flow was started. At 10 ml/hr, about 67% was lost from the effluent. More rapid flow reduced the extent of loss. Analysis of clinical samples of parenteral nutrition solutions showed losses of 21 to 57% after 20 hours. Because losses after five hours were of the same magnitude, the authors concluded that the loss occurs fairly rapidly and is not due to gradual decomposition (1049).

McKenna and Bieri reported that 40% retinol losses occurred in two hours and 60% in five hours from parenteral nutrition solutions pumped at 10 ml/hr through standard infusion sets at room temperature. The retinol concentration in the bottle remained constant while the retinol in the effluent decreased. Antioxidants had no effect. Much of the vitamin A was recoverable from hexane washings of the tubing (1050).

Interestingly, no loss of vitamin A to PVC delivery systems of *enteral* feeding solutions, after six hours of storage without protection from light and with exposure to ambient temperature, was reported by Bryant and Neufeld. The authors attributed this result to the presence of other (undefined) substances in the enteral feeding mixtures (1051).

To minimize the importance of this sorption, Allwood suggested using vitamin A palmitate instead of acetate; he stated that vitamin A palmitate does not sorb to PVC. However, this does not alter the problem of degradation from exposure to light. Alternatively, an excess of vitamin A could be used (1033).

Plasticizer Leaching— Multivitamins (Lyphomed) 1 ml in 50 ml of dextrose 5% in water leached insignificant amounts of diethylhexyl phthalate (DEHP) plasticizer. This leaching was due to the surfactant polysorbate 80 in the formulation. This finding is consistent with the low surfactant concentration (0.032%) in the final admixture solution (1683).

NAFCILLIN SODIUM
AHFS 8:12.16

Apothecon

Products— Nafcillin sodium is available in vials containing the equivalent of 500 mg, 1 g, and 2 g of nafcillin. Reconstitute the vials with sterile water for injection, sodium chloride 0.9%, or bacteriostatic water for injection with parabens or benzyl alcohol in the following amounts (4; 154):

Vial Size	Volume of Diluent
500 mg	1.7 ml
1 g	3.4 ml
2 g	6.8 ml

The solution then contains nafcillin sodium equivalent to nafcillin 250 mg/ml with sodium citrate buffer. The final volumes of the 500-mg, 1- and 2-g vials are 2, 4, and 8 ml, respectively (4; 154).

Nafcillin sodium is also available in 1- and 2-g piggyback units buffered with 40 mg of sodium citrate per gram of drug. Reconstitute the piggyback units with a compatible diluent according to the manufacturer's directions and shake well (4).

A 10-g pharmacy bulk vial is also available and is reconstituted with 93 ml of sterile water for injection or sodium chloride 0.9% to yield a 100-mg/ml solution with sodium citrate buffer 4 mg/ml (4).

Nafcillin sodium is also available as frozen premixed solutions containing 1 and 2 g of nafcillin per minibag in dextrose 3.6% or 2%, respectively (4; 29).

pH— The pH of the reconstituted solution and frozen premixed solution is 6 to 8.5 (17).

Osmolality— The osmolality of nafcillin sodium (Wyeth) 250 mg/ml in sterile water for injection was determined to be 709 mOsm/kg by freezing-point depression and 665 mOsm/kg by vapor pressure (1071).

The frozen premixed solutions have an osmolality of 300 mOsm/kg (4).

The osmolality of nafcillin sodium (Wyeth) 40 mg/ml was determined to be 403 mOsm/kg in dextrose 5% in water and 402 mOsm/kg in sodium chloride 0.9% (1375).

The osmolality of nafcillin sodium was calculated for the following dilutions (1054):

Diluent	Osmolality (mOsm/kg)	
	50 ml	100 ml
2 g		
Dextrose 5% in water	399	334
Sodium chloride 0.9%	425	361
3 g		
Dextrose 5% in water	458	371
Sodium chloride 0.9%	485	398

Robinson et al. recommended the following maximum nafcillin sodium concentrations to achieve osmolalities suitable for peripheral infusion in fluid-restricted patients (1180):

Diluent	Maximum Concentration (mg/ml)	Osmolality (mOsm/kg)
Dextrose 5% in water	71	491
Sodium chloride 0.9%	64	470
Sterile water for injection	128	319

Sodium Content— Each gram of nafcillin sodium with sodium citrate buffer contains 2.9 mEq (66 mg) of sodium (4; 27).

Administration— Nafcillin sodium may be administered intramuscularly by deep intragluteal injection, by direct intravenous injection, or by intermittent intravenous infusion. For direct intravenous injection, the dose should be diluted with 15 to 30 ml of sterile water for injection or sodium chloride 0.45 or 0.9% and given over five to 10 minutes into the tubing of a running intravenous infusion. Intermittent intravenous infusion in a concentration between 2 and 40 mg/ml should be administered slowly, over 30 to 60 minutes (4).

Stability— Intact containers should be stored at controlled room temperature or lower (4). When reconstituted to a concentration of 250 mg/ml, nafcillin sodium is stable for three days at room temperature or seven days when refrigerated at 2 to 8 °C (4; 27). For the piggyback concentrations of 2 to 40 mg/ml, nafcillin sodium is stable for 24 hours at room temperature or 96 hours under refrigeration, although longer periods have also been cited (4).

Commercially available frozen premixed nafcillin sodium solutions, thawed at room temperature or under refrigeration, are stable for 72 hours at 25 °C and 21 days at 5 °C (4).

pH Effects— The stability of nafcillin sodium is pH dependent, with a maximum stability at pH 6 and a preferred range of pH 5 to 8. Drug decomposition is rapidly increased as pH values vary from this range (27).

Freezing Solutions— At a concentration of 250 mg/ml in sterile water for injection and frozen at −20 °C, the drug is stable for up to three months (27; 123).

In one study, however, when nafcillin sodium (Wyeth) 1 g/4 ml was frozen at −20 °C in glass syringes (Hy-Pod), the potency was retained for nine months (532).

In another study, nafcillin sodium (Wyeth) 1 g/50 ml of dextrose 5% in water in PVC bags frozen at −20 °C for 30 days and then thawed by exposure to ambient temperature or microwave radiation showed no evidence of precipitation or color change but had a 2 to 3% loss of potency as determined microbiologically. Subsequent storage of the admixture at room temperature for 24 hours also yielded physically compatible solutions with no additional loss of activity (555).

Nafcillin sodium (Wyeth) 20 mg/ml in dextrose 5% in water and sodium chloride 0.9% frozen at −20 °C for 12 weeks exhibited little or no loss of potency by HPLC analysis in latex elastomeric reservoirs (Secure Medical) and in glass containers (1970).

Portable Pumps— Stiles et al. evaluated the stability of nafcillin sodium (Wyeth) 80 mg/ml in sterile water for injection and sodium chloride 0.9% in 100-ml portable pump reservoirs (Pharmacia Deltec) during simulated administration for 48 hours. The drug solutions were tested by HPLC analysis immediately after preparation and after storage for 24 hours at 5 °C before 48-hour simulated administration. During simulated administration, some reservoirs were kept at 30 °C; others were placed in insulated pouches with frozen (−20 °C) gel packs to keep them chilled below the ambient temperature. The nafcillin sodium solutions exhibited a 5% or less loss by HPLC under all study conditions during 24 hours of simulated administration and an 8% or less loss during 48 hours of such administration. Chilling of the drug reservoirs was not necessary to complete the infusions, nor did it enhance stability substantially during the study period (1779).

Nafcillin sodium (Marsam) 20 mg/ml in sterile water for injection in PVC portable pump reservoirs (Pharmacia Deltec) exhibited no loss by HPLC analysis in three days stored at 25 °C and in 14 days at 5 °C. However, at a concentration of 120 mg/ml, 6% loss was found in three days at 25 °C, and 2% loss occurred in 14 days at 5 °C (2080).

Elastomeric Reservoir Pumps— Nafcillin sodium (Wyeth) 20 mg/ml in 100 ml of dextrose 5% in water and sodium chloride 0.9% was packaged in latex elastomeric reservoirs (Secure Medical). Little or no loss by HPLC analysis occurred in 24 hours at 25 °C and in four days at 5 °C (1970).

Compatibility Information

Solution Compatibility

Nafcillin sodium

Solution	Mfr	Mfr	Conc/L	Remarks	Ref	C/I
Alcohol 5% in dextrose 5%	AB	WY	2 and 30 g	Physically compatible and potency retained for 24 hr at 25 °C	27	C
Dextran 40 10% in dextrose 5%	PH	WY	2 and 30 g	Physically compatible and potency retained for 24 hr at 25 °C	27	C
Dextrose 5% in Ringer's injection	AB	WY	2 and 30 g	Physically compatible and potency retained for 24 hr at 25 °C	27	C
Dextrose 5% in half-strength Ringer's injection, lactated	AB	WY	2 and 30 g	Physically compatible	27	C

Solution Compatibility (Cont.)

Nafcillin sodium

Solution	Mfr	Mfr	Conc/L	Remarks	Ref	C/I
Dextrose 5% in Ringer's injection, lactated	AB	WY	2 and 30 g	Physically compatible	27	C
Dextrose 5% in sodium chloride 0.225%	AB	WY	2 and 30 g	Physically compatible	27	C
Dextrose 5% in sodium chloride 0.45%	AB	WY	2 and 30 g	Physically compatible and potency retained for 24 hr at 25 °C	27	C
Dextrose 5% in sodium chloride 0.9%	AB	WY	2 and 30 g	Physically compatible and potency retained for 24 hr at 25 °C	27	C
Dextrose 5% in water		WY	1 g	Potency retained for 24 hr	109	C
	AB	WY	2 and 30 g	Physically compatible and potency retained for 24 hr at 25 °C	27	C
	TR[a]	WY	20 g	Physically compatible and no loss of potency in 24 hr at room temperature	555	C
	AB[b]	WY	20 g	4% or less nafcillin loss by HPLC in 24 hr at 25 °C and in 4 days at 5 °C	1970	C
Dextrose 10% in sodium chloride 0.9%	AB	WY	2 and 30 g	Physically compatible	27	C
Dextrose 10% in water	AB	WY	2 and 30 g	Physically compatible	27	C
Ionosol T with dextrose 5%	AB	WY	2 and 30 g	Physically compatible	27	C
Normosol M in dextrose 5% in water	AB	WY	2 and 30 g	Physically compatible and potency retained for 24 hr at 25 °C	27	C
Normosol M, 900 cal	AB	WY	2 and 30 g	Physically compatible	27	C
Normosol R	AB	WY	2 and 30 g	Physically compatible	27	C
Normosol R in dextrose 5% in water	AB	WY	2 and 30 g	Physically compatible	27	C
Normosol R, pH 7.4	AB	WY	2 and 30 g	Physically compatible	27	C
Polysal M in dextrose 5% in water	CU	WY	30 g	Physically compatible and potency retained for 24 hr at 25 °C	27	C
Ringer's injection	AB	WY	2 and 30 g	Physically compatible and potency retained for 24 hr at 25 °C	27	C
Ringer's injection, lactated	AB	WY	2 and 30 g	Physically compatible and potency retained for 24 hr at 25 °C	27	C
Sodium chloride 0.9%		WY	1 g	Potency retained for 24 hr	109	C
	AB	WY	2 and 30 g	Physically compatible and potency retained for 24 hr at 25 °C	27	C
	AB[c]	WY	80 g	5% or less loss by HPLC with 24-hr storage at 5 °C followed by 48-hr simulated administration at 30 °C via portable pump	1779	C
	AB[b]	WY	20 g	4% or less nafcillin loss by HPLC in 24 hr at 25 °C and in 4 days at 5 °C	1970	C
Sodium lactate ⅙ M	AB	WY	2 and 30 g	Physically compatible and potency retained for 24 hr at 25 °C	27	C

Solution Compatibility (Cont.)

Nafcillin sodium

Solution	Mfr	Mfr	Conc/L	Remarks	Ref	C/I
TPN #107[d]			1 and 2 g	Physically compatible and nafcillin activity retained for 24 hr at 21 °C by microbiological assay	1326	C

[a]Tested in PVC containers.
[b]Tested in glass containers and latex elastomeric reservoirs (Secure Medical).
[c]Tested in portable pump reservoirs (Pharmacia Deltec).
[d]Refer to Appendix I for the composition of parenteral nutrition solutions. TPN indicates a 2-in-1 admixture.

Additive Compatibility

Nafcillin sodium

Drug	Mfr	Conc/L	Mfr	Conc/L	Test Soln	Remarks	Ref	C/I
Aminophylline	SE	500 mg	WY	30 g	D5W	Nafcillin potency retained for 24 hr at 25 °C	27	C
	SE	500 mg	WY	2 g	D5W	14% nafcillin decomposition in 24 hr at 25 °C	27	I
Ascorbic acid injection	UP	500 mg	WY	5 g	D5W	Physically incompatible	15	I
Aztreonam	SQ	20 g	BR	20 g	D5W, NS[a]	Cloudiness with a fine precipitate forms gradually. 6 to 7% aztreonam loss and 10 to 11% nafcillin loss in 24 hr at room temperature	1028	I
Bleomycin sulfate	BR	20 and 30 units	BR	2.5 g	NS	Substantial loss of bleomycin activity in 1 week at 4 °C	763	I
Chloramphenicol sodium succinate	PD	1 g	WY	500 mg		Physically compatible	27	C
Chlorothiazide sodium	MSD	500 mg	WY	500 mg		Physically compatible	27	C
Cytarabine	UP	100 mg		4 g	D5W	Heavy crystalline precipitation	174	I
Dexamethasone sodium phosphate	MSD	4 mg	WY	500 mg		Physically compatible	27	C
Diphenhydramine HCl	PD	50 mg	WY	500 mg		Physically compatible	27	C
Ephedrine sulfate		50 mg	WY	500 mg		Physically compatible	27	C
Gentamicin sulfate		75 mg		1 g	TPN #107[b]	10% gentamicin loss in 24 hr at 21 °C by microbiological assay	1326	I
Heparin sodium	AB, WY	20,000 units	WY	500 mg		Physically compatible	27	C
	AB	20,000 units	WY	500 mg		Physically compatible	21	C
Hydrocortisone sodium succinate	UP	250 mg	WY	500 mg		Precipitate forms within 1 hr	27	I
Hydroxyzine HCl	PF	100 mg	WY	500 mg		Physically compatible	27	C
Lidocaine HCl	AST	0.6 g	AP	20 g	D5W[a], NS[c]	Visually compatible with little or no nafcillin loss by HPLC in 48 hr at 23 °C. Lidocaine not tested	1806	C
Methylprednisolone sodium succinate	UP	125 mg	WY	500 mg	D5W	Precipitate forms	329	I
Potassium chloride	TR	40 mEq	WY	30 g	NS	Nafcillin potency retained for 24 hr at 25 °C	27	C
	AB	40 mEq	WY	500 mg		Physically compatible	27	C

Additive Compatibility (Cont.)

Nafcillin sodium

Drug	Mfr	Conc/L	Mfr	Conc/L	Test Soln	Remarks	Ref	C/I
Prochlorperazine edisylate	SKF	10 mg	WY	500 mg		Physically compatible	27	C
Promazine HCl	WY	100 mg	WY	500 mg		Physically compatible for only 6 hr	27	I
Sodium bicarbonate	AB	40 mEq	WY	500 mg		Physically compatible	27	C
Sodium lactate	AB	50 mEq	WY	500 mg		Physically compatible	27	C
Verapamil HCl	KN	80 mg	WY	4 g	D5W, NS	Physically compatible for 24 hr	764	C
	SE	[d]	WY	40 g	D5W, NS	Cloudy solution clears with agitation	1166	?
Vitamin B complex with C	WY	2 ml	WY	2 and 30 g	D5W	Nafcillin potency retained for 24 hr at 25 °C	27	C
	WY	2 ml	WY	2 g	NS	Nafcillin potency retained for 24 hr at 25 °C	27	C
	AB	5 ml	WY	5 g	D5W	Physically incompatible	15	I

[a]Tested in PVC containers.
[b]Refer to Appendix I for the composition of parenteral nutrition solutions. TPN indicates a 2-in-1 admixture.
[c]Tested in polyolefin containers.
[d]Final concentration unspecified.

Drugs in Syringe Compatibility

Nafcillin sodium

Drug (in syringe)	Mfr	Amt	Mfr	Amt	Remarks	Ref	C/I
Cimetidine HCl	SKF	300 mg/ 2 ml		1 g/5 ml	Physically compatible for 48 hr at room temperature	516	C
Heparin sodium	AB	20,000 units/ 1 ml	WY	500 mg	Physically compatible for at least 30 min	21	C

Y-Site Injection Compatibility (1:1 Mixture)

Nafcillin sodium

Drug	Mfr	Conc	Mfr	Conc	Remarks	Ref	C/I
Acyclovir sodium	BW	5 mg/ml[a]	WY	20 mg/ml[a]	Physically compatible for 4 hr at 25 °C	1157	C
Atropine sulfate		0.4 mg/ml	WY	33 mg/ml[b]	No precipitation	547	C
Cyclophosphamide	MJ	20 mg/ml[a]	WY	20 mg/ml[a]	Physically compatible for 4 hr at 25 °C	1194	C
Diazepam		5 mg/ml	WY	33 mg/ml[b]	No precipitation	547	C
Diltiazem HCl	MMD	5 mg/ml	WY	10 mg/ml[b]	Cloudiness forms and persists	1807	I
	MMD	5 mg/ml	WY	200 mg/ml[b]	Cloudiness forms but clears with swirling	1807	?
	MMD	1 mg/ml[b]	WY	10 and 200 mg/ml[b]	Visually compatible	1807	C
Droperidol		2.5 mg/ml	WY	33 mg/ml[b]	Precipitate forms, probably free nafcillin	547	I
Enalaprilat	MSD	0.05 mg/ml[b]	BR	10 mg/ml[a]	Physically compatible for 24 hr at room temperature under fluorescent light	1355	C
Esmolol HCl	DCC	10 mg/ml[a]	BR	10 mg/ml[a]	Physically compatible for 24 hr at 22 °C	1169	C
Famotidine	MSD	0.2 mg/ml[a]	WY	15 mg/ml[b]	Physically compatible for 14 hr	1196	C
Fentanyl citrate		0.05 mg/ml	WY	33 mg/ml[b]	No precipitation	547	C
Fentanyl citrate and droperidol (Innovar)		0.05 + 2.5 mg/ml	WY	33 mg/ml[b]	Precipitate forms, probably free nafcillin	547	I

Y-Site Injection Compatibility (1:1 Mixture) (Cont.)

		Nafcillin sodium					
Drug	Mfr	Conc	Mfr	Conc	Remarks	Ref	C/I
Fluconazole	RR	2 mg/ml	BR	20 mg/ml	Physically compatible for 24 hr at 25 °C	1407	C
Foscarnet sodium	AST	24 mg/ml	BR	20 mg/ml[c]	Physically compatible for 24 hr at 25 °C under fluorescent light by visual and microscopic examination	1393	C
Hydromorphone HCl	WY	0.2 mg/ml[a]	WY	20 mg/ml[a]	Physically compatible for at least 4 hr at 25 °C under fluorescent light	987	C
Insulin, regular	LI	0.2 unit/ml[b]	BA	20 and 40 mg/ml[a]	Immediate precipitation	1395	I
Labetalol HCl	SC	1 mg/ml[a]	BR	10 mg/ml[a]	Cloudiness and fine precipitate form immediately	1171	I
Magnesium sulfate	IX	16.7, 33.3, 66.7, 100 mg/ml[a]	WY	20 mg/ml[a]	Physically compatible for at least 4 hr at 32 °C	813	C
Meperidine HCl	WY	10 mg/ml[a]	WY	20 mg/ml[a]	Cloudy haze cleared on mixing and remained clear for 4 hr at 25 °C	987	C
	WY	10 mg/ml[b]	WY	20 and 30 mg/ml[a]	Cloudy solution formed immediately and persisted for at least 1 hr at 25 °C	1338	I
Midazolam HCl	RC	1 mg/ml[a]	WY	20 mg/ml[a]	Haze forms immediately. Particles form in 4 hr	1847	I
Morphine sulfate	WI	1 mg/ml[a]	WY	20 mg/ml[a]	Physically compatible for at least 4 hr at 25 °C under fluorescent light	987	C
	ES	1 mg/ml[b]	WY	30 mg/ml[a]	Physically compatible for 1 hr at 25 °C	1338	C
Nalbuphine HCl		10 mg/ml	WY	33 mg/ml[b]	Precipitate forms, probably free nafcillin	547	I
Pentazocine lactate		30 mg/ml	WY	33 mg/ml[b]	Precipitate forms, probably free nafcillin	547	I
Perphenazine	SC	0.02 mg/ml[a]	WY	20 mg/ml[a]	Physically compatible for 4 hr at 25 °C	1155	C
Propofol	ZEN	10 mg/ml	MAR	20 mg/ml[a]	Physically compatible for 1 hr at 23 °C with no increase in particle content	2066	C
Theophylline	TR	4 mg/ml	WY	20 mg/ml[a]	Visually compatible for 6 hr at 25 °C	1793	C
TNA #218 to #226[d]			BE, APC	20 mg/ml[a]	Visually compatible with no precipitate or emulsion damage apparent in 4 hr at 23 °C	2215	C
TPN #54[d]				250 mg/ml	Physically compatible and nafcillin activity retained over 6 hr at 22 °C by microbiological assay	1045	C
TPN #61[d]		[e]	WY	250 mg/1 ml[f]	Physically compatible	1012	C
		[g]	WY	1.5 g/6 ml[f]	Physically compatible	1012	C
TPN #212 to #215[d]			BE	20 mg/ml[a]	Physically compatible with no change in measured turbidity or increase in particle content in 4 hr at 23 °C	2109	C
Vancomycin HCl	AB	20 mg/ml[a]	BE	250 mg/ml[i]	Transient precipitate forms followed by a visibly hazy solution	2189	I
	AB	20 mg/ml[a]	BE	10 and 50 mg/ml[b]	Gross white precipitate forms immediately	2189	I
	AB	20 mg/ml[a]	BE	1 mg/ml[b]	Physically compatible with no change in measured turbidity or increase in particle content in 4 hr at 23 °C	2189	C
	AB	2 mg/ml[a]	BE	10[b], 50[b], 250[i] mg/ml	Subvisual measured haze forms immediately	2189	I

Y-Site Injection Compatibility (1:1 Mixture) (Cont.)

Nafcillin sodium

Drug	Mfr	Conc	Mfr	Conc	Remarks	Ref	C/I
	AB	2 mg/ml[a]	BE	1 mg/ml[b]	Physically compatible with no change in measured turbidity or increase in particle content in 4 hr at 23 °C	2189	**C**
Verapamil HCl		[h]			White milky precipitate forms immediately	840	**I**
	SE	2.5 mg/ml	WY	40 mg/ml[c]	White milky precipitate forms immediately and persists. 20% of verapamil precipitated	1166	**I**
Zidovudine	BW	4 mg/ml[a]	BR	20 mg/ml[a]	Physically compatible for 4 hr at 25 °C under fluorescent light by visual and microscopic examination	1193	**C**

[a]*Tested in dextrose 5% in water.*
[b]*Tested in sodium chloride 0.9%.*
[c]*Tested in both dextrose 5% in water and sodium chloride 0.9%.*
[d]*Refer to Appendix I for the composition of parenteral nutrition solutions. TNA indicates a 3-in-1 admixture, and TPN indicates a 2-in-1 admixture.*
[e]*Run at 21 ml/hr.*
[f]*Given over five minutes by syringe pump.*
[g]*Run at 94 ml/hr.*
[h]*Injected into a line being used to infuse nafcillin sodium.*
[i]*Tested in sterile water for injection.*

Additional Compatibility Information

Solutions—— Nafcillin sodium (Wyeth) 500 mg/L is physically compatible with most Abbott infusion solutions. A precipitate forms within several hours when nafcillin sodium is mixed with infusion solutions containing vitamin B complex or vitamin C (27).

It is stated that nafcillin sodium, at concentrations of 2 to 40 mg/ml, will lose less than 10% potency in 24 hours at room temperature or 96 hours under refrigeration in the following infusion solutions (4):

Dextrose 5% in sodium chloride 0.45%
Dextrose 5% in water
Ringer's injection
Sodium chloride 0.9%
Sodium lactate ⅙ M

However, individual package labeling should be consulted because manufacturers' recommended stability periods for nafcillin sodium vary (4).

Care should be exercised when mixing nafcillin sodium (Wyeth) at concentrations of 500 mg/L or less in dextrose–polyelectrolyte solutions. These solutions have their pH adjusted to maintain dextrose stability and have a relatively high buffer capacity. Small amounts of nafcillin sodium may not have enough buffer capability to adjust the pH adequately (27).

Peritoneal Dialysis Solutions—— The activity of nafcillin 100 mg/L was evaluated in peritoneal dialysis fluids containing dextrose 1.5 or 4.25% (Dianeal 137, Travenol). Storage at 25 °C resulted in no loss of antimicrobial activity in 24 hours (515).

The stability of nafcillin sodium (Wyeth) 100 mg/L in peritoneal dialysis solutions (Dianeal 137 and PD2) with heparin sodium 500 units/L was evaluated by microbiological assay. Approximately 98 ± 7% activity remained after 24 hours at 25 °C (1228).

Acidic and Alkaline Additives—— Additives that may result in a final pH of above 8 or below 5 should not be mixed with nafcillin sodium. These additives include metaraminol bitartrate, succinylcholine chloride, and ascorbic acid (22; 27).

Nafcillin sodium (Wyeth) 500 mg/L has been reported to be conditionally compatible with norepinephrine bitartrate (Winthrop) 8 mg/L. The admixture is physically compatible for 24 hours, but the pH is 5.3 and the solution should therefore be used within six hours (27).

Vancomycin—— The compatibility or incompatibility of vancomycin HCl mixed with or administered simultaneously with nafcillin sodium is concentration dependent (2189). See Y-Site Compatibility above. Vancomycin HCl has a low pH and is variably compatible with drugs having neutral to mildly alkaline pH, including cephalosporins and penicillins. The compatibility may depend on a number of factors, including concentration of each drug, dilution vehicle, actual pH of solutions, and completeness of mixing during administration. Combinations that are compatible when well mixed may result in precipitation if only partially mixed, presumably due to regionally different concentrations and pH values. If attempting to administer vancomycin HCl with nafcillin sodium, take care to ensure that the specific combination and the concentrations are compatible under the exact administration conditions to be used. An inline filter should be used as a final safety measure (2189).

Aminoglycosides—— Lundergan et al. studied the interaction of tobramycin sulfate with several penicillins in vitro in human serum under clinical laboratory conditions. Tobramycin sulfate 10 μg/ml was combined with carbenicillin disodium 200 μg/ml, oxacillin sodium (Bristol) 50 μg/ml, and nafcillin sodium (Wyeth) 50 μg/ml. Samples were evaluated over 72 hours at −23, 6, and 23 °C. Although results were somewhat variable, only the carbenicillin sample at 23 °C exhibited substantial decomposition after 72 hours. None of the other carbenicillin, oxacillin, and nafcillin samples showed significant differences over the study period (814).

To determine if spurious aminoglycoside levels could result from a delay in assaying blood samples, Tindula et al. evaluated the inactivation of amikacin 35 μg/ml and gentamicin and tobramycin 10 μg/ml in human serum by 400-μg/ml concentrations of several penicillins and cephalosporins. Samples were stored for 24 hours at room temperature or frozen at −20 °C. For the room temperature samples, cefazolin and cefamandole caused relatively little inactivation. Nafcillin, cephapirin, and cefoxitin caused moderate inactivation, 20% or less. Penicillin, ampicillin, carbenicillin, and ticarcillin generally caused 25% or more inactivation of gentamicin and tobramycin. Amikacin was somewhat less affected. Freezing samples at −20 °C prevented significant inactivation of amikacin and gentamicin by any of the drugs. Freezing the tobramycin samples was satisfactory for most of the drugs except penicillin, ampicillin,

and carbenicillin, which still exhibited a 15 to 20% loss in 24 hours (824).

The clinical significance of these interactions in patients appears to be confined primarily to those with renal failure (218; 334; 361; 364; 616; 847). Literature reports of greatly reduced aminoglycoside levels in such patients have appeared frequently (363; 365–367; 614; 615; 962). In addition, the interaction may be clinically important if assays for aminoglycoside levels in serum are sufficiently delayed (517; 618; 824; 832; 847; 1052).

Verapamil— A milky white precipitate formed immediately when verapamil HCl was given by intravenous push into an infusion line being used for nafcillin sodium (840).

NALBUPHINE HCL
AHFS 28:08.12

Nubain   **Endo**
                                           Abbott

Products— Nalbuphine HCl (Endo) is available as a 10-mg/ml concentration in 1-ml ampuls and 10-ml vials and as a 20-mg/ml concentration in 1-ml ampuls and 10-ml vials. Each milliliter of solution in vials contains (2):

Nalbuphine HCl	10 mg	20 mg
Sodium chloride	0.2%	
Sodium citrate hydrous	0.94%	0.94%
Citric acid anhydrous	1.26%	1.26%
Methyl- and propylparabens (9:1)	0.2%	0.2%
Hydrochloric acid	to adjust pH	to adjust pH

Nalbuphine HCl in ampuls is provided without the parabens (2).

pH— The pH is adjusted to 3.5 to 3.7 (2; 4).

Osmolality— Nalbuphine HCl (Abbott) 10 mg/ml has an osmolality of 290 mOsm/kg (2043).

Administration— Nalbuphine HCl is administered by subcutaneous, intramuscular, or intravenous injection (2; 4).

Stability— Intact vials and ampuls should be protected from excessive light and stored at 15 to 30 °C (2; 4).

Compatibility Information

Drugs in Syringe Compatibility

Nalbuphine HCl

Drug (in syringe)	Mfr	Amt	Mfr	Amt	Remarks	Ref	C/I
Atropine sulfate	WY	0.2 mg	EN	10 mg/ 1 ml	Physically compatible for 36 hr at 27 °C	762	**C**
	WY	0.2 mg	EN	5 mg/ 0.5 ml	Physically compatible for 36 hr at 27 °C	762	**C**
	WY	0.5 mg	EN	10 mg/ 1 ml	Physically compatible for 36 hr at 27 °C	762	**C**
	WY	0.5 mg	EN	5 mg/ 0.5 ml	Physically compatible for 36 hr at 27 °C	762	**C**
		0.4 and 1 mg	DU	10 mg/ 1 ml	Physically compatible for 48 hr	128	**C**
		0.4 and 1 mg	DU	20 mg/ 1 ml	Physically compatible for 48 hr	128	**C**
Cimetidine HCl	SKF	300 mg/ 2 ml	EN	10 mg/ 1 ml	Physically compatible for 4 hr at 25 °C	25	**C**
		300 mg/ 2 ml	DU	10 mg/ 1 ml	Physically compatible for 48 hr	128	**C**
		300 mg/ 2 ml	DU	20 mg/ 1 ml	Physically compatible for 48 hr	128	**C**

Drugs in Syringe Compatibility (Cont.)

Nalbuphine HCl

Drug (in syringe)	Mfr	Amt	Mfr	Amt	Remarks	Ref	C/I
Diazepam	RC	5 mg/ 1 ml	EN	10 mg/ 1 ml	Immediate white milky precipitate that persists for 36 hr at 27 °C	762	I
	RC	5 mg/ 1 ml	EN	5 mg/ 0.5 ml	Immediate white milky precipitate that clears upon vigorous shaking. Remains clear for 36 hr at 27 °C	762	I
	RC	5 mg/ 1 ml	EN	2.5 mg/ 0.25 ml	Immediate white milky precipitate that clears upon vigorous shaking. Remains clear for 36 hr at 27 °C	762	I
	RC	10 mg/ 2 ml	DU	10 mg/ 1 ml	Physically incompatible	128	I
	RC	10 mg/ 2 ml	DU	20 mg/ 1 ml	Physically incompatible	128	I
Diphenhydramine HCl	PD	50 mg/ 1 ml	DU	10 mg/ 1 ml	Physically compatible for 48 hr	128	C
	PD	50 mg/ 1 ml	DU	20 mg/ 1 ml	Physically compatible for 48 hr	128	C
Droperidol	JN	5 mg/ 2 ml	EN	5 mg/ 0.5 ml	Physically compatible for 36 hr at 27 °C	762	C
	JN	2.5 mg/ 1 ml	EN	10 mg/ 1 ml	Physically compatible for 36 hr at 27 °C	762	C
	JN	2.5 mg/ 1 ml	EN	5 mg/ 0.5 ml	Physically compatible for 36 hr at 27 °C	762	C
	JN	5 mg/ 2 ml	DU	10 mg/ 1 ml	Physically compatible for 48 hr	128	C
	JN	5 mg/ 2 ml	DU	20 mg/ 1 ml	Physically compatible for 48 hr	128	C
Glycopyrrolate	RB	0.2 mg/ 1 ml	DU	10 mg/ 1 ml	Physically compatible for 48 hr	128	C
	RB	0.2 mg/ 1 ml	DU	20 mg/ 1 ml	Physically compatible for 48 hr	128	C
Hydroxyzine HCl	PF	50 mg	EN	10 mg/ 1 ml	Physically compatible for 36 hr at 27 °C	762	C
	PF	50 mg	EN	5 mg/ 0.5 ml	Physically compatible for 36 hr at 27 °C	762	C
	PF	50 mg	EN	2.5 mg/ 0.25 ml	Physically compatible for 36 hr at 27 °C	762	C
	PF	25 mg/ 1 ml	DU	10 mg/ 1 ml	Physically compatible for 48 hr	128	C
	PF	25 mg/ 1 ml	DU	20 mg/ 1 ml	Physically compatible for 48 hr	128	C
Ketorolac tromethamine	SY	180 mg/ 6 ml	DU	30 mg/ 3 ml	White solid precipitate forms immediately and settles to bottom	1703	I
Lidocaine HCl		40 mg	DU	10 mg/ 1 ml	Physically compatible for 48 hr	128	C
		40 mg	DU	20 mg/ 1 ml	Physically compatible for 48 hr	128	C
Midazolam HCl	RC	5 mg/ 1 ml	DU	10 mg/ 1 ml	Physically compatible for 4 hr at 25 °C under fluorescent light	1145	C
Pentobarbital sodium	WY	50 mg/ 1 ml	EN	10 mg/ 1 ml	Immediate white milky precipitate that persists for 36 hr at 27 °C	762	I
	WY	50 mg/ 1 ml	EN	2.5 mg/ 0.25 ml	Immediate white milky precipitate that clears upon vigorous shaking	762	I

Drugs in Syringe Compatibility (Cont.)

Nalbuphine HCl

Drug (in syringe)	Mfr	Amt	Mfr	Amt	Remarks	Ref	C/I
	WY	50 mg/ 1 ml	EN	5 mg/ 0.5 ml	Immediate white milky precipitate that persists for 36 hr at 27 °C	762	**I**
Prochlorperazine edisylate	WY	5 mg/ 0.5 ml	EN	10 mg/ 1 ml	Physically compatible for 36 hr at 27 °C	762	**C**
	WY	5 mg/ 1 ml	EN	5 mg/ 0.5 ml	Physically compatible for 36 hr at 27 °C	762	**C**
	WY	5 mg/ 1 ml	EN	2.5 mg/ 0.25 ml	Physically compatible for 36 hr at 27 °C	762	**C**
	SKF	10 mg/ 2 ml	DU	10 mg/ ml	Physically compatible for 48 hr	128	**C**
	SKF	10 mg/ 2 ml	DU	20 mg/ 1 ml	Physically compatible for 48 hr	128	**C**
Promethazine HCl	ES	25 mg	EN	10 mg/ 1 ml	Physically compatible for 36 hr at 27 °C	762	**C**
	ES	25 mg	EN	5 mg/ 0.5 ml	Physically compatible for 36 hr at 27 °C	762	**C**
	ES	12.5 mg	EN	10 mg/ 1 ml	Physically compatible for 36 hr at 27 °C	762	**C**
	WY	25 and 50 mg	DU	10 mg/ 1 ml	Physically incompatible	128	**I**
	WY	25 and 50 mg	DU	20 mg/ 1 ml	Physically incompatible	128	**I**
	WY	25 mg/ 1 ml	DU	10 mg/ 1 ml	White flocculent precipitate forms immediately	1183	**I**
	ES	25 mg/ 1 ml	DU	10 mg/ 1 ml	Physically compatible for 24 hr at room temperature	1183	**C**
Ranitidine HCl	GL	50 mg/ 2 ml	EN	10 mg/ 1 ml	Physically compatible for 1 hr at 25 °C both macroscopically and microscopically	978	**C**
Scopolamine HBr	BW	0.86 mg/ 1 ml	EN	10 mg/ 1 ml	Physically compatible for 36 hr at 27 °C	762	**C**
	BW	0.86 mg/ 1 ml	EN	5 mg/ 0.5 ml	Physically compatible for 36 hr at 27 °C	762	**C**
	BW	0.43 mg/ 0.5 ml	EN	10 mg/ 1 ml	Physically compatible for 36 hr at 27 °C	762	**C**
		0.4 mg	DU	10 mg/ 1 ml	Physically compatible for 48 hr	128	**C**
		0.4 mg	DU	20 mg/ 1 ml	Physically compatible for 48 hr	128	**C**
Thiethylperazine malate	BI	5 mg/ 1 ml	EN	10 mg/ 1 ml	Physically compatible for 36 hr at 27 °C	762	**C**
	BI	5 mg/ 1 ml	EN	5 mg/ 0.5 ml	Crystals form in 24 hr at 27 °C. Physically compatible for at least 12 hr	762	**I**
	BI	5 mg/ 1 ml	EN	2.5 mg/ 0.25 ml	Crystals form in 24 hr at 27 °C. Physically compatible for at least 12 hr	762	**I**
		10 mg/ 2 ml	DU	10 mg/ 1 ml	Physically compatible for 48 hr	128	**C**
		10 mg/ 2 ml	DU	20 mg/ 1 ml	Physically compatible for 48 hr	128	**C**
Trimethobenzamide HCl	BE	100 mg/ 1 ml	EN	10 mg/ 1 ml	Physically compatible for 36 hr at 27 °C	762	**C**
	BE	100 mg/ 1 ml	EN	5 mg/ 0.5 ml	Physically compatible for 36 hr at 27 °C	762	**C**

Drugs in Syringe Compatibility (Cont.)

Nalbuphine HCl

Drug (in syringe)	Mfr	Amt	Mfr	Amt	Remarks	Ref	C/I
	BE	100 mg/ 1 ml	EN	2.5 mg/ 0.25 ml	Physically compatible for 36 hr at 27 °C	762	C
		200 mg/ 2 ml	DU	10 mg/ 1 ml	Physically compatible for 48 hr	128	C
		200 mg/ 2 ml	DU	20 mg/ 1 ml	Physically compatible for 48 hr	128	C

Y-Site Injection Compatibility (1:1 Mixture)

Nalbuphine HCl

Drug	Mfr	Conc	Mfr	Conc	Remarks	Ref	C/I
Allopurinol sodium	BW	3 mg/ml[b]	DU	10 mg/ml	Tiny particles form in 1 hr, becoming numerous crystals in 4 hr	1686	I
Amifostine	USB	10 mg/ml[a]	AST	10 mg/ml	Physically compatible with no change in measured turbidity or increase in particle content in 4 hr at 23 °C	1845	C
Amphotericin B cholesteryl sulfate complex	SEQ	0.83 mg/ml[a]	AST	10 mg/ml	Gross precipitate forms	2117	I
Aztreonam	SQ	40 mg/ml[a]	AST	10 mg/ml	Physically compatible with no subvisual haze or particle formation in 4 hr at 23 °C	1758	C
Cefepime HCl	BR	20 mg/ml[a]	DU	10 mg/ml	Haze forms immediately and becomes flocculent precipitate in 4 hr	1689	I
Cisatracurium besylate	GW	0.1, 2, 5 mg/ml[a]	AST	10 mg/ml	Physically compatible with no change in measured turbidity or increase in particle content in 4 hr at 23 °C	2074	C
Cladribine	ORT	0.015[b] and 0.5[c] mg/ml	AST	10 mg/ml	Physically compatible with no change in measured turbidity or increase in particle content in 4 hr at 23 °C	1969	C
Docetaxel	RPR	0.9 mg/ml[a]	AST	10 mg/ml	Increase in measured subvisual turbidity occurs immediately	2224	I
Etoposide phosphate	BR	5 mg/ml[a]	AST	10 mg/ml	Physically compatible with no change in measured turbidity or increase in particle content in 4 hr at 23 °C	2218	C
Filgrastim	AMG	30 μg/ml[a]	DU	10 mg/ml	Physically compatible with no change in measured turbidity or increase in particle content in 4 hr at 22 °C	1687	C
Fludarabine phosphate	BX	1 mg/ml[a]	DU	10 mg/ml[a]	Physically compatible for 4 hr at room temperature under fluorescent light	1439	C
Gemcitabine HCl	LI	10 mg/ml[b]	AST	10 mg/ml	Physically compatible with no change in measured turbidity or increase in particle content in 4 hr at 23 °C	2226	C
Granisetron HCl	SKB	0.05 mg/ml[a]	AB	10 mg/ml	Physically compatible with no change in measured turbidity or increase in particle content in 4 hr at 23 °C	2000	C
Melphalan HCl	BW	0.1 mg/ml[b]	AST	10 mg/ml	Physically compatible with no change in measured turbidity or increase in particle content in 3 hr at 22 °C	1557	C

Y-Site Injection Compatibility (1:1 Mixture) (Cont.)

Nalbuphine HCl

Drug	Mfr	Conc	Mfr	Conc	Remarks	Ref	C/I
Methotrexate sodium		30 mg/ml	DU	10 mg/ml	Heavy yellow precipitate forms immediately	1788	I
Nafcillin sodium	WY	33 mg/ml[b]		10 mg/ml	Precipitate forms, probably free nafcillin	547	I
Paclitaxel	NCI	1.2 mg/ml[a]	AST	10 mg/ml	Physically compatible with no change in measured turbidity in 4 hr at 22 °C	1556	C
Piperacillin sodium–tazobactam sodium	LE	40 + 5 mg/ml[a]	DU	10 mg/ml	Heavy white turbidity forms immediately and particles form in 4 hr	1688	I
Propofol	ZEN	10 mg/ml	AB	10 mg/ml	Physically compatible for 1 hr at 23 °C with no increase in particle content	2066	C
Remifentanil HCl	GW	0.025 and 0.25 mg/ml[b]	AST	10 mg/ml	Physically compatible with no change in measured turbidity or increase in particle content in 4 hr at 23 °C	2075	C
Sargramostim	IMM	10 μg/ml[b]	DU	10 mg/ml[b]	Slight haze, visible with high intensity light, formed in 30 min. Filament formed in 4 hr in one of two samples	1436	I
Sodium bicarbonate		1.4%	DU	10 mg/ml	Gas evolves	1788	I
Teniposide	BR	0.1 mg/ml[a]	DU	10 mg/ml	Physically compatible with no subvisual haze or particle formation in 4 hr at 23 °C	1725	C
Thiotepa	IMM[d]	1 mg/ml[b]	AST	10 mg/ml	Physically compatible with no change in measured turbidity or increase in particle content in 4 hr at 23 °C	1861	C
TNA #218 to #226[e]			AB, AST	10 mg/ml	Damage to emulsion integrity occurs immediately with free oil formation possible	2215	I
TPN #212 to #215[e]			AB	10 mg/ml	Physically compatible with no change in measured turbidity or increase in particle content in 4 hr at 23 °C	2109	C
Vinorelbine tartrate	BW	1 mg/ml[b]	AST	10 mg/ml	Physically compatible with no change in measured turbidity or increase in particle content in 4 hr at 22 °C	1558	C

[a]*Tested in dextrose 5% in water.*
[b]*Tested in sodium chloride 0.9%.*
[c]*Tested in bacteriostatic sodium chloride 0.9% preserved with benzyl alcohol 0.9%.*
[d]*Lyophilized formulation tested.*
[e]*Refer to Appendix I for the composition of parenteral nutrition solutions. TNA indicates a 3-in-1 admixture, and TPN indicates a 2-in-1 admixture.*

Additional Compatibility Information

Solutions— Nalbuphine HCl (DuPont) 10 and 20 mg/ml was physically compatible for 48 hours when diluted in 1:1 and 1:2 ratios with the following diluents (128):

> Dextrose 5% in sodium chloride 0.9%
> Dextrose 10% in water
> Ringer's injection, lactated
> Sodium chloride 0.9%

Promethazine— The compatibility of nalbuphine HCl with promethazine HCl appears to be conditional on the specific formulation of promethazine HCl being used. When Elkins-Sinn promethazine HCl is combined with nalbuphine HCl, the admixture is compatible. However, if the Wyeth promethazine HCl is combined, a precipitate forms immediately (128; 762; 1183).

NALMEFENE HCL
AHFS 28:10

Revex   **Baxter**

Products— Nalmefene HCl (Baxter) is available as 100 µg/ml (of nalmefene) in 1-ml ampuls and as 1 mg/ml (of nalmefene) in 2-ml ampuls and syringes. Both concentrations also contain sodium chloride 9 mg/ml and hydrochloric acid to adjust the pH (2).

pH— Adjusted to pH 3.9 (2).

Osmolality— Nalmefene HCl injections are made nearly isotonic by the presence of sodium chloride 9 mg/ml (2134).

Administration— Nalmefene HCl injection may be administered by subcutaneous, intramuscular, or intravenous injection (4).

Stability— Intact containers of nalmefene HCl should be stored at controlled room temperature (2).

Nalmefene HCl has been determined to be extremely stable in solution, with significant decomposition occurring only at elevated temperatures. For solutions containing 0.1 or 1 mg/ml, essentially no decomposition occurred when stored at 4 °C, and very little loss occurred after 35 months stored at 30 °C. Significant losses were found if either concentration was stored exposed to temperatures of 40 °C and above. In addition, the decomposition product of nalmefene HCl is less toxic than nalmefene itself (2134).

Compatibility Information

Solution Compatibility

Nalmefene HCl

Solution	Mfr	Mfr	Conc/L	Remarks	Ref	C/I
Dextrose 5% in Ringer's injection, lactated	AB[a]	OHM	10 mg	Little or no loss by HPLC in 72 hr at 4, 21, and 40 °C	1962	C
Dextrose 5% in sodium chloride 0.45%	AB[a]	OHM	10 mg	Little or no loss by HPLC in 72 hr at 4, 21, and 40 °C	1962	C
Dextrose 5% in water	AB[a]	OHM	10 mg	Little or no loss by HPLC in 72 hr at 4, 21, and 40 °C	1962	C
Ringer's injection, lactated	AB[a]	OHM	10 mg	Little or no loss by HPLC in 72 hr at 4, 21, and 40 °C	1962	C
Sodium bicarbonate 5%	AB[a]	OHM	10 mg	Little or no loss by HPLC in 72 hr at 4, 21, and 40 °C	1962	C
Sodium chloride 0.45%	AB[a]	OHM	10 mg	Little or no loss by HPLC in 72 hr at 4, 21, and 40 °C	1962	C
Sodium chloride 0.9%	AB[a]	OHM	10 mg	Little or no loss by HPLC in 72 hr at 4, 21, and 40 °C	1962	C

[a]*Tested in glass containers.*

NALOXONE HCL
AHFS 28:10

Narcan   **Endo**

Products— Naloxone HCl (Endo) is available in the following formulations (2):

Component	Preserved (mg/ml)		Paraben-Free (mg/ml)		
Naloxone HCl	1	0.4	1	0.4	0.02
Sodium chloride	8.35	8.6	9	9	9
Methyl- and propylparabens (9:1)	2	2			
Sizes (ml)	10	10	2	1	2

pH— The pH is adjusted to 3 to 4 with hydrochloric acid (2).

Osmolality— The osmolality of the 0.02-mg/ml concentration was determined to be 293 mOsm/kg by freezing-point depression and 289 mOsm/kg by vapor pressure (1071).

The osmolality of naloxone HCl 0.4 mg/ml was determined to be 301 mOsm/kg (1233).

Administration— Naloxone HCl may be administered by subcutaneous, intramuscular, or intravenous injection or by continuous intravenous infusion. Solutions for continuous intravenous infusion may be prepared as 2 mg/500 ml (4 µg/ml) of sodium chloride 0.9% or dextrose 5% in water (2; 4).

Stability— Naloxone HCl should be stored at room temperature and protected from excessive light. It is stable at pH 2.5 to 5. It should not be mixed with any alkaline solutions. Naloxone HCl solutions diluted in infusion solutions for administration should be discarded after 24 hours (2; 4).

Syringes— Naloxone HCl (Astra) 0.133 mg/ml in sodium chloride 0.9% packaged in polypropylene syringes (Sherwood) was physi-

cally stable and exhibited little or no loss by stability-indicating HPLC analysis in 24 hours stored at 4 and 23 °C (2199).

Compatibility Information

Additive Compatibility

Naloxone HCl

Drug	Mfr	Conc/L	Mfr	Conc/L	Test Soln	Remarks	Ref	C/I
Verapamil HCl	KN	80 mg	EN	0.8 mg	D5W, NS	Physically compatible for 24 hr	764	C

Drugs in Syringe Compatibility

Naloxone HCl

Drug (in syringe)	Mfr	Amt	Mfr	Amt	Remarks	Ref	C/I
Heparin sodium		2500 units/ 1 ml	DU	0.4 mg/ 1 ml	Physically compatible for at least 5 min	1053	C
Ondansetron HCl	GW	1.33 mg/ ml[a]	AST	0.133 mg/ ml[a]	Physically compatible with no measured increase in particulates and 6% or less loss of ondansetron and 5% or less loss of naloxone by HPLC in 24 hr at 4 or 23 °C	2199	C

[a]*Tested in sodium chloride 0.9%.*

Y-Site Injection Compatibility (1:1 Mixture)

Naloxone HCl

Drug	Mfr	Conc	Mfr	Conc	Remarks	Ref	C/I
Amphotericin B cholesteryl sulfate complex	SEQ	0.83 mg/ml[a]	AST	0.4 mg/ml	Gross precipitate forms	2117	I
Propofol	ZEN	10 mg/ml	AST	0.4 mg/ml	Physically compatible for 1 hr at 23 °C with no increase in particle content	2066	C

[a]*Tested in dextrose 5% in water.*

Additional Compatibility Information

Solutions— Sterile water for injection is recommended as a diluent for naloxone HCl. For intravenous infusion, dextrose 5% in water and sodium chloride 0.9% are recommended as vehicles (2; 4).

Miscellaneous— It has been stated that naloxone HCl should not be mixed with bisulfite, sulfite, or long-chain or high molecular weight anions or any solution with an alkaline pH (2; 4).

NEOSTIGMINE METHYLSULFATE
AHFS 12:04

Prostigmin   **ICN Pharmaceuticals**

Products— Neostigmine methylsulfate (ICN) is available in a concentration of 1:2000 in 1-ml ampuls and in concentrations of 1:1000

and 1:2000 in 10-ml multiple-dose vials. Each milliliter of these products contains (2):

Ampuls	1:2000
Neostigmine methylsulfate	0.5 mg
Methyl- and propylparabens	0.2%

Vials	1:1000	1:2000
Neostigmine methylsulfate	1 mg	0.5 mg
Phenol	0.45%	0.45%
Sodium acetate	0.2 mg	0.2 mg

In addition, these products contain sodium hydroxide (ampuls) or acetic acid and sodium hydroxide (vials) to adjust the pH (2).

pH— The pH is adjusted to approximately 5.9 (2).

Osmolality— The osmolality of neostigmine (salt form unspecified) 0.5 mg/ml was determined to be 251 mOsm/kg (1233).

Administration— Neostigmine methylsulfate may be administered intramuscularly, subcutaneously, or slowly intravenously (2; 4).

Stability— Neostigmine methylsulfate in intact containers should be stored at controlled room temperature and protected from light, freezing, and temperatures of 40 °C or more (4).

Syringes— The stability of neostigmine (salt form unspecified) 0.5 mg/ml repackaged in polypropylene syringes was evaluated by spectrophotometric and potentiometric methods. Little or no change in concentration was found after four weeks of storage at room temperature not exposed to direct light (2164).

Neostigmine methylsulfate (Elkins-Sinn) 0.167 mg/ml in sodium chloride 0.9% packaged in polypropylene syringes (Sherwood) was physically stable and exhibited no loss by stability-indicating HPLC analysis in 24 hours stored at 4 and 23 °C (2199).

Compatibility Information

Additive Compatibility

Neostigmine methylsulfate

Drug	Mfr	Conc/L	Mfr	Conc/L	Test Soln	Remarks	Ref	C/I
Netilmicin sulfate	SC	3 g	RC	40 mg	D5S	Physically compatible and netilmicin chemically stable for 3 days at 4 and 25 °C. Neostigmine not tested	558	C

Drugs in Syringe Compatibility

Neostigmine methylsulfate

Drug (in syringe)	Mfr	Amt	Mfr	Amt	Remarks	Ref	C/I
Glycopyrrolate	RB	0.2 mg/ 1 ml	RC	0.5 mg/ 1 ml	Physically compatible and pH in stability range for glycopyrrolate for 48 hr at 25 °C	331	C
	RB	0.2 mg/ 1 ml	RC	1 mg/ 2 ml	Physically compatible and pH in stability range for glycopyrrolate for 48 hr at 25 °C	331	C
	RB	0.4 mg/ 2 ml	RC	0.5 mg/ 1 ml	Physically compatible and pH in stability range for glycopyrrolate for 48 hr at 25 °C	331	C
Heparin sodium		2500 units/ 1 ml	RC	0.5 mg/ 1 ml	Physically compatible for at least 5 min	1053	C
Ondansetron HCl	GW	1.33 mg/ ml[a]	ES	0.167 mg/ ml[a]	Physically compatible with no measured increase in particulates and less than 3% loss of ondansetron and less than 5% loss of neostigmine by HPLC in 24 hr at 4 or 23 °C	2199	C
Pentobarbital sodium	AB	500 mg/ 10 ml	RC	0.5 mg/ 1 ml	Physically compatible	55	C
Thiopental sodium	AB	75 mg/ 3 ml	RC	0.5 mg/ 1 ml	Physically compatible	55	C

[a]*Tested in sodium chloride 0.9%.*

Y-Site Injection Compatibility (1:1 Mixture)

Neostigmine methylsulfate

Drug	Mfr	Conc	Mfr	Conc	Remarks	Ref	C/I
Heparin sodium	UP	1000 units/L[a]	RC	0.5 mg/ml	Physically compatible for at least 4 hr at room temperature by visual and microscopic examination	534	C
Hydrocortisone sodium succinate	UP	10 mg/L[a]	RC	0.5 mg/ml	Physically compatible for at least 4 hr at room temperature by visual and microscopic examination	534	C
Potassium chloride	AB	40 mEq/L[a]	RC	0.5 mg/ml	Physically compatible for at least 4 hr at room temperature by visual and microscopic examination	534	C
Vitamin B complex with C	RC	2 ml/L[a]	RC	0.5 mg/ml	Physically compatible for at least 4 hr at room temperature by visual and microscopic examination	534	C

[a]*Tested in dextrose 5% in Ringer's injection, dextrose 5% in Ringer's injection, lactated, dextrose 5% in water, Ringer's injection, lactated, and sodium chloride 0.9%.*

NETILMICIN SULFATE
AHFS 8:12.02

Netromycin   **Schering**

Products— Netilmicin sulfate (Schering) is available in a concentration of 100 mg/ml in 1.5-ml vials. Each milliliter of the solution contains (2):

Netilmicin (as sulfate)	100 mg
Sodium metabisulfite	2.4 mg
Sodium sulfite	0.8 mg
Edetate disodium	0.1 mg
Benzyl alcohol	10 mg
Water for injection	qs 1 ml

pH— From 3.5 to 6 (2; 4).

Osmolality— Netilmicin sulfate (Schering) 100 mg/ml has an osmolality of 430 mOsm/kg (2043).

Administration— Netilmicin sulfate may be administered by intramuscular or intravenous infusion. For intravenous administration to adults, the dose is added to 50 to 200 ml of a compatible infusion solution and infused over 30 to 120 minutes. The volume of solution should be less for pediatric patients, based on the patient's fluid requirements (2; 4).

Stability— Netilmicin sulfate injection is a clear, colorless to pale yellow solution. It should be stored between 2 and 30 °C, i.e., at room temperature or under refrigeration, and should be protected from freezing (2; 4).

Compatibility Information

Solution Compatibility

Netilmicin sulfate

Solution	Mfr	Mfr	Conc/L	Remarks	Ref	C/I
Amino acids 8.5%	MG	SC	3 g	Physically compatible and chemically stable for 7 days at 4 and 25 °C	558	C
Dextran 6% in dextrose 5%	AB	SC	3 g	Physically compatible and chemically stable for 7 days at 4 and 25 °C	558	C
Dextran 40 10% in dextrose 5%	PH, TR	SC	3 g	Physically compatible and chemically stable for 7 days at 4 and 25 °C	558	C
Dextrose 50%	TR	SC	3 g	Physically compatible and chemically stable for 7 days at 4 and 25 °C	558	C

Solution Compatibility (Cont.)

Netilmicin sulfate

Solution	Mfr	Mfr	Conc/L	Remarks	Ref	C/I
Dextrose 5% in Electrolyte #48	TR	SC	3 g	Physically compatible and chemically stable for 7 days at 4 and 25 °C	558	**C**
Dextrose 5% in Ringer's injection, lactated	TR	SC	3 g	Physically compatible and chemically stable for 7 days at 4 and 25 °C	558	**C**
Dextrose 5% in sodium chloride 0.9%	TR	SC	3 g	Physically compatible and chemically stable for 7 days at 4 and 25 °C	558	**C**
Dextrose 5% in water	TR	SC	3 g	Physically compatible and chemically stable for 7 days at 4 and 25 °C	558	**C**
	AB[a]	SC	3 g	Physically compatible with no netilmicin loss in 24 hr at 25 °C	994	**C**
Dextrose 10% in water	TR	SC	3 g	Physically compatible and chemically stable for 7 days at 4 and 25 °C	558	**C**
Fructose 10% in water	TR	SC	3 g	Physically compatible and chemically stable for 7 days at 4 and 25 °C	558	**C**
Invert sugar 10% in Electrolyte #2	TR	SC	3 g	Physically compatible and chemically stable for 7 days at 4 and 25 °C	558	**C**
Invert sugar 10% in Electrolyte #3	TR	SC	3 g	Physically compatible and chemically stable for 7 days at 4 and 25 °C	558	**C**
Ionosol B in dextrose 5%	AB	SC	3 g	Physically compatible and chemically stable for 7 days at 4 and 25 °C	558	**C**
Ionosol T in dextrose 5%	AB	SC	3 g	Physically compatible and chemically stable for 7 days at 4 and 25 °C	558	**C**
Isolyte E with dextrose 5%	MG	SC	3 g	Physically compatible and chemically stable for 7 days at 4 and 25 °C	558	**C**
Isolyte M with dextrose 5%	MG	SC	3 g	Physically compatible and chemically stable for 7 days at 4 and 25 °C	558	**C**
Isolyte P with dextrose 5%	MG	SC	3 g	Physically compatible and chemically stable for 7 days at 4 and 25 °C	558	**C**
Mannitol 10%	TR	SC	3 g	Physically compatible and chemically stable for 7 days at 4 and 25 °C	558	**C**
Mannitol 20%	TR	SC	3 g	Physically compatible and chemically stable for 7 days at 4 and 25 °C	558	**C**
Normosol R	AB	SC	3 g	Physically compatible and chemically stable for 7 days at 4 and 25 °C	558	**C**
Normosol R, pH 7.4	AB	SC	3 g	Physically compatible and chemically stable for 7 days at 4 and 25 °C	558	**C**
Plasma-Lyte 56 in dextrose 5%	TR	SC	3 g	Physically compatible and chemically stable for 7 days at 4 and 25 °C	558	**C**
Plasma-Lyte 148 in dextrose 5%	TR	SC	3 g	Physically compatible and chemically stable for 7 days at 4 and 25 °C	558	**C**
Plasma-Lyte M in dextrose 5%	TR	SC	3 g	Physically compatible and chemically stable for 7 days at 4 and 25 °C	558	**C**
Polysal	CU	SC	3 g	Physically compatible and chemically stable for 7 days at 4 and 25 °C	558	**C**
Polysal in dextrose 5%	CU	SC	3 g	Physically compatible and chemically stable for 7 days at 4 and 25 °C	558	**C**

Solution Compatibility (Cont.)

Netilmicin sulfate

Solution	Mfr	Mfr	Conc/L	Remarks	Ref	C/I
Ringer's injection	TR	SC	3 g	Physically compatible and chemically stable for 7 days at 4 and 25 °C	558	C
Ringer's injection, lactated	CU	SC	3 g	Physically compatible and chemically stable for 7 days at 4 and 25 °C	558	C
Sodium bicarbonate 5%	TR	SC	3 g	Physically compatible and chemically stable for 7 days at 4 and 25 °C	558	C
Sodium chloride 0.9%	TR	SC	3 g	Physically compatible and chemically stable for 7 days at 4 and 25 °C	558	C
	AB[a]	SC	3 g	Physically compatible with no netilmicin loss in 24 hr at 25 °C	994	C
TPN #107[b]			75 mg	Physically compatible and netilmicin activity retained for 24 hr at 21 °C by microbiological assay	1326	C

[a]Tested in both glass and PVC containers.
[b]Refer to Appendix I for the composition of parenteral nutrition solutions. TPN indicates a 2-in-1 admixture.

Additive Compatibility

Netilmicin sulfate

Drug	Mfr	Conc/L	Mfr	Conc/L	Test Soln	Remarks	Ref	C/I
Aminocaproic acid	LE	10 g	SC	3 g	D5S	Physically compatible and netilmicin chemically stable for 7 days at 25 and 4 °C. Aminocaproic acid not tested	558	C
Atropine sulfate	BW	40 mg	SC	3 g	D5S	Physically compatible and netilmicin chemically stable for 7 days at 4 and 25 °C. Atropine sulfate not tested	558	C
Cefepime HCl	BR	40 g	SC	1 g	D5W, NS	Cloudiness forms immediately	1682	I
	BR	2.5 g	SC	5 g	D5W, NS	Cloudiness forms immediately	1682	I
Cefuroxime sodium	GL	7.5 g	EX	1 g	D5W, NS[a]	Physically compatible with no loss of either drug in 1 hr	1036	C
Chlorpromazine HCl	SKF	100 mg	SC	3 g	D5S	Physically compatible and netilmicin chemically stable for 7 days at 4 and 25 °C. Chlorpromazine not tested	558	C
Ciprofloxacin	BAY	2 g	SC	2.5 g	NS	Visually compatible with little or no ciprofloxacin loss by HPLC in 24 hr at 25 °C. Netilmicin not tested	1934	C
Clindamycin phosphate	UP	9 g	SC	3 g	D5W, NS[b]	Physically compatible with no clindamycin loss and 2 to 5% netilmicin loss in 24 hr at 25 °C	994	C
Dexamethasone sodium phosphate	MSD	80 mg	SC	3 g	D5S	Physically compatible and netilmicin chemically stable for 7 days at 4 and 25 °C. Dexamethasone not tested	558	C
Diazepam	RC	40 mg	SC	3 g	D5S	Physically compatible and netilmicin chemically stable for 7 days at 4 and 25 °C. Diazepam not tested	558	C

Additive Compatibility (Cont.)

Netilmicin sulfate

Drug	Mfr	Conc/L	Mfr	Conc/L	Test Soln	Remarks	Ref	C/I
Diphenhydramine HCl	PD	400 mg	SC	3 g	D5S	Physically compatible and netilmicin chemically stable for 3 days at 4 and 25 °C. 17% loss after 7 days at 25 °C. Diphenhydramine not tested	558	**C**
Edetate calcium disodium	RI	4 g	SC	3 g	D5S	Physically compatible and netilmicin chemically stable for 7 days at 4 and 25 °C. Edetate not tested	558	**C**
Fibrinolysin and deoxyribonuclease combined	PD	40 ml	SC	3 g	D5S	Physically compatible and netilmicin chemically stable for 7 days at 4 and 25 °C. Enzymes not tested	558	**C**
Floxacillin sodium	BE	10 g	EX	1 g	NS	Physically compatible for 48 hr. Potency of both drugs retained when assayed after 1 hr at room temperature	1036	**C**
	BE	10 g	EX	1 g	D5W	Immediate precipitation	1036	**I**
Furosemide	HO	400 mg	SC	1.5 g	D5W, NS	Immediate precipitation of furosemide	876	**I**
Hydrocortisone sodium succinate	UP	400 mg	SC	3 g	D5S	Physically compatible and netilmicin chemically stable for 7 days at 4 and 25 °C. Hydrocortisone not tested	558	**C**
Hydrocortisone sodium succinate with potassium chloride	UP AB	400 mg 160 mEq	SC	3 g	D5S	Physically compatible and netilmicin chemically stable for 7 days at 4 and 25 °C. Other drugs not tested	558	**C**
Iron dextran	MRN	8 ml	SC	3 g	D5S	Physically compatible and netilmicin chemically stable for 7 days at 4 and 25 °C. Iron dextran not tested	558	**C**
Isoproterenol HCl	WI	400 mg[c]	SC	3 g	D5S	Physically compatible and netilmicin chemically stable for 7 days at 4 and 25 °C. Isoproterenol not tested	558	**C**
Methyldopate HCl	MSD	1 g	SC	3 g	D5S	Physically compatible and netilmicin chemically stable for 7 days at 4 and 25 °C. Methyldopate not tested	558	**C**
Metronidazole	RP	5 g[d]	SC	1.4 g		Physically compatible with little or no pH change for at least 24 hr at 23 °C and 72 hr at 4 °C	807	**C**
		5 g	EX	1 g	[a]	Physically compatible with no loss of either drug in 1 hr	1036	**C**
Multivitamins	USV	40 ml	SC	3 g	D5S	Physically compatible and netilmicin chemically stable for 24 hr at 4 and 25 °C. 20% loss after 3 days. Multivitamins not tested	558	**C**
Neostigmine methylsulfate	RC	40 mg	SC	3 g	D5S	Physically compatible and netilmicin chemically stable for 3 days at 4 and 25 °C. Neostigmine not tested	558	**C**
Norepinephrine bitartrate	WI	64 mg	SC	3 g	D5S	Physically compatible and netilmicin chemically stable for 7 days at 4 and 25 °C. Norepinephrine not tested	558	**C**
Oxytocin	PD	4 ml	SC	3 g	D5S	Physically compatible and netilmicin chemically stable for 7 days at 4 and 25 °C. Oxytocin not tested	558	**C**

Additive Compatibility (Cont.)

Netilmicin sulfate

Drug	Mfr	Conc/L	Mfr	Conc/L	Test Soln	Remarks	Ref	C/I
Phytonadione	MSD	100 mg	SC	3 g	D5S	Physically compatible and netilmicin chemically stable for 7 days at 4 and 25 °C. Phytonadione not tested	558	C
Potassium chloride	AB	160 mEq	SC	3 g	D5S	Physically compatible and netilmicin chemically stable for 7 days at 4 and 25 °C. Potassium chloride not tested	558	C
Potassium chloride with hydrocortisone sodium succinate	AB UP	160 mEq 400 mg	SC	3 g	D5S	Physically compatible and netilmicin chemically stable for 7 days at 4 and 25 °C. Other drugs not tested	558	C
Procainamide HCl	SQ	4 g	SC	3 g	D5S	Physically compatible and netilmicin chemically stable for 7 days at 4 and 25 °C. Procainamide not tested	558	C
Promethazine HCl	WY	100 mg	SC	3 g	D5S	Physically compatible and netilmicin chemically stable for 7 days at 4 and 25 °C. Promethazine not tested	558	C
Triflupromazine HCl	SQ	400 mg	SC	3 g	D5S	Physically compatible and netilmicin chemically stable for 7 days at 4 and 25 °C. Triflupromazine not tested	558	C
Vitamin B complex	PD	40 ml	SC	3 g	D5S	Physically compatible and netilmicin chemically stable for 7 days at 4 and 25 °C. Vitamins not tested	558	C
	UP	8 ml	SC	3 g	D5S	Physically compatible with 10 to 12% netilmicin loss in 24 hr at 4 and 25 °C. Vitamins not tested	558	I
Vitamin B complex with C	LI	40 ml	SC	3 g	D5S	Physically compatible and netilmicin chemically stable for 7 days at 4 and 25 °C. Vitamins not tested	558	C
	RC	8 ml	SC	3 g	D5S	Physically compatible and netilmicin chemically stable for 7 days at 4 and 25 °C. Vitamins not tested	558	C

[a]*Tested in PVC containers.*
[b]*Tested in both glass and PVC containers.*
[c]*Isoproterenol HCl 1% inhalation solution tested. Injection is also expected to be compatible.*
[d]*Minibags (100 ml) containing metronidazole 500 mg with disodium phosphate 150 mg, citric acid 44 mg, and sodium chloride 740 mg. This product differs from the Searle product.*

Drugs in Syringe Compatibility

Netilmicin sulfate

Drug (in syringe)	Mfr	Amt	Mfr	Amt	Remarks	Ref	C/I
Doxapram HCl	RB	400 mg/ 20 ml		100 mg/ 2 ml	Physically compatible with 2% decomposition in 24 hr	1177	C
Heparin sodium		2500 units/ 1 ml		150 mg	Turbidity or precipitate forms within 5 min	1053	I

Y-Site Injection Compatibility (1:1 Mixture)

Netilmicin sulfate

Drug	Mfr	Conc	Mfr	Conc	Remarks	Ref	C/I
Allopurinol sodium	BW	3 mg/ml[b]	SC	5 mg/ml[b]	Haze increases and flakes form in 1 hr	1686	**I**
Amifostine	USB	10 mg/ml[a]	SC	5 mg/ml[a]	Physically compatible with no change in measured turbidity or increase in particle content in 4 hr at 23 °C	1845	**C**
Aminophylline	ES	800 μg/ml[c]	SC	5 mg/ml[c]	Physically compatible and no netilmicin loss in 2 hr at 24 °C	1021	**C**
Amphotericin B cholesteryl sulfate complex	SEQ	0.83 mg/ml[a]	SC	5 mg/ml[a]	Gross precipitate forms	2117	**I**
Aztreonam	SQ	40 mg/ml[c]	SCH	5 mg/ml[c]	Physically compatible with no subvisual haze or particle formation in 4 hr at 23 °C	1758	**C**
Calcium gluconate	WY	40 mg/ml[c]	SC	5 mg/ml[c]	Physically compatible and no netilmicin loss in 2 hr at 24 °C	1021	**C**
Cisatracurium besylate	GW	0.1, 2, 5 mg/ml[a]	SC	5 mg/ml[a]	Physically compatible with no change in measured turbidity or increase in particle content in 4 hr at 23 °C	2074	**C**
Docetaxel	RPR	0.9 mg/ml[a]	SCH	5 mg/ml[a]	Physically compatible with no change in measured turbidity or increase in particle content in 4 hr at 23 °C	2224	**C**
Doxorubicin HCl liposome injection	SEQ	0.4 mg/ml[a]	SC	5 mg/ml[a]	Physically compatible with little or no change in measured turbidity and no increase in particle content in 4 hr at 23 °C	2087	**C**
Etoposide phosphate	BR	5 mg/ml[a]	SCH	5 mg/ml[a]	Physically compatible with no change in measured turbidity or increase in particle content in 4 hr at 23 °C	2218	**C**
Filgrastim	AMG	30 μg/ml[a]	SC	5 mg/ml[a]	Physically compatible with no change in measured turbidity or increase in particle content in 4 hr at 22 °C	1687	**C**
Fludarabine phosphate	BX	1 mg/ml[a]	SC	5 mg/ml[a]	Physically compatible for 4 hr at room temperature under fluorescent light	1439	**C**
Furosemide	HO	10 mg/ml	SC	1.5 mg/ml[d]	White precipitate of furosemide forms immediately	876	**I**
Gemcitabine HCl	LI	10 mg/ml[b]	SCH	5 mg/ml[b]	Physically compatible with no change in measured turbidity or increase in particle content in 4 hr at 23 °C	2226	**C**
Granisetron HCl	SKB	0.05 mg/ml[a]	SCH	5 mg/ml[a]	Physically compatible with no change in measured turbidity or increase in particle content in 4 hr at 23 °C	2000	**C**
Melphalan HCl	BW	0.1 mg/ml[b]	SC	5 mg/ml[b]	Physically compatible with no change in measured turbidity or increase in particle content in 3 hr at 22 °C	1557	**C**
Propofol	ZEN	10 mg/ml	SC	5 mg/ml[a]	Precipitate forms immediately	2066	**I**
Remifentanil HCl	GW	0.025 and 0.25 mg/ml[b]	SC	5 mg/ml[a]	Physically compatible with no change in measured turbidity or increase in particle content in 4 hr at 23 °C	2075	**C**
Sargramostim	IMM	10 μg/ml[b]	SC	5 mg/ml[b]	Physically compatible for 4 hr at 22 °C	1436	**C**

Y-Site Injection Compatibility (1:1 Mixture) (Cont.)

Netilmicin sulfate

Drug	Mfr	Conc	Mfr	Conc	Remarks	Ref	C/I
Teniposide	BR	0.1 mg/ml[a]	SC	5 mg/ml[a]	Physically compatible with no subvisual haze or particle formation in 4 hr at 23 °C	1725	C
Thiotepa	IMM[e]	1 mg/ml[b]	SC	5 mg/ml[b]	Physically compatible with no change in measured turbidity or increase in particle content in 4 hr at 23 °C	1861	C
TNA #218 to #226[f]			SC	5 mg/ml[a]	Visually compatible with no precipitate or emulsion damage apparent in 4 hr at 23 °C	2215	C
TPN #61[f]		[g]	SC	12.5 mg/ 0.13 ml[h]	Physically compatible	1012	C
		[i]	SC	75 mg/ 0.75 ml[h]	Physically compatible	1012	C
TPN #212 to #215[f]			SC	5 mg/ml[a]	Physically compatible with no change in measured turbidity or increase in particle content in 4 hr at 23 °C	2109	C
Vinorelbine tartrate	BW	1 mg/ml[b]	SC	5 mg/ml[b]	Physically compatible with no change in measured turbidity or increase in particle content in 4 hr at 22 °C	1558	C

[a]*Tested in dextrose 5% in water.*
[b]*Tested in sodium chloride 0.9%.*
[c]*Tested in dextrose 5% in sodium chloride 0.2%.*
[d]*Tested in both dextrose 5% in water and sodium chloride 0.9%.*
[e]*Lyophilized formulation tested.*
[f]*Refer to Appendix I for the composition of parenteral nutrition solutions. TNA indicates a 3-in-1 admixture, and TPN indicates a 2-in-1 admixture.*
[g]*Run at 21 ml/hr.*
[h]*Given over 30 minutes by syringe pump.*
[i]*Run at 94 ml/hr.*

Additional Compatibility Information

Solutions—— The manufacturer indicates that netilmicin sulfate 2.1 to 3 mg/ml is stable in most infusion solutions in glass containers for up to 72 hours stored at room temperature or under refrigeration (2). Published information (see table above) indicates that the drug may be stable for up to seven days under these conditions (558).

Peritoneal Dialysis Solutions—— Netilmicin sulfate (Schering) 3 and 10 mg/L in peritoneal dialysis concentrate with dextrose 50% (Mc-Gaw) retained about 90% of its initial activity for seven hours and about 80% for 24 hours at room temperature as determined by microbiological assay (1044).

β-Lactam Antibiotics—— In common with other aminoglycoside antibiotics, netilmicin activity may be impaired by the β-lactam antibiotics (penicillins or cephalosporins) (4). This inactivation is dependent on concentration, temperature, and time of exposure.

Netilmicin sulfate 5 and 10 μg/ml dissolved in human serum and incubated with carbenicillin and ticarcillin 100 to 600 μg/ml at 37 °C demonstrated greater rates of netilmicin decomposition at the higher concentrations of the penicillins. In 24 hours, little or no loss of netilmicin activity occurred at 100 μg/ml but about a 25% loss occurred at 600 μg/ml of carbenicillin. Approximately 5% loss at 100 μg/ml to 60% loss at 600 μg/ml occurred in 72 hours with carbenicillin. Ticarcillin affected netilmicin less under these conditions. Little or no loss of netilmicin activity occurred at 100 μg/ml, but about a 17% loss occurred at 600 μg/ml in 72 hours (575).

Pickering and Rutherford evaluated several aminoglycosides combined with a number of penicillins. Gentamicin sulfate, netilmicin sulfate, and tobramycin sulfate 5 and 10 μg/ml and amikacin 10 and 20 μg/ml were combined in human serum with 125, 250, and 500 μg/ml of azlocillin, carbenicillin disodium, amdinocillin, mezlocillin, and piperacillin individually. Tobramycin and gentamicin sustained greater losses than netilmicin and amikacin at each of the penicillin concentrations. Significant decomposition of all aminoglycosides occurred in 24 hours at 37 °C at a penicillin concentration of 500 μg/ml. Tobramycin and gentamicin had losses of 40 to 60%, while 15 to 30% losses occurred for netilmicin. Amikacin sustained the least inactivation with losses of about 10 to 20%. At penicillin concentrations of 125 to 250 μg/ml, smaller losses of aminoglycosides were observed (68).

Several aminoglycosides were evaluated in combination with several penicillins. Gentamicin sulfate, netilmicin sulfate, and tobramycin sulfate 5 μg/ml were combined with carbenicillin disodium, azlocillin sodium, and mezlocillin sodium 50, 250, and 500 μg/ml in human plasma. Samples were evaluated over nine days at 27 and 37 °C. All of the aminoglycosides underwent significant inactivation during the evaluation. Aminoglycoside decomposition of 17 to 61% in 24 hours occurred at the higher two concentrations of penicillins—the highest inactivation was sustained by tobramycin and the lowest by netilmicin. Little if any aminoglycoside inactivation occurred at 50 μg/ml of penicillin. Carbenicillin caused a greater degree of aminoglycoside decomposition than did azlocillin or mezlocillin (616).

Flournoy noted the relative degree of inactivation of tobramycin, gentamicin, netilmicin, and amikacin 10 mg/L in serum when combined with carbenicillin 125 to 1000 mg/L over temperatures ranging from −20 to 42 °C. Tobramycin was more susceptible to inactivation than the others. Amikacin was the least susceptible, and gentamicin and netilmicin were similar in intermediate susceptibility to inactivation (617).

Although piperacillin sodium and aminoglycosides act synergistically and have been used successfully when recommended doses of each drug were administered, mixing piperacillin sodium directly in a syringe or infusion bottle with an aminoglycoside can result in substantial inactivation of the aminoglycoside (740).

The comparative inactivation of five aminoglycosides by seven β-lactam antibiotics in human serum at 37 °C was reported by Riff and Thomason. Amikacin, followed by netilmicin, had the lowest degree of inactivation; tobramycin sustained the most pronounced losses. Gentamicin and kanamycin were intermediate in the extent of losses. The six penicillins that were tested all produced aminoglycoside inactivation; the greatest extent of inactivation was caused by carbenicillin followed by ticarcillin, penicillin G, oxacillin, methicillin, and ampicillin, in approximate descending order. Cephalothin produced minimal inactivation (5 to 10% in 24 hours). The rate of inactivation could be reduced by storage at 4 °C and further reduced by storage at −20 °C. The authors suggested processing blood samples rapidly to avoid inaccurate serum determinations. Storage of specimens at low temperature until analysis may be helpful (1052).

Roberts et al. studied the stability of azlocillin sodium 500 mg/L combined with the aminoglycosides amikacin sulfate 20 mg/L, gentamicin sulfate 8 mg/L, and netilmicin sulfate 7.5 mg/L in peritoneal dialysis solution (Dianeal 1.36%) stored at 37 °C. No azlocillin sodium loss occurred by HPLC during the eight-hour study period. However, the aminoglycosides tested by the enzyme-multiplied immunoassay technique (EMIT) showed 10% losses in about six hours for gentamicin sulfate and netilmicin sulfate and in about 30 minutes for amikacin sulfate (1179).

Cefotetan disodium is stated to be physically incompatible with aminoglycosides (4), including netilmicin sulfate (283).

Cefotaxime sodium (Hoechst-Roussel) should not be mixed with aminoglycosides in the same solution, but they may be administered to the same patient separately (792).

The clinical significance of these interactions in patients appears to be confined primarily to those with renal failure (218; 334; 361; 364; 616; 847). Literature reports of greatly reduced aminoglycoside levels in such patients have appeared frequently (303; 365–367; 614; 615; 962). In addition, the interaction may be clinically important if assays for aminoglycoside levels in serum are sufficiently delayed (576; 618; 847; 1052).

Most authors believe that in vitro mixing of penicillins such as ticarcillin disodium with aminoglycoside antibiotics should be avoided but that clinical use of the drugs in combination can be of great value. It is generally recommended that the drugs be given separately in such combined therapy (157; 218; 222; 224; 361; 364; 368–370).

Heparin— A white precipitate may result from the administration of netilmicin sulfate through a heparinized intravenous cannula (976). Flushing heparin locks with sterile water for injection or sodium chloride 0.9% before and after administering drugs incompatible with heparin has been recommended (4).

NICARDIPINE HCL
AHFS 24:04

Cardene I.V.   **Wyeth-Ayerst**

Products— Nicardipine HCl (Wyeth-Ayerst) is available as a 2.5-mg/ml concentrate in 10-ml ampuls. Each milliliter also contains sorbitol 48 mg, citric acid monohydrate 0.525 mg, and sodium hydroxide 0.09 mg in water for injection. Additional citric acid and/or sodium hydroxide may have been added to adjust solution pH (2).

pH— Buffered to pH 3.5 (2).

Administration— Nicardipine HCl must be diluted for use. It is administered as a slow continuous intravenous infusion at a concentration of 0.1 mg/ml. The infusion is prepared by adding 10 ml of nicardipine HCl (25 mg) to 240 ml of compatible infusion solution, making 250 ml of a 0.1-mg/ml solution. If nicardipine HCl is administered via a peripheral vein, the infusion site should be changed every 12 hours to avoid venous irritation (2; 4).

Stability— Intact ampuls of the clear, yellow solution should be stored at controlled room temperature between 15 and 30 °C and protected from light. Elevated temperatures should be avoided (2).

Deliberate exposure of a 0.1-mg/ml nicardipine HCl solution to daylight resulted in about 8% loss in seven hours and 21% loss in 14 hours by HPLC analysis. The authors recommended that protection from light be considered for pharmaceutical dosage forms (2193).

Compatibility Information

Y-Site Injection Compatibility (1:1 Mixture)

Nicardipine HCl

Drug	Mfr	Conc	Mfr	Conc	Remarks	Ref	C/I
Diltiazem HCl	MMD	1 mg/ml[a]	WY	1 mg/ml[a]	Visually compatible for 4 hr at 27 °C	2062	C

Y-Site Injection Compatibility (1:1 Mixture) (Cont.)

Nicardipine HCl

Drug	Mfr	Conc	Mfr	Conc	Remarks	Ref	C/I
Dobutamine HCl	LI	4 mg/ml[a]	WY	1 mg/ml[a]	Visually compatible for 4 hr at 27 °C	2062	C
Dopamine HCl	AB	3.2 mg/ml[a]	WY	1 mg/ml[a]	Visually compatible for 4 hr at 27 °C	2062	C
Epinephrine HCl	AB	0.02 mg/ml[a]	WY	1 mg/ml[a]	Visually compatible for 4 hr at 27 °C	2062	C
Fentanyl citrate	ES	0.05 mg/ml	WY	1 mg/ml[a]	Visually compatible for 4 hr at 27 °C	2062	C
Furosemide	AMR	10 mg/ml	WY	1 mg/ml[a]	Precipitate forms immediately	2062	I
Heparin sodium	ES	100 units/ml[a]	WY	1 mg/ml[a]	Precipitate forms immediately	2062	I
Hydromorphone HCl	KN	1 mg/ml	WY	1 mg/ml[a]	Visually compatible for 4 hr at 27 °C	2062	C
Labetalol HCl	AH	2 mg/ml[a]	WY	1 mg/ml[a]	Visually compatible for 4 hr at 27 °C	2062	C
Lorazepam	WY	0.5 mg/ml[a]	WY	1 mg/ml[a]	Visually compatible for 4 hr at 27 °C	2062	C
Midazolam HCl	RC	2 mg/ml[a]	WY	1 mg/ml[a]	Visually compatible for 4 hr at 27 °C	2062	C
Milrinone lactate	SW	0.2 mg/ml[a]	WY	1 mg/ml[a]	Visually compatible for 4 hr at 27 °C	2062	C
Morphine sulfate	SCN	2 mg/ml[a]	WY	1 mg/ml[a]	Visually compatible for 4 hr at 27 °C	2062	C
Nitroglycerin	AB	0.4 mg/ml[a]	WY	1 mg/ml[a]	Visually compatible for 4 hr at 27 °C	2062	C
Norepinephrine bitartrate	AB	0.128 mg/ml[a]	WY	1 mg/ml[a]	Visually compatible for 4 hr at 27 °C	2062	C
Ranitidine HCl	GL	1 mg/ml[a]	WY	1 mg/ml[a]	Visually compatible for 4 hr at 27 °C	2062	C
Thiopental sodium	AB	25 mg/ml[b]	WY	1 mg/ml[a]	Precipitate forms immediately	2062	I
Vecuronium bromide	OR	1 mg/ml	WY	1 mg/ml[a]	Visually compatible for 4 hr at 27 °C	2062	C

[a]*Tested in dextrose 5% in water.*
[b]*Tested in sterile water for injection.*

Additional Compatibility Information

Infusion Solutions— The manufacturer states that nicardipine HCl is stable for 24 hours at room temperature diluted to a 0.1-mg/ml concentration in glass and PVC containers in the following infusion solutions (2):

> Dextrose 5% with potassium chloride 40 mEq

> Dextrose 5% in sodium chloride 0.45%
> Dextrose 5% in sodium chloride 0.9%
> Dextrose 5% in water
> Sodium chloride 0.45%
> Sodium chloride 0.9%

Nicardipine HCl is incompatible with Ringer's injection, lactated, and sodium bicarbonate 5% (2).

NITROGLYCERIN
AHFS 24:12

Products— Nitroglycerin injections are available in concentrations of 0.5 and 5 mg/ml (4). Care must be taken to ensure that the proper dilution and dosage are utilized.

Nitro-Bid (Hoechst Marion Roussel) is available as a 5-mg/ml concentration in 1-, 5-, and 10-ml vials. Each milliliter of solution also contains propylene glycol 45 mg in ethanol 70% (2).

Nitroglycerin injections must be diluted before use (2; 4).

Nitroglycerin (Abbott) is available premixed in dextrose 5% in water at concentrations of 100, 200, and 400 μg/ml in 250- and 500-ml containers. In addition, each milliliter contains propylene glycol 0.9, 1.8, and 3.6 mg, respectively. Nitric acid may be used to adjust the pH, if necessary (1-3/95).

pH— From 3 to 6.5 (4).

Osmotic Values— The osmolality of nitroglycerin 1 mg/ml was determined to be 281 mOsm/kg (1233). The osmolarities of the premixed infusion solutions in dextrose 5% in water (Abbott) are 264, 277, and 301 mOsm/L for the 100-, 200-, and 400-μg/ml concentrations, respectively (1-3/95).

Administration— Nitroglycerin injection is administered by intravenous infusion after dilution in dextrose 5% in water or sodium chloride 0.9% contained in glass bottles, using an infusion control device. The use of filters should be avoided. Various concentrations and administration rates are utilized, depending on the fluid requirements of the patient and the duration of therapy. An initial concentration of 50 to 100 μg/ml, with adjustment to the concentration if necessary, has been recommended. The concentration should not exceed 400 μg/ml (2; 4).

Because of nitroglycerin sorption into PVC plastic, dosing is higher with standard PVC administration sets and should be reduced when nonabsorbing administration sets are used (2; 4).

Inaccurate nitroglycerin dosing may occur with nonabsorbing high-density polyethylene plastic administration sets. Such tubing is less pliable than PVC and may not work well with some infusion control devices designed for PVC tubing, resulting in overinfusion (729–731; 1120).

Stability— Nitroglycerin injections are practically colorless and stable in the intact containers. The solutions are not explosive. Storage should be at controlled room temperature; the containers should be protected from freezing (2; 4). Exposure to light, even high intensity light, does not adversely affect nitroglycerin stability (506; 510; 928; 930; 1941). Dilution of the nitroglycerin injections with dextrose 5% in water or sodium chloride 0.9% in glass containers results in physically and chemically stable solutions for 48 hours at room temperature and seven days under refrigeration (4).

pH Effects— The rate of nitroglycerin hydrolysis becomes significant at low pH values and is also quite rapid in alkaline solutions (933). In neutral to weakly acidic solutions, the drug is stable. No loss was observed over 136 days at room temperature at pH 3 to 5 (1072).

Filtration— Some filters absorb nitroglycerin and should be avoided (2). In one study, a filter material specially treated with a proprietary agent was evaluated for a possible reduction in nitroglycerin binding. Nitroglycerin (Abbott) 62.5 mg/250 ml in dextrose 5% in water and sodium chloride 0.9% was run through an administration set with a treated 0.22-μm cellulose ester inline filter at a rate of 3 ml/min. Cumulative nitroglycerin losses of less than 6% occurred from 200 ml of either solution. However, equilibrium binding studies showed no significant differences in drug affinity between treated and untreated filter material in either solution (904). All Ivex integral filter and extension sets (Abbott) currently use the treated filter material (1074).

Repackaging in Syringes— Nitroglycerin concentrate 5 mg/ml from four manufacturers (Abbott, DuPont, Goldline, Marion) was filled as 10 ml in 10-ml glass syringes (Becton-Dickinson) and in 10-ml (Becton-Dickinson) and 12-ml (Monoject) polypropylene plastic syringes. No loss of nitroglycerin content by HPLC analysis occurred in 23 hours when stored at 25 °C protected from light. Mean nitroglycerin concentrations were greater than 99% and were the same for both the glass and plastic syringes (2055).

Sorption to Plastics— Nitroglycerin readily undergoes sorption to many soft plastics (943), especially PVC which is commonly used to make infusion solution bags and intravenous tubing.

Hard solid plastics such as polyethylene and polypropylene generally do not absorb nitroglycerin. Consequently, it is recommended that only infusion solution containers made from glass or a plastic known to be compatible with nitroglycerin (i.e., polyolefin) be used for mixing infusions.

To circumvent the significant loss to PVC tubing, use of the special high-density polyethylene administration sets provided by the various nitroglycerin injection manufacturers is recommended. Nitroglycerin is not significantly sorbed to these special sets, but the rate of loss to conventional PVC sets is significant (40 to 80%), although not constant nor self-limiting. Many factors including flow rate, concentration, and length of the set affect the extent of sorption. The greatest amount of sorption occurs early in the infusion. A slow rate of flow and long tubing length increase the loss. Simple calculations or corrections cannot be applied to this complex phenomenon to determine or control the actual amount of nitroglycerin delivered through PVC tubing (2; 4).

Numerous articles have described or evaluated nitroglycerin sorption characteristics.

Sturek et al. reported the stability of a 0.4-mg/ml solution in sterile water for injection prepared from solubilized sublingual tablets. The solution was sterilized by filtration through a 0.22-μm filter and stored in 10-ml glass ampuls or rubber-stoppered vials at room temperature. While the authors did not feel an adequate prediction of the stability of aqueous nitroglycerin solutions could be made from their data, they did note a significantly increased rate of loss of nitroglycerin in the rubber-stoppered vials. About 10% of the nitroglycerin was lost over eight days in glass ampuls, while about 25% was lost in the vials stored in the inverted position. The solution also appeared to reach an equilibrium after four weeks of storage in ampuls or vials at about 75 or 55%, respectively. The presence or absence of light had no apparent effect on the loss of the drug (506).

These authors also found no difference in the stability of nitroglycerin 46.5 mg/100 ml in dextrose 5% in water or sodium chloride 0.9% in 500-ml glass bottles. A loss of about 13% was noted in 50 hours at room temperature (506).

A profound impact of the container size and type on the loss of nitroglycerin was reported in this article, however. Compared with the 13% loss mentioned above, the same solutions in 150-ml PVC bags exhibited an 83.5% loss. At the other end of the spectrum, a 5.35-mg/10 ml solution in 10-ml glass ampuls showed about a 3% loss. The differences were attributed to variations in the amount of sorption occurring among the different containers. The authors recommended the use of only glass containers for injections of nitroglycerin (506).

This work supports other reports that indicated substantial sorption of nitroglycerin by plastics.

Crouthamel et al. prepared nitroglycerin 50 μg/ml in dextrose 5% in water in PVC bags and glass bottles. Using HPLC analysis, they determined that nearly half of the drug had disappeared from solution within two hours when stored in PVC bags. In glass bottles, little change was noted. Because degradation products were not observed, it was concluded that sorption of nitroglycerin to the plastic was occurring. Upon testing nitroglycerin solutions infused through PVC infusion sets (Travenol, 2.4 m), a similar effect was noted. At a rate of 2 ml/min from a glass bottle, a 20% loss of nitroglycerin was noted (508).

Cossum et al. noted this effect of infusion sets on nitroglycerin 0.01% in dextrose 5% in water in glass bottles. The nitroglycerin content decreased rapidly during the first hour and then reached a plateau. The level of the plateau varied from 20 to 70% of the initial amount for flow rates from 0.07 to 0.91 ml/min, respectively. However, little nitroglycerin was lost from the solution when a glass syringe pump system fitted with a high-density polyethylene cannula was used to deliver a constant flow rate of 0.05 ml/min (509).

Boylan et al. reported a 50% loss of nitroglycerin in 24 hours at room temperature from a solution stored in PVC bags that originally contained 32 μg/ml in dextrose 5% in water. Potency loss was negligible upon storing the solution in glass bottles (510).

McNiff et al. found little or no loss in nitroglycerin solutions prepared from sublingual tablets and stored in glass bottles. The solutions varied in initial concentration from about 35 to 87 μg/ml in dextrose 5% in water and sodium chloride 0.9% and were stored in closed-system or open-airway type bottles for about 70 days at room temperature or under refrigeration. However, solutions of about 35 μg/ml in dextrose 5% in water in PVC bags exhibited approximately 10% loss during the first hour. Further, solutions stored at room temperature exhibited a greater loss of drug after seven days (55%) than those stored under refrigeration (30%). The drug lost in the PVC containers could be recovered by methanol extraction over 13 days, indicating that a reversible adsorption phenomenon was occurring (503).

The work of Ludwig and Ueda, however, did not support a difference between glass and plastic containers. Using solutions of approximately 10 μg/ml in dextrose 5% in water, they found essentially similar rates of drug loss for both glass bottles and PVC bags. About 10% was lost in one hour and about 25% in five hours at room temperature. Refrigeration of the solutions resulted in about a 20% loss in five hours in both (511). However, in light of both previous and subsequent work, this anomalous result is questionable.

Yuen et al. evaluated the type of sorption that occurs. Aqueous solutions of nitroglycerin in concentrations of 61 to 473 μg/ml were tested with PVC test strips from Viaflex bags. The authors believed that their results showed that the nitroglycerin loss was primarily an absorption or partitioning process into the matrix of the plastic. However, the results did not rule out some adsorption (723).

Baaske et al. evaluated the extent of nitroglycerin sorption to various filters, sets, and containers. Filtration of 250 ml of a 485-μg/ml aqueous solution through three different 142-mm, 0.2-μm filters was performed. A loss of 55% resulted with the Gelman GA filter composed of cellulose triacetate. Losses of only 5% occurred with a Millipore GS filter (a mixture of cellulose acetate and cellulose nitrate), and 2% losses occurred with a Gelman Tuffryn filter (a high-temperature aromatic polymer) (724).

Baaske et al. also found extensive sorption to PVC bags (Travenol) from nitroglycerin 50 μg/ml in dextrose 5% in water and sodium chloride 0.9%. The sorption process was quite rapid and interfered with obtaining accurate time-zero assays. After 24 hours, the solutions had lost 43 to 45% at 4 °C and 54 to 64% at 25 °C, indicating that increases in temperature also increased the loss of nitroglycerin. Varying the PVC bag size and, therefore, surface area impacted on the loss of nitroglycerin from solutions. The larger the volume of the bags, the slower was the rate of sorption. However, over a seven-day period, the total amount of drug lost increased with the increasing size of the PVC bag. The authors stated that neither small nor large PVC bags of infusion solutions are suitable for the infusion of nitroglycerin (724).

Eight different intravenous infusion sets were tested with a nitroglycerin 100-μg/ml aqueous solution at a flow rate of 1 ml/min. Four of the sets were obtained from the United States and four came from Europe, but all were believed to be manufactured from PVC. All of the sets caused a substantial fall in the amount of nitroglycerin delivered, to about 50 to 70% of the nominal concentration during the first 25 minutes. After that time, the rate of loss gradually became less and delivery of approximately 60 to 90% of the nom-

inal concentration occurred after about 120 minutes of infusion. The authors indicated that this result was consistent with an initial rapid adsorption which soon saturated available sites. This was then followed by an absorption into the plastic matrix at a slower rate. Differences in sorption characteristics between sets were attributed to differences in plastic formulations, tubing length and size, and composition of the drip chamber (724). A theoretical treatment of these data and a model consisting of surface adsorption followed by partitioning into the plastic have been developed (944; 945).

The rate of infusion (and, therefore, the contact time with the PVC tubing) also is an important factor. Delivered amounts of nitroglycerin were much lower at a flow rate of 0.5 ml/min (20 to 30%) than at 2 ml/min (60 to 70%). The authors noted that small adjustments in flow rates could greatly increase or decrease the concentration of the solution delivered to the patient. Moreover, control of the flow rate did not actually provide accurate control of the amount of nitroglycerin delivered through PVC tubing. It was speculated that this result could be a factor in the variability of responses (724).

Roberts et al. noted significant sorption to PVC bags and tubing and, in addition, to cellulose propionate burette chambers from Buretrol sets. In static experiments with each, nitroglycerin from a 200-μg/ml solution in water, sodium chloride 0.9%, or dextrose 5% in water was initially lost rapidly but then leveled and became constant, indicating sorption to the plastic. The most rapid and extensive sorption occurred with the tubing, which yielded only 8% of the initial amount of nitroglycerin after five hours. Roberts et al. also confirmed that the loss of nitroglycerin from solution is related to the surface area of plastic in contact with the solution. For the PVC bags, nitroglycerin was lost at a more rapid rate from smaller volumes. However, the rate of loss appeared to be independent of the nitroglycerin concentration (725).

In addition, Roberts et al. simulated infusions of nitroglycerin 200 μg/ml in sodium chloride 0.9% from glass containers through Buretrol sets. The delivered concentration of nitroglycerin dropped to about 50 to 60% of the initial concentration during the first hour of infusion. Thereafter, the delivered concentration gradually increased until nitroglycerin accumulated in the plastic to such an extent that sorption from the solution diminished. Flow rate was an important factor in determining the amount of delivered nitroglycerin. The slower flow rates provided the greatest contact time with the plastic and delivered the lowest concentrations of nitroglycerin during the first 24 hours. Given sufficient time, the delivered concentration eventually returned to the initial concentration with any flow rate. Also, the total cumulative amount of drug that was sorbed was independent of flow rate (725).

One comparison of nitroglycerin sorption characteristics by Amann et al. involved glass, PVC, and polyolefin containers. Nitroglycerin (American Critical Care) 50 μg/ml in both dextrose 5% in water and sodium chloride 0.9% was tested for 48 hours at 25 and 4 °C in containers made of the three different materials. Nitroglycerin in both glass and polyolefin containers remained stable for the study period, exhibiting less than a 6% loss. However, in the PVC bags, losses of 38 to 44% at 4 °C and of up to 68 to 70% at 25 °C occurred. Polyolefin containers appeared to work equally as well as glass containers for nitroglycerin administration (721).

Christiansen et al. tested the delivered concentration of nitroglycerin from a 100-μg/ml solution in dextrose 5% in water in glass, polyethylene, and PVC containers. They found a rapid fall during the first hour, followed by a continual decline in nitroglycerin content to about 65% of the initial amount after eight hours of storage in the PVC bag. In the glass container, no loss was apparent; in the polyethylene containers, about a 5% loss occurred during the first two hours with no further decline thereafter. These authors also confirmed that the concentration of nitroglycerin delivered through an infusion set declines rapidly during the first hour to about 50% of the initial amount and then begins to increase gradually until equilibrium is reached after about four hours. Attempts to presaturate the tubing by rinsing it with a nitroglycerin solution yielded a more quickly achieved equilibrium (within one hour) but still only delivered about half of the intended amount. The authors also confirmed the greater extent of sorption at slower flow rates (726).

Sokoloski et al. attempted to define the mechanism and quantitate the rate of sorption to PVC intravenous infusion tubing. The mechanism was described as a highly complex adsorption process. Complicating factors include the existence of different solid forms of nitroglycerin, temperature, and the complex composition of the plastic, including not only PVC but also plasticizers, fillers, and other ingredients, as well as its complex surface characteristics. Therefore, precise quantitative kinetic and equilibrium characterization was not possible. However, the rate of nitroglycerin sorption by PVC tubing was quite rapid. At 21 °C, the observed half-life to the attainment of equilibrium with nitroglycerin solutions was 2.8 minutes (727).

The lack of significant sorption of nitroglycerin by high-density polyethylene has been observed (509; 726). An administration set made of polyethylene (Tridilset) was tested by Baaske et al. Evaluation of the delivered concentration of nitroglycerin 100 µg/ml in sodium chloride 0.9% showed little or no sorption at flow rates of 0.2, 0.6, and 1 ml/min over three hours. When conventional PVC sets were used, variable and unpredictable amounts of nitroglycerin were delivered, although the greatest losses occurred at the slower rates. When a 24-hour infusion of the 100-µg/ml solution (flow rate of 0.17 ml/min) through polyethylene tubing was evaluated, delivered concentrations were 94% or greater at all time intervals (728).

Although the presaturation of PVC intravenous infusion sets has been suggested (935), other work shows that such attempts complicate the titration of nitroglycerin infusions, leading to greater variation in the delivered amount of nitroglycerin (936).

Kowaluk et al. also found negligible nitroglycerin sorption using a polyethylene administration set (Tridilset). Nitroglycerin 50 mg/L in sodium chloride 0.9% in a glass bottle was delivered at 1 ml/min through the set over eight hours at 15 to 20 °C (769).

The sorption of nitroglycerin 200 mg/L in sodium chloride 0.9% was evaluated in 100-ml PVC infusion bags (Travenol). After eight hours at 20 to 24 °C, 54% of the nitroglycerin was lost. Nitroglycerin showed a negligible (less than 3%) loss if the aqueous solution was stored in polypropylene infusion bags (770).

Plastic syringes having polypropylene barrels and polyethylene plungers (Pharma-Plast, AHS Australia) and all-glass containers were compared in an investigation of the possible sorption of nitroglycerin. After 24 hours of storage of aqueous nitroglycerin solutions (concentrations unspecified), no drug loss was found in either the plastic syringes or glass containers. The authors indicated that these plastic syringes could be substituted for glass syringes for use with syringe pumps (782).

Yliruusi et al. found a negligible loss of nitroglycerin to glass or polyethylene containers from 90-mg/L concentrations in dextrose 5% in water or sodium chloride 0.9%. However, in PVC containers, drug losses of around 28% occurred in 24 hours at 25 °C (797).

Scheife et al. found nitroglycerin losses of 38 to 44% from solutions of 200 mg/L in sodium chloride 0.9% in PVC bags after 52 hours at 29 °C. Losses were reduced to 14% when the solutions

were stored at 6 °C. Similar solutions stored in glass bottles exhibited no loss of nitroglycerin. Losses to PVC tubing during simulated infusion ranged up to 50%. However, two one-minute exposures of a 1-mg/ml nitroglycerin solution to a 50-ml plastic syringe resulted in no loss (930).

Ingram and Miller reported no loss of nitroglycerin from 50- and 200-µg/ml solutions after storage for five hours in both glass and polypropylene (Monoject) syringes. However, PVC bags and tubing and cellulose propionate drip chambers caused nitroglycerin losses of 40 to 80%. Slower infusion rates caused greater decrements in the nitroglycerin concentration (931).

Using a solution of nitroglycerin 0.625 mg/ml in dextrose 5% in water, Mathot et al. also noted no nitroglycerin loss from a delivery system consisting of a syringe pump, polypropylene syringe, and polyethylene tubing. This result was contrasted with a PVC bag and tubing system in which losses of up to 75% were found. When silicone rubber tubing was tested, only 14% of the nitroglycerin was delivered (932).

Cavello and Bonn demonstrated the difference in sorption of nitroglycerin by PVC and polyethylene tubing. At slow rates of infusion through PVC, losses of up to 60% were observed. Polyethylene tubing did not show this reduction in concentration (934).

The comparative sorption of nitroglycerin 50 mg/500 ml in sodium chloride 0.9% from PVC and polybutadiene (PBD) administration sets (Avon Medicals, U.K.) has been reported. The nitroglycerin admixture in glass bottles was run through PVC administration sets, with and without a cellulose propionate burette chamber, and through PBD sets, with and without a methacrylate butadiene styrene (MBS) burette chamber. At a flow rate of 1 ml/min, the delivered concentration was about 50% of the expected amount initially, climbing to about 70 to 75% after four hours. Slowing the flow rate to 0.5 ml/min decreased the delivered concentration at four hours to about 60 to 65%. If a cellulose propionate burette chamber was used to prepare the admixture, 10 to 15% sorption occurred in the burette. Conversely, use of the PBD set, with or without the MBS burette chamber, resulted in no detectable loss of nitroglycerin potency (1027).

Nix et al. reported on a solution of nitroglycerin 50 mg/500 ml in dextrose 5% in water in glass bottles. When the solution was infused at rates of 6, 12, and 24 ml/hr through PVC sets over 24 hours, delivered nitroglycerin was about 42, 63, and 76%, respectively. Polyethylene administration sets delivered about 97% in 24 hours at all of the infusion rates (1121).

Schaber et al. compared the sorption of nitroglycerin, from a solution of 100 mg/L in dextrose 5% in water, to sets of plain PVC tubing and a set lined with 87% of polyethylene/ethylene vinyl acetate (AVI 290). Nitroglycerin was absorbed by all sets, but the extent of sorption was considerably less with the set lined with polyethylene/ethylene vinyl acetate. At a rate of 12 ml/hr, the delivered concentration dropped to about 50% at about 90 minutes and then increased to about 70 to 80% over 24 hr through the lined set. The delivered concentration through the plain PVC sets initially fell to about 20% at 90 minutes and then increased to about 25 to 50% over 24 hours. Increasing the flow rate to 60 ml/hr and flushing the sets with nitroglycerin solution immediately prior to use increased the amount of drug delivered (1122).

Martens et al. reported that nitroglycerin 100 µg/ml in sodium chloride 0.9% in PVC containers exhibited a 10% loss in one hour and a 51% loss in 24 hr at 21 °C due to sorption. Only a 2% loss occurred in glass bottles and a 5% loss occurred in polyethylene-lined laminated bags in 24 hours under the study conditions (1392).

DeRudder et al. evaluated several infusion sets and burettes, composed of various plastic materials, for the sorption of nitroglycerin from a solution of 250 µg/ml in dextrose 5% in water. In cellulose propionate (Travenol) and polystyrolbutadiene (Braun) burettes, losses of about 70 and 50%, respectively, occurred in five hours; in a high density polyethylene burette (Miramed), no loss was observed. Similarly, PVC infusion sets from various manufacturers showed losses of about 50 to 70% when run at 15 and 3 ml/min (1512).

Tracy et al. compared the nitroglycerin (Parke-Davis) losses from solutions of 50, 125, and 200 µg/ml in sodium chloride 0.9% in glass bottles run through PVC sets and polyethylene-lined administration sets (IMED) over 24 hours at 24 °C at 12 and 60 ml/hr. Nitroglycerin sorption losses to the PVC sets were approximately 40%; losses to the polyethylene-lined sets were about 2% (1510).

Nitroglycerin (DuPont) (concentration unspecified) was filled into 3-ml plastic syringes (Becton-Dickinson, Sherwood Monoject, and Terumo) and stored at −20, 4, and 25 °C in the dark. Nitroglycerin losses by spectroscopy in one day ranged from 10 to 15% at 25 °C, to 2 to 3% at 4 °C, to 2% or less at −20 °C. Long-term storage for seven days at 4 °C and 30 days at −20 °C resulted in losses of 5 to 7% and 2% or less, respectively. The losses were presumably due to sorption to surfaces and/or the elastomeric plunger (1562).

Nitroglycerin (DuPont) 50 mg/50 ml in dextrose 5% in water exhibited no change in appearance and about a 3.6% loss in potency by HPLC when stored in 60-ml plastic syringes (Becton-Dickinson) for 24 hours at 25 °C (1579).

Loucas et al. determined the effect of the diluent and ionic strength on nitroglycerin sorption from a 0.4-mg/ml solution delivered at 100 ml/hr through a PVC set. During the initial 10 minutes, the greatest losses (about 40%) were observed when dextrose 5% in water was the diluent; slightly lower losses (about 35%) occurred from a sodium chloride 0.9% solution. After 18 minutes, the pattern reversed, with higher losses for sodium chloride 0.9% and lower losses for dextrose 5% in water. When sodium chloride solutions of 0.25, 0.9, and 5% were the diluents, the losses appeared as an inverse function of ionic strength. The highest losses occurred with the 0.25% solution and the lowest with the 5% solution (1511).

Nitroglycerin 0.5 mg/ml was delivered at 5 ml per hour by syringe pump through Terumo administration sets 100 cm in length with an internal diameter of 2.1 mm. HPLC analysis of the effluent found about 90% loss during the first hour, gradually changing to about 70% loss over eight hours (2143).

In addition to PVC bags and infusion tubing, nitroglycerin has been demonstrated to undergo similar sorption to PVC pulmonary artery catheters (937) and central venous pressure catheters (Intracath, Deseret) (938), a polyurethane sponge used to defoam blood in a bubble oxygenator (939), a silicone rubber membrane in a membrane oxygenator (940), an infusion pump cassette (Accuset C-924, IMED) (941), and silicone rubber microbore intravenous infusion tubing (942).

Nitroglycerin (Orion) 100 µg/ml in sodium chloride 0.9% exhibited no loss due to sorption by HPLC analysis in 120 hours at 21 °C in glass bottles and polypropylene trilayer bags (Softbag, Orion). However, about a 75% loss due to sorption occurred under these conditions in PVC bags (1796).

However, the clinical importance of the sorption to PVC has been questioned because nitroglycerin administration is titrated to clinical response, not in a fixed dosage (1120; 1123; 2015; 2016; 2054). Young et al. reported 25 to 35% loss to PVC tubing at rates of nitroglycerin administration of 80 and 60 µg/min, respectively. Polyethylene tubing delivered essentially 100% of the nitroglycerin. Nevertheless, there was no statistically significant difference in physiologic response in patients when a variety of parameters were evaluated. The authors concluded that the type of tubing used does not influence the ultimate hemodynamic responses significantly, because even the PVC delivered a significant amount of the drug. The authors advised that physiologic endpoints be monitored in patients on intravenous nitroglycerin (1120).

Similar results were reported by McCollom et al. (2015), Altavela et al. (2016), and Haas et al. (2054). Adequate clinical response was achieved using PVC containers and tubing. However, changes in patient hemodynamic status could occur if containers for nitroglycerin infusions were changed during the treatment course; switching from PVC to glass or vice versa could require substantial adjustment in the rate of administration to achieve a similar clinical response (2016).

Compatibility Information

Solution Compatibility

Nitroglycerin

Solution	Mfr	Mfr	Conc/L	Remarks	Ref	C/I
Dextrose 5% in Ringer's injection, lactated	MG	ACC	200 and 400 mg	Physically compatible with little or no loss after 28 days at 4 °C and room temperature in glass and polyolefin containers	928	C
Dextrose 5% in sodium chloride 0.45%	MG	ACC	200 and 400 mg	Physically compatible with little or no loss after 28 days at 4 °C and room temperature in glass and polyolefin containers	928	C
Dextrose 5% in sodium chloride 0.9%	MG	ACC	200 and 400 mg	Physically compatible with little or no loss after 28 days at 4 °C and room temperature in glass and polyolefin containers	928	C
Dextrose 5% in water		LI	32 mg	Negligible loss over 24 hr at room temperature in glass bottles	510	C
		[a]	100 mg	Less than 1% loss of nitroglycerin in 24 hr at room temperature in glass bottles	509	C

Solution Compatibility (Cont.)

Nitroglycerin

Solution	Mfr	Mfr	Conc/L	Remarks	Ref	C/I
	TR		50 mg	Little change in 2 hr in glass containers	508	C
	TR	a	465 mg	About 8% loss in 24 hr and 13% in 50 hr at room temperature in glass containers	506	C
		a	35 to 87 mg	Little or no loss after 70 days at room temperature or under refrigeration in glass bottles	503	C
	MG	ACC	50 mg	0 to 3% loss in 48 hr at 4 and 25 °C in glass bottles	721	C
	MG	ACC	50 mg	1 to 6% loss in 48 hr at 4 and 25 °C in polyolefin containers	721	C
	MG	a	50 mg	Nitroglycerin stable for 48 hr at 4 and 25 °C in glass containers	724	C
			100 mg	Little or no loss in 8 hr in glass containers	726	C
	ON	a	90 mg	No precipitate and negligible drug loss in 24 hr at 25 °C in glass and polyethylene containers	797	C
	MG	ACC	200 and 400 mg	Physically compatible with little or no loss after 28 days at 4 °C and room temperature in glass and polyolefin containers	928	C
	TR	a	200 mg	No loss of nitroglycerin after 52 hr at 29 °C in glass bottles	930	C
			200 to 800 mg	Physically compatible with 4% or less loss in 24 hr in glass bottles exposed to light	1412	C
			250 mg	3% or less loss in 24 hr at 6, 20, and 40 °C in glass containers exposed to light or in the dark	1512	C
	TR	LI	32 mg	Approximately 50% loss in 24 hr at room temperature in PVC containers	510	I
	TR		50 mg	Almost 50% loss in 2 hr in PVC containers	508	I
	TR	a	465 mg	Over 50% loss in 8 hr and over 83% in 50 hr at room temperature in PVC containers	506	I
		a	35 mg	Approximately 10% loss in 1 hr in PVC bags. In 7 days, 55% loss at room temperature and 30% under refrigeration	503	I
	TR	ACC	50 mg	Rapid loss in PVC bags with approximately 44% loss in 48 hr at 4 °C and about 70% loss at 25 °C	721	I
	TR	a	50 mg	Approximately 43% loss at 4 °C and 64% at 25 °C in 24 hr in PVC bags	724	I
	TR	a	100 and 500 mg	Approximately 50% loss in 24 hr at 20 to 24 °C in PVC bags	725	I
	TR		100 mg	Approximately 20% loss in 1 hr and 35% in 8 hr in PVC bags	726	I
		a	90 mg	No precipitate but 10% potency loss in 3 hr and 27% loss in 24 hr at 25 °C in PVC containers	797	I
	BA[b]	AMR	800 mg	No nitroglycerin loss by HPLC in 24 hr at 23 °C	2085	C
Ringer's injection, lactated	MG	ACC	200 and 400 mg	Physically compatible with little or no loss after 28 days at 4 °C and room temperature in glass and polyolefin containers	928	C
Sodium chloride 0.45%	MG	ACC	200 and 400 mg	Physically compatible with little or no loss after 28 days at 4 °C and room temperature in glass and polyolefin containers	928	C
Sodium chloride 0.9%	TR	a	465 mg	About 8% loss in 24 hr and 13% in 50 hr at room temperature in glass containers	506	C

Solution Compatibility (Cont.)

Nitroglycerin

Solution	Mfr	Mfr	Conc/L	Remarks	Ref	C/I
		a	35 to 87 mg	Little or no loss after 70 days of storage at room temperature or under refrigeration in glass bottles	503	C
	MG	ACC	50 mg	Approximately 5% loss in 48 hr at 4 and 25 °C in glass bottles	721	C
	MG	ACC	50 mg	No loss in 48 hr at 4 and 25 °C in polyolefin containers	721	C
		a	200 mg	No loss in 24 hr and about 5% loss in 3 months in glass bottles stored at room temperature or under refrigeration	722	C
		a	3.6 to 95 mg	Little or no loss in 48 hr at 35 °C in glass flasks	723	C
		a	0.2 mg	About 10% loss in 24 hr and 13% in 48 hr at 35 °C in glass flasks	723	C
	MG	a	50 mg	Nitroglycerin stable for 48 hr at 4 and 25 °C in glass containers	724	C
	ON	a	90 mg	No precipitate and 2 to 3% drug loss in 24 hr at 25 °C in glass and polyethylene containers	797	C
	MG	ACC	200 and 400 mg	Physically compatible with little or no loss after 28 days at 4 °C and room temperature in glass and polyolefin containers	928	C
	TR	a	200 mg	No loss of nitroglycerin after 52 hr at 29 °C in glass bottles	930	C
			200 to 800 mg	Physically compatible with 8% or less loss in 24 hr in glass bottles exposed to light	1412	C
			100 mg	Physically compatible with 2% loss in glass bottles and 5% loss in polyethylene-lined bags in 24 hr at 21 °C in the dark	1392	C
			250 mg	4% loss at 6 °C and 7% loss at 40 °C in 6 hr in glass bottles; no further loss in 24 hr	1512	C
	TR	a	465 mg	Over 50% loss in 8 hr and over 83% in 50 hr at room temperature in PVC containers	506	I
	TR	ACC	50 mg	Rapid loss in PVC bags with approximately 38% loss in 48 hr at 4 °C and about 68% at 25 °C	721	I
	TR	a	50 mg	Approximately 45% loss at 4 °C and 54% at 25 °C in 24 hr in PVC bags	724	I
	TR	a	100 and 500 mg	Approximately 50% loss in 24 hr at 20 to 24 °C in PVC bags	725	I
		a	90 mg	No precipitate but 10% potency loss in 3 hr and 28% loss in 24 hr at 25 °C in PVC containers	797	I
	TR	a	200 mg	38 to 44% nitroglycerin loss in 8 hr at 29 °C in PVC bags. At 6 °C, 14% loss in 8 hr	930	I
			100 mg	10% loss in 1 hr and 51% loss in 24 hr at 21 °C in PVC containers in the dark	1392	I
		PD	50, 125, 200 mg	About 14% loss in 24 hr at 24 °C in glass bottles	1510	I
	ON	ON	100 mg	Visually compatible with no loss by UV and HPLC in 24 hr at 21 °C in glass and polypropylene trilayer containers	1796	C
	ON	ON	100 mg	Visually compatible but 50% loss in 24 hr and 75% loss in 120 hr by HPLC at 21 °C in PVC bags due to sorption	1796	I

Solution Compatibility (Cont.)

Nitroglycerin

Solution	Mfr	Mfr	Conc/L	Remarks	Ref	C/I
Sodium lactate ⅙ M	MG	ACC	200 and 400 mg	Physically compatible with little or no loss after 28 days at 4 °C and room temperature in glass and polyolefin containers	928	**C**

[a]An extemporaneous preparation was tested.
[b]Tested in PVC containers.

Additive Compatibility

Nitroglycerin

Drug	Mfr	Conc/L	Mfr	Conc/L	Test Soln	Remarks	Ref	C/I
Alteplase	GEN	0.5 g	ACC	400 mg	D5W, NS	Visually compatible with 2% or less alteplase clot-lysis activity loss in 24 hr at 25 °C	1856	**C**
Aminophylline	IX	1 g	ACC	400 mg	D5W[a]	Physically compatible with 4% nitroglycerin loss in 24 hr and 6% loss in 48 hr at 23 °C. Aminophylline not tested	929	**C**
	IX	1 g	ACC	400 mg	NS[a]	Physically compatible with no nitroglycerin loss in 24 hr and 5% loss in 48 hr at 23 °C. Aminophylline not tested	929	**C**
Bretylium tosylate	ACC	10 g	ACC	400 mg	D5W, NS[a]	Physically compatible with little or no nitroglycerin loss in 48 hr at 23 °C. Bretylium not tested	929	**C**
	ACC	10 g	ACC	100 mg	D5S[a]	Physically compatible and both drugs chemically stable for 48 hr at room temperature and 7 days at 4 °C	522	**C**
	ACC	10 g	ACC	100 mg	D5S[b]	Physically compatible and bretylium chemically stable for 48 hr at room temperature and 7 days at 4 °C. 40% loss of nitroglycerin at room temperature and 10% loss at 4 °C in 24 hr due to sorption to PVC	522	**I**
Cibenzoline succinate		2 g	ACC	500 mg	D5W, NS	Physically compatible for 24 hr at 25 °C by visual and microscopic examination	1182	**C**
Dobutamine HCl	LI	1 g	AB	120 mg	D5W, NS	Physically compatible for 24 hr at 21 °C	812	**C**
	LI	500 mg	ACC	100 mg	D5S	Chemically stable with no loss of either drug after 24 hr at 25 °C. Pale pink color developed after 4 hr	990	**C**
Dobutamine HCl with sodium nitroprusside		2 to 8 g 200 to 800 mg		200 to 800 mg	D5W[a]	Pale pink discoloration with small amount of dark brown precipitate and 11 to 19% sodium nitroprusside loss in 24 hr exposed to light	1412	**I**
Dobutamine HCl with sodium nitroprusside		2 to 8 g 200 to 800 mg		200 to 800 mg	NS[a]	Pale pink discoloration with all drugs remaining stable for 24 hr exposed to light. Not more than 8% loss for either drug	1412	**C**
Dopamine HCl	ACC	800 mg	ACC	400 mg	D5W, NS[a]	Physically compatible with little or no nitroglycerin loss in 48 hr at 23 °C. Dopamine not tested	929	**C**

Additive Compatibility (Cont.)

Nitroglycerin

Drug	Mfr	Conc/L	Mfr	Conc/L	Test Soln	Remarks	Ref	C/I
Enalaprilat	MSD	12 mg	DU	200 mg	D5W[a]	Visually compatible with about 4% enalaprilat loss by HPLC in 24 hr at room temperature under fluorescent light. Nitroglycerin not tested	1572	C
Furosemide	HO	1 g	ACC	400 mg	D5W[a]	Physically compatible with no nitroglycerin loss in 48 hr at 23 °C. Furosemide not tested	929	C
	HO	1 g	ACC	400 mg	NS[a]	Physically compatible with 3% nitroglycerin loss in 48 hr at 23 °C. Furosemide not tested	929	C
Hydralazine HCl	CI	1 g	ACC	400 mg	D5W[a]	Deep yellow color produced. 4% nitroglycerin loss in 48 hr at 23 °C. Hydralazine not tested	929	I
	CI	1 g	ACC	400 mg	NS[a]	Pale yellow color produced. No nitroglycerin loss in 48 hr at 23 °C. Hydralazine not tested.	929	I
Lidocaine HCl	IMS	4 g	ACC	400 mg	D5W, NS[a]	Physically compatible with no nitroglycerin loss in 48 hr at 23 °C. Lidocaine not tested	929	C
Phenytoin sodium	PD	1 g	ACC	400 mg	D5W, NS[a]	Phenytoin crystals produced in 24 hr. 3 to 4% nitroglycerin loss in 24 hr and 9% loss in 48 hr at 23 °C. Phenytoin not tested	929	I
Verapamil HCl	KN	80 mg	ACC	100 mg	D5W, NS	Physically compatible for 24 hr	764	C

[a]*Tested in glass containers.*
[b]*Tested in PVC containers.*

Drugs in Syringe Compatibility

Nitroglycerin

Drug (in syringe)	Mfr	Amt	Mfr	Amt	Remarks	Ref	C/I
Heparin sodium		2500 units/ 1 ml		25 mg/ 25 ml	Physically compatible for at least 5 min	1053	C

Y-Site Injection Compatibility (1:1 Mixture)

Nitroglycerin

Drug	Mfr	Conc	Mfr	Conc	Remarks	Ref	C/I
Alteplase	GEN	1 mg/ml	DU	0.2 mg/ml[a]	Haze noted in 24 hr by visual examination. Erratic spectrophotometer readings	1340	I
Amiodarone HCl	LZ	4 mg/ml[c]	AB	0.24 mg/ml[c]	Physically compatible for 24 hr at 21 °C	1032	C
Amphotericin B cholesteryl sulfate complex	SEQ	0.83 mg/ml[a]	AMR	0.4 mg/ml[a]	Physically compatible with little or no change in measured turbidity or increase in particle content in 4 hr at 23 °C under fluorescent light	2117	C
Amrinone lactate	WB	3 mg/ml[b]		0.8 mg/ml[a]	Physically compatible for at least 4 hr at 25 °C under fluorescent light	992	C

Y-Site Injection Compatibility (1:1 Mixture) (Cont.)

				Nitroglycerin			
Drug	*Mfr*	*Conc*	*Mfr*	*Conc*	*Remarks*	*Ref*	*C/I*
Atracurium besylate	BW	0.5 mg/ml[a]	SO	0.4 mg/ml[a]	Physically compatible for 24 hr at 28 °C	1337	C
Cisatracurium besylate	GW	0.1, 2, 5 mg/ml[a]	DU	0.4 mg/ml[a]	Physically compatible with no change in measured turbidity or increase in particle content in 4 hr at 23 °C	2074	C
Diltiazem HCl	MMD	1 mg/ml[a]	DU	0.032 mg/ml[a]	Visually compatible for 24 hr at 25 °C	1530	C
	MMD	1[b] and 5 mg/ml	DU	400 μg/ml[b]	Visually compatible	1807	C
	MMD	5 mg/ml	DU	400 μg/ml[a]	Visually compatible	1807	C
	MMD	1 mg/ml[a]	AB	0.4 mg/ml[a]	Visually compatible for 4 hr at 27 °C	2062	C
Dobutamine HCl	LI	4 mg/ml[c]	LY	0.4 mg/ml[c]	Physically compatible for 3 hr	1316	C
	LI	4 mg/ml[c]	AB	0.4 mg/ml[c]	Visually compatible for 4 hr at 27 °C	2062	C
Dobutamine HCl with dopamine HCl	LI DCC	4 mg/ml[c] 3.2 mg/ml[c]	LY	0.4 mg/ml[c]	Physically compatible for 3 hr	1316	C
Dobutamine HCl with lidocaine HCl	LI AB	4 mg/ml[c] 8 mg/ml[c]	LY	0.4 mg/ml[c]	Physically compatible for 3 hr	1316	C
Dobutamine HCl with sodium nitroprusside	LI ES	4 mg/ml[c] 0.4 mg/ml[c]	LY	0.4 mg/ml[c]	Physically compatible for 3 hr	1316	C
Dopamine HCl	DCC	3.2 mg/ml[c]	LY	0.4 mg/ml[c]	Physically compatible for 3 hr	1316	C
	AB	3.2 mg/ml[a]	AB	0.4 mg/ml[a]	Visually compatible for 4 hr at 27 °C	2062	C
Dopamine HCl with dobutamine HCl	DCC LI	3.2 mg/ml[c] 4 mg/ml[c]	LY	0.4 mg/ml[c]	Physically compatible for 3 hr	1316	C
Dopamine HCl with lidocaine HCl	DCC AB	3.2 mg/ml[c] 8 mg/ml[c]	LY	0.4 mg/ml[c]	Physically compatible for 3 hr	1316	C
Dopamine HCl with sodium nitroprusside	DCC ES	3.2 mg/ml[c] 0.4 mg/ml[c]	LY	0.4 mg/ml[c]	Physically compatible for 3 hr	1316	C
Epinephrine HCl	AB	0.02 mg/ml[a]	AB	0.4 mg/ml[a]	Visually compatible for 4 hr at 27 °C	2062	C
Esmolol HCl	DU	40 mg/ml[a]	OM	0.2 mg/ml[a]	Visually compatible for 24 hr at 23 °C	1877	C
Famotidine	MSD	0.2 mg/ml[a]	IMS	0.8 mg/ml[a]	Physically compatible for 4 hr at 25 °C	1188	C
	MSD	0.2 mg/ml[a]	PD	85 μg/ml[b]	Physically compatible for 14 hr	1196	C
Fentanyl citrate	ES	0.05 mg/ml	AB	0.4 mg/ml[a]	Visually compatible for 4 hr at 27 °C	2062	C
Fluconazole	RR	2 mg/ml	AMR	0.2 mg/ml[a]	Visually compatible for 24 hr at 28 °C under fluorescent light	1760	C
Furosemide	AMR	10 mg/ml	AB	0.4 mg/ml[a]	Visually compatible for 4 hr at 27 °C	2062	C
Haloperidol lactate	MN	0.5[a] and 5 mg/ml	DU	0.4 mg/ml[a]	Visually compatible for 24 hr at 21 °C	1523	C
Heparin sodium	OR	100 units/ml[a]	OM	0.2 mg/ml[a]	Visually compatible for 24 hr at 23 °C	1877	C
	ES	100 units/ml[a]	AB	0.4 mg/ml[a]	Visually compatible for 4 hr at 27 °C	2062	C
Hydralazine HCl	SO	1 mg/ml[a]	LY	0.4 mg/ml[a]	Physically compatible for 3 hr	1316	C
	SO	1 mg/ml[b]	LY	0.4 mg/ml[b]	Slight precipitate in 3 hr	1316	I
Hydromorphone HCl	KN	1 mg/ml	AB	0.4 mg/ml[a]	Visually compatible for 4 hr at 27 °C	2062	C
Insulin, regular	LI	1 unit/ml[a]	OM	0.2 mg/ml[a]	Visually compatible for 24 hr at 23 °C	1877	C
Labetalol HCl	GL	1 mg/ml[a]	DU	0.2 mg/ml[a]	Visually compatible with no labetalol loss and 6% nitroglycerin loss by HPLC in 4 hr at room temperature	1762	C
	GL	5 mg/ml	OM	0.2 mg/ml[a]	Visually compatible for 24 hr at 23 °C	1877	C
	AH	2 mg/ml[a]	AB	0.4 mg/ml[a]	Visually compatible for 4 hr at 27 °C	2062	C

Y-Site Injection Compatibility (1:1 Mixture) (Cont.)

			Nitroglycerin				
Drug	*Mfr*	*Conc*	*Mfr*	*Conc*	*Remarks*	*Ref*	*C/I*
Lidocaine HCl	AB	8 mg/ml[c]	LY	0.4 mg/ml[c]	Physically compatible for 3 hr	1316	**C**
Lidocaine HCl with dobutamine HCl	AB LI	8 mg/ml[c] 4 mg/ml[c]	LY	0.4 mg/ml[c]	Physically compatible for 3 hr	1316	**C**
Lidocaine HCl with dopamine HCl	AB DCC	8 mg/ml[c] 3.2 mg/ml[c]	LY	0.4 mg/ml[c]	Physically compatible for 3 hr	1316	**C**
Lidocaine HCl with sodium nitroprusside	AB ES	8 mg/ml[c] 0.4 mg/ml[c]	LY	0.4 mg/ml[c]	Physically compatible for 3 hr	1316	**C**
Lorazepam	WY	0.5 mg/ml[a]	AB	0.4 mg/ml[a]	Visually compatible for 4 hr at 27 °C	2062	**C**
Midazolam HCl	RC RC RC	1 mg/ml[a] 1 mg/ml[a] 2 mg/ml[a]	SO OM AB	0.2 mg/ml[a] 0.2 mg/ml[a] 0.4 mg/ml[a]	Visually compatible for 24 hr at 23 °C Visually compatible for 24 hr at 23 °C Visually compatible for 4 hr at 27 °C	1847 1877 2062	**C** **C** **C**
Milrinone lactate	SW SW	0.2 mg/ml[a] 0.4 mg/ml[a]	AB SO	0.4 mg/ml[a] 0.8 mg/ml[a]	Visually compatible for 4 hr at 27 °C Visually compatible with little or no loss of either drug by HPLC in 4 hr at 23 °C	2062 2214	**C** **C**
Morphine sulfate	SCN	2 mg/ml[a]	AB	0.4 mg/ml[a]	Visually compatible for 4 hr at 27 °C	2062	**C**
Nicardipine HCl	WY	1 mg/ml[a]	AB	0.4 mg/ml[a]	Visually compatible for 4 hr at 27 °C	2062	**C**
Norepinephrine bitartrate	AB	0.128 mg/ml[a]	AB	0.4 mg/ml[a]	Visually compatible for 4 hr at 27 °C	2062	**C**
Pancuronium bromide	ES	0.05 mg/ml[a]	SO	0.4 mg/ml[a]	Physically compatible for 24 hr at 28 °C	1337	**C**
Propofol	ZEN	10 mg/ml	DU	0.4 mg/ml[a]	Physically compatible for 1 hr at 23 °C with no increase in particle content	2066	**C**
Ranitidine HCl	GL GL	0.5 mg/ml[e] 1 mg/ml[a]	SO AB	0.2 mg/ml[a] 0.4 mg/ml[a]	Physically compatible for 24 hr Visually compatible for 4 hr at 27 °C	1323 2062	**C** **C**
Remifentanil HCl	GW	0.025 and 0.25 mg/ml[b]	DU	0.4 mg/ml[a]	Physically compatible with no change in measured turbidity or increase in particle content in 4 hr at 23 °C	2075	**C**
Sodium nitroprusside	ES	0.4 mg/ml[c]	LY	0.4 mg/ml[c]	Physically compatible for 3 hr	1316	**C**
Sodium nitroprusside with dobutamine HCl	ES LI	0.4 mg/ml[c] 4 mg/ml[c]	LY	0.4 mg/ml[c]	Physically compatible for 3 hr	1316	**C**
Sodium nitroprusside with dopamine HCl	ES DCC	0.4 mg/ml[c] 3.2 mg/ml[c]	LY	0.4 mg/ml[c]	Physically compatible for 3 hr	1316	**C**
Sodium nitroprusside with lidocaine HCl	ES AB	0.4 mg/ml[c] 8 mg/ml[c]	LY	0.4 mg/ml[c]	Physically compatible for 3 hr	1316	**C**
Streptokinase	HO	30,000 units/ml[a]	DU	0.2 mg/ml[a]	Physically compatible for at least 5 days by visual examination	1340	**C**
Tacrolimus	FUJ	1 mg/ml[b]	DU	0.1 mg/ml[a]	Visually compatible for 24 hr at 25 °C	1630	**C**
Theophylline	TR	4 mg/ml	LY	0.2 mg/ml[a]	Visually compatible for 6 hr at 25 °C	1793	**C**
Thiopental sodium	AB	25 mg/ml[d]	AB	0.4 mg/ml[a]	Visually compatible for 4 hr at 27 °C	2062	**C**
TNA #218 to #226[f]			DU	0.4 mg/ml[a]	Visually compatible with no precipitate or emulsion damage apparent in 4 hr at 23 °C	2215	**C**
TPN #212 to #215[f]			DU	0.4 mg/ml[a]	Physically compatible with no change in measured turbidity or increase in particle content in 4 hr at 23 °C	2109	**C**
Vecuronium bromide	OR	0.1 mg/ml[a]	SO	0.4 mg/ml[a]	Physically compatible for 24 hr at 28 °C	1337	**C**

Y-Site Injection Compatibility (1:1 Mixture) (Cont.)

Nitroglycerin

Drug	Mfr	Conc	Mfr	Conc	Remarks	Ref	C/I
	OR	1 mg/ml	AB	0.4 mg/ml[a]	Visually compatible for 4 hr at 27 °C	2062	C
Warfarin sodium	DU	2 mg/ml[d]	FAU	0.4 mg/ml[a]	Visually compatible with no warfarin loss by HPLC in 30 min	2010	C
	DME	2 mg/ml[d]	DU	0.4 mg/ml[a]	Visually compatible for 24 hr at 24 °C	2078	C

[a]*Tested in dextrose 5% in water.*
[b]*Tested in sodium chloride 0.9%.*
[c]*Tested in both dextrose 5% in water and sodium chloride 0.9%.*
[d]*Tested in sterile water for injection.*
[e]*Premixed infusion solution.*
[f]*Refer to Appendix I for the composition of parenteral nutrition solutions. TNA indicates a 3-in-1 admixture, and TPN indicates a 2-in-1 admixture.*

Additional Compatibility Information

Dextrose 5% in water or sodium chloride 0.9% is recommended for dilution (2; 4). It is also recommended that no other drug be admixed with nitroglycerin (1-3/95; 2).

Dobutamine, Dopamine, Lidocaine, and Nitroprusside— Dobutamine HCl (Lilly) 4 mg/ml, dopamine HCl (Dupont Critical Care) 3.2 mg/ml, lidocaine HCl (Abbott) 8 mg/ml, nitroglycerin (Lyphomed) 0.4 mg/ml, and sodium nitroprusside (Elkins-Sinn) 0.4 mg/ml, prepared in dextrose 5% in water and sodium chloride 0.9%, were combined in equal quantities in all possible combinations of two, three, four, and five drugs and then evaluated for physical compatibility. No physical incompatibility was observed in any combination within the three-hour study period (1316).

NOREPINEPHRINE BITARTRATE (NORADRENALINE ACID TARTRATE)
AHFS 12:12

Levophed   **Abbott**

Products— Norepinephrine bitartrate (Levophed, Abbott) is available in 4-ml ampuls. Each milliliter of solution contains (29; 77):

Norepinephrine base (as norepinephrine bitartrate, 2 mg)	1 mg
Sodium chloride	~7.4 mg
Sodium metabisulfite	2 mg
Water for injection	qs 1 ml

Abbott also makes a generic norepinephrine bitartrate injection available in 4-ml ampuls that has a different formulation. Each milliliter of the generic norepinephrine bitartrate injection contains (1-10/92):

Norepinephrine base (as bitartrate)	1 mg
Sodium chloride	8.2 mg
Sodium metabisulfite	0.46 mg
Citric acid, anhydrous	1.3 mg
Sodium citrate, dihydrate	0.9 mg
Water for injection	qs 1 ml

pH— From 3 to 4.5 (4; 77).

Osmolality— The osmolality of norepinephrine (salt form unspecified) 1 mg/ml was determined to be 319 mOsm/kg (1233).

Administration— Norepinephrine bitartrate is administered by intravenous infusion into a large vein, using a pump or other flow rate control device. Extravasation may cause tissue damage and should be avoided. A 4-μg/ml dilution of norepinephrine base for infusion is usually prepared by adding 4 mg of base (4 ml) to 1000 ml of dextrose 5% in water with or without sodium chloride. The concentration and infusion rate depend on the patient's requirements (4).

Stability— Norepinephrine bitartrate in intact containers should be stored at controlled room temperature and protected from light (4). The drug gradually darkens upon exposure to light or air and must not be used if it is discolored or has a precipitate (4). It is stable at pH 3.6 to 6 in dextrose 5% in water (48; 77). The pH of a solution is the primary determinant of catecholamine stability in intravenous admixtures (527). At a concentration of 5 mg/L in dextrose 5% in water at pH 6.5, norepinephrine bitartrate loses 5% potency in six hours; at pH 7.5, it loses 5% potency in four hours (77). The rate of decomposition also increases with exposure to increasing temperatures (1929).

Filtration— Norepinephrine bitartrate (Winthrop) 4 mg/L in dextrose 5% in water and sodium chloride 0.9% was filtered at a rate of 120 ml/hr for six hours through a 0.22-μm cellulose ester membrane filter (Ivex-2). No significant reduction in potency due to binding to the filter was noted (533).

Compatibility Information

Solution Compatibility

Norepinephrine bitartrate

Solution	Mfr	Mfr	Conc/L	Remarks	Ref	C/I
Amino acids 4.25%, dextrose 25%	MG	WI	4 mg	No increase in particulate matter in 24 hr at 5 °C	349	C
Dextrose 5% in sodium chloride 0.9%		WI	8 mg	Physically compatible	74	C
Dextrose 5% in water		WI	8 mg	Physically compatible	74	C
	AB	WI	8 mg	Physically compatible and chemically stable. 10% decomposition is calculated to occur in 2500 hr at 25 °C	527	C
	TR[a]	WI	4 and 8 mg	2 to 4% loss in 24 hr at room temperature exposed to light	1163	C
	BA[a]	WI	16 mg	5% loss by HPLC in 47.2 days at 5 °C protected from light	1610	C
	BA[a]	WI	40 mg	5% loss by HPLC in 87.7 days at 5 °C protected from light	1610	C
	TR[a]	RC	4 and 8 mg	Visually compatible with no norepinephrine loss by HPLC in 48 hr at room temperature	1802	C
	BA[a]	SW	42 mg	No norepinephrine loss by HPLC in 24 hr at 23 °C protected from light	2085	C
Ringer's injection, lactated		WI	8 mg	Physically compatible	74	C
Sodium chloride 0.9%		WI	8 mg	Physically compatible	74	C
	TR[a]	WI	4 and 8 mg	2% loss in 24 hr at room temperature exposed to light	1163	C

[a]Tested in PVC containers.

Additive Compatibility

Norepinephrine bitartrate

Drug	Mfr	Conc/L	Mfr	Conc/L	Test Soln	Remarks	Ref	C/I
Amikacin sulfate	BR	5 g	WI	8 mg	D5LR, D5R, D5S, D5W, D10W, IS10, LR, NS, R, SL	Physically compatible and potency of both retained for 24 hr at 25 °C	294	C
Aminophylline	SE	500 mg	WI	8 mg	D5W	10% norepinephrine decomposition in 3.6 hr at 25 °C	527	I
Amobarbital sodium			WI			Physically incompatible	9	I
	LI	1 g	WI	2 mg	D5W	Physically incompatible	15	I
Blood, whole			WI			Physically incompatible	9	I
Calcium chloride	UP	1 g	WI	8 mg	D, D–S, S	Physically compatible	77	C
Calcium gluconate		1 g	WI	8 mg	D5W	Physically compatible	74	C
Chlorothiazide sodium	MSD		WI			Physically incompatible	9	I
Chlorpheniramine maleate			WI			Physically incompatible	9	I
	SC	100 mg	WI	2 mg	D5W	Physically incompatible	15	I
Cibenzoline succinate		2 g	WB	80 mg	D5W, NS	Physically compatible for 24 hr at 25 °C by visual and microscopic examination	1182	C

Additive Compatibility (Cont.)

Norepinephrine bitartrate

Drug	Mfr	Conc/L	Mfr	Conc/L	Test Soln	Remarks	Ref	C/I
Cimetidine HCl	SKF	3 g	WI	40 mg	D5W	Physically compatible and cimetidine chemically stable for 24 hr at room temperature. Norepinephrine not tested	551	**C**
Corticotropin		500 units	WI	8 mg	D5W	Physically compatible	74	**C**
Dimenhydrinate	SE	50 mg	WI	8 mg	D5W	Physically compatible	74	**C**
Dobutamine HCl	LI	1 g	BN	32 mg	D5W, NS	Physically compatible for 24 hr at 21 °C	812	**C**
Heparin sodium		12,000 units	WI	8 mg	D5W	Physically compatible	74	**C**
	AB	20,000 units	WI	8 mg	D, D–S, S	Physically compatible	77	**C**
Hydrocortisone sodium succinate	UP	100 mg	WI	8 mg	D5W	Physically compatible	74	**C**
Magnesium sulfate		1 g	WI	8 mg	D, D–S, S	Physically compatible	77	**C**
Meropenem	ZEN	1 and 20 g	WI	8 g	NS	Visually compatible for 4 hr at room temperature	1994	**C**
Methylprednisolone sodium succinate	UP	40 mg	WI	8 mg	D5S	Physically compatible	329	**C**
Multivitamins	USV	10 ml	WI	8 mg	D, D–S, S	Physically compatible	77	**C**
Netilmicin sulfate	SC	3 g	WI	64 mg	D5S	Physically compatible and netilmicin chemically stable for 7 days at 4 and 25 °C. Norepinephrine not tested	558	**C**
Pentobarbital sodium			WI			Physically incompatible	9	**I**
Phenobarbital sodium	WI		WI			Physically incompatible	9	**I**
Phenytoin sodium	PD		WI			Physically incompatible	9	**I**
Potassium chloride		3 g	WI	8 mg	D5W	Physically compatible	74	**C**
	AB	40 mEq	WI	8 mg	D, D–S, S	Physically compatible	77	**C**
Ranitidine HCl	GL	2 g	WI	4 and 8 mg	D5W, NS[a]	Physically compatible with no ranitidine loss in 48 hr at room temperature under fluorescent light. Norepinephrine not tested	1361	**C**
	GL	50 mg	WI	4 and 8 mg	D5W, NS[a]	Physically compatible with 2 to 6% ranitidine loss in 48 hr at room temperature under fluorescent light. Norepinephrine not tested	1361	**C**
	GL	50 mg and 2 g		4 mg	D5W	Physically compatible and ranitidine chemically stable by HPLC for 24 hr at 25 °C. Norepinephrine not tested	1515	**C**
	GL	50 mg	RC	4 and 8 mg	D5W[a]	Visually compatible with 5 to 7% ranitidine loss and little or no norepinephrine loss by HPLC in 48 hr at room temperature	1802	**C**
	GL	2 g	RC	4 mg	D5W[a]	Visually compatible but 7% norepinephrine loss in 4 hr and 13% loss in 12 hr by HPLC at room temperature. No ranitidine loss in 48 hr	1802	**I**
	GL	2 g	RC	8 mg	D5W[a]	Visually compatible but 6% norepinephrine loss in 12 hr and 11% loss in 24 hr by HPLC at room temperature. No ranitidine loss in 48 hr	1802	**I**

Additive Compatibility (Cont.)

Norepinephrine bitartrate

Drug	Mfr	Conc/L	Mfr	Conc/L	Test Soln	Remarks	Ref	C/I
Sodium bicarbonate			WI			Physically incompatible	9	I
	AB	80 mEq	WI	2 mg	D5W	Physically incompatible	15	I
	AB	2.4 mEq[b]	BN	8 mg	D5W	Norepinephrine inactivated	772	I
Streptomycin sulfate			WI			Physically incompatible	9	I
Succinylcholine chloride	AB	2 g	WI	8 mg	D, D–S, S	Physically compatible	77	C
Thiopental sodium	AB		WI			Physically incompatible	9	I
Verapamil HCl	KN	80 mg	BN	8 mg	D5W, NS	Physically compatible for 24 hr	764	C
Vitamin B complex with C		1 vial	WI	8 mg	D5W	Physically compatible	74	C
	AB	10 ml	WI	8 mg	D, D–S, S	Physically compatible	77	C
	UP	10 ml	WI	8 mg	D, D–S, S	Physically compatible	77	C

[a]Tested in PVC containers.
[b]One vial of Neut added to a liter of admixture.

Drugs in Syringe Compatibility

Norepinephrine bitartrate

Drug (in syringe)	Mfr	Amt	Mfr	Amt	Remarks	Ref	C/I
Heparin sodium		2500 units/ 1 ml	HO[a]	1 mg/ 1 ml	Physically compatible for at least 5 min	1053	C

[a]Tested as the hydrochloride salt.

Y-Site Injection Compatibility (1:1 Mixture)

Norepinephrine bitartrate

Drug	Mfr	Conc	Mfr	Conc	Remarks	Ref	C/I
Amiodarone HCl	LZ	4 mg/ml[c]	BN	0.064 mg/ml[c]	Physically compatible for 24 hr at 21 °C	1032	C
Amrinone lactate	WB	3 mg/ml[b]	BN	0.004 mg/ml[a]	Physically compatible for at least 4 hr at 25 °C under fluorescent light	992	C
Cisatracurium besylate	GW	0.1, 2, 5 mg/ml[a]	SW	0.12 mg/ml[a]	Physically compatible with no change in measured turbidity or increase in particle content in 4 hr at 23 °C	2074	C
Diltiazem HCl	MMD	1 mg/ml[a]	WI	0.12 mg/ml[a]	Visually compatible for 24 hr at 25 °C	1530	C
	MMD	1 mg/ml[a]	AB	0.128 mg/ml[a]	Visually compatible for 4 hr at 27 °C	2062	C
Dobutamine HCl	LI	4 mg/ml[a]	AB	0.128 mg/ml[a]	Visually compatible for 4 hr at 27 °C	2062	C
Dopamine HCl	DU	3.2 mg/ml[a]	STR	0.064 mg/ml[a]	Visually compatible for 24 hr at 23 °C	1877	C
	AB	3.2 mg/ml[a]	AB	0.128 mg/ml[a]	Visually compatible for 4 hr at 27 °C	2062	C
Epinephrine HCl	AB	0.02 mg/ml[a]	AB	0.128 mg/ml[a]	Visually compatible for 4 hr at 27 °C	2062	C
Esmolol HCl	DU	40 mg/ml[a]	STR	0.064 mg/ml[a]	Visually compatible for 24 hr at 23 °C	1877	C
Famotidine	MSD	0.2 mg/ml[a]	WI	0.004 mg/ml[a]	Physically compatible for 4 hr at 25 °C	1188	C
Fentanyl citrate	ES	0.05 mg/ml	AB	0.128 mg/ml[a]	Visually compatible for 4 hr at 27 °C	2062	C
Furosemide	AMR	10 mg/ml	AB	0.128 mg/ml[a]	Visually compatible for 4 hr at 27 °C	2062	C
Haloperidol lactate	MN	0.5[a] and 5 mg/ml	WI	0.032 mg/ml[a]	Visually compatible for 24 hr at 21 °C	1523	C

Y-Site Injection Compatibility (1:1 Mixture) (Cont.)

Norepinephrine bitartrate

Drug	Mfr	Conc	Mfr	Conc	Remarks	Ref	C/I
Heparin sodium	UP	1000 units/L[d]	WI	1 mg/ml	Physically compatible for at least 4 hr at room temperature by visual and microscopic examination	534	**C**
	ES	100 units/ml[a]	AB	0.128 mg/ml[a]	Visually compatible for 4 hr at 27 °C	2062	**C**
Hydrocortisone sodium succinate	UP	10 mg/L[d]	WI	1 mg/ml	Physically compatible for at least 4 hr at room temperature by visual and microscopic examination	534	**C**
Hydromorphone HCl	KN	1 mg/ml	AB	0.128 mg/ml[a]	Visually compatible for 4 hr at 27 °C	2062	**C**
Insulin, regular	LI	1 unit/ml[a]	STR	0.064 mg/ml[a]	White precipitate forms immediately	1877	**I**
Labetalol HCl	GL	5 mg/ml	STR	0.064 mg/ml[a]	Visually compatible for 24 hr at 23 °C	1877	**C**
	AH	2 mg/ml[a]	AB	0.128 mg/ml[a]	Visually compatible for 4 hr at 27 °C	2062	**C**
Lorazepam	WY	0.5 mg/ml[a]	AB	0.128 mg/ml[a]	Visually compatible for 4 hr at 27 °C	2062	**C**
Meropenem	ZEN	1 and 50 mg/ml[b]	WI	1 mg/ml[e]	Visually compatible for 4 hr at room temperature	1994	**C**
Midazolam HCl	RC	1 mg/ml[a]	STR	0.064 mg/ml[a]	Visually compatible for 24 hr at 23 °C	1877	**C**
	RC	2 mg/ml[a]	AB	0.128 mg/ml[a]	Visually compatible for 4 hr at 27 °C	2062	**C**
Milrinone lactate	SW	0.2 mg/ml[a]	AB	0.128 mg/ml[a]	Visually compatible for 4 hr at 27 °C	2062	**C**
	SW	0.4 mg/ml[a]	SW	0.064 mg/ml[a]	Visually compatible with little or no loss of either drug by HPLC in 4 hr at 23 °C	2214	**C**
Morphine sulfate	SX	1 mg/ml[a]	STR	0.064 mg/ml[a]	Visually compatible for 24 hr at 23 °C	1877	**C**
	SCN	2 mg/ml[a]	AB	0.128 mg/ml[a]	Visually compatible for 4 hr at 27 °C	2062	**C**
Nicardipine HCl	WY	1 mg/ml[a]	AB	0.128 mg/ml[a]	Visually compatible for 4 hr at 27 °C	2062	**C**
Nitroglycerin	AB	0.4 mg/ml[a]	AB	0.128 mg/ml[a]	Visually compatible for 4 hr at 27 °C	2062	**C**
Potassium chloride	AB	40 mEq/L[d]	WI	1 mg/ml	Physically compatible for at least 4 hr at room temperature by visual and microscopic examination	534	**C**
Propofol	ZEN	10 mg/ml	AB	0.016 mg/ml[a]	Physically compatible for 1 hr at 23 °C with no increase in particle content	2066	**C**
Ranitidine HCl	GL	1 mg/ml[a]	AB	0.128 mg/ml[a]	Visually compatible for 4 hr at 27 °C	2062	**C**
Remifentanil HCl	GW	0.025 and 0.25 mg/ml[b]	SW	0.12 mg/ml[a]	Physically compatible with no change in measured turbidity or increase in particle content in 4 hr at 23 °C	2075	**C**
Thiopental sodium	AB	25 mg/ml[e]	AB	0.128 mg/ml[a]	Precipitate forms in 4 hr at 27 °C	2062	**I**
TNA #73[f]			BN	0.4 mg/50 ml[c]	Physically compatible for 4 hr by visual observation	1009	**C**
TPN #212 to #215[f]			AB	0.016 mg/ml[a]	Physically compatible with no change in measured turbidity or increase in particle content in 4 hr at 23 °C	2109	**C**
Vecuronium bromide	OR	1 mg/ml	AB	0.128 mg/ml[a]	Visually compatible for 4 hr at 27 °C	2062	**C**

Y-Site Injection Compatibility (1:1 Mixture) (Cont.)

Norepinephrine bitartrate

Drug	Mfr	Conc	Mfr	Conc	Remarks	Ref	C/I
Vitamin B complex with C	RC	2 ml/L[d]	WI	1 mg/ml	Physically compatible for at least 4 hr at room temperature by visual and microscopic examination	534	C

[a]*Tested in dextrose 5% in water.*
[b]*Tested in sodium chloride 0.9%.*
[c]*Tested in both dextrose 5% in water and sodium chloride 0.9%.*
[d]*Tested in dextrose 5% in Ringer's injection, dextrose 5% in Ringer's injection, lactated, dextrose 5% in water, Ringer's injection, lactated, and sodium chloride 0.9%.*
[e]*Tested in sterile water for injection.*
[f]*Refer to Appendix I for the composition of parenteral nutrition solutions. TNA indicates a 3-in-1 admixture, and TPN indicates a 2-in-1 admixture.*

Additional Compatibility Information

Miscellaneous— If whole blood or plasma is indicated, it should be administered from a separate flask through a Y-tube (2; 4).

Solutions— At a concentration of 8 mg/L, norepinephrine bitartrate is stated to be compatible with all Abbott infusion solutions (77). However, dextrose 5% in water and dextrose 5% in sodium chloride 0.9% are the recommended diluents for infusion because their dextrose content provides protection against significant loss of potency due to oxidation. Administration of norepinephrine bitartrate in sodium chloride 0.9% is not recommended because of the lack of oxidation protection (2). However, other information indicates that norepinephrine bitartrate may be stable in sodium chloride 0.9% (1163). (See the Solution Compatibility table.)

Alkaline Solutions— Caution should be employed in mixing additives that may result in a final pH above 6 since norepinephrine bitartrate is alkali labile. These additives include sodium bicarbonate, barbiturates, alkaline-buffered antibiotics (77), lidocaine HCl (24), and aminophylline (6). Such admixtures should be administered immediately after preparation to assure full potency of norepinephrine bitartrate (77), or separate administration should be considered (24).

Visual inspection for color change may be inadequate to assess compatibility of admixtures. In one evaluation with aminophylline stored at 25 °C, a color change was not noted until 48 hours had elapsed. However, no intact norepinephrine bitartrate was present in the admixture at 48 hours (527).

Nafcillin Sodium— Norepinephrine bitartrate (Winthrop) 8 mg/L has been reported to be conditionally compatible with nafcillin sodium (Wyeth) 500 mg/L. The admixture is physically compatible for 24 hours, but the pH is 5.3 and the solution should therefore be used within six hours (27).

OCTREOTIDE ACETATE
AHFS 92:00

Sandostatin   **Novartis**

Products— Octreotide acetate (Novartis) is available in 1-ml ampuls containing 0.05, 0.1, or 0.5 mg of octreotide and in 5-ml multiple-dose vials containing 0.2 or 1 mg/ml of octreotide. Each milliliter also contains (2):

	Ampul	Vial
Lactic acid	3.4 mg	3.4 mg
Mannitol	45 mg	45 mg
Phenol		5 mg
Sodium bicarbonate	to adjust pH	to adjust pH
Water for injection	qs 1 ml	qs 1 ml

pH— From 3.9 to 4.5 (2).

Osmolality— Octreotide acetate 0.5 mg/ml has an osmolality of 279 mOsm/kg (1689).

Administration— Octreotide acetate is usually administered by subcutaneous injection in the smallest volume that will deliver the dose. Subcutaneous injection sites should be rotated. Multiple subcutaneous injections at the same site within a short time should be avoided. Administration by intravenous injection over three minutes or by infusion over 15 to 30 minutes after further dilution with 50 to 200 ml of dextrose 5% in water or sodium chloride 0.9% also has been recommended (2; 4).

Stability— Octreotide acetate is a clear solution. Ampuls and vials should be stored under refrigeration and protected from light. However, octreotide acetate can be stored at room temperature for up to 14 days when protected from light (2; 4).

Syringes— When stored in Travenol, Minimed, and Becton-Dickinson (Plastipak) plastic syringes of polypropylene and natural rubber, octreotide 100 and 500 µg/ml as the acetate retained its potency for 30 days (1370).

The stability of octreotide acetate (Sandoz) 0.2 mg/ml packaged 1 ml in 3-ml polypropylene syringes (Becton-Dickinson) sealed with tip caps (Becton-Dickinson) was evaluated at 3 and 23 °C both exposed to and protected from normal room light. Using HPLC analysis, the authors found no octreotide acetate loss in 29 days stored at 3 °C protected from light but about 7 to 9% loss in 15 to 22 days exposed to light. At 23 °C, the drug was less stable. Although results were somewhat variable, more than 10% loss occurred in about two weeks. The authors recommended a maximum storage time of one week at 23 °C, whether protected from light or not (2020).

In a similar study, the stability of octreotide acetate (Sandoz) 0.2 mg/ml was evaluated for 60 days stored at 5 and −20 °C (light conditions were not stated). The undiluted octreotide acetate injection was packaged 1 ml in 3-ml polypropylene syringes (Terumo) and sealed with a cap. HPLC analysis found losses of about 6% at both storage conditions after 60 days (2021).

Sorption— The manufacturer indicates that octreotide, a peptide, has the potential for adsorption to plastic and, possibly, glass (1540). However, in both static and dynamic tests, octreotide did not adsorb to Travenol, Minimed, and Becton-Dickinson (Plastipak) syringes of polypropylene and natural rubber, Travenol 3-ml insulin pump containers of polypropylene and polycarbonate, and Microflex PVC and Minimed polyolefin-lined PVC administration tubing (1370). Neither was it adsorbed to glass infusion bottles or a PVC administration set at a concentration of 5 µg/ml in sodium chloride 0.9% (1371).

Compatibility Information

Solution Compatibility

Octreotide acetate

Solution	Mfr	Mfr	Conc/L	Remarks	Ref	C/I
Fat emulsion 10%, intravenous	KV	SZ	1.5 mg	Octreotide content unstable with time	1373	**I**
Sodium chloride 0.9%	TR[a]	SZ	1.5 mg	Little octreotide loss over 48 hr at room temperature in ambient room light	1373	**C**
TNA #139[b]	[c]	SZ	450 µg	Physically compatible with no change in lipid particle size in 48 hr at 22 °C under fluorescent light and 7 days at 4 °C. Octreotide activity highly variable by radioimmunoassay	1540	**?**
TPN #119 and #120[b]	[a]	SZ	1.5 mg	Little octreotide loss over 48 hr at room temperature in ambient room light	1373	**C**

[a]*Tested in PVC containers.*
[b]*Refer to Appendix I for the composition of parenteral nutrition solutions. TNA indicates a 3-in-1 admixture, and TPN indicates a 2-in-1 admixture.*
[c]*Tested in both glass and ethylene vinyl acetate (EVA) containers.*

Additive Compatibility

Octreotide acetate

Drug	Mfr	Conc/L	Mfr	Conc/L	Test Soln	Remarks	Ref	C/I
Heparin sodium	ES	1000 units	SZ	1.5 mg	TPN #120[a]	Little octreotide loss over 48 hr at room temperature in ambient light	1373	**C**

[a]*Refer to Appendix I for the composition of parenteral nutrition solutions. TPN indicates a 2-in-1 admixture.*

Y-Site Injection Compatibility (1:1 Mixture)

Octreotide acetate

Drug	Mfr	Conc	Mfr	Conc	Remarks	Ref	C/I
TNA #218 to #226[b]			SZ	0.01 mg/ml[a]	Visually compatible with no precipitate or emulsion damage apparent in 4 hr at 23 °C	2215	**C**
TPN #212 to #215[b]			SZ	0.01 mg/ml[a]	Physically compatible with no change in measured turbidity or increase in particle content in 4 hr at 23 °C	2109	**C**

[a]*Tested in dextrose 5% in water.*
[b]*Refer to Appendix I for the composition of parenteral nutrition solutions. TNA indicates a 3-in-1 admixture, and TPN indicates a 2-in-1 admixture.*

Additional Compatibility Information

Diluents— Octreotide acetate (Sandoz) is physically compatible and chemically stable in concentrations of 5, 50, and 100 μg/ml in sodium chloride 0.9%, exhibiting no decomposition in 96 hours at room temperature when exposed to light (1372).

The manufacturer states that octreotide acetate should not be added to total parenteral nutrition solutions because of the formation of a glycosyl octreotide conjugate that may decrease the product's efficacy (2), although the clinical value of this administration approach continues to be debated (2136).

Insulin— Radioimmunoassays of insulin levels in 3-L bags of parenteral nutrition solutions showed a marked reduction when octreotide 150 μg was added. Sample parenteral nutrition solutions, with and without octreotide, were prepared with regular insulin 15 units/3-L bag. Subsequent analysis found an insulin level of 3.5 units/L in the plain parenteral nutrition solution, an amount consistent with losses occurring due to surface adsorption. However, in the parenteral nutrition solution containing octreotide, the insulin level was only 0.6 unit/L. The reason for this incompatibility is not known (1377).

OFLOXACIN
AHFS 8:22

Floxin I.V.   **Ortho-McNeil**

Products— Ofloxacin (Ortho-McNeil) is available as a concentrate in 10-ml single-use vials containing 40 mg/ml of drug in water for injection. Before use, the concentrate must be diluted to 4 mg/ml in a compatible intravenous infusion solution. The manufacturer provides the following information to aid in the preparation (2):

Dose	40 mg/ml in 10-ml vial	Volume of Diluent
200 mg	5 ml	qs 50 ml
300 mg	7.5 ml	qs 75 ml
400 mg	10 ml	qs 100 ml

Ofloxacin (Ortho-McNeil) also is available as a premixed single-use solution of 400 mg/100 ml of dextrose 5% in water in bottles and of 200 mg/50 ml and 400 mg/100 ml in dextrose 5% in water in flexible containers. No further dilution of the premixed solutions is necessary (2).

Hydrochloric acid and sodium hydroxide may have been added to adjust the pH (2).

pH— The concentrate has a pH of 3.5 to 5.5. For pH values of the concentrate after dilution in various infusion solutions, see the Solutions section under Additional Compatibility Information. The premixed forms in dextrose 5% in water have a pH of 3.8 to 5.8 (2).

Osmolality— The osmolality of ofloxacin (Ortho-McNeil) 0.4 and 4 mg/ml in several infusion solutions has been reported (1636):

Diluent	Osmolality (mOsm/kg)	
	0.4 mg/ml	4 mg/ml
Dextrose 5% in Ringer's injection, lactated	523	489
Dextrose 5% in sodium chloride 0.9%	547	512
Dextrose 5% in sodium chloride 0.45% with potassium chloride 0.15%	439	412
Dextrose 5% in water	259	252
Mannitol 20%	1303	1196
Plasma-Lyte 56 with dextrose 5%	372	353
Sodium chloride 0.9%	281	270
Sodium lactate ⅙ M	311	294

The premixed products in dextrose 5% in water are stated to be nearly isotonic (4).

Administration— Ofloxacin is administered by intravenous infusion over at least 60 minutes. Bolus injection or more rapid intravenous infusion is not recommended. The concentrate must be diluted with a compatible infusion solution to a concentration of 4 mg/ml before administration. If given intermittently via Y-site, the primary solution should be temporarily discontinued. If the set is used to administer other drugs, the tubing should be flushed with a compatible infusion solution both before and after ofloxacin administration (2; 4).

Stability— Ofloxacin solutions are light yellow to amber; the color intensity is not reflective of potency. Both the concentrate and premix solution in bottles should be stored at controlled room temperature (15 to 30 °C) and protected from light. The premix solution in flexible containers should be stored at 25 °C or lower and protected from light, but brief exposure to temperatures above 40 °C does not adversely affect it (2).

Ofloxacin has aqueous solubilities of 60 mg/ml at pH 2 to 5, 4 mg/ml at pH 7, and 303 mg/ml at pH 9.8 (2; 4).

Ofloxacin 0.4 to 4 mg/ml, diluted in a compatible infusion solution in glass and plastic containers, is stable for 72 hours at or below 24 °C, for 14 days under refrigeration at 5 °C, or for six months when frozen at −20 °C. The frozen solution is stable for an additional 14 days if it is refrigerated after thawing. Frozen solutions should be thawed at room temperature or in a refrigerator—not by microwave irradiation or water bath immersion. Thawed solutions should not be refrozen (2).

Sorption— Ofloxacin (Diamant) 200 mg/250 ml in dextrose 5% in water and sodium chloride 0.9% in PVC bags was infused through infusion sets at about 4 ml/min. No drug loss due to sorption was detected by HPLC (1698).

Compatibility Information

Solution Compatibility

Ofloxacin

Solution	Mfr	Mfr	Conc/L	Remarks	Ref	C/I
Dextrose 5% in Ringer's injection, lactated	BA[a]	ORT	0.4 and 4 g	Physically compatible with little or no ofloxacin loss by HPLC in 3 days at 24 °C or 14 days at 5 °C	1636	C
Dextrose 5% in sodium chloride 0.9%	BA[a]	ORT	0.4 and 4 g	Physically compatible with little or no ofloxacin loss by HPLC in 3 days at 24 °C or 14 days at 5 °C	1636	C
Dextrose 5% in sodium chloride 0.45% with potassium chloride 0.15%	BA[a]	ORT	0.4 and 4 g	Physically compatible with little or no ofloxacin loss by HPLC in 3 days at 24 °C or 14 days at 5 °C	1636	C
Dextrose 5% in water	BA[a]	ORT	0.4 and 4 g	Physically compatible with little or no ofloxacin loss by HPLC in 3 days at 24 °C or 14 days at 5 °C	1636	C
	[a]	DIA	800 mg	Visually compatible with no significant ofloxacin loss by HPLC in 6 hr at 22 °C exposed to light	1698	C
Mannitol 20%	BA[a]	ORT	0.4 and 4 g	Physically compatible with little or no ofloxacin loss by HPLC in 3 days at 24 °C. White mannitol crystals form upon refrigeration at 5 °C or freezing at −20 °C but disappear upon warming	1636	C
Plasma-Lyte 56 with dextrose 5%	BA[a]	ORT	0.4 and 4 g	Physically compatible with little or no ofloxacin loss by HPLC in 3 days at 24 °C or 14 days at 5 °C	1636	C
Sodium bicarbonate 5%	BA[a]	ORT	0.4 and 4 g	Physically compatible with little or no ofloxacin loss by HPLC in 3 days at 24 °C or 14 days at 5 °C	1636	C
Sodium chloride 0.9%	BA[a]	ORT	0.4 and 4 g	Physically compatible with little or no ofloxacin loss by HPLC in 3 days at 24 °C or 14 days at 5 °C	1636	C
	[a]	DIA	800 mg	Visually compatible with no significant ofloxacin loss by HPLC in 6 hr at 22 °C exposed to light	1698	C
Sodium lactate ⅙ M	BA[a]	ORT	0.4 and 4 g	Physically compatible with little or no ofloxacin loss by HPLC in 3 days at 24 °C or 14 days at 5 °C	1636	C

[a]Tested in PVC containers.

Additive Compatibility

Ofloxacin

Drug	Mfr	Conc/L	Mfr	Conc/L	Test Soln	Remarks	Ref	C/I
Amoxicillin sodium	BE	8.3 g	HO	1.67 g	W	Visually compatible with little or no loss of either drug by HPLC in 48 hr	1613	C
Amoxicillin sodium–clavulanic acid	BE	8.33 + 1.67 g	HO	1.67 g	W	Visually compatible with little or no loss of either drug by HPLC in 48 hr	1613	C
Ceftazidime	GL[a]	8.3 g	HO	1.67 g	W	Visually compatible with little or no loss of either drug by HPLC in 48 hr	1613	C

Additive Compatibility (Cont.)

			Ofloxacin					
Drug	Mfr	Conc/L	Mfr	Conc/L	Test Soln	Remarks	Ref	C/I
Clindamycin phosphate	UP	6 g	HO	2 g	W	Visually compatible with little or no loss of either drug by HPLC in 48 hr	1613	C
Flucloxacillin sodium	BE	8.3 g	HO	1.67 g	W	Visually compatible for 7 hr. Precipitate forms by 24 hr with about 75% ofloxacin loss and 20% flucloxacillin loss by HPLC	1613	I
Gentamicin sulfate	ESX	800 mg	HO	2 g	W	Visually compatible with little or no loss of either drug by HPLC in 48 hr	1613	C
Piperacillin sodium	LE	16.7 g	HO	1.67 g	W	Visually compatible with little or no loss of either drug by HPLC in 48 hr	1613	C
Tobramycin sulfate	LI	800 mg	HO	2 g	W	Visually compatible with little or no loss of either drug by HPLC in 48 hr	1613	C
Vancomycin HCl	LI	4.2 g	HO	1.67 g	W	Visually compatible with little or no loss of either drug by HPLC in 48 hr	1613	C

[a]Sodium carbonate–containing formulation tested.

Drugs in Syringe Compatibility

			Ofloxacin				
Drug (in syringe)	Mfr	Amt	Mfr	Amt	Remarks	Ref	C/I
Cefotaxime sodium	HO	2 g	HO	200 mg	Visually compatible with no loss of either drug by HPLC in 4 hr at room temperature	1735	C

Y-Site Injection Compatibility (1:1 Mixture)

			Ofloxacin				
Drug	Mfr	Conc	Mfr	Conc	Remarks	Ref	C/I
Amphotericin B cholesteryl sulfate complex	SEQ	0.83 mg/ml[a]	ORT	4 mg/ml[a]	Gross precipitate forms	2117	I
Ampicillin sodium	HO	21.3 mg/ml	HO	2.2 mg/ml	Visually compatible with no loss of either drug by HPLC in 2 hr at room temperature	1734	C
Cefepime HCl	BR	20 mg/ml[a]	ORT	4 mg/ml[a]	Haze forms immediately and becomes flocculent precipitate in 4 hr	1689	I
Cisatracurium besylate	GW	0.1, 2, 5 mg/ml[a]	ORT	4 mg/ml[a]	Physically compatible with no change in measured turbidity or increase in particle content in 4 hr at 23 °C	2074	C
Docetaxel	RPR	0.9 mg/ml[a]	MN	4 mg/ml[a]	Physically compatible with no change in measured turbidity or increase in particle content in 4 hr at 23 °C	2224	C
Doxorubicin HCl liposome injection	SEQ	0.4 mg/ml[a]	ORT	4 mg/ml[a]	Increase in measured turbidity	2087	I
Etoposide phosphate	BR	5 mg/ml[a]	MN	4 mg/ml[a]	Physically compatible with no change in measured turbidity or increase in particle content in 4 hr at 23 °C	2218	C

Y-Site Injection Compatibility (1:1 Mixture) (Cont.)

Drug	Mfr	Conc	Mfr	Conc	Remarks	Ref	C/I
			Ofloxacin				
Gemcitabine HCl	LI	10 mg/ml[b]	MN	4 mg/ml[b]	Physically compatible with no change in measured turbidity or increase in particle content in 4 hr at 23 °C	2226	**C**
Granisetron HCl	SKB	0.05 mg/ml[a]	ORT	4 mg/ml[a]	Physically compatible with no change in measured turbidity or increase in particle content in 4 hr at 23 °C	2000	**C**
Propofol	ZEN	10 mg/ml	ORT	4 mg/ml[a]	Physically compatible for 1 hr at 23 °C with no increase in particle content	2066	**C**
Remifentanil HCl	GW	0.025 and 0.25 mg/ml[b]	ORT	4 mg/ml[a]	Physically compatible with no change in measured turbidity or increase in particle content in 4 hr at 23 °C	2075	**C**
Thiotepa	IMM[c]	1 mg/ml[a]	ORT	4 mg/ml	Physically compatible with no change in measured turbidity or increase in particle content in 4 hr at 23 °C	1861	**C**
TNA #218 to #226[d]			ORT	4 mg/ml[a]	Visually compatible with no precipitate or emulsion damage apparent in 4 hr at 23 °C	2215	**C**
TPN #212 to #215[d]			ORT	4 mg/ml[a]	Physically compatible with no change in measured turbidity or increase in particle content in 4 hr at 23 °C	2109	**C**

[a]*Tested in dextrose 5% in water.*
[b]*Tested in sodium chloride 0.9%.*
[c]*Lyophilized formulation tested.*
[d]*Refer to Appendix I for the composition of parenteral nutrition solutions. TNA indicates a 3-in-1 admixture, and TPN indicates a 2-in-1 admixture.*

Additional Compatibility Information

Solutions— The manufacturer states that ofloxacin 4 mg/ml is compatible and stable for 72 hours at or below 24 °C, for 14 days under refrigeration at 5 °C, or for six months when frozen at −20 °C in the following infusion solutions (2):

Infusion Solution	pH at 4 mg/ml
Dextrose 5% in Ringer's injection, lactated	4.94
Dextrose 5% in sodium chloride 0.9%	4.56
Dextrose 5% in sodium chloride 0.45% with potassium chloride 0.15%	4.64
Dextrose 5% in water	4.57
Plasma-Lyte 56 with dextrose 5%	5.02
Sodium bicarbonate 5%	7.95
Sodium chloride 0.9%	4.69
Sodium lactate ⅙ M	5.64

Metal Ions— Ofloxacin may chelate with metal ions including Ca^{+2}, Cu^{+2}, Fe^{+3}, Mg^{+2}, and Zn^{+2} (2).

ONDANSETRON HCL
AHFS 56:22

Zofran **Glaxo Wellcome**

Products— Ondansetron HCl (Glaxo Wellcome) is available in 20-ml multiple-dose vials and 2-ml single-dose vials. Each milliliter of solution in multiple-dose vials contains ondansetron (as the hydrochloride dihydrate) 2 mg with sodium chloride 8.3 mg, citric acid monohydrate 0.5 mg, sodium citrate dihydrate 0.25 mg, methylparaben 1.2 mg, and propylparaben 0.15 mg. Each milliliter of solution in single-dose vials contains ondansetron (as the hydrochloride dihydrate) 2 mg with sodium chloride 9 mg, citric acid monohydrate 0.5 mg, and sodium citrate dihydrate 0.25 mg (2).

Ondansetron HCl (Glaxo Wellcome) is also available as a premixed infusion solution in dextrose 5% containing in each 50 ml of solution ondansetron 32 mg (as the hydrochloride dihydrate), dextrose 2.5 g, citric acid 26 mg, and sodium citrate 11.5 mg in water for injection (2).

pH— From 3.3 to 4 (2).

Osmolality— Ondansetron HCl 2 mg/ml has an osmolality of 281 mOsm/kg (1689). The osmolarity of the premixed ondansetron HCl 32 mg/50 ml solution is 270 mOsm/L (2).

Administration— Ondansetron hydrochloride is administered intravenously over 15 minutes after further dilution with 50 ml of sodium chloride 0.9% or dextrose 5% in water. By intravenous injection, it is administered undiluted over at least 30 seconds and preferably over two to five minutes (2; 4).

Stability— Ondansetron HCl is a clear, colorless solution. It should be stored at room temperature or under refrigeration and protected from light and from freezing (2). Although ondansetron HCl is unstable under intense light, it is stable for about a month in daylight with added fluorescent light (1366).

When diluted with compatible infusion solutions, ondansetron HCl is stable for up to seven days at room temperature or under refrigeration in polypropylene–neoprene syringes (Plastipak, Becton-Dickinson) with syringe caps (1366).

Ondansetron HCl (Glaxo) 0.03 and 0.3 mg/ml in dextrose 5% in water or sodium chloride 0.9% was stable when frozen at −20 °C, exhibiting a 10% or less loss in three months (1642).

pH Effects— The natural pH of ondansetron HCl solutions is about 4.5 to 4.6 (1366; 1367). If the pH is increased, a precipitate of ondansetron free base has been reported to develop at pH 5.7 (1366) and pH 7 (1513). Redissolution of the ondansetron precipitate occurs at pH 6.2 when titrated with hydrochloric acid (1513). Precipitation by combination with alkaline drugs has been observed (1365; 1513).

Filtration— Ondansetron HCl (Glaxo) 30 and 200 µg/ml in sodium chloride 0.9% was delivered over 15 minutes through five 0.2-µm inline filters: Continu-Flo Solution Set (Baxter, 2C5561S), Filtered Extension Sets (Burron, PFE-2007 and FE-2024), Universal Primary infusion set (IVAC, 52023), and Ivex-HP Filterset-SL (Abbott, 4524). Little or no ondansetron loss was determined by HPLC (1678).

Repackaging in Syringes— Casto reported the stability of ondansetron HCl undiluted at 2 mg/ml and diluted in dextrose 5% in water and sodium chloride 0.9% at 1, 0.5, and 0.25 mg/ml packaged in polypropylene syringes. Representative syringes were stored at 24 °C for 48 hours, 4 °C for 14 days, and frozen at −20 °C for 90 days. Visually, the solutions exhibited no precipitate or color or clarity changes. HPLC analysis found ondansetron HCl concentrations in all samples remained above 90% throughout the study periods; most samples were above 95%. Sequentially storing sample syringes for 90 days at −20 °C followed by 14 days at 4 °C followed by 48 hours at 24 °C did not alter the stability (2056).

Portable Infusion Pumps— Ondansetron HCl (Glaxo) 2 mg/ml in medication cassette reservoirs (Pharmacia Deltec CADD-1) was pumped by portable infusion pumps (CADD-Plus) and maintained at 30 °C to simulate use conditions. Approximately 95% of the initial concentration was retained by HPLC after seven days (1553).

Compatibility Information

Solution Compatibility

Ondansetron HCl

Solution	Mfr	Mfr	Conc/L	Remarks	Ref	C/I
Dextrose 5% in water	BP[a]	GL	16 and 80 mg	Physically compatible and chemically stable for 7 days at room temperature exposed to light and at 4 °C	1366	C
		GL	24 and 96 mg	Visually compatible with no loss by HPLC in 14 days at 24 °C or 14 days at 5 °C followed by 2 days at 24 °C	1560	C
	BA[a]	GL	30 and 300 mg	Visually compatible with 5% or less loss by HPLC in 48 hr at 25 °C or 14 days at 5 °C	1642	C
	MG[b]	GL	0.03 and 0.3 g	Visually compatible with no ondansetron loss by HPLC in 14 days at 4 °C under fluorescent light and no microbial growth	1722	C
Dextrose 5% in water with potassium chloride 0.3%	BP[a]	GL	16 mg	Physically compatible and chemically stable for 7 days at room temperature exposed to light and at 4 °C	1366	C
Mannitol 10%	BP[a]	GL	16 mg	Physically compatible and chemically stable for 7 days at room temperature exposed to light and at 4 °C	1366	C
Ringer's injection	BP[a]	GL	16 mg	Physically compatible and chemically stable for 7 days at room temperature exposed to light and at 4 °C	1366	C

Solution Compatibility (Cont.)

Ondansetron HCl

Solution	Mfr	Mfr	Conc/L	Remarks	Ref	C/I
Ringer's injection, lactated		GL	24 and 96 mg	Visually compatible with no loss by HPLC in 14 days at 24 °C or 14 days at 5 °C followed by 2 days at 24 °C	1560	C
Sodium chloride 0.9%	BP[a]	GL	16 and 80 mg	Physically compatible and chemically stable for 7 days at room temperature exposed to light and at 4 °C	1366	C
		GL	24 and 96 mg	Visually compatible with no loss by HPLC in 14 days at 24 °C or 14 days at 5 °C followed by 2 days at 24 °C	1560	C
	BA[c]	GL	240 mg	No loss by HPLC in 24 hr at 30 °C or 30 days at 3 °C followed by 24 hr at 30 °C	1553	C
	BA[a]	GL	30 and 300 mg	Visually compatible with 4% or less loss by HPLC in 48 hr at 25 °C or 14 days at 5 °C	1642	C
	MG[b]	GL	0.03 and 0.3 g	Visually compatible with no ondansetron loss by HPLC in 14 days at 4 °C under fluorescent light and no microbial growth	1722	C
	BA[a]	CER	100 mg	Visually compatible with about 6 to 7% loss by HPLC after 30 days at 4 °C followed by 2 days at 23 °C	1882	C
	BA[a]	CER	200, 400, 640 mg	Visually compatible with not more than 4% loss by HPLC after 30 days at 4 °C followed by 2 days at 23 °C	1882	C
Sodium chloride 0.9% with potassium chloride 0.3%	BP[a]	GL	16 mg	Physically compatible and chemically stable for 7 days at room temperature exposed to light and at 4 °C	1366	C
TNA #190[d]		GL	0.03 and 0.3 g	Physically compatible with little or no ondansetron loss by HPLC in 48 hr at 24 °C under fluorescent light	1766	C

[a]Tested in PVC containers.
[b]Tested in a Kraton polymer elastomeric infusion device (Homepump, Block).
[c]Tested in a medication cassette reservoir (Pharmacia Deltec CADD-1).
[d]Refer to Appendix I for the composition of parenteral nutrition solutions. TNA indicates a 3-in-1 admixture.

Additive Compatibility

Ondansetron HCl

Drug	Mfr	Conc/L	Mfr	Conc/L	Test Soln	Remarks	Ref	C/I
Cisplatin	BR	485 mg	GL	1.031 g	NS[a]	Physically compatible with little or no loss of either drug by HPLC in 24 hr at 4 °C followed by 7 days at 30 °C	1846	C
	BR	219 mg	GL	479 mg	NS[b]	Physically compatible with little or no loss of either drug by HPLC in 24 hr at 4 °C followed by 7 days at 30 °C	1846	C
Cyclophosphamide	MJ	300 mg	GL	50 mg	D5W[a], NS[a]	Visually compatible with 9 to 10% cyclophosphamide loss and no ondansetron loss by HPLC in 5 days at 24 °C. No loss of either drug in 8 days at 4 °C	1812	C
	MJ	2 g	GL	400 mg	D5W[a], NS[a]	Visually compatible with 10% cyclophosphamide loss and no ondansetron loss by HPLC in 5 days at 24 °C. No loss of either drug in 8 days at 4 °C	1812	C

Additive Compatibility (Cont.)

Ondansetron HCl

Drug	Mfr	Conc/L	Mfr	Conc/L	Test Soln	Remarks	Ref	C/I
Cytarabine	UP	200 mg	GL	30 and 300 mg	D5W[a]	Physically compatible with little or no loss of either drug by HPLC in 48 hr at 23 °C	1876	**C**
	UP	40 g	GL	30 and 300 mg	D5W[a]	Physically compatible with little or no loss of either drug by HPLC in 48 hr at 23 °C	1876	**C**
Dacarbazine	MI	1 g	GL	30 and 300 mg	D5W[a]	Physically compatible with little or no loss of ondansetron by HPLC in 48 hr at 23 °C. 8 to 12% dacarbazine loss in 24 hr and 20% loss in 48 hr at 23 °C	1876	**C**
	MI	3 g	GL	30 and 300 mg	D5W[a]	Physically compatible with little or no loss of ondansetron by HPLC in 48 hr at 23 °C. 8% dacarbazine loss in 24 hr and 15% loss in 48 hr at 23 °C	1876	**C**
Dacarbazine with doxorubicin HCl	LY AD	8 g 800 mg	GL	640 mg	D5W[a]	Visually compatible with greater than 90% ondansetron and doxorubicin potency by HPLC over 24 hr at 30 °C and after 7 days at 4 °C followed by 24 hr at 30 °C. Dacarbazine stable for 8 hr but up to 13% loss in 24 hr	2092	**I**
Dacarbazine with doxorubicin HCl	LY AD	20 g 1.5 g	GL	640 mg	D5W[a]	Visually compatible with greater than 90% potency of all drugs by HPLC over 24 hr at 30 °C and after 7 days at 4 °C followed by 24 hr at 30 °C.	2092	**C**
Dacarbazine with doxorubicin HCl	LY AD	8 g 800 mg	GL	640 mg	D5W[b]	Visually compatible with greater than 90% potency of all drugs by HPLC over 24 hr at 30 °C and after 7 days at 4 °C followed by 24 hr at 30 °C.	2092	**C**
Dacarbazine with doxorubicin HCl	LY AD	20 g 1.5 g	GL	640 mg	D5W[b]	Visually compatible with greater than 90% potency of all drugs by HPLC over 24 hr at 30 °C and after 7 days at 4 °C followed by 24 hr at 30 °C.	2092	**C**
Dexamethasone sodium phosphate		20 and 40 mg	GL	48 mg	D5W, NS	Visually compatible for 24 hr at 22 °C	1608	**C**
		200 and 400 mg	GL	160 mg	NS	Visually compatible for 24 hr at 22 °C	1608	**C**
	ES	200 mg	CER	100 mg	NS[a]	Visually compatible with no dexamethasone loss and 8% ondansetron loss by HPLC after 30 days at 4 °C followed by 2 days at 23 °C	1882	**C**
	ES	400 mg	CER	100 and 200 mg	NS[a]	Visually compatible with no dexamethasone loss and 7 to 10% ondansetron loss by HPLC after 30 days at 4 °C followed by 2 days at 23 °C	1882	**C**
	ES	200 mg	CER	200, 400, and 640 mg	NS[a]	Visually compatible with no dexamethasone loss and not more than 5% ondansetron loss by HPLC after 30 days at 4 °C followed by 2 days at 23 °C	1882	**C**
	ES	400 mg	CER	400 and 640 mg	NS[a]	Visually compatible with no dexamethasone loss and not more than 3% ondansetron loss by HPLC after 30 days at 4 °C followed by 2 days at 23 °C	1882	**C**

Additive Compatibility (Cont.)

Ondansetron HCl

Drug	Mfr	Conc/L	Mfr	Conc/L	Test Soln	Remarks	Ref	C/I
	ES	200 and 400 mg	CER	640 mg	D5W[c]	Visually compatible with 7% dexamethasone loss and no ondansetron loss by HPLC after 30 days at 4 °C followed by 2 days at 23 °C	1882	C
	MSD	400 mg	GL	150 mg	NS[a]	Visually compatible with 4% or less loss of either drug by HPLC in 28 days at 4 and 22 °C	2084	C
	MSD	400 mg	GL	150 mg	D5W[a]	Visually compatible with 4% or less loss of either drug by HPLC in 28 days at 4 °C. Up to 10% ondansetron loss in 3 days at 22 °C	2084	C
	MSD	230 mg	GL	750 mg	NS[a]	Visually compatible with 4% or less loss of either drug by HPLC in 28 days at 4 °C. Up to 10% ondansetron loss in 7 days at 22 °C	2084	C
	MSD	230 mg	GL	750 mg	D5W[a]	Visually compatible with up to 13% ondansetron loss by HPLC in 3 days at 4 and 22 °C	2084	?
Doxorubicin HCl	MJ	100 mg	GL	30 and 300 mg	D5W[a]	Physically compatible with little or no loss of either drug by HPLC in 48 hr at 23 °C	1876	C
	MJ	2 g	GL	30 and 300 mg	D5W[a]	Physically compatible with little or no loss of either drug by HPLC in 48 hr at 23 °C	1876	C
Doxorubicin HCl with vincristine sulfate	AD LI	400 mg 14 mg	GL	480 mg	D5W[b]	Visually compatible with greater than 90% potency of all drugs by HPLC after 5 days at 4 °C followed by 24 hr at 30 °C	2092	C
Doxorubicin HCl with vincristine sulfate	AD LI	800 mg 28 mg	GL	960 mg	D5W[a]	Visually compatible with greater than 90% potency of all drugs by HPLC after 120 hr at 30 °C	2092	C
Etoposide	BR	100 mg	GL	30 and 300 mg	D5W[a]	Physically compatible with little or no loss of ondansetron by HPLC in 48 hr at 23 °C. 4% etoposide loss in 24 hr and 6% loss in 48 hr at 23 °C	1876	C
	BR	400 mg	GL	30 and 300 mg	D5W[a]	Physically compatible with little or no loss of either drug by HPLC in 48 hr at 23 °C	1876	C
Fluconazole with ranitidine HCl	RR GL	2 g 500 mg	GL	100 mg	[a]	Visually compatible with no loss of any drug by HPLC in 4 hr	1730	C
Hydromorphone HCl	ES	500 mg	GL	100 mg and 1 g	NS	Physically compatible with no loss of either drug by HPLC in 7 days at 32 °C or 31 days at 4 and 22 °C protected from light	1690	C
Meperidine HCl	WY	4 g	GL	100 mg and 1 g	NS[a]	Physically compatible with no change in measured turbidity or increase in particle content and no loss of either drug by HPLC in 31 days at 4 and 22 °C and in 7 days at 32 °C	1862	C
Meropenem	ZEN	1 g	GL	1 g	NS	Visually compatible for 4 hr at room temperature	1994	C
	ZEN	20 g	GL	1 g	NS	White precipitate forms immediately	1994	I

Additive Compatibility (Cont.)

		Ondansetron HCl						
Drug	Mfr	Conc/L	Mfr	Conc/L	Test Soln	Remarks	Ref	C/I
Methotrexate sodium	LE	500 mg	GL	30 and 300 mg	D5W[a]	Physically compatible with little or no loss of either drug by HPLC in 48 hr at 23 °C	1876	**C**
	LE	6 g	GL	30 and 300 mg	D5W[a]	Physically compatible with little or no loss of either drug by HPLC in 48 hr at 23 °C	1876	**C**
Morphine sulfate	AST	1 g	GL	100 mg and 1 g	NS	Physically compatible with no ondansetron loss and 5% or less morphine loss by HPLC in 7 days at 32 °C or 31 days at 4 and 22 °C protected from light	1690	**C**

[a]Tested in PVC containers.
[b]Tested in polyisoprene reservoirs (Travenol Infusors).
[c]Tested in ondansetron HCl ready-to-use CR3 polyester bags.

Drugs in Syringe Compatibility

		Ondansetron HCl					
Drug (in syringe)	Mfr	Amt	Mfr	Amt	Remarks	Ref	C/I
Alfentanil HCl	JN	0.167 mg/ml[b]	GW	1.33 mg/ml[b]	Physically compatible with no measured increase in particulates and little or no loss of either drug by HPLC in 24 hr at 4 or 23 °C	2199	**C**
Atropine sulfate	GNS	0.133 mg/ml[b]	GW	1.33 mg/ml[b]	Physically compatible with no measured increase in particulates and less than 6% loss of ondansetron and less than 7% loss of atropine by HPLC in 24 hr at 4 or 23 °C	2199	**C**
Dexamethasone sodium phosphate	ES	0.5 and 1 mg/ml[a]	CER	0.17 mg/ml[a]	Visually compatible with no loss of either drug by HPLC after 30 days at 4 °C followed by 2 days at 23 °C	1882	**C**
	ES	0.5 mg/ml[a]	CER	0.25 mg/ml[a]	Visually compatible with no loss of either drug by HPLC after 30 days at 4 °C followed by 2 days at 23 °C	1882	**C**
	ES	1 mg/ml[a]	CER	0.25 mg/ml[a]	Visually compatible for 3 days at 4 °C. Precipitation of ondansetron observed at 7 days as opaque white ring	1882	**C**
	ES	0.33 and 0.67 mg/ml[a]	CER	0.33 mg/ml[a]	Visually compatible with no loss of either drug by HPLC after 30 days at 4 °C followed by 2 days at 23 °C	1882	**C**
	ES	0.5 mg/ml[a]	CER	0.5 mg/ml[a]	Visually compatible with no loss of either drug by HPLC after 30 days at 4 °C followed by 2 days at 23 °C	1882	**C**
	ES	1 mg/ml[a]	CER	0.5 mg/ml[a]	Visually compatible for 3 days at 4 °C. Precipitation of ondansetron observed at 7 days as opaque white ring	1882	**C**
	ES	0.33 and 0.67 mg/ml[a]	CER	0.67 mg/ml[a]	Visually compatible with no loss of either drug by HPLC after 30 days at 4 °C followed by 2 days at 23 °C	1882	**C**
	ES	0.33 mg/ml[a]	CER	1.07 mg/ml[a]	Visually compatible with no loss of either drug by HPLC after 30 days at 4 °C followed by 2 days at 23 °C	1882	**C**

Drugs in Syringe Compatibility (Cont.)

Ondansetron HCl

Drug (in syringe)	Mfr	Amt	Mfr	Amt	Remarks	Ref	C/I
	ES	0.67 mg/ ml[a]	CER	1.07 mg/ ml[a]	Heavy white flocculent precipitate within 72 hr at 4 °C. 25 to 30% loss of both drugs by HPLC	1882	I
Droperidol	AMR	1.25 mg/ ml[b]	GW	1 mg/ml[b]	Droperidol precipitates in less than 4 hr at 4 °C. At 23 °C, little or no loss of either drug by HPLC in 8 hr, but droperidol precipitates after that time	2199	I
Fentanyl citrate	ES	0.0167 mg/ml[b]	GW	1.33 mg/ ml[b]	Physically compatible with no measured increase in particulates and little or no loss of either drug by HPLC in 24 hr at 4 or 23 °C	2199	C
Glycopyrrolate	AMR	0.1 mg/ ml[b]	GW	1 mg/ml[b]	Physically compatible with no measured increase in particulates and little or no loss of either drug by HPLC in 24 hr at 4 or 23 °C	2199	C
Meperidine HCl	ES	8.33 mg/ ml[b]	GW	1.33 mg/ ml[b]	Physically compatible with no measured increase in particulates and little or no loss of either drug by HPLC in 24 hr at 4 or 23 °C	2199	C
Metoclopramide HCl	SO	2.5 mg/ ml[b]	GW	1 mg/ml[b]	Physically compatible with no measured increase in particulates and less than 6% loss of ondansetron and less than 5% loss of metoclopramide by HPLC in 24 hr at 4 or 23 °C	2199	C
Midazolam HCl	RC	1.66 mg/ ml[b]	GW	1.33 mg/ ml[b]	Physically compatible with no measured increase in particulates and less than 4% loss of ondansetron and less than 7% loss of midazolam by HPLC in 24 hr at 4 or 23 °C	2199	C
Morphine sulfate	ES	2.67 mg/ ml[b]	GW	1.33 mg/ ml[b]	Physically compatible with no measured increase in particulates and less than 5% loss of ondansetron and less than 4% loss of morphine by HPLC in 24 hr at 4 or 23 °C	2199	C
Naloxone HCl	AST	0.133 mg/ ml[b]	GW	1.33 mg/ ml[b]	Physically compatible with no measured increase in particulates and 6% or less loss of ondansetron and 5% or less loss of naloxone by HPLC in 24 hr at 4 or 23 °C	2199	C
Neostigmine methylsulfate	ES	0.167 mg/ ml[b]	GW	1.33 mg/ ml[b]	Physically compatible with no measured increase in particulates and less than 3% loss of ondansetron and less than 5% loss of neostigmine by HPLC in 24 hr at 4 or 23 °C	2199	C
Propofol	STU	1 and 5 mg/ml[b]	GW	1 mg/ml[b]	Physically compatible with no measured increase in particulates and little or no loss of either drug by HPLC in 4 hr at 23 °C	2199	C

[a]*Diluted with sodium chloride 0.9% drawn into a syringe prior to drugs to yield the concentrations cited.*
[b]*Tested in sodium chloride 0.9%.*

Y-Site Injection Compatibility (1:1 Mixture)

Ondansetron HCl

Drug	Mfr	Conc	Mfr	Conc	Remarks	Ref	C/I
Acyclovir sodium	BW	7 mg/ml[a]	GL	1 mg/ml[b]	Immediate precipitation	1365	**I**
Aldesleukin	CHI	33,800 I.U./ml[a]	GL	0.7 mg/ml[a]	Visually compatible with little or no loss of aldesleukin activity by bioassay	1857	**C**
Allopurinol sodium	BW	3 mg/ml[b]	GL	1 mg/ml[b]	Heavy turbidity forms immediately, becoming white flocculent precipitate	1686	**I**
Amifostine	USB	10 mg/ml[a]	GL	1 mg/ml[a]	Physically compatible with no change in measured turbidity or increase in particle content in 4 hr at 23 °C	1845	**C**
Amikacin sulfate	BR	5 mg/ml[a]	GL	1 mg/ml[b]	Physically compatible for 4 hr at 22 °C	1365	**C**
Aminophylline	AMR	2.5 mg/ml[a]	GL	1 mg/ml[b]	Immediate turbidity and precipitation	1365	**I**
Amphotericin B	SQ	0.6 mg/ml[a]	GL	1 mg/ml[a]	Immediate pale yellow turbidity and precipitation	1365	**I**
Amphotericin B cholesteryl sulfate complex	SEQ	0.83 mg/ml[a]	CER	1 mg/ml[a]	Gross precipitate forms	2117	**I**
Ampicillin sodium	BR	20 mg/ml[b]	GL	1 mg/ml[b]	Immediate turbidity and precipitation	1365	**I**
Ampicillin sodium–sulbactam sodium	RR	20 + 10 mg/ml[b]	GL	1 mg/ml[b]	Immediate turbidity and precipitation	1365	**I**
Amsacrine	NCI	1 mg/ml[a]	GL	1 mg/ml[a]	Orange precipitate forms within 30 min	1365	**I**
Aztreonam	SQ	40 mg/ml[a]	GL	1 mg/ml[b]	Physically compatible for 4 hr at 22 °C	1365	**C**
	SQ	40 mg/ml[a]	GL	0.03 and 0.3 mg/ml[a]	Visually compatible with little or no loss of either drug by HPLC in 4 hr at 25 °C	1732	**C**
	SQ	40 mg/ml[a]	GL	1 mg/ml[a]	Physically compatible with no subvisual haze or particle formation in 4 hr at 23 °C	1758	**C**
Bleomycin sulfate	BR	1 unit/ml[b]	GL	1 mg/ml[b]	Physically compatible for 4 hr at 22 °C	1365	**C**
Carboplatin	BR	5 mg/ml[a]	GL	1 mg/ml[b]	Physically compatible for 4 hr at 22 °C	1365	**C**
		0.18 to 9.9 mg/ml	GL	16 to 160 µg/ml	Physically compatible when carboplatin given over 10 to 60 min via Y-site	1366	**C**
Carmustine	BR	1.5 mg/ml[a]	GL	1 mg/ml[b]	Physically compatible for 4 hr at 22 °C	1365	**C**
Cefazolin sodium	LEM	20 mg/ml[a]	GL	1 mg/ml[b]	Physically compatible for 4 hr at 22 °C	1365	**C**
	LI	20 mg/ml[a]	GL	0.03 and 0.3 mg/ml[a]	Visually compatible with little or no loss of either drug by HPLC in 4 hr at 25 °C	1732	**C**
Cefepime HCl	BR	20 mg/ml[a]	GL	1 mg/ml[a]	Haze forms immediately	1689	**I**
Cefoperazone sodium	RR	40 mg/ml[a]	GL	1 mg/ml[b]	Immediate turbidity and precipitation	1365	**I**
Cefotaxime sodium	HO	20 mg/ml[a]	GL	1 mg/ml[b]	Physically compatible for 4 hr at 22 °C	1365	**C**
Cefoxitin sodium	MSD	20 mg/ml[a]	GL	1 mg/ml[b]	Physically compatible for 4 hr at 22 °C	1365	**C**
Ceftazidime	GL[i]	40 mg/ml[a]	GL	1 mg/ml[b]	Physically compatible for 4 hr at 22 °C	1365	**C**
	[i]	100 to 200 mg/ml	GL	16 to 160 µg/ml	Physically compatible when ceftazidime given as 5-min bolus via Y-site	1366	**C**
	LI[i]	40 mg/ml[a]	GL	0.03 and 0.3 mg/ml[a]	Visually compatible with less than 10% loss of either drug by HPLC in 4 hr at 25 °C	1732	**C**
	GL[h]	40 mg/ml[a]	GL	1 mg/ml[b]	Physically compatible for 4 hr at 22 °C	1365	**C**
Ceftizoxime sodium	FUJ	20 mg/ml[a]	GL	1 mg/ml[b]	Physically compatible for 4 hr at 22 °C	1365	**C**

Y-Site Injection Compatibility (1:1 Mixture) (Cont.)

Ondansetron HCl

Drug	Mfr	Conc	Mfr	Conc	Remarks	Ref	C/I
Cefuroxime sodium	LI	30 mg/ml[a]	GL	1 mg/ml[b]	Physically compatible for 4 hr at 22 °C	1365	C
Chlorpromazine HCl	ES	2 mg/ml[a]	GL	1 mg/ml[b]	Physically compatible for 4 hr at 22 °C	1365	C
Cimetidine HCl	SKF	12 mg/ml[a]	GL	1 mg/ml[b]	Physically compatible for 4 hr at 22 °C	1365	C
Cisatracurium besylate	GW	0.1, 2, 5 mg/ml[a]	CER	1 mg/ml[a]	Physically compatible with no change in measured turbidity or increase in particle content in 4 hr at 23 °C	2074	C
Cisplatin	BR	1 mg/ml 0.48 mg/ml	GL GL	1 mg/ml[b] 16 to 160 μg/ml	Physically compatible for 4 hr at 22 °C Physically compatible when cisplatin given over 1 to 8 hr via Y-site	1365 1366	C C
Cladribine	ORT	0.015[b] and 0.5[d] mg/ml	CER	1 mg/ml[b]	Physically compatible with no change in measured turbidity or increase in particle content in 4 hr at 23 °C	1969	C
Clindamycin phosphate	LY	10 mg/ml[a]	GL	1 mg/ml[b]	Physically compatible for 4 hr at 22 °C	1365	C
Cyclophosphamide	MJ	10 mg/ml[a] 20 mg/ml	GL GL	1 mg/ml[b] 16 to 160 μg/ml	Physically compatible for 4 hr at 22 °C Physically compatible when cyclophosphamide given as 5-min bolus via Y-site	1365 1366	C C
Cytarabine	UP	50 mg/ml	GL	1 mg/ml[b]	Physically compatible for 4 hr at 22 °C	1365	C
Dacarbazine	MI	4 mg/ml[a]	GL	1 mg/ml[b]	Physically compatible for 4 hr at 22 °C	1365	C
Dactinomycin	MSD	0.01 mg/ml[a]	GL	1 mg/ml[b]	Physically compatible for 4 hr at 22 °C	1365	C
Daunorubicin HCl	WY	2 mg/ml[a]	GL	1 mg/ml[b]	Physically compatible for 4 hr at 22 °C	1365	C
Dexamethasone sodium phosphate	MSD	1 mg/ml[a]	GL	1 mg/ml[b]	Physically compatible for 4 hr at 22 °C	1365	C
Diphenhydramine HCl	PD	2 mg/ml[a]	GL	1 mg/ml[b]	Physically compatible for 4 hr at 22 °C	1365	C
Docetaxel	RPR	0.9 mg/ml[a]	GW	1 mg/ml[a]	Physically compatible with no change in measured turbidity or increase in particle content in 4 hr at 23 °C	2224	C
Dopamine HCl	AB	0.8 mg/ml[a]	GL	0.32 mg/ml[c]	Visually compatible for 24 hr at room temperature in test tubes. No precipitate found on filter from Y-site delivery	2063	C
Doxorubicin HCl	CET	2 mg/ml 2 mg/ml	GL GL	1 mg/ml[b] 16 to 160 μg/ml	Physically compatible for 4 hr at 22 °C Physically compatible when doxorubicin given as 5-min bolus via Y-site	1365 1366	C C
Doxorubicin HCl liposome injection	SEQ	0.4 mg/ml[a]	CER	1 mg/ml[a]	Physically compatible with little or no change in measured turbidity and no increase in particle content in 4 hr at 23 °C	2087	C
Doxycycline hyclate	ES	1 mg/ml[a]	GL	1 mg/ml[b]	Physically compatible for 4 hr at 22 °C	1365	C
Droperidol	JN	0.4 mg/ml[a]	GL	1 mg/ml[b]	Physically compatible for 4 hr at 22 °C	1365	C
Etoposide	BR	0.4 mg/ml[a] 0.144 to 0.25 mg/ml	GL GL	1 mg/ml[b] 16 to 160 μg/ml	Physically compatible for 4 hr at 22 °C Physically compatible when etoposide given over 30 to 60 min via Y-site	1365 1366	C C
Etoposide phosphate	BR	5 mg/ml[a]	GW	1 mg/ml[a]	Physically compatible with no change in measured turbidity or increase in particle content in 4 hr at 23 °C	2218	C
Famotidine	MSD	2 mg/ml[a]	GL	1 mg/ml[b]	Physically compatible for 4 hr at 22 °C	1365	C

Y-Site Injection Compatibility (1:1 Mixture) (Cont.)

Ondansetron HCl

Drug	Mfr	Conc	Mfr	Conc	Remarks	Ref	C/I
Filgrastim	AMG	30 μg/ml[a]	GL	1 mg/ml[a]	Physically compatible with no change in measured turbidity or increase in particle content in 4 hr at 22 °C	1687	**C**
Floxuridine	RC	3 mg/ml[a]	GL	1 mg/ml[b]	Physically compatible for 4 hr at 22 °C	1365	**C**
Fluconazole	PF	2 mg/ml	GL	1 mg/ml[b]	Physically compatible for 4 hr at 22 °C	1365	**C**
	RR	2 mg/ml[b]	GL	0.03 and 0.3 mg/ml[a]	Visually compatible with little or no loss of either drug by HPLC in 4 hr at 25 °C	1732	**C**
	RR	2 mg/ml	GL	0.03, 0.1, 0.3 mg/ml[a,b]	Visually compatible with little or no ondansetron or fluconazole loss by HPLC in 4 hr and 5% or less loss of both drugs in 12 hr at room temperature	2168	**C**
Fludarabine phosphate	BX	1 mg/ml[a]	GL	0.5 mg/ml[a]	Physically compatible for 4 hr at room temperature under fluorescent light	1439	**C**
Fluorouracil	SO	16 mg/ml[a]	GL	1 mg/ml[b]	Immediate precipitation	1365	**I**
		≦0.8 mg/ml	GL	16 to 160 μg/ml	Physically compatible when fluorouracil given at 20 ml/hr via Y-site	1366	**C**
Furosemide	AB	3 mg/ml[a]	GL	1 mg/ml[b]	Immediate turbidity and precipitation	1365	**I**
Ganciclovir sodium	SY	20 mg/ml[a]	GL	1 mg/ml[b]	Immediate turbidity and precipitation	1365	**I**
Gemcitabine HCl	LI	10 mg/ml[b]	GW	1 mg/ml[b]	Physically compatible with no change in measured turbidity or increase in particle content in 4 hr at 23 °C	2226	**C**
Gentamicin sulfate	ES	5 mg/ml[a]	GL	1 mg/ml[b]	Physically compatible for 4 hr at 22 °C	1365	**C**
Haloperidol lactate	LY	0.2 mg/ml[a]	GL	1 mg/ml[b]	Physically compatible for 4 hr at 22 °C	1365	**C**
Heparin sodium	SO	40 units/ml[a]	GL	1 mg/ml[b]	Physically compatible for 4 hr at 22 °C	1365	**C**
Hydrocortisone sodium phosphate	MSD	1 mg/ml[a]	GL	1 mg/ml[b]	Physically compatible for 4 hr at 22 °C	1365	**C**
Hydrocortisone sodium succinate	UP	1 mg/ml[a]	GL	1 mg/ml[b]	Physically compatible for 4 hr at 22 °C	1365	**C**
Hydromorphone HCl	KN	0.5 mg/ml[a]	GL	1 mg/ml[b]	Physically compatible for 4 hr at 22 °C	1365	**C**
Hydroxyzine HCl	WI	4 mg/ml[a]	GL	1 mg/ml[b]	Physically compatible for 4 hr at 22 °C	1365	**C**
Ifosfamide	MJ	25 mg/ml[a]	GL	1 mg/ml[b]	Physically compatible for 4 hr at 22 °C	1365	**C**
Imipenem–cilastatin sodium	MSD	5 mg/ml[b]	GL	1 mg/ml[b]	Physically compatible for 4 hr at 22 °C	1365	**C**
Lorazepam	WY	0.1 mg/ml[a]	GL	1 mg/ml[b]	Light haze develops immediately	1365	**I**
Magnesium sulfate	SO	100 mg/ml[a]	GL	1 mg/ml[b]	Physically compatible for 4 hr at 22 °C	1365	**C**
Mannitol	BA	15%	GL	1 mg/ml[b]	Physically compatible for 4 hr at 22 °C	1365	**C**
Mechlorethamine HCl	MSD	1 mg/ml	GL	1 mg/ml[b]	Physically compatible for 4 hr at 22 °C	1365	**C**
Melphalan HCl	BW	0.1 mg/ml[b]	GL	1 mg/ml[b]	Physically compatible with no change in measured turbidity or increase in particle content in 3 hr at 22 °C	1557	**C**
Meperidine HCl	WI	4 mg/ml[a]	GL	1 mg/ml[b]	Physically compatible for 4 hr at 22 °C	1365	**C**
Meropenem	ZEN	1 mg/ml[b]	GL	1 mg/ml[c]	Visually compatible for 4 hr at room temperature	1994	**C**
	ZEN	50 mg/ml[b]	GL	1 mg/ml[c]	White precipitate forms immediately	1994	**I**
Mesna	BR	10 mg/ml[a]	GL	1 mg/ml[b]	Physically compatible for 4 hr at 22 °C	1365	**C**
Methotrexate sodium	CET	15 mg/ml[a]	GL	1 mg/ml[b]	Physically compatible for 4 hr at 22 °C	1365	**C**

Y-Site Injection Compatibility (1:1 Mixture) (Cont.)

Ondansetron HCl

Drug	Mfr	Conc	Mfr	Conc	Remarks	Ref	C/I
		30 mg/ml	GL	2 mg/ml	Visually compatible for 4 hr at room temperature	1788	C
Methylprednisolone sodium succinate	UP	5 mg/ml[a]	GL	1 mg/ml[b]	Light haze develops in 30 min	1365	I
Metoclopramide HCl	DU	5 mg/ml	GL	1 mg/ml[b]	Physically compatible for 4 hr at 22 °C	1365	C
Mitomycin	BR	0.5 mg/ml	GL	1 mg/ml[b]	Physically compatible for 4 hr at 22 °C	1365	C
Mitoxantrone HCl	LE	0.5 mg/ml[a]	GL	1 mg/ml[b]	Physically compatible for 4 hr at 22 °C	1365	C
Morphine sulfate	WI	1 mg/ml[a]	GL	1 mg/ml[b]	Physically compatible for 4 hr at 22 °C	1365	C
Paclitaxel	NCI	1.2 mg/ml[a]	GL	0.5 mg/ml[a]	Physically compatible with no change in measured turbidity in 4 hr at 22 °C	1556	C
	BR	0.3 mg/ml[a]	GL	0.03 and 0.3 mg/ml[a]	Visually compatible with no loss of either drug in 4 hr at 23 °C	1741	C
	BR	1.2 mg/ml[a]	GL	0.03 and 0.3 mg/ml[a]	Visually compatible with no loss of either drug in 4 hr at 23 °C	1741	C
Paclitaxel with ranitidine HCl	BR GL	1.2 mg/ml[a] 2 mg/ml[a]	GL	0.3 mg/ml[a]	Visually compatible with no loss of any drug by HPLC in 4 hr at 23 °C	1741	C
Pentostatin	NCI	0.4 mg/ml[b]	GL	1 mg/ml[b]	Physically compatible for 4 hr at 22 °C	1365	C
Piperacillin sodium	LE	40 mg/ml[a]	GL	1 mg/ml[b]	Slight turbidity appears in 30 min	1365	I
Piperacillin sodium–tazobactam sodium	LE	40 + 5 mg/ml[a]	GL	1 mg/ml[a]	Physically compatible with no change in measured turbidity or increase in particle content in 4 hr at 22 °C	1688	C
	LE	40 + 5 mg/ml[b]	GL	0.03, 0.1, 0.3 mg/ml[b]	Visually compatible with no loss of any component by HPLC in 4 hr	1751	C
	LE	80 + 10 mg/ml[b]	GL	0.03, 0.1, 0.3 mg/ml[b]	Visually compatible with no loss of any component by HPLC in 4 hr	1751	C
Potassium chloride	AB	0.1 mEq/ml[a]	GL	1 mg/ml[b]	Physically compatible for 4 hr at 22 °C	1365	C
Prochlorperazine edisylate	SKF	0.5 mg/ml[a]	GL	1 mg/ml[b]	Physically compatible for 4 hr at 22 °C	1365	C
Promethazine HCl	ES	2 mg/ml[a]	GL	1 mg/ml[b]	Physically compatible for 4 hr at 22 °C	1365	C
Ranitidine HCl	GL	2 mg/ml[a]	GL	1 mg/ml[b]	Physically compatible for 4 hr at 22 °C	1365	C
	GL	0.5 mg/ml[a]	GL	0.03, 0.1, 0.3 mg/ml[a]	Visually compatible with no loss of either drug by HPLC in 4 hr	1730	C
	GL	2 mg/ml[a]	GL	0.03, 0.1, 0.3 mg/ml[a]	Visually compatible with no loss of either drug by HPLC in 4 hr	1730	C
Remifentanil HCl	GW	0.025 and 0.25 mg/ml[b]	CER	1 mg/ml[a]	Physically compatible with no change in measured turbidity or increase in particle content in 4 hr at 23 °C	2075	C
Sargramostim	IMM	10 μg/ml[b]	GL	0.5 mg/ml[b]	Filaments form in 30 to 60 min	1436	I
Sodium acetate		0.1 and 1 mEq/ml[a]	GL	0.1 mg/ml[a]	Visually compatible with no increase in 10-, 25-, and 50-μm particles in 4 hr at room temperature	1661	C
Sodium bicarbonate		0.05 mM/ml[e]	GL	0.32 mg/ml[a]	White precipitate forms immediately	1513	I
		0.1 mEq/ml[a]	GL	0.1 mg/ml[a]	Large increase in 10-, 25-, and 50-μm particles. Visible particles in 30 to 60 min at room temperature	1661	I
		1.4%	GL	2 mg/ml	Heavy white precipitate forms immediately	1788	I
Streptozocin	UP	30 mg/ml[a]	GL	1 mg/ml[b]	Physically compatible for 4 hr at 22 °C	1365	C

Y-Site Injection Compatibility (1:1 Mixture) (Cont.)

Ondansetron HCl

Drug	Mfr	Conc	Mfr	Conc	Remarks	Ref	C/I
Teniposide	BR	0.1 mg/ml[a]	GL	1 mg/ml[b]	Physically compatible for 4 hr at 22 °C	1365	C
	BR	0.1 mg/ml[a]	GL	1 mg/ml[a]	Physically compatible with no subvisual haze or particle formation in 4 hr at 23 °C	1725	C
Thiotepa	IMM[f]	1 mg/ml[a]	GL	1 mg/ml[a]	Physically compatible with no change in measured turbidity or increase in particle content in 4 hr at 23 °C	1861	C
Ticarcillin disodium	BE	30 mg/ml[a]	GL	1 mg/ml[b]	Physically compatible for 4 hr at 22 °C	1365	C
Ticarcillin disodium–clavulanate potassium	BE	31 mg/ml[a]	GL	1 mg/ml[b]	Physically compatible for 4 hr at 22 °C	1365	C
TNA #218 to #226[g]			CER	1 mg/ml[a]	Damage to emulsion integrity occurs immediately with free oil formation possible	2215	I
TPN #212 to #215[g]			GL	1 mg/ml[a]	Physically compatible with no change in measured turbidity or increase in particle content in 4 hr at 23 °C	2109	C
Vancomycin HCl	LI	10 mg/ml[a]	GL	1 mg/ml[b]	Physically compatible for 4 hr at 22 °C	1365	C
Vinblastine sulfate	LY	0.12 mg/ml[a]	GL	1 mg/ml[b]	Physically compatible for 4 hr at 22 °C	1365	C
Vincristine sulfate	LY	0.05 mg/ml[a]	GL	1 mg/ml[b]	Physically compatible for 4 hr at 22 °C	1365	C
Vinorelbine tartrate	BW	1 mg/ml[b]	GL	1 mg/ml[b]	Physically compatible with no change in measured turbidity or increase in particle content in 4 hr at 22 °C	1558	C
Zidovudine	BW	4 mg/ml[a]	GL	1 mg/ml[b]	Physically compatible for 4 hr at 22 °C	1365	C

[a]*Tested in dextrose 5% in water.*
[b]*Tested in sodium chloride 0.9%.*
[c]*Tested in sterile water for injection.*
[d]*Tested in bacteriostatic sodium chloride 0.9% preserved with benzyl alcohol 0.9%.*
[e]*Tested in dextrose 5% in water with potassium chloride 0.02 mM/ml.*
[f]*Lyophilized formulation tested.*
[g]*Refer to Appendix I for the composition of parenteral nutrition solutions. TNA indicates a 3-in-1 admixture, and TPN indicates a 2-in-1 admixture.*
[h]*Arginine-containing formulation tested.*
[i]*Sodium carbonate–containing formulation tested.*

Additional Compatibility Information

Solutions— The manufacturer states that ondansetron HCl is stable at room temperature and exposed to normal light for 48 hours when diluted in the following infusion solutions (2):

Dextrose 5% in sodium chloride 0.45%
Dextrose 5% in sodium chloride 0.9%
Dextrose 5% in water
Sodium chloride 0.9%
Sodium chloride 3%

OXACILLIN SODIUM
AHFS 8:12.16

Products— Oxacillin sodium is available in vials containing the equivalent of oxacillin 500 mg, 1 g, 2 g, and 4 g. A 10-g hospital bulk package also is available. The products also contain dibasic sodium phosphate 40 mg/g of drug (4).

For intramuscular use, reconstitute the vials with the appropriate amount of sterile water for injection or sodium chloride 0.45 or 0.9% as listed below and shake until a clear solution is obtained. A 250-mg/1.5 ml (167 mg/ml) solution results (4).

Vial Size	Volume of Diluent
500 mg	2.8 ml
1 g	5.7 ml
2 g	11.4 ml
4 g	21.8 ml

For direct intravenous injection, reconstitute the 500-mg, 1-, 2-, and 4-g vials with 5, 10, 20, or 40 ml, respectively, of sterile water for injection, sodium chloride 0.45%, or sodium chloride 0.9% and shake until a clear solution is obtained to yield a 100-mg/ml concentration (4).

The 10-g hospital bulk package is reconstituted with 93 ml of sterile water for injection to yield a 100-mg/ml solution (4).

Frozen premixed solutions of oxacillin 1 g/50 ml in dextrose 3% and 2 g/50 ml in dextrose 0.6% are also available. The solutions also contain sodium citrate buffer and hydrochloric acid and/or sodium hydroxide to adjust the pH (4).

pH— From 6 to 8.5 (4). At a concentration of 10 g/L in dextrose 5% in water, the pH has been variously reported as 7.4 (149) and 7.94 (153). At this concentration in sodium chloride 0.9%, the pH has been reported as 7.73 (153).

Osmolality— The osmolality of oxacillin sodium (Bristol) 250 mg/1.5 ml in sterile water for injection was determined to be 596 mOsm/kg by freezing-point depression and 657 mOsm/kg by vapor pressure (1071).

The osmolality of oxacillin sodium (Beecham) 50 mg/ml was determined to be 381 mOsm/kg in dextrose 5% in water and 396 mOsm/kg in sodium chloride 0.9% (1375).

The osmolality of oxacillin sodium was calculated for the following dilutions (1054):

| | Osmolality (mOsm/kg) | |
Diluent	50 ml	100 ml
1 g		
Dextrose 5% in water	326	295
Sodium chloride 0.9%	353	321
2 g		
Dextrose 5% in water	379	329
Sodium chloride 0.9%	406	356

Robinson et al. recommended the following maximum oxacillin sodium concentrations to achieve osmolalities suitable for peripheral infusion in fluid-restricted patients (1180):

Diluent	Maximum Concentration (mg/ml)	Osmolality (mOsm/kg)
Dextrose 5% in water	59	530
Sodium chloride 0.9%	53	519
Sterile water for injection	106	422

The frozen premixed solutions are iso-osmotic, having an osmolality of about 300 mOsm/kg (4).

Sodium Content— Each gram of oxacillin sodium powder contains approximately 2.5 to 3.1 mEq of sodium (4; 154).

Administration— Oxacillin sodium may be administered by deep intramuscular injection, direct intravenous injection, or by continuous or intermittent intravenous infusion. By direct intravenous injection, the dose should be given over a 10-minute period. For intermittent infusion, the drug should be further diluted with a compatible solution to a concentration of 0.5 to 40 mg/ml (4).

Stability— Oxacillin sodium in intact vials should be stored at controlled room temperature. After reconstitution, oxacillin sodium is stable for three days at room temperature and for one week under refrigeration at concentrations used for intramuscular or direct intravenous injection. In ADD-Vantage vials, oxacillin sodium reconstituted with sodium chloride 0.9% or dextrose 5% in water is stated to be stable for 24 hours or three days, respectively, at room temperature. The reconstituted hospital bulk package is stable for 24 hours at room temperature (4).

The frozen premixed injection is stable at −20 °C for at least 90 days after shipping. The frozen premixed infusions should be thawed at room temperature or under refrigeration and should not be refrozen after being thawed initially. The thawed solutions are stated to be stable for 48 hours at room temperature and 21 days under refrigeration (4).

Freezing Solutions— Oxacillin sodium (Bristol), 500 mg/2.5 ml and 1 g/5 ml in sterile water for injection packaged in glass and plastic syringes and 200 mg/ml in the original vial, was frozen at −20 °C. Chemical analysis indicated that adequate stability was maintained over three months of storage (303).

In another study, oxacillin sodium (Bristol) 1 g/100 ml of dextrose 5% in water in PVC bags was frozen at −20 °C for 30 days. The bags were then thawed by exposure to ambient temperature or microwave radiation. The solutions showed no evidence of precipitation or color change and no loss of potency as determined microbiologically. Subsequent storage of the admixture at room temperature for 24 hours yielded a physically compatible solution, which exhibited a 3 to 4% loss of potency (554).

Portable Infusion Pumps— The stability of oxacillin sodium (Marsam) 120 mg/ml in sterile water for injection was evaluated in PVC portable infusion pump reservoirs (Pharmacia Deltec). HPLC analysis found no oxacillin loss in three days at 25 °C and 5% loss in 14 days at 5 °C (2080).

Sorption— Picard et al. reported little or no loss due to sorption of oxacillin sodium (Bristol) 1 g/100 ml in dextrose 5% in water and sodium chloride 0.9% in trilayer solution bags (Bieffe Medital) composed of polyethylene, polyamide, and polypropylene. The admixtures were evaluated by HPLC analysis up to two hours after preparation. Similarly, no loss was found during a one-hour simulated infusion (1918).

Compatibility Information

Solution Compatibility

Oxacillin sodium

Solution	Mfr	Mfr	Conc/L	Remarks	Ref	C/I
Amino acids 4.25%, dextrose 25%	MG	BR	500 mg	No increase in particulate matter in 24 hr at 5 °C	349	C
Dextran 70 6% in dextrose 5%			4 g	Approximately 1 to 3% decomposition in 24 hr at 20 °C	834	C
Dextran 40 10% in dextrose 5%			4 g	3% decomposition in 24 hr at 20 °C	834	C
Dextrose 5% in Ringer's injection, lactated	TR[a]	BR	1 g	Potency retained for 24 hr at 5 °C	282	C
Dextrose 5% in sodium chloride 0.9%	TR[a]	BR	1 g	Potency retained for 24 hr at 5 °C	282	C
		BR	2 g	12% decomposition in 12 hr and 14% in 24 hr	109	I
Dextrose 5% in water		BR	2 g	Potency retained for 24 hr	109	C
		BR	1, 10, 50 g	4 to 9% oxacillin decomposition in 24 hr at 23 °C	153	C
	TR[a]	BR	1 g	Potency retained for 24 hr at 5 °C	282	C
	TR[b]	BR	10 g	Physically compatible with approximately 8% potency loss in 24 hr at room temperature	554	C
			4 g	8% loss in 6 hr and 14% loss in 24 hr at room temperature	768	I
	b	BR	20 g	No drug loss by HPLC during 2-hr storage and 1-hr simulated infusion	1774	C
Dextrose 10% in water		BR	2 g	Potency retained for 24 hr	109	C
Hetastarch 6%			4 g	1% decomposition in 24 hr at 20 °C	834	C
Ringer's injection, lactated	TR[a]	BR	1 g	Potency retained for 24 hr at 5 °C	282	C
Sodium chloride 0.9%		BR	2 g	Potency retained for 24 hr	109	C
		BR	1, 10, 50 g	2 to 4% oxacillin decomposition in 24 hr at 23 °C	153	C
	TR[a]	BR	1 g	Potency retained for 24 hr at 5 °C	282	C
			4 g	10% loss in 8 hr and 12% loss in 24 hr at room temperature	768	I
	b	BR	20 g	No drug loss by HPLC during 2-hr storage and 1-hr simulated infusion	1774	C

[a]Tests performed in both glass and PVC containers.
[b]Tested in PVC containers.

Additive Compatibility

Oxacillin sodium

Drug	Mfr	Conc/L	Mfr	Conc/L	Test Soln	Remarks	Ref	C/I
Amikacin sulfate	BR	5 g	BR	2 g	D5LR, D5R, D5S, D5W, D10W, IS10, LR, NS, R	Physically compatible and potency of both retained for 24 hr at 25 °C	293	C
	BR	5 g	BR	2 g	NR, SL	Oxacillin potency retained through 8 hr at 25 °C. Greater than 10% decomposition in 24 hr	293	I
Chloramphenicol sodium succinate	PD	500 mg	BR	500 mg	D5S, D5W	Therapeutic availability maintained	110	C
	PD	1 g	BR	2 g	D5S, D5W	Therapeutic availability maintained	110	C

Additive Compatibility (Cont.)

Oxacillin sodium

Drug	Mfr	Conc/L	Mfr	Conc/L	Test Soln	Remarks	Ref	C/I
	PD	1 g	BR	2 g		Physically compatible	6	C
Cytarabine	UP	100 mg		2 g	D5W	pH outside stability range for oxacillin	174	I
Dopamine HCl	AS	800 mg	BR	2 g	D5W	No dopamine decomposition and 2% oxacillin decomposition in 24 hr at 25 °C	312	C
Potassium chloride		20, 40, 80 mEq	BR	1, 2.5, 4 g	D5S, D5W	Therapeutic availability maintained	110	C
Sodium bicarbonate	AB	2.4 mEq[a]	BR	500 mg	D5W	Physically compatible for 24 hr	772	C
Verapamil HCl	KN	80 mg	BR	4 g	D5W, NS	Physically compatible for 24 hr	764	C
	SE	[b]	BR	40 g	D5W, NS	Cloudy solution clears with agitation	1166	?

[a]One vial of Neut added to a liter of admixture.
[b]Final concentration unspecified.

Y-Site Injection Compatibility (1:1 Mixture)

Oxacillin sodium

Drug	Mfr	Conc	Mfr	Conc	Remarks	Ref	C/I
Acyclovir sodium	BW	5 mg/ml[a]	BE	20 mg/ml[a]	Physically compatible for 4 hr at 25 °C	1157	C
Cyclophosphamide	MJ	20 mg/ml[a]	BE	20 mg/ml[a]	Physically compatible for 4 hr at 25 °C	1194	C
Diltiazem HCl	MMD	1[b] and 5 mg/ml		100 mg/ml[b]	Visually compatible	1807	C
	MMD	5 mg/ml		10 mg/L[b]	Visually compatible	1807	C
Famotidine	MSD	0.2 mg/ml[a]	BE	20 mg/ml[b]	Physically compatible for 14 hr	1196	C
Fluconazole	RR	2 mg/ml	BE	40 mg/ml	Physically compatible for 24 hr at 25 °C	1407	C
Foscarnet sodium	AST	24 mg/ml	BR	40 mg/ml	Physically compatible for 24 hr at room temperature under fluorescent light	1335	C
	AST	24 mg/ml	BE	20 mg/ml[c]	Physically compatible for 24 hr at 25 °C under fluorescent light by visual and microscopic examination	1393	C
Heparin sodium	UP	1000 units/L[d]	BR	100 mg/ml	Physically compatible for at least 4 hr at room temperature by visual and microscopic examination	534	C
Hydrocortisone sodium succinate	UP	10 mg/L[d]	BR	100 mg/ml	Physically compatible for at least 4 hr at room temperature by visual and microscopic examination	534	C
Hydromorphone HCl	WY	0.2 mg/ml[a]	BE	20 mg/ml[a]	Physically compatible for at least 4 hr at 25 °C under fluorescent light	987	C
Labetalol HCl	SC	1 mg/ml[a]	BR	10 mg/ml[a]	Physically compatible for 24 hr at 18 °C	1171	C
Magnesium sulfate	IX	16.7, 33.3, 66.7, 100 mg/ml[a]	BE	20 mg/ml[a]	Physically compatible for at least 4 hr at 32 °C	813	C
Meperidine HCl	WY	10 mg/ml[a]	BE	20 mg/ml[a]	Physically compatible for at least 4 hr at 25 °C under fluorescent light	987	C
Methotrexate sodium		30 mg/ml	BR	250 mg/ml	Visually compatible for 4 hr at room temperature	1788	C
Morphine sulfate	WI	1 mg/ml[a]	BE	20 mg/ml[a]	Physically compatible for at least 4 hr at 25 °C under fluorescent light	987	C

Y-Site Injection Compatibility (1:1 Mixture) (Cont.)

Oxacillin sodium

Drug	Mfr	Conc	Mfr	Conc	Remarks	Ref	C/I
Perphenazine	SC	0.02 mg/ml[a]	BE	20 mg/ml[a]	Physically compatible for 4 hr at 25 °C	1155	C
Potassium chloride	AB	40 mEq/L[d]	BR	100 mg/ml	Physically compatible for at least 4 hr at room temperature by visual and microscopic examination	534	C
Sodium bicarbonate		1.4%	BR	250 mg/ml	Gas evolves	1788	I
Tacrolimus	FUJ	1 mg/ml[b]	BR	40 mg/ml[a]	Visually compatible for 24 hr at 25 °C	1630	C
TNA #73[e]		32.5 ml[f]	BE	1 g/50 ml[a]	Physically compatible by visual observation for 4 hr at 25 °C	1008	C
TPN #54[e]				100 and 150 mg/ml	Physically compatible with 88 to 94% oxacillin activity retained over 6 hr at 22 °C by microbiological assay	1045	C
TPN #61[e]		[g]	BE	250 mg/ 1.5 ml[h]	Physically compatible	1012	C
		[i]	BE	1.5 g/9 ml[h]	Physically compatible	1012	C
Verapamil HCl	SE	2.5 mg/ml	BR	40 mg/ml[c]	White milky precipitate forms immediately and persists. 39% of verapamil precipitated	1166	I
Vitamin B complex with C	RC	2 ml/L[d]	BR	100 mg/ml	Physically compatible for at least 4 hr at room temperature by visual and microscopic examination	534	C
Zidovudine	BW	4 mg/ml[a]	BR	20 mg/ml[a]	Physically compatible for 4 hr at 25 °C under fluorescent light by visual and microscopic examination	1193	C

[a]*Tested in dextrose 5% in water.*
[b]*Tested in sodium chloride 0.9%.*
[c]*Tested in both dextrose 5% in water and sodium chloride 0.9%.*
[d]*Tested in dextrose 5% in Ringer's injection, dextrose 5% in Ringer's injection, lactated, dextrose 5% in water, Ringer's injection, lactated, and sodium chloride 0.9%.*
[e]*Refer to Appendix I for the composition of parenteral nutrition solutions. TNA indicates a 3-in-1 admixture, and TPN indicates a 2-in-1 admixture.*
[f]*A 32.5-ml sample of parenteral nutrition solution mixed with 50 ml of antibiotic solution.*
[g]*Run at 21 ml/hr.*
[h]*Given over five minutes by syringe pump.*
[i]*Run at 94 ml/hr.*

Additional Compatibility Information

Acidic Additives— Acid-labile drugs such as oxacillin sodium may degrade in infusion solutions containing acidic additives (22).

Infusion Solutions— Oxacillin sodium in concentrations of 0.5 to 40 mg/ml loses less than 10% activity at room temperature in six hours in the following infusion solutions (4):

Dextrose 5% in sodium chloride 0.9%
Dextrose 5% in water
Fructose 10% in sodium chloride 0.9%
Fructose 10% in water
Invert sugar 10% in Electrolyte #1
Invert sugar 10% in Electrolyte #2
Invert sugar 10% in Electrolyte #3
Invert sugar 10% and potassium chloride 0.3%
Invert sugar 10% in sodium chloride 0.9%
Invert sugar 10% in water
Ringer's injection, lactated
Sodium chloride 0.9%

It has been stated that the decomposition of oxacillin sodium in solutions is independent of concentration. However, dextrose has a catalytic effect on the hydrolysis of the drug. It was predicted that oxacillin sodium in solutions with dextrose 5% or less would be stable for at least 24 hours at room temperature. In higher dextrose concentrations, the drug would not be stable for 24 hours at room temperature (153).

Aminoglycosides— Lundergan et al. studied, in vitro, the interaction of tobramycin sulfate with several penicillins in human serum under clinical laboratory conditions. Tobramycin sulfate 10 μg/ml was combined with carbenicillin disodium 200 μg/ml, oxacillin sodium (Bristol) 50 μg/ml, and nafcillin sodium (Wyeth) 50 μg/ml. Samples were evaluated over 72 hours at −23, 6, and 23 °C. Although the results were somewhat variable, only the carbenicillin sample at 23 °C exhibited substantial decomposition after 72 hours. None of the other carbenicillin, oxacillin, or nafcillin samples showed significant differences over the study period (814).

The comparative inactivation of five aminoglycosides by seven β-lactam antibiotics in human serum at 37 °C was reported by Riff and Thomason. Amikacin, followed by netilmicin, had the lowest degree of inactivation; tobramycin sustained the most pronounced losses. Gentamicin and kanamycin were intermediate in the extent of losses. The six penicillins that were tested all produced aminoglycoside inactivation; the greatest extent of inactivation was caused by carbenicillin followed by ticarcillin, penicillin G, oxacillin, methicillin, and ampicillin, in approximate descending order. Ceph-

alothin produced minimal inactivation (5 to 10% in 24 hours). The rate of inactivation could be reduced by storage at 4 °C and further reduced by storage at −20 °C. The authors suggested processing blood samples rapidly to avoid inaccurate serum determinations. Storage of specimens at low temperature until analysis may be helpful (1052).

Plastic Container Component Extraction— Oxacillin sodium as the frozen premixed infusion solutions may leach small amounts of container components from the PL 2040 (Galaxy) plastic containers. However, it is stated that the safety of the products has been confirmed by biological testing (4).

OXYMORPHONE HCL
AHFS 28:08.08

Numorphan   **Endo**

Products— Oxymorphone HCl (Endo) is available in a concentration of 1 mg/ml in 1-ml ampuls. It is also available in a concentration of 1.5 mg/ml in 10-ml vials. Each milliliter of solution contains (2):

	1-ml Ampul	10-ml Vial
Oxymorphone HCl	1 mg	1.5 mg
Sodium chloride	8 mg	8 mg

Methylparaben		1.8 mg
Propylparaben		0.2 mg
Hydrochloric acid	to adjust pH	to adjust pH

pH— From 2.7 to 4.5 (4).

Administration— Oxymorphone HCl may be administered by subcutaneous, intramuscular, or intravenous injection (2; 4).

Stability— Intact containers of oxymorphone HCl should be stored at controlled room temperature and protected from light and freezing (2; 4).

Compatibility Information

Drugs in Syringe Compatibility

Oxymorphone HCl

Drug (in syringe)	Mfr	Amt	Mfr	Amt	Remarks	Ref	C/I
Glycopyrrolate	RB	0.2 mg/ 1 ml	EN	1 mg/ 1 ml	Physically compatible and pH in stability range for glycopyrrolate for 48 hr at 25 °C	331	C
	RB	0.2 mg/ 1 ml	EN	2 mg/ 2 ml	Physically compatible and pH in stability range for glycopyrrolate for 48 hr at 25 °C	331	C
	RB	0.4 mg/ 2 ml	EN	1 mg/ 1 ml	Physically compatible and pH in stability range for glycopyrrolate for 48 hr at 25 °C	331	C
	RB	0.2 mg/ 1 ml	EN	1.5 mg/ 1 ml	Physically compatible and pH in stability range for glycopyrrolate for 48 hr at 25 °C	331	C
	RB	0.2 mg/ 1 ml	EN	3 mg/ 2 ml	Physically compatible and pH in stability range for glycopyrrolate for 48 hr at 25 °C	331	C
	RB	0.4 mg/ 2 ml	EN	1.5 mg/ 1 ml	Physically compatible and pH in stability range for glycopyrrolate for 48 hr at 25 °C	331	C
Hydroxyzine HCl	PF	100 mg/ 2 ml	EN	0.75 mg/ 0.5 ml	Physically compatible	771	C
Ranitidine HCl	GL	50 mg/ 2 ml	EN	1.5 mg/ 1 ml	Physically compatible for 1 hr at 25 °C both macroscopically and microscopically	978	C

OXYTOCIN
AHFS 76:00

Syntocinon **Novartis**
Pitocin **Monarch**
 Fujisawa

Products— Oxytocin is available in 1-ml ampuls, 1-ml disposable syringes, and 1- and 10-ml vials. Each milliliter contains oxytocin 10 units with chlorobutanol 0.5%. Oxytocin (Syntocinon, Novartis) also incorporates ethanol 0.61% into the formulation. Acetic acid may have been added to adjust the pH during manufacture (1-2/97; 4; 29).

Units— One unit of oxytocin is equivalent to 2 to 2.2 μg of pure oxytocin (4).

pH— The USP cites the official pH range as 3 to 5 (17), and the commercial products from Fujisawa are also listed as pH 3 to 5 (1-2/97). The AHFS cites the pH range as being 2.5 to 4.5 (4).

Osmolality— Oxytocin 10 units/ml has an osmolality of 24 mOsm/kg (1689).

Administration— Oxytocin is administered by intravenous infusion using an infusion control device (1-2/97; 4) or intramuscular injection (1-2/97). For intravenous administration the injection should be diluted to a usual concentration of 10 milliunits/ml by adding 10 units (1 ml) to 1000 ml of dextrose 5% in water, Ringer's injection, lactated, or sodium chloride 0.9% (1-2/97; 4). A higher concentration range of 10 to 40 milliunits/ml has been cited to control postpartum uterine bleeding (1-2/97).

Stability— Oxytocin injection should be stored at room temperature (15 to 25 °C) and protected from freezing. Do not use the solution if it is discolored or contains a precipitate (1-2/97; 4).

Filtration— Oxytocin (Parke-Davis) 25 units/100 ml in dextrose 5% in water and sodium chloride 0.9% was filtered at about 3 ml/min through a 0.22-μm cellulose ester membrane filter (Ivex-2). At this concentration, 25 times higher than normally used, oxytocin appeared to bind initially to the filter from the sodium chloride 0.9% solution. Results in dextrose 5% in water were equivocal. From these data, it is not possible to draw a definite conclusion regarding substantial binding of oxytocin during normal usage (533).

Compatibility Information

Solution Compatibility

Oxytocin

Solution	Mfr	Mfr	Conc/L	Remarks	Ref	C/I
Dextran 6% in dextrose 5%	AB	PD	5 units	Physically compatible	3	C
Dextran 6% in sodium chloride 0.9%	AB	PD	5 units	Physically compatible	3	C
Dextrose–Ringer's injection combinations	AB	PD	5 units	Physically compatible	3	C
Dextrose–Ringer's injection, lactated, combinations	AB	PD	5 units	Physically compatible	3	C
Dextrose–saline combinations	AB	PD	5 units	Physically compatible	3	C
Dextrose 2½% in water	AB	PD	5 units	Physically compatible	3	C
Dextrose 5% in water	AB	PD	5 units	Physically compatible	3	C
	CN		10.4 units	Stable for at least 6 hr at room temperature	333	C
Dextrose 10% in water	AB	PD	5 units	Physically compatible	3	C
Fructose 10% in sodium chloride 0.9%	AB	PD	5 units	Physically compatible	3	C
Fructose 10% in water	AB	PD	5 units	Physically compatible	3	C
Invert sugar 5 and 10% in sodium chloride 0.9%	AB	PD	5 units	Physically compatible	3	C
Invert sugar 5 and 10% in water	AB	PD	5 units	Physically compatible	3	C
Ionosol products	AB	PD	5 units	Physically compatible	3	C
Ringer's injection	AB	PD	5 units	Physically compatible	3	C
Ringer's injection, lactated	AB	PD	5 units	Physically compatible	3	C
Sodium chloride 0.45%	AB	PD	5 units	Physically compatible	3	C
Sodium chloride 0.9%	AB	PD	5 units	Physically compatible	3	C
Sodium lactate ⅙ M	AB	PD	5 units	Physically compatible	3	C

Additive Compatibility

Oxytocin

Drug	Mfr	Conc/L	Mfr	Conc/L	Test Soln	Remarks	Ref	C/I
Chloramphenicol sodium succinate	PD	1 g	PD	5 units		Physically compatible	6	**C**
Fibrinolysin, human	MSD	2 g	PD	5 units	D5W	Physically incompatible	11	**I**
Metaraminol bitartrate	MSD	100 mg	PD	5 units		Physically compatible	7	**C**
Netilmicin sulfate	SC	3 g	PD	4 ml	D5S	Physically compatible and netilmicin chemically stable for 7 days at 4 and 25 °C. Oxytocin not tested	558	**C**
Sodium bicarbonate	AB	2.4 mEq[a]	PD	5 units	D5W	Physically compatible for 24 hr	772	**C**
Thiopental sodium	AB	2.5 g	PD	5 units	D5W	Physically compatible	21	**C**
Verapamil HCl	KN	80 mg	SZ	40 units	D5W, NS	Physically compatible for 24 hr	764	**C**

[a]One vial of Neut added to a liter of admixture.

Y-Site Injection Compatibility (1:1 Mixture)

Oxytocin

Drug	Mfr	Conc	Mfr	Conc	Remarks	Ref	C/I
Heparin sodium	UP	1000 units/L[d]	SZ	1 mg/ml	Physically compatible for at least 4 hr at room temperature by visual and microscopic examination	534	**C**
Hydrocortisone sodium succinate	UP	10 mg/L[d]	SZ	1 mg/ml	Physically compatible for at least 4 hr at room temperature by visual and microscopic examination	534	**C**
Insulin, regular	LI	0.2 unit/ml[b]	PD	0.02 unit/ml[c]	Physically compatible for 2 hr at 25 °C	1395	**C**
Meperidine HCl	WY	10 mg/ml[b]	PD	0.02 mg/ml[c]	Physically compatible for 1 hr at 25 °C	1338	**C**
Morphine sulfate	ES	1 mg/ml[b]	PD	0.02 mg/ml[c]	Physically compatible for 1 hr at 25 °C	1338	**C**
Potassium chloride	AB	40 mEq/L[d]	SZ	1 mg/ml	Physically compatible for at least 4 hr at room temperature by visual and microscopic examination	534	**C**
Vitamin B complex with C	RC	2 ml/L[d]	SZ	1 mg/ml	Physically compatible for at least 4 hr at room temperature by visual and microscopic examination	534	**C**
Warfarin sodium	DU	0.1[a,b] and 2[e] mg/ml	FUJ	1 unit/ml[a,b]	Physically compatible with no change in measured turbidity or increase in particle content in 24 hr at 23 °C	2011	**C**

[a]Tested in dextrose 5% in water.
[b]Tested in sodium chloride 0.9%.
[c]Tested in dextrose 5% in Ringer's injection, lactated.
[d]Tested in dextrose 5% in Ringer's injection, dextrose 5% in Ringer's injection, lactated, dextrose 5% in water, Ringer's injection, lactated, and sodium chloride 0.9%.
[e]Tested in sterile water for injection.

Additional Compatibility Information

Sodium chloride 0.9% and dextrose 5% in water have been recommended as diluents for oxytocin infusion (4).

Oxytocin appears to be rapidly decomposed in the presence of sodium bisulfite (333).

Oxytocin is stated to be incompatible with fibrinolysin, norepi-nephrine bitartrate, prochlorperazine edisylate, and warfarin sodium (4).

Phytonadione— Oxytocin (Parke-Davis) 5 units/L has been reported to be conditionally compatible with phytonadione (Abbott) 50 mg/L. The mixture is physically compatible in most Abbott infusion solutions except dextran 12%, in which a haze or precipitate forms within one hour (3).

PACLITAXEL
AHFS 10:00

Taxol   **Bristol-Myers Squibb**

Products— Paclitaxel (Bristol-Myers Squibb) is available in a non-aqueous solution in 5-, 16.7-, and 50-ml multidose vials containing 30, 100, and 300 mg of paclitaxel, respectively. Each milliliter of solution contains paclitaxel 6 mg, polyoxyethylated castor oil (Cremophor EL) 527 mg, and dehydrated alcohol 49.7% (v/v). The product is a concentrate that must be diluted for use (2).

Administration— Paclitaxel is administered by intravenous infusion. The concentrate must be diluted to a final paclitaxel concentration of 0.3 to 1.2 mg/ml in dextrose 5% in water, sodium chloride 0.9%, dextrose 5% in sodium chloride 0.9%, or dextrose 5% in lactated Ringer's injection. Administration over three hours is often recommended (2; 4), although other duration periods have been used (4). An inline 0.22-μm filter should be used for administration. The intravenous solution containers and administration sets should be free of the plasticizer diethylhexyl phthalate (DEHP) (2). See Plasticizer Extraction under Additional Compatibility Information below.

Use of self-venting sets spiked into glass bottles of paclitaxel admixtures has occasionally resulted in solution dripping from the air vent. Presumably, the surfactant content wetted the hydrophobic filter, allowing the solution to drip (1843). In another observation, the spikes of administration sets were made sufficiently slippery by surfactant in the paclitaxel formulation that the spike slipped out after it had been seated through the rubber bung of the glass bottle. The admixture also leaked due to a poor seal. The authors recommend use of non-PVC plastic solution containers (Excel, McGaw) to avoid the problem (2052).

Stability— Intact vials should be stored between 20 and 25 °C and protected from light. Stability is not adversely affected by refrigeration or freezing. Refrigeration may result in the precipitation of formulation components. However, warming to room temperature redissolves the material and does not adversely affect the product. If a precipitate is insoluble, the product should be discarded (2).

Turbidity— Paclitaxel concentrate is a clear, colorless to slightly yellow viscous liquid. After dilution in an infusion solution, the drug may exhibit haziness because of the surfactant content of the formulation (2; 1528). This haziness increases until the maximum turbidity of around 6 to 8 nephelometric turbidity units occurs between 0.3 and 0.9 mg/ml. This level of haze may be visible in normal room light. Continued dilution below 0.3 mg/ml results in a con-tinual decline of measured turbidity through 0.01 mg/ml, the lowest concentration evaluated (1528).

Sorption— No paclitaxel loss due to sorption to containers or sets has been observed (1520; 2230–2232).

Filtration— The manufacturer recommends the use of a 0.22-μm in-line filter for paclitaxel administration (2). No loss of paclitaxel due to filtration through 0.22-μm filters has been observed (2; 1520).

The acceptability of the 0.22-μm IV Express Filter Unit (Millipore) for the administration of paclitaxel was evaluated. Paclitaxel vehicle equivalent to paclitaxel 1.2 mg/ml (for plasticizer leaching) and paclitaxel 0.3 mg/ml (for sorption potential) in 500 ml of dextrose 5% in water in polyolefin containers (McGaw) was delivered through the filter units over a three-hour period at a rate of 167 ml/hr at about 23 °C to simulate paclitaxel administration. HPLC analysis found no leached plasticizer and no loss of paclitaxel due to sorption. The filter unit was determined to be acceptable for the administration of paclitaxel infusions (2231).

Central Venous Catheter— The acceptability of the Arrow-Howes triple-lumen, 7 French, 30-cm polyurethane central catheter (Arrow International) for the administration of paclitaxel was evaluated. Paclitaxel vehicle equivalent to paclitaxel 0.3 and 1.2 mg/ml (for catheter component leaching) and paclitaxel 0.3 mg/ml (for sorption potential) were prepared in polyolefin bags of dextrose 5% in water (McGaw). The solutions were delivered through the polyurethane central venous catheters for periods of three hours and of 24 hours at 23 °C to simulate rapid and slow administration. HPLC analysis found no leached catheter components in the effluent solution and no loss of paclitaxel due to sorption. The Arrow-Howes polyurethane central venous catheter was determined to be acceptable for the administration of paclitaxel infusions in the concentration range of 0.3 to 1.2 mg/ml over short or long delivery periods (2230).

Precipitation— Although paclitaxel in aqueous solutions is chemically stable for 27 hours (2) or longer (1746; 1842), precipitation has occurred irregularly and unpredictably. Such precipitation occurs within the recommended range of 0.3 to 1.2 mg/ml and at even lower paclitaxel concentrations. These precipitates often have been observed in the infusion tubing distal to the pump chamber (1716). Although the precipitation of insoluble drugs in an aqueous medium is a forgone conclusion, the time to precipitation is irregular. It may be accelerated by various factors including the presence or formation of crystallization nuclei, agitation, and contact with incompatible drugs or materials (1374; 1521). Since the mechanism of this irregular paclitaxel precipitation has not been identified (1739), care and vigilance throughout its infusion are required.

Compatibility Information

Solution Compatibility

Paclitaxel

Solution	Mfr	Mfr	Conc/L	Remarks	Ref	C/I
Dextrose 5% in water	MG, TR[a]	NCI	0.3, 0.6, 0.9 g	Visually compatible with no paclitaxel loss by HPLC over 12 hr at 22 °C	1520	**C**
	MG[b]	NCI	0.6 g	Visually compatible with no paclitaxel loss by HPLC over 25 hr at 22 °C	1520	**C**
	MG, TR[c]	NCI	1.2 g	Visually compatible with no paclitaxel loss by HPLC over 12 hr at 22 °C	1520	**C**
		BR	0.2 to 0.58 g	Fluffy, white precipitate forms occasionally in administration set just distal to pump chamber	1716	**I**
	MG[b]	BR	0.1 and 1 g	Physically compatible with no change in subvisual haze or particle content and stable by HPLC for 3 days at 4, 22, and 32 °C. Small, needlelike crystals form after 3 days	1746	**C**
	MG[b]	BR	0.3 and 1.2 g	Physically compatible and chemically stable for 48 hr at 22 °C	1842	**C**
	BA[d]	FAU	0.3 and 1.2 g	Physically compatible with no change in subvisual haze or particle content and stable by HPLC for 3 days at 25 and 32 °C. Unknown material leached from EVA container by 24 hr	2182	**?**
Sodium chloride 0.9%	MG, TR[a]	NCI	0.3, 0.6, 0.9, 1.2 g	Visually compatible with no paclitaxel loss by HPLC over 12 hr at 22 °C	1520	**C**
	MG[b]	NCI	0.6 and 1.2 g	Visually compatible with no paclitaxel loss by HPLC over 26 hr at 22 °C	1520	**C**
	MG[b]	BR	0.1 and 1 g	Physically compatible with no change in subvisual haze or particle content and stable by HPLC for 3 days at 4, 22, and 32 °C. Small, needlelike crystals form after 3 days	1746	**C**
	MG[b]	BR	0.3 and 1.2 g	Physically compatible and chemically stable for 48 hr at 22 °C	1842	**C**
	BA[d]	FAU	0.3 and 1.2 g	Physically compatible with no change in subvisual haze or particle content and stable by HPLC for 3 days at 25 and 32 °C. Unknown material leached from EVA container by 24 hr	2182	**?**

[a]Tested in both glass and PVC containers.
[b]Tested in polyolefin containers.
[c]Tested in glass, PVC, and polyolefin containers.
[d]Tested in Baxter ethylene vinyl acetate (EVA) containers.

Additive Compatibility

Paclitaxel

Drug	Mfr	Conc/L	Mfr	Conc/L	Test Soln	Remarks	Ref	C/I
Carboplatin	BMS	2 g	BMS	300 mg and 1.2 g	NS	No paclitaxel loss but carboplatin losses of 2, 5, and 7% at 4, 24, and 32 °C, respectively, in 24 hr by HPLC. Physically compatible for 24 hr but subvisual particulates of paclitaxel form after 3 to 5 days	2094	**C**

Additive Compatibility (Cont.)

Paclitaxel

Drug	Mfr	Conc/L	Mfr	Conc/L	Test Soln	Remarks	Ref	C/I
	BMS	2 g	BMS	300 mg and 1.2 g	D5W	No paclitaxel and carboplatin loss by HPLC at 4, 24, and 32 °C in 24 hr. Physically compatible for 24 hr but subvisual particulates of paclitaxel form after 3 to 5 days	2094	**C**
Cisplatin	BMS	200 mg	BMS	300 mg	NS	No paclitaxel loss and cisplatin losses of 1, 4, and 5% at 4, 24 and 32 °C, respectively, in 24 hr by HPLC. Physically compatible for 24 hr but subvisual particulates of paclitaxel form after 3 to 5 days	2094	**C**
	BMS	200 mg	BMS	1.2 g	NS	No paclitaxel loss but cisplatin losses of 10, 19, and 22% at 4, 24, and 32 °C, respectively, in 24 hr by HPLC. Physically compatible for 24 hr but subvisual particulates of paclitaxel form after 3 to 5 days	2094	**I**

Y-Site Injection Compatibility (1:1 Mixture)

Paclitaxel

Drug	Mfr	Conc	Mfr	Conc	Remarks	Ref	C/I
Acyclovir sodium	BW	7 mg/ml[a]	NCI	1.2 mg/ml[a]	Physically compatible with no change in measured turbidity in 4 hr at 22 °C	1556	**C**
Amikacin sulfate	BR	5 mg/ml[a]	NCI	1.2 mg/ml[a]	Physically compatible with no change in measured turbidity in 4 hr at 22 °C	1556	**C**
Aminophylline	AB	2.5 mg/ml[a]	NCI	1.2 mg/ml[a]	Physically compatible with no change in measured turbidity in 4 hr at 22 °C	1556	**C**
Amphotericin B	SQ	0.6 mg/ml[a]	NCI	1.2 mg/ml[a]	Immediate increase in measured turbidity followed by separation into two layers in 24 hr at 22 °C	1556	**I**
Amphotericin B cholesteryl sulfate complex	SEQ	0.83 mg/ml[a]	MJ	0.6 mg/ml[a]	Decreased natural turbidity occurs immediately	2117	**I**
Ampicillin sodium–sulbactam sodium	RR	20 + 10 mg/ml[b]	NCI	1.2 mg/ml[a]	Physically compatible with no change in measured turbidity in 4 hr at 22 °C	1556	**C**
Bleomycin sulfate	MJ	1 unit/ml[a]	NCI	1.2 mg/ml[a]	Physically compatible with no change in measured turbidity in 4 hr at 22 °C	1556	**C**
Butorphanol tartrate	BR	0.04 mg/ml[a]	NCI	1.2 mg/ml[a]	Physically compatible with no change in measured turbidity in 4 hr at 22 °C	1556	**C**
Calcium chloride	AST	20 mg/ml[a]	NCI	1.2 mg/ml[a]	Physically compatible with no change in measured turbidity in 4 hr at 22 °C	1556	**C**
Carboplatin		5 mg/ml[a]	NCI	1.2 mg/ml[a]	Physically compatible with no change in measured turbidity in 4 hr at 22 °C	1528	**C**
Cefepime HCl	BR	20 mg/ml[a]	BR	0.6 mg/ml[a]	Physically compatible with no change in measured turbidity or increase in particle content in 4 hr at 22 °C	1689	**C**
Cefotetan disodium	STU	20 mg/ml[a]	NCI	1.2 mg/ml[a]	Physically compatible with no change in measured turbidity in 4 hr at 22 °C	1556	**C**

Y-Site Injection Compatibility (1:1 Mixture) (Cont.)

Paclitaxel

Drug	Mfr	Conc	Mfr	Conc	Remarks	Ref	C/I
Ceftazidime	LI[f]	40 mg/ml[a]	NCI	1.2 mg/ml[a]	Physically compatible with no change in measured turbidity in 4 hr at 22 °C	1556	C
Ceftriaxone sodium	RC	20 mg/ml[a]	NCI	1.2 mg/ml[a]	Physically compatible with no change in measured turbidity in 4 hr at 22 °C	1556	C
Chlorpromazine HCl	ES	2 mg/ml[a]	NCI	1.2 mg/ml[a]	Normal inherent haze from paclitaxel decreases immediately	1556	I
Cimetidine HCl		12 mg/ml[a]	NCI	1.2 mg/ml[a]	Physically compatible with no change in measured turbidity in 4 hr at 22 °C	1528	C
Cisplatin		1 mg/ml	NCI	1.2 mg/ml[a]	Physically compatible with no change in measured turbidity in 4 hr at 22 °C	1528	C
Cladribine	ORT	0.015[b] and 0.5[c] mg/ml	BR	0.6 mg/ml[b]	Physically compatible with no change in measured turbidity or increase in particle content in 4 hr at 23 °C	1969	C
Cyclophosphamide		10 mg/ml[a]	NCI	1.2 mg/ml[a]	Physically compatible with no change in measured turbidity in 4 hr at 22 °C	1528	C
Cytarabine		50 mg/ml	NCI	1.2 mg/ml[a]	Physically compatible with no change in measured turbidity in 4 hr at 22 °C	1528	C
Dacarbazine	MI	4 mg/ml[a]	NCI	1.2 mg/ml[a]	Physically compatible with no change in measured turbidity in 4 hr at 22 °C	1556	C
Dexamethasone sodium phosphate		1 mg/ml[a]	NCI	1.2 mg/ml[a]	Physically compatible with no change in measured turbidity in 4 hr at 22 °C	1528	C
Diphenhydramine HCl		2 mg/ml[a]	NCI	1.2 mg/ml[a]	Physically compatible with no change in measured turbidity in 4 hr at 22 °C	1528	C
Doxorubicin HCl		2 mg/ml	NCI	1.2 mg/ml[a]	Physically compatible with no change in measured turbidity in 4 hr at 22 °C	1528	C
Doxorubicin HCl liposome injection	SEQ	0.4 mg/ml[a]	MJ	0.6 mg/ml[a]	Partial loss of measured natural turbidity	2087	I
Droperidol	JN	0.4 mg/ml[a]	NCI	1.2 mg/ml[a]	Physically compatible with no change in measured turbidity in 4 hr at 22 °C	1556	C
Etoposide		0.4 mg/ml[a]	NCI	1.2 mg/ml[a]	Physically compatible with no change in measured turbidity in 4 hr at 22 °C	1528	C
Etoposide phosphate	BR	5 mg/ml[a]	MJ	1.2 mg/ml[a]	Physically compatible with no change in measured turbidity or increase in particle content in 4 hr at 23 °C	2218	C
Famotidine	MSD	2 mg/ml[a]	NCI	1.2 mg/ml[a]	Physically compatible with no change in measured turbidity in 4 hr at 22 °C	1556	C
Floxuridine	RC	3 mg/ml[a]	NCI	1.2 mg/ml[a]	Physically compatible with no change in measured turbidity in 4 hr at 22 °C	1556	C
Fluconazole	RR	2 mg/ml	NCI	1.2 mg/ml[a]	Physically compatible with no change in measured turbidity in 4 hr at 22 °C	1556	C
	PF	2 mg/ml	BR	0.3 and 1.2 mg/ml[a]	Visually compatible with no loss of either drug by HPLC in 4 hr at 23 °C	1790	C
Fluorouracil		16 mg/ml[a]	NCI	1.2 mg/ml[a]	Physically compatible with no change in measured turbidity in 4 hr at 22 °C	1528	C
Furosemide	AST	3 mg/ml[a]	NCI	1.2 mg/ml[a]	Physically compatible with no change in measured turbidity in 4 hr at 22 °C	1556	C

Y-Site Injection Compatibility (1:1 Mixture) (Cont.)

Paclitaxel

Drug	Mfr	Conc	Mfr	Conc	Remarks	Ref	C/I
Ganciclovir sodium	SY	20 mg/ml[a]	NCI	1.2 mg/ml[a]	Physically compatible with no change in measured turbidity in 4 hr at 22 °C	1556	**C**
Gemcitabine HCl	LI	10 mg/ml[b]	MJ	1.2 mg/ml[a]	Physically compatible with no change in measured turbidity or increase in particle content in 4 hr at 23 °C	2226	**C**
Gentamicin sulfate	ES	5 mg/ml[a]	NCI	1.2 mg/ml[a]	Physically compatible with no change in measured turbidity in 4 hr at 22 °C	1556	**C**
Granisetron HCl	SKB	1 mg/ml	MJ	0.3 mg/ml[b]	Physically compatible with little or no loss of either drug by HPLC in 4 hr at 22 °C	1883	**C**
	SKB	0.05 mg/ml[a]	MJ	1.2 mg/ml[a]	Physically compatible with no change in measured turbidity or increase in particle content in 4 hr at 23 °C	2000	**C**
Haloperidol lactate		0.2 mg/ml[a]	NCI	1.2 mg/ml[a]	Physically compatible with no change in measured turbidity in 4 hr at 22 °C	1528	**C**
Heparin sodium	WY	100 units/ml[a]	NCI	1.2 mg/ml[a]	Physically compatible with no change in measured turbidity in 4 hr at 22 °C	1556	**C**
Hydrocortisone sodium phosphate	MSD	1 mg/ml[a]	NCI	1.2 mg/ml[a]	Physically compatible with no change in measured turbidity in 4 hr at 22 °C	1556	**C**
Hydrocortisone sodium succinate	AB	1 mg/ml[a]	NCI	1.2 mg/ml[a]	Physically compatible with no change in measured turbidity in 4 hr at 22 °C	1556	**C**
Hydromorphone HCl	KN	0.5 mg/ml[a]	NCI	1.2 mg/ml[a]	Physically compatible with no change in measured turbidity in 4 hr at 22 °C	1556	**C**
Hydroxyzine HCl	ES	4 mg/ml[a]	NCI	1.2 mg/ml[a]	Normal inherent haze from paclitaxel decreases immediately	1556	**I**
Ifosfamide	BR	25 mg/ml[a]	NCI	1.2 mg/ml[a]	Physically compatible with no change in measured turbidity in 4 hr at 22 °C	1556	**C**
Lorazepam		0.1 mg/ml[a]	NCI	1.2 mg/ml[a]	Physically compatible with no change in measured turbidity in 4 hr at 22 °C	1528	**C**
Magnesium sulfate	AST	100 mg/ml[a]	NCI	1.2 mg/ml[a]	Physically compatible with no change in measured turbidity in 4 hr at 22 °C	1556	**C**
Mannitol	BA	15%	NCI	1.2 mg/ml[a]	Physically compatible with no change in measured turbidity in 4 hr at 22 °C	1556	**C**
Meperidine HCl	WY	4 mg/ml[a]	NCI	1.2 mg/ml[a]	Physically compatible with no change in measured turbidity in 4 hr at 22 °C	1556	**C**
Mesna	MJ	10 mg/ml[a]	NCI	1.2 mg/ml[a]	Physically compatible with no change in measured turbidity in 4 hr at 22 °C	1556	**C**
Methotrexate sodium		15 mg/ml[a]	NCI	1.2 mg/ml[a]	Physically compatible with no change in measured turbidity in 4 hr at 22 °C	1528	**C**
Methylprednisolone sodium succinate	UP	5 mg/ml[a]	NCI	1.2 mg/ml[a]	Normal inherent haze from paclitaxel decreases immediately	1556	**I**
Metoclopramide HCl		5 mg/ml	NCI	1.2 mg/ml[a]	Physically compatible with no change in measured turbidity in 4 hr at 22 °C	1528	**C**
Mitoxantrone HCl	LE	0.5 mg/ml[a]	NCI	1.2 mg/ml[a]	Normal inherent haze from paclitaxel decreases immediately	1556	**I**
Morphine sulfate	WY	1 mg/ml[a]	NCI	1.2 mg/ml[a]	Physically compatible with no change in measured turbidity in 4 hr at 22 °C	1556	**C**

Y-Site Injection Compatibility (1:1 Mixture) (Cont.)

Paclitaxel

Drug	Mfr	Conc	Mfr	Conc	Remarks	Ref	C/I
Nalbuphine HCl	AST	10 mg/ml	NCI	1.2 mg/ml[a]	Physically compatible with no change in measured turbidity in 4 hr at 22 °C	1556	**C**
Ondansetron HCl	GL	0.5 mg/ml[a]	NCI	1.2 mg/ml[a]	Physically compatible with no change in measured turbidity in 4 hr at 22 °C	1556	**C**
	GL	0.03 and 0.3 mg/ml[a]	BR	0.3 mg/ml[a]	Visually compatible with no loss of either drug in 4 hr at 23 °C	1741	**C**
	GL	0.03 and 0.3 mg/ml[a]	BR	1.2 mg/ml[a]	Visually compatible with no loss of either drug in 4 hr at 23 °C	1741	**C**
Ondansetron HCl with ranitidine HCl	GL GL	0.3 mg/ml[a] 2 mg/ml[a]	BR	1.2 mg/ml[a]	Visually compatible with no loss of any drug by HPLC in 4 hr at 23 °C	1741	**C**
Pentostatin	NCI	0.4 mg/ml[b]	NCI	1.2 mg/ml[a]	Physically compatible with no change in measured turbidity in 4 hr at 22 °C	1556	**C**
Potassium chloride	AB	0.1 mEq/ml[a]	NCI	1.2 mg/ml[a]	Physically compatible with no change in measured turbidity in 4 hr at 22 °C	1556	**C**
Prochlorperazine edisylate		0.5 mg/ml[a]	NCI	1.2 mg/ml[a]	Physically compatible with no change in measured turbidity in 4 hr at 22 °C	1528	**C**
Propofol	ZEN	10 mg/ml	MJ	1.2 mg/ml[a]	Physically compatible for 1 hr at 23 °C with no increase in particle content	2066	**C**
Ranitidine HCl		2 mg/ml[a]	NCI	1.2 mg/ml[a]	Physically compatible with no change in measured turbidity in 4 hr at 22 °C	1528	**C**
	GL	0.5 and 2 mg/ml[a]	BR	0.3 mg/ml[a]	Visually compatible with no loss of either drug in 4 hr at 23 °C	1741	**C**
	GL	0.5 and 2 mg/ml[a]	BR	1.2 mg/ml[a]	Visually compatible with no loss of either drug in 4 hr at 23 °C	1741	**C**
Sodium bicarbonate	LY	1 mEq/ml	NCI	1.2 mg/ml[a]	Physically compatible with no change in measured turbidity in 4 hr at 22 °C	1556	**C**
Thiotepa	IMM[d]	1 mg/ml[a]	MJ	0.6 mg/ml[a]	Physically compatible with no change in measured turbidity or increase in particle content in 4 hr at 23 °C	1861	**C**
TNA #218 to #226[e]			MJ	1.2 mg/ml[a]	Visually compatible with no precipitate or emulsion damage apparent in 4 hr at 23 °C	2215	**C**
TPN #212 to #215[e]			MJ	1.2 mg/ml[a]	Physically compatible with no change in measured turbidity or increase in particle content in 4 hr at 23 °C	2109	**C**
Vancomycin HCl		10 mg/ml[a]	NCI	1.2 mg/ml[a]	Physically compatible with no change in measured turbidity in 4 hr at 22 °C	1528	**C**
Vinblastine sulfate	LI	0.12 mg/ml[b]	NCI	1.2 mg/ml[a]	Physically compatible with no change in measured turbidity in 4 hr at 22 °C	1556	**C**
Vincristine sulfate	LI	0.05 mg/ml[a]	NCI	1.2 mg/ml[a]	Physically compatible with no change in measured turbidity in 4 hr at 22 °C	1556	**C**
Zidovudine	BW	4 mg/ml[a]	NCI	1.2 mg/ml[a]	Physically compatible with no change in measured turbidity in 4 hr at 22 °C	1556	**C**

[a]*Tested in dextrose 5% in water.*
[b]*Tested in sodium chloride 0.9%.*
[c]*Tested in bacteriostatic sodium chloride 0.9% preserved with benzyl alcohol 0.9%.*
[d]*Lyophilized formulation tested.*
[e]*Refer to Appendix I for the composition of parenteral nutrition solutions. TNA indicates a 3-in-1 admixture, and TPN indicates a 2-in-1 admixture.*
[f]*Sodium carbonate–containing formulation tested.*

Additional Compatibility Information

Solutions— The manufacturer recommends dilution of paclitaxel to a concentration between 0.3 and 1.2 mg/ml in dextrose 5% in water, dextrose 5% in sodium chloride 0.9%, dextrose 5% in Ringer's injection, or sodium chloride 0.9%. These solutions are stated to be physically and chemically stable for up to 27 hours at room temperature (about 25 °C) under normal room light (2).

Plasticizer Extraction— Contact of undiluted paclitaxel concentrate with plasticized PVC equipment and devices is not recommended (2).

Table 1. Administration Sets Compatible with Paclitaxel Infusions by Manufacturer (1843)

Abbott
  LifeCare 5000 Plum PVC specialty set (11594)
  Life Shield anesthesia pump set OL with cartridge (13503)
  LifeCare model 4P specialty set, non-PVC (11434)
  Omni-Flow universal primary intravenous pump short minibore patient line (40527)

Baxter
  Vented volumetric pump nitroglycerin set (2C1042)

Block Medical
  Verifuse nonvented administration set with 0.22-μm filter, check valve, injection site, and non-DEHP PVC tubing (V021015)

I-Flow
  Vivus-4000 polyethylene-lined infusion set (5000-784)

IMED
  Standard PVC set (9215)
  Closed-system non-PVC fluid path nonvented quick-spike administration set (9635)
  Non-PVC set with inline filter (9986)
  Gemini 20 nonvented primary administration set for nitroglycerin and emulsions (2262)

IVAC
  Universal set with low-sorbing tubing (52053, 59953, and S75053)

Ivion/Medex
  WalkMed spike set (SP-06) with pump set (PS-401, PS-360, FPS-560, or FPX-560)

Siemens
  Reduced-PVC full set MiniMed Uni-Set macrobore (28-60-190)

Paclitaxel itself does not contribute to the extraction of the plasticizer DEHP (1520). However, the surfactant, Cremophor EL, in the paclitaxel formulation extracts DEHP from PVC containers and sets. The amount of DEHP extracted increases with time and drug concentration (2; 1520; 1683; 1912; 2146). Consequently, the use of DEHP-plasticized PVC containers and sets is not recommended for infusion of paclitaxel solutions. Instead, the manufacturer recommends the use of glass, polypropylene, or polyolefin containers and non-PVC administration sets such as those that are polyethylene lined (2).

The use of inline filters, such as the Ivex-2 filter set that incorporates about 10 inches of PVC inlet and outlet tubing, has resulted

Table 2. Extension Sets Compatible with Paclitaxel Infusions by Manufacturer (1843)

Abbott
  Ivex-HP filter set (4524)
  Ivex-2 filter set (2679)

Becton-Dickinson
  Intima intravenous catheter placement set (38-6918-1)
  J-loop connector (38-1252-2)
  E-Z infusion set shorty (38-53741)
  E-Z infusion set (38-53121)

Baxter
  Polyethylene-lined extension set with 0.22-μm air-eliminating filter (1C8363)

Braun
  0.2-μm filter extension set (FE-2012L)
  Small-bore 0.2-μm filter extension set (PFE-2007)
  Whin-winged extension set with 90° Huber needle (HW-2267)
  Whin extension set with Y-site and Huber needle (HW-2276 YHR)
  Y-extension set with valve (ET-08-YL)
  Small-bore extension set with T-fitting (ET-04T)
  Small-bore extension set with reflux valve (ET-116L)

Gish Biomedical
  VasTack noncoring portal-access needle system (VT-2022)

IMED
  0.2-μm add-on filter set (9400 XL)

IVAC
  Spec-Sets extension set with 0.22-μm inline filter (C20028 and C20350)

Ivion/Medex
  Extension set with 0.22-μm filter (IV4A07-IV3)

PALL
  SetSaver extended-life disposable set with 0.2-μm filter (ELD-96P and ELD-96LL)
  SetSaver extended-life disposable microbore extension tubing with 0.2-μm Posidyne filter (ELD-96LYL and ELD-96LYLN)

Pfizer/Strato Medical
  Lifeport vascular-access system infusion set with Y-site (LPS 3009)

---

in a small amount of DEHP extraction. Since the extracted DEHP is at a sufficiently low level, however, the manufacturer considers the Ivex-2 filter set to be acceptable (2).

A study was performed on the compatibility of paclitaxel 0.3- and 1.2-mg/ml infusions with various non-PVC infusion sets. The paclitaxel infusions were run through the study sets, and the effluent was then analyzed by HPLC for leached DEHP plasticizer. The following sets had significant and unacceptable amounts of leached DEHP: Baxter vented nitroglycerin (2C7552S), Baxter vented basic solution (1C8355S), McGaw Horizon pump vented nitroglycerin (V7450), and McGaw Intelligent pump vented nitroglycerin (V7150). Although these sets were largely non-PVC, their highly plasticized pumping segments contributed the DEHP. The administration and extension sets cited in Tables 1 and 2 exhibited no more leached DEHP than the Ivex-2 filter set specified in the product labeling (1843).

Mazzo et al. evaluated the leaching of DEHP plasticizer by paclitaxel 0.3 and 1.2 mg/ml in dextrose 5% in water and in sodium chloride 0.9%. PVC bags of the solutions were used to prepare the admixtures. The leaching of the plasticizer was found to be time and concentration dependent; however, there was little difference between the two infusion solutions. After storage for eight hours at 21 °C, HPLC analysis found leached DEHP in the range from 73 to 108 µg/ml for the 1.2 mg/ml concentration and from 21 to 30 µg/ml for the 0.3 mg/ml concentration. During a simulated one-hour infusion using DEHP plasticized administration sets, the amount of leached DEHP did not exceed 18 µg/ml at the 0.3 mg/ml paclitaxel concentration but resulted in a maximum of 114 µg/ml with the 1.2 mg/ml concentration (1825).

Allwood and Martin confirmed the leaching of DEHP plasticizer from PVC containers and administration sets, and the amount of DEHP leached was again found to depend on surfactant concentration and length of contact period. They also reported leaching of up to 30 mg of DEHP per dose from Flo-Gard Low Adsorption Sets (Baxter), a set with a reduced amount of PVC present in its construction (2146).

An acceptability limit of no more than 5 parts per million (5 µg/ml) for DEHP plasticizer released from PVC containers, administration sets, and other equipment has been proposed. The limit was proposed based on a review of metabolic and toxicologic considerations (2185).

The acceptability of two reduced-phthalate administration sets for the Acclaim (Abbott) pump was evaluated. Administration set model 11993-48 (Abbott) is composed of polyethylene tubing but has a DEHP-plasticized pumping segment. Administration set model L-12060 (Abbott) is composed of tris(2-ethylhexyl)trimellitate (TOTM)–plasticized PVC tubing and a DEHP-plasticized pumping segment. Paclitaxel diluent at concentrations equivalent to 0.3 and 1.2 mg/ml in dextrose 5% in water delivered rapidly over three hours at 23 °C did not leach detectable levels of TOTM from model L-12060 or DEHP from either set using HPLC analysis. Similarly, slow delivery over four days of the 0.3-mg/ml concentration yielded detectable but not quantifiable amounts of plasticizer. However, slow delivery of the equivalent of 1.2 mg/ml over four days yielded large but variable amounts of DEHP from both sets; DEHP concentrations ranged from 30 to 150 µg/ml. Consequently, these two reduced-phthalate sets are suitable for short-term delivery up to three hours of paclitaxel at concentrations up to 1.2 mg/ml. However, these sets should not be used for slow delivery of higher concentrations (2198).

The admonition of the paclitaxel labeling (2) to avoid PVC administration sets was found not to extend to a TOTM-plasticized PVC set (SoloPak). Paclitaxel vehicle equivalent to paclitaxel 0.3 and 1.2 mg/ml in dextrose 5% in water did not leach TOTM plasticizer from the set during simulated three-hour administration. During extremely slow delivery at 5.2 ml/hr for four days, no detectable TOTM was found in the 0.3-mg/ml equivalent concentration, and only a barely detectable, unquantifiable, trace amount of TOTM was found with the 1.2-mg/ml equivalent solution (2232).

Paclitaxel (Faulding) 0.3 and 1.2 mg/ml in dextrose 5% in water or in sodium chloride 0.9% in ethylene vinyl acetate (EVA) plastic containers was found to leach an unknown material after storage at 25 and 32 °C for 24 hours (2182).

Other Information

Bacterial Challenge— Paclitaxel (Bristol) 0.7 mg/ml diluted in sodium chloride 0.9% did not exhibit an antimicrobial effect on the growth of three of four organisms (*Enterococcus faecium, Staphylococcus aureus, Pseudomonas aeruginosa,* and *Candida albicans*) inoculated into the solution. *S. aureus* remained viable for 4 hours. *E. faecium* and *P. aeruginosa* remained viable for 48 hours, and *C. albicans* remained viable to the end of the study at 120 hours. The author recommended that diluted solutions of paclitaxel be stored under refrigeration whenever possible and that the potential for microbiological growth be considered when assigning expiration periods (2160).

PANCURONIUM BROMIDE
AHFS 12:20

Baxter
Organon

Pavulon

Products— Pancuronium bromide (Baxter) is available in 2- and 5-ml vials containing 2 mg/ml of drug. It is also available in 10-ml vials at a concentration of 1 mg/ml. Each milliliter also contains sodium acetate anhydrous 2 mg, benzyl alcohol 1%, and sodium chloride 4 mg for isotonicity. Acetic acid and/or sodium hydroxide is added to adjust the pH (1-9/98; 4).

pH— The solution has been adjusted to pH 3.8 to 4.2 by the manufacturer (1-9/98; 4).

Osmolality— The osmolality of pancuronium bromide (Organon) 1 mg/ml was determined to be 277 mOsm/kg by freezing-point depression and 273 mOsm/kg by vapor pressure (1071).

The osmolality of pancuronium bromide 2 mg/ml was determined to be 338 mOsm/kg (1233).

Administration— Pancuronium bromide is administered intravenously (1-9/98; 4).

Stability— Pancuronium bromide should be stored under refrigeration at 2 to 8 °C (4). However, the manufacturer indicates that the drug is stable for six months at room temperature (1-9/98; 853; 1181; 1433).

Sorption— The manufacturer indicates that pancuronium bromide in compatible infusion solutions does not undergo sorption to glass or plastic containers during short-term storage over 48 hours at room temperature (1-9/98; 4). However, the drug may exhibit sorption to plastic containers with prolonged contact (4).

Compatibility Information

Additive Compatibility

		Pancuronium bromide						
Drug	Mfr	Conc/L	Mfr	Conc/L	Test Soln	Remarks	Ref	C/I
Verapamil HCl	KN	80 mg	OR	8 mg	D5W, NS	Physically compatible for 24 hr	764	C

Drugs in Syringe Compatibility

		Pancuronium bromide					
Drug (in syringe)	Mfr	Amt	Mfr	Amt	Remarks	Ref	C/I
Heparin sodium		2500 units/ 1 ml		4 mg/ 2 ml	Physically compatible for at least 5 min	1053	C

Y-Site Injection Compatibility (1:1 Mixture)

		Pancuronium bromide					
Drug	Mfr	Conc	Mfr	Conc	Remarks	Ref	C/I
Aminophylline	AB	1 mg/ml[a]	ES	0.05 mg/ml[a]	Physically compatible for 24 hr at 28 °C	1337	C
Cefazolin sodium	LY	10 mg/ml[a]	ES	0.05 mg/ml[a]	Physically compatible for 24 hr at 28 °C	1337	C
Cefuroxime sodium	GL	7.5 mg/ml[a]	ES	0.05 mg/ml[a]	Physically compatible for 24 hr at 28 °C	1337	C
Cimetidine HCl	SKF	6 mg/ml[a]	ES	0.05 mg/ml[a]	Physically compatible for 24 hr at 28 °C	1337	C
Diazepam	ES	5 mg/ml[a]	ES	0.05 mg/ml[a]	Cloudy solution forms immediately	1337	I
Dobutamine HCl	LI	1 mg/ml[a]	ES	0.05 mg/ml[a]	Physically compatible for 24 hr at 28 °C	1337	C
Dopamine HCl	SO	1.6 mg/ml[a]	ES	0.05 mg/ml[a]	Physically compatible for 24 hr at 28 °C	1337	C
Epinephrine HCl	AB	4 μg/ml[a]	ES	0.05 mg/ml[a]	Physically compatible for 24 hr at 28 °C	1337	C
Esmolol HCl	DCC	10 mg/ml[a]	ES	0.05 mg/ml[a]	Physically compatible for 24 hr at 28 °C	1337	C
Etomidate	AB	2 mg/ml	GNS	2 mg/ml	Visually compatible for up to 7 days at 25 °C	1801	C
Fentanyl citrate	ES	10 μg/ml[a]	ES	0.05 mg/ml[a]	Physically compatible for 24 hr at 28 °C	1337	C
Fluconazole	RR	2 mg/ml	GNS	0.5 mg/ml[b]	Visually compatible for 24 hr at 28 °C	1760	C
Gentamicin sulfate	ES	2 mg/ml[a]	ES	0.05 mg/ml[a]	Physically compatible for 24 hr at 28 °C	1337	C
Heparin sodium	SO	40 units/ml[a]	ES	0.05 mg/ml[a]	Physically compatible for 24 hr at 28 °C	1337	C
Hydrocortisone sodium succinate	AB	1 mg/ml[a]	ES	0.05 mg/ml[a]	Physically compatible for 24 hr at 28 °C	1337	C
Isoproterenol HCl	ES	4 μg/ml	ES	0.05 mg/ml[a]	Physically compatible for 24 hr at 28 °C	1337	C
Lorazepam	WY	0.5 mg/ml[a]	ES	0.05 mg/ml[a]	Physically compatible for 24 hr at 28 °C	1337	C
Midazolam HCl	RC	0.05 mg/ml[a]	ES	0.05 mg/ml[a]	Physically compatible for 24 hr at 28 °C	1337	C
Milrinone lactate	SW	0.4 mg/ml[a]	GEN	1 mg/ml	Visually compatible with little or no loss of either drug by HPLC in 4 hr at 23 °C	2214	C
Morphine sulfate	WY	1 mg/ml[a]	ES	0.05 mg/ml[a]	Physically compatible for 24 hr at 28 °C	1337	C
Nitroglycerin	SO	0.4 mg/ml[a]	ES	0.05 mg/ml[a]	Physically compatible for 24 hr at 28 °C	1337	C
Propofol	STU	2 mg/ml	GNS	2 mg/ml	Oil droplets form within 7 days at 25 °C. No visible change in 24 hr	1801	?

Y-Site Injection Compatibility (1:1 Mixture) (Cont.)

Pancuronium bromide

Drug	Mfr	Conc	Mfr	Conc	Remarks	Ref	C/I
	ZEN	10 mg/ml	AST	1 mg/ml	Physically compatible for 1 hr at 23 °C with no increase in particle content	2066	C
Ranitidine HCl	GL	0.5 mg/ml[a]	ES	0.05 mg/ml[a]	Physically compatible for 24 hr at 28 °C	1337	C
Sodium nitroprusside	ES	0.2 mg/ml[a]	ES	0.05 mg/ml[a]	Physically compatible for 24 hr at 28 °C	1337	C
Thiopental sodium	AB	25 mg/ml	GNS	2 mg/ml	White precipitate forms immediately	1801	I
Trimethoprim–sulfamethoxazole	ES	0.64 + 3.2 mg/ml[a]	ES	0.05 mg/ml[a]	Physically compatible for 24 hr at 28 °C	1337	C
Vancomycin HCl	ES	5 mg/ml[a]	ES	0.05 mg/ml[a]	Physically compatible for 24 hr at 28 °C	1337	C

[a]*Tested in dextrose 5% in water.*
[b]*Tested in sodium chloride 0.9%.*

Additional Compatibility Information

The manufacturer states that pancuronium bromide exhibits no decomposition for 48 hours mixed in the following infusion solutions (1-9/98):

    Dextrose 5% in sodium chloride 0.9%
    Dextrose 5% in water

    Ringer's injection, lactated
    Sodium chloride 0.9%

It is stated that a precipitate may be formed if pancuronium bromide is mixed with barbiturates (4). However, a precipitate was not visible when pancuronium bromide was mixed in a syringe with thiopental or methohexital as well as succinylcholine, meperidine, opium alkaloids HCl, neostigmine, gallamine, tubocurarine, alcuronium, hydrocortisone, or promethazine (134).

PAPAVERINE HCL
AHFS 24:12

Bedford

Products— Papaverine HCl (Bedford) is available in 2-ml ampuls and 10-ml vials. Each milliliter of solution contains 30 mg of papaverine as the hydrochloride with edetate disodium 0.005% and sodium hydroxide to adjust the pH. The vials also contain chlorobutanol 0.5% (1-7/98).

pH— Not below 3 (17). A 2% solution in water has a pH of 3 to 4 (5).

Osmolality— Papaverine HCl 30 mg/ml has an osmolality of 99 mOsm/kg (1689).

Administration— Papaverine HCl may be administered by intramuscular or slow intravenous injection over one to two minutes (2; 4).

Stability— Papaverine HCl injection should be stored at room temperature and protected from temperatures of 40 °C or higher and from freezing (4). It should not be refrigerated because of a reduction in solubility with possible precipitation (593). The solutions should be clear and colorless to pale yellow (1-7/98). The yellow discoloration of papaverine HCl injection does not appear to be related to drug decomposition. HPLC analysis of a yellow injection found nearly 100% of the labeled potency. Furthermore, yellow discoloration is not produced by intentional degradation from boiling with acid or base (1996).

Compatibility Information

Solution Compatibility

Papaverine HCl

Solution	Mfr	Mfr	Conc/L	Remarks	Ref	C/I
Dextran 6% in dextrose 5%	AB		96 mg	Physically compatible	3	C
Dextran 6% in sodium chloride 0.9%	AB		96 mg	Physically compatible	3	C
Dextrose–Ringer's injection combinations	AB		96 mg	Physically compatible	3	C

Solution Compatibility (Cont.)

Papaverine HCl

Solution	Mfr	Mfr	Conc/L	Remarks	Ref	C/I
Dextrose–saline combinations	AB		96 mg	Physically compatible	3	C
Dextrose 2½% in water	AB		96 mg	Physically compatible	3	C
Dextrose 5% in water	AB		96 mg	Physically compatible	3	C
Dextrose 10% in water	AB		96 mg	Physically compatible	3	C
Fructose 10% in sodium chloride 0.9%	AB		96 mg	Physically compatible	3	C
Fructose 10% in water	AB		96 mg	Physically compatible	3	C
Invert sugar 5 and 10% in sodium chloride 0.9%	AB		96 mg	Physically compatible	3	C
Invert sugar 5 and 10% in water	AB		96 mg	Physically compatible	3	C
Ionosol products	AB		96 mg	Physically compatible	3	C
Ringer's injection	AB		96 mg	Physically compatible	3	C
Sodium chloride 0.45%	AB		96 mg	Physically compatible	3	C
Sodium chloride 0.9%	AB		96 mg	Physically compatible	3	C
Sodium lactate ⅙ M	AB		96 mg	Physically compatible	3	C

Additive Compatibility

Papaverine HCl

Drug	Mfr	Conc/L	Mfr	Conc/L	Test Soln	Remarks	Ref	C/I
Aminophylline with trimecaine HCl		480 mg 600 mg		120 mg	D5W	Papaverine precipitates within 3 hr due to alkaline pH	835	I
Theophylline		2 g		160 mg	D5W	Visually compatible with little or no loss of either drug in 48 hr	1909	C

Drugs in Syringe Compatibility

Papaverine HCl

Drug (in syringe)	Mfr	Amt	Mfr	Amt	Remarks	Ref	C/I
Diatrizoate meglumine 66%, diatrizoate sodium 10%	SQ	3 ml	LI	30 mg/ 1 ml	White precipitate disappears after 1 to 2 min	1437	?
Diatrizoate meglumine 52%, diatrizoate sodium 8%	MA	5 ml	ME	32 mg/ 1 ml	Transient precipitate clears and then reforms after 2 hr	1438	I
Diatrizoate sodium 60%	WI	5 ml	ME	32 mg/ 1 ml	Transient precipitate clears within 5 min	1438	?
Iohexol 64.7%	WI	5 ml	LI	30 mg/ 1 ml	Physically compatible for at least 2 hr	1438	C
Iopamidol 61%	SQ	5 ml	LI	30 mg/ 1 ml	Physically compatible for at least 2 hr	1438	C
Iothalamate sodium 60%	MA	3 ml	LI	30 mg/ 1 ml	Physically compatible	1437	C
Ioxaglate meglumine 39.3%, ioxaglate sodium 19.6%	MA	5 ml	LI	32 mg/ 1 ml	Precipitate forms immediately and persists for at least 2 hr	1438	I

Drugs in Syringe Compatibility (Cont.)

Papaverine HCl

Drug (in syringe)	Mfr	Amt	Mfr	Amt	Remarks	Ref	C/I
	MA	3 and 5 ml	LI	30 mg/ 1 ml	White amorphous precipitate forms immediately and persists for 24 hr. If shaken, it redissolves in 20 to 30 min	1437	I
	MA	5 ml	LI	30 mg/2 to 6 ml[a]	Precipitate forms	1437	I
	MA	5 ml	LI	30 mg/ 11 and 16 ml[a]	Precipitate forms and then redissolves	1437	?
	MA	5 ml	LI	30 mg/ 21 ml[a]	Physically compatible	1437	C
	MA	15 and 30 ml	LI	30 mg/ 11 ml[a]	Physically compatible	1437	C
	MA	5 ml	LI	60 mg/ 12 and 17 ml[a]	Precipitate forms	1437	I
	MA	5 ml	LI	60 mg/ 22 ml[a]	Precipitate forms and then redissolves	1437	?
Metrizamide 48.25%	WI	3 ml	LI	30 mg/ 1 ml	Physically compatible	1437	C
Phentolamine mesylate	BV, CI	0.5 mg/ ml[b]	LI	30 mg/ ml	Physically compatible with virtually no papaverine loss at 5 and 25 °C and 1 to 3% phentolamine loss at 5 °C and 4 to 5% loss at 25 °C in 30 days	1161	C

[a]Diluted in sodium chloride 0.9%.
[b]Reconstituted with the papaverine HCl injection.

Additional Compatibility Information

Papaverine HCl should not be added to Ringer's injection, lactated, because precipitation results (1-7/98; 4).

PENICILLIN G POTASSIUM (BENZYLPENICILLIN POTASSIUM) AHFS 8:12.16

Pfizerpen **Pfizer Pharmaceuticals Apothecon**

Products— Penicillin G potassium is available from several manufacturers in vial sizes ranging from 1 to 20 million units (4; 29). The commercial products contain sodium citrate and citric acid as buffers. Depending on the route of administration, reconstitute the vials with sterile water for injection, dextrose 5% in water, or sodium chloride 0.9%. The recommended reconstitution volumes vary slightly among manufacturers; the amount of diluent recommended by the manufacturer should be used for reconstitution. To reconstitute the product, loosen the powder in the vials. While holding the vial horizontally, rotate it and add the diluent slowly, directing the stream against the wall of the vial. Shake the vial vigorously. When the required volume of solvent is greater than the capacity of the vial, a portion of the total volume of diluent may be added to the vial first to dissolve the drug. The resulting solution should then be withdrawn and mixed with the remainder of the needed diluent in a larger container (2; 4).

Penicillin G potassium is also available as frozen premixed infusion solutions of 1, 2, and 3 million units in 50 ml of dextrose 4, 2.3, and 0.7%, respectively (4; 29).

pH— From 5.5 to 8.5 (4; 17).

Osmolality— The osmolality of penicillin G potassium (Pfizer) 250,000 units/ml in sterile water for injection was determined to be 776 mOsm/kg by freezing-point depression and 767 mOsm/kg by vapor pressure (1071). Another report cited the osmolality of this concentration as 749 mOsm/kg (50).

The osmolality of penicillin G potassium (Roerig) 50,000 units/ml was determined to be 402 mOsm/kg in dextrose 5% in water and 414 mOsm/kg in sodium chloride 0.9%. At 100,000 units/ml, the osmolality was determined to be 535 mOsm/kg in dextrose 5% in water and 554 mOsm/kg in sodium chloride 0.9% (1375).

The osmolality of penicillin G potassium was calculated for the following dilutions (1054):

Diluent	Osmolality (mOsm/kg)	
	50 ml	100 ml
3 million units		
Dextrose 5% in water	411	340
Sodium chloride 0.9%	437	367
5 million units		
Dextrose 5% in water	501	394
Sodium chloride 0.9%	527	420

Robinson et al. recommended the following maximum penicillin G potassium concentrations to achieve osmolalities suitable for peripheral infusion in fluid-restricted patients (1180):

Diluent	Maximum Concentration (units/ml)	Osmolality (mOsm/kg)
Dextrose 5% in water	81,568	566
Sodium chloride 0.9%	73,455	545
Sterile water for injection	147,205	513

Sodium and Potassium Content— Penicillin G potassium contains, in each million units, 1.7 mEq of potassium and 0.3 mEq of sodium (4).

Equivalency— Each milligram of penicillin G potassium has a potency of 1440 to 1680 USP units. Each milligram of the powder for injection (which contains sodium citrate buffer) has a potency of 1355 to 1595 USP units (4).

Administration— NOTE: Do not confuse other forms of penicillin G with penicillin G potassium.

Penicillin G potassium is administered by intramuscular injection or continuous or intermittent intravenous infusion (2). It may also be administered by intrathecal, intra-articular, and intrapleural injections and other local instillations. Vials containing 10 or 20 million units are intended for intravenous administration. For intramuscular injections, concentrations of up to 100,000 units/ml will cause a minimum of discomfort. Higher concentrations may be used when needed (2; 4).

In high doses, intravenous administration should be performed slowly to avoid electrolyte imbalance from the potassium content. For daily doses of 10 million units or more, the drug may be diluted in 1 or 2 L of infusion solution and administered in a 24-hour period (2; 4). By intermittent intravenous infusion, one-fourth or one-sixth of the daily dose may be given over one to two hours and repeated every six to four hours, respectively. Divided doses are generally infused over 15 to 30 minutes in children and neonates (4).

Stability— The dry powder is stable when stored at room temperature (4). After reconstitution, penicillin G potassium is stable for seven days under refrigeration at 2 to 8 °C (4; 47).

However, penicillin G potassium approximately 500,000 units/ml was stored at room temperature and 4 °C. After 24 hours at room temperature, HPLC analysis revealed a new peak, which increased in size by 72 hours. Storage at 4 °C significantly reduced the rate of formation of this new compound. Although the therapeutic potency of penicillin G potassium was retained over the time period studied, the authors indicated that its potential as an antigen may change due to possible formation of polymers or conjugation products that may cause allergic sensitization reactions. It was recommended that the drug be freshly prepared before use or refrigerated during interim storage (785).

Another study found increased formation of specific antipenicillin antibodies in patients administered aged penicillin solutions, not only at room temperature but also 4 °C. The authors indicated that the causative antigens were degradation or transformation products of penicillin G. Freshly prepared solutions did not seem to be immunogenic (946).

pH Effects— The stability of penicillin G potassium 500,000 units/ml is greatest at pH 7 (160). Penicillin G activity rapidly declines at pH 5.5 and below. Penicillin inactivation also occurs at pH values above 8 (47).

Freezing Solutions— Frozen premixed infusion solutions of penicillin G potassium are stable for at least 90 days from shipping stored at −20 °C. The frozen solutions should be thawed at room temperature or under refrigeration and, once thawed, should not be refrozen. Thawing should not be performed using a warm water bath or microwave radiation. Thawed solutions are stated to be stable for 24 hours at room temperature and for 14 days under refrigeration (4).

Shoup and Thur reported that penicillin G potassium 1 million units/ml is stable for 12 weeks when frozen at −18 °C (161). Aisenstein and Kahn reported penicillin G potassium (Lilly), reconstituted to a concentration of 500,000 units/ml with sterile water for injection, to be stable for at least 35 days (325). However, the validity of these results has been questioned because the highly inaccurate serial dilution method was employed (162; 299). Boylan et al. cited a report by Grant et al. that showed a loss of penicillin G in 17 hours when frozen at −18 °C with imidazole or histidine (163). However, other reports indicate that the freezing of penicillin G potassium may be satisfactory. One report showed that penicillin G potassium in concentrations of 1 to 10%, buffered to pH 6.85, lost no more than 1% potency in one month when frozen at −20 °C (99). Another study of penicillin G potassium at a concentration of 5 million units in 50 ml of dextrose 5% in water, in PVC containers frozen at −20 °C, showed no loss of potency after 14 days of storage. It was noted, however, that this study was not conclusive evidence of the safety of using such a technique (155). Additional information has come from a report of penicillin G potassium 2 million units/50 ml of dextrose 5% in water and sodium chloride 0.9% in PVC containers frozen at −20 °C for 30 days. The results indicate that potency was retained for the duration of the study (299).

Penicillin G potassium (Squibb) 1 million units/100 ml of dextrose 5% in water in PVC bags was also frozen at −20 °C for 30 days and then thawed by exposure to ambient temperature or microwave radiation. No evidence of precipitation or color change was observed, and a 3 to 4% loss of potency, as determined microbiologically, was reported. Subsequent storage of the thawed admixture at room temperature for 24 hours yielded a physically compatible solution, which exhibited no further loss of potency (554).

Miller and Pesko reported an approximate fivefold increase in particles of 2 to 60 μm produced by freezing and thawing penicillin G potassium (Squibb) 2 million units/100 ml of dextrose 5% in water (Travenol). The constituted drug was filtered through a 0.45-μm filter into PVC bags of solution and frozen for seven days at −20 °C. Thawing was performed at 29 °C for 12 hours. Although the total number of particles increased significantly, no particles greater than 60 μm were observed; the solutions complied with USP standards for particle sizes and numbers in large volume parenteral solutions (822).

Penicillin G potassium (Parke-Davis) 1 million units/50 ml of sodium chloride 0.9% lost 5% in 16 days and 7% in 25 days (by HPLC) when frozen at −7 °C. However, samples of the same solution stored at 4 °C showed similar results, indicating a lack of advantage for frozen storage (1035).

Filtration— Filtering penicillin G potassium (Pfizer) through 5-μm stainless steel and 0.22-μm cellulose ester inline filters resulted in no significant reduction in activity under conditions of varying doses, temperatures, flow rates, and administration methods (167).

Elastomeric Reservoir Pumps— Penicillin G potassium (Pfizer) 40,000 units/ml in both dextrose 5% in water and sodium chloride 0.9% was evaluated for binding potential to natural rubber elastomeric reservoirs (Baxter). No loss was found after storage for two weeks at 35 °C with gentle agitation (2014).

Portable Infusion Pumps— The stability of penicillin G potassium (Marsam) 100,000 and 200,000 units/ml in sterile water for injection was evaluated in PVC portable pump reservoirs (Pharmacia Deltec). HPLC analysis found 6% loss in three days at 25 °C. The 200,000-unit/ml concentration was also tested stored at 5 °C. About 3% loss occurred in 14 days (2080).

Compatibility Information

Solution Compatibility

Penicillin G potassium

Solution	Mfr	Mfr	Conc/L	Remarks	Ref	C/I
Alcohol 5%, dextrose 5%	AB		1 MU[b]	34% decomposition in 24 hr. Potency retained for 6 hr	46	I
Amino acids 4.25%, dextrose 25%	MG	LI	1 MU[b]	No increase in particulate matter in 24 hr at 5 °C	349	C
Dextran 6% in dextrose 5%	AB		1 MU[b]	Physically compatible	3	C
Dextran 6% in sodium chloride 0.9%	AB		1 MU[b]	Physically compatible	3	C
Dextran 70 6% in dextrose 5%			~6 MU[b]	7% decomposition in 6 hr and 18% in 24 hr at 20 °C	834	I
Dextran 40 10% in dextrose 5%			~6 MU[b]	34% decomposition in 24 hr at 20 °C	834	I
Dextrose–Ringer's injection combinations	AB		1 MU[b]	Physically compatible	3	C
Dextrose–Ringer's injection, lactated, combinations	AB		1 MU[b]	Physically compatible	3	C
Dextrose 5% in Ringer's injection, lactated	TR[c]	SQ	10 MU[b]	Potency retained for 24 hr at 5 °C	282	C
Dextrose–saline combinations	AB		1 MU[b]	Physically compatible	3	C
Dextrose 5% in sodium chloride 0.9%	MG	SQ	5 MU[b]	Potency retained for 24 hr at 4 and 25 °C	105	C
		SQ	2 MU[b]	Potency retained for 24 hr	109	C
	AB, BA, CU	(B)	5 MU[b]	Potency retained for 48 hr at 25 °C	164	C
			1 MU[b]	Physically compatible	74	C
	TR[c]	SQ	10 MU[b]	Potency retained for 24 hr at 5 °C	282	C
Dextrose 2½% in water	AB		1 MU[b]	Physically compatible	3	C
Dextrose 5% in water	AB		1 MU[b]	Physically compatible	3	C
			10 MU[b]	No decomposition in 12 hr	165	C
			100 MU[b]	7.5% decomposition in 48 hr at 25 °C and none at 5 °C	141	C
	MG	SQ	5 MU[b]	Potency retained for 24 hr at 4 and 25 °C	105	C
		SQ	2 MU[b]	Potency retained for 24 hr	109	C
		(B)	900,000 units	Potency retained for 24 hr at 25 °C	48	C
			1 MU[b]	Physically compatible	74	C
	TR[c]	SQ	10 MU[b]	Potency retained for 24 hr at 5 °C	282	C
	BA[c], TR	AY	40 MU[b]	Potency retained for 24 hr at 5 and 22 °C	298	C
	TR[d]	SQ	10 MU[b]	Physically compatible with approximately 5% potency loss in 24 hr at room temperature	554	C

Solution Compatibility (Cont.)

Penicillin G potassium

Solution	Mfr	Mfr	Conc/L	Remarks	Ref	C/I
Dextrose 10% in water	AB		1 MU[b]	Physically compatible	3	**C**
	MG	SQ	5 MU[b]	Potency retained for 24 hr at 4 and 25 °C	105	**C**
		SQ	2 MU[b]	Potency retained for 24 hr	109	**C**
Fat emulsion 10%, intravenous	VT	SQ	10 MU[b]	Physically compatible for 48 hr at 4 °C and room temperature	32	**C**
	VT		2 MU[b]	Microscopic globule coalescence in 24 hr at 8 and 25 °C	825	**I**
Fructose 10% in sodium chloride 0.9%	AB		1 MU[b]	Physically compatible	3	**C**
Fructose 10% in water	AB		1 MU[b]	Physically compatible	3	**C**
Hetastarch 6%			~6 MU[b]	7% decomposition in 24 hr at 20 °C	834	**C**
Invert sugar 5 and 10% in sodium chloride 0.9%	AB		1 MU[b]	Physically compatible	3	**C**
Invert sugar 5 and 10% in water	AB		1 MU[b]	Physically compatible	3	**C**
Isolyte M with dextrose 5%	MG	SQ	5 MU[b]	Potency retained for 24 hr at 4 and 25 °C	105	**C**
Isolyte P with dextrose 5%	MG	SQ	5 MU[b]	Potency retained for 24 hr at 4 and 25 °C	105	**C**
Ionosol products	AB		1 MU[b]	Physically compatible	3	**C**
Ringer's injection	AB		1 MU[b]	Physically compatible	3	**C**
Ringer's injection, lactated	AB		1 MU[b]	Physically compatible	3	**C**
	MG	SQ	5 MU[b]	Potency retained for 24 hr at 4 and 25 °C	105	**C**
			1 MU[b]	Physically compatible	74	**C**
	TR[c]	SQ	10 MU[b]	Potency retained for 24 hr at 5 °C	282	**C**
Sodium chloride 0.45%	AB		1 MU[b]	Physically compatible	3	**C**
Sodium chloride 0.9%	AB		1 MU[b]	Physically compatible	3	**C**
			100 MU[b]	Potency retained for 48 hr at 5 °C	141	**C**
	MG	SQ	5 MU[b]	Potency retained for 24 hr at 4 and 25 °C	105	**C**
		SQ	2 MU[b]	Potency retained for 24 hr	109	**C**
	AB, BA, CU	(B)	5 MU[b]	Potency retained for 48 hr at 25 °C	164	**C**
			1 MU[b]	Physically compatible	74	**C**
	TR[c]	SQ	10 MU[b]	Potency retained for 24 hr at 5 °C	282	**C**
	BA[c], TR	AY	40 MU[b]	Potency retained for 24 hr at 5 and 22 °C	298	**C**
	TR[d]	PD	20 MU[b]	5% penicillin loss at 24 °C and no loss at 4 °C in 4 days	1035	**C**
TPN #21[e]		SQ	5 MU[b]	Antibiotic potency retained for 24 hr at 4 and 25 °C	87	**C**
TPN #22[e]		AY	25 MU[b]	Physically compatible with no activity loss by microbiological assay in 24 hr at 22 °C in the dark	837	**C**
TPN #107[e]			2 g	Physically compatible and penicillin G activity retained for 24 hr at 21 °C by microbiological assay	1326	**C**

[a]*Citations with the notation "(B)" in the penicillin G potassium manufacturer's column specified a buffered preparation.*
[b]*Million units.*
[c]*Tested in both glass and PVC containers.*
[d]*Tested in PVC containers.*
[e]*Refer to Appendix I for the composition of parenteral nutrition solutions. TPN indicates a 2-in-1 admixture.*

Additive Compatibility

Penicillin G potassium

Drug	Mfr	Conc/L	Mfr	Conc/L	Test Soln	Remarks	Ref	C/I
Amikacin sulfate	BR	5 g	LI	20 MU[b]	D5LR, D5R, D5S, D5W, D10W, LR, NS, R, SL	Physically compatible and potency of both retained for 24 hr at 25 °C	293	**C**
	BR	5 g	LI	20 MU[b]	IG–D5W, IS10	Potency of penicillin retained through 8 hr at 25 °C. Greater than 10% decomposition in 24 hr	293	**I**
Aminophylline	SE	500 mg	(B)	900,000 units	D5W	22% penicillin decomposition in 6 hr at 25 °C	48	**I**
	SE	500 mg	SQ	1 MU[b]	D5W	44% penicillin decomposition in 24 hr at 25 °C	47	**I**
Amphotericin B		200 mg	BP	10 MU[b]	D5W	Haze develops over 3 hr	26	**I**
	SQ	50 mg	SQ	5 MU[b]		Precipitate forms within 1 hr	47	**I**
	SQ	100 mg	SQ	20 MU[b]	D5W	Physically incompatible	15	**I**
Ascorbic acid injection	AB	1 g		1 MU[b]		Physically compatible	3	**C**
	PD	500 mg	SQ	10 MU[b]	D5W	99% penicillin potency retained for at least 8 hr	166	**C**
Calcium chloride	UP	1 g	SQ	20 MU[b]	D5W	Physically compatible	15	**C**
	UP	1 g	SQ	5 MU[b]	D	Physically compatible	47	**C**
Calcium gluconate	UP	1 g	SQ	20 MU[b]	D5W	Physically compatible	15	**C**
		1 g		1 MU[b]	D5W	Physically compatible	74	**C**
Chloramphenicol sodium succinate	PD	10 g	SQ	20 MU[b]	D5W	Physically compatible	15	**C**
	PD	1 g	SQ	5 MU[b]		Physically compatible	47	**C**
	PD	500 mg	SQ	1 MU[b]	D5S, D5W	Therapeutic availability maintained	110	**C**
	PD	1 g	SQ	5 and 10 MU[b]	D5S, D5W	Therapeutic availability maintained	110	**C**
	PD	1 g		1 MU[b]		Physically compatible	3	**C**
	PD	1 g	SQ	10 MU[b]		Physically compatible	6	**C**
Chlorpromazine HCl	BP	200 mg	BP	10 MU[b]	NS	Haze develops over 3 hr	26	**I**
Cimetidine HCl	SKF	1.2 and 5 g	LI	2.4 MU[b]	D5W, NS	Physically compatible and cimetidine chemically stable for 24 hr at room temperature. Penicillin not tested	551	**C**
Clindamycin phosphate	UP	1.2 g		10 MU[b]	D5W	Physically compatible and clindamycin potency retained for 24 hr at room temperature	104	**C**
	UP	2.4 g		20 MU[b]	D5W	Physically compatible and clindamycin potency retained for 24 hr at room temperature	104	**C**
Colistimethate sodium	WC	500 mg	SQ	20 MU[b]	D5W	Physically compatible	15	**C**
	WC	500 mg	SQ	5 MU[b]	D	Physically compatible	47	**C**
Corticotropin		500 units		1 MU[b]	D5W	Physically compatible	74	**C**
Dimenhydrinate	SE	50 mg		1 MU[b]	D5W	Physically compatible	74	**C**
Diphenhydramine HCl	PD	80 mg	SQ	20 MU[b]	D5W	Physically compatible	15	**C**
	PD	50 mg	SQ	1 MU[b]	D5W	Physically compatible. Penicillin potency retained for 24 hr at 25 °C	47	**C**

Additive Compatibility (Cont.)

Penicillin G potassium

Drug	Mfr	Conc/L	Mfr	Conc/L	Test Soln	Remarks	Ref	C/I
Dopamine HCl	AS	800 mg	LI	20 MU[b]	D5W	14% penicillin decomposition in 24 hr at 23 to 25 °C. Dopamine potency retained for 24 hr	78	I
Ephedrine sulfate		50 mg		1 MU[b]		Physically compatible	3	C
	AB	50 mg	SQ	5 MU[b]		Physically compatible	47	C
Erythromycin lactobionate	AB	5 g	SQ	20 MU[b]	D5W	Physically compatible	15	C
	AB	1 g	SQ	5 MU[b]		Physically compatible	20;47	C
	AB	1 g		1 MU[b]		Physically compatible	3	C
Floxacillin sodium	BE	20 g	GL	12 g[c]	NS	Haze forms in 24 hr and precipitate forms in 48 hr at 30 °C. No change at 15 °C	1479	I
Furosemide	HO	1 g	GL	12 g[c]	NS	Physically compatible for 24 hr at 15 and 30 °C. Precipitate forms in 48 to 72 hr at 30 °C. No change at 15 °C	1479	C
Heparin sodium		12,000 units		1 MU[b]	D5W	Physically compatible	74	C
	AB	20,000 units	SQ	1 MU[b]	D5W	Penicillin potency retained for 24 hr at 25 °C	47	C
		32,000 units		20 MU[b]	NS	Physically compatible and heparin activity retained for 24 hr	57	C
	UP	4000 units	SQ	20 MU[b]	D5W	Physically incompatible	15	I
Hydrocortisone sodium succinate	UP	500 mg	SQ	20 MU[b]	D5W	Physically compatible	15	C
	UP	250 mg	SQ	5 MU[b]	D	Physically compatible	47	C
	UP	100 mg		1 MU[b]	D5W	Physically compatible	74	C
Hydroxyzine HCl	RR	250 mg	SQ	20 MU[b]	D5W	Physically incompatible	15	I
Kanamycin sulfate	BR	4 g	SQ	20 MU[b]	D5W	Physically compatible	15	C
	BR	4 g	SQ	5 MU[b]	D	Physically compatible	47	C
Lidocaine HCl	AST	2 g	SQ	1 MU[b]		Physically compatible	24	C
Lincomycin HCl	UP	6 g	SQ	20 MU[b]	D5W	Physically compatible	15	C
	UP	600 mg	SQ	5 MU[b]	D	Physically compatible	47	C
	UP					Physically incompatible	9	I
Magnesium sulfate		1 g	PF	500 mg	W	5% penicillin loss in 1 day and 13% in 2 days at 24 °C	999	C
		2 to 8 g	PF	500 mg	W	7 to 8% penicillin loss in 1 day and 20 to 25% in 2 days at 24 °C	999	C
Metaraminol bitartrate	MSD	100 mg	SQ	1 MU[b]	D5W	59% penicillin decomposition in 24 hr at 25 °C	47	I
	MSD	100 mg	(B)	900,000 units	D5W	17% penicillin decomposition in 6 hr at 25 °C	48	I
Methylprednisolone sodium succinate	UP	80 mg		2 to 10 MU[b]	D5S, D5W, LR	Clear solution for 24 hr	329	C
Metronidazole	RP	5 g[d]	AY	12 MU[b]		Physically compatible for at least 72 hr at 23 °C, but pH changed significantly	807	?
	SE	5 g[e]	PF	200 MU[b]		5% penicillin loss in 22 hr and 8% in 72 hr at 25 °C. 2% penicillin loss in 12 days at 5 °C. No metronidazole loss	993	C
Metronidazole HCl with sodium bicarbonate	SE	5 g	SQ	5 MU[b]	D5W, NS	Physically compatible for 48 hr	765	C
	AB	50 mEq						

Additive Compatibility (Cont.)

Penicillin G potassium

Drug	Mfr	Conc/L	Mfr	Conc/L	Test Soln	Remarks	Ref	C/I
Pentobarbital sodium	AB	500 mg	(B)	900,000 units	D5W	17% penicillin decomposition in 6 hr at 25 °C	48	I
	AB	500 mg	SQ	1 MU[b]	D5W	42% penicillin decomposition in 24 hr at 25 °C	47	I
Polymyxin B sulfate	BW	200 mg	SQ	20 MU[b]	D5W	Physically compatible	15	C
	BW	200 mg	SQ	5 MU[b]	D	Physically compatible	47	C
Potassium chloride		20 mEq	SQ	1 MU[b]	D5S, D5W	Therapeutic availability maintained	110	C
		40 mEq	SQ	5 MU[b]	D5S, D5W	Therapeutic availability maintained	110	C
	AB	40 mEq	SQ	5 MU[b]		Physically compatible	47	C
Potassium chloride with vitamin B complex with C	TR	20 mEq 1 ampul	SQ	2 MU[b]	D5S, D5W	Therapeutic availability maintained	110	C
Potassium chloride with vitamin B complex with C	TR	40 mEq 1 ampul	SQ	8 MU[b]	D5S, D5W	Therapeutic availability maintained	110	C
Procaine HCl	WI	1 g	SQ	20 MU[b]	D5W	Physically compatible	15	C
		1 g		1 MU[b]		Physically compatible	3	C
Prochlorperazine edisylate	SKF	10 mg	SQ	5 MU[b]	D5W	Physically compatible. Penicillin potency retained for 24 hr at 25 °C	47	C
	SKF	10 mg	(B)	900,000 units	D5W	Penicillin potency retained for 24 hr at 25 °C	48	C
Prochlorperazine mesylate	BP	100 mg	BP	10 MU[b]	NS	Haze develops over 3 hr	26	I
Promethazine HCl	WY	100 mg	SQ	5 MU[b]		Physically compatible	47	C
	WY	100 mg		1 MU[b]		Physically compatible	3	C
	WY	250 mg		20 MU[b]	D5W	Physically incompatible	15	I
Ranitidine HCl	GL	50 mg and 2 g		24 MU[b]	D5W, NS	Physically compatible and ranitidine chemically stable by HPLC for 24 hr at 25 °C. Penicillin not tested	1515	C
Sodium bicarbonate		0.5 and 0.75 g	SQ	1 MU[b]	D5W	Penicillin decomposition at 20 °C due to pH	135	I
		3.75 g	(B)	900,000 units	D5W	26% penicillin decomposition in 24 hr at 25 °C	48	I
	AB	3.75 g	SQ	1 MU[b]	D5W	26% penicillin decomposition in 24 hr at 25 °C	47	I
	AB	2.4 mEq[f]		100 MU[b]	D5W	Physically compatible for 24 hr	772	C
Thiopental sodium	AB	2.5 g	SQ	20 MU[b]	D5W	Precipitate forms within 1 hr	21	I
	AB	2.5 g	PF	20 MU[b]	D5W	Physically incompatible	11	I
Verapamil HCl	KN	80 mg	SQ	10 MU[b]	D5W, NS	Physically compatible for 24 hr	764	C
	SE	[g]	PD	62.5 g	D5W, NS	Physically compatible for 24 hr at 21 °C under fluorescent light	1166	C
Vitamin B complex with C	AB	5 ml	SQ	20 MU[b]	D5W	Physically compatible	15	C
	TR	1 ampul	SQ	2 and 8 MU[b]	D5S, D5W	Therapeutic availability maintained	110	C
	AB	2 ml		1 MU[b]		Physically compatible	3	C
		1 vial		1 MU[b]	D5W	Physically compatible	74	C
		10 ml	(B)	900,000 units	D5W	37% penicillin decomposition in 6 hr at 25 °C	48	I
	AB	10 ml	SQ	1 MU[b]	D5W	86% penicillin decomposition in 24 hr at 25 °C	47	I

Additive Compatibility (Cont.)

Penicillin G potassium

Drug	Mfr	Conc/L	Mfr	Conc/L	Test Soln	Remarks	Ref	C/I
Vitamin B complex with C with oxytetracycline HCl	TR PF	1 ampul 500 mg and 1 g	SQ	5 MU[b]	D5W, NS	Therapeutic availability lost	110	**I**
Vitamin B complex with C with potassium chloride	TR	1 ampul 20 mEq	SQ	2 MU[b]	D5S, D5W	Therapeutic availability maintained	110	**C**
Vitamin B complex with C with potassium chloride	TR	1 ampul 40 mEq	SQ	8 MU[b]	D5S, D5W	Therapeutic availability maintained	110	**C**

[a]Citations with the notation "(B)" in the penicillin G potassium manufacturer's column specified a buffered preparation.
[b]Million units.
[c]Salt form unspecified.
[d]Minibags (100 ml) containing metronidazole 500 mg with disodium phosphate 150 mg, citric acid 44 mg, and sodium chloride 740 mg. This product differs from the Searle product.
[e]Searle's ready-to-use formulation tested.
[f]One vial of Neut added to a liter of admixture.
[g]Final concentration unspecified.

Drugs in Syringe Compatibility

Penicillin G potassium

Drug (in syringe)	Mfr	Amt	Mfr	Amt	Remarks	Ref	C/I
Heparin sodium		2500 units/ 1 ml		10 million units	Physically compatible for at least 5 min	1053	**C**
Metoclopramide HCl	RB	10 mg/ 2 ml	SQ	250,000 units/ 1 ml	Incompatible. If mixed, use immediately	924	**I**
	RB	10 mg/ 2 ml	SQ	1 million units/ 4 ml	Incompatible. If mixed, use immediately	924	**I**
	RB	10 mg/ 2 ml	SQ	250,000 units/ 1 ml	Incompatible. If mixed, use immediately	1167	**I**
	RB	10 mg/ 2 ml	SQ	1 million units/ 4 ml	Incompatible. If mixed, use immediately	1167	**I**
	RB	160 mg/ 32 ml	SQ	1 million units/ 4 ml	Incompatible. If mixed, use immediately	1167	**I**

Y-Site Injection Compatibility (1:1 Mixture)

Penicillin G potassium

Drug	Mfr	Conc	Mfr	Conc	Remarks	Ref	C/I
Acyclovir sodium	BW	5 mg/ml[a]	PF	40,000 units/ ml[a]	Physically compatible for 4 hr at 25 °C	1157	**C**
Amiodarone HCl	LZ	4 mg/ml[c]	PF	100,000 units/ ml[c]	Physically compatible for 4 hr at room temperature	1444	**C**
Cyclophosphamide	MJ	20 mg/ml[a]	PF	100,000 units/ ml[a]	Physically compatible for 4 hr at 25 °C	1194	**C**

Y-Site Injection Compatibility (1:1 Mixture) (Cont.)

Penicillin G potassium

Drug	Mfr	Conc	Mfr	Conc	Remarks	Ref	C/I
Diltiazem HCl	MMD	1[b] and 5 mg/ ml	RR	1 million units/ml	Visually compatible	1807	C
	MMD	5 mg/ml	RR	100,000 units/ ml[b]	Visually compatible	1807	C
Enalaprilat	MSD	0.05 mg/ml[b]	PF	50,000 units/ ml[a]	Physically compatible for 24 hr at room temperature under fluorescent light	1355	C
Esmolol HCl	DCC	10 mg/ml[a]	PF	50,000 units/ ml[a]	Physically compatible for 24 hr at 22 °C	1169	C
Fluconazole	RR	2 mg/ml	RR	100,000 units/ ml	Physically compatible for 24 hr at 25 °C	1407	C
Foscarnet sodium	AST	24 mg/ml	SQ	100,000 units/ ml	Physically compatible for 24 hr at room temperature under fluorescent light	1335	C
Heparin sodium	TR	50 units/ml	RR	40,000 units/ ml[b]	Visually compatible for 6 hr at 25 °C	1793	C
Heparin sodium with hydrocortisone sodium succinate	RI UP	1000 units + 100 mg/L[d]	LI	200,000 units/ ml	Physically compatible for at least 4 hr at room temperature by visual and micro-scopic examination	322	C
Hydromorphone HCl	WY	0.2 mg/ml[a]	PF	100,000 units/ ml[a]	Physically compatible for at least 4 hr at 25 °C under fluorescent light	987	C
Labetalol HCl	SC	1 mg/ml[a]	PF	50,000 units/ ml[a]	Physically compatible for 24 hr at 18 °C	1171	C
Magnesium sulfate	IX	16.7, 33.3, 66.7, 100 mg/ml[a]	SQ	100,000 units/ ml[a]	Physically compatible for at least 4 hr at 32 °C	813	C
Meperidine HCl	WY	10 mg/ml[a]	PF	100,000 units/ ml[a]	Physically compatible for at least 4 hr at 25 °C under fluorescent light	987	C
Morphine sulfate	WI	1 mg/ml[a]	PF	100,000 units/ ml[a]	Physically compatible for at least 4 hr at 25 °C under fluorescent light	987	C
Perphenazine	SC	0.02 mg/ml[a]	PF	100,000 units/ ml[a]	Physically compatible for 4 hr at 25 °C	1155	C
Potassium chloride		40 mEq/L[d]	LI	200,000 units/ ml	Physically compatible for at least 4 hr at room temperature by visual and micro-scopic examination	322	C
Tacrolimus	FUJ	1 mg/ml[b]	BR	100,000 units/ ml[a]	Visually compatible for 24 hr at 25 °C	1630	C
Theophylline	TR	4 mg/ml	RR	40,000 units/ ml[b]	Visually compatible for 6 hr at 25 °C	1793	C
TNA #73[e]		32.5 ml[f]	SQ	2 million units/50 ml[a]	Physically compatible for 4 hr at 25 °C by visual observation	1008	C
TPN #54[e]				320,000 and 500,000 units/ ml	Physically compatible and 88% penicillin activity retained over 6 hr at 22 °C by microbiological assay	1045	C
TPN #61[e]		[g]	PF	200,000 units/ 2 ml[h]	Physically compatible	1012	C
		[i]	PF	1.2 million units/1.2 ml[h]	Physically compatible	1012	C
TPN #189[e]				300 mg/ml[b]	Visually compatible for 24 hr at 22 °C	1767	C

Y-Site Injection Compatibility (1:1 Mixture) (Cont.)

Penicillin G potassium

Drug	Mfr	Conc	Mfr	Conc	Remarks	Ref	C/I
Verapamil HCl	SE	2.5 mg/ml	PD	62.5 mg/ml[c]	Physically compatible for 15 min at 21 °C under fluorescent light	1166	C
Vitamin B complex with C	RC	2 ml/L[d]	LI	200,000 units/ml	Physically compatible for at least 4 hr at room temperature by visual and microscopic examination	322	C

[a]Tested in dextrose 5% in water.
[b]Tested in sodium chloride 0.9%.
[c]Tested in both dextrose 5% in water and sodium chloride 0.9%.
[d]Tested in dextrose 5% in water, Ringer's injection, lactated, and sodium chloride 0.9%.
[e]Refer to Appendix I for the composition of parenteral nutrition solutions. TNA indicates a 3-in-1 admixture, and TPN indicates a 2-in-1 admixture.
[f]A 32.5-ml sample of parenteral nutrition solution mixed with 50 ml of antibiotic solution.
[g]Run at 21 ml/hr.
[h]Given over five minutes by syringe pump.
[i]Run at 94 ml/hr.

Additional Compatibility Information

Miscellaneous— Penicillin G potassium is rapidly inactivated by oxidizing and reducing agents, alcohols, and glycols (281). High concentrations of penicillin G in combination with vancomycin HCl may result in a precipitate. Five to 10 million units of penicillin G added to vancomycin HCl, especially in dextrose solutions, will cause precipitation (143). The degradation of penicillin G may be accelerated by the presence of zinc, copper, chromium, manganese, and, especially, iron ions in solutions (81).

Solutions— Penicillin G potassium (Squibb) in concentrations up to 5 million units/L is stated to be physically compatible in all Abbott infusion solutions. Although physical compatibility does not indicate nonvisual deterioration, the citrate buffer is sufficient to adjust the pH of most intravenous solutions to the optimum pH range (47).

Although the stability of penicillin G potassium (buffered) in dextrose 5% in water and sodium chloride 0.9% has been reported to be 60 days at 5 °C (144), studies using more accurate assay methods indicate substantial (as much as 30% in 28 days) potency losses during this period (141).

Peritoneal Dialysis Solutions— The activity of penicillin G 6 mg/L was evaluated in peritoneal dialysis fluids containing dextrose 1.5 and 4.25% (Dianeal 137, Travenol). Storage at 25 °C resulted in about a 25% loss of antimicrobial activity in 24 hours. The loss of activity was attributed to the pH (5.2) of the dialysis fluids (515).

Aminoglycosides— Penicillin G 100 μg/ml mixed with gentamicin 5 μg/ml in distilled water had no appreciable effect on gentamicin potency over 72 hours at 20 °C (362).

To determine if spurious aminoglycoside levels could result from a delay in assaying blood samples, Tindula et al. evaluated the inactivation of amikacin 35 μg/ml and gentamicin and tobramycin 10 μg/ml in human serum by 400-μg/ml concentrations of several penicillins and cephalosporins. Samples were stored for 24 hours at room temperature and frozen at -20 °C. For the room temperature samples, cefazolin and cefamandole caused relatively little inactivation. Nafcillin, cephapirin, and cefoxitin caused moderate inactivation, 20% or less. Penicillin, ampicillin, carbenicillin, and ticarcillin generally caused 25% or more inactivation of gentamicin and

tobramycin. Amikacin was somewhat less affected. Freezing samples at -20 °C prevented significant inactivation of amikacin and gentamicin by any of the drugs. Freezing the tobramycin samples was satisfactory for most of the drugs except penicillin, ampicillin, and carbenicillin, which still exhibited a 15 to 20% loss in 24 hours (824).

The inactivation of tobramycin sulfate 8 μg/ml in human serum by ampicillin, carbenicillin disodium, and penicillin G potassium, each at 200 μg/ml, was studied at 0, 23, and 37 °C by O'Bey et al. For the tobramycin–ampicillin mixture, essentially no differences were observed at the various temperatures. The t_{90} values were 19, 16.5, and 20 hours at 0, 23, and 37 °C, respectively. Carbenicillin displayed a temperature-dependent inactivation of tobramycin. At 0 °C, the t_{90} was 36 hours; but at 23 and 37 °C, the t_{90} values were 10 and 12 hours, respectively. With penicillin G potassium, the t_{90} values for tobramycin inactivation at 0, 23, and 37 °C were 48, 44, and 16 hours, respectively. Inaccurate pharmacokinetic dosing of tobramycin may occur if serum samples are not properly handled (832).

The inactivation of tobramycin, gentamicin, and amikacin 10 μg/ml in sterile distilled water by penicillin G 500 and 100 μg/ml stored at 37 °C was investigated by Jorgensen and Crawford. Penicillin G 500 μg/ml caused a 23% tobramycin loss in six hours, but no significant loss occurred at the 100-μg/ml concentration. Gentamicin and amikacin were not inactivated in either concentration of penicillin G. No loss of penicillin G activity was detected in any combination (973).

The comparative inactivation of five aminoglycosides by seven β-lactam antibiotics in human serum at 37 °C was reported by Riff and Thomason. Amikacin, followed by netilmicin, had the lowest degree of inactivation; tobramycin sustained the most pronounced losses. Gentamicin and kanamycin were intermediate in the extent of losses. The six penicillins that were tested all produced aminoglycoside inactivation; the greatest extent of inactivation was caused by carbenicillin followed by ticarcillin, penicillin G, oxacillin, methicillin, and ampicillin, in approximate descending order. Cephalothin produced minimal inactivation (5 to 10% in 24 hours). The rate of inactivation could be reduced by storage at 4 °C and further reduced by storage at -20 °C. The authors suggested processing blood samples rapidly to avoid inaccurate serum determinations.

Storage of specimens at low temperature until analysis may be helpful (1052).

Acidic and Alkaline Additives— Penicillin G potassium is both an acid- and alkali-labile drug. It should not be mixed with drugs that may result in a final pH outside of its stability range of pH 5.5 to 8 (47). Unfortunately, the citrate buffer is of little value in the presence of strongly acidic or alkaline drugs (48). These drugs include the acidic drugs metaraminol bitartrate and ascorbic acid (not ascorbate sodium) and the alkaline drugs aminophylline, sodium bicarbonate, sodium salts of barbituric acid derivatives, and THAM (6; 7; 22; 47).

Hydrocortisone— Penicillin G potassium 1 million units/L has also been reported to be conditionally compatible with hydrocortisone sodium succinate (Upjohn) 250 mg/L. The mixture is physically compatible in most Abbott infusion solutions except as noted here (3):

Ionosol B with invert sugar 10%	Haze or precipitate forms within 24 hr
Ionosol D-CM with dextrose 5%	Haze or precipitate forms within 24 hr
Ionosol D with invert sugar 10%	Haze or precipitate forms within 24 hr
Ionosol G with invert sugar 10%	Haze or precipitate forms within 24 hr

Vitamins— Penicillin G potassium is inactivated by the low pH of ascorbic acid in solution. However, it is compatible with ascorbic acid injection, which has a pH of 5.5 to 7 (166).

The times to 10% decomposition of combinations of penicillin G potassium buffered (Lilly, Pfizer, and Squibb) with multivitamin infusion concentrate (USV) or vitamin B complex with C (Betalin

Table 1. Time to 10% Decomposition of Penicillin G Potassium with Vitamin Products (304)

Penicillin G Potassium	Multi-vitamin Infusion Concentrate	or	Vitamin B Complex with C	pH	Time to 10% Decomposition
1 million units/L	1 ml/L	or	2 ml/L	5.1	6.51 hr
	5 ml/L	or	10 ml/L	4.9	4.56 hr
3 million units/L	1 ml/L	or	2 ml/L	5.4	13.56 hr
	5 ml/L	or	10 ml/L	5.0	6.38 hr
5 million units/L	1 ml/L	or	2 ml/L	5.7	22.01 hr
	5 ml/L	or	10 ml/L	5.1	6.51 hr
10 million units/L	1 ml/L	or	2 ml/L	5.9	>24 hr
	5 ml/L	or	10 ml/L	5.4	13.54 hr

Complex F.C., Lilly) in dextrose 5% in water and sodium chloride 0.9% have been mathematically predicted on the basis of the final pH of the admixture (Table 1) (304).

Concentrated Solutions— The following incompatibility determinations were performed with concentrated solutions. The drugs in dry form were constituted according to manufacturers' recommendations. One milliliter of penicillin G potassium was added to 5 ml of sterile distilled water along with 1 ml of each of the following drugs. Particulate matter was noted within two hours (28):

Hydroxyzine HCl (Pfizer)
Metaraminol bitartrate (MSD)
Phenytoin sodium (Parke-Davis)
Prochlorperazine edisylate (SKF)
Promazine HCl (Wyeth)
Promethazine HCl (Wyeth)
Vancomycin HCl (Lilly)

PENICILLIN G SODIUM (BENZYLPENICILLIN SODIUM) AHFS 8:12.16

Marsam

Products— Penicillin G sodium (Marsam) is available in vials containing 5 million units of drug with sodium citrate and citric acid as buffers. Depending on the route of administration, reconstitute the vials with sterile water for injection, dextrose 5% in water, or sodium chloride 0.9% in the following amounts (1-12/92; 4; 154):

Volume of Diluent (ml)	Concentration (units/ml)
23	200,000
18	250,000
8	500,000
3	1 million

Loosen the powder. While holding the vial horizontally, rotate it and add the diluent slowly, directing the stream against the wall of the vial. Shake the vial vigorously (1-12/92; 4).

pH— The USP cites the official pH range as 5 to 7.5 (17). The AHFS cites the pH range as being 6 to 7.5 (4).

Osmolality— Penicillin G sodium (Squibb) 250,000 units/ml in sterile water for injection has an osmolality of 795 mOsm/kg (50).

The osmolality of penicillin G sodium was calculated for the following dilutions (1054):

Diluent	Osmolality (mOsm/kg)	
	50 ml	100 ml
3 million units		
Dextrose 5% in water	413	341
Sodium chloride 0.9%	439	368
5 million units		
Dextrose 5% in water	502	394
Sodium chloride 0.9%	529	421

Robinson et al. recommended the following maximum penicillin G sodium concentrations to achieve osmolalities suitable for peripheral infusion in fluid-restricted patients (1180):

Diluent	Maximum Concentration (units/ml)	Osmolality (mOsm/kg)
Dextrose 5% in water	85,383	573
Sodium chloride 0.9%	76,891	563
Sterile water for injection	154,091	545

Sodium Content— Penicillin G sodium contains 2 mEq of sodium per million units (4).

Equivalency— Each milligram of penicillin G sodium has a potency of 1500 to 1750 USP units. Each milligram of the powder for injection (which contains sodium citrate buffer) has a potency of 1420 to 1667 USP units (4).

Administration— NOTE: Do not confuse other forms of penicillin G with penicillin G sodium.

Penicillin G sodium is administered by intramuscular injection or by continuous or intermittent intravenous infusion. For intramuscular injections, concentrations of up to 100,000 units/ml will cause a minimum of discomfort. Higher concentrations may be used when needed. In high doses, intravenous administration should be performed slowly to avoid electrolyte imbalance from the sodium content. For daily doses of 10 million units or more, the drug may be diluted in 1 or 2 L of infusion solution and administered in a 24-hour period. By intermittent intravenous infusion, one-fourth or one-sixth of the daily dose may be given over one to two hours and repeated every six to four hours, respectively. Divided doses are generally infused over 15 to 30 minutes in children and neonates (4).

Stability— The dry powder may be stored at room temperature without significant potency loss. After reconstitution, solutions may be stored for one week under refrigeration. Intravenous infusions containing this drug are stable at room temperature for at least 24 hours (4).

Exposure of penicillin G sodium (Squibb-Marsam) 180,000 units/ml in sterile water for injection to 37 °C for 24 hours, to simulate the use of a portable infusion pump, resulted in a 10 to 13% penicillin loss (1391).

Freezing Solutions— It has been shown that penicillin G sodium in concentrations of 1 to 10%, buffered to pH 6.85, loses not more than 1% potency in one month when frozen at −20 °C (99). Another report stated that solutions of penicillin G sodium at a concentration of 50,000 units/ml in water, sodium chloride 0.9%, and 0.05 M citrate buffer and also at a concentration of 500,000 units/ml with sodium citrate 15 mg are stable for at least 12 weeks when frozen at −25 °C. At −5 °C in the citrate buffer, the rate of decomposition is considerably higher than at either −25 or 5 °C (156).

Rayani et al. reported that penicillin G sodium 2.5 million units/ 50 ml of dextrose 5% in water in PVC containers was physically compatible and chemically stable for 39 days when frozen at −20 °C. Subsequent thawing and storage at 4 °C resulted in a 3 to 4% loss in 10 to 15 days and up to a 10% loss in 31 days (1125).

Stiles et al. reported little or no penicillin G sodium loss from a solution containing 180,000 units/ml in sterile water for injection in PVC and glass containers after 30 days at −20 °C. Subsequent thawing and storage for four days at 5 °C, followed by 24 hours at 37 °C to simulate the use of a portable infusion pump, resulted in about a 12 to 16% penicillin loss (1391).

pH Effects— At 25 °C, the maximum stability of penicillin G sodium is attained at pH 6.8 (131), but little difference in the rate of decomposition occurs in the pH range of 6.5 to 7.5 (1947). Not more than 10% loss of activity occurs in 24 hours in a pH range of approximately 5.4 to 8.5 (131). Unbuffered penicillin G sodium injection 12 and 48 mg/ml in sodium chloride 0.9% had an initial pH between 5.4 and 5.8. Approximately 7% loss determined by HPLC analysis occurred in two days in samples stored at 5 °C. However, reconstituting with citrate buffers having pH values of 6.5, 7.0, and 7.5 resulted in great stability improvement. At these same concentrations in sodium chloride 0.9% in minibags stored at 5 °C, losses of 5 to 7% occurred in 28 days and 10% in 56 days (1947).

Portable Infusion Pumps— The stability of penicillin G sodium (Marsam) 100,000 and 200,000 units/ml in sterile water for injection was evaluated in PVC portable pump reservoirs (Pharmacia Deltec). HPLC analysis found about 4 to 6% loss in three days at 25 °C (2080).

Compatibility Information

Solution Compatibility

Penicillin G sodium

Solution	Mfr	Mfr	Conc/L	Remarks	Ref	C/I
Dextran 40 10%	PH	KA	6 MU[a]	Potency retained for 24 hr at 25 °C	131	C
Dextrose 5% in water		KA	6 MU[a]	Potency retained for 24 hr at 25 °C	131	C
		BE	20 MU[a]	25% decomposition in 24 hr at 25 °C	113	I
			4 MU[a,b]	7% loss in 6 hr and 29% loss in 24 hr at room temperature	768	I
	TR[c]	AY	50 MU[a]	No penicillin loss in 39 days at −20 °C. Up to 10% loss on subsequent storage for 31 days at 5 °C	1125	C
Fat emulsion 10%, intravenous	VT		2 MU[a]	Microscopic globule coalescence in 24 hr at 8 and 25 °C	825	I

Solution Compatibility (Cont.)

Penicillin G sodium

Solution	Mfr	Mfr	Conc/L	Remarks	Ref	C/I
Invert sugar 10%		KA	6 MU[a]	10% decomposition in 6 to 12 hr at 25 °C	131	I
Sodium chloride 0.9%		BE	20 MU[a]	Potency retained for 24 hr at 25 °C	131	C
			4 MU[a,b]	10% loss in 8 hr and 16% loss in 24 hr at room temperature	768	I
	TR[c]	GL	20 and 80 MU[a]	In unbuffered solution. 7 to 8% loss by HPLC in 48 hr and 18% loss in 96 hr at 5 °C	1671	C
	TR[c]	GL	20 MU[a]	Reconstituted with citrate buffer (pH 6.5 to 7.5). 5% loss by HPLC in 28 days and 10% loss in 56 days at 5 °C	1671	C
TPN #107[e]			2 g	Physically compatible and penicillin G activity retained for 24 hr at 21 °C by microbiological assay	1326	C
TPN #189[e]			300 mg/ml[f]	Visually compatible for 24 hr at 22 °C	1767	C

[a]Million units.
[b]An unbuffered preparation was specified.
[c]Tested in PVC containers.
[d]Tested in both PVC and glass containers.
[e]Refer to Appendix I for the composition of parenteral nutrition solutions. TPN indicates a 2-in-1 admixture.
[f]Tested in sodium chloride 0.9%.

Additive Compatibility

Penicillin G sodium

Drug	Mfr	Conc/L	Mfr	Conc/L	Test Soln	Remarks	Ref	C/I
Amphotericin B	SQ	100 mg	UP	20 MU[a]	D5W	Physically incompatible	15	I
		200 mg	BP	10 MU[a]	D5W	Haze develops over 3 hr	26	I
Bleomycin sulfate	BR	20 and 30 units	SQ	2 MU[a]	NS	77% loss of bleomycin activity in 1 week at 4 °C	763	I
	BR	20 and 30 units	SQ	5 MU[a]	NS	41% loss of bleomycin activity in 1 week at 4 °C	763	I
Calcium chloride	UP	1 g	UP	20 MU[a]	D5W	Physically compatible	15	C
Calcium gluconate	UP	1 g	UP	20 MU[a]	D5W	Physically compatible	15	C
Chloramphenicol sodium succinate	PD	10 g	UP	20 MU[a]	D5W	Physically compatible	15	C
Chlorpromazine HCl	BP	200 mg	BP	10 MU[a]	NS	Haze develops over 3 hr	26	I
Clindamycin phosphate	UP	1.2 g		10 MU[a]	D5W	Physically compatible and clindamycin potency retained for 24 hr at room temperature	104	C
	UP	2.4 g		20 MU[a]	D5W	Physically compatible and clindamycin potency retained for 24 hr at room temperature	104	C
Colistimethate sodium	WC	500 mg	UP	20 MU[a]	D5W	Physically compatible	15	C
Cytarabine	UP	200 mg		2 MU[a]	D5W	pH outside stability range for penicillin G	174	I
Diphenhydramine HCl	PD	80 mg	UP	20 MU[a]	D5W	Physically compatible	15	C
Erythromycin lactobionate	AB	5 g	UP	20 MU[a]	D5W	Physically compatible	15	C
Floxacillin sodium	BE	20 g	GL	12 g[b]	NS	Haze forms in 24 hr and precipitate forms in 48 hr at 30 °C. No change at 15 °C	1479	I

Additive Compatibility (Cont.)

Penicillin G sodium

Drug	Mfr	Conc/L	Mfr	Conc/L	Test Soln	Remarks	Ref	C/I
Furosemide	HO	1 g	GL	12 g[b]	NS	Physically compatible for 24 hr at 15 and 30 °C. Precipitate forms in 48 to 72 hr at 30 °C. No change at 15 °C	1479	C
Gentamicin sulfate	RS	160 mg	GL	13 and 40 MU[a]	D5¼S, D5W, NS	Gentamicin potency retained for 24 hr at room temperature	157	C
Heparin sodium	OR	20,000 units	BE	20 MU[a]	NS	Potency of both retained for 24 hr at 25 °C	113	C
		32,000 units		20 MU[a]	NS	Physically compatible and heparin activity retained for 24 hr	57	C
	UP	4000 units	UP	20 MU[a]	D5W	Physically incompatible	15	I
Hydrocortisone sodium succinate	UP	500 mg	UP	20 MU[a]	D5W	Physically compatible	15	C
Hydroxyzine HCl	RR	250 mg	UP	20 MU[a]	D5W	Physically incompatible	15	I
Kanamycin sulfate	BR	4 g	UP	20 MU[a]	D5W	Physically compatible	15	C
Lincomycin HCl	UP	6 g	UP	20 MU[a]	D5W	Physically compatible	15	C
	UP					Physically incompatible	9	I
Methylprednisolone sodium succinate	UP	125 mg		5 MU[a]	D5W, LR	Precipitate forms	329	I
Polymyxin B sulfate	BW	200 mg	UP	20 MU[a]	D5W	Physically compatible	15	C
Potassium chloride		40 mEq	KA	6 MU[a]	D5W	Penicillin potency retained for at least 24 hr at 25 °C	131	C
		40 mEq	KA	5 MU[a]	IS10	pH outside stability range for penicillin	131	I
Procaine HCl	WI	1 g	UP	20 MU[a]	D5W	Physically compatible	15	C
Prochlorperazine mesylate	BP	100 mg	BP	10 MU[a]	NS	Haze develops over 3 hr	26	I
Promethazine HCl	WY	25 mg	UP	20 MU[a]	D5W	Physically incompatible	15	I
Ranitidine HCl	GL	100 mg		2.4 MU[a]	D5W	Physically compatible for 24 hr at ambient temperature under fluorescent light	1151	C
Verapamil HCl	KN	80 mg	SQ	10 MU[a]	D5W, NS	Physically compatible for 24 hr	764	C
Vitamin B complex with C	AB	5 ml	UP	20 MU[a]	D5W	Physically compatible	15	C

[a]Million units.
[b]Salt form unspecified.

Drugs in Syringe Compatibility

Penicillin G sodium

Drug (in syringe)	Mfr	Amt	Mfr	Amt	Remarks	Ref	C/I
Chloramphenicol sodium succinate	PD	250 and 400 mg/ 1.5 to 2 ml		1 million units	No precipitate or color change within 1 hr at room temperature	99	C
Cimetidine HCl	SKF	300 mg/ 2 ml		1 million units/ 5 ml	Precipitate forms between 36 and 48 hr at room temperature	516	C
Colistimethate sodium	PX	40 mg/ 2 ml		1 million units	No precipitate or color change within 1 hr at room temperature	99	C

Drugs in Syringe Compatibility (Cont.)

Penicillin G sodium

Drug (in syringe)	Mfr	Amt	Mfr	Amt	Remarks	Ref	C/I
Gentamicin sulfate		80 mg/ 2 ml		1 million units	No precipitate or color change within 1 hr at room temperature	99	C
Heparin sodium		2500 units/ 1 ml		10 million units	Physically compatible for at least 15 min	1053	C
Kanamycin sulfate		1 g/4 ml		1 million units	No precipitate or color change within 1 hr at room temperature	99	C
Lincomycin HCl	UP	600 mg/ 2 ml		1 million units	No precipitate or color change within 1 hr at room temperature	99	C
Polymyxin B sulfate	BW	25 mg/ 1.5 to 2 ml		1 million units	No precipitate or color change within 1 hr at room temperature	99	C
Streptomycin sulfate		1 g/2 ml		1 million units	No precipitate or color change within 1 hr at room temperature	99	C

Y-Site Injection Compatibility (1:1 Mixture)

Penicillin G sodium

Drug (in syringe)	Mfr	Amt	Mfr	Amt	Remarks	Ref	C/I
Clarithromycin	AB	4 mg/ml[a]	BRT	24 mg/ ml[a]	Visually compatible for 72 hr at both 30 and 17 °C	2174	C
TPN #54[e]				320,000 and 500,000 units/ml	Physically compatible and 88% penicillin activity retained over 6 hr at 22 °C by microbiological assay	1045	C
TPN #61[e]		[b]	PF	200,000 units/ 2 ml[c]	Physically compatible	1012	C
		[d]	PF	1.2 million units/ 12 ml[c]	Physically compatible	1012	C

[a]*Tested in dextrose 5% in water.*
[b]*Run at 21 ml/hr.*
[c]*Given over five minutes by syringe pump.*
[d]*Run at 94 ml/hr.*
[e]*Refer to Appendix I for the composition of parenteral nutrition solutions. TPN indicates a 2-in-1 admixture.*

Additional Compatibility Information

Miscellaneous— High concentrations of penicillin G in combination with vancomycin HCl may result in a precipitate. Five to 10 million units of penicillin G added to vancomycin HCl, especially in dextrose solutions, will cause precipitation (143). Also, lincomycin HCl is reported to be physically compatible for only four hours in infusion solutions (154).

In addition, penicillin G is inactivated by oxidizing and reducing agents, alcohols, and glycols (281). Also, the degradation of penicillin G may be accelerated by the presence of zinc, copper, chromium, manganese, and, especially, iron ions in solutions (81).

Solutions— Penicillin G sodium degradation was unaffected by the presence of dextrose 5 and 10%, fructose 5 and 15%, invert sugar 4 and 8%, or ethanol 2.5, 5, 10, and 20% in solutions at 25 °C at a constant pH of 5.4 (131).

Peritoneal Dialysis Solutions— The activity of penicillin G 6 mg/L was evaluated in peritoneal dialysis fluids containing dextrose 1.5 and 4.25% (Dianeal 137, Travenol). Storage at 25 °C resulted in about a 25% loss of antimicrobial activity in 24 hours. The loss of activity was attributed to the pH (5.2) of the dialysis fluids (515).

Aminoglycosides— Penicillin G 100 μg/ml mixed with gentamicin 5 μg/ml in distilled water had no appreciable effect on gentamicin potency over 72 hours at 20 °C (362).

Rank et al. evaluated the inactivation of tobramycin 6 μg/ml in human serum with the sodium salts of cloxacillin and piperacillin 150 and 300 µg/ml, ampicillin 100 and 200 µg/ml, and penicillin G 75 and 150 I.U./ml at 25 and 37 °C for up to 12 hours. Piperacillin induced the greatest inactivation among the penicillins, with up to a 15% loss in 12 hours at 37 °C in the 300-µg/ml concentration. Cloxacillin and ampicillin had an intermediate effect, causing about a 5% loss in 12 hours at 37 °C in the highest concentrations. Penicillin G did not yield significant tobramycin inactivation (817).

To determine if spurious aminoglycoside levels could result from a delay in assaying blood samples, Tindula et al. evaluated the inactivation of amikacin 35 µg/ml and gentamicin and tobramycin 10 µg/ml in human serum by 400-µg/ml concentrations of several penicillins and cephalosporins. Samples were stored for 24 hours at room temperature and frozen at −20 °C. For the room temperature samples, cefazolin and cefamandole caused relatively little inactivation. Nafcillin, cephapirin, and cefoxitin caused moderate inactivation, 20% or less. Penicillin, ampicillin, carbenicillin, and ticarcillin generally caused 25% or more inactivation of gentamicin and tobramycin. Amikacin was somewhat less affected. Freezing samples at −20 °C prevented significant inactivation of amikacin and gentamicin by any of the drugs. Freezing the tobramycin sample was satisfactory for most of the drugs except penicillin, ampicillin, and carbenicillin, which still exhibited a 15 to 20% loss in 24 hours (824).

The inactivation of tobramycin, gentamicin, and amikacin 10 µg/ml in sterile distilled water by penicillin G 500 and 100 µg/ml

stored at 37 °C was investigated by Jorgensen and Crawford. Penicillin G 500 µg/ml caused a 23% tobramycin loss in six hours, but no significant loss occurred at the 100-µg/ml concentration. Gentamicin and amikacin were not inactivated in either concentration of penicillin G. No loss of penicillin G activity was detected in any combination (973).

The comparative inactivation of five aminoglycosides by seven β-lactam antibiotics in human serum at 37 °C was reported by Riff and Thomason. Amikacin, followed by netilmicin, had the lowest degree of inactivation; tobramycin sustained the most pronounced losses. Gentamicin and kanamycin were intermediate in the extent of losses. The six penicillins that were tested all produced aminoglycoside inactivation; the greatest extent of inactivation was caused by carbenicillin followed by ticarcillin, penicillin G, oxacillin, methicillin, and ampicillin, in approximate descending order. Cephalothin produced minimal inactivation (5 to 10% in 24 hours). The rate of inactivation could be reduced by storage at 4 °C and further reduced by storage at −20 °C. The authors suggested processing blood samples rapidly to avoid inaccurate serum determinations. Storage of specimens at low temperature until analysis may be helpful (1052).

Acidic Additives— The rate of decomposition of acid-sensitive drugs such as penicillin G sodium may be increased by mixing with acidic additives such as metaraminol bitartrate, oxytetracycline HCl, and tetracycline HCl (7; 22).

PENTAMIDINE ISETHIONATE
AHFS 8:40

Pentam 300   **Abbott**

Products— Pentamidine isethionate (Abbott) is available in vials containing 300 mg in lyophilized form. For intramuscular injection, the contents of a vial should be reconstituted with 3 ml of sterile water for injection to yield a 100-mg/ml concentration. For intravenous injection, the contents of a vial should be reconstituted with 3, 4, or 5 ml of sterile water for injection or dextrose 5% in water to yield solutions containing 100, 75, or 60 mg/ml, respectively. The dose should be withdrawn and further diluted in 50 to 250 ml of dextrose 5% in water for administration (4).

pH— Reconstituted solutions of 60 to 100 mg/ml have a pH of approximately 5.4 in sterile water for injection and of 4.09 to 4.38 in dextrose 5% in water (4).

Osmolality— At a concentration of 100 mg/ml in sterile water for injection and dextrose 5% in water, the osmolalities are 160 and 455 mOsm/kg, respectively (4).

Equivalency— Pentamidine isethionate 1.74 mg is equivalent to pentamidine 1 mg (4).

Administration— Pentamidine isethionate injection may be administered by slow intravenous infusion or deep intramuscular injection.

Intravenously, the calculated dose should be diluted in 50 to 250 ml of dextrose 5% in water and infused over at least one hour. The drug should not be administered by rapid intravenous injection or infusion (4).

Stability— The sterile dry powder should be stored at controlled room temperature and protected from light (4).

Reconstituted solutions containing 60 to 100 mg/ml are stable for 48 hours at room temperature protected from light (4). Because the product does not contain a preservative, the manufacturer recommends discarding any unused portion of the solution (4).

Pentamidine isethionate at concentrations of 1 and 2.5 mg/ml in dextrose 5% in water is stated to be stable at room temperature for up to 24 hours (4), but other information indicates that the drug may be stable for a longer period at room temperature exposed to fluorescent light. See Compatibility Information.

Elastomeric Reservoir Pumps— Pentamidine isethionate (Fujisawa) 3 mg/ml in dextrose 5% in water and 2 mg/ml in sodium chloride 0.9% was evaluated for binding potential to natural rubber elastomeric reservoirs (Baxter). No loss was found after storage for two weeks at 35 °C with gentle agitation (2014).

Sorption— The possible sorption of small amounts of pentamidine isethionate to PVC tubing has been reported (1142). However, other work indicated that no significant loss occurs due to sorption to PVC containers and tubing (1311).

Compatibility Information

Solution Compatibility

Pentamidine isethionate

Solution	Mfr	Mfr	Conc/L	Remarks	Ref	C/I
Dextrose 5% in water	TR[a]	LY	1 g	Physically compatible with 3% loss in 48 hr at 24 °C under fluorescent light	1142	**C**
	TR[a]	LY	2 g	Physically compatible with 1% loss in 48 hr at 24 °C under fluorescent light	1142	**C**
	TR[a]	MB	2 g	Physically compatible with little or no loss in 24 hr at 20 °C	1311	**C**
Sodium chloride 0.9%	TR[a]	LY	1 g	Physically compatible with 2% loss in 48 hr at 24 °C under fluorescent light	1142	**C**
	TR[a]	LY	2 g	Physically compatible with no loss in 48 hr at 24 °C under fluorescent light	1142	**C**
	TR[a]	MB	2 g	Physically compatible with little or no loss in 24 hr at 20 °C	1311	**C**

[a]Tested in PVC containers.

Y-Site Injection Compatibility (1:1 Mixture)

Pentamidine isethionate

Drug	Mfr	Conc	Mfr	Conc	Remarks	Ref	C/I
Aldesleukin	CHI	33,800 I.U./ml[a]	FUJ	6 mg/ml[a]	Aldesleukin bioactivity inhibited	1857	**I**
Cefazolin sodium	SKB	20 mg/ml[a]	FUJ	3 mg/ml[a]	Cloudiness and gelatin-like precipitate form immediately	1880	**I**
Cefoperazone sodium	RR	20 mg/ml[e]	FUJ	3 mg/ml[a]	Heavy white precipitate forms immediately	1880	**I**
Cefotaxime sodium	HO	20 mg/ml[a]	FUJ	3 mg/ml[a]	Fine precipitate, difficult to see, forms immediately	1880	**I**
Cefoxitin sodium	ME	20 mg/ml[c]	FUJ	3 mg/ml[a]	Cloudiness and powder-like precipitate form immediately	1880	**I**
Ceftazidime	LI[d]	20 mg/ml[a]	FUJ	3 mg/ml[a]	Fine precipitate, difficult to see, forms immediately	1880	**I**
Ceftriaxone sodium	RC	20 mg/ml[a]	FUJ	3 mg/ml[a]	Heavy white precipitate forms immediately	1880	**I**
Diltiazem HCl	MMD	5 mg/ml	LY	6 and 30 mg/ml[a]	Visually compatible	1807	**C**
Fluconazole	RR	2 mg/ml	LY	6 mg/ml	Cloudiness develops	1407	**I**
Foscarnet sodium	AST	24 mg/ml	LY	6 mg/ml	Immediate precipitation	1335	**I**
	AST	24 mg/ml	LY	6 mg/ml[a,b]	Pentamidine crystals form immediately	1393	**I**
Zidovudine	BW	4 mg/ml[a]	LY	6 mg/ml[a]	Physically compatible for 4 hr at 25 °C under fluorescent light by visual and microscopic examination	1193	**C**

[a]Tested in dextrose 5% in water.
[b]Tested in sodium chloride 0.9%.
[c]Tested in dextrose 4% in water.
[d]Sodium carbonate-containing formulation tested.
[e]Tested in dextrose 4.6% in water.

PENTAZOCINE LACTATE
AHFS 28:08.12

Talwin   **Abbott**

Products— Pentazocine lactate (Abbott) is supplied in 1-, 1.5-, and 2-ml ampuls and disposable cartridge-needle units as well as 10-ml multiple-dose vials. Each milliliter of solution contains (1-2/94):

Component	Ampul	Cartridge Unit	Vial
Pentazocine (as lactate)	30 mg	30 mg	30 mg
Sodium chloride	2.8 mg	2.2 mg	1.5 mg
Acetone sodium bisulfite		1 mg	2 mg
Methylparaben			1 mg
Water for injection	qs 1 ml	qs 1 ml	qs 1 ml

pH— The pH is adjusted to between 4 and 5 with lactic acid or sodium hydroxide (1-2/94).

Osmolality— The osmolality of pentazocine lactate 30 mg/ml was determined to be 307 mOsm/kg (1233).

Administration— Pentazocine lactate may be administered by intramuscular, subcutaneous, or intravenous injection. For repeated administration, the drug should be given by intramuscular injection with constant rotation of the injection sites. Subcutaneous injection should be used only when necessary because of possible tissue damage (1-2/94; 4).

Stability— Pentazocine lactate injection should be stored at room temperature and protected from temperatures of 40 °C or above and from freezing (4).

Pentazocine lactate (Winthrop) 30 mg/ml was found to retain potency for three months at room temperature when 1 ml of solution was packaged in Tubex cartridges (13).

Pentazocine lactate (Winthrop) 30 mg/1 ml, repackaged in 3-ml clear glass syringes (Hy-Pod) and stored at 25 °C, exhibited no significant changes in pH, physical appearance, or drug concentration during 360 days of storage (535).

Compatibility Information

Additive Compatibility

Pentazocine lactate

Drug	Mfr	Conc/L	Mfr	Conc/L	Test Soln	Remarks	Ref	C/I
Aminophylline	SE	1 g	WI	300 mg	D5W	Physically incompatible	15	I
Amobarbital sodium	LI	1 g	WI	300 mg	D5W	Physically incompatible	15	I
Pentobarbital sodium	AB	1 g	WI	300 mg	D5W	Physically incompatible	15	I
Phenobarbital sodium	WI	200 mg	WI	300 mg	D5W	Physically incompatible	15	I
Sodium bicarbonate	AB	80 mEq	WI	300 mg	D5W	Physically incompatible	15	I

Drugs in Syringe Compatibility

Pentazocine lactate

Drug (in syringe)	Mfr	Amt	Mfr	Amt	Remarks	Ref	C/I
Atropine sulfate		0.6 mg/ 1.5 ml	WI	30 mg/ 1 ml	Physically compatible for at least 15 min	14	C
	ST	0.4 mg/ 1 ml	WI	30 mg/ 1 ml	Physically compatible for at least 15 min	326	C
Butorphanol tartrate	BR	4 mg/ 2 ml	WI	30 mg/ 1 ml	Physically compatible both macroscopically and microscopically for 30 min at room temperature	566	C
Chlorpromazine HCl	SKF	50 mg/ 2 ml	WI	30 mg/ 1 ml	Physically compatible for at least 15 min	14	C
	PO	50 mg/ 2 ml	WI	30 mg/ 1 ml	Physically compatible for at least 15 min	326	C
Cimetidine HCl	SKF	300 mg/ 2 ml	WI	60 mg/ 2 ml	Physically compatible for 4 hr at 25 °C	25	C
Dimenhydrinate	HR	50 mg/ 1 ml	WI	30 mg/ 1 ml	Physically compatible for at least 15 min	326	C

Drugs in Syringe Compatibility (Cont.)

Pentazocine lactate

Drug (in syringe)	Mfr	Amt	Mfr	Amt	Remarks	Ref	C/I
Diphenhydramine HCl	PD	50 mg/ 1 ml	WI	30 mg/ 1 ml	Physically compatible for at least 15 min	326	**C**
Droperidol	MN	2.5 mg/ 1 ml	WI	30 mg/ 1 ml	Physically compatible for at least 15 min	326	**C**
Fentanyl citrate	MN	0.05 mg/ 1 ml	WI	30 mg/ 1 ml	Physically compatible for at least 15 min	326	**C**
Glycopyrrolate	RB	0.2 mg/ 1 ml	WI	30 mg/ 1 ml	Immediate precipitation	331	**I**
	RB	0.2 mg/ 1 ml	WI	60 mg/ 2 ml	Immediate precipitation	331	**I**
	RB	0.4 mg/ 2 ml	WI	30 mg/ 1 ml	Immediate precipitation	331	**I**
Heparin sodium		2500 units/ 1 ml	WI	30 mg/ 1 ml	Turbidity or precipitate forms within 5 min	1053	**I**
Hydromorphone HCl	KN	4 mg/ 2 ml	WI	30 mg/ 1 ml	Physically compatible for 30 min	517	**C**
Hydroxyzine HCl	PF	100 mg/ 4 ml	WI	30 mg/ 1 ml	Physically compatible for at least 15 min	14	**C**
	PF	50 mg/ 1 ml	WI	30 mg/ 1 ml	Physically compatible for at least 15 min	326	**C**
	PF	50 mg/ 1 ml	WI	60 mg/ 2 ml	Physically compatible	771	**C**
	PF	100 mg/ 2 ml	WI	30 mg/ 1 ml	Physically compatible	771	**C**
Meperidine HCl	WI	50 mg/ 1 ml	WI	30 mg/ 1 ml	Physically compatible for at least 15 min	326	**C**
Meperidine HCl with perphenazine		150 mg 5 mg		15 mg	Physically compatible for at least 15 min	815	**C**
Metoclopramide HCl	NO	10 mg/ 2 ml	WI	30 mg/ 1 ml	Physically compatible both macroscopically and microscopically for 15 min at room temperature	565	**C**
Morphine sulfate	ST	15 mg/ 1 ml	WI	30 mg/ 1 ml	Physically compatible for at least 15 min	326	**C**
Pentobarbital sodium	WY	100 mg/ 2 ml	WI	30 mg/ 1 ml	Precipitate forms within 15 min	14	**I**
	AB	50 mg/ 1 ml	WI	30 mg/ 1 ml	Physically incompatible within 15 min	326	**I**
Perphenazine	SC	5 mg/ 1 ml	WI	30 mg/ 1 ml	Physically compatible both macroscopically and microscopically for 30 min at room temperature	566	**C**
Perphenazine with meperidine HCl		5 mg 150 mg		15 mg	Physically compatible for at least 15 min	815	**C**
Prochlorperazine edisylate	PO	5 mg/ 1 ml	WI	30 mg/ 1 ml	Physically compatible for at least 15 min	326	**C**
Promazine HCl	WY	25 mg/ 1 ml	WI	30 mg/ 1 ml	Potency retained for 3 months at room temperature in Tubex	13	**C**
	WY	50 mg/ 1 ml	WI	30 mg/ 1 ml	Potency retained for 3 months at room temperature in Tubex	13	**C**

Drugs in Syringe Compatibility (Cont.)

Pentazocine lactate

Drug (in syringe)	Mfr	Amt	Mfr	Amt	Remarks	Ref	C/I
	WY	50 mg/ 1 ml	WI	30 mg/ 1 ml	Physically compatible for at least 15 min	326	C
Promethazine HCl	WY	50 mg/ 2 ml	WI	30 mg/ 1 ml	Physically compatible for at least 15 min	14	C
	WY	25 mg/ 0.5 ml	WI	30 mg/ 1 ml	Potency retained for 3 months at room temperature in Tubex	13	C
	WY	25 mg/ 1 ml	WI	30 mg/ 1 ml	Potency retained for 3 months at room temperature in Tubex	13	C
	WY	50 mg/ 1 ml	WI	30 mg/ 1 ml	Potency retained for 3 months at room temperature in Tubex	13	C
	WY	25 mg/ 0.5 ml	WI	45 mg/ 1.5 ml	Potency retained for 3 months at room temperature in Tubex	13	C
	PO	50 mg/ 2 ml	WI	30 mg/ 1 ml	Physically compatible for at least 15 min	326	C
Propiomazine HCl	WY	20 mg/ 1 ml	WI	30 mg/ 1 ml	Potency retained for 3 months at room temperature in Tubex	13	C
	WY	10 mg/ 0.5 ml	WI	30 mg/ 1 ml	Potency retained for 3 months at room temperature in Tubex	13	C
Ranitidine HCl	GL	50 mg/ 2 ml	WI	60 mg/ 2 ml	Physically compatible for 1 hr at 25 °C both macroscopically and microscopically	978	C
Scopolamine HBr		0.6 mg/ 1.5 ml	WI	30 mg/ 1 ml	Physically compatible for at least 15 min	14	C
	ST	0.4 mg/ 1 ml	WI	30 mg/ 1 ml	Physically compatible for at least 15 min	326	C

Y-Site Injection Compatibility (1:1 Mixture)

Pentazocine lactate

Drug	Mfr	Conc	Mfr	Conc	Remarks	Ref	C/I
Heparin sodium	UP	1000 units/L[a]	WI	30 mg/ml	Physically compatible for at least 4 hr at room temperature by visual and microscopic examination	534	C
Hydrocortisone sodium succinate	UP	10 mg/L[a]	WI	30 mg/ml	Physically compatible for at least 4 hr at room temperature by visual and microscopic examination	534	C
Nafcillin sodium	WY	33 mg/ml[b]		30 mg/ml	Precipitate forms, probably free nafcillin	547	I
Potassium chloride	AB	40 mEq/L[a]	WI	30 mg/ml	Physically compatible for at least 4 hr at room temperature by visual and microscopic examination	534	C
Vitamin B complex with C	RC	2 ml/L[a]	WI	30 mg/ml	Physically compatible for at least 4 hr at room temperature by visual and microscopic examination	534	C

[a]Tested in dextrose 5% in Ringer's injection, dextrose 5% in Ringer's injection, lactated, dextrose 5% in water, Ringer's injection, lactated, and sodium chloride 0.9%.
[b]Tested in sodium chloride 0.9%.

Additional Compatibility Information

Pentazocine lactate is incompatible with alkaline substances such as aminophylline and barbiturates (4). Mixing pentazocine lactate and barbiturates in the same syringe may result in precipitation (1-2/94).

PENTOBARBITAL SODIUM
AHFS 28:24.04

Nembutal   **Abbott**

Products— Pentobarbital sodium (Abbott) is available in 20-ml (1 g) and 50-ml (2.5 g) multiple-dose vials. Each milliliter of solution contains (2):

Pentobarbital sodium	50 mg
Propylene glycol	40% (v/v)
Alcohol	10%
Hydrochloric acid and/or sodium hydroxide	to adjust pH
Water for injection	qs

pH— Adjusted to approximately 9.5 (2); range 9 to 10.5 (4).

Administration— Pentobarbital sodium may be administered by deep intramuscular injection into a large muscle or by slow intravenous injection. It is usually administered in a concentration of 50 mg/ml. The rate of intravenous administration should not exceed 50 mg/min. No more than 5 ml of solution (250 mg) should be injected intramuscularly at any one site (2; 4).

Stability— Intact vials of pentobarbital sodium should be stored at room temperature and protected from excessive heat and freezing. Brief exposures to temperatures up to 40 °C does not adversely affect the product (2).

Aqueous solutions of pentobarbital sodium are not stable. The commercially available pentobarbital sodium in a propylene glycol vehicle is more stable. In an acidic medium, pentobarbital sodium may precipitate (4). No solution containing a precipitate or that is cloudy should be used (2; 4).

Sorption— Pentobarbital sodium (Abbott) 25 mg/L did not display significant sorption to a PVC plastic test strip in 24 hours (12).

The sorption of pentobarbital sodium 30 mg/L in sodium chloride 0.9% was evaluated in 100-ml PVC infusion bags (Travenol). After eight hours at 20 to 24 °C, no loss of pentobarbital had occurred (770).

Filtration— Pentobarbital sodium (Abbott) 600 mg/L and 1.25 g/L in dextrose 5% in water and also sodium chloride 0.9% was filtered through a 0.45-μm filter. The delivered concentration did not decrease (754).

Compatibility Information

Solution Compatibility

Pentobarbital sodium

Solution	Mfr	Mfr	Conc/L	Remarks	Ref	C/I
Dextran 6% in dextrose 5%	AB	AB	500 mg	Physically compatible	3	**C**
Dextran 6% in sodium chloride 0.9%	AB	AB	500 mg	Physically compatible	3	**C**
Dextrose–Ringer's injection combinations	AB	AB	500 mg	Physically compatible	3	**C**
Dextrose–Ringer's injection, lactated, combinations	AB	AB	500 mg	Physically compatible	3	**C**
Dextrose–saline combinations	AB	AB	500 mg	Physically compatible	3	**C**
Dextrose 2½% in water	AB	AB	500 mg	Physically compatible	3	**C**
Dextrose 5% in water	AB	AB	500 mg	Physically compatible	3	**C**
	MG[a]	AB	600 mg and 1.25 g	Physically compatible and chemically stable for 12-hr study period	754	**C**
	BA[b]	AB	4 and 8 g	Visually compatible with no loss by HPLC in 24 hr	1590	**C**
	BA[b]	AB	>8 g	Occasional visible precipitation	1590	**I**

Solution Compatibility (Cont.)

Pentobarbital sodium

Solution	Mfr	Mfr	Conc/L	Remarks	Ref	C/I
Dextrose 10% in water	AB	AB	500 mg	Physically compatible	3	C
Fructose 10% in sodium chloride 0.9%	AB	AB	500 mg	Physically compatible	3	C
Fructose 10% in water	AB	AB	500 mg	Physically compatible	3	C
Invert sugar 5 and 10% in sodium chloride 0.9%	AB	AB	500 mg	Physically compatible	3	C
Invert sugar 5 and 10% in water	AB	AB	500 mg	Physically compatible	3	C
Ionosol products	AB	AB	500 mg	Physically compatible	3	C
Ringer's injection	AB	AB	500 mg	Physically compatible	3	C
Ringer's injection, lactated	AB	AB	500 mg	Physically compatible	3	C
Sodium chloride 0.45%	AB	AB	500 mg	Physically compatible	3	C
Sodium chloride 0.9%	AB	AB	500 mg	Physically compatible	3	C
	MG[a]	AB	600 mg and 1.25 g	Physically compatible and chemically stable for 12-hr study period	754	C
	BA[b]	AB	4 and 8 g	Visually compatible with no loss by HPLC in 24 hr	1590	C
	BA[b]	AB	>8 g	Occasional visible precipitation	1590	I
Sodium lactate ⅙ M	AB	AB	500 mg	Physically compatible	3	C

[a]Tested in polyolefin containers.
[b]Tested in PVC containers.

Additive Compatibility

Pentobarbital sodium

Drug	Mfr	Conc/L	Mfr	Conc/L	Test Soln	Remarks	Ref	C/I
Amikacin sulfate	BR	5 g	AB	100 mg	D5LR, D5R, D5S, D5W, D10W, IS10, LR, NS, R, SL	Physically compatible and potency of both drugs retained for 24 hr at 25 °C	294	C
Aminophylline		500 mg	AB	500 mg		Physically compatible	3	C
	SE	500 mg	AB	500 mg		Physically compatible	6	C
	SE	1 g	AB	1 g	D5W	Physically compatible	15	C
Calcium chloride	UP	1 g	AB	1 g	D5W	Physically compatible	15	C
Chloramphenicol sodium succinate	PD	1 g	AB	200 mg		Physically compatible	6	C
Chlorpheniramine maleate						Physically incompatible	9	I
	SC	100 mg	AB	1 g	D5W	Physically incompatible	15	I
Dimenhydrinate	SE	500 mg	AB	1 g	D5W	Physically compatible	15	C
Ephedrine sulfate						Physically incompatible	9	I
	LI	250 mg	AB	1 g	D5W	Physically incompatible	15	I
Erythromycin lactobionate	AB	1 g	AB	500 mg		Physically compatible. Erythromycin stable for 24 hr at 25 °C	20	C
Hydrocortisone sodium succinate						Physically incompatible	9	I
	UP	500 mg	AB	1 g	D5W	Physically incompatible	15	I

Additive Compatibility (Cont.)

Pentobarbital sodium

Drug	Mfr	Conc/L	Mfr	Conc/L	Test Soln	Remarks	Ref	C/I
Hydroxyzine HCl	PF					Physically incompatible	9	I
	RR	250 mg	AB	1 g	D5W	Physically incompatible	15	I
Insulin, regular[a]						Physically incompatible	9	I
Levorphanol bitartrate	RC					Physically incompatible	9	I
Lidocaine HCl	AST	2 g	AB	500 mg		Physically compatible	24	C
Norepinephrine bitartrate	WI					Physically incompatible	9	I
Penicillin G potassium	(B)[b]	900,000 units	AB	500 mg	D5W	17% penicillin decomposition in 6 hr at 25 °C	48	I
	SQ	1 million units	AB	500 mg	D5W	42% penicillin decomposition in 24 hr at 25 °C	47	I
Pentazocine lactate	WI	300 mg	AB	1 g	D5W	Physically incompatible	15	I
Phenytoin sodium	PD					Physically incompatible	9	I
Promazine HCl	WY	1 g	AB	200 mg	D5W	Physically incompatible	11	I
Promethazine HCl	WY	250 mg	AB	1 g	D5W	Physically incompatible	15	I
Sodium bicarbonate						Physically incompatible	9	I
	AB	80 mEq	AB	1 g	D5W	Physically incompatible	15	I
	AB	2.4 mEq[c]	AB	500 mg	D5W	Physically compatible for 24 hr	772	C
Streptomycin sulfate						Physically incompatible	9	I
Succinylcholine chloride	AB	2 g	AB	500 mg		Physically compatible	3	C
						Physically incompatible	9	I
Thiopental sodium	AB	2.5 g	AB	200 mg	D5W	Physically compatible	21	C
Triflupromazine HCl	SQ					Precipitate forms	40	I
Vancomycin HCl	LI					Physically incompatible	9	I
Verapamil HCl	KN	80 mg	AB	200 mg	D5W, NS	Physically compatible for 24 hr	764	C

[a]*Test performed prior to availability of neutral regular insulin.*
[b]*A buffered preparation was specified.*
[c]*One vial of Neut added to a liter of admixture.*

Drugs in Syringe Compatibility

Pentobarbital sodium

Drug (in syringe)	Mfr	Amt	Mfr	Amt	Remarks	Ref	C/I
Aminophylline		500 mg/ 2 ml	AB	500 mg/ 10 ml	Physically compatible	55	C
Atropine sulfate		0.6 mg/ 1.5 ml	WY	100 mg/ 2 ml	Physically compatible for at least 15 min	14	C
	ST	0.4 mg/ 1 ml	AB	50 mg/ 1 ml	Physically compatible for at least 15 min	326	C
	LI	0.6 mg/ 1.5 ml	AB	100 mg/ 2 ml	Precipitate forms within 24 hr at room temperature	542	I
Atropine sulfate with cimetidine HCl	LI	0.6 mg/ 1.5 ml	AB	100 mg/ 2 ml	Immediate precipitation	542	I
	SKF	300 mg/ 2 ml					

Drugs in Syringe Compatibility (Cont.)

Pentobarbital sodium

Drug (in syringe)	Mfr	Amt	Mfr	Amt	Remarks	Ref	C/I
Butorphanol tartrate	BR	4 mg/ 2 ml	AB	50 mg/ 1 ml	Immediate precipitation	761	I
Chlorpromazine HCl	SKF	50 mg/ 2 ml	AB	500 mg/ 10 ml	Physically incompatible	55	I
	SKF	50 mg/ 2 ml	WY	100 mg/ 2 ml	Precipitate forms within 15 min	14	I
	PO	50 mg/ 2 ml	AB	50 mg/ 1 ml	Physically incompatible within 15 min	326	I
Cimetidine HCl	SKF	300 mg/ 2 ml	AB	100 mg/ 2 ml	Immediate precipitation	542	I
Cimetidine HCl with atropine sulfate	SKF LI	300 mg/ 2 ml 0.6 mg/ 1.5 ml	AB	100 mg/ 2 ml	Immediate precipitation	542	I
Dimenhydrinate	SE	50 mg/ 1 ml	AB	500 mg/ 10 ml	Physically incompatible	55	I
	HR	50 mg/ 1 ml	AB	50 mg/ 1 ml	Physically incompatible within 15 min	326	I
Diphenhydramine HCl	PD	50 mg/ 1 ml	AB	500 mg/ 10 ml	Physically incompatible	55	I
	PD	50 mg/ 1 ml	AB	50 mg/ 1 ml	Physically incompatible within 15 min	326	I
Droperidol	MN	2.5 mg/ 1 ml	AB	50 mg/ 1 ml	Physically incompatible within 15 min	326	I
Ephedrine sulfate		50 mg/ 1 ml	AB	500 mg/ 10 ml	Physically compatible	55	C
Fentanyl citrate	MN	0.05 mg/ 1 ml	AB	50 mg/ 1 ml	Physically incompatible within 15 min	326	I
Glycopyrrolate	RB	0.2 mg/ 1 ml	AB	50 mg/ 1 ml	Immediate precipitation	331	I
	RB	0.4 mg/ 2 ml	AB	50 mg/ 1 ml	Immediate precipitation	331	I
	RB	0.2 mg/ 1 ml	AB	100 mg/ 2 ml	Immediate precipitation	331	I
Hyaluronidase		150 units	AB	500 mg/ 10 ml	Physically compatible	55	C
Hydromorphone HCl	KN	4 mg/ 2 ml[a]	AB	50 mg/ 1 ml	Physically compatible for 30 min	517	C
	KN	4 mg/ 2 ml[b]	AB	50 mg/ 1 ml	Transient precipitate dissipates after mixing. Physically compatible for 30 min	517	C
Hydroxyzine HCl	PF	100 mg/ 4 ml	WY	100 mg/ 2 ml	Precipitate forms within 15 min	14	I
	PF	50 mg/ 1 ml	AB	50 mg/ 1 ml	Physically incompatible within 15 min	326	I
Meperidine HCl	WI	100 mg/ 2 ml	AB	500 mg/ 10 ml	Physically incompatible	55	I
	WY	100 mg/ 1 ml	WY	100 mg/ 2 ml	Precipitate forms within 15 min	14	I
	WI	50 mg/ 1 ml	AB	50 mg/ 1 ml	Physically incompatible within 15 min	326	I

Drugs in Syringe Compatibility (Cont.)

Pentobarbital sodium

Drug (in syringe)	Mfr	Amt	Mfr	Amt	Remarks	Ref	C/I
Midazolam HCl	RC	5 mg/ 1 ml	WY	100 mg/ 2 ml	White precipitate forms immediately	1145	**I**
Morphine sulfate		16.2 mg/ 1 ml	AB	500 mg/ 10 ml	Physically compatible	55	**C**
	WY	15 mg/ 1 ml	WY	100 mg/ 2 ml	Precipitate forms within 15 min	14	**I**
	ST	15 mg/ 1 ml	AB	50 mg/ 1 ml	Physically incompatible within 15 min	326	**I**
Nalbuphine HCl	EN	10 mg/ 1 ml	WY	50 mg/ 1 ml	Immediate white milky precipitate that persists for 36 hr at 27 °C	762	**I**
	EN	2.5 mg/ 0.25 ml	WY	50 mg/ 1 ml	Immediate white milky precipitate that clears upon vigorous shaking	762	**I**
	EN	5 mg/ 0.5 ml	WY	50 mg/ 1 ml	Immediate white milky precipitate that persists for 36 hr at 27 °C	762	**I**
Neostigmine methylsulfate	RC	0.5 mg/ 1 ml	AB	500 mg/ 10 ml	Physically compatible	55	**C**
Pentazocine lactate	WI	30 mg/ 1 ml	WY	100 mg/ 2 ml	Precipitate forms within 15 min	14	**I**
	WI	30 mg/ 1 ml	AB	50 mg/ 1 ml	Physically incompatible within 15 min	326	**I**
Perphenazine	SC	5 mg/ 1 ml	AB	50 mg/ 1 ml	Immediate precipitation	761	**I**
Prochlorperazine edisylate	SKF	10 mg/ 2 ml	AB	500 mg/ 10 ml	Physically incompatible	55	**I**
	SKF		WY	100 mg/ 2 ml	Precipitate forms within 15 min	14	**I**
	PO	5 mg/ 1 ml	AB	50 mg/ 1 ml	Physically incompatible within 15 min	326	**I**
Promazine HCl	WY	50 mg/ 1 ml	AB	50 mg/ 1 ml	Physically incompatible within 15 min	326	**I**
Promethazine HCl	WY	100 mg/ 4 ml	AB	500 mg/ 10 ml	Physically incompatible	55	**I**
	WY	50 mg/ 2 ml	WY	100 mg/ 2 ml	Precipitate forms within 15 min	14	**I**
	PO	50 mg/ 2 ml	AB	50 mg/ 1 ml	Physically incompatible within 15 min	326	**I**
Ranitidine HCl	GL	50 mg/ 5 ml	AB	100 mg	Immediate precipitation	1151	**I**
Scopolamine HBr		0.6 mg/ 1.5 ml	WY	100 mg/ 2 ml	Physically compatible for at least 15 min	14	**C**
		0.13 mg/ 0.26 ml	AB	500 mg/ 10 ml	Physically compatible	55	**C**
	ST	0.4 mg/ 1 ml	AB	50 mg/ 1 ml	Physically compatible for at least 15 min	326	**C**
Sodium bicarbonate		3.75 g/ 50 ml	AB	500 mg/ 10 ml	Physically compatible	55	**C**
Thiopental sodium	AB	75 mg/ 3 ml	AB	50 mg/ 1 ml	Physically compatible for at least 30 min	21	**C**

Drugs in Syringe Compatibility (Cont.)

Pentobarbital sodium

Drug (in syringe)	Mfr	Amt	Mfr	Amt	Remarks	Ref	C/I
	AB	75 mg/ 3 ml	AB	37.5 mg/ 0.75 ml	Physically compatible	55	**C**

[a]Vial formulation was tested.
[b]Ampul formulation was tested.

Y-Site Injection Compatibility (1:1 Mixture)

Pentobarbital sodium

Drug	Mfr	Conc	Mfr	Conc	Remarks	Ref	C/I
Acyclovir sodium	BW	5 mg/ml[a]	WY	2 mg/ml[a]	Physically compatible for 4 hr at 25 °C	1157	**C**
Amphotericin B cholesteryl sulfate complex	SEQ	0.83 mg/ml[a]	AB	5 mg/ml[a]	Decreased natural turbidity occurs immediately	2117	**I**
Insulin, regular (Humulin R) (beef, pork)	LI LI	1 unit/ml[b] 1 unit/ml[b]	WY WY	2 mg/ml[b] 2 mg/ml[b]	Physically compatible for 3 hr Physically compatible for 3 hr	1316 1316	**C** **C**
Propofol	ZEN	10 mg/ml	WY	5 mg/ml[a]	Physically compatible for 1 hr at 23 °C with no increase in particle content	2066	**C**
TNA #218 to #226[c]			AB	5 mg/ml[a]	Damage to emulsion integrity occurs immediately with free oil formation possible	2215	**I**
TPN #212 to #215[c]			AB	5 mg/ml[a]	Physically compatible with no change in measured turbidity or increase in particle content in 4 hr at 23 °C	2109	**C**

[a]Tested in dextrose 5% in water.
[b]Tested in sodium chloride 0.9%.
[c]Refer to Appendix I for the composition of parenteral nutrition solutions. TNA indicates a 3-in-1 admixture, and TPN indicates a 2-in-1 admixture.

Additional Compatibility Information

Miscellaneous— The manufacturer recommends that pentobarbital sodium be mixed with no other medication or solution (2). Drugs stated to be incompatible with pentobarbital sodium or barbiturate salts include clindamycin phosphate (106), cefazolin sodium (278), fentanyl citrate (4), pancuronium bromide (4), droperidol (4), and cimetidine HCl (360).

Pentobarbital sodium should not be mixed in the same syringe with pentazocine lactate because precipitation occurs (4).

Acidic Additives— Drugs such as pentobarbital sodium that exhibit poor solubility in an acidic medium may precipitate in solutions containing acidic additives (4; 22). Metaraminol bitartrate is acidic and may cause precipitation, depending on the concentrations of the additives (7). Also, the acidic methyldopate HCl imparts some buffer capacity to admixtures and may pose solubility problems with barbiturate salts (23).

Alkali-Labile Drugs— Pentobarbital sodium may raise the pH of admixture solutions to the alkaline range and, therefore, should not be mixed with alkali-labile drugs such as penicillin G (47). Significant decomposition of isoproterenol HCl and norepinephrine bitartrate may also occur. If either of these two drugs is mixed with pentobarbital sodium, the admixture should be used immediately after preparation (59; 77).

Atracurium besylate also may be inactivated by alkaline solutions such as barbiturates; precipitation of a free acid of the admixed drug may occur, depending on the resultant pH of the admixture (4).

Succinylcholine Chloride— When barbiturates are mixed with succinylcholine chloride, either the free barbiturate will precipitate or the succinylcholine chloride will be hydrolyzed, depending on the final pH of the admixture (4; 21).

Promethazine and Chlorpromazine— Pentobarbital sodium (Abbott) 500 mg/L has been reported to be conditionally compatible with promethazine HCl (Wyeth) 100 mg/L and chlorpromazine HCl 50 mg/L. The mixtures are physically incompatible in most Abbott infusion solutions except as noted below (3):

Ionosol MB with dextrose 5%	Physically compatible
Ionosol T with dextrose 5%	Physically compatible

Hydrocortisone— Pentobarbital sodium (Abbott) has also been reported to be conditionally compatible with hydrocortisone sodium succinate (Upjohn) 250 mg/L. The mixture is physically compatible in most Abbott infusion solutions except Ionosol G with invert sugar 10%, in which a haze or precipitate forms within six hours (3).

Plasticizer Leaching— Pentobarbital sodium (Abbott) 2 mg/ml in dextrose 5% in water did not leach diethylhexyl phthalate (DEHP) plasticizer from 50-ml PVC bags in 24 hours at 24 °C (1683).

PENTOSTATIN
AHFS 10:00

Nipent   **SuperGen**

Products—— Pentostatin (SuperGen) is available as a lyophilized powder in vials containing 10 mg of drug. Also present are 50 mg of mannitol and sodium hydroxide or hydrochloric acid to adjust the pH. Reconstitute the vial contents with 5 ml of sterile water for injection and shake well to yield a 2-mg/ml solution (2).

pH—— From 7 to 8.5 (2).

Administration—— Pentostatin is administered intravenously by injection over five minutes or by infusion over 20 to 30 minutes when diluted in 25 to 50 ml of dextrose 5% in water or sodium chloride 0.9%. Adequate hydration is necessary prior to administering pentostatin. Administration of 500 to 1000 ml of dextrose 5% in sodium chloride 0.45% or similar solution prior to drug administration with an additional 500 ml of dextrose 5% in water or similar solution after drug administration is recommended (2; 4).

Stability—— The manufacturer recommends that pentostatin be stored under refrigeration (2), but other information indicates that the drug in intact vials is stable for at least three years at room temperature (234).

The white to off-white powder yields a colorless solution when reconstituted. The manufacturer states that reconstituted pentostatin solutions are stable at room temperature for up to eight hours only because of the absence of antibacterial preservatives (2). Other information indicates that the reconstituted solution is stable for 72 hours at room temperature, exhibiting a 2 to 4% loss (234; 1453).

pH Effects—— Pentostatin displays greater decomposition under acidic conditions compared to alkaline conditions. The pH range of maximum stability is about 6.5 to 11.5. At pH 6 to 8, hydrolysis is not sensitive to the ionic strength of the solution (1453).

Sorption—— Pentostatin does not undergo sorption to PVC containers or administration sets at concentrations between 0.18 and 0.33 mg/ml in dextrose 5% water or sodium chloride 0.9% (2).

Compatibility Information

Solution Compatibility

				Pentostatin		
Solution	Mfr	Mfr	Conc/L	Remarks	Ref	C/I
Dextrose 5% in water		NCI	20 mg	Approximately 2% loss in 24 hr and 8 to 10% loss in 48 hr at room temperature. No loss in 96 hr under refrigeration	234	C
	TRᵃ, BAᵇ NCI		20 mg	10% loss in 54 hr at 23 °C	1453	C
	TRᵃ, BAᵇ NCI		2 mg	10% loss in 11 hr at 23 °C	1453	I
Ringer's injection, lactated		NCI	20 mg	Approximately 0 to 4% loss in 48 hr at room temperature	234	C
Sodium chloride 0.9%		NCI	20 mg	Approximately 0 to 4% loss in 48 hr at room temperature. No loss in 96 hr under refrigeration	234	C
	ABᵃ, BAᵇ NCI		20 mg	1 to 4% loss in about 49 hr at 23 °C	1453	C
	ABᵃ, BAᵇ NCI		2 mg	3 to 6% loss in 48 hr at 23 °C	1453	C

ᵃTested in glass containers.
ᵇTested in PVC containers.

Y-Site Injection Compatibility (1:1 Mixture)

				Pentostatin		
Drug	Mfr	Conc	Mfr	Conc	Remarks	Ref	C/I
Fludarabine phosphate	BX	1 mg/mlᵃ	NCI	0.4 mg/mlᵇ	Physically compatible for 4 hr at room temperature under fluorescent light	1439	C
Melphalan HCl	BW	0.1 mg/mlᵇ	PD	0.4 mg/mlᵇ	Physically compatible with no change in measured turbidity or increase in particle content in 3 hr at 22 °C under fluorescent light	1557	C
Ondansetron HCl	GL	1 mg/mlᵇ	NCI	0.4 mg/mlᵇ	Physically compatible for 4 hr at 22 °C	1365	C
Paclitaxel	NCI	1.2 mg/mlᵃ	NCI	0.4 mg/mlᵇ	Physically compatible with no change in measured turbidity in 4 hr at 22 °C	1556	C

Y-Site Injection Compatibility (1:1 Mixture) (Cont.)

					Pentostatin		
Drug	Mfr	Conc	Mfr	Conc	Remarks	Ref	C/I
Sargramostim	IMM	10 μg/ml[b]	NCI	0.4 mg/ml[b]	Physically compatible for 4 hr at 22 °C	1436	C

[a]*Tested in dextrose 5% in water.*
[b]*Tested in sodium chloride 0.9%.*

Additional Compatibility Information

Solutions— Dextrose 5% in water and sodium chloride 0.9% are recommended as diluents for the infusion of pentostatin. The manufacturer recommends use within eight hours (2).

Other information indicates that the drug is stable for much longer periods (234; 1453) except in very low concentrations (approximately 0.002 mg/ml) in dextrose 5% in water when buffering to neutral pH may be desirable (1453). (See Solution Compatibility.)

Other Information

Bacterial Challenge— Pentostatin (Parke-Davis) 0.03 mg/ml diluted in sodium chloride 0.9% and stored at 22 °C did not exhibit a substantial antimicrobial effect on the growth of four organisms (*Enterococcus faecium, Staphylococcus aureus, Pseudomonas aeruginosa,* and *Candida albicans*) inoculated into the solution. *C. albicans* maintained viability for 24 hours, and the others were viable for 48 to 120 hours. The author recommended that diluted solutions of pentostatin be stored under refrigeration whenever possible and that the potential for microbiological growth be considered when assigning expiration periods (2160).

PERPHENAZINE
AHFS 28:16.08

Trilafon   **Schering**

Products— Perphenazine (Schering) is available as a 5-mg/ml solution in 1-ml ampuls. Each milliliter also contains citric acid, sodium bisulfite, and water for injection (2).

pH— From 4.2 to 5.6 (4).

Osmolality— Perphenazine 5 mg/ml has an osmolality of 263 mOsm/kg (1689).

Administration— Perphenazine is given by deep intramuscular injection or, rarely, by fractional intravenous injection or slow intravenous infusion. The intravenous route is used only when necessary in severe cases and limited to recumbent hospitalized adult patients. By fractional intravenous injection, a 0.5-mg/ml dilution in sodium chloride 0.9% is administered; a maximum of 1 mg per injection should be given slowly at intervals of at least one to two minutes (2; 4).

Stability— Perphenazine should be stored at room temperature and protected from temperatures above 40 °C and from freezing (4). Perphenazine is light sensitive and should be protected from light. Exposure to light may cause a discoloration. Potency or therapeutic efficacy is not altered by a slight yellowish discoloration, but the drug should be discarded if a marked discoloration appears (2).

Compatibility Information

Drugs in Syringe Compatibility

					Perphenazine		
Drug (in syringe)	Mfr	Amt	Mfr	Amt	Remarks	Ref	C/I
Atropine sulfate	ST	0.4 mg/ 1 ml	SC	5 mg/ 1 ml	Physically compatible both macroscopically and microscopically for 30 min at room temperature	566	C
Benztropine mesylate	MSD	2 mg/ 2 ml	SC	10 mg/ 2 ml	Visually compatible for 60 min	1784	C
Butorphanol tartrate	BR	4 mg/ 2 ml	SC	5 mg/ 1 ml	Physically compatible both macroscopically and microscopically for 30 min at room temperature	761	C

Drugs in Syringe Compatibility (Cont.)

Perphenazine

Drug (in syringe)	Mfr	Amt	Mfr	Amt	Remarks	Ref	C/I
Chlorpromazine HCl	MB	25 mg/ 1 ml	SC	5 mg/ 1 ml	Physically compatible both macroscopically and microscopically for 30 min at room temperature	566	C
Cimetidine HCl	SKF	300 mg/ 2 ml	SC	5 mg/ 1 ml	Physically compatible for 4 hr at 25 °C	25	C
Dimenhydrinate	HR	50 mg/ 1 ml	SC	5 mg/ 1 ml	Physically compatible both macroscopically and microscopically for 30 min at room temperature	761	C
Diphenhydramine HCl	PD	50 mg/ 1 ml	SC	5 mg/ 1 ml	Physically compatible both macroscopically and microscopically for 30 min at room temperature	566	C
	ES	100 mg/ 2 ml	SC	10 mg/ 2 ml	Visually compatible for 60 min	1784	C
Droperidol	MN	5 mg/ 2 ml	SC	5 mg/ 1 ml	Physically compatible both macroscopically and microscopically for 30 min at room temperature	566	C
Fentanyl citrate	MN	0.1 mg/ 2 ml	SC	5 mg/ 1 ml	Physically compatible both macroscopically and microscopically for 30 min at room temperature	566	C
Hydroxyzine HCl	ES	100 mg/ 2 ml	SC	10 mg/ 2 ml	Visually compatible for 60 min	1784	C
Meperidine HCl	WI	50 mg/ 1 ml	SC	5 mg/ 1 ml	Physically compatible both macroscopically and microscopically for 30 min at room temperature	566	C
Meperidine HCl with pentazocine lactate		150 mg 15 mg		5 mg	Physically compatible for at least 15 min	815	C
Methotrimeprazine		25 mg/ 1 ml	SC	5 mg/ 1 ml	Physically compatible for 30 min at room temperature both macroscopically and microscopically	566	C
Metoclopramide HCl	NO	10 mg/ 2 ml	SC	5 mg/ 1 ml	Physically compatible both macroscopically and microscopically for 30 min at room temperature	565; 566	C
Midazolam HCl	RC	5 mg/ 1 ml	SC	5 mg/ 1 ml	White precipitate forms immediately	1145	I
Morphine sulfate	AH	15 mg/ 1 ml	SC	5 mg/ 1 ml	Physically compatible both macroscopically and microscopically for 30 min at room temperature	566	C
Pentazocine lactate	WI	30 mg/ 1 ml	SC	5 mg/ 1 ml	Physically compatible both macroscopically and microscopically for 30 min at room temperature	566	C
Pentazocine lactate with meperidine HCl		15 mg 150 mg		5 mg	Physically compatible for at least 15 min	815	C
Pentobarbital sodium	AB	50 mg/ 1 ml	SC	5 mg/ 1 ml	Immediate precipitation	761	I
Prochlorperazine edisylate	MB	5 mg/ 1 ml	SC	5 mg/ 1 ml	Physically compatible both macroscopically and microscopically for 30 min at room temperature	566	C

Drugs in Syringe Compatibility (Cont.)

Perphenazine

Drug (in syringe)	Mfr	Amt	Mfr	Amt	Remarks	Ref	C/I
Promethazine HCl	WY	25 mg/ 1 ml	SC	5 mg/ 1 ml	Physically compatible both macroscopically and microscopically for 30 min at room temperature	566	C
Ranitidine HCl	GL	50 mg/ 2 ml	SC	5 mg/ 1 ml	Physically compatible for 1 hr at 25 °C both macroscopically and microscopically	978	C
Scopolamine HBr	ST	0.4 mg/ 1 ml	SC	5 mg/ 1 ml	Physically compatible both macroscopically and microscopically for 30 min at room temperature	566	C
Thiethylperazine malate	BI	10 mg/ 1 ml	SC	5 mg/ 1 ml	Yellow discoloration within 15 min	761	I

Y-Site Injection Compatibility (1:1 Mixture)

Perphenazine

Drug	Mfr	Conc	Mfr	Conc	Remarks	Ref	C/I
Acyclovir sodium	BW	5 mg/ml[a]	SC	0.1 mg/ml[a]	Physically compatible for 4 hr at 25 °C	1157	C
Amikacin sulfate	BR	5 mg/ml[a]	SC	0.02 mg/ml[a]	Physically compatible for 4 hr at 25 °C	1155	C
Ampicillin sodium	BR	20 mg/ml[b]	SC	0.02 mg/ml[a]	Physically compatible for 4 hr at 25 °C	1155	C
Azlocillin sodium	MI	20 mg/ml[a]	SC	0.02 mg/ml[a]	Physically compatible for 4 hr at 25 °C	1155	C
Cefamandole nafate	LI	20 mg/ml[a]	SC	0.02 mg/ml[a]	Physically compatible for 4 hr at 25 °C	1155	C
Cefazolin sodium	SKF	20 mg/ml[c]	SC	0.02 mg/ml[a]	Physically compatible for 4 hr at 25 °C	1155	C
Cefoperazone sodium	RR	20 mg/ml[a]	SC	0.02 mg/ml[a]	Cloudy solution forms immediately with fine precipitate persisting for 4 hr at 25 °C	1155	I
Cefotaxime sodium	HO	20 mg/ml[a]	SC	0.02 mg/ml[a]	Physically compatible for 4 hr at 25 °C	1155	C
Cefoxitin sodium	MSD	20 mg/ml[c]	SC	0.02 mg/ml[a]	Physically compatible for 4 hr at 25 °C	1155	C
Cefuroxime sodium	GL	30 mg/ml[a]	SC	0.02 mg/ml[a]	Physically compatible for 4 hr at 25 °C	1155	C
Chloramphenicol sodium succinate	ES	20 mg/ml[a]	SC	0.02 mg/ml[a]	Physically compatible for 4 hr at 25 °C	1155	C
Clindamycin phosphate	UP	12 mg/ml[a]	SC	0.02 mg/ml[a]	Physically compatible for 4 hr at 25 °C	1155	C
Doxycycline hyclate	ES	1 mg/ml[a]	SC	0.02 mg/ml[a]	Physically compatible for 4 hr at 25 °C	1155	C
Erythromycin lactobionate	AB	5 mg/ml[a]	SC	0.02 mg/ml[a]	Physically compatible for 4 hr at 25 °C	1155	C
Famotidine	MSD	0.2 mg/ml[a]	SC	0.04 mg/ml[a]	Physically compatible for 4 hr at 25 °C	1188	C
Gentamicin sulfate	TR	1.6 mg/ml[c]	SC	0.02 mg/ml[a]	Physically compatible for 4 hr at 25 °C	1155	C
Kanamycin sulfate	BR	2.5 mg/ml[a]	SC	0.02 mg/ml[a]	Physically compatible for 4 hr at 25 °C	1155	C
Metronidazole	SE	5 mg/ml[c]	SC	0.02 mg/ml[a]	Physically compatible for 4 hr at 25 °C	1155	C
Minocycline HCl	LE	0.2 mg/ml[a]	SC	0.02 mg/ml[a]	Physically compatible for 4 hr at 25 °C	1155	C
Nafcillin sodium	WY	20 mg/ml[a]	SC	0.02 mg/ml[a]	Physically compatible for 4 hr at 25 °C	1155	C
Oxacillin sodium	BE	20 mg/ml[a]	SC	0.02 mg/ml[a]	Physically compatible for 4 hr at 25 °C	1155	C
Penicillin G potassium	PF	100,000 units/ml[a]	SC	0.02 mg/ml[a]	Physically compatible for 4 hr at 25 °C	1155	C
Piperacillin sodium	LE	60 mg/ml[a]	SC	0.02 mg/ml[a]	Physically compatible for 4 hr at 25 °C	1155	C
Tacrolimus	FUJ	1 mg/ml[b]	SC	2.5 mg/ml[a]	Visually compatible for 24 hr at 25 °C	1630	C

Y-Site Injection Compatibility (1:1 Mixture) (Cont.)

				Perphenazine			
Drug	*Mfr*	*Conc*	*Mfr*	*Conc*	*Remarks*	*Ref*	*C/I*
Ticarcillin disodium	BE	30 mg/ml[a]	SC	0.02 mg/ml[a]	Physically compatible for 4 hr at 25 °C	1155	C
Ticarcillin disodium–clavulanate potassium	BE	31 mg/ml[a]	SC	0.02 mg/ml[a]	Physically compatible for 4 hr at 25 °C	1155	C
Tobramycin sulfate	DI	0.8 mg/ml[a]	SC	0.02 mg/ml[a]	Physically compatible for 4 hr at 25 °C	1155	C
Trimethoprim–sulfamethoxazole	BW	0.8 + 4 mg/ ml[a]	SC	0.02 mg/ml[a]	Physically compatible for 4 hr at 25 °C	1155	C
Vancomycin HCl	LI	5 mg/ml[a]	SC	0.02 mg/ml[a]	Physically compatible for 4 hr at 25 °C	1155	C

[a]Tested in dextrose 5% in water.
[b]Tested in sodium chloride 0.9%.

PHENOBARBITAL SODIUM
AHFS 28:12.04 and 28:24.04

Products— Phenobarbital sodium injection is available in various dosage forms and sizes, including 30, 60, 65, and 130 mg/ml, from several manufacturers (4; 29).

Phenobarbital sodium (Wyeth-Ayerst) is available in 1-ml Tubex cartridge units in concentrations of 30, 60, and 130 mg/ml. Each milliliter also contains ethanol 10% and propylene glycol approximately 75%. When needed, pH may have been adjusted using hydrochloric acid (1-4/13/95).

Phenobarbital sodium (Elkins-Sinn) is available as 65- and 130-mg/ml solutions in 1-ml vials. Each milliliter of solution also contains alcohol 10%, benzyl alcohol 1.5%, and propylene glycol 67.8% in water for injection; hydrochloric acid may have been added to adjust the pH (1-6/93; 4).

pH— The USP cites the official pH range as 9.2 to 10.2 (17). The AHFS cites the pH range as being 8.5 to 10.5 (4).

Osmolality— The osmolality of phenobarbital sodium (Elkins-Sinn) 65 mg/ml was determined to be 15,570 mOsm/kg by freezing-point depression and 9285 mOsm/kg by vapor pressure (1071).

The osmolality of phenobarbital sodium 200 mg/ml was determined to be 10,800 mOsm/kg (1233).

The osmolality of phenobarbital sodium 100 mg was calculated for the following dilutions (1054):

	Osmolality (mOsm/kg)	
Diluent	50 ml	100 ml
Dextrose 5% in water	296	289
Sodium chloride 0.9%	325	317

Administration— Phenobarbital sodium is administered by intramuscular injection into a large muscle and slow intravenous injection. The commercial injection is highly alkaline and may cause local tissue damage (1-4/13/95; 1-6/93; 4). Intramuscular injection should be limited to 5 ml at any one site (1-6/93; 1-4/13/95). When given intravenously, the rate of injection should not exceed 60 mg/min (1-6/93; 1-4/13/95; 4).

Stability— Phenobarbital sodium injection in intact containers should be stored at controlled room temperature (1-4/13/95; 17).

Phenobarbital sodium is not generally considered stable in aqueous solutions (4). However, a test of phenobarbital sodium 10% (w/v) in aqueous solution showed 7% decomposition in four weeks when stored at 20 °C. There was no measurable decomposition in eight weeks with storage at −25 °C (233).

In addition, Nahata et al. studied the stability of phenobarbital sodium (Elkins-Sinn) diluted to a 10-mg/ml concentration in sodium chloride 0.9% for use in infants. When stored at 4 °C, the dilution was physically compatible with no loss of phenobarbital during the 28-day test period (1294).

Phenobarbital sodium in the special propylene glycol base is more stable (4).

Phenobarbital may be precipitated from solutions of phenobarbital sodium, depending on the concentration and pH (29):

Concentration	pH at which Precipitate Forms
3 mg/ml	7.5 or below
6 mg/ml	7.9 or below
10 mg/ml	8.3 or below
20 mg/ml	8.6 or below

No solution containing a precipitate or that is more than slightly discolored should be used (1-4/13/95; 1-6/93; 4).

Filtration— Phenobarbital sodium (Mallinckrodt) 130 mg/L in dextrose 5% in water, sodium chloride 0.9%, and Ringer's injection, lactated, filtered over 12 hours through a 5-μm stainless steel depth filter (Argyle Filter Connector), a 0.22-μm cellulose ester membrane filter (Ivex-2 Filter Set), and a 0.22-μm polycarbonate membrane filter (In-Sure Filter Set), showed no significant potency loss due to binding to the filters (320).

Compatibility Information

Solution Compatibility

Phenobarbital sodium

Solution	Mfr	Mfr	Conc/L	Remarks	Ref	C/I
Alcohol 5%, dextrose 5%	AB		320 mg	Color changes	3	**I**
Dextran 6% in dextrose 5%	AB		320 mg	Physically compatible	3	**C**
Dextran 6% in sodium chloride 0.9%	AB		320 mg	Physically compatible	3	**C**
Dextrose–Ringer's injection combinations	AB		320 mg	Physically compatible	3	**C**
Dextrose–Ringer's injection, lactated, combinations	AB		320 mg	Physically compatible	3	**C**
Dextrose–saline combinations	AB		320 mg	Physically compatible	3	**C**
Dextrose 2½% in water	AB		320 mg	Physically compatible	3	**C**
Dextrose 5% in water	AB		320 mg	Physically compatible	3	**C**
Dextrose 10% in water	AB		320 mg	Physically compatible	3	**C**
Fructose 10% in sodium chloride 0.9%	AB		320 mg	Physically compatible	3	**C**
Fructose 10% in water	AB		320 mg	Physically compatible	3	**C**
Invert sugar 5 and 10% in sodium chloride 0.9%	AB		320 mg	Physically compatible	3	**C**
Invert sugar 5 and 10% in water	AB		320 mg	Physically compatible	3	**C**
Ionosol products	AB		320 mg	Physically compatible	3	**C**
Ringer's injection	AB		320 mg	Physically compatible	3	**C**
Ringer's injection, lactated	AB		320 mg	Physically compatible	3	**C**
Sodium chloride 0.45%	AB		320 mg	Physically compatible	3	**C**
Sodium chloride 0.9%	AB		320 mg	Physically compatible	3	**C**
Sodium lactate ⅙ M	AB		320 mg	Physically compatible	3	**C**

Additive Compatibility

Phenobarbital sodium

Drug	Mfr	Conc/L	Mfr	Conc/L	Test Soln	Remarks	Ref	C/I
Amikacin sulfate	BR	5 g	LI	300 mg	D5LR, D5R, D5S, D5W, D10W, IS10, LR, NS, R, SL	Physically compatible and potency of both retained for 24 hr at 25 °C	294	**C**
Aminophylline	SE	500 mg	AB	100 mg		Physically compatible	6	**C**
	SE	1 g	WI	200 mg	D5W	Physically compatible	15	**C**
Calcium chloride	UP	1 g	WI	200 mg	D5W	Physically compatible	15	**C**
Calcium gluconate	UP	1 g	WI	200 mg	D5W	Physically compatible	15	**C**
Chlorpromazine HCl	BP	200 mg	BP	800 mg	D5W, NS	Immediate precipitation	26	**I**
Colistimethate sodium	WC	500 mg	WI	200 mg	D5W	Physically compatible	15	**C**
Dimenhydrinate	SE	500 mg	WI	200 mg	D5W	Physically compatible	15	**C**
Ephedrine HCl			WI			Physically incompatible	9	**I**
	LI	250 mg	WI	200 mg	D5W	Physically incompatible	15	**I**

Additive Compatibility (Cont.)

Phenobarbital sodium

Drug	Mfr	Conc/L	Mfr	Conc/L	Test Soln	Remarks	Ref	C/I
Hydralazine HCl	BP	80 mg	BP	800 mg	D5W	Yellow color and precipitate forms within 3 hr	26	I
Hydrocortisone sodium succinate			WI			Physically incompatible	9	I
	UP	500 mg	WI	200 mg	D5W	Physically incompatible	15	I
Hydroxyzine HCl	RR	250 mg	WI	200 mg	D5W	Physically incompatible	15	I
Insulin, regular[a]			WI			Physically incompatible	9	I
Levorphanol bitartrate	RC		WI			Physically incompatible	9	I
Meperidine HCl	WI		WI			Physically incompatible	9	I
Meropenem	ZEN	1 and 20 g	ES	200 mg	NS	Visually compatible for 4 hr at room temperature	1994	C
Morphine sulfate			WI			Physically incompatible	9	I
Norepinephrine bitartrate	WI		WI			Physically incompatible	9	I
Pentazocine lactate	WI	300 mg	WI	200 mg	D5W	Physically incompatible	15	I
Polymyxin B sulfate	BW	200 mg	WI	200 mg	D5W	Physically compatible	15	C
Procaine HCl			WI			Physically incompatible	9	I
Prochlorperazine mesylate	BP	100 mg	BP	800 mg	D5W	Haze develops over 3 hr	26	I
	BP	100 mg	BP	800 mg	NS	Immediate precipitation	26	I
Promazine HCl	BP	200 mg	BP	800 mg	NS	Immediate precipitation	26	I
Promethazine HCl	WY	250 mg	WI	200 mg	D5W	Physically incompatible	15	I
	BP	100 mg	BP	800 mg	D5W	Haze develops over 3 hr	26	I
	BP	100 mg	BP	800 mg	NS	Immediate precipitation	26	I
Sodium bicarbonate	AB	2.4 mEq[b]		320 mg	D5W	Physically compatible for 24 hr	772	C
Streptomycin sulfate			WI			Physically incompatible	9	I
Thiopental sodium	AB	2.5 g	AB	100 mg	D5W	Physically compatible	21	C
Vancomycin HCl	LI		WI			Physically incompatible	9	I
Verapamil HCl	KN	80 mg	ES	260 mg	D5W, NS	Physically compatible for 24 hr	764	C

[a]*Test performed prior to availability of neutral regular insulin.*
[b]*One vial of Neut added to a liter of admixture.*

Drugs in Syringe Compatibility

Phenobarbital sodium

Drug (in syringe)	Mfr	Amt	Mfr	Amt	Remarks	Ref	C/I
Heparin sodium		2500 units/ 1 ml		200 mg/ 1 ml	Physically compatible for at least 5 min	1053	C
Hydromorphone HCl	KN	2, 10, 40 mg/ 1 ml	AB	120 mg/ 1 ml	Precipitate forms immediately but dissipates with shaking. A white precipitate of phenobarbital re-forms after 6 hr at room temperature	2082	I
Ranitidine HCl	GL	50 mg/ 2 ml	AB	120 mg/ 1 ml	Immediate white haze	978	I
Sufentanil citrate	JN	50 μg/ml	WY	60 mg/ ml	Haze forms immediately and particles form in 24 hr at 23 °C	1711	I

Y-Site Injection Compatibility (1:1 Mixture)

Phenobarbital sodium

Drug	Mfr	Conc	Mfr	Conc	Remarks	Ref	C/I
Amphotericin B cholesteryl sulfate complex	SEQ	0.83 mg/ml[a]	WY	5 mg/ml[a]	Increased turbidity forms immediately	2117	I
Enalaprilat	MSD	1.25 mg/ml	WY	0.32 mg/ml[a,b]	Physically compatible for 4 hr at 21 °C under fluorescent light by microscopic and macroscopic examination	1409	C
Fosphenytoin sodium	PD	10 mg PE/ml[b,e]		130 mg/ml	Visually compatible wtih no loss of either drug by HPLC in 8 hr at room temperature	2212	C
Hydromorphone HCl	KN	2, 10, 40 mg/ml	AB	120 mg/ml	Turbidity forms immediately but dissipates; phenobarbital precipitate develops in 6 hr	1532	I
Meropenem	ZEN	1 and 50 mg/ml[b]	ES	0.32 mg/ml[c]	Visually compatible for 4 hr at room temperature	1994	C
Propofol	ZEN	10 mg/ml	WY	5 mg/ml[a]	Physically compatible for 1 hr at 23 °C with no increase in particle content	2066	C
Sufentanil citrate	JN	12.5 µg/ml[a]	WY	2 mg/ml[a]	Physically compatible with no subvisual haze or particle formation in 24 hr at 23 °C	1711	C
TNA #218 to #226[d]			WY	5 mg/ml[a]	Damage to emulsion integrity occurs immediately with free oil formation possible	2215	I
TPN #212 to #215[d]			WY	5 mg/ml[a]	Physically compatible with no change in measured turbidity or increase in particle content in 4 hr at 23 °C	2109	C

[a]Tested in dextrose 5% in water.
[b]Tested in sodium chloride 0.9%.
[c]Tested in sterile water for injection.
[d]Refer to Appendix I for the composition of parenteral nutrition solutions. TNA indicates a 3-in-1 admixture, and TPN indicates a 2-in-1 admixture.
[e]Concentration expressed in milligrams of phenytoin sodium equivalents (PE) per milliliter.

Additional Compatibility Information

Miscellaneous— Drugs stated to be incompatible with barbiturate salts include clindamycin phosphate (106), droperidol (4), pancuronium bromide (4), and cimetidine HCl (360).

Phenobarbital sodium should not be mixed in the same syringe with pentazocine lactate because precipitation occurs (4).

Heating plasma samples to 56 °C for one hour to inactivate potential HIV content resulted in no phenobarbital loss as determined by fluorescence polarization immunoassay (1615).

Acidic Additives— Drugs such as phenobarbital sodium that exhibit poor solubility in an acidic medium may precipitate in solutions containing acidic additives (4; 22). Metaraminol bitartrate is acidic and may cause precipitation, depending on the concentration of the additives (7). Also, the acidic methyldopate HCl imparts some buffer capacity to admixtures and may pose solubility problems with barbiturate salts (23).

Alkali-Labile Drugs— Phenobarbital sodium may raise the pH of admixture solutions to the alkaline range and, therefore, should not be mixed with alkali-labile drugs such as penicillin G (47). Signif-

icant decomposition of isoproterenol HCl and norepinephrine bitartrate may also occur. If either of these two drugs is mixed with phenobarbital sodium, the admixture should be used immediately after preparation (59; 77).

Atracurium besylate also may be inactivated by alkaline solutions such as barbiturates; precipitation of a free acid of the admixed drug may occur, depending on the resultant pH of the admixture (4).

Succinylcholine Chloride— When barbiturates are mixed with succinylcholine chloride, either the free barbiturate will precipitate or the succinylcholine chloride will be hydrolyzed, depending on the final pH of the admixture (4; 21).

Ephedrine— Titration of 50 ml of a 0.5 M aqueous solution of ephedrine HCl (BP) with 30.8 ml or more of a 0.5 M aqueous solution of phenobarbital sodium (BP) resulted in precipitation of an ephedrine–phenobarbital complex. The point at which precipitation began corresponded to the point at which the pH of the ephedrine HCl solution had been increased from its initial pH 7 to 8.5. Further addition of phenobarbital sodium resulted in additional precipitation but did not alter the pH (322).

Concentrated Solutions— The following incompatibility determinations were performed with concentrated solutions. The drugs in dry form were constituted according to manufacturer's recommendations. One milliliter of phenobarbital sodium (Winthrop) was added to 5 ml of sterile distilled water along with 1 ml of each of the following drugs. Particulate matter was noted within two hours (28):

Dimenhydrinate (Searle)
Diphenhydramine HCl (Parke-Davis)
Hydroxyzine HCl (Pfizer)
Kanamycin sulfate (Bristol)

Phenytoin sodium (Parke-Davis)
Prochlorperazine edisylate (SKF)
Promazine HCl (Wyeth)
Promethazine HCl (Wyeth)

Plasticizer Leaching— Phenobarbital sodium (Wyeth-Ayerst) 6 mg/ml in dextrose 5% in water did not leach diethylhexyl phthalate (DEHP) plasticizer from 50-ml PVC bags in 24 hours at 24 °C (1683).

PHENTOLAMINE MESYLATE
AHFS 12:16

Regitine   **Novartis**

Products— Phentolamine mesylate (Novartis) is available in vials containing 5 mg of drug with 25 mg of mannitol. Reconstitution with 1 ml of sterile water for injection results in a 5-mg/ml solution (2; 4).

pH— From 4.5 to 6.5 (4).

Osmolality— Phentolamine mesylate 5 mg/ml has an osmolality of 169 mOsm/kg (1689).

Administration— Phentolamine mesylate may be administered by intramuscular or intravenous injection (2; 4).

Stability— The intact vials should be stored at controlled room temperature (2; 4). Although the manufacturer recommends that reconstituted solutions be used immediately and not stored (2), other information indicates that such solutions are stable for 48 hours at room temperature and one week at 2 to 8 °C (4).

Sorption— Phentolamine mesylate (Novartis) 18 mg/L in sodium chloride 0.9% (Travenol) in PVC bags did not exhibit significant sorption to the plastic during one week of storage at room temperature (15 to 20 °C) (536).

In another study, phentolamine mesylate (Novartis) 18 mg/L in sodium chloride 0.9% did not exhibit any loss due to sorption during a seven-hour simulated infusion through an infusion set (Travenol) consisting of a cellulose propionate burette chamber and 170 cm of PVC tubing (606).

The drug was also tested as a simulated infusion over at least one hour by a syringe pump system. A glass syringe on a syringe pump was fitted with 20 cm of polyethylene tubing or 50 cm of Silastic tubing. No loss of drug due to sorption was observed with either tubing (606).

A 25-ml aliquot of phentolamine mesylate (Novartis) 18 mg/L in sodium chloride 0.9% was stored in all-plastic syringes composed of polypropylene barrels and polyethylene plungers for 24 hours at room temperature in the dark. No loss due to sorption occurred (606).

Compatibility Information

Additive Compatibility

Phentolamine mesylate

Drug	Mfr	Conc/L	Mfr	Conc/L	Test Soln	Remarks	Ref	C/I
Cibenzoline succinate		2 g	CI	40 mg	D5W, NS	Physically compatible for 24 hr at 25 °C by visual and microscopic examination	1182	C
Dobutamine HCl	LI	1 g	CI	20 mg	D5W, NS	Physically compatible for 24 hr at 21 °C	812	C
Verapamil HCl	KN	80 mg	CI	10 mg	D5W, NS	Physically compatible for 24 hr	764	C

Drugs in Syringe Compatibility

Phentolamine mesylate

Drug (in syringe)	Mfr	Amt	Mfr	Amt	Remarks	Ref	C/I
Papaverine HCl	LI	30 mg/ml	BV, CI	0.5 mg/ml[a]	Physically compatible with virtually no papaverine loss at 5 and 25 °C and 1 to 3% phentolamine loss at 5 °C and 4 to 5% loss at 25 °C in 30 days	1161	C

[a]Constituted with the papaverine HCl injection.

Y-Site Injection Compatibility (1:1 Mixture)

Phentolamine mesylate

Drug	Mfr	Conc	Mfr	Conc	Remarks	Ref	C/I
Amiodarone HCl	LZ	4 mg/ml[a]	CI	0.04 mg/ml[a]	Physically compatible for 24 hr at 21 °C under fluorescent light	1032	C

[a]*Tested in both dextrose 5% in water and sodium chloride 0.9%.*

Additional Compatibility Information

Sodium chloride 0.9% has been recommended for the dilution of phentolamine mesylate (2; 4).

The admixture of 10 mg/L of phentolamine mesylate with norepinephrine has been stated to not affect the pressor ability of norepinephrine (2; 4).

PHENYLEPHRINE HCL
AHFS 12:12

Products— Phenylephrine HCl is available as a 1% solution in 1-ml ampuls and 1- and 5-ml vials (154). Each milliliter of solution contains (2):

Phenylephrine HCl	10 mg
Sodium chloride	3.5 mg
Sodium citrate dihydrate	4.56 mg
Citric acid monohydrate	1 mg
Sodium metabisulfite	not more than 2 mg

Sodium hydroxide and/or hydrochloric acid may have been added during manufacture to adjust pH (2).

pH— From 3 to 6.5 (2; 4).

Osmolality— Phenylephrine HCl 10 mg/ml has an osmolality of 284 mOsm/kg (1689).

Administration— Phenylephrine HCl is administered by subcutaneous, intramuscular, or direct slow intravenous injection or by intravenous infusion. For direct intravenous injection, a 0.1% solution (1 mg/ml) may be prepared by diluting 1 ml of phenylephrine HCl with 9 ml of sterile water for injection. Solutions for intravenous infusion are usually prepared by adding 10 mg of drug to 500 ml of dextrose 5% in water or sodium chloride 0.9% (2; 4).

Stability— Intact containers of phenylephrine HCl should be stored at controlled room temperature and protected from light (2; 4). Solutions of the drug must not be used if they are brown or contain a precipitate. However, oxidation may occur, resulting in loss of activity even though no color change is evident (4).

Phenylephrine HCl (Winthrop) was stable for up to 84 days at 60 °C in a 250-mg/100 ml concentration in sterile water for injection (132). At pH 2, no loss of potency occurred in 10 days at 97 °C. A rise in pH, especially above 9, increased decomposition (29).

Phenylephrine HCl in dextrose 5% in water is stated to be stable for at least 48 hours at pH 3.5 to 7.5 (4).

Compatibility Information

Solution Compatibility

Phenylephrine HCl

Solution	Mfr	Mfr	Conc/L	Remarks	Ref	C/I
Dextran 6% in dextrose 5%	AB	WI	1 mg	Physically compatible	3	C
Dextran 6% in sodium chloride 0.9%	AB	WI	1 mg	Physically compatible	3	C
Dextrose–Ringer's injection combinations	AB	WI	1 mg	Physically compatible	3	C
Dextrose–Ringer's injection, lactated, combinations	AB	WI	1 mg	Physically compatible	3	C
Dextrose–saline combinations	AB	WI	1 mg	Physically compatible	3	C
Dextrose 2½% in water	AB	WI	1 mg	Physically compatible	3	C
Dextrose 5% in water	AB	WI	1 mg	Physically compatible	3	C

Solution Compatibility (Cont.)

Phenylephrine HCl

Solution	Mfr	Mfr	Conc/L	Remarks	Ref	C/I
Dextrose 10% in water	AB	WI	1 mg	Physically compatible	3	C
Fructose 10% in sodium chloride 0.9%	AB	WI	1 mg	Physically compatible	3	C
Fructose 10% in water	AB	WI	1 mg	Physically compatible	3	C
Invert sugar 5 and 10% in sodium chloride 0.9%	AB	WI	1 mg	Physically compatible	3	C
Invert sugar 5 and 10% in water	AB	WI	1 mg	Physically compatible	3	C
Ionosol products	AB	WI	1 mg	Physically compatible	3	C
Ringer's injection	AB	WI	1 mg	Physically compatible	3	C
Ringer's injection, lactated	AB	WI	1 mg	Physically compatible	3	C
Sodium bicarbonate 5%		WI	20 mg	Potency retained for 24 hr at 25 °C	48	C
Sodium chloride 0.45%	AB	WI	1 mg	Physically compatible	3	C
Sodium chloride 0.9%		WI	2.5 g	Potency retained for 24 hr at 22 °C	132	C
	AB	WI	1 mg	Physically compatible	3	C
Sodium lactate ⅙ M	AB	WI	1 mg	Physically compatible	3	C

Additive Compatibility

Phenylephrine HCl

Drug	Mfr	Conc/L	Mfr	Conc/L	Test Soln	Remarks	Ref	C/I
Chloramphenicol sodium succinate	PD	500 mg	WI	2.5 g	D5W, NS	Phenylephrine potency retained for over 24 hr at 22 °C	132	C
Chloramphenicol sodium succinate with sodium bicarbonate	PD AB	500 mg 7.5 g	WI	2.5 g	D5W	Phenylephrine potency retained for over 24 hr at 22 °C	132	C
Cibenzoline succinate		2 g	WB	40 mg	D5W, NS	Physically compatible for 24 hr at 25 °C by visual and microscopic examination	1182	C
Dobutamine HCl	LI	1 g	WI	20 mg	D5W, NS	Physically compatible for 24 hr at 21 °C	812	C
Lidocaine HCl	AST	2 g	WI	20 mg		Physically compatible	24	C
Potassium chloride	AB	40 mEq	WI	2.5 g	D5W	Phenylephrine potency retained for over 24 hr at 22 °C	132	C
Sodium bicarbonate	AB	2.4 mEq[a]	WI	10 mg	D5W	Physically compatible for 24 hr	772	C
Sodium bicarbonate with chloramphenicol sodium succinate	AB PD	7.5 g 500 mg	WI	2.5 g	D5W	Phenylephrine potency retained for over 24 hr at 22 °C	132	C

[a]One vial of Neut added to a liter of admixture.

Y-Site Injection Compatibility (1:1 Mixture)

Phenylephrine HCl

Drug	Mfr	Conc	Mfr	Conc	Remarks	Ref	C/I
Amiodarone HCl	LZ	4 mg/ml[a,b]	WI	0.04 mg/ml[a,b]	Physically compatible for 24 hr at 21 °C	1032	C
Amrinone lactate	WB	3 mg/ml[b]	WI	0.02 mg/ml[a]	Physically compatible for at least 4 hr at 25 °C under fluorescent light	992	C

Y-Site Injection Compatibility (1:1 Mixture) (Cont.)

Phenylephrine HCl

Drug	Mfr	Conc	Mfr	Conc	Remarks	Ref	C/I
Cisatracurium besylate	GW	0.1, 2, 5 mg/ml[a]	GNS	1 mg/ml[a]	Physically compatible with no change in measured turbidity or increase in particle content in 4 hr at 23 °C	2074	C
Etomidate	AB	2 mg/ml	ES	10 mg/ml	Visually compatible for up to 7 days at 25 °C	1801	C
Famotidine	MSD	0.2 mg/ml[a]	WI	0.02 mg/ml[a]	Physically compatible for 4 hr at 25 °C	1188	C
Haloperidol lactate	MN	0.5[a] and 5 mg/ml	WB	0.02 mg/ml[a]	Visually compatible for 24 hr at 21 °C	1523	C
Propofol	STU	2 mg/ml	ES	10 mg/ml	Bright yellow discoloration forms within 7 days at 25 °C. No visible change in 24 hr	1801	?
	ZEN	10 mg/ml	ES	0.1 mg/ml[a]	Physically compatible for 1 hr at 23 °C with no increase in particle content	2066	C
Remifentanil HCl	GW	0.025 and 0.25 mg/ml[b]	AMR	1 mg/ml[a]	Physically compatible with no change in measured turbidity or increase in particle content in 4 hr at 23 °C	2075	C
Thiopental sodium	AB	25 mg/ml	ES	10 mg/ml	White precipitate forms immediately	1801	I
Zidovudine	BW	4 mg/ml[a]	WI	1 mg/ml[a]	Physically compatible for 4 hr at 25 °C under fluorescent light by visual and microscopic examination	1193	C

[a]*Tested in dextrose 5% in water.*
[b]*Tested in sodium chloride 0.9%.*

Additional Compatibility Information

Dextrose 5% in water and sodium chloride 0.9% have been recommended as diluents for infusion solutions. Phenylephrine HCl may be added to anesthetics for local or spinal anesthesia (2; 4).

Phenylephrine HCl has been stated to be incompatible with alkalies, ferric salts, and other metals (4).

The following incompatibility determination was performed with concentrated solutions. One milliliter of phenylephrine HCl (Winthrop) was added to 5 ml of sterile distilled water along with 1 ml of phenytoin sodium (Parke-Davis). Particulate matter was noted within two hours (28).

Lidocaine— Lidocaine HCl 2% in combination with phenylephrine HCl 0.25% was stable for at least 66 days at 25 °C. No loss of either drug was found by HPLC analysis, and little change in pH occurred during the test period (1278).

PHENYTOIN SODIUM
AHFS 28:12.12

Elkins-Sinn

Products— Phenytoin sodium (Elkins-Sinn) is available as a ready-mixed solution in 100-mg (2 ml) vials and ampuls and 250-mg (5 ml) vials. Each milliliter of solution contains (1-9/98):

Phenytoin sodium	50 mg
Propylene glycol	40%
Alcohol	10%
Sodium hydroxide	to adjust pH
Water for injection	qs

CAUTION: Care should be taken to avoid confusion between phenytoin sodium and fosphenytoin sodium to prevent dosing errors.

pH— From 10 to 12.3 (1-9/98; 17). The pH is adjusted to about 12 during manufacture (4).

The apparent pH of multiple lots of phenytoin sodium from several manufacturers was evaluated. The lower apparent pH of some products may play a role in microcrystal formation on dilution (1514):

Manufacturer	Apparent pH
Elkins-Sinn	11.39 ± 0.21
Lyphomed	11.68 ± 0.36
Parke-Davis	12.00 ± 0.06
SoloPak	11.38 ± 0.33

Osmolality— The osmolality of phenytoin sodium (Parke-Davis) 50 mg/ml was determined to be 9740 mOsm/kg by freezing-point depression and 6175 mOsm/kg by vapor pressure (1071).

Another report indicated that the osmolality of phenytoin sodium 50 mg/ml was 3035 mOsm/kg by freezing-point depression (1233).

The osmolality of phenytoin sodium 500 mg was calculated for the following dilutions (1054):

Diluent	Osmolality (mOsm/kg)	
	50 ml	100 ml
Sodium chloride 0.9%	336	312

Sodium Content— Each milliliter of phenytoin sodium injection contains 0.2 mEq of sodium (4).

Administration— Phenytoin sodium is preferably administered by direct intravenous injection into a large vein through a large-gauge needle or intravenous catheter. Although intramuscular injection can be used, erratic or delayed absorption may occur. Subcutaneous injection should be avoided because of the possibility of local tissue damage (1-9/98; 4). The rate of intravenous injection should not exceed 50 mg/min in adults or 1 to 3 mg/kg/min in neonates. Following intravenous injection, sodium chloride 0.9% should be injected through the same needle or catheter to reduce irritation (1-9/98; 4).

Because of the drug's low solubility and possible precipitation (1-9/98; 4), intravenous infusion is usually not recommended. How-ever, some clinicians have suggested that intravenous infusion is reasonable in an appropriately diluted, compatible infusion solution for short periods using inline filtration; they have advocated infusion to circumvent the adverse effects associated with direct intravenous injection. (See Additional Compatibility Information.)

Stability— Intact containers should be stored at controlled room temperature and protected from freezing. Phenytoin sodium is stable as long as it remains free of haziness and precipitation. If refrigerated or frozen, a precipitate may form, but it dissolves on standing at room temperature. On dissolution of the precipitate, the product is still suitable for use. Also, a faint yellow color, which has no effect on potency, may sometimes develop in the injection (1-9/98; 4).

Precipitation of free phenytoin occurs at pH 11.5 or less (4).

Sorption— Phenytoin sodium (Sigma) 114 mg/L in sodium chloride 0.9% (Travenol) in PVC bags did not exhibit significant sorption to the plastic during one week of storage at room temperature (15 to 20 °C) (536).

In another study, phenytoin sodium (Sigma) 114 mg/L in sodium chloride 0.9% did not exhibit any loss due to sorption during a seven-hour simulated infusion through an infusion set (Travenol) consisting of a cellulose propionate burette chamber and 170 cm of PVC tubing (606).

The drug was also tested as a simulated infusion over at least one hour by a syringe pump system. A glass syringe on a syringe pump was fitted with 20 cm of polyethylene tubing or 50 cm of Silastic tubing. No loss of drug due to sorption was observed with either tubing (606).

A 25-ml aliquot of phenytoin sodium (Sigma) 114 mg/L in sodium chloride 0.9% was stored in all-plastic syringes composed of polypropylene barrels and polyethylene plungers for 24 hours at room temperature in the dark. No loss due to sorption occurred (606).

Filtration— Phenytoin sodium (Parke-Davis) 250 mg/5 ml in a 5-ml syringe was filtered at a rate of 1 ml/min through a 5-μm stainless steel depth filter (Argyle Filter Connector). No significant reduction in potency due to binding to the filter was observed (320).

Compatibility Information

Solution Compatibility

Phenytoin sodium

Solution	Mfr	Mfr	Conc/L	Remarks	Ref	C/I
Dextrose 5% in sodium chloride 0.9%	TR	PD	1 g	Visible crystals in minutes. 21% crystallized in 8 hr and 38% in 24 hr	306	I
Dextrose 5% in water	TR	PD	1 g	Visible crystals in minutes. 15% crystallized in 8 hr and 36% in 24 hr	306	I
	TR	PD	4.6, 9.2, 18.4 g	Phenytoin crystal formation. Erratic concentrations delivered through 0.2-μm filter over 24 hr at 29 °C	305	I
	MG	PD	1 g	No visible precipitate or reduction in phenytoin in 8 hr at room temperature. Precipitate forms within 24 hr with 15% loss of phenytoin	446	I
	TR	PD	1 g	Substantial crystal formation in 1 hr found upon filtration	450; 451	I
	AB	PD	1 g	Visible crystals in less than 12 min. 18% loss of phenytoin in 14 hr and 22% in 24 hr	452	I

Solution Compatibility (Cont.)

Phenytoin sodium

Solution	Mfr	Mfr	Conc/L	Remarks	Ref	C/I
			1 g	10% of phenytoin removed by filtration in 2 hr and 15 to 18% in 4 hr	453	**I**
		PD	670 mg to 4 g	Phenytoin crystals within 5 to 25 min. Reduced phenytoin concentration	708	**I**
	AB, CU, MG, TR	ES, PD	0.4 to 4.55 g	Visible precipitate forms within 10 to 60 min with significant reduction in phenytoin concentration in 20 to 45 min	710	**I**
	TR	PD	1, 1.5, 2, 4, 10 g	Visible crystals in 30 min. 12 to 20% crystallized in 4 hr	951	**I**
Fat emulsion 10%, intravenous	VT	PD	1 g	Phenytoin crystal formation	32	**I**
Ringer's injection, lactated	TR	PD	4.6, 9.2, 18.4 g	Phenytoin crystal formation. Erratic concentration delivered through 0.2-μm filter over 24 hr at 29 °C	305	**I**
	TR	PD	1 g	Visible crystals in 6 to 9 hr. Approximately 0.8% crystallized in 8 hr and 7% in 24 hr	306	**I**
	TR	ES, PD	0.4 to 4.55 g	No significant reduction in phenytoin concentration for 12 to 24 hr at 23 °C. Visible precipitate inconsistently formed	710	**I**
Sodium chloride 0.45%	TR	PD	4.6, 9.2, 18.4 g	Phenytoin crystal formation. Less than 10% phenytoin reduction delivered through 0.2-μm filter over 24 hr at 29 °C	305	**I**
Sodium chloride 0.9%		PD	1 to 10 g	Phenytoin crystal formation in 20 to 30 min	63	**I**
		PD	200 mg to 10 g	Phenytoin crystal formation in 30 min	65;447	**I**
		PD	2 and 4 g	Phenytoin crystal formation in 10 to 15 min	66	**I**
	TR	PD	1 g	Visible crystals in 6 to 9 hr. Approximately 0.8% crystallized in 8 hr and 7% in 24 hr	306	**I**
	TR	PD	4.6, 9.2, 18.4 g	Phenytoin crystal formation. Less than 10% phenytoin reduction delivered through 0.2-μm filter over 24 hr at 29 °C	305	**I**
	TR	PD	100 mg	No visible precipitation in approximately 24 hr	449	**C**
			1 g	10% of phenytoin removed by filtration in 4 hr	453	**I**
		PD	670 mg to 4 g	No crystals observed during 1-hr study period	708	**C**
	TR	PD	1 to 10 g	Crystals formed in unfiltered solutions in 18 hr. Filtered solutions stored at 6 °C had no crystals and no reduction in phenytoin in 24 hr	709	**I**
	TR	ES, PD	0.4 to 4.55 g	No significant reduction in phenytoin for 8 to 24 hr at 23 °C. Visible precipitate inconsistently formed	710	**I**
	TR	PD	1, 1.5, 2, 4, 10 g	Physically compatible for 24 hr	951	**C**
	TR	PD	9.2 and 18.4 g	Physically compatible for 2 hr by microscopic and macroscopic examination. Filtration did not significantly reduce phenytoin concentration	1514	**C**
	TR	ES, LY, SO	9.2 and 18.4 g	Microcrystals formed repeatedly, but inconsistently, over 2 hr. Filtration did not significantly reduce phenytoin concentration	1514	**?**

Additive Compatibility

Phenytoin sodium

Drug	Mfr	Conc/L	Mfr	Conc/L	Test Soln	Remarks	Ref	C/I
Amikacin sulfate	BR	5 g	PD	250 mg	D5LR, D5R, D5S, D5W, D10W, IS10, LR, NS, R, SL	Immediate precipitation	294	I
Bleomycin sulfate	BR	20 and 30 units	PD	500 mg	NS	Physically compatible and bleomycin activity retained for 1 week at 4 °C. Phenytoin not tested	763	C
Bretylium tosylate	ACC	1 g	PD	2 g	D5W, NS	Immediate precipitation	756	I
Dobutamine HCl	LI	1 g	ES	1 g	D5W, NS	White precipitate forms within 5 to 10 min	789	I
	LI	1 g	AHP	25 g	D5W, NS	White precipitate forms rapidly, with brown solution in 6 hr at 21 °C	812	I
Insulin, regular[a]			PD			Physically incompatible	9	I
Levorphanol bitartrate	RC		PD			Physically incompatible	9	I
Lidocaine HCl	AST	2 g	ES	1 g	D5W, LR, NS	Immediate formation of white cloudy precipitate	775	I
Lincomycin HCl	UP		PD			Physically incompatible	9	I
Meperidine HCl	WI		PD			Physically incompatible	9	I
Metaraminol bitartrate	MSD		PD			Physically incompatible	9	I
Morphine sulfate			PD			Physically incompatible	9	I
Nitroglycerin	ACC	400 mg	PD	1 g	D5W, NS[b]	Phenytoin crystal formation in 24 hr. 3 to 4% nitroglycerin loss in 24 hr and 9% loss in 48 hr at 23 °C. Phenytoin not tested	929	I
Norepinephrine bitartrate	WI		PD			Physically incompatible	9	I
Pentobarbital sodium			PD			Physically incompatible	9	I
Procaine HCl			PD			Physically incompatible	9	I
Sodium bicarbonate	AB	2.4 mEq[c]	PD	250 mg	D5W	Physically compatible for 24 hr	772	C
Streptomycin sulfate			PD			Physically incompatible	9	I
Verapamil HCl	KN	80 mg	PD	500 mg	D5W, NS	Physically compatible for 48 hr	739	C

[a]*Test performed prior to availability of neutral regular insulin.*
[b]*Tested in glass containers.*
[c]*One vial of Neut added to a liter of admixture.*

Drugs in Syringe Compatibility

Phenytoin sodium

Drug (in syringe)	Mfr	Amt	Mfr	Amt	Remarks	Ref	C/I
Hydromorphone HCl	KN	2, 10, 40 mg/1 ml	AB	50 mg/1 ml	White precipitate of phenytoin forms immediately	2082	I
Sufentanil citrate	JN	50 μg/ml	SO	50 mg/ml	Small crystals form immediately. Large crystals settle to bottom in 24 hr at 23 °C	1711	I

Y-Site Injection Compatibility (1:1 Mixture)

Phenytoin sodium

Drug	Mfr	Conc	Mfr	Conc	Remarks	Ref	C/I
Amphotericin B cholesteryl sulfate complex	SEQ	0.83 mg/ml[a]	ES	50 mg/ml[a]	Gross precipitate forms	2117	I
Ciprofloxacin	MI	2 mg/ml[c]	PD	50 mg/ml	Immediate crystal formation	1655	I
Clarithromycin	AB	4 mg/ml[a]	ANT	20 mg/ml[a]	White cloudiness forms immediately, becoming a white precipitate in 1 hr at both 30 and 17 °C	2174	I
Diltiazem HCl	MMD	1 mg/ml[b]	PD	50 mg/ml	Precipitate forms	1807	I
Enalaprilat	MSD	1.25 mg/ml	PD	1 mg/ml[b]	Crystalline precipitate forms immediately	1409	I
Esmolol HCl	DCC	10 mg/ml[a]	IX	1 mg/ml[a]	Physically compatible for 24 hr at 22 °C	1169	C
Famotidine	MSD	0.2 mg/ml[a]	PD	50 mg/ml	Physically compatible for 14 hr	1196	C
Fluconazole	RR	2 mg/ml	PD	50 mg/ml	Physically compatible for 24 hr at 25 °C	1407	C
Foscarnet sodium	AST	24 mg/ml	PD	50 mg/ml	Physically compatible for 24 hr at room temperature under fluorescent light	1335	C
Heparin sodium	TR	50 units/ml	ES	2 mg/ml[b]	Cloudiness forms immediately and becomes dense, white, flocculent precipitate in 6 hr at 25 °C	1793	I
Heparin sodium with hydrocortisone sodium succinate	RI UP	1000 units + 100 mg/L[d]	PD	50 mg/ml	Immediate formation of phenytoin crystals	322	I
Hydromorphone HCl	KN	2, 10, 40 mg/ml	AB	50 mg/ml	Turbidity forms immediately and phenytoin precipitate develops	1532	I
Potassium chloride		40 mEq/L[a]	PD	50 mg/ml	Immediate formation of phenytoin crystals	322	I
		40 mEq/L[e]	PD	50 mg/ml	Phenytoin crystals form within 4 hr at room temperature	322	I
Propofol	ZEN	10 mg/ml	ES	50 mg/ml	Needle-like crystals form immediately	2066	I
Sufentanil citrate	JN	12.5 μg/ml[a]	ES	2 mg/ml[a]	Numerous tiny crystals form immediately and become larger over 24 hr at 23 °C under fluorescent light	1711	I
Tacrolimus	FUJ	1 mg/ml[b]	ES	5 mg/ml[a]	Visually compatible for 4 hr at 25 °C. White haze forms by 24 hr	1630	C
Theophylline	TR	4 mg/ml	ES	2 mg/ml[b]	Cloudiness forms immediately and becomes dense, flocculent precipitate in 6 hr at 25 °C	1793	I
TPN #189[f]			PD	50 mg/ml	Heavy white precipitate forms immediately	1767	I
Vitamin B complex with C	RC	2 ml/L[g]	PD	50 mg/ml	Phenytoin crystals form within 4 hr at room temperature	322	I
	RC	2 ml/L[c]	PD	50 mg/ml	Immediate formation of phenytoin crystals	322	I

[a]Tested in dextrose 5% in water.
[b]Tested in sodium chloride 0.9%.
[c]Tested in both dextrose 5% in water and sodium chloride 0.9%.
[d]Tested in dextrose 5% in water, Ringer's injection, lactated, and sodium chloride 0.9%.
[e]Tested in both Ringer's injection, lactated, and sodium chloride 0.9%.
[f]Refer to Appendix I for the composition of parenteral nutrition solutions. TPN indicates a 2-in-1 admixture.
[g]Tested in Ringer's injection, lactated.

Additional Compatibility Information

Clindamycin phosphate (Upjohn) (2p2462) has been stated to be physically incompatible with phenytoin sodium.

Solutions— The mixing of phenytoin sodium with other drugs or with intravenous infusion solutions is not recommended (1-9/98; 4) because the solubility of phenytoin sodium is such that crystallization or precipitation may result if the special vehicle is altered or the pH is lowered (62; 63; 613). Unfortunately, direct intravenous injection of phenytoin sodium is inconvenient and is occasionally associated with significant cardiovascular side effects (1-9/98; 4). In spite of the caveat against dilution, some clinicians have advocated the infusion of phenytoin sodium (443; 444; 448; 611; 947–950; 1295) or administration into the tubing of a running infusion solution (63; 65; 338; 445).

Reports of phenytoin crystallization in infusion solutions are numerous. Tobias and Kellick microscopically examined solutions composed of 10 mg of phenytoin sodium in 1 to 50 ml of sodium chloride 0.9% 30 minutes after mixing. They found rod-shaped crystals in all concentrations. They did not find crystals when phenytoin was injected into a running sodium chloride 0.9% infusion (65). Frank repeated the experiment and confirmed the results (447). However, a more recent study pointed out that this crystallization may have occurred from evaporation and the consequent increase in concentration of free phenytoin (306).

Chan noted that the addition of 100 mg of phenytoin sodium to 25 to 50 ml of sodium chloride 0.9% resulted in immediate microcrystal formation with subsequent visually apparent macrocrystal formation in 10 to 15 minutes (66).

In contrast, Bighley et al. added phenytoin sodium 100 mg/L to sodium chloride 0.9% in PVC bags and, by visual observation, did not detect any precipitate formation (449).

Furthermore, Greenblatt and Shader added 500 mg of phenytoin sodium (Parke-Davis) to 490 ml of dextrose 5% in water and, by visual inspection, found no precipitation for at least eight hours at room temperature. Analysis of the solution showed the phenytoin concentration to be 105% of the predicted concentration. They did note a fine crystalline precipitate after 24 hours. Also, the concentration had declined to 85% at that time (446).

Using this same 500-mg/500 ml in dextrose 5% in water admixture, both Schondelmeyer et al. (450) and Baumann et al. (451) found substantial crystal formation in one hour by filtering the solution through 0.45- and 0.22-μm filters, respectively. Crystals could be detected in as little as five minutes, and the quantity increased with time.

More recent studies examined the problem in depth. Baumann et al. (306) evaluated phenytoin sodium at a concentration of 1 g/L in dextrose 5% in water, sodium chloride 0.9%, dextrose 5% in sodium chloride 0.9%, and Ringer's injection, lactated. At various time intervals, samples were withdrawn and filtered through a 0.22-μm filter. The filtrate was then analyzed for phenytoin content. In both sodium chloride 0.9% and Ringer's injection, lactated, there was no detected crystallization in four hours and only 0.8% crystallization in eight hours. Visible crystal formation did not occur until six to nine hours after admixture. In contrast, the dextrose solutions had 5 to 9% and 15 to 21% crystallization in one and eight hours, respectively. Visible crystals were observed within minutes. The authors suggested that, at a concentration of 1 mg/ml, the critical pH for

aqueous solubility of phenytoin is 10. It would, therefore, be expected that phenytoin solubility would increase as this pH is approached. Their results were consistent with the pH values of the four admixtures:

Solution	pH of Phenytoin Sodium 1 mg/ml
Ringer's injection, lactated	10.4
Sodium chloride 0.9%	10.0
Dextrose 5% in water	9.3
Dextrose 5% in sodium chloride 0.9%	9.3

It was noted that the pH of infusion solutions may vary (as may the pH of the drug) (452), and it is not possible to predict the final pH of the admixture accurately. The authors concluded that intravenous infusion of phenytoin sodium was feasible at a concentration of 1 mg/ml in sodium chloride 0.9% or Ringer's injection, lactated, provided the administration of the solutions was started immediately after preparation and watched carefully (306).

Subsequent studies, performed by Sistare and Greene (452) and Biberdorf and Spurbeck (453), tended to corroborate this result.

Cloyd et al. also studied phenytoin sodium in infusion solutions but in higher concentrations. The concentrations tested were 4.6, 9.2, and 18.4 mg/ml in sodium chloride 0.45 and 0.9%, dextrose 5% in water, and Ringer's injection, lactated. The test was conducted over 24 hours at 29 °C, and the pH values of all solutions were between 10.15 and 11.50. Crystallization was observed in all admixtures but was not sufficient to permit precise quantitation. Analysis of the admixtures yielded rather erratic results, but it was felt that phenytoin sodium retained sufficient potency for 24 hours in both sodium chloride solutions. The extent of crystallization was not believed to be large enough to reduce significantly the phenytoin concentration when an inline filter was used (305).

Carmichael et al. diluted phenytoin sodium 100 mg in 25, 50, 100, and 150 ml of dextrose 5% in water and sodium chloride 0.9%. The dextrose admixtures were noted to have consistently lower pH values than those in sodium chloride. Further, as the volume of diluent increased, the pH decreased. In the dextrose 5% in water admixtures, visible crystals were observed within five to 25 minutes. In sodium chloride 0.9%, no crystals were visually apparent within the one-hour study period. During simulated infusion of a 100-mg/50 ml solution in dextrose 5% in water or sodium chloride 0.9% through a burette administration set, a reduced concentration of phenytoin sodium was delivered in the dextrose solution, but no significant reduction occurred in the sodium chloride solution. The use of a 1-μm inline filter had no significant effect on the delivered concentrations. The authors concluded that dextrose 5% in water was an unacceptable diluent for phenytoin sodium infusion. However, they indicated that sodium chloride 0.9% could be acceptable as a diluent if the phenytoin sodium concentration was no less than 100 mg/100 ml and, preferably, at 100 mg/25 or 50 ml. Moreover, such solutions should be prepared immediately before use and infused within one hour, and an inline filter should be used because of the possibility of microcrystal formation (708).

Salem et al. evaluated the compatibility of phenytoin sodium at concentrations of 1, 2.5, 5, 7.5, and 10 mg/ml in sodium chloride 0.9% over 24 hours at 6 °C. At the one-hour interval in all concentrations, a small increase in concentration was observed and attributed to supersaturation. But at eight through 24 hours, the phenytoin concentrations had returned to expected values and remained consistent. Observation of additional 1- and 10-mg/ml concentrations for the Tyndall effect demonstrated light scattering, which the authors indicated would suggest a colloidal dispersion rather than a true solution. Also crystals formed in those solutions within 18 hours. However, unlike the initial test solutions, these latter two solutions were unfiltered. In filtered solutions, crystal formation took up to three days to occur, which the authors indicated explained why no crystals appeared in the original dilutions in 24 hours. It was noted that while the time to crystal formation may be variable and difficult to predict, it was nonetheless inevitable. The authors recommended using phenytoin sodium infusions as soon as possible after preparation, observing closely for particulate matter, and avoiding conditions that would enhance precipitation such as refrigeration (709).

Phenytoin sodium concentrations of 0.40, 0.98, 2.38, and 4.55 mg/ml in dextrose 5% in water, sodium chloride 0.9%, and Ringer's injection, lactated, were evaluated by Pfeifle et al. Concentrations of the drug in sodium chloride 0.9% or Ringer's injection, lactated, did not significantly vary from the initial amount for at least eight hours and usually for 12 to 24 hours at 23 °C. In dextrose 5% in water, however, significant reductions in concentration appeared in as little as 20 minutes. Further, visible precipitation occurred within 10 minutes at all concentrations in dextrose 5% in water, except 0.4 mg/ml in which 15 to 60 minutes elapsed before crystallization occurred. With phenytoin sodium from Elkins-Sinn, the precipitate flocculated and sank or floated; the Parke-Davis product produced a precipitate that remained suspended. In sodium chloride 0.9% and Ringer's injection, lactated, visible precipitation was not consistently observed. However, nephelometer determinations indicated that some particulate matter was present in all admixtures. Although not precisely predictable, the authors concluded that formation of a visible precipitate did coincide with a phenytoin concentration decline but did not correlate with the differences in pH observed in this study. While dextrose 5% in water was determined to be unacceptable for phenytoin sodium dilution, the authors indicated that sodium chloride 0.9% and Ringer's injection, lactated, were suitable (710).

In a paper by Newton and Kluza, the relationship of phenytoin sodium solubility to various solution characteristics was explored. It was noted that the effect of the special solvent system could be disregarded in dilutions of 1:5 or more. The pH of the admixture was stated to be the primary determinant of the occurrence or absence of crystallization. With a given solution, the pH is dependent on the volume of dilution, with a lower pH resulting from greater dilution. Phenytoin becomes less soluble in aqueous solution as the pH drops. Equations for predicting the compatibility of phenytoin sodium in admixture solutions were presented, but the authors noted that it is not possible to predict the time required to develop precipitation (713).

Giacona et al. evaluated phenytoin sodium (Parke-Davis) and two European preparations of phenytoin utilizing tromethamine in dextrose 5% in water and sodium chloride 0.9% (Travenol) in PVC bags. Phenytoin concentrations ranged from 1 to 10 mg/ml. The two European preparations did not develop visually apparent crystals for four or five days in either solution. Microscopic examination revealed no crystals in 24 hours in either solution. Phenytoin sodium (Parke-Davis) in dextrose 5% in water developed visible particles in 30 minutes, with 12 to 20% of the phenytoin crystallizing in four hours. In sodium chloride 0.9%, macroscopic and microscopic examination showed that phenytoin crystals did not develop within 24

hours when the solution was sealed from the atmosphere. However, in an open container, crystals formed in three hours. This result was attributed to the absorption of atmospheric carbon dioxide decreasing the solution pH (951).

Markowsky et al. evaluated the pH variability among six lots each of phenytoin sodium from four suppliers (Elkins-Sinn, Lyphomed, Parke-Davis, and SoloPak) and the impact on microcrystal formation on dilution. The Parke-Davis product had the highest apparent pH and the least variability. At concentrations of 9.2 and 18.4 mg/ml in sodium chloride 0.9% over two hours, the Parke-Davis lots had no microcrystal formation while the other products had inconsistent but repeated episodes. Microcrystallization was observed most frequently when the apparent pH of the initial product was less than 11.35 and the admixture apparent pH was less than 10.8. Filtration did not remove significant amounts of phenytoin even from the solutions containing microcrystals (1514).

Collins and Lutz demonstrated that phenytoin sodium 50 mg/ml precipitated when injected simultaneously with a total parenteral nutrition solution through a double-lumen catheter using separate ports in a simulated venous flow model. White clouds of precipitated phenytoin and clumps of phenytoin crystals were observed. With a triple-lumen catheter, no clumps were noted, but a white coating formed on the catheter (1421).

Although some feel that infusion of phenytoin sodium is, perhaps, too dangerous to perform clinically (452), others indicate that such administration may be feasible provided proper precautions are taken such as using a suitable vehicle (i.e., sodium chloride 0.9% or Ringer's injection, lactated), using a sufficiently concentrated solution, starting the infusion immediately after preparation and completing administration within a relatively short time, using a 0.22-μm inline filter, and watching the admixture very carefully (305; 306; 453; 611–613; 708–710; 947–950; 1295).

Gentamicin— A 2-ml fluid barrier of dextrose 5% in water in a microbore retrograde infusion set failed to prevent precipitation between gentamicin sulfate 5 mg/0.5 ml and phenytoin sodium 5 mg/0.1 ml (1385).

Concentrated Solutions— The following incompatibility determinations were performed with concentrated solutions. The drugs in dry form were constituted according to manufacturers' recommendations. One milliliter of phenytoin sodium was added to 5 ml of sterile distilled water along with 1 ml of each of the following drugs. Particulate matter was noted within two hours (28):

Aminophylline
Chloramphenicol sodium succinate (Parke-Davis)
Dimenhydrinate (Searle)
Diphenhydramine HCl (Parke-Davis)
Hydroxyzine HCl (Pfizer)
Kanamycin sulfate (Bristol)
Metaraminol bitartrate (MSD)
Penicillin G potassium
Phenobarbital sodium (Winthrop)
Phenylephrine HCl (Winthrop)
Phytonadione (MSD)
Procainamide HCl (Squibb)
Prochlorperazine edisylate (SKF)
Promazine HCl (Wyeth)
Promethazine HCl (Wyeth)
Vancomycin HCl (Lilly)
Vitamin B complex with C (Lederle)

Plasticizer Leaching— Phenytoin sodium (Elkins-Sinn) 10 mg/ml in sodium chloride 0.9% did not leach diethylhexyl phthalate (DEHP) plasticizer from 50-ml PVC bags in 24 hours at 24 °C (1683).

Miscellaneous— Heating plasma samples to 56 °C for one hour to inactivate potential HIV content resulted in no phenytoin loss as determined by fluorescence polarization immunoassay (1615).

PHYTONADIONE
(PHYTOMENADIONE)
AHFS 88:24

AquaMEPHYTON   **Merck**

Products— Phytonadione (Merck) is available as a 2-mg/ml aqueous dispersion in 0.5-ml ampuls and as a 10-mg/ml aqueous dispersion in 1-ml ampuls and 2.5- and 5-ml vials. Each milliliter contains (2):

Phytonadione	2 or 10 mg
Polyoxyethylated fatty acid	70 mg
Dextrose	37.5 mg
Benzyl alcohol	0.9%
Water for injection	qs 1 ml

pH— The USP cites the official pH range as 3.5 to 7 (17). Phytonadione (Merck) has a pH of 5 to 7 (2).

Osmolality— The osmolality of phytonadione (MSD) 10 mg/ml was determined to be 325 mOsm/kg by freezing-point depression and 303 mOsm/kg by vapor pressure (1071).

Administration— The intramuscular or subcutaneous routes are preferred for phytonadione (Merck). If intravenous injection is unavoidable, phytonadione (Merck) may be given by direct intravenous injection at a rate not exceeding 1 mg/min or by intravenous infusion (2; 4).

Stability— Phytonadione injection is available as an essentially clear yellow liquid. Phytonadione is stable in the presence of heat and moisture and may be autoclaved (4), but it is photosensitive and should be protected from light at all times (2; 4). When dilutions are indicated, administration should start immediately after mixing with the diluent; unused portions of the dilution, as well as unused contents of the ampul, should be discarded (2; 4).

Phytonadione (MSD) 10 mg/ml was found to retain potency for three weeks at room temperature when 1 and 2 ml were packaged in Tubex cartridges. After one month, however, an insoluble precipitate was noted (13).

Effects of Light— A study of phytonadione in intravenous solutions showed 50% decomposition in 15 days under fluorescent light and 43 to 63% in three hours on exposure to sunlight (463). The manufacturer indicates that about a 10 to 15% loss occurs over 24 hours on exposure to fluorescent light or sunlight (854). It has been recommended that infusion solutions containing phytonadione require wrapping the container with aluminum foil or other opaque material for light protection (4).

Martinelli et al. evaluated the loss of phytonadione (Roche) 0.05 to 0.1 mg/ml from solutions in glass and polypropylene containers unprotected or packaged in light-protective overwraps when exposed to neon light and daylight. HPLC evaluation found losses approached 80% in one day unprotected from light exposure. A brown polyethylene light protection bag (specific mass 6.6 g/cm^2) provided the best protection, yielding no phytonadione loss during a seven-day exposure period. A white "light-tight" light-protective overwrap (6 g/cm^2) and a black plastic waste disposal bag (2.7 g/cm^2) failed to protect the phytonadione completely. In the black bag, phytonadione losses of over 30% occurred in seven days; the white light-protective overwrap was worse, allowing loss of nearly half of the phytonadione in one day. The authors concluded that substantial differences in light protection are afforded by the different materials and that the efficacy of purported light-protection barriers for light-sensitive drugs should be validated prior to use (1923).

Filtration— The manufacturer states that phytonadione passes through an inline filter (porosity and filter media unspecified) with negligible loss occurring (854).

Compatibility Information

Solution Compatibility

Phytonadione

Solution	Mfr	Mfr	Conc/L	Remarks	Ref	C/I
Amino acids 2%, dextrose 12.5%		ROR	5 ml[a]	7% phytonadione loss in 4 hr and 27% loss in 24 hr by HPLC under ambient temperature and light	1815	**I**
Amino acids 4.25%, dextrose 25%	MG	MSD	10 mg	No increase in particulate matter in 24 hr at 4 °C	349	**C**
Dextran 12%	AB	AB	50 mg	Haze or precipitate forms within 1 hr	3	**I**
Dextran 6% in dextrose 5%	AB	AB	50 mg	Physically compatible	3	**C**
Dextran 6% in sodium chloride 0.9%	AB	AB	50 mg	Physically compatible	3	**C**

Solution Compatibility (Cont.)

Phytonadione

Solution	Mfr	Mfr	Conc/L	Remarks	Ref	C/I
Dextrose 2½% in water	AB	AB	50 mg	Physically compatible	3	C
Dextrose 5% in water	AB	AB	50 mg	Physically compatible	3	C
Dextrose 10% in water	AB	AB	50 mg	Physically compatible	3	C
Dextrose–Ringer's injection combinations	AB	AB	50 mg	Physically compatible	3	C
Dextrose–Ringer's injection, lactated, combinations	AB	AB	50 mg	Physically compatible	3	C
Dextrose–saline combinations	AB	AB	50 mg	Physically compatible	3	C
Fat emulsion 10%, intravenous	KA	KA[a]	16 mg	Physically compatible for 24 hr at 26 °C with little loss of phytonadione and of most other vitamins by HPLC; up to 52% ascorbate loss	2050	C
Fructose 10% in sodium chloride 0.9%	AB	AB	50 mg	Physically compatible	3	C
Fructose 10% in water	AB	AB	50 mg	Physically compatible	3	C
Invert sugar 5 and 10% in sodium chloride 0.9%	AB	AB	50 mg	Physically compatible	3	C
Invert sugar 5 and 10% in water	AB	AB	50 mg	Physically compatible	3	C
Ionosol products	AB	AB	50 mg	Physically compatible	3	C
Ringer's injection	AB	AB	50 mg	Physically compatible	3	C
Ringer's injection, lactated	AB	AB	50 mg	Physically compatible	3	C
Sodium chloride 0.45%	AB	AB	50 mg	Physically compatible	3	C
Sodium chloride 0.9%	AB	AB	50 mg	Physically compatible	3	C
Sodium lactate ⅙ M	AB	AB	50 mg	Physically compatible	3	C
TPN #11 to #15[b]		MSD	5 and 10 mg	Physically compatible for 24 hr at 22 °C. TLC changes of amino acids in similar solutions attributed to M.V.I. or vitamin B complex with C	313	C
TPN #16 to #20[b]		MSD	5 and 10 mg	Physically compatible for 24 hr at 22 °C. UV spectra for amino acids solution unaltered	313	C

[a]From multivitamins.
[b]Refer to Appendix I for the composition of parenteral nutrition solutions. TPN indicates a 2-in-1 admixture.

Additive Compatibility

Phytonadione

Drug	Mfr	Conc/L	Mfr	Conc/L	Test Soln	Remarks	Ref	C/I
Amikacin sulfate	BR	5 g	MSD	200 mg	D5LR, D5R, D5S, D5W, D10W, IS10, LR, NS, R, SL	Physically compatible and amikacin potency retained for 24 hr at 25 °C. Phytonadione not analyzed	294	C
Chloramphenicol sodium succinate	PD	1 g	MSD	50 mg		Physically compatible	6	C
Cimetidine HCl	SKF	3 g	MSD	100 mg	D5W	Physically compatible and cimetidine chemically stable for 24 hr at room temperature. Phytonadione not tested	551	C

Additive Compatibility (Cont.)

Drug	Mfr	Conc/L	Mfr	Conc/L	Test Soln	Remarks	Ref	C/I
Netilmicin sulfate	SC	3 g	MSD	100 mg	D5S	Physically compatible and netilmicin chemically stable for 7 days at 4 and 25 °C. Phytonadione not tested	558	C
Ranitidine HCl	GL	50 mg and 2 g		100 mg	D5W	Ranitidine chemically stable by HPLC for only 6 hr at 25 °C. Phytonadione not tested	1515	I
Sodium bicarbonate	AB	2.4 mEq[a]	MSD	10 mg	D5W	Physically compatible for 24 hr	772	C

[a]One vial of Neut added to a liter of admixture.

Drugs in Syringe Compatibility

Drug (in syringe)	Mfr	Amt	Mfr	Amt	Remarks	Ref	C/I
Doxapram HCl	RB	400 mg/ 20 ml		10 mg/ 1 ml	Physically compatible with no doxapram loss in 24 hr	1177	C

Y-Site Injection Compatibility (1:1 Mixture)

Drug	Mfr	Conc	Mfr	Conc	Remarks	Ref	C/I
Ampicillin sodium	WY	40 mg/ml[a]	MSD	0.4 mg/ml[b]	Physically compatible for 3 hr	1316	C
Dobutamine HCl	LI	4 mg/ml[b]	MSD	0.4 mg/ml[b]	Slight haze in 3 hr	1316	I
Epinephrine HCl	ES	0.032 mg/ ml[b]	MSD	0.4 mg/ml[b]	Physically compatible for 3 hr	1316	C
Famotidine	MSD	0.2 mg/ml[c]	MSD	2 mg/ml	Physically compatible for 14 hr	1196	C
Heparin sodium	UP	1000 units/L[d]	RC	10 mg/ml	Physically compatible for at least 4 hr at room temperature by visual and microscopic examination	534	C
Hydrocortisone sodium succinate	UP	10 mg/L[d]	RC	10 mg/ml	Physically compatible for at least 4 hr at room temperature by visual and microscopic examination	534	C
Potassium chloride	AB	40 mEq/L[d]	RC	10 mg/ml	Physically compatible for at least 4 hr at room temperature by visual and microscopic examination	534	C
Tolazoline HCl		0.1 mg/ml[c]	MSD	2 mg/ml	Physically compatible for 24 hr at 22 °C	1363	C
Vitamin B complex with C	RC	2 ml/L[d]	RC	10 mg/ml	Physically compatible for at least 4 hr at room temperature by visual and microscopic examination	534	C

[a]Tested in sodium chloride 0.9%.
[b]Tested in both dextrose 5% in water and sodium chloride 0.9%.
[c]Tested in dextrose 5% in water.
[d]Tested in dextrose 5% in Ringer's injection, dextrose 5% in Ringer's injection, lactated, dextrose 5% in water, Ringer's injection, lactated, and sodium chloride 0.9%.

Additional Compatibility Information

Solutions— If intravenous infusion is necessary, preservative-free solutions only should be used; dextrose 5% in water, sodium chloride 0.9%, and dextrose 5% in sodium chloride 0.9% have been recommended as diluents. Other diluents are not recommended by the manufacturer (2).

The stability of phytonadione was evaluated in a TPN solution containing amino acids 2%, dextrose 12.5%, "standard" electrolytes, and multivitamins (M.V.I. Pediatric) by HPLC analysis over 24 hours while exposed to light. Vitamin losses were about 7 and 27% in four and 24 hours, respectively. Some loss was attributed to the light sensitivity of phytonadione (1815).

Billion-Rey et al. reported substantial loss by HPLC analysis of retinol all-*trans* palmitate and phytonadione from both TPN and TNA admixtures due to exposure to sunlight. In three hours of exposure to sunlight, essentially total loss of retinol and 50% loss of phytonadione had occurred. The presence or absence of lipids did not affect stability. In contrast, tocopherol concentrations remained essentially unchanged by exposure to sunlight through 12 hours. The container material used to store the nutrition admixtures affected the concentration of the vitamins as well. Losses were greatest (10 to 25%) in PVC containers and were slightly better in EVA and glass containers (2049).

See Effects of Light above.

Oxytocin— Phytonadione (Abbott) 50 mg/L has been reported to be conditionally compatible with oxytocin (Parke-Davis) 5 USP units/L. The mixture is physically compatible in most Abbott infusion solutions except dextran 12% in which a haze or precipitate forms within one hour (3).

Phenytoin Sodium— Phytonadione (MSD) has been reported to be incompatible with phenytoin sodium (Parke-Davis) in concentrated solutions. Phenytoin sodium was constituted according to the manufacturer's directions, and 1 ml was added to a solution of 5 ml of sterile distilled water along with 1 ml of phytonadione. Particulate matter was noted within two hours (28).

PIPERACILLIN SODIUM
AHFS 8:12.16

Pipracil   **Lederle**

Products— Piperacillin sodium (Lederle) is available in 2-, 3-, and 4-g vials and infusion bottles and 40-g bulk packages (2).

For intramuscular use, reconstitute the appropriate vial with sterile water for injection, sodium chloride 0.9%, bacteriostatic sterile water for injection or bacteriostatic sodium chloride 0.9% (preserved with parabens or benzyl alcohol), dextrose 5% in sodium chloride 0.9%, dextrose 5% in water, or lidocaine HCl 0.5 to 1% (without epinephrine) and shake well until dissolved. Reconstitute the 2-, 3-, and 4-g vials with 4, 6, and 8 ml of diluent, respectively, to yield solutions containing 1 g/2.5 ml (2; 4).

For intravenous use, each gram of piperacillin sodium should be reconstituted with at least 5 ml of sterile water for injection, sodium chloride 0.9%, bacteriostatic sterile water for injection, bacteriostatic sodium chloride 0.9% (preserved with parabens or benzyl alcohol), dextrose 5% in water, or dextrose 5% in sodium chloride 0.9%. Shake well until dissolved. This solution may be administered by direct intravenous injection, or it may be further diluted with at least 50 ml of compatible infusion solution for intermittent intravenous infusion (2; 4).

The 40-g bulk pharmacy package is reconstituted with 172 ml of a compatible diluent (except lidocaine HCl) to provide a 200-mg/ml concentration (2; 4).

pH— The pH of the reconstituted solution is 5.5 to 7.5 (2).

Osmolality— The osmolality of piperacillin sodium (Lederle) 45 mg/ml was determined to be 346 mOsm/kg in dextrose 5% in water and 361 mOsm/kg in sodium chloride 0.9%. At 70 mg/ml, the osmolality was determined to be 389 mOsm/kg in dextrose 5% in water and 399 mOsm/kg in sodium chloride 0.9% (1375).

The osmolality of piperacillin sodium was calculated for the following dilutions (1054):

Diluent	Osmolality (mOsm/kg)	
	50 ml	100 ml
3 g		
Dextrose 5% in water	425	348
Sodium chloride 0.9%	452	375
4 g		
Dextrose 5% in water	475	377
Sodium chloride 0.9%	502	404

Robinson et al. recommended the following maximum piperacillin sodium concentrations to achieve osmolalities suitable for peripheral infusion in fluid-restricted patients (1180):

Diluent	Maximum Concentration (mg/ml)	Osmolality (mOsm/kg)
Dextrose 5% in water	91	536
Sodium chloride 0.9%	81	515
Sterile water for injection	163	439

Sodium Content— Each gram of piperacillin sodium contains 1.85 mEq (42.5 mg) of sodium (2).

Administration— Piperacillin sodium may be administered by direct intravenous injection slowly over three to five minutes, by intermittent intravenous infusion diluted in at least 50 ml of compatible diluent and given over about 20 to 30 minutes, or by intramuscular injection, preferably into the upper outer quadrant of the buttock. No more than 2 g should be administered intramuscularly at any one site (2; 4).

Stability— Piperacillin sodium is a white to off-white powder which may be stored at controlled room temperature (2). Storage of the powder for two months at 56 °C and for four months at 2 °C resulted in retention of at least 95% potency. Exposure of the powder to sunlight for one month resulted in a slight darkening of the powder but no loss of potency (740).

Reconstitution yields a colorless to pale yellow solution which is chemically stable and remains clear for at least 24 hours at room temperature, one week under refrigeration, and one month if frozen. (Pharmacy bulk packages should not be frozen, and ADD-Vantage vials should not be refrigerated or frozen.) Slight darkening of the solution does not indicate a potency loss. Shorter storage periods of 24 hours at room temperature and 48 hours under refrigeration may be appropriate when aseptic technique and sterility considerations indicate (2; 4). In solution the drug is stable over a pH range of 4.5 to 8.5 (740).

Piperacillin sodium reconstituted to a 40% (2 g/5 ml) concentration with sterile water for injection retains chemical stability for at least 32 days when frozen in both glass (Glaspak) and plastic (Plastipak) syringes (740).

Dilution of the piggyback infusion bottles to a 12% (6 g/50 ml) concentration with the following infusion diluents also results in solutions that are chemically stable for at least 24 hours at room temperature, one week under refrigeration, and one month if frozen (740):

Dextran 6% in sodium chloride 0.9%
Dextrose 5% in sodium chloride 0.9%
Dextrose 5% in water
Ringer's injection, lactated
Sodium chloride 0.9%

Piperacillin sodium in a concentration of 0.2% in various admixture solutions has been shown to be stable in both glass and PVC containers for 24 hours at room temperature, 48 hours under refrigeration, and one month if frozen (740).

Borst et al. reported that piperacillin sodium (Lederle) 2 and 3 g/10 ml in sterile water for injection, packaged in plastic syringes (Monoject), exhibited a 10% piperacillin loss in two days at 24 °C and 10 days at 4 °C as determined by HPLC. Frozen at −15 °C, the

drug exhibited less than a 10% loss during the three-month study period (1178).

Das Gupta et al. evaluated the stability of piperacillin sodium (Lederle) 10 g/L in dextrose 5% in water and sodium chloride 0.9% when frozen at −10 °C. After 71 days of storage, the solutions were thawed by warming under tap water and by microwave exposure for four minutes. No loss of potency was noted with either thawing technique (1126).

Piperacillin sodium (Lederle) 41.5 mg/ml in dextrose 5% in water was visually compatible and showed no potency loss by HPLC after frozen storage (−20 °C) for 30 days followed by seven days of refrigeration at 4 °C (1539).

Elastomeric Reservoir Pumps— Piperacillin sodium (Lederle) 30 mg/ml in dextrose 5% in water and sodium chloride 0.9% 100 ml was packaged in latex elastomeric reservoirs (Secure Medical). Little or no loss by HPLC analysis occurred in 24 hours at 25 °C, 4% or less loss occurred in seven days at 5 °C, and 7% or less loss occurred in 12 weeks frozen at −20 °C (1970).

Piperacillin sodium (Lederle) 16 mg/ml in both dextrose 5% in water and sodium chloride 0.9% was evaluated for binding potential to natural rubber elastomeric reservoirs (Baxter). No loss was found after storage for two weeks at 35 °C with gentle agitation (2014).

Sorption— Picard et al. reported little or no loss due to sorption of piperacillin sodium (Lederle) 4 g/100 ml in dextrose 5% in water and sodium chloride 0.9% in trilayer solution bags (Bieffe Medital) composed of polyethylene, polyamide, and polypropylene. The admixtures were evaluated by HPLC analysis up to two hours after preparation. Similarly, no loss was found during one-hour simulated infusion (1918).

Filtration— Piggyback infusions at a 4% (2 g/50 ml) concentration in dextrose 5% in sodium chloride 0.9%, Ringer's injection, lactated, and sodium chloride 0.9% exhibited no changes in potency or pH when passed through an intravenous administration set with a 0.45-μm inline final filter (Abbott) (740).

Compatibility Information

Solution Compatibility

Piperacillin sodium

Solution	Mfr	Mfr	Conc/L	Remarks	Ref	C/I
Dextran 6% in sodium chloride 0.9%		LE	120 g[a]	Physically compatible and chemically stable for 24 hr at room temperature and 1 week under refrigeration	740	C
Dextrose 5% in sodium chloride 0.9%		LE	120 g[a]	Physically compatible and chemically stable for 24 hr at room temperature and 1 week under refrigeration	740	C
Dextrose 5% in water		LE	120 g[a]	Physically compatible and chemically stable for 24 hr at room temperature and 1 week under refrigeration	740	C
	TR[b]	LE	2 g	Physically compatible and chemically stable for 24 hr at room temperature and 48 hr under refrigeration	740	C
	MG[c]	LE	40 g	Physically compatible and less than 2% drug loss in 48 hr at 25 °C under fluorescent light	1026	C

Solution Compatibility (Cont.)

Piperacillin sodium

Solution	Mfr	Mfr	Conc/L	Remarks	Ref	C/I
	TR[b]	LE	10 g	Physically compatible with 4% loss in 48 hr and 9% in 5 days at 25 °C. 3% loss in 28 days and 8% in 49 days at 5 °C. No loss in 71 days at −10 °C	1126	**C**
	MG[d]	LE	41.5 g	Visually compatible with no piperacillin loss by HPLC after 30 days at −20 °C followed by 7 days at 4 °C	1539	**C**
	[b]	LE	80 g	No drug loss by HPLC during 2-hr storage and 1-hr simulated infusion	1774	**C**
	AB[e]	LE	30 g	7% or less drug loss by HPLC in 24 hr at 25 °C and in 7 days at 5 °C	1970	**C**
Ringer's injection, lactated		LE	120 g[a]	Physically compatible and chemically stable for 24 hr at room temperature and 1 week under refrigeration	740	**C**
	TR[b]	LE	2 g	Physically compatible and chemically stable for 24 hr at room temperature and 48 hr under refrigeration	740	**C**
Sodium chloride 0.9%		LE	120 g[a]	Physically compatible and chemically stable for 24 hr at room temperature and 1 week under refrigeration	740	**C**
	TR[b]	LE	2 g	Physically compatible and chemically stable for 24 hr at room temperature and 48 hr under refrigeration	740	**C**
	MG[c]	LE	40 g	Physically compatible and less than 2% drug loss in 48 hr at 25 °C under fluorescent light	1026	**C**
	TR[b]	LE	10 g	Physically compatible with 3.5% loss in 48 hr and 8% in 5 days at 25 °C. 2% loss in 28 days and 6% in 49 days at 5 °C. No loss in 71 days at −10 °C	1126	**C**
	[b]	LE	80 g	No drug loss by HPLC during 2-hr storage and 1-hr simulated infusion	1774	**C**
	AB[e]	LE	30 g	Little or no drug loss by HPLC in 24 hr at 25 °C and in 7 days at 5 °C	1970	**C**
TPN #107[f]			2 g	43% piperacillin loss in 24 hr at 21 °C by microbiological assay	1326	**I**

[a]*The piggyback concentration of 12% (6 g/50 ml).*
[b]*Tested in PVC containers.*
[c]*Tested in glass containers.*
[d]*Tested in polyolefin containers.*
[e]*Tested in glass containers and latex elastomeric reservoirs (Secure Medical).*
[f]*Refer to Appendix I for the composition of parenteral nutrition solutions. TPN indicates a 2-in-1 admixture.*

Additive Compatibility

Piperacillin sodium

Drug	Mfr	Conc/L	Mfr	Conc/L	Test Soln	Remarks	Ref	C/I
Ciprofloxacin	MI	1 g	LE	40 g	D5W, NS	Physically compatible for 24 hr at 22 °C	1189	**C**
Clindamycin phosphate	UP	9 g	LE	40 g	D5W, NS	Physically compatible with 2% clindamycin loss and 3 to 5% piperacillin loss in 48 hr at 25 °C under fluorescent light	1026	**C**

Additive Compatibility (Cont.)

Piperacillin sodium

Drug	Mfr	Conc/L	Mfr	Conc/L	Test Soln	Remarks	Ref	C/I
Flucloxacillin sodium	BE	50 g	LE	120 g	W	10% piperacillin loss and 6% flucloxacillin loss by HPLC in 12 days at 5 °C. 3% piperacillin loss and 6% flucloxacillin loss by HPLC in 1 day at 30 °C	1748	C
Fluconazole	PF	1 g	LE	40 g	D5W	Visually compatible with no fluconazole loss by HPLC in 72 hr at 25 °C under fluorescent light. Piperacillin not tested	1677	C
Hydrocortisone sodium succinate	UP	40 mg	LE	40 g	D5S[a]	Physically compatible and piperacillin chemically stable for 24 hr at room temperature and 1 week under refrigeration. Hydrocortisone not tested	740	C
Ofloxacin	HO	1.67 g	LE	16.7 g	W	Visually compatible with little or no loss of either drug by HPLC in 48 hr	1613	C
Potassium chloride		40 mEq	LE	2 g	D5S, D5W, LR, R, NS	Physically compatible and piperacillin chemically stable for 24 hr at room temperature and 48 hr under refrigeration	740	C
Verapamil HCl	SE	[b]	LE	40 g	D5W, NS	Physically compatible for 24 hr at 21 °C	1166	C

[a]*Tested in PVC containers.*
[b]*Final concentration unspecified.*

Drugs in Syringe Compatibility

Piperacillin sodium

Drug (in syringe)	Mfr	Amt	Mfr	Amt	Remarks	Ref	C/I
Heparin sodium		2500 units/ 1 ml	LE	2 g	Physically compatible for at least 5 min	1053	C

Y-Site Injection Compatibility (1:1 Mixture)

Piperacillin sodium

Drug	Mfr	Conc	Mfr	Conc	Remarks	Ref	C/I
Acyclovir sodium	BW	5 mg/ml[a]	LE	60 mg/ml[a]	Physically compatible for 4 hr at 25 °C	1157	C
Allopurinol sodium	BW	3 mg/ml[b]	LE	40 mg/ml[b]	Physically compatible with no change in measured turbidity or increase in particle content in 4 hr at 22 °C	1686	C
Amifostine	USB	10 mg/ml[a]	LE	40 mg/ml[a]	Physically compatible with no change in measured turbidity or increase in particle content in 4 hr at 23 °C	1845	C
Amphotericin B cholesteryl sulfate complex	SEQ	0.83 mg/ml[a]	LE	40 mg/ml[a]	Microprecipitate forms in 4 hr at 23 °C under fluorescent light	2117	I
Aztreonam	SQ	40 mg/ml[a]	LE	40 mg/ml[a]	Physically compatible with no subvisual haze or particle formation in 4 hr at 23 °C	1758	C
Ciprofloxacin	MI	1 mg/ml[a]	LE	40 mg/ml[c]	Physically compatible for 24 hr at 22 °C	1189	C
Cisatracurium besylate	GW	0.1 mg/ml[a]	LE	40 mg/ml[a]	Physically compatible with no change in measured turbidity or increase in particle content in 4 hr at 23 °C	2074	C

Y-Site Injection Compatibility (1:1 Mixture) (Cont.)

Piperacillin sodium

Drug	Mfr	Conc	Mfr	Conc	Remarks	Ref	C/I
	GW	2 mg/ml[a]	LE	40 mg/ml[a]	Subvisual haze forms immediately	2074	**I**
	GW	5 mg/ml[a]	LE	40 mg/ml[a]	Haze forms immediately	2074	**I**
Cyclophosphamide	MJ	20 mg/ml[a]	LE	60 mg/ml[a]	Physically compatible for 4 hr at 25 °C	1194	**C**
Diltiazem HCl	MMD	1[b] and 5 mg/ml	LE	200 mg/ml[b]	Visually compatible	1807	**C**
	MMD	5 mg/ml	LE	20 mg/ml[b]	Visually compatible	1807	**C**
Docetaxel	RPR	0.9 mg/ml[a]	LE	40 mg/ml[a]	Physically compatible with no change in measured turbidity or increase in particle content in 4 hr at 23 °C	2224	**C**
Doxorubicin HCl liposome injection	SEQ	0.4 mg/ml[a]	LE	40 mg/ml[a]	Physically compatible with little or no change in measured turbidity and no increase in particle content in 4 hr at 23 °C	2087	**C**
Enalaprilat	MSD	0.05 mg/ml[b]	LE	12 mg/ml[a]	Physically compatible for 24 hr at room temperature under fluorescent light	1355	**C**
Esmolol HCl	DCC	10 mg/ml[a]	LE	30 mg/ml[a]	Physically compatible for 24 hr at 22 °C	1169	**C**
Etoposide phosphate	BR	5 mg/ml[a]	LE	40 mg/ml[a]	Physically compatible with no change in measured turbidity or increase in particle content in 4 hr at 23 °C	2218	**C**
Famotidine	MSD	0.2 mg/ml[a]	LE	40 mg/ml[b]	Physically compatible for 14 hr	1196	**C**
	ME	2 mg/ml[b]		40 mg/ml[a]	Visually compatible for 4 hr at 22 °C	1936	**C**
Filgrastim	AMG	30 μg/ml[a]	LE	40 mg/ml[a]	Particles and filaments form immediately	1687	**I**
Fluconazole	RR	2 mg/ml	LE	80 mg/ml	Viscous gel-like substance forms	1407	**I**
Fludarabine phosphate	BX	1 mg/ml[a]	LE	40 mg/ml[a]	Physically compatible for 4 hr at room temperature under fluorescent light	1439	**C**
Foscarnet sodium	AST	24 mg/ml	LE	80 mg/ml	Physically compatible for 24 hr at room temperature under fluorescent light	1335	**C**
Gemcitabine HCl	LI	10 mg/ml[b]	LE	40 mg/ml[b]	Cloudiness forms immediately, becoming precipitated clumps in 4 hr	2226	**I**
Granisetron HCl	SKB	0.05 mg/ml[a]	LE	40 mg/ml[a]	Physically compatible with no change in measured turbidity or increase in particle content in 4 hr at 23 °C	2000	**C**
Heparin sodium	TR	50 units/ml	LE	60 mg/ml[a]	Visually compatible for 6 hr at 25 °C	1793	**C**
Hydromorphone HCl	WY	0.2 mg/ml[a]	LE	60 mg/ml[a]	Physically compatible for at least 4 hr at 25 °C under fluorescent light	987	**C**
IL-2	RC	4800 I.U./ml[b]	LE	200 mg/ml	Visually compatible and IL-2 activity by bioassay retained. Piperacillin not tested	1552	**C**
Labetalol HCl	SC	1 mg/ml[a]	LE	10 mg/ml[a]	Physically compatible for 24 hr at 18 °C	1171	**C**
Lorazepam	WY	0.33 mg/ml[b]	LE	150 mg/ml	Visually compatible for 24 hr at 22 °C	1855	**C**
Magnesium sulfate	IX	16.7, 33.3, 66.7, 100 mg/ml[a]	LE	60 mg/ml[a]	Physically compatible for at least 4 hr at 32 °C	813	**C**
Melphalan HCl	BW	0.1 mg/ml[b]	LE	40 mg/ml[b]	Physically compatible with no change in measured turbidity or increase in particle content in 3 hr at 22 °C	1557	**C**

Y-Site Injection Compatibility (1:1 Mixture) (Cont.)

Piperacillin sodium

Drug	Mfr	Conc	Mfr	Conc	Remarks	Ref	C/I
Meperidine HCl	WY	10 mg/ml[a]	LE	60 mg/ml[a]	Physically compatible for at least 4 hr at 25 °C under fluorescent light	987	**C**
Midazolam HCl	RC	5 mg/ml	LE	150 mg/ml	Visually compatible for 24 hr at 22 °C	1855	**C**
Morphine sulfate	WI	1 mg/ml[a]	LE	60 mg/ml[a]	Physically compatible for at least 4 hr at 25 °C under fluorescent light	987	**C**
Ondansetron HCl	GL	1 mg/ml[b]	LE	40 mg/ml[a]	Slight turbidity appears in 30 min	1365	**I**
Perphenazine	SC	0.02 mg/ml[a]	LE	60 mg/ml[a]	Physically compatible for 4 hr at 25 °C	1155	**C**
Propofol	ZEN	10 mg/ml	LE	40 mg/ml[a]	Physically compatible for 1 hr at 23 °C with no increase in particle content	2066	**C**
Ranitidine HCl	GL	1 mg/ml[b]	LE	30 mg/ml[a]	Little or no loss of either drug by HPLC in 4 hr at 22 °C under fluorescent light	1632	**C**
Remifentanil HCl	GW	0.025 and 0.25 mg/ml[b]	LE	40 mg/ml[a]	Physically compatible with no change in measured turbidity or increase in particle content in 4 hr at 23 °C	2075	**C**
Sargramostim	IMM	10 μg/ml[b]	LE	40 mg/ml[b]	Small amount of particles form in 4 hr	1436	**I**
Tacrolimus	FUJ	1 mg/ml[b]	LE	80 mg/ml[a]	Visually compatible for 24 hr at 25 °C	1630	**C**
Teniposide	BR	0.1 mg/ml[a]	LE	40 mg/ml[a]	Physically compatible with no subvisual haze or particle formation in 4 hr at 23 °C	1725	**C**
Theophylline	TR	4 mg/ml	LE	60 mg/ml[a]	Visually compatible for 6 hr at 25 °C	1793	**C**
Thiotepa	IMM[d]	1 mg/ml[a]	LE	40 mg/ml[a]	Physically compatible with no change in measured turbidity or increase in particle content in 4 hr at 23 °C	1861	**C**
TNA #218 to #226[e]			LE	40 mg/ml[a]	Visually compatible with no precipitate or emulsion damage apparent in 4 hr at 23 °C	2215	**C**
TPN #54[e]				133 and 200 mg/ml	Physically compatible and 90 to 100% piperacillin activity retained over 6 hr at 22 °C by microbiological assay	1045	**C**
TPN #61[e]		f	LE	250 mg/ 1.25 ml[g]	Physically compatible	1012	**C**
		h	LE	1.5 g/7.5 ml[g]	Physically compatible	1012	**C**
TPN #212 to #215[e]			LE	40 mg/ml[a]	Physically compatible with no change in measured turbidity or increase in particle content in 4 hr at 23 °C	2109	**C**
Vancomycin HCl	AB	20 mg/ml[a]	LE	200 mg/ml[i]	Transient precipitate forms, followed by clear solution	2189	**?**
	AB	20 mg/ml[a]	LE	10 and 50 mg/ml[a]	Gross white precipitate forms immediately	2189	**I**
	AB	20 mg/ml[a]	LE	1 mg/ml[a]	Physically comptible with no change in measured turbidity or increase in particle content in 4 hr at 23 °C	2189	**C**
	AB	2 mg/ml[a]	LE	1[a], 10[a], 50[a], 200[i] mg/ml	Physically compatible with no change in measured turbidity or increase in particle content in 4 hr at 23 °C	2189	**C**
Verapamil HCl	SE	2.5 mg/ml	LE	40 mg/ml[c]	Physically compatible for 15 min at 21 °C under fluorescent light	1166	**C**

Y-Site Injection Compatibility (1:1 Mixture) (Cont.)

Piperacillin sodium

Drug	Mfr	Conc	Mfr	Conc	Remarks	Ref	C/I
Vinorelbine tartrate	BW	1 mg/ml[b]	LE	40 mg/ml[b]	Heavy white turbidity forms immediately, becoming white flocculent precipitate in 4 hr at 22 °C	1558	I
Zidovudine	BW	4 mg/ml[a]	LE	4 mg/ml[a]	Physically compatible for 4 hr at 25 °C under fluorescent light by visual and microscopic examination	1193	C

[a]*Tested in dextrose 5% in water.*
[b]*Tested in sodium chloride 0.9%.*
[c]*Tested in both dextrose 5% in water and sodium chloride 0.9%.*
[d]*Lyophilized formulation tested.*
[e]*Refer to Appendix I for the composition of parenteral nutrition solutions. TNA indicates a 3-in-1 admixture, and TPN indicates a 2-in-1 admixture.*
[f]*Run at 21 ml/hr.*
[g]*Given over five minutes by syringe pump.*
[h]*Run at 94 ml/hr.*
[i]*Tested in sterile water for injection.*

Additional Compatibility Information

Aminoglycosides— Although piperacillin sodium and aminoglycosides act synergistically and have been used successfully clinically when recommended doses of each drug were administered, mixing piperacillin sodium directly in a syringe or infusion bottle with an aminoglycoside can result in substantial inactivation of the aminoglycoside (740).

Using bioassay and radioimmunoassay, Hale et al. evaluated piperacillin and carbenicillin at concentrations of 62.5 to 1000 μg/ml in human serum in combination with amikacin, gentamicin, or tobramycin 10 μg/ml at 37 °C for up to 24 hours. Penicillin concentrations of 62.5 and 125 μg/ml had relatively little effect on the aminoglycoside concentration, even after 24 hours. However, increasing the penicillin concentration to 250 or 500 μg/ml greatly increased decomposition. After 24 hours with carbenicillin 500 μg/ml, the amounts of aminoglycosides remaining were: amikacin, 82%; gentamicin, 43%; and tobramycin, 27%. After 24 hours with piperacillin 500 μg/ml, the remaining concentrations were 95, 45, and 52%, respectively. Even greater inactivation occurred at 1000 μg/ml of the penicillins, including the essentially complete loss of tobramycin in 24 hours. The authors concluded that amikacin is much more resistant to inactivation than the other aminoglycosides tested and that carbenicillin is more aggressive in its inactivation than piperacillin (816).

Pickering and Rutherford evaluated several aminoglycosides combined with a number of penicillins. Gentamicin sulfate, netilmicin sulfate, and tobramycin sulfate 5 and 10 μg/ml and amikacin 10 and 20 μg/ml were combined in human serum with 125, 250, and 500 μg/ml of azlocillin, carbenicillin disodium, amdinocillin, mezlocillin, and piperacillin individually. Tobramycin and gentamicin sustained greater losses than netilmicin and amikacin at each of the penicillin concentrations. Significant decomposition of all aminoglycosides occurred in 24 hours at 37 °C at a penicillin concentration of 500 μg/ml. Tobramycin and gentamicin had losses of 40 to 60%, while 15 to 30% losses occurred for netilmicin. Amikacin sustained the least inactivation with losses of about 10 to 20%. At penicillin concentrations of 125 to 250 μg/ml, smaller losses of aminoglycosides were observed (68).

Rank et al. evaluated the inactivation of tobramycin 6 μg/ml in human serum with the sodium salts of cloxacillin and piperacillin 150 and 300 μg/ml, ampicillin 100 and 200 μg/ml, and penicillin G 75 and 150 I.U./ml at 25 and 37 °C for up to 12 hours. Piperacillin induced the greatest inactivation among the penicillins, with up to a 15% loss in 12 hours at 37 °C in the 300-μg/ml concentration. Cloxacillin and ampicillin had an intermediate effect, causing about a 5% loss in 12 hours at 37 °C in the highest concentrations. Penicillin G did not yield significant tobramycin inactivation (817).

The inactivation of gentamicin, tobramycin, and amikacin, each 5 μg/ml, by seven β-lactam antibiotics, 250 and 500 μg/ml, in serum at 25 °C over 24 hours was studied using bioassay, enzyme-mediated immunoassay technique (EMIT), fluorescence polarization immunoassay (TDx), and radioimmunoassay. Results with the penicillins varied, depending on the assay technique used. The bioassay was the most sensitive to loss, TDx and radioimmunoassay were intermediate, and EMIT was the least sensitive. Azlocillin, carbenicillin, mezlocillin, and piperacillin all caused variable but extensive inactivation (up to 70%) of gentamicin and tobramycin in 24 hours. Amikacin, however, had only minor losses compared to the other aminoglycosides (654).

The clinical significance of these interactions in patients appears to be confined primarily to those with renal failure (218; 334; 361; 364; 616; 816; 847; 952). Literature reports of greatly reduced aminoglycoside levels in such patients have appeared frequently (363; 365–367; 614; 615; 962). In addition, the interaction may be clinically important if assays for aminoglycoside levels in serum are sufficiently delayed (576; 618; 735; 814; 824; 832; 847; 1052).

Most authors believe that in vitro mixing of penicillins, such as piperacillin sodium, with aminoglycoside antibiotics should be avoided but that clinical use of the drugs in combination can be of great value. It is generally recommended that the drugs be given separately in such combined therapy (157; 218; 222; 224; 361; 364; 368–370).

Vancomycin— The compatibility or incompatibility of vancomycin HCl mixed with or administered simultaneously with piperacillin sodium is concentration dependent (2189). See Y-Site Compatibility above. Vancomycin HCl has a low pH and is variably compatible with drugs having neutral to mildly alkaline pH, including cephalosporins and penicillins. The compatibility may depend on a number of factors, including concentration of each drug, dilution vehicle, actual pH of solutions, and completeness of mixing during administration. Combinations that are compatible when well mixed may result in precipitation if only partially mixed, presumably because of regionally different concentrations and pH values. If attempting to administer vancomycin HCl with piperacillin sodium, take care to ensure that the specific combination and the concentrations are compatible under the exact administration conditions to be used. An inline filter should be used as a final safety measure (2189).

Peritoneal Dialysis Solutions—— The stability of piperacillin sodium (Lederle) 200 mg/L in peritoneal dialysis solutions (Dianeal 137 and PD2) with heparin sodium 500 units/L was evaluated at 25 °C by microbiological assay. Approximately 94 ± 11% activity remained after 24 hours (1228).

PIPERACILLIN SODIUM–TAZOBACTAM SODIUM
AHFS 8:12.16

Zosyn   **Lederle**

Products—— Piperacillin sodium–tazobactam sodium (Lederle) is available in vials containing 2.25 g (piperacillin 2 g plus tazobactam 250 mg), 3.375 g (piperacillin 3 g plus tazobactam 375 mg), and 4.5 g (piperacillin 4 g plus tazobactam 500 mg) as sodium salts. The drug is also available in a pharmacy bulk package containing 40.5 g (piperacillin 36 plus tazobactam 4.5) as sodium salts. The products contain no preservatives. The pH may have been adjusted during manufacture with sodium bicarbonate or hydrochloric acid (2; 4).

Each gram of piperacillin should be reconstituted with at least 5 ml of sterile water for injection, sodium chloride 0.9%, bacteriostatic water for injection (preserved with benzyl alcohol or parabens), bacteriostatic sodium chloride 0.9% (preserved with benzyl alcohol or parabens), or dextrose 5% in water and shaken well until dissolved. The solution should be diluted in at least 50 ml of compatible infusion solution for intermittent infusion (2).

The pharmacy bulk package is reconstituted with 152 ml of compatible diluent to yield a solution containing 200 mg/ml of piperacillin and 25 mg/ml of tazobactam. The reconstituted pharmacy bulk package solution must be diluted further for use (4).

Piperacillin sodium–tazobactam sodium (Lederle) is also available as frozen iso-osmotic injections containing piperacillin sodium 40 mg/ml with tazobactam 5 mg/ml and piperacillin sodium 60 mg/ml with tazobactam sodium 7.5 mg/ml (2; 4).

pH— From 4.5 to 6.8 (4).

Sodium Content— The combination product contains 2.35 mEq (54 mg) of sodium per gram of piperacillin (2).

Administration—— Piperacillin sodium–tazobactam sodium should be administered by intravenous infusion over at least 30 minutes after dilution to at least 50 ml in a compatible diluent. It can also be infused using ambulatory infusion pumps (2; 4).

Stability—— The white to off-white lyophilized powder in intact vials should be stored at controlled room temperature (2).

Single-dose vials of the solution should be used immediately after reconstitution. Any remaining portion should be discarded after 24 hours at room temperature or 48 hours under refrigeration at 2 to 8 °C. In ADD-Vantage vials, the product has been found to be stable for 24 hours at room temperature but should not be refrigerated or frozen (2; 4).

In compatible infusion solutions, the drug is stable for up to 24 hours at room temperature or one week under refrigeration. Glass and plastic (including syringes, intravenous solution bags, and tubing) do not affect stability (2).

The product was shown to be stable for up to 12 hours in an ambulatory infusion pump. Each dose was diluted to 25 or 37.5 ml, and stability was not affected (2).

The commercially available frozen injections should be stored at or below −20 °C. The frozen solutions should be thawed at room temperature or under refrigeration but should not be thawed in a warm water bath or by exposure to microwave radiation. Thawed solutions should not be refrozen. After thawing, the solutions are stable for 24 hours at room temperature or 14 days under refrigeration (4).

Freezing Solutions— Piperacillin sodium–tazobactam sodium (American Cyanamid) 80 + 10 mg/ml in PVC bags of dextrose 5% in water and sodium chloride 0.9% was frozen at −15 °C for 30 days and thawed by microwave radiation for 45 seconds. HPLC analysis showed no loss of either component (1768).

Piperacillin sodium–tazobactam sodium (American Cyanamid) 150 + 18.75 mg/ml and 200 + 25 mg/ml in dextrose 5% in water and sodium chloride 0.9% was drawn as 20-ml aliquots into polypropylene syringes (Becton-Dickinson). The syringes were frozen at −15 °C for 30 days and then stored at 4 °C for seven days. HPLC analysis showed no loss of either component (1768).

Syringes— Piperacillin sodium–tazobactam sodium (American Cyanamid) 150 + 18.75 mg/ml and 200 + 25 mg/ml in dextrose 5% in water and sodium chloride 0.9% was drawn as 20-ml aliquots into polypropylene syringes (Becton-Dickinson). The syringes were stored at 25 °C for one day and at 4 °C for seven days. HPLC analysis showed no loss of either drug in the dextrose 5% in water samples. Similarly, no tazobactam loss occurred in the sodium chloride 0.9% solutions. However, piperacillin losses of 7% in one day at 25 °C and 4% in seven days at 4 °C were found in the sodium chloride 0.9% solutions (1768).

Compatibility Information

Y-Site Injection Compatibility (1:1 Mixture)

Piperacillin sodium–tazobactam sodium

Drug	Mfr	Conc	Mfr	Conc	Remarks	Ref	C/I
Acyclovir sodium	BW	7 mg/ml[a]	LE	40 + 5 mg/ml[a]	Particles form in 1 hr	1688	I
Aminophylline	AB	2.5 mg/ml[a]	LE	40 + 5 mg/ml[a]	Physically compatible with no change in measured turbidity or increase in particle content in 4 hr at 22 °C	1688	C
Amphotericin B	SQ	0.6 mg/ml[a]	LE	40 + 5 mg/ml[a]	Heavy yellow flocculent precipitate forms immediately	1688	I
Amphotericin B cholesteryl sulfate complex	SEQ	0.83 mg/ml[a]	CY	40 + 5 mg/ml[a]	Microprecipitate forms immediately	2117	I
Aztreonam	SQ	40 mg/ml[a]	LE	40 + 5 mg/ml[a]	Physically compatible with no change in measured turbidity or increase in particle content in 4 hr at 22 °C	1688	C
Bleomycin sulfate	BR	1 unit/ml[b]	LE	40 + 5 mg/ml[a]	Physically compatible with no change in measured turbidity or increase in particle content in 4 hr at 22 °C	1688	C
Bumetanide	RC	0.04 mg/ml[a]	LE	40 + 5 mg/ml[a]	Physically compatible with no change in measured turbidity or increase in particle content in 4 hr at 22 °C	1688	C
Buprenorphine HCl	RKC	0.04 mg/ml[a]	LE	40 + 5 mg/ml[a]	Physically compatible with no change in measured turbidity or increase in particle content in 4 hr at 22 °C	1688	C
Butorphanol tartrate	BR	0.04 mg/ml[a]	LE	40 + 5 mg/ml[a]	Physically compatible with no change in measured turbidity or increase in particle content in 4 hr at 22 °C	1688	C
Calcium gluconate	AMR	40 mg/ml[a]	LE	40 + 5 mg/ml[a]	Physically compatible with no change in measured turbidity or increase in particle content in 4 hr at 22 °C	1688	C
Carboplatin	BR	5 mg/ml[a]	LE	40 + 5 mg/ml[a]	Physically compatible with no change in measured turbidity or increase in particle content in 4 hr at 22 °C	1688	C
Carmustine	BR	1.5 mg/ml[a]	LE	40 + 5 mg/ml[a]	Physically compatible with no change in measured turbidity or increase in particle content in 4 hr at 22 °C	1688	C
Cefepime HCl	BR	20 mg/ml[a]	LE	40 + 5 mg/ml[a]	Physically compatible with no change in measured turbidity or increase in particle content in 4 hr at 22 °C	1689	C
Chlorpromazine HCl	RU	2 mg/ml[a]	LE	40 + 5 mg/ml[a]	Heavy white turbidity forms immediately. White precipitate forms in 4 hr	1688	I
Cimetidine HCl	SKB	12 mg/ml[a]	LE	40 + 5 mg/ml[a]	Physically compatible with no change in measured turbidity or increase in particle content in 4 hr at 22 °C	1688	C
Cisatracurium besylate	GW	0.1 and 2 mg/ml[a]	CY	40 + 5 mg/ml[a]	Physically compatible with no change in measured turbidity or increase in particle content in 4 hr at 23 °C	2074	C
	GW	5 mg/ml[a]	CY	40 + 5 mg/ml[a]	Tiny particles and subvisual haze within 4 hr	2074	I
Cisplatin	BR	1 mg/ml	LE	40 + 5 mg/ml[a]	Haze and particles form in 1 hr	1688	I

Y-Site Injection Compatibility (1:1 Mixture) (Cont.)

Piperacillin sodium–tazobactam sodium

Drug	Mfr	Conc	Mfr	Conc	Remarks	Ref	C/I
Clindamycin phosphate	AB	10 mg/ml[a]	LE	40 + 5 mg/ml[a]	Physically compatible with no change in measured turbidity or increase in particle content in 4 hr at 22 °C	1688	C
Cyclophosphamide	MJ	10 mg/ml[a]	LE	40 + 5 mg/ml[a]	Physically compatible with no change in measured turbidity or increase in particle content in 4 hr at 22 °C	1688	C
Cytarabine	SCN	50 mg/ml	LE	40 + 5 mg/ml[a]	Physically compatible with no change in measured turbidity or increase in particle content in 4 hr at 22 °C	1688	C
Dacarbazine	MI	4 mg/ml[a]	LE	40 + 5 mg/ml[a]	Turbidity and particles form immediately and increase over 4 hr	1688	I
Daunorubicin HCl	WY	1 mg/ml[a]	LE	40 + 5 mg/ml[a]	Turbidity increases immediately	1688	I
Dexamethasone sodium phosphate	LY	1 mg/ml[a]	LE	40 + 5 mg/ml[a]	Physically compatible with no change in measured turbidity or increase in particle content in 4 hr at 22 °C	1688	C
Diphenhydramine HCl	WY	2 mg/ml[a]	LE	40 + 5 mg/ml[a]	Physically compatible with no change in measured turbidity or increase in particle content in 4 hr at 22 °C	1688	C
Dobutamine HCl	LI	4 mg/ml[a]	LE	40 + 5 mg/ml[a]	Heavy white turbidity forms immediately	1688	I
Docetaxel	RPR	0.9 mg/ml[a]	CY	40 + 5 mg/ml[a]	Physically compatible with no change in measured turbidity or increase in particle content in 4 hr at 23 °C	2224	C
Dopamine HCl	AST	3.2 mg/ml[a]	LE	40 + 5 mg/ml[a]	Physically compatible with no change in measured turbidity or increase in particle content in 4 hr at 22 °C	1688	C
Doxorubicin HCl	CET	2 mg/ml	LE	40 + 5 mg/ml[a]	Turbidity forms immediately	1688	I
Doxorubicin HCl liposome injection	SEQ	0.4 mg/ml[a]	CY	40 + 5 mg/ml[a]	Partial loss of measured natural turbidity	2087	I
Doxycycline hyclate	ES	1 mg/ml[a]	LE	40 + 5 mg/ml[a]	Heavy white turbidity forms immediately	1688	I
Droperidol	JN	0.4 mg/ml[a]	LE	40 + 5 mg/ml[a]	Heavy white turbidity with white precipitate forms immediately	1688	I
Enalaprilat	MSD	0.1 mg/ml[a]	LE	40 + 5 mg/ml[a]	Physically compatible with no change in measured turbidity or increase in particle content in 4 hr at 22 °C	1688	C
Etoposide	BR	0.4 mg/ml[a]	LE	40 + 5 mg/ml[a]	Physically compatible with no change in measured turbidity or increase in particle content in 4 hr at 22 °C	1688	C
Etoposide phosphate	BR	5 mg/ml[a]	LE	40 + 5 mg/ml[b]	Physically compatible with no change in measured turbidity or increase in particle content in 4 hr at 23 °C	2218	C
Famotidine	MSD	2 mg/ml[a]	LE	40 + 5 mg/ml[a]	Particles form immediately	1688	I

Y-Site Injection Compatibility (1:1 Mixture) (Cont.)

Piperacillin sodium–tazobactam sodium

Drug	Mfr	Conc	Mfr	Conc	Remarks	Ref	C/I
Floxuridine	RC	3 mg/ml[a]	LE	40 + 5 mg/ml[a]	Physically compatible with no change in measured turbidity or increase in particle content in 4 hr at 22 °C	1688	C
Fluconazole	RR	2 mg/ml	LE	40 + 5 mg/ml[a]	Physically compatible with no change in measured turbidity or increase in particle content in 4 hr at 22 °C	1688	C
Fludarabine phosphate	BX	1 mg/ml[a]	LE	40 + 5 mg/ml[a]	Physically compatible with no change in measured turbidity or increase in particle content in 4 hr at 22 °C	1688	C
Fluorouracil	LY	16 mg/ml[a]	LE	40 + 5 mg/ml[a]	Physically compatible with no change in measured turbidity or increase in particle content in 4 hr at 22 °C	1688	C
Furosemide	AB	3 mg/ml[a]	LE	40 + 5 mg/ml[a]	Physically compatible with no change in measured turbidity or increase in particle content in 4 hr at 22 °C	1688	C
Ganciclovir sodium	SY	20 mg/ml[a]	LE	40 + 5 mg/ml[a]	Large crystals form in 1 hr and become heavy white precipitate in 4 hr	1688	I
Gemcitabine HCl	LI	10 mg/ml[b]	LE	40 + 5 mg/ml[b]	Cloudiness forms immediately, becoming flocculent precipitate in 1 hr	2226	I
Granisetron HCl	SKB	0.05 mg/ml[a]	CY	40 + 5 mg/ml[a]	Physically compatible with no change in measured turbidity or increase in particle content in 4 hr at 23 °C	2000	C
Haloperidol lactate	MN	0.2 mg/ml[a]	LE	40 + 5 mg/ml[a]	White turbidity and particles form immediately	1688	I
Heparin sodium	ES	100 units/ml[a]	LE	40 + 5 mg/ml[a]	Physically compatible with no change in measured turbidity or increase in particle content in 4 hr at 22 °C	1688	C
Hydrocortisone sodium phosphate	MSD	1 mg/ml[a]	LE	40 + 5 mg/ml[a]	Physically compatible with no change in measured turbidity or increase in particle content in 4 hr at 22 °C	1688	C
Hydrocortisone sodium succinate	UP	1 mg/ml[a]	LE	40 + 5 mg/ml[a]	Physically compatible with no change in measured turbidity or increase in particle content in 4 hr at 22 °C	1688	C
Hydromorphone HCl	ES	0.5 mg/ml[a]	LE	40 + 5 mg/ml[a]	Physically compatible with no change in measured turbidity or increase in particle content in 4 hr at 22 °C	1688	C
Hydroxyzine HCl	WI	4 mg/ml[a]	LE	40 + 5 mg/ml[a]	Haze and particles form immediately	1688	I
Idarubicin HCl	AD	0.5 mg/ml[a]	LE	40 + 5 mg/ml[a]	Immediate increase in haze much larger than from simple dilution alone	1688	I
Ifosfamide	MJ	25 mg/ml[a]	LE	40 + 5 mg/ml[a]	Physically compatible with no change in measured turbidity or increase in particle content in 4 hr at 22 °C	1688	C
Leucovorin calcium	LE	2 mg/ml[a]	LE	40 + 5 mg/ml[a]	Physically compatible with no change in measured turbidity or increase in particle content in 4 hr at 22 °C	1688	C
Lorazepam	WY	0.1 mg/ml[a]	LE	40 + 5 mg/ml[a]	Physically compatible with no change in measured turbidity or increase in particle content in 4 hr at 22 °C	1688	C

Y-Site Injection Compatibility (1:1 Mixture) (Cont.)

Piperacillin sodium–tazobactam sodium

Drug	Mfr	Conc	Mfr	Conc	Remarks	Ref	C/I
Magnesium sulfate	AST	100 mg/ml	LE	40 + 5 mg/ml[a]	Physically compatible with no change in measured turbidity or increase in particle content in 4 hr at 22 °C	1688	C
Mannitol	BA	15%	LE	40 + 5 mg/ml[a]	Physically compatible with no change in measured turbidity or increase in particle content in 4 hr at 22 °C	1688	C
Meperidine HCl	WY	4 mg/ml[a]	LE	40 + 5 mg/ml[a]	Physically compatible with no change in measured turbidity or increase in particle content in 4 hr at 22 °C	1688	C
Mesna	MJ	10 mg/ml[a]	LE	40 + 5 mg/ml[a]	Physically compatible with no change in measured turbidity or increase in particle content in 4 hr at 22 °C	1688	C
Methotrexate sodium	LE	15 mg/ml[a]	LE	40 + 5 mg/ml[a]	Physically compatible with no change in measured turbidity or increase in particle content in 4 hr at 22 °C	1688	C
Methylprednisolone sodium succinate	AB	5 mg/ml[a]	LE	40 + 5 mg/ml[a]	Physically compatible with no change in measured turbidity or increase in particle content in 4 hr at 22 °C	1688	C
Metoclopramide HCl	RB	5 mg/ml	LE	40 + 5 mg/ml[a]	Physically compatible with no change in measured turbidity or increase in particle content in 4 hr at 22 °C	1688	C
Metronidazole	BA	5 mg/ml	LE	40 + 5 mg/ml[a]	Physically compatible with no change in measured turbidity or increase in particle content in 4 hr at 22 °C	1688	C
Minocycline HCl	LE	1 mg/ml[a]	LE	40 + 5 mg/ml[a]	Particles form immediately, becoming numerous in 4 hr	1688	I
Mitomycin	BR	0.5 mg/ml	LE	40 + 5 mg/ml[a]	Blue color darkens in 4 hr, becoming reddish purple in 24 hr	1688	I
Mitoxantrone HCl	LE	0.5 mg/ml[a]	LE	40 + 5 mg/ml[a]	Haze and particles form immediately. Large particles form in 4 hr	1688	I
Morphine sulfate	WY	1 mg/ml[a]	LE	40 + 5 mg/ml[a]	Physically compatible with no change in measured turbidity or increase in particle content in 4 hr at 22 °C	1688	C
Nalbuphine HCl	DU	10 mg/ml	LE	40 + 5 mg/ml[a]	Heavy white turbidity forms immediately. Particles form in 4 hr	1688	I
Ondansetron HCl	GL	1 mg/ml[a]	LE	40 + 5 mg/ml[a]	Physically compatible with no change in measured turbidity or increase in particle content in 4 hr at 22 °C	1688	C
	GL	0.03, 0.1, 0.3 mg/ml[b]	LE	40 + 5 mg/ml[b]	Visually compatible with no loss of any component by HPLC in 4 hr	1751	C
	GL	0.03, 0.1, 0.3 mg/ml[b]	LE	80 + 10 mg/ml[b]	Visually compatible with no loss of any component by HPLC in 4 hr	1751	C
Plicamycin	MI	0.01 mg/ml[a]	LE	40 + 5 mg/ml[a]	Physically compatible with no change in measured turbidity or increase in particle content in 4 hr at 22 °C	1688	C
Potassium chloride	AB	0.1 mEq/ml[a]	LE	40 + 5 mg/ml[a]	Physically compatible with no change in measured turbidity or increase in particle content in 4 hr at 22 °C	1688	C

Y-Site Injection Compatibility (1:1 Mixture) (Cont.)

Drug	Mfr	Conc	Mfr	Conc	Remarks	Ref	C/I
				Piperacillin sodium–tazobactam sodium			
Prochlorperazine edisylate	SCN	0.5 mg/ml[a]	LE	40 + 5 mg/ml[a]	White turbidity forms immediately	1688	**I**
Promethazine HCl	SCN	2 mg/ml[a]	LE	40 + 5 mg/ml[a]	Heavy white turbidity forms immediately. Particles form in 4 hr	1688	**I**
Ranitidine HCl	GL	2 mg/ml[a]	LE	40 + 5 mg/ml[a]	Physically compatible with no change in measured turbidity or increase in particle content in 4 hr at 22 °C	1688	**C**
	GL	0.5 and 2 mg/ml[b]	LE	80 + 10 mg/ml[b]	Visually compatible with little or no loss of any component by HPLC in 4 hr at 23 °C	1759	**C**
	GL	0.5 and 2 mg/ml[b]	LE	40 + 5 mg/ml[b]	Visually compatible with little or no loss of ranitidine and tazobactam by HPLC in 4 hr at 23 °C. Piperacillin not tested	1759	**C**
Remifentanil HCl	GW	0.025 and 0.25 mg/ml[b]	CY	40 + 5 mg/ml[a]	Physically compatible with no change in measured turbidity or increase in particle content in 4 hr at 23 °C	2075	**C**
Sargramostim	HO	10 μg/ml[a]	LE	40 + 5 mg/ml[a]	Physically compatible with no change in measured turbidity or increase in particle content in 4 hr at 22 °C	1688	**C**
Sodium bicarbonate	AB	1 mEq/ml	LE	40 + 5 mg/ml[a]	Physically compatible with no change in measured turbidity or increase in particle content in 4 hr at 22 °C	1688	**C**
Streptozocin	UP	40 mg/ml[a]	LE	40 + 5 mg/ml[a]	Particles form in 1 hr	1688	**I**
Thiotepa	LE	1 mg/ml[a]	LE	40 + 5 mg/ml[a]	Physically compatible with no change in measured turbidity or increase in particle content in 4 hr at 22 °C	1688	**C**
TNA #218 to #226[c]			LE	40 + 5 mg/ml[a]	Visually compatible with no precipitate or emulsion damage apparent in 4 hr at 23 °C	2215	**C**
TPN #212 to #215[c]			CY	40 + 5 mg/ml[a]	Physically compatible with no change in measured turbidity or increase in particle content in 4 hr at 23 °C	2109	**C**
Trimethoprim–sulfamethoxazole	ES	0.8 + 4 mg/ml[a]	LE	40 + 5 mg/ml[a]	Physically compatible with no change in measured turbidity or increase in particle content in 4 hr at 22 °C	1688	**C**
Vancomycin HCl	AB	10 mg/ml[a]	LE	40 + 5 mg/ml[a]	White turbidity forms immediately. White precipitate forms in 4 hr	1688	**I**
	AB	20 mg/ml[a]	LE	200 + 25 mg/ml[d]	Transient precipitate forms, followed by clear solution	2189	**?**
	AB	20 mg/ml[a]	LE	50 + 6.25 and 10 + 1.25 mg/ml[a]	Gross white precipitate forms immediately	2189	**I**
	AB	20 mg/ml[a]	LE	1 + 0.125 mg/ml[a]	Physically compatible with no change in measured turbidity or increase in particle content in 4 hr at 23 °C	2189	**C**
	AB	2 mg/ml[a]	LE	1 + 0.125[a], 10 + 1.25[a], 50 + 6.25[a], and 200 + 25[d] mg/ml	Physically compatible with no change in measured turbidity or increase in particle content in 4 hr at 23 °C	2189	**C**

Y-Site Injection Compatibility (1:1 Mixture) (Cont.)

Piperacillin sodium–tazobactam sodium

Drug	Mfr	Conc	Mfr	Conc	Remarks	Ref	C/I
Vinblastine sulfate	LI	0.12 mg/ml[a]	LE	40 + 5 mg/ml[a]	Physically compatible with no change in measured turbidity or increase in particle content in 4 hr at 22 °C	1688	**C**
Vincristine sulfate	LI	0.05 mg/ml[a]	LE	40 + 5 mg/ml[a]	Physically compatible with no change in measured turbidity or increase in particle content in 4 hr at 22 °C	1688	**C**
Zidovudine	BW	4 mg/ml[a]	LE	40 + 5 mg/ml[a]	Physically compatible with no change in measured turbidity or increase in particle content in 4 hr at 22 °C	1688	**C**

[a]*Tested in dextrose 5% in water.*
[b]*Tested in sodium chloride 0.9%.*
[c]*Refer to Appendix I for the composition of parenteral nutrition solutions. TNA indicates a 3-in-1 admixture, and TPN indicates a 2-in-1 admixture.*
[d]*Tested in sterile water for injection.*

Additional Compatibility Information

Also see Piperacillin Sodium monograph.

Solutions—— The manufacturer states that the following intravenous solutions are compatible with piperacillin sodium–tazobactam sodium (2):

Bacteriostatic sodium chloride 0.9% (benzyl alcohol or parabens)
Bacteriostatic water for injection (benzyl alcohol or parabens)
Dextran 6% in sodium chloride 0.9%
Dextrose 5% in water
Sodium chloride 0.9%
Sterile water for injection

The manufacturer also states that piperacillin sodium–tazobactam sodium is incompatible with Ringer's injection, lactated (2).

Peritoneal Dialysis Solutions—— The physical and chemical stability of piperacillin sodium–tazobactam sodium (Lederle) at concentrations of 200 and 25 µg/ml, respectively, were evaluated in Dianeal PD-2 with dextrose 1.5% and Dianeal PD-2 with dextrose 4.25% (Baxter). Samples were stored at 4 °C for 14 days, 23 °C for seven days, and 37 °C for one day. The samples were physically and chemically stable. Little or no loss of either component occurred in the 4 °C samples throughout the 14-day period. At 23 °C, losses of each component were in the range of 3 to 6% in seven days. The one-day losses at 37 °C were similarly small (2018).

Vancomycin—— The compatibility or incompatibility of vancomycin HCl mixed with or administered simultaneously with piperacillin sodium–tazobactam sodium is concentration dependent (2189). See Y-Site Compatibility above. Vancomycin HCl has a low pH and is variably compatible with drugs having neutral to mildly alkaline pH, including cephalosporins and penicillins. The compatibility may depend on a number of factors, including concentration of each drug, dilution vehicle, actual pH of solutions, and completeness of mixing during administration. Combinations that are compatible when well mixed may result in precipitation if only partially mixed, presumably because of regionally different concentrations and pH values. If attempting to administer vancomycin HCl with piperacillin sodium–tazobactam sodium, take care to ensure that the specific combination and the concentrations are compatible under the exact administration conditions to be used. An inline filter should be used as a final safety measure (2189).

Miscellaneous—— Potassium chloride injection in stated to be compatible with piperacillin sodium–tazobactam sodium (2).

Aminoglycosides should not be combined with piperacillin sodium–tazobactam sodium because substantial aminoglycoside inactivation may occur. Concomitant therapy should be performed with separate administration (2).

PLICAMYCIN
(MITHRAMYCIN)
AHFS 10:00

Mithracin   **Bayer**

Products—— Plicamycin (Bayer) is available in vials containing 2500 µg (2.5 mg) of the drug in a freeze-dried preparation. Also present are mannitol 100 mg and disodium phosphate to adjust the pH (2).

Reconstitute with 4.9 ml of water for injection and shake to dissolve the drug. The vials contain an excess of drug so that the concentration of reconstituted vials is 500 µg/ml (2; 4).

pH—— The pH is adjusted to 7 (2).

Osmolality—— Plicamycin (Bayer) 0.5 mg/ml in sterile water for injection has an osmolality of 104 mOsm/kg (2043).

Administration— Plicamycin is administered by intravenous infusion. The appropriate dose is added to 1000 ml of dextrose 5% in water or sodium chloride 0.9% and administered over four to six hours. Extravasation should be avoided because of local tissue irritation and cellulitis. Rapid direct intravenous push administration is associated with a higher incidence and greater severity of side effects and is not recommended (2; 4).

Stability— The intact vials should be stored at 2 to 8 °C (2). Although refrigeration is recommended, intact vials of plicamycin have been variously reported by the manufacturer to be stable at room temperatures less than 25 °C for five days (1433) or longer (60; 1369).

Plicamycin contains no antibacterial preservative. The manufacturer recommends that the plicamycin solution be prepared freshly each day of therapy and that any remaining unused solution be discarded (2). Reconstituting the solution immediately before injection has also been recommended (4). However, reconstituted solutions have been found to be chemically stable for two days under refrigeration (1369).

pH Effects— Plicamycin is rapidly hydrolyzed in acidic solutions below pH 4 (4). At pH 4 to 5, 13% losses in 24 hours have been reported. At pH 5 to 7.5, the drug is stable in solution for at least two days at 2 to 6 °C (1369).

Filtration— Plicamycin (Pfizer) 2.5 mg/L in dextrose 5% in water and sodium chloride 0.9% was filtered at 120 ml/hr for six hours through a 0.22-μm cellulose ester membrane filter (Ivex-2). Significant losses of plicamycin due to binding to the filters were noted with both solutions. In dextrose 5% in water, a total of 14.3% of the dose was bound over the six-hour period; a 9.9% loss occurred over this time from the sodium chloride 0.9% solution (533).

In static equilibrium experiments, 100 mg of 0.22-μm cellulose ester membrane filter (Ivex-2) was soaked in 25 ml of plicamycin (Pfizer) 25 and 50 μg/ml in both dextrose 5% in water and sodium chloride 0.9%. In dextrose 5% in water, about 60 and 40% were bound to the filter for each strength, respectively, in 24 hours. In sodium chloride 0.9%, about 33 to 39% was bound for both strengths in the same time (533).

In a followup study, a filter material specially treated with a proprietary agent was evaluated for a reduction in plicamycin binding. Plicamycin (Miles) 2.5 mg/L in dextrose 5% in water and sodium chloride 0.9% was run through an administration set with a treated 0.22-μm cellulose ester inline filter at a rate of 2 ml/min. Cumulative plicamycin losses of about 4% occurred from both solutions compared to the much higher losses previously reported for untreated cellulose ester filter material. Furthermore, equilibrium binding studies showed five- and sevenfold reductions in binding from sodium chloride 0.9% and dextrose 5% in water, respectively (904). All Abbott Ivex integral filter and extension sets currently use this treated filter material (1074).

Compatibility Information

Y-Site Injection Compatibility (1:1 Mixture)

Plicamycin

Drug	Mfr	Conc	Mfr	Conc	Remarks	Ref	C/I
Allopurinol sodium	BW	3 mg/ml[b]	MI	0.01 mg/ml[b]	Physically compatible with no change in measured turbidity or increase in particle content in 4 hr at 22 °C	1686	C
Amifostine	USB	10 mg/ml[a]	MI	0.01 mg/ml[a]	Physically compatible with no change in measured turbidity or increase in particle content in 4 hr at 23 °C	1845	C
Aztreonam	SQ	40 mg/ml[a]	MI	0.01 mg/ml[a]	Physically compatible with no subvisual haze or particle formation in 4 hr at 23 °C	1758	C
Cefepime HCl	BR	20 mg/ml[a]	MI	0.01 mg/ml[a]	Haze forms immediately. Particles form in 1 hr	1689	I
Etoposide phosphate	BR	5 mg/ml[a]	MI	0.01 mg/ml[a]	Physically compatible with no change in measured turbidity or increase in particle content in 4 hr at 23 °C	2218	C
Filgrastim	AMG	30 μg/ml[a]	MI	0.01 mg/ml[a]	Physically compatible with no change in measured turbidity or increase in particle content in 4 hr at 22 °C	1687	C
Gemcitabine HCl	LI	10 mg/ml[b]	BAY	0.01 mg/ml[b]	Physically compatible with no change in measured turbidity or increase in particle content in 4 hr at 23 °C	2226	C
Granisetron HCl	SKB	0.05 mg/ml[a]	BAY	0.01 mg/ml[a]	Physically compatible with no change in measured turbidity or increase in particle content in 4 hr at 23 °C	2000	C

Y-Site Injection Compatibility (1:1 Mixture) (Cont.)

		Plicamycin					
Drug	*Mfr*	*Conc*	*Mfr*	*Conc*	*Remarks*	*Ref*	*C/I*
Melphalan HCl	BW	0.1 mg/ml[b]	MI	0.01 mg/ml[b]	Physically compatible with no change in measured turbidity or increase in particle content in 3 hr at 22 °C	1557	C
Piperacillin sodium–tazobactam sodium	LE	40 + 5 mg/ml[a]	MI	0.01 mg/ml[a]	Physically compatible with no change in measured turbidity or increase in particle content in 4 hr at 22 °C	1688	C
Teniposide	BR	0.1 mg/ml[a]	MI	0.01 mg/ml[a]	Physically compatible with no subvisual haze or particle formation in 4 hr at 23 °C	1725	C
Thiotepa	IMM[c]	1 mg/ml[a]	MI	0.01 mg/ml[a]	Physically compatible with no change in measured turbidity or increase in particle content in 4 hr at 23 °C	1861	C
Vinorelbine tartrate	BW	1 mg/ml[b]	MI	0.01 mg/ml[b]	Physically compatible with no change in measured turbidity or increase in particle content in 4 hr at 22 °C	1558	C

[a]*Tested in dextrose 5% in water.*
[b]*Tested in sodium chloride 0.9%.*
[c]*Lyophilized formulation tested.*

Additional Compatibility Information

Plicamycin has a strong ability to chelate metal ions, especially iron (4; 1369).

Solutions—— Dextrose 5% in water and sodium chloride 0.9% have been recommended as appropriate infusion solutions for plicamycin (2; 4). In a study of plicamycin (Dome) 23.8 μg/ml in dextrose 5% in water (Travenol) in both glass and PVC containers, less than a 10% decrease in plicamycin content occurred in 24 hours at room temperature (519).

Other Information

Inactivation—— In the event of spills or leaks, Miles recommends the use of trisodium phosphate 10%, in contact for 24 hours, to inactivate plicamycin (1200).

POLYMYXIN B SULFATE
AHFS 8:12.28

Products—— Polymyxin B sulfate is available in 10-ml vials containing 500,000 units of polymyxin B. For intramuscular injection, reconstitute the vial with 2 ml of sterile water for injection, sodium chloride 0.9%, or procaine HCl 1% solution. For intravenous infusion, dilute 500,000 units in 300 to 500 ml of dextrose 5% in water. For intrathecal administration, reconstitute the vial with 10 ml of sodium chloride 0.9%. Procaine HCl should not be used for intrathecal injection (4; 29).

pH—— From 5 to 7.5 (4; 54).

Osmolality—— Polymyxin B sulfate 50,000 units/ml in sterile water for injection has an osmolality of 10 mOsm/kg (1689).

Equivalency—— Each milligram of polymyxin base is equivalent to 10,000 units. Each microgram is equivalent to 10 units (4).

Administration—— Polymyxin B sulfate is usually administered by intravenous infusion; 500,000 units is added to 300 to 500 ml of dextrose 5% in water (providing 1667 to 1000 units/ml) and is administered over 60 to 90 minutes. The drug may also be administered intrathecally as a 50,000-units/ml solution in sodium chloride 0.9%. Although it may be administered by deep intramuscular injection in the upper outer quadrant of the gluteal muscles, this route is generally not recommended, because severe pain at the injection site results (4).

Stability—— Intact vials should be stored at temperatures not exceeding 30 °C and protected from light. Aqueous solutions of polymyxin B sulfate in the pH range of 5 to 7.5 are stable for six to 12 months under refrigeration. However, it is recommended that unused portions of the reconstituted solution be discarded after 72 hours. Polymyxin B sulfate is inactivated in strongly acidic or alkaline solutions (4). In the pH range of 2 to 7, pH has little effect on the rate of decomposition. However, as pH values become more alkaline, the rate of decomposition increases markedly (1946).

Compatibility Information

Solution Compatibility

Polymyxin B sulfate

Solution	Mfr	Mfr	Conc/L	Remarks	Ref	C/I
Invert sugar 7.5% with electrolytes		NOV	40 mg	Physically compatible with no polymyxin B loss in 24 hr at 29 °C by microbiological assay	440	C
TPN #52 and #53[a]		NOV	40 mg	Physically compatible with no polymyxin B loss in 24 hr at 29 °C by microbiological assay	440	C

[a]*Refer to Appendix I for the composition of parenteral nutrition solutions. TPN indicates a 2-in-1 admixture.*

Additive Compatibility

Polymyxin B sulfate

Drug	Mfr	Conc/L	Mfr	Conc/L	Test Soln	Remarks	Ref	C/I
Amikacin sulfate	BR	5 g	BW	200 mg	D5LR, D5R, D5S, D5W, D10W, IS10, LR, NS, R, SL	Physically compatible and amikacin potency retained for 24 hr at 25 °C. Polymyxin not analyzed	293	C
Amphotericin B		200 mg	BP	20 mg	D5W	Haze develops over 3 hr	26	I
Ascorbic acid injection	UP	500 mg	BW	200 mg	D5W	Physically compatible	15	C
Chloramphenicol sodium succinate	PD	10 g	BW	200 mg	D5W	Physically incompatible	15	I
	PD	10 g	BW	200 mg		Precipitate forms within 1 hr	6	I
Chlorothiazide sodium	BP	2 g	BP	20 mg	D5W	Yellow color produced	26	I
Colistimethate sodium	WC	500 mg	BW	200 mg	D5W	Physically compatible	15	C
Diphenhydramine HCl	PD	80 mg	BW	200 mg	D5W	Physically compatible	15	C
Erythromycin lactobionate	AB	5 g	BW	200 mg	D5W	Physically compatible	15	C
Heparin sodium	BP	20,000 units	BP	20 mg	D5W	Immediate precipitation	26	I
	BP	20,000 units	BP	20 mg	NS	Haze develops over 3 hr	26	I
Hydrocortisone sodium succinate	UP	500 mg	BW	200 mg	D5W	Physically compatible	15	C
Kanamycin sulfate	BR	4 g	BW	200 mg	D5W	Physically compatible	15	C
Magnesium sulfate	LI	16 mEq	BW	200 mg	D5W	Physically incompatible	15	I
Penicillin G potassium	SQ	20 million units	BW	200 mg	D5W	Physically compatible	15	C
	SQ	5 million units	BW	200 mg	D	Physically compatible	47	C
Penicillin G sodium	UP	20 million units	BW	200 mg	D5W	Physically compatible	15	C
Phenobarbital sodium	WI	200 mg	BW	200 mg	D5W	Physically compatible	15	C
Ranitidine HCl	GL	50 mg and 2 g		1 million units	D5W	Physically compatible and ranitidine chemically stable by HPLC for 24 hr at 25 °C. Polymyxin B not tested	1515	C

Additive Compatibility (Cont.)

Polymyxin B sulfate

Drug	Mfr	Conc/L	Mfr	Conc/L	Test Soln	Remarks	Ref	C/I
Vitamin B complex with C	AB	5 ml	BW	200 mg	D5W	Physically compatible	15	C

Drugs in Syringe Compatibility

Polymyxin B sulfate

Drug (in syringe)	Mfr	Amt	Mfr	Amt	Remarks	Ref	C/I
Ampicillin sodium	AY	500 mg	BW	25 mg/ 1.5 ml	Physically compatible for 1 hr at room temperature	300	C
	AY	250 mg	BW	25 mg/ 1.5 ml	Precipitate forms within 1 hr at room temperature	300	I
Penicillin G sodium		1 million units	BW	25 mg/ 1.5 to 2 ml	No precipitate or color change within 1 hr at room temperature	99	C

Y-Site Injection Compatibility (1:1 Mixture)

Polymyxin B sulfate

Drug	Mfr	Conc	Mfr	Conc	Remarks	Ref	C/I
Esmolol HCl	DCC	10 mg/ml[a]	PF	0.005 unit/ ml[a]	Physically compatible for 24 hr at 22 °C	1169	C

[a]*Tested in dextrose 5% in water.*

Additional Compatibility Information

Miscellaneous— Polymyxin B sulfate has been reported to be visually compatible and stable for 24 hours at 29 °C in a parenteral nutrition solution (854).

Polymyxin B sulfate is stated to be physically compatible for 24 hours at room temperature with lincomycin HCl in infusion solutions (154).

Solutions of polymyxin B sulfate are stated to be inactivated by alkalies and strong acids (4). Cefazolin sodium also appears to be incompatible with polymyxin B sulfate (278) as are calcium and magnesium salts (4).

POTASSIUM ACETATE
AHFS 40:12

Abbott
Fujisawa

Products— Potassium acetate additive solution is available in 20-, 50-, and 100-ml vials at a concentration of 2 mEq/ml in water for injection. Each milliliter provides potassium acetate 196 mg. It is also available in 50-ml vials at a concentration of 4 mEq/ml in water for injection. Each milliliter provides 392 mg of potassium acetate. The pH of the solutions may have been adjusted with acetic acid when necessary. These concentrated solutions must be diluted for administration (1-10/93; 29).

pH— The pH of potassium acetate additive solution has been stated to be approximately 7.1 to 7.7 (4) and around 6.2 to 6.3 with a range of 5.5 to 8 (1-10/93).

Osmolarity— The calculated osmolarity of the 2-mEq/ml solution is 4000 mOsm/L and for the 4-mEq/ml solution is 8000 mOsm/L (1-10/93).

Administration— Potassium acetate is administered as a dilute solution by slow intravenous infusion (1-10/93; 4). In most cases, the maximum recommended concentration is 40 mEq/L. Solutions generally may be infused at a rate up to 20 mEq/hr (4).

Stability— Potassium acetate additive solution should be stored at room temperature and protected from freezing. It should not be administered unless the solution is clear (1-10/93).

Compatibility Information

Additive Compatibility

Potassium acetate

Drug	Mfr	Conc/L	Mfr	Conc/L	Test Soln	Remarks	Ref	C/I
Metoclopramide HCl	RB	10 and 160 mg	IX	20 mEq	NS	Physically compatible for 48 hr at room temperature	924	**C**
	RB	10 and 160 mg	IX	20 mEq		Physically compatible for 48 hr at 25 °C	1167	**C**

Y-Site Injection Compatibility (1:1 Mixture)

Potassium acetate

Drug	Mfr	Conc	Mfr	Conc	Remarks	Ref	C/I
Ciprofloxacin	MI	2 mg/ml[a]	LY	2 mEq/ml	Visually compatible for 2 hr at 25 °C	1628	**C**

[a]*Tested in dextrose 5% in water.*

POTASSIUM CHLORIDE
AHFS 40:12

Abbott

Products— Potassium chloride (Abbott) is available as concentrated solutions of 1.5 and 2 mEq/ml in 10-, 20-, 30-, and 40-mEq sizes in water for injection in ampuls, vials, and syringes. It is also available in 250-ml pharmacy bulk packages (29). The pH may have been adjusted with hydrochloric acid. The concentrated solutions must be diluted before use (1-8/95).

Potassium chloride is also available premixed in infusion solutions in concentrations of 10, 20, 30, and 40 mEq/L (4).

pH— From 4 to 8 (4). The Abbott products have a target pH of 5.4 for the syringe and of 4.6 for the other dosage forms (1-8/95).

Osmotic Values— The manufacturer states that the approximate osmolarities of the 1.5- and 2-mEq/ml concentrations are 3000 and 4000 mOsm/L, respectively (1-8/95).

The osmolality of potassium chloride (Abbott) 2 mEq/ml was determined to be 4355 mOsm/kg by freezing-point depression and 3440 mOsm/kg by vapor pressure (1071).

The osmolality of a potassium chloride 7.5% solution was determined to be 1895 mOsm/kg (1233).

Administration— Potassium chloride in the concentrated injections must be diluted before administration. Mix potassium chloride injection thoroughly with the infusion solution before administration. See Other Information below. The usual maximum concentration is 40 mEq/L. Extravasation should be avoided (1-8/95; 4)

Stability— The solution should be stored at controlled room temperature and used only if it is clear (1-8/95).

Potassium chloride injection 80 mEq/L added to dextrose 5% in water contained in glass bottles results in a leaching of precipitates consisting of silica and alumina (129).

Compatibility Information

Solution Compatibility

Potassium chloride

Solution	Mfr	Mfr	Conc/L	Remarks	Ref	C/I
Alcohol 5% and dextrose 5%	BA	LI	80 mEq	Physically compatible for 24 hr	315	**C**
Dextran 6% in dextrose 5%	AB	AB	160 mEq	Physically compatible	3	**C**
Dextran 6% in sodium chloride 0.9%	AB	AB	160 mEq	Physically compatible	3	**C**
Dextrose–Ringer's injection combinations	AB	AB	160 mEq	Physically compatible	3	**C**
Dextrose–Ringer's injection, lactated, combinations	AB	AB	160 mEq	Physically compatible	3	**C**

Solution Compatibility (Cont.)

Potassium chloride

Solution	Mfr	Mfr	Conc/L	Remarks	Ref	C/I
Dextrose 5% in Ringer's injection, lactated	BA	LI	80 mEq	Physically compatible for 24 hr	315	C
Dextrose–saline combinations	AB	AB	160 mEq	Physically compatible	3	C
Dextrose 5% in sodium chloride 0.9%			3 g	Physically compatible	74	C
	BA	LI	80 mEq	Physically compatible for 24 hr	315	C
Dextrose 2½% in water	AB	AB	160 mEq	Physically compatible	3	C
Dextrose 5% in water			3 g	Physically compatible	74	C
	AB	AB	160 mEq	Physically compatible	3	C
	BA	LI	80 mEq	Physically compatible for 24 hr	315	C
Dextrose 10% in water	AB	AB	160 mEq	Physically compatible	3	C
	BA	LI	80 mEq	Physically compatible for 24 hr	315	C
Dextrose 20% in water	BA	LI	80 mEq	Physically compatible for 24 hr	315	C
Fat emulsion 10%, intravenous	VT		7.5 g	Physically compatible for 48 hr at 4 °C and room temperature	32	C
	CU		200 mEq	Globule coalescence with noticeable surface creaming in 4 hr at room temperature. Oil globules noted on surface at 48 hr	656	I
	CU		100 mEq	No significant change in emulsion for 24 hr at room temperature. Significant globule coalescence noted at 48 hr	656	C
	VT	DB	4 g	Microscopic globule coalescence in 24 hr at 8 and 25 °C	825	I
Fructose 10% in sodium chloride 0.9%	AB	AB	160 mEq	Physically compatible	3	C
Fructose 10% in water	AB	AB	160 mEq	Physically compatible	3	C
	BA	LI	80 mEq	Physically compatible for 24 hr	315	C
Invert sugar 10% in Electrolyte #1	BA	LI	80 mEq	Physically compatible for 24 hr	315	C
Invert sugar 10% in Electrolyte #2	BA	LI	80 mEq	Physically compatible for 24 hr	315	C
Invert sugar 5 and 10% in sodium chloride 0.9%	AB	AB	160 mEq	Physically compatible	3	C
Invert sugar 5 and 10% in water	AB	AB	160 mEq	Physically compatible	3	C
Ionosol products	AB	AB	160 mEq	Physically compatible	3	C
Polysal M with dextrose 5%	CU	LI	80 mEq	Physically compatible for 24 hr	315	C
Ringer's injection	AB	AB	160 mEq	Physically compatible	3	C
			3 g	Physically compatible	74	C
Ringer's injection, lactated	AB	AB	160 mEq	Physically compatible	3	C
	BA	LI	80 mEq	Physically compatible for 24 hr	315	C
Sodium chloride 0.45%	AB	AB	160 mEq	Physically compatible	3	C
Sodium chloride 0.9%			3 g	Physically compatible	74	C
	AB	AB	160 mEq	Physically compatible	3	C
	BA	LI	80 mEq	Physically compatible for 24 hr	315	C
Sodium chloride 3%	BA	LI	80 mEq	Physically compatible for 24 hr	315	C
Sodium lactate ⅙ M	AB	AB	160 mEq	Physically compatible	3	C
	BA	LI	80 mEq	Physically compatible for 24 hr	315	C

Additive Compatibility

Potassium chloride

Drug	Mfr	Conc/L	Mfr	Conc/L	Test Soln	Remarks	Ref	C/I
Amikacin sulfate	BR	5 g	LI	3 g	D5LR, D5R, D5S, D5W, D10W, IS10, LR, NS, R, SL	Physically compatible and potency of both retained for 24 hr at 25 °C	294	C
	BR	5 g	LI	3 g	DXN–S	14% amikacin decomposition in 4 hr at 25 °C	294	I
Aminophylline		250 mg		3 g	D5W	Physically compatible	74	C
	SE	500 mg	AB	40 mEq		Physically compatible	6	C
Amiodarone HCl	LZ	1.8 g	AB	40 mEq	D5W, NS[a]	Physically compatible with no amiodarone loss in 24 hr at 24 °C under fluorescent light	1031	C
Amoxicillin sodium		10, 20, 50 g		0.3%	NS	4 and 9% amoxicillin losses in 8 hr at 10 and 20 g/L, respectively, and 9% loss in 3 hr at 50 g/L at 25 °C	1469	I
Amphotericin B		200 mg	BP	4 g	D5W	Haze develops over 3 hr	26	I
	SQ	100 mg	AB	100 mEq	D5W	Physically incompatible	15	I
Atracurium besylate	BW	500 mg		80 mEq	D5W	Physically compatible and atracurium chemically stable for 24 hr at 5 and 30 °C	1694	C
Bretylium tosylate	ACC	10 g	AB	40 mEq	D5W[b]	Physically compatible and chemically stable for 48 hr at room temperature and 7 days at 4 °C	541	C
Calcium gluconate		1 g		3 g	D5W	Physically compatible	74	C
Cefepime HCl	BR	4 g	AB	40 mEq	D5W, NS	Visually compatible with 2% cefepime loss by HPLC in 24 hr at room temperature or 7 days at 5 °C	1681	C
	BR	4 g	AB	10 mEq	D5W	Visually compatible with 2% cefepime loss by HPLC in 24 hr at room temperature or 7 days at 5 °C	1681	C
Chloramphenicol sodium succinate	PD	500 mg		3 g	D5W	Physically compatible	74	C
	PD	1 g	AB	40 mEq		Physically compatible	6	C
	PD	500 mg and 1 g		20 and 40 mEq	D2.5½S, D5W	Therapeutic availability maintained	110	C
Cibenzoline succinate		2 g	IX	160 mEq	D5W, NS	Physically compatible for 24 hr at 25 °C by visual and microscopic examination	1182	C
Cimetidine HCl	SKF	1.2 and 5 g	SKF	20 mEq	D5S, D5W, NS	Physically compatible and cimetidine chemically stable for 24 hr at room temperature. Potassium chloride not tested	551	C
	SKF	1.2 and 5 g	SKF	80 mEq	D5S, D5W, NS	Physically compatible and cimetidine chemically stable for 24 hr at room temperature. Potassium chloride not tested	551	C
Ciprofloxacin	BAY	2 g	AB	40 mEq	NS	Visually compatible with little or no ciprofloxacin loss by HPLC in 24 hr at 25 °C	1934	C

Additive Compatibility (Cont.)

Potassium chloride

Drug	Mfr	Conc/L	Mfr	Conc/L	Test Soln	Remarks	Ref	C/I
Clindamycin phosphate	UP	600 mg		40 mEq	D5½S	Physically compatible and clindamycin potency retained for 24 hr at room temperature	104	**C**
	UP	600 mg		100 mEq	D5W, NS	Physically compatible	101	**C**
	UP	6 g		400 mEq	D5½S	Clindamycin stability maintained for 24 hr	101	**C**
Corticotropin		500 units		3 g	D5W	Physically compatible	74	**C**
Cytarabine	UP	2 g		100 mEq	D5S	Physically compatible and chemically stable for 8 days	174	**C**
	UP	170 mg		80 mEq	D5S	Physically compatible for 24 hr	174	**C**
Dimenhydrinate	SE	50 mg		3 g	D5W	Physically compatible	74	**C**
Dobutamine HCl	LI	1 g	ES	160 mEq	D5W, NS	Slightly pink in 24 hr at 25 °C	789	**I**
	LI	1 g	AB	20 mEq	D5W, NS	Physically compatible for 24 hr at 21 °C	812	**C**
Dopamine HCl	AS	800 mg	MG		D5W	No dopamine decomposition in 24 hr at 25 °C	312	**C**
Enalaprilat	MSD	12 mg	AB	3 g	D5W[a]	Visually compatible with little or no enalaprilat loss by HPLC in 24 hr at room temperature under fluorescent light. Potassium chloride not tested	1572	**C**
Erythromycin lactobionate	AB	1 g	AB	40 mEq		Physically compatible	20	**C**
Etoposide with cisplatin and mannitol	BR BR LY	400 mg 200 mg 1.875%	LY	20 mEq	NS[b]	Physically compatible and etoposide and cisplatin chemically stable for 8 hr at 22 °C. Precipitate forms within 24 hr	1329	**I**
Etoposide with cisplatin and mannitol	BR BR LY	400 mg 200 mg 1.875%	BR	20 mEq	D5½S[b]	Physically compatible and etoposide and cisplatin chemically stable for 24 hr at 22 °C. Precipitate forms within 48 hr	1329	**C**
Floxacillin sodium	BE	20 g	ANT	40 mM	W	Physically compatible for 72 hr at 15 and 30 °C	1479	**C**
Fluconazole	PF	1 g	AB	10 mEq	D5W[a]	Fluconazole chemically stable by gas chromatography for at least 24 hr at 25 °C under fluorescent light	1676	**C**
Foscarnet sodium	AST	12 g		20, 40, 60, 80, 120 mmol	NS	Foscarnet stability was maintained for at least 65 hr. UV analysis found concentrations of 93 to 99% throughout	2156	**C**
Fosphenytoin sodium	PD	1, 8, 20 mg PE/ml[e]	BA	20 and 40 mEq	D5½S[a]	Visually compatible with little or no loss of fosphenytoin by HPLC in 7 days at 25 °C under fluorescent light	2083	**C**
Furosemide	HO	1 g	ANT	40 mmol	W	Physically compatible for 72 hr at 15 and 30 °C	1479	**C**
Heparin sodium		12,000 units		3 g	D5W	Physically compatible	74	**C**
	AB	20,000 units	AB	40 mEq		Physically compatible	21	**C**
		32,000 units		80 mEq	NS	Physically compatible and heparin activity retained for 24 hr	57	**C**
Hydrocortisone sodium succinate	UP	100 mg		3 g	D5W	Physically compatible	74	**C**

Additive Compatibility (Cont.)

Potassium chloride

Drug	Mfr	Conc/L	Mfr	Conc/L	Test Soln	Remarks	Ref	C/I
Hydrocortisone sodium succinate with netilmicin sulfate	UP SC	400 mg 3 g	AB	160 mEq	D5S	Physically compatible and netilmicin chemically stable for 7 days at 4 and 25 °C. Other drugs not tested	558	C
Isoproterenol HCl	WI	4 mg	AB	40 mEq		Physically compatible	59	C
Lidocaine HCl	AST	2 g	AB	40 mEq		Physically compatible	24	C
Metaraminol bitartrate	MSD	100 mg	AB	40 mEq		Physically compatible	7	C
Methyldopate HCl	MSD	1 g		40 mEq	D, D–S, S	Physically compatible	23	C
Metoclopramide HCl	RB	10 and 160 mg	ES	30 mEq	NS	Physically compatible for 48 hr at room temperature	924	C
	RB	10 and 160 mg	ES	30 mEq		Physically compatible for 48 hr at 25 °C	1167	C
Mitoxantrone HCl	LE	500 mg		50 mEq	D5W	Visually compatible and mitoxantrone potency by HPLC retained for 24 hr at room temperature. Potassium chloride not tested	1531	C
Nafcillin sodium	WY	500 mg	AB	40 mEq		Physically compatible	27	C
	WY	30 g	TR	40 mEq	NS	Nafcillin potency retained for 24 hr at 25 °C	27	C
Netilmicin sulfate	SC	3 g	AB	160 mEq	D5S	Physically compatible and netilmicin chemically stable for 7 days at 4 and 25 °C. Potassium chloride not tested	558	C
Netilmicin sulfate with hydrocortisone sodium succinate	SC UP	3 g 400 mg	AB	160 mEq	D5S	Physically compatible and netilmicin chemically stable for 7 days at 4 and 25 °C. Other drugs not tested	558	C
Norepinephrine bitartrate	WI	8 mg		3 g	D5W	Physically compatible	74	C
	WI	8 mg	AB	40 mEq	D, D–S, S	Physically compatible	77	C
Oxacillin sodium	BR	1, 2.5, 4 g		20, 40, 80 mEq	D5S, D5W	Therapeutic availability maintained	110	C
Penicillin G potassium	SQ	5 million units	AB	40 mEq		Physically compatible	47	C
	SQ	5 million units		40 mEq	D5S, D5W	Therapeutic availability maintained	110	C
	SQ	1 million units		20 mEq	D5S, D5W	Therapeutic availability maintained	110	C
Penicillin G potassium with vitamin B complex with C	SQ TR	2 million units 1 ampul		20 mEq	D5S, D5W	Therapeutic availability maintained	110	C
Penicillin G potassium with vitamin B complex with C	SQ TR	8 million units 1 ampul		40 mEq	D5S, D5W	Therapeutic availability maintained	110	C
Penicillin G sodium	KA	6 million units		40 mEq	D5W	Penicillin potency retained for at least 24 hr at 25 °C	131	C

Additive Compatibility (Cont.)

Potassium chloride

Drug	Mfr	Conc/L	Mfr	Conc/L	Test Soln	Remarks	Ref	C/I
	KA	5 million units		40 mEq	IS10	pH outside stability range for penicillin	131	**I**
Phenylephrine HCl	WI	2.5 g	AB	40 mEq	D5W	Phenylephrine potency retained for over 24 hr at 22 °C	132	**C**
Piperacillin sodium	LE	2 g		40 mEq	D5S, D5W, LR, R, NS	Physically compatible and piperacillin chemically stable for 24 hr at room temperature and 48 hr under refrigeration	740	**C**
Propafenone HCl	KN	0.54 g	AST	18 mmol[f]	D5W	Visually compatible for 24 hr at 22 °C exposed to fluorescent light	412	**C**
Ranitidine HCl	GL	2 g	LY	10 and 60 mEq	D5W, NS[a]	Physically compatible with 2% or less ranitidine loss in 48 hr at room temperature under fluorescent light	1361	**C**
	GL	50 mg	LY	10 and 60 mEq	NS[a]	Physically compatible with no ranitidine loss in 48 hr at room temperature under fluorescent light	1361	**C**
	GL	50 mg	LY	10 and 60 mEq	D5W[a]	Physically compatible with 7% ranitidine loss in 48 hr at room temperature under fluorescent light	1361	**C**
	GL	50 mg and 2 g		80 mEq	D5S, D5W, NS	Physically compatible and ranitidine chemically stable by HPLC for 24 hr at 25 °C. Potassium chloride not tested	1515	**C**
Sodium bicarbonate	AB	2.4 mEq[d]		120 mEq	D5W	Physically compatible for 24 hr	772	**C**
Thiopental sodium	AB	2.5 g	AB	40 mEq	D5W	Physically compatible	21	**C**
Vancomycin HCl	LI	1 g		3 g	D5W	Physically compatible	74	**C**
Verapamil HCl	KN	80 mg	TR	80 mEq	D5W, NS	Physically compatible for 24 hr	764	**C**
Vitamin B complex with C		1 vial		3 g	D5W	Physically compatible	74	**C**
Vitamin B complex with C with penicillin G potassium	TR SQ	1 ampul 2 million units		20 mEq	D5S, D5W	Therapeutic availability maintained	110	**C**
Vitamin B complex with C with penicillin G potassium	TR SQ	1 ampul 8 million units		40 mEq	D5S, D5W	Therapeutic availability maintained	110	**C**

[a]*Tested in PVC containers.*
[b]*Tested in both glass and PVC containers.*
[c]*Tested in both polyolefin and PVC containers.*
[d]*One vial of Neut added to a liter of admixture.*
[e]*Concentration expressed in milligrams of phenytoin sodium equivalents (PE) per milliliter.*
[f]*Approximate concentration.*

Y-Site Injection Compatibility (1:1 Mixture)

Potassium chloride

Drug	Mfr	Conc	Mfr	Conc	Remarks	Ref	C/I
Acyclovir sodium	BW	5 mg/ml[a]	IX	0.04 mEq/ml[a]	Physically compatible for 4 hr at 25 °C	1157	**C**
Aldesleukin	CHI	33,800 I.U./ml[a]	AB	0.2 mEq/ml	Visually compatible with little or no loss of aldesleukin activity by bioassay	1857	**C**

Y-Site Injection Compatibility (1:1 Mixture) (Cont.)

Potassium chloride

Drug	Mfr	Conc	Mfr	Conc	Remarks	Ref	C/I
Allopurinol sodium	BW	3 mg/ml[b]	AB	0.1 mEq/ml[b]	Physically compatible with no change in measured turbidity or increase in particle content in 4 hr at 22 °C	1686	**C**
Amifostine	USB	10 mg/ml[a]	AB	0.1 mEq/ml[a]	Physically compatible with no change in measured turbidity or increase in particle content in 4 hr at 23 °C	1845	**C**
Aminophylline	SE	25 mg/ml		40 mEq/L[c]	Physically compatible for at least 4 hr at room temperature by visual and microscopic examination	322	**C**
Amiodarone HCl	LZ	4 mg/ml[d]	AB	0.04 mg/ml[d]	Physically compatible for 24 hr at 21 °C	1032	**C**
Amphotericin B cholesteryl sulfate complex	SEQ	0.83 mg/ml[a]	AB	0.1 mEq/ml[a]	Gross precipitate forms	2117	**I**
Ampicillin sodium	BR	25, 50, 100, 125 mg/ml		40 mEq/L[c]	Physically compatible for at least 4 hr at room temperature by visual and microscopic examination	322	**C**
Amrinone lactate	WB	3 mg/ml[b]	IX	0.04 mEq/ml[a]	Physically compatible for at least 4 hr at 25 °C under fluorescent light	992	**C**
	WI	5 mg/ml	LY	80 mEq/L[e]	Physically compatible with little or no loss of either drug in 4 hr at 22 °C	1419	**C**
	WI	2.5 mg/ml[e]	LY	80 mEq/L[e]	Physically compatible with little or no loss of either drug in 4 hr at 22 °C	1419	**C**
Atropine sulfate	BW	0.5 mg/ml	AB	40 mEq/L[f]	Physically compatible for at least 4 hr at room temperature by visual and microscopic examination	534	**C**
Aztreonam	SQ	40 mg/ml[a]	AB	0.1 mEq/ml[a]	Physically compatible with no subvisual haze or particle formation in 4 hr at 23 °C	1758	**C**
Betamethasone sodium phosphate	SC	3 mg/ml	AB	40 mEq/L[f]	Physically compatible for at least 4 hr at room temperature by visual and microscopic examination	534	**C**
Calcium gluconate	UP	100 mg/ml		40 mEq/L[c]	Physically compatible for at least 4 hr at room temperature by visual and microscopic examination	322	**C**
Chlordiazepoxide HCl	RC	10 mg/ml	AB	40 mEq/L[f]	Physically compatible for at least 4 hr at room temperature by visual and microscopic examination	534	**C**
Chlorpromazine HCl	SKF	25 mg/ml	AB	40 mEq/L[f]	Physically compatible for at least 4 hr at room temperature by visual and microscopic examination	534	**C**
Ciprofloxacin	MI	2 mg/ml[d]	LY	0.04 mEq/ml	Visually compatible for 24 hr at 24 °C	1655	**C**
	MI	2 mg/ml[a]	AMR	2 mEq/ml	Visually compatible for 2 hr at 25 °C	1628	**C**
Cisatracurium besylate	GW	0.1, 2, 5 mg/ml[a]	AB	0.1 mEq/ml[a]	Physically compatible with no change in measured turbidity or increase in particle content in 4 hr at 23 °C	2074	**C**
Cladribine	ORT	0.015[b] and 0.5[h] mg/ml	AB	0.1 mEq/ml[b]	Physically compatible with no change in measured turbidity or increase in particle content in 4 hr at 23 °C	1969	**C**
Clarithromycin	AB	4 mg/ml[a]	ANT	0.08 mmol/ml[a]	Visually compatible for 72 hr at both 30 and 17 °C	2174	**C**

Y-Site Injection Compatibility (1:1 Mixture) (Cont.)

Potassium chloride

Drug	Mfr	Conc	Mfr	Conc	Remarks	Ref	C/I
Cyanocobalamin	PD	0.1 mg/ml	AB	40 mEq/L[f]	Physically compatible for at least 4 hr at room temperature by visual and microscopic examination	534	C
Dexamethasone sodium phosphate	MSD	4 mg/ml		40 mEq/L[c]	Physically compatible for at least 4 hr at room temperature by visual and microscopic examination	322	C
Diazepam	RC	5 mg/ml		40 mEq/L[c]	Immediate haziness and globule formation	322	I
Digoxin	BW	0.25 mg/ml		40 mEq/L[c]	Physically compatible for at least 4 hr at room temperature by visual and microscopic examination	322	C
Diltiazem HCl	MMD	5 mg/ml	LY	0.08[a] and 2 mEq/ml	Visually compatible	1807	C
Diphenhydramine HCl	PD	50 mg/ml	AB	40 mEq/L[f]	Physically compatible for at least 4 hr at room temperature by visual and microscopic examination	534	C
Dobutamine HCl	LI	4 mg/ml[d]	AB	0.06 mEq/ml[d]	Physically compatible for 3 hr	1316	C
Docetaxel	RPR	0.9 mg/ml[a]	AB	0.1 mEq/ml[a]	Physically compatible with no change in measured turbidity or increase in particle content in 4 hr at 23 °C	2224	C
Dopamine HCl	ACC	40 mg/ml	AB	40 mEq/L[f]	Physically compatible for at least 4 hr at room temperature by visual and microscopic examination	534	C
Doxorubicin HCl liposome injection	SEQ	0.4 mg/ml[a]	AB	0.1 mEq/ml[a]	Physically compatible with little or no change in measured turbidity and no increase in particle content in 4 hr at 23 °C	2087	C
Droperidol	CR	1.25 mg/ml	AB	40 mEq/L[f]	Physically compatible for at least 4 hr at room temperature by visual and microscopic examination	534	C
Edrophonium chloride	RC	10 mg/ml	AB	40 mEq/L[f]	Physically compatible for at least 4 hr at room temperature by visual and microscopic examination	534	C
Enalaprilat	MSD	0.05 mg/ml[b]	LY	0.4 mEq/ml[a]	Physically compatible for 24 hr at room temperature under fluorescent light	1355	C
Epinephrine HCl	AB	0.1 mg/ml	AB	40 mEq/L[f]	Physically compatible for at least 4 hr at room temperature by visual and microscopic examination	534	C
Ergotamine tartrate	SZ	0.5 mg/ml	AB	40 mEq/L[f]	Crystal formation and brown discoloration in 4 hr at room temperature	534	I
Esmolol HCl	DCC	10 mg/ml[a]	IX	0.4 mEq/ml[a]	Physically compatible for 24 hr at 22 °C	1169	C
Estrogens, conjugated	AY	5 mg/ml		40 mEq/L[c]	Physically compatible for at least 4 hr at room temperature by visual and microscopic examination	322	C
Ethacrynate sodium	MSD	1 mg/ml		40 mEq/L[c]	Physically compatible for at least 4 hr at room temperature by visual and microscopic examination	322	C

Y-Site Injection Compatibility (1:1 Mixture) (Cont.)

Potassium chloride

Drug	Mfr	Conc	Mfr	Conc	Remarks	Ref	C/I
Etoposide phosphate	BR	5 mg/ml[a]	AB	0.1 mEq/ml[a]	Physically compatible with no change in measured turbidity or increase in particle content in 4 hr at 23 °C	2218	**C**
Famotidine	MSD ME	0.2 mg/ml[a] 2 mg/ml[b]	AB	0.04 mEq/ml[a] 0.1 mEq/ml[a]	Physically compatible for 4 hr at 25 °C Visually compatible for 4 hr at 22 °C	1188 1936	**C** **C**
Fentanyl citrate	MN	0.05 mg/ml	AB	40 mEq/L[f]	Physically compatible for at least 4 hr at room temperature by visual and microscopic examination	534	**C**
Fentanyl citrate and droperidol	MN	0.05 + 2.5 mg/ml	AB	40 mEq/L[f]	Physically compatible for at least 4 hr at room temperature by visual and microscopic examination	534	**C**
Filgrastim	AMG	30 μg/ml[a]	AB	0.1 mEq/ml[a]	Physically compatible with no change in measured turbidity or increase in particle content in 4 hr at 22 °C	1687	**C**
Fludarabine phosphate	BX	1 mg/ml[a]	AB	0.1 mEq/ml[a]	Physically compatible for 4 hr at room temperature under fluorescent light	1439	**C**
Fluorouracil	RC	50 mg/ml	AB	40 mEq/L[f]	Physically compatible for at least 4 hr at room temperature by visual and microscopic examination	534	**C**
Furosemide	HO	10 mg/ml	AB	40 mEq/L[f]	Physically compatible for at least 4 hr at room temperature by visual and microscopic examination	534	**C**
Gemcitabine HCl	LI	10 mg/ml[b]	AB	0.1 mEq/ml[b]	Physically compatible with no change in measured turbidity or increase in particle content in 4 hr at 23 °C	2226	**C**
Granisetron HCl	SKB	1 mg/ml	LY	0.04 mEq/ml[b]	Physically compatible with little or no loss of granisetron by HPLC in 4 hr at 22 °C	1883	**C**
Heparin sodium	TR	50 units/ml	AB	0.2 mEq/ml[a]	Visually compatible for 6 hr at 25 °C	1793	**C**
Hydralazine HCl	CI	20 mg/ml	AB	40 mEq/L[f]	Physically compatible for at least 4 hr at room temperature by visual and microscopic examination	534	**C**
Idarubicin HCl	AD	1 mg/ml[b]	AB	0.03 mEq/ml[b]	Visually compatible for 24 hr at 25 °C	1525	**C**
Indomethacin sodium trihydrate	MSD	1 mg/ml[b]	AB	0.2 mEq/ml[a]	Visually compatible for 24 hr at 28 °C	1527	**C**
Insulin, regular	LI	40 units/ml		40 mEq/L[c]	Physically compatible for at least 4 hr at room temperature by visual and microscopic examination	322	**C**
Isoproterenol HCl	WI	0.2 mg/ml	AB	40 mEq/L[f]	Physically compatible for at least 4 hr at room temperature by visual and microscopic examination	534	**C**
Kanamycin sulfate	BR	250 mg/ml		40 mEq/L[c]	Physically compatible for at least 4 hr at room temperature by visual and microscopic examination	322	**C**
Labetalol HCl	SC	1 mg/ml[a]	IX	0.4 mEq/ml[a]	Physically compatible for 24 hr at 18 °C	1171	**C**
Lidocaine HCl	AST	20 mg/ml		40 mEq/L[c]	Physically compatible for at least 4 hr at room temperature by visual and microscopic examination	322	**C**
Lorazepam	WY	0.33 mg/ml[b]	BRN	1 mEq/ml	Visually compatible for 24 hr at 22 °C	1855	**C**

Y-Site Injection Compatibility (1:1 Mixture) (Cont.)

Potassium chloride

Drug	Mfr	Conc	Mfr	Conc	Remarks	Ref	C/I
Magnesium sulfate	AB	500 mg/ml	AB	40 mEq/L[f]	Physically compatible for at least 4 hr at room temperature by visual and microscopic examination	534	**C**
Melphalan HCl	BW	0.1 mg/ml[b]	AB	0.1 mEq/ml[b]	Physically compatible with no change in measured turbidity or increase in particle content in 3 hr at 22 °C	1557	**C**
Menadiol sodium diphosphate	RC	5 mg/ml	AB	40 mEq/L[f]	Physically compatible for at least 4 hr at room temperature by visual and microscopic examination	534	**C**
Meperidine HCl	AB	10 mg/ml	AB	0.4 mEq/ml[a]	Physically compatible for 4 hr at 25 °C	1397	**C**
Methoxamine HCl	BW	10 mg/ml	AB	40 mEq/L[f]	Physically compatible for at least 4 hr at room temperature by visual and microscopic examination	534	**C**
Methylergonovine maleate	SZ	0.2 mg/ml	AB	40 mEq/L[f]	Physically compatible for at least 4 hr at room temperature by visual and microscopic examination	534	**C**
Methylprednisolone sodium succinate	UP	40 mg/ml		40 mEq/L[a]	Physically compatible for at least 4 hr at room temperature by visual and microscopic examination	322	**C**
	UP	40 mg/ml		40 mEq/L[b]	Physically compatible initially but haze forms within 4 hr at room temperature	322	**I**
	UP	40 mg/ml		40 mEq/L[i]	Immediate haze formation	322	**I**
Midazolam HCl	RC	5 mg/ml	BRN	1 mEq/ml	Visually compatible for 24 hr at 22 °C	1855	**C**
Milrinone lactate	SW	0.4 mg/ml[a]	AB	1 mEq/ml[a]	Visually compatible with no loss of milrinone by HPLC in 4 hr at 23 °C	2214	**C**
Minocycline HCl	LE	50 mg/ml	AB	40 mEq/L[f]	Physically compatible for at least 4 hr at room temperature by visual and microscopic examination	534	**C**
Morphine sulfate	WY	15 mg/ml	AB	40 mEq/L[f]	Physically compatible for at least 4 hr at room temperature by visual and microscopic examination	534	**C**
Neostigmine methylsulfate	RC	0.5 mg/ml	AB	40 mEq/L[f]	Physically compatible for at least 4 hr at room temperature by visual and microscopic examination	534	**C**
Norepinephrine bitartrate	WI	1 mg/ml	AB	40 mEq/L[f]	Physically compatible for at least 4 hr at room temperature by visual and microscopic examination	534	**C**
Ondansetron HCl	GL	1 mg/ml[b]	AB	0.1 mEq/ml[a]	Physically compatible for 4 hr at 22 °C	1365	**C**
Oxacillin sodium	BR	100 mg/ml	AB	40 mEq/L[f]	Physically compatible for at least 4 hr at room temperature by visual and microscopic examination	534	**C**
Oxytocin	SZ	1 mg/ml	AB	40 mEq/L[f]	Physically compatible for at least 4 hr at room temperature by visual and microscopic examination	534	**C**
Paclitaxel	NCI	1.2 mg/ml[a]	AB	0.1 mEq/ml[a]	Physically compatible with no change in measured turbidity in 4 hr at 22 °C	1556	**C**
Penicillin G potassium	LI	200,000 units		40 mEq/L[c]	Physically compatible for at least 4 hr at room temperature by visual and microscopic examination	322	**C**

Y-Site Injection Compatibility (1:1 Mixture) (Cont.)

Potassium chloride

Drug	Mfr	Conc	Mfr	Conc	Remarks	Ref	C/I
Pentazocine lactate	WI	30 mg/ml	AB	40 mEq/L[f]	Physically compatible for at least 4 hr at room temperature by visual and microscopic examination	534	**C**
Phenytoin sodium	PD	50 mg/ml		40 mEq/L[a]	Immediate formation of phenytoin crystals	322	**I**
	PD	50 mg/ml		40 mEq/L[b,i]	Phenytoin crystals form in 4 hr at room temperature	322	**I**
Phytonadione	RC	10 mg/ml	AB	40 mEq/L[f]	Physically compatible for at least 4 hr at room temperature by visual and microscopic examination	534	**C**
Piperacillin sodium–tazobactam sodium	LE	40 + 5 mg/ml[a]	AB	0.1 mEq/ml[a]	Physically compatible with no change in measured turbidity or increase in particle content in 4 hr at 22 °C	1688	**C**
Procainamide HCl	SQ	100 mg/ml	AB	40 mEq/L[f]	Physically compatible for at least 4 hr at room temperature by visual and microscopic examination	534	**C**
Prochlorperazine edisylate	SKF	5 mg/ml	AB	40 mEq/L[f]	Physically compatible for at least 4 hr at room temperature by visual and microscopic examination	534	**C**
Promethazine HCl	SV	50 mg/ml	AB	40 mEq/L[j]	Physically compatible initially, but cloudiness developed in 4 hr at room temperature	534	**I**
	SV	50 mg/ml	AB	40 mEq/L[k]	Physically compatible for at least 4 hr at room temperature by visual and microscopic examination	534	**C**
Propofol	ZEN	10 mg/ml	AB	0.1 mEq/ml[a]	Physically compatible for 1 hr at 23 °C with no increase in particle content	2066	**C**
Propranolol HCl	AY	1 mg/ml	AB	40 mEq/L[f]	Physically compatible for at least 4 hr at room temperature by visual and microscopic examination	534	**C**
Pyridostigmine bromide	RC	5 mg/ml	AB	40 mEq/L[f]	Physically compatible for at least 4 hr at room temperature by visual and microscopic examination	534	**C**
Remifentanil HCl	GW	0.025 and 0.25 mg/ml[b]	AB	0.1 mEq/ml[a]	Physically compatible with no change in measured turbidity or increase in particle content in 4 hr at 23 °C	2075	**C**
Sargramostim	IMM	10 μg/ml[b]	AB	0.1 mEq/ml[b]	Physically compatible for 4 hr at 22 °C under fluorescent light	1436	**C**
Scopolamine HBr	BW	0.86 mg/ml	AB	40 mEq/L[f]	Physically compatible for at least 4 hr at room temperature by visual and microscopic examination	534	**C**
Sodium bicarbonate	BR	75 mg/ml		40 mEq/L[c]	Physically compatible for at least 4 hr at room temperature by visual and microscopic examination	322	**C**
Succinylcholine chloride	BW	20 mg/ml		40 mEq/L[c]	Physically compatible for at least 4 hr at room temperature by visual and microscopic examination	322	**C**
Tacrolimus	FUJ	1 mg/ml[b]	AB	2 mEq/ml	Visually compatible for 24 hr at 25 °C	1630	**C**

Y-Site Injection Compatibility (1:1 Mixture) (Cont.)

Potassium chloride

Drug	Mfr	Conc	Mfr	Conc	Remarks	Ref	C/I
Teniposide	BR	0.1 mg/ml[a]	AB	0.1 mEq/ml[a]	Physically compatible with no subvisual haze or particle formation in 4 hr at 23 °C	1725	**C**
Theophylline	TR	4 mg/ml	AB	0.2 mEq/ml[a]	Visually compatible for 6 hr at 25 °C	1793	**C**
Thiotepa	IMM[l]	1 mg/ml[a]	AMR	0.1 mEq/ml[a]	Physically compatible with no change in measured turbidity or increase in particle content in 4 hr at 23 °C	1861	**C**
TNA #218 to #226[m]			AB	0.1 mEq/ml[a]	Visually compatible with no precipitate or emulsion damage apparent in 4 hr at 23 °C	2215	**C**
TPN #189[m]			AST	30 mg/ml[b]	Visually compatible for 24 hr at 22 °C	1767	**C**
TPN #212 to #215[m]			AB	0.1 mEq/ml[a]	Physically compatible with no change in measured turbidity or increase in particle content in 4 hr at 23 °C	2109	**C**
Trimethaphan camsylate	RC	50 mg/ml	AB	40 mEq/L[f]	Physically compatible for at least 4 hr at room temperature by visual and microscopic examination	534	**C**
Trimethobenzamide HCl	RC	100 mg/ml	AB	40 mEq/L[f]	Physically compatible for at least 4 hr at room temperature by visual and microscopic examination	534	**C**
Vinorelbine tartrate	BW	1 mg/ml[b]	AB	0.1 mEq/ml[b]	Physically compatible with no change in measured turbidity or increase in particle content in 4 hr at 22 °C	1558	**C**
Warfarin sodium	DME	2 mg/ml[g]	BA	0.04 mEq/ml[n]	Visually compatible for 24 hr at 24 °C	2078	**C**
Zidovudine	BW	4 mg/ml[a]	IMS	0.67 mEq/ml[a]	Physically compatible for 4 hr at 25 °C under fluorescent light by visual and microscopic examination	1193	**C**

[a]*Tested in dextrose 5% in water.*
[b]*Tested in sodium chloride 0.9%.*
[c]*Tested in dextrose 5% in water, sodium chloride 0.9%, and Ringer's injection, lactated.*
[d]*Tested in both dextrose 5% in water and sodium chloride 0.9%.*
[e]*Tested in sodium chloride 0.45%.*
[f]*Tested in dextrose 5% in Ringer's injection, dextrose 5% in Ringer's injection, lactated, dextrose 5% in water, Ringer's injection, lactated, and sodium chloride 0.9%.*
[g]*Tested in sterile water for injection.*
[h]*Tested in bacteriostatic sodium chloride 0.9% preserved with benzyl alcohol 0.9%.*
[i]*Tested in Ringer's injection, lactated.*
[j]*Tested in dextrose 5% in Ringer's injection.*
[k]*Tested in dextrose 5% in Ringer's injection, lactated, dextrose 5% in water, Ringer's injection, lactated, and sodium chloride 0.9%.*
[l]*Lyophilized formulation tested.*
[m]*Refer to Appendix I for the composition of parenteral nutrition solutions. TNA indicates a 3-in-1 admixture, and TPN indicates a 2-in-1 admixture.*
[n]*Tested in dextrose 5% in sodium chloride 0.45%.*

Additional Compatibility Information

Miscellaneous— Potassium chloride appears to be physically compatible with ceftazidime (4).

The addition of potassium chloride to mannitol 20 or 25% solutions may cause precipitation of the mannitol (38).

Methylprednisolone—— The compatibility of methylprednisolone sodium succinate (Upjohn) with potassium chloride added to an auxiliary medication infusion unit has been studied. Primary admixtures were prepared by adding potassium chloride 40 mEq/L to dextrose 5% in water, dextrose 5% in sodium chloride 0.9%, and Ringer's injection, lactated. The primary admixture was added along with methylprednisolone sodium succinate (Upjohn) to the auxiliary medication infusion unit with the following results (329):

Methylprednisolone Sodium Succinate	Potassium Chloride 40 mEq/L Primary Solution	Results
500 mg	D5S, D5W, LR qs 100 ml	Clear solution for 24 hr
1000 mg	D5W qs 100 ml	Clear solution for 24 hr
	D5S, LR qs 100 ml	Clear solution for 6 hr
2000 mg	D5S, D5W, LR qs 100 ml	Clear solution for 24 hr

Other Information

Great care is required when adding potassium chloride to infusion solutions, whether in flexible plastic containers or in rigid bottles. Adding potassium chloride to running infusion solutions hanging in the use position, especially in flexible containers, has resulted in the pooling of potassium chloride and a resultant high-concentration bolus of the drug being administered to patients, with serious and even fatal consequences. Attempts to mix adequately the potassium chloride in flexible containers by squeezing the container in the hanging position were unsuccessful. It is recommended that drugs be admixed with solutions in flexible containers when positioned with the injection arm of the container uppermost. With both rigid bottles and flexible containers, subsequent repeated inversion and agitation to effect thorough mixture are necessary (85; 130; 454–456; 714; 715; 1127; 1778; 2151).

POTASSIUM PHOSPHATES
AHFS 40:12

American Pharmaceutical Partners
Abbott

Products— Potassium phosphates injection is available from several manufacturers in flip-top vials containing 5 or 15 ml of solution and 50-ml bulk additive solution containers (29). Each milliliter of solution contains monobasic potassium phosphate 224 mg and dibasic potassium phosphate 236 mg in water for injection. The phosphate concentration of the solution is 3 mmol/ml, and the potassium content is 4.4 mEq/ml. This concentrated solution must be diluted for use (1-11/98; 4).

pH— Potassium phosphates injection is stated to have a pH of approximately 7 to 7.8 (4). However, some products cite a pH range of 6.2 to 6.8 (1-11/98).

Osmolarity— The osmolarity of potassium phosphates injection has been variously cited as 12 mOsm/ml (1-2/94) and 7.4 mOsm/ml (1-11/98).

Administration— Potassium phosphates injection is administered slowly intravenously diluted in infusion solutions (4).

The relationship between milliequivalents and millimoles of phosphate is expressed in the following equation:

$$\text{mEq phosphate} = \text{mmol phosphate} \times \text{valence}$$

However, the average valence of phosphate changes with changes in pH. Consequently, it is necessary to specify a pH before the valence, and therefore the milliequivalents, can be determined. To avoid this problem, it has been suggested that doses of phosphate be expressed in terms of millimoles, which is independent of valence (178; 716–718). Alternatively, the dose may be expressed in terms of milligrams of phosphorus. One millimole of phosphorus equals 31 mg (205; 717).

Stability— Potassium phosphates injection should be stored at controlled room temperature. The solutions should be clear and free of particulate matter (1-11/98).

Compatibility Information

Solution Compatibility

Potassium phosphates

Solution	Mfr	Mfr	Conc/L	Remarks	Ref	C/I
Amino acids 4%, dextrose 25%	CU	MG	100 mEq	Physically compatible for 24 hr at 22 °C	313	C
Dextran 6% in dextrose 5%	AB	AB	160 mEq	Physically compatible	3	C
Dextran 6% in sodium chloride 0.9%	AB	AB	160 mEq	Physically compatible	3	C

Solution Compatibility (Cont.)

Potassium phosphates

Solution	Mfr	Mfr	Conc/L	Remarks	Ref	C/I
Dextrose 2½% in half-strength Ringer's injection	AB	AB	160 mEq	Haze or precipitate forms within 1 hr	3	I
Dextrose 5% in Ringer's injection	AB	AB	160 mEq	Haze or precipitate forms within 1 hr	3	I
Dextrose 2½% in half-strength Ringer's injection, lactated	AB	AB	160 mEq	Haze or precipitate forms within 24 hr	3	I
Dextrose 5% in Ringer's injection, lactated	AB	AB	160 mEq	Haze or precipitate forms within 24 hr	3	I
Dextrose 10% in Ringer's injection	AB	AB	160 mEq	Physically compatible	3	C
Dextrose 10% in Ringer's injection, lactated	AB	AB	160 mEq	Physically compatible	3	C
Dextrose–saline combinations (except as noted below)	AB	AB	160 mEq	Physically compatible	3	C
Dextrose 10% in sodium chloride 0.9%	AB	AB	160 mEq	Haze or precipitate forms within 24 hr	3	I
Dextrose 2½% in water	AB	AB	160 mEq	Physically compatible	3	C
Dextrose 5% in water	AB	AB	160 mEq	Physically compatible	3	C
Dextrose 10% in water	AB	AB	160 mEq	Physically compatible	3	C
Fructose 10% in sodium chloride 0.9%	AB	AB	160 mEq	Physically compatible	3	C
Fructose 10% in water	AB	AB	160 mEq	Physically compatible	3	C
Invert sugar 5 and 10% in sodium chloride 0.9%	AB	AB	160 mEq	Physically compatible	3	C
Invert sugar 5 and 10% in water	AB	AB	160 mEq	Physically compatible	3	C
Ionosol products (except as noted below)	AB	AB	160 mEq	Physically compatible	3	C
Ionosol D-CM	AB	AB	160 mEq	Haze or precipitate forms within 1 hr	3	I
Ionosol D-CM with dextrose 5%	AB	AB	160 mEq	Haze or precipitate forms within 6 hr	3	I
Ionosol D with invert sugar 10%	AB	AB	160 mEq	Color change	3	I
Ionosol D modified with invert sugar 10%	AB	AB	160 mEq	Haze or precipitate forms within 24 hr	3	I
Ringer's injection	AB	AB	160 mEq	Haze or precipitate forms within 1 hr	3	I
Ringer's injection, lactated	AB	AB	160 mEq	Haze or precipitate forms within 24 hr	3	I
Sodium chloride 0.45%	AB	AB	160 mEq	Physically compatible	3	C
Sodium chloride 0.9%	AB	AB	160 mEq	Physically compatible	3	C
Sodium lactate ⅙ M	AB	AB	160 mEq	Physically compatible	3	C
TPN #11 to #15[a]		MG	10 to 40 mEq	Physically compatible for 24 hr at 22 °C. TLC changes of amino acids in similar solutions attributed to M.V.I. or vitamin B complex with C	313	C
TPN #81 to #85[a]		MG	10 to 40 mEq	Physically compatible for 24 hr at 22 °C. Changes in UV spectra of amino acids and vitamins in solutions with M.V.I. and vitamin B complex with C. TLC changes in similar solutions attributed to vitamins	313	C

[a]*Refer to Appendix I for the composition of parenteral nutrition solutions. TPN indicates a 2-in-1 admixture.*

Additive Compatibility

Potassium phosphates

Drug	Mfr	Conc/L	Mfr	Conc/L	Test Soln	Remarks	Ref	C/I
Dobutamine HCl	LI	200 mg	AB	100 mmol	NS	Small particles form after 1 hr. White precipitate noted after 15 hr	552	I
Magnesium sulfate	LI	1, 2, 3, 4 mEq	MG	10, 20, 30, 40 mEq	AA 4%, D 25%	Physically compatible for 24 hr at 22 °C	313	C
Metoclopramide HCl	RB	10 and 160 mg	IX	15 mmol	NS	Physically compatible for 48 hr at room temperature	924	C
	RB	10 and 160 mg	IX	15 mmol		Physically compatible for 48 hr at 25 °C	1167	C
Verapamil HCl	KN	80 mg	AB	88 mEq	D5W, NS	Physically compatible for 24 hr	764	C

Y-Site Injection Compatibility (1:1 Mixture)

Potassium phosphates

Drug	Mfr	Conc	Mfr	Conc	Remarks	Ref	C/I
Ciprofloxacin	MI	2 mg/ml[a]	LY	3 mmol/ml	Visually compatible for 2 hr at 25 °C	1628	C
Diltiazem HCl	MMD	5 mg/ml	AMR	0.015 mmol/ml	Visually compatible	1807	C
Enalaprilat	MSD	0.05 mg/ml[b]	LY	0.44 mEq/ml[a]	Physically compatible for 24 hr at room temperature under fluorescent light	1355	C
Esmolol HCl	DCC	10 mg/ml[a]	LY	0.44 mEq/ml[a]	Physically compatible for 24 hr at 22 °C	1169	C
Famotidine	MSD	0.2 mg/ml[a]	LY	3 mmol/ml[a]	Physically compatible for 14 hr	1196	C
Labetalol HCl	SC	1 mg/ml[a]	LY	0.44 mEq/ml[a]	Physically compatible for 24 hr at 18 °C	1171	C
TNA #218 to #226[c]			AB	3 mmol/ml	Damage to emulsion integrity occurs immediately with free oil formation possible	2215	I
TPN #212 to #215[c]			AB	3 mmol/ml	Increased turbidity forms immediately	2109	I

[a]*Tested in dextrose 5% in water.*
[b]*Tested in sodium chloride 0.9%.*
[c]*Refer to Appendix I for the composition of parenteral nutrition solutions. TNA indicates a 3-in-1 admixture, and TPN indicates a 2-in-1 admixture.*

Additional Compatibility Information

Calcium and Phosphate— UNRECOGNIZED CALCIUM PHOSPHATE PRECIPITATION IN A 3-IN-1 PARENTERAL NUTRITION MIXTURE RESULTED IN PATIENT DEATH.

The potential for the formation of a calcium phosphate precipitate in parenteral nutrition solutions is well studied and documented (1771; 1777), but the information is complex and difficult to apply to the clinical situation (1770; 1772; 1777). The incorporation of fat emulsion in 3-in-1 parenteral nutrition solutions obscures any precipitate that is present which has led to substantial debate on the dangers associated with 3-in-1 parenteral nutrition mixtures and when or if the danger to the patient is warranted therapeutically (1770–1772; 2031–2036). Because such precipitation may be life-threatening to patients (2037), the Food and Drug Administration issued a Safety Alert containing the following recommendations (1769):

"1. The amounts of phosphorus and of calcium added to the admixture are critical. The solubility of the added calcium should be calculated from the volume at the time the calcium is added. It should not be based upon the final volume.

Some amino acid injections for TPN admixtures contain phosphate ions (as a phosphoric acid buffer). These phosphate ions and the volume at the time the phosphate is added should be considered when calculating the concentration of phosphate additives. Also, when adding calcium and phosphate to an admixture, the phosphate should be added first.

The line should be flushed between the addition of any potentially incompatible components.

2. A lipid emulsion in a three-in-one admixture obscures the presence of a precipitate. Therefore, if a lipid emulsion is needed, either (1) use a two-in-one admixture with the lipid infused separately, or (2) if a three-in-one admixture is

medically necessary, then add the calcium before the lipid emulsion and according to the recommendations in number 1 above.

If the amount of calcium or phosphate which must be added is likely to cause a precipitate, some or all of the calcium should be administered separately. Such separate infusions must be properly diluted and slowly infused to avoid serious adverse events related to the calcium.

3. When using an automated compounding device, the above steps should be considered when programming the device. In addition, automated compounders should be maintained and operated according to the manufacturer's recommendations.

Any printout should be checked against the programmed admixture and weight of components.

4. During the mixing process, pharmacists who mix parenteral nutrition admixtures should periodically agitate the admixture and check for precipitates. Medical or home care personnel who start and monitor these infusions should carefully inspect for the presence of precipitates both before and during infusion. Patients and care givers should be trained to visually inspect for signs of precipitation. They also should be advised to stop the infusion and seek medical assistance if precipitates are noted.

5. A filter should be used when infusing either central or peripheral parenteral nutrition admixtures. At this time, data have not been submitted to document which size filter is most effective in trapping precipitates.

Standards of practice vary, but the following is suggested: a 1.2-μm air-eliminating filter for lipid-containing admixtures and a 0.22-μm air-eliminating filter for non-lipid-containing admixtures.

6. Parenteral nutrition admixtures should be administered within the following time frames: if stored at room temperature, the infusion should be started within 24 hours after mixing; if stored at refrigerated temperatures, the infusion should be started within 24 hours of rewarming. Because warming parenteral nutrition admixtures may contribute to the formation of precipitates, once administration begins, care should be taken to avoid excessive warming of the admixture.

Persons administering home care parenteral nutrition admixtures may need to deviate from these time frames. Pharmacists who initially prepare these admixtures should check a reserve sample for precipitates over the duration and under the conditions of storage.

7. If symptoms of acute respiratory distress, pulmonary emboli, or interstitial pneumonitis develop, the infusion should be stopped immediately and thoroughly checked for precipitates. Appropriate medical interventions should be instituted. Home care personnel and patients should immediately seek medical assistance."

Calcium Phosphate Precipitation Fatalities— Hill et al. reported fatal cases of paroxysmal respiratory failure in two previously healthy women receiving peripheral vein parenteral nutrition. The patients experienced sudden cardiopulmonary arrest consistent with pulmonary emboli. The authors used in vitro simulations and an animal model to conclude that unrecognized calcium phosphate precipitation in a 3-in-1 total nutrition admixture caused the fatalities. The precipitation resulted during compounding by introducing calcium and phosphate near to one another in the compounding sequence and

Table 1. Parenteral Nutrition Solutions Evaluated by Eggert et al. (609)

Component	Solution Number			
	#1	#2	#3	#4
FreAmine III	4%	2%	1%	1%
Dextrose	25%	20%	10%	10%
pH	6.3	6.4	6.6	7.0[a]

[a]*Adjusted with sodium hydroxide.*

prior to complete fluid addition. This resulted in a temporarily high concentration of the drugs and precipitation of calcium phosphate. Observation of the precipitate was obscured by the incorporation of 20% fat emulsion, intravenous into the nutrition mixture. No filter was used during infusion of the fatal nutrition admixtures (2037).

Calcium salts are conditionally compatible with potassium phosphate in parenteral nutrition solutions. The incompatibility is dependent on a solubility and concentration phenomenon and is not entirely predictable. Precipitation may occur during compounding or at some time after compounding is completed.

NOTE: Some amino acids solutions inherently contain calcium and phosphate, which must be considered in any projection of compatibility. See the Amino Acid Injection monograph, Table 1.

It has been noted that the order of mixing of calcium gluconate and potassium phosphate may affect compatibility at elevated concentrations. Addition of potassium phosphate should precede calcium gluconate (313).

Eggert et al. (609) evaluated the compatibility of calcium and phosphate in several parenteral nutrition formulas for newborn infants. Calcium gluconate 10% (Cutter) and potassium phosphate (Abbott) were used to achieve concentrations of 2.5 to 100 mEq/L of calcium and 2.5 to 100 mmol/L of phosphorus added. The parenteral nutrition solutions evaluated were as shown in Table 1.

Eggert et al. noted the pH dependence of the phosphate–calcium precipitation. Dibasic calcium phosphate is very insoluble while monobasic calcium phosphate is relatively soluble. At low pH, the soluble monobasic form predominates; but as the pH increases, more dibasic phosphate becomes available to bind with calcium and precipitate. Therefore, the lower the pH of the parenteral nutrition solution, the more calcium and phosphate can be solubilized. Once again, the effects of temperature were also observed. As the temperature is increased, more calcium ion becomes available and more dibasic calcium phosphate is formed. Therefore, temperature increases increase the amount of precipitate (609).

Fitzgerald and MacKay reported calcium and phosphate solubility curves for neonatal parenteral nutrition solutions using TrophAmine (McGaw) 2, 1.5, and 0.8% as the sources of amino acids. The solutions also contained dextrose 10%, with cysteine and pH adjustment in some admixtures. Calcium and phosphate solubility followed the patterns reported by Eggert et al. (609). A slightly greater concentration of phosphate could be used in some mixtures, but this finding was not consistent (1024).

Using a similar study design, Fitzgerald and MacKay also studied six neonatal parenteral nutrition solutions based on Aminosyn-PF (Abbott) 2, 1.5, and 0.8%, with and without added cysteine HCl and dextrose 10%. Calcium concentrations ranged from 2.5 to 50 mEq/L, and phosphate concentrations ranged from 2.5 to 50 mmol/L. Solutions sat for 18 hours at 25 °C and then were warmed to 37 °C in a water bath to simulate the clinical situation of warming prior to infusion into a child. Solubility curves were markedly different than those for TrophAmine in the previous study (1024). Solubilities were reported to decrease by 15 mEq/L for calcium and

15 mmol/L for phosphate. The solutions remained clear during room temperature storage, but crystals often formed on warming to 37 °C (1211).

However, these data were questioned by Mikrut, who noted the similarities between the Aminosyn-PF and TrophAmine products and found little difference in calcium and phosphate solubilities in a preliminary report (1212). In the full report (1213), parenteral nutrition solutions containing Aminosyn-PF or TrophAmine 1 or 2.5% with dextrose 10 or 25%, respectively, plus electrolytes and trace metals, with or without cysteine HCl, were evaluated under the same conditions used by Fitzgerald and MacKay. Calcium concentrations ranged from 2.5 to 50 mEq/L, and phosphate concentrations ranged from 5 to 50 mmol/L. In contrast to the results of Fitzgerald and MacKay, the solubility curves were very similar for the Aminosyn-PF and TrophAmine parenteral nutrition solutions but very different from those of the previous Aminosyn-PF study (1211). The authors again showed that the solubility of calcium and phosphate is greater in solutions containing higher concentrations of amino acids and dextrose (1213).

Dunham et al. also reported calcium and phosphate solubility curves for TrophAmine 1 and 2% with dextrose 10% and electrolytes, vitamins, heparin, and trace elements. Calcium concentrations ranged from 10 to 60 mEq/L, and phosphorus concentrations ranged from 10 to 40 mmol/L. Calcium and phosphate solubilities were assessed by analysis of the calcium concentrations and followed patterns similar to those reported by Henry et al. (608) and Eggert et al. (609). The higher percentage of amino acids (TrophAmine 2%) permitted a slightly greater solubility of calcium and phosphate, especially in the 10 to 50 mEq/L and 10 to 35 mmol/L ranges, respectively (1614).

Knight et al. reported the maximal product of the amount of calcium (as gluconate) times phosphate (as potassium) that can be added to a parenteral nutrition solution, composed of amino acids 1% (Travenol) and dextrose 10%, for preterm infants. Turbidity was observed on initial mixing when the solubility product was around 115 to 130 mmol^2 or greater. After storage at 7 °C for 20 hours, visible precipitates formed at solubility products of 130 mmol^2 or greater. If the solution was administered through a barium-impregnated silicone rubber catheter, crystalline precipitates obstructed the catheters in 12 hours at a solubility product of 100 mmol^2 and in 10 days at 79 mmol^2, much lower than the in vitro results (1041).

Alexander and Arena evaluated the compatibility of calcium gluconate (American Quinine) and potassium phosphate (Lyphomed) in a parenteral nutrition solution, composed of dextrose 12.5% and amino acid injection (FreAmine III, McGaw) 1.33% and having a pH of 6.6, for premature infants. Potassium phosphate was added in varying amounts to samples of this solution. The samples were then titrated with calcium gluconate 10%. From the resulting data, an equation was derived to predict when precipitation would occur:

$$Y = -0.455X + 2.951$$

where Y is the Log_{10} of the calcium gluconate concentration (as mg/100 ml) and X is the phosphate concentration (as mmol/100 ml). The equation can be solved to determine the maximum concentration of calcium gluconate for a given phosphate concentration or vice versa. If either additive is sufficiently dilute, then the other can be added in high concentrations without precipitation occurring, obviating the need for the equation. These lower limits were set at 60 mg/100 ml for calcium gluconate and 0.6 mmol/100 ml for phosphate (1004).

While the authors noted that this equation technically applies to the specific solution being tested and that other variables such as temperature can affect precipitation, in practice they found it applicable to a variety of parenteral nutrition solutions, having similar components and pH values, for premature infants. The equation is *not* applicable to parenteral nutrition solutions with amino acid and dextrose concentrations, other components, or pH values that are much different (1004).

Venkataraman et al. evaluated the solubility of calcium and phosphorus in neonatal parenteral nutrition solutions composed of amino acids (Abbott) 1.25 and 2.5% with dextrose 5 and 10%, respectively. Also present were multivitamins and trace elements. The solutions contained calcium (as gluconate) in amounts ranging from 25 to 200 mg/100 ml. The phosphorus (as potassium phosphate) concentrations evaluated ranged from 25 to 150 mg/100 ml. If calcium gluconate was added first, cloudiness occurred immediately. If potassium phosphate was added first, substantial quantities could be added with no precipitate formation in 48 hours at 4 °C (Table 2). However, if stored at 22 °C, the solutions were stable for only 24 hours, and all contained precipitates after 48 hours (1210).

Kirkpatrick et al. reported the physical compatibility of calcium gluconate 10 to 40 mEq/L and potassium phosphates 10 to 40 mmol/L in three neonatal parenteral nutrition solutions (TPN #123 to #125 in Appendix I), alone and with retrograde administration of aminophylline 7.5 mg diluted with 1.5 ml of sterile water for injection. Contact of the alkaline aminophylline solution with the parenteral nutrition solutions resulted in the precipitation of calcium phosphate at much lower concentrations than were compatible in the parenteral nutrition solutions alone (1404).

Koorenhof and Timmer reported the maximum allowable concentrations of calcium and phosphate in a 3-in-1 parenteral nutrition mixture for children (TNA #192 in Appendix I). Added calcium was varied from 1.5 to 150 mmol/L, while added phosphate was varied from 21 to 300 mmol/L. The mixtures were stable for 48 hours at 22 and 37 °C as long as the pH was not greater than 5.7, the calcium concentration was below 16 mmol/L, the phosphate concentration was below 52 mmol/L, and the product of the calcium and phosphate concentrations was below 250 mmol^2/L^2 (1773).

MacKay et al. reported additional calcium and phosphate solubility curves for specialty parenteral nutrition solutions based on NephrAmine and also HepatAmine at concentrations of 0.8, 1.5, and 2% as the sources of amino acids. The solutions also contained dextrose 10%, with cysteine and pH adjustment to simulate addition of fat emulsion used in some admixtures. Calcium and phosphate solubility followed the hyperbolic patterns reported by Eggert et al. (609). Temperature, time, and pH affected calcium and phosphate solubility, with pH having the greatest effect (2038).

Table 2. Maximum Calcium and Phosphorus Concentrations Physically Compatible for 48 Hours at 4 °C (1210)

| Calcium (mg/100 ml) | Phosphorus (mg/100 ml) | |
	Amino Acids 1.25% + Dextrose 5%[a]	Amino Acids 2.5% + Dextrose 10%[a]
200[b]	50	75
150	50	100
100	75	100
50	100	125
25	150[b]	150[b]

[a]*Plus multivitamins and trace elements.*
[b]*Maximum concentration tested.*

Shatsky et al. reported the maximum sodium phosphate concentrations for given amounts of calcium gluconate that could be admixed in parenteral nutrition solutions containing TrophAmine in varying quantities (with cysteine HCl 40 mg/g of amino acid) and dextrose 10%. The solutions also contained magnesium sulfate 4 mEq/L, potassium acetate 24 mEq/L, sodium chloride 32 mEq/L, pediatric multivitamins, and trace elements. The presence of cysteine HCl reduces the solution pH and increases the amount of calcium and phosphate that can be incorporated before precipitation occurs. The results of this study cannot be safely extrapolated to TPN solutions with compositions other than the ones tested. The admixtures were compounded with the sodium phosphate added last, after thorough mixing of all other components. The authors noted this is not the preferred order of mixing (usually phosphate is added first and thoroughly mixed before adding calcium last); however, they believed this reversed order of mixing would provide a margin of error in cases in which the proper order is not followed. After compounding, the solutions were stored for 24 hours at 40 °C. The maximum calcium and phosphate amounts that could be mixed in the various solutions were reported tabularly and are shown in Table 3 (2039). However, these results are not entirely consistent with the study of Hoie and Narducci (2196). See below.

The temperature dependence of the calcium–phosphate precipitation has resulted in the occlusion of a subclavian catheter by a solution apparently free of precipitation. The parenteral nutrition solution consisted of FreAmine III 500 ml, dextrose 70% 500 ml, sodium chloride 50 mEq, sodium phosphate 40 mmol, potassium acetate 10 mEq, potassium phosphate 40 mmol, calcium gluconate 10 mEq, magnesium sulfate 10 mEq, and Shil's trace metals solution 1 ml. Although there was no evidence of precipitation in the bottle, tubing and pump cassette, and filter (all at approximately 26 °C) during administration, the occluded catheter and Vicra Loop Lock (next to the patient's body at 37 °C) had numerous crystals identified as calcium phosphate. In vitro, it was found that this parenteral nutrition solution had a precipitate in 12 hours at 37 °C but was clear for 24 hours at 26 °C (610).

Similarly, a parenteral nutrition solution that was clear and free of particulates after two weeks under refrigeration developed a precipitate in four to six hours when stored at room temperature. When the solution was warmed in a 37 °C water bath, precipitation occurred in one hour. Administration of the solution before the precipitate was noticed led to interstitial pneumonitis due to deposition of calcium phosphate crystals (1427).

Fausel et al. evaluated calcium phosphate precipitation phenomena in a series of parenteral nutrition admixtures composed of dextrose 22%, amino acids (FreAmine III) 2.7%, and fat emulsion (Abbott) 0, 1, and 3.2%. Incorporation of calcium gluconate 19 to 24 mEq/L and phosphate (as sodium) 22 to 28 mmol/L resulted in visible precipitation in the fat-free admixtures. New precipitate continued to form over 14 days, even after repeated filtrations of the solutions through 0.2-μm filters. The presence of the amino acids increased calcium and phosphate solubility compared to simple aqueous solutions. However, the incorporation of the fat emulsion did not result in a statistically significant increase in calcium and phosphate solubility. The authors noted that the pharmacokinetics of calcium phosphate precipitate formation do not appear to be entirely predictable; both transient and permanent precipitation can occur either during the compounding process or at some time afterward. Because calcium phosphate precipitation can be clinically very dangerous, the use of inline filters was recommended. The filters should have a porosity appropriate to the parenteral nutrition admixture: 1.2

Table 3. Maximum Amount of Phosphate (as Sodium) (mmol/L) Not Resulting in Precipitation According to the Study of Shatsky et al. (2039). See CAUTION below[a]

Calcium	Amino Acid (as TrophAmine) with Cysteine HCl 40 mg/g of Amino Acid				
(as gluconate)	0%	0.4%	1%	2%	3%
9.8 mEq/L	0	27	42	60	66
14.7 mEq/L	0	15	18	30	36
19.6 mEq/L	0	6	15	27	30
29.4 mEq/L	0	3	6	21	24

[a]CAUTION: The results cannot be safely extrapolated to other solutions. See text.

Table 4. Maximum Amount of Phosphate (as Potassium) (mmol/L) Not Resulting in Precipitation According to the Study of Hoie and Narducci (2196). See CAUTION below.[a]

Calcium (as Gluconate) (mEq/L)	Amino Acid (as TrophAmine) plus Cysteine HCl 1 g/L					
	0.5%	1%	1.5%	2%	2.5%	3%
10	22	28	38	38	38	43
14	18	18	18	38	38	43
19	18	18	18	33	33	38
24	12	18	18	22	28	28
28	12	18	18	18	18	18
33	12	12	12	12	12	12
37	12	12	12	12	12	12
41	9	9	9	12	12	12
45	0	9	9	12	12	12
49	0	9	9	9	12	12
53	0	9	9	9	9	9

[a]CAUTION: The results cannot be safely extrapolated to solutions with formulas other than the ones tested. See text.

μm for fat-containing and 0.2 or 0.45 μm for fat-free, nutrition mixtures (2061).

Hoie and Narducci used laser particle analysis to evaluate the formation of calcium phosphate precipitation in pediatric TPN solutions containing TrophAmine in concentrations ranging from 0.5 to 3% and also containing L-cysteine HCl 1 g/L. The solutions also contained in each liter sodium chloride 20 mEq, sodium acetate 20 mEq, magnesium sulfate 3 mEq, trace elements 3 ml, and heparin sodium 500 units. The presence of L-cysteine HCl reduces the solution pH and increases the amount of calcium and phosphate that can be incorporated before precipitation occurs. The results of this study cannot be safely extrapolated to TPN solutions with compositions other than the ones tested. The maximum amounts of phosphate that were incorporated without the appearance of a measurable increase in particulates in 24 hours at 37 °C for each of the amino acid concentrations is shown in Table 4 (2196). These results are not entirely consistent with those of Shatsky et al. See above. The use of more sensitive electronic particle measurement for the formation of subvisual particulates in this study may contribute to the differences in the results.

The presence of magnesium in solutions may also influence the reaction between calcium and phosphate, including the nature and extent of precipitation (158; 159).

The interaction of calcium and phosphate in parenteral nutrition solutions is a complex phenomenon. Various factors have been identified as playing a role in the solubility or precipitation of a given combination, including (608; 609; 1042; 1063; 1404; 1427):

1. Concentration of calcium
2. Salt form of calcium
3. Concentration of phosphate
4. Concentration of amino acids
5. Amino acids composition
6. Concentration of dextrose
7. Temperature of solution
8. pH of solution
9. Presence of other additives
10. Order of mixing

Enhanced precipitate formation would be expected from such factors as high concentrations of calcium and phosphate, increases in solution pH, decreased amino acid concentrations, increases in temperature, addition of calcium prior to the phosphate, lengthy standing times or slow infusion rates, and use of calcium as the chloride salt (854).

Even if precipitation does not occur in the bottle, it has been reported that crystallization of calcium phosphate may occur in a Silastic infusion pump chamber or tubing if the rate of administration is slow, as for premature infants. Water vapor may be transmitted outward and be replaced by air rapidly enough to produce supersaturation (202). Several other cases of catheter occlusion have been reported (610; 1427–1429).

The UV spectrum of an equal parts mixture of amino acids 8%–dextrose 50% solution was not altered in 24 hours at 22 °C by the addition of calcium gluconate 20 mEq and potassium phosphate 25 mEq (313).

Also see the monograph on sodium phosphates.

Ciprofloxacin— Admixing ciprofloxacin with sodium phosphates has resulted in reports of both compatibility and incompatibility. (See the Sodium Phosphates monograph.) Combining the two drugs in sodium chloride 0.45 or 0.9% can result in a large amount of white crystalline precipitate forming (1971; 1972), while the same concentrations in dextrose 5% in water result in little or no precipitate formation (1628; 1972). This dependency of precipitation on the nature of the infusion solution may extend to potassium phosphates as well. Although ciprofloxacin has been reported to be compatible with potassium phosphates in dextrose 5% in water (1628), the manufacturer has had reports of precipitation of these two drugs. Unfortunately, the infusion solution vehicles involved in the precipitations were not identified (2009).

PROCAINAMIDE HCL
AHFS 24:04

Products— Procainamide HCl is available in 10-ml vials providing 100 mg/ml or 2-ml vials and 2- and 4-ml prefilled syringes providing 500 mg/ml. The 100-mg/ml form also contains benzyl alcohol 0.9% (w/v) and sodium metabisulfite not more than 0.09%. The 500-mg/ml form contains methylparaben 0.1% and sodium metabisulfite not more than 0.2%. In both forms, the pH is adjusted with hydrochloric acid and/or sodium hydroxide (4; 154).

pH— From 4 to 6 (4).

Osmolality— Procainamide HCl 500 mg/ml has an osmolality exceeding 2000 mOsm/kg (1689).

Administration— Procainamide HCl may be administered by intramuscular or direct intravenous injection or intravenous infusion (4; 8). Both the 100- and 500-mg/ml forms must be diluted prior to intravenous use. The intravenous rate of administration should not exceed 25 to 50 mg/min (4).

Stability— Procainamide HCl may be stored at room temperatures up to 27 °C. However, refrigeration retards oxidation, which causes color formation. The solution is initially colorless but may turn slightly yellow on standing. Injection of air into the vial causes the solution to darken. Solutions darker than a light amber should be discarded (4).

Sorption— Procainamide HCl (Sigma) 8 mg/L in sodium chloride 0.9% (Travenol) in PVC bags did not exhibit significant sorption to the plastic during one week of storage at room temperature (15 to 20 °C) (536).

In another study, procainamide HCl (Sigma) 8 mg/L in sodium chloride 0.9% did not exhibit any loss due to sorption during a seven-hour simulated infusion through an infusion set (Travenol) consisting of a cellulose propionate burette chamber and 170 cm of PVC tubing (606).

The drug was also tested as a simulated infusion over at least one hour by a syringe pump system. A glass syringe on a syringe pump was fitted with 20 cm of polyethylene tubing or 50 cm of Silastic tubing. No loss of drug due to sorption was observed with either tubing (606).

A 25-ml aliquot of procainamide HCl (Sigma) 8 mg/L in sodium chloride 0.9% was stored in all-plastic syringes composed of polypropylene barrels and polyethylene plungers for 24 hours at room temperature in the dark. No loss due to sorption occurred (606).

Compatibility Information

Solution Compatibility

Procainamide HCl

Solution	Mfr	Mfr	Conc/L	Remarks	Ref	C/I
Dextrose 5% in sodium chloride 0.9%	MGª	SQ	4 g	Approximately 17% decomposition in 24 hr at room temperature	522	**I**

Solution Compatibility (Cont.)

Procainamide HCl

Solution	Mfr	Mfr	Conc/L	Remarks	Ref	C/I
	MG[a]	SQ	4 g	Approximately 5% decomposition in 24 hr at 4 °C	522	**C**
	TR[b]	SQ	4 g	Approximately 17% decomposition in 24 hr at room temperature	522	**I**
	TR[b]	SQ	4 g	Approximately 5% decomposition in 24 hr at 4 °C	522	**C**
	MG[a]	SQ	4 g	Approximately 20% decomposition in 24 hr at room temperature	546	**I**
	MG[a]	SQ	4 g	Approximately 5% decomposition in 24 hr at 4 °C	546	**C**
Dextrose 5% in water	TR[a]	SQ	1 g	No decomposition in 8 hr but 12% loss in 24 hr at room temperature	545	**I**
	BA[b]	ASC	4 and 8 g	12 to 14% loss in 12 hr at room temperature. 6 to 10% loss in 24 hr under refrigeration	1327	**I**
(neutralized)[c]	BA[b]	ASC	4 g	10% or less loss in 24 hr at room temperature and under refrigeration	1327	**C**
(neutralized)[c]	BA[b]	ASC	8 g	Little or no loss in 24 hr at room temperature and under refrigeration	1327	**C**
	TR	ES	4 g	24% loss in 24 hr at room temperature under fluorescent light	1358	**I**
		LY	4 and 10 g	Physically compatible with 14 to 15% loss in 4 hr at 22 °C	1419	**I**
	AB	SQ	2 g	10% procainamide loss in 5 hr and 30% loss in 24 hr at 25 °C by HPLC due to reaction with dextrose	1896	**I**
Sodium chloride 0.45%		LY	4 and 10 g	Physically compatible with no loss in 4 hr at 22 °C	1419	**C**
Sodium chloride 0.9%	TR[a]	SQ	1 g	No decomposition in 24 hr at room temperature	545	**C**

[a]Tested in glass containers.
[b]Tested in PVC containers.
[c]With pH adjusted to approximately 7.5 with sodium bicarbonate 8.4%.

Additive Compatibility

Procainamide HCl

Drug	Mfr	Conc/L	Mfr	Conc/L	Test Soln	Remarks	Ref	C/I
Amiodarone HCl	LZ	1.8 g	SQ	4 g	D5W, NS[a]	Physically compatible with amiodarone losses of 5% or less in 24 hr at 24 °C under fluorescent light	1031	**C**
Atracurium besylate	BW	500 mg		4 g	D5W	Physically compatible	1694	**C**
Bretylium tosylate	ACC	10 g	SQ	4 g	D5S[b]	Physically compatible and bretylium chemically stable for 48 hr at room temperature. Approximately 14% procainamide loss in 24 hr	522	**I**
	ACC	10 g	SQ	4 g	D5S[b]	Physically compatible and bretylium chemically stable for 7 days at 4 °C. Approximately 7% procainamide loss in 24 hr	522	**C**
	ACC	1 g	SQ	1 g	D5W, NS	Physically compatible for 48 hr at 25 °C	756	**C**
Cibenzoline succinate		2 g	SQ	8 g	D5W, NS	Physically compatible for 24 hr at 25 °C by visual and microscopic examination	1182	**C**

Additive Compatibility (Cont.)

Procainamide HCl

Drug	Mfr	Conc/L	Mfr	Conc/L	Test Soln	Remarks	Ref	C/I
Dobutamine HCl	LI	1 g	SQ	1 g	D5W, NS	Physically compatible with no color change in 24 hr at 25 °C	789	C
	LI	1 g	AHP	4 and 50 g	D5W, NS	Physically compatible for 24 hr at 21 °C	812	C
Esmolol HCl	DU	6 g	ES	4 g	D5W	43% procainamide loss in 24 hr at room temperature under fluorescent light	1358	I
Ethacrynate sodium	MSD	50 mg	SQ	1 g	NS	Altered UV spectra for both drugs at room temperature	16	I
Flumazenil	RC	20 mg	ES	4 g	D5W[c]	Visually compatible with no flumazenil loss by HPLC in 24 hr at 23 °C under fluorescent light. Procainamide not tested	1710	C
Lidocaine HCl	AST	2 g	SQ	1 g	D5W, LR, NS	Physically compatible for 24 hr at 25 °C	775	C
Milrinone lactate	WI	200 mg	SQ	2 and 4 g	D5W	2 to 3% procainamide loss in 1 hr and 10 to 11% in 4 hr at 23 °C. No milrinone loss	1191	I
Netilmicin sulfate	SC	3 g	SQ	4 g	D5S	Physically compatible and netilmicin chemically stable for 7 days at 4 and 25 °C. Procainamide not tested	558	C
Verapamil HCl	KN	80 mg	SQ	2 g	D5W, NS	Physically compatible for 48 hr	739	C

[a]Tested in both polyolefin and PVC containers.
[b]Tested in both glass and PVC containers.
[c]Tested in PVC containers.

Y-Site Injection Compatibility (1:1 Mixture)

Procainamide HCl

Drug	Mfr	Conc	Mfr	Conc	Remarks	Ref	C/I
Amiodarone HCl	LZ	4 mg/ml[c]	AHP	8 mg/ml[c]	Physically compatible for 24 hr at 21 °C	1032	C
Amrinone lactate	WB	3 mg/ml[b]	SQ	4 mg/ml[a]	Physically compatible for at least 4 hr at 25 °C under fluorescent light	992	C
	WI	2.5 mg/ml[d]	LY	20 mg/ml[d]	Physically compatible with little or no loss of either drug in 4 hr at 22 °C	1419	C
	WI	2.5 mg/ml[a]	LY	20 mg/ml[a]	18% procainamide loss and 10% amrinone loss in 4 hr at 22 °C due to dextrose diluent	1419	I
	WI	5 mg/ml	LY	4 mg/ml[d]	Physically compatible with little or no loss of either drug in 4 hr at 22 °C	1419	C
	WI	5 mg/ml	LY	4 mg/ml[a]	20% procainamide loss and 8% amrinone loss in 4 hr at 22 °C due to dextrose diluent	1419	I
	WI	2.5 mg/ml[d]	LY	4 mg/ml[d]	Physically compatible with little or no loss of either drug in 4 hr at 22 °C	1419	C
	WI	2.5 mg/ml[a]	LY	4 mg/ml[a]	17% procainamide loss in 4 hr at 22 °C due to dextrose diluent	1419	I
Cisatracurium besylate	GW	0.1, 2, 5 mg/ml[a]	ES	10 mg/ml[a]	Pysically compatible with no change in measured turbidity or increase in particle content in 4 hr at 23 °C	2074	C
Diltiazem HCl	MMD	5 mg/ml	ES	500 mg/ml	Cloudiness forms but clears within 2 min	1807	?
	MMD	1 mg/ml[b]	ES	50 mg/ml[a]	Visually compatible	1807	C

Y-Site Injection Compatibility (1:1 Mixture) (Cont.)

Procainamide HCl

Drug	Mfr	Conc	Mfr	Conc	Remarks	Ref	C/I
	MMD	5 mg/ml	ES	2 mg/ml[a]	Visually compatible	1807	C
Famotidine	MSD	0.2 mg/ml[a]	ASC	5 mg/ml[a]	Physically compatible for 4 hr at 25 °C	1188	C
Heparin sodium	UP	1000 units/L[e]	SQ	100 mg/ml	Physically compatible for at least 4 hr at room temperature by visual and microscopic examination	534	C
Hydrocortisone sodium succinate	UP	10 mg/L[e]	SQ	100 mg/ml	Physically compatible for at least 4 hr at room temperature by visual and microscopic examination	534	C
Milrinone	WI	350 µg/ml[a]	SQ	2 and 4 mg/ml[a]	3 to 6% procainamide loss in 1 hr and 10 to 13% in 4 hr at 23 °C. No milrinone loss	1191	I
Potassium chloride	AB	40 mEq/L[e]	SQ	100 mg/ml	Physically compatible for at least 4 hr at room temperature by visual and microscopic examination	534	C
Ranitidine HCl	GL	0.5 mg/ml[f]	BA	4 mg/ml[a]	Physically compatible for 24 hr	1323	C
Remifentanil HCl	GW	0.025 and 0.25 mg/ml[b]	ES	10 mg/ml[a]	Physically compatible with no change in measured turbidity or increase in particle content in 4 hr at 23 °C	2075	C
Vitamin B complex with C	RC	2 ml/L[e]	SQ	100 mg/ml	Physically compatible for at least 4 hr at room temperature by visual and microscopic examination	534	C

[a]Tested in dextrose 5% in water.
[b]Tested in sodium chloride 0.9%.
[c]Tested in dextrose 5% in water and sodium chloride 0.9%.
[d]Tested in sodium chloride 0.45%.
[e]Tested in dextrose 5% in Ringer's injection, dextrose 5% in Ringer's injection, lactated, dextrose 5% in water, Ringer's injection, lactated, and sodium chloride 0.9%.
[f]Premixed infusion solution.

Additional Compatibility Information

Oxidizing agents may cause discoloration, though usually without a significant loss of potency (40).

Solutions— Procainamide HCl 2 to 4 mg/ml in sodium chloride 0.9% or sterile water for injection is stated to be stable for 24 hours at room temperature or seven days under refrigeration (4).

Similarly, procainamide HCl in dextrose 5% in water has been stated to be stable for 24 hours at room temperature or seven days under refrigeration. However, other information indicates that procainamide HCl may be subject to greater decomposition in dextrose 5% in water unless the admixture is refrigerated (1327) or the pH is adjusted (1327; 1358; 1422; 1423).

Raymond et al. found that neutralization of the acidic pH of procainamide HCl 0.4 and 0.8% in dextrose 5% in water to approximately pH 7.5 with sodium bicarbonate 8.4% increased stability. The neutralized admixtures maintained their stability for at least 24 hours at 24 °C; the acidic admixtures lost greater than 10% procainamide HCl in six to 12 hours at 24 °C. Similar increased stability could be obtained by refrigeration (1327).

Procainamide HCl forms α- and β-glucosylamine compounds with dextrose. The reaction proceeds rapidly, with about 10% procainamide loss in dextrose 5% in water occurring in about five hours and 30% loss in 24 hours at 25 °C. Equilibrium is achieved with about 62% of the procainamide present as glucosylamines (1896). The bioavailability, activity, and metabolic fate of these compounds is not known (546; 1896). The α- and β-glucosylamine compounds that form are reversible (1422; 1896), although the extent of reversibility in plasma has been questioned (2051). The rate and extent of complex formation are dependent on the dextrose concentration and the solution pH but are independent of the procainamide HCl concentration (1422). In dextrose concentrations ranging from 1 to 5%, the extent of procainamide complex formation ranged from 6% in two days in dextrose 1% up to 35% (1422) to 60% (1896) in dextrose 5%. Lowering the pH from the normal 4.5 to 1.4 with 0.01 *N* hydrochloric acid completely prevented complex formation (1422). Similarly, increasing the solution pH to 8 is reported to block complexation (1423). Maximum complex formation occurred at pH 3 to 5 (1423) or 4 to 5.2 (1358), the natural pH of procainamide HCl admixtures in dextrose 5% in water.

The clinical importance of this complexation, if any, is uncertain. Consequently, the manufacturer continues to state that procainamide HCl 2 to 4 mg/ml in dextrose 5% in water can be considered stable for 24 hours at room temperature or seven days under refrigeration (4).

Phenytoin— The following incompatibility determination was performed with concentrated solutions. One milliliter of procainamide HCl (Squibb) was added to 5 ml of sterile distilled water along with 1 ml of phenytoin sodium (Parke-Davis). Particulate matter was observed within two hours (28).

PROCAINE HCL
AHFS 72:00

Novocain   **Abbott**

Products— Procaine HCl (Abbott) is available as a 2% solution in 30-ml vials. This solution is made isotonic with sodium chloride and contains not more than 2 mg/ml of acetone sodium bisulfite and chlorobutanol 0.25%. It is also available as a 1% solution in 2- and 6-ml ampuls and in 30-ml vials. The solutions are made isotonic with sodium chloride. The ampuls contain not more than 1 mg/ml of acetone sodium bisulfite. The vials contain not more than 2 mg/ml of acetone sodium bisulfite and chlorobutanol 0.25% (1-10/98; 4).

Procaine HCl (Abbott) is also provided as a 10% solution in 2-ml ampuls for spinal anesthesia. Each milliliter contains 100 mg of drug and not more than 1 mg of acetone sodium bisulfite (4; 29; 154).

pH— From 3 to 5.5 (4).

Osmolality— Procaine HCl 10 mg/ml has an osmolality of 279 mOsm/kg (1689).

Administration— Procaine HCl may be administered by infiltration, peripheral or sympathetic nerve block, or subarachnoid block. Less concentrated solutions may be prepared by diluting the 1% solution (1-10/98; 4).

For intraspinal use, doses of the 10% solution are diluted with 0.5 to 1 ml of appropriate diluent, depending on site of injection, and are delivered at a rate of injection of 1 ml/5 sec. For spinal anesthesia, sodium chloride 0.9%, sterile water for injection, spinal fluid, and (for hyperbaric technique) dextrose injection may be used as diluents (4).

Stability— Intact containers should be stored at controlled room temperature and protected from exposure to temperatures of 40 °C or more, from freezing, and from exposure to light. The solutions may be autoclaved at 121 °C and 15 psi for 15 minutes, but reautoclaving increases the possibility of crystal formation. Solutions of procaine HCl should not be used if crystal formation, cloudiness, or discoloration is observed (1-10/98; 4).

pH Effects— The pH of maximum stability is 3.5, with the best range being approximately 3 to 5. Procaine HCl solutions are subject to acid and base catalysis at pH values outside of this range (1072).

Compatibility Information

Solution Compatibility

Procaine HCl

Solution	Mfr	Mfr	Conc/L	Remarks	Ref	C/I
Dextran 6% in dextrose 5%	AB		1 g	Physically compatible	3	C
Dextran 6% in sodium chloride 0.9%	AB		1 g	Physically compatible	3	C
Dextrose–Ringer's injection combinations	AB		1 g	Physically compatible	3	C
Dextrose–Ringer's injection, lactated, combinations	AB		1 g	Physically compatible	3	C
Dextrose–saline combinations	AB		1 g	Physically compatible	3	C
Dextrose 2½% in water	AB		1 g	Physically compatible	3	C
Dextrose 5% in water	AB		1 g	Physically compatible	3	C
Dextrose 10% in water	AB		1 g	Physically compatible	3	C
Fructose 10% in sodium chloride 0.9%	AB		1 g	Physically compatible	3	C
Fructose 10% in water	AB		1 g	Physically compatible	3	C
Invert sugar 5 and 10% in sodium chloride 0.9%	AB		1 g	Physically compatible	3	C
Invert sugar 5 and 10% in water	AB		1 g	Physically compatible	3	C
Ionosol products	AB		1 g	Physically compatible	3	C
Ringer's injection	AB		1 g	Physically compatible	3	C

Solution Compatibility (Cont.)

Procaine HCl

Solution	Mfr	Mfr	Conc/L	Remarks	Ref	C/I
Ringer's injection, lactated	AB		1 g	Physically compatible	3	**C**
Sodium chloride 0.45%	AB		1 g	Physically compatible	3	**C**
Sodium chloride 0.9%	AB		1 g	Physically compatible	3	**C**
Sodium lactate ⅙ M	AB		1 g	Physically compatible	3	**C**

Additive Compatibility

Procaine HCl

Drug	Mfr	Conc/L	Mfr	Conc/L	Test Soln	Remarks	Ref	C/I
Aminophylline	SE	500 mg	AB	1 g		Physically compatible	6	**C**
						Physically incompatible	9	**I**
	SE	1 g	WI	1 g	D5W	Physically incompatible	15	**I**
Amobarbital sodium						Physically incompatible	9	**I**
	LI	1 g	WI	1 g	D5W	Physically incompatible	15	**I**
Ascorbic acid injection	UP	500 mg	WI	1 g	D5W	Physically compatible	15	**C**
Chlorothiazide sodium	MSD					Physically incompatible	9	**I**
Hydrocortisone sodium succinate	UP	500 mg	WI	1 g	D5W	Physically compatible	15	**C**
Magnesium sulfate						Physically incompatible	9	**I**
	LI	16 mEq	WI	1 g	D5W	Physically incompatible	15	**I**
Penicillin G potassium		1 million units		1 g		Physically compatible	3	**C**
	SQ	20 million units	WI	1 g	D5W	Physically compatible	15	**C**
Penicillin G sodium	UP	20 million units	WI	1 g	D5W	Physically compatible	15	**C**
Phenobarbital sodium	WI					Physically incompatible	9	**I**
Phenytoin sodium	PD					Physically incompatible	9	**I**
Sodium bicarbonate						Physically incompatible	9	**I**
	AB	80 mEq	WI	1 g	D5W	Physically incompatible	15	**I**
Vitamin B complex with C	AB	2 ml		1 g		Physically compatible	3	**C**
	AB	5 ml	WI	1 g	D5W	Physically compatible	15	**C**

Drugs in Syringe Compatibility

Procaine HCl

Drug (in syringe)	Mfr	Amt	Mfr	Amt	Remarks	Ref	C/I
Ampicillin sodium	BE				Physically compatible	89	**C**
Glycopyrrolate	RB	0.2 mg/ 1 ml	ES	10 mg/ 1 ml	Physically compatible and pH in stability range for glycopyrrolate for 48 hr at 25 °C	331	**C**
	RB	0.2 mg/ 1 ml	ES	20 mg/ 2 ml	Physically compatible and pH in stability range for glycopyrrolate for 48 hr at 25 °C	331	**C**
	RB	0.4 mg/ 2 ml	ES	10 mg/ 1 ml	Physically compatible and pH in stability range for glycopyrrolate for 48 hr at 25 °C	331	**C**

Drugs in Syringe Compatibility (Cont.)

Procaine HCl

Drug (in syringe)	Mfr	Amt	Mfr	Amt	Remarks	Ref	C/I
	RB	0.2 mg/ 1 ml	ES	20 mg/ 1 ml	Physically compatible and pH in stability range for glycopyrrolate for 48 hr at 25 °C	331	C
	RB	0.2 mg/ 1 ml	ES	40 mg/ 2 ml	Physically compatible and pH in stability range for glycopyrrolate for 48 hr at 25 °C	331	C
	RB	0.4 mg/ 2 ml	ES	20 mg/ 1 ml	Physically compatible and pH in stability range for glycopyrrolate for 48 hr at 25 °C	331	C
Hydroxyzine HCl	PF	50 mg/ 2 ml	WI	2%/2 ml	Physically compatible	771	C
	PF	100 mg/ 2 ml	WI	2%/2 ml	Physically compatible	771	C

Additional Compatibility Information

Miscellaneous— Local anesthetics such as procaine HCl cause precipitation of amphotericin B (107). Procaine HCl is incompatible with alkali hydroxides and their carbonates (4).

Hydrocortisone— Procaine HCl 1 g/L has been reported to be conditionally compatible with hydrocortisone sodium succinate (Upjohn) 250 mg/L. The mixture is physically compatible in most Abbott infusion solutions except as noted below (3):

Beclysyl 5 and 10%	Haze or precipitate forms within 24 hr
Ionosol B with invert sugar 10%	Haze or precipitate forms within 24 hr
Ionosol G with invert sugar 10%	Haze or precipitate forms within 24 hr

Cardioplegia Solutions— The stability of procaine HCl in cardioplegia solutions composed of Ringer's injection with added increments of potassium and magnesium was assessed. The procaine HCl underwent little or no decomposition after 101 days of storage (719).

In another study, the cardioplegia solutions were similarly formulated except that the pH was buffered with tromethamine from the inherent pH 5 to a physiological pH of 7.3 to 7.6. The procaine HCl underwent 10% decomposition in 10 days when stored under refrigeration. It was calculated that a 10% loss would occur in about two days at room temperature. The authors recommended that if the cardioplegia solution is to be buffered to the physiological range, then the procaine HCl should be added to the formulation at the time of dispensing to permit a minimal loss of the drug (720).

Synave et al. evaluated the stability of procaine HCl 270 mg/L in cardioplegia solutions containing sodium bicarbonate (pH 7.6) and stored at 37, 21, 6, and −10 °C. At 37 °C, 70% of the procaine HCl was lost in one week. At 21 and 6 °C, 10% was lost in one and five weeks, respectively. When frozen at −10 °C, the solutions lost less than 10% in nine weeks. However, thawing in a microwave oven resulted in the formation of a white crystalline precipitate. Exposure to light did not affect the rate of procaine hydrolysis (1128).

PROCHLORPERAZINE EDISYLATE
AHFS 28:16.08 and 56:22

Compazine   **SmithKline Beecham**

Products— Prochlorperazine edisylate (SmithKline Beecham) is available in 2-ml vials and disposable syringes and 10-ml multiple-dose vials. Each milliliter of solution contains (2):

Prochlorperazine as edisylate	5 mg
Sodium biphosphate	5 mg
Sodium tartrate	12 mg
Sodium saccharin	0.9 mg
Benzyl alcohol	0.75%

pH— From 4.2 to 6.2 (4).

Osmolality— Prochlorperazine edisylate 5 mg/ml has an osmolality of 282 mOsm/kg (1689).

Administration— Prochlorperazine edisylate may be given intramuscularly deep into the upper outer quadrant of the buttock. It may also be given by direct intravenous injection at a rate not exceeding 5 mg/min. It can be given undiluted or diluted in a compatible diluent. It should not be given as a bolus intravenous injection (2; 4). For intravenous infusion, dilution of 20 mg in a liter of compatible infusion solution is recommended (4). Because the drug causes local irritation subcutaneous injection is not recommended (2; 4).

Stability— Intact containers should be stored at controlled room temperature and protected from temperatures of 40 °C or more and from freezing. Solutions of prochlorperazine edisylate are light sensitive and, therefore, should be protected from light. A slightly yellow solution has not had its potency altered. However, a markedly discolored solution should be discarded (2; 4).

Prochlorperazine edisylate (SKF) 5 mg/ml retained potency for three months at room temperature when 1 and 2 ml of solution were packaged in Tubex cartridges (13).

Filtration— Prochlorperazine edisylate (SKF) 5 mg/L in dextrose 5%

in water and sodium chloride 0.9% did not display significant sorption to a 0.45-μm cellulose membrane filter during an eight-hour simulated infusion (567).

Compatibility Information

Solution Compatibility

Prochlorperazine edisylate

Solution	Mfr	Mfr	Conc/L	Remarks	Ref	C/I
Dextran 6% in dextrose 5%	AB	SKF	10 mg	Physically compatible	3	C
Dextran 6% in sodium chloride 0.9%	AB	SKF	10 mg	Physically compatible	3	C
Dextrose–Ringer's injection combinations	AB	SKF	10 mg	Physically compatible	3	C
Dextrose–Ringer's injection, lactated, combinations	AB	SKF	10 mg	Physically compatible	3	C
Dextrose–saline combinations	AB	SKF	10 mg	Physically compatible	3	C
Dextrose 2½% in water	AB	SKF	10 mg	Physically compatible	3	C
Dextrose 5% in water	AB	SKF	10 mg	Physically compatible	3	C
Dextrose 10% in water	AB	SKF	10 mg	Physically compatible	3	C
Fructose 10% in sodium chloride 0.9%	AB	SKF	10 mg	Physically compatible	3	C
Fructose 10% in water	AB	SKF	10 mg	Physically compatible	3	C
Invert sugar 5 and 10% in sodium chloride 0.9%	AB	SKF	10 mg	Physically compatible	3	C
Invert sugar 5 and 10% in water	AB	SKF	10 mg	Physically compatible	3	C
Ionosol products	AB	SKF	10 mg	Physically compatible	3	C
Ringer's injection	AB	SKF	10 mg	Physically compatible	3	C
Ringer's injection, lactated	AB	SKF	10 mg	Physically compatible	3	C
Sodium chloride 0.45%	AB	SKF	10 mg	Physically compatible	3	C
Sodium chloride 0.9%	AB	SKF	10 mg	Physically compatible	3	C
Sodium lactate ⅙ M	AB	SKF	10 mg	Physically compatible	3	C

Additive Compatibility

Prochlorperazine edisylate[a]

Drug	Mfr	Conc/L	Mfr	Conc/L	Test Soln	Remarks	Ref	C/I
Amikacin sulfate	BR	5 g	SKF	20 mg	D5LR, D5R, D5S, D5W, D10W, IS10, LR, NS, R, SL	Physically compatible and potency of both drugs retained for 24 hr at 25 °C	294	C
Aminophylline	SE	1 g	SKF	100 mg	D5W	Physically incompatible	15	I
	BP	1 g	BP	100 mg (M)	D5W, NS	Immediate precipitation	26	I
Amphotericin B		200 mg	BP	100 mg (M)	D5W	Haze develops over 3 hr	26	I
Ampicillin sodium	BP	2 g	BP	100 mg (M)	D5W, NS	Immediate precipitation	26	I

Additive Compatibility (Cont.)

Prochlorperazine edisylate[a]

Drug	Mfr	Conc/L	Mfr	Conc/L	Test Soln	Remarks	Ref	C/I
Ascorbic acid injection	UP	500 mg	SKF	100 mg	D5W	Physically compatible	15	C
Calcium gluconate			SKF			Physically incompatible	9	I
	UP	1 g	SKF	100 mg	D5W	Physically compatible	15	C
Chloramphenicol sodium succinate	PD	10 g	SKF	100 mg	D5W	Physically incompatible	15	I
	BP	4 g	BP	100 mg (M)	NS	Haze develops over 3 hr	26	I
Chlorothiazide sodium	MSD		SKF			Physically incompatible	9	I
	BP	2 g	BP	100 mg (M)	D5W	Immediate precipitation	26	I
	BP	2 g	BP	100 mg (M)	NS	Haze develops over 3 hr	26	I
Dexamethasone sodium phosphate	MSD	20 mg	SKF	100 mg	D5W	Physically compatible	15	C
Dimenhydrinate	SE	500 mg	SKF	100 mg	D5W	Physically compatible	15	C
Erythromycin lactobionate	AB	1 g	SKF	10 mg		Physically compatible. Erythromycin potency retained for 24 hr at 25 °C	20	C
Ethacrynate sodium	MSD	80 mg	SKF	20 mg	NS	Little alteration of UV spectra within 8 hr at room temperature	16	C
Floxacillin sodium	BE	20 g	MB	1.25 g	W	Precipitate forms immediately	1479	I
Furosemide	HO	1 g	MB	1.25 g	W	Yellow globular precipitate forms immediately	1479	I
Hydrocortisone sodium succinate			SKF			Physically incompatible	9	I
Lidocaine HCl	AST	2 g	SKF	10 mg		Physically compatible	24	C
Methohexital sodium	BP	2 g	BP	100 mg (M)	D5W	Haze develops over 3 hr	26	I
Nafcillin sodium	WY	500 mg	SKF	10 mg		Physically compatible	27	C
Penicillin G potassium	SQ	1 million units	SKF	10 mg	D5W	Physically compatible. Penicillin potency retained for 24 hr at 25 °C	47	C
	(B)[b]	900,000 units	SKF	10 mg	D5W	Penicillin potency retained for 24 hr at 25 °C	48	C
	BP	10 million units	BP	100 mg (M)	NS	Haze develops over 3 hr	26	I
Penicillin G sodium	BP	10 million units	BP	100 mg (M)	NS	Haze develops over 3 hr	26	I
Phenobarbital sodium	BP	800 mg	BP	100 mg (M)	D5W	Haze develops over 3 hr	26	I
	BP	800 mg	BP	100 mg (M)	NS	Immediate precipitation	26	I
Sodium bicarbonate	AB	2.4 mEq[c]	SKF	10 mg	D5W	Physically compatible for 24 hr	772	C
Thiopental sodium	AB		SKF			Physically incompatible	9	I

Additive Compatibility (Cont.)

Prochlorperazine edisylate[a]

Drug	Mfr	Conc/L	Mfr	Conc/L	Test Soln	Remarks	Ref	C/I
Vitamin B complex with C	AB	5 ml	SKF	100 mg	D5W	Physically compatible	15	**C**

[a]Entries with the notation "(M)" in the prochlorperazine Conc/L column were tested as the mesylate salt.
[b]A buffered preparation was specified.
[c]One vial of Neut added to a liter of admixture.

Drugs in Syringe Compatibility

Prochlorperazine edisylate

Drug (in syringe)	Mfr	Amt	Mfr	Amt	Remarks	Ref	C/I
Atropine sulfate		0.6 mg/ 1.5 ml	SKF		Physically compatible for at least 15 min	14	**C**
	ST	0.4 mg/ 1 ml	PO	5 mg/ 1 ml	Physically compatible for at least 15 min	326	**C**
Butorphanol tartrate	BR	4 mg/ 2 ml	MB	5 mg/ 1 ml	Physically compatible both macroscopically and microscopically for 30 min at room temperature	566	**C**
Chlorpromazine HCl	SKF	50 mg/ 2 ml	SKF		Physically compatible for at least 15 min	14	**C**
	PO	50 mg/ 2 ml	PO	5 mg/ 1 ml	Physically compatible for at least 15 min	326	**C**
Cimetidine HCl	SKF	300 mg/ 2 ml	SKF	10 mg/ 2 ml	Physically compatible for 4 hr at 25 °C	25	**C**
Diamorphine HCl	MB	10, 25, 50 mg/ 1 ml	MB	1.25 mg/ 1 ml[a]	Physically compatible and diamorphine content retained for 24 hr at room temperature	1454	**C**
Dimenhydrinate	HR	50 mg/ 1 ml	PO	5 mg/ 1 ml	Physically incompatible within 15 min	326	**I**
Diphenhydramine HCl	PD	50 mg/ 1 ml	PO	5 mg/ 1 ml	Physically compatible for at least 15 min	326	**C**
Droperidol	MN	2.5 mg/ 1 ml	PO	5 mg/ 1 ml	Physically compatible for at least 15 min	326	**C**
Fentanyl citrate	MN	0.05 mg/ 1 ml	PO	5 mg/ 1 ml	Physically compatible for at least 15 min	326	**C**
Glycopyrrolate	RB	0.2 mg/ 1 ml	SKF	5 mg/ 1 ml	Physically compatible and pH in stability range for glycopyrrolate for 48 hr at 25 °C	331	**C**
	RB	0.2 mg/ 1 ml	SKF	10 mg/ 2 ml	Physically compatible and pH in stability range for glycopyrrolate for 48 hr at 25 °C	331	**C**
	RB	0.4 mg/ 2 ml	SKF	5 mg/ 1 ml	Physically compatible and pH in stability range for glycopyrrolate for 48 hr at 25 °C	331	**C**
Hydromorphone HCl	KN	4 mg/ 2 ml[b]	SKF	5 mg/ 1 ml	Immediate precipitation	517	**I**
	KN	4 mg/ 2 ml[c]	SKF	5 mg/ 1 ml	Physically compatible for 30 min	517	**C**
	KN	1, 10, 40 mg/ 1 ml	RP	5 mg/ 1 ml[d]	Visually compatible with little or no loss of either drug by HPLC in 7 days at 4, 23, and 37 °C	1776	**C**
	SX	0.5 mg/ ml[f]	RP	1.5 mg/ ml[d,f]	Visually and microscopically compatible for 96 hr at room temperature exposed to light	2171	**C**

Drugs in Syringe Compatibility (Cont.)

Prochlorperazine edisylate

Drug (in syringe)	Mfr	Amt	Mfr	Amt	Remarks	Ref	C/I
Hydroxyzine HCl	PF	50 mg/ 1 ml	PO	5 mg/ 1 ml	Physically compatible for at least 15 min	326	C
Ketorolac tromethamine	SY	180 mg/ 6 ml	STS	15 mg/ 3 ml	Heavy white precipitate forms immediately, separating into two layers over time	1703	I
Meperidine HCl	WY	100 mg/ 1 ml	SKF		Physically compatible for at least 15 min	14	C
	WI	50 mg/ 1 ml	PO	5 mg/ 1 ml	Physically compatible for at least 15 min	326	C
Metoclopramide HCl	NO	10 mg/ 2 ml	MB	10 mg/ 2 ml	Physically compatible both macroscopically and microscopically for 15 min at room temperature	565	C
Midazolam HCl	RC	5 mg/ 1 ml	SKF	10 mg/ 2 ml	White precipitate forms immediately	1145	I
Morphine sulfate	WY	15 mg/ 1 ml	SKF		Physically compatible for at least 15 min	14	C
	ST	15 mg/ 1 ml	PO	5 mg/ 1 ml	Physically compatible for at least 15 min	326	C
	WB	10 mg/ 1 ml	ES, SKF	10 mg/ 2 ml	Immediate precipitation, probably due to phenol in morphine formulation	1006	I
	WY	8, 10, 15 mg/ 1 ml	SKF	5 mg/ 1 ml	Physically compatible for 24 hr at 25 °C	1086	C
Morphine tartrate	DB	e	DB	10 mg/ 2 ml	Visually discolored with 22% morphine loss by HPLC in 48 hr at room temperature protected from light. Prochlorperazine not tested	1599	I
Nalbuphine HCl	EN	10 mg/ 1 ml	WY	5 mg/ 1 ml	Physically compatible for 36 hr at 27 °C	762	C
	EN	5 mg/ 0.5 ml	WY	5 mg/ 1 ml	Physically compatible for 36 hr at 27 °C	762	C
	EN	2.5 mg/ 0.25 ml	WY	5 mg/ 1 ml	Physically compatible for 36 hr at 27 °C	762	C
	DU	10 mg/ 1 ml	SKF	10 mg/ 2 ml	Physically compatible for 48 hr	128	C
	DU	20 mg/ 1 ml	SKF	10 mg/ 2 ml	Physically compatible for 48 hr	128	C
Pentazocine lactate	WI	30 mg/ 1 ml	PO	5 mg/ 1 ml	Physically compatible for at least 15 min	326	C
Pentobarbital sodium	WY	100 mg/ 2 ml	SKF		Precipitate forms within 15 min	14	I
	AB	500 mg/ 10 ml	SKF	10 mg/ 2 ml	Physically incompatible	55	I
	AB	50 mg/ 1 ml	PO	5 mg/ 1 ml	Physically incompatible within 15 min	326	I
Perphenazine	SC	5 mg/ 1 ml	MB	5 mg/ 1 ml	Physically compatible both macroscopically and microscopically for 30 min at room temperature	566	C
Promazine HCl	WY	50 mg/ 1 ml	PO	5 mg/ 1 ml	Physically compatible for at least 15 min	326	C
Promethazine HCl	PO	50 mg/ 2 ml	PO	5 mg/ 1 ml	Physically compatible for at least 15 min	326	C

Drugs in Syringe Compatibility (Cont.)

Prochlorperazine edisylate

Drug (in syringe)	Mfr	Amt	Mfr	Amt	Remarks	Ref	C/I
Ranitidine HCl	GL	50 mg/ 2 ml	RP	10 mg/ 2 ml	Physically compatible for 1 hr at 25 °C both macroscopically and microscopically	978	C
Scopolamine HBr		0.6 mg/ 1.5 ml	SKF		Physically compatible for at least 15 min	14	C
	ST	0.4 mg/ 1 ml	PO	5 mg/ 1 ml	Physically compatible for at least 15 min	326	C
Sufentanil citrate	JN	50 μg/ml	SCN	5 mg/ml	Physically compatible with no subvisual haze or particle formation in 24 hr at 23 °C	1711	C
Thiopental sodium	AB	75 mg/ 3 ml	SKF	10 mg/ 2 ml	Physically incompatible	21	I

[a]*Diluted with sterile water for injection.*
[b]*The vial formulation was tested.*
[c]*The ampul formulation was tested.*
[d]*Tested as the mesylate salt.*
[e]*Amount unspecified.*
[f]*Diluted in sodium chloride 0.9%.*

Y-Site Injection Compatibility (1:1 Mixture)

Prochlorperazine edisylate

Drug	Mfr	Conc	Mfr	Conc	Remarks	Ref	C/I
Aldesleukin	CHI	33,800 I.U./ ml[a]	SKB	5 mg/ml	Aldesleukin bioactivity inhibited	1857	I
Allopurinol sodium	BW	3 mg/ml[b]	SKB	0.5 mg/ml[b]	Heavy turbidity forms immediately	1686	I
Amifostine	USB	10 mg/ml[a]	SN	0.5 mg/ml[a]	Immediate increase in subvisual haze	1845	I
Amphotericin B cholesteryl sulfate complex	SEQ	0.83 mg/ml[a]	SKB	0.5 mg/ml[a]	Gross precipitate forms	2117	I
Amsacrine	NCI	1 mg/ml[a]	SKF	0.5 mg/ml[a]	Physically compatible for 4 hr at room temperature under fluorescent light	1381	C
Aztreonam	SQ	40 mg/ml[a]	ES	0.5 mg/ml[a]	Haze and tiny particles form within 4 hr	1758	I
Calcium gluconate	AMR	10 mg/ml[b]	SCN	5 mg/ml	Visually compatible for 24 hr at room temperature in test tubes. No precipitate found on filter from Y-site delivery	2063	C
Cefepime HCl	BR	20 mg/ml[a]	SN	0.5 mg/ml[a]	Haze forms immediately. Flocculent precipitate forms in 4 hr	1689	I
Cisatracurium besylate	GW	0.1, 2, 5 mg/ml[a]	SO	0.5 mg/ml[a]	Physically compatible with no change in measured turbidity or increase in particle content in 4 hr at 23 °C	2074	C
Cisplatin	BR	1 mg/ml	SKF	0.5 mg/ml[a]	Visually compatible for 4 hr at room temperature under fluorescent light	1685	C
Cladribine	ORT	0.015[b] and 0.5[d] mg/ml	SCN	0.5 mg/ml[b]	Physically compatible with no change in measured turbidity or increase in particle content in 4 hr at 23 °C	1969	C
Clarithromycin	AB	4 mg/ml[a]	ANT[i]	12.5 mg/ml	Visually compatible for 72 hr at both 30 and 17 °C	2174	C
Cyclophosphamide	MJ	10 mg/ml	SKF	0.5 mg/ml[a]	Visually compatible for 4 hr at room temperature under fluorescent light	1685	C

Y-Site Injection Compatibility (1:1 Mixture) (Cont.)

Prochlorperazine edisylate

Drug	Mfr	Conc	Mfr	Conc	Remarks	Ref	C/I
Cytarabine	UP	50 mg/ml	SKF	0.5 mg/ml[a]	Visually compatible for 4 hr at room temperature under fluorescent light	1685	C
Docetaxel	RPR	0.9 mg/ml[a]	SO	0.5 mg/ml[a]	Physically compatible with no change in measured turbidity or increase in particle content in 4 hr at 23 °C	2224	C
Doxorubicin HCl	AD	0.2 mg/ml[a]	SKF	0.5 mg/ml[a]	Visually compatible for 4 hr at room temperature under fluorescent light	1685	C
Doxorubicin HCl liposome injection	SEQ	0.4 mg/ml[a]	SO	0.5 mg/ml[a]	Physically compatible with little or no change in measured turbidity and no increase in particle content in 4 hr at 23 °C	2087	C
Etoposide phosphate	BR	5 mg/ml[a]	ES	0.5 mg/ml[a]	White cloudy solution forms immediately with precipitate in 4 hr	2218	I
Fluconazole	RR	2 mg/ml	SKF	5 mg/ml	Physically compatible for 24 hr at 25 °C	1407	C
Fludarabine phosphate	BX	1 mg/ml[a]	WY	0.5 mg/ml[a]	Slight haze forms within 30 min	1439	I
Foscarnet sodium	AST	24 mg/ml	SKF	5 mg/ml	Cloudy brown solution	1335	I
Filgrastim	AMG	30 μg/ml[a]	SCN	0.5 mg/ml[a]	Particles form immediately. Filaments form in 1 hr	1687	I
Gemcitabine HCl	LI	10 mg/ml[b]	SCN	0.5 mg/ml[b]	Subvisual haze forms immediately and increases over 4 hr	2226	I
Granisetron HCl	SKB	0.05 mg/ml[a]	SCN	0.5 mg/ml[a]	Physically compatible with no change in measured turbidity or increase in particle content in 4 hr at 23 °C	2000	C
Heparin sodium	UP	1000 units/L[e]	SKF	5 mg/ml	Physically compatible for at least 4 hr at room temperature by visual and microscopic examination	534	C
Hydrocortisone sodium succinate	UP	10 mg/L[e]	SKF	5 mg/ml	Physically compatible for at least 4 hr at room temperature by visual and microscopic examination	534	C
Melphalan HCl	BW	0.1 mg/ml[b]	SKB	0.5 mg/ml[b]	Physically compatible with no change in measured turbidity or increase in particle content in 3 hr at 22 °C	1557	C
Methotrexate sodium	AD	15 mg/ml[f]	SKF	0.5 mg/ml[a]	Visually compatible for 4 hr at room temperature under fluorescent light	1685	C
Ondansetron HCl	GL	1 mg/ml[b]	SKF	0.5 mg/ml[a]	Physically compatible for 4 hr at 22 °C	1365	C
Paclitaxel	NCI	1.2 mg/ml[a]		0.5 mg/ml[a]	Physically compatible with no change in measured turbidity in 4 hr at 22 °C	1528	C
Piperacillin sodium–tazobactam sodium	LE	40 + 5 mg/ml[a]	SCN	0.5 mg/ml[a]	White turbidity forms immediately	1688	I
Potassium chloride	AB	40 mEq/L[e]	SKF	5 mg/ml	Physically compatible for at least 4 hr at room temperature by visual and microscopic examination	534	C
Propofol	ZEN	10 mg/ml	SCN	0.5 mg/ml[a]	Physically compatible for 1 hr at 23 °C with no increase in particle content	2066	C
Remifentanil HCl	GW	0.025 and 0.25 mg/ml[b]	SO	0.5 mg/ml[a]	Physically compatible with no change in measured turbidity or increase in particle content in 4 hr at 23 °C	2075	C

Y-Site Injection Compatibility (1:1 Mixture) (Cont.)

Prochlorperazine edisylate

Drug	Mfr	Conc	Mfr	Conc	Remarks	Ref	C/I
Sargramostim	IMM	10 μg/ml[b]	ES	0.5 mg/ml[b]	Physically compatible for 4 hr at 22 °C	1436	**C**
Sufentanil citrate	JN	12.5 μg/ml[a]	SCN	0.5 mg/ml[a]	Physically compatible with little subvisual haze or particle formation in 24 hr at 23 °C	1711	**C**
Teniposide	BR	0.1 mg/ml[a]	SCN	0.5 mg/ml[a]	Physically compatible with no subvisual haze or particle formation in 4 hr at 23 °C	1725	**C**
Thiotepa	IMM[g]	1 mg/ml[a]	SCN	0.5 mg/ml[a]	Physically compatible with no change in measured turbidity or increase in particle content in 4 hr at 23 °C	1861	**C**
TNA #218 to #226[h]			SCN, SO	0.5 mg/ml[a]	Visually compatible with no precipitate or emulsion damage apparent in 4 hr at 23 °C	2215	**C**
TPN #212 to #215[h]			SCN	0.5 mg/ml[a]	Physically compatible with no change in measured turbidity or increase in particle content in 4 hr at 23 °C	2109	**C**
Vinorelbine tartrate	BW	1 mg/ml[b]	SKB	0.5 mg/ml[b]	Physically compatible with no change in measured turbidity or increase in particle content in 4 hr at 22 °C	1558	**C**
Vitamin B complex with C	RC	2 ml/L[e]	SKF	5 mg/ml	Physically compatible for at least 4 hr at room temperature by visual and microscopic examination	534	**C**

[a]*Tested in dextrose 5% in water.*
[b]*Tested in sodium chloride 0.9%.*
[c]*Tested in sterile water for injection.*
[d]*Tested in bacteriostatic sodium chloride 0.9% preserved with benzyl alcohol 0.9%.*
[e]*Tested in dextrose 5% in Ringer's injection, dextrose 5% in Ringer's injection, lactated, dextrose 5% in water, Ringer's injection, lactated, and sodium chloride 0.9%.*
[f]*Tested in dextrose 5% in water with sodium bicarbonate 0.05 mEq/ml.*
[g]*Lyophilized formulation tested.*
[h]*Refer to Appendix I for the composition of parenteral nutrition solutions. TNA indicates a 3-in-1 admixture, and TPN indicates a 2-in-1 admixture.*
[i]*Salt form unspecified.*

Additional Compatibility Information

The manufacturer recommends that other agents not be mixed in a syringe with prochlorperazine edisylate (2).

Diamorphine HCl—— Prochlorperazine edisylate is stated to be compatible with diamorphine HCl (1442).

Parabens—— Dilution of prochlorperazine edisylate (SKF) to a 1-mg/ml concentration with bacteriostatic sodium chloride 0.9% containing methyl- and propylparabens resulted in a distinctly cloudy solution. This cloudiness did not occur when sodium chloride 0.9% preserved with benzyl alcohol was used for the dilution (752).

Concentrated Solutions—— The following incompatibility determinations were performed with concentrated solutions. The drugs in dry form were reconstituted according to manufacturers' recommendations. One milliliter of prochlorperazine edisylate (SKF) was added to 5 ml of sterile distilled water along with 1 ml of each of the following drugs. Particulate matter was noted within two hours (28):

Aminophylline
Chloramphenicol sodium succinate (Parke-Davis)
Dexamethasone sodium phosphate (MSD)
Dimenhydrinate (Searle)
Heparin sodium
Penicillin G potassium
Phenobarbital sodium (Winthrop)
Phenytoin sodium (Parke-Davis)
Vitamin B complex with C (Lederle)

PROMETHAZINE HCL
AHFS 4:00 and 28:24.92

Phenergan   **Wyeth-Ayerst**

Products— Promethazine HCl (Wyeth-Ayerst) is available in 1-ml ampuls and Tubex disposable cartridge units. Each milliliter of solution contains (2):

Component	Ampul	Tubex
Promethazine HCl	25 or 50 mg	25 or 50 mg
Disodium edetate	0.1 mg	0.1 mg
Calcium chloride	0.04 mg	0.04 mg
Sodium metabisulfite	0.25 mg	
Monothioglycerol		≦5 mg
Phenol	5 mg	5 mg

Both the ampul and Tubex formulations also contain a sodium acetate–acetic acid buffer (2).

pH— From 4 to 5.5 (4).

Osmolality— The osmolality of promethazine HCl 25 mg/ml was determined to be 291 mOsm/kg (1233).

Administration— Promethazine HCl is administered by deep intramuscular or intravenous injection. It should not be given subcutaneously or intra-arterially. When given by intravenous injection, a concentration not exceeding 25 mg/ml should be given into the tubing of a running infusion solution at a rate not exceeding 25 mg/min (2; 4). Extravasation should be avoided (4).

Stability— The product should be stored at controlled room temperature and protected from freezing and light. The injection should be inspected prior to administration for particulate matter formation and discoloration; the injection should be discarded if particulate matter or discoloration is observed (2; 4). In general, promethazine HCl exhibits increasing stability with decreasing pH (1072).

Repackaging in Syringes— Promethazine HCl (Fellows) 25 mg/1 ml repackaged in 3-ml amber glass syringes (Hy-Pod) and stored at 25 °C exhibited no significant changes in pH or physical appearance during 360 days of storage. A possible reduction in drug concentration to about 95% of initial was noted during this period (535).

Sorption— Promethazine HCl (May & Baker) 8 mg/L in sodium chloride 0.9% (Travenol) in PVC bags exhibited only about 5% sorption to the plastic during one week of storage at room temperature (15 to 20 °C). However, when the solution was buffered from its initial pH of 5 to 7.4, approximately 59% of the drug was lost in one week due to sorption (536).

In another study, promethazine HCl (May & Baker) 8 mg/L in sodium chloride 0.9% exhibited a cumulative 22% loss during a seven-hour simulated infusion through an infusion set (Travenol) consisting of a cellulose propionate burette chamber and 170 cm of PVC tubing due to sorption. Both the burette and the tubing contributed to the loss. The extent of sorption was found to be independent of concentration (606).

The drug was also tested as a simulated infusion over at least one hour by a syringe pump system. A glass syringe on a syringe pump was fitted with 20 cm of polyethylene tubing or 50 cm of Silastic tubing. Only 5% of the drug was lost with the polyethylene tubing, but a cumulative loss of 72% occurred during the one-hour infusion through the Silastic tubing (606).

A 25-ml aliquot of promethazine HCl (May & Baker) 8 mg/L in sodium chloride 0.9% was stored in all-plastic syringes composed of polypropylene barrels and polyethylene plungers for 24 hours at room temperature in the dark. No loss due to sorption occurred (606).

Martens et al. reported that promethazine HCl 100 µg/ml in sodium chloride 0.9% in PVC, glass, and polyethylene-lined laminated containers exhibited little or no loss due to sorption in 24 hours at 21 °C when protected from light (1392).

Compatibility Information

Solution Compatibility

Promethazine HCl

Solution	Mfr	Mfr	Conc/L	Remarks	Ref	C/I
Dextran 6% in dextrose 5%	AB	WY	100 mg	Physically compatible	3	C
Dextran 6% in sodium chloride 0.9%	AB	WY	100 mg	Physically compatible	3	C
Dextrose–Ringer's injection combinations	AB	WY	100 mg	Physically compatible	3	C
Dextrose–Ringer's injection, lactated, combinations	AB	WY	100 mg	Physically compatible	3	C
Dextrose–saline combinations	AB	WY	100 mg	Physically compatible	3	C
Dextrose 2½% in water	AB	WY	100 mg	Physically compatible	3	C
Dextrose 5% in water	AB	WY	100 mg	Physically compatible	3	C
Dextrose 10% in water	AB	WY	100 mg	Physically compatible	3	C
Fructose 10% in sodium chloride 0.9%	AB	WY	100 mg	Physically compatible	3	C
Fructose 10% in water	AB	WY	100 mg	Physically compatible	3	C
Invert sugar 5 and 10% in sodium chloride 0.9%	AB	WY	100 mg	Physically compatible	3	C

Solution Compatibility (Cont.)

Promethazine HCl

Solution	Mfr	Mfr	Conc/L	Remarks	Ref	C/I
Invert sugar 5 and 10% in water	AB	WY	100 mg	Physically compatible	3	C
Ionosol products	AB	WY	100 mg	Physically compatible	3	C
Ringer's injection	AB	WY	100 mg	Physically compatible	3	C
Ringer's injection, lactated	AB	WY	100 mg	Physically compatible	3	C
Sodium chloride 0.45%	AB	WY	100 mg	Physically compatible	3	C
Sodium chloride 0.9%	AB	WY	100 mg	Physically compatible	3	C
	a		100 mg	Physically compatible with little or no drug loss in 24 hr at 21 °C in the dark	1392	C
Sodium lactate ⅙ M	AB	WY	100 mg	Physically compatible	3	C

[a]Tested in PVC, glass, and polyethylene-lined laminated containers.

Additive Compatibility

Promethazine HCl

Drug	Mfr	Conc/L	Mfr	Conc/L	Test Soln	Remarks	Ref	C/I
Amikacin sulfate	BR	5 g	WY	100 mg	D5LR, D5R, D5S, D5W, D10W, IS10, LR, NS, R, SL	Physically compatible and potency of both drugs retained for 24 hr at 25 °C	294	C
Aminophylline	SE	1 g	WY	250 mg	D5W	Physically incompatible	15	I
	BP	1 g	BP	100 mg	D5W, NS	Immediate precipitation	26	I
Ascorbic acid injection	UP	500 mg	WY	250 mg	D5W	Physically compatible	15	C
Chloramphenicol sodium succinate	PD	10 g	WY	250 mg	D5W	Physically incompatible	15	I
Chloroquine phosphate		5 mg		5 mg	W	Visually compatible with no change in UV spectra	1745	C
		25 mg		5 mg	W	Visually compatible with no change in UV spectra	1745	C
		5 mg		25 mg	W	Visually compatible with no change in UV spectra	1745	C
Chlorothiazide sodium	MSD		WY			Physically incompatible	9	I
	BP	2 g	BP	100 mg	D5W, NS	Immediate precipitation	26	I
Floxacillin sodium	BE	20 g	MB	5 g	W	White precipitate forms immediately	1479	I
Furosemide	HO	1 g	MB	5 g	W	White precipitate forms immediately	1479	I
Heparin sodium	UP	4000 units	WY	250 mg	D5W	Physically incompatible	15	I
Hydrocortisone sodium succinate	UP	500 mg	WY	250 mg	D5W	Physically incompatible	15	I
Hydromorphone HCl	KN	1 g	ES	300 mg	NS[a]	Visually compatible for 21 days at 4 and 25 °C	1992	C
Methohexital sodium	BP	2 g	BP	100 mg	D5W	Immediate precipitation	26	I
Netilmicin sulfate	SC	3 g	WY	100 mg	D5S	Physically compatible and netilmicin chemically stable for 7 days at 4 and 25 °C. Promethazine not tested	558	C

Additive Compatibility (Cont.)

Promethazine HCl

Drug	Mfr	Conc/L	Mfr	Conc/L	Test Soln	Remarks	Ref	C/I
Penicillin G potassium	SQ	20 million units	WY	250 mg	D5W	Physically incompatible	15	I
		1 million units	WY	100 mg		Physically compatible	3	C
	SQ	5 million units	WY	100 mg		Physically compatible	47	C
Penicillin G sodium	UP	20 million units	WY	250 mg	D5W	Physically incompatible	15	I
Pentobarbital sodium	AB	1 g	WY	250 mg	D5W	Physically incompatible	15	I
Phenobarbital sodium	WI	200 mg	WY	250 mg	D5W	Physically incompatible	15	I
	BP	800 mg	BP	100 mg	D5W	Haze develops over 3 hr	26	I
	BP	800 mg	BP	100 mg	NS	Immediate precipitation	26	I
Thiopental sodium	AB		WY			Physically incompatible	9	I
Vitamin B complex with C	AB	2 ml	WY	100 mg		Physically compatible	3	C
	AB	5 ml	WY	250 mg	D5W	Physically compatible	15	C

[a]Tested in PVC containers.

Drugs in Syringe Compatibility

Promethazine HCl

Drug (in syringe)	Mfr	Amt	Mfr	Amt	Remarks	Ref	C/I
Atropine sulfate		0.6 mg/ 1.5 ml	WY	50 mg/ 2 ml	Physically compatible for at least 15 min	14	C
	ST	0.4 mg/ 1 ml	PO	50 mg/ 2 ml	Physically compatible for at least 15 min	326	C
Atropine sulfate with meperidine HCl	WY	0.6 mg/ 1.5 ml 100 mg/ 1 ml	WY	50 mg/ 2 ml	Physically compatible	14	C
Atropine sulfate with meperidine HCl	LI WI	0.4 mg/ 1 ml 50 mg/ 1 ml	WY	25 mg/ 1 ml	No loss of any drug in 24 hr at 25 °C. Slight haze not present at 6 hr but developed by 24 hr	991	C
Butorphanol tartrate	BR	4 mg/ 2 ml	WY	25 mg/ 1 ml	Physically compatible both macroscopically and microscopically for 30 min at room temperature	566	C
Cefotetan disodium	ZE	10 mg/ ml[a]	ES	25 mg/ 1 ml	White precipitate, resembling cottage cheese, forms immediately	1753	I
Chloroquine phosphate		250 mg/ 5 ml		50 mg/ 2 ml	Greenish-yellow discoloration becomes precipitate in 22 hr	1745	I
		50 mg/ 1 ml		50 mg/ 2 ml	Greenish-yellow discoloration becomes precipitate in 17 hr	1745	I
Chlorpromazine HCl	PO	50 mg/ 2 ml	PO	50 mg/ 2 ml	Physically compatible for at least 15 min	326	C

Drugs in Syringe Compatibility (Cont.)

Promethazine HCl

Drug (in syringe)	Mfr	Amt	Mfr	Amt	Remarks	Ref	C/I
Cimetidine HCl	SKF	300 mg/ 2 ml	WY	25 mg/ 1 ml	Physically compatible for 4 hr at 25 °C	25	**C**
Diatrizoate sodium 75% (Hypaque)	WI	40 to 1 ml	WY	1 ml[b]	Immediate precipitation	530	**I**
Diatrizoate meglumine 52%, diatrizoate sodium 8% (Renografin-60)	SQ	40 to 1 ml	WY	1 ml[b]	Immediate precipitation	530	**I**
Diatrizoate meglumine 34.3%, diatrizoate sodium 35% (Renovist)	SQ	40 to 1 ml	WY	1 ml[b]	Immediate precipitation	530	**I**
Dimenhydrinate	HR	50 mg/ 1 ml	PO	50 mg/ 2 ml	Physically incompatible within 15 min	326	**I**
Diphenhydramine HCl	PD	50 mg/ 1 ml	WY	50 mg/ 2 ml	Physically compatible for at least 15 min	14	**C**
	PD	50 mg/ 1 ml	PO	50 mg/ 2 ml	Physically compatible for at least 15 min	326	**C**
Droperidol	MN	2.5 mg/ 1 ml	PO	50 mg/ 2 ml	Physically compatible for at least 15 min	326	**C**
Fentanyl citrate	MN	0.05 mg/ 1 ml	PO	50 mg/ 2 ml	Physically compatible for at least 15 min	326	**C**
Glycopyrrolate	RB	0.2 mg/ 1 ml	WY	25 mg/ 1 ml	Physically compatible and pH in stability range for glycopyrrolate for 48 hr at 25 °C	331	**C**
	RB	0.2 mg/ 1 ml	WY	50 mg/ 2 ml	Physically compatible and pH in stability range for glycopyrrolate for 48 hr at 25 °C	331	**C**
	RB	0.4 mg/ 2 ml	WY	25 mg/ 1 ml	Physically compatible and pH in stability range for glycopyrrolate for 48 hr at 25 °C	331	**C**
Heparin sodium		2500 units/ 1 ml		50 mg/ 2 ml	Turbidity or precipitate forms within 5 min	1053	**I**
Hydromorphone HCl	KN	4 mg/ 2 ml	WY	50 mg/ 1 ml	Physically compatible for 30 min	517	**C**
	KN	4 mg/ 2 ml	WY	25 mg/ 1 ml	Physically compatible for 30 min	517	**C**
Hydroxyzine HCl	PF	100 mg/ 4 ml	WY	50 mg/ 2 ml	Physically compatible for at least 15 min	14	**C**
	PF	50 mg/ 1 ml	PO	50 mg/ 2 ml	Physically compatible for at least 15 min	326	**C**
Iodipamide meglumine 52% (Cholografin)	SQ	40 and 20 ml	WY	1 ml[b]	Forms a precipitate initially but clears within 1 hr and remains clear for 48 hr	530	**I**
	SQ	10 to 1 ml	WY	1 ml[b]	Immediate precipitation	530	**I**
Iothalamate meglumine 60% (Conray)	MA	40 to 1 ml	WY	1 ml[b]	Immediate precipitation	530	**I**
Iothalamate sodium 80% (Angio-Conray)	MA	40 to 1 ml	WY	1 ml[b]	Immediate precipitation	530	**I**
Ketorolac tromethamine	SY	180 mg/ 6 ml	ES	75 mg/ 3 ml	Heavy white precipitate forms immediately, separating into two layers over time	1703	**I**
Meperidine HCl	WY	100 mg/ 1 ml	WY	50 mg/ 2 ml	Physically compatible for at least 15 min	14	**C**

Drugs in Syringe Compatibility (Cont.)

Promethazine HCl

Drug (in syringe)	Mfr	Amt	Mfr	Amt	Remarks	Ref	C/I
	WI	50 mg/ 1 ml	PO	50 mg/ 2 ml	Physically compatible for at least 15 min	326	**C**
Meperidine HCl with atropine sulfate	WY	100 mg/ 1 ml 0.6 mg/ 1.5 ml	WY	50 mg/ 2 ml	Physically compatible	14	**C**
Meperidine HCl with atropine sulfate	WI LI	50 mg/ 1 ml 0.4 mg/ 1 ml	WY	25 mg/ 1 ml	No loss of any drug in 24 hr at 25 °C. Slight haze not present at 6 hr but developed by 24 hr	991	**C**
Metoclopramide HCl	NO	10 mg/ 2 ml	WY	25 mg/ 1 ml	Physically compatible both macroscopically and microscopically for 30 min at room temperature	565	**C**
Midazolam HCl	RC	5 mg/ 1 ml	WY	25 mg/ 1 ml	Physically compatible for 4 hr at 25 °C under fluorescent light	1145	**C**
Morphine sulfate	WY	15 mg/ 1 ml	WY	50 mg/ 2 ml	Physically compatible for at least 15 min	14	**C**
	ST	15 mg/ 1 ml	PO	50 mg/ 2 ml	Physically compatible for at least 15 min	326	**C**
	WY	8 mg	WY	12.5 mg	Cloudiness develops	98	**I**
Nalbuphine HCl	EN	10 mg/ 1 ml	ES	25 mg	Physically compatible for 36 hr at 27 °C	762	**C**
	EN	5 mg/ 0.5 ml	ES	25 mg	Physically compatible for 36 hr at 27 °C	762	**C**
	EN	10 mg/ 1 ml	ES	12.5 mg	Physically compatible for 36 hr at 27 °C	762	**C**
	DU	10 mg/ 1 ml	WY	25 and 50 mg	Physically incompatible	128	**I**
	DU	20 mg/ 1 ml	WY	25 and 50 mg	Physically incompatible	128	**I**
	DU	10 mg/ 1 ml	WY	25 mg/ 1 ml	White flocculent precipitate forms immediately	1183	**I**
	DU	10 mg/ 1 ml	ES	25 mg/ 1 ml	Physically compatible for 24 hr at room temperature	1183	**C**
Pentazocine lactate	WI	30 mg/ 1 ml	WY	50 mg/ 2 ml	Physically compatible for at least 15 min	14	**C**
	WI	30 mg/ 1 ml	WY	25 mg/ 0.5 or 1 ml	Potency retained for 3 months at room temperature in Tubex	13	**C**
	WI	30 mg/ 1 ml	WY	50 mg/ 1 ml	Potency retained for 3 months at room temperature in Tubex	13	**C**
	WI	45 mg/ 1.5 ml	WY	25 mg/ 0.5 ml	Potency retained for 3 months at room temperature in Tubex	13	**C**
	WI	30 mg/ 1 ml	PO	50 mg/ 2 ml	Physically compatible for at least 15 min	326	**C**
Pentobarbital sodium	AB	500 mg/ 10 ml	WY	100 mg/ 4 ml	Physically incompatible	55	**I**
	WY	100 mg/ 2 ml	WY	50 mg/ 2 ml	Precipitate forms within 15 min	14	**I**
	AB	50 mg/ 1 ml	PO	50 mg/ 2 ml	Physically incompatible within 15 min	326	**I**

Drugs in Syringe Compatibility (Cont.)

Promethazine HCl

Drug (in syringe)	Mfr	Amt	Mfr	Amt	Remarks	Ref	C/I
Perphenazine	SC	5 mg/ 1 ml	WY	25 mg/ 1 ml	Physically compatible both macroscopically and microscopically for 30 min at room temperature	566	C
Prochlorperazine edisylate	PO	5 mg/ 1 ml	PO	50 mg/ 2 ml	Physically compatible for at least 15 min	326	C
Promazine HCl	WY	50 mg/ 1 ml	PO	50 mg/ 2 ml	Physically compatible for at least 15 min	326	C
Ranitidine HCl	GL	50 mg/ 2 ml	RP	25 mg/ 1 ml	Physically compatible for 1 hr at 25 °C both macroscopically and microscopically	978	C
	GL	50 mg/ 5 ml	RP	25 mg	Physically compatible for 4 hr at ambient temperature under fluorescent light	1151	C
Scopolamine HBr		0.6 mg/ 1.5 ml	WY	50 mg/ 2 ml	Physically compatible for at least 15 min	14	C
	ST	0.4 mg/ 1 ml	PO	50 mg/ 2 ml	Physically compatible for at least 15 min	326	C
Thiopental sodium	AB	75 mg/ 3 ml	WY	100 mg/ 4 ml	Physically incompatible	21	I

[a]Tested in dextrose 5% in water.
[b]Promethazine HCl concentration unspecified.

Y-Site Injection Compatibility (1:1 Mixture)

Promethazine HCl

Drug	Mfr	Conc	Mfr	Conc	Remarks	Ref	C/I
Aldesleukin	CHI	33,800 I.U./ ml[a]	ES	25 mg/ml	Aldesleukin bioactivity inhibited	1857	I
Allopurinol sodium	BW	3 mg/ml[b]	WY	2 mg/ml[b]	Heavy turbidity forms immediately, developing white particles in 4 hr	1686	I
Amifostine	USB	10 mg/ml[a]	ES	2 mg/ml[a]	Physically compatible with no change in measured turbidity or increase in particle content in 4 hr at 23 °C	1845	C
Amphotericin B cholesteryl sulfate complex	SEQ	0.83 mg/ml[a]	ES	2 mg/ml[a]	Gross precipitate forms	2117	I
Amsacrine	NCI	1 mg/ml[a]	ES	2 mg/ml[a]	Physically compatible for 4 hr at room temperature under fluorescent light	1381	C
Aztreonam	SQ	40 mg/ml[a]	SCN	2 mg/ml[a]	Physically compatible with no subvisual haze or particle formation in 4 hr at 23 °C	1758	C
Cefazolin sodium	LI	10 mg/ml[a]	ES	25 mg	Fine cloudy precipitate forms immediately and dissolves in seconds	1753	?
Cefepime HCl	BR	20 mg/ml[a]	WY	2 mg/ml[a]	Haze forms immediately and becomes flocculent precipitate in 4 hr	1689	I
Cefoperazone sodium	RR	[a,d]		6.25 mg	White precipitate forms due to ionic complex formation	1336	I
Cefotetan disodium	ZE	10 mg/ml[a]	ES	25 mg	White lumpy precipitate forms immediately but dissipates after several minutes of agitation	1753	I

Y-Site Injection Compatibility (1:1 Mixture) (Cont.)

Promethazine HCl

Drug	Mfr	Conc	Mfr	Conc	Remarks	Ref	C/I
Ceftizoxime sodium	FUJ	10 mg/ml[a]	ES	25 mg	Fine cloudy precipitate forms immediately and dissolves in seconds	1753	?
Ciprofloxacin	MI	2 mg/ml[e]	ES	25 mg/ml	Visually compatible for 24 hr at 24 °C	1655	C
Cisatracurium besylate	GW	0.1, 2, 5 mg/ml[a]	ES	2 mg/ml[a]	Physically compatible with no change in measured turbidity or increase in particle content in 4 hr at 23 °C	2074	C
Cisplatin	BR	1 mg/ml	WY	2 mg/ml[a]	Visually compatible for 4 hr at room temperature under fluorescent light	1685	C
Cladribine	ORT	0.015[b] and 0.5[f] mg/ml	SCN	2 mg/ml[b]	Physically compatible with no change in measured turbidity or increase in particle content in 4 hr at 23 °C	1969	C
Cyclophosphamide	MJ	10 mg/ml	WY	2 mg/ml[a]	Visually compatible for 4 hr at room temperature under fluorescent light	1685	C
Cytarabine	UP	50 mg/ml	WY	2 mg/ml[a]	Visually compatible for 4 hr at room temperature under fluorescent light	1685	C
Docetaxel	RPR	0.9 mg/ml[a]	SCN	2 mg/ml[a]	Physically compatible with no change in measured turbidity or increase in particle content in 4 hr at 23 °C	2224	C
Doxorubicin HCl	AD	0.2 mg/ml[a]	WY	2 mg/ml[a]	Visually compatible for 4 hr at room temperature under fluorescent light	1685	C
Doxorubicin HCl liposome injection	SEQ	0.4 mg/ml[a]	ES	2 mg/ml[a]	Increase in measured turbidity	2087	I
Etoposide phosphate	BR	5 mg/ml[a]	SCN	2 mg/ml[a]	Physically compatible with no change in measured turbidity or increase in particle content in 4 hr at 23 °C	2218	C
Filgrastim	AMG	30 μg/ml[a]	SCN	2 mg/ml[a]	Physically compatible with no change in measured turbidity or increase in particle content in 4 hr at 22 °C	1687	C
Fluconazole	RR	2 mg/ml	ES	50 mg/ml	Physically compatible for 24 hr at 25 °C	1407	C
Fludarabine phosphate	BX	1 mg/ml[a]	WY	2 mg/ml[a]	Physically compatible for 4 hr at room temperature under fluorescent light	1439	C
Foscarnet sodium	AST	24 mg/ml	ES	50 mg/ml	Gas production	1335	I
Gemcitabine HCl	LI	10 mg/ml[b]	SCN	2 mg/ml[b]	Physically compatible with no change in measured turbidity or increase in particle content in 4 hr at 23 °C	2226	C
Granisetron HCl	SKB	0.05 mg/ml[a]	WY	2 mg/ml[a]	Physically compatible with no change in measured turbidity or increase in particle content in 4 hr at 23 °C	2000	C
Heparin sodium		50 units/ml/min[b]		50 mg/2 ml[g]	Distinct turbidity	1053	I
	UP	1000 units/L[h]	SV	50 mg/ml	Physically compatible for at least 4 hr at room temperature by visual and microscopic examination	534	C
	UP	1000 units/L[i]	SV	50 mg/ml	Physically compatible initially, but cloudiness developed within 4 hr at room temperature	534	I

Y-Site Injection Compatibility (1:1 Mixture) (Cont.)

Promethazine HCl

Drug	Mfr	Conc	Mfr	Conc	Remarks	Ref	C/I
Hydrocortisone sodium succinate	UP	10 mg/L[h]	SV	50 mg/ml	Physically compatible for at least 4 hr at room temperature by visual and microscopic examination	534	C
	UP	10 mg/L[i]	SV	50 mg/ml	Physically compatible initially, but cloudiness developed within 4 hr at room temperature	534	I
Melphalan HCl	BW	0.1 mg/ml[b]	WY	2 mg/ml[b]	Physically compatible with no change in measured turbidity or increase in particle content in 3 hr at 22 °C	1557	C
Methotrexate sodium	AD	15 mg/ml[j]	WY	2 mg/ml[a]	Turbidity forms within 30 min	1685	I
Ondansetron HCl	GL	1 mg/ml[b]	ES	2 mg/ml[a]	Physically compatible for 4 hr at 22 °C	1365	C
Piperacillin sodium–tazobactam sodium	LE	40 + 5 mg/ml[a]	SCN	2 mg/ml[a]	Heavy white turbidity forms immediately. Particles form in 4 hr	1688	I
Potassium chloride	AB	40 mEq/L[h]	SV	50 mg/ml	Physically compatible for at least 4 hr at room temperature by visual and microscopic examination	534	C
	AB	40 mEq/L[i]	SV	50 mg/ml	Physically compatible initially, but cloudiness developed within 4 hr at room temperature	534	I
Remifentanil HCl	GW	0.025 and 0.25 mg/ml[b]	SCN	2 mg/ml[a]	Physically compatible with no change in measured turbidity or increase in particle content in 4 hr at 23 °C	2075	C
Sargramostim	IMM	10 μg/ml[b]	ES	2 mg/ml[b]	Physically compatible for 4 hr at 22 °C	1436	C
Teniposide	BR	0.1 mg/ml[a]	WY	2 mg/ml[a]	Physically compatible with no subvisual haze or particle formation in 4 hr at 23 °C	1725	C
Thiotepa	IMM[k]	1 mg/ml[a]	WY	2 mg/ml[a]	Physically compatible with no change in measured turbidity or increase in particle content in 4 hr at 23 °C	1861	C
TNA #218 to #226[l]			SCN	2 mg/ml[a]	Visually compatible with no precipitate or emulsion damage apparent in 4 hr at 23 °C	2215	C
TPN #212 and #214[l]			SCN	2 mg/ml[a]	Physically compatible with no change in measured turbidity or increase in particle content in 4 hr at 23 °C	2109	C
TPN #213 and #215[l]			SCN	2 mg/ml[a]	Amber discoloration forms in 4 hr	2109	I
Vinorelbine tartrate	BW	1 mg/ml[b]	ES	2 mg/ml[b]	Physically compatible with no change in measured turbidity or increase in particle content in 4 hr at 22 °C	1558	C
Vitamin B complex with C	RC	2 ml/L[h]	SV	50 mg/ml	Physically compatible for at least 4 hr at room temperature by visual and microscopic examination	534	C

Y-Site Injection Compatibility (1:1 Mixture) (Cont.)

Promethazine HCl

Drug	Mfr	Conc	Mfr	Conc	Remarks	Ref	C/I
	RC	2 ml/L[i]	SV	50 mg/ml	Physically compatible initially, but cloudiness developed within 4 hr at room temperature	534	I

[a]*Tested in dextrose 5% in water.*
[b]*Tested in sterile water for injection.*
[c]*Tested in sodium chloride 0.9%.*
[d]*Concentration unspecified.*
[e]*Tested in both dextrose 5% in water and sodium chloride 0.9%.*
[f]*Tested in bacteriostatic sodium chloride 0.9% preserved with benzyl alcohol 0.9%.*
[g]*Given over three minutes into running infusion solution.*
[h]*Tested in dextrose 5% in Ringer's injection, lactated, dextrose 5% in water, Ringer's injection, lactated, and sodium chloride 0.9%.*
[i]*Tested in dextrose 5% in Ringer's injection.*
[j]*Tested in dextrose 5% in water with sodium bicarbonate 0.05 mEq/ml.*
[k]*Lyophilized formulation tested.*
[l]*Refer to Appendix I for the composition of parenteral nutrition solutions. TNA indicates a 3-in-1 admixture, and TPN indicates a 2-in-1 admixture.*

Additional Compatibility Information

Miscellaneous— Promethazine HCl has been stated to be physically and chemically compatible with butorphanol tartrate (Bristol) (481) and buprenorphine HCl (4). However, promethazine HCl is stated to be incompatible with diatrizoate meglumine products (Squibb) and iodipamide meglumine (Squibb) (40). Metal ions such as iron and especially copper, even in trace quantities, accelerate the degradation rate of promethazine HCl (1072).

Promethazine HCl (Wyeth) 50 mg/2 ml, meperidine HCl (Wyeth) 100 mg/1 ml, and scopolamine HBr 0.6 mg/1.5 ml have been reported to be conditionally compatible when packaged in syringes. The mixture is physically compatible when the order of mixing is as listed above (14).

Nalbuphine— The compatibility of nalbuphine HCl with promethazine HCl appears to be conditional on the specific formulation of promethazine HCl being used. When Elkins-Sinn's promethazine HCl is combined with nalbuphine HCl, the admixture is compatible. However, if Wyeth's promethazine HCl is combined, a precipitate forms immediately (128; 762; 1183).

Chlorpromazine and Meperidine— Chlorpromazine HCl (Elkins-Sinn), meperidine HCl (Winthrop), and promethazine HCl (Elkins-Sinn), combined as an extemporaneous mixture for preoperative sedation, developed a brownish-yellow color after two weeks of storage with protection from light. The discoloration was attributed to the metacresol preservative content of Winthrop's meperidine HCl. Use of Wyeth's meperidine HCl instead, which contains a different preservative, resulted in a solution that remained clear and colorless for at least three months when protected from light (1148).

Heparin Lock— It has been reported that if promethazine HCl is injected into a heparinized scalp vein infusion set, a precipitate will form. It has been suggested that these heparinized sets be flushed with sterile water for injection or sodium chloride 0.9% both before and after drug administration. A heparin lock flush solution may then be reinjected into the device (4; 97).

Pentobarbital— Promethazine HCl (Wyeth) 100 mg/L has been reported to be conditionally compatible with pentobarbital sodium (Abbott) 500 mg/L. The mixture is physically incompatible in most Abbott infusion solutions except as noted below (3):

Ionosol MB with dextrose 5%	Physically compatible
Ionosol T with dextrose 5%	Physically compatible

Concentrated Solutions— The following incompatibility determinations were performed with concentrated solutions. The drugs in dry form were reconstituted according to manufacturers' recommendations. One milliliter of promethazine HCl (Wyeth) was added to 5 ml of sterile distilled water along with 1 ml of each of the following drugs. Particulate matter was noted within two hours (28):

Aminophylline
Chloramphenicol sodium succinate (Parke-Davis)
Dimenhydrinate (Searle)
Heparin sodium
Hydrocortisone sodium succinate (Upjohn)
Penicillin G potassium
Phenobarbital sodium (Winthrop)
Phenytoin sodium (Parke-Davis)
Vitamin B complex with C (Lederle)

PROPOFOL
AHFS 28:04

Diprivan   **AstraZeneca**
                                                                 Baxter

Products—— Propofol (AstraZeneca) 1% is available as a ready-to-use oil-in-water emulsion in 20-ml ampuls, 50-ml prefilled syringes, and 50- and 100-ml infusion vials. Each milliliter contains propofol 10 mg along with soybean oil 100 mg, glycerol 22.5 mg, egg lecithin 12 mg, and disodium edetate 0.005% with sodium hydroxide to adjust the pH (2).

Propofol (Baxter) 1% is also available as a ready-to-use oil-in-water emulsion in 20-ml vials and 50- and 100-ml infusion vials. However, the product differs from the Diprivan formulation. Each milliliter contains propofol 10 mg along with soybean oil 100 mg, glycerol 22.5 mg, and egg yolk phospholipid 12 mg, but incorporates sodium metabisulfite 0.25 mg. Sodium hydroxide is used to adjust the pH during manufacture (1-4/99). See pH section below for the differing pH ranges for these two products.

NOTE: Compatibility information for propofol with other drug products has been developed using Diprivan from AstraZeneca and cannot be automatically extrapolated to the other product because of the formulation differences.

pH—— The AstraZeneca formulation has a pH of 7 to 8.5 (2). The Baxter formulation has a pH of 4.5 to 6.4 (1-4/99) but appears to be usually near the lower range limit.

Tonicity—— Propofol 1% injectable emulsion from both suppliers is isotonic (1-4/99; 2).

Administration—— Before use, propofol should be shaken well. It may be administered undiluted by intravenous injection or infusion or diluted with dextrose 5% in water to no less than 2 mg/ml (1-4/99; 2).

Numerous outbreaks of serious postoperative infections have resulted from inadvertent contamination of propofol during preparation. The contamination resulted from risky preparation practices and lapses in aseptic technique. The product's lipid base supports microbiological growth (1-4/99; 2; 1930). The disodium edetate and sodium bisulfite in the AstraZeneca and Baxter formulations, respectively, retard the growth of microorganisms, but the products can still support growth and are not antimicrobially preserved. Strict aseptic procedures are required during preparation (1-4/99; 2).

Stability—— Propofol 1% injection is a white, oil-in-water emulsion. Intact containers should be stored between 4 and 22 °C and protected from freezing. The emulsion should not be used if phase separation is evident (1-4/99; 2).

Propofol is subject to oxidative degradation when exposed to oxygen. Intact containers are packaged using nitrogen to avoid oxygen exposure. If propofol is administered directly from the vial, administration should be completed within 12 hours after the vial is spiked. The tubing and any unused propofol should be discarded after 12 hours (1-4/99; 2).

If propofol emulsion is transferred to a syringe or other container prior to use, administration should be begun promptly and completed within six hours after the container is opened. After six hours, the product should be discarded and the lines should be flushed or discarded (1-4/99; 2).

Propofol emulsion is a single-use product and can support the growth of microorganisms (1-4/99; 2; 1930). Strict aseptic procedures, including wiping of the ampul neck or vial stopper with isopropanol 70%, are essential (1-4/99; 2).

Repackaging in Syringes—— Propofol (Zeneca) 10 mg/ml was repackaged into 60-ml polypropylene syringes (Monoject, Sherwood Medical) and stored at 23 °C under fluorescent light and at 4 °C protected from light. No visually apparent changes occurred to the emulsion under either storage condition. Propofol losses by HPLC analysis were 7% in five days and 12% in seven days in the room-temperature samples. No propofol losses occurred in 13 days in the refrigerated samples (1984). Propofol supports microbial growth; see Administration.

Propofol (Zeneca) 1% was repackaged into 2- and 10-ml Plastipak (Becton-Dickinson) and 2-ml Inject (B. Braun) plastic syringes and was stored at 5 °C. Propofol losses by HPLC analysis were about 7 to 8% in the Plastipak syringes and about 2% in the Inject syringes after 28 days of refrigerated storage (2118).

Filtration—— The manufacturer recommends that filters with a pore size less than 5 μm should not be used with propofol emulsion. These filters may restrict its administration and/or cause the breakdown of the emulsion (2). However, Bailey et al. reported that 10 ml of propofol injection (Stuart) 10 mg/ml filtered through a 5-μm filter needle (Burron Medical) underwent no potency loss by HPLC analysis (2057). Whether this also applies to other filters is not known.

Plastic and Glass Containers—— As the diluted product, propofol has been shown to be more stable in glass than in plastic containers. The manufacturer indicates that the potency is only 95% after only two hours in plastic (1-4/99; 2).

In a study by Bailey et al., propofol injection (Stuart) was diluted to 2 mg/ml with dextrose 5% in water and stored in polyvinyl chloride tubing (Kendall-McGaw). HPLC analysis showed a loss in propofol concentration exceeding 31% after static storage for two hours. In simulated infusions using the same initial concentration, administration through 72-inch PVC administration sets at a rate of 1.75 ml/min resulted in an average propofol loss of 7.7% over the two-hour period (2057).

Compatibility Information

Drugs in Syringe Compatibility

					Propofol		
Drug (in syringe)	*Mfr*	*Amt*	*Mfr*	*Amt*	*Remarks*	*Ref*	*C/I*
Ondansetron HCl	GW	1 mg/ml[b]	STU	1 and 5 mg/ml[b]	Physically compatible with no measured increase in particulates and little or no loss of either drug by HPLC in 4 hr at 23 °C	2199	C

Drugs in Syringe Compatibility (Cont.)

Drug (in syringe)	Mfr	Amt	Mfr	Amt	Remarks	Ref	C/I
				Propofol			
Thiopental sodium	AB	12.5 mg/ml[a]	ZEN	5 mg/ml[a]	Visually compatible. 10% loss by HPLC of thiopental in 10 days and of propofol in 5 days at 23 °C under fluorescent light. No thiopental loss and 4% propofol loss in 13 days at 4 °C protected from light	1984	C
	AB	37.5 mg/1.5 ml	ICI	5 mg/0.5 ml	Little or no increase in measured emulsion droplet size in 24 hr at 25 °C.	1985	C
	AB	31.25 mg/1.25 ml	ICI	7.5 mg/0.75 ml	Little or no increase in measured emulsion droplet size in 24 hr at 25 °C.	1985	C
	AB	25 mg/1 ml	ICI	10 mg/1 ml	Little or no increase in measured emulsion droplet size in 24 hr at 25 °C. Little or no loss of either drug by HPLC in 24 hr at 25 °C	1985	C
	AB	18.75 mg/0.75 ml	ICI	12.5 mg/1.25 ml	Little or no increase in measured emulsion droplet size in 24 hr at 25 °C.	1985	C
	AB	12.5 mg/0.5 ml	ICI	15 mg/1.5 ml	Little or no increase in measured emulsion droplet size in 24 hr at 25 °C.	1985	C

[a]*Final concentrations after mixing.*
[b]*Tested in sodium chloride 0.9%.*

Y-Site Injection Compatibility (1:1 Mixture)

Drug	Mfr	Conc	Mfr	Conc	Remarks	Ref	C/I
				Propofol			
Acyclovir sodium	BW	7 mg/ml[a]	ZEN	10 mg/ml	Physically compatible for 1 hr at 23 °C with no increase in particle content	2066	C
Alfentanil HCl	JN	0.5 mg/ml	ZEN	10 mg/ml	Physically compatible for 1 hr at 23 °C with no increase in particle content	2066	C
Amikacin sulfate	DU	5 mg/ml[a]	ZEN	10 mg/ml	White precipitate and yellow color form immediately	2066	I
Aminophylline	AMR	2.5 mg/ml[a]	ZEN	10 mg/ml	Physically compatible for 1 hr at 23 °C with no increase in particle content	2066	C
Amphotericin B	APC	0.6 mg/ml[a]	ZEN	10 mg/ml	Gel-like precipitate forms immediately	2066	I
Ampicillin sodium	WY	20 mg/ml[b]	ZEN	10 mg/ml	Physically compatible for 1 hr at 23 °C with no increase in particle content	2066	C
Amrinone lactate	WI	1 mg/ml[a]	ZEN	10 mg/ml	Physically compatible for 1 hr at 23 °C with no increase in particle content	2066	C
Ascorbic acid	AB	500 mg/ml	STU	2 mg/ml	Yellow discoloration forms within 7 days at 25 °C	1801	?
Atracurium besylate	BW	10 mg/ml	STU	2 mg/ml	Oil droplets form within 24 hr, followed by phase separation at 25 °C	1801	I
	BW	10 mg/ml	ZEN	10 mg/ml	Emulsion broke and oiled out	2066	I
Atropine sulfate	GNS	0.4 mg/ml	STU	2 mg/ml	Oil droplets form within 7 days at 25 °C	1801	?
	AST	0.1 mg/ml[a]	ZEN	10 mg/ml	Physically compatible for 1 hr at 23 °C with no increase in particle content	2066	C
Aztreonam	SQ	40 mg/ml[a]	ZEN	10 mg/ml	Physically compatible for 1 hr at 23 °C with no increase in particle content	2066	C
Bretylium tosylate	AST	50 mg/ml	ZEN	10 mg/ml	Emulsion broke and oiled out	2066	I
Bumetanide	RC	0.04 mg/ml[a]	ZEN	10 mg/ml	Physically compatible for 1 hr at 23 °C with no increase in particle content	2066	C

Y-Site Injection Compatibility (1:1 Mixture) (Cont.)

			Propofol				
Drug	*Mfr*	*Conc*	*Mfr*	*Conc*	*Remarks*	*Ref*	*C/I*
Buprenorphine HCl	RKC	0.04 mg/ml[a]	ZEN	10 mg/ml	Physically compatible for 1 hr at 23 °C with no increase in particle content	2066	**C**
Butorphanol tartrate	APC	0.04 mg/ml[a]	ZEN	10 mg/ml	Physically compatible for 1 hr at 23 °C with no increase in particle content	2066	**C**
Calcium chloride	AST	40 mg/ml[a]	ZEN	10 mg/ml	White precipitate formed in 1 hr	2066	**I**
Calcium gluconate	AMR	40 mg/ml[a]	ZEN	10 mg/ml	Physically compatible for 1 hr at 23 °C with no increase in particle content	2066	**C**
Carboplatin	BR	5 mg/ml[a]	ZEN	10 mg/ml	Physically compatible for 1 hr at 23 °C with no increase in particle content	2066	**C**
Cefazolin sodium	MAR	20 mg/ml[a]	ZEN	10 mg/ml	Physically compatible for 1 hr at 23 °C with no increase in particle content	2066	**C**
Cefoperazone sodium	RR	40 mg/ml[a]	ZEN	10 mg/ml	Physically compatible for 1 hr at 23 °C with no increase in particle content	2066	**C**
Cefotaxime sodium	HO	20 mg/ml[a]	ZEN	10 mg/ml	Physically compatible for 1 hr at 23 °C with no increase in particle content	2066	**C**
Cefotetan disodium	STU	20 mg/ml[a]	ZEN	10 mg/ml	Physically compatible for 1 hr at 23 °C with no increase in particle content	2066	**C**
Cefoxitin sodium	ME	20 mg/ml[a]	ZEN	10 mg/ml	Physically compatible for 1 hr at 23 °C with no increase in particle content	2066	**C**
Ceftazidime[c]	SKB	40 mg/ml[a]	ZEN	10 mg/ml	Physically compatible for 1 hr at 23 °C with no increase in particle content	2066	**C**
Ceftizoxime sodium	FUJ	20 mg/ml[a]	ZEN	10 mg/ml	Physically compatible for 1 hr at 23 °C with no increase in particle content	2066	**C**
Ceftriaxone sodium	RC	20 mg/ml[a]	ZEN	10 mg/ml	Physically compatible for 1 hr at 23 °C with no increase in particle content	2066	**C**
Cefuroxime sodium	LI	30 mg/ml[a]	ZEN	10 mg/ml	Physically compatible for 1 hr at 23 °C with no increase in particle content	2066	**C**
Chlorpromazine HCl	SCN	2 mg/ml[a]	ZEN	10 mg/ml	Physically compatible for 1 hr at 23 °C with no increase in particle content	2066	**C**
Cimetidine HCl	SKB	12 mg/ml[a]	ZEN	10 mg/ml	Physically compatible for 1 hr at 23 °C with no increase in particle content	2066	**C**
Ciprofloxacin	MI	1 mg/ml[a]	ZEN	10 mg/ml	Emulsion broke and oiled out	1916	**I**
Cisplatin	BR	1 mg/ml	ZEN	10 mg/ml	Physically compatible for 1 hr at 23 °C with no increase in particle content	2066	**C**
Clindamycin phosphate	AST	10 mg/ml[a]	ZEN	10 mg/ml	Physically compatible for 1 hr at 23 °C with no increase in particle content	2066	**C**
Cyclophosphamide	MJ	10 mg/ml[a]	ZEN	10 mg/ml	Physically compatible for 1 hr at 23 °C with no increase in particle content	2066	**C**
Cyclosporine	SZ	5 mg/ml[a]	ZEN	10 mg/ml	Physically compatible for 1 hr at 23 °C with no increase in particle content	2066	**C**
Cytarabine	CHI	50 mg/ml	ZEN	10 mg/ml	Physically compatible for 1 hr at 23 °C with no increase in particle content	2066	**C**
Dexamethasone sodium phosphate	AMR	1 mg/ml[a]	ZEN	10 mg/ml	Physically compatible for 1 hr at 23 °C with no increase in particle content	2066	**C**
Diazepam	ES	5 mg/ml	ZEN	10 mg/ml	Emulsion broke and oiled out	2066	**I**
Digoxin	ES	0.25 mg/ml	ZEN	10 mg/ml	Emulsion broke and oiled out	1916	**I**

Y-Site Injection Compatibility (1:1 Mixture) (Cont.)

		Propofol					
Drug	*Mfr*	*Conc*	*Mfr*	*Conc*	*Remarks*	*Ref*	*C/I*
Diphenhydramine HCl	SCN	2 mg/ml[a]	ZEN	10 mg/ml	Physically compatible for 1 hr at 23 °C with no increase in particle content	2066	C
Dobutamine HCl	LI	4 mg/ml[a]	ZEN	10 mg/ml	Physically compatible for 1 hr at 23 °C with no increase in particle content	2066	C
Dopamine HCl	AST	3.2 mg/ml[a]	ZEN	10 mg/ml	Physically compatible for 1 hr at 23 °C with no increase in particle content	2066	C
Doxacurium chloride	BW	1 mg/ml	STU	2 mg/ml	Separation into layers occurs within 7 days at 25 °C	1801	?
Doxorubicin HCl	CHI	2 mg/ml	ZEN	10 mg/ml	Emulsion broke and oiled out	1916	I
Doxycycline hyclate	LY	1 mg/ml[a]	ZEN	10 mg/ml	Physically compatible for 1 hr at 23 °C with no increase in particle content	2066	C
Droperidol	JN	0.4 mg/ml[a]	ZEN	10 mg/ml	Physically compatible for 1 hr at 23 °C with no increase in particle content	2066	C
Enalaprilat	MSD	0.1 mg/ml[a]	ZEN	10 mg/ml	Physically compatible for 1 hr at 23 °C with no increase in particle content	2066	C
Ephedrine HCl	AB	5 mg/ml[a]	ZEN	10 mg/ml	Physically compatible for 1 hr at 23 °C with no increase in particle content	2066	C
Epinephrine HCl	AMR	0.1 mg/ml	ZEN	10 mg/ml	Physically compatible for 1 hr at 23 °C with no increase in particle content	2066	C
Esmolol HCl	OHM	10 mg/ml	ZEN	10 mg/ml	Physically compatible for 1 hr at 23 °C with no increase in particle content	2066	C
Famotidine	AB	2 mg/ml[a]	ZEN	10 mg/ml	Physically compatible for 1 hr at 23 °C with no increase in particle content	2066	C
Fentanyl citrate	AB	0.05 mg/ml	ZEN	10 mg/ml	Physically compatible for 1 hr at 23 °C with no increase in particle content	2066	C
Fluconazole	PF	2 mg/ml[a]	ZEN	10 mg/ml	Physically compatible for 1 hr at 23 °C with no increase in particle content	2066	C
Fluorouracil	AD	16 mg/ml[a]	ZEN	10 mg/ml	Physically compatible for 1 hr at 23 °C with no increase in particle content	2066	C
Furosemide	AB	3 mg/ml[a]	ZEN	10 mg/ml	Physically compatible for 1 hr at 23 °C with no increase in particle content	2066	C
Ganciclovir sodium	SY	20 mg/ml[a]	ZEN	10 mg/ml	Physically compatible for 1 hr at 23 °C with no increase in particle content	2066	C
Gentamicin sulfate	ES	5 mg/ml[a]	ZEN	10 mg/ml	White precipitate forms immediately	2066	I
Glycopyrrolate	RB	0.2 mg/ml	ZEN	10 mg/ml	Physically compatible for 1 hr at 23 °C with no increase in particle content	2066	C
Granisetron HCl	SKB	0.05 mg/ml[a]	ZEN	10 mg/ml	Physically compatible for 1 hr at 23 °C with no increase in particle content	2066	C
Haloperidol lactate	MN	0.2 mg/ml[a]	ZEN	10 mg/ml	Physically compatible for 1 hr at 23 °C with no increase in particle content	2066	C
Heparin sodium	ES	100 units/ml[a]	ZEN	10 mg/ml	Physically compatible for 1 hr at 23 °C with no increase in particle content	2066	C
Hydrocortisone sodium succinate	UP	1 mg/ml[a]	ZEN	10 mg/ml	Physically compatible for 1 hr at 23 °C with no increase in particle content	2066	C
Hydromorphone HCl	AST	0.5 mg/ml[a]	ZEN	10 mg/ml	Physically compatible for 1 hr at 23 °C with no increase in particle content	2066	C

Y-Site Injection Compatibility (1:1 Mixture) (Cont.)

		Propofol					
Drug	*Mfr*	*Conc*	*Mfr*	*Conc*	*Remarks*	*Ref*	*C/I*
Hydroxyzine HCl	ES	2 mg/ml[a]	ZEN	10 mg/ml	Physically compatible for 1 hr at 23 °C with no increase in particle content	2066	**C**
Ifosfamide	MJ	25 mg/ml[a]	ZEN	10 mg/ml	Physically compatible for 1 hr at 23 °C with no increase in particle content	2066	**C**
Imipenem–cilastatin sodium	ME	10 mg/ml[b]	ZEN	10 mg/ml	Physically compatible for 1 hr at 23 °C with no increase in particle content	2066	**C**
Insulin	NOV	1 unit/ml[a]	ZEN	10 mg/ml	Physically compatible for 1 hr at 23 °C with no increase in particle content	2066	**C**
Isoproterenol HCl	AB	0.004 mg/ml[a]	ZEN	10 mg/ml	Physically compatible for 1 hr at 23 °C with no increase in particle content	2066	**C**
Ketamine HCl	PD	10 mg/ml	ZEN	10 mg/ml	Physically compatible for 1 hr at 23 °C with no increase in particle content	2066	**C**
Labetalol HCl	AH	5 mg/ml	ZEN	10 mg/ml	Physically compatible for 1 hr at 23 °C with no increase in particle content	2066	**C**
Levorphanol tartrate	RC	0.5 mg/ml[a]	ZEN	10 mg/ml	Physically compatible for 1 hr at 23 °C with no increase in particle content	2066	**C**
Lidocaine HCl	AST	10 mg/ml	ZEN	10 mg/ml	Physically compatible for 1 hr at 23 °C with no increase in particle content	2066	**C**
Lorazepam	WY	0.1 mg/ml[a]	ZEN	10 mg/ml	Physically compatible for 1 hr at 23 °C with no increase in particle content	2066	**C**
Magnesium sulfate	AST	100 mg/ml[a]	ZEN	10 mg/ml	Physically compatible for 1 hr at 23 °C with no increase in particle content	2066	**C**
Mannitol	BA	15%	ZEN	10 mg/ml	Physically compatible for 1 hr at 23 °C with no increase in particle content	2066	**C**
Meperidine HCl	WY	4 mg/ml[a]	ZEN	10 mg/ml	Physically compatible for 1 hr at 23 °C with no increase in particle content	2066	**C**
Methotrexate sodium	LE	15 mg/ml[a]	ZEN	10 mg/ml	Small amount of white precipitate forms in 1 hr	2066	**I**
Methylprednisolone sodium succinate	AB	5 mg/ml[a]	ZEN	10 mg/ml	Small amount of white precipitate forms immediately	2066	**I**
Metoclopramide HCl	RB	5 mg/ml	ZEN	10 mg/ml	Emulsion broke and oiled out	1916	**I**
Midazolam HCl	RC	5 mg/ml	STU	2 mg/ml	Oil droplets form within 7 days at 25 °C	1801	**?**
	RC	2 mg/ml[a]	ZEN	10 mg/ml	Physically compatible for 1 hr at 23 °C with no increase in particle content	2066	**C**
Milrinone lactate	SW	0.4 mg/ml[a]	ZEN	10 mg/ml	Little or no loss of either drug by HPLC in 4 hr at 23 °C	2214	**C**
Minocycline HCl	LE	0.2 mg/ml[a]	ZEN	10 mg/ml	Small amount of white particles forms immediately	2066	**I**
Mitoxantrone HCl	IMM	0.5 mg/ml[a]	ZEN	10 mg/ml	Small amount of particles forms immediately	2066	**I**
Morphine sulfate	AST	1 mg/ml[a]	ZEN	10 mg/ml	Physically compatible for 1 hr at 23 °C with no increase in particle content	2066	**C**
Nafcillin sodium	MAR	20 mg/ml[a]	ZEN	10 mg/ml	Physically compatible for 1 hr at 23 °C with no increase in particle content	2066	**C**
Nalbuphine HCl	AB	10 mg/ml	ZEN	10 mg/ml	Physically compatible for 1 hr at 23 °C with no increase in particle content	2066	**C**

Y-Site Injection Compatibility (1:1 Mixture) (Cont.)

			Propofol				
Drug	*Mfr*	*Conc*	*Mfr*	*Conc*	*Remarks*	*Ref*	*C/I*
Naloxone HCl	AST	0.4 mg/ml	ZEN	10 mg/ml	Physically compatible for 1 hr at 23 °C with no increase in particle content	2066	C
Netilmicin sulfate	SC	5 mg/ml[a]	ZEN	10 mg/ml	Precipitate forms immediately	2066	I
Nitroglycerin	DU	0.4 mg/ml[a]	ZEN	10 mg/ml	Physically compatible for 1 hr at 23 °C with no increase in particle content	2066	C
Norepinephrine bitartrate	AB	0.016 mg/ml[a]	ZEN	10 mg/ml	Physically compatible for 1 hr at 23 °C with no increase in particle content	2066	C
Ofloxacin	ORT	4 mg/ml[a]	ZEN	10 mg/ml	Physically compatible for 1 hr at 23 °C with no increase in particle content	2066	C
Paclitaxel	MJ	1.2 mg/ml[a]	ZEN	10 mg/ml	Physically compatible for 1 hr at 23 °C with no increase in particle content	2066	C
Pancuronium bromide	GNS	2 mg/ml	STU	2 mg/ml	Oil droplets form within 7 days at 25 °C	1801	?
	AST	1 mg/ml	ZEN	10 mg/ml	Physically compatible for 1 hr at 23 °C with no increase in particle content	2066	C
Pentobarbital sodium	WY	5 mg/ml[a]	ZEN	10 mg/ml	Physically compatible for 1 hr at 23 °C with no increase in particle content	2066	C
Phenobarbital sodium	WY	5 mg/ml[a]	ZEN	10 mg/ml	Physically compatible for 1 hr at 23 °C with no increase in particle content	2066	C
Phenylephrine HCl	ES	10 mg/ml	STU	2 mg/ml	Bright yellow discoloration forms within 7 days at 25 °C	1801	?
	ES	0.1 mg/ml[a]	ZEN	10 mg/ml	Physically compatible for 1 hr at 23 °C with no increase in particle content	2066	C
Phenytoin sodium	ES	50 mg/ml	ZEN	10 mg/ml	Needle-like crystals form immediately	2066	I
Piperacillin sodium	LE	40 mg/ml[a]	ZEN	10 mg/ml	Physically compatible for 1 hr at 23 °C with no increase in particle content	2066	C
Potassium chloride	AB	0.1 mEq/ml[a]	ZEN	10 mg/ml	Physically compatible for 1 hr at 23 °C with no increase in particle content	2066	C
Prochlorperazine edisylate	SCN	0.5 mg/ml[a]	ZEN	10 mg/ml	Physically compatible for 1 hr at 23 °C with no increase in particle content	2066	C
Propranolol HCl	SO	1 mg/ml	ZEN	10 mg/ml	Physically compatible for 1 hr at 23 °C with no increase in particle content	2066	C
Ranitidine HCl	GL	2 mg/ml[a]	ZEN	10 mg/ml	Physically compatible for 1 hr at 23 °C with no increase in particle content	2066	C
Scopolamine hydrobromide	LY	0.4 mg/ml	ZEN	10 mg/ml	Physically compatible for 1 hr at 23 °C with no increase in particle content	2066	C
Sodium bicarbonate	AB	1 mEq/ml	ZEN	10 mg/ml	Physically compatible for 1 hr at 23 °C with no increase in particle content	2066	C
Sodium nitroprusside	ES	0.4 mg/ml[a]	ZEN	10 mg/ml	Physically compatible for 1 hr at 23 °C with no increase in particle content	2066	C
Succinylcholine chloride	AB	20 mg/ml[a]	ZEN	10 mg/ml	Physically compatible for 1 hr at 23 °C with no increase in particle content	2066	C
Sufentanil citrate	JN	0.05 mg/ml	ZEN	10 mg/ml	Physically compatible for 1 hr at 23 °C with no increase in particle content	2066	C
Ticarcillin disodium	SKB	30 mg/ml[a]	ZEN	10 mg/ml	Physically compatible for 1 hr at 23 °C with no increase in particle content	2066	C

Y-Site Injection Compatibility (1:1 Mixture) (Cont.)

Drug	Mfr	Conc	Propofol Mfr	Conc	Remarks	Ref	C/I
Ticarcillin disodium–clavulanate potassium	SKB	31 mg/ml[a]	ZEN	10 mg/ml	Physically compatible for 1 hr at 23 °C with no increase in particle content	2066	**C**
Tobramycin sulfate	AB	5 mg/ml[a]	ZEN	10 mg/ml	Precipitate forms immediately	2066	**I**
TPN #186[d]			STU	500 mg	Physically compatible with no change in particle size distribution but 28% propofol loss by HPLC in 5 hr at 22 °C	1805	**I**
TPN #187 and #188[d]			STU	500 mg	Physically compatible with no change in particle size distribution and 6% or less propofol loss by HPLC in 5 hr at 22 °C	1805	**C**
TPN #186 to #188[d]			STU	2 and 3 g	Physically compatible with no change in particle size distribution and 6% or less propofol loss by HPLC in 5 hr at 22 °C	1805	**C**
Vancomycin HCl	AB	10 mg/ml[a]	ZEN	10 mg/ml	Physically compatible for 1 hr at 23 °C with no increase in particle content	2066	**C**
Vecuronium bromide	OR	1 mg/ml	ZEN	10 mg/ml	Physically compatible for 1 hr at 23 °C with no increase in particle content	2066	**C**
Verapamil HCl	AMR	2.5 mg/ml	ZEN	10 mg/ml	Emulsion broke and oiled out	1916	**I**

[a]*Tested in dextrose 5% in water.*
[b]*Tested in sodium chloride 0.9%.*
[c]*Sodium carbonate-containing formulation.*
[d]*Refer to Appendix I for the composition of parenteral nutrition solutions. TPN indicates a 2-in-1 admixture.*

Additional Compatibility Information

Compatibility information for propofol with other drug products has been developed using Diprivan from AstraZeneca and cannot be automatically extrapolated to the other product because of the formulation differences.

The manufacturers recommend that propofol not be mixed with other therapeutic agents or with blood, plasma, or serum. Aggregates of the emulsion have been found when propofol has been in contact with blood, plasma, and serum (1-4/99; 2).

Solutions— The propofol emulsions are compatible with the following infusion solutions (1-4/99; 2):

Dextrose 5% in Ringer's injection, lactated
Dextrose 5% in sodium chloride 0.2%
Dextrose 5% in sodium chloride 0.45%
Dextrose 5% in water
Ringer's injection, lactated

The manufacturers recommend that only dextrose 5% in water be used to dilute propofol and that the concentration not be less than 2 mg/ml (1-4/99; 2).

PROPRANOLOL HCL
AHFS 24:04

Inderal   **Wyeth-Ayerst**

Products— Propranolol HCl (Wyeth-Ayerst) is available in 1-ml ampuls containing 1 mg of the drug with citric acid to adjust the pH in water for injection (2).

pH— From 2.8 to 3.5 (4).

Osmolality— The osmolality of propranolol HCl 1 mg/ml was determined to be 12 mOsm/kg (1233).

Administration— Propranolol HCl is administered by intravenous injection at a rate not exceeding 1 mg/min for life-threatening arrhythmias or those occurring during anesthesia (2; 4).

Stability— Propranolol HCl should be stored at controlled room temperature around 25 °C and protected from light, freezing, or excessive heat (2; 4). Solutions of the drug have maximum stability at pH 3 and decompose rapidly at alkaline pH. Decomposition in aqueous solutions is accompanied by a lowered pH and discoloration. Solutions fluoresce at pH 4 to 5 (4).

Sorption— Propranolol HCl (Sigma) 20 mg/L in sodium chloride 0.9% (Travenol) in PVC bags did not exhibit significant sorption to the plastic during one week of storage at room temperature (15 to 20 °C) (536).

In another study, propranolol HCl (Sigma) 20 mg/L in sodium chloride 0.9% did not exhibit any loss due to sorption during a seven-hour simulated infusion through an infusion set (Travenol) consisting of a cellulose propionate burette chamber and 170 cm of PVC tubing (606).

The drug was also tested as a simulated infusion over at least one hour by a syringe pump system. A glass syringe on a syringe pump was fitted with 20 cm of polyethylene tubing or 50 cm of Silastic tubing. No loss of drug due to sorption was observed with either tubing (606).

A 25-ml aliquot of propranolol HCl (Sigma) 20 mg/L in sodium chloride 0.9% was stored in all-plastic syringes composed of polypropylene barrels and polyethylene plungers for 24 hours at room temperature in the dark. No loss due to sorption occurred (606).

Propranolol HCl (Ayerst) 0.5 and 20 mg/L was evaluated for 24 hours at room temperature in PVC (Abbott and Travenol) and polyolefin (McGaw) containers of the following solutions:

> Dextrose 5% in sodium chloride 0.45 and 0.9%
> Dextrose 5% in water
> Ringer's injection, lactated
> Sodium chloride 0.9%

Samples for HPLC analysis were taken through administration sets and 0.2-μm filters attached to the admixture containers. The results indicated no sorption of propranolol HCl to the plastic solution containers, sets, or filters (746).

Compatibility Information

Solution Compatibility

Propranolol HCl

Solution	Mfr	Mfr	Conc/L	Remarks	Ref	C/I
Dextrose 5% in sodium chloride 0.45%	AB[a], TR[a]	AY	0.5 and 20 mg	Physically compatible and chemically stable for 24 hr at room temperature	746	C
	MG[b]	AY	0.5 and 20 mg	Physically compatible and chemically stable for 24 hr at room temperature	746	C
Dextrose 5% in sodium chloride 0.9%	AB[a], TR[a]	AY	0.5 and 20 mg	Physically compatible and chemically stable for 24 hr at room temperature	746	C
	MG[b]	AY	0.5 and 20 mg	Physically compatible and chemically stable for 24 hr at room temperature	746	C
Dextrose 5% in water	AB[a], TR[a]	AY	0.5 and 20 mg	Physically compatible and chemically stable for 24 hr at room temperature	746	C
	MG[b]	AY	0.5 and 20 mg	Physically compatible and chemically stable for 24 hr at room temperature	746	C
Ringer's injection, lactated	AB[a], TR[a]	AY	0.5 and 20 mg	Physically compatible and chemically stable for 24 hr at room temperature	746	C
	MG[b]	AY	0.5 and 20 mg	Physically compatible and chemically stable for 24 hr at room temperature	746	C
Sodium chloride 0.45%		LY	500 mg	Physically compatible with no loss in 4 hr at 22 °C	1419	C
Sodium chloride 0.9%	AB[a], TR[a]	AY	0.5 and 20 mg	Physically compatible and chemically stable for 24 hr at room temperature	746	C
	MG[b]	AY	0.5 and 20 mg	Physically compatible and chemically stable for 24 hr at room temperature	746	C

[a]*Tested in PVC containers.*
[b]*Tested in polyolefin containers.*

Additive Compatibility

Propranolol HCl

Drug	Mfr	Conc/L	Mfr	Conc/L	Test Soln	Remarks	Ref	C/I
Dobutamine HCl	LI	1 g	AY	50 mg	D5W, NS	Physically compatible for 24 hr at 21 °C	812	C
Verapamil HCl	KN	80 mg	AY	4 mg	D5W, NS	Physically compatible for 24 hr	764	C

Drugs in Syringe Compatibility

			Propranolol HCl				
Drug (in syringe)	Mfr	Amt	Mfr	Amt	Remarks	Ref	C/I
Amrinone lactate	WI	5 mg/ 1 ml	LY	1 mg/ 1 ml	Physically compatible with little or no loss of either drug in 4 hr at 22 °C	1419	C
Milrinone lactate	WI	3.5 mg/ 3.5 ml	AY	3 mg/ 3 ml	Brought to 10-ml total volume with D5W. Physically compatible with no loss of either drug in 4 hr at 23 °C	1191	C

Y-Site Injection Compatibility (1:1 Mixture)

			Propranolol HCl				
Drug	Mfr	Conc	Mfr	Conc	Remarks	Ref	C/I
Alteplase	GEN	1 mg/ml	AY	1 mg/ml	Visually compatible with 2% or less alteplase clot-lysis activity loss in 24 hr at 25 °C	1856	C
Amphotericin B cholesteryl sulfate complex	SEQ	0.83 mg/ml[a]	WY	1 mg/ml	Gross precipitate forms	2117	I
Amrinone lactate	WI	2.5 mg/ml[c]	LY	1 mg/ml	Physically compatible with little or no loss of either drug in 4 hr at 22 °C	1419	C
Diazoxide	SC	15 mg/ml[a]	AY	0.08 mg/ml[a]	Moderate precipitate and slight color change in 1 hr	1316	I
	SC	15 mg/ml[b]	AY	0.08 mg/ml[b]	Moderate precipitate in 1 hr	1316	I
Heparin sodium	UP	1000 units/ L[d]	AY	1 mg/ml	Physically compatible for at least 4 hr at room temperature by visual and microscopic examination	534	C
Hydrocortisone sodium succinate	UP	10 mg/L[d]	AY	1 mg/ml	Physically compatible for at least 4 hr at room temperature by visual and microscopic examination	534	C
Meperidine HCl	AB	10 mg/ml	WY	1 mg/ml	Physically compatible for 4 hr at 25 °C	1397	C
Milrinone lactate	WI	200 μg/ml[a]	AY	1 mg/ml	Physically compatible with no loss of either drug in 4 hr at 23 °C	1191	C
Morphine sulfate	AB	1 mg/ml	WY	1 mg/ml	Physically compatible for 4 hr at 25 °C	1397	C
Potassium chloride	AB	40 mEq/L[d]	AY	1 mg/ml	Physically compatible for at least 4 hr at room temperature by visual and microscopic examination	534	C
Propofol	ZEN	10 mg/ml	SO	1 mg/ml	Physically compatible for 1 hr at 23 °C with no increase in particle content	2066	C
Tacrolimus	FUJ	1 mg/ml[b]	AY	1 mg/ml	Visually compatible for 24 hr at 25 °C	1630	C
Vitamin B complex with C	RC	2 ml/L[d]	AY	1 mg/ml	Physically compatible for at least 4 hr at room temperature by visual and microscopic examination	534	C

[a]Tested in dextrose 5% in water.
[b]Tested in sodium chloride 0.9%.
[c]Tested in sodium chloride 0.45%.
[d]Tested in dextrose 5% in Ringer's injection, dextrose 5% in Ringer's injection, lactated, dextrose 5% in water, Ringer's injection, lactated, and sodium chloride 0.9%.

Additional Compatibility Information

Alteplase— Propranolol HCl is stated to be physically compatible with alteplase when administered by Y-site injection into a running alteplase solution (4).

PROTAMINE SULFATE
AHFS 20:12.08

Lilly

Products— Protamine sulfate (Lilly) is available in 25-ml vials. Each milliliter contains 10 mg of protamine sulfate with sodium chloride 0.9% and sodium phosphate and/or sulfuric acid to adjust the pH (2). It is also available in 5- and 25-ml ampuls and 5-, 10-, and 25-ml vials from other manufacturers (154).

pH— From 6 to 7 (2).

Osmolality— The osmolality of protamine sulfate (Lilly) 10 mg/ml was determined to be 290 mOsm/kg by freezing-point depression and 292 mOsm/kg by vapor pressure (1071).

Administration— Protamine sulfate is administered by slow intravenous injection undiluted as the 10-mg/ml concentration given over one to three minutes. No more than 50 mg should be administered in any 10-minute period. It has also been given by intravenous infusion after dilution in sodium chloride 0.9% or dextrose 5% in water (2; 4).

Stability— Protamine sulfate (Lilly) should be stored under refrigeration; freezing should be avoided (2). However, protamine sulfate has been stated to be stable for 10 days (1433) to two weeks (853) at room temperature.

Filtration— Protamine sulfate (Fournier Freres) 0.2 mg/ml in dextrose 5% in water and sodium chloride 0.9% was filtered through a 0.22-µm cellulose ester membrane filter (Ivex-HP, Millipore) over six hours. No significant drug loss due to binding to the filter was noted (1034).

Compatibility Information

Additive Compatibility

						Protamine sulfate		
Drug	Mfr	Conc/L	Mfr	Conc/L	Test Soln	Remarks	Ref	C/I
Cimetidine HCl	SKF	3 g	LI	500 mg	D5W	Physically compatible and cimetidine chemically stable for 24 hr at room temperature. Protamine not tested	551	C
Ranitidine HCl	GL	50 mg and 2 g		500 mg	D5W	Physically compatible and ranitidine chemically stable by HPLC for 24 hr at 25 °C. Protamine not tested	1515	C
Verapamil HCl	KN	80 mg	LI	100 mg	D5W, NS	Physically compatible for 24 hr	764	C

Drugs in Syringe Compatibility

					Protamine sulfate		
Drug (in syringe)	Mfr	Amt	Mfr	Amt	Remarks	Ref	C/I
Diatrizoate meglumine 52%, diatrizoate sodium 8%	MA	5 ml	LI	10 mg/ 1 ml	Precipitate forms immediately and persists for at least 2 hr	1438	I
Diatrizoate sodium 60%	WI	5 ml	LI	10 mg/ 1 ml	Precipitate forms immediately and persists for at least 2 hr	1438	I
Iohexol 64.7%	WI	5 ml	LI	10 mg/ 1 ml	Physically compatible for at least 2 hr	1438	C
Iopamidol 61%	SQ	5 ml	LI	10 mg/ 1 ml	Physically compatible for at least 2 hr	1438	C

Drugs in Syringe Compatibility (Cont.)

Protamine sulfate

Drug (in syringe)	Mfr	Amt	Mfr	Amt	Remarks	Ref	C/I
Iothalamate meglumine 60%	MA	5 ml	LI	10 mg/ 1 ml	Physically compatible for at least 2 hr	1438	C
Ioxaglate meglumine 39.3%, ioxaglate sodium 19.6%	MA	5 ml	LI	10 mg/ 1 ml	Precipitate forms immediately and persists for at least 2 hr	1438	I

Additional Compatibility Information

Dextrose 5% in water and sodium chloride 0.9% have been recommended for the infusion of protamine sulfate (2; 4).

The manufacturer recommends that protamine sulfate not be mixed with other drugs unless their compatibility is known. Protamine sulfate is incompatible with some antibiotics including several cephalosporins and penicillins (2).

PYRIDOSTIGMINE BROMIDE
AHFS 12:04

Mestinon   **ICN Pharmaceuticals**

Products— Pyridostigmine bromide (ICN Pharmaceuticals) is available in 2-ml ampuls. Each milliliter of solution contains (2):

Pyridostigmine bromide	5 mg
Methyl- and propylparabens	0.2%
Sodium citrate	0.02%
Citric acid and sodium hydroxide	to adjust pH

pH— Approximately 5 (2; 4).

Osmolality— Pyridostigmine bromide 5 mg/ml has an osmolality of 132 mOsm/kg (1689).

Administration— Pyridostigmine bromide is administered intramuscularly or by very slow intravenous injection (2; 4).

Stability— Pyridostigmine bromide is unstable in alkaline solutions (4).

Compatibility Information

Drugs in Syringe Compatibility

Pyridostigmine bromide

Drug (in syringe)	Mfr	Amt	Mfr	Amt	Remarks	Ref	C/I
Glycopyrrolate	RB	0.2 mg/ 1 ml	RC	5 mg/ 1 ml	Physically compatible and pH in stability range for glycopyrrolate for 48 hr at 25 °C	331	C
	RB	0.2 mg/ 1 ml	RC	10 mg/ 2 ml	Physically compatible and pH in stability range for glycopyrrolate for 48 hr at 25 °C	331	C
	RB	0.4 mg/ 2 ml	RC	5 mg/ 1 ml	Physically compatible and pH in stability range for glycopyrrolate for 48 hr at 25 °C	331	C

Y-Site Injection Compatibility (1:1 Mixture)

Pyridostigmine bromide

Drug	Mfr	Conc	Mfr	Conc	Remarks	Ref	C/I
Heparin sodium	UP	1000 units/ L[a]	RC	5 mg/ml	Physically compatible for at least 4 hr at room temperature by visual and microscopic examination	534	C

Y-Site Injection Compatibility (1:1 Mixture) (Cont.)

Pyridostigmine bromide

Drug	Mfr	Conc	Mfr	Conc	Remarks	Ref	C/I
Hydrocortisone sodium succinate	UP	10 mg/L[a]	RC	5 mg/ml	Physically compatible for at least 4 hr at room temperature by visual and microscopic examination	534	**C**
Potassium chloride	AB	40 mEq/L[a]	RC	5 mg/ml	Physically compatible for at least 4 hr at room temperature by visual and microscopic examination	534	**C**
Vitamin B complex with C	RC	2 ml/L[a]	RC	5 mg/ml	Physically compatible for at least 4 hr at room temperature by visual and microscopic examination	534	**C**

[a]*Tested in dextrose 5% in Ringer's injection, dextrose 5% in Ringer's injection, lactated, dextrose 5% in water, Ringer's injection, lactated, and sodium chloride 0.9%.*

PYRIDOXINE HCL
AHFS 88:08

Products— Pyridoxine HCl injection is available from several manufacturers in 1-, 10-, and 30-ml multiple-dose vials as an aqueous solution providing 100 mg/ml. Also present are antimicrobial preservatives, such as benzyl alcohol 1.5% or chlorobutanol 0.5%. Sodium hydroxide and/or hydrochloric acid may have been used to adjust pH (1-1/99; 4; 29; 154).

pH— From 2 to 3.8 (1-1/99; 4).

Osmolality— The osmolality of pyridoxine HCl (Lilly) 100 mg/ml was determined to be 870 mOsm/kg by freezing-point depression and 852 mOsm/kg by vapor pressure (1071).

Administration— Pyridoxine HCl may be administered by intramuscular, subcutaneous, or intravenous injection (4).

Stability— The product should be stored at controlled room temperature and protected from freezing and from light (1-1/99; 4).

Because pyridoxine HCl is photosensitive and degrades slowly when exposed to light, protection from light has been recommended (4).

Sorption— Pyridoxine HCl (Sigma) 40 mg/L did not display significant sorption to a PVC plastic test strip in 24 hours (12).

Compatibility Information

Solution Compatibility

Pyridoxine HCl

Solution	Mfr	Mfr	Conc/L	Remarks	Ref	C/I
Fat emulsion 10%, intravenous	KA	KA[a]	98 mg	Physically compatible for 24 hr at 26 °C with little loss of pyridoxine HCl and of most other vitamins by HPLC; up to 52% ascorbate loss	2050	**C**

[a]*From multivitamins.*

Drugs in Syringe Compatibility

Pyridoxine HCl

Drug (in syringe)	Mfr	Amt	Mfr	Amt	Remarks	Ref	C/I
Doxapram HCl	RB	400 mg/ 20 ml		10 mg/ 1 ml	Physically compatible with 6% doxapram loss in 24 hr	1177	**C**

Pyridoxine HCl is stated to be incompatible with alkaline solutions, iron salts, and oxidizing agents (4; 18).

Antibiotics— In vitro testing of pyridoxine HCl at a concentration of 0.1% with the following antibiotics at a concentration of 0.025% in sterile distilled water showed significant reduction in antibiotic activity in one hour at 25 °C (314):

Erythromycin (as estolate)
Kanamycin sulfate
Streptomycin sulfate

Solutions— Pyridoxine HCl in infusion solutions under hospital conditions is reported to be stable. However, addition of riboflavin phosphate sodium promoted decomposition of the pyridoxine so that approximately 8% remained after three hours in the light. Addition of an antioxidant such as ascorbic acid or protection from light reduced the rate of degradation of pyridoxine (563).

Parenteral Nutrition Solutions— The stability of pyridoxine HCl 15 mg/L was studied in representative parenteral nutrition solutions exposed to fluorescent light, indirect sunlight, and direct sunlight for eight hours. One 5-ml vial of multivitamin concentrate (Lyphomed) containing 15 mg of pyridoxine HCl and also 1 mg of folic acid (Lederle) was added to a liter of parenteral nutrition solution composed of amino acids 4.25%–dextrose 25% (Travenol) with standard electrolytes and trace elements. Pyridoxine HCl was stable over the eight-hour study at room temperature under fluorescent light and indirect sunlight. However, eight hours of exposure to direct sunlight caused an 86% loss of pyridoxine HCl (842).

Dahl et al. reported the stability of numerous vitamins in parenteral nutrition solutions composed of amino acids (Kabi-Vitrum), dextrose 30%, and fat emulsion 20% (Kabi-Vitrum) in a 2:1:1 ratio with electrolytes, trace elements, and both fat- and water-soluble vitamins. The admixtures were stored in darkness at 2 to 8 °C for 96 hours with no significant loss of retinyl palmitate, alpha-tocopherol, thiamine mononitrate, sodium riboflavin-5′-phosphate, pyridoxine HCl, nicotinamide, folic acid, biotin, sodium pantothenate, and cyanocobalamin. Sodium ascorbate and its biologically active degradation product, dehydroascorbic acid, totaled 59 and 42% of the nominal starting concentration at 24 and 96 hours, respectively. However, the actual initial concentration was only 66% of the nominal concentration (1225).

QUINIDINE GLUCONATE
AHFS 24:04

Lilly

Products— Quinidine gluconate (Lilly) is available in 10-ml vials. Each milliliter contains 80 mg of drug with edetate disodium 0.005% and phenol 0.25% in sterile water for injection. D-gluconic acid delta-lactone may have been added to adjust the pH (1-3/12/98).

pH— Quinidine gluconate injection has a pH of 5.5 to 7 (4).

Osmolality— Quinidine gluconate 80 mg/ml has an osmolality of 220 mOsm/kg (1689).

Equivalency— Quinidine gluconate 800 mg is equivalent to 500 mg of anhydrous quinidine (1-3/12/98).

Administration— Quinidine gluconate injection may be administered by intermittent or continuous intravenous infusion (4). For intravenous administration in treating arrhythmias, 800 mg (10 ml) is diluted with 40 ml of dextrose 5% in water for a total of 50 ml to yield a 16-mg/ml solution. The drug has also been given by intramuscular injection, but this route is not recommended because of variable absorption (1-3/12/98; 4).

For the treatment of malaria, continuous and intermittent infusion regimens have been used. A loading dose is prepared as a dilution in about 250 ml of sodium chloride 0.9% and given as a one- or two-hour (continuous regimen) or four-hour (intermittent regimen) infusion. This is followed by continuous or intermittent intravenous infusions (4).

Infusions of quinidine gluconate must be delivered slowly at a rate no faster than 0.25 mg/kg/min, preferably using a volumetric pump to control the rate of administration (1-3/12/98).

Stability— Quinidine gluconate should be stored at controlled room temperature. Quinidine salts slowly discolor on exposure to light, acquiring a brownish tint. Only clear, colorless solutions are suitable for injection (4).

Sorption— Quinidine (as the sulfate) 4.5 mg/L in sodium chloride 0.9% (Travenol) in PVC bags did not exhibit significant sorption to the plastic during one week of storage at room temperature (15 to 20 °C) (536).

In another study, quinidine (as the sulfate) 4.5 mg/L in sodium chloride 0.9% did not exhibit any loss due to sorption during a seven-hour simulated infusion through an infusion set (Travenol) consisting of a cellulose propionate burette chamber and 170 cm of PVC tubing (606).

The drug was also tested as a simulated infusion over at least one hour by a syringe pump system. A glass syringe on a syringe pump was fitted with 20 cm of polyethylene tubing or 50 cm of Silastic tubing. No loss of drug due to sorption was observed with either tubing (606).

In addition, a 25-ml aliquot of quinidine (as the sulfate) 4.5 mg/L in sodium chloride 0.9% was stored in all-plastic syringes composed of polypropylene barrels and polyethylene plungers for 24 hours at room temperature in the dark. No loss due to sorption occurred (606).

Darbar et al. noted a substantial loss of quinidine gluconate due to sorption to PVC containers and administration sets. Quinidine gluconate (Lilly) 6 mg/ml in dextrose 5% in water in 100-ml PVC bags (Baxter) exhibited about 5 to 7% loss determined by UV spectroscopy. Administration of the solution over 30 minutes through

112-inch PVC administration sets (Gemini, IMED) resulted in an additional loss of over 30% of the quinidine gluconate from the delivered solution. Losses totaled over 40% for both bag and catheter. Use of a glass syringe on a syringe pump and a winged administration catheter having only 12 inches of PVC tubing reduced the loss to about 3% (2005).

However, quinidine as the sulfate salt has been reported not to exhibit sorption to PVC.

Compatibility Information

Additive Compatibility

		Quinidine gluconate						
Drug	Mfr	Conc/L	Mfr	Conc/L	Test Soln	Remarks	Ref	C/I
Amiodarone HCl	LZ	1.8 g	LI	1 g	D5W[a]	Precipitation caused a milky appearance. 13% amiodarone loss in 6 hr and 23% in 24 hr at 24 °C under fluorescent light	1031	**I**
	LZ	1.8 g	LI	1 g	D5W[b]	Precipitation caused a milky appearance. No amiodarone loss in 24 hr at 24 °C under fluorescent light	1031	**I**
	LZ	1.8 g	LI	1 g	NS[a]	Physically compatible but 4% amiodarone loss in 6 hr and 13% in 24 hr at 24 °C under fluorescent light	1031	**I**
	LZ	1.8 g	LI	1 g	NS[b]	Physically compatible with no amiodarone loss in 24 hr at 24 °C under fluorescent light	1031	**C**
Atracurium besylate	BW	500 mg		8.3 g	D5W	Particles form and atracurium chemically unstable at 5 and 30 °C	1694	**I**
Bretylium tosylate	ACC	1 g	LI	800 mg	D5W, NS	Physically compatible for 48 hr at 25 °C	756	**C**
Cimetidine HCl	SKF	3 g	LI	3.2 g	D5W	Physically compatible and cimetidine chemically stable for 24 hr at room temperature. Quinidine not tested	551	**C**
Milrinone lactate	WI	200 mg	LI	16 g	D5W	Physically compatible with no loss of either drug in 4 hr at 23 °C	1191	**C**
Ranitidine HCl	GL	50 mg and 2 g		3.2 mg	D5W	Physically compatible and ranitidine chemically stable by HPLC for 24 hr at 25 °C. Quinidine not tested	1515	**C**
Verapamil HCl	KN	80 mg	LI	800 mg	D5W, NS	Physically compatible for 48 hr	739	**C**

[a]Tested in PVC containers.
[b]Tested in polyolefin containers.

Y-Site Injection Compatibility (1:1 Mixture)

		Quinidine gluconate					
Drug	Mfr	Conc	Mfr	Conc	Remarks	Ref	C/I
Diazepam	ES	0.2 mg/ml[a]	LI	6 mg/ml[a]	Physically compatible for 3 hr	1316	**C**
Furosemide	ES	4 mg/ml[a]	LI	6 mg/ml[a]	Immediate gross precipitation	1316	**I**
Heparin sodium	ES	50 units/ml[b]	LI	6 mg/ml[b]	Physically compatible for 3 hr	1316	**C**
	ES	50 units/ml[c]	LI	6 mg/ml[c]	Immediate gross haze	1316	**I**
Milrinone lactate	WI	350 μg/ml[c]	LI	16 mg/ml[c]	Physically compatible with no loss of either drug in 4 hr at 23 °C	1191	**C**

[a]Tested in both dextrose 5% in water and sodium chloride 0.9%.
[b]Tested in sodium chloride 0.9%.
[c]Tested in dextrose 5% in water.

Additional Compatibility Information

At a concentration of 16 mg/ml in dextrose 5% in water, quinidine gluconate is reported to be stable for 24 hours at room temperature and for 48 hours under refrigeration (4).

RANITIDINE HCL
AHFS 56:40

Zantac   **Glaxo Wellcome**

Products— Ranitidine HCl (Glaxo Wellcome) is available in 2-ml single-dose vials, 6-ml multiple-dose vials, and 40-ml pharmacy bulk packages. Each milliliter of solution contains (2):

Ranitidine (as the hydrochloride)	25 mg
Phenol	5 mg
Dibasic sodium phosphate	2.4 mg
Monobasic potassium phosphate	0.96 mg

Ranitidine HCl (Glaxo Wellcome) is also available at a 1-mg/ml concentration in 50-ml (50 mg) plastic containers premixed in sodium chloride 0.45%. The solution also contains citric acid 15 mg and dibasic sodium phosphate 90 mg as buffers (2).

pH— From 6.7 to 7.3 (2; 4).

Osmolality— The osmolality of ranitidine HCl 10 mg/ml was determined to be 59 mOsm/kg (1233).

The osmolality of ranitidine HCl (Glaxo) 1 mg/ml was determined to be 260 mOsm/kg in dextrose 5% in water and 302 mOsm/kg in sodium chloride 0.9%. At 2 mg/ml, the osmolality was determined to be 257 mOsm/kg in dextrose 5% in water and 294 mOsm/kg in sodium chloride 0.9% (1375).

The premixed ranitidine 1-mg/ml solution (Glaxo Wellcome) in sodium chloride 0.45% has an osmolarity of 180 mOsm/L (2).

Equivalency— Ranitidine HCl 168 mg is approximately equivalent to 150 mg of ranitidine (4).

Administration— Ranitidine HCl is administered intramuscularly undiluted or slowly intravenously after dilution. For direct intravenous injection, 50 mg is usually diluted to a total of at least 20 ml with a compatible intravenous infusion fluid and given over at least five minutes (4 ml/min). For intermittent intravenous infusion, 50 mg may be added to at least 100 ml of appropriate intravenous solution and infused over 15 to 20 minutes. For continuous intravenous infusion, 150 mg of ranitidine HCl may be diluted in 250 ml of intravenous fluid and infused at 6.25 mg/hr for 24 hours (2; 4).

Stability— Ranitidine HCl injection should be stored between 4 and 30 °C and protected from light and excessive heat. Brief exposure to temperatures up to 40 °C will not adversely affect the stability of the injection. The product is a clear, colorless to yellow solution.

Slight darkening does not affect potency. The pharmacy bulk package should be used as soon as possible after initial entry; unused portions should be discarded within 24 hours. The premixed infusion solution should be stored between 2 and 25 °C (2; 4).

Ranitidine HCl (Glaxo) was diluted to a concentration of 2.5 mg/ml with bacteriostatic water for injection and repackaged in 30-ml glass vials and 10-ml polypropylene syringes (Becton-Dickinson) (closure not specified). The vials and syringes were stored at 4 °C for 91 days. Approximately 5 to 6% ranitidine loss determined by HPLC analysis occurred after 91 days of storage under refrigeration. Freshly prepared syringes and syringes stored at 4 °C for 91 days were also stored at 22 °C for 72 hours. No ranitidine loss was found in the freshly prepared syringes, and about 2% additional loss was found in syringes stored under refrigeration for 91 days (1965).

Freezing Solutions— Ranitidine HCl (Glaxo) 0.5, 1, and 2 mg/ml in dextrose 5% in water and sodium chloride 0.9% in PVC bags showed no significant change in appearance or potency when frozen for 30 days at −30 °C. An additional 14 days of refrigerated storage at 4 °C for these previously frozen solutions also resulted in no potency loss (1143).

At a concentration of 2 mg/ml in dextrose 5% in water and sodium chloride 0.9% in PVC containers, no significant change in appearance or potency occurred even after 100 days of frozen storage at −30 °C (1143).

Ranitidine HCl (Glaxo) 441 μg/ml in dextrose 5% in water was visually compatible and showed no potency loss by HPLC after frozen storage (−20 °C) for 30 days followed by 10 days of refrigeration at 4 °C (1539).

Stewart et al. studied the stability of ranitidine HCl (Glaxo) 0.5, 1, and 2 mg/ml in several infusion fluids when frozen at −20 °C for 60 days followed by seven days at 23 °C or 14 days at 4 °C. In dextrose 5% in sodium chloride 0.45%, dextrose 5% in water, dextrose 10% in water, and sodium chloride 0.9%, ranitidine was physically compatible and chemically stable, retaining more than 90% of the initial concentration under these storage conditions. However, in dextrose 5% in Ringer's injection, lactated, the thawed solutions were slightly yellow with ranitidine HCl losses of up to 25% at 0.5 mg/ml and 16% at 1 mg/ml. At 2 mg/ml, losses were 9% or less (1516).

Ranitidine HCl (Glaxo) 1.5 mg/ml in dextrose 5% in water or in sodium chloride 0.9% was packaged in PVC infusion pump reservoirs. The reservoirs were frozen at −20 °C and stored for 30 days. The frozen solutions were then thawed by storing at 3 °C for 24 hours followed by 24 hours at 30 °C to simulate use conditions. No loss of ranitidine HCl was found by HPLC analysis of the solutions (1865).

Filtration— Filtration of ranitidine HCl (Glaxo) 0.25, 0.5, and 2.5 mg/ml in sodium chloride 0.9% through 0.2-μm polysulfone filters (IVS Set-P Supor Filter, Codan) at a rate of 4 ml/hr for five hours did not result in any loss of drug due to sorption to the filter (2229).

Compatibility Information

Solution Compatibility

Ranitidine HCl

Solution	Mfr	Mfr	Conc/L	Remarks	Ref	C/I
Amino acids 8.5%	TR	GL	50 mg and 2 g	Physically compatible and ranitidine chemically stable by HPLC for 24 hr at 25 °C	1515	C
Dextrose 5% in Ringer's injection, lactated	TR[a]	GL	50 mg	15% ranitidine loss in 2 days at room temperature under fluorescent light	1362	I
	TR[a]	GL	500 mg, 1 g, 2 g	Physically compatible with 5% or less ranitidine loss in 7 days at 23 °C and 8% or less loss in 30 days at 4 °C	1516	C
Dextrose 5% in sodium chloride 0.45%	TR[a]	GL	50 mg	8 to 10% ranitidine loss in 7 days at room temperature under fluorescent light	1362	C
	TR[a]	GL	500 mg, 1 g, 2 g	Physically compatible with 5% or less ranitidine loss in 7 days at 23 °C and 8% or less loss in 30 days at 4 °C	1516	C
Dextrose 5% in water	TR[a]	GL	1 g	Little or no ranitidine loss in 10 days at 4 °C	1143	C
	TR[a]		1 g	Physically compatible with 8% loss in 18 days at 25 °C and 3% loss in 66 days at 5 °C	1342	C
	TR[a]	GL	1 g	Physically compatible with no loss in 92 days at 4 °C	1350	C
	TR[a]	GL	50 mg	Physically compatible with 6% loss in 48 hr at room temperature under fluorescent light	1361	C
	TR[a]	GL	2 g	Physically compatible with 2% loss in 48 hr at room temperature under fluorescent light	1361	C
	TR[a]	GL	500 mg, 1 g, 2 g	5% or less ranitidine loss in 28 days at room temperature under fluorescent light	1362	C
	TR[a]	GL	50 mg	8 to 10% ranitidine loss in 7 days at room temperature under fluorescent light	1362	C
	TR[a]	GL	500 mg, 1 g, 2 g	Physically compatible with 5% or less ranitidine loss in 7 days at 23 °C and 6% or less loss in 30 days at 4 °C	1516	C
	MG	GL	441 mg	Visually compatible with no ranitidine loss by HPLC after 30 days at −20 °C followed by 10 days at 4 °C	1539	C
	TR[a]	GL	2 g	Visually compatible with little or no ranitidine loss by HPLC in 48 hr at room temperature	1802	C
	TR[a]	GL	50 mg	Visually compatible with 6% ranitidine loss by HPLC in 48 hr at room temperature	1802	C
	AB[a]	GL	1.5 g	Little or no ranitidine loss by HPLC in 24 hr at 30 °C and for 7 days at 3 °C followed by 24 hr at 30 °C	1865	C
Dextrose 10% in water	TR[a]	GL	50 mg	7% ranitidine loss in 2 days at room temperature under fluorescent light	1362	C
	TR[a]	GL	500 mg, 1 g, 2 g	Physically compatible with 4% or less ranitidine loss in 7 days at 23 °C and 8% or less loss in 30 days at 4 °C	1516	C
Fat emulsion 10%, intravenous	KV	GL	50 mg	Physically compatible with no effect on emulsion stability and 2 to 4% ranitidine loss in 48 hr at 25 °C with or without light protection	1360	C

Solution Compatibility (Cont.)

Ranitidine HCl

Solution	Mfr	Mfr	Conc/L	Remarks	Ref	C/I
	KV	GL	100 mg	Physically compatible with no effect on emulsion stability and no ranitidine loss in 48 hr under refrigeration and at 25 °C with or without light protection	1360	**C**
Sodium chloride 0.9%	TR	GL	50 and 100 mg	No ranitidine loss in 48 hr at 24 °C under fluorescent light	1010	**C**
	TR[a]	GL	1 g	Little or no ranitidine loss in 10 days at 4 °C	1143	**C**
	TR[a]		1 g	Physically compatible with no loss in 18 days at 25 °C and in 66 days at 5 °C	1342	**C**
	TR[a]	GL	1 g	Physically compatible with no loss in 92 days at 4 °C	1350	**C**
	TR	GL	50 mg	Physically compatible with no loss in 48 hr at 25 °C protected from light	1360	**C**
	TR	GL	100 mg	Physically compatible with no loss in 48 hr at 25 °C with or without light protection and under refrigeration for 24 hr followed by 24 hr at 25 °C with or without light protection	1360	**C**
	TR[a]	GL	50 mg and 2 g	Physically compatible with no loss in 48 hr at room temperature under fluorescent light	1361	**C**
	TR[a]	GL	500 mg, 1 g, 2 g	No ranitidine loss in 28 days at room temperature under fluorescent light	1362	**C**
	TR[a]	GL	50 mg	3% or less ranitidine loss in 28 days at room temperature under fluorescent light	1362	**C**
	TR[a]	GL	500 mg, 1 g, 2 g	Physically compatible with no ranitidine loss in 7 days at 23 °C and 3% or less loss in 30 days at 4 °C	1516	**C**
	TR[a]	GL	50 mg and 2 g	Visually compatible with little or no ranitidine loss in 48 hr at room temperature	1802	**C**
	AB[a]	GL	1.5 g	Little or no ranitidine loss by HPLC in 24 hr at 30 °C and for 7 days at 3 °C followed by 24 hr at 30 °C	1865	**C**
	BA[a]	GL	600 mg	Visually compatible with little or no loss of ranitidine by HPLC in 24 hr at ambient temperature	2079	**C**
	BA[a]	GL	1 g	Visually compatible with little or no loss of ranitidine by HPLC in 4 hr at ambient temperature	2079	**C**
TNA #92[b]	[c]	GL	50 and 100 mg	7 to 10% ranitidine loss in 12 hr and 20 to 28% in 24 hr at 23 °C under fluorescent light	1183	**I**
TNA #118[b]		GL	50 and 100 mg	Physically compatible with no effect on emulsion stability and about 6 to 10% ranitidine loss in 36 hr under refrigeration and at 25 °C with or without light protection	1360	**C**
TNA #197 to #200[b]		GL	75 mg	Physically compatible with 7% or less ranitidine loss by HPLC in 24 hr at 22 °C exposed to light. About 15% loss in 48 hr	1921	**C**
TPN #58[b]		GL	83, 167, 250 mg	10% ranitidine loss in 48 hr at 23 °C	997	**C**
TPN #59 and #60[b]	[a]	GL	50 and 100 mg	No color change and 7 to 9% ranitidine loss in 24 hr at 24 °C under fluorescent light. Amino acids not substantially affected. Darkened color and 10 to 12% ranitidine loss in 48 hr	1010	**C**
TPN #117[b]		GL	50 and 100 mg	Physically compatible and 5% or less ranitidine loss in 48 hr at 25 °C and under refrigeration	1360	**C**

Solution Compatibility (Cont.)

Ranitidine HCl

Solution	Mfr	Mfr	Conc/L	Remarks	Ref	C/I
TPN #196[b]		GL	75 mg	Physically compatible with 7% or less ranitidine loss by HPLC in 24 hr at 22 °C exposed to light. About 12% loss in 48 hr	1921	C

[a]Tested in PVC containers.
[b]Refer to Appendix I for the composition of parenteral nutrition solutions. TNA indicates a 3-in-1 admixture, and TPN indicates a 2-in-1 admixture.
[c]Tested in ethylene vinyl acetate containers.

Additive Compatibility

Ranitidine HCl

Drug	Mfr	Conc/L	Mfr	Conc/L	Test Soln	Remarks	Ref	C/I
Acetazolamide sodium		5 g	GL	50 mg and 2 g	D5W	Physically compatible and ranitidine chemically stable by HPLC for 24 hr at 25 °C. Acetazolamide not tested	1515	C
Amikacin sulfate	BR	1 g	GL	100 mg	D5W	Physically compatible for 24 hr at ambient temperature under fluorescent light	1151	C
		2.5 g	GL	50 mg and 2 g	D5W	Physically compatible and ranitidine chemically stable by HPLC for 24 hr at 25 °C. Amikacin not tested	1515	C
Aminophylline	ES	500 mg and 2 g	GL	50 mg and 2 g	D5W, NS[a]	Physically compatible with 4% or less ranitidine loss in 24 hr at room temperature under fluorescent light. Aminophylline not tested	1361	C
	ES	0.5 and 2 g	GL	50 mg and 2 g	D5W, NS[a]	Visually compatible with little or no loss of either drug by HPLC in 48 hr at room temperature	1802	C
Amphotericin B	SQ	200 mg	GL	100 mg	D5W	Color change and particle formation	1151	I
Ampicillin sodium		2 g	GL	100 mg	D5W	Physically compatible for 24 hr at ambient temperature under fluorescent light. Ampicillin instability is determining factor	1151	?
		1 g	GL	50 mg and 2 g	NS	Physically compatible and ranitidine chemically stable by HPLC for 24 hr at 25 °C. Ampicillin not tested	1515	C
Atracurium besylate	BW	500 mg		500 mg	D5W	Atracurium chemically unstable due to high pH	1694	I
Cefamandole nafate		1 g	GL	50 mg and 2 g	D5W	Ranitidine chemically stable by HPLC for only 6 hr at 25 °C. Cefamandole not tested	1515	I
Cefazolin sodium		2 g	GL	100 mg	D5W	Color change within 24 hr at ambient temperature under fluorescent light	1151	?
		1 g	GL	50 mg and 2 g	D5W	Ranitidine chemically stable by HPLC for only 6 hr at 25 °C. Cefazolin not tested	1515	I
Cefoxitin sodium		10 g	GL	50 mg and 2 g	D5W	Ranitidine chemically stable by HPLC for only 4 hr at 25 °C. Cefoxitin not tested	1515	I
Ceftazidime	GL[c]	10 g	GL	500 mg	D2.5½S	8% ranitidine loss in 4 hr and 39% loss in 24 hr by HPLC at 22 °C	1632	I
Cefuroxime sodium	GL	1.5 g	GL	100 mg	D5W	Color change within 24 hr at ambient temperature under fluorescent light	1151	?

Additive Compatibility (Cont.)

Ranitidine HCl

Drug	Mfr	Conc/L	Mfr	Conc/L	Test Soln	Remarks	Ref	C/I
		6 g	GL	50 mg and 2 g	D5W	Ranitidine chemically stable by HPLC for only 6 hr at 25 °C. Cefuroxime not tested	1515	**I**
Chloramphenicol sodium succinate		2 g	GL	100 mg	D5W	Physically compatible for 24 hr at ambient temperature	1151	**C**
Chlorothiazide sodium		5 g	GL	50 mg and 2 g	D5W	Physically compatible and ranitidine chemically stable by HPLC for 24 hr at 25 °C. Chlorothiazide not tested	1515	**C**
Ciprofloxacin	BAY	2 g	GL	500 mg and 1 g	NS	Visually compatible with little or no ciprofloxacin loss by HPLC in 24 hr at 25 °C. Ranitidine not tested	1934	**C**
Clindamycin phosphate	UP	1.2 g	GL	100 mg	D5W	Color change and gas formation	1151	**I**
		1.2 g	GL	50 mg and 2 g	D5W, NS	Physically compatible and ranitidine chemically stable by HPLC for 24 hr at 25 °C. Clindamycin not tested	1515	**C**
Colistimethate sodium		1.5 g	GL	50 mg and 2 g	D5W	Physically compatible and ranitidine chemically stable by HPLC for 24 hr at 25 °C. Colistimethate not tested	1515	**C**
Dexamethasone sodium phosphate		40 mg	GL	50 mg and 2 g	D5W	Physically compatible and ranitidine chemically stable by HPLC for 24 hr at 25 °C. Dexamethasone not tested	1515	**C**
Digoxin		2.5 mg	GL	50 mg and 2 g	D5W	Physically compatible and ranitidine chemically stable by HPLC for 24 hr at 25 °C. Digoxin not tested	1515	**C**
Dobutamine HCl	LI	250 mg and 1 g	GL	2 g	D5W, NS[a]	Physically compatible with no ranitidine loss in 48 hr at room temperature under fluorescent light. Dobutamine not tested	1361	**C**
	LI	250 mg and 1 g	GL	50 mg	D5W[a]	Physically compatible with 5 to 7% ranitidine loss in 48 hr at room temperature under fluorescent light. Dobutamine not tested	1361	**C**
	LI	250 mg and 1 g	GL	50 mg	NS[a]	Physically compatible with no ranitidine loss in 48 hr at room temperature under fluorescent light. Dobutamine not tested	1361	**C**
	LI	0.25 to 1 g	GL	50 mg and 2 g	D5W, NS[a]	Visually compatible with little or no loss of either drug by HPLC in 48 hr at room temperature	1802	**C**
Dopamine HCl	ES	400 mg and 3.2 g	GL	50 mg and 2 g	D5W, NS[a]	Physically compatible with 6% or less ranitidine loss in 48 hr at room temperature under fluorescent light. Dopamine not tested	1361	**C**
	ES	0.4 and 3.2 g	GL	50 mg and 2 g	D5W, NS[a]	Visually compatible with 5 to 7% ranitidine loss and little or no dopamine loss by HPLC in 48 hr at room temperature	1802	**C**
Doxycycline hyclate	PF	200 mg	GL	100 mg	D5W	Physically compatible for 24 hr at ambient temperature under fluorescent light	1151	**C**
Epinephrine HCl		50 mg	GL	50 mg and 2 g	D5W	Physically compatible and ranitidine chemically stable by HPLC for 24 hr at 25 °C. Epinephrine not tested	1515	**C**

Additive Compatibility (Cont.)

Ranitidine HCl

Drug	Mfr	Conc/L	Mfr	Conc/L	Test Soln	Remarks	Ref	C/I
Erythromycin lactobionate		5 g	GL	50 mg and 2 g	NS	Physically compatible and ranitidine chemically stable by HPLC for 24 hr at 25 °C. Erythromycin not tested	1515	C
Ethacrynate sodium		500 mg	GL	50 mg and 2 g	D5W	Ranitidine chemically stable by HPLC for only 6 hr at 25 °C. Ethacrynate not tested	1515	I
Floxacillin sodium	BE	20 g	GL	500 mg	NS	Physically compatible for 72 hr at 15 and 30 °C	1479	C
Fluconazole with ondansetron HCl	RR GL	2 g 100 mg	GL	500 mg	[a]	Visually compatible with no loss of any drug by HPLC in 4 hr	1730	C
Flumazenil	RC	20 mg	GL	300 mg	D5W[a]	Visually compatible with 3% flumazenil loss by HPLC in 24 hr at 23 °C under fluorescent light. Ranitidine not tested	1710	C
Furosemide	HO	1 g	GL	500 mg	NS	Physically compatible for 72 hr at 15 and 30 °C	1479	C
		400 mg	GL	50 mg and 2 g	D5W	Physically compatible and ranitidine chemically stable by HPLC for 24 hr at 25 °C. Furosemide not tested	1515	C
Gentamicin sulfate		160 mg	GL	100 mg	D5W	Physically compatible for 24 hr at ambient temperature under fluorescent light	1151	C
		80 mg	GL	50 mg and 2 g	D5W, NS	Physically compatible and ranitidine chemically stable by HPLC for 24 hr at 25 °C. Gentamicin not tested	1515	C
Heparin sodium	ES	10,000 and 40,000 units	GL	2 g	D5W, NS[a]	Physically compatible with 2% or less ranitidine loss in 48 hr at room temperature under fluorescent light. Heparin not tested	1361	C
	ES	10,000 and 40,000 units	GL	50 mg	NS[a]	Physically compatible with no ranitidine loss in 48 hr at room temperature under fluorescent light. Heparin not tested	1361	C
	ES	10,000 and 40,000 units	GL	50 mg	D5W[a]	Physically compatible with 7% ranitidine loss in 24 hr and about 12% loss in 48 hr at room temperature under fluorescent light. Heparin not tested	1361	C
Insulin, regular		100 units	GL	50 mg and 2 g	NS	Physically compatible and ranitidine chemically stable by HPLC for 24 hr at 25 °C. Insulin not tested	1515	C
	LI[b]	1000 units	GL	600 mg	NS[a]	Visually compatible with little or no loss by HPLC of ranitidine in 24 hr at ambient temperature but insulin losses of 9% in 4 hr and 14% in 24 hr presumably due to sorption	2079	I
Isoproterenol HCl		20 mg	GL	50 mg and 2 g	D5W	Physically compatible and ranitidine chemically stable by HPLC for 24 hr at 25 °C. Isoproterenol not tested	1515	C
Lidocaine HCl	AST	1 and 8 g	GL	50 mg and 2 g	D5W, NS[a]	Physically compatible with 3% or less ranitidine loss in 24 hr at room temperature under fluorescent light. Lidocaine not tested	1361	C

Additive Compatibility (Cont.)

Ranitidine HCl

Drug	Mfr	Conc/L	Mfr	Conc/L	Test Soln	Remarks	Ref	C/I
		2.5 g	GL	50 mg and 2 g	D5W	Physically compatible and ranitidine chemically stable by HPLC for 24 hr at 25 °C. Lidocaine not tested	1515	C
	AST	1 and 8 g	GL	50 mg and 2 g	D5W, NS[a]	Visually compatible with little or no loss of either drug by HPLC in 48 hr at room temperature	1802	C
Lincomycin HCl		2.4 g	GL	50 mg and 2 g	D5W	Physically compatible and ranitidine chemically stable by HPLC for 24 hr at 25 °C. Lincomycin not tested	1515	C
Meropenem	ZEN	1 and 20 g	GL	100 mg	NS	Visually compatible for 4 hr at room temperature	1994	C
Methylprednisolone sodium succinate	UP	40 mg	GL	50 mg	D5W[a]	Visually compatible with 7% ranitidine loss and no methylprednisolone loss by HPLC in 48 hr at room temperature	1802	C
	UP	2 g	GL	50 mg	D5W[a]	Visually compatible with 6% ranitidine loss and 10% methylprednisolone loss by HPLC in 48 hr at room temperature	1802	C
	UP	40 mg and 2 g	GL	2 g	D5W[a]	Visually compatible with no loss of either drug by HPLC in 48 hr at room temperature	1802	C
	UP	40 mg and 2 g	GL	50 mg and 2 g	NS[a]	Visually compatible with no ranitidine loss and about 10% methylprednisolone loss by HPLC in 48 hr at room temperature	1802	C
Norepinephrine bitartrate	WI	4 and 8 mg	GL	2 g	D5W, NS[a]	Physically compatible with no ranitidine loss in 48 hr at room temperature under fluorescent light. Norepinephrine not tested	1361	C
	WI	4 and 8 mg	GL	50 mg	D5W, NS[a]	Physically compatible with 2 to 6% ranitidine loss in 48 hr at room temperature under fluorescent light. Norepinephrine not tested	1361	C
		4 mg	GL	50 mg and 2 g	D5W	Physically compatible and ranitidine chemically stable by HPLC for 24 hr at 25 °C. Norepinephrine not tested	1515	C
	RC	4 and 8 mg	GL	50 mg	D5W[a]	Visually compatible with 5 to 7% ranitidine loss and little or no norepinephrine loss by HPLC in 48 hr at room temperature	1802	C
	RC	4 mg	GL	2 g	D5W[a]	Visually compatible but 7% norepinephrine loss in 4 hr and 13% loss in 12 hr by HPLC at room temperature. No ranitidine loss in 48 hr	1802	I
	RC	8 mg	GL	2 g	D5W[a]	Visually compatible but 6% norepinephrine loss in 12 hr and 11% loss in 24 hr by HPLC at room temperature. No ranitidine loss in 48 hr	1802	I
Penicillin G potassium		24 million units	GL	50 mg and 2 g	D5W, NS	Physically compatible and ranitidine chemically stable by HPLC for 24 hr at 25 °C. Penicillin not tested	1515	C

Additive Compatibility (Cont.)

Ranitidine HCl

Drug	Mfr	Conc/L	Mfr	Conc/L	Test Soln	Remarks	Ref	C/I
Penicillin G sodium		2.4 million units	GL	100 mg	D5W	Physically compatible for 24 hr at ambient temperature under fluorescent light	1151	**C**
Phytonadione		100 mg	GL	50 mg and 2 g	D5W	Ranitidine chemically stable by HPLC for only 6 hr at 25 °C. Phytonadione not tested	1515	**I**
Polymyxin B sulfate		1 million units	GL	50 mg and 2 g	D5W	Physically compatible and ranitidine chemically stable by HPLC for 24 hr at 25 °C. Polymyxin B not tested	1515	**C**
Potassium chloride	LY	10 and 60 mEq	GL	2 g	D5W, NS[a]	Physically compatible with 2% or less ranitidine loss in 48 hr at room temperature under fluorescent light	1361	**C**
	LY	10 and 60 mEq	GL	50 mg	NS[a]	Physically compatible with no ranitidine loss in 48 hr at room temperature under fluorescent light	1361	**C**
	LY	10 and 60 mEq	GL	50 mg	D5W[a]	Physically compatible with 7% ranitidine loss in 48 hr at room temperature under fluorescent light	1361	**C**
		80 mEq	GL	50 mg and 2 g	D5S, D5W, NS	Physically compatible and ranitidine chemically stable by HPLC for 24 hr at 25 °C. Potassium chloride not tested	1515	**C**
Protamine sulfate		500 mg	GL	50 mg and 2 g	D5W	Physically compatible and ranitidine chemically stable by HPLC for 24 hr at 25 °C. Protamine not tested	1515	**C**
Quinidine gluconate		3.2 g	GL	50 mg and 2 g	D5W	Physically compatible and ranitidine chemically stable by HPLC for 24 hr at 25 °C. Quinidine not tested	1515	**C**
Sodium nitroprusside	RC	50 and 400 mg	GL	2 g	D5W, NS[a]	Physically compatible with no ranitidine loss in 48 hr at room temperature protected from light. Nitroprusside not tested	1361	**C**
	RC	50 and 400 mg	GL	50 mg	NS[a]	Physically compatible with no ranitidine loss in 48 hr at room temperature protected from light. Nitroprusside not tested	1361	**C**
	RC	50 and 400 mg	GL	50 mg	D5W[a]	Physically compatible with 7% or less ranitidine loss in 48 hr protected from light. Nitroprusside not tested	1361	**C**
		50 mg and 1 g	GL	50 mg and 2 g	D5W, NS	Physically compatible and both drugs chemically stable for 48 hr at room temperature protected from light	1515	**C**
		100 mg	GL	50 mg and 2 g	D5W	Physically compatible and ranitidine chemically stable by HPLC for 24 hr at 25 °C. Sodium nitroprusside not tested	1515	**C**
	RC	50 and 400 mg	GL	50 mg and 2 g	D5W[a]	Visually compatible with 5 to 7% ranitidine loss and 8% or less nitroprusside loss in 48 hr at room temperature protected from light	1802	**C**
	RC	50 and 400 mg	GL	50 mg and 2 g	NS[a]	Visually compatible with no loss of either drug by HPLC in 48 hr at room temperature protected from light	1802	**C**

Additive Compatibility (Cont.)

Ranitidine HCl

Drug	Mfr	Conc/L	Mfr	Conc/L	Test Soln	Remarks	Ref	C/I
Ticarcillin disodium	BE	10 g	GL	100 mg	D5W	Physically compatible for 24 hr at ambient temperature under fluorescent light	1151	C
Tobramycin sulfate	DI	200 mg	GL	100 mg	D5W	Physically compatible for 24 hr at ambient temperature under fluorescent light	1151	C
Vancomycin HCl	DI	1 g	GL	100 mg	D5W	Physically compatible for 24 hr at ambient temperature under fluorescent light	1151	C
		5 g	GL	50 mg and 2 g	D5W	Physically compatible and ranitidine chemically stable by HPLC for 24 hr at 25 °C. Vancomycin not tested	1515	C

[a]Tested in PVC containers.
[b]Regular human insulin.
[c]Sodium carbonate–containing formulation tested.

Drugs in Syringe Compatibility

Ranitidine HCl

Drug (in syringe)	Mfr	Amt	Mfr	Amt	Remarks	Ref	C/I
Atropine sulfate	GL	0.4 mg/ 1 ml	GL	50 mg/ 2 ml	Physically compatible for 1 hr at 25 °C both macroscopically and microscopically	978	C
Chlorpromazine HCl	RP	25 mg/ 1 ml	GL	50 mg/ 2 ml	Physically compatible for 1 hr at 25 °C both macroscopically and microscopically	978	C
	RP	25 mg	GL	50 mg/ 5 ml	Gas formation	1151	I
Cyclizine lactate	CA	50 mg/ 1 ml	GL	50 mg/ 2 ml	Physically compatible for 1 hr at 25 °C both macroscopically and microscopically	978	C
Dexamethasone sodium phosphate	ME	4 mg	GL	50 mg/ 5 ml	Physically compatible for 4 hr at ambient temperature under fluorescent light	1151	C
Diazepam	RC	10 mg/ 2 ml	GL	50 mg/ 2 ml	Immediate white haze which disappeared following vortex mixing	978	I
		10 mg	GL	50 mg/ 5 ml	Physically compatible for 4 hr at ambient temperature under fluorescent light	1151	C
Dimenhydrinate	HR	50 mg/ 1 ml	GL	50 mg/ 2 ml	Physically compatible for 1 hr at 25 °C both macroscopically and microscopically	978	C
Diphenhydramine HCl	PD	50 mg/ 1 ml	GL	50 mg/ 2 ml	Physically compatible for 1 hr at 25 °C both macroscopically and microscopically	978	C
Dobutamine HCl	LI	25 mg	GL	50 mg/ 5 ml	Physically compatible for 4 hr at ambient temperature under fluorescent light	1151	C
Dopamine HCl		40 mg	GL	50 mg/ 5 ml	Physically compatible for 4 hr at ambient temperature under fluorescent light	1151	C
Fentanyl citrate	JN	0.1 mg/ 2 ml	GL	50 mg/ 2 ml	Physically compatible for 1 hr at 25 °C both macroscopically and microscopically	978	C
Glycopyrrolate	RB	0.2 mg/ 1 ml	GL	50 mg/ 2 ml	Physically compatible for 1 hr at 25 °C both macroscopically and microscopically	978	C
Hydromorphone HCl		2 mg/ 1 ml	GL	50 mg/ 2 ml	Physically compatible for 1 hr at 25 °C both macroscopically and microscopically	978	C
Hydroxyzine HCl	PF	50 mg/ 1 ml	GL	50 mg/ 2 ml	Immediate white haze which disappeared following vortex mixing	978	I

Drugs in Syringe Compatibility (Cont.)

Ranitidine HCl

Drug (in syringe)	Mfr	Amt	Mfr	Amt	Remarks	Ref	C/I
Isoproterenol sulfate	BI	0.2 mg	GL	50 mg/ 5 ml	Physically compatible for 4 hr at ambient temperature under fluorescent light	1151	**C**
Lorazepam	WY	4 mg/ 1 ml	GL	50 mg/ 2 ml	Lorazepam viscosity caused poor mixing and layering which disappeared following vortex mixing	978	**?**
Meperidine HCl	WI	100 mg/ 1 ml	GL	50 mg/ 2 ml	Physically compatible for 1 hr at 25 °C both macroscopically and microscopically	978	**C**
Methotrimeprazine	RP	25 mg/ 1 ml	GL	50 mg/ 2 ml	Immediate white turbidity	978	**I**
Metoclopramide HCl	RB	10 mg/ 1 ml	GL	50 mg/ 2 ml	Physically compatible for 1 hr at 25 °C both macroscopically and microscopically	978	**C**
Midazolam HCl	RC	5 mg/ 1 ml	GL	50 mg/ 2 ml	White precipitate forms immediately	1145	**I**
Morphine sulfate	AH	10 mg/ 1 ml	GL	50 mg/ 2 ml	Physically compatible for 1 hr at 25 °C both macroscopically and microscopically	978	**C**
Nalbuphine HCl	EN	10 mg/ 1 ml	GL	50 mg/ 2 ml	Physically compatible for 1 hr at 25 °C both macroscopically and microscopically	978	**C**
Oxymorphone HCl	EN	1.5 mg/ 1 ml	GL	50 mg/ 2 ml	Physically compatible for 1 hr at 25 °C both macroscopically and microscopically	978	**C**
Pentazocine lactate	WI	60 mg/ 2 ml	GL	50 mg/ 2 ml	Physically compatible for 1 hr at 25 °C both macroscopically and microscopically	978	**C**
Pentobarbital sodium	AB	100 mg	GL	50 mg/ 5 ml	Immediate precipitation	1151	**I**
Perphenazine	SC	5 mg/ 1 ml	GL	50 mg/ 2 ml	Physically compatible for 1 hr at 25 °C both macroscopically and microscopically	978	**C**
Phenobarbital sodium	AB	120 mg/ 1 ml	GL	50 mg/ 2 ml	Immediate white haze	978	**I**
Prochlorperazine edisylate	RP	10 mg/ 2 ml	GL	50 mg/ 2 ml	Physically compatible for 1 hr at 25 °C both macroscopically and microscopically	978	**C**
Promethazine HCl	RP	25 mg/ 1 ml	GL	50 mg/ 2 ml	Physically compatible for 1 hr at 25 °C both macroscopically and microscopically	978	**C**
	RP	25 mg	GL	50 mg/ 5 ml	Physically compatible for 4 hr at ambient temperature under fluorescent light	1151	**C**
Scopolamine HBr	AB	0.4 mg/ 1 ml	GL	50 mg/ 2 ml	Physically compatible for 1 hr at 25 °C both macroscopically and microscopically	978	**C**
		0.5 mg	GL	50 mg/ 5 ml	Physically compatible for 4 hr at ambient temperature under fluorescent light	1151	**C**
Thiethylperazine malate	SZ	10 mg/ 1 ml	GL	50 mg/ 2 ml	Physically compatible for 1 hr at 25 °C both macroscopically and microscopically	978	**C**

Y-Site Injection Compatibility (1:1 Mixture)

Ranitidine HCl

Drug	Mfr	Conc	Mfr	Conc	Remarks	Ref	C/I
Acyclovir sodium	BW	5 mg/ml[a]	GL	1 mg/ml[a]	Physically compatible for 4 hr at 25 °C	1157	**C**
Aldesleukin	CHI	33,800 I.U./ ml[a]	AB	1 mg/ml[c]	Visually compatible with little or no loss of aldesleukin activity by bioassay	1857	**C**

Y-Site Injection Compatibility (1:1 Mixture) (Cont.)

Ranitidine HCl

Drug	Mfr	Conc	Mfr	Conc	Remarks	Ref	C/I
Allopurinol sodium	BW	3 mg/ml[b]	GL	2 mg/ml[b]	Physically compatible with no change in measured turbidity or increase in particle content in 4 hr at 22 °C	1686	**C**
Amifostine	USB	10 mg/ml[a]	GL	2 mg/ml[a]	Physically compatible with no change in measured turbidity or increase in particle content in 4 hr at 23 °C	1845	**C**
Aminophylline	LY	4 mg/ml[a]	GL	0.5 mg/ml[d]	Physically compatible for 24 hr	1323	**C**
Amphotericin B cholesteryl sulfate complex	SEQ	0.83 mg/ml[a]	GL	2 mg/ml[a]	Microprecipitate and increased turbidity form immediately	2117	**I**
Amsacrine	NCI	1 mg/ml[a]	GL	2 mg/ml[a]	Physically compatible for 4 hr at room temperature under fluorescent light	1381	**C**
Atracurium besylate	BW	0.5 mg/ml[a]	GL	0.5 mg/ml[a]	Physically compatible for 24 hr at 28 °C	1337	**C**
Aztreonam	SQ	16.7 mg/ml[b]	GL	1 mg/ml[b]	No loss of either drug by HPLC in 4 hr at 22 °C under fluorescent light	1632	**C**
	SQ	40 mg/ml[a]	GL	2 mg/ml[a]	Physically compatible with no subvisual haze or particle formation in 4 hr at 23 °C	1758	**C**
Bretylium tosylate	LY	4 mg/ml[a]	GL	0.5 mg/ml[d]	Physically compatible for 24 hr	1323	**C**
Cefepime HCl	BR	20 mg/ml[a]	GL	2 mg/ml[a]	Physically compatible with no change in measured turbidity or increase in particle content in 4 hr at 22 °C	1689	**C**
Cefoperazone sodium	TAK	20 mg/ml[b]	GL	1 mg/ml[b]	Visually compatible with no loss of either drug by HPLC in 4 hr at 25 °C	2209	**C**
Ceftazidime	GL[k]	20 mg/ml[a]	GL	1 mg/ml[b]	No ceftazidime loss and 8% ranitidine loss by HPLC in 4 hr at 22 °C	1632	**C**
Ceftizoxime sodium	FUJ	20 mg/ml[b]	GL	1 mg/ml[b]	Visually compatible with no loss of either drug by HPLC in 4 hr 25 °C	2209	**C**
Ciprofloxacin	MI	2 mg/ml[e]	GL	0.5 mg/ml[e]	Visually compatible for 24 hr at 24 °C	1655	**C**
Cisatracurium besylate	GW	0.1, 2, 5 mg/ml[a]	GL	2 mg/ml[a]	Physically compatible with no change in measured turbidity or increase in particle content in 4 hr at 23 °C	2074	**C**
Cisplatin	BR	1 mg/ml	GL	1 mg/ml[a]	Visually compatible for 4 hr at room temperature under fluorescent light	1685	**C**
Cladribine	ORT	0.015[b] and 0.5[f] mg/ml	GL	2 mg/ml[b]	Physically compatible with no change in measured turbidity or increase in particle content in 4 hr at 23 °C	1969	**C**
Clarithromycin	AB	4 mg/ml[a]	GW	5 mg/ml[a]	Visually compatible for 72 hr at both 30 and 17 °C	2174	**C**
Cyclophosphamide	MJ	10 mg/ml	GL	1 mg/ml[a]	Visually compatible for 4 hr at room temperature under fluorescent light	1685	**C**
Cytarabine	UP	50 mg/ml	GL	1 mg/ml[a]	Visually compatible for 4 hr at room temperature under fluorescent light	1685	**C**
Diltiazem HCl	MMD	1[c] and 5 mg/ml	GL	25 mg/ml	Visually compatible	1807	**C**
	MMD	5 mg/ml	GL	0.5[c] and 1[b] mg/ml	Visually compatible	1807	**C**
	MMD	1 mg/ml[a]	GL	1 mg/ml[a]	Visually compatible for 4 hr at 27 °C	2062	**C**

Y-Site Injection Compatibility (1:1 Mixture) (Cont.)

		Ranitidine HCl					
Drug	*Mfr*	*Conc*	*Mfr*	*Conc*	*Remarks*	*Ref*	*C/I*
Dobutamine HCl	LI	1 mg/ml[a]	GL	0.5 mg/ml[d]	Physically compatible for 24 hr	1323	C
	LI	4 mg/ml[a]	GL	1 mg/ml[a]	Visually compatible for 4 hr at 27 °C	2062	C
Docetaxel	RPR	0.9 mg/ml[a]	GL	2 mg/ml[a]	Physically compatible with no change in measured turbidity or increase in particle content in 4 hr at 23 °C	2224	C
Dopamine HCl	ES	1.6 mg/ml[a]	GL	0.5 mg/ml[d]	Physically compatible for 24 hr	1323	C
	AB	3.2 mg/ml[a]	GL	1 mg/ml[a]	Visually compatible for 4 hr at 27 °C	2062	C
Doxorubicin HCl	AD	0.2 mg/ml[a]	GL	1 mg/ml[a]	Visually compatible for 4 hr at room temperature under fluorescent light	1685	C
Doxorubicin HCl liposome injection	SEQ	0.4 mg/ml[a]	GL	2 mg/ml[a]	Physically compatible with little or no change in measured turbidity and no increase in particle content in 4 hr at 23 °C	2087	C
Enalaprilat	MSD	0.05 mg/ml[b]	GL	0.5 mg/ml[a]	Physically compatible for 24 hr at room temperature under fluorescent light	1355	C
Epinephrine HCl	AB	0.02 mg/ml[a]	GL	1 mg/ml[a]	Visually compatible for 4 hr at 27 °C	2062	C
Esmolol HCl	DCC	10 mg/ml[a]	GL	0.5 mg/ml[a]	Physically compatible for 24 hr at 22 °C	1169	C
Etoposide phosphate	BR	5 mg/ml[a]	GL	2 mg/ml[a]	Physically compatible with no change in measured turbidity or increase in particle content in 4 hr at 23 °C	2218	C
Fentanyl citrate	ES	0.05 mg/ml	GL	1 mg/ml[a]	Visually compatible for 4 hr at 27 °C	2062	C
Filgrastim	AMG	30 μg/ml[a]	GL	2 mg/ml[a]	Physically compatible with no change in measured turbidity or increase in particle content in 4 hr at 22 °C	1687	C
Fluconazole	BR	2 mg/ml[b]	GL	0.5 and 2 mg/ml[a]	Visually compatible with no loss of either drug by HPLC in 4 hr	1730	C
Fludarabine phosphate	BX	1 mg/ml[a]	GL	2 mg/ml[a]	Physically compatible for 4 hr at room temperature under fluorescent light	1439	C
Foscarnet sodium	AST	24 mg/ml	GL	2 mg/ml[e]	Physically compatible for 24 hr at 25 °C under fluorescent light by visual and microscopic examination	1393	C
Furosemide	AMR	10 mg/ml	GL	1 mg/ml[a]	Visually compatible for 4 hr at 27 °C	2062	C
Gemcitabine HCl	LI	10 mg/ml[b]	GL	2 mg/ml[b]	Physically compatible with no change in measured turbidity or increase in particle content in 4 hr at 23 °C	2226	C
Granisetron HCl	SKB	0.05 mg/ml[a]	GL	2 mg/ml[a]	Physically compatible with no change in measured turbidity or increase in particle content in 4 hr at 23 °C	2000	C
Heparin sodium	LY	50 units/ml[a]	GL	0.5 mg/ml[d]	Physically compatible for 24 hr	1323	C
	TR	50 units/ml	GL	1 mg/ml	Visually compatible for 6 hr at 25 °C	1793	C
	ES	100 units/ml[a]	GL	1 mg/ml[a]	Visually compatible for 4 hr at 27 °C	2062	C
Hetastarch	DCC	6%	GL	0.5 mg/ml[d]	Barely visible single particle appeared after 1 hr but disappeared when vial was rotated	1313	?
	DCC	6%	GL	0.5 mg/ml[d]	Barely visible particles appeared and disappeared in three of five vials	1314	I

Y-Site Injection Compatibility (1:1 Mixture) (Cont.)

Drug	Mfr	Conc	Mfr	Conc	Remarks	Ref	C/I
	DCC	6%	GL	0.5 mg/ml[d]	Small white particle in two of five test vials. Small white fiber formed on needle during Y-site infusion	1315	I
Hydromorphone HCl	KN	1 mg/ml	GL	1 mg/ml[a]	Visually compatible for 4 hr at 27 °C	2062	C
Idarubicin HCl	AD	1 mg/ml[b]	GL	1 mg/ml[a]	Visually compatible for 24 hr at 25 °C	1525	C
Insulin, regular	LI[l]	1 unit/ml[b]	GL	1 mg/ml[b]	Visually compatible with little or no loss by HPLC of ranitidine in 4 hr at ambient temperature but insulin losses of 10% in 1 hr and 22% in 4 hr presumably due to sorption	2079	I
Labetalol HCl	SC	1 mg/ml[a]	GL	0.5 mg/ml[a]	Physically compatible for 24 hr at 18 °C	1171	C
	GL	1 mg/ml[a]	GL	0.6 mg/ml[a]	Visually compatible with 5% labetalol loss and little or no ranitidine loss by HPLC in 4 hr at room temperature	1762	C
	AH	2 mg/ml[a]	GL	1 mg/ml[a]	Visually compatible for 4 hr at 27 °C	2062	C
Lorazepam	WY	0.33 mg/ml[b]	GL	0.5 mg/ml	Visually compatible for 24 hr at 22 °C	1855	C
	WY	0.5 mg/ml[a]	GL	1 mg/ml[a]	Visually compatible for 4 hr at 27 °C	2062	C
Melphalan HCl	BW	0.1 mg/ml[b]	GL	2 mg/ml[b]	Physically compatible with no change in measured turbidity or increase in particle content in 3 hr at 22 °C	1557	C
Meperidine HCl	WY	10 mg/ml[b]	GL	0.5 mg/ml[c]	Physically compatible for 1 hr at 25 °C	1338	C
Methotrexate sodium	AD	15 mg/ml[g]	GL	1 mg/ml[a]	Visually compatible for 4 hr at room temperature under fluorescent light	1685	C
Midazolam HCl	RC	5 mg/ml	GL	0.5 mg/ml	Visually compatible for 24 hr at 22 °C	1855	C
	RC	2 mg/ml[a]	GL	1 mg/ml[a]	Visually compatible for 4 hr at 27 °C	2062	C
Milrinone lactate	SW	0.2 mg/ml[a]	GL	1 mg/ml[a]	Visually compatible for 4 hr at 27 °C	2062	C
	SW	0.4 mg/ml[a]	GL	2 mg/ml[a]	Visually compatible with little or no loss of either drug by HPLC in 4 hr at 23 °C	2214	C
Morphine sulfate	ES	1 mg/ml[b]	GL	0.5 mg/ml[c]	Physically compatible for 1 hr at 25 °C	1338	C
	SCN	2 mg/ml[a]	GL	1 mg/ml[a]	Visually compatible for 4 hr at 27 °C	2062	C
Nicardipine HCl	WY	1 mg/ml[a]	GL	1 mg/ml[a]	Visually compatible for 4 hr at 27 °C	2062	C
Nitroglycerin	SO	0.2 mg/ml[a]	GL	0.5 mg/ml[d]	Physically compatible for 24 hr	1323	C
	AB	0.4 mg/ml[a]	GL	1 mg/ml[a]	Visually compatible for 4 hr at 27 °C	2062	C
Norepinephrine bitartrate	AB	0.128 mg/ml[a]	GL	1 mg/ml[a]	Visually compatible for 4 hr at 27 °C	2062	C
Ondansetron HCl	GL	1 mg/ml[b]	GL	2 mg/ml[a]	Physically compatible for 4 hr at 22 °C	1365	C
	GL	0.03, 0.1, 0.3 mg/ml[a]	GL	0.5 mg/ml[a]	Visually compatible with no loss of either drug by HPLC in 4 hr	1730	C
	GL	0.03, 0.1, 0.3 mg/ml[a]	GL	2 mg/ml[a]	Visually compatible with no loss of either drug by HPLC in 4 hr	1730	C
Ondansetron HCl with paclitaxel	GL	0.3 mg/ml[a]	GL	2 mg/ml[a]	Visually compatible with no loss of any drug by HPLC in 4 hr at 23 °C under fluorescent light	1741	C
	BR	1.2 mg/ml[a]					
Paclitaxel	NCI	1.2 mg/ml[a]		2 mg/ml[a]	Physically compatible with no change in measured turbidity in 4 hr at 22 °C	1528	C
	BR	0.3 mg/ml[a]	GL	0.5 and 2 mg/ml[a]	Visually compatible with no loss of either drug in 4 hr at 23 °C under fluorescent light	1741	C

Y-Site Injection Compatibility (1:1 Mixture) (Cont.)

Drug	Mfr	Conc	Mfr	Conc	Remarks	Ref	C/I
	BR	1.2 mg/ml[a]	GL	0.5 and 2 mg/ml[a]	Visually compatible with no loss of either drug in 4 hr at 23 °C under fluorescent light	1741	C
Pancuronium bromide	ES	0.05 mg/ml[a]	GL	0.5 mg/ml[a]	Physically compatible for 24 hr at 28 °C	1337	C
Piperacillin sodium	LE	30 mg/ml[a]	GL	1 mg/ml[b]	Little or no loss of either drug by HPLC in 4 hr at 22 °C under fluorescent light	1632	C
Piperacillin sodium–tazobactam sodium	LE	40 + 5 mg/ml[a]	GL	2 mg/ml[a]	Physically compatible with no change in measured turbidity or increase in particle content in 4 hr at 22 °C	1688	C
	LE	80 + 10 mg/ml[b]	GL	0.5 and 2 mg/ml[b]	Visually compatible with little or no loss of any component by HPLC in 4 hr at 23 °C under fluorescent light	1759	C
	LE	40 + 5 mg/ml[b]	GL	0.5 and 2 mg/ml[b]	Visually compatible with little or no loss of ranitidine and tazobactam by HPLC in 4 hr at 23 °C under fluorescent light. Piperacillin not tested	1759	C
Procainamide HCl	BA	4 mg/ml[a]	GL	0.5 mg/ml[d]	Physically compatible for 24 hr	1323	C
Propofol	ZEN	10 mg/ml	GL	2 mg/ml[a]	Physically compatible for 1 hr at 23 °C with no increase in particle content	2066	C
Remifentanil HCl	GW	0.025 and 0.25 mg/ml[b]	GL	2 mg/ml[a]	Physically compatible with no change in measured turbidity or increase in particle content in 4 hr at 23 °C	2075	C
Sargramostim	IMM	10 μg/ml[b]	GL	2 mg/ml[b]	Physically compatible for 4 hr at 22 °C	1436	C
Tacrolimus	FUJ	1 mg/ml[b]	GL	25 mg/ml[a]	Visually compatible for 24 hr at 25 °C	1630	C
Teniposide	BR	0.1 mg/ml[a]	GL	2 mg/ml[a]	Physically compatible with no subvisual haze or particle formation in 4 hr at 23 °C	1725	C
Theophylline	TR	4 mg/ml	GL	1 mg/ml	Visually compatible for 6 hr at 25 °C	1793	C
Thiopental sodium	AB	25 mg/ml[h]	GL	1 mg/ml[a]	Visually compatible for 4 hr at 27 °C	2062	C
Thiotepa	IMM[i]	1 mg/ml[a]	GL	20 mg/ml[a]	Physically compatible with no change in measured turbidity or increase in particle content in 4 hr at 23 °C	1861	C
TNA #218 to #226[j]			GL	2 mg/ml[a]	Visually compatible with no precipitate or emulsion damage apparent in 4 hr at 23 °C	2215	C
TPN #189[j]			GL	2.5 mg/ml[b]	Visually compatible for 24 hr at 22 °C	1767	C
TPN #203 and #204[j]			GL	25 mg/ml	Visually compatible for 2 hr at 23 °C	1974	C
TPN #212 to #215[j]			GL	2 mg/ml[a]	Physically compatible with no change in measured turbidity or increase in particle content in 4 hr at 23 °C	2109	C
Vecuronium bromide	OR	0.1 mg/ml[a]	GL	0.5 mg/ml[a]	Physically compatible for 24 hr at 28 °C	1337	C
	OR	1 mg/ml	GL	1 mg/ml[a]	Visually compatible for 4 hr at 27 °C	2062	C
Vinorelbine tartrate	BW	1 mg/ml[b]	GL	2 mg/ml[b]	Physically compatible with no change in measured turbidity or increase in particle content in 4 hr at 22 °C	1558	C
Warfarin sodium	DU	2 mg/ml[h]	GL	1 mg/ml[a]	Visually compatible with no warfarin loss by HPLC in 30 min	2010	C
	DME	2 mg/ml[h]	GL	1 mg/ml[a]	Visually compatible for 24 hr at 24 °C	2078	C

Y-Site Injection Compatibility (1:1 Mixture) (Cont.)

Ranitidine HCl

Drug	Mfr	Conc	Mfr	Conc	Remarks	Ref	C/I
Zidovudine	BW	4 mg/ml[a]	GL	1 mg/ml[a]	Physically compatible for 4 hr at 25 °C under fluorescent light by visual and microscopic examination	1193	C

[a]*Tested in dextrose 5% in water.*
[b]*Tested in sodium chloride 0.9%.*
[c]*Tested in sodium chloride 0.45%.*
[d]*Premixed infusion solution.*
[e]*Tested in both dextrose 5% in water and sodium chloride 0.9%.*
[f]*Tested in bacteriostatic sodium chloride 0.9% preserved with benzyl alcohol 0.9%.*
[g]*Tested in dextrose 5% in water with sodium bicarbonate 0.05 mEq/ml.*
[h]*Tested in sterile water for injection.*
[i]*Lyophilized formulation tested.*
[j]*Refer to Appendix I for the composition of parenteral nutrition solutions. TNA indicates a 3-in-1 admixture, and TPN indicates a 2-in-1 admixture.*
[k]*Sodium carbonate–containing formulation tested.*
[l]*Regular human insulin.*

Additional Compatibility Information

Solutions— The manufacturer states that ranitidine HCl is stable for 48 hours at room temperature in most infusion solutions such as dextrose 5 and 10% in water, Ringer's injection, lactated, sodium bicarbonate 5%, and sodium chloride 0.9% (2; 4).

Parenteral Nutrition Solutions— The stability of ranitidine HCl has been evaluated in a number of TPN solutions with variable results. See Solution Compatibility table above. The major mechanism of ranitidine HCl decomposition is oxidation. A number of factors have been found to contribute to ranitidine HCl instability in TPN solutions including the presence or absence of antioxidants (such as sodium metabisulfite) in the amino acids, the addition of trace elements (which can catalyze ranitidine oxidation), solution pH, and the type of plastic container used. In a study of rantidine HCl stability in several TPN solutions stored at 5 °C, the drug was most stable in FreAmine III–based (contains sodium metabisulfite) admixtures with additives when packaged in multilayer, gas-impermeable plastic containers (Ultrastab), with about 8% ranitidine HCl loss by HPLC in 28 days. In contrast, in ethylene vinyl acetate (EVA) bags, which are permeable to oxygen, ranitidine HCl losses of approximately 50% occurred in this time period. If Vamin 14 with no antioxidant present was used as the amino acid source and the solution was packaged in EVA bags, ranitidine HCl losses of approximately 65% occurred in 28 days. Similarly, the addition of air to the bags during compounding increased rantidine HCl oxidation substantially (2195).

Miscellaneous— Ranitidine HCl is stated to be incompatible with amphotericin B and metaraminol bitartrate (1515).

REMIFENTANIL HCL
AHFS 28:08.08

Ultiva   **Glaxo Wellcome**

Products— Remifentanil HCl (Glaxo Wellcome) is available in vials containing 1, 2, or 5 mg of remifentanil base present as the hydrochloride. Each vial also contains glycine 15 mg and hydrochloric acid for pH adjustment. The contents of the vials should be reconstituted with 1 ml of compatible diluent per milligram of remifentanil to yield a 1-mg/ml solution (2).

pH— From 2.5 to 3.5 (2).

Administration— Remifentanil HCl is administered intravenously only. Single doses may be given over 30 to 60 seconds. Remifentanil HCl may also be given by continuous intravenous infusion using an infusion device. The manufacturer recommends that the injection site be near the venous cannula and that all tubing be cleared at the time the infusion is discontinued. Bolus doses and continuous infusion should not be administered simultaneously to spontaneously breathing patients (2).

For intravenous administration, remifentanil HCl should be diluted to a final concentration of 25, 50, or 250 µg/ml. It should not be administered without dilution (2).

Stability— Remifentanil HCl is a white to off-white lyophilized powder that forms a clear, colorless solution upon reconstitution. Intact vials should be stored between 2 and 25 °C (2).

Compatibility Information

Y-Site Injection Compatibility (1:1 Mixture)

Remifentanil HCl

Drug	Mfr	Conc	Mfr	Conc	Remarks	Ref	C/I
Acyclovir sodium	BW	7 mg/ml[a]	GW	0.025 and 0.25 mg/ml[b]	Physically compatible with no change in measured turbidity or increase in particle content in 4 hr at 23 °C	2075	**C**
Alfentanil HCl	JN	0.125 mg/ml[a]	GW	0.025 and 0.25 mg/ml[b]	Physically compatible with no change in measured turbidity or increase in particle content in 4 hr at 23 °C	2075	**C**
Amikacin sulfate	AB	5 mg/ml[a]	GW	0.025 and 0.25 mg/ml[b]	Physically compatible with no change in measured turbidity or increase in particle content in 4 hr at 23 °C	2075	**C**
Aminophylline	AB	2.5 mg/ml[a]	GW	0.025 and 0.25 mg/ml[b]	Physically compatible with no change in measured turbidity or increase in particle content in 4 hr at 23 °C	2075	**C**
Amphotericin B	PHT	0.6 mg/ml[a]	GW	0.025 mg/ml[a]	Physically compatible with no change in measured turbidity or increase in particle content in 4 hr at 23 °C	2075	**C**
	PHT	0.6 mg/ml[a]	GW	0.25 mg/ml[a]	Yellow precipitate forms immediately	2075	**I**
Amphotericin B cholesteryl sulfate complex	SEQ	0.83 mg/ml[a]	GW	0.5 mg/ml[a]	Gross precipitate forms	2117	**I**
Ampicillin sodium	SKB	20 mg/ml[b]	GW	0.025 and 0.25 mg/ml[b]	Physically compatible with no change in measured turbidity or increase in particle content in 4 hr at 23 °C	2075	**C**
Ampicillin sodium–sulbactam sodium	RR	20 + 10 mg/ml[b]	GW	0.025 and 0.25 mg/ml[b]	Physically compatible with no change in measured turbidity or increase in particle content in 4 hr at 23 °C	2075	**C**
Amrinone lactate	SW	2.5 mg/ml[a]	GW	0.025 and 0.25 mg/ml[b]	Physically compatible with no change in measured turbidity or increase in particle content in 4 hr at 23 °C	2075	**C**
Aztreonam	SQ	40 mg/ml[a]	GW	0.025 and 0.25 mg/ml[b]	Physically compatible with no change in measured turbidity or increase in particle content in 4 hr at 23 °C	2075	**C**
Bretylium tosylate	AST	4 mg/ml[a]	GW	0.025 and 0.25 mg/ml[b]	Physically compatible with no change in measured turbidity or increase in particle content in 4 hr at 23 °C	2075	**C**
Bumetanide	RC	0.04 mg/ml[a]	GW	0.025 and 0.25 mg/ml[b]	Physically compatible with no change in measured turbidity or increase in particle content in 4 hr at 23 °C	2075	**C**
Buprenorphine HCl	RKC	0.04 mg/ml[a]	GW	0.025 and 0.25 mg/ml[b]	Physically compatible with no change in measured turbidity or increase in particle content in 4 hr at 23 °C	2075	**C**
Butorphanol tartrate	APC	0.04 mg/ml[a]	GW	0.025 and 0.25 mg/ml[b]	Physically compatible with no change in measured turbidity or increase in particle content in 4 hr at 23 °C	2075	**C**
Calcium gluconate	AB	40 mg/ml[a]	GW	0.025 and 0.25 mg/ml[b]	Physically compatible with no change in measured turbidity or increase in particle content in 4 hr at 23 °C	2075	**C**
Cefazolin sodium	SKB	20 mg/ml[a]	GW	0.025 and 0.25 mg/ml[b]	Physically compatible with no change in measured turbidity or increase in particle content in 4 hr at 23 °C	2075	**C**

Y-Site Injection Compatibility (1:1 Mixture) (Cont.)

Remifentanil HCl

Drug	Mfr	Conc	Mfr	Conc	Remarks	Ref	C/I
Cefoperazone sodium	RR	40 mg/ml[a]	GW	0.025 mg/ml[b]	Physically compatible with no change in measured turbidity or increase in particle content in 4 hr at 23 °C	2075	C
	RR	40 mg/ml[a]	GW	0.25 mg/ml[b]	Subvisual haze forms in 1 hr	2075	I
Cefotaxime sodium	HO	20 mg/ml[a]	GW	0.025 and 0.25 mg/ml[b]	Physically compatible with no change in measured turbidity or increase in particle content in 4 hr at 23 °C	2075	C
Cefotetan sodium	ZEN	20 mg/ml[a]	GW	0.025 and 0.25 mg/ml[b]	Physically compatible with no change in measured turbidity or increase in particle content in 4 hr at 23 °C	2075	C
Cefoxitin sodium	ME	20 mg/ml[a]	GW	0.025 and 0.25 mg/ml[b]	Physically compatible with no change in measured turbidity or increase in particle content in 4 hr at 23 °C	2075	C
Ceftazidime	GW[c]	40 mg/ml[a]	GW	0.025 and 0.25 mg/ml[b]	Physically compatible with no change in measured turbidity or increase in particle content in 4 hr at 23 °C	2075	C
Ceftizoxime sodium	FUJ	20 mg/ml[a]	GW	0.025 and 0.25 mg/ml[b]	Physically compatible with no change in measured turbidity or increase in particle content in 4 hr at 23 °C	2075	C
Ceftriaxone sodium	RC	20 mg/ml[a]	GW	0.025 and 0.25 mg/ml[b]	Physically compatible with no change in measured turbidity or increase in particle content in 4 hr at 23 °C	2075	C
Cefuroxime sodium	LI	30 mg/ml[a]	GW	0.025 and 0.25 mg/ml[b]	Physically compatible with no change in measured turbidity or increase in particle content in 4 hr at 23 °C	2075	C
Chlorpromazine HCl	SCN	2 mg/ml[a]	GW	0.025 mg/ml[b]	Slight subvisual haze forms in 1 hr	2075	I
	SCN	2 mg/ml[a]	GW	0.25 mg/ml[b]	Physically compatible with no change in measured turbidity or increase in particle content in 4 hr at 23 °C	2075	C
Cimetidine HCl	SKB	12 mg/ml[a]	GW	0.025 and 0.25 mg/ml[b]	Physically compatible with no change in measured turbidity or increase in particle content in 4 hr at 23 °C	2075	C
Ciprofloxacin	BAY	1 mg/ml[a]	GW	0.025 and 0.25 mg/ml[b]	Physically compatible with no change in measured turbidity or increase in particle content in 4 hr at 23 °C	2075	C
Cisatracurium besylate	GW	2 mg/ml[a]	GW	0.025 and 0.25 mg/ml[b]	Physically compatible with no change in measured turbidity or increase in particle content in 4 hr at 23 °C	2075	C
Clindamycin phosphate	AST	10 mg/ml[a]	GW	0.025 and 0.25 mg/ml[b]	Physically compatible with no change in measured turbidity or increase in particle content in 4 hr at 23 °C	2075	C
Dexamethasone sodium phosphate	FUJ	2 mg/ml[a]	GW	0.025 and 0.25 mg/ml[b]	Physically compatible with no change in measured turbidity or increase in particle content in 4 hr at 23 °C	2075	C
Diazepam	ES	5 mg/ml	GW	0.025 and 0.25 mg/ml[b]	White turbidity forms immediately	2075	I
	ES	0.25 mg/ml[a]	GW	0.025 and 0.25 mg/ml[b]	Physically compatible with no change in measured turbidity or increase in particle content in 4 hr at 23 °C	2075	C

Y-Site Injection Compatibility (1:1 Mixture) (Cont.)

Remifentanil HCl

Drug	Mfr	Conc	Mfr	Conc	Remarks	Ref	C/I
Digoxin	ES	0.25 mg/ml	GW	0.025 and 0.25 mg/ml[b]	Physically compatible with no change in measured turbidity or increase in particle content in 4 hr at 23 °C	2075	C
Diphenhydramine HCl	SCN	2 mg/ml[a]	GW	0.025 and 0.25 mg/ml[b]	Physically compatible with no change in measured turbidity or increase in particle content in 4 hr at 23 °C	2075	C
Dobutamine HCl	LI	4 mg/ml[a]	GW	0.025 and 0.25 mg/ml[b]	Physically compatible with no change in measured turbidity or increase in particle content in 4 hr at 23 °C	2075	C
Dopamine HCl	AB	3.2 mg/ml[a]	GW	0.025 and 0.25 mg/ml[b]	Physically compatible with no change in measured turbidity or increase in particle content in 4 hr at 23 °C	2075	C
Doxycycline hyclate	FUJ	1 mg/ml[a]	GW	0.025 and 0.25 mg/ml[b]	Physically compatible with no change in measured turbidity or increase in particle content in 4 hr at 23 °C	2075	C
Droperidol	AST	2.5 mg/ml	GW	0.025 and 0.25 mg/ml[b]	Physically compatible with no change in measured turbidity or increase in particle content in 4 hr at 23 °C	2075	C
Enalaprilat	ME	0.1 mg/ml[a]	GW	0.025 and 0.25 mg/ml[b]	Physically compatible with no change in measured turbidity or increase in particle content in 4 hr at 23 °C	2075	C
Epinephrine HCl	AMR	0.05 mg/ml[a]	GW	0.025 and 0.25 mg/ml[b]	Physically compatible with no change in measured turbidity or increase in particle content in 4 hr at 23 °C	2075	C
Esmolol HCl	OHM	10 mg/ml[a]	GW	0.025 and 0.25 mg/ml[b]	Physically compatible with no change in measured turbidity or increase in particle content in 4 hr at 23 °C	2075	C
Famotidine	MSD	2 mg/ml[a]	GW	0.025 and 0.25 mg/ml[b]	Physically compatible with no change in measured turbidity or increase in particle content in 4 hr at 23 °C	2075	C
Fentanyl citrate	ES	0.0125 mg/ml[a]	GW	0.025 and 0.25 mg/ml[b]	Physically compatible with no change in measured turbidity or increase in particle content in 4 hr at 23 °C	2075	C
Fluconazole	RR	2 mg/ml	GW	0.025 and 0.25 mg/ml[b]	Physically compatible with no change in measured turbidity or increase in particle content in 4 hr at 23 °C	2075	C
Furosemide	AMR	3 mg/ml[a]	GW	0.025 and 0.25 mg/ml[b]	Physically compatible with no change in measured turbidity or increase in particle content in 4 hr at 23 °C	2075	C
Ganciclovir sodium	SY	20 mg/ml[a]	GW	0.025 and 0.25 mg/ml[b]	Physically compatible with no change in measured turbidity or increase in particle content in 4 hr at 23 °C	2075	C
Gentamicin sulfate	ES	5 mg/ml[a]	GW	0.025 and 0.25 mg/ml[b]	Physically compatible with no change in measured turbidity or increase in particle content in 4 hr at 23 °C	2075	C
Haloperidol lactate	MN	0.2 mg/ml[a]	GW	0.025 and 0.25 mg/ml[b]	Physically compatible with no change in measured turbidity or increase in particle content in 4 hr at 23 °C	2075	C

Y-Site Injection Compatibility (1:1 Mixture) (Cont.)

Remifentanil HCl

Drug	Mfr	Conc	Mfr	Conc	Remarks	Ref	C/I
Heparin sodium	AB	100 units/ml	GW	0.025 and 0.25 mg/ml[b]	Physically compatible with no change in measured turbidity or increase in particle content in 4 hr at 23 °C	2075	C
Hydrocortisone sodium succinate	AB	1 mg/ml[a]	GW	0.025 and 0.25 mg/ml[b]	Physically compatible with no change in measured turbidity or increase in particle content in 4 hr at 23 °C	2075	C
Hydromorphone HCl	ES	0.5 mg/ml[a]	GW	0.025 and 0.25 mg/ml[b]	Physically compatible with no change in measured turbidity or increase in particle content in 4 hr at 23 °C	2075	C
Hydroxyzine HCl	ES	2 mg/ml[a]	GW	0.025 and 0.25 mg/ml[b]	Physically compatible with no change in measured turbidity or increase in particle content in 4 hr at 23 °C	2075	C
Imipenem–cilastatin sodium	ME	10 mg/ml[a]	GW	0.025 and 0.25 mg/ml[b]	Physically compatible with no change in measured turbidity or increase in particle content in 4 hr at 23 °C	2075	C
Isoproterenol HCl	SW	0.02 mg/ml[a]	GW	0.025 and 0.25 mg/ml[b]	Physically compatible with no change in measured turbidity or increase in particle content in 4 hr at 23 °C	2075	C
Ketorolac tromethamine	RC	15 mg/ml[a]	GW	0.025 and 0.25 mg/ml[b]	Physically compatible with no change in measured turbidity or increase in particle content in 4 hr at 23 °C	2075	C
Lidocaine HCl	AST	8 mg/ml[a]	GW	0.025 and 0.25 mg/ml[b]	Physically compatible with no change in measured turbidity or increase in particle content in 4 hr at 23 °C	2075	C
Lorazepam	WY	0.5 mg/ml[a]	GW	0.025 and 0.25 mg/ml[b]	Physically compatible with no change in measured turbidity or increase in particle content in 4 hr at 23 °C	2075	C
Magnesium sulfate	AB	100 mg/ml[a]	GW	0.025 and 0.25 mg/ml[b]	Physically compatible with no change in measured turbidity or increase in particle content in 4 hr at 23 °C	2075	C
Mannitol	BA	15%	GW	0.025 and 0.25 mg/ml[b]	Physically compatible with no change in measured turbidity or increase in particle content in 4 hr at 23 °C	2075	C
Meperidine HCl	AST	4 mg/ml[a]	GW	0.025 and 0.25 mg/ml[b]	Physically compatible with no change in measured turbidity or increase in particle content in 4 hr at 23 °C	2075	C
Methylprednisolone sodium succinate	AB	5 mg/ml[a]	GW	0.025 and 0.25 mg/ml[b]	Physically compatible with no change in measured turbidity or increase in particle content in 4 hr at 23 °C	2075	C
Metoclopramide HCl	AB	5 mg/ml	GW	0.025 and 0.25 mg/ml[b]	Physically compatible with no change in measured turbidity or increase in particle content in 4 hr at 23 °C	2075	C
Metronidazole	AB	5 mg/ml	GW	0.025 and 0.25 mg/ml[b]	Physically compatible with no change in measured turbidity or increase in particle content in 4 hr at 23 °C	2075	C
Mezlocillin disodium	MI	40 mg/ml[a]	GW	0.025 and 0.25 mg/ml[b]	Physically compatible with no change in measured turbidity or increase in particle content in 4 hr at 23 °C	2075	C

Y-Site Injection Compatibility (1:1 Mixture) (Cont.)

Remifentanil HCl

Drug	Mfr	Conc	Mfr	Conc	Remarks	Ref	C/I
Midazolam HCl	RC	1 mg/ml[a]	GW	0.025 and 0.25 mg/ml[b]	Physically compatible with no change in measured turbidity or increase in particle content in 4 hr at 23 °C	2075	C
Minocycline HCl	LE	0.2 mg/ml[a]	GW	0.025 and 0.25 mg/ml[b]	Physically compatible with no change in measured turbidity or increase in particle content in 4 hr at 23 °C	2075	C
Morphine sulfate	AST	1 mg/ml[a]	GW	0.025 and 0.25 mg/ml[b]	Physically compatible with no change in measured turbidity or increase in particle content in 4 hr at 23 °C	2075	C
Nalbuphine HCl	AST	10 mg/ml	GW	0.025 and 0.25 mg/ml[b]	Physically compatible with no change in measured turbidity or increase in particle content in 4 hr at 23 °C	2075	C
Netilmicin sulfate	SC	5 mg/ml[a]	GW	0.025 and 0.25 mg/ml[b]	Physically compatible with no change in measured turbidity or increase in particle content in 4 hr at 23 °C	2075	C
Nitroglycerin	DU	0.4 mg/ml[a]	GW	0.025 and 0.25 mg/ml[b]	Physically compatible with no change in measured turbidity or increase in particle content in 4 hr at 23 °C	2075	C
Norepinephrine bitartrate	SW	0.12 mg/ml[a]	GW	0.025 and 0.25 mg/ml[b]	Physically compatible with no change in measured turbidity or increase in particle content in 4 hr at 23 °C	2075	C
Ofloxacin	ORT	4 mg/ml[a]	GW	0.025 and 0.25 mg/ml[b]	Physically compatible with no change in measured turbidity or increase in particle content in 4 hr at 23 °C	2075	C
Ondansetron HCl	CER	1 mg/ml[a]	GW	0.025 and 0.25 mg/ml[b]	Physically compatible with no change in measured turbidity or increase in particle content in 4 hr at 23 °C	2075	C
Phenylephrine HCl	AMR	1 mg/ml[a]	GW	0.025 and 0.25 mg/ml[b]	Physically compatible with no change in measured turbidity or increase in particle content in 4 hr at 23 °C	2075	C
Piperacillin sodium	LE	40 mg/ml[a]	GW	0.025 and 0.25 mg/ml[b]	Physically compatible with no change in measured turbidity or increase in particle content in 4 hr at 23 °C	2075	C
Piperacillin sodium–tazobactam sodium	CY	40 + 5 mg/ml[a]	GW	0.025 and 0.25 mg/ml[b]	Physically compatible with no change in measured turbidity or increase in particle content in 4 hr at 23 °C	2075	C
Potassium chloride	AB	0.1 mg/ml[a]	GW	0.025 and 0.25 mg/ml[b]	Physically compatible with no change in measured turbidity or increase in particle content in 4 hr at 23 °C	2075	C
Procainamide HCl	ES	10 mg/ml[a]	GW	0.025 and 0.25 mg/ml[b]	Physically compatible with no change in measured turbidity or increase in particle content in 4 hr at 23 °C	2075	C
Prochlorperazine edisylate	SO	0.5 mg/ml[a]	GW	0.025 and 0.25 mg/ml[b]	Physically compatible with no change in measured turbidity or increase in particle content in 4 hr at 23 °C	2075	C
Promethazine HCl	SCN	2 mg/ml[a]	GW	0.025 and 0.25 mg/ml[b]	Physically compatible with no change in measured turbidity or increase in particle content in 4 hr at 23 °C	2075	C

Y-Site Injection Compatibility (1:1 Mixture) (Cont.)

Remifentanil HCl

Drug	Mfr	Conc	Mfr	Conc	Remarks	Ref	C/I
Ranitidine HCl	GL	2 mg/ml[a]	GW	0.025 and 0.25 mg/ml[b]	Physically compatible with no change in measured turbidity or increase in particle content in 4 hr at 23 °C	2075	C
Sodium bicarbonate	AB	1 mEq/ml	GW	0.025 and 0.25 mg/ml[b]	Physically compatible with no change in measured turbidity or increase in particle content in 4 hr at 23 °C	2075	C
Sufentanil citrate	ES	0.0125 mg/ml[a]	GW	0.025 and 0.25 mg/ml[b]	Physically compatible with no change in measured turbidity or increase in particle content in 4 hr at 23 °C	2075	C
Theophylline	AB	3.2 mg/ml[a]	GW	0.025 and 0.25 mg/ml[b]	Physically compatible with no change in measured turbidity or increase in particle content in 4 hr at 23 °C	2075	C
Thiopental sodium	AB	50 mg/ml[a]	GW	0.025 and 0.25 mg/ml[b]	Physically compatible with no change in measured turbidity or increase in particle content in 4 hr at 23 °C	2075	C
Ticarcillin disodium	SKB	30 mg/ml[a]	GW	0.025 and 0.25 mg/ml[b]	Physically compatible with no change in measured turbidity or increase in particle content in 4 hr at 23 °C	2075	C
Ticarcillin disodium–clavulanate potassium	SKB	31 mg/ml[a]	GW	0.025 and 0.25 mg/ml[b]	Physically compatible with no change in measured turbidity or increase in particle content in 4 hr at 23 °C	2075	C
Tobramycin sulfate	AB	5 mg/ml[a]	GW	0.025 and 0.25 mg/ml[b]	Physically compatible with no change in measured turbidity or increase in particle content in 4 hr at 23 °C	2075	C
Trimethoprim–sulfamethoxazole	ES	0.8 + 4 mg/ml[a]	GW	0.025 and 0.25 mg/ml[b]	Physically compatible with no change in measured turbidity or increase in particle content in 4 hr at 23 °C	2075	C
Vancomycin HCl	AB	10 mg/ml[a]	GW	0.025 and 0.25 mg/ml[b]	Physically compatible with no change in measured turbidity or increase in particle content in 4 hr at 23 °C	2075	C
Zidovudine	BW	4 mg/ml[a]	GW	0.025 and 0.25 mg/ml[b]	Physically compatible with no change in measured turbidity or increase in particle content in 4 hr at 23 °C	2075	C

[a]Tested in dextrose 5% in water.
[b]Tested in sodium chloride 0.9%.
[c]L-Arginine–containing formulation tested.

Additional Compatibility Information

Solutions— Remifentanil HCl is compatible and stable for 24 hours after reconstitution and dilution to concentrations from 20 to 250 μg/ml in the following diluents:

Dextrose 5% in Ringer's injection, lactated
Dextrose 5% in sodium chloride 0.9%
Dextrose 5% in water
Sodium chloride 0.45%

Sodium chloride 0.9%
Sterile water for injection

In Ringer's injection, lactated, remifentanil HCl is stable for four hours at room temperature (2).

Other Drugs— Propofol (Zeneca) has been stated to be compatible with remifentanil HCl. However, administration of remifentanil HCl into the same tubing with blood is not recommended, because of the possibility of hydrolysis (2).

RIFAMPIN
AHFS 8:16

Rifadin I.V.   **Aventis**

Products—— Rifampin (Aventis) is available as a lyophilized powder in vials containing rifampin 600 mg, sodium formaldehyde sulfoxylate 10 mg, and sodium hydroxide to adjust the pH. Reconstitute with 10 ml of sterile water for injection; swirl gently to dissolve the vial contents for a 60-mg/ml solution (2).

Administration—— Rifampin is administered by intravenous infusion. It must not be given intramuscularly or subcutaneously, and extravasation should be avoided. The reconstituted solution may be diluted in 500 ml of dextrose 5% in water or sodium chloride 0.9% and infused over three hours. Alternatively, the desired dose may be diluted in 100 ml and administered over 30 minutes (2; 4).

Stability—— Rifampin powder is reddish brown. Intact vials should be stored at room temperature and protected from excessive heat and light (2).

The reconstituted solution is stable for 24 hours at room temperature (2).

Compatibility Information

Solution Compatibility

	Rifampin					
Solution	Mfr	Mfr	Conc/L	Remarks	Ref	C/I
Dextrose 5% in water	AB	MMD	6 g	Gelatinous precipitate adhered to PVC container wall after overnight room temperature storage protected from light	1543	I
	AB	MMD	1.2 g	Clear with no visible precipitation during 3-hr administration period	1543	C
	BA[a]	MMD	0.1 g	Brownish color appears in 4 hr and darkens over 3 days. 5% rifampin loss in 8 hr and 15 to 17% loss in 24 hr at 24 °C by HPLC. 8% loss in 3 days at 4 °C	1559	I[b]
Sodium chloride 0.9%	BA[a]	MMD	0.1 g	Brownish color appears in 4 hr and darkens over 3 days. 5 to 7% rifampin loss in 8 hr and 11 to 13% loss in 24 hr at 24 °C by HPLC. 7% loss in 3 days at 4 °C	1559	I[b]

[a]Tested in PVC containers.
[b]Incompatible by conventional standards. May be used in shorter time periods.

Additive Compatibility

	Rifampin							
Drug	Mfr	Conc/L	Mfr	Conc/L	Test Soln	Remarks	Ref	C/I
Minocycline HCl	LE	0.1 g	MMD	0.1 g	NS	Brownish color appears in 4 hr at 37 and 24 °C and 8 hr at 4 °C. 10% rifampin loss by HPLC in 3 days at 4 °C and 8 hr at 24 °C; 14% loss in 4 hr at 37 °C. Less than 2% minocycline loss by HPLC under these conditions	1559	I

Y-Site Injection Compatibility (1:1 Mixture)

	Rifampin					
Drug	Mfr	Conc	Mfr	Conc	Remarks	Ref	C/I
Diltiazem HCl	MMD	1[a] and 5 mg/ml	MMD	6 mg/ml[a]	Precipitate forms	1807	I

[a]Tested in sodium chloride 0.9%.

Additional Compatibility Information

Solutions— The manufacturer recommends use of rifampin dilutions in dextrose 5% in water within four hours due to the potential for precipitation beyond this time period (2). However, the manufacturer recommends use of rifampin diluted in sodium chloride 0.9% within 24 hours (2) although other information indicates substantial (11 to 13%) rifampin decomposition occurs in 24 hours at room temperature in this infusion solution (1559). The administration of rifampin admixtures in either infusion solution within three hours of preparation seems to be a reasonable time frame based on both precipitation potential and drug decomposition.

SARGRAMOSTIM
AHFS 20:16

Leukine   **Immunex**

Products— Sargramostim (Immunex) is available in single-dose vials labeled as 250 μg. Reconstitute the vial with 1 ml of sterile water for injection or bacteriostatic water for injection containing benzyl alcohol 0.9% directed at the sides of the vial. Gently swirl to avoid foaming during dissolution, and do not shake. Each milliliter of the reconstituted solution contains sargramostim 250 μg, mannitol 40 mg, sucrose 10 mg, and tromethamine 1.2 mg (2; 4). The contents of vials reconstituted with different diluents should not be mixed (2).

Sargramostim (Immunex) is also available as an preserved liquid formulation in 1-ml vials containing in each milliliter sargramostim 500 μg along with mannitol 40 mg, sucrose 10 mg, tromethamine 1.2 mg, and benzyl alcohol 1.1% as an antimicrobial preservative (2; 4).

pH— From 7.1 to 7.7 (17).

Administration— Sargramostim may be administered by subcutaneous injection undiluted or by intravenous infusion usually over two to four hours after dilution in sodium chloride 0.9% (2; 4). Intravenous infusion also has been performed over 30 to 60 minutes, over five to 12 hours, and as a continuous infusion over 24 hours (4). For infusion concentrations below 10 μg/ml, normal human serum albumin at a final concentration of 0.1% should be added to the intravenous solution prior to the addition of sargramostim to prevent adsorption (2; 4).

The preparations containing benzyl alcohol (Leukine liquid, and lyophilized Leukine reconstituted with bacteriostatic water for injection containing benzyl alcohol) should not be used in neonates (2).

Stability— Intact vials, reconstituted solutions, and sargramostim diluted in sodium chloride 0.9% should be stored under refrigeration. Solutions should be protected from freezing and not shaken. The liquid formulation is a clear, colorless solution. The white lyophilized powder forms a clear, colorless solution on reconstitution. The manufacturer recommends administration within six hours following reconstitution with sterile water for injection and/or dilution in an infusion solution and discarding any unused solution. When reconstituted with bacteriostatic water for injection preserved with benzyl alcohol 0.9%, the manufacturer states that the solution may be stored for up to 20 days under refrigeration (2).

Other information indicates that sargramostim reconstituted with sterile water for injection or bacteriostatic water for injection retains potency for 30 days at room temperature (25 °C) or under refrigeration (4).

Repackaging in Syringes— Sargramostim reconstituted with bacteriostatic water for injection preserved with benzyl alcohol 0.9% and repackaged into 1-ml tuberculin syringes remained sterile for 14 days under refrigeration (1764). However, because of the limited nature of the tests performed, the results may apply to a single institution only. Other institutions that repackage sargramostim injection need to establish specific testing results for their own sterile facilities, equipment, procedures, and personnel (1765).

Sorption— Sargramostim will adsorb to containers and tubing if the concentration is below 10 μg/ml. Albumin 0.1% should be added to the intravenous solution to prevent this adsorption (2).

Filtration— Sargramostim should not be infused through an inline filter because of possible absorption (2; 4).

Compatibility Information

Y-Site Injection Compatibility (1:1 Mixture)

Sargramostim

Drug	Mfr	Conc	Mfr	Conc	Remarks	Ref	C/I
Acyclovir sodium	BW	7 mg/ml[b]	IMM	10 μg/ml[b]	Few small white particles in 4 hr	1436	**I**
Amikacin sulfate	BR	5 mg/ml[b]	IMM	10 μg/ml[b]	Physically compatible for 4 hr at 22 °C	1436	**C**
Aminophylline	ES	2.5 mg/ml[b]	IMM	10 μg/ml[b]	Physically compatible for 4 hr at 22 °C	1436	**C**

Y-Site Injection Compatibility (1:1 Mixture) (Cont.)

Sargramostim

Drug	Mfr	Conc	Mfr	Conc	Remarks	Ref	C/I
Amphotericin B	SQ	0.6 mg/ml[a]	IMM	10 μg/ml[b]	Moderately heavy yellow precipitate forms immediately	1436	I
	SQ	0.6 mg/ml[a]	IMM	10 μg/ml[a]	Physically compatible for 4 hr at 22 °C	1436	C
Ampicillin sodium	BR	20 mg/ml[b]	IMM	10 μg/ml[b]	Few small particles in 4 hr	1436	I
Ampicillin sodium–sulbactam sodium	RR	20 + 10 mg/ml[b]	IMM	10 μg/ml[b]	Few small particles in 4 hr in one of two samples	1436	I
Amsacrine	NCI	1 mg/ml[a]	IMM	10 μg/ml[b]	Immediate haze with heavy yellow flocculent precipitate in 30 min	1436	I
	NCI	1 mg/ml[a]	IMM	10 μg/ml[a]	Physically compatible for 4 hr at 22 °C	1436	C
Aztreonam	SQ	40 mg/ml[b]	IMM	10 μg/ml[b]	Physically compatible for 4 hr at 22 °C	1436	C
	SQ	40 mg/ml[a]	IMM	10 μg/ml[b]	Physically compatible with no subvisual haze or particle formation in 4 hr at 23 °C	1758	C
Bleomycin sulfate	MJ	1 unit/ml[b]	IMM	10 μg/ml[b]	Physically compatible for 4 hr at 22 °C	1436	C
Butorphanol tartrate	BR	0.04 mg/ml[b]	IMM	10 μg/ml[b]	Physically compatible for 4 hr at 22 °C	1436	C
Calcium gluconate	AMR	40 mg/ml[b]	IMM	10 μg/ml[b]	Physically compatible for 4 hr at 22 °C	1436	C
Carboplatin	BR	5 mg/ml[b]	IMM	10 μg/ml[b]	Physically compatible for 4 hr at 22 °C	1436	C
Carmustine	BR	1.5 mg/ml[b]	IMM	10 μg/ml[b]	Physically compatible for 4 hr at 22 °C	1436	C
Cefazolin sodium	LEM	20 mg/ml[b]	IMM	10 μg/ml[b]	Physically compatible for 4 hr at 22 °C	1436	C
Cefepime HCl	BR	20 mg/ml[a]	IMM	10 μg/ml[b]	Physically compatible with no change in measured turbidity or increase in particle content in 4 hr at 22 °C	1689	C
Cefoperazone sodium	RR	40 mg/ml[b]	IMM	10 μg/ml[b]	Slight haze, visible with high intensity light, forms immediately	1436	I
Cefotaxime sodium	HO	20 mg/ml[b]	IMM	10 μg/ml[b]	Physically compatible for 4 hr at 22 °C	1436	C
Cefotetan disodium	STU	20 mg/ml[b]	IMM	10 μg/ml[b]	Physically compatible for 4 hr at 22 °C	1436	C
Ceftazidime	GL[c]	40 mg/ml[b]	IMM	10 μg/ml[b]	Particles and filaments form in 4 hr	1436	I
	LI[c]	40 mg/ml[d]	IMM	6[b,e] and 15[b] μg/ml	Visually compatible for 2 hr	1618	C
Ceftizoxime sodium	FUJ	20 mg/ml[b]	IMM	10 μg/ml[b]	Physically compatible for 4 hr at 22 °C	1436	C
Ceftriaxone sodium	RC	20 mg/ml[b]	IMM	10 μg/ml[b]	Physically compatible for 4 hr at 22 °C	1436	C
Cefuroxime sodium	GL	30 mg/ml[b]	IMM	10 μg/ml[b]	Physically compatible for 4 hr at 22 °C	1436	C
Chlorpromazine HCl	ES	2 mg/ml[b]	IMM	10 μg/ml[b]	Slight haze, visible with high intensity light, forms immediately	1436	I
Cimetidine HCl	SKF	12 mg/ml[b]	IMM	10 μg/ml[b]	Physically compatible for 4 hr at 22 °C	1436	C
Cisplatin	BR	1 mg/ml	IMM	10 μg/ml[b]	Physically compatible for 4 hr at 22 °C	1436	C
Clindamycin phosphate	LY	10 mg/ml[b]	IMM	10 μg/ml[b]	Physically compatible for 4 hr at 22 °C	1436	C
Cyclophosphamide	MJ	10 mg/ml[b]	IMM	10 μg/ml[b]	Physically compatible for 4 hr at 22 °C	1436	C
Cyclosporine	SZ	5 mg/ml[b]	IMM	6[b,e] and 15[b] μg/ml	Visually compatible for 2 hr	1618	C
Cytarabine	SCN	50 mg/ml	IMM	10 μg/ml[b]	Physically compatible for 4 hr at 22 °C	1436	C
Dacarbazine	MI	4 mg/ml[b]	IMM	10 μg/ml[b]	Physically compatible for 4 hr at 22 °C	1436	C
Dactinomycin	MSD	0.01 mg/ml[b]	IMM	10 μg/ml[b]	Physically compatible for 4 hr at 22 °C	1436	C

Y-Site Injection Compatibility (1:1 Mixture) (Cont.)

Sargramostim

Drug	Mfr	Conc	Mfr	Conc	Remarks	Ref	C/I
Dexamethasone sodium phosphate	ES	1 mg/ml[b]	IMM	10 µg/ml[b]	Physically compatible for 4 hr at 22 °C	1436	C
Diphenhydramine HCl	RU	1 mg/ml[b]	IMM	10 µg/ml[b]	Physically compatible for 4 hr at 22 °C	1436	C
Dopamine HCl	DU	1.6 mg/ml[d]	IMM	6[b,e] and 15[b] µg/ml	Visually compatible for 2 hr	1618	C
Doxorubicin HCl	CET	2 mg/ml	IMM	10 µg/ml[b]	Physically compatible for 4 hr at 22 °C	1436	C
Doxycycline hyclate	LY	1 mg/ml[b]	IMM	10 µg/ml[b]	Physically compatible for 4 hr at 22 °C	1436	C
Droperidol	DU	0.4 mg/ml[b]	IMM	10 µg/ml[b]	Physically compatible for 4 hr at 22 °C	1436	C
Etoposide	BR	0.4 mg/ml[b]	IMM	10 µg/ml[b]	Physically compatible for 4 hr at 22 °C	1436	C
Famotidine	MSD	2 mg/ml	IMM	10 µg/ml[b]	Physically compatible for 4 hr at 22 °C	1436	C
Fentanyl citrate	ES	50 µg/ml	IMM	6[b,e] and 15[b] µg/ml	Visually compatible for 2 hr	1618	C
Floxuridine	RC	3 mg/ml[b]	IMM	10 µg/ml[b]	Physically compatible for 4 hr at 22 °C	1436	C
Fluconazole	PF	2 mg/ml	IMM	10 µg/ml[b]	Physically compatible for 4 hr at 22 °C	1436	C
Fluorouracil	SO	16 mg/ml	IMM	10 µg/ml[b]	Physically compatible for 4 hr at 22 °C	1436	C
Furosemide	AB	3 mg/ml[b]	IMM	10 µg/ml[b]	Physically compatible for 4 hr at 22 °C	1436	C
Ganciclovir sodium	SY	20 mg/ml[b]	IMM	10 µg/ml[b]	Very small amount of particles formed in 4 hr in one of two samples	1436	I
Gentamicin sulfate	SO	5 mg/ml[b]	IMM	10 µg/ml[b]	Physically compatible for 4 hr at 22 °C	1436	C
Granisetron HCl	SKB	0.05 mg/ml[a]	IMM	10 µg/ml[b]	Physically compatible with no change in measured turbidity or increase in particle content in 4 hr at 23 °C	2000	C
Haloperidol lactate	LY	0.2 mg/ml[b]	IMM	10 µg/ml[b]	Small particles formed in 4 hr in one of two samples	1436	I
Heparin sodium	WY	100 units/ml[b]	IMM	10 µg/ml[b]	Physically compatible for 4 hr at 22 °C	1436	C
	ES	100 units/ml[d]	IMM	6[b,e] and 15[b] µg/ml	Visually compatible for 2 hr	1618	C
Hydrocortisone sodium phosphate	MSD	1 mg/ml[b]	IMM	10 µg/ml[b]	Filament formed in 4 hr in one of two samples	1436	I
Hydrocortisone sodium succinate	UP	1 mg/ml[b]	IMM	10 µg/ml[b]	Few small particles in 1 hr	1436	I
Hydromorphone HCl	WI	0.5 mg/ml[b]	IMM	10 µg/ml[b]	Few small particles in 30 min	1436	I
Hydroxyzine HCl	ES	4 mg/ml[b]	IMM	10 µg/ml[b]	Slight haze, visible with high intensity light, and small flake-like particles formed in 4 hr in one of two samples	1436	I
Idarubicin HCl	AD	0.5 mg/ml[b]	IMM	10 µg/ml[b]	Increase in measured turbidity no greater than dilution of idarubicin with sodium chloride 0.9%	1675	C
Ifosfamide	MJ	25 mg/ml[b]	IMM	10 µg/ml[b]	Physically compatible for 4 hr at 22 °C	1436	C
Imipenem–cilastatin sodium	MSD	5 mg/ml[b]	IMM	10 µg/ml[b]	Large particle and fibrous clump form in 4 hr	1436	I
Immune globulin intravenous	CU	50 mg/ml	IMM	6[b,e] and 15[b] µg/ml	Visually compatible for 2 hr	1618	C
Lorazepam	WY	0.1 mg/ml[b]	IMM	10 µg/ml[b]	Slightly bluish haze, visible with high intensity light, forms in 1 hr	1436	I

Y-Site Injection Compatibility (1:1 Mixture) (Cont.)

Sargramostim

Drug	Mfr	Conc	Mfr	Conc	Remarks	Ref	C/I
Magnesium sulfate	LY	100 mg/ml[b]	IMM	10 μg/ml[b]	Physically compatible for 4 hr at 22 °C	1436	C
Mannitol	BA	15%	IMM	10 μg/ml[b]	Physically compatible for 4 hr at 22 °C	1436	C
Mechlorethamine HCl	MSD	1 mg/ml	IMM	10 μg/ml[b]	Physically compatible for 4 hr at 22 °C	1436	C
Meperidine HCl	WI	4 mg/ml[b]	IMM	10 μg/ml[b]	Physically compatible for 4 hr at 22 °C	1436	C
Mesna	MJ	10 mg/ml[b]	IMM	10 μg/ml[b]	Physically compatible for 4 hr at 22 °C	1436	C
Methotrexate sodium	CET	15 mg/ml[b]	IMM	10 μg/ml[b]	Physically compatible for 4 hr at 22 °C	1436	C
Methylprednisolone sodium succinate	UP	5 mg/ml[b]	IMM	10 μg/ml[b]	Small amounts of particles and filaments form in 4 hr	1436	I
Metoclopramide HCl	DU	5 mg/ml[b]	IMM	10 μg/ml[b]	Physically compatible for 4 hr at 22 °C	1436	C
Metronidazole	MG	5 mg/ml	IMM	10 μg/ml[b]	Physically compatible for 4 hr at 22 °C	1436	C
Minocycline HCl	LE	0.2 mg/ml[b]	IMM	10 μg/ml[b]	Physically compatible for 4 hr at 22 °C	1436	C
Mitomycin	BR	0.5 mg/ml	IMM	10 μg/ml[b]	Slight haze, visible with high intensity light, forms in 30 min	1436	I
Mitoxantrone HCl	LE	0.5 mg/ml[b]	IMM	10 μg/ml[b]	Physically compatible for 4 hr at 22 °C	1436	C
Morphine sulfate	WI	1 mg/ml[b]	IMM	10 μg/ml[b]	Slight haze, visible with high intensity light, and small amount of particles formed in 1 hr in one of two samples	1436	I
Nalbuphine HCl	DU	10 mg/ml[b]	IMM	10 μg/ml[b]	Slight haze, visible with high intensity light, forms in 30 min. Filament formed in 4 hr in one of two samples	1436	I
Netilmicin sulfate	SC	5 mg/ml[b]	IMM	10 μg/ml[b]	Physically compatible for 4 hr at 22 °C	1436	C
Ondansetron HCl	GL	0.5 mg/ml[b]	IMM	10 μg/ml[b]	Filaments form in 30 to 60 min	1436	I
Pentostatin	NCI	0.4 mg/ml[b]	IMM	10 μg/ml[b]	Physically compatible for 4 hr at 22 °C	1436	C
Piperacillin sodium	LE	40 mg/ml[b]	IMM	10 μg/ml[b]	Small amount of particles forms in 4 hr	1436	I
Piperacillin sodium–tazobactam sodium	LE	40 + 5 mg/ml[a]	HO	10 μg/ml[a]	Physically compatible with no change in measured turbidity or increase in particle content in 4 hr at 22 °C	1688	C
Potassium chloride	AB	0.1 mEq/ml[b]	IMM	10 μg/ml[b]	Physically compatible for 4 hr at 22 °C	1436	C
Prochlorperazine edisylate	ES	0.5 mg/ml[b]	IMM	10 μg/ml[b]	Physically compatible for 4 hr at 22 °C	1436	C
Promethazine HCl	ES	2 mg/ml[b]	IMM	10 μg/ml[b]	Physically compatible for 4 hr at 22 °C	1436	C
Ranitidine HCl	GL	2 mg/ml[b]	IMM	10 μg/ml[b]	Physically compatible for 4 hr at 22 °C	1436	C
Sodium bicarbonate	LY	1 mEq/ml	IMM	10 μg/ml[b]	Small amount of particles forms in 4 hr	1436	I
Teniposide	BR	0.1 mg/ml[b]	IMM	10 μg/ml[b]	Physically compatible for 4 hr at 22 °C	1436	C
Ticarcillin disodium	BE	30 mg/ml[b]	IMM	10 μg/ml[b]	Physically compatible for 4 hr at 22 °C	1436	C
Ticarcillin disodium–clavulanate potassium	BE	31 mg/ml[b]	IMM	10 μg/ml[b]	Physically compatible for 4 hr at 22 °C	1436	C
Tobramycin sulfate	LI	5 mg/ml[b]	IMM	10 μg/ml[b]	Particles and filaments form in 4 hr	1436	I
TPN #133[f]			IMM	10 μg/ml[b]	Physically compatible for 4 hr at 22 °C	1436	C
TPN #181[f]			IMM	6[b,e] and 15[b] μg/ml	Visually compatible for 2 hr	1618	C
Trimethoprim–sulfamethoxazole	ES	0.8 + 4 mg/ml[b]	IMM	10 μg/ml[b]	Physically compatible for 4 hr at 22 °C	1436	C
Vancomycin HCl	LI	10 mg/ml[b]	IMM	10 μg/ml[b]	Physically compatible for 4 hr at 22 °C	1436	C

Y-Site Injection Compatibility (1:1 Mixture) (Cont.)

					Sargramostim		
Drug	*Mfr*	*Conc*	*Mfr*	*Conc*	*Remarks*	*Ref*	*C/I*
	LI	20 mg/ml[d]	IMM	15 μg/ml[b]	Visually compatible for 2 hr	1618	**C**
	LI	20 mg/ml[d]	IMM	6 μg/ml[b,e]	Haze forms within 15 min and increases due to vancomycin incompatibility with albumin	1618; 1701	**I**
Vinblastine sulfate	LY	0.12 mg/ml[b]	IMM	10 μg/ml[b]	Physically compatible for 4 hr at 22 °C	1436	**C**
Vincristine sulfate	LY	0.05 mg/ml[b]	IMM	10 μg/ml[b]	Physically compatible for 4 hr at 22 °C	1436	**C**
Zidovudine	BW	4 mg/ml[b]	IMM	10 μg/ml[b]	Physically compatible for 4 hr at 22 °C	1436	**C**

[a]Tested in dextrose 5% in water.
[b]Tested in sodium chloride 0.9%.
[c]Sodium carbonate-containing formulation tested.
[d]Tested in both dextrose 5% in water and sodium chloride 0.9%.
[e]Tested with 0.1% albumin (human) added.
[f]Refer to Appendix I for the composition of parenteral nutrition solutions. TPN indicates a 2-in-1 admixture.

Additional Compatibility Information

The manufacturer recommends that no other medication be added to sargramostim infusions in the absence of compatibility and stability information (2).

Solutions— The manufacturer recommends that only sodium chloride 0.9% be used for dilution of sargramostim for infusion (2). When diluted for infusion, sargramostim is stable for 48 hours at room temperature or under refrigeration (4). The manufacturer recommends use within six hours due to microbiological concerns (2; 4).

Sargramostim concentrations below 10 μg/ml require normal human serum albumin 0.1% to prevent adsorption. This albumin concentration may be obtained by adding 1 mg of albumin per 1 ml of solution. For example, 1 ml of normal human serum albumin 5% is added to 50 ml of sodium chloride 0.9% (2).

Other Information

Specific Activity— The specific activity is approximately 5.6×10^6 units per milligram (2).

SCOPOLAMINE HYDROBROMIDE (HYOSCINE HYDROBROMIDE) AHFS 12:08.08

Fujisawa

Products— Scopolamine hydrobromide (Fujisawa) is available in 1-ml multiple-dose vials containing 0.4- and 1-mg/ml concentrations. Also present in the products are methylparaben 0.18% and propylparaben 0.02%. Hydrobromic acid may have been used to adjust the pH (1-10/96; 4).

pH— From 3.5 to 6.5 (4).

Osmolality— The osmolality of scopolamine hydrobromide 0.5 mg/ml was determined to be 303 mOsm/kg (1233).

Administration— Scopolamine hydrobromide may be administered subcutaneously, intramuscularly, or intravenously by direct intravenous injection after dilution with sterile water for injection (4).

Stability— The product should be stored at controlled room temperature and protected from light (1-10/96). Scopolamine hydrobromide decomposition is primarily due to hydrolysis below pH 3 and to both hydrolysis and inversion about the chiral carbon above pH 3. The minimum rate of decomposition occurs at pH 3.5 (1071).

Compatibility Information

Additive Compatibility

			Scopolamine HBr					
Drug	*Mfr*	*Conc/L*	*Mfr*	*Conc/L*	*Test Soln*	*Remarks*	*Ref*	*C/I*
Floxacillin sodium	BE	20 g	BI	2 g[a]	W	Physically compatible for 24 hr at 15 and 30 °C. Precipitate forms in 48 hr at 30 °C. No change at 15 °C in 48 hr	1479	C
Furosemide	HO	1 g	BI	2 g[a]	W	Physically compatible for 72 hr at 15 and 30 °C	1479	C
Meperidine HCl	WI	100 mg		0.43 mg		Physically compatible	3	C
Succinylcholine chloride	AB	2 g		0.43 mg		Physically compatible	3	C

[a]*Present as the butylbromide salt.*

Drugs in Syringe Compatibility

			Scopolamine HBr				
Drug (in syringe)	*Mfr*	*Amt*	*Mfr*	*Amt*	*Remarks*	*Ref*	*C/I*
Atropine sulfate	ST	0.4 mg/ 1 ml	ST	0.4 mg/ 1 ml	Physically compatible for at least 15 min	326	C
Butorphanol tartrate	BR	4 mg/ 2 ml	ST	0.4 mg/ 1 ml	Physically compatible both macroscopically and microscopically for 30 min at room temperature	566	C
Chlorpromazine HCl	SKF	50 mg/ 2 ml		0.6 mg/ 1.5 ml	Physically compatible for at least 15 min	14	C
	PO	50 mg/ 2 ml	ST	0.4 mg/ 1 ml	Physically compatible for at least 15 min	326	C
Cimetidine HCl	SKF	300 mg/ 2 ml	BW	0.43 mg/ 0.5 ml	Physically compatible for 4 hr at 25 °C	25	C
Diamorphine HCl	MB	10, 25, 50 mg/ 1 ml	EV	60 μg/ 1 ml[a]	Physically compatible and diamorphine potency retained for 24 hr at room temperature	1454	C
	EV	50 and 150 mg/ 1 ml	EV	0.4 mg/ 1 ml	Physically compatible with 7% diamorphine loss in 7 days at room temperature	1455	C
	EV	50 and 150 mg/ 1 ml	BI	20 mg/ 1 ml[b]	Physically compatible with no scopolamine loss and 4% diamorphine loss in 7 days at room temperature	1455	C
Dimenhydrinate	HR	50 mg/ 1 ml	ST	0.4 mg/ 1 ml	Physically compatible for at least 15 min	326	C
Diphenhydramine HCl	PD	50 mg/ 1 ml	ST	0.4 mg/ 1 ml	Physically compatible for at least 15 min	326	C
Droperidol	MN	2.5 mg/ 1 ml	ST	0.4 mg/ 1 ml	Physically compatible for at least 15 min	326	C
Fentanyl citrate	MN	100 μg/ 1 ml		0.6 mg/ 1.5 ml	Physically compatible for at least 15 min	14	C
	MN	0.05 mg/ 1 ml	ST	0.4 mg/ 1 ml	Physically compatible for at least 15 min	326	C
Glycopyrrolate	RB	0.2 mg/ 1 ml	ES	0.4 mg/ 1 ml	Physically compatible and pH in stability range for glycopyrrolate for 48 hr at 25 °C	331	C
	RB	0.2 mg/ 1 ml	ES	0.8 mg/ 2 ml	Physically compatible and pH in stability range for glycopyrrolate for 48 hr at 25 °C	331	C

Drugs in Syringe Compatibility (Cont.)

Scopolamine HBr

Drug (in syringe)	Mfr	Amt	Mfr	Amt	Remarks	Ref	C/I
	RB	0.4 mg/ 2 ml	ES	0.4 mg/ 1 ml	Physically compatible and pH in stability range for glycopyrrolate for 48 hr at 25 °C	331	C
Hydromorphone HCl	KN	4 mg/ 2 ml	BW	0.43 mg/ 0.5 ml	Physically compatible for 30 min	517	C
Hydroxyzine HCl	PF	100 mg/ 4 ml		0.6 mg/ 1.5 ml	Physically compatible for at least 15 min	14	C
	PF	50 mg/ 1 ml	ST	0.4 mg/ 1 ml	Physically compatible for at least 15 min	326	C
	PF	100 mg/ 2 ml		0.65 mg/ 1 ml	Physically compatible	771	C
	PF	50 mg/ 1 ml		0.65 mg/ 1 ml	Physically compatible	771	C
Meperidine HCl	WY	100 mg/ 1 ml		0.6 mg/ 1.5 ml	Physically compatible for at least 15 min	14	C
	WI	50 mg/ 1 ml	ST	0.4 mg/ 1 ml	Physically compatible for at least 15 min	326	C
Metoclopramide HCl	NO	10 mg/ 2 ml	ST	0.4 mg/ 1 ml	Physically compatible both macroscopically and microscopically for 15 min at room temperature	565	C
Midazolam HCl	RC	5 mg/ 1 ml	BW	0.43 mg/ 0.5 ml	Physically compatible for 4 hr at 25 °C under fluorescent light	1145	C
Morphine HCl	BP	500 mg/ 5 ml	BP	5 mg/ 5 ml	Little or no scopolamine loss by HPLC in 14 days at room temperature or 37 °C. Morphine not tested	1609	C
Morphine sulfate	WY	15 mg/ 1 ml		0.6 mg/ 1.5 ml	Physically compatible for at least 15 min	14	C
	ST	15 mg/ 1 ml	ST	0.4 mg/ 1 ml	Physically compatible for at least 15 min	326	C
	BP	500 mg/ 5 ml	BP	5 mg/ 5 ml	Little or no scopolamine loss by HPLC in 14 days at room temperature or 37 °C. Morphine not tested	1609	C
Nalbuphine HCl	EN	10 mg/ 1 ml	BW	0.86 mg/ 1 ml	Physically compatible for 36 hr at 27 °C	762	C
	EN	5 mg/ 0.5 ml	BW	0.86 mg/ 1 ml	Physically compatible for 36 hr at 27 °C	762	C
	EN	10 mg/ 1 ml	BW	0.43 mg/ 0.5 ml	Physically compatible for 36 hr at 27 °C	762	C
	DU	10 mg/ 1 ml		0.4 mg	Physically compatible for 48 hr	128	C
	DU	20 mg/ 1 ml		0.4 mg	Physically compatible for 48 hr	128	C
Pentazocine lactate	WI	30 mg/ 1 ml		0.6 mg/ 1.5 ml	Physically compatible for at least 15 min	14	C
	WI	30 mg/ 1 ml	ST	0.4 mg/ 1 ml	Physically compatible for at least 15 min	326	C
Pentobarbital sodium	AB	500 mg/ 10 ml		0.13 mg/ 0.26 ml	Physically compatible	55	C
	WY	100 mg/ 2 ml		0.6 mg/ 1.5 ml	Physically compatible for at least 15 min	14	C
	AB	50 mg/ 1 ml	ST	0.4 mg/ 1 ml	Physically compatible for at least 15 min	326	C

Drugs in Syringe Compatibility (Cont.)

Scopolamine HBr

Drug (in syringe)	Mfr	Amt	Mfr	Amt	Remarks	Ref	C/I
Perphenazine	SC	5 mg/ 1 ml	ST	0.4 mg/ 1 ml	Physically compatible both macroscopically and microscopically for 30 min at room temperature	566	C
Prochlorperazine edisylate	SKF			0.6 mg/ 1.5 ml	Physically compatible for at least 15 min	14	C
	PO	5 mg/ 1 ml	ST	0.4 mg/ 1 ml	Physically compatible for at least 15 min	326	C
Promazine HCl	WY	50 mg/ 1 ml	ST	0.4 mg/ 1 ml	Physically compatible for at least 15 min	326	C
Promethazine HCl	WY	50 mg/ 2 ml		0.6 mg/ 1.5 ml	Physically compatible for at least 15 min	14	C
	PO	50 mg/ 2 ml	ST	0.4 mg/ 1 ml	Physically compatible for at least 15 min	326	C
Ranitidine HCl	GL	50 mg/ 2 ml	AB	0.4 mg/ 1 ml	Physically compatible for 1 hr at 25 °C both macroscopically and microscopically	978	C
	GL	50 mg/ 5 ml		0.5 mg	Physically compatible for 4 hr at ambient temperature under fluorescent light	1151	C
Sufentanil citrate	JN	50 μg/ml	LY	0.43 mg/ ml	Physically compatible with no subvisual haze or particle formation in 24 hr at 23 °C	1711	C
Thiopental sodium	AB	75 mg/ 3 ml		0.13 mg/ 0.26 ml	Physically compatible for at least 30 min	21	C
	AB	75 mg/ 3 ml		0.13 mg/ 0.26 ml	Physically compatible	55	C

[a]*Diluted with sterile water for injection.*
[b]*Present as the butylbromide salt.*

Y-Site Injection Compatibility (1:1 Mixture)

Scopolamine HBr

Drug	Mfr	Conc	Mfr	Conc	Remarks	Ref	C/I
Heparin sodium	UP	1000 units/L[a]	BW	0.86 mg/ml	Physically compatible for at least 4 hr at room temperature by visual and microscopic examination	534	C
Hydrocortisone sodium succinate	UP	10 mg/L[a]	BW	0.86 mg/ml	Physically compatible for at least 4 hr at room temperature by visual and microscopic examination	534	C
Potassium chloride	AB	40 mEq/L[a]	BW	0.86 mg/ml	Physically compatible for at least 4 hr at room temperature by visual and microscopic examination	534	C
Propofol	ZEN	10 mg/ml	LY	0.4 mg/ml	Physically compatible for 1 hr at 23 °C with no increase in particle content	2066	C
Sufentanil citrate	JN	12.5 μg/ml[b]	LY	0.05 mg/ml[b]	Physically compatible with no subvisual haze or particle formation in 24 hr at 23 °C	1711	C
Vitamin B complex with C	RC	2 ml/L[a]	BW	0.86 mg/ml	Physically compatible for at least 4 hr at room temperature by visual and microscopic examination	534	C

[a]*Tested in dextrose 5% in Ringer's injection, dextrose 5% in Ringer's injection, lactated, dextrose 5% in water, Ringer's injection, lactated, and sodium chloride 0.9%.*
[b]*Tested in dextrose 5% in water.*

Additional Compatibility Information

Scopolamine hydrobromide is stated to be physically and chemically compatible with buprenorphine HCl (4) and diamorphine HCl (1442).

Scopolamine hydrobromide is stated to be incompatible with alkalies (4). A haze forms in one hour when scopolamine hydrobromide is mixed with methohexital sodium (4).

A mixture of promethazine HCl (Wyeth) 50 mg/2 ml, meperidine HCl (Wyeth) 100 mg/1 ml, and scopolamine hydrobromide 0.6 mg/1.5 ml has been reported to be conditionally compatible when packaged in syringes. The mixture is physically compatible when the order of mixing is as stated above (14).

SODIUM ACETATE
AHFS 40:08

American Regent

Products— Sodium acetate is available as a 16.4% solution in 20-, 50-, and 100-ml vials. Each milliliter of solution contains 2 mEq of sodium acetate in water for injection. Sodium acetate is also available as a 32.8% solution in 50- and 100-ml vials. Each milliliter of solution contains 4 mEq of sodium acetate in water for injection (154). The pH may have been adjusted with acetic acid (1-11/95).

pH— From 6 to 7 (1-11/95).

Osmolarity— Sodium acetate injection has a calculated osmolarity of 4 mOsm/ml (1-11/95).

Administration— Sodium acetate is administered by slow intravenous infusion after addition to a larger volume of fluid. It must not be given undiluted (1-11/95).

Stability— The product should be stored at controlled room temperature and protected from freezing and excessive heat. Discarding the vials four hours after initial entry has been recommended (1-11/95).

Compatibility Information

Drugs in Syringe Compatibility

Sodium acetate

Drug (in syringe)	Mfr	Amt	Mfr	Amt	Remarks	Ref	C/I
Cimetidine HCl	SKF	300 mg/ 2 ml		10 mEq/ 5 ml	Physically compatible for 48 hr at room temperature	516	C

Y-Site Injection Compatibility (1:1 Mixture)

Sodium acetate

Drug	Mfr	Conc	Mfr	Conc	Remarks	Ref	C/I
Enalaprilat	MSD	0.05 mg/ml[a]	LY	0.4 mEq/ml[b]	Physically compatible for 24 hr at room temperature under fluorescent light	1355	C
Esmolol HCl	DCC	10 mg/ml[b]	LY	0.4 mEq/ml[b]	Physically compatible for 24 hr at 22 °C	1169	C
Labetalol HCl	SC	1 mg/ml[b]	LY	0.4 mEq/ml[b]	Physically compatible for 24 hr at 18 °C	1171	C
Ondansetron HCl	GL	0.1 mg/ml[b]		0.1 and 1 mEq/ml[b]	Visually compatible with no increase in 10-, 25-, and 50-μm particles in 4 hr at room temperature	1661	C

[a]*Tested in sodium chloride 0.9%.*
[b]*Tested in dextrose 5% in water.*

SODIUM BICARBONATE
AHFS 40:08

Products— Sodium bicarbonate injections are available from various manufacturers in vials, ampuls, bottles, and disposable syringes as aqueous solutions in concentrations ranging from 4.2% to 8.4% (1-7/98; 4; 29).

Concentration	Bicarbonate (and Sodium) Concentration	Total Container Content	Osmolarity
8.4%	1 mEq/ml	10 mEq/10 ml	2000 mOsm/L
		50 mEq/50 ml	
7.5%	0.892 mEq/ml	44.6 mEq/50 ml	1790 mOsm/L
5.0%	0.595 mEq/ml	297.5 mEq/500 ml	1200 mOsm/L
4.2%	0.5 mEq/ml	5 mEq/10 ml	1000 mOsm/L

The osmolality of sodium bicarbonate (Invenex) 1 mEq/ml was determined to be 1555 mOsm/kg by freezing-point depression and 1538 mOsm/kg by vapor pressure (1071).

The osmolalities of sodium bicarbonate solutions were determined to be 815, 1095, and 1815 mOsm/kg for concentrations of 4.2, 6, and 8.4%, respectively (1233).

Sodium bicarbonate injection is available in a 5% concentration as a large volume parenteral in 500-ml bottles. The solution provides 0.6 mEq/ml or 297.5 mEq/500 ml of bicarbonate and sodium and also contains 0.9 mg/ml of edetate disodium. It has an osmolarity of about 1190 to 1203 mOsm/L (4; 29).

Sodium bicarbonate 4% neutralizing additive solution (Neut, Abbott) is available in 10-ml vials. Each milliliter of solution provides 0.48 mEq of bicarbonate and sodium. Sodium bicarbonate 4.2% neutralizing additive solution (American Pharmaceutical Partners) is available in 5-ml vials. Each milliliter of solution provides 0.5 mEq of bicarbonate and sodium (1-9/98; 4; 29). The sodium bicarbonate-neutralizing additive solutions are used to raise the pH of acidic solutions.

pH— From 7 to 8.5 (4).

Equivalency— Each 84 mg of sodium bicarbonate provides 1 mEq of sodium and bicarbonate ions. Each gram of sodium bicarbonate provides about 12 mEq of sodium and bicarbonate ions (4).

Administration— Sodium bicarbonate is administered intravenously, either undiluted or diluted in other fluids. It may also be given subcutaneously if diluted to isotonicity (1.5%) (4).

Stability— Sodium bicarbonate injection should be stored at controlled room temperature and protected from freezing and excessive temperatures of 40 °C or above. Do not use a solution that is unclear or that contains a precipitate (4).

Combining sodium bicarbonate with acids in aqueous solutions results in the liberation of carbon dioxide gas. The bubbles can be evolved in sufficient quantity to cause effervescence (4).

The stability of sodium bicarbonate 7.5% in polypropylene syringes is inversely related to the storage temperature (136). Estimates of room temperature stability range from one week (137) to one month (136). Refrigeration may increase the stability to 60 (137) to 90 days (136). Stability may also be increased by refrigerating the sodium bicarbonate injection and the syringes before preparation, rinsing the syringes twice with refrigerated sterile water for injection, minimizing the contact of the solution with the air by expelling the air from the syringes, and taping the plunger in place to minimize its movement from escaping carbon dioxide (137).

Compatibility Information

Solution Compatibility

Sodium bicarbonate

Solution	Mfr	Mfr	Conc/L	Remarks	Ref	C/I
Alcohol 5%, dextrose 5%	AB		3.75 g	Color change	3	**I**
Dextran 6% in dextrose 5%	AB		3.75 g	Physically compatible	3	**C**
Dextran 6% in sodium chloride 0.9%	AB		3.75 g	Physically compatible	3	**C**
Dextrose–Ringer's injection combinations	AB		3.75 g	Physically compatible	3	**C**
Dextrose–Ringer's injection, lactated, combinations	AB		3.75 g	Physically compatible	3	**C**
Dextrose 5% in Ringer's injection, lactated	AB	AB	80 mEq	Physically incompatible	15	**I**
Dextrose–saline combinations	AB		3.75 g	Physically compatible	3	**C**
Dextrose 5% in sodium chloride 0.9%	TR[a]	AB	4 g	Potency retained for 24 hr at 5 °C	282	**C**
Dextrose 2½% in water	AB		3.75 g	Physically compatible	3	**C**
Dextrose 5% in water	AB		3.75 g	Physically compatible	3	**C**
	TR[a]	AB	4 g	Potency retained for 24 hr at 5 °C	282	**C**
Dextrose 10% in water	AB		3.75 g	Physically compatible	3	**C**
Fat emulsion 10%, intravenous	VT	BR	7.5 g	Physically compatible for 48 hr at 4 °C and room temperature	32	**C**

Solution Compatibility (Cont.)

Sodium bicarbonate

Solution	Mfr	Mfr	Conc/L	Remarks	Ref	C/I
	VT		3.4 g	Microscopic globule coalescence in 24 hr at 8 and 25 °C	825	I
Fructose 10% in sodium chloride 0.9%	AB		3.75 g	Physically compatible	3	C
Fructose 10% in water	AB		3.75 g	Physically compatible	3	C
Invert sugar 5 and 10% in sodium chloride 0.9%	AB		3.75 g	Physically compatible	3	C
Invert sugar 5 and 10% in water	AB		3.75 g	Physically compatible	3	C
Ionosol products (except as noted below)	AB		3.75 g	Physically compatible	3	C
Ionosol B with invert sugar 10%	AB		3.75 g	Color change	3	I
Ionosol D with invert sugar 10%	AB		3.75 g	Color change	3	I
Ionosol D modified with invert sugar 10%	AB		3.75 g	Color change	3	I
Ionosol G with invert sugar 10%	AB		3.75 g	Color change	3	I
Ringer's injection	AB		3.75 g	Physically compatible	3	C
				Physically incompatible	9	I
Ringer's injection, lactated	AB		3.75 g	Physically compatible	3	C
				Physically incompatible	9	I
	AB	AB	80 mEq	Physically incompatible	15	I
Sodium chloride 0.45%	AB		3.75 g	Physically compatible	3	C
Sodium chloride 0.9%	AB		3.75 g	Physically compatible	3	C
	TR[a]	AB	4 g	Potency retained for 24 hr at 5 °C	282	C
Sodium lactate ⅙ M	AB		3.75 g	Physically compatible	3	C
				Physically incompatible	9	I
TNA #66 to #68[b]			50 and 150 mEq	Physically compatible with 10% or less carbon dioxide loss and unchanged pH in 7 days at 25 °C protected from light	1011	C
TPN #62 to #65[b]			50 and 150 mEq	Physically compatible with 10% or less carbon dioxide loss and unchanged pH in 7 days at 25 °C protected from light	1011	C

[a]Tested in both glass and PVC containers.
[b]Refer to Appendix I for the composition of parenteral nutrition solutions. TNA indicates a 3-in-1 admixture, and TPN indicates a 2-in-1 admixture.

Additive Compatibility

Sodium bicarbonate

Drug	Mfr	Conc/L	Mfr	Conc/L	Test Soln	Remarks	Ref	C/I
Amikacin sulfate	BR	5 g	BR	15 g	D5LR, D5R, D5S, D5W, D10W, IS10, LR, NS, R, SL	Physically compatible and potency of both drugs retained for 24 hr at 25 °C	294	C
Aminophylline	SE	1 g	AB	80 mEq	D5W	Physically compatible	15	C
	SE	500 mg	AB	40 mEq		Physically compatible	6	C
		500 mg	AB	2.4 mEq[a]	D5W	Physically compatible for 24 hr	772	C
Amobarbital sodium	LI	500 mg	AB	2.4 mEq[a]	D5W	Physically compatible for 24 hr	772	C

Additive Compatibility (Cont.)

Sodium bicarbonate

Drug	Mfr	Conc/L	Mfr	Conc/L	Test Soln	Remarks	Ref	C/I
Amoxicillin sodium		10, 20, 50 g		2.74%		9% amoxicillin loss in 6 and 4 hr at 10 and 20 g/L, respectively, and 15% loss in 4 hr at 50 g/L at 25 °C	1469	I
		10, 20, 50 g		8.4%		10 and 13% amoxicillin loss in 4 hr at 10 and 20 g/L, respectively, and 17% loss in 3 hr at 50 g/L at 25 °C	1469	I
Amphotericin B	SQ	50 mg	AB	2.4 mEq[a]	D5W	Physically compatible for 24 hr	772	C
Ampicillin sodium	BR	500 mg	AB	2.4 mEq[a]	D5W	Physically compatible for 24 hr. Ampicillin instability is determining factor	772	?
Ascorbic acid injection	UP	500 mg	AB	80 mEq	D5W	Physically incompatible	15	I
Atropine sulfate		0.4 mg	AB	2.4 mEq[a]	D5W	Physically compatible for 24 hr	772	C
Bretylium tosylate	ACC	10 g	MG	5%		Physically compatible and chemically stable for 48 hr at room temperature and 7 days at 4 °C	541	C
Calcium chloride		1 g	AB	2.4 mEq[a]	D5W	Physically compatible for 24 hr	772	C
Carboplatin		7 g		200 mM		13% carboplatin loss in 24 hr at 27 °C	1379	I
Carmustine	BR	100 mg	AB	100 mEq	D5W, NS	10% carmustine decomposition in 15 min and 27% in 90 min	523	I
Cefoxitin sodium	MSD	1, 2, 10, 20 g	AB	200 mg/ g cefoxitin	W	5 to 6% cefoxitin decomposition in 24 hr and 11 to 12% in 48 hr at 25 °C. 2 to 3% decomposition in 7 days at 5 °C	308	C
Ceftazidime	GL[i]	20 g		4.2%		3% ceftazidime loss in 6 hr and 11% in 24 hr at 25 °C. 1% loss in 24 hr and 3% in 48 hr at 4 °C	1136	C
Chloramphenicol sodium succinate	PD PD	10 g 1 g	AB AB	80 mEq 80 mEq	D5W	Physically compatible Physically compatible	15 6	C C
Chlorothiazide sodium	MSD	500 mg	AB	2.4 mEq[a]	D5W	Physically compatible for 24 hr	772	C
Cimetidine HCl	SKF	1.2 and 5 g	TR	5%		Physically compatible and chemically stable for 1 week at room temperature	549	C
Cisplatin		50 and 500 mg		5%		Bright gold precipitate forms in 8 to 24 hr at 25 °C	635	I
Clindamycin phosphate	UP	1.2 g		44 mEq	D5S, D5W	Clindamycin stability maintained for 24 hr	101	C
Corticotropin	AR	250 units	AB	80 mEq	D5W	Physically incompatible	15	I
	AR	40 units	AB	2.4 mEq[a]	D5W	Physically compatible for 24 hr	772	C
Cytarabine	UP	200 mg and 1 g	AB	50 mEq	D5W[b]	Physically compatible with no cytarabine loss in 7 days at 8 and 22 °C	748	C
	UP	200 mg	AB	50 mEq	D5¼S[b]	Physically compatible with no cytarabine loss in 7 days at 8 and 22 °C	748	C
Dobutamine HCl	LI	1 g	MG	5%		Cloudy brownish solution with precipitate forms within 3 hr at 25 °C. 18% dobutamine loss with dense precipitate in 24 hr	789	I
	LI	1 g	IX	500 mEq	D5W, NS	White precipitate forms within 6 hr at 21 °C	812	I

Additive Compatibility (Cont.)

Sodium bicarbonate

Drug	Mfr	Conc/L	Mfr	Conc/L	Test Soln	Remarks	Ref	C/I
Dopamine HCl	AS	800 mg	MG	5%		Color change 5 min after mixing. Also second spot appeared on TLC	79	I
Epinephrine HCl		4 mg	AB	2.4 mEq[a] D5W		Epinephrine inactivated	772	I
Ergonovine maleate		0.2 mg	AB	2.4 mEq[a] D5W		Physically compatible for 24 hr	772	C
Erythromycin lactobionate	AB	1 g	AB	3.75 g		Physically compatible. Erythromycin potency retained for 24 hr at 25 °C	20	C
	AB	1 g	AB	2.4 mEq[a] D5W		Physically compatible for 24 hr	772	C
Esmolol HCl	ACC	10 g	MG[c]	5%		Visually compatible with 5 and 8% esmolol losses by HPLC in 7 days at 4 and 27 °C, respectively. 9 and 4% losses in 24 hr at 40 °C and under intense light, respectively	1831	C
Fentanyl citrate and droperidol (Innovar)	JN	0.05 + 2.5 mg	AB	2.4 mEq[a] D5W		Physically compatible for 24 hr	772	C
Floxacillin sodium	BE	20 g	IMS	8.4%		Physically compatible for 72 hr at 15 and 30 °C	1479	C
Furosemide	HO	1 g	IMS	8.4%		Physically compatible for 72 hr at 15 and 30 °C	1479	C
Heparin sodium	AB	20,000 units	AB	2.4 mEq[a] D5W		Physically compatible for 24 hr	772	C
Hyaluronidase	WY	150 units	AB	2.4 mEq[a] D5W		Physically compatible for 24 hr	772	C
Hydrocortisone sodium phosphate	MSD	100 mg	AB	2.4 mEq[a] D5W		Physically compatible for 24 hr	772	C
Hydrocortisone sodium succinate	UP	250 mg	AB	2.4 mEq[a] D5W		Physically compatible for 24 hr	772	C
Hydromorphone HCl						Physically incompatible	9	I
Imipenem–cilastatin sodium	MSD	2.5 g	AB	5%		43% imipenem loss in 3 hr at 25 °C and 52% in 24 hr at 4 °C	1141	I
	MSD	5 g	AB	5%		45% imipenem loss in 3 hr at 25 °C and 50% in 24 hr at 4 °C	1141	I
Isoproterenol HCl	BN	1 mg	AB	2.4 mEq[a] D5W		Isoproterenol inactivated	772	I
Kanamycin sulfate	BR	4 g	AB	80 mEq D5W		Physically compatible	15	C
Labetalol HCl	SC	1.25, 2.5, 3.75 g	TR	5%		White precipitate forms within 6 hr after mixing at 4 and 25 °C	757	I
Levorphanol bitartrate	RC					Physically incompatible	9	I
Lidocaine HCl	AST	2 g	AB	40 mEq		Physically compatible	24	C
		1 g	AB	2.4 mEq[a] D5W		Physically compatible for 24 hr	772	C
Magnesium sulfate						Physically incompatible	9	I
	LI	16 mEq	AB	80 mEq D5W		Physically incompatible	15	I
Mannitol	AMR	25 g	AB	44.6 mEq	D5LR, D5¼S, D5½S, D5S, D5W, D10W, NS, ½S[d]	Visually compatible for 24 hr at 24 °C	1853; 1973	C

Additive Compatibility (Cont.)

Sodium bicarbonate

Drug	Mfr	Conc/L	Mfr	Conc/L	Test Soln	Remarks	Ref	C/I
Meperidine HCl	WI					Physically incompatible	9	I
	WI	100 mg	AB	2.4 mEq[a]	D5W	Physically compatible for 24 hr	772	C
Meropenem	ZEN	1 g	BA[f]	5%		10% meropenem loss by HPLC in 4 hr at 24 °C and 18 hr at 4 °C	2089	I[h]
	ZEN	20 g	BA[f]	5%		9 to 10% meropenem loss by HPLC in 3 hr at 24 °C and 18 hr at 4 °C	2089	I[h]
Metaraminol bitartrate	MSD	100 mg	AB	3.75 g		Physically compatible	7	C
	MSD	100 mg	AB	4.8 mEq[e]	D5W	Physically compatible for 24 hr	772	C
Methotrexate sodium	LE	750 mg		50 mEq	D5W	1.4% methotrexate decomposition in 72 hr and 6% in 1 week at 5 °C protected from light. At 23 °C exposed to light, 6% methotrexate decomposition in 72 hr and 15% in 1 week	465	C
Methyldopate HCl	MSD	1 g		50 mEq	D, D–S, S	Physically compatible	23	C
Morphine sulfate						Physically incompatible	9	I
Multivitamins	USV	10 ml	AB	4.8 mEq[e]	D5W	Physically compatible for 24 hr	772	C
Nafcillin sodium	WY	500 mg	AB	40 mEq		Physically compatible	27	C
Nalmefene HCl	OHM	10 mg	AB	5%[c]		Little or no nalmefene loss by HPLC in 72 hr at 4, 21, and 40 °C	1962	C
Netilmicin sulfate	SC	3 g	TR	5%		Physically compatible and chemically stable for 7 days at 4 and 25 °C	558	C
Nizatidine	LI	0.75, 1.5, 3 g	MG[c]	5%		Visually compatible and nizatidine potency by HPLC retained for 7 days at 4 and 25 °C	1533	C
Norepinephrine bitartrate	WI					Physically incompatible	9	I
	WI	2 mg	AB	80 mEq	D5W	Physically incompatible	15	I
	BN	8 mg	AB	2.4 mEq[a]	D5W	Norepinephrine inactivated	772	I
Ofloxacin	ORT	0.4 and 4 g	BA[f]	5%		Physically compatible with little or no ofloxacin loss by HPLC in 3 days at 24 °C and 14 days at 5 °C	1636	C
Oxacillin sodium	BR	500 mg	AB	2.4 mEq[a]	D5W	Physically compatible for 24 hr	772	C
Oxytocin	PD	5 units	AB	2.4 mEq[a]	D5W	Physically compatible for 24 hr	772	C
Penicillin G potassium		100 million units	AB	2.4 mEq[a]	D5W	Physically compatible for 24 hr	772	C
	SQ	1 million units	AB	3.75 g	D5W	26% penicillin decomposition in 24 hr at 25 °C	47	I
	SQ	1 million units		0.5 and 0.75 g	D5W	Penicillin decomposition at 20 °C due to pH	135	I
	[g]	900,000 units		3.75 g	D5W	26% penicillin decomposition in 24 hr at 25 °C	48	I
Pentazocine lactate	WI	300 mg	AB	80 mEq	D5W	Physically incompatible	15	I
Pentobarbital sodium						Physically incompatible	9	I
	AB	1 g	AB	80 mEq	D5W	Physically incompatible	15	I
	AB	500 mg	AB	2.4 mEq[a]	D5W	Physically compatible for 24 hr	772	C

Additive Compatibility (Cont.)

Sodium bicarbonate

Drug	Mfr	Conc/L	Mfr	Conc/L	Test Soln	Remarks	Ref	C/I
Phenobarbital sodium		320 mg	AB	2.4 mEq[a]	D5W	Physically compatible for 24 hr	772	C
Phenylephrine HCl	WI	10 mg	AB	2.4 mEq[a]	D5W	Physically compatible for 24 hr	772	C
	WI	20 mg		5%		Potency retained for 24 hr at 25 °C	48	C
Phenytoin sodium	PD	250 mg	AB	2.4 mEq[a]	D5W	Physically compatible for 24 hr	772	C
Phytonadione	MSD	10 mg	AB	2.4 mEq[a]	D5W	Physically compatible for 24 hr	772	C
Potassium chloride		120 mEq	AB	2.4 mEq[a]	D5W	Physically compatible for 24 hr	772	C
Procaine HCl						Physically incompatible	9	I
	WI	1 g	AB	80 mEq	D5W	Physically incompatible	15	I
Prochlorperazine edisylate	SKF	10 mg	AB	2.4 mEq[a]	D5W	Physically compatible for 24 hr	772	C
Promazine HCl	WY	100 mg	AB	2.4 mEq[a]	D5W	Physically compatible for 24 hr	772	C
	WY	1 g	AB	3.75 g	D5W	Physically incompatible	11	I
Streptomycin sulfate						Physically incompatible	9	I
Succinylcholine chloride	AB	1 g	AB	2.4 mEq[a]	D5W	Succinylcholine inactivated	772	I
Thiopental sodium	AB	2.5 g	AB	40 mEq	D5W	Physically compatible	21	C
	AB	1 g	AB	2.4 mEq[a]	D5W	Physically compatible for 24 hr	772	C
Vancomycin HCl	LI					Physically incompatible	9	I
	LI	500 mg	AB	2.4 mEq[a]	D5W	Physically compatible for 24 hr	772	C
Verapamil HCl	KN	80 mg	BR	89.2 mEq	D5W, NS	Physically compatible for 24 hr	764	C
Vitamin B complex with C	LE					Physically incompatible	9	I
	AB	5 ml	AB	80 mEq	D5W	Physically incompatible	15	I

[a]One vial of Neut added to a liter of admixture.
[b]Tested in both glass and PVC containers.
[c]Tested in glass containers.
[d]Tested in polyolefin containers.
[e]Two vials of Neut added to a liter of admixture.
[f]Tested in PVC bags.
[g]A buffered preparation was specified.
[h]Incompatible by conventional standards but may be used in shorter periods of time.
[i]Sodium carbonate–containing formulation tested.

Drugs in Syringe Compatibility

Sodium bicarbonate

Drug (in syringe)	Mfr	Amt	Mfr	Amt	Remarks	Ref	C/I
Bupivacaine HCl	AST, WI	0.25, 0.5[a], 0.75%[a]; 20 ml	AB	4%, 0.05 to 0.6 ml	Precipitate forms in 1 to 2 min up to 2 hr at lowest amount of bicarbonate	1724	I
	BEL	0.5%[b], 20 ml		1.4%, 1.5 ml	Little or no epinephrine loss by HPLC in 7 days at room temperature. Bupivacaine not tested	1743	C
	BEL	0.5%[b], 20 ml		4.2 and 8.4%, 1.5 ml	5 to 7% epinephrine loss by HPLC in 7 days at room temperature. Bupivacaine not tested	1743	C
Chlorprocaine HCl	AST	2 and 3%, 20 ml	AST	8.4%, 0.5 and 1 ml	Visually compatible for up to 5 hr at room temperature	1724	C

Drugs in Syringe Compatibility (Cont.)

Drug (in syringe)	Mfr	Amt	Mfr	Amt	Remarks	Ref	C/I
				Sodium bicarbonate			
	AST	2 and 3%, 20 ml	AST	8.4%, 2 ml	Haze forms but clarifies with gentle agitation	1724	?
	AST	2 and 3%, 20 ml	AB	4%, 1 and 2 ml	Visually compatible for up to 5 hr at room temperature	1724	C
	AST	2 and 3%, 20 ml	AB	4%, 4 ml	Haze forms but clarifies with gentle agitation	1724	?
Etidocaine HCl	AST	1 and 1.5%[a], 20 ml	AB	4%, 0.015 to 0.2 ml	Precipitate forms in 1 to 2 min to over 4 hr at lowest amount of bicarbonate	1724	I
Glycopyrrolate	RB	0.2 mg/ 1 ml	AB	75 mg/ 1 ml	Gas evolves	331	I
	RB	0.2 mg/ 1 ml	AB	150 mg/ 2 ml	Gas evolves	331	I
	RB	0.4 mg/ 2 ml	AB	75 mg/ 1 ml	Gas evolves	331	I
Lidocaine HCl	ES	2%[c], 30 ml	ES	3 mEq/ 3 ml	11% lidocaine loss in 1 week and 22% loss in 2 weeks at 25 °C by GC. 28% epinephrine loss by HPLC in 1 week at 25 °C	1712	I
	ES	2%[c], 30 ml	AB	3 mEq/ 3 ml	6% lidocaine loss by GC in 4 weeks at 4 °C. 2% epinephrine loss in 1 week and 12% loss in 3 weeks at 4 °C by HPLC	1712	C
	AST	1%[c], 30 ml	LY	0.1 mEq/ml	25% epinephrine loss by HPLC in 1 week at room temperature. Lidocaine not tested	1713	I
		0.9%		0.088 mEq/ml	11% lidocaine loss by fluorescence polarization immunoassay in 7 days at room temperature	1723	C
	AST	1 and 1.5%[a], 20 ml	AST	8.4%, 2 ml	Visually compatible for up to 5 hr at room temperature	1724	C
	AST	2%[a], 20 ml	AST	8.4%, 2 ml	Haze forms but clarifies with gentle agitation	1724	?
	AST	1 and 1.5%[a], 20 ml	AB	4%, 4 ml	Visually compatible for up to 5 hr at room temperature	1724	C
	AST	2%[a], 20 ml	AB	4%, 4 ml	Haze forms but clarifies with gentle agitation	1724	?
	BEL	2%[d], 20 ml		1.4 and 8.4%, 1.5 ml	8% epinephrine loss by HPLC in 7 days at room temperature. Lidocaine not tested	1743	C
Mepivacaine HCl	AST, WI	1 and 1.5%, 20 ml	AST	8.4%; 0.5, 1, 2 ml	Precipitate forms within approximately 1 hr	1724	I
	AST, WI	1 and 1.5%, 20 ml	AB	4%; 1, 2, 4 ml	Precipitate forms within approximately 1 hr	1724	I
Metoclopramide HCl	RB	10 mg/ 2 ml	AB	100 mEq/ 100 ml	Incompatible. Do not mix	924	I
	RB	10 mg/ 2 ml	AB	100 mEq/ 100 ml	Gas evolves	1167	I

Drugs in Syringe Compatibility (Cont.)

Sodium bicarbonate

Drug (in syringe)	Mfr	Amt	Mfr	Amt	Remarks	Ref	C/I
	RB	160 mg/ 32 ml	AB	100 mEq/ 100 ml	Gas evolves	1167	**I**
Milrinone lactate	WI	5.25 mg/ 5.25 ml	AB	3.75 g/ 50 ml	Physically compatible with no milrinone loss in 20 min at 23 °C under fluorescent light	1410	**C**
Pentobarbital sodium	AB	500 mg/ 10 ml	AB	3.75 g/ 50 ml	Physically compatible	55	**C**
Thiopental sodium	AB	75 mg/ 3 ml	AB	3.75 g/ 50 ml	Physically incompatible	55	**I**

[a]Tested with and without epinephrine HCl 1:200,000 added.
[b]Tested with epinephrine HCl 1:200,000 added.
[c]Tested with epinephrine HCl 1:100,000 added.
[d]Tested with epinephrine HCl 1:80,000 added.

Y-Site Injection Compatibility (1:1 Mixture)

Sodium bicarbonate

Drug	Mfr	Conc	Mfr	Conc	Remarks	Ref	C/I
Acyclovir sodium	BW	5 mg/ml[a]	IX	0.5 mEq/ml[a]	Physically compatible for 4 hr at 25 °C	1157	**C**
Allopurinol sodium	BW	3 mg/ml[b]	AB	1 mEq/ml	Small and large crystals form in 1 hr	1686	**I**
Amifostine	USB	10 mg/ml[a]	AST	1 mEq/ml	Physically compatible with no change in measured turbidity or increase in particle content in 4 hr at 23 °C	1845	**C**
Amiodarone HCl	WY	3 mg/ml[a]	AB	1 mEq/ml	Precipitate forms immediately	1851	**I**
Amphotericin B cholesteryl sulfate complex	SEQ	0.83 mg/ml[a]	AB	1 mEq/ml	Gross precipitate forms	2117	**I**
Amrinone lactate	WB	3 mg/ml[b]	AB	1 mEq/ml	Immediate change from yellow to colorless	992	**I**
	WI	5 mg/ml	AST	75 mg/ml	Immediate precipitation	1419	**I**
	WI	2.5 mg/ml[c]	AST	75 mg/ml	Precipitate forms in 10 min	1419	**I**
Asparaginase	BEL	120 I.U./ml[a]		1.4%	Visually compatible for 4 hr at room temperature	1788	**C**
Aztreonam	SQ	40 mg/ml[a]	AB	1 mEq/ml	Physically compatible with no subvisual haze or particle formation in 4 hr at 23 °C	1758	**C**
Calcium chloride	AB	4 mg/ml[d]	AB	1 mEq/ml[d]	Slight haze or precipitate in 1 hr	1316	**I**
Cefepime HCl	BR	20 mg/ml[a]	AB	1 mEq/ml	Physically compatible with no change in measured turbidity or increase in particle content in 4 hr at 22 °C	1689	**C**
Ceftriaxone sodium	RC	100 mg/ml		1.4%	Visually compatible for 4 hr at room temperature	1788	**C**
Ciprofloxacin	MI	2 mg/ml[a]	AB	1 mEq/ml	Visually compatible for 24 hr at 24 °C	1655	**C**
	MI	2 mg/ml[b]	AB	1 mEq/ml	Very fine crystals form in 20 min in NS	1655	**I**
	MI	2 mg/ml[a]	AB	1 mEq/ml	Physically compatible with no change in measured turbidity or increase in particle content in 4 hr at 23 °C	1869	**C**
	MI	2 mg/ml[a]	AB	0.1 mEq/ml[a]	Subvisual haze forms immediately, becoming a white crystalline precipitate in 4 hr at 23 °C	1869	**I**

Y-Site Injection Compatibility (1:1 Mixture) (Cont.)

Sodium bicarbonate

Drug	Mfr	Conc	Mfr	Conc	Remarks	Ref	C/I
	BAY	1 and 2 mg/ml[a]	AB	1 and 0.75[a] mEq/ml	Physically compatible with no change in measured turbidity or increase in particle content in 4 hr at 23 °C	2065	**C**
	BAY	1 mg/ml[b]	AB	1 and 0.75[b] mEq/ml	Physically compatible with no change in measured turbidity or increase in particle content in 4 hr at 23 °C	2065	**C**
	BAY	2 mg/ml[b]	AB	1 and 0.75[b] mEq/ml	Small amount of particles forms immediately, becoming more numerous over 4 hr at 23 °C	2065	**I**
	BAY	1 and 2 mg/ml[a]	AB	0.5, 0.25, 0.1 mEq/ml[a]	Small amount of particles forms immediately, becoming more numerous over 4 hr at 23 °C	2065	**I**
	BAY	1 mg/ml[b]	AB	0.5, 0.25, 0.1 mEq/ml[b]	Small amount of particles forms in 1 hr, becoming more numerous over 4 hr at 23 °C	2065	**I**
	BAY	2 mg/ml[b]	AB	0.5, 0.25, 0.1 mEq/ml[b]	Precipitate forms immediately	2065	**I**
Cisatracurium besylate	GW	0.1 mg/ml[a]	AB	1 mEq/ml	Physically compatible with no change in measured turbidity or increase in particle content in 4 hr at 23 °C	2074	**C**
	GW	2 mg/ml[a]	AB	1 mEq/ml	Subvisual light brown discoloration with subvisual haze in 1 hr	2074	**I**
	GW	5 mg/ml[a]	AB	1 mEq/ml	Subvisual haze forms immediately; subvisual light brown discoloration with turbidity forms in 4 hr	2074	**I**
Cladribine	ORT	0.015[b] and 0.5[f] mg/ml	AB	1 mEq/ml	Physically compatible with no change in measured turbidity or increase in particle content in 4 hr at 23 °C	1969	**C**
Cyclophosphamide		20 mg/ml[a]		1.4%	Visually compatible for 4 hr at room temperature	1788	**C**
Cytarabine	UP	0.6 mg/ml[a]		1.4%	Visually compatible for 4 hr at room temperature	1788	**C**
Daunorubicin HCl	BEL	0.52 mg/ml[a]		1.4%	Visually compatible for 4 hr at room temperature	1788	**C**
Dexamethasone sodium phosphate	MSD	4 mg/ml		1.4%	Visually compatible for 4 hr at room temperature	1788	**C**
Dexchlorpheniramine maleate		5 mg/ml		1.4%	Visually compatible for 4 hr at room temperature	1788	**C**
Diltiazem HCl	MMD	5 mg/ml	LY	1 mEq/ml	Precipitate forms	1807	**I**
	MMD	1 mg/ml[b]	LY	1 mEq/ml	Visually compatible	1807	**C**
	MMD	5 mg/ml	LY	0.05 mEq/ml[a]	Visually compatible	1807	**C**
Docetaxel	RPR	0.9 mg/ml[a]	AB	1 mEq/ml	Physically compatible with no change in measured turbidity or increase in particle content in 4 hr at 23 °C	2224	**C**
Doxorubicin HCl	FA	0.4 mg/ml[a]		1.4%	Visually compatible for 2 hr at room temperature	1788	**C**
Doxorubicin HCl liposome injection	SEQ	0.4 mg/ml[a]	AB	1 mEq/ml	Partial loss of measured natural turbidity	2087	**I**
Etoposide	BR	0.6 mg/ml[b]		1.4%	Visually compatible for 4 hr at room temperature	1788	**C**

Y-Site Injection Compatibility (1:1 Mixture) (Cont.)

			Sodium bicarbonate				
Drug	Mfr	Conc	Mfr	Conc	Remarks	Ref	C/I
Etoposide phosphate	BR	5 mg/ml[a]	AB	1 mEq/ml	Physically compatible with no change in measured turbidity or increase in partical content in 4 hr at 23 °C	2218	C
Famotidine	MSD	0.2 mg/ml[a]	AB	1 mEq/ml[a]	Physically compatible for 4 hr at 25 °C	1188	C
Filgrastim	AMG	30 μg/ml[a]	AB	1 mEq/ml	Physically compatible with no change in measured turbidity or increase in particle content in 4 hr at 22 °C	1687	C
Fludarabine phosphate	BX	1 mg/ml[a]	AB	1 mEq/ml	Physically compatible for 4 hr at room temperature under fluorescent light	1439	C
Gemcitabine HCl	LI	10 mg/ml[b]	AB	1 mEq/ml	Physically compatible with no change in measured turbidity or increase in particle content in 4 hr at 23 °C	2226	C
Granisetron HCl	SKB	0.05 mg/ml[a]	AB	1 mEq/ml	Physically compatible with no subvisual haze or particle formation in 4 hr at 23 °C	1804	C
	SKB	1 mg/ml	AB	0.33 mEq/ml[b]	Physically compatible with 8% loss of granisetron by HPLC in 4 hr at 22 °C	1883	C
	SKB	0.05 mg/ml[a]	AB	1 mEq/ml	Physically compatible with no change in measured turbidity or increase in particle content in 4 hr at 23 °C	2000	C
Heparin[g]	CH	500 units/ml[b]		1.4%	Visually compatible for 4 hr at room temperature	1788	C
Heparin sodium with hydrocortisone sodium succinate	RI UP	1000 units + 100 mg/L[h]	BR	75 mg/ml	Physically compatible for at least 4 hr at room temperature by visual and microscopic examination	322	C
Idarubicin HCl	AD	1 mg/ml[b]	AB	0.09 mEq/ml[a]	Haze forms and color changes immediately. Precipitate forms in 20 min	1525	I
Ifosfamide		36 mg/ml[a]		1.4%	Visually compatible for 4 hr at room temperature	1788	C
Imipenem–cilastatin sodium	MSD	5 mg/ml[a]		1.4%	Pale yellow precipitate forms in 1 hr at room temperature	1788	I
Indomethacin sodium trihydrate	MSD	1 mg/ml[b]	AB	0.5 mEq/ml[a]	Visually compatible for 24 hr at 28 °C	1527	C
Insulin, regular (Humulin R) (beef, pork)	LI LI	1 unit/ml[d] 1 unit/ml[d]	AB AB	1 mEq/ml[d] 1 mEq/ml[d]	Physically compatible for 3 hr Physically compatible for 3 hr	1316 1316	C C
Leucovorin calcium	LE	10 mg/ml		1.4%	Yellow precipitate forms in 0.5 hr at room temperature	1788	I
Melphalan HCl	BW	0.1 mg/ml[b]	AB	1 mEq/ml	Physically compatible with no change in measured turbidity or increase in particle content in 3 hr at 22 °C	1557	C
Mesna		1.8 mg/ml[a]		1.4%	Visually compatible for 4 hr at room temperature	1788	C
Methylprednisolone sodium succinate	UP	20 mg/ml		1.4%	Visually compatible for 4 hr at room temperature	1788	C
Midazolam HCl	RC RC	5 mg/ml 1 mg/ml[a]	IMS	1.4% 1 mEq/ml	White precipitate forms immediately Haze forms immediately. Precipitate forms in 2 hr	1788 1847	I I
Milrinone lactate	SW	0.4 mg/ml[a]	AB	1 mEq/ml	Visually compatible with 4% loss of milrinone by HPLC in 4 hr at 23 °C	2214	C

Y-Site Injection Compatibility (1:1 Mixture) (Cont.)

					Sodium bicarbonate		
Drug	*Mfr*	*Conc*	*Mfr*	*Conc*	*Remarks*	*Ref*	*C/I*
Morphine sulfate	WY	0.2 mg/ml[d]	AB	1 mEq/ml[d]	Physically compatible for 3 hr	1316	C
Nalbuphine HCl	DU	10 mg/ml		1.4%	Gas evolves	1788	I
Ondansetron HCl	GL	0.32 mg/ml[a]		0.05 mM/ml[i]	White precipitate forms immediately	1513	I
	GL	0.1 mg/ml[a]		0.1 mEq/ml[a]	Large increase in 10-, 25-, and 50-μm particles. Visible particles in 30 to 60 min at room temperature	1661	I
	GL	2 mg/ml		1.4%	Heavy white precipitate forms immediately	1788	I
Oxacillin sodium	BR	250 mg/ml		1.4%	Gas evolves	1788	I
Paclitaxel	NCI	1.2 mg/ml[a]	LY	1 mEq/ml	Physically compatible with no change in measured turbidity in 4 hr at 22 °C	1556	C
Piperacillin sodium–tazobactam sodium	LE	40 + 5 mg/ml[a]	AB	1 mEq/ml	Physically compatible with no change in measured turbidity or increase in particle content in 4 hr at 22 °C	1688	C
Potassium chloride		40 mEq/L[h]	BR	75 mg/ml	Physically compatible for at least 4 hr at room temperature by visual and microscopic examination	322	C
Propofol	ZEN	10 mg/ml	AB	1 mEq/ml	Physically compatible for 1 hr at 23 °C with no increase in particle content	2066	C
Remifentanil HCl	GW	0.025 and 0.25 mg/ml[b]	AB	1 mEq/ml	Physically compatible with no change in measured turbidity or increase in particle content in 4 hr at 23 °C	2075	C
Sargramostim	IMM	10 μg/ml[b]	LY	1 mEq/ml	Small amount of particles forms in 4 hr	1436	I
Tacrolimus	FUJ	1 mg/ml[b]	AB	1 mEq/ml	Visually compatible for 24 hr at 25 °C	1630	C
Teniposide	BR	0.1 mg/ml[a]	AB	1 mEq/ml	Physically compatible with no subvisual haze or particle formation in 4 hr at 23 °C	1725	C
Thiotepa	IMM[j]	1 mg/ml[a]	AB	1 mEq/ml	Physically compatible with no change in measured turbidity or increase in particle content in 4 hr at 23 °C	1861	C
TNA #218 to #226[k]			AB	1 mEq/ml	Visually compatible with no precipitate or emulsion damage apparent in 4 hr at 23 °C	2215	C
Tolazoline HCl		0.1 mg/ml[a]	AB	0.5 mEq/ml	Physically compatible for 24 hr at 22 °C	1363	C
TPN #212 and #214[k]			AB	1 mEq/ml	Small amount of hazy subvisual precipitate forms in 1 hr and settles	2109	I
TPN #213 and #215[k]			AB	1 mEq/ml	Physically compatible with no change in measured turbidity or increase in particle content in 4 hr at 23 °C	2109	C
Vancomycin HCl		5 mg/ml[a]		1.4%	Visually compatible for 4 hr at room temperature	1788	C
Verapamil HCl	SE	5 mg/2 ml		88 mEq/L[c]	Crystalline precipitate forms when verapamil injected into infusion line	839	I
Vincristine sulfate	LI	0.1 mg/ml		1.4%	White precipitate forms in 0.5 hr at room temperature	1788	I
Vindesine sulfate	LI	0.1 mg/ml		1.4%	White precipitate forms in 0.5 hr at room temperature	1788	I

Y-Site Injection Compatibility (1:1 Mixture) (Cont.)

Sodium bicarbonate

Drug	Mfr	Conc	Mfr	Conc	Remarks	Ref	C/I
Vinorelbine tartrate	BW	1 mg/ml[b]	AB	1 mEq/ml	Tiny particles and light blue haze form immediately, developing into large particles in 4 hr at 22 °C	1558	I
Vitamin B complex with C	RC	2 ml/L[h]	BR	75 mg/ml	Physically compatible for at least 4 hr at room temperature by visual and microscopic examination	322	C

[a]*Tested in dextrose 5% in water.*
[b]*Tested in sodium chloride 0.9%.*
[c]*Tested in sodium chloride 0.45%.*
[d]*Tested in both dextrose 5% in water and sodium chloride 0.9%.*
[e]*Tested in sterile water for injection.*
[f]*Tested in bacteriostatic sodium chloride 0.9% preserved with benzyl alcohol 0.9%.*
[g]*Salt form not specified.*
[h]*Tested in dextrose 5% in water, sodium chloride 0.9%, and Ringer's injection, lactated.*
[i]*Tested in dextrose 5% in water with potassium chloride 0.02 mM/ml.*
[j]*Lyophilized formulation tested.*
[k]*Refer to Appendix I for the composition of parenteral nutrition solutions. TNA indicates a 3-in-1 admixture, and TPN indicates a 2-in-1 admixture.*

Additional Compatibility Information

Sodium bicarbonate is stated to be incompatible with acids, acidic salts, and many alkaloidal salts (4).

Alkali-Labile Drugs— Drugs such as sodium bicarbonate that may raise the pH of an admixture above 6 may cause significant decomposition of isoproterenol HCl and norepinephrine bitartrate. If they are combined, the mixture should be administered immediately after preparation (59; 77). Also, dopamine HCl is inactivated in alkaline solutions such as sodium bicarbonate 5% (79).

Ciprofloxacin— Ciprofloxacin mixed with sodium bicarbonate in lower concentrations has resulted in the formation of a haze and precipitate, while 10-fold higher concentrations of sodium bicarbonate appear to be physically compatible with the same amount of ciprofloxacin (1869). Although not unprecedented, it is less common for high concentrations of drugs to be compatible while lower concentrations are incompatible. The differing compatibility results have been ascribed to pH dependency of ciprofloxacin solubility (2012). However, a thorough evaluation of the compatibility of ciprofloxacin with a wide range of sodium bicarbonate concentrations found that incompatibility cannot be predicted by pH of the solutions alone; the solutions were generally in a very narrow pH range (8.0 to 8.3). Because the interaction between ciprofloxacin and sodium bicarbonate appears to be complex and variable, simultaneous administration of these drugs should be avoided (2065).

Amiodarone HCl— The manufacturer states that amiodarone HCl may precipitate if mixed with sodium bicarbonate (2p3288).

Cefotaxime— Cefotaxime sodium should not be mixed in alkaline solutions such as sodium bicarbonate injection (4).

Dobutamine HCl— Dobutamine HCl has been stated to be incompatible with alkaline solutions and should not be mixed with sodium bicarbonate 5% or other alkaline solutions (4).

Timentin— Ticarcillin disodium–clavulanate potassium (SmithKline Beecham) is stated to be incompatible with sodium bicarbonate (4).

Calcium Salts— The manufacturer recommends avoiding the addition of sodium bicarbonate to infusion solutions that contain calcium unless compatibility has been established. Haze formation or precipitation may result from such combinations (4).

Sodium bicarbonate (Abbott) in dextrose 5% in water has been reported to be conditionally compatible with calcium chloride (Upjohn) and calcium gluconate (Upjohn). The incompatibility is dependent on the concentration of the additives. Therefore, if attempting to combine sodium bicarbonate with either of these drugs, mix the solution thoroughly and observe it closely for any sign of incompatibility (15). A white precipitate and turbidity were found in concentrated solutions (845).

Amino Acids— Because of the acidity of amino acid injection, the addition of bicarbonate ion may result in the loss of some of this ion as carbon dioxide. Moreover, adding bicarbonate ion to solutions containing calcium or magnesium may result in the precipitation of insoluble carbonates (189).

Methylprednisolone— The compatibility of methylprednisolone sodium succinate (Upjohn) with sodium bicarbonate added to an auxiliary medication infusion unit has been studied. Primary admixtures were prepared by adding sodium bicarbonate 44.6 mEq/L to dextrose 5% in water, dextrose 5% in sodium chloride 0.9%, and Ringer's injection, lactated. Up to 100 ml of the primary admixture was added along with methylprednisolone sodium succinate (Upjohn) to the auxiliary medication infusion unit with the following results (329):

Methylprednisolone Sodium Succinate	Sodium Bicarbonate 44.6 mEq/L Primary Solution	Results
500 mg	D5S, D5W qs 100 ml	Clear solution for 24 hr
	LR qs 100 ml or added to 100 ml LR	Clear solution for 1 hr
1000 mg	D5W qs 100 ml	Clear solution for 24 hr
	D5S qs 100 ml or added to 100 ml D5S	Clear solution for 24 hr
	LR qs 100 ml	Clear solution for 1 hr
	Added to 100 ml LR	Clear solution for 4 hr
2000 mg	D5S, D5W qs 100 ml	Clear solution for 24 hr
	LR qs 100 ml	Clear solution for 30 min
	Added to 100 ml LR	Clear solution for 4 hr

Solutions— Raymond and DeGennaro reported the change in pH that occurred when 5 ml of Neut was added to a liter of 10 common infusion solutions. The results were as follows:

Solution	Initial pH	pH after Neut Added	pH Increase
Dextrose 5% in Electrolyte #48	5.0	6.1	1.1
Dextrose 5% in Electrolyte #75	4.7	5.5	0.8
Dextrose 5% in Ringer's injection	4.3	7.3	3.0
Dextrose 5% in Ringer's injection, lactated	5.0	6.2	1.2
Dextrose 5% in water	4.4	7.5	3.1
Dextrose 10% in water	3.9	7.1	3.2
Ringer's injection	5.6	7.5	1.9
Ringer's injection, lactated	6.3	7.4	1.1
Sodium chloride 0.45%	5.6	7.8	2.2
Sodium chloride 0.9%	5.4	7.6	2.2

The observed pH increase persisted over the 24-hour study period. Solutions with a low buffer capacity exhibited pH increases of about two to three pH units. Solutions with a higher buffer capacity showed pH changes of approximately one pH unit (1129).

Other Information

Preparing Isotonic Solutions— An isotonic 1.5% sodium bicarbonate solution may be prepared by diluting the concentrated injections with sterile water for injection in the following amounts:

Sodium Bicarbonate Concentration (%)	Amount of Sodium Bicarbonate Concentrate (ml)	Amount of Sterile Water for Injection (ml)
8.4	1	4.61
7.5	1	4
4.2	1	1.8

SODIUM CHLORIDE
AHFS 40:12

Products— Sodium chloride additive solution is available in various size containers in concentrations of 14.6 and 23.4%. The 14.6% concentration contains sodium chloride 146 mg/ml and provides 2.5 mEq/ml of sodium and chloride ions. The 23.4% concentration contains sodium chloride 234 mg/ml and provides 4 mEq/ml of sodium and chloride ions (4; 29).

pH— From 4.5 to 7 (4).

Osmotic Values— The osmolarities of the 14.6 and 23.4% concentrations are about 5000 and 8000 mOsm/L, respectively (4). The osmolality of the 14.6% concentration was determined to be 5370 mOsm/kg by freezing-point depression and 4783 mOsm/kg by vapor pressure (1071). A 0.9% sodium chloride solution is isotonic, having an osmolarity of 308 mOsm/L (4).

Administration— Sodium chloride additive solutions of 14.6 and 23.4% are administered by intravenous infusion only after dilution in a larger volume of fluid. When concentrations of 3 or 5% are indicated, these hypertonic solutions should be administered into a large vein, at a rate not exceeding 100 ml/hr. Infiltration should be avoided (4).

Stability— Sodium chloride additive solution should be stored at controlled room temperature and protected from excessive heat and freezing (17).

Elastomeric Reservoir Pumps— Sodium chloride 0.9% (Baxter) 250 ml was filled into Intermate LV 250 (Baxter) elastomeric infusion devices and stored at 5 and 23 °C for 90 days. The solution remained visually compatible with no change in pH and sodium or chloride concentration and less than 0.1% water loss (1993).

Compatibility Information

Solution Compatibility

Sodium chloride

Solution	Mfr	Mfr	Conc/L	Remarks	Ref	C/I
Dextran 6% in dextrose 5%	AB	AB	200 mEq	Physically compatible	3	**C**
Dextran 6% in sodium chloride 0.9%	AB	AB	200 mEq	Physically compatible	3	**C**
Dextrose–Ringer's injection combinations	AB	AB	200 mEq	Physically compatible	3	**C**
Dextrose–Ringer's injection, lactated, combinations	AB	AB	200 mEq	Physically compatible	3	**C**
Dextrose–saline combinations	AB	AB	200 mEq	Physically compatible	3	**C**
Dextrose 2½% in water	AB	AB	200 mEq	Physically compatible	3	**C**
Dextrose 5% in water	AB	AB	200 mEq	Physically compatible	3	**C**
Dextrose 10% in water	AB	AB	200 mEq	Physically compatible	3	**C**
Fat emulsion 10%, intravenous	CU		200 mEq	Globule coalescence with noticeable surface creaming in 4 hr at room temperature. Oil globules noted on surface at 48 hr	656	**I**
	CU		100 mEq	No significant change in emulsion for 24 hr at room temperature. Significant emulsion globule coalescence noted at 48 hr	656	**C**
Fructose 10% in sodium chloride 0.9%	AB	AB	200 mEq	Physically compatible	3	**C**
Fructose 10% in water	AB	AB	200 mEq	Physically compatible	3	**C**
Invert sugar 5 and 10% in sodium chloride 0.9%	AB	AB	200 mEq	Physically compatible	3	**C**
Invert sugar 5 and 10% in water	AB	AB	200 mEq	Physically compatible	3	**C**
Ionosol products	AB	AB	200 mEq	Physically compatible	3	**C**
Ringer's injection	AB	AB	200 mEq	Physically compatible	3	**C**
Ringer's injection, lactated	AB	AB	200 mEq	Physically compatible	3	**C**
Sodium chloride 0.45%	AB	AB	200 mEq	Physically compatible	3	**C**
Sodium chloride 0.9%	AB	AB	200 mEq	Physically compatible	3	**C**
Sodium lactate ⅙ M	AB	AB	200 mEq	Physically compatible	3	**C**

Drugs in Syringe Compatibility

Sodium chloride

Drug (in syringe)	Mfr	Amt	Mfr	Amt	Remarks	Ref	C/I
Cimetidine HCl	SKF	300 mg/ 2 ml		12.5 mEq/ 5 ml	Precipitate forms between 36 and 48 hr at room temperature	516	**C**

Y-Site Injection Compatibility (1:1 Mixture)

Sodium chloride

Drug	Mfr	Conc	Mfr	Conc	Remarks	Ref	C/I
Ciprofloxacin	MI	2 mg/ml[a]	AMR	4 mEq/ml	Visually compatible for 2 hr at 25 °C	1628	**C**

[a]Tested in dextrose 5% in water.

Additional Compatibility Information

The addition of sodium chloride to mannitol 20 or 25% may cause precipitation of the mannitol (4; 38).

SODIUM LACTATE
AHFS 40:08

Products— Sodium lactate additive solution is available in 10-ml vials (29). Each milliliter of solution contains 5 mEq of sodium lactate. The 10-ml vial contains a total of 50 mEq each of Na$^+$ and lactate ion (5.6 g of sodium lactate). The pH is adjusted with hydrochloric acid, lactic acid, or sodium hydroxide if necessary (4).

pH— From 6 to 7.3 (4).

Osmotic Values— Sodium lactate additive solution osmolality was determined to be 11,490 mOsm/kg by freezing-point depression and 10,665 mOsm/kg by vapor pressure (1071).

Sodium lactate ⅙ M (1.9%) is approximately isotonic with a calculated osmolarity of 330 mOsm/L (4).

Administration— Sodium lactate additive solution is administered by intravenous infusion after dilution in a larger volume of fluid. A ⅙M (1.9%) solution may be prepared by diluting 50 mEq of the additive solution to 300 ml with a nonelectrolyte solution or sterile water for injection. The rate of infusion should not exceed 300 ml/hr in adults (4).

Stability— Sodium lactate additive solution should be stored at room temperature and protected from freezing and excessive temperatures of 40 °C or more (4).

Compatibility Information

Solution Compatibility

Sodium lactate

Solution	Mfr	Mfr	Conc/L	Remarks	Ref	C/I
Dextran 6% in dextrose 5%	AB	AB	200 mEq	Physically compatible	3	C
Dextran 6% in sodium chloride 0.9%	AB	AB	200 mEq	Physically compatible	3	C
Dextrose–Ringer's injection combinations	AB	AB	200 mEq	Physically compatible	3	C
Dextrose–Ringer's injection, lactated, combinations	AB	AB	200 mEq	Physically compatible	3	C
Dextrose–saline combinations	AB	AB	200 mEq	Physically compatible	3	C
Dextrose 2½% in water	AB	AB	200 mEq	Physically compatible	3	C
Dextrose 5% in water	AB	AB	200 mEq	Physically compatible	3	C
Dextrose 10% in water	AB	AB	200 mEq	Physically compatible	3	C
Fructose 10% in sodium chloride 0.9%	AB	AB	200 mEq	Physically compatible	3	C
Fructose 10% in water	AB	AB	200 mEq	Physically compatible	3	C
Invert sugar 5 and 10% in sodium chloride 0.9%	AB	AB	200 mEq	Physically compatible	3	C
Invert sugar 5 and 10% in water	AB	AB	200 mEq	Physically compatible	3	C
Ionosol products	AB	AB	200 mEq	Physically compatible	3	C
Ringer's injection	AB	AB	200 mEq	Physically compatible	3	C
Ringer's injection, lactated	AB	AB	200 mEq	Physically compatible	3	C
Sodium chloride 0.45%	AB	AB	200 mEq	Physically compatible	3	C
Sodium chloride 0.9%	AB	AB	200 mEq	Physically compatible	3	C

Additive Compatibility

Sodium lactate

Drug	Mfr	Conc/L	Mfr	Conc/L	Test Soln	Remarks	Ref	C/I
Lidocaine HCl	AST	2 g	AB	50 mEq		Physically compatible	24	**C**
Nafcillin sodium	WY	500 mg	AB	50 mEq		Physically compatible	27	**C**
Sodium bicarbonate						Physically incompatible	9	**I**

Drugs in Syringe Compatibility

Sodium lactate

Drug (in syringe)	Mfr	Amt	Mfr	Amt	Remarks	Ref	C/I
Cimetidine HCl	SKF	300 mg/ 2 ml		25 mEq/ 5 ml	Physically compatible for 48 hr at room temperature	516	**C**

SODIUM NITROPRUSSIDE
AHFS 24:08

Nitropress   **Abbott**
                                                          Baxter

Products— Sodium nitroprusside (Abbott) is available in vials containing 50 mg of sodium nitroprusside dihydrate. Reconstitute with 2 to 3 ml of dextrose 5% in water (4) or sterile water for injection (without preservative) (4; 457). Bacteriostatic water for injection should not be used, because preservatives increase the rate of decomposition (4).

Sodium nitroprusside (Baxter) is available in 2-ml vials as a 25-mg/ml solution of sodium nitroprusside dihydrate in sterile water for injection (1-9/98).

For administration, dilute the reconstituted solution or the liquid form in dextrose 5% in water. Sodium nitroprusside 50 mg added to 250, 500, and 1000 ml of dextrose 5% in water results in concentrations of 200, 100, and 50 μg/ml, respectively. The infusion containers should be wrapped in aluminum foil or other opaque material for light protection. It is not necessary to cover the infusion drip chamber or tubing (1-9/98; 4).

pH— The pH of sodium nitroprusside diluted with dextrose 5% in water is 3.5 to 6 (4).

Osmolality— Sodium nitroprusside 25 mg/ml in sterile water for injection has an osmolality of 214 mOsm/kg (1689).

Sodium Content— Sodium nitroprusside contains 0.335 mEq of sodium per 50 mg of drug (846).

Administration— Sodium nitroprusside is administered only as an intravenous infusion by freshly reconstituting the drug and diluting 50 mg in 250 to 1000 ml of dextrose 5% in water. An infusion pump, microdrip regulator, or similar device should be used to control the flow rate precisely. Extravasation should be avoided (1-9/98; 4).

Stability— Sodium nitroprusside is a reddish-brown color. Sodium nitroprusside in intact containers should be stored at controlled room temperature and protected from light and heat (1-9/98; 4) and from freezing for the liquid product (1-9/98).

It was previously stated that solutions of sodium nitroprusside should be discarded four hours after reconstitution (4; 90). However, numerous studies reported the stability, protected from light, to be from 12 to 24 hours (93; 460; 1296; 1579), to 48 hours (958), to 13 days (95), or even longer (94; 458; 459; 732). It is now recommended that reconstituted sodium nitroprusside solutions be used within 24 hours when stored adequately protected from light (4). Similarly, the freshly diluted liquid injection is stated to be stable for 24 hours when protected from light (1-9/98).

Light Sensitivity— Solutions of sodium nitroprusside exhibit a color variously described as brownish (4), brown (90), brownish-pink (91), light orange (95), and straw (92). These solutions are highly sensitive to light. Exposure to light causes decomposition, resulting in a highly colored solution of orange (92), dark brown (91), or blue (4; 90–92). A blue color indicates almost complete degradation (92).

The rate of decomposition of sodium nitroprusside when exposed to light is dependent on such factors as the wavelength and intensity of light, temperature, infusion fluid, pH, and container material. The amount of loss occurring in the administration tubing can be affected additionally by the nature and thickness of the tubing wall, duration of light exposure, volume of fluid, and flow rate (1297).

In one study, sodium nitroprusside 0.01% in both water and dextrose 5% in water in glass bottles exhibited 9 to 10% decomposition in two hours and 18 to 20% decomposition in four hours on exposure to fluorescent light. No decomposition was detected in either solution in 24 hours when protected from light. In PVC bags, even greater decomposition occurred on exposure to light (460).

In another study, 10-mg/ml aqueous solutions of sodium nitroprusside lost 3% in 24 hours on exposure to fluorescent light and 10% in 24 hours when exposed to both fluorescent light and indirect daylight. At a concentration of 200 mg/L in infusion solutions, exposure to bright daylight increased the loss to approximately 15 to 30% in five hours. The rate of breakdown was related to the amount of illumination. When the containers were protected from light by wrapping with foil, no decomposition was observed in infusion solutions for seven days at room temperature and for two years at 10 mg/ml in glass tubes at room temperature or 4 °C (732).

Davidson and Lyall studied the rate of decomposition of sodium nitroprusside (David Bull Laboratories) 1 mg/ml in dextrose 5% in water when exposed to fluorescent light and natural daylight. The solutions were stored at 23 °C in the burette chambers of an amber light-protective set, a clear colorless set, and a clear set covered with a foil overwrap. With exposure to fluorescent light, losses in the clear burette chamber totaled 11% in 150 minutes and 100% in 24 hours. Both the amber and foil-wrapped clear sets sustained virtually no loss in four hours and about a 3 to 4% loss in 24 hours. Natural daylight caused a more rapid drug loss in the unprotected burette; essentially all drug was lost in 30 to 150 minutes, depending on the daylight intensity. The amber set slowed the degradation rate, but 32% was still lost in two hours with exposure to intense direct sunlight (1296).

Solutions of sodium nitroprusside should be protected from light by wrapping the container with aluminum foil or some other opaque material (1-9/98; 4; 90; 91; 1297). The container should be wrapped as soon as practical without delaying therapy (959). Amber plastic bags, which are often used for light protection, have been stated not to provide sufficient protection for sodium nitroprusside against photodegradation. Only opaque materials should be used (733).

The effect of the light exposure that sodium nitroprusside infusions receive while flowing through a 3-m long PVC infusion set tubing was evaluated. Sodium nitroprusside infusions in dextrose 5% in water, sodium chloride 0.9%, and Ringer's injection, lactated, were studied for 24 and eight hours at flow rates of 10 and 50 ml/hr, respectively. The delivered amount of sodium nitroprusside was not reduced (958).

Baaske et al. evaluated the stability of sodium nitroprusside (Roche) 100 μg/ml in dextrose 5% in water when delivered through tubing exposed to normal room light. No degradation occurred in the infusion container wrapped in foil, but concentration differences in the delivered solution of about 2% were noted at each time point sampled over the five-hour study. When the effects of different light sources on a 50-μg/ml solution in dextrose 5% in water were compared, about a 7% loss occurred on exposure to fluorescent light for six hours but a 32% loss occurred in one hour on exposure to direct sunlight (1131).

Sewell et al. evaluated the stability of sodium nitroprusside (Roche) 0.5 and 1.67 mg/ml in dextrose 5% in water administered by a syringe pump system. In polypropylene syringes (Sherwood Medical) exposed to both artificial and daylight, sodium nitroprus-

side losses after 24 hours were 26.0 and 18.7% at 0.5 and 1.67 mg/ml, respectively. The level of free cyanide exceeded 2 μg/ml. The time to 10% decomposition was about four hours. Syringes wrapped in foil exhibited less than a 5% loss in 24 hours. A comparison of the decomposition occurring in the delivery tubing showed that about 10.3 and 3.7% were lost from the 0.5- and 1.67-mg/ml concentrations, respectively, when delivered by pumps at 3 ml/hr through tubing exposed to the light. Wrapping the line with foil prevented any decomposition over the 24-hour study (1130).

Sodium nitroprusside (Roche) 50 mg/50 ml in dextrose 5% in water exhibited no change in appearance and no loss in potency by HPLC when stored for 24 hours at 25 °C in 60-ml plastic syringes (Becton-Dickinson) wrapped in foil. However, if the syringes were not wrapped in foil for light protection, the solution turned yellow in 12 hours and had 11 and 17% losses in six and 12 hours, respectively (1579).

Heat Sensitivity— Sodium nitroprusside solutions are also heat sensitive. Autoclaving a solution of 100 mg/250 ml in dextrose 5% in water at 115 °C for 30 minutes results in decomposition to a pale blue-green precipitate (458). It has been stated that autoclaving is less deleterious than even moderate exposure to light (94).

Sorption— Sodium nitroprusside (May & Baker) 5 g/L in dextrose 5% in water (Travenol) in PVC bags wrapped in aluminum foil for light protection did not exhibit significant sorption to the plastic during one week of storage at room temperature (15 to 20 °C) (536).

In another study, sodium nitroprusside (May & Baker) 5 g/L in dextrose 5% in water did not exhibit any loss due to sorption during a seven-hour simulated infusion through an infusion set (Travenol) consisting of a cellulose propionate burette chamber and 170 cm of PVC tubing (606).

The drug was also tested as a simulated infusion over at least one hour by a syringe pump system. A glass syringe on a syringe pump was fitted with 20 cm of polyethylene tubing or 50 cm of Silastic tubing. No loss of drug due to sorption was observed with either tubing (606).

In addition, a 25-ml aliquot of sodium nitroprusside (May & Baker) 5 g/L in dextrose 5% in water was stored in all-plastic syringes composed of polypropylene barrels and polyethylene plungers for 24 hours at room temperature in the dark. No loss due to sorption was observed (606).

Baaske et al. noted a 2% loss of sodium nitroprusside (Roche) 50 μg/ml when delivered through administration sets exposed to normal room light. Examination of the HPLC chromatogram showed the loss to be due to photodecomposition. No evidence of any sorption to the plastic was noted (1131).

Compatibility Information

Solution Compatibility

Sodium nitroprusside

Solution	Mfr	Mfr	Conc/L		Remarks	Ref	C/I
Dextrose 4% in sodium chloride 0.18%	TR		200	mg	No decomposition in 7 days at room temperature in foil-wrapped bottles	732	**C**
	TR		200	mg	20 to 25% decomposition in 5 hr exposed to bright daylight	732	**I**
Dextrose 5% in water			100	mg	No decomposition in 24 hr protected from light	460	**C**

Solution Compatibility (Cont.)

Sodium nitroprusside

Solution	Mfr	Mfr	Conc/L	Remarks	Ref	C/I
			100 mg	9 to 10% decomposition in 2 hr exposed to light	460	I
	TR		200 mg	No decomposition in 7 days at room temperature in foil-wrapped bottles	732	C
	TR		200 mg	14 to 16% decomposition in 5 hr exposed to bright daylight	732	I
	TR[a]		88 mg	18% loss in 24 hr when bag was hung adjacent to a window exposed to both daylight and fluorescent light	732	I
	TR	RC	165 mg	4% loss in 65 min in bright daylight	732	I
	AB[b]	RC	50 and 100 mg	No decomposition in 48 hr in foil-wrapped bottles and bags at room temperature	958	C
	MG	RC	50 mg	Little or no loss over 6 days at room temperature protected from light	1131	C
	MG	RC	50 mg	10% loss in 7 hr at room temperature exposed to fluorescent light. 32% loss in 1 hr exposed to direct sunlight	1131	I
	BT[c]	DB	100 mg	11% loss in 2.5 hr and 100% in 24 hr at 23 °C under fluorescent light. 100% loss in 0.5 to 2.5 hr in daylight	1296	I
	BT[c]	DB	100 mg	3 to 4% loss in 24 hr at 23 °C protected from light with foil wrapping or amber light-protective set	1296	C
	BT[c]	DB	100 mg	32% loss in 2 hr at 23 °C in intense daylight in amber light-protective set	1296	I
	d		200 to 800 mg	Physically compatible with 7% or less loss in 24 hr exposed to light	1412	C
	TR[a]	RC	50 and 400 mg	Visually compatible with little or no drug loss in 48 hr at room temperature	1802	C
Ringer's injection, lactated	AB[b]	RC	50 and 100 mg	No decomposition in 48 hr in foil-wrapped bottles and bags at room temperature	958	C
Sodium chloride 0.9%	TR		200 mg	No decomposition in 7 days at room temperature in foil-wrapped bottles	732	C
	TR		200 mg	24 to 28% decomposition in 5 hr exposed to bright daylight	732	I
	TR		289 mg	4% loss in 3 hr exposed to both daylight and fluorescent light	732	I
	TR		206 mg	2% loss in 60 min exposed to both daylight and fluorescent light	732	I
	TR		183 mg	1% loss in 2 hr in fluorescent light only	732	I
	AB[b]	RC	50 and 100 mg	No decomposition in 48 hr in foil-wrapped bottles and bags at room temperature	958	C
	d		200 to 800 mg	Physically compatible with 8% or less loss in 24 hr exposed to light	1412	C
	TR[a]	RC	50 and 400 mg	Visually compatible with little or no drug loss in 48 hr at room temperature	1802	C

[a]*Tested in PVC containers.*
[b]*Tested in both glass and PVC containers.*
[c]*Tested in burette chambers of administration sets.*
[d]*Tested in glass containers.*

Additive Compatibility

				Sodium nitroprusside				
Drug	*Mfr*	*Conc/L*	*Mfr*	*Conc/L*	*Test Soln*	*Remarks*	*Ref*	*C/I*
Atracurium besylate	BW	500 mg		2 g	D5W	Physically incompatible. Haze, particles, and yellow color form	1694	**I**
Cimetidine HCl	SKF	3 g	RC	500 mg	D5W	Physically compatible and cimetidine chemically stable for 24 hr at room temperature. Sodium nitroprusside not tested	551	**C**
Dobutamine HCl with nitroglycerin		2 to 8 g 200 to 800 mg		200 to 800 mg	D5W[a]	Pale pink discoloration with small amount of dark brown precipitate and 11 to 19% nitroprusside loss in 24 hr exposed to light	1412	**I**
Dobutamine HCl with nitroglycerin		2 to 8 g 200 to 800 mg		200 to 800 mg	NS[a]	Pale pink discoloration with all drugs stable for 24 hr exposed to light. 8% or less loss for any drug in any combination	1412	**C**
Enalaprilat	MSD	12 mg	ES	1 g	D5W[b]	Visually compatible with little or no enalaprilat loss by HPLC in 24 hr at room temperature protected from light. Sodium nitroprusside not tested	1572	**C**
Ranitidine HCl	GL	2 g	RC	50 and 400 mg	D5W, NS[b]	Physically compatible with no ranitidine loss in 48 hr at room temperature protected from light. Nitroprusside not tested	1361	**C**
	GL	50 mg	RC	50 and 400 mg	NS[b]	Physically compatible with no ranitidine loss in 48 hr at room temperature protected from light. Nitroprusside not tested	1361	**C**
	GL	50 mg	RC	50 and 400 mg	D5W[b]	Physically compatible with 7% or less ranitidine loss in 48 hr protected from light. Nitroprusside not tested	1361	**C**
	GL	50 mg and 2 g		50 mg and 1 g	D5W, NS	Physically compatible and both drugs chemically stable for 48 hr at room temperature protected from light	1515	**C**
	GL	50 mg and 2 g		100 mg	D5W	Physically compatible and ranitidine chemically stable by HPLC for 24 hr at 25 °C. Sodium nitroprusside not tested	1515	**C**
	GL	50 mg and 2 g	RC	50 and 400 mg	D5W[a]	Visually compatible with 5 to 7% ranitidine losses and 8% or less nitroprusside loss by HPLC in 48 hr at room temperature protected from light	1802	**C**
	GL	50 mg and 2 g	RC	50 and 400 mg	NS[a]	Visually compatible with no loss of either drug by HPLC in 48 hr at room temperature protected from light	1802	**C**
Verapamil HCl	KN	80 mg	RC	100 mg	D5W, NS	Physically compatible for 24 hr	764	**C**

[a]*Tested in glass containers.*
[b]*Tested in PVC containers.*

Drugs in Syringe Compatibility

Sodium nitroprusside

Drug (in syringe)	Mfr	Amt	Mfr	Amt	Remarks	Ref	C/I
Heparin sodium		2500 units/ 1 ml		60 mg/ 5 ml	Physically compatible for at least 5 min	1053	**C**

Y-Site Injection Compatibility (1:1 Mixture)

Sodium nitroprusside

Drug	Mfr	Conc	Mfr	Conc	Remarks	Ref	C/I
Amrinone lactate	WB	3 mg/ml[b]	AB	0.2 mg/ml[a]	Physically compatible for at least 4 hr at 25 °C under fluorescent light	992	**C**
Atracurium besylate	BW	0.5 mg/ml[a]	ES	0.2 mg/ml[a]	Physically compatible for 24 hr at 28 °C	1337	**C**
Cisatracurium besylate	GW	0.1 mg/ml[a]	AB	2 mg/ml[a]	Physically compatible with no change in measured turbidity or increase in particle content in 4 hr at 23 °C protected from light	2074	**C**
	GW	2 and 5 mg/ ml[a]	AB	2 mg/ml[a]	White cloudiness forms immediately	2074	**I**
Diltiazem HCl	MMD	5 mg/ml	AB	0.2 mg/ml[a]	Visually compatible	1807	**C**
Dobutamine HCl	LI	4 mg/ml[c]	ES	0.4 mg/ml[c]	Physically compatible for 3 hr	1316	**C**
Dobutamine HCl with dopamine HCl	LI DCC	4 mg/ml[c] 3.2 mg/ml[c]	ES	0.4 mg/ml[c]	Physically compatible for 3 hr	1316	**C**
Dobutamine HCl with lidocaine HCl	LI AB	4 mg/ml[c] 8 mg/ml[c]	ES	0.4 mg/ml[c]	Physically compatible for 3 hr	1316	**C**
Dobutamine HCl with nitroglycerin	LI LY	4 mg/ml[c] 0.4 mg/ml[c]	ES	0.4 mg/ml[c]	Physically compatible for 3 hr	1316	**C**
Dopamine HCl	DCC	3.2 mg/ml[c]	ES	0.4 mg/ml[c]	Physically compatible for 3 hr	1316	**C**
Dopamine HCl with dobutamine HCl	DCC LI	3.2 mg/ml[c] 4 mg/ml[c]	ES	0.4 mg/ml[c]	Physically compatible for 3 hr	1316	**C**
Dopamine HCl with lidocaine HCl	DCC AB	3.2 mg/ml[c] 8 mg/ml[c]	ES	0.4 mg/ml[c]	Physically compatible for 3 hr	1316	**C**
Dopamine HCl with nitroglycerin	DCC LY	3.2 mg/ml[c] 0.4 mg/ml[c]	ES	0.4 mg/ml[c]	Physically compatible for 3 hr	1316	**C**
Enalaprilat	MSD	0.05 mg/ml[b]	LY	0.2 mg/ml[a]	Physically compatible for 24 hr at room temperature under fluorescent light	1355	**C**
Esmolol HCl	DU	40 mg/ml[a]	RC	0.2 mg/ml[a]	Visually compatible for 24 hr at 23 °C	1877	**C**
Famotidine	MSD	0.2 mg/ml[a]	ES	0.2 mg/ml[a]	Physically compatible for 4 hr at 25 °C protected from light	1188	**C**
Haloperidol lactate	MN	5 mg/ml	AB	0.2 mg/ml[d]	Turbidity forms immediately and persists, developing fine precipitate in 24 hr at 21 °C under fluorescent light	1523	**I**
	MN	0.5 mg/ml[a]	AB	0.2 mg/ml[d]	Visually compatible for 24 hr at 21 °C	1523	**C**
Heparin sodium	TR	50 units/ml	ES	0.2 mg/ml[a]	Visually compatible for 6 hr at 25 °C protected from light	1793	**C**
	OR	100 units/ml[a]	RC	0.2 mg/ml[a]	Visually compatible for 24 hr at 23 °C	1877	**C**
Indomethacin sodium trihydrate	MSD	1 mg/ml[b]	AB	0.2 mg/ml[a]	Visually compatible for 24 hr at 28 °C	1527	**C**
Insulin, regular	LI	1 unit/ml[a]	RC	0.2 mg/ml[a]	Visually compatible for 24 hr at 23 °C	1877	**C**

Y-Site Injection Compatibility (1:1 Mixture) (Cont.)

Sodium nitroprusside

Drug	Mfr	Conc	Mfr	Conc	Remarks	Ref	C/I
Labetalol HCl	GL	5 mg/ml	RC	0.2 mg/ml[a]	Visually compatible for 24 hr at 23 °C	1877	C
Lidocaine HCl	AB	8 mg/ml[c]	ES	0.4 mg/ml[c]	Physically compatible for 3 hr	1316	C
Lidocaine HCl with dobutamine HCl	AB LI	8 mg/ml[c] 4 mg/ml[c]	ES	0.4 mg/ml[c]	Physically compatible for 3 hr	1316	C
Lidocaine HCl with dopamine HCl	AB DCC	8 mg/ml[c] 3.2 mg/ml[c]	ES	0.4 mg/ml[c]	Physically compatible for 3 hr	1316	C
Lidocaine HCl with nitroglycerin	AB LY	8 mg/ml[c] 0.4 mg/ml[a]	ES	0.4 mg/ml[c]	Physically compatible for 3 hr	1316	C
Midazolam HCl	RC RC	1 mg/ml[a] 1 mg/ml[a]	ES RC	0.2 mg/ml[a] 0.2 mg/ml[a]	Visually compatible for 24 hr at 23 °C Visually compatible for 24 hr at 23 °C	1847 1877	C C
Milrinone lactate	SW	0.4 mg/ml[a]	AB	0.8 mg/ml[a]	Visually compatible with little or no loss of either drug by HPLC in 4 hr at 23 °C protected from light	2214	C
Morphine sulfate	SX	1 mg/ml[a]	RC	0.2 mg/ml[a]	Visually compatible for 24 hr at 23 °C	1877	C
Nitroglycerin	LY	0.4 mg/ml[c]	ES	0.4 mg/ml[c]	Physically compatible for 3 hr	1316	C
Nitroglycerin with dobutamine HCl	LY LI	0.4 mg/ml[c] 4 mg/ml[c]	ES	0.4 mg/ml[c]	Physically compatible for 3 hr	1316	C
Nitroglycerin with dopamine HCl	LY DCC	0.4 mg/ml[c] 3.2 mg/ml[c]	ES	0.4 mg/ml[c]	Physically compatible for 3 hr	1316	C
Nitroglycerin with lidocaine HCl	LY AB	0.4 mg/ml[c] 8 mg/ml[c]	ES	0.4 mg/ml[c]	Physically compatible for 3 hr	1316	C
Pancuronium bromide	ES	0.05 mg/ml[a]	ES	0.2 mg/ml[a]	Physically compatible for 24 hr at 28 °C	1337	C
Propofol	ZEN	10 mg/ml	ES	0.4 mg/ml[a]	Physically compatible for 1 hr at 23 °C with no increase in particle content	2066	C
Tacrolimus	FUJ	1 mg/ml[b]	ES	0.004 mg/ml[a]	Visually compatible for 24 hr at 25 °C	1630	C
Theophylline	TR	4 mg/ml	ES	0.2 mg/ml[a]	Visually compatible for 6 hr at 25 °C protected from light	1793	C
TNA #218 to #226[e]			AB	0.4 mg/ml[a]	Visually compatible with no precipitate or emulsion damage apparent in 4 hr at 23 °C protected from light	2215	C
TPN #212 to #215[e]			AB	0.4 mg/ml[a]	Physically compatible with no change in measured turbidity or increase in particle content in 4 hr at 23 °C protected from light	2109	C
Vecuronium bromide	OR	0.1 mg/ml[a]	ES	0.2 mg/ml[a]	Physically compatible for 24 hr at 28 °C	1337	C

[a]*Tested in dextrose 5% in water.*
[b]*Tested in sodium chloride 0.9%.*
[c]*Tested in both dextrose 5% in water and sodium chloride 0.9%.*
[d]*Tested in sterile water for injection.*
[e]*Refer to Appendix I for the composition of parenteral nutrition solutions. TNA indicates a 3-in-1 admixture, and TPN indicates a 2-in-1 admixture.*

Additional Compatibility Information

Solutions— Dextrose 5% in water is the recommended infusion solution for admixture (1-9/98; 4; 90; 91). However, it has been reported that solutions of sodium nitroprusside in either dextrose or saline exposed to light exhibit decomposition similar in rate and degree. The dextrose admixture turns blue more rapidly than the drug in saline solution (732).

Another study found no decomposition of sodium nitroprusside 50 and 100 mg/L in dextrose 5% in water, sodium chloride 0.9%, and Ringer's injection, lactated, after 48 hours of storage when protected from light. The authors concluded that there was no factual basis for the restriction of sodium nitroprusside infusions to dextrose 5% in water (958).

Sodium nitroprusside 1 mg/ml in six solutions in PVC bags was evaluated for production of cyanide, produced by sodium nitroprusside degradation from exposure to 300 foot-candles of light for 72 hours. The solutions tested included three nonelectrolyte solutions (dextrose 5% in water, dextrose 10% in water, distilled water) and three electrolyte solutions (sodium chloride 0.9%, Ringer's injection, lactated, Ringer's injection, lactated, with dextrose 5%). Analysis was performed with a cyanide ion-specific electrode. There was no difference in the amount of cyanide produced among the solutions throughout the first 24 hours. However, the electrolyte solutions exhibited statistically significant lower mean cyanide ion concentrations, about 2 to 5 ppm, than the nonelectrolyte solutions (about 7 to 9 ppm). These levels of cyanide are an order of magnitude greater than in light-protected solutions. The authors concluded that electrolyte solutions may be preferable to dextrose 5% in water for sodium nitroprusside administration and that all doses should be prepared as fresh as possible and protected from light (2023).

Additives and Trace Contaminants— Sodium nitroprusside reacts with even minute quantities of a wide variety of inorganic and organic substances, forming highly colored reaction products (usually blue, green, or dark red). Such solutions should not be used. It is, therefore, recommended that no drug or preservative be added to sodium nitroprusside solutions (1-9/98; 4).

Dobutamine, Dopamine, Lidocaine, and Nitroglycerin— Dobutamine HCl (Lilly) 4 mg/ml, dopamine HCl (Dupont Critical Care) 3.2 mg/ml, lidocaine HCl (Abbott) 8 mg/ml, nitroglycerin (Lyphomed) 0.4 mg/ml, and sodium nitroprusside (Elkins-Sinn) 0.4 mg/ml, prepared in dextrose 5% in water and sodium chloride 0.9%, were combined in equal quantities in all possible combinations of two, three, four, and five drugs and then evaluated for physical compatibility. No physical incompatibility was observed in any combination within the three-hour study period (1316).

SODIUM PHOSPHATES
AHFS 40:12

American Pharmaceutical Partners

Products— Sodium phosphates additive solution (American Pharmaceutical Partners) is available in 5-, 15-, and 50-ml vials. Each milliliter contains monobasic sodium phosphate monohydrate 276 mg and dibasic sodium phosphate anhydrous 142 mg. The phosphorus concentration is 3 mmol/ml (93 mg/ml), and the sodium content is 4 mEq/ml (92 mg/ml) (1-9/98).

The additive solution is a concentrate and must be diluted for use (1-9/98).

pH— Approximately 5.7 (1-9/98).

Osmolarity— The osmolarity of sodium phosphates additive solution is calculated to be about 12 mOsm/ml (1-9/98).

Administration— Sodium phosphates additive solution must be diluted and thoroughly mixed in a larger volume of fluid before use. It should be infused slowly to avoid phosphate intoxication (1-4/95).

Stability— Sodium phosphates additive solution should be stored at controlled room temperature. The solution should be inspected for discoloration or particulate matter prior to use and should be used only if it is clear. The injection contains no antibacterial preservative. After the vials have been entered, discard any unused portions (1-9/98).

Compatibility Information

Y-Site Injection Compatibility (1:1 Mixture)

Sodium phosphates

Drug	Mfr	Conc	Mfr	Conc	Remarks	Ref	C/I
Ciprofloxacin	BAY	2 mg/ml[a]	AB	3 mmol/ml[a]	Subvisual microcrystals form in 1 hr at 23 °C	1972	**I**
	BAY	2 mg/ml[b]	AB	3 mmol/ml[b]	White crystalline precipitate forms immediately	1971; 1972	**I**
TNA #218 to #226[c]			AB	3 mmol/ml	Damage to emulsion integrity occurs immediately with free oil formation possible	2215	**I**
TPN #212 to #215[c]			AB	3 mmol/ml	Increased turbidity forms immediately	2109	**I**

[a]*Tested in dextrose 5% in water.*
[b]*Tested in both sodium chloride 0.9% and 0.45%.*
[c]*Refer to Appendix I for the composition of parenteral nutrition solutions. TNA indicates a 3-in-1 admixture, and TPN indicates a 2-in-1 admixture.*

Additional Compatibility Information

Metal Ions— Phosphates may be incompatible with metal ions such as magnesium and calcium. A number of studies using potassium phosphate have been performed. For additional information, refer to the potassium phosphate monograph.

UNRECOGNIZED CALCIUM PHOSPHATE PRECIPITATION IN A 3-IN-1 PARENTERAL NUTRITION MIXTURE RESULTED IN PATIENT DEATH.

The potential for the formation of a calcium phosphate precipitate in parenteral nutrition solutions is well studied and documented (1771; 1777), but the information is complex and difficult to apply to the clinical situation (1770; 1772; 1777). The incorporation of fat emulsion in 3-in-1 parenteral nutrition solutions obscures any precipitate that is present, which has led to substantial debate on the dangers associated with 3-in-1 parenteral nutrition mixtures and when or if the danger to the patient is warranted therapeutically (1770-1772; 2031-2036). Because such precipitation may be life-threatening to patients (2037), the Food and Drug Administration issued a Safety Alert containing the following recommendations (1769):

"1. The amounts of phosphorus and of calcium added to the admixture are critical. The solubility of the added calcium should be calculated from the volume at the time the calcium is added. It should not be based upon the final volume.

Some amino acid injections for TPN admixtures contain phosphate ions (as a phosphoric acid buffer). These phosphate ions and the volume at the time the phosphate is added should be considered when calculating the concentration of phosphate additives. Also, when adding calcium and phosphate to an admixture, the phosphate should be added first.

The line should be flushed between the addition of any potentially incompatible components.

2. A lipid emulsion in a three-in-one admixture obscures the presence of a precipitate. Therefore, if a lipid emulsion is needed, either (1) use a two-in-one admixture with the lipid infused separately, or (2) if a three-in-one admixture is medically necessary, then add the calcium before the lipid emulsion and according to the recommendations in number 1 above.

If the amount of calcium or phosphate which must be added is likely to cause a precipitate, some or all of the calcium should be administered separately. Such separate infusions must be properly diluted and slowly infused to avoid serious adverse events related to the calcium.

3. When using an automated compounding device, the above steps should be considered when programming the device. In addition, automated compounders should be maintained and operated according to the manufacturer's recommendations.

Any printout should be checked against the programmed admixture and weight of components.

4. During the mixing process, pharmacists who mix parenteral nutrition admixtures should periodically agitate the admixture and check for precipitates. Medical or home care personnel who start and monitor these infusions should carefully inspect for the presence of precipitates both before and during infusion. Patients and care givers should be trained to visually inspect for signs of precipitation. They also should be advised to stop the infusion and seek medical assistance if precipitates are noted.

5. A filter should be used when infusing either central or peripheral parenteral nutrition admixtures. At this time, data have not been submitted to document which size filter is most effective in trapping precipitates.

Standards of practice vary, but the following is suggested: a 1.2-μm air-eliminating filter for lipid-containing admixtures and a 0.22-μm air-eliminating filter for non-lipid-containing admixtures.

6. Parenteral nutrition admixtures should be administered within the following time frames: if stored at room temperature, the infusion should be started within 24 hours after mixing; if stored at refrigerated temperatures, the infusion should be started within 24 hours of rewarming. Because warming parenteral nutrition admixtures may contribute to the formation of precipitates, once administration begins, care should be taken to avoid excessive warming of the admixture.

Persons administering home care parenteral nutrition admixtures may need to deviate from these time frames. Pharmacists who initially prepare these admixtures should check a reserve sample for precipitates over the duration and under the conditions of storage.

7. If symptoms of acute respiratory distress, pulmonary emboli, or interstitial pneumonitis develop, the infusion should be stopped immediately and thoroughly checked for precipitates. Appropriate medical interventions should be instituted. Home care personnel and patients should immediately seek medical assistance."

Calcium Phosphate Precipitation Fatalities— Hill et al. reported fatal cases of paroxysmal respiratory failure in two previously healthy women receiving peripheral vein parenteral nutrition. The patients experienced sudden cardiopulmonary arrest consistent with pulmonary emboli. The authors used in vitro simulations and an animal model to conclude that unrecognized calcium phosphate precipitation in a 3-in-1 total nutrition admixture caused the fatalities. The precipitation resulted during compounding by introducing calcium and phosphate near to one another in the compounding sequence and prior to complete fluid addition. This resulted in a temporarily high concentration of the drugs and precipitation of calcium phosphate. Observation of the precipitate was obscured by the incorporation of 20% fat emulsion, intravenous into the nutrition mixture. No filter was used during infusion of the fatal nutrition admixtures (2037).

Calcium salts are conditionally compatible with phosphates in parenteral nutrition solutions. The incompatibility is dependent on a solubility and concentration phenomenon and is not entirely predictable. Precipitation may occur during compounding or at some time after compounding is completed.

NOTE: Some amino acid solutions inherently contain calcium and phosphate, which must be considered in any projection of compatibility. See the amino acid injection monograph, Table 1.

It has been noted that the order of mixing of calcium and phosphate may affect compatibility at elevated concentrations. Addition of phosphate should precede calcium (313).

Sodium phosphate was used in a study by Henry et al. (608). The maximum concentrations of calcium (as chloride and gluconate) and phosphate that can be maintained without precipitation in a parenteral nutrition solution consisting of FreAmine II 4.25% and dextrose 25% for 24 hours at 30 °C were determined. The results are depicted in Figure 1.

Henry et al. noted that the amino acids in parenteral nutrition solutions form soluble complexes with calcium and phosphate, reducing the available free calcium and phosphate that can form insoluble precipitates. The concentration of calcium available for precipitation is greater with the chloride salt compared to the gluconate salt, at least in part because of differences in dissociation characteristics. This can be seen in Figure 1 by the greater concentration of calcium gluconate that can be mixed with sodium phosphate (608).

In addition to the concentrations of phosphate and calcium and the salt form of the calcium, Henry et al. noted that the concentration of amino acids and the time and temperature of storage altered the formation of calcium phosphate in parenteral nutrition solutions. As the temperature was increased, the incidence of precipitate formation also increased. This result was attributed, at least in part, to a greater degree of dissociation of the calcium and phosphate complexes and the decreased solubility of calcium phosphate. Therefore, it is possible for a solution to be stored at 4 °C with no precipitation but, on warming to room temperature, a precipitate will form over time (608).

Poole et al. determined the solubility characteristics of calcium and phosphate in pediatric parenteral nutrition solutions composed of Aminosyn 0.5, 2, and 4% with dextrose 10 to 25%. Also present were electrolytes and vitamins. Sodium phosphate was added sequentially in phosphorus concentrations from 10 to 30 mmol/L. Calcium gluconate was added last in amounts ranging from 1 to 10 g/L. The solutions were stored at 25 °C for 30 hours and examined visually and microscopically for precipitation. The authors found that higher concentrations of Aminosyn increased the solubility of calcium and phosphate. Precipitation occurred at lower calcium and phosphate concentrations in the 0.5% solution compared to the 2 and 4% solutions. For example, at a phosphorus concentration of 30 mmol/L, precipitation occurred at calcium gluconate concentrations of about 1, 2, and 4 g/L in the 0.5, 2, and 4% Aminosyn mixtures, respectively. Similarly, at a calcium gluconate concentration of 8 g/L and above, precipitation occurred at phosphorus concentrations of about 13, 17, and 22 mmol/L in the 0.5, 2, and 4% solutions, respectively. The dextrose concentration did not appear to affect the calcium and phosphate solubility significantly (1042).

Koorenhof and Timmer reported the maximum allowable concentrations of calcium and phosphate in a 3-in-1 parenteral nutrition mixture for children (TNA #192 in Appendix I). Added calcium was varied from 1.5 to 150 mmol/L, while added phosphate was varied from 21 to 300 mmol/L. The mixtures were stable for 48 hours at 22 and 37 °C as long as the pH was not greater than 5.7, the calcium concentration was below 16 mmol/L, the phosphate concentration was below 52 mmol/L, and the product of the calcium and phosphate concentrations was below 250 $mmol^2/L^2$ (1773).

MacKay et al. reported additional calcium and phosphate solubility curves for specialty parenteral nutrition solutions based on NephrAmine and also HepatAmine at concentrations of 0.8, 1.5, and 2% as the sources of amino acids. The solutions also contained dextrose 10%, with cysteine and pH adjustment to simulate addition of fat emulsion used in some admixtures. Calcium and phosphate solubility followed the hyperbolic patterns reported by Eggert et al. (609). Temperature, time, and pH affected calcium and phosphate solubility, with pH having the greatest effect (2038).

Shatsky et al. reported the maximum sodium phosphate concentrations for given amounts of calcium gluconate that could be ad-

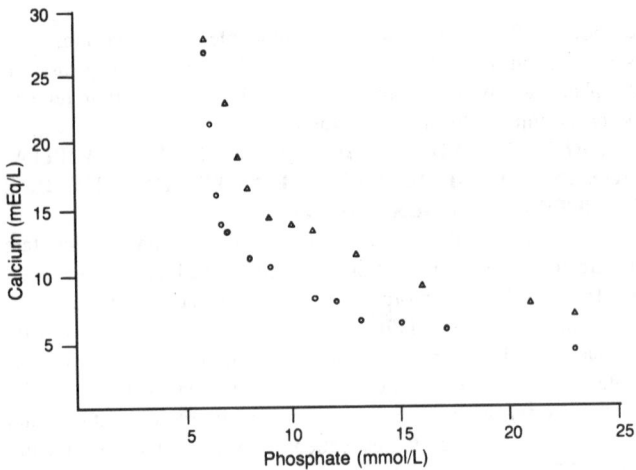

Figure 1. *Maximum solubilities of calcium chloride (○) and calcium gluconate (△) with sodium phosphate in an amino acid 4.25% – dextrose 25% solution at 30 °C*

mixed in parenteral nutrition solutions containing TrophAmine in varying quantities (with cysteine HCl 40 mg/g of amino acid) and dextrose 10%. The solutions also contained magnesium sulfate 4 mEq/L, potassium acetate 24 mEq/L, sodium chloride 32 mEq/L, pediatric multivitamins, and trace elements. The presence of cysteine HCl reduces the solution pH and increases the amount of calcium and phosphate that can be incorporated before precipitation occurs. The results of this study cannot be safely extrapolated to TPN solutions with compositions other than the ones tested. The admixtures were compounded with the sodium phosphate added last after thorough mixing of all other components. The authors noted this is not the preferred order of mixing (usually phosphate is added first and thoroughly mixed before adding calcium last); however, they believed this reversed order of mixing would provide a margin of error in cases where the proper order is not followed. After compounding, the solutions were stored for 24 hours at 40 °C. The maximum calcium and phosphate amounts that could be mixed in the various solutions were reported tabularly and are shown in Table 1 (2039). However, these results are not entirely consistent with the study of Hoie and Narducci using potassium phosphates (2196). See Potassium Phosphates monograph.

Fausel et al. evaluated calcium phosphate precipitation phenomena in a series of parenteral nutrition admixtures composed of dextrose 22%, amino acids (FreAmine III) 2.7%, and fat emulsion (Abbott) 0, 1, and 3.2%. Incorporation of calcium gluconate 19 to 24 mEq/L and phosphate (as sodium) 22 to 28 mmol/L resulted in visible precipitation in the fat-free admixtures. New precipitate continued to form over 14 days, even after repeated filtrations of the solutions through 0.2-μm filters. The presence of the amino acids increased calcium and phosphate solubility compared with simple aqueous solutions. However, the incorporation of the fat emulsion did not result in a statistically significant increase in calcium and phosphate solubility. The authors noted that the kinetics of calcium phosphate precipitate formation do not appear to be entirely predictable; both transient and permanent precipitation can occur either during the compounding process or at some time afterward. Because calcium phosphate precipitation can be clinically very dangerous, the use of inline filters was recommended. The filters should have a porosity appropriate to the parenteral nutrition admixture—1.2 μm for fat-containing and 0.2 or 0.45 μm for fat-free nutrition mixtures (2061).

A 2-ml fluid barrier of dextrose 5% in water in a microbore

Table 1. Maximum Amount of Phosphate (as Sodium) (mmol/L) Not Resulting in Precipitation According to the Study of Shatsky et al (2039). See CAUTION below.[a]

Calcium (as gluconate)	Amino Acid (as TrophAmine) plus Cysteine HCl 40 mg/g of Amino Acid				
	0%	0.4%	1%	2%	3%
9.8 mEq/L	0	27	42	60	66
14.7 mEq/L	0	15	18	30	36
19.6 mEq/L	0	6	15	27	30
29.4 mEq/L	0	3	6	21	24

[a]*CAUTION: The results cannot be safely extrapolated to solutions with formulas other than the ones tested. See text.*

retrograde infusion set failed to prevent precipitation when used between calcium gluconate 200 mg/2 ml and sodium phosphate 0.3 mmol/0.1 ml (1385).

The presence of magnesium in solutions may also influence the reaction between calcium and phosphate, including the nature and extent of precipitation (158; 159).

The interaction of calcium and phosphate in parenteral nutrition solutions is a complex phenomenon. Various factors have been identified as playing a role in the solubility or precipitation of a given combination, including (608, 609; 1042; 1063; 1427):

1. Concentration of calcium
2. Salt form of calcium
3. Concentration of phosphate
4. Concentration of amino acids
5. Amino acids composition
6. Concentration of dextrose
7. Temperature of solution
8. pH of solution
9. Presence of other additives
10. Order of mixing

Enhanced precipitate formation would be expected from such factors as high concentrations of calcium and phosphate, increases in solution pH, decreased amino acid concentrations, increases in temperature, addition of calcium prior to phosphate, lengthy standing times or slow infusion rates, and use of calcium as the chloride salt (854).

Ciprofloxacin— Admixing ciprofloxacin with sodium phosphates has resulted in reports of both compatibility and incompatibility (see table above.) Combining the two drugs in sodium chloride 0.45% or 0.9% can result in a large amount of white crystalline precipitate forming (1971; 1972), while the same concentrations in dextrose 5% in water result in little or no precipitate formation (1628; 1972). This dependency of precipitation on the nature of the infusion solution may extend to potassium phosphates as well. Although ciprofloxacin has been reported to be compatible with potassium phosphates in dextrose 5% in water (1628), the manufacturer has had reports of precipitation of these two drugs. Unfortunately, the infusion solution vehicles involved in the precipitations were not identified (2009).

STREPTOKINASE
AHFS 20:40

Streptase   **Astra**

Products— Streptokinase (Astra) is available as a lyophilized powder in 6.5-ml vials containing 250,000, 750,000, or 1,500,000 I.U. and in 50-ml infusion bottles containing 1,500,000 I.U. Each vial or infusion bottle of the products also contains cross-linked gelatin polypeptides 25 mg, sodium L-glutamate 25 mg, and human albumin 100 mg as stabilizers with sodium hydroxide to adjust pH (2).

Reconstitute streptokinase (Astra) in vials or in the infusion bottles with 5 ml of sodium chloride 0.9% or dextrose 5% in water, directing the diluent against the sides of the vials rather than the drug powder. Roll and tilt the vials gently to effect dissolution; do not shake, to avoid foam formation. The reconstituted solution may be diluted further for administration; the contents of the vials may be diluted up to 500 ml in glass bottles or 50 ml in plastic bags, while the streptokinase infusion bottle may have an additional 40 ml added after reconstitution yielding a total volume of 45 ml (2).

pH— The pH of the reconstituted solution is dependent on the diluent used (4).

Administration— Streptokinase is administered by intravenous, intra-arterial, or intracoronary infusion after dilution with sodium chloride 0.9% or dextrose 5% in water, using a volumetric infusion control device (2; 4). Reconstituted streptokinase solutions may adversely affect the accuracy of drop-counting infusion devices (both manual and instrument controlled) by altering drop size. Consequently, use of volumetric infusion control devices or syringe pumps is recommended for administration of streptokinase (4).

To clear an occluded intravenous cannula, streptokinase 250,000 I.U. is administered over 25 to 35 minutes in 2 ml of solution. The drug is infused directly into the cannula, which is then clamped for 2 hours, aspirated, and flushed with sodium chloride solution (2; 4).

Stability— Streptokinase, a white lyophilized powder, may have a slight yellow color in solution due to the presence of albumin (4). Intact vials should be stored at room temperature. Reconstituted solutions should be refrigerated and are stable for 24 hours (4). However, the manufacturers recommend use within eight hours (2).

Streptokinase is most stable in solution at pH 6 to 8. Small amounts of flocculation may occur; solutions with large amounts of flocculation should be discarded. Streptokinase may be filtered through a 0.8-μm or larger filter (2; 4).

Streptokinase flocculation was observed after transfer to 250-ml evacuated glass bottles. The flocculation was delayed in some cases but was always visible within 10 to 15 minutes. Although filtration removed the filaments, more flocculation occurred afterward. The flocculation was attributed to the acetic acid–sodium acetate buffer present in the evacuated glass bottles for glass preservation during sterilization (1517).

Compatibility Information

Y-Site Injection Compatibility (1:1 Mixture)

Streptokinase

Drug	Mfr	Conc	Mfr	Conc	Remarks	Ref	C/I
Dobutamine HCl	LI	2 mg/ml[a]	HO	30,000 units/ml[a]	Physically compatible for at least 48 hr by spectrophotometric and visual examination	1340	**C**
Dopamine HCl	DU	8 mg/ml[a]	HO	30,000 units/ml[a]	Physically compatible for at least 4 days by visual examination	1340	**C**
Heparin sodium	ES	100 units/ml[a]	HO	30,000 units/ml[a]	Physically compatible for at least 5 days by visual examination	1340	**C**
Lidocaine HCl	AB	8 mg/ml[a]	HO	30,000 units/ml[a]	Physically compatible for at least 3 days by visual examination	1340	**C**
Nitroglycerin	DU	0.2 mg/ml[a]	HO	30,000 units/ml[a]	Physically compatible for at least 5 days by visual examination	1340	**C**

[a]*Tested in dextrose 5% in water.*

Additional Compatibility Information

Solutions— Sodium chloride 0.9% is the preferred diluent for streptokinase, although dextrose 5% in water may be used. Solutions are stable for 24 hours under refrigeration (4).

Dextrans— Streptokinase is reported to be incompatible with dextrans (4).

Other Information

Units— One International Unit (I.U.) is equivalent to one Christensen Unit, which is the amount of streptokinase that activates sufficient human plasminogen to lyse a standard fibrin clot within 10 minutes in vitro (4).

STREPTOMYCIN SULFATE
AHFS 8:12.02

Pfizer
Pharma-Tek

Products— Streptomycin sulfate (Pfizer) is available as a solution in ampuls containing 1 g/2.5 ml (400 mg/ml). Each milliliter also contains sodium citrate dihydrate 12 mg, phenol 0.25% (w/v), and sodium metabisulfite 2 mg in water for injection (2).

Streptomycin sulfate (Pharma-Tek) is available as a lyophilized powder for injection in vials containing 1 g of drug with no preservatives. Reconstitute with 4.2, 3.2, or 1.8 ml of sterile water for injection to yield solutions containing 200, 250, or 400 mg/ml, respectively (4; 29).

pH— The injection from Pfizer has a pH of 5 to 8 (2). The reconstituted Pharma-Tek injection at a concentration of 200 mg/ml has a pH of 4.5 to 7 (4).

Administration— Streptomycin sulfate is administered by deep intramuscular injection well within the body of a relatively large muscle, such as the upper outer quadrant of the buttock in adults or the midlateral thigh in adults or children. Injection sites should be alternated (2; 4). Intravenous injection is not recommended (4), although it has been performed (1603).

Stability— Intact containers of streptomycin sulfate injection (Pfizer) should be stored under refrigeration at 2 to 8 °C. Intact vials of streptomycin sulfate lyophilized powder (Pharma-Tek) should be stored at controlled room temperature and protected from light (4).

Reconstituted solutions of streptomycin sulfate are stated to be stable for one week at room temperature and protected from light. However, no preservatives are present and the possibility of microbiological contamination must be considered (4).

Compatibility Information

Additive Compatibility

Streptomycin sulfate

Drug	Mfr	Conc/L	Mfr	Conc/L	Test Soln	Remarks	Ref	C/I
Amobarbital sodium						Physically incompatible	9	I
Amphotericin B		200 mg	BP	4 g	D5W	Haze develops over 3 hr	26	I
Bleomycin sulfate	BR	20 and 30 units	PF	4 g	NS	Physically compatible and bleomycin activity retained for 1 week at 4 °C. Streptomycin not tested	763	C
Chlorothiazide sodium	MSD					Physically incompatible	9	I
Heparin sodium						Physically incompatible	9	I
	AB	20,000 units		1 g		Precipitate forms within 1 hr	21	I
	BP	20,000 units	BP	4 g	D5W, NS	Immediate precipitation	26	I
Methohexital sodium	BP	2 g	BP	4 g	NS	Crystals produced	26	I
Norepinephrine bitartrate	WI					Physically incompatible	9	I
Pentobarbital sodium						Physically incompatible	9	I
Phenobarbital sodium	WI					Physically incompatible	9	I
Phenytoin sodium	PD					Physically incompatible	9	I
Sodium bicarbonate						Physically incompatible	9	I

Drugs in Syringe Compatibility

Streptomycin sulfate

Drug (in syringe)	Mfr	Amt	Mfr	Amt	Remarks	Ref	C/I
Ampicillin sodium	AY	500 mg		1 g/2 ml	No precipitate or color change within 1 hr at room temperature	99	C
	AY	500 mg	BP	1 g/2 ml	Physically compatible for 1 hr at room temperature	300	C
	AY	500 mg	BP[a]	0.75 g/1.5 ml	Precipitate forms within 1 hr at room temperature	300	I
	AY	500 mg	BP	1 g/1.5 ml	Syrupy solution forms	300	I
Heparin sodium	AB	20,000 units/1 ml		1 g	Physically incompatible	21	I
Penicillin G sodium		1 million units		1 g/2 ml	No precipitate or color change within 1 hr at room temperature	99	C

[a]Stabilized injection.

Y-Site Injection Compatibility (1:1 Mixture)

Streptomycin sulfate

Drug	Mfr	Conc	Mfr	Conc	Remarks	Ref	C/I
Esmolol HCl	DCC	10 mg/ml[a]	PF	10 mg/ml[a]	Physically compatible for 24 hr at 22 °C	1169	C

[a]Tested in dextrose 5% in water.

Additional Compatibility Information

In vitro testing of thiamine HCl, riboflavin-5'-phosphate, pyridoxine HCl, niacinamide, and ascorbic acid individually at concentrations of 0.1% with streptomycin sulfate 0.025% in sterile distilled water showed significant reduction in antibiotic activity in one hour at 25 °C (314).

Although piperacillin sodium and aminoglycosides act synergistically and have been used successfully clinically when recommended doses of each drug were administered, mixing piperacillin sodium directly in a syringe or infusion bottle with an aminoglycoside can result in substantial inactivation of the aminoglycoside (740).

STREPTOZOCIN
AHFS 10:00

Zanosar   **Pharmacia & Upjohn**

Products— Streptozocin (Pharmacia & Upjohn) is available in single-dose vials containing 1 g of drug and 220 mg of citric acid anhydrous. Sodium hydroxide may have been used to adjust the pH (2).

Reconstitute with 9.5 ml of sodium chloride 0.9% or dextrose 5% in water to provide a 100-mg/ml solution (2; 4).

pH— From 3.5 to 4.5 (2).

Administration— Streptozocin may be administered by rapid intravenous injection or intravenous infusion over 15 minutes to six hours (2; 4). Streptozocin has also been administered intra-arterially (4).

Stability— Intact vials containing a pale yellow powder should be refrigerated and protected from light (2; 4).

The pale gold reconstituted solution is stable for 48 hours at room temperature or 96 hours under refrigeration (4). However, the manufacturer recommends use within 12 hours because the product does not contain an antibacterial preservative (2; 4).

Filtration— Streptozocin 10 to 200 μg/ml exhibited no loss due to sorption to either cellulose nitrate/cellulose acetate ester (Millex OR) or Teflon (Millex FG) filters (1415; 1416).

Compatibility Information

Y-Site Injection Compatibility (1:1 Mixture)

Streptozocin

Drug	Mfr	Conc	Mfr	Conc	Remarks	Ref	C/I
Allopurinol sodium	BW	3 mg/ml[b]	UP	40 mg/ml[b]	Haze and small particles form in 1 hr and increase in 4 hr	1686	I
Amifostine	USB	10 mg/ml[a]	UP	40 mg/ml[a]	Physically compatible with no change in measured turbidity or increase in particle content in 4 hr at 23 °C	1845	C
Aztreonam	SQ	40 mg/ml[a]	UP	40 mg/ml[a]	Color changes from pale gold to red in 1 hr	1758	I
Cefepime HCl	BR	20 mg/ml[a]	UP	40 mg/ml[a]	Haze forms immediately and particles form in 1 hr. Deep red color forms in 4 hr	1689	I
Etoposide phosphate	BR	5 mg/ml[a]	UP	40 mg/ml[a]	Physically compatible with no change in measured turbidity or increase in particle content in 4 hr at 23 °C	2218	C
Filgrastim	AMG	30 μg/ml[a]	UP	40 mg/ml[a]	Physically compatible with no change in measured turbidity or increase in particle content in 4 hr at 22 °C	1687	C
Gemcitabine	LI	10 mg/ml[b]	UP	40 mg/ml[b]	Physically compatible with no change in measured turbidity or increase in particle content in 4 hr at 23 °C	2226	C
Granisetron HCl	SKB	1 mg/ml	UP	9.1 mg/ml[b]	Physically compatible with little or no loss of either drug by HPLC in 4 hr at 22 °C	1883	C

Y-Site Injection Compatibility (1:1 Mixture) (Cont.)

Streptozocin

Drug	Mfr	Conc	Mfr	Conc	Remarks	Ref	C/I
Melphalan HCl	BW	0.1 mg/ml[b]	UP	40 mg/ml[b]	Physically compatible with no change in measured turbidity or increase in particle content in 3 hr at 22 °C	1557	C
Ondansetron HCl	GL	1 mg/ml[b]	UP	30 mg/ml[a]	Physically compatible for 4 hr at 22 °C	1365	C
Piperacillin sodium–tazobactam sodium	LE	40 + 5 mg/ml[a]	UP	40 mg/ml[a]	Particles form in 1 hr	1688	I
Teniposide	BR	0.1 mg/ml[a]	UP	40 mg/ml[a]	Physically compatible with no subvisual haze or particle formation in 4 hr at 23 °C	1725	C
Thiotepa	IMM[c]	1 mg/ml[a]	UP	40 mg/ml[a]	Physically compatible with no change in measured turbidity or increase in particle content in 4 hr at 23 °C	1861	C
Vinorelbine tartrate	BW	1 mg/ml[b]	UP	40 mg/ml[b]	Physically compatible with no change in measured turbidity or increase in particle content in 4 hr at 22 °C	1558	C

[a]*Tested in dextrose 5% in water.*
[b]*Tested in sodium chloride 0.9%.*
[c]*Lyophilized formulation tested.*

Additional Compatibility Information

Solutions— Dextrose 5% in water and sodium chloride 0.9% are recommended for dilution of streptozocin for infusion (2). In these solutions, streptozocin 2 mg/ml is stable for at least 48 hours at room temperature or 96 hours under refrigeration (4). The manufacturer recommends use within 12 hours, however, because the product does not contain an antibacterial preservative (2; 4).

SUCCINYLCHOLINE CHLORIDE
AHFS 12:20

Anectine   **Glaxo Wellcome**

Products— Succinylcholine chloride (Glaxo Wellcome) is available in 10-ml multiple-dose vials. Each milliliter contains 20 mg of drug along with methylparaben 0.1%, sodium chloride for isotonicity, and hydrochloric acid for pH adjustment (2). Also available are 50- and 100-mg/ml concentrations from other manufacturers (29).

pH— From 3 to 4.5 (4). Glaxo Wellcome indicates that the pH is adjusted to 3.5 (2).

Osmolality— The osmolality of succinylcholine chloride 50 mg/ml was determined to be 409 mOsm/kg (1233).

Administration— Succinylcholine chloride is usually administered by direct intermittent intravenous injection or intravenous infusion. For continuous intravenous infusion, a 1- to 2-mg/ml (0.1 to 0.2%) solution is prepared, usually in 250 to 1000 ml of compatible fluid. If necessary, when a suitable vein is inaccessible, a maximum of 150 mg of the drug may be administered by deep intramuscular injection, preferably high into the deltoid muscle (2; 4).

Stability— Commercially available injections of succinylcholine chloride should be stored at 2 to 8 °C to retard potency loss (2; 4). Glaxo Wellcome indicates that the drug is stable for up to 14 days at room temperature (2; 1433). Abbott indicates that its product is stable for three months at temperatures up to 25 °C. Squibb cites a three-month stability period for its 100-mg/ml concentration and a six-month stability period for the 20- and 50-mg/ml concentrations at room temperature (1239). In one study, storage for seven days at 40 °C followed by storage at 25 °C for four weeks was used to simulate the worst case of shipping followed by storage on an emergency cart. Calculated loss of potency at room temperature was 1%/week; at 40 °C, it was 3.2%/week. Therefore, the loss was estimated to be about 7% under such conditions (960).

The dry powder form of succinylcholine chloride (Glaxo Wellcome) is stable at room temperature in an unopened container. After dilution to a concentration of 0.1 or 0.2%, the solution is stable for four weeks at 5 °C and one week at 25 °C (4). However, the product contains no antibacterial preservatives; the manufacturer recommends that unused solutions be discarded after 24 hours (2).

Succinylcholine chloride is unstable in alkaline solutions (2; 4) and decomposes in solutions with a pH greater than 4.5 (4). It is relatively stable in acidic solutions (2). The pH of maximum stability was found to be 3.75 to 4.50 (960).

Repackaging in Syringes— Succinylcholine chloride (Abbott) 20 mg/ml was packaged in both glass and polypropylene syringes (Becton-Dickinson) sealed with rubber luer-tip caps (Becton-Dickinson). The syringes were stored for 45 days at 4 °C, 22 °C and 50% relative humidity, and 37 °C and 85% relative humidity. At 4 °C, there was little or no succinylcholine chloride loss after 45 days in either glass or plastic syringes. At 22 °C and 50% relative humidity, about a 5% loss occurred in 45 days. However, at 37 °C and 85% relative humidity, the drug concentration fell below the acceptable USP limit after about 30 days (1209).

Succinylcholine chloride (Burroughs Wellcome) 20 mg/ml in dextrose 5% in water and in sodium chloride 0.9% (Baxter) was packaged as 10 ml in 12-ml plastic syringes (Monoject) and wrapped in aluminum foil. Samples were evaluated by HPLC analysis. Little or no loss of succinylcholine chloride occurred during 107 days of storage at 5 °C. At 25 °C, about 5 to 6% loss occurred in 100 days. Samples at an elevated temperature of 40 °C were stable through 22 days with only 3 to 4% loss but exhibited 12 to 14% loss at the next assay point of 63 days (1892).

Compatibility Information

Solution Compatibility

Succinylcholine chloride

Solution	Mfr	Mfr	Conc/L	Remarks	Ref	C/I
Dextran 6% in dextrose 5%	AB	AB	2 g	Physically compatible	3	C
Dextran 6% in sodium chloride 0.9%	AB	AB	2 g	Physically compatible	3	C
Dextrose–Ringer's injection combinations	AB	AB	2 g	Physically compatible	3	C
Dextrose–Ringer's injection, lactated, combinations	AB	AB	2 g	Physically compatible	3	C
Dextrose 5% in Ringer's injection, lactated	TR[a]	TR	1 g	Potency retained for 24 hr at 5 °C	282	C
Dextrose–saline combinations	AB	AB	2 g	Physically compatible	3	C
Dextrose 5% in sodium chloride 0.9%	TR[a]	TR	1 g	Potency retained for 24 hr at 5 °C	282	C
Dextrose 2½% in water	AB	AB	2 g	Physically compatible	3	C
Dextrose 5% in water	AB	AB	2 g	Physically compatible	3	C
	TR[a]	TR	1 g	Potency retained for 24 hr at 5 °C	282	C
Dextrose 10% in water	AB	AB	2 g	Physically compatible	3	C
Fructose 10% in sodium chloride 0.9%	AB	AB	2 g	Physically compatible	3	C
Fructose 10% in water	AB	AB	2 g	Physically compatible	3	C
Invert sugar 5 and 10% in sodium chloride 0.9%	AB	AB	2 g	Physically compatible	3	C
Invert sugar 5 and 10% in water	AB	AB	2 g	Physically compatible	3	C
Ionosol products	AB	AB	2 g	Physically compatible	3	C
Ringer's injection	AB	AB	2 g	Physically compatible	3	C
Ringer's injection, lactated	AB	AB	2 g	Physically compatible	3	C
	TR[a]	TR	1 g	Potency retained for 24 hr at 5 °C	282	C
Sodium chloride 0.45%	AB	AB	2 g	Physically compatible	3	C
Sodium chloride 0.9%	AB	AB	2 g	Physically compatible	3	C
	TR[a]	TR	1 g	Potency retained for 24 hr at 5 °C	282	C
Sodium lactate ⅙ M	AB	AB	2 g	Physically compatible	3	C

[a]*Tested in both glass and PVC containers.*

Additive Compatibility

Succinylcholine chloride

Drug	Mfr	Conc/L	Mfr	Conc/L	Test Soln	Remarks	Ref	C/I
Amikacin sulfate	BR	5 g	SQ	2 g	D5LR, D5R, D5S, D5W, D10W, IS10, LR, NS, R, SL	Physically compatible and potency of both retained for 24 hr at 25 °C	294	C
Isoproterenol HCl	WI	4 mg	AB	2 g		Physically compatible	59	C
Meperidine HCl	WI	100 mg	AB	2 g		Physically compatible	3	C
Methyldopate HCl	MSD	1 g	AB	2 g	D, D–S, S	Physically compatible	23	C
Morphine sulfate		16.2 mg	AB	2 g		Physically compatible	3	C
Norepinephrine bitartrate	WI	8 mg	AB	2 g	D, D–S, S	Physically compatible	77	C
Pentobarbital sodium						Physically incompatible	9	I
	AB	500 mg	AB	2 g		Physically compatible	3	C
Scopolamine HBr		0.43 mg	AB	2 g		Physically compatible	3	C
Sodium bicarbonate	AB	2.4 mEq[a]	AB	1 g	D5W	Succinylcholine inactivated	772	I
Thiopental sodium	AB	25 g	AB	2 g		Haze or precipitate forms within 1 to 6 hr	3	I

[a]*One vial of Neut added to a liter of admixture.*

Drugs in Syringe Compatibility

Succinylcholine chloride

Drug (in syringe)	Mfr	Amt	Mfr	Amt	Remarks	Ref	C/I
Heparin sodium		2500 units/ 1 ml		100 mg/ 5 ml	Physically compatible for at least 5 min	1053	C

Y-Site Injection Compatibility (1:1 Mixture)

Succinylcholine chloride

Drug	Mfr	Conc	Mfr	Conc	Remarks	Ref	C/I
Etomidate	AB	2 mg/ml	AB	20 mg/ml	Visually compatible for up to 7 days at 25 °C	1801	C
Heparin sodium with hydrocortisone sodium succinate	RI UP	1000 units + 100 mg/L[a]	BW	20 mg/ml	Physically compatible for at least 4 hr at room temperature by visual and microscopic examination	322	C
Potassium chloride		40 mEq/L[a]	BW	20 mg/ml	Physically compatible for at least 4 hr at room temperature by visual and microscopic examination	322	C
Propofol	ZEN	10 mg/ml	AB	20 mg/ml[b]	Physically compatible for 1 hr at 23 °C with no increase in particle content	2066	C
Thiopental sodium	AB	25 mg/ml	AB	20 mg/ml	White cloudiness forms immediately followed by fine crystalline particles	1801	I

Y-Site Injection Compatibility (1:1 Mixture) (Cont.)

Succinylcholine chloride

Drug	Mfr	Conc	Mfr	Conc	Remarks	Ref	C/I
Vitamin B complex with C	RC	2 ml/L[a]	BW	20 mg/ml	Physically compatible for at least 4 hr at room temperature by visual and microscopic examination	322	C

[a]Tested in dextrose 5% in water, sodium chloride 0.9%, and Ringer's injection, lactated.
[b]Tested in dextrose 5% in water.

Additional Compatibility Information

Solutions— Dextrose 5% in water, sodium chloride 0.9% (2; 4), dextrose 5% in sodium chloride 0.9%, and sodium lactate ⅙ M have been recommended as diluents for infusing succinylcholine chloride (4).

Barbiturates— Succinylcholine chloride is unstable in alkaline solutions (2; 4) and decomposes in solutions with a pH greater than 4.5 (4). In combination with barbiturates, either free barbituric acid will precipitate or the succinylcholine chloride will be hydrolyzed, depending on the final pH of the admixture (2; 4; 21). Succinylcholine chloride should not be mixed with barbiturates in the same syringe or given simultaneously through the same needle (2).

A haze forms in 30 minutes when succinylcholine chloride is mixed with methohexital sodium (4).

Nafcillin— Additives, such as succinylcholine chloride, that may result in a final admixture pH below 5 should not be mixed with nafcillin sodium because of an increased rate of nafcillin decomposition (27).

SUFENTANIL CITRATE
AHFS 28:08.08

Products— Sufentanil citrate is available as a preservative-free aqueous injection in 1-, 2-, and 5-ml ampuls from several manufacturers. Each milliliter of solution contains sufentanil citrate equivalent to 50 μg of sufentanil base. Citric acid may have been used to adjust pH during manufacture (1-12/97).

pH— From 3.5 to 6 (17).

Administration— Sufentanil citrate is administered intravenously by slow injection or infusion. For labor and delivery, it may be administered epidurally. The drug has also been given intramuscularly (4).

Stability— Sufentanil citrate is a stable, clear, aqueous, preservative-free injection. The product should be stored at controlled room temperature and protected from light. It is hydrolyzed in acidic solutions (4).

pH Effects— Sufentanil citrate 5 μg/ml in a solution with a pH greater than 3 lost less than 1% potency in 48 weeks at 90 °C. However, at a pH of less than 2, the drug loss was 14% at 60 °C and 32% at 90 °C in 48 weeks (1755).

Freezing Solutions— Sufentanil citrate (Janssen) 5 μg/ml in sodium chloride 0.9% became nonhomogeneous and difficult to restore to homogeneity when frozen at −20 °C. The authors cautioned against freezing these solutions (1755).

Syringes— Sufentanil citrate (Janssen) 2 μg/ml in sodium chloride 0.9% was packaged in 50-ml polypropylene syringes (Omnifix, B. Braun) and stored at 21 °C. HPLC analysis, although variable, reported less than 10% sufentanil loss in 24 hours (2201).

Sorption— Sufentanil citrate (Janssen) 5 μg/ml in sodium chloride 0.9% in PVC/Kalex 3000 (phthalate ester) CADD pump reservoirs (Pharmacia) exhibited a 13% drug loss in two days at 32 °C due to sorption to the container. A slight white precipitate also formed in several containers. However, little or no loss occurred in reservoirs stored at 4 °C. In glass and polyethylene containers, the drug was stable by HPLC for at least 21 days at 4 and 32 °C (1755).

Sufentanil citrate (Janssen) at concentrations near 5 μg/ml in dextrose 5% in water in PVC/Kalex 3000 CADD pump reservoirs (Pharmacia) also sorbed to the container, although to a lesser extent than the sodium chloride 0.9% solution. HPLC analysis found losses of 5 to 6% in 7 days and 10% in 30 days at 32 °C. At 4 °C, little or no loss occurred in 30 days. In simulated epidural administration, losses in the first 5 ml of priming solution were 25 to 30%, but the concentration returned to about 94% after two hours and 99% after 48 hours (1756).

Sufentanil citrate (Janssen) 20 μg/ml in sodium chloride 0.9% in PVC/Kalex 3000 CADD pump reservoirs (Pharmacia) lost approximately 10 and 18% potency after 24 hours at 26 and 37 °C, respectively. Losses increased to about 22 and 30% after 10 days at 26 and 37 °C, respectively. In contrast, only about a 5% loss occurred after 10 days at 5 °C. The sufentanil losses, determined by HPLC analysis, were attributed to sorption to the container. The addition of bupivacaine HCl 3 mg/ml reduced sufentanil losses to no more than 5% at any of the three temperatures during 10 days of storage (1751).

The extent of sufentanil citrate sorption into PVC containers from aqueous solutions is influenced by the pH of the solution. Sufentanil citrate 5 μg/ml in sodium chloride 0.9% exhibited about 30% loss due to sorption to a PVC/phthalate ester container (CADD pump reservoir, Pharmacia Deltec) in one day at its natural pH of about 6. The extent of loss increased to 80% after 21 days of storage. However, combined with pH 4.6 citrate buffer, about 5% loss due to sorption occurred initially with little change thereafter (2042).

Sufentanil citrate (Janssen) 2 μg/ml in sodium chloride 0.9% was delivered from 50-ml polypropylene syringes (Omnifix, B. Braun) by a syringe pump (JMS-Syringe-Pump Model SP-100, Japan Medical Supply Company) through polyethylene extension sets (Original-Perfusor-Leitung, Type PE, B. Braun) or polyvinyl chloride extension sets (Original-Perfusor-Leitung, Type N, B. Braun), 0.2-μm epidural filters (Sterifix, B. Braun), and epidural catheters (Perifix, B. Braun) over 24 hours. The pump, syringes, and extension sets were kept at 21 °C while the filters and epidural catheters were kept at 36 °C. Running at 1 ml/hr, the delivered sufentanil concentration using PVC tubing was about 7 to 10% below the theoretical concentration throughout 24 hours. Using polyethylene tubing, losses were about 16% initially but the concentration re-

turned to expected levels within one to two hours and remained stable throughout the 24-hour delivery (2201).

Filtration— Sufentanil citrate (Janssen) 50 μg/10 ml in sodium chloride 0.9% was evaluated for drug loss when administered through filters or epidural catheters; 2.5-g cellulose acetate/cellulose nitrate 0.2-μm filters (Millex, Millipore) were utilized. Approximately 20% of the sufentanil was lost to the void volume and/or adsorption. This loss should be considered when a new filter is used (1667).

Sufentanil citrate (Janssen) 2 μg/ml in sodium chloride 0.9% delivered at 1 ml/hr through 0.2-μm epidural filters (Sterifix, B. Braun) during the first hour was 83% of the theoretical concentration and remained at reduced concentrations of 85 to 89% of theoretical through at least six hours. By 24 hours the concentration was near 96% of theoretical. The authors attributed the lower concentrations to sorption of sufentanil onto the filter (2201).

Compatibility Information

Solution Compatibility

Sufentanil citrate

Solution	Mfr	Mfr	Conc/L	Remarks	Ref	C/I
Dextrose 5% in water	[a]	JN	5 mg	10% sufentanil loss by HPLC in 30 days at 32 °C and little or no loss in 30 days at 4 °C	1756	C
Sodium chloride 0.9%	[a]	JN	20 mg	10 and 18% sufentanil losses by HPLC in 24 hr at 26 and 37 °C, respectively, due to sorption. 5% loss in 10 days at 5 °C	1751	I
	[a]	JN	5 mg	13% sufentanil loss by HPLC in 2 days at 32 °C due to sorption. Little or no loss in 25 days at 4 °C. Slight white precipitate forms within 6 days in some containers	1755	I
	FRE[b]	JN	5 mg	No sufentanil loss by HPLC in 21 days at 4 and 32 °C	1755	C
	[c]	JN	5 mg	No sufentanil loss by HPLC in 21 days at 4 and 32 °C	1755	C
	[a]	JN	5 mg	Visually compatible with 11% sufentanil loss in 48 hr at 32 °C. No loss in 48 hr when buffered to pH 4.6	2042	C

[a]Tested in PVC/Kalex 3000 (phthalate ester) CADD pump reservoirs.
[b]Tested in glass bottles.
[c]Tested in high-density polyethylene containers.

Additive Compatibility

Sufentanil citrate

Drug	Mfr	Conc/L	Mfr	Conc/L	Test Soln	Remarks	Ref	C/I
Bupivacaine HCl		3 g	JN	20 mg	NS[a]	5% sufentanil loss and no bupivacaine loss by HPLC in 10 days at 5, 26, and 37 °C	1751	C
	AST	2 g	JN	5 mg	D5W[a]	9% sufentanil loss and 5% bupivacaine loss by HPLC in 30 days at 32 °C. Little or no loss of either drug in 30 days at 4 °C	1756	C

Additive Compatibility (Cont.)

Sufentanil citrate

Drug	Mfr	Conc/L	Mfr	Conc/L	Test Soln	Remarks	Ref	C/I
	AST	2 g	JN	5 mg	NS[a]	Buffered with pH 4.6 citrate buffer. Visually compatible with little or no loss of either drug by HPLC in 48 hr at 32 °C	2042	**C**

[a]*Tested in PVC/Kalex 3000 (phthalate ester) CADD pump reservoirs.*

Drugs in Syringe Compatibility

Sufentanil citrate

Drug (in syringe)	Mfr	Amt	Mfr	Amt	Remarks	Ref	C/I
Atracurium besylate	BW	10 mg/ml		50 µg/ml	Physically compatible and atracurium chemically stable for 24 hr at 5 and 25 °C	1694	**C**
Atropine sulfate	LY	0.4 mg/ml	JN	50 µg/ml	Physically compatible with no subvisual haze or particle formation in 24 hr at 23 °C	1711	**C**
Dexamethasone sodium phosphate	AMR	4 mg/ml	JN	50 µg/ml	Physically compatible with no subvisual haze or particle formation in 24 hr at 23 °C	1711	**C**
Diazepam	ES	5 mg/ml	JN	50 µg/ml	White turbidity forms immediately. Precipitate forms in 24 hr at 23 °C	1711	**I**
Diphenhydramine HCl	SCN	50 mg/ml	JN	50 µg/ml	Physically compatible with no subvisual haze or particle formation in 24 hr at 23 °C	1711	**C**
Haloperidol lactate	MN	5 mg/ml	JN	50 µg/ml	Physically compatible with no subvisual haze or particle formation in 24 hr at 23 °C	1711	**C**
Hydroxyzine HCl	ES	50 mg/ml	JN	50 µg/ml	Physically compatible with no subvisual haze or particle formation in 24 hr at 23 °C	1711	**C**
Ketorolac tromethamine	SY	30 mg/ml	JN	50 µg/ml	Physically compatible with no subvisual haze or particle formation in 24 hr at 23 °C	1711	**C**
Lorazepam	WY	2 mg/ml	JN	50 µg/ml	Turbidity increases within 0.5 hr and continues to increase over 24 hr at 23 °C	1711	**I**
Methotrimeprazine	LE	20 mg/ml	JN	50 µg/ml	Physically compatible with no subvisual haze or particle formation in 24 hr at 23 °C	1711	**C**
Metoclopramide HCl	RB	5 mg/ml	JN	50 µg/ml	Physically compatible with no subvisual haze or particle formation in 24 hr at 23 °C	1711	**C**
Midazolam HCl	RC	5 mg/ml	JN	50 µg/ml	Physically compatible with no subvisual haze or particle formation in 24 hr at 23 °C	1711	**C**
Phenobarbital sodium	WY	60 mg/ml	JN	50 µg/ml	Haze forms immediately and particles form in 24 hr at 23 °C	1711	**I**
Phenytoin sodium	SO	50 mg/ml	JN	50 µg/ml	Small crystals form immediately. Large crystals settle to bottom in 24 hr at 23 °C	1711	**I**
Prochlorperazine edisylate	SCN	5 mg/ml	JN	50 µg/ml	Physically compatible with no subvisual haze or particle formation in 24 hr at 23 °C	1711	**C**
Scopolamine HBr	LY	0.43 mg/ml	JN	50 µg/ml	Physically compatible with no subvisual haze or particle formation in 24 hr at 23 °C	1711	**C**

Y-Site Injection Compatibility (1:1 Mixture)

				Sufentanil citrate			
Drug	*Mfr*	*Conc*	*Mfr*	*Conc*	*Remarks*	*Ref*	*C/I*
Amphotericin B cholesteryl sulfate complex	SEQ	0.83 mg/ml[a]	JN	0.05 mg/ml	Physically compatible with little or no change in measured turbidity or increase in particle content in 4 hr at 23 °C under fluorescent light	2117	**C**
Atropine sulfate	LY	0.4 mg/ml[a]	JN	12.5 μg/ml[a]	Physically compatible with no subvisual haze or particle formation in 24 hr at 23 °C	1711	**C**
Cisatracurium besylate	GW	0.1, 2, 5 mg/ml[a]	ES	0.0125 mg/ml[a]	Physically compatible with no change in measured turbidity or increase in particle content in 4 hr at 23 °C	2074	**C**
Dexamethasone sodium phosphate	AMR	1 mg/ml[a]	JN	12.5 μg/ml[a]	Physically compatible with no subvisual haze or particle formation in 24 hr at 23 °C	1711	**C**
Diazepam	ES	0.5 mg/ml[a]	JN	12.5 μg/ml[a]	Physically compatible with no subvisual haze or particle formation in 24 hr at 23 °C	1711	**C**
Diphenhydramine HCl	SCN	2 mg/ml[a]	JN	12.5 μg/ml[a]	Physically compatible with no subvisual haze or particle formation in 24 hr at 23 °C	1711	**C**
Etomidate	AB	2 mg/ml	JN	0.05 mg/ml	Visually compatible for up to 7 days at 25 °C	1801	**C**
Haloperidol lactate	MN	0.2 mg/ml[a]	JN	12.5 μg/ml[a]	Physically compatible with no subvisual haze or particle formation in 24 hr at 23 °C	1711	**C**
Hydroxyzine HCl	ES	4 mg/ml[a]	JN	12.5 μg/ml[a]	Physically compatible with little subvisual haze or particle formation in 24 hr at 23 °C	1711	**C**
Ketorolac tromethamine	SY	1 mg/ml[a]	JN	12.5 μg/ml[a]	Physically compatible with no subvisual haze or particle formation in 24 hr at 23 °C	1711	**C**
Lorazepam	WY	0.1 mg/ml[a]	JN	12.5 μg/ml[a]	Large increase in measured turbidity occurs immediately and persists for 24 hr at 23 °C under fluorescent light	1711	**I**
Methotrimeprazine	LE	0.2 mg/ml[a]	JN	12.5 μg/ml[a]	Physically compatible with no subvisual haze or particle formation in 24 hr at 23 °C	1711	**C**
Metoclopramide HCl	RB	5 mg/ml	JN	12.5 μg/ml[a]	Physically compatible with no subvisual haze or particle formation in 24 hr at 23 °C	1711	**C**
Midazolam HCl	RC	0.2 mg/ml[a]	JN	12.5 μg/ml[a]	Physically compatible with no subvisual haze or particle formation in 24 hr at 23 °C	1711	**C**
Phenobarbital sodium	WY	2 mg/ml[a]	JN	12.5 μg/ml[a]	Physically compatible with no subvisual haze or particle formation in 24 hr at 23 °C	1711	**C**
Phenytoin sodium	ES	2 mg/ml[a]	JN	12.5 μg/ml[a]	Numerous tiny crystals form immediately and become larger over 24 hr at 23 °C under fluorescent light	1711	**I**

Y-Site Injection Compatibility (1:1 Mixture) (Cont.)

Sufentanil citrate

Drug	Mfr	Conc	Mfr	Conc	Remarks	Ref	C/I
Prochlorperazine edisylate	SCN	0.5 mg/ml[a]	JN	12.5 μg/ml[a]	Physically compatible with little subvisual haze or particle formation in 24 hr at 23 °C	1711	C
Propofol	ZEN	10 mg/ml	JN	0.05 mg/ml	Physically compatible for 1 hr at 23 °C with no increase in particle content	2066	C
Remifentanil HCl	GW	0.025 and 0.25 mg/ml[b]	ES	0.0125 mg/ml[a]	Physically compatible with no change in measured turbidity or increase in particle content in 4 hr at 23 °C	2075	C
Scopolamine HBr	LY	0.05 mg/ml[a]	JN	12.5 μg/ml[a]	Physically compatible with no subvisual haze or particle formation in 24 hr at 23 °C	1711	C
Thiopental sodium	AB	25 mg/ml	JN	0.05 mg/ml	White pellets form within 24 hr at 25 °C	1801	I

[a]*Tested in dextrose 5% in water.*
[b]*Tested in sodium chloride 0.9%.*

TACROLIMUS
AHFS 92:00

Prograf   **Fujisawa**

Products— Tacrolimus injection (Fujisawa) is available in 1-ml ampuls containing the equivalent of 5 mg of anhydrous tacrolimus per milliliter. In addition to tacrolimus, each milliliter contains polyoxyl 60 hydrogenated castor oil (surfactant) 200 mg and dehydrated alcohol, USP, 80% (v/v). The product is a concentrate that must be diluted for use in dextrose 5% in water or sodium chloride 0.9% (2).

Administration— Tacrolimus is administered by intravenous infusion diluted to a final concentration of 0.004 to 0.02 mg/ml (4 to 20 μg/ml) in dextrose 5% in water or sodium chloride 0.9%. Intravenous solution containers should be made of glass or polyethylene; PVC containers plasticized with diethylhexyl phthalate (DEHP) should be avoided due to leaching of plasticizer and decreased stability. For dilute solutions of tacrolimus, non-PVC tubing should also be used to minimize the potential for significant drug sorption (2).

Stability— Intact ampuls should be stored at temperatures between 5 and 25 °C (2). Tacrolimus exhibits a minimum rate of decomposition at pH values between 2 and 6; the rate of decomposition increases substantially at higher pH values (1926) and is unstable above pH 9 (2216). The manufacturer recommends that tacrolimus not be mixed with or even co-infused with solutions having a pH of 9 or greater (2).

Syringes— Tacrolimus (Fujisawa) 100 μg/ml in sodium chloride 0.9% was packaged 20 ml in 30-ml plastic syringes (Becton-Dickinson) and stored at 24 °C exposed to normal room light and protected from light. No decrease in tacrolimus concentration was found by HPLC analysis after storage for 24 hours (1864).

Sorption— Tacrolimus (Fujisawa) 100 μg/ml in dextrose 5% in water was delivered through PVC anesthesia extension tubing (Abbott), PVC intravenous administration set tubing (Venoset, Abbott), and fat emulsion tubing (Abbott). HPLC analysis of the delivered solutions found no loss of tacrolimus using the PVC administration set tubing and the fat emulsion tubing and only 2.5% drug loss from the PVC anesthesia extension tubing (1864).

However, tacrolimus has demonstrated drug loss in PVC containers that did not occur with other container materials (1864). See Solution Compatibility below. The manufacturer recommends that non-PVC tubing be used for low concentrations of tacrolimus to minimize the potential for significant drug sorption (2).

Compatibility Information

Solution Compatibility

Tacrolimus

Solution	Mfr	Mfr	Conc/L	Remarks	Ref	C/I
Dextrose 5% in water	AB[a]	FUJ	100 mg	5 to 8% loss by HPLC in 48 hr at 24 °C	1864	C

Solution Compatibility (Cont.)

Tacrolimus

Solution	Mfr	Mfr	Conc/L	Remarks	Ref	C/I
	AB[b]	FUJ	100 mg	15% loss in 6 hr and 19% loss in 24 hr by HPLC at 24 °C	1864	I
Sodium chloride 0.9%	BA[c]	FUJ	10 mg	Visually compatible with 4% loss by HPLC in 48 hr	1854	C
	AB[c]	FUJ	100 mg	10 to 12% loss by HPLC in 24 hr at 24 °C	1864	C
	AB[b]	FUJ	100 mg	12% loss in 6 hr and 16% loss in 24 hr by HPLC at 24 °C	1864	I
TPN #201[d]	c	FUJ	100 mg	Visually compatible with no loss by HPLC in 24 hr at 24 °C	1922	C

[a]Tested in glass and polyolefin containers.
[b]Tested in PVC containers.
[c]Tested in glass containers.
[d]Refer to Appendix I for the composition of parenteral nutrition solutions. TPN indicates a 2-in-1 admixture.

Additive Compatibility

Tacrolimus

Drug	Mfr	Conc/L	Mfr	Conc/L	Test Soln	Remarks	Ref	C/I
Cimetidine HCl	SKB	600 mg	FUJ	10 mg	NS[a]	Visually compatible with no cimetidine loss and 3% tacrolimus loss by HPLC in 48 hr at 24 °C	1854	C

[a]Tested in glass containers.

Y-Site Injection Compatibility (1:1 Mixture)

Tacrolimus

Drug	Mfr	Conc	Mfr	Conc	Remarks	Ref	C/I
Acyclovir sodium	BW	10 mg/ml[a]	FUJ	1 mg/ml[b]	Visually compatible for 24 hr at 25 °C	1630	C
Aminophylline	ES	2 mg/ml[a]	FUJ	1 mg/ml[b]	Visually compatible for 24 hr at 25 °C	1630	C
Amphotericin B	LY	5 mg/ml[a]	FUJ	1 mg/ml[c]	Visually compatible for 24 hr at 25 °C	1630	C
Ampicillin sodium	WY	20 mg/ml[a]	FUJ	1 mg/ml[b]	Visually compatible for 24 hr at 25 °C	1630	C
Ampicillin sodium–sulbactam sodium	RR	33.3 + 16.7 mg/ml[a]	FUJ	1 mg/ml[b]	Visually compatible for 24 hr at 25 °C	1630	C
Benztropine mesylate	MSD	1 mg/ml[a]	FUJ	1 mg/ml[b]	Visually compatible for 24 hr at 25 °C	1630	C
Calcium gluconate	ES	100 mg/ml	FUJ	1 mg/ml[b]	Visually compatible for 24 hr at 25 °C	1630	C
Cefazolin sodium	BR	40 mg/ml[a]	FUJ	1 mg/ml[b]	Visually compatible for 24 hr at 25 °C	1630	C
Cefotetan disodium	STU	40 mg/ml[a]	FUJ	1 mg/ml[b]	Visually compatible for 24 hr at 25 °C	1630	C
Ceftazidime	GL[e]	20 mg/ml[a]	FUJ	1 mg/ml[b]	Visually compatible for 24 hr at 25 °C	1630	C
	GW[e]	40 mg/ml[a]	FUJ	10 and 40 μg/ml[a]	Visually compatible with no loss of either drug by HPLC in 4 hr at 24 °C under fluorescent light	2216	C
	GW[e]	200 mg/ml[a]	FUJ	10 and 40 μg/ml[a]	Visually compatible with no loss of either drug by HPLC in 4 hr at 24 °C under fluorescent light	2216	C
Ceftriaxone sodium	RC	40 mg/ml[a]	FUJ	1 mg/ml[b]	Visually compatible for 24 hr at 25 °C	1630	C
Cefuroxime sodium	LI	30 mg/ml[a]	FUJ	1 mg/ml[b]	Visually compatible for 24 hr at 25 °C	1630	C

Y-Site Injection Compatibility (1:1 Mixture) (Cont.)

Tacrolimus

Drug	Mfr	Conc	Mfr	Conc	Remarks	Ref	C/I
Chloramphenicol sodium succinate	PD	20 mg/ml[a]	FUJ	1 mg/ml[b]	Visually compatible for 24 hr at 25 °C	1630	C
Cimetidine HCl	SKB	150 mg/ml[a]	FUJ	1 mg/ml[b]	Visually compatible for 24 hr at 25 °C	1630	C
Ciprofloxacin	MI	1 mg/ml[a]	FUJ	1 mg/ml[b]	Visually compatible for 24 hr at 25 °C	1630	C
Clindamycin phosphate	ES	12 mg/ml[a]	FUJ	1 mg/ml[b]	Visually compatible for 24 hr at 25 °C	1630	C
Dexamethasone sodium phosphate	ES	4 mg/ml[a]	FUJ	1 mg/ml[b]	Visually compatible for 24 hr at 25 °C	1630	C
Digoxin	WY	0.25 mg/ml	FUJ	1 mg/ml[b]	Visually compatible for 24 hr at 25 °C	1630	C
Diphenhydramine HCl	ES	1 mg/ml[a]	FUJ	1 mg/ml[b]	Visually compatible for 24 hr at 25 °C	1630	C
Dobutamine HCl	LI	1 mg/ml[a]	FUJ	1 mg/ml[b]	Visually compatible for 24 hr at 25 °C	1630	C
Dopamine HCl	ES	1.6 mg/ml[a]	FUJ	1 mg/ml[b]	Visually compatible for 24 hr at 25 °C	1630	C
Doxycycline hyclate	RR	5 mg/ml[a]	FUJ	1 mg/ml[b]	Visually compatible for 24 hr at 25 °C	1630	C
Erythromycin lactobionate	AB	20 mg/ml[a]	FUJ	1 mg/ml[b]	Visually compatible for 24 hr at 25 °C	1630	C
Esmolol HCl	DU	10 mg/ml[a]	FUJ	1 mg/ml[b]	Visually compatible for 24 hr at 25 °C	1630	C
Fluconazole	RR	2 mg/ml[a]	FUJ	1 mg/ml[b]	Visually compatible for 24 hr at 25 °C	1630	C
	PF	1 mg/ml[b]	FUJ	10 and 40 μg/ml[b]	Visually compatible with no loss of either drug by HPLC in 3 hr at 24 °C under fluorescent light	2225	C
	PF	15 mg/ 7.5 ml[b]	FUJ	50 and 200 μg/2.5 ml[b]	Mixed in the amounts indicated.[f] Visually compatible with no loss of either drug by HPLC in 3 hr at 24 °C under fluorescent light	2225	C
Furosemide	ES	10 mg/ml	FUJ	1 mg/ml[b]	Visually compatible for 24 hr at 25 °C	1630	C
Ganciclovir sodium	SY	50 mg/ml[a]	FUJ	1 mg/ml[b]	Visually compatible for 24 hr at 25 °C	1630	C
Gentamicin sulfate	SCN	4 mg/ml[a]	FUJ	1 mg/ml[b]	Visually compatible for 24 hr at 25 °C	1630	C
Haloperidol lactate	SO	2.5 mg/ml[a]	FUJ	1 mg/ml[b]	Visually compatible for 24 hr at 25 °C	1630	C
Heparin sodium	ES	10 units/ml[a]	FUJ	1 mg/ml[b]	Visually compatible for 24 hr at 25 °C	1630	C
Hydrocortisone sodium succinate	AB	50 mg/ml[a]	FUJ	1 mg/ml[b]	Visually compatible for 24 hr at 25 °C	1630	C
Hydromorphone HCl	KN	200 μg/ml[a]	FUJ	10 and 40 μg/ml[a]	Visually compatible with no loss of either drug by HPLC in 4 hr at 24 °C under fluorescent light	2216	C
	KN	2 mg/ml[a]	FUJ	10 and 40 μg/ml[a]	Visually compatible with no loss of either drug by HPLC in 4 hr at 24 °C under fluorescent light	2216	C
Imipenem–cilastatin sodium	MSD	10 mg/ml[b]	FUJ	1 mg/ml[b]	Visually compatible for 24 hr at 25 °C	1630	C
Insulin, regular	LI	0.1 unit/ml[a]	FUJ	1 mg/ml[b]	Visually compatible for 24 hr at 25 °C	1630	C
Isoproterenol HCl	ES	0.04 mg/ml[a]	FUJ	1 mg/ml[b]	Visually compatible for 24 hr at 25 °C	1630	C
Leucovorin calcium	ES	10 mg/ml[a]	FUJ	1 mg/ml[b]	Visually compatible for 24 hr at 25 °C	1630	C
Lorazepam	WY	1 mg/ml[a]	FUJ	1 mg/ml[b]	Visually compatible for 24 hr at 25 °C	1630	C
Methylprednisolone sodium succinate	UP	0.8 mg/ml[a]	FUJ	1 mg/ml[b]	Visually compatible for 24 hr at 25 °C	1630	C
Metoclopramide HCl	DU	0.2 mg/ml[a]	FUJ	1 mg/ml[b]	Visually compatible for 24 hr at 25 °C	1630	C
Metronidazole	AB	5 mg/ml	FUJ	1 mg/ml[b]	Visually compatible for 24 hr at 25 °C	1630	C

Y-Site Injection Compatibility (1:1 Mixture) (Cont.)

Tacrolimus

Drug	Mfr	Conc	Mfr	Conc	Remarks	Ref	C/I
Morphine sulfate	SCN	1 mg/ml[b]	FUJ	10 and 40 μg/ml[b]	Visually compatible with no loss of either drug by HPLC in 4 hr at 24 °C under fluorescent light	2216	C
	SCN	3 mg/ml[b]	FUJ	10 and 40 μg/ml[b]	Visually compatible with no loss of either drug by HPLC in 4 hr at 24 °C under fluorescent light	2216	C
Multivitamins	LY	0.001 ml/ml[a]	FUJ	1 mg/ml[b]	Visually compatible for 24 hr at 25 °C	1630	C
Nitroglycerin	DU	0.1 mg/ml[a]	FUJ	1 mg/ml[b]	Visually compatible for 24 hr at 25 °C	1630	C
Oxacillin sodium	BR	40 mg/ml[a]	FUJ	1 mg/ml[b]	Visually compatible for 24 hr at 25 °C	1630	C
Penicillin G potassium	BR	100,000 units/ml[a]	FUJ	1 mg/ml[b]	Visually compatible for 24 hr at 25 °C	1630	C
Perphenazine	SC	2.5 mg/ml[a]	FUJ	1 mg/ml[b]	Visually compatible for 24 hr at 25 °C	1630	C
Phenytoin sodium	ES	5 mg/ml[a]	FUJ	1 mg/ml[b]	Visually compatible for 4 hr at 25 °C. White haze forms by 24 hr	1630	C
Piperacillin sodium	LE	80 mg/ml[a]	FUJ	1 mg/ml[b]	Visually compatible for 24 hr at 25 °C	1630	C
Potassium chloride	AB	2 mEq/ml	FUJ	1 mg/ml[b]	Visually compatible for 24 hr at 25 °C	1630	C
Propranolol HCl	AY	1 mg/ml	FUJ	1 mg/ml[b]	Visually compatible for 24 hr at 25 °C	1630	C
Ranitidine HCl	GL	25 mg/ml[a]	FUJ	1 mg/ml[b]	Visually compatible for 24 hr at 25 °C	1630	C
Sodium bicarbonate	AB	1 mEq/ml	FUJ	1 mg/ml[b]	Visually compatible for 24 hr at 25 °C	1630	C
Sodium nitroprusside	ES	0.004 mg/ml[a]	FUJ	1 mg/ml[b]	Visually compatible for 24 hr at 25 °C	1630	C
Sodium tetradecyl sulfate	ES	10 mg/ml	FUJ	1 mg/ml[b]	Visually compatible for 24 hr at 25 °C	1630	C
TNA #218 to #226[d]			FUJ	1 mg/ml[a]	Visually compatible with no precipitate or emulsion damage apparent in 4 hr at 23 °C	2215	C
Tobramycin sulfate	BR	40 mg/ml	FUJ	1 mg/ml[b]	Visually compatible for 24 hr at 25 °C	1630	C
TPN #212 to #215[d]			FUJ	1 mg/ml[a]	Physically compatible with no change in measured turbidity or increase in particle content in 4 hr at 23 °C	2109	C
Trimethoprim–sulfamethoxazole	RC	1.6 + 8 mg/ml[a]	FUJ	1 mg/ml[b]	Visually compatible for 24 hr at 25 °C	1630	C
Vancomycin HCl	LI	5 mg/ml[a]	FUJ	1 mg/ml[b]	Visually compatible for 24 hr at 25 °C	1630	C

[a]Tested in dextrose 5% in water.
[b]Tested in sodium chloride 0.9%.
[c]Diluted with sterile water for injection.
[d]Refer to Appendix I for the composition of parenteral nutrition solutions. TNA indicates a 3-in-1 admixture, and TPN indicates a 2-in-1 admixture.
[e]Sodium carbonate–containing formulation tested.
[f]Final concentrations were 1.5 mg/ml of fluconazole and 5 and 20 μg/ml of tacrolimus.

Additional Compatibility Information

Solutions— The manufacturer recommends dilution of tacrolimus to 0.004 to 0.02 mg/ml in dextrose 5% in water or sodium chloride 0.9%. These solutions are reported to be stable for 24 hours (2).

Plasticizer Extraction— Parenteral products containing a large amount of a surfactant will extract the plasticizer DEHP from PVC containers and administration sets. Consequently, their use should be avoided. Instead, glass or polyethylene containers and non-DEHP plasticized administration sets are recommended (2; 4; 1683).

TENIPOSIDE
AHFS 10:00

Vumon   **Bristol-Myers Squibb**

Products— Teniposide (Bristol-Myers Squibb) is available in a non-aqueous solution in 5-ml ampuls containing 50 mg of drug. Each milliliter of solution contains teniposide 10 mg, benzyl alcohol 30 mg, N,N-dimethylacetamide 60 mg, polyoxyethylated castor oil (Cremophor EL) 500 mg, and dehydrated alcohol 42.7%. The pH is adjusted with maleic acid (2).

The product is a concentrate that must be diluted for use (2).

pH— Approximately 5 (2).

Administration— Teniposide is administered by slow intravenous infusion over at least 30 to 60 minutes after dilution in dextrose 5% in water or sodium chloride 0.9% to a final concentration of 0.1, 0.2, 0.4, or 1 mg/ml (2). Extended infusions of 0.1- and 0.2-mg/ml solutions over 24 hours have resulted in precipitation (2; 1502; 1521). The intravenous solution containers and sets used to administer teniposide should not contain the plasticizer diethylhexyl phthalate (DEHP) (2; 4). Extravasation should be avoided because of local tissue irritation and phlebitis. Tissue necrosis is unlikely (2; 4; 1561; 1562).

Stability— The teniposide concentrate is clear (2) but may exhibit a slight opalescence when diluted in infusion solutions due to the surfactant content (234).

Intact ampuls should be stored under refrigeration. Teniposide stability is not adversely affected by freezing (2) or exposure to normal room fluorescent light (1374).

The manufacturer does not recommend refrigeration of teniposide diluted in infusion solutions (2).

Sorption— No teniposide loss due to sorption to PVC containers has been observed (1374; 2053). See Additional Compatibility Information.

Precipitation— Although teniposide is chemically stable for at least 24 hours, precipitation from aqueous solutions has occurred irregularly and unpredictably even at 0.1 and 0.2 mg/ml, the lowest recommended concentrations (2; 1502; 1521). The precipitation rate depends on the formation of crystallization nuclei. Precipitation then proceeds rapidly. The formation of crystallization nuclei may be accelerated by agitation, contact with incompatible drugs or material surfaces, and, possibly, other factors (1374; 1502; 1521). The manufacturer recommends avoiding an inordinate amount of agitation during preparation, minimizing storage time prior to administration, and avoiding contact with other drugs and solutions. Even the compatibility of teniposide infusions with some infusion set materials and pumps cannot be assured (2; 1502; 1521).

Compatibility Information

Solution Compatibility

Teniposide

Solution	Mfr	Mfr	Conc/L	Remarks	Ref	C/I
Dextrose 5% in water	a	BR	400 mg	Physically compatible with up to 6% teniposide loss in 4 days at 21 °C under fluorescent light or in the dark	1374	C
Ringer's injection, lactated	a	BR	400 mg	Physically compatible with 1 to 3% teniposide loss in 4 days at 21 °C under fluorescent light or in the dark	1374	C
Sodium chloride 0.9%	b	BR	400 mg	Physically compatible with 2 to 4% teniposide loss in 4 days at 21 °C under fluorescent light or in the dark	1374	C
	a	BR	500, 600, 700 mg	Physically compatible for 4 days at 21 °C	1374	C

ªTested in glass containers.
ᵇTested in both glass and PVC containers.

Y-Site Injection Compatibility (1:1 Mixture)

Teniposide

Drug	Mfr	Conc	Mfr	Conc	Remarks	Ref	C/I
Acyclovir sodium	BW	7 mg/mlª	BR	0.1 mg/mlª	Physically compatible with no subvisual haze or particle formation in 4 hr at 23 °C	1725	C
Allopurinol	BW	3 mg/mlª	BR	0.1 mg/mlª	Physically compatible with no subvisual haze or particle formation in 4 hr at 23 °C	1725	C

Y-Site Injection Compatibility (1:1 Mixture) (Cont.)

Teniposide

Drug	Mfr	Conc	Mfr	Conc	Remarks	Ref	C/I
Amifostine	USB	10 mg/ml[a]	BR	0.1 mg/ml[a]	Physically compatible with no change in measured turbidity or increase in particle content in 4 hr at 23 °C	1845	C
Amikacin sulfate	BR	5 mg/ml[a]	BR	0.1 mg/ml[a]	Physically compatible with no subvisual haze or particle formation in 4 hr at 23 °C	1725	C
Aminophylline	AB	2.5 mg/ml[a]	BR	0.1 mg/ml[a]	Physically compatible with no subvisual haze or particle formation in 4 hr at 23 °C	1725	C
Amphotericin B	SQ	0.6 mg/ml[a]	BR	0.1 mg/ml[a]	Physically compatible with no subvisual haze or particle formation in 4 hr at 23 °C	1725	C
Ampicillin sodium	WY	20 mg/ml[b]	BR	0.1 mg/ml[a]	Physically compatible with no subvisual haze or particle formation in 4 hr at 23 °C	1725	C
Ampicillin sodium–sulbactam sodium	RR	20 + 10 mg/ ml[b]	BR	0.1 mg/ml[a]	Physically compatible with no subvisual haze or particle formation in 4 hr at 23 °C	1725	C
Aztreonam	SQ	40 mg/ml[a]	BR	0.1 mg/ml[a]	Physically compatible with no subvisual haze or particle formation in 4 hr at 23 °C	1725	C
Bleomycin sulfate	BR	1 unit/ml[b]	BR	0.1 mg/ml[a]	Physically compatible with no subvisual haze or particle formation in 4 hr at 23 °C	1725	C
Bumetanide	RC	0.04 mg/ml[a]	BR	0.1 mg/ml[a]	Physically compatible with no subvisual haze or particle formation in 4 hr at 23 °C	1725	C
Buprenorphine HCl	RKC	0.04 mg/ml[a]	BR	0.1 mg/ml[a]	Physically compatible with no subvisual haze or particle formation in 4 hr at 23 °C	1725	C
Butorphanol tartrate	BR	0.04 mg/ml[a]	BR	0.1 mg/ml[a]	Physically compatible with no subvisual haze or particle formation in 4 hr at 23 °C	1725	C
Calcium gluconate	AMR	40 mg/ml[a]	BR	0.1 mg/ml[a]	Physically compatible with no subvisual haze or particle formation in 4 hr at 23 °C	1725	C
Carboplatin	BR	5 mg/ml[a]	BR	0.1 mg/ml[a]	Physically compatible with no subvisual haze or particle formation in 4 hr at 23 °C	1725	C
Carmustine	BR	1.5 mg/ml[a]	BR	0.1 mg/ml[a]	Physically compatible with no subvisual haze or particle formation in 4 hr at 23 °C	1725	C
Cefazolin sodium	MAR	20 mg/ml[a]	BR	0.1 mg/ml[a]	Physically compatible with no subvisual haze or particle formation in 4 hr at 23 °C	1725	C
Cefoperazone sodium	RR	40 mg/ml[a]	BR	0.1 mg/ml[a]	Physically compatible with no subvisual haze or particle formation in 4 hr at 23 °C	1725	C

Y-Site Injection Compatibility (1:1 Mixture) (Cont.)

Teniposide

Drug	Mfr	Conc	Mfr	Conc	Remarks	Ref	C/I
Cefotaxime sodium	HO	20 mg/ml[a]	BR	0.1 mg/ml[a]	Physically compatible with no subvisual haze or particle formation in 4 hr at 23 °C	1725	**C**
Cefotetan disodium	STU	20 mg/ml[a]	BR	0.1 mg/ml[a]	Physically compatible with no subvisual haze or particle formation in 4 hr at 23 °C	1725	**C**
Cefoxitin sodium	MSD	20 mg/ml[a]	BR	0.1 mg/ml[a]	Physically compatible with no subvisual haze or particle formation in 4 hr at 23 °C	1725	**C**
Ceftazidime	LI[d]	40 mg/ml[a]	BR	0.1 mg/ml[a]	Physically compatible with no subvisual haze or particle formation in 4 hr at 23 °C	1725	**C**
Ceftizoxime sodium	FUJ	20 mg/ml[a]	BR	0.1 mg/ml[a]	Physically compatible with no subvisual haze or particle formation in 4 hr at 23 °C	1725	**C**
Ceftriaxone sodium	RC	20 mg/ml[a]	BR	0.1 mg/ml[a]	Physically compatible with no subvisual haze or particle formation in 4 hr at 23 °C	1725	**C**
Cefuroxime sodium	GL	20 mg/ml[a]	BR	0.1 mg/ml[a]	Physically compatible with no subvisual haze or particle formation in 4 hr at 23 °C	1725	**C**
Chlorpromazine HCl	SCN	2 mg/ml[a]	BR	0.1 mg/ml[a]	Physically compatible with no subvisual haze or particle formation in 4 hr at 23 °C	1725	**C**
Cimetidine HCl	SKB	12 mg/ml[a]	BR	0.1 mg/ml[a]	Physically compatible with no subvisual haze or particle formation in 4 hr at 23 °C	1725	**C**
Ciprofloxacin	MI	2 mg/ml[a]	BR	0.1 mg/ml[a]	Physically compatible with no subvisual haze or particle formation in 4 hr at 23 °C	1725	**C**
Cisplatin	BR	1 mg/ml	BR	0.1 mg/ml[a]	Physically compatible with no subvisual haze or particle formation in 4 hr at 23 °C	1725	**C**
Cladribine	ORT	0.015[b] and 0.5[c] mg/ml	BR	0.1 mg/ml[b]	Physically compatible with no change in measured turbidity or increase in particle content in 4 hr at 23 °C	1969	**C**
Clindamycin phosphate	AST	10 mg/ml[a]	BR	0.1 mg/ml[a]	Physically compatible with no subvisual haze or particle formation in 4 hr at 23 °C	1725	**C**
Cyclophosphamide	MJ	10 mg/ml[a]	BR	0.1 mg/ml[a]	Physically compatible with no subvisual haze or particle formation in 4 hr at 23 °C	1725	**C**
Cytarabine	CET	50 mg/ml	BR	0.1 mg/ml[a]	Physically compatible with no subvisual haze or particle formation in 4 hr at 23 °C	1725	**C**
Dacarbazine	MI	4 mg/ml[a]	BR	0.1 mg/ml[a]	Physically compatible with no subvisual haze or particle formation in 4 hr at 23 °C	1725	**C**

Y-Site Injection Compatibility (1:1 Mixture) (Cont.)

Teniposide

Drug	Mfr	Conc	Mfr	Conc	Remarks	Ref	C/I
Dactinomycin	MSD	0.01 mg/ml[a]	BR	0.1 mg/ml[a]	Physically compatible with no subvisual haze or particle formation in 4 hr at 23 °C	1725	**C**
Daunorubicin HCl	WY	1 mg/ml[a]	BR	0.1 mg/ml[a]	Physically compatible with no subvisual haze or particle formation in 4 hr at 23 °C	1725	**C**
Dexamethasone sodium phosphate	LY	1 mg/ml[a]	BR	0.1 mg/ml[a]	Physically compatible with no subvisual haze or particle formation in 4 hr at 23 °C	1725	**C**
Diphenhydramine HCl	ES	2 mg/ml[a]	BR	0.1 mg/ml[a]	Physically compatible with no subvisual haze or particle formation in 4 hr at 23 °C	1725	**C**
Doxorubicin HCl	CET	2 mg/ml	BR	0.1 mg/ml[a]	Physically compatible with no subvisual haze or particle formation in 4 hr at 23 °C	1725	**C**
Doxycycline hyclate	LY	1 mg/ml[a]	BR	0.1 mg/ml[a]	Physically compatible with no subvisual haze or particle formation in 4 hr at 23 °C	1725	**C**
Droperidol	JN	0.4 mg/ml[a]	BR	0.1 mg/ml[a]	Physically compatible with no subvisual haze or particle formation in 4 hr at 23 °C	1725	**C**
Enalaprilat	MSD	0.1 mg/ml[a]	BR	0.1 mg/ml[a]	Physically compatible with no subvisual haze or particle formation in 4 hr at 23 °C	1725	**C**
Etoposide	BR	0.4 mg/ml[a]	BR	0.1 mg/ml[a]	Physically compatible with no subvisual haze or particle formation in 4 hr at 23 °C	1725	**C**
Etoposide phosphate	BR	5 mg/ml[a]	BR	0.1 mg/ml[a]	Physically compatible with no change in measured turbidity or increase in particle content in 4 hr at 23 °C	2218	**C**
Famotidine	MSD	2 mg/ml[a]	BR	0.1 mg/ml[a]	Physically compatible with no subvisual haze or particle formation in 4 hr at 23 °C	1725	**C**
Floxuridine	RC	3 mg/ml[a]	BR	0.1 mg/ml[a]	Physically compatible with no subvisual haze or particle formation in 4 hr at 23 °C	1725	**C**
Fluconazole	RR	2 mg/ml	BR	0.1 mg/ml[a]	Physically compatible with no subvisual haze or particle formation in 4 hr at 23 °C	1725	**C**
Fludarabine phosphate	BX	1 mg/ml[a]	BR	0.1 mg/ml[a]	Physically compatible with no subvisual haze or particle formation in 4 hr at 23 °C	1725	**C**
Fluorouracil	AD	16 mg/ml[a]	BR	0.1 mg/ml[a]	Physically compatible with no subvisual haze or particle formation in 4 hr at 23 °C	1725	**C**
Furosemide	AB	3 mg/ml[a]	BR	0.1 mg/ml[a]	Physically compatible with no subvisual haze or particle formation in 4 hr at 23 °C	1725	**C**

Y-Site Injection Compatibility (1:1 Mixture) (Cont.)

Teniposide

Drug	Mfr	Conc	Mfr	Conc	Remarks	Ref	C/I
Ganciclovir sodium	SY	20 mg/ml[a]	BR	0.1 mg/ml[a]	Physically compatible with no subvisual haze or particle formation in 4 hr at 23 °C	1725	**C**
Gemcitabine HCl	LI	10 mg/ml[b]	BR	0.1 mg/ml[a]	Physically compatible with no change in measured turbidity or increase in particle content in 4 hr at 23 °C	2226	**C**
Gentamicin sulfate	LY	5 mg/ml[a]	BR	0.1 mg/ml[a]	Physically compatible with no subvisual haze or particle formation in 4 hr at 23 °C	1725	**C**
Granisetron HCl	SKB	0.05 mg/ml[a]	BMS	0.1 mg/ml[a]	Physically compatible with no change in measured turbidity or increase in particle content in 4 hr at 23 °C	2000	**C**
Haloperidol lactate	MN	0.2 mg/ml[a]	BR	0.1 mg/ml[a]	Physically compatible with no subvisual haze or particle formation in 4 hr at 23 °C	1725	**C**
Hydrocortisone sodium phosphate	MSD	1 mg/ml[a]	BR	0.1 mg/ml[a]	Physically compatible with no subvisual haze or particle formation in 4 hr at 23 °C	1725	**C**
Hydrocortisone sodium succinate	UP	1 mg/ml[a]	BR	0.1 mg/ml[a]	Physically compatible with no subvisual haze or particle formation in 4 hr at 23 °C	1725	**C**
Hydromorphone HCl	KN	0.5 mg/ml[a]	BR	0.1 mg/ml[a]	Physically compatible with no subvisual haze or particle formation in 4 hr at 23 °C	1725	**C**
Hydroxyzine HCl	WI	4 mg/ml[a]	BR	0.1 mg/ml[a]	Physically compatible with no subvisual haze or particle formation in 4 hr at 23 °C	1725	**C**
Idarubicin HCl	AD	0.5 mg/ml[a]	BR	0.1 mg/ml[a]	Unacceptable increase in turbidity occurs immediately	1725	**I**
Ifosfamide	MJ	25 mg/ml[a]	BR	0.1 mg/ml[a]	Physically compatible with no subvisual haze or particle formation in 4 hr at 23 °C	1725	**C**
Imipenem–cilastatin sodium	MSD	10 mg/ml[b]	BR	0.1 mg/ml[a]	Physically compatible with no subvisual haze or particle formation in 4 hr at 23 °C	1725	**C**
Leucovorin calcium	LE	2 mg/ml[a]	BR	0.1 mg/ml[a]	Physically compatible with no subvisual haze or particle formation in 4 hr at 23 °C	1725	**C**
Lorazepam	WY	0.1 mg/ml[a]	BR	0.1 mg/ml[a]	Physically compatible with no subvisual haze or particle formation in 4 hr at 23 °C	1725	**C**
Mannitol	WY	15%	BR	0.1 mg/ml[a]	Physically compatible with no subvisual haze or particle formation in 4 hr at 23 °C	1725	**C**
Mechlorethamine HCl	MSD	1 mg/ml	BR	0.1 mg/ml[a]	Physically compatible with no subvisual haze or particle formation in 4 hr at 23 °C	1725	**C**

Y-Site Injection Compatibility (1:1 Mixture) (Cont.)

Teniposide

Drug	Mfr	Conc	Mfr	Conc	Remarks	Ref	C/I
Melphalan HCl	BW	0.1 mg/ml[a]	BR	0.1 mg/ml[a]	Physically compatible with no subvisual haze or particle formation in 4 hr at 23 °C	1725	C
Meperidine HCl	WY	4 mg/ml[a]	BR	0.1 mg/ml[a]	Physically compatible with no subvisual haze or particle formation in 4 hr at 23 °C	1725	C
Mesna	MJ	10 mg/ml[a]	BR	0.1 mg/ml[a]	Physically compatible with no subvisual haze or particle formation in 4 hr at 23 °C	1725	C
Methotrexate sodium	LE	15 mg/ml[a]	BR	0.1 mg/ml[a]	Physically compatible with no subvisual haze or particle formation in 4 hr at 23 °C	1725	C
Methylprednisolone sodium succinate	AB	5 mg/ml[a]	BR	0.1 mg/ml[a]	Physically compatible with no subvisual haze or particle formation in 4 hr at 23 °C	1725	C
Metoclopramide HCl	ES	5 mg/ml	BR	0.1 mg/ml[a]	Physically compatible with no subvisual haze or particle formation in 4 hr at 23 °C	1725	C
Metronidazole	BA	5 mg/ml	BR	0.1 mg/ml[a]	Physically compatible with no subvisual haze or particle formation in 4 hr at 23 °C	1725	C
Minocycline HCl	LE	0.2 mg/ml[a]	BR	0.1 mg/ml[a]	Physically compatible with no subvisual haze or particle formation in 4 hr at 23 °C	1725	C
Mitomycin	BR	0.5 mg/ml	BR	0.1 mg/ml[a]	Physically compatible with no subvisual haze or particle formation in 4 hr at 23 °C	1725	C
Mitoxantrone HCl	LE	0.5 mg/ml[a]	BR	0.1 mg/ml[a]	Physically compatible with no subvisual haze or particle formation in 4 hr at 23 °C	1725	C
Morphine sulfate	AST	1 mg/ml[a]	BR	0.1 mg/ml[a]	Physically compatible with no subvisual haze or particle formation in 4 hr at 23 °C	1725	C
Nalbuphine HCl	DU	10 mg/ml	BR	0.1 mg/ml[a]	Physically compatible with no subvisual haze or particle formation in 4 hr at 23 °C	1725	C
Netilmicin sulfate	SC	5 mg/ml[a]	BR	0.1 mg/ml[a]	Physically compatible with no subvisual haze or particle formation in 4 hr at 23 °C	1725	C
Ondansetron HCl	GL	1 mg/ml[b]	BR	0.1 mg/ml[a]	Physically compatible for 4 hr at 22 °C	1365	C
	GL	1 mg/ml[a]	BR	0.1 mg/ml[a]	Physically compatible with no subvisual haze or particle formation in 4 hr at 23 °C	1725	C
Piperacillin sodium	LE	40 mg/ml[a]	BR	0.1 mg/ml[a]	Physically compatible with no subvisual haze or particle formation in 4 hr at 23 °C	1725	C
Plicamycin	MI	0.01 mg/ml[a]	BR	0.1 mg/ml[a]	Physically compatible with no subvisual haze or particle formation in 4 hr at 23 °C	1725	C

Y-Site Injection Compatibility (1:1 Mixture) (Cont.)

Teniposide

Drug	Mfr	Conc	Mfr	Conc	Remarks	Ref	C/I
Potassium chloride	AB	0.1 mEq/ml[a]	BR	0.1 mg/ml[a]	Physically compatible with no subvisual haze or particle formation in 4 hr at 23 °C	1725	C
Prochlorperazine edisylate	SCN	0.5 mg/ml[a]	BR	0.1 mg/ml[a]	Physically compatible with no subvisual haze or particle formation in 4 hr at 23 °C	1725	C
Promethazine HCl	WY	2 mg/ml[a]	BR	0.1 mg/ml[a]	Physically compatible with no subvisual haze or particle formation in 4 hr at 23 °C	1725	C
Ranitidine HCl	GL	2 mg/ml[a]	BR	0.1 mg/ml[a]	Physically compatible with no subvisual haze or particle formation in 4 hr at 23 °C	1725	C
Sargramostim	IMM	10 μg/ml[b]	BR	0.1 mg/ml[b]	Physically compatible for 4 hr at 22 °C	1436	C
Sodium bicarbonate	AB	1 mEq/ml	BR	0.1 mg/ml[a]	Physically compatible with no subvisual haze or particle formation in 4 hr at 23 °C	1725	C
Streptozocin	UP	40 mg/ml[a]	BR	0.1 mg/ml[a]	Physically compatible with no subvisual haze or particle formation in 4 hr at 23 °C	1725	C
Thiotepa	LE	1 mg/ml[a]	BR	0.1 mg/ml[a]	Physically compatible with no subvisual haze or particle formation in 4 hr at 23 °C	1725	C
Ticarcillin disodium	BE	30 mg/ml[a]	BR	0.1 mg/ml[a]	Physically compatible with no subvisual haze or particle formation in 4 hr at 23 °C	1725	C
Ticarcillin disodium–clavulanate potassium	SKB	31 mg/ml[a]	BR	0.1 mg/ml[a]	Physically compatible with no subvisual haze or particle formation in 4 hr at 23 °C	1725	C
Tobramycin sulfate	LI	5 mg/ml[a]	BR	0.1 mg/ml[a]	Physically compatible with no subvisual haze or particle formation in 4 hr at 23 °C	1725	C
Trimethoprim–sulfamethoxazole	ES	0.8 + 4 mg/ml[a]	BR	0.1 mg/ml[a]	Physically compatible with no subvisual haze or particle formation in 4 hr at 23 °C	1725	C
Vancomycin HCl	AB	10 mg/ml[a]	BR	0.1 mg/ml[a]	Physically compatible with no subvisual haze or particle formation in 4 hr at 23 °C	1725	C
Vinblastine sulfate	LI	0.12 mg/ml[a]	BR	0.1 mg/ml[a]	Physically compatible with no subvisual haze or particle formation in 4 hr at 23 °C	1725	C
Vincristine sulfate	LI	0.05 mg/ml[a]	BR	0.1 mg/ml[a]	Physically compatible with no subvisual haze or particle formation in 4 hr at 23 °C	1725	C
Vinorelbine tartrate	BW	1 mg/ml[a]	BR	0.1 mg/ml[a]	Physically compatible with no subvisual haze or particle formation in 4 hr at 23 °C	1725	C

Y-Site Injection Compatibility (1:1 Mixture) (Cont.)

Teniposide

Drug	Mfr	Conc	Mfr	Conc	Remarks	Ref	C/I
Zidovudine	BW	4 mg/ml[a]	BR	0.1 mg/ml[a]	Physically compatible with no subvisual haze or particle formation in 4 hr at 23 °C	1725	C

[a]*Tested in dextrose 5% in water.*
[b]*Tested in sodium chloride 0.9%.*
[c]*Tested in bacteriostatic sodium chloride 0.9% preserved with benzyl alcohol 0.9%.*
[d]*Sodium carbonate–containing formulation tested.*

Additional Compatibility Information

Solutions— Dextrose 5% in water and sodium chloride 0.9% are recommended for dilution of teniposide. Concentrations of 0.1, 0.2, and 0.4 mg/ml in these solutions are stable for 24 hours at room temperature. At 1 mg/ml, teniposide administration should be completed within four hours because of the potential for precipitation. Solutions should not be refrigerated (2).

Plastic— Contact of the undiluted teniposide concentrate with plastic equipment and devices during preparation has resulted in softening of the plastic, cracking, and leakage. Damage to plastic equipment has not been reported with diluted solutions (2).

Plasticizer Extraction— The surfactant, Cremophor EL, in the teniposide formulation extracts the plasticizer DEHP from PVC containers and sets. The amount extracted increases with time and drug concentration and is similar for sodium chloride 0.9% and dextrose 5% in water. Consequently, the manufacturer recommends the use of non-PVC containers, such as glass bottles and polyolefin plastic bags, and non-PVC administration sets, such as lipid administration sets and nitroglycerin sets (2).

Teniposide (Bristol) 0.1 mg/ml in dextrose 5% in water leached relatively large amounts of DEHP from PVC bags due to the Cremophor EL in the formulation. After eight hours at 24 °C, the DEHP concentration in 50-ml bags of infusion solution was as much as 7.5 μg/ml; it continued to increase through 24 hours to 22.2 μg/ml. This finding is consistent with the surfactant concentration (1%) of the final admixture solution. The actual amount of DEHP leached from PVC containers and administration sets may vary in clinical situations, depending on surfactant concentration, bag size, and contact time (1683).

Faouzi et al. reported substantial leaching of DEHP plasticizer from PVC bags of dextrose 5% in water and sodium chloride 0.9% and PVC administration sets by teniposide admixtures containing 0.4 mg/ml of drug by the Cremophor EL surfactant used in the formulation. DEHP levels increased throughout the one hour of infusion to over 20 μg/ml from both the bags and sets. There was no difference in plasticizer leaching between the two infusion solutions. Storage of the teniposide 0.4-mg/ml admixtures for 48 hours at both 4 and 24 °C resulted in substantially greater DEHP leaching. DEHP concentrations ranged from about 60 μg/ml in the refrigerated samples to over 200 μg/ml (a total of 52 mg) in the room temperature samples. The authors noted that the actual amount of DEHP a patient will receive is dependent on a number of factors, including Cremophor EL concentration, temperature, and contact time. No plasticizer was leached from glass bottles or polyolefin infusion containers. To minimize plasticizer leaching if PVC containers and sets must be used, it is recommended that teniposide admixtures be used immediately after preparation and administered over no more than one hour (2053).

Heparin— Heparin sodium can cause precipitation of teniposide. Administration apparatus should be thoroughly flushed before and after teniposide administration with dextrose 5% in water or sodium chloride 0.9% (2; 1502).

TERBUTALINE SULFATE
AHFS 12:12

Brethine   **Novartis**
Bricanyl   **Aventis**

Products— Terbutaline sulfate is available in 1-ml ampuls. Each milliliter contains terbutaline sulfate 1 mg, sodium chloride 8.9 mg, and hydrochloric acid to adjust the pH (2).

pH— The pH is adjusted to 3 to 5 (2).

Osmolality— The injection is isotonic (2). Terbutaline sulfate 1 mg/ml has an osmolality of 283 mOsm/kg (1689).

Administration— Terbutaline sulfate injection is administered subcutaneously only, usually into the lateral deltoid area (2; 4).

Stability— Although relatively stable compared to corresponding catecholamines (738), terbutaline sulfate is nonetheless sensitive to light and excessive heat. The injection should be stored at controlled room temperature and protected from light. Discolored solutions should not be used (2; 4). Terbutaline sulfate is stated to be stable over the pH range of 1 to 7 (4).

Syringes— Glascock et al. studied the stability of terbutaline sulfate (Geigy) 1 mg/ml packaged in polypropylene syringes (Becton-Dickinson) fitted with luer-tip caps (Becton-Dickinson). The samples were stored at 4 °C in the dark, 25 °C in the dark, and 25 °C with exposure to fluorescent light. Samples stored in the dark at both temperatures were stable, exhibiting a 5 to 6% drug loss in 60 days. The 25 °C samples exposed to light showed a 5% loss in 28 days and an 11% loss in 60 days, with a yellow discoloration at the latter time point (1298).

Raymond (1299) also evaluated the stability of terbutaline sulfate (Geigy) 1 mg/ml repackaged in syringes. A 0.25-ml sample was drawn into each plastic tuberculin syringe (Becton-Dickinson) and sealed with a luer-tip cap (Becton-Dickinson). Samples were stored at 4 and 24 °C with exposure to light and light protection. Little difference was reported in the terbutaline sulfate content among the four storage conditions. Drug losses of 5% or less were observed after seven weeks of storage. Although no discoloration was reported, as found by Glascock et al. (1298), it may not have been observed in the small sample present in the tuberculin syringe.

Compatibility Information

Solution Compatibility

Terbutaline sulfate

Solution	Mfr	Mfr	Conc/L	Remarks	Ref	C/I
Dextrose 5% in water	AB	CI	4 mg	Physically compatible and chemically stable exposed to light. 10% decomposition calculated to occur in 328 hr at 25 °C	527	C
	TR[a]	MRD	30 mg	Less than 10% terbutaline loss in 7 days at 25 °C under fluorescent light	1133	C
Sodium chloride 0.45%	TR[a]	MRD	30 mg	Less than 10% terbutaline loss in 7 days at 25 °C under fluorescent light or at 4 °C	1133	C
Sodium chloride 0.9%	TR[a]	MRD	30 mg	Less than 10% terbutaline loss in 7 days at 25 °C under fluorescent light	1133	C

[a]Tested in PVC containers.

Additive Compatibility

Terbutaline sulfate

Drug	Mfr	Conc/L	Mfr	Conc/L	Test Soln	Remarks	Ref	C/I
Aminophylline	SE	500 mg	CI	4 mg	D5W	Physically compatible. 10% terbutaline decomposition in 44 hr at 25 °C exposed to light	527	C
Bleomycin sulfate	BR	20 and 30 units	GG	7.5 mg	NS	36% loss of bleomycin activity in 1 week at 4 °C	763	I

Drugs in Syringe Compatibility

Terbutaline sulfate

Drug (in syringe)	Mfr	Amt	Mfr	Amt	Remarks	Ref	C/I
Doxapram HCl	RB	400 mg/ 20 ml		0.2 mg/ 1 ml	Physically compatible with 6% doxapram loss in 24 hr	1177	C

Y-Site Injection Compatibility (1:1 Mixture)

Terbutaline sulfate

Drug	Mfr	Conc	Mfr	Conc	Remarks	Ref	C/I
Insulin, regular	LI	0.2 unit/ml[a]	CI	0.02 mg/ml[b]	Physically compatible for 2 hr at 25 °C under fluorescent light	1395	C

[a]Tested in sodium chloride 0.9%.
[b]Tested in dextrose 5% in water.

THEOPHYLLINE
AHFS 86:16

Products— Theophylline is available, premixed in dextrose 5% in water, in various concentrations (expressed as anhydrous theophylline) and container sizes (4; 154):

Concentration	Container Size	Total Theophylline
4 mg/ml	50 ml	200 mg
	100 ml	400 mg
3.2 mg/ml	250 ml	800 mg
2 mg/ml	100 ml	200 mg
1.6 mg/ml	250 ml	400 mg
	500 ml	800 mg
0.8 mg/ml	500 ml	400 mg
	1000 ml	800 mg
0.4 mg/ml	1000 ml	400 mg

pH— From 3.5 to 6.5 (17).

Administration— Theophylline may be administered by continuous or intermittent intravenous infusion. Slow administration, not exceeding 20 mg/min, has been recommended. Loading doses are usually given over 20 to 30 minutes (4).

Stability— Theophylline injection should be stored at controlled room temperature and protected from freezing. Avoid excessive heat (17).

At a concentration of 1 g/L in dextrose 5% in water, theophylline was stable during autoclaving for 20 minutes at 120 °C. No decrease in the theophylline content was detected (1173).

Compatibility Information

Additive Compatibility

						Theophylline		
Drug	Mfr	Conc/L	Mfr	Conc/L	Test Soln	Remarks	Ref	C/I
Ascorbic acid injection		1.9 g		2 g	D5W	Yellow discoloration with 8% ascorbic acid loss in 6 hr and 15% in 24 hr. No loss of theophylline	1909	I
Cefepime HCl	BR	4 g	BA	800 mg	D5W	Visually compatible with 3% cefepime loss by HPLC in 24 hr at room temperature and 7 days at 5 °C. No theophylline loss	1681	C
Ceftriaxone sodium	RC	40 g	BA[a]	4 g		Yellow color forms immediately. 14% ceftriaxone loss and no theophylline loss by HPLC in 24 hr	1727	I
Chlorpromazine HCl		200 mg		2 g	D5W	Visually compatible with little or no theophylline loss and 7% chlorpromazine loss in 48 hr	1909	C
Deslanoside		1.6 mg		2 g	D5W	Visually compatible with little or no theophylline loss and 4% deslanoside loss in 48 hr	1909	C
Fluconazole	PF	1 g	BA	0.4 g	D5W[a,b]	Fluconazole chemically stable by gas chromatography for at least 72 hr at 25 °C under fluorescent light. Theophylline not tested	1676	C
Furosemide		330 mg		2 g	D5W	Visually compatible with little or no theophylline loss and 10% furosemide loss in 48 hr	1909	C
Hydrocortisone hemisuccinate		390 mg		2 g	D5W	Visually compatible with little or no loss of either drug in 48 hr	1909	C
Lidocaine HCl		380 mg		2 g	D5W	Visually compatible with little or no loss of either drug in 48 hr	1909	C

Additive Compatibility (Cont.)

Theophylline

Drug	Mfr	Conc/L	Mfr	Conc/L	Test Soln	Remarks	Ref	C/I
Methylprednisolone sodium succinate	UP	500 mg and 2 g	AB	4 g	D5W[b]	Physically compatible with little or no theophylline or methylprednisolone alcohol loss in 24 hr at room temperature. 8% ester hydrolysis termed not clinically important	1150	C
	UP	500 mg and 2 g	AB	400 mg	D5W[b]	Physically compatible with little or no theophylline or methylprednisolone alcohol loss in 24 hr at room temperature. 11% ester hydrolysis termed not clinically important	1150	C
Papaverine HCl		160 mg		2 g	D5W	Visually compatible with little or no loss of either drug in 48 hr	1909	C
Verapamil HCl	KN	100 and 400 mg	AB	400 mg and 4 g	D5W[b]	Physically compatible both visually and microscopically with little or no loss of either drug in 24 hr at 24 °C under fluorescent light	1172	C

[a]*Tested in PVC containers.*
[b]*Premixed theophylline infusion.*

Y-Site Injection Compatibility (1:1 Mixture)

Theophylline

Drug	Mfr	Conc	Mfr	Conc	Remarks	Ref	C/I
Acyclovir sodium	BW	5 mg/ml[a]	TR	1.6 mg/ml[a]	Physically compatible for 4 hr at 25 °C	1157	C
Ampicillin sodium	WY	20 mg/ml[b]	TR	4 mg/ml	Visually compatible for 6 hr at 25 °C	1793	C
Ampicillin sodium–sulbactam sodium	PF	20 + 10 mg/ml[b]	TR	4 mg/ml	Visually compatible for 6 hr at 25 °C	1793	C
Aztreonam	BV	20 mg/ml[a]	TR	4 mg/ml	Visually compatible for 6 hr at 25 °C	1793	C
Cefazolin sodium	SKB	20 mg/ml	TR	4 mg/ml	Visually compatible for 6 hr at 25 °C	1793	C
Cefotetan disodium	STU	40 mg/ml[a]	TR	4 mg/ml	Visually compatible for 6 hr at 25 °C	1793	C
Ceftazidime	LI[d]	20 mg/ml	TR	4 mg/ml	Visually compatible for 6 hr at 25 °C	1793	C
Ceftriaxone sodium	RC	20 mg/ml	TR	4 mg/ml	Visually compatible for 6 hr at 25 °C	1793	C
Cimetidine HCl	SKB	6 mg/ml[a]	TR	4 mg/ml	Visually compatible for 6 hr at 25 °C	1793	C
Cisatracurium besylate	GW	0.1, 2, 5 mg/ml[a]	AB	3.2 mg/ml	Physically compatible with no change in measured turbidity or increase in particle content in 4 hr at 23 °C	2074	C
Clindamycin phosphate	UP	12 mg/ml[a]	TR	4 mg/ml	Visually compatible for 6 hr at 25 °C	1793	C
Dexamethasone sodium phosphate	ES	0.08 mg/ml[a]	TR	4 mg/ml	Visually compatible for 6 hr at 25 °C	1793	C
Diltiazem HCl	MMD	5 mg/ml	AB	0.8 mg/ml[a]	Visually compatible	1807	C
Dobutamine HCl	LI	1 mg/ml[a]	TR	4 mg/ml	Visually compatible for 6 hr at 25 °C	1793	C
Dopamine HCl	BA	1.6 mg/ml	TR	4 mg/ml	Visually compatible for 6 hr at 25 °C	1793	C
Doxycycline hyclate	ES	1 mg/ml[a]	TR	4 mg/ml	Visually compatible for 6 hr at 25 °C	1793	C
Erythromycin lactobionate	AB	3.3 mg/ml[b]	TR	4 mg/ml	Visually compatible for 6 hr at 25 °C	1793	C

Y-Site Injection Compatibility (1:1 Mixture) (Cont.)

Theophylline

Drug	Mfr	Conc	Mfr	Conc	Remarks	Ref	C/I
Famotidine	MSD	0.2 mg/ml[a]	TR	1.6 mg/ml[a]	Physically compatible for 4 hr at 25 °C	1188	**C**
Fluconazole	RR	2 mg/ml	AMR	1.6 mg/ml[a]	Visually compatible for 24 hr at 28 °C under fluorescent light	1760	**C**
	PF	2 mg/ml	TR	4 mg/ml	Visually compatible for 6 hr at 25 °C	1793	**C**
Gentamicin sulfate	TR	2 mg/ml	TR	4 mg/ml	Visually compatible for 6 hr at 25 °C	1793	**C**
Haloperidol lactate	MN	0.5[a] and 5 mg/ml	TR	1.6 mg/ml[a]	Visually compatible for 24 hr at 21 °C	1523	**C**
Heparin sodium	TR	50 units/ml	TR	4 mg/ml	Visually compatible for 6 hr at 25 °C	1793	**C**
Hetastarch	DCC	6%	TR	4 mg/ml[c]	Precipitation after 2 hr at room temperature	1313	**I**
Hydrocortisone sodium succinate	UP	2 mg/ml[a]	TR	4 mg/ml	Visually compatible for 6 hr at 25 °C	1793	**C**
Lidocaine HCl	TR	4 mg/ml	TR	4 mg/ml	Visually compatible for 6 hr at 25 °C	1793	**C**
Methyldopate HCl	ES	5 mg/ml[a]	TR	4 mg/ml	Visually compatible for 6 hr at 25 °C	1793	**C**
Methylprednisolone sodium succinate	UP	2.5 mg/ml[a]	TR	4 mg/ml	Visually compatible for 6 hr at 25 °C	1793	**C**
Metronidazole	MG	5 mg/ml	TR	4 mg/ml	Visually compatible for 6 hr at 25 °C	1793	**C**
Midazolam HCl	RC	1 mg/ml[a]	BA	1.6 mg/ml[a]	Visually compatible for 24 hr at 23 °C	1847	**C**
Milrinone lactate	SW	0.4 mg/ml[a]	AB	1.6 mg/ml[a]	Visually compatible with little or no loss of milrinone by HPLC and theophylline by immunoassay in 4 hr at 23 °C	2214	**C**
Nafcillin sodium	WY	20 mg/ml[a]	TR	4 mg/ml	Visually compatible for 6 hr at 25 °C	1793	**C**
Nitroglycerin	LY	0.2 mg/ml[a]	TR	4 mg/ml	Visually compatible for 6 hr at 25 °C	1793	**C**
Penicillin G potassium	RR	40,000 units/ml[a]	TR	4 mg/ml	Visually compatible for 6 hr at 25 °C	1793	**C**
Phenytoin sodium	ES	2 mg/ml[b]	TR	4 mg/ml	Cloudiness forms immediately and becomes dense, flocculent precipitate in 6 hr at 25 °C	1793	**I**
Piperacillin sodium	LE	60 mg/ml[a]	TR	4 mg/ml	Visually compatible for 6 hr at 25 °C	1793	**C**
Potassium chloride	AB	0.2 mEq/ml[a]	TR	4 mg/ml	Visually compatible for 6 hr at 25 °C	1793	**C**
Ranitidine HCl	GL	1 mg/ml	TR	4 mg/ml	Visually compatible for 6 hr at 25 °C	1793	**C**
Remifentanil HCl	GW	0.025 and 0.25 mg/ml[b]	AB	3.2 mg/ml[a]	Physically compatible with no change in measured turbidity or increase in particle content in 4 hr at 23 °C	2075	**C**
Sodium nitroprusside	ES	0.2 mg/ml[a]	TR	4 mg/ml	Visually compatible for 6 hr at 25 °C protected from light	1793	**C**
Ticarcillin disodium	BE	20 mg/ml[a]	TR	4 mg/ml	Visually compatible for 6 hr at 25 °C	1793	**C**
Ticarcillin disodium–clavulanate potassium	BE	31 mg/ml[a]	TR	4 mg/ml	Visually compatible for 6 hr at 25 °C	1793	**C**
Tobramycin sulfate	LI	0.8 mg/ml[a]	TR	4 mg/ml	Visually compatible for 6 hr at 25 °C	1793	**C**
Vancomycin HCl	LI	6.6 mg/ml[a]	TR	4 mg/ml	Visually compatible for 6 hr at 25 °C	1793	**C**

[a]*Tested in dextrose 5% in water.*
[b]*Tested in sodium chloride 0.9%.*
[c]*Premixed infusion solution.*
[d]*Sodium carbonate–containing formulation tested.*

Cimetidine— Complex formation between cimetidine and theophylline was noted in pH 7.4 phosphate buffer solution and human plasma (1043).

Heating Plasma— Heating plasma samples to 56 °C for one hour to inactivate potential HIV content resulted in no theophylline loss as determined by fluorescence polarization immunoassay (1615).

THIAMINE HCL
AHFS 88:08

Elkins-Sinn

Products— Thiamine HCl (Elkins-Sinn) is available in 1-ml vials. Each milliliter of solution contains 100 mg of thiamine HCl along with sodium formaldehyde sulfoxylate 1 mg and chlorobutanol 3.5 mg in water for injection. Sodium hydroxide may be added for pH adjustment (1-3/91).

pH— From 2.5 to 4.5 (17).

Osmolality— Thiamine HCl 100 mg/ml has an osmolality of 777 mOsm/kg (1689).

Administration— Thiamine HCl injection may be administered by intramuscular or slow intravenous injection. An intradermal test dose has been recommended for patients with suspected thiamine sensitivity (1-3/91; 4).

Stability— Thiamine HCl in intact containers should be stored at controlled room temperature and protected from light and freezing (4).

pH Effects— Thiamine HCl is stable in acid solutions (1-3/91), losing activity very slowly at pH 4 or less. It is maximally stable at pH 2 (1072). Thiamine HCl is unstable in neutral or alkaline solutions (1-3/91; 4; 1072).

Syringes— Thiamine HCl (Lilly) 100 mg/ml was repackaged in glass syringes (Glaspak), back-fill glass syringes (Hy-Pod), and plastic syringes (Stylex). Half of the syringes were filled with thiamine HCl injection filtered through 5-μm stainless steel depth filters (Extemp filter pin), and the rest were filled with unfiltered drug. The syringes containing 1 ml of thiamine HCl injection were stored protected from light (amber UV-light-inhibiting plastic bags) at 22 to 24 °C for 84 days. No color changes were observed, and changes in pH were minimal. Furthermore, no differences between filtered or unfiltered samples occurred, with all solutions retaining approximately 100% of the initial potency over the 84 days (734).

Sorption— Thiamine HCl (Merck) 30 mg/L did not display significant sorption to a PVC plastic test strip in 24 hours (12).

Compatibility Information

Solution Compatibility

Thiamine HCl

Solution	Mfr	Mfr	Conc/L	Remarks	Ref	C/I
Dextran 6% in dextrose 5%	AB		100 mg	Physically compatible	3	C
Dextran 6% in sodium chloride 0.9%	AB		100 mg	Physically compatible	3	C
Dextrose–Ringer's injection combinations	AB		100 mg	Physically compatible	3	C
Dextrose–Ringer's injection, lactated, combinations	AB		100 mg	Physically compatible	3	C
Dextrose–saline combinations	AB		100 mg	Physically compatible	3	C
Dextrose 2½% in water	AB		100 mg	Physically compatible	3	C
Dextrose 5% in water	AB		100 mg	Physically compatible	3	C
Dextrose 10% in water	AB		100 mg	Physically compatible	3	C
Fat emulsion 10%, intravenous	KA	KA[a]	118 mg	Physically compatible for 24 hr at 26 °C with little loss of thiamine HCl and of most other vitamins by HPLC; up to 52% ascorbate loss	2050	C
Fructose 10% in sodium chloride 0.9%	AB		100 mg	Physically compatible	3	C
Fructose 10% in water	AB		100 mg	Physically compatible	3	C

Solution Compatibility (Cont.)

Thiamine HCl

Solution	Mfr	Mfr	Conc/L		Remarks	Ref	C/I
Invert sugar 5 and 10% in sodium chloride 0.9%	AB		100	mg	Physically compatible	3	C
Invert sugar 5 and 10% in water	AB		100	mg	Physically compatible	3	C
Ionosol products	AB		100	mg	Physically compatible	3	C
Ringer's injection	AB		100	mg	Physically compatible	3	C
Ringer's injection, lactated	AB		100	mg	Physically compatible	3	C
Sodium chloride 0.45%	AB		100	mg	Physically compatible	3	C
Sodium chloride 0.9%	AB		100	mg	Physically compatible	3	C
Sodium lactate ⅙ M	AB		100	mg	Physically compatible	3	C

[a]*From multivitamins.*

Drugs in Syringe Compatibility

Thiamine HCl

Drug (in syringe)	Mfr	Amt	Mfr	Amt	Remarks	Ref	C/I
Doxapram HCl	RB	400 mg/ 20 ml		10 mg/ 2 ml	Physically compatible with 6% doxapram loss in 24 hr	1177	C

Y-Site Injection Compatibility (1:1 Mixture)

Thiamine HCl

Drug	Mfr	Conc	Mfr	Conc	Remarks	Ref	C/I
Famotidine	MSD	0.2 mg/ml[a]	ES	100 mg/ml	Physically compatible for 14 hr	1196	C

[a]*Tested in dextrose 5% in water.*

Additional Compatibility Information

Thiamine HCl is stated to be incompatible with alkaline or neutral solutions (4) (i.e., barbiturates, carbonates and bicarbonates, etc.) and with copper ions (461).

Thiamine HCl is also stated to be incompatible with oxidizing and reducing agents (4). In solutions with sulfites or bisulfites, it is rapidly inactivated (52; 1072; 1925). Oxidation of thiamine HCl results in the formation of the highly blue-colored and biologically inactive compound thiochrome (734; 1072).

Solutions— A study of the stability of thiamine HCl in the multivitamin products Berocca-PN (Roche), Multivitamin Additive (Abbott), and M.V.I.-12 (USV) showed extensive decomposition when these products were admixed in infusion solutions containing sodium bisulfite. After 24 hours at 23 °C, thiamine losses ranged from 70% in Travasol 5.5% (pH 5.5) to 97% in FreAmine III 8.5% (pH 6.5). The extent of decomposition increased as the pH neared neutrality. The rate of decomposition could be slowed, but not eliminated, by refrigeration. When admixed in solutions without bisulfite, the thiamine was much more stable, showing losses of 0 to 11% in 24 hours at 23 °C. The authors noted that if bisulfite-containing solutions are necessary to administer multivitamin preparations, the admixtures should be used immediately after preparation and pa-

tients on long-term therapy should be monitored for thiamine deficiency (774).

The stability of thiamine HCl 50 mg/L was studied in representative parenteral nutrition solutions exposed to fluorescent light, indirect sunlight, and direct sunlight for eight hours. One 5-ml vial of multivitamin concentrate (Lyphomed) containing 50 mg of thiamine HCl and also 1 mg of folic acid (Lederle) were added to a liter of parenteral nutrition solution composed of amino acids 4.25%–dextrose 25% (Travenol) with standard electrolytes and trace elements. Thiamine HCl was stable over the eight-hour study period at room temperature under fluorescent light and indirect sunlight, but direct sunlight caused a 26% loss (842).

Samples from 24 1-L and four 2-L parenteral nutrition solutions containing one vial each of multivitamin concentrate (USV) were evaluated for thiamine HCl content 48 to 72 hours after mixing. The parenteral nutrition solutions contained amino acids 2.75 to 5%, dextrose 15 to 25%, and electrolytes. Thiamine HCl was stable in all of the solutions tested in spite of an approximately 0.05% sulfite content (843).

In another experiment, multivitamin concentrate (USV) was added to 500-ml glass bottles of amino acids 10% (Travenol) containing 0.1% sulfite and also 1000-ml PVC bags containing amino acids 4.25%–dextrose 25% (Travenol) with about 0.05% sulfite. After 22 hours at 30 °C, a 40% loss of thiamine HCl occurred in the amino acid 10% solution, but no loss occurred in the PVC bags of parenteral nutrition solution. The authors concluded that the thiamine HCl content is retained in usual clinical parenteral nutrition solutions, probably because of the dilution of the sulfite and buffering of pH. However, direct addition to solutions with a high sulfite content (0.1%) may result in significant decomposition (843).

Shine and Farwell reported a 50% initial drop in thiamine concentration immediately after admixture of multivitamins in a parenteral nutrition solution composed of amino acids, dextrose, electrolytes, and trace elements in PVC bags. The thiamine concentration then remained relatively constant for 120 hours when stored at both 4 and 25 °C (1063).

Dahl et al. reported the stability of numerous vitamins in parenteral nutrition solutions composed of amino acids (Kabi-Vitrum), dextrose 30%, and fat emulsion 20% (Kabi-Vitrum) in a 2:1:1 ratio with electrolytes, trace elements, and both fat- and water-soluble vitamins. The admixtures were stored in darkness at 2 to 8 °C for 96 hours with no significant loss of retinyl palmitate, alpha-tocopherol, thiamine mononitrate, sodium riboflavin-5′-phosphate, pyridoxine HCl, nicotinamide, folic acid, biotin, sodium pantothenate, and cyanocobalamin. Sodium ascorbate and its biologically active degradation product, dehydroascorbic acid, totaled 59 and 42% of the nominal starting concentration at 24 and 96 hours, respectively. However, the actual initial concentration was only 66% of the nominal concentration (1225).

Smith et al. reported the stability of several vitamins from M.V.I.-12 (Armour) admixed in parenteral nutrition solutions composed of different amino acid products, with or without Intralipid 10%, when stored in glass bottles and PVC bags at 25 and 5 °C for 48 hours. Thiamine HCl was stable in the parenteral nutrition solutions prepared with amino acid products without bisulfite. However, amino acid products containing bisulfite (Travasol and FreAmine III) had a 25% thiamine loss in 12 hours and a 50% loss in 24 hours when the solutions were stored at 25 °C; no loss occurred when the solutions were stored at 5 °C (1431).

The stability of thiamine HCl from a multiple vitamin product in dextrose 5% in water and sodium chloride 0.9% in PVC and Clear-Flex containers was evaluated. HPLC analysis showed that thiamine HCl was stable at 23 °C when exposed to or protected from light, exhibiting losses of 11% or less in 24 hours (1509).

Antibiotics— In vitro testing of thiamine HCl at a concentration of 0.1% with the following antibiotics at a concentration of 0.025% in sterile distilled water showed significant reduction in antibiotic activity in one hour at 25 °C (314):

Erythromycin (as estolate)
Kanamycin sulfate
Streptomycin sulfate

THIETHYLPERAZINE MALATE
AHFS 56:22

Torecan   **Roxane**

Products— Thiethylperazine malate (Roxane) is available in 2-ml ampuls. Each milliliter of solution contains (2):

Thiethylperazine malate	5 mg
Sodium metabisulfite	0.25 mg
Ascorbic acid	1 mg
Sorbitol	20 mg
Carbon dioxide	qs
Water for injection	qs 1 ml

pH— From 3 to 4 (4).

Administration— Thiethylperazine malate is administered by deep intramuscular injection. Subcutaneous or intravenous injection is not recommended (2; 4).

Stability— The solution should be stored in light-resistant containers below 30 °C and used only if clear and colorless (2).

Thiethylperazine malate (Sandoz) 5 mg/ml was found to retain potency for two weeks under refrigeration when 2 ml of solution was packaged in Tubex cartridges. Room temperature storage for one week and refrigerated storage for three weeks resulted in a darkening in color (13).

Compatibility Information

Drugs in Syringe Compatibility

Thiethylperazine malate

Drug (in syringe)	Mfr	Amt	Mfr	Amt	Remarks	Ref	C/I
Butorphanol tartrate	BR	4 mg/ 2 ml	BI	10 mg/ 1 ml	Physically compatible both macroscopically and microscopically for 30 min at room temperature	761	C
Hydromorphone HCl	KN	4 mg/ 2 ml	SZ	5 mg/ 1 ml	Physically compatible for 30 min	517	C
Ketorolac tromethamine	SY	30 mg/ 1 ml	ROX	5 mg/ 1 ml	White crystalline precipitate forms immediately	1785	I

Drugs in Syringe Compatibility (Cont.)

Thiethylperazine malate

Drug (in syringe)	Mfr	Amt	Mfr	Amt	Remarks	Ref	C/I
Midazolam HCl	RC	5 mg/ 1 ml	BI	10 mg/ 2 ml	Physically compatible for 4 hr at 25 °C under fluorescent light	1145	C
Nalbuphine HCl	EN	10 mg/ 1 ml	BI	5 mg/ 1 ml	Physically compatible for 36 hr at 27 °C	762	C
	EN	5 mg/ 0.5 ml	BI	5 mg/ 1 ml	Crystals form within 24 hr at 27 °C. Physically compatible for at least 12 hr	762	I
	EN	2.5 mg/ 0.25 ml	BI	5 mg/ 1 ml	Crystals form within 24 hr at 27 °C. Physically compatible for at at least 12 hr	762	I
	DU	10 mg/ 1 ml		10 mg/ 2 ml	Physically compatible for 48 hr	128	C
	DU	20 mg/ 1 ml		10 mg/ 2 ml	Physically compatible for 48 hr	128	C
Perphenazine	SC	5 mg/ 1 ml	BI	10 mg/ 1 ml	Yellow discoloration within 15 min	761	I
Ranitidine HCl	GL	50 mg/ 2 ml	SZ	10 mg/ 1 ml	Physically compatible for 1 hr at 25 °C both macroscopically and microscopically	978	C

Y-Site Injection Compatibility (1:1 Mixture)

Thiethylperazine malate

Drug	Mfr	Conc	Mfr	Conc	Remarks	Ref	C/I
Aldesleukin	CHI	33,800 I.U./ ml[a]	SZ	0.4 mg/ml[a]	Visually compatible with little or no loss of aldesleukin activity by bioassay	1857	C

[a]*Tested in dextrose 5% in water.*

THIOPENTAL SODIUM
AHFS 28:24.04

Pentothal Sodium   **Abbott**

Products— Thiopental sodium is available in 250-, 400-, and 500-mg syringes, 500-mg and 1-g vials, and 1-, 2.5-, and 5-g containers in kits (29; 154). The products also contain anhydrous sodium carbonate as a buffer (1-8/96; 17). Reconstitute only with sterile water for injection, sodium chloride 0.9%, or dextrose 5% in water for solutions in the 2 to 5% range or with dextrose 5% in water, sodium chloride 0.9%, or Normosol R, pH 7.4, for solutions of 0.2 or 0.4%. Do not use sterile water for injection to prepare thiopental sodium solutions less than 2% because such solutions would be very hypotonic and would cause hemolysis (1-8/96; 21; 154).

Thiopental Sodium	Volume of Diluent	Concentration
1 g	500 ml	2 mg/ml (0.2%)
1 g	250 ml	4 mg/ml (0.4%)
2 g	500 ml	4 mg/ml (0.4%)
5 g	250 ml	20 mg/ml (2.0%)
10 g	500 ml	20 mg/ml (2.0%)
1 g	40 ml	25 mg/ml (2.5%)
5 g	200 ml	25 mg/ml (2.5%)
1 g	20 ml	50 mg/ml (5.0%)
5 g	100 ml	50 mg/ml (5.0%)

pH— A thiopental sodium 80 mg/ml solution in water has an official pH range of 10.2 to 11.2 (17). The pH of a 2.5% solution in sterile water for injection is 10 to 11 (21).

Osmolality— The osmolality of thiopental sodium 25 and 100 mg/ml was determined to be 215 and 942 mOsm/kg, respectively (1233). A 3.4% solution in sterile water for injection is isotonic. A thiopental sodium concentration less than 2% in sterile water for injection is very hypotonic and will cause hemolysis (1-8/96; 154). Sterile water for injection should not be used to prepare thiopental sodium solutions less than 2%.

Sodium Content— Each gram of thiopental sodium contains 4.9 mEq of sodium (846).

Administration— Thiopental sodium is given by slow intravenous infusion only. For intermittent intravenous administration, the concentrations used range between 2 and 5% in sterile water for injection, dextrose 5% in water, or sodium chloride 0.9%, with 2 or 2.5%

being the most common. By continuous intravenous drip, concentrations of 0.2 or 0.4% in dextrose 5% in water, sodium chloride 0.9%, or a pH 7.4 combined electrolyte solution such as Normosol R are used. Sterile water for injection should not be used for these concentrations, because of resulting hemolysis from the hypotonic solution. Extravasation and intra-arterial administration should be avoided because of the high alkalinity of the solutions (1-8/96).

Stability—— Thiopental sodium is a yellowish-colored powder. Intact containers should be stored at controlled room temperature. Factors that affect the stability of solutions of thiopental sodium include the diluent, storage temperature, and the amount of carbon dioxide from room air that gains access to the solution and combines with water to form carbonic acid, lowering the pH of the solution. The drug is most stable when reconstituted with sterile water for injection or sodium chloride 0.9%, stored under refrigeration, and tightly sealed (1-8/96). Reconstituted solutions are stated to be stable for three days at room temperature (18 to 22 °C) and for seven days under refrigeration (5 to 6 °C) (108). Since no preservative is present, however, use within 24 hours is recommended (1-8/96; 21). Also, glass attack has been noted in 48 hours (46). Sterilization by heating should not be attempted (1-8/96).

The pH of thiopental sodium must be very alkaline or the insoluble acid form will precipitate (21).

Syringes—— Thiopental sodium (Abbott) 25 mg/ml (2.5%) in water for injection, repackaged in 20-ml syringes (Monoject and Becton-Dickinson), was stable for up to five days at 25 °C and 45 days at 5 °C, sustaining potency losses of 6 to 7%. No physical changes occurred during the study period (1300).

Thiopental sodium (Abbott) 25 mg/ml was repackaged into 60-ml polypropylene syringes (Monoject, Sherwood Medical) and stored at 23 °C under fluorescent light and at 4 °C protected from light. No visually apparent changes occurred under either storage condition. Thiopental sodium losses by HPLC analysis were 9% in 10 days in the room temperature samples. No thiopental sodium losses occurred in 13 days in the refrigerated samples (1984).

The stability of thiopental sodium 25 mg/ml repackaged in polypropylene syringes was evaluated by spectrophotometric and potentiometric methods. About 7% loss of drug concentration was found after four weeks of storage at room temperature not exposed to direct light (2164).

Sorption—— Thiopental sodium (May & Baker) 7 mg/L in sodium chloride 0.9% (Travenol) in PVC bags exhibited approximately 23% loss in 24 hours and 37% loss in one week at room temperature (15 to 20 °C) due to sorption (536).

In another study, thiopental sodium (May & Baker) 7 mg/L in sodium chloride 0.9%, buffered to pH 6.1, exhibited a cumulative 16% loss during a seven-hour simulated infusion through an infusion set (Travenol) consisting of a cellulose propionate burette chamber and 170 cm of PVC tubing due to sorption. Thiopental sorption was attributed mainly to the burette. The extent of sorption was dependent on the pH of the solution. As the pH decreased, the percentage of unionized drug increased. In turn, the extent of sorption also increased (606).

The drug was also tested as a simulated infusion over at least one hour by a syringe pump system. A glass syringe on a syringe pump was fitted with 20 cm of polyethylene tubing or 50 cm of Silastic tubing. Only 5% of the drug was lost with the polyethylene tubing, but a cumulative loss of 50% occurred during the one-hour infusion through the Silastic tubing (606).

In contrast, a 25-ml aliquot of thiopental sodium (May & Baker) 7 mg/L in sodium chloride 0.9% was stored in all-plastic syringes composed of polypropylene barrels and polyethylene plungers for 24 hours at room temperature in the dark. No loss due to sorption occurred (606).

In a continuation of this work, thiopental sodium (May & Baker) 9 mg/L in sodium chloride 0.9% in a glass bottle was delivered through a polyethylene administration set (Tridilset) over eight hours at 15 to 20 °C. The flow rate was set at 1 ml/min. No appreciable loss because of sorption occurred (769). This finding is in contrast to the 16% loss with a conventional administration set (606).

The sorption of thiopental sodium 30 mg/L in sodium chloride 0.9% (pH 4 and 7.2) was evaluated in 100-ml PVC infusion bags (Travenol). After eight hours at 20 to 24 °C, 25% of the thiopental was lost. Thiopental sodium showed a negligible (less than 3%) loss if the aqueous solution was stored in polypropylene infusion bags (770).

Martens et al. (1392) reported that thiopental sodium 2 mg/ml in sodium chloride 0.9% in PVC, glass, and polyethylene-lined laminated containers exhibited no loss due to sorption in 24 hours at 21 °C when protected from light. This finding differs from that of Kowaluk et al. who reported a significant loss in PVC containers (536). Martens et al. attribute the difference to their use of a much higher concentration, representing a therapeutic dosage, which resulted in a sharply different solution pH (pH 9.1); the more dilute solution in the Kowaluk et al. study had a pH of 6. At lower pH, more drug remains unionized, increasing the rate of sorption (1392).

Compatibility Information

Solution Compatibility

Thiopental sodium

Solution	Mfr	Mfr	Conc/L	Remarks	Ref	C/I
Alcohol 5%, dextrose 5%	AB	AB	25 g	Physically compatible	21	**C**
Beclysyl products	AB	AB	25 g	Haze or precipitate forms within 1 hr	3; 21	**I**
Dextran 6% in dextrose 5%	AB	AB	25 g	Physically compatible	3; 21	**C**
Dextran 6% in sodium chloride 0.9%	AB	AB	25 g	Physically compatible	3; 21	**C**
Dextrose–Ringer's injection combinations	AB	AB	25 g	Haze or precipitate forms within 1 hr	3; 21	**I**

Solution Compatibility (Cont.)

Thiopental sodium

Solution	Mfr	Mfr	Conc/L	Remarks	Ref	C/I
Dextrose–Ringer's injection, lactated, combinations	AB	AB	25 g	Haze or precipitate forms within 1 hr	3; 21	I
Dextrose 5% in Ringer's injection, lactated	TR	AB		Precipitate forms within variable time periods	544	I
Dextrose 2½% in sodium chloride 0.45%	AB	AB	25 g	Physically compatible	3	C
Dextrose 2½% in sodium chloride 0.9%	AB	AB	25 g	Physically compatible	3	C
Dextrose 5% in sodium chloride 0.225%	AB	AB	25 g	Physically compatible	3; 21	C
Dextrose 5% in sodium chloride 0.45%	AB	AB	25 g	Physically compatible	3; 21	C
Dextrose 5% in sodium chloride 0.9%	AB	AB	2 g	Potency retained for 48 hr	46	C
	TR[a]	AB	2 g	Potency retained for 24 hr at 5 °C	282	C
	AB	AB	25 g	Haze or precipitate forms within 24 hr. Physically compatible for 6 hr	3; 21	I
Dextrose 10% in sodium chloride 0.9%		AB		Physically incompatible	9	I
	AB	AB	25 g	Haze or precipitate forms within 1 hr	3; 21	I
Dextrose 2½% in water	AB	AB	25 g	Physically compatible	3	C
Dextrose 5% in water	AB	AB	25 g	Physically compatible	3; 21	C
	AB	AB	2 g	Potency retained for 48 hr	46	C
	TR[a]	AB	2 g	Potency retained for 24 hr at 5 °C	282	C
Dextrose 10% in water	AB	AB	25 g	Haze or precipitate forms within 1 hr	3; 21	I
Fructose 10% in sodium chloride 0.9%	AB	AB	25 g	Haze or precipitate forms within 1 hr	3	I
Fructose 10% solutions	AB	AB	25 g	Precipitate forms within 1 hr	21	I
Fructose 10% in water	BA	AB	1 g	Physically incompatible	10	I
Invert sugar 5 and 10% in sodium chloride 0.9%	AB	AB	25 g	Haze or precipitate forms within 1 to 6 hr	3	I
	AB	AB	25 g	Precipitate forms within 1 hr	21	I
Invert sugar 5 and 10% in water	AB	AB	25 g	Haze or precipitate forms within 1 to 6 hr	3	I
	AB	AB	25 g	Precipitate forms within 1 hr	21	I
Ionosol products (except PSL)	AB	AB	25 g	Haze or precipitate forms within 1 hr	3; 21	I
Ionosol PSL	AB	AB	25 g	Physically compatible	3; 21	C
Multielectrolyte solution	AB	AB	2 g	Potency retained for 48 hr	46	C
Normosol solutions (except R)	AB	AB	25 g	Precipitate forms within 1 hr	21	I
Normosol R	AB	AB	25 g	Physically compatible	21	C
Ringer's injection	AB	AB	25 g	Haze or precipitate forms within 1 hr	3	I
Ringer's injection, lactated		AB		Physically incompatible	9	I
	AB	AB	25 g	Haze or precipitate forms within 1 hr	3	I
Sodium chloride 0.45%	AB	AB	25 g	Physically compatible	3	C
Sodium chloride 0.9%	AB	AB	25 g	Physically compatible	3; 21	C
	AB	AB	2 g	Potency retained for 48 hr	46	C
	TR[a]	AB	2 g	Potency retained for 24 hr at 5 °C	282	C
	[b]		2 g	Physically compatible with little or no drug loss in 24 hr at 21 °C in the dark	1392	C
Sodium lactate ⅙ M	AB	AB	25 g	Physically compatible	3; 21	C

[a]Tested in both glass and PVC containers.
[b]Tested in PVC, glass, and polyethylene-lined laminated containers.

Additive Compatibility

Thiopental sodium

Drug	Mfr	Conc/L	Mfr	Conc/L	Test Soln	Remarks	Ref	C/I
Amikacin sulfate	BR	5 g	AB	4 g	D5LR, D5R, D5S, D5W, D10W, IS10, LR, NS, R, SL	Immediate precipitation	294	I
Chloramphenicol sodium succinate	PD	1 g	AB	2.5 g	D5W	Physically compatible	21	C
Dimenhydrinate	SE		AB			Physically incompatible	9	I
Diphenhydramine HCl	PD		AB			Physically incompatible	9	I
Ephedrine sulfate			AB			Physically incompatible	9	I
	AB	50 mg	AB	2.5 g	D5W	Physically compatible	21	C
Fibrinolysin, human	MSD	2 g	AB	2.5 g	D5W	Physically incompatible	11	I
Hydrocortisone sodium succinate	UP	100 mg	AB	2.5 g	D5W	Physically compatible	21	C
Hydromorphone HCl			AB			Physically incompatible	9	I
Insulin, regular[a]			AB			Physically incompatible	9	I
Levorphanol bitartrate	RC		AB			Physically incompatible	9	I
Meperidine HCl	WI		AB			Physically incompatible	9	I
Metaraminol bitartrate	MSD	100 mg	AB	2.5 g		Precipitate forms within 1 hr	7	I
	MSD	200 mg	AB	2.5 g	D5W	Physically incompatible	11	I
	MSD	200 mg	AB	2.5 g	D5W	Precipitate forms within 1 hr	21	I
Morphine sulfate			AB			Physically incompatible	9	I
Norepinephrine bitartrate	WI		AB			Physically incompatible	9	I
Oxytocin	PD	5 units	AB	2.5 g	D5W	Physically compatible	21	C
Penicillin G potassium	SQ	20 million units	AB	2.5 g	D5W	Precipitate forms within 1 hr	21	I
	PF	20 million units	AB	2.5 g	D5W	Physically incompatible	11	I
Pentobarbital sodium	AB	200 mg	AB	2.5 g	D5W	Physically compatible	21	C
Phenobarbital sodium	AB	100 mg	AB	2.5 g	D5W	Physically compatible	21	C
Potassium chloride	AB	40 mEq	AB	2.5 g	D5W	Physically compatible	21	C
Prochlorperazine edisylate	SKF		AB			Physically incompatible	9	I
Promazine HCl	WY	100 mg	AB	2.5 g	D5W	Precipitate forms within 1 hr	21	I
	WI	1 g	AB	2.5 g	D5W	Physically incompatible	11	I
Promethazine HCl	WY		AB			Physically incompatible	9	I
Sodium bicarbonate	AB	40 mEq	AB	2.5 g	D5W	Physically compatible	21	C
	AB	2.4 mEq[b]	AB	1 g	D5W	Physically compatible for 24 hr	772	C
Succinylcholine chloride	AB	2 g	AB	25 g		Haze or precipitate forms within 1 to 6 hr	3	I

[a]*Test performed prior to availability of neutral regular insulin.*
[b]*One vial of Neut added to a liter of admixture.*

Drugs in Syringe Compatibility

Thiopental sodium

Drug (in syringe)	Mfr	Amt	Mfr	Amt	Remarks	Ref	C/I
Aminophylline	SE	500 mg/ 2 ml	AB	75 mg/ 3 ml	Physically compatible for at least 30 min	21	C
		500 mg/ 2 ml	AB	75 mg/ 3 ml	Physically compatible	55	C
Chlorpromazine HCl	SKF	50 mg/ 2 ml	AB	75 mg/ 3 ml	Physically incompatible	21	I
Dimenhydrinate	SE	50 mg/ 1 ml	AB	75 mg/ 3 ml	Physically incompatible	21	I
Diphenhydramine HCl	PD	50 mg/ 1 ml	AB	75 mg/ 3 ml	Physically incompatible	21	I
Doxapram HCl	RB	400 mg/ 20 ml		300 mg/ 12 ml	Immediate precipitation	1177	I
Ephedrine sulfate	AB	50 mg/ 1 ml	AB	75 mg/ 3 ml	Physically incompatible	21	I
Glycopyrrolate	RB	0.2 mg/ 1 ml	AB	25 mg/ 1 ml	Immediate precipitation	331	I
	RB	0.2 mg/ 1 ml	AB	50 mg/ 2 ml	Immediate precipitation	331	I
	RB	0.4 mg/ 2 ml	AB	25 mg/ 1 ml	Immediate precipitation	331	I
Hyaluronidase	AB	150 units	AB	75 mg/ 3 ml	Physically compatible	55	C
Hydrocortisone sodium succinate	UP	250 mg/ 2 ml	AB	75 mg/ 3 ml	Physically compatible for at least 30 min	21	C
Meperidine HCl	WI	100 mg/ 2 ml	AB	75 mg/ 3 ml	Physically incompatible	21	I
Morphine sulfate	LI	16.2 mg/ 1 ml	AB	75 mg/ 3 ml	Physically incompatible	21	I
Neostigmine methylsulfate	RC	0.5 mg/ 1 ml	AB	75 mg/ 3 ml	Physically compatible	55	C
Pentobarbital sodium	AB	50 mg/ 1 ml	AB	75 mg/ 3 ml	Physically compatible for at least 30 min	21	C
	AB	37.5 mg/ 0.75 ml	AB	75 mg/ 3 ml	Physically compatible	55	C
Prochlorperazine edisylate	SKF	10 mg/ 2 ml	AB	75 mg/ 3 ml	Physically incompatible	21	I
Promethazine HCl	WY	100 mg/ 4 ml	AB	75 mg/ 3 ml	Physically incompatible	21	I
Propofol	ZEN	5 mg/ml[a]	AB	12.5 mg/ ml[a]	Visually compatible with 10% loss by HPLC of thiopental in 10 days and of propofol in 5 days at 23 °C under fluorescent light. No thiopental loss and 4% propofol loss in 13 days at 4 °C protected from light	1984	C
	ICI	5 mg/ 0.5 ml	AB	37.5 mg/ 1.5 ml	Little or no increase in measured emulsion droplet size in 24 hr at 25 °C.	1985	C
	ICI	7.5 mg/ 0.75 ml	AB	31.25 mg/ 1.25 ml	Little or no increase in measured emulsion droplet size in 24 hr at 25 °C.	1985	C

Drugs in Syringe Compatibility (Cont.)

Thiopental sodium

Drug (in syringe)	Mfr	Amt	Mfr	Amt	Remarks	Ref	C/I
	ICI	10 mg/ 1 ml	AB	25 mg/ 1 ml	Little or no increase in measured emulsion droplet size in 24 hr at 25 °C. Little or no loss of either drug by HPLC in 24 hr at 25 °C	1985	**C**
	ICI	12.5 mg/ 1.25 ml	AB	18.75 mg/ 0.75 ml	Little or no increase in measured emulsion droplet size in 24 hr at 25 °C.	1985	**C**
	ICI	15 mg/ 1.5 ml	AB	12.5 mg/ 0.5 ml	Little or no increase in measured emulsion droplet size in 24 hr at 25 °C.	1985	**C**
Scopolamine HBr		0.13 mg/ 0.26 ml	AB	75 mg/ 3 ml	Physically compatible for at least 30 min	21	**C**
		0.13 mg/ 0.26 ml	AB	75 mg/ 3 ml	Physically compatible	55	**C**
Sodium bicarbonate		3.75 g/ 50 ml	AB	75 mg/ 3 ml	Physically incompatible	55	**I**
Tubocurarine chloride		2.25 mg/ 0.15 ml	AB	75 mg/ 3 ml	Physically compatible for at least 30 min	21	**C**
		2.25 mg/ 0.15 ml	AB	75 mg/ 3 ml	Physically compatible	55	**C**

[a]*Final concentrations after mixing.*

Y-Site Injection Compatibility (1:1 Mixture)

Thiopental sodium

Drug	Mfr	Conc	Mfr	Conc	Remarks	Ref	C/I
Alfentanil HCl	JN	0.5 mg/ml	AB	25 mg/ml	White pellets form within 24 hr at 25 °C	1801	**I**
Ascorbic acid	AB	500 mg/ml	AB	25 mg/ml	Yellow discoloration and fine precipitate form in 24 hr	1801	**I**
Atracurium besylate	BW	10 mg/ml	AB	25 mg/ml	White cloudiness forms immediately but clears within 24 hr at 25 °C	1801	**I**
Atropine sulfate	GNS	0.4 mg/ml	AB	25 mg/ml	White particles form immediately and yellow discoloration forms within 24 hr at 25 °C	1801	**I**
Cisatracurium besylate	GW	0.1 mg/ml[a]	AB	25 mg/ml[a]	Physically compatible with no change in measured turbidity or increase in particle content in 4 hr at 23 °C	2074	**C**
	GW	2 mg/ml[a]	AB	25 mg/ml[a]	White turbidity forms immediately but dissipates within 1 min; subvisual haze remains	2074	**I**
	GW	5 mg/ml[a]	AB	25 mg/ml[a]	White cloudiness forms immediately	2074	**I**
Diltiazem HCl	MMD	1 mg/ml[a]	AB	25 mg/ml[c]	Precipitate forms immediately	2062	**I**
Dobutamine HCl	LI	4 mg/ml[a]	AB	25 mg/ml[c]	Precipitate forms immediately	2062	**I**
Dopamine HCl	AB	3.2 mg/ml[a]	AB	25 mg/ml[c]	Precipitate forms immediately	2062	**I**
Doxacurium chloride	BW	1 mg/ml	AB	25 mg/ml	Visually compatible for up to 7 days at 25 °C	1801	**C**
Ephedrine sulfate	AB	50 mg/ml	AB	25 mg/ml	White cloudiness forms immediately, followed by fine crystalline particles	1801	**I**
Epinephrine HCl	AB	0.02 mg/ml[a]	AB	25 mg/ml[c]	Yellow color forms in 4 hr at 27 °C	2062	**I**

Y-Site Injection Compatibility (1:1 Mixture) (Cont.)

Thiopental sodium

Drug	Mfr	Conc	Mfr	Conc	Remarks	Ref	C/I
Fentanyl citrate	ES	0.05 mg/ml	AB	25 mg/ml	Visually compatible for up to 7 days at 25 °C	1801	**C**
	ES	0.05 mg/ml	AB	25 mg/ml[c]	Visually compatible for 4 hr at 27 °C	2062	**C**
Furosemide	AMR	10 mg/ml	AB	25 mg/ml[c]	Precipitate forms immediately	2062	**I**
Heparin sodium	ES	100 units/ml[a]	AB	25 mg/ml[c]	Visually compatible for 4 hr at 27 °C	2062	**C**
Hydromorphone HCl	KN	1 mg/ml	AB	25 mg/ml[c]	Precipitate forms in 4 hr at 27 °C	2062	**I**
Labetalol HCl	AH	2 mg/ml[a]	AB	25 mg/ml[c]	Precipitate forms immediately	2062	**I**
Lidocaine HCl	AST	20 mg/ml	AB	25 mg/ml	White cloudiness forms immediately but clears within 24 hr at 25 °C	1801	**I**
Lorazepam	WY	2 mg/ml	AB	25 mg/ml	Yellow discoloration forms	1801	**I**
	WY	0.5 mg/ml[a]	AB	25 mg/ml[c]	Visually compatible for 4 hr at 27 °C	2062	**C**
Midazolam HCl	RC	5 mg/ml	AB	25 mg/ml	White precipitate forms immediately	1801	**I**
	RC	2 mg/ml[a]	AB	25 mg/ml[c]	Precipitate forms immediately	2062	**I**
Milrinone lactate	SW	0.2 mg/ml[a]	AB	25 mg/ml[c]	Visually compatible for 4 hr at 27 °C	2062	**C**
Mivacurium chloride	BW	2 mg/ml	AB	25 mg/ml	Visually compatible for up to 7 days at 25 °C	1801	**C**
Morphine sulfate	ES	10 mg/ml	AB	25 mg/ml	White precipitate forms immediately	1801	**I**
	SCN	2 mg/ml[a]	AB	25 mg/ml[c]	Visually compatible for 4 hr at 27 °C	2062	**C**
Nicardipine HCl	WY	1 mg/ml[a]	AB	25 mg/ml[c]	Precipitate forms immediately	2062	**I**
Nitroglycerin	AB	0.4 mg/ml[a]	AB	25 mg/ml[c]	Visually compatible for 4 hr at 27 °C	2062	**C**
Norepinephrine bitartrate	AB	0.128 mg/ml[a]	AB	25 mg/ml[c]	Precipitate forms in 4 hr at 27 °C	2062	**I**
Pancuronium bromide	GNS	2 mg/ml	AB	25 mg/ml	White precipitate forms immediately	1801	**I**
Phenylephrine HCl	ES	10 mg/ml	AB	25 mg/ml	White precipitate forms immediately	1801	**I**
Ranitidine HCl	GL	1 mg/ml[a]	AB	25 mg/ml[c]	Visually compatible for 4 hr at 27 °C	2062	**C**
Remifentanil HCl	GW	0.025 and 0.25 mg/ml[b]	AB	50 mg/ml[a]	Physically compatible with no change in measured turbidity or increase in particle content in 4 hr at 23 °C	2075	**C**
Succinylcholine chloride	AB	20 mg/ml	AB	25 mg/ml	White cloudiness forms immediately, followed by fine crystalline particles	1801	**I**
Sufentanil citrate	JN	0.05 mg/ml	AB	25 mg/ml	White pellets form within 24 hr at 25 °C	1801	**I**
Vecuronium bromide	OR	1 mg/ml	AB	25 mg/ml	White particles form immediately	1801	**I**
	OR	1 mg/ml	AB	25 mg/ml[c]	Precipitate forms immediately	2062	**I**

[a]*Tested in dextrose 5% in water.*
[b]*Tested in sodium chloride 0.9%.*
[c]*Tested in sterile water for injection.*

Additional Compatibility Information

Any thiopental sodium solution containing a visible precipitate should not be administered (1-8/96; 21).

The physical incompatibilities of thiopental sodium are of three types (21):

1. Acid solutions that precipitate thiopental acid
2. Calcium and magnesium solutions that form insoluble carbonates
3. Amine salts that liberate the insoluble free base in alkaline solution

Solutions— Dextrose 5% in water, sodium chloride 0.9%, and Normosol R, pH 7.4, have been recommended as diluents for the continuous infusion of thiopental sodium (1-8/96).

Thiopental sodium is incompatible or possesses limited compatibility with solutions containing sugars in concentrations above 5%. This is due to the relatively high titratable acidity of the solutions, which converts part of the thiopental sodium to the insoluble acid form. The acidity of dextrose–multielectrolyte solutions and vitamin infusion solutions (pH adjusted with hydrochloric acid) also causes such precipitation (21). The absorption of carbon dioxide, which can combine with water to form carbonic acid, may also lower the pH of the solution and cause precipitation (1-8/96).

In addition, calcium ions in solutions such as Ringer's injection and Ringer's injection, lactated, may form insoluble carbonates. Thiopental sodium may sometimes be administered into the tubing of the administration set of these solutions, although the titratable acidity of each lot of solution, the rate of injection, and the amount of thiopental sodium will affect the outcome (21).

Acidic Additives— The acidity of various additives may also result in an incompatibility. Drugs such as thiopental sodium that exhibit poor solubility in an acidic medium may precipitate in solutions containing acidic additives (4; 22). Metaraminol bitartrate is acidic and may cause precipitation, depending on the concentration of the additives (7). In addition, the acidic methyldopa HCl imparts some buffer capacity to admixtures and may pose solubility problems for barbiturate salts (23).

Alkali-Sensitive Drugs— Thiopental sodium may raise the pH of admixture solutions to the alkaline range and, therefore, should not be mixed with alkali-labile drugs such as penicillin G (47). Significant decomposition of isoproterenol HCl and norepinephrine bitartrate may also occur. If either of these two drugs is mixed with thiopental sodium, the admixture should be administered immediately after preparation (59; 77).

Succinylcholine Chloride— When barbiturates are mixed in combination with succinylcholine chloride, either the free barbiturate precipitates (4) or the succinylcholine chloride is hydrolyzed, depending on the final pH of the admixture (4; 21).

Atracurium Besylate— Atracurium besylate also may be inactivated by alkaline solutions, such as barbiturates, and precipitation of a free acid of the admixed drug may occur, depending on the resultant pH of the admixture (4).

Pancuronium Bromide— It is stated that a visible precipitate may form if pancuronium bromide is mixed with barbiturates (4). However, a precipitate was not visible when pancuronium bromide was mixed in a syringe with thiopental or methohexital (134).

Tubocurarine Chloride— Tubocurarine chloride 15 mg/ml has been reported to be conditionally compatible with thiopental sodium 2.5% in a 1:19 ratio. This mixture is usually satisfactory, but occasional precipitation does occur if the pH of the tubocurarine chloride is at its lower limit. The overall pH of the mixture is then reduced below 9.7, resulting in thiopental precipitation. As long as the final pH is above 9.7, there is no precipitate over 48 hours (40).

In infusion solutions, tubocurarine chloride 9 mg/L has also been reported to be conditionally compatible with thiopental sodium (Abbott) 25 g/L. The mixture is physically incompatible in most Abbott infusion solutions except as noted below (3):

Dextran 6% in dextrose 5%	Physically compatible
Dextran 6% in sodium chloride 0.9%	Physically compatible
Dextrose 2½% in sodium chloride 0.45%	Physically compatible
Dextrose 2½% in sodium chloride 0.9%	Physically compatible
Dextrose 5% in sodium chloride 0.225%	Physically compatible
Dextrose 5% in sodium chloride 0.45%	Physically compatible
Dextrose 2½% in water	Physically compatible
Dextrose 5% in water	Physically compatible
Ionosol PSL	Physically compatible
Sodium chloride 0.45%	Physically compatible
Sodium chloride 0.9%	Physically compatible
Sodium lactate ⅙ M	Physically compatible

Other Drugs— Other drugs stated to be incompatible with thiopental sodium or barbiturate salts include clindamycin phosphate (106), fentanyl citrate (4), droperidol (4), and cimetidine HCl (360). In addition, thiopental sodium should not be mixed in the same syringe with pentazocine lactate because precipitation will occur (4).

THIOTEPA
AHFS 10:00

Thioplex   **Immunex**

Products— Thiotepa (Immunex) is available in vials containing 15 mg of drug as a lyophilized powder. Reconstitute the vials with 1.5 ml of sterile water for injection. The approximate withdrawable volume is 1.4 ml. Because of a small excess of drug, the reconstituted solution contains thiotepa 10.4 mg/ml, yielding a withdrawable amount of approximately 14.7 mg from each vial (2).

pH— Approximately 5.5 to 7.5 (2).

Tonicity— Reconstitution with sterile water for injection results in a hypotonic solution; it should be diluted in sodium chloride 0.9% prior to use (2).

Thiotepa concentrations, 0.5 and 1 mg/ml diluted in sodium chloride 0.9%, are nearly isotonic, having osmolalities of 277 and 269 mOsm/kg, respectively. However, thiotepa concentrations of 3 and 5 mg/ml in sodium chloride 0.9% are hypotonic (2006).

Administration— Thiotepa is usually given by rapid intravenous administration but may also be given by the intracavitary or intravesical route (2; 4). The drug has also been given by intramuscular, intrathecal, and intratumoral administration (4).

Stability— Intact vials should be stored under refrigeration and protected from light at all times. Reconstituted solutions are clear to slightly opaque and should be stored under refrigeration and protected from light until used (2; 4). The reconstituted solution in sterile water for injection is stated to be stable for up to 28 days stored under refrigeration or frozen and seven days at room temperature (1369). However, the manufacturer recommends storage under refrigeration and use within eight hours because of the absence of an antimicrobial preservative (2; 4). Thiotepa may undergo polymerization forming inactive and insoluble polymeric derivatives

(1369), especially at high temperatures (4). Solutions that are grossly opaque or contain a precipitate should not be used (2; 4).

Thiotepa is stable in alkaline media but unstable in acidic media (2; 4), undergoing increased rates of hydrolysis (1389).

In sodium chloride–containing solutions, thiotepa reacts to form a chloro-adduct product. The amount and rate of chloro-adduct formation are inversely related to the thiotepa concentration. Refrigerated storage slows but does not eliminate chloro-adduct formation. Substantial chloro-adduct formation occurred in as little as eight hours in a 0.5 mg/ml solution at room temperature but did not occur until 24 hours or more than 48 hours in 1 and 3 mg/ml solutions, respectively (2077).

Syringes— Thiotepa reconstituted to a concentration of 10 mg/ml with sterile water for injection was found to be stable for 24 hours under refrigeration at 8 °C and at room temperature of 23 °C in both the original vials and transferred to plastic syringes (2006).

Filtration— The manufacturer recommends that thiotepa solutions be filtered through a 0.22-μm filter, either a polysulfone membrane (Sterile Acrodisc, Gelman) or mixed ester of cellulose and PVC (Millex-GS, Millipore). The filtering reduces haze but not potency. Solutions should be clear for use. Solutions that remain opaque or contain a precipitate after filtration should not be used (2).

Thiotepa 10 to 300 μg/ml exhibited no loss due to sorption to either cellulose nitrate/cellulose acetate ester (Millex OR) or Teflon (Millex FG) filters (1415; 1416).

Sorption— An evaluation of the stability of thiotepa (Immunex) 0.5 and 5 mg/ml in dextrose 5% in water in both PVC and polyolefin containers found no difference in concentration between the two containers, indicating no loss due to sorption to PVC (2007).

Compatibility Information

Solution Compatibility

Thiotepa

Solution	Mfr	Mfr	Conc/L	Remarks	Ref	C/I
Dextrose 5% in water	BA[a], MG[b]	IMM	0.5 g	Physically stable with losses of 10% or less by HPLC in 8 hr at 4 and 23 °C. Losses ranged up to 17% in 24 hr	2007	I
	BA[a], MG[b]	IMM	5 g	Physically stable with losses of less than 10% by HPLC in 14 days at 4 °C and in 3 days at 23 °C	2007	C
Sodium chloride 0.9%	BA[a]	IMM	1 and 3 g	Physically stable with 7 to 10% loss by HPLC in 24 hr at 25 °C and 4% or less in 48 hr at 4 °C	2077	C
	BA[a]	IMM	0.5 g	Physically stable but up to 7% loss by HPLC in 8 hr with substantial chloro-adduct formation. Up to 13% loss in 24 hr at 25 °C	2077	I
	BA[a]	IMM	0.5 g	Physically stable with 4% or less loss by HPLC in 48 hr at 8 °C	2077	C

[a]Tested in PVC containers.
[b]Tested in polyolefin containers.

Additive Compatibility

Thiotepa

Drug	Mfr	Conc/L	Mfr	Conc/L	Test Soln	Remarks	Ref	C/I
Cisplatin		200 mg		1 g	NS	Yellow precipitation	1379	I

Y-Site Injection Compatibility (1:1 Mixture)

Thiotepa

Drug	Mfr	Conc	Mfr	Conc	Remarks	Ref	C/I
Acyclovir sodium	BW	7 mg/ml[a]	IMM[c]	1 mg/ml[a]	Physically compatible with no change in measured turbidity or increase in particle content in 4 hr at 23 °C	1861	C

Y-Site Injection Compatibility (1:1 Mixture) (Cont.)

		Thiotepa					
Drug	*Mfr*	*Conc*	*Mfr*	*Conc*	*Remarks*	*Ref*	*C/I*
Allopurinol sodium	BW	3 mg/ml[b]	LE[d]	1 mg/ml[c]	Physically compatible with no change in measured turbidity or increase in particle content in 4 hr at 22 °C	1686	**C**
Amifostine	USB	10 mg/ml[a]	LE[d]	1 mg/ml[a]	Physically compatible with no change in measured turbidity or increase in particle content in 4 hr at 23 °C	1845	**C**
Amikacin sulfate	DU	5 mg/ml[a]	IMM[c]	1 mg/ml[a]	Physically compatible with no change in measured turbidity or increase in particle content in 4 hr at 23 °C	1861	**C**
Aminophylline	AMR	2.5 mg/ml[a]	IMM[c]	1 mg/ml[a]	Physically compatible with no change in measured turbidity or increase in particle content in 4 hr at 23 °C	1861	**C**
Amphotericin B	APC	0.6 mg/ml[a]	IMM[c]	1 mg/ml[a]	Physically compatible with no change in measured turbidity or increase in particle content in 4 hr at 23 °C	1861	**C**
Ampicillin sodium	WY	20 mg/ml[b]	IMM[c]	1 mg/ml[a]	Physically compatible with no change in measured turbidity or increase in particle content in 4 hr at 23 °C	1861	**C**
Ampicillin sodium–sulbactam sodium	RR	20 + 10 mg/ml[b]	IMM[c]	1 mg/ml[a]	Physically compatible with no change in measured turbidity or increase in particle content in 4 hr at 23 °C	1861	**C**
Aztreonam	SQ	40 mg/ml[a]	LE[d]	1 mg/ml[a]	Physically compatible with no subvisual haze or particle formation in 4 hr at 23 °C	1758	**C**
	SQ	40 mg/ml[a]	IMM[c]	1 mg/ml[a]	Physically compatible with no change in measured turbidity or increase in particle content in 4 hr at 23 °C	1861	**C**
Bleomycin sulfate	MJ	1 unit/ml[b]	IMM[c]	1 mg/ml[a]	Physically compatible with no change in measured turbidity or increase in particle content in 4 hr at 23 °C	1861	**C**
Bumetanide	RC	0.04 mg/ml[a]	IMM[c]	1 mg/ml[a]	Physically compatible with no change in measured turbidity or increase in particle content in 4 hr at 23 °C	1861	**C**
Buprenorphine HCl	RKC	0.04 mg/ml[a]	IMM[c]	1 mg/ml[a]	Physically compatible with no change in measured turbidity or increase in particle content in 4 hr at 23 °C	1861	**C**
Butorphanol tartrate	APC	0.04 mg/ml[a]	IMM[c]	1 mg/ml[a]	Physically compatible with no change in measured turbidity or increase in particle content in 4 hr at 23 °C	1861	**C**
Calcium gluconate	AMR	40 mg/ml[a]	IMM[c]	1 mg/ml[a]	Physically compatible with no change in measured turbidity or increase in particle content in 4 hr at 23 °C	1861	**C**
Carboplatin	BMS	5 mg/ml[a]	IMM[c]	1 mg/ml[a]	Physically compatible with no change in measured turbidity or increase in particle content in 4 hr at 23 °C	1861	**C**
Carmustine	BMS	1.5 mg/ml[a]	IMM[c]	1 mg/ml[a]	Physically compatible with no change in measured turbidity or increase in particle content in 4 hr at 23 °C	1861	**C**

Y-Site Injection Compatibility (1:1 Mixture) (Cont.)

Thiotepa

Drug	Mfr	Conc	Mfr	Conc	Remarks	Ref	C/I
Cefazolin sodium	MAR	20 mg/ml[a]	IMM[c]	1 mg/ml[a]	Physically compatible with no change in measured turbidity or increase in particle content in 4 hr at 23 °C	1861	C
Cefepime HCl	BR	20 mg/ml[a]	LE[d]	1 mg/ml[a]	Physically compatible with no change in measured turbidity or increase in particle content in 4 hr at 22 °C	1689	C
Cefoperazone sodium	RR	40 mg/ml[a]	IMM[c]	1 mg/ml[a]	Physically compatible with no change in measured turbidity or increase in particle content in 4 hr at 23 °C	1861	C
Cefotaxime sodium	HO	20 mg/ml[a]	IMM[c]	1 mg/ml[a]	Physically compatible with no change in measured turbidity or increase in particle content in 4 hr at 23 °C	1861	C
Cefotetan sodium	STU	20 mg/ml[a]	IMM[c]	1 mg/ml[a]	Physically compatible with no change in measured turbidity or increase in particle content in 4 hr at 23 °C	1861	C
Cefoxitin sodium	ME	20 mg/ml[a]	IMM[c]	1 mg/ml[a]	Physically compatible with no change in measured turbidity or increase in particle content in 4 hr at 23 °C	1861	C
Ceftazidime	LI[e]	40 mg/ml[a]	IMM[c]	1 mg/ml[a]	Physically compatible with no change in measured turbidity or increase in particle content in 4 hr at 23 °C	1861	C
Ceftizoxime sodium	FUJ	20 mg/ml[a]	IMM[c]	1 mg/ml[a]	Physically compatible with no change in measured turbidity or increase in particle content in 4 hr at 23 °C	1861	C
Ceftriaxone sodium	RC	20 mg/ml[a]	IMM[c]	1 mg/ml[a]	Physically compatible with no change in measured turbidity or increase in particle content in 4 hr at 23 °C	1861	C
Cefuroxime sodium	MI	30 mg/ml[a]	IMM[c]	1 mg/ml[a]	Physically compatible with no change in measured turbidity or increase in particle content in 4 hr at 23 °C	1861	C
Chlorpromazine HCl	SCN	2 mg/ml[a]	IMM[c]	1 mg/ml[a]	Physically compatible with no change in measured turbidity or increase in particle content in 4 hr at 23 °C	1861	C
Cimetidine HCl	SKB	12 mg/ml[a]	IMM[c]	1 mg/ml[a]	Physically compatible with no change in measured turbidity or increase in particle content in 4 hr at 23 °C	1861	C
Ciprofloxacin	MI	1 mg/ml[a]	IMM[c]	1 mg/ml[a]	Physically compatible with no change in measured turbidity or increase in particle content in 4 hr at 23 °C	1861	C
Cisplatin	BMS	1 mg/ml	IMM[c]	1 mg/ml[a]	White cloudiness appears in 4 hr at 23 °C	1861	I
Clindamycin phosphate	AST	10 mg/ml[a]	IMM[c]	1 mg/ml[a]	Physically compatible with no change in measured turbidity or increase in particle content in 4 hr at 23 °C	1861	C
Cyclophosphamide	MJ	10 mg/ml[a]	IMM[c]	1 mg/ml[a]	Physically compatible with no change in measured turbidity or increase in particle content in 4 hr at 23 °C	1861	C

Y-Site Injection Compatibility (1:1 Mixture) (Cont.)

			Thiotepa				
Drug	*Mfr*	*Conc*	*Mfr*	*Conc*	*Remarks*	*Ref*	*C/I*
Cytarabine	CET	50 mg/ml	IMM[c]	1 mg/ml[a]	Physically compatible with no change in measured turbidity or increase in particle content in 4 hr at 23 °C	1861	**C**
Dacarbazine	MI	4 mg/ml[a]	IMM[c]	1 mg/ml[a]	Physically compatible with no change in measured turbidity or increase in particle content in 4 hr at 23 °C	1861	**C**
Dactinomycin	ME	0.01 mg/ml[a]	IMM[c]	1 mg/ml[a]	Physically compatible with no change in measured turbidity or increase in particle content in 4 hr at 23 °C	1861	**C**
Daunorubicin HCl	WY	1 mg/ml[a]	IMM[c]	1 mg/ml[a]	Physically compatible with no change in measured turbidity or increase in particle content in 4 hr at 23 °C	1861	**C**
Dexamethasone sodium phosphate	AMR	1 mg/ml[a]	IMM[c]	1 mg/ml[a]	Physically compatible with no change in measured turbidity or increase in particle content in 4 hr at 23 °C	1861	**C**
Diphenhydramine HCl	WY	2 mg/ml[a]	IMM[c]	1 mg/ml[a]	Physically compatible with no change in measured turbidity or increase in particle content in 4 hr at 23 °C	1861	**C**
Dobutamine HCl	LI	4 mg/ml[a]	IMM[c]	1 mg/ml[a]	Physically compatible with no change in measured turbidity or increase in particle content in 4 hr at 23 °C	1861	**C**
Dopamine HCl	AST	3.2 mg/ml[a]	IMM[c]	1 mg/ml[a]	Physically compatible with no change in measured turbidity or increase in particle content in 4 hr at 23 °C	1861	**C**
Doxorubicin HCl	CHI	2 mg/ml	IMM[c]	1 mg/ml[a]	Physically compatible with no change in measured turbidity or increase in particle content in 4 hr at 23 °C	1861	**C**
Doxycycline hyclate	LY	1 mg/ml[a]	IMM[c]	1 mg/ml[a]	Physically compatible with no change in measured turbidity or increase in particle content in 4 hr at 23 °C	1861	**C**
Droperidol	JN	0.4 mg/ml[a]	IMM[c]	1 mg/ml[a]	Physically compatible with no change in measured turbidity or increase in particle content in 4 hr at 23 °C	1861	**C**
Enalaprilat	ME	0.1 mg/ml[a]	IMM[c]	1 mg/ml[a]	Physically compatible with no change in measured turbidity or increase in particle content in 4 hr at 23 °C	1861	**C**
Etoposide	BMS	0.4 mg/ml[a]	IMM[c]	1 mg/ml[a]	Physically compatible with no change in measured turbidity or increase in particle content in 4 hr at 23 °C	1861	**C**
Etoposide phosphate	BR	5 mg/ml[a]	IMM[c]	1 mg/ml[a]	Physically compatible with no change in measured turbidity or increase in particle content in 4 hr at 23 °C	2218	**C**
Famotidine	ME	2 mg/ml[a]	IMM[c]	1 mg/ml[a]	Physically compatible with no change in measured turbidity or increase in particle content in 4 hr at 23 °C	1861	**C**
Filgrastim	AMG	30 µg/ml[a]	LE[d]	1 mg/ml[a]	Particles and filaments form immediately	1687	**I**
Floxuridine	RC	3 mg/ml[a]	IMM[c]	1 mg/ml[a]	Physically compatible with no change in measured turbidity or increase in particle content in 4 hr at 23 °C	1861	**C**

Y-Site Injection Compatibility (1:1 Mixture) (Cont.)

Drug	Mfr	Conc	Mfr	Conc	Remarks	Ref	C/I
				Thiotepa			
Fluconazole	RR	2 mg/ml	IMM[c]	1 mg/ml[a]	Physically compatible with no change in measured turbidity or increase in particle content in 4 hr at 23 °C	1861	C
Fludarabine phosphate	BX	1 mg/ml[a]	IMM[c]	1 mg/ml[a]	Physically compatible with no change in measured turbidity or increase in particle content in 4 hr at 23 °C	1861	C
Fluorouracil	AD	16 mg/ml[a]	IMM[c]	1 mg/ml[a]	Physically compatible with no change in measured turbidity or increase in particle content in 4 hr at 23 °C	1861	C
Furosemide	AMR	3 mg/ml[a]	IMM[c]	1 mg/ml[a]	Physically compatible with no change in measured turbidity or increase in particle content in 4 hr at 23 °C	1861	C
Ganciclovir sodium	SY	20 mg/ml[a]	IMM[c]	1 mg/ml[a]	Physically compatible with no change in measured turbidity or increase in particle content in 4 hr at 23 °C	1861	C
Gemcitabine HCl	LI	10 mg/ml[b]	IMM[c]	1 mg/ml[b]	Physically compatible with no change in measured turbidity or increase in particle content in 4 hr at 23 °C	2226	C
Gentamicin sulfate	ES	5 mg/ml[a]	IMM[c]	1 mg/ml[a]	Physically compatible with no change in measured turbidity or increase in particle content in 4 hr at 23 °C	1861	C
Granisetron HCl	SKB	0.05 mg/ml[a]	IMM[c]	1 mg/ml[a]	Physically compatible with no change in measured turbidity or increase in particle content in 4 hr at 23 °C	1861; 2000	C
Haloperidol lactate	MN	0.2 mg/ml[a]	IMM[c]	1 mg/ml[a]	Physically compatible with no change in measured turbidity or increase in particle content in 4 hr at 23 °C	1861	C
Heparin sodium	ES	100 units/ml[a]	IMM[c]	1 mg/ml[a]	Physically compatible with no change in measured turbidity or increase in particle content in 4 hr at 23 °C	1861	C
Hydrocortisone sodium phosphate	MSD	1 mg/ml[a]	IMM[c]	1 mg/ml[a]	Physically compatible with no change in measured turbidity or increase in particle content in 4 hr at 23 °C	1861	C
Hydrocortisone sodium succinate	UP	1 mg/ml[a]	IMM[c]	1 mg/ml[a]	Physically compatible with no change in measured turbidity or increase in particle content in 4 hr at 23 °C	1861	C
Hydromorphone HCl	AST	0.5 mg/ml[a]	IMM[c]	1 mg/ml[a]	Physically compatible with no change in measured turbidity or increase in particle content in 4 hr at 23 °C	1861	C
Hydroxyzine HCl	ES	4 mg/ml[a]	IMM[c]	1 mg/ml[a]	Physically compatible with no change in measured turbidity or increase in particle content in 4 hr at 23 °C	1861	C
Idarubicin HCl	AD	0.5 mg/ml[a]	IMM[c]	1 mg/ml[a]	Increase in turbidity no greater than dilution with D5W alone. No increase in particle content in 4 hr at 23 °C	1861	C
Ifosfamide	MJ	25 mg/ml[a]	IMM[c]	1 mg/ml[a]	Physically compatible with no change in measured turbidity or increase in particle content in 4 hr at 23 °C	1861	C

Y-Site Injection Compatibility (1:1 Mixture) (Cont.)

Thiotepa

Drug	Mfr	Conc	Mfr	Conc	Remarks	Ref	C/I
Imipenem–cilastatin sodium	ME	10 mg/ml[a]	IMM[c]	1 mg/ml[a]	Physically compatible with no change in measured turbidity or increase in particle content in 4 hr at 23 °C	1861	C
Leucovorin calcium	LE	2 mg/ml[a]	IMM[c]	1 mg/ml[a]	Physically compatible with no change in measured turbidity or increase in particle content in 4 hr at 23 °C	1861	C
Lorazepam	WY	0.1 mg/ml[a]	IMM[c]	1 mg/ml[a]	Physically compatible with no change in measured turbidity or increase in particle content in 4 hr at 23 °C	1861	C
Magnesium sulfate	AST	100 mg/ml[a]	IMM[c]	1 mg/ml[a]	Physically compatible with no change in measured turbidity or increase in particle content in 4 hr at 23 °C	1861	C
Mannitol	BA	15%	IMM[c]	1 mg/ml[a]	Physically compatible with no change in measured turbidity or increase in particle content in 4 hr at 23 °C	1861	C
Melphalan HCl	BW	0.1 mg/ml[b]	LE[d]	10 mg/ml[b]	Physically compatible with no change in measured turbidity or increase in particle content in 3 hr at 22 °C	1557	C
Meperidine HCl	WY	4 mg/ml[a]	IMM[c]	1 mg/ml[a]	Physically compatible with no change in measured turbidity or increase in particle content in 4 hr at 23 °C	1861	C
Mesna	MJ	10 mg/ml[a]	IMM[c]	1 mg/ml[a]	Physically compatible with no change in measured turbidity or increase in particle content in 4 hr at 23 °C	1861	C
Methotrexate sodium	LE	15 mg/ml[a]	IMM[c]	1 mg/ml[a]	Physically compatible with no change in measured turbidity or increase in particle content in 4 hr at 23 °C	1861	C
Methylprednisolone sodium succinate	AB	5 mg/ml[a]	IMM[c]	1 mg/ml[a]	Physically compatible with no change in measured turbidity or increase in particle content in 4 hr at 23 °C	1861	C
Metoclopramide HCl	RB	5 mg/ml	IMM[c]	1 mg/ml[a]	Physically compatible with no change in measured turbidity or increase in particle content in 4 hr at 23 °C	1861	C
Metronidazole	BA	5 mg/ml	IMM[c]	1 mg/ml[a]	Physically compatible with no change in measured turbidity or increase in particle content in 4 hr at 23 °C	1861	C
Minocycline HCl	LE	0.2 mg/ml[a]	IMM[c]	1 mg/ml[a]	Yellow-green discoloration forms in 1 hr at 23 °C	1861	I
Mitomycin	BMS	0.5 mg/ml	IMM[c]	1 mg/ml[a]	Physically compatible with no change in measured turbidity or increase in particle content in 4 hr at 23 °C	1861	C
Mitoxantrone HCl	IMM	0.5 mg/ml[a]	IMM[c]	1 mg/ml[a]	Physically compatible with no change in measured turbidity or increase in particle content in 4 hr at 23 °C	1861	C
Morphine sulfate	AST	1 mg/ml[a]	IMM[c]	1 mg/ml[a]	Physically compatible with no change in measured turbidity or increase in particle content in 4 hr at 23 °C	1861	C

Y-Site Injection Compatibility (1:1 Mixture) (Cont.)

		Thiotepa					
Drug	*Mfr*	*Conc*	*Mfr*	*Conc*	*Remarks*	*Ref*	*C/I*
Nalbuphine HCl	AST	10 mg/ml	IMM[c]	1 mg/ml[a]	Physically compatible with no change in measured turbidity or increase in particle content in 4 hr at 23 °C	1861	**C**
Netilmicin sulfate	SC	5 mg/ml[a]	IMM[c]	1 mg/ml[a]	Physically compatible with no change in measured turbidity or increase in particle content in 4 hr at 23 °C	1861	**C**
Ofloxacin	ORT	4 mg/ml	IMM[c]	1 mg/ml[a]	Physically compatible with no change in measured turbidity or increase in particle content in 4 hr at 23 °C	1861	**C**
Ondansetron HCl	GL	1 mg/ml[a]	IMM[c]	1 mg/ml[a]	Physically compatible with no change in measured turbidity or increase in particle content in 4 hr at 23 °C	1861	**C**
Paclitaxel	MJ	0.6 mg/ml[a]	IMM[c]	1 mg/ml[a]	Physically compatible with no change in measured turbidity or increase in particle content in 4 hr at 23 °C	1861	**C**
Piperacillin sodium	LE	40 mg/ml[a]	IMM[c]	1 mg/ml[a]	Physically compatible with no change in measured turbidity or increase in particle content in 4 hr at 23 °C	1861	**C**
Piperacillin sodium–tazobactam sodium	LE	40 + 5 mg/ml[a]	LE[d]	1 mg/ml[a]	Physically compatible with no change in measured turbidity or increase in particle content in 4 hr at 22 °C	1688	**C**
Plicamycin	MI	0.01 mg/ml[a]	IMM[c]	1 mg/ml[a]	Physically compatible with no change in measured turbidity or increase in particle content in 4 hr at 23 °C	1861	**C**
Potassium chloride	AMR	0.1 mEq/ml[a]	IMM[c]	1 mg/ml[a]	Physically compatible with no change in measured turbidity or increase in particle content in 4 hr at 23 °C	1861	**C**
Prochlorperazine edisylate	SCN	0.5 mg/ml[a]	IMM[c]	1 mg/ml[a]	Physically compatible with no change in measured turbidity or increase in particle content in 4 hr at 23 °C	1861	**C**
Promethazine HCl	WY	2 mg/ml[a]	IMM[c]	1 mg/ml[a]	Physically compatible with no change in measured turbidity or increase in particle content in 4 hr at 23 °C	1861	**C**
Ranitidine HCl	GL	20 mg/ml[a]	IMM[c]	1 mg/ml[a]	Physically compatible with no change in measured turbidity or increase in particle content in 4 hr at 23 °C	1861	**C**
Sodium bicarbonate	AB	1 mEq/ml	IMM[c]	1 mg/ml[a]	Physically compatible with no change in measured turbidity or increase in particle content in 4 hr at 23 °C	1861	**C**
Streptozocin	UP	40 mg/ml[a]	IMM[c]	1 mg/ml[a]	Physically compatible with no change in measured turbidity or increase in particle content in 4 hr at 23 °C	1861	**C**
Teniposide	BR	0.1 mg/ml[a]	LE[d]	1 mg/ml[a]	Physically compatible with no subvisual haze or particle formation in 4 hr at 23 °C	1725	**C**
Ticarcillin disodium	SKB	30 mg/ml[a]	IMM[c]	1 mg/ml[a]	Physically compatible with no change in measured turbidity or increase in particle content in 4 hr at 23 °C	1861	**C**

Y-Site Injection Compatibility (1:1 Mixture) (Cont.)

Drug	Mfr	Conc	Mfr	Conc	Remarks	Ref	C/I
				Thiotepa			
Ticarcillin disodium–clavulanate potassium	SKB	31 mg/ml[a]	IMM[c]	1 mg/ml[a]	Physically compatible with no change in measured turbidity or increase in particle content in 4 hr at 23 °C	1861	**C**
Tobramycin sulfate	LI	5 mg/ml[a]	IMM[c]	1 mg/ml[a]	Physically compatible with no change in measured turbidity or increase in particle content in 4 hr at 23 °C	1861	**C**
TPN #193[f]			IMM[c]	1 mg/ml[a]	Physically compatible with no change in measured turbidity or increase in particle content in 4 hr at 23 °C	1861	**C**
Trimethoprim–sulfamethoxazole	ES	0.8 + 4 mg/ml[a]	IMM[c]	1 mg/ml[a]	Physically compatible with no change in measured turbidity or increase in particle content in 4 hr at 23 °C	1861	**C**
Vancomycin sulfate	AB	10 mg/ml[a]	IMM[c]	1 mg/ml[a]	Physically compatible with no change in measured turbidity or increase in particle content in 4 hr at 23 °C	1861	**C**
Vinblastine sulfate	LI	0.12 mg/ml[a]	IMM[c]	1 mg/ml[a]	Physically compatible with no change in measured turbidity or increase in particle content in 4 hr at 23 °C	1861	**C**
Vincristine sulfate	LI	0.05 mg/ml[a]	IMM[c]	1 mg/ml[a]	Physically compatible with no change in measured turbidity or increase in particle content in 4 hr at 23 °C	1861	**C**
Vinorelbine tartrate	BW	1 mg/ml[b]	LE[d]	10 mg/ml[b]	Cloudy solution with particles forms immediately	1558	**I**
Zidovudine	BW	4 mg/ml[a]	IMM[c]	1 mg/ml[a]	Physically compatible with no change in measured turbidity or increase in particle content in 4 hr at 23 °C	1861	**C**

[a]*Tested in dextrose 5% in water.*
[b]*Tested in sodium chloride 0.9%.*
[c]*Lyophilized formulation tested.*
[d]*Powder fill formulation tested.*
[e]*Sodium carbonate–containing formulation tested.*
[f]*Refer to Appendix I for the composition of parenteral nutrition solutions. TPN indicates a 2-in-1 admixture.*

Additional Compatibility Information

Solutions— The reconstituted thiotepa solution may be diluted for administration with dextrose or dextrose and sodium chloride injections, sodium chloride injection, Ringer's injection, or lactated Ringer's injection if larger volumes of fluid are desired (4).

The manufacturer has stated that thiotepa 1 and 3 mg/ml in sodium chloride 0.9% in PVC containers is stable for up to 24 hours at 25 °C and up to 48 hours at 8 °C, while at a concentration of 5 mg/ml in sodium chloride 0.9% thiotepa is stable for 24 hours at either 8 or 23 °C. However, thiotepa 0.5 mg/ml in sodium chloride 0.9% is unstable and should be used immediately if mixed at this concentration (2006). Similar results have been reported for admixtures in dextrose 5% in water (2007). See Compatibility Information above.

Miscellaneous— Reconstituted thiotepa may be mixed with 2% procaine HCl and/or 0.1% epinephrine HCl for local administration (4).

TICARCILLIN DISODIUM
AHFS 8:12.16

Ticar   **SmithKline Beecham**

Products— Ticarcillin disodium (SmithKline Beecham) is available in 1-, 3-, and 6-g standard vials, 3-g piggyback bottles, and 20- and 30-g bulk pharmacy packages (2; 4).

For intramuscular injections, each gram of ticarcillin disodium in standard vials should be reconstituted with 2 ml of sterile water for injection, sodium chloride 0.9%, lidocaine HCl 1% (without epinephrine), or another compatible intravenous infusion solution to yield a solution containing ticarcillin 1 g/2.6 ml (385 mg/ml) (2; 4).

For intravenous use, each gram of drug in standard vials should be reconstituted with at least 4 ml of sodium chloride 0.9%, dextrose 5% in water, or lactated Ringer's injection to yield a solution containing ticarcillin approximately 200 mg/ml (2; 4).

The 3-g piggyback bottles should be reconstituted with a compatible intravenous infusion solution in the following amounts (2; 4):

Amount of Diluent	Solution Concentration
100 ml	1 g/34 ml
60 ml	1 g/20 ml
30 ml	1 g/10 ml

The 20- or 30-g bulk pharmacy packages should be reconstituted with 85 or 75 ml, respectively, of sodium chloride 0.9%, dextrose 5% in water, or lactated Ringer's injection (added in two portions, with shaking after each addition) to yield a 200- or 300-mg/ml ticarcillin concentration, respectively. This concentrated solution must be diluted further in a compatible infusion solution for administration (2; 4).

pH— From 6 to 8 (2; 4).

Osmolality— The osmolality of ticarcillin disodium 3 g was calculated for the following dilutions (1054):

Diluent	Osmolality (mOsm/kg)	
	50 ml	100 ml
Dextrose 5% in water	558	420
Sodium chloride 0.9%	579	442

Robinson et al. recommended the following maximum ticarcillin disodium concentrations to achieve osmolalities suitable for peripheral infusion in fluid-restricted patients (1180):

Diluent	Maximum Concentration (mg/ml)	Osmolality (mOsm/kg)
Dextrose 5% in water	50	558
Sodium chloride 0.9%	45	538
Sterile water for injection	90	541

Sodium Content— Each gram of ticarcillin disodium contains 5.2 (120 mg) to 6.5 mEq of sodium (4; 371; 462; 846).

Administration— Ticarcillin disodium is administered by deep intramuscular injection or direct intravenous injection as slowly as possible or by continuous or intermittent intravenous infusion (2; 4; 8). Intramuscular injection should be made well within the body of a relatively large muscle. Doses should not exceed 2 g per injection by this route. By direct intravenous injection, concentrations of 50 mg/ml or less should be administered to minimize vein irritation. For intravenous infusion, the reconstituted solution is diluted with an appropriate volume of a suitable diluent to a concentration of 10 to 100 mg/ml and administered continuously or intermittently over 30 to 120 minutes in adults or over 10 to 20 minutes in neonates (2; 4).

Stability— Intact vials of ticarcillin disodium may be stored at controlled room temperature or below. The manufacturer recommends that intramuscular solutions be used promptly (2). Storage of ticarcillin disodium solutions, especially high concentrations at room temperature, may form polymer conjugation products that play a role in hypersensitivity reactions even though the potency remains acceptable. Consequently, refrigeration or use within 30 minutes of reconstituting solutions has been recommended by some clinicians (4).

Nicholas et al. reported on ticarcillin disodium 250 mg/ml stored at room temperature and 4 °C. After 24 hours at room temperature, HPLC analysis revealed a new peak, which increased in size by 72 hours. Storage at 4 °C significantly reduced the formation rate of this new compound. Although the therapeutic potency of ticarcillin disodium is retained over the time period studied, the potential as an antigen may change because of the possible formation of polymers or conjugation products that may cause allergic sensitization reactions. The authors recommended that the drug be freshly prepared before use or refrigerated during interim storage (785).

Lynn reported on the chemical stability of a ticarcillin disodium concentration of 500 mg/ml in sterile water for injection. Approximately 3% decomposition occurred at 5 °C and 7% at 25 °C in 24 hours. When stored at 5 °C for seven days, 9% decomposition occurred. However, at 25 °C for only three days, 27% decomposition was noted (334).

Reconstitution of the bulk pharmacy package to a 200- or 300-mg/ml concentration results in a solution that should be used or discarded within 24 hours at room temperature or 72 hours under refrigeration (4).

Syringes— Borst et al. reported that ticarcillin disodium (Beecham) 2 and 3 g/10 ml in sterile water for injection, packaged in plastic syringes (Monoject), exhibited 10% ticarcillin loss in four days at 24 °C and six days at 4 °C as determined by HPLC (1178).

Ticarcillin disodium (Beecham) 100 mg/ml in sterile water for injection and 25 mg/ml in sodium chloride 0.45% was packaged as 10 ml in 12-ml polypropylene syringes (Sherwood) and sealed with syringe tip caps (Sherwood). Samples were stored at 24 °C for one day, 4 °C for seven days, and −20 °C for 30 days. All samples at all three temperatures remained physically and chemically stable throughout the study. HPLC analysis found no loss of ticarcillin disodium (2019).

Freezing Solutions— Ticarcillin disodium (Beecham) 3 g/50 ml of dextrose 5% in water, in PVC bags frozen at −20 °C for 30 days and then thawed by exposure to ambient temperature or microwave radiation, showed no evidence of precipitation or color change and showed no loss of potency as determined microbiologically. Subsequent storage of the admixture at room temperature for 24 hours also yielded a physically compatible solution which exhibited little or no additional loss of activity (555).

Solutions of ticarcillin disodium 1.5 g/50 ml in dextrose 5% in water and sodium chloride 0.9% in PVC containers were stored at −27 °C for 270 days and then thawed in a microwave oven for 2.5

minutes. Both solutions retained their ticarcillin potency for the 270 days. Some loss of ticarcillin was observed during further storage of the thawed solutions for 24 hours at 4 °C, usually between 2 and 7%, but no sample fell below 90% of the labeled concentration (1176).

Borst et al. reported that ticarcillin disodium (Beecham) 2 and 3 g/10 ml in sterile water for injection, packaged in plastic syringes (Monoject) and frozen at −15 °C, was stable for the three-month study period, exhibiting less than a 10% loss as determined by HPLC (1178).

Ticarcillin disodium (Beecham) 100 mg/ml in sterile water for injection and 25 mg/ml in sodium chloride 0.45% in polypropylene syringes was physically and chemically stable for 30 days when frozen at −20 °C (2019).

At concentrations of 10 to 100 mg/ml in the following infusion solutions, ticarcillin disodium will not lose potency for up to 30 days when frozen immediately after preparation (2; 4):

> Dextrose 5% in water
> Ringer's injection
> Ringer's injection, lactated
> Sodium chloride 0.9%
> Sterile water for injection

The stabilities of thawed solutions are identical with those of solutions that have not been frozen, although use within 24 hours of thawing is recommended (2; 4). (See Additional Compatibility Information.)

Compatibility Information

Solution Compatibility

Ticarcillin disodium

Solution	Mfr	Mfr	Conc/L	Remarks	Ref	C/I
Dextrose 4.3% in sodium chloride 0.18%		BE	20 g	No decomposition in 24 hr at 25 °C	334	C
Dextrose 5% in water		BE	20 g	3% decomposition in 24 hr at 25 °C	334	C
	TR[a]	BE	30 g	Physically compatible and potency retained for 24 hr at room temperature	518	C
	TR[a]	BE	60 g	Physically compatible and no potency loss in 24 hr at room temperature	565	C
Sodium chloride 0.9%		BE	20 g	6% decomposition in 24 hr at 25 °C	334	C
	TR[a]	BE	30 g	Physically compatible and potency retained for 24 hr at room temperature	518	C
Sodium lactate ⅙ M		BE	20 g	11% decomposition in 24 hr at 25 °C	334	C
TPN #86 to #88[b]		BE	10 mg	10% ticarcillin loss in 24 hr at room temperature exposed to light	1160	C
		BE	20 mg	12 to 15% ticarcillin loss in 4 hr at room temperature exposed to light	1160	I
TPN #107[b]			2 g	50% ticarcillin loss in 24 hr at 21 °C by microbiological assay	1326	I

[a]Tested in PVC containers.
[b]Refer to Appendix I for the composition of parenteral nutrition solutions. TPN indicates a 2-in-1 admixture.

Additive Compatibility

Ticarcillin disodium

Drug	Mfr	Conc/L	Mfr	Conc/L	Test Soln	Remarks	Ref	C/I
Gentamicin sulfate		100 mg		2 g	TPN #107[a]	Over 98% gentamicin loss in 24 hr at 21 °C by microbiological assay	1326	I
Ranitidine HCl	GL	100 mg	BE	10 g	D5W	Physically compatible for 24 hr at ambient temperature under fluorescent light	1151	C
Verapamil HCl	KN	80 mg	BE	6 g	D5W, NS	Physically compatible for 24 hr	764	C
	SE	[b]	BE	40 g	D5W, NS	Physically compatible for 24 hr at 21 °C	1166	C

[a]Refer to Appendix I for the composition of parenteral nutrition solutions. TPN indicates a 2-in-1 admixture.
[b]Final concentration unspecified.

Drugs in Syringe Compatibility

			Ticarcillin disodium				
Drug (in syringe)	*Mfr*	*Amt*	*Mfr*	*Amt*	*Remarks*	*Ref*	*C/I*
Doxapram HCl	RB	400 mg/ 20 ml		1 g/ 20 ml	18% doxapram loss in 3 hr	1177	**I**

Y-Site Injection Compatibility (1:1 Mixture)

			Ticarcillin disodium				
Drug	*Mfr*	*Conc*	*Mfr*	*Conc*	*Remarks*	*Ref*	*C/I*
Acyclovir sodium	BW	5 mg/ml[a]	TR	30 mg/ml[a]	Physically compatible for 4 hr at 25 °C	1157	**C**
Allopurinol sodium	BW	3 mg/ml[b]	BE	30 mg/ml[b]	Physically compatible with no change in measured turbidity or increase in particle content in 4 hr at 22 °C	1686	**C**
Amifostine	USB	10 mg/ml[a]	BE	30 mg/ml[a]	Physically compatible with no change in measured turbidity or increase in particle content in 4 hr at 23 °C	1845	**C**
Amphotericin B cholesteryl sulfate complex	SEQ	0.83 mg/ml[a]	SKB	30 mg/ml[a]	Microprecipitate forms immediately	2117	**I**
Aztreonam	SQ	40 mg/ml[a]	BE	30 mg/ml[a]	Physically compatible with no subvisual haze or particle formation in 4 hr at 23 °C	1758	**C**
Cisatracurium besylate	GW	0.1, 2, 5 mg/ml[a]	SKB	30 mg/ml[a]	Physically compatible with no change in measured turbidity or increase in particle content in 4 hr at 23 °C	2074	**C**
Cyclophosphamide	MJ	20 mg/ml[a]	BE	30 mg/ml[a]	Physically compatible for 4 hr at 25 °C	1194	**C**
Diltiazem HCl	MMD	1[b] and 5 mg/ml	BE	200 mg/ml[b]	Visually compatible	1807	**C**
	MMD	5 mg/ml	BE	10 mg/ml[b]	Visually compatible	1807	**C**
Docetaxel	RPR	0.9 mg/ml[a]	SKB	30 mg/ml[a]	Physically compatible with no change in measured turbidity or increase in particle content in 4 hr at 23 °C	2224	**C**
Doxorubicin HCl liposome injection	SEQ	0.4 mg/ml[a]	SKB	30 mg/ml[a]	Physically compatible with little or no change in measured turbidity and no increase in particle content in 4 hr at 23 °C	2087	**C**
Etoposide phosphate	BR	5 mg/ml[a]	SKB	30 mg/ml[a]	Physically compatible with no change in measured turbidity or increase in particle content in 4 hr at 23 °C	2218	**C**
Famotidine	MSD	0.2 mg/ml[a]	BE	30 mg/ml[b]	Physically compatible for 14 hr	1196	**C**
Filgrastim	AMG	30 μg/ml[a]	BE	30 mg/ml[a]	Physically compatible with no change in measured turbidity or increase in particle content in 4 hr at 22 °C	1687	**C**
Fluconazole	RR	2 mg/ml	BE	15 mg/ml	Viscous gel-like substance forms	1407	**I**
Fludarabine phosphate	BX	1 mg/ml[a]	BE	30 mg/ml[a]	Physically compatible for 4 hr at room temperature under fluorescent light	1439	**C**
Gemcitabine HCl	LI	10 mg/ml[b]	SKB	30 mg/ml[b]	Physically compatible with no change in measured turbidity or increase in particle content in 4 hr at 23 °C	2226	**C**

Y-Site Injection Compatibility (1:1 Mixture) (Cont.)

Ticarcillin disodium

Drug	Mfr	Conc	Mfr	Conc	Remarks	Ref	C/I
Granisetron HCl	SKB	0.05 mg/ml[a]	SKB	30 mg/ml[a]	Physically compatible with no change in measured turbidity or increase in particle content in 4 hr at 23 °C	2000	C
Heparin sodium	TR	50 units/ml	BE	20 mg/ml[a]	Visually compatible for 6 hr at 25 °C	1793	C
Hydromorphone HCl	WY	0.2 mg/ml[a]	BE	60 mg/ml[a]	Physically compatible for at least 4 hr at 25 °C under fluorescent light	987	C
IL-2	RC	4800 I.U./ml[b]	BE	200 mg/ml	Visually compatible and IL-2 activity by bioassay retained. Ticarcillin not tested	1552	C
Insulin, regular	LI	0.2 unit/ml[b]	BE	30 mg/ml[b]	Physically compatible for 2 hr at 25 °C	1395	C
Magnesium sulfate	IX	16.7, 33.3, 66.7, 100 mg/ml[a]	BE	60 mg/ml[a]	Physically compatible for at least 4 hr at 32 °C	813	C
Melphalan HCl	BW	0.1 mg/ml[b]	BE	30 mg/ml[b]	Physically compatible with no change in measured turbidity or increase in particle content in 3 hr at 22 °C	1557	C
Meperidine HCl	WY	10 mg/ml[a]	BE	60 mg/ml[a]	Physically compatible for at least 4 hr at 25 °C under fluorescent light	987	C
Morphine sulfate	WI	1 mg/ml[a]	BE	60 mg/ml[a]	Physically compatible for at least 4 hr at 25 °C under fluorescent light	987	C
Ondansetron HCl	GL	1 mg/ml[b]	BE	30 mg/ml[a]	Physically compatible for 4 hr at 22 °C	1365	C
Perphenazine	SC	0.02 mg/ml[a]	BE	30 mg/ml[a]	Physically compatible for 4 hr at 25 °C	1155	C
Propofol	ZEN	10 mg/ml	SKB	30 mg/ml[a]	Physically compatible for 1 hr at 23 °C with no increase in particle content	2066	C
Remifentanil HCl	GW	0.025 and 0.25 mg/ml[b]	SKB	30 mg/ml[a]	Physically compatible with no change in measured turbidity or increase in particle content in 4 hr at 23 °C	2075	C
Sargramostim	IMM	10 μg/ml[b]	BE	30 mg/ml[b]	Physically compatible for 4 hr at 22 °C	1436	C
Teniposide	BR	0.1 mg/ml[a]	BE	30 mg/ml[a]	Physically compatible with no subvisual haze or particle formation in 4 hr at 23 °C	1725	C
Theophylline	TR	4 mg/ml	BE	20 mg/ml[a]	Visually compatible for 6 hr at 25 °C	1793	C
Thiotepa	IMM[c]	1 mg/ml[a]	SKB	30 mg/ml[a]	Physically compatible with no change in measured turbidity or increase in particle content in 4 hr at 23 °C	1861	C
TNA #73[d]		32.5 ml[e]	BE	3 g/50 ml[a]	Physically compatible for 4 hr at 25 °C by visual observation	1008	C
TNA #218 to #226[d]			SKB	30 mg/ml[a]	Visually compatible with no precipitate or emulsion damage apparent in 4 hr at 23 °C	2215	C
TPN #54[d]				267 and 400 mg/ml	Physically compatible and 89 to 94% ticarcillin activity retained over 6 hr at 22 °C by microbiological assay	1045	C
TPN #61[d]		[f]	BE	250 mg/ 1 ml[g]	Physically compatible	1012	C
		[h]	BE	1.5 g/6 ml[g]	Physically compatible	1012	C

Y-Site Injection Compatibility (1:1 Mixture) (Cont.)

Ticarcillin disodium

Drug	Mfr	Conc	Mfr	Conc	Remarks	Ref	C/I
TPN #212 to #215[d]			SKB	30 mg/ml[a]	Physically compatible with no change in measured turbidity or increase in particle content in 4 hr at 23 °C	2109	**C**
Vancomycin HCl	AB	20 mg/ml[a]	SKB	50[a] and 200[j] mg/ml	Transient precipitate forms followed by clear solution	2189	**?**
	AB	20 mg/ml[a]	SKB	1 and 10 mg/ml[a]	Gross white precipitate forms immediately	2189	**I**
	AB	2 mg/ml[a]	SKB	1[a], 10[a], 50[a], and 200[j] mg/ml	Physically compatible with no change in measured turbidity or increase in particle content in 4 hr at 23 °C	2189	**C**
Verapamil HCl	SE	2.5 mg/ml	BE	40 mg/ml[i]	Physically compatible for 15 min at 21 °C under fluorescent light	1166	**C**
Vinorelbine tartrate	BW	1 mg/ml[b]	BE	30 mg/ml[b]	Physically compatible with no change in measured turbidity or increase in particle content in 4 hr at 22 °C	1558	**C**

[a]*Tested in dextrose 5% in water.*
[b]*Tested in sodium chloride 0.9%.*
[c]*Lyophilized formulation tested.*
[d]*Refer to Appendix I for the composition of parenteral nutrition solutions. TNA indicates a 3-in-1 admixture, and TPN indicates a 2-in-1 admixture.*
[e]*A 32.5-ml sample of parenteral nutrition solution mixed with 50 ml of antibiotic solution.*
[f]*Run at 21 ml/hr.*
[g]*Given over five minutes by syringe pump.*
[h]*Run at 94 ml/hr.*
[i]*Tested in both dextrose 5% in water and sodium chloride 0.9%.*
[j]*Tested in sterile water for injection.*

Additional Compatibility Information

Solutions— The manufacturer indicates that ticarcillin disodium in the following infusion solutions will provide sufficient activity at room temperature in the indicated concentrations and time periods (4):

Solution	Time Period
Between 10 and 100 mg/ml	
Dextrose 5% in water	72 hr
Ringer's injection	48 hr
Ringer's injection, lactated	48 hr
Sodium chloride 0.9%	72 hr
Sterile water for injection	72 hr
Between 10 and 50 mg/ml	
Alcohol 5%, dextrose 5% in sodium chloride 0.9%	72 hr
Dextrose 5% in Electrolyte #48	48 hr
Dextrose 5% in Electrolyte #75	48 hr
Dextrose 5% in sodium chloride 0.225%	72 hr
Dextrose 5% in sodium chloride 0.45%	72 hr
Fructose 5% in Electrolyte #75	48 hr
Invert sugar 10% in water	48 hr

These solutions are stable for 14 days when stored at 4 °C but should not be used for multidose purposes (2; 4).

Peritoneal Dialysis Solutions— The activity of ticarcillin 200 mg/L was evaluated in peritoneal dialysis fluids containing 1.5 or 4.25% dextrose (Dianeal 137, Travenol). Storage at 25 °C resulted in virtually no loss of antimicrobial activity in 24 hours (515).

Aminoglycosides— Like carbenicillin, ticarcillin disodium is incompatible with gentamicin sulfate, tobramycin sulfate, and other aminoglycoside antibiotics. Inactivation of aminoglycosides is dependent on the concentration of ticarcillin, temperature, and time of exposure (2; 4).

In vitro, a 50% reduction in gentamicin activity results in 15 to 20 hours when ticarcillin 200 µg/ml is incubated with gentamicin 10 µg/ml at 37 °C in phosphate-buffered saline (pH 7.3) (365).

In a study by Holt et al., ticarcillin 500 mg/L in sodium chloride 0.9% was incubated at 37 °C for 24 hours with amikacin, sisomicin, gentamicin sulfate, and tobramycin sulfate individually at concentrations of 10 mg/L. Aminoglycoside activity was reduced by about 50 to 70% for all except amikacin, which showed a 25% reduction. Substituting serum for the sodium chloride solution slowed the loss of activity, but the loss of activity was accentuated when buffered to pH 7.4 in aqueous solution (574).

In another study, ticarcillin 100 to 600 µg/ml was combined with amikacin 10 and 20 µg/ml, netilmicin sulfate 5 and 10 µg/ml, gentamicin sulfate 5 and 10 µg/ml, and tobramycin sulfate 5 and 10 µg/ml, individually in human serum. Incubation at 37 °C demonstrated greater rates of aminoglycoside decomposition with higher concentrations of ticarcillin. In 72 hours, little or no loss of amikacin, netilmicin, or gentamicin occurred when combined with ticarcillin 100 µg/ml. Tobramycin lost about 11% of its initial activity with this concentration of ticarcillin. At 600 µg/ml of ticarcillin, however, losses were increased to 10% for amikacin, 17% for netilmicin, and about 70% for gentamicin and tobramycin. In general, ticarcillin exerted a less severe adverse effect on aminoglycoside activity than did carbenicillin under these conditions (575).

Murillo et al. determined that lower serum levels of gentamicin occurred in patients with normal renal function when concomitant ticarcillin disodium was administered compared to cephalothin sodium. The dose of ticarcillin disodium was 12 g/m^2/day while cephalothin sodium was given at 7 g/m^2/day. The gentamicin sulfate dose was 180 mg/m^2/day. In one hour, gentamicin serum levels of 3.1 µg/ml resulted in patients receiving cephalothin while only 2 µg/ml was achieved in patients on ticarcillin. Ticarcillin levels were also substantially reduced (667).

To determine if spurious aminoglycoside levels could result from a delay in assaying blood samples, Tindula et al. evaluated the inactivation of amikacin 35 µg/ml and gentamicin and tobramycin 10 µg/ml in human serum by 400-µg/ml concentrations of several penicillins and cephalosporins. Samples were stored for 24 hours at room temperature or frozen at −20 °C. For the room temperature samples, cefazolin and cefamandole caused relatively little inactivation. Nafcillin, cephapirin, and cefoxitin caused moderate inactivation, 20% or less. Penicillin, ampicillin, carbenicillin, and ticarcillin generally caused 25% or more inactivation of gentamicin and tobramycin. Amikacin was somewhat less affected. Freezing samples at −20 °C prevented significant inactivation of amikacin and gentamicin by any of the drugs. Freezing the tobramycin samples was satisfactory for most of the drugs except penicillin, ampicillin, and carbenicillin, which still exhibited a 15 to 20% loss in 24 hours (824).

The inactivation of tobramycin, gentamicin, and amikacin 10 µg/ml in sterile distilled water by ticarcillin 500 and 100 µg/ml stored at 37 °C was reported by Jorgensen and Crawford. Ticarcillin 500 µg/ml caused about a 45% tobramycin loss in two hours and a 75% loss in six hours. At 100 µg/ml, 47% tobramycin inactivation occurred in six hours. The gentamicin loss was 34 and 15% in six hours for ticarcillin 500- and 100-µg/ml concentrations, respectively. The amikacin loss was 16% in six hours with ticarcillin 500 µg/ml but was insignificant with the 100-µg/ml concentration. No loss of ticarcillin activity was detected in any combination (973).

The comparative inactivation of five aminoglycosides by seven β-lactam antibiotics in human serum at 37 °C was reported by Riff and Thomason. Amikacin, followed by netilmicin, had the lowest degree of inactivation; tobramycin sustained the most pronounced losses. Gentamicin and kanamycin were intermediate in the extent of losses. The six penicillins that were tested all produced aminoglycoside inactivation; the greatest extent of inactivation was caused by carbenicillin followed by ticarcillin, penicillin G, oxacillin, methicillin, and ampicillin, in approximate descending order. Cephalothin produced minimal inactivation (5 to 10% in 24 hours). The rate of inactivation could be reduced by storage at 4 °C and further reduced by storage at −20 °C. The authors suggested processing blood samples rapidly to avoid inaccurate serum determinations. Storage of specimens at low temperature until analysis may be helpful (1052).

The clinical significance of these interactions in patients appears to be primarily confined to those with renal failure (218; 334; 361; 364; 616; 847). Literature reports of greatly reduced aminoglycoside levels in such patients have appeared frequently (363; 365–367; 614; 615; 962). In addition, the interaction may be clinically important if assays for aminoglycoside levels in serum are sufficiently delayed (576; 618; 824; 847; 1052).

Most authors believe that in vitro mixing of penicillins such as ticarcillin disodium with aminoglycoside antibiotics should be avoided but that clinical use of the drugs in combination can be of great value. In such combined therapy, it is generally recommended that the drugs be given separately (2; 157; 218; 222; 224; 361; 364; 368–370).

Methylprednisolone— The compatibility of methylprednisolone sodium succinate (Upjohn) with ticarcillin disodium added to an auxiliary medication infusion unit has been studied. Primary admixtures were prepared by adding ticarcillin disodium 6 g/L to dextrose 5% in water, dextrose 5% in sodium chloride 0.9%, and Ringer's injection, lactated. Up to 100 ml of the primary admixture was added, along with the methylprednisolone sodium succinate (Upjohn), to the auxiliary medication infusion unit with the following results (329):

Methylprednisolone Sodium Succinate	Ticarcillin Disodium 6 g/L Primary Solution	Results
500 mg	D5S, D5W qs 100 ml	Clear solution for 24 hr
	LR qs 100 ml	Clear solution for 6 hr
	Added to 100 ml LR	Clear solution for 24 hr
1000 mg	D5W qs 100 ml	Clear solution for 24 hr
	D5S qs 100 ml or added to 100 ml D5S	Clear solution for 6 hr
	LR qs 100 ml	Clear solution for 1 hr
	Added to 100 ml LR	Clear solution for 6 hr

Vancomycin— Direct mixture of vancomycin HCl and ticarcillin disodium reportedly does not result in precipitate formation. However, sequential administration of ticarcillin disodium 4.25 g/50 ml and then vancomycin HCl 500 mg/50 ml in dextrose 5% in sodium chloride 0.3% through a calibrated chamber set (Buretrol) can result in a white precipitate. In that study, the precipitate did not appear during the initial infusion but formed after repeated administration through the same set. The sequence of administration (ticarcillin first, followed by vancomycin), drug concentrations, and repetitive administration all appear to affect the appearance of the precipitate (972).

The compatibility or incompatibility of vancomycin HCl mixed with or administered simultaneously with ticarcillin disodium is concentration dependent (2189). See Y-Site Injection Compatibility above. Vancomycin HCl has a low pH and is variably compatible with drugs having neutral to mildly alkaline pH, including cephalosporins and penicillins. The compatibility may depend on a number of factors, including concentration of each drug, dilution vehicle, actual pH of solutions, and completeness of mixing during administration. Combinations that are compatible when well mixed may result in precipitation if only partially mixed, presumably because of regionally different concentrations and pH values. If attempting to administer vancomycin HCl with ticarcillin disodium, care should be taken to ensure that the specific combination and the concentrations are compatible under the exact administration conditions to be used. An inline filter should be used as a final safety measure (2189).

TICARCILLIN DISODIUM–CLAVULANATE POTASSIUM
AHFS 8:12.16

Timentin   **SmithKline Beecham**

Products— Ticarcillin disodium–clavulanate potassium (SmithKline Beecham) is available in vials and piggyback bottles containing 3.1 g (ticarcillin 3 g as the disodium salt plus clavulanic acid 100 mg as the potassium salt) (2). Reconstitute the vials with 13 ml of sterile water for injection or sodium chloride 0.9% and shake well. When dissolution is completed, the solution will contain ticarcillin 200 mg/ml with clavulanic acid 6.7 mg/ml (2).

The 3.1-g piggyback bottles may be reconstituted with 50 to 100 ml of sodium chloride 0.9%, dextrose 5% in water, or lactated Ringer's injection (4).

The product is also available in a pharmacy bulk package containing 31 g (ticarcillin 30 g as the disodium salt plus clavulanic acid 1 g as the potassium salt). It should be reconstituted with 76 ml of sterile water for injection or sodium chloride 0.9%, added in two portions, and shaken well. Each milliliter of this concentrate contains ticarcillin 300 mg plus clavulanic acid 10 mg (4).

Ticarcillin disodium–clavulanate potassium is available as a frozen premixed infusion containing 3.1 g in 100 ml of water (30 mg/ml of ticarcillin plus 1 mg/ml of clavulanic acid) with sodium citrate buffer and hydrochloric acid or sodium hydroxide to adjust pH. Thawing for use should be performed at room temperature or under refrigeration and not by warming in a water bath or by exposure to microwave radiation. Any precipitate that has formed during freezing should redissolve upon reaching room temperature. The container and ports should be checked for leaking by squeezing the bag (4).

pH— From 5.5 to 7.5 (2).

Osmolality— Robinson et al. recommended the following maximum ticarcillin disodium–clavulanate potassium concentrations to achieve osmolalities suitable for peripheral infusion in fluid-restricted patients (1180):

Diluent	Maximum Concentration[a] (mg/ml)	Osmolality (mOsm/kg)
Dextrose 5% in water	48	562
Sodium chloride 0.9%	43	546
Sterile water for injection	86	573

[a]*Ticarcillin concentration.*

Sodium and Potassium Content— Each gram of this combination product contains 4.75 mEq of sodium. The 3.1-g vial contains 0.15 mEq of potassium (2).

The 3.1 g/100 ml frozen injection contains 0.187 mEq of sodium and 0.005 mEq of potassium (4).

Administration— Reconstituted ticarcillin disodium–clavulanate potassium solutions should be further diluted to concentrations of 10 to 100 mg/ml of ticarcillin and given over 30 minutes by intermittent intravenous infusion directly into a vein or through a Y-type administration set. Other solutions should be temporarily discontinued during the infusion of ticarcillin disodium–clavulanate potassium (2; 4).

Stability— The commercially available combination product as a powder is white to pale yellow. It should be stored at 24 °C or less. Higher temperatures may cause darkening, an indication of clavulanate potassium degradation (4).

The concentrated reconstituted solutions, which are colorless to pale yellow, are stable for up to six hours after reconstitution when stored at room temperatures of 21 to 24 °C or for up to 72 hours when refrigerated at 4 °C (2; 4).

pH Effects— Clavulanic acid exhibits maximum stability at pH 6.4 (1797).

Freezing Solutions— Ticarcillin disodium–clavulanate potassium solutions of 10 to 100 mg/ml (based on ticarcillin content) in sodium chloride 0.9% or Ringer's injection, lactated, are stable for up to 30 days when frozen at −18 °C. Diluted to this concentration range in dextrose 5% in water, the drug is stable for up to seven days when frozen. Frozen solutions should be thawed at room temperature, and thawed solutions should be used within eight hours and not be refrozen (2; 4).

The frozen premixed infusion solutions should be stored at −20 °C. After thawing at room temperature or under refrigeration, the solutions are stable for 24 hours at room temperature or seven days under refrigeration. Thawed solutions should not be refrozen (4).

Elastomeric Reservoir Pumps— Ticarcillin disodium–clavulanate potassium (Beecham) 15 mg/ml in both dextrose 5% in water and sodium chloride 0.9% was evaluated for binding potential to natural rubber elastomeric reservoirs (Baxter). No loss was found after storage for two weeks at 35 °C with gentle agitation (2014).

Compatibility Information

Y-Site Injection Compatibility (1:1 Mixture)

Ticarcillin disodium–clavulanate potassium

Drug	Mfr	Conc	Mfr	Conc	Remarks	Ref	C/I
Allopurinol sodium	BW	3 mg/ml[b]	SKB	31 mg/ml[b]	Physically compatible with no change in measured turbidity or increase in particle content in 4 hr at 22 °C	1686	C

Y-Site Injection Compatibility (1:1 Mixture) (Cont.)

Ticarcillin disodium–clavulanate potassium

Drug	Mfr	Conc	Mfr	Conc	Remarks	Ref	C/I
Amifostine	USB	10 mg/ml[a]	SKB	31 mg/ml[a]	Physically compatible with no change in measured turbidity or increase in particle content in 4 hr at 23 °C	1845	C
Amphotericin B cholesteryl sulfate complex	SEQ	0.83 mg/ml[a]	SKB	31 mg/ml[a]	Gross precipitate forms	2117	I
Aztreonam	SQ	40 mg/ml[a]	SKB	31 mg/ml[a]	Physically compatible with no subvisual haze or particle formation in 4 hr at 23 °C	1758	C
Cefepime HCl	BR	20 mg/ml[a]	SKB	31 mg/ml[a]	Physically compatible with no change in measured turbidity or increase in particle content in 4 hr at 22 °C	1689	C
Cisatracurium besylate	GW	0.1 and 2 mg/ml[a]	SKB	31 mg/ml[a]	Physically compatible with no change in measured turbidity or increase in particle content in 4 hr at 23 °C	2074	C
	GW	5 mg/ml[a]	SKB	31 mg/ml[a]	Subvisual haze forms immediately	2074	I
Clarithromycin	AB	4 mg/ml[a]	BE	32 mg/ml[a]	Visually compatible for 72 hr at both 30 and 17 °C	2174	C
Cyclophosphamide	MJ	20 mg/ml[a]	BE	31 mg/ml[a]	Physically compatible for 4 hr at 25 °C	1194	C
Diltiazem HCl	MMD	1[b] and 5 mg/ml	BE	200 mg/ml[b]	Visually compatible	1807	C
	MMD	5 mg/ml	BE	10 mg/ml[b]	Visually compatible	1807	C
Docetaxel	RPR	0.9 mg/ml[a]	SKB	31 mg/ml[a]	Physically compatible with no change in measured turbidity or increase in particle content in 4 hr at 23 °C	2224	C
Doxorubicin HCl liposome injection	SEQ	0.4 mg/ml[a]	SKB	31 mg/ml[a]	Physically compatible with little or no change in measured turbidity and no increase in particle content in 4 hr at 23 °C	2087	C
Etoposide phosphate	BR	5 mg/ml[a]	SKB	31 mg/ml[a]	Physically compatible with no change in measured turbidity or increase in particle content in 4 hr at 23 °C	2218	C
Famotidine	MSD	0.2 mg/ml[a]	BE	31 mg/ml[b]	Physically compatible for 14 hr	1196	C
Filgrastim	AMG	30 μg/ml[a]	SKB	31 mg/ml[a]	Physically compatible with no change in measured turbidity or increase in particle content in 4 hr at 22 °C	1687	C
Fluconazole	RR	2 mg/ml	BE	60 mg/ml	Physically compatible for 24 hr at 25 °C	1407	C
Fludarabine phosphate	BX	1 mg/ml[a]	BE	31 mg/ml[a]	Physically compatible for 4 hr at room temperature under fluorescent light	1439	C
Foscarnet sodium	AST	24 mg/ml	BE	100 mg/ml[c]	Physically compatible for 24 hr at 25 °C under fluorescent light by visual and microscopic examination	1393	C
Gemcitabine	LI	10 mg/ml[b]	SKB	31 mg/ml[b]	Physically compatible with no change in measured turbidity or increase in particle content in 4 hr at 23 °C	2226	C
Granisetron HCl	SKB	1 mg/ml	SKB	27 mg/ml[b]	Physically compatible with little or no loss of either drug by HPLC in 4 hr at 22 °C	1883	C

Y-Site Injection Compatibility (1:1 Mixture) (Cont.)

Ticarcillin disodium–clavulanate potassium

Drug	Mfr	Conc	Mfr	Conc	Remarks	Ref	C/I
	SKB	0.05 mg/ml[a]	SKB	31 mg/ml[a]	Physically compatible with no change in measured turbidity or increase in particle content in 4 hr at 23 °C	2000	C
Heparin sodium	TR	50 units/ml	BE	31 mg/ml[b]	Visually compatible for 6 hr at 25 °C	1793	C
Insulin, regular	LI	0.2 unit/ml[b]	BE	31 mg/ml[b]	Physically compatible for 2 hr at 25 °C	1395	C
Melphalan HCl	BW	0.1 mg/ml[b]	SKB	31 mg/ml[b]	Physically compatible with no change in measured turbidity or increase in particle content in 3 hr at 22 °C	1557	C
Meperidine HCl	WY	10 mg/ml[b]	BE	31 mg/ml[b]	Physically compatible for 1 hr at 25 °C	1338	C
Morphine sulfate	ES	1 mg/ml[b]	BE	31 mg/ml[b]	Physically compatible for 1 hr at 25 °C	1338	C
Ondansetron HCl	GL	1 mg/ml[b]	BE	31 mg/ml[a]	Physically compatible for 4 hr at 22 °C	1365	C
Perphenazine	SC	0.02 mg/ml[a]	BE	31 mg/ml[a]	Physically compatible for 4 hr at 25 °C	1155	C
Propofol	ZEN	10 mg/ml	SKB	31 mg/ml[a]	Physically compatible for 1 hr at 23 °C with no increase in particle content	2066	C
Remifentanil HCl	GW	0.025 and 0.25 mg/ml[b]	SKB	31 mg/ml[a]	Physically compatible with no change in measured turbidity or increase in particle content in 4 hr at 23 °C	2075	C
Sargramostim	IMM	10 μg/ml[b]	BE	31 mg/ml[b]	Physically compatible for 4 hr at 22 °C	1436	C
Teniposide	BR	0.1 mg/ml[a]	SKB	31 mg/ml[a]	Physically compatible with no subvisual haze or particle formation in 4 hr at 23 °C	1725	C
Theophylline	TR	4 mg/ml	BE	31 mg/ml[b]	Visually compatible for 6 hr at 25 °C	1793	C
Thiotepa	IMM[d]	1 mg/ml[a]	SKB	31 mg/ml[a]	Physically compatible with no change in measured turbidity or increase in particle content in 4 hr at 23 °C	1861	C
TNA #218 to #226[e]			SKB	31 mg/ml[a]	Visually compatible with no precipitate or emulsion damage apparent in 4 hr at 23 °C	2215	C
TPN #189[e]			BE	30 mg/ml[b]	Visually compatible for 24 hr at 22 °C	1767	C
TPN #212 to #215[e]			SKB	31 mg/ml[a]	Physically compatible with no change in measured turbidity or increase in particle content in 4 hr at 23 °C	2109	C
Vancomycin HCl	AB	20 mg/ml[a]	SKB	206.7 mg/ml[f]	Transient precipitate forms followed by clear solution	2189	?
	AB	20 mg/ml[a]	SKB	1.034, 10.335, and 51.675 mg/ml[a]	Gross white precipitate forms	2189	I
		5 mg/ml[b]	SKB	31 mg/ml[b]	White precipitate formed sporadically	2167	I
	AB	2 mg/ml[a]	SKB	1.034[a], 10.335[a], 51.675[a], and 206.7[f] mg/ml	Physically compatible with no change in measured turbidity or increase in particle content in 4 hr at 23 °C	2189	C

Y-Site Injection Compatibility (1:1 Mixture) (Cont.)

Ticarcillin disodium–clavulanate potassium

Drug	Mfr	Conc	Mfr	Conc	Remarks	Ref	C/I
Vinorelbine tartrate	BW	1 mg/ml[b]	SKB	31 mg/ml[b]	Physically compatible with no change in measured turbidity or increase in particle content in 4 hr at 22 °C	1558	C

[a]*Tested in dextrose 5% in water.*
[b]*Tested in sodium chloride 0.9%.*
[c]*Tested in both dextrose 5% in water and sodium chloride 0.9%.*
[d]*Lyophilized formulation tested.*
[e]*Refer to Appendix I for the composition of parenteral nutrition solutions. TNA indicates a 3-in-1 admixture, and TPN indicates a 2-in-1 admixture.*
[f]*Tested in sterile water for injection.*

Additional Compatibility Information

The compatibility information on ticarcillin disodium should be considered. See previous monograph.

Solutions— Dextrose 5% in water, Ringer's injection, lactated, sodium chloride 0.9%, and sterile water for injection are recommended for dilution of ticarcillin disodium–clavulanate potassium (2; 4).

The manufacturer indicates that storage of the 200-mg/ml (based on ticarcillin content) reconstituted solution for up to six hours at room temperature, followed by dilution to 10 to 100 mg/ml in the following infusion solutions, results in the stability periods noted (2):

Solution	Room Temperature	Refrigeration
Dextrose 5% in water	24 hr	3 days
Ringer's injection, lactated	24 hr	7 days
Sodium chloride 0.9%	24 hr	7 days

If the 300-mg/ml (based on ticarcillin content) reconstituted solution in the pharmacy bulk package is stored for six hours at room temperature, followed by dilution to 10 to 100 mg/ml, the following stability periods result (2):

Solution	Room Temperature	Refrigeration
Dextrose 5% in water	24 hr	3 days
Ringer's injection, lactated	24 hr	4 days
Sodium chloride 0.9%	24 hr	4 days
Sterile water for injection	24 hr	4 days

Additives— Ticarcillin disodium–clavulanate potassium is incompatible with sodium bicarbonate (2; 4). Because of the potential for incompatibility, the manufacturer recommends that other anti-infectives, such as aminoglycosides, not be admixed with ticarcillin disodium–clavulanate potassium (2).

Vancomycin HCl— Ticarcillin disodium–clavulanate potassium when admixed with vancomycin HCl has been reported to exhibit occasional precipitate formation. This observation from practice was made with a combination of vancomycin HCl 5 mg/ml and ticarcillin disodium–clavulanate potassium 30 + 1 mg/ml and also with combinations at variable but unrecorded concentrations. The occurrence of precipitate formation was characterized as sporadic and unpredictable (2167).

The compatibility or incompatibility of vancomycin HCl mixed with or administered simultaneously with ticarcillin disodium–clavulanate potassium is concentration dependent (2189). See Y-Site Injection Compatibility above. Vancomycin HCl has a low pH and is variably compatible with drugs having neutral to mildly alkaline pH, including cephalosporins and penicillins. The compatibility may depend on a number of factors, including concentration of each drug, dilution vehicle, actual pH of solutions, and completeness of mixing during administration. Combinations that are compatible when well mixed may result in precipitation if only partially mixed, presumably because of regionally different concentrations and pH values. If attempting to administer vancomycin HCl with ticarcillin disodium–clavulanate potassium, take care to ensure that the specific combination and the concentrations are compatible under the exact administration conditions to be used. An inline filter should be used as a final safety measure (2189).

TOBRAMYCIN SULFATE
AHFS 8:12.02

Nebcin   **Lilly**
                                                   Abbott

Products— Tobramycin sulfate (Lilly) is available in a concentration equivalent to tobramycin base 40 mg/ml in 2-ml (80 mg) and 30-ml (1.2 g) vials and 1.5-ml (60 mg) and 2-ml (80 mg) disposable syringes. It is also available as a pediatric injection in 2-ml vials containing tobramycin sulfate equivalent to tobramycin base 10 mg/ml. Each milliliter of solution contains phenol 5 mg, sodium bisulfite 3.2 mg, and disodium edetate 0.1 mg in water for injection. Sodium hydroxide and/or sulfuric acid may have been added during manufacture for pH adjustment (2).

The drug is also supplied in 60- and 80-mg ADD-Vantage vials with phenol 1.25 mg, sodium bisulfite 1.6 mg, and edetate disodium 0.1 mg in water for injection. Sodium hydroxide and/or sulfuric acid may have been added during manufacture for pH adjustment (2).

Tobramycin sulfate (Abbott) also is available premixed in sodium chloride 0.9% in 0.8-mg/ml (80 mg), 1.2-mg/ml (60 mg), and 1.6-mg/ml (80 mg) concentrations (4).

Tobramycin sulfate (Lilly) is also available in a pharmacy bulk package as a dry powder in vials containing the equivalent of tobramycin 1.2 g (2). The vial contents should be diluted with 30 ml of sterile water for injection to yield a 40-mg/ml solution. The reconstituted solution is intended to be diluted in a suitable intravenous infusion solution for administration (4).

pH— The pH of the injection is adjusted to 3 to 6.5. The reconstituted solution from powder has a pH of 6 to 8 (4).

Osmotic Values— The osmolality of tobramycin sulfate (Dista) 10 mg/ml was determined to be 133 mOsm/kg by freezing-point depression and 213 mOsm/kg by vapor pressure (1071).

The osmolality of tobramycin sulfate (Lilly) 1 mg/ml was determined to be 254 mOsm/kg in dextrose 5% in water and 288 mOsm/kg in sodium chloride 0.9%. At 2.5 mg/ml, the osmolality was determined to be 261 mOsm/kg in dextrose 5% in water and 283 mOsm/kg in sodium chloride 0.9% (1375).

The osmolality of tobramycin sulfate 80 mg was calculated for the following dilutions (1054):

	Osmolality (mOsm/kg)	
Diluent	50 ml	100 ml
Dextrose 5% in water	289	285
Sodium chloride 0.9%	319	315

The premixed products in sodium chloride 0.9% have an osmolarity of approximately 316 mOsm/kg (4).

Sodium Content— The premixed products contain about 15.4 mEq of sodium per 100 ml of solution (4).

Administration— Tobramycin sulfate may be administered by intramuscular injection or intermittent intravenous infusion. Intramuscular doses should be withdrawn only from multiple-dose vials; alternatively, the commercial prefilled syringes may be used. When given by intravenous infusion, the dose should be added to 50 to 100 ml of infusion solution and administered over 20 to 60 minutes. In children, the volume should be proportionately less but should allow an infusion period of 20 to 60 minutes. Infusion periods should not be less than 20 minutes; such shorter periods could result in excessive peak serum concentrations (2; 4).

Stability— Tobramycin sulfate is stable at room temperature both as the clear, colorless solution and as the dry powder. Intact containers should be stored at controlled room temperature between 15 and 30 °C; premixed infusion solutions may be stored at temperatures up to 25 °C. Freezing and excessive temperatures above 40 °C should be avoided. The injections should not be used if they are discolored. The manufacturer recommends use of the 40-mg/ml reconstituted solution within 24 hours when stored at room temperature or 96 hours if refrigerated (2; 4). Tobramycin sulfate is stable for several weeks at pH 1 to 11 at temperatures from 5 to 27 °C. It can be autoclaved without loss of potency (145).

Freezing Solutions— Tobramycin sulfate reconstituted to a concentration of 40 mg/ml and immediately frozen in the original container is stable for up to 12 weeks when stored at −10 to −20 °C (4).

Holmes et al. evaluated tobramycin sulfate (Lilly) 160 mg/50 ml of dextrose 5% in water in PVC bags frozen at −20 °C for 30 days and then thawed by exposure to ambient temperature or microwave radiation. The solutions showed no evidence of precipitation or color change and showed 6% or less loss of potency determined microbiologically. Subsequent storage of the admixture at room temperature for 24 hours also yielded a physically compatible solution which exhibited little or no additional loss of activity (555).

Marble et al. reported that tobramycin sulfate (Dista) 120 mg/50 ml in dextrose 5% in water and sodium chloride 0.9% in PVC bags lost 9% activity in 28 days when frozen at −20 °C (981).

Minibags of tobramycin sulfate in dextrose 5% in water or sodium chloride 0.9%, frozen at −20 °C for up to 35 days, were thawed at room temperature and in a microwave oven, with care taken that the thawed solution temperature never exceeded 25 °C. No significant differences in tobramycin sulfate concentrations occurred between the two thawing methods (1192).

Syringes— Samples of a 40-mg/ml solution of tobramycin sulfate (Lilly) from a reconstituted 1.2-g vial were stored in Monoject plastic syringes at both 25 and 4 °C. After two months, no significant change in potency was detected in samples at either storage temperature. The authors did note that the manufacturer does not recommend storage in plastic syringes because of possible incompatibility with the plunger heads (736).

Tobramycin sulfate (Dista) 120 mg diluted with 1 ml of sodium chloride 0.9% to a final volume of 4 ml was stable (less than a 10% loss) when stored in polypropylene syringes (Becton-Dickinson) for 48 hours at 25 °C under fluorescent light (1159).

Elastomeric Reservoir Pumps— Tobramycin sulfate (Lilly) 0.8 mg/ml in sodium chloride 0.9% 100 ml was packaged in latex elastomeric reservoirs (Secure Medical). Little or no loss by HPLC analysis occurred in 24 hours at 25 °C (1970).

Tobramycin sulfate (Lilly) 0.8 mg/ml in both dextrose 5% in water and sodium chloride 0.9% was evaluated for binding potential to natural rubber elastomeric reservoirs (Baxter). No loss was found after storage for two weeks at 35 °C with gentle agitation (2014).

Sorption— Tobramycin sulfate (Lilly) 20 mg/L in sodium chloride 0.9% (Travenol) in PVC bags did not exhibit significant sorption to the plastic during one week of storage at room temperature (15 to 20 °C) (536).

In another study, tobramycin sulfate (Lilly) 20 mg/L in sodium chloride 0.9% did not exhibit any loss due to sorption during a seven-hour simulated infusion through an infusion set (Travenol) consisting of a cellulose propionate burette chamber and 170 cm of PVC tubing (606).

The drug was also tested as a simulated infusion over at least one hour by a syringe pump system. A glass syringe on a syringe pump was fitted with 20 cm of polyethylene tubing or 50 cm of Silastic tubing. No loss of drug due to sorption was observed with either tubing (606).

Furthermore, a 25-ml aliquot of tobramycin sulfate (Lilly) 20 mg/L in sodium chloride 0.9% was stored in all-plastic syringes composed of polypropylene barrels and polyethylene plungers for 24 hours at room temperature in the dark. No loss due to sorption occurred (606).

Filtration— Tobramycin sulfate (Lilly) 0.3 mg/ml in dextrose 5% in water and sodium chloride 0.9% was filtered through a 0.22-μm cellulose ester membrane filter (Ivex-HP, Millipore) over six hours.

No significant drug loss due to binding to the filter was noted (1034).

Thompson et al. evaluated tobramycin sulfate 5 and 10 mg/55 ml in dextrose 5% in water and sodium chloride 0.9% filtered over 20 minutes through a 0.22-μm cellulose ester filter set (Ivex-2, Millipore). Enzyme-mediated immunoassays showed that little or no binding of the drug to the filter occurred (1003).

Elenbaas et al. found no significant loss due to sorption to a 0.22-μm cellulose ester filter (Continu-Flo 2C0252s, Travenol) from a solution containing tobramycin sulfate (Dista) 80 mg/100 ml of dextrose 5% in water administered over 30 minutes. An enzyme immunoassay found no difference in drug recovery between filtered and unfiltered solutions. However, the authors did note that 10% or more of the solution may remain in the tubing unless the sets are flushed (1132).

Compatibility Information

Solution Compatibility

Tobramycin sulfate

Solution	Mfr	Mfr	Conc/L	Remarks	Ref	C/I
Alcohol 5% in dextrose 5%		LI	200 mg and 1 g	Opalescent haze develops immediately	147	I
Amino acids 4.25%, dextrose 25%	MG	LI	80 mg	No increase in particulate matter in 24 hr at 25 °C	349	C
Dextran 40 10% in dextrose 5% in water	TR	LI	200 mg and 1 g	Physically compatible and chemically stable for 24 hr at 25 °C. Not more than 9% loss occurs	147	C
Dextrose 5% in Polysal	CU	LI	200 mg and 1 g	12 to 15% decomposition in 24 hr at 25 °C. Potency retained through 4 hr	147	I
Dextrose 5% in Polysal M	CU	LI	200 mg and 1 g	11% decomposition in 24 hr at 25 °C. Potency retained through 4 hr	147	I
Dextrose 5% in sodium chloride 0.9%	TR[a]	LI	200 mg and 1 g	Physically compatible and chemically stable for 48 hr at 25 °C. Not more than 7% loss occurs	147	C
Dextrose 5% in water	TR[a]	LI	200 mg and 1 g	Physically compatible and chemically stable for 48 hr at 25 °C. Not more than 4% loss occurs	147	C
	TR[a]	LI	3.2 g	Physically compatible and no potency loss in 24 hr at room temperature	555	C
		LI	1 and 5 g	Physically compatible with no loss of tobramycin activity in 60 min at room temperature	984	C
	AB[a]	DI	1.2 g	Visually compatible and potency by immunoassay retained for 48 hr at 25 °C under fluorescent light and 4 °C in the dark	1541	C
Dextrose 10% in water	TR[a]	LI	200 mg and 1 g	Physically compatible and chemically stable for 48 hr at 25 °C. Not more than 4% loss occurs	147	C
	SO	LI	60 mg/ 21.5 ml[b]	Visually compatible with little or no tobramycin loss by TDx in 30 days at 5 °C in the dark	1731	C
	SO	LI	60 mg/ 18.5 ml[b]	Visually compatible with little or no tobramycin loss by TDx in 30 days at 5 °C in the dark	1731	C
	SO	LI	120 mg/ 23 ml[b]	Visually compatible with little or no tobramycin loss by TDx in 30 days at 5 °C in the dark	1731	C
	SO	LI	120 mg/ 20 ml[b]	Visually compatible with little or no tobramycin loss by TDx in 30 days at 5 °C in the dark	1731	C
Invert sugar 5% in Electrolyte #2	TR	LI	200 mg and 1 g	Physically compatible and chemically stable for 24 hr at 25 °C. Not more than 2% loss occurs	147	C

Solution Compatibility (Cont.)

Tobramycin sulfate

Solution	Mfr	Mfr	Conc/L	Remarks	Ref	C/I
Invert sugar 10% in Electrolyte #3	TR	LI	200 mg and 1 g	Physically compatible and chemically stable for 24 hr at 25 °C	147	**C**
Isolyte E in dextrose 5% in water	MG	LI	1 g	12% decomposition in 24 hr at 25 °C. Potency retained through 4 hr	147	**I**
Isolyte M in dextrose 5% in water	MG	LI	200 mg and 1 g	12% decomposition in 24 hr at 25 °C. Potency retained through 4 hr	147	**I**
Isolyte P in dextrose 5% in water	MG	LI	200 mg and 1 g	11 to 12% decomposition in 24 hr at 25 °C. Potency retained through 4 hr	147	**I**
Mannitol 15%, dextrose 5% in sodium chloride 0.45%		LI	200 mg and 1 g	Physically compatible and chemically stable for 48 hr at 25 °C. Not more than 6% loss occurs	147	**C**
Mannitol 20%		LI	200 mg and 1 g	Physically compatible and chemically stable for 48 hr at 25 °C	147	**C**
Normosol M in dextrose 5% in water	AB	LI	200 mg and 1 g	Physically compatible and chemically stable for 24 hr at 25 °C. Not more than 10% loss occurs	147	**C**
Normosol R	AB	LI	200 mg and 1 g	Physically compatible and chemically stable for 24 hr at 25 °C	147	**C**
Normosol R in dextrose 5% in water	AB	LI	200 mg and 1 g	Physically compatible and chemically stable for 24 hr at 25 °C. Not more than 8% loss occurs	147	**C**
Normosol R, pH 7.4	AB	LI	200 mg and 1 g	Physically compatible and chemically stable for 24 hr at 25 °C	147	**C**
Ringer's injection	TR[a]	LI	200 mg and 1 g	Physically compatible and chemically stable for 24 hr at 25 °C	147	**C**
Ringer's injection, lactated		LI	200 mg and 1 g	Physically compatible and chemically stable for 24 hr at 25 °C	147	**C**
Sodium chloride 0.9%	TR[a]	LI	200 mg and 1 g	Physically compatible and chemically stable for 48 hr at 25 °C	147	**C**
	AB[a]	DI	1.2 g	Visually compatible and potency by immunoassay retained for 48 hr at 25 °C under fluorescent light and 4 °C in the dark	1541	**C**
	AB[c]	LI	800 mg	Little or no loss of drug by HPLC in 24 hr at 25 °C	1970	**C**
	AB[d]	MAR	1 and 10 g	Little or no loss by HPLC in 3 days at 25 °C and 14 days at 5 °C in PVC portable infusion pump reservoirs	2080	**C**
Sodium lactate ⅙ M		LI	200 mg and 1 g	Physically compatible and chemically stable for 48 hr at 25 °C	147	**C**

[a]*Tested in PVC containers.*
[b]*Tested in glass vials as a concentrate.*
[c]*Tested in glass containers and latex elastomeric reservoirs (Secure Medical).*
[d]*Tested in PVC portable pump reservoirs (Pharmacia Deltec).*

Additive Compatibility

Tobramycin sulfate

Drug	Mfr	Conc/L	Mfr	Conc/L	Test Soln	Remarks	Ref	C/I
Aztreonam	SQ	10 and 20 g	LI	200 and 800 mg	D5W, NS	Little or no loss of either drug in 48 hr at 25 °C and 7 days at 4 °C	1023	**C**

Additive Compatibility (Cont.)

Tobramycin sulfate

Drug	Mfr	Conc/L	Mfr	Conc/L	Test Soln	Remarks	Ref	C/I
Bleomycin sulfate	BR	20 and 30 units	LI	500 mg	NS	Physically compatible and bleomycin activity retained for 1 week at 4 °C. Tobramycin not tested	763	**C**
Calcium gluconate		16 g	LI	5 g	D5W	Physically compatible with no loss of tobramycin activity in 60 min at room temperature	984	**C**
		33 g	LI	1 g	D5W	Physically compatible with no loss of tobramycin activity in 60 min at room temperature	984	**C**
Cefamandole nafate	LI	2 and 20 g	LI	80 mg	D5W, NS, W	Haze or precipitate forms within 4 hr	376; 788	**I**
Cefepime HCl	BR	40 g	AB	0.4 g	D5W, NS	Cloudiness forms immediately	1682	**I**
	BR	2.5 g	AB	2 g	D5W, NS, W	Cloudiness forms immediately	1682	**I**
Cefoxitin sodium	MSD	5 g	LI	400 mg	D5S	5% cefoxitin decomposition in 24 hr and 13% in 48 hr at 25 °C. 3% in 48 hr at 5 °C. 8% tobramycin decomposition in 24 hr and 37% in 48 hr at 25 °C. 3% in 48 hr at 5 °C	308	**C**
Ciprofloxacin	MI	1 g	LI	1.6 g	D5W, NS	Physically compatible for 24 hr at 22 °C under fluorescent light	1189	**C**
	MI	1.6 g	LI	1 g	D5W, NS	Visually compatible and ciprofloxacin potency by HPLC and tobramycin potency by immunoassay retained for 48 hr at 25 °C under fluorescent light and 4 °C in the dark	1541	**C**
Clindamycin phosphate	UP	18 g	DI	2.4 g	D5W[a]	8% tobramycin activity lost in 14 days and 17% in 28 days frozen at −20 °C. Clindamycin potency retained	981	**C**
	UP	18 g	DI	2.4 g	NS[a]	Potency of both drugs retained for 28 days frozen at −20 °C	981	**C**
	UP	9 g	DI	1 g	D5W, NS[b]	Physically compatible and potency of both drugs retained for 48 hr at room temperature exposed to light and for 1 week frozen	174	**C**
	UP	9 g	DI	1.2 g	D5W[c]	Physically compatible and potency of clindamycin retained for 28 days frozen. About 8% tobramycin loss in 14 days and 17% in 28 days	174	**C**
	UP	9 g	DI	1.2 g	NS[c]	Physically compatible and potency of both drugs retained for 28 days frozen	174	**C**
Floxacillin sodium	BE	20 g	LI	8 g	NS	White precipitate forms in 7 hr	1479	**I**
Furosemide	HO	1 g	LI	8 g	NS	Physically compatible for 72 hr at 15 and 30 °C	1479	**C**
	HO	800 mg	DI	1.6 g	D5W, NS	Transient cloudiness during admixture; then physically compatible for 24 hr at 21 °C	876	**C**
Metronidazole	RP	5 g[d]	LI	800 mg		Physically compatible with little or no pH change for at least 72 hr at 23 °C	807	**C**

Additive Compatibility (Cont.)

Tobramycin sulfate

Drug	Mfr	Conc/L	Mfr	Conc/L	Test Soln	Remarks	Ref	C/I
	RP	5 g[e]	LI	1 g		Visually compatible with no loss of metronidazole by HPLC in 15 days at 5 and 25 °C. 10% tobramycin loss by immunoassay in 73 hr at 25 °C and 12.1 days at 5 °C	1931	**C**
Metronidazole HCl with sodium bicarbonate	SE AB	5 g 50 mEq	LI	700 mg	D5W, NS	Physically compatible for 48 hr	765	**C**
Ofloxacin	HO	2 g	LI	800 mg	W	Visually compatible with little or no loss of either drug by HPLC in 48 hr	1613	**C**
Ranitidine HCl	GL	100 mg	DI	200 mg	D5W	Physically compatible for 24 hr at ambient temperature under fluorescent light	1151	**C**
Verapamil HCl	KN	80 mg	LI	160 mg	D5W, NS	Physically compatible for 24 hr	764	**C**

[a]Tested in PVC containers.
[b]Tested in both glass and PVC containers.
[c]Tested in glass containers.
[d]Minibags (100 ml) containing metronidazole 500 mg with disodium phosphate 150 mg, citric acid 44 mg, and sodium chloride 740 mg. This product differs from the Searle product.
[e]Tested in ready-to-use metronidazole injection.

Drugs in Syringe Compatibility

Tobramycin sulfate

Drug (in syringe)	Mfr	Amt	Mfr	Amt	Remarks	Ref	C/I
Cefamandole nafate	LI	1 g/ 10 ml	LI	80 mg/ 2 ml	Haze or precipitate forms within 4 hr	376; 788	**I**
	LI	1 g/3 ml	LI	80 mg/ 2 ml	Haze or precipitate forms within 4 hr	376; 788	**I**
Clindamycin phosphate	UP	900 mg/ 6 ml	DI	120 mg/ 4 ml[a]	Cloudy white precipitate forms immediately and changes to gel-like precipitate	1159	**I**
Doxapram HCl	RB	400 mg/ 20 ml		60 mg/ 1.5 ml	Physically compatible with no doxapram loss in 24 hr	1177	**C**
Heparin sodium		10 units/ 1 ml		80 mg/ 2 ml	Turbidity or fine white precipitate due to formation of an insoluble salt	845	**I**
		2500 units/ 1 ml	LI	40 mg	Turbidity or precipitate forms within 5 min	1053	**I**

[a]Diluted to 4 ml with 1 ml of sodium chloride 0.9%.

Y-Site Injection Compatibility (1:1 Mixture)

Tobramycin sulfate

Drug	Mfr	Conc	Mfr	Conc	Remarks	Ref	C/I
Acyclovir sodium	BW	5 mg/ml[a]	DI	1.6 mg/ml[a]	Physically compatible for 4 hr at 25 °C	1157	**C**
Allopurinol sodium	BW	3 mg/ml[b]	LI	5 mg/ml[b]	Haze and crystals form in 1 hr	1686	**I**
Amifostine	USB	10 mg/ml[a]	LI	5 mg/ml[a]	Physically compatible with no change in measured turbidity or increase in particle content in 4 hr at 23 °C	1845	**C**
Amiodarone HCl	LZ	4 mg/ml[c]	LI	0.8 mg/ml[c]	Physically compatible for 4 hr at room temperature	1441	**C**

Y-Site Injection Compatibility (1:1 Mixture) (Cont.)

					Tobramycin sulfate		
Drug	*Mfr*	*Conc*	*Mfr*	*Conc*	*Remarks*	*Ref*	*C/I*
Amphotericin B cholesteryl sulfate complex	SEQ	0.83 mg/ml[a]	AB	5 mg/ml[a]	Gross precipitate forms	2117	I
Amsacrine	NCI	1 mg/ml[a]	LI	5 mg/ml[a]	Physically compatible for 4 hr at room temperature under fluorescent light	1381	C
Aztreonam	SQ	40 mg/ml[a]	LI	5 mg/ml[a]	Physically compatible with no subvisual haze or particle formation in 4 hr at 23 °C	1758	C
Ciprofloxacin	MI	1 mg/ml[a]	LI	1.6 mg/ml[c]	Physically compatible for 24 hr at 22 °C	1189	C
Cisatracurium besylate	GW	0.1, 2, 5 mg/ml[a]	AB	5 mg/ml[a]	Physically compatible with no change in measured turbidity or increase in particle content in 4 hr at 23 °C	2074	C
Cyclophosphamide	MJ	20 mg/ml[a]	DI	0.8 mg/ml[a]	Physically compatible for 4 hr at 25 °C	1194	C
Diltiazem HCl	MMD	5 mg/ml	LI	2.4[b] and 40 mg/ml	Visually compatible	1807	C
Docetaxel	RPR	0.9 mg/ml[a]	LI	5 mg/ml[a]	Physically compatible with no change in measured turbidity or increase in particle content in 4 hr at 23 °C	2224	C
Doxorubicin HCl liposome injection	SEQ	0.4 mg/ml[a]	AB	5 mg/ml[a]	Physically compatible with little or no change in measured turbidity and no increase in particle content in 4 hr at 23 °C	2087	C
Enalaprilat	MSD	0.05 mg/ml[b]	LI	0.8 mg/ml[a]	Physically compatible for 24 hr at room temperature under fluorescent light	1355	C
Esmolol HCl	DCC	10 mg/ml[a]	LI	0.8 mg/ml[a]	Physically compatible for 24 hr at 22 °C	1169	C
Etoposide phosphate	BR	5 mg/ml[a]	LI	5 mg/ml[a]	Physically compatible with no change in measured turbidity or increase in particle content in 4 hr at 23 °C	2218	C
Filgrastim	AMG	30 µg/ml[a]	LI	5 mg/ml[a]	Physically compatible with no change in measured turbidity or increase in particle content in 4 hr at 22 °C	1687	C
	AMG	10[d] and 40[a] µg/ml	LI	1.6 mg/ml[a]	Visually compatible with little or no loss of filgrastim activity by bioassay and tobramycin by immunoassay in 4 hr at 25 °C	2060	C
Fluconazole	RR	2 mg/ml	LI	40 mg/ml	Physically compatible for 24 hr at 25 °C	1407	C
Fludarabine phosphate	BX	1 mg/ml[a]	LI	5 mg/ml[a]	Physically compatible for 4 hr at room temperature under fluorescent light	1439	C
Foscarnet sodium	AST	24 mg/ml	LI	40 mg/ml	Physically compatible for 24 hr at room temperature under fluorescent light	1335	C
Furosemide	HO	10 mg/ml	DI	1.6 mg/ml[a]	Physically compatible for 24 hr at 21 °C	876	C
Gemcitabine HCl	LI	10 mg/ml[b]	LI	5 mg/ml[b]	Physically compatible with no change in measured turbidity or increase in particle content in 4 hr at 23 °C	2226	C
Granisetron HCl	SKB	0.05 mg/ml[a]	AB	5 mg/ml[a]	Physically compatible with no change in measured turbidity or increase in particle content in 4 hr at 23 °C	2000	C
Heparin sodium	ES	50 units/ml[c]	LI	3.2 mg/ml[c]	Immediate gross haze	1316	I

Y-Site Injection Compatibility (1:1 Mixture) (Cont.)

Tobramycin sulfate

Drug	Mfr	Conc	Mfr	Conc	Remarks	Ref	C/I
	TR	50 units/ml	LI	0.8 mg/ml[a]	Visually incompatible within 6 hr at 25 °C	1793	**I**
Hetastarch	DCC	6%	LI	0.8 mg/ml[e]	Small crystals formed immediately after mixing and persisted for 4 hr	1313	**I**
Hydromorphone HCl	WY	0.2 mg/ml[a]	DI	0.8 mg/ml[a]	Physically compatible for at least 4 hr at 25 °C under fluorescent light	987	**C**
IL-2	RC	4800 I.U./ml[b]	LI	40 mg/ml	Visually compatible and IL-2 activity by bioassay retained. Tobramycin not tested	1552	**C**
Indomethacin sodium trihydrate	MSD	0.5 and 1 mg/ml[a]		1 mg/ml[a]	White turbidity forms immediately and becomes white flakes in 1 hr	1550	**I**
Insulin, regular	LI	0.2 unit/ml[b]	LI	1.6 and 2 mg/ml[a]	Physically compatible for 2 hr at 25 °C	1395	**C**
Labetalol HCl	SC	1 mg/ml[a]	LI	0.8 mg/ml[a]	Physically compatible for 24 hr at 18 °C	1171	**C**
Magnesium sulfate	IX	16.7, 33.3, 66.7, 100 mg/ml[a]	DI	0.8 mg/ml[a]	Physically compatible for at least 4 hr at 32 °C	813	**C**
Melphalan HCl	BW	0.1 mg/ml[b]	LI	5 mg/ml[b]	Physically compatible with no change in measured turbidity or increase in particle content in 3 hr at 22 °C	1557	**C**
Meperidine HCl	WY	10 mg/ml[a]	DI	0.8 mg/ml[a]	Physically compatible for at least 4 hr at 25 °C under fluorescent light	987	**C**
	WY	10 mg/ml[b]	LI	1.6, 2, 2.4 mg/ml[a]	Physically compatible for 1 hr at 25 °C	1338	**C**
Midazolam HCl	RC	1 mg/ml[a]	LI	10 mg/ml	Visually compatible for 24 hr at 23 °C	1847	**C**
Morphine sulfate	WI	1 mg/ml[a]	DI	0.8 mg/ml[a]	Physically compatible for at least 4 hr at 25 °C under fluorescent light	987	**C**
	ES	1 mg/ml[b]	LI	1.6, 2, 2.4 mg/ml[a]	Physically compatible for 1 hr at 25 °C	1338	**C**
Perphenazine	SC	0.02 mg/ml[a]	DI	0.8 mg/ml[a]	Physically compatible for 4 hr at 25 °C	1155	**C**
Propofol	ZEN	10 mg/ml	AB	5 mg/ml[a]	Precipitate forms immediately	2066	**I**
Remifentanil HCl	GW	0.025 and 0.25 mg/ml[b]	AB	5 mg/ml[a]	Physically compatible with no change in measured turbidity or increase in particle content in 4 hr at 23 °C	2075	**C**
Sargramostim	IMM	10 μg/ml[b]	LI	5 mg/ml[b]	Particles and filaments form in 4 hr	1436	**I**
Tacrolimus	FUJ	1 mg/ml[b]	BR	40 mg/ml	Visually compatible for 24 hr at 25 °C	1630	**C**
Teniposide	BR	0.1 mg/ml[a]	LI	5 mg/ml[a]	Physically compatible with no subvisual haze or particle formation in 4 hr at 23 °C	1725	**C**
Theophylline	TR	4 mg/ml	LI	0.8 mg/ml[a]	Visually compatible for 6 hr at 25 °C	1793	**C**
Thiotepa	IMM[c]	1 mg/ml[a]	LI	5 mg/ml[a]	Physically compatible with no change in measured turbidity or increase in particle content in 4 hr at 23 °C	1861	**C**
TNA #73[g]		32.5 ml[h]	LI	80 mg/ 50 ml[a]	Physically compatible by visual observation for 4 hr at 25 °C	1008	**C**

Y-Site Injection Compatibility (1:1 Mixture) (Cont.)

Tobramycin sulfate

Drug	Mfr	Conc	Mfr	Conc	Remarks	Ref	C/I
TNA #97 to #104[g]			LI	40 mg/ml	Physically compatible and tobramycin content retained for 6 hr at 21 °C by TDx	1324	**C**
TNA #218 to #226[g]			AB	5 mg/ml[a]	Visually compatible with no precipitate or emulsion damage apparent in 4 hr at 23 °C	2215	**C**
Tolazoline HCl		0.1 mg/ml[a]	LI	10 mg/ml[a]	Physically compatible for 24 hr at 22 °C	1363	**C**
TPN #54[g]				20 mg/ml	Physically compatible and tobramycin activity retained over 6 hr at 22 °C by microbiological assay	1045	**C**
TPN #61[g]	[i]		DI	12.5 mg/1.25 ml[j]	Physically compatible	1012	**C**
	[k]		DI	75 mg/1.9 ml[j]	Physically compatible	1012	**C**
TPN #91[g]	[l]		LI	5 mg[m]	Physically compatible	1170	**C**
TPN #212 to #215[g]			AB	5 mg/ml[a]	Physically compatible with no change in measured turbidity or increase in particle content in 4 hr at 23 °C	2109	**C**
Vinorelbine tartrate	BW	1 mg/ml[b]	LI	5 mg/ml[b]	Physically compatible with no change in measured turbidity or increase in particle content in 4 hr at 22 °C	1558	**C**
Zidovudine	BW	4 mg/ml[a]	LI	2 mg/ml[a]	Physically compatible for 4 hr at 25 °C under fluorescent light by visual and microscopic examination	1193	**C**

[a]*Tested in dextrose 5% in water.*
[b]*Tested in sodium chloride 0.9%.*
[c]*Tested in both dextrose 5% in water and sodium chloride 0.9%.*
[d]*Tested in dextrose 5% in water with human albumin 2 mg/ml.*
[e]*Premixed infusion solution.*
[f]*Lyophilized formulation tested.*
[g]*Refer to Appendix I for the composition of parenteral nutrition solutions. TNA indicates a 3-in-1 admixture, and TPN indicates a 2-in-1 admixture.*
[h]*A 32.5-ml sample of parenteral nutrition solution mixed with 50 ml of antibiotic solution.*
[i]*Run at 21 ml/hr.*
[j]*Given over 30 minutes by syringe pump.*
[k]*Run at 94 ml/hr.*
[l]*Run at 10 ml/hr.*
[m]*Given over one hour by syringe pump.*

Additional Compatibility Information

The manufacturer recommends that other drugs not be mixed with tobramycin sulfate (2).

Tobramycin sulfate is stated to be physically incompatible with heparin sodium (147). In addition, its activity appears to be inhibited by calcium and magnesium ions (145).

Peritoneal Dialysis Solutions— Tobramycin base (Lilly) 3 and 10 mg/L in peritoneal dialysis concentrate with dextrose 50% (Mc-Gaw) retained about 50 to 60% of initial activity in seven hours and about 15 to 30% in 24 hours at room temperature as determined by microbiological assay (1044).

The stability of tobramycin sulfate (Lilly) 10 mg/L in peritoneal dialysis solutions (Dianeal 137 and PD2) with heparin sodium 500 units/L was evaluated by microbiological assay. Approximately 102 ± 20% activity remained after 24 hours at 25 °C (1228).

In another study, the stability of tobramycin sulfate (Lilly) was evaluated in peritoneal dialysis concentrates containing dextrose 30 and 50% (Dianeal) as well as in a diluted solution containing dextrose 2.5%. The tobramycin sulfate concentrations were 100 and 160 mg/L in the peritoneal dialysate concentrates and 5 and 8 mg/L in the diluted solution. With immunoassay techniques, tobramycin sulfate was found to be stable in the diluted peritoneal dialysis solution for at least 24 hours at 23 °C. However, greater decomposition occurred in the concentrates, with a 10% loss in as little as 9 to 15 hours (1229).

Drake et al., using a disc diffusion bioassay, evaluated the retention of antimicrobial activity of tobramycin sulfate (Lilly) 120 mg/L alone and with vancomycin HCl (Lilly) 1 g/L in Dianeal PD-2 (Travenol) with dextrose 1.5%. Little or no loss of either antibiotic occurred in eight hours at 37 °C. Tobramycin sulfate alone retained activity for at least 48 hours at 4 and 25 °C. With vancomycin HCl, the antimicrobial activity of both antibiotics was retained for up to 48 hours; however, the authors recommended refrigeration at 4 °C for storage longer than 24 hours (1414).

Ceftazidime (Fortaz) 125 mg/L and tobramycin sulfate (Lilly) 8 mg/L in Dianeal PD-2 with dextrose 2.5% (Baxter) were visually compatible and chemically stable by HPLC (ceftazidime) and fluorescence polarization immunoassay (tobramycin). After 16 hours of storage at 25 °C under fluorescent light, the loss of both drugs was less than 3%. Additional storage for eight hours at 37 °C, to simulate the maximum peritoneal dwell time, showed tobramycin sulfate concentrations of 96% and ceftazidime concentrations of 92 to 96% (1652).

Tobramycin sulfate (Lilly) 25 μg/ml combined separately with the cephalosporins cefazolin sodium (Lilly), cefamandole nafate (Lilly), and cefoxitin sodium (MSD) at a concentration of 125 μg/ml in peritoneal dialysis solution (Dianeal 1.5%) exhibited enhanced rates of lethality to *Staphylococcus aureus*, *Escherichia coli*, and *Pseudomonas aeruginosa* compared to any of the drugs alone (1623).

Heparin— A white precipitate may result from the administration of tobramycin sulfate through a heparinized intravenous cannula (976). Flushing heparin locks with sterile water for injection or sodium chloride 0.9% before and after administering drugs incompatible with heparin has been recommended (4).

Clindamycin— Clindamycin phosphate (Upjohn) 600 mg/L has been reported to be conditionally compatible with tobramycin sulfate 80 mg/L. Clindamycin stability is maintained for 24 hours in sodium chloride 0.9%, but an unstable mixture results in dextrose 5% in water (101).

β-Lactam Antibiotics— In common with other aminoglycoside antibiotics, tobramycin sulfate activity may be impaired by the β-lactam antibiotics. The inactivation is dependent on concentration, temperature, and time of exposure.

Levison et al. evaluated tobramycin 10 μg/ml in combination with carbenicillin in concentrations ranging from 200 to 800 μg/ml in a bacterial growth medium incubated at 37 °C for 24 hours. At carbenicillin concentrations of 200 to 400 μg/ml, no loss of tobramycin activity (determined microbiologically) occurred over the 24-hour period. However, at a carbenicillin concentration of 600 μg/ml, tobramycin activity was retained for only six hours. The solution had lost 90% of the activity by 24 hours. At 800 μg/ml, 50% of the tobramycin concentration was lost in two hours (737).

Holt et al. found that tobramycin sulfate 10 mg/L in sodium chloride 0.9%, incubated with 500 mg/L of carbenicillin or ticarcillin at 37 °C for 24 hours, resulted in about a 60 to 70% reduction in tobramycin activity. When serum was substituted for the sodium chloride solution, a 40 to 50% reduction in activity was reported. However, about 80% of the activity was lost when buffered to pH 7.4 in aqueous solution (574).

In another study, tobramycin sulfate 5 and 10 μg/ml, dissolved in human serum and incubated with carbenicillin and ticarcillin 100 to 600 μg/ml at 37 °C, demonstrated greater decomposition rates at the higher penicillin concentrations. In 24 hours, about a 3 to 7% loss of tobramycin activity occurred at 100 μg/ml and about a 70% loss occurred at 600 μg/ml of carbenicillin. Approximately a 12% loss at 100 μg/ml to a 90% loss at 600 μg/ml occurred in 72 hours with carbenicillin. When tobramycin sulfate was combined with

ticarcillin under these conditions, about an 11% loss of tobramycin activity occurred at 100 μg/ml of ticarcillin in 72 hours. The tobramycin loss increased to 25% at 300 μg/ml and to 75% at 600 μg/ml of ticarcillin in 72 hours (575).

Several aminoglycosides in combination with several penicillins were evaluated by Henderson et al. Gentamicin sulfate, netilmicin sulfate, and tobramycin sulfate 5 μg/ml were combined with carbenicillin disodium, azlocillin sodium, and mezlocillin sodium 50, 250, and 500 μg/ml in human plasma. Samples were evaluated over nine days at 27 and 37 °C. All of the aminoglycosides underwent significant inactivation during the evaluation. Aminoglycoside decomposition of 17 to 61% in 24 hours occurred at the higher two concentrations of penicillins—the highest inactivation was sustained by tobramycin and the lowest by netilmicin. Little if any aminoglycoside inactivation occurred at 50 μg/ml of penicillin. Carbenicillin caused a greater degree of aminoglycoside decomposition than did azlocillin or mezlocillin (616).

Flournoy noted the relative degree of inactivation of tobramycin, gentamicin, netilmicin, and amikacin 10 mg/L in serum when combined with carbenicillin 125 to 1000 mg/L over temperatures ranging from −20 to 42 °C. Tobramycin was more susceptible to inactivation than the others. Amikacin was the least susceptible, and gentamicin and netilmicin were similar in intermediate susceptibility to inactivation (617).

Although piperacillin sodium and aminoglycosides act synergistically and have been used successfully clinically when recommended doses of each drug were administered, mixing piperacillin sodium directly in a syringe or infusion bottle with an aminoglycoside can result in substantial inactivation of the aminoglycoside (740).

While most evaluations of aminoglycoside and penicillin combinations have centered on aminoglycoside decomposition, Das Gupta and Stewart evaluated the stability of carbenicillin in the presence of tobramycin. Carbenicillin disodium (Roerig) 100 to 1000 μg/ml was combined with tobramycin sulfate (Lilly) 40 to 160 μg/ml in dextrose 5% in water, sodium chloride 0.9%, and pH 6.6 phosphate buffer. At 24 °C, the rate of decomposition of carbenicillin increased by 0.5% for each microgram per milliliter of tobramycin. The decomposition of tobramycin apparently is dependent on the carbenicillin concentration, and the decomposition of carbenicillin apparently is dependent on the tobramycin concentration (783).

The inactivation of tobramycin 10 μg/ml in sterile distilled water by several β-lactam antibiotics stored at 37 °C was reported by Jorgensen and Crawford. Ticarcillin and carbenicillin 500 μg/ml caused about a 45% tobramycin loss in two hours and a 75% loss in six hours, while 100 μg/ml caused a 47 and 39% loss, respectively, after six hours. Penicillin G 500 μg/ml caused a 23% tobramycin loss in six hours, but no significant loss occurred at 100 μg/ml. Tobramycin was not inactivated by 500- or 100-μg/ml concentrations of cephalothin, cefotaxime, and moxalactam. No loss of β-lactam antibiotic activity was detected in any combination (973).

Pickering and Rutherford evaluated several aminoglycosides combined with a number of penicillins. Gentamicin sulfate, netilmicin sulfate, and tobramycin sulfate 5 and 10 μg/ml and amikacin 10 and 20 μg/ml were combined in human serum with 125, 250, and 500 μg/ml of azlocillin, carbenicillin disodium, amdinocillin, mezlocillin, and piperacillin individually. Tobramycin and gentamicin sustained greater losses than netilmicin and amikacin at each of the penicillin concentrations. Significant decomposition of all aminoglycosides occurred in 24 hours at 37 °C at a penicillin concentration of 500 μg/ml. Tobramycin and gentamicin had losses of 40 to

60%, while 15 to 30% losses occurred for netilmicin. Amikacin sustained the least inactivation with losses of about 10 to 20%. At penicillin concentrations of 125 to 250 μg/ml, smaller losses of aminoglycosides were observed (68).

Lundergan et al. studied, in vitro, the interaction of tobramycin sulfate with several penicillins in human serum under clinical laboratory conditions. Tobramycin sulfate 10 μg/ml was combined with carbenicillin disodium 200 μg/ml, oxacillin sodium (Bristol) 50 μg/ml, and nafcillin sodium (Wyeth) 50 μg/ml. Samples were evaluated over 72 hours at −23, 6, and 23 °C. Although results were variable, only the carbenicillin sample at 23 °C exhibited substantial decomposition after 72 hours. None of the other samples of carbenicillin, oxacillin, or nafcillin showed significant differences over the study period (814).

Using bioassay and radioimmunoassay, Hale et al. evaluated piperacillin and carbenicillin at concentrations of 62.5 to 1000 μg/ml in human serum in combination with amikacin, gentamicin, or tobramycin 10 μg/ml at 37 °C for up to 24 hours. Penicillin concentrations of 62.5 and 125 μg/ml had relatively little effect on the aminoglycoside concentration, even after 24 hours. However, increasing the penicillin concentration to 250 or 500 μg/ml greatly increased decomposition. After 24 hours with carbenicillin 500 μg/ml, the amounts of aminoglycosides remaining were amikacin 82%, gentamicin 43%, and tobramycin 27%. After 24 hours with piperacillin 500 μg/ml, the remaining concentrations were 95, 45, and 52%, respectively. Even greater inactivation occurred at 1000 μg/ml of the penicillins, including the essentially complete loss of tobramycin in 24 hours. The authors concluded that amikacin is much more resistant to inactivation than the other aminoglycosides tested and that carbenicillin is somewhat more aggressive in its inactivation than piperacillin (816).

Rank et al. evaluated the inactivation of tobramycin 6 μg/ml in human serum with the sodium salts of cloxacillin and piperacillin 150 and 300 μg/ml, ampicillin 100 and 200 μg/ml, and penicillin G 75 and 150 I.U./ml at 25 and 37 °C for up to 12 hours. Piperacillin induced the greatest inactivation among the penicillins, with up to a 15% loss in 12 hours at 37 °C in the 300-μg/ml concentration. Cloxacillin and ampicillin had an intermediate effect, causing about a 5% loss in 12 hours at 37 °C in the highest concentrations. Penicillin G did not yield significant tobramycin inactivation (817).

The inactivation of tobramycin sulfate 8 μg/ml in human serum by ampicillin, carbenicillin disodium, and penicillin G potassium, each at 200 μg/ml, was studied at 0, 23, and 37 °C by O'Bey et al. For the tobramycin–ampicillin mixture, essentially no differences were observed at the various temperatures. The t_{90} values were 19, 16.5, and 20 hours at 0, 23, and 37 °C, respectively. Carbenicillin displayed a temperature-dependent inactivation of tobramycin. At 0 °C, the t_{90} was 36 hours; but at 23 and 37 °C, the t_{90} values were 10 and 12 hours, respectively. With penicillin G potassium, the t_{90} values for tobramycin inactivation at 0, 23, and 37 °C were 48, 44, and 16 hours, respectively. Inaccurate pharmacokinetic dosing of tobramycin may occur if serum samples are not handled properly (832).

The comparative inactivation of five aminoglycosides by seven β-lactam antibiotics in human serum at 37 °C was reported by Riff and Thomason. Amikacin, followed by netilmicin, had the lowest degree of inactivation; tobramycin sustained the most pronounced losses. Gentamicin and kanamycin were intermediate in the extent of losses. The six penicillins that were tested all produced aminoglycoside inactivation; the greatest extent of inactivation was caused by carbenicillin followed by ticarcillin, penicillin G, oxacillin,

methicillin, and ampicillin, in approximate descending order. Cephalothin produced minimal inactivation (5 to 10% in 24 hours). The rate of inactivation could be reduced by storage at 4 °C and further reduced by storage at −20 °C. The authors suggested processing blood samples rapidly to avoid inaccurate serum determinations. Storage of specimens at low temperature until analysis may be helpful (1052).

Spruill et al. evaluated the effect of various cephalosporins on tobramycin sulfate 7.7 μg/ml in human serum. At concentrations of 250 and 1000 μg/ml, cefazolin, cefoxitin, cefamandole, cefoperazone, and cefotaxime caused about a 10 to 15% loss of tobramycin over 48 hours at 0 and 21 °C. Moxalactam caused about a 15% loss at 0 °C and a 20 to 30% loss at 21 °C over 48 hours (1005).

Pennell et al. evaluated the potential for inactivation of tobramycin sulfate (Lilly) 9 μg/ml with 100- and 200-μg/ml concentrations of ceftazidime (Lilly), cefoperazone sodium (Roerig), and cefotaxime sodium (Hoechst-Roussel) in human serum. No loss of tobramycin sulfate was determined by TDx fluorescence polarization immunoassay over 48 hours when stored at 4, 24, and 37 °C (1420).

To determine if spurious aminoglycoside levels could result from a delay in assaying blood samples, Tindula et al. evaluated the inactivation of amikacin 35 μg/ml and gentamicin and tobramycin 10 μg/ml in human serum by 400-μg/ml concentrations of several penicillins and cephalosporins. Samples were stored for 24 hours at room temperature or frozen at −20 °C. For the room temperature samples, cefazolin and cefamandole caused relatively little inactivation. Nafcillin, cephapirin, and cefoxitin caused moderate inactivation, 20% or less. Penicillin, ampicillin, carbenicillin, and ticarcillin generally caused 25% or more inactivation of gentamicin and tobramycin. Amikacin was somewhat less affected. Freezing samples at −20 °C prevented significant inactivation of amikacin and gentamicin by any of the drugs. Freezing the tobramycin samples was satisfactory for most of the drugs except penicillin, ampicillin, and carbenicillin, which still exhibited a 15 to 20% tobramycin loss in 24 hours (824).

The inactivation of gentamicin, tobramycin, and amikacin, each 5 μg/ml, by seven β-lactam antibiotics, 250 and 500 μg/ml, in serum at 25 °C over 24 hours was studied using bioassay, enzyme-mediated immunoassay technique (EMIT), TDx, and radioimmunoassay. No inactivation of any aminoglycoside by the cephalosporins moxalactam, cefotaxime, and cefazolin occurred within the study period. Results with the penicillins varied, depending on the assay technique used. The bioassay was the most sensitive to loss, TDx and radioimmunoassay were intermediate, and EMIT was the least sensitive. Azlocillin, carbenicillin, mezlocillin, and piperacillin all caused variable but extensive inactivation (up to 70%) of gentamicin and tobramycin in 24 hours. Amikacin, however, had only minor losses compared to the other aminoglycosides (654).

The clinical significance of these interactions appears to be primarily confined to patients with renal failure (218; 334; 361; 364; 616; 737; 816; 847; 952). Literature reports of greatly reduced aminoglycoside levels in such patients have appeared frequently (363; 365–367; 614; 615; 962). In addition, the interaction may be clinically important if assays for aminoglycoside levels in serum are sufficiently delayed (576; 618; 735; 824; 832; 847; 1052).

Most authors believe that in vitro mixing of penicillins such as ticarcillin disodium with aminoglycoside antibiotics should be avoided but that clinical use of the drugs in combination can be of great value. It is generally recommended that the drugs be given separately in such combined therapy (157; 218; 222; 224; 361; 364; 368–370).

Cephalosporins— Cefotaxime sodium should not be mixed with aminoglycosides in the same solution, but they may be administered to the same patient separately (2; 792).

When tobramycin sulfate (Lilly) 80 mg/100 ml in dextrose 5% in water was run through an administration set previously used to administer cefoperazone (Roerig) 4 g/100 ml in dextrose 5% in water, an immediate precipitate formed in the infusion tubing where the two solutions mixed. A retest using cefoperazone 1 g/100 ml produced the same result (831).

Cefotetan is stated to be physically incompatible with tobramycin sulfate (4).

Imipenem— The potential for inactivation of tobramycin sulfate by the carbapenem antibiotic imipenem–cilastatin sodium was investigated by Ariano et al. Tobramycin sulfate 10 μg/ml was incubated at 37 °C for five days with imipenem–cilastatin sodium concentrations ranging from 10 to 40 μg/ml in human serum. Degradation rates of tobramycin sulfate determined by fluorescence polarization immunoassay were not enhanced by the presence of imipenem–cilastatin sodium (2013).

Other Information

Heating Plasma— Heating plasma samples to 56 °C for one hour to inactivate potential HIV content resulted in no tobramycin loss as determined by TDx (1615).

TOLAZOLINE HCL
AHFS 24:12

Priscoline Hydrochloride   **Novartis**

Products— Tolazoline HCl (Novartis) is supplied in 4-ml ampuls containing tolazoline HCl 25 mg/ml. Also present in each milliliter of solution are tartaric acid, hydrous sodium citrate, and 0.5% chlorobutanol (4; 29).

pH— From 3 to 4 (4).

Osmolality— The osmolality of tolazoline HCl (Ciba) 25 mg/ml was determined to be 402 mOsm/kg by freezing-point depression and 353 mOsm/kg by vapor pressure (1071).

Administration— Tolazoline HCl may be administered intravenously. It has also been given by subcutaneous, intramuscular, or intra-arterial injection (4).

Stability— Intact ampuls of tolazoline HCl should be stored at controlled room temperature and protected from light (2; 4).

Compatibility Information

Solution Compatibility

Tolazoline HCl

Solution	Mfr	Mfr	Conc/L	Remarks	Ref	C/I
Dextran 6% in dextrose 5%	AB	CI	50 mg	Physically compatible	3	C
Dextran 6% in sodium chloride 0.9%	AB	CI	50 mg	Physically compatible	3	C
Dextrose–Ringer's injection combinations	AB	CI	50 mg	Physically compatible	3	C
Dextrose–Ringer's injection, lactated, combinations	AB	CI	50 mg	Physically compatible	3	C
Dextrose–saline combinations	AB	CI	50 mg	Physically compatible	3	C
Dextrose 2½% in water	AB	CI	50 mg	Physically compatible	3	C
Dextrose 5% in water	AB	CI	50 mg	Physically compatible	3	C
Dextrose 10% in water	AB	CI	50 mg	Physically compatible	3	C
Fructose 10% in sodium chloride 0.9%	AB	CI	50 mg	Physically compatible	3	C
Fructose 10% in water	AB	CI	50 mg	Physically compatible	3	C
Invert sugar 5 and 10% in sodium chloride 0.9%	AB	CI	50 mg	Physically compatible	3	C
Invert sugar 5 and 10% in water	AB	CI	50 mg	Physically compatible	3	C
Ionosol products	AB	CI	50 mg	Physically compatible	3	C
Ringer's injection	AB	CI	50 mg	Physically compatible	3	C
Ringer's injection, lactated	AB	CI	50 mg	Physically compatible	3	C

Solution Compatibility (Cont.)

Tolazoline HCl

Solution	Mfr	Mfr	Conc/L	Remarks	Ref	C/I
Sodium chloride 0.45%	AB	CI	50 mg	Physically compatible	3	C
Sodium chloride 0.9%	AB	CI	50 mg	Physically compatible	3	C
Sodium lactate ⅙ M	AB	CI	50 mg	Physically compatible	3	C

Additive Compatibility

Tolazoline HCl

Drug	Mfr	Conc/L	Mfr	Conc/L	Test Soln	Remarks	Ref	C/I
Ethacrynate sodium	MSD	50 mg	CI	400 mg	NS	Altered UV spectra for both at room temperature	16	I
Verapamil HCl	KN	80 mg	CI	160 mg	D5W, NS	Physically compatible for 24 hr	764	C

Y-Site Injection Compatibility (1:1 Mixture)

Tolazoline HCl

Drug	Mfr	Conc	Mfr	Conc	Remarks	Ref	C/I
Aminophylline	AB	5[a] and 25 mg/ml		0.1 mg/ml[a]	Physically compatible for 24 hr at 22 °C	1363	C
Ampicillin sodium	WY	30 mg/ml[b]		0.1 mg/ml[a]	Physically compatible for 24 hr at 22 °C	1363	C
Calcium gluconate	AMR	100 mg/ml		0.1 mg/ml[a]	Physically compatible for 24 hr at 22 °C	1363	C
Cefotaxime sodium	HO	60 mg/ml[a]		0.1 mg/ml[a]	Physically compatible for 24 hr at 22 °C	1363	C
Cimetidine HCl	SKF	15 mg/ml[a]		0.1 mg/ml[a]	Physically compatible for 24 hr at 22 °C	1363	C
Dobutamine HCl	LI	1.2 mg/ml[a]		0.1 mg/ml[a]	Physically compatible for 24 hr at 22 °C	1363	C
Dopamine HCl	AB	1.2 mg/ml[a]		0.1 mg/ml[a]	Physically compatible for 24 hr at 22 °C	1363	C
Furosemide	AB	10 mg/ml		0.1 mg/ml[a]	Physically compatible for 24 hr at 22 °C	1363	C
Gentamicin sulfate	ES	10 mg/ml[a]		0.1 mg/ml[a]	Physically compatible for 24 hr at 22 °C	1363	C
Indomethacin sodium trihydrate	MSD	1 mg/ml		0.1 mg/ml[a]	White precipitate forms within 30 min	1363	I
Phytonadione	MSD	2 mg/ml		0.1 mg/ml[a]	Physically compatible for 24 hr at 22 °C	1363	C
Sodium bicarbonate	AB	0.5 mEq/ml		0.1 mg/ml[a]	Physically compatible for 24 hr at 22 °C	1363	C
Tobramycin sulfate	LI	10 mg/ml[a]		0.1 mg/ml[a]	Physically compatible for 24 hr at 22 °C	1363	C
Vancomycin HCl	LE	5 mg/ml[a]		0.1 mg/ml[a]	Physically compatible for 24 hr at 22 °C	1363	C

[a]Tested in dextrose 5% in water.
[b]Tested in sodium chloride 0.9%.

TOPOTECAN HCL
AHFS 10:00

Hycamtin   **SmithKline Beecham**

Products— Topotecan HCl (SmithKline Beecham) is available in vials containing 4 mg of topotecan base (present as the hydrochloride) as a lyophilized powder. Reconstitute with 4 ml of sterile water for injection to yield a 1-mg/ml topotecan (as the hydrochloride) solution. In addition to topotecan HCl, each milliliter of the reconstituted solution contains mannitol 12 mg and tartaric acid 5 mg. Hydrochloric acid and sodium hydroxide may have been used during manufacture to adjust the pH. The reconstituted solution must be diluted for use (2).

pH— From 2.5 to 3.5 (2).

Administration— Topotecan HCl is administered by intravenous infusion over 30 minutes after dilution in 50 to 250 ml of either sodium chloride 0.9% or dextrose 5% in water. Extravasation should be avoided; local reactions including erythema and bruising may result (2; 4).

Stability— Topotecan HCl in intact vials should be stored in the original cartons at controlled room temperature and protected from light. The lyophilized drug is a light yellow to greenish powder. The reconstituted solution is yellow to yellow-green in color (2). The reconstituted solution should be inspected for particulate matter in the vial and again in the transferring syringe prior to preparing admixtures. As for all parenteral products, the admixtures should also be inspected for particulate matter and discoloration prior to administration (4).

Reconstituted topotecan HCl is stated to be stable for 24 hours at 20 to 25 °C exposed to ambient light (4). However, the manufacturer recommends use immediately after reconstitution because the product contains no antibacterial preservative (2).

Other information indicates the reconstituted drug may be stable for longer periods. Vials of reconstituted topotecan HCl (SmithKline Beecham) at a concentration of 1 mg/ml were stored at 5, 25, and 30 °C both upright and inverted for 28 days. The solutions remained visually clear with no change in color, and HPLC analysis found little or no loss of topotecan HCl at any condition (2211).

pH Effects— Topotecan HCl has a pH near 3 maintained with tartaric acid to ensure adequate solubility of greater than 2.5 mg/ml. The solubility decreases as the pH increases, becoming virtually insoluble at pH 4.5 (1747). Hydrolysis of the topotecan HCl lactone ring is known to occur at pH values above 4 (2140).

Compatibility Information

Solution Compatibility

Topotecan HCl

Solution	Mfr	Mfr	Conc/L	Remarks	Ref	C/I
Dextrose 5% in water	BA[a], MG[b], MG[c]	SKB	50 mg	Visually compatible with no loss by HPLC in 24 hr at 24 °C exposed to light and 7 days at 5 °C protected from light	2140	C
	BA[a]	SKB	25 mg	Visually compatible with no loss by HPLC in 24 hr at 24 °C exposed to light and 7 days at 5 °C protected from light	2140	C
Sodium chloride 0.9%	BA[a], MG[b], MG[c]	SKB	50 mg	Visually compatible with no loss by HPLC in 24 hr at 24 °C exposed to light and 7 days at 5 °C protected from light	2140	C
	BA[a]	SKB	25 mg	Visually compatible with no loss by HPLC in 24 hr at 24 °C exposed to light and 7 days at 5 °C protected from light	2140	C

[a]*Tested in PVC containers.*
[b]*Tested in polyolefin containers.*
[c]*Tested in glass containers.*

Y-Site Injection Compatibility (1:1 Mixture)

Topotecan HCl

Drug	Mfr	Conc	Mfr	Conc	Remarks	Ref	C/I
Gemcitabine HCl	SKB	0.1 mg/ml[b]	LI	10 mg/ml[b]	Physically compatible with no change in measured turbidity or increase in particle content in 4 hr at 23 °C	2226	C

[b]*Tested in sodium chloride 0.9%.*

Additional Compatibility Information

Solutions— The manufacturer states that topotecan HCl reconstituted and further diluted for infusion is stable for 24 hours stored at 20 to 25 °C under ambient lighting conditions (2). However, other information indicates that topotecan HCl diluted for infusion in dextrose 5% in water or sodium chloride 0.9% in PVC bags at concentrations of 10 to 500 µg/ml is stable for up to four days at room temperature (4).

Plasticizer Leaching— Topotecan HCl (SmithKline Beecham) 0.025 and 0.05 mg/ml in dextrose 5% in water or in sodium chloride 0.9% did not result in measureable amounts of diethylhexyl phthalate leached from PVC containers (2140).

Other Information

Bacterial Challenge— Whether any antimicrobial effect of topotecan HCl exists is uncertain but could be concentration dependent. Two studies that have been performed seem to have different results, perhaps due to the very different topotecan HCl concentrations being tested.

Topotecan HCl (SmithKline Beecham) 0.01 mg/ml diluted in sodium chloride 0.9% and stored at 22 °C did not exhibit an antimicrobial effect on the growth of four organisms (*Enterococcus faecium*, *Staphylococcus aureus*, *Pseudomonas aeruginosa*, and *Candida albicans*) inoculated into the solution. The author recommended that diluted solutions of topotecan HCl be stored under refrigeration whenever possible and that the potential for microbiological growth be considered when assigning expiration periods (2160).

Topotecan HCl (SmithKline Beecham) 1 mg/ml reconstituted with sterile water did not support the growth of five organisms inoculated into the solution. The USP Preservative Effectiveness Test found that *Pseudomonas aeruginosa*, *Staphylococcus aureus*, and *Escherichia coli* were not viable after 16 hours, 24 hours, and 28 days, respectively. *Candida albicans* and *Aspergillus niger* did not lose viability but did not exhibit growth during the test (2211).

Handling Precautions— As for other toxic drugs, topotecan HCl should be prepared using protective measures to avoid inadvertent contact with the drug. The use of gloves, protective clothing, and vertical laminar flow hoods or biological safety cabinets is recommended. If skin contact with the drug does occur, wash the area thoroughly with soap and water. For mucous membrane contact, flush thoroughly with water. Disposal should also be performed safely to avoid inadvertent exposure (2; 4).

TORSEMIDE
AHFS 40:28

Demadex   **Roche**

Products— Torsemide (Roche) is available in 2- and 5-ml ampuls. Each milliliter of solution contains torsemide 10 mg along with polyethylene glycol 400, tromethamine, water for injection, and sodium hydroxide if needed to adjust pH during manufacture (2).

pH— Approximately 8.3 (2).

Administration— Torsemide is administered intravenously either slowly as a bolus over two minutes or as a continuous infusion. If given through an intravenous line, flushing with sodium chloride 0.9% before and after torsemide administration is recommended (2).

Stability— Intact containers of torsemide should be stored at controlled room temperature and protected from freezing. At concentrations of 0.1 and 0.8 mg/ml in dextrose 5% in water and sodium chloride 0.9% and at concentrations of 0.1 and 0.4 mg/ml in sodium chloride 0.45%, torsemide is stated to be stable for 24 hours at room temperature (2).

Compatibility Information

Solution Compatibility

Torsemide

Solution	Mfr	Mfr	Conc/L	Remarks	Ref	C/I
Dextrose 5% in water	AB[a]	BM	200 mg	6% loss by HPLC occurs in 72 hr at 24 °C	2108	C
	AB[a]	BM	5 g	3% loss by HPLC occurs in 72 hr at 24 °C	2108	C

[a]*Tested in PVC containers.*

Y-Site Injection Compatibility (1:1 Mixture)

					Torsemide		
Drug	*Mfr*	*Conc*	*Mfr*	*Conc*	*Remarks*	*Ref*	*C/I*
Milrinone lactate	BM	10 mg/ml	SW	0.4 mg/ml[a]	Visually compatible with little or no loss of either drug by HPLC in 4 hr at 23 °C	2214	C

[a]*Tested in dextrose 5% in water.*

TRIFLUOPERAZINE HCL
AHFS 28:16.08

Stelazine   **SmithKline Beecham**

Products— Trifluoperazine HCl (SmithKline Beecham) is available in 10-ml multiple-dose vials. Each milliliter of the aqueous solution contains trifluoperazine 2 mg as the hydrochloride, sodium tartrate 4.75 mg, sodium biphosphate 11.6 mg, sodium saccharin 0.3 mg, and benzyl alcohol 0.75% as a preservative (2).

pH— From 4 to 5 (4).

Osmolality— Trifluoperazine HCl 2 mg/ml has an osmolality of 288 mOsm/kg (1689).

Administration— Trifluoperazine HCl is administered by deep intramuscular injection (2; 4).

Stability— Trifluoperazine HCl should be stored at controlled room temperature and protected from light and freezing (2; 4). Exposure to ultraviolet light results in discoloration; trifluoperazine HCl solutions gradually become yellowish-red and then reddish-brown, depending on the length of exposure time (1957). A slight yellowish color does not indicate significant alteration in potency, but a markedly discolored solution should not be used (2; 4).

Sorption— Trifluoperazine HCl (SKF) 10 mg/L in sodium chloride 0.9% (Travenol) in PVC bags did not exhibit significant sorption to the plastic during one week of storage at room temperature (15 to 20 °C). However, when the solution was buffered from its initial pH of 5 to 7.4, approximately 91% of the drug was lost in one week due to sorption (536).

In another study, trifluoperazine HCl (SKF) 10 mg/L in sodium chloride 0.9% exhibited a cumulative 45% loss during a seven-hour simulated infusion through an infusion set (Travenol) consisting of a cellulose propionate burette chamber and 170 cm of PVC tubing due to sorption. Both the burette and the tubing contributed to the loss. The extent of sorption was found to be independent of concentration (606).

The drug was also tested as a simulated infusion over at least one hour by a syringe pump system. A glass syringe on a syringe pump was fitted with 20 cm of polyethylene tubing or 50 cm of Silastic tubing. Only 5% of the drug was lost with the polyethylene tubing, but a cumulative loss of 78% occurred during the one-hour infusion through the Silastic tubing (606).

In addition, a 25-ml aliquot of trifluoperazine HCl (SKF) 10 mg/L in sodium chloride 0.9% was stored in all-plastic syringes composed of polypropylene barrels and polyethylene plungers for 24 hours at room temperature in the dark. No loss due to sorption occurred (606).

TRIFLUPROMAZINE HCL
AHFS 28:16.08

Vesprin   **Apothecon**

Products— Triflupromazine HCl (Apothecon) is available in multiple-dose vials providing 10 or 20 mg/ml of drug. Also present are benzyl alcohol 1.5% (w/v), sodium chloride for isotonicity, and sodium hydroxide or hydrochloric acid for pH adjustment (1-4/94; 29).

pH— The pH has been adjusted to 3.5 to 5.2 (1-4/94).

Osmolality— Triflupromazine HCl 10 mg/ml has an osmolality of 253 mOsm/kg (1689).

Administration— Triflupromazine HCl may be administered by intramuscular or intravenous injection; intravenous injection is not recommended for children (1-4/94; 4).

Stability— Triflupromazine HCl should be stored at controlled room temperature, protected from light, and kept from freezing. Parenteral solutions may vary from colorless to light amber or faintly yellowish green. Markedly discolored solutions or solutions discolored in any other way should not be used (1-4/94; 4). The pH of maximum stability was stated to be 5.5 (67). Precipitation of free triflupromazine may occur at pH 6.4 and above (4).

Compatibility Information

Additive Compatibility

Triflupromazine HCl

Drug	Mfr	Conc/L	Mfr	Conc/L	Test Soln	Remarks	Ref	C/I
Chlorothiazide sodium			SQ			Precipitate forms	40	I
Ethacrynate sodium	MSD		SQ		NS	Occasional gas bubble formation	16	I
Meperidine HCl			SQ			Physically compatible	40	C
Netilmicin sulfate	SC	3 g	SQ	400 mg	D5S	Physically compatible and netilmicin chemically stable for 7 days at 4 and 25 °C. Triflupromazine not tested	558	C
Pentobarbital sodium			SQ			Precipitate forms	40	I

Drugs in Syringe Compatibility

Triflupromazine HCl

Drug (in syringe)	Mfr	Amt	Mfr	Amt	Remarks	Ref	C/I
Glycopyrrolate	RB	0.2 mg/ 1 ml	SQ	10 mg/ 1 ml	Physically compatible and pH in stability range for glycopyrrolate for 48 hr at 25 °C	331	C
	RB	0.2 mg/ 1 ml	SQ	20 mg/ 2 ml	Physically compatible and pH in stability range for glycopyrrolate for 48 hr at 25 °C	331	C
	RB	0.4 mg/ 2 ml	SQ	10 mg/ 1 ml	Physically compatible and pH in stability range for glycopyrrolate for 48 hr at 25 °C	331	C
	RB	0.2 mg/ 1 ml	SQ	20 mg/ 1 ml	Physically compatible and pH in stability range for glycopyrrolate for 48 hr at 25 °C	331	C
	RB	0.2 mg/ 1 ml	SQ	40 mg/ 2 ml	Physically compatible and pH in stability range for glycopyrrolate for 48 hr at 25 °C	331	C
	RB	0.4 mg/ 2 ml	SQ	20 mg/ 1 ml	Physically compatible and pH in stability range for glycopyrrolate for 48 hr at 25 °C	331	C
Heparin sodium		2500 units/ 1 ml		10 mg/ 1 ml	Turbidity or precipitate forms within 5 min	1053	I

Y-Site Injection Compatibility (1:1 Mixture)

Triflupromazine HCl

Drug	Mfr	Conc	Mfr	Conc	Remarks	Ref	C/I
Heparin sodium		50 units/ml/ min[a]	SQ	10 mg/ 1 ml[b]	White precipitation	1053	I

[a]Tested in sodium chloride 0.9%.
[b]Given over three minutes via a Y-site into the running heparin infusion solution.

TRIMETHOBENZAMIDE HCL
AHFS 56:22

Tigan   **Monarch**

Products— Trimethobenzamide HCl (Monarch) is available in 2-ml (200 mg) ampuls and disposable syringes and 20-ml (100 mg/ml) multiple-dose vials. Each milliliter of solution contains (2):

Component	Ampul	Syringe	Vial
Trimethobenzamide HCl	100 mg	100 mg	100 mg
Methyl- and propylparabens	0.2%		
Phenol		0.45%	0.45%
Sodium citrate	0.5 mg	0.5 mg	0.5 mg
Citric acid	0.2 mg	0.2 mg	0.2 mg
Edetate disodium		0.1 mg	
Sodium hydroxide	to adjust pH	to adjust pH	to adjust pH

pH— The official pH range is 4.5 to 5.5 (17). The manufacturer indicates the actual pH is approximately 5 (2).

Osmolality— Trimethobenzamide HCl 100 mg/ml has an osmolality of 244 mOsm/kg (1689).

Administration— Trimethobenzamide HCl is administered by intramuscular injection deep into the upper outer quadrant of the gluteal region. Intravenous and subcutaneous injections are not recommended (2; 4).

Stability— Trimethobenzamide HCl should be stored at controlled room temperature and protected from freezing (4).

Trimethobenzamide HCl (Roche) 100 mg/ml was found to retain potency for three months at room temperature when 1 or 2 ml of solution was packaged in Tubex cartridges (13).

Compatibility Information

Drugs in Syringe Compatibility

Trimethobenzamide HCl

Drug (in syringe)	Mfr	Amt	Mfr	Amt	Remarks	Ref	C/I
Glycopyrrolate	RB	0.2 mg/ 1 ml	BE	100 mg/ 1 ml	Physically compatible and pH in stability range for glycopyrrolate for 48 hr at 25 °C	331	C
	RB	0.2 mg/ 1 ml	BE	200 mg/ 2 ml	Physically compatible and pH in stability range for glycopyrrolate for 48 hr at 25 °C	331	C
	RB	0.4 mg/ 2 ml	BE	100 mg/ 1 ml	Physically compatible and pH in stability range for glycopyrrolate for 48 hr at 25 °C	331	C
Hydromorphone HCl	KN	4 mg/ 2 ml	BE	100 mg/ 1 ml	Physically compatible for 30 min	517	C
Midazolam HCl	RC	5 mg/ 1 ml	BE	200 mg/ 2 ml	Physically compatible for 4 hr at 25 °C under fluorescent light	1145	C
Nalbuphine HCl	EN	10 mg/ 1 ml	BE	100 mg/ 1 ml	Physically compatible for 36 hr at 27 °C	762	C
	EN	5 mg/ 0.5 ml	BE	100 mg/ 1 ml	Physically compatible for 36 hr at 27 °C	762	C
	EN	2.5 mg/ 0.25 ml	BE	100 mg/ 1 ml	Physically compatible for 36 hr at 27 °C	762	C
	DU	10 mg/ 1 ml		200 mg/ 2 ml	Physically compatible for 48 hr	128	C
	DU	20 mg/ 1 ml		200 mg/ 2 ml	Physically compatible for 48 hr	128	C

Y-Site Injection Compatibility (1:1 Mixture)

Trimethobenzamide HCl

Drug	Mfr	Conc	Mfr	Conc	Remarks	Ref	C/I
Heparin sodium	UP	1000 units/L[a]	RC	100 mg/ml	Physically compatible for at least 4 hr at room temperature by visual and microscopic examination	534	C
Hydrocortisone sodium succinate	UP	10 mg/L[a]	RC	100 mg/ml	Physically compatible for at least 4 hr at room temperature by visual and microscopic examination	534	C
Potassium chloride	AB	40 mEq/L[a]	RC	100 mg/ml	Physically compatible for at least 4 hr at room temperature by visual and microscopic examination	534	C
Vitamin B complex with C	RC	2 ml/L[a]	RC	100 mg/ml	Physically compatible for at least 4 hr at room temperature by visual and microscopic examination	534	C

[a]*Tested in dextrose 5% in Ringer's injection, dextrose 5% in Ringer's injection, lactated, dextrose 5% in water, Ringer's injection, lactated, and sodium chloride 0.9%.*

TRIMETHOPRIM–SULFAMETHOXAZOLE (CO-TRIMOXAZOLE)
AHFS 8:40

Septra   **Monarch**
Bactrim   **Roche**

Products— Trimethoprim–sulfamethoxazole is available in 5-, 10-, and 20-ml vials. Each milliliter contains (2):

Trimethoprim	16 mg
Sulfamethoxazole	80 mg
Propylene glycol	40%
Ethyl alcohol	10%
Diethanolamine	0.3%
Benzyl alcohol	1%
Sodium metabisulfite	0.1%
Sodium hydroxide	to adjust pH
Water for injection	qs

pH— Approximately 10 (2).

Osmolality— The osmolalities of trimethoprim–sulfamethoxazole (Burroughs Wellcome) in concentrations of 0.8 + 4, 1.1 + 5.5, and 1.6 + 8 mg/ml in dextrose 5% in water were determined to be 541, 669, and 798 mOsm/kg, respectively. At 1.6 + 8 mg/ml in sodium chloride 0.9%, the osmolality was determined to be 833 mOsm/kg (1375).

Administration— Trimethoprim–sulfamethoxazole is administered by intravenous infusion only after dilution in dextrose 5% in water. The drug should not be injected intramuscularly. Infusion over 60 to 90 minutes is recommended; rapid or direct intravenous injection must not be used. It is recommended that each 5-ml vial be diluted in 100 to 125 ml or, if fluid restriction is required, in 75 ml of dextrose 5% in water. Infusion admixtures should be inspected for cloudiness or crystallization before and during administration (2; 4).

Stability— Trimethoprim–sulfamethoxazole in intact vials should be stored at controlled room temperature between 15 and 25 °C and not refrigerated. The multiple-dose vials should be used within 48 hours of initial entry (2).

The solubility of trimethoprim in aqueous solutions is partially dependent on the pH of the solution. Trimethoprim is a weak base, and its solubility is lower in solutions with a more alkaline pH (553).

Syringes— Undiluted trimethoprim–sulfamethoxazole (Elkins-Sinn) (16 + 80 mg/ml) was stored in polypropylene syringes (Becton-Dickinson) for 2.5 days at room temperature. The syringes were exposed to fluorescent light during the day but kept in the dark at night. No loss by HPLC was observed (1582).

Sorption— Trimethoprim (Sigma) 25 mg/L in sodium chloride 0.9% (Travenol) in PVC bags did not exhibit significant sorption to the plastic during one week of storage at room temperature (15 to 20 °C) (536).

In another study, trimethoprim (Sigma) 25 mg/L in sodium chloride 0.9% did not exhibit any loss due to sorption during a seven-hour simulated infusion through an infusion set (Travenol) consisting of a cellulose propionate burette chamber and 170 cm of PVC tubing (606).

The drug was also tested as a simulated infusion over at least one hour by a syringe pump system. A glass syringe on a syringe pump was fitted with 20 cm of polyethylene tubing or 50 cm of Silastic tubing. No loss of drug due to sorption was observed with either tubing (606).

In addition, a 25-ml aliquot of trimethoprim (Sigma) 25 mg/L in sodium chloride 0.9% was stored in all-plastic syringes composed of polypropylene barrels and polyethylene plungers for 24 hours at room temperature in the dark. No loss due to sorption occurred (606).

A 1:10 (v/v) dilution of trimethoprim–sulfamethoxazole (Roche) in dextrose 5% in water prepared in a glass container and also in a burette chamber administration set (Travenol) showed no loss of either drug because of sorption during 24 hours at 23 to 25 °C (747).

Filtration— Filtration of dilutions of trimethoprim–sulfamethoxazole (Roche), ranging from 1:25 (v/v) to 1:10 (v/v) in several common intravenous infusion solutions, did not appear to result in loss of either drug because of sorption to the filter. Filtration of a visibly precipitated solution resulted in a substantial loss of trimethoprim (747).

Trimethoprim–sulfamethoxazole (Roche) 1.88 mg/ml in dextrose 5% in water and sodium chloride 0.9% was filtered through a 0.22-μm cellulose ester membrane filter (Ivex-HP, Millipore) over six hours. No significant drug loss due to binding to the filter was noted (1034).

Compatibility Information

Solution Compatibility

Trimethoprim + Sulfamethoxazole

Solution	Mfr	Mfr	Conc/L	Remarks	Ref	C/I
Dextrose 5% in sodium chloride 0.45%	AB	RC	640 mg + 3.2 g	Physically compatible with 6% trimethoprim loss and little or no sulfamethoxazole loss in 24 hr at 23 to 25 °C	747	**C**
	AB	RC	800 mg + 4 g	Physically compatible with 4% trimethoprim loss and little or no sulfamethoxazole loss in 24 hr at 23 to 25 °C	747	**C**
Dextrose 5% in water	AB	RC	640 mg + 3.2 g	Physically compatible with little or no trimethoprim and sulfamethoxazole loss in 24 hr at 23 to 25 °C	747	**C**
	AB	RC	800 mg + 4 g	Physically compatible with little or no trimethoprim and sulfamethoxazole loss in 24 hr at 23 to 25 °C	747	**C**
	TR	RC	640 mg + 3.2 g	Admixture clear and colorless for 4 hr at 22 °C. Turbidity and precipitation appear after this time. 5% trimethoprim loss in 4 hr and 28% in 24 hr. About 1% sulfamethoxazole loss in 24 hr	553	**I**[a]
	TR	RC	1.6 + 8 g	Admixture clear and colorless for 2 hr at 22 °C. Turbidity and precipitation appear after this time. 5% trimethoprim loss in 2 hr and 64% in 24 hr. About 3% sulfamethoxazole loss in 24 hr	553	**I**[a]
	TR	RC	3.2 + 16 g	Rapid precipitation and 32% trimethoprim loss in 1 hr. 9% sulfamethoxazole loss in 24 hr	553	**I**
	AB[b]	BW, RC	640 mg + 3.2 g	Physically compatible with little or no trimethoprim and sulfamethoxazole loss in 48 hr at 24 °C	1201	**C**
	AB[b]	BW, RC	800 mg + 4 g	Physically compatible with little or no trimethoprim and sulfamethoxazole loss in 24 hr at 24 °C. Precipitate forms within 48 hr	1201	**C**
	AB[b]	BW, RC	1.07 + 5.33 g	Physically compatible with little or no trimethoprim and sulfamethoxazole loss in 4 hr at 24 °C. Precipitate forms within 8 hr	1201	**I**[a]
	AB[b]	BW, RC	1.6 + 8 g	Precipitate forms as early as 2 hr at 24 °C. Up to 75% trimethoprim loss in 4 hr	1201	**I**
Ringer's injection, lactated	AB	RC	640 mg + 3.2 g	Physically compatible with 4% trimethoprim loss and little or no sulfamethoxazole loss in 24 hr at 23 to 25 °C	747	**C**
	AB	RC	800 mg + 4 g	Physically compatible with little or no trimethoprim loss and about 4% sulfamethoxazole loss in 24 hr at 23 to 25 °C	747	**C**

Solution Compatibility (Cont.)

Trimethoprim + Sulfamethoxazole

Solution	Mfr	Mfr	Conc/L	Remarks	Ref	C/I
Sodium chloride 0.45%	AB	RC	640 mg + 3.2 g	Physically compatible with little or no trimethoprim and sulfamethoxazole loss in 24 hr at 23 to 25 °C	747	C
	AB	RC	800 mg + 4 g	Physically compatible with 4% trimethoprim loss and little or no sulfamethoxazole loss in 24 hr at 23 to 25 °C	747	C
Sodium chloride 0.9%	AB	RC	640 mg + 3.2 g	Physically compatible with 5% trimethoprim loss and 4% sulfamethoxazole loss in 24 hr at 23 to 25 °C	747	C
	AB	RC	800 mg + 4 g	Physically compatible with little or no trimethoprim and sulfamethoxazole loss in 24 hr at 23 to 25 °C	747	C
	TR	RC	640 mg + 3.2 g	Admixture clear and colorless for 4 hr at 22 °C. Turbidity and precipitation appear after this time. 1% trimethoprim loss in 4 hr and 36% in 24 hr. No sulfamethoxazole loss in 24 hr	553	I[a]
	TR	RC	1.6 + 8 g	Admixture clear and colorless for 1 to 2 hr at 22 °C. Turbidity appears after this time. 15% trimethoprim loss in 2 hr and 76% in 24 hr. 5% sulfamethoxazole loss in 24 hr	553	I
	TR	RC	3.2 + 16 g	Rapid precipitation and 74% trimethoprim loss in 1 hr. 6% sulfamethoxazole loss in 24 hr	553	I
	AB[b]	BW, RC	640 mg + 3.2 g	Physically compatible with little or no trimethoprim and sulfamethoxazole loss in 48 hr at 24 °C	1201	C
	AB[b]	BW, RC	800 mg + 4 g	Physically compatible with little or no trimethoprim and sulfamethoxazole loss in 14 hr at 24 °C. Precipitate forms within 24 hr	1201	I[a]
	AB[b]	BW, RC	1.07 + 5.33 g	Physically compatible with little or no trimethoprim and sulfamethoxazole loss in 2 hr at 24 °C. Precipitate forms within 4 hr	1201	I[a]
	AB[b]	BW, RC	1.6 + 8 g	Precipitate forms as early as 2 hr at 24 °C. Up to 18% trimethoprim loss in 4 hr	1201	I
	[b]	BW	1.6 + 8 g	Precipitate forms in 1.5 hr at 20 °C. 10% trimethoprim loss by HPLC in 1.5 hr, 21% loss in 3 hr, and 60% loss in 24 hr	1555	I

[a]Incompatible by conventional standards. May be used in shorter time periods.
[b]Tested in glass containers.

Additive Compatibility

Trimethoprim + Sulfamethoxazole

Drug	Mfr	Conc/L	Mfr	Conc/L	Test Soln	Remarks	Ref	C/I
Fluconazole	PF	1 g	ES	0.4 + 2 g	D5W	Delayed cloudiness and precipitation. No fluconazole loss by HPLC in 72 hr at 25 °C under fluorescent light	1677	I
Verapamil HCl	KN	80 mg	BW	160 + 800 mg	D5W, NS	Transient precipitate	764	I

Drugs in Syringe Compatibility

Trimethoprim + Sulfamethoxazole

Drug (in syringe)	Mfr	Amt	Mfr	Amt	Remarks	Ref	C/I
Heparin sodium		2500 units/ 1 ml		80 + 400 mg/ 5 ml	Physically compatible for at least 5 min	1053	**C**

Y-Site Injection Compatibility (1:1 Mixture)

Trimethoprim + Sulfamethoxazole

Drug	Mfr	Conc	Mfr	Conc	Remarks	Ref	C/I
Acyclovir sodium	BW	5 mg/ml[a]	RC	0.8 + 4 mg/ ml[a]	Physically compatible for 4 hr at 25 °C	1157	**C**
Aldesleukin	CHI	33,800 I.U./ ml[a]	BW	1.6 + 8 mg/ ml[a]	Visually compatible with little or no loss of aldesleukin activity by bioassay	1857	**C**
Allopurinol sodium	BW	3 mg/ml[b]	ES	0.8 + 4 mg/ ml[b]	Physically compatible with no change in measured turbidity or increase in particle content in 4 hr at 22 °C	1686	**C**
Amifostine	USB	10 mg/ml[a]	ES	0.8 + 4 mg/ ml[a]	Physically compatible with no change in measured turbidity or increase in particle content in 4 hr at 23 °C	1845	**C**
Amphotericin B cholesteryl sulfate complex	SEQ	0.83 mg/ml[a]	ES	0.8 + 4 mg/ ml[a]	Physically compatible with little or no change in measured turbidity or increase in particle content in 4 hr at 23 °C under fluorescent light	2117	**C**
Atracurium besylate	BW	0.5 mg/ml[a]	ES	0.64 + 3.2 mg/ml[a]	Physically compatible for 24 hr at 28 °C	1337	**C**
Aztreonam	SQ	40 mg/ml[a]	ES	0.8 + 4 mg/ ml[a]	Physically compatible with no subvisual haze or particle formation in 4 hr at 23 °C	1758	**C**
Cefepime HCl	BR	20 mg/ml[a]	ES	0.8 + 4 mg/ ml[a]	Physically compatible with no change in measured turbidity or increase in particle content in 4 hr at 22 °C	1689	**C**
Cisatracurium besylate	GW	0.1 mg/ml[a]	ES	0.8 + 4 mg/ ml[a]	Physically compatible with no change in measured turbidity or increase in particle content in 4 hr at 23 °C	2074	**C**
	GW	2 mg/ml[a]	ES	0.8 + 4 mg/ ml[a]	Subvisual haze forms in 1 hr	2074	**I**
	GW	5 mg/ml[a]	ES	0.8 + 4 mg/ ml[a]	Subvisual haze forms immediately	2074	**I**
Cyclophosphamide	MJ	20 mg/ml[a]	BW	0.8 + 4 mg/ ml[a]	Physically compatible for 4 hr at 25 °C	1194	**C**
Diltiazem HCl	MMD	5 mg/ml	BW, RC	0.21 + 1 mg/ml[a] and 0.63 + 3.2 mg/ml[a]	Visually compatible	1807	**C**
Docetaxel	RPR	0.9 mg/ml[a]	ES	0.8 + 4 mg/ ml[a]	Physically compatible with no change in measured turbidity or increase in particle content in 4 hr at 23 °C	2224	**C**

Y-Site Injection Compatibility (1:1 Mixture) (Cont.)

Trimethoprim + Sulfamethoxazole

Drug	Mfr	Conc	Mfr	Conc	Remarks	Ref	C/I
Doxorubicin HCl liposome injection	SEQ	0.4 mg/ml[a]	ES	0.8 + 4 mg/ml[a]	Physically compatible with little or no change in measured turbidity and no increase in particle content in 4 hr at 23 °C	2087	C
Enalaprilat	MSD	0.05 mg/ml[b]	QU	0.8 + 1.6 mg/ml[a]	Physically compatible for 24 hr at room temperature under fluorescent light	1355	C
Esmolol HCl	DCC	10 mg/ml[a]	BW	0.64 + 3.2 mg/ml[a]	Physically compatible for 24 hr at 22 °C	1169	C
Etoposide phosphate	BR	5 mg/ml[a]	ES	0.8 + 4 mg/ml[a]	Physically compatible with no change in measured turbidity or increase in particle content in 4 hr at 23 °C	2218	C
Filgrastim	AMG	30 μg/ml[a]	ES	0.8 + 4 mg/ml[a]	Physically compatible with no change in measured turbidity or increase in particle content in 4 hr at 22 °C	1687	C
Fluconazole	RR	2 mg/ml	BW	16 + 80 mg/ml	Viscous gel-like substance forms	1407	I
Fludarabine phosphate	BX	1 mg/ml[a]	ES	0.8 + 4 mg/ml[a]	Physically compatible for 4 hr at room temperature under fluorescent light	1439	C
Foscarnet sodium	AST	24 mg/ml	RC	16 + 80 mg/ml	Immediate precipitation and gas production	1335	I
	AST	24 mg/ml	BW	0.53 + 2.6 mg/ml[a]	Physically compatible for 24 hr at 25 °C under fluorescent light by visual and microscopic examination	1393	C
Gemcitabine HCl	LI	10 mg/ml[b]	ES	0.8 + 4 mg/ml[b]	Physically compatible with no change in measured turbidity or increase in particle content in 4 hr at 23 °C	2226	C
Granisetron HCl	SKB	0.05 mg/ml[a]	ES	0.8 + 4 mg/ml[a]	Physically compatible with no change in measured turbidity or increase in particle content in 4 hr at 23 °C	2000	C
Hydromorphone HCl	WY	0.2 mg/ml[a]	BW	0.8 + 4 mg/ml[a]	Physically compatible for at least 4 hr at 25 °C under fluorescent light	987	C
Labetalol HCl	SC	1 mg/ml[a]	BW	0.8 + 4 mg/ml[a]	Physically compatible for 24 hr at 18 °C	1171	C
Lorazepam	WY	0.33 mg/ml[b]	RC	0.8 + 4 mg/ml	Visually compatible for 24 hr at 22 °C	1855	C
Magnesium sulfate	IX	16.7, 33.3, 66.7, 100 mg/ml[a]	RC	0.8 + 4 mg/ml[a]	Physically compatible for at least 4 hr at 32 °C	813	C
Melphalan HCl	BW	0.1 mg/ml[b]	ES	0.8 + 4 mg/ml[b]	Physically compatible with no change in measured turbidity or increase in particle content in 3 hr at 22 °C	1557	C
Meperidine HCl	WY	10 mg/ml[a]	BW	0.8 + 4 mg/ml[a]	Physically compatible for at least 4 hr at 25 °C under fluorescent light	987	C
Midazolam HCl	RC	5 mg/ml	RC	0.8 + 4 mg/ml	White precipitate forms immediately	1855	I
Morphine sulfate	WI	1 mg/ml[a]	BW	0.8 + 4 mg/ml[a]	Physically compatible for at least 4 hr at 25 °C under fluorescent light	987	C

Y-Site Injection Compatibility (1:1 Mixture) (Cont.)

Trimethoprim + Sulfamethoxazole

Drug	Mfr	Conc	Mfr	Conc	Remarks	Ref	C/I
Pancuronium bromide	ES	0.05 mg/ml[a]	ES	0.64 + 3.2 mg/ml[a]	Physically compatible for 24 hr at 28 °C	1337	**C**
Perphenazine	SC	0.02 mg/ml[a]	BW	0.8 + 4 mg/ml[a]	Physically compatible for 4 hr at 25 °C	1155	**C**
Piperacillin sodium–tazobactam sodium	LE	40 + 5 mg/ml[a]	ES	0.8 + 4 mg/ml[a]	Physically compatible with no change in measured turbidity or increase in particle content in 4 hr at 22 °C	1688	**C**
Remifentanil HCl	GW	0.025 and 0.25 mg/ml[b]	ES	0.8 + 4 mg/ml[a]	Physically compatible with no change in measured turbidity or increase in particle content in 4 hr at 23 °C	2075	**C**
Sargramostim	IMM	10 μg/ml[b]	ES	0.8 + 4 mg/ml[b]	Physically compatible for 4 hr at 22 °C	1436	**C**
Tacrolimus	FUJ	1 mg/ml[b]	RC	1.6 + 8 mg/ml[a]	Visually compatible for 24 hr at 25 °C	1630	**C**
Teniposide	BR	0.1 mg/ml[a]	ES	0.8 + 4 mg/ml[a]	Physically compatible with no subvisual haze or particle formation in 4 hr at 23 °C	1725	**C**
Thiotepa	IMM[c]	1 mg/ml[a]	ES	0.8 + 4 mg/ml[a]	Physically compatible with no change in measured turbidity or increase in particle content in 4 hr at 23 °C	1861	**C**
TNA #218 to #226[d]			ES	0.8 + 4 mg/ml[a]	Visually compatible with no precipitate or emulsion damage apparent in 4 hr at 23 °C	2215	**C**
TPN #212 to #215[d]			ES	0.8 + 4 mg/ml[a]	Physically compatible with no change in measured turbidity or increase in particle content in 4 hr at 23 °C	2109	**C**
Vecuronium bromide	OR	0.1 mg/ml[a]	ES	0.64 + 3.2 mg/ml[a]	Physically compatible for 24 hr at 28 °C	1337	**C**
Vinorelbine tartrate	BW	1 mg/ml[b]	ES	0.8 + 4 mg/ml[b]	Heavy white turbidity forms immediately, developing particles in 1 hr	1558	**I**
Zidovudine	BW	4 mg/ml[a]	BW	0.53 + 2.6 mg/ml[a]	Physically compatible for 4 hr at 25 °C under fluorescent light by visual and microscopic examination	1193	**C**

[a]*Tested in dextrose 5% in water.*
[b]*Tested in sodium chloride 0.9%.*
[c]*Lyophilized formulation tested.*
[d]*Refer to Appendix I for the composition of parenteral nutrition solutions. TNA indicates a 3-in-1 admixture, and TPN indicates a 2-in-1 admixture.*

Additional Compatibility Information

Solutions— The manufacturers recommend only dextrose 5% in water for dilution and infusion of trimethoprim–sulfamethoxazole. No other drugs or solutions should be mixed with the product (2).

Precipitation occurs in the diluted infusion solution in varying time periods, depending on the final concentration. For dilutions of 5 ml per 125 ml of dextrose 5% in water (trimethoprim 640 mg/L, sulfamethoxazole 3.2 g/L), use within six hours is recommended (2). However, precipitation within four hours has been observed at this concentration (553). For dilutions of 5 ml per 100 ml of dex-

trose 5% in water (trimethoprim 800 mg/L, sulfamethoxazole 4 g/L), use within four hours is recommended. For dilutions of 5 ml per 75 ml of dextrose 5% in water (trimethoprim 1.067 g/L, sulfamethoxazole 5.33 g/L), use within two hours is recommended. All infusions should be inspected carefully and watched closely for turbidity and precipitation. Infusion admixtures in dextrose 5% in water should not be refrigerated (2; 4).

Lesko et al. (553) and Deans et al. (747) reported dramatically different results for the compatibility of trimethoprim–sulfamethoxazole in aqueous solution, and Jarosinski et al. (1201) showed results between these two reports. Highly concentrated admixtures, at 1:15 or greater, apparently precipitate in only two to four hours (553; 1201). For more dilute trimethoprim–

sulfamethoxazole admixtures, caution and close inspection are still warranted.

The use of trimethoprim–sulfamethoxazole in glass, PVC, and polyolefin containers was found to be satisfactory (2).

Precipitation has also been found in intravenous infusion set tubing that was not flushed or changed after administration of a trimethoprim–sulfamethoxazole infusion. The authors recommended thorough flushing of the total infusion tubing or replacement after drug administration (963).

Giordano et al. evaluated the nature of the precipitate that forms from seven infusion solutions containing trimethoprim–sulfamethoxazole (Roche). In all cases, the sulfamethoxazole concentrations were within 5% of expected values, but the trimethoprim concentrations dropped to about 30% of the initial values. Further evaluation of the solid phases showed them to be trimethoprim alone or with trimethoprim monohydrate (1895).

Plasticizer Leaching— Trimethoprim–sulfamethoxazole (Elkins-Sinn) 0.8 + 4 mg/ml in dextrose 5% in water did not leach diethylhexyl phthalate (DEHP) plasticizer from 50-ml PVC bags in 24 hours at 24 °C (1683).

TRIMETREXATE GLUCURONATE
AHFS 8:40

Neutrexin   **U.S. Bioscience**

Products— Trimetrexate glucuronate (U.S. Bioscience) is available in 5-ml vials containing the equivalent of trimetrexate 25 mg and 30-ml vials containing the equivalent of trimetrexate 200 mg. Reconstitute the 25-mg vials with 2 ml of sterile water for injection or dextrose 5% in water. Reconstitute the 200-mg vials in accordance with the label instructions with dextrose 5% in water or sterile water for injection. The reconstituted vials yield a solution containing trimetrexate 12.5 mg/ml as the glucuronate. Complete dissolution should occur within 30 seconds. Do not reconstitute or dilute with chloride-containing solutions or with leucovorin because precipitate forms immediately. The reconstituted solution should be passed through a 0.22-μm filter prior to further dilution. It should not be used if cloudiness or precipitate is observed before or after filtration (2; 4).

pH— From 3.5 to 5.5 (234).

Administration— Trimetrexate glucuronate is administered by intravenous infusion at a concentration of 0.25 to 2 mg/ml in dextrose 5% in water. Do not dilute in chloride-containing infusion solutions. Flush the intravenous line with at least 10 ml of dextrose 5% in water both before and after administering trimetrexate glucuronate. The diluted trimetrexate glucuronate solution is infused intravenously over 60 to 90 minutes. Leucovorin calcium must also be administered to avoid serious, even life-threatening, toxicities (2; 4).

Stability— Intact vials of trimetrexate glucuronate should be stored at controlled room temperature and protected from exposure to light. Trimetrexate glucuronate is a pale greenish-yellow cake or powder; the reconstituted solution is a pale greenish-yellow clear solution. Do not use if cloudiness or precipitate is present. The drug is stable after reconstitution for 48 hours at room temperature, five days under refrigeration at 2 to 8 °C, and eight days frozen at −10 to −20 °C (2).

Chloride-Containing Solutions— Precipitation will occur immediately if trimetrexate glucuronate is reconstituted or diluted with chloride-containing solutions (2; 4).

Compatibility Information

Y-Site Injection Compatibility (1:1 Mixture)

Trimetrexate glucuronate

Drug	Mfr	Conc	Mfr	Conc	Remarks	Ref	C/I
Amifostine	USB	10 mg/ml[a]	USB	2 mg/ml[a]	Physically compatible with no change in measured turbidity or increase in particle content in 4 hr at 23 °C	1845	C
Foscarnet	AST	24 mg/ml	WL	1 mg/ml[a]	Trimetrexate crystals form immediately	1393	I
Indomethacin sodium trihydrate	MSD	0.5 and 1 mg/ml[a]		1 mg/ml[a]	White turbidity forms immediately, becoming white flakes in 1 hr	1550	I
Zidovudine	BW	4 mg/ml[a]	WL	1 mg/ml[a]	Physically compatible for 4 hr at 25 °C under fluorescent light by visual and microscopic examination	1193	C

[a]*Tested in dextrose 5% in water.*

Additional Compatibility Information

Solutions— Trimetrexate glucuronate reconstituted as directed and further diluted in dextrose 5% in water to a concentration of 0.25 to 2 mg/ml is stable for 24 hours at room temperature or under refrigeration. Discard any unused solution after 24 hours. Diluted solutions for infusion should not be frozen. Precipitation will occur immediately if admixed in any chloride-containing infusion solution (2; 4).

Leucovorin— Trimetrexate glucuronate will precipitate immediately if reconstituted or mixed with leucovorin calcium. The manufacturer recommends flushing the intravenous line with at least 10 ml of dextrose 5% in water both before and after trimetrexate glucuronate, particularly if leucovorin is to be administered through the same line (2; 4).

Other Information

Handling Precautions— If contact with the drug occurs, wash the area thoroughly with soap and water. Disposal should also be performed safely to avoid inadvertent exposure (2).

TUBOCURARINE CHLORIDE
AHFS 12:20

Abbott

Products— Tubocurarine chloride is available as a 3-mg/ml solution in 10- and 20-ml multiple-dose vials and 5-ml syringes (4; 29). Each milliliter of solution contains (1-11/90):

Component	Amount
Tubocurarine chloride	3 mg
Benzyl alcohol	9 mg
Sodium metabisulfite	1 mg
Sodium chloride	qs[a]
Sodium citrate, dihydrate	0.3 mg
Citric acid, anhydrous	1 mg
Water for injection	qs

[a]*Sufficient to adjust tonicity.*

pH— From 2.5 to 5 (4).

Osmolality— The osmolality of tubocurarine chloride 3 mg/ml was determined to be 296 mOsm/kg (1233).

Equivalency— Each 3 mg of tubocurarine chloride is equivalent to approximately 20 units of crude curare extract (4).

Administration— Tubocurarine chloride is usually administered intravenously, although intramuscular injection may be performed for infants or other patients if a suitable vein is not available. Undiluted at a concentration of 3 mg/ml, tubocurarine chloride should be given over approximately 60 to 90 seconds when administered by direct intravenous injection (4).

Stability— Store this product at controlled room temperature. Freezing and excessive heat of 40 °C or more should be avoided. The drug should not be used if it is more than faintly discolored (4).

Sorption— Tubocurarine chloride (Abbott) 80 mg/L did not display significant sorption to a PVC plastic test strip in 24 hours (12).

Compatibility Information

Solution Compatibility

Tubocurarine chloride

Solution	Mfr	Mfr	Conc/L	Remarks	Ref	C/I
Dextran 6% in dextrose 5%	AB		9 mg	Physically compatible	3	**C**
Dextran 6% in sodium chloride 0.9%	AB		9 mg	Physically compatible	3	**C**
Dextrose–Ringer's injection combinations	AB		9 mg	Physically compatible	3	**C**
Dextrose–Ringer's injection, lactated, combinations	AB		9 mg	Physically compatible	3	**C**
Dextrose–saline combinations	AB		9 mg	Physically compatible	3	**C**

Solution Compatibility (Cont.)

Tubocurarine chloride

Solution	Mfr	Mfr	Conc/L	Remarks	Ref	C/I
Dextrose 2½% in water	AB		9 mg	Physically compatible	3	**C**
Dextrose 5% in water	AB		9 mg	Physically compatible	3	**C**
Dextrose 10% in water	AB		9 mg	Physically compatible	3	**C**
Fructose 10% in sodium chloride 0.9%	AB		9 mg	Physically compatible	3	**C**
Fructose 10% in water	AB		9 mg	Physically compatible	3	**C**
Invert sugar 5 and 10% in sodium chloride 0.9%	AB		9 mg	Physically compatible	3	**C**
Invert sugar 5 and 10% in water	AB		9 mg	Physically compatible	3	**C**
Ionosol products	AB		9 mg	Physically compatible	3	**C**
Ringer's injection	AB		9 mg	Physically compatible	3	**C**
Ringer's injection, lactated	AB		9 mg	Physically compatible	3	**C**
Sodium chloride 0.45%	AB		9 mg	Physically compatible	3	**C**
Sodium chloride 0.9%	AB		9 mg	Physically compatible	3	**C**
Sodium lactate ⅙ M	AB		9 mg	Physically compatible	3	**C**

Additive Compatibility

Tubocurarine chloride

Drug	Mfr	Conc/L	Mfr	Conc/L	Test Soln	Remarks	Ref	C/I
Trimethaphan camsylate	BP	1 g	BP	60 mg	D5W	Haze develops within 3 hr	26	**I**

Drugs in Syringe Compatibility

Tubocurarine chloride

Drug (in syringe)	Mfr	Amt	Mfr	Amt	Remarks	Ref	C/I
Pentobarbital sodium	AB	500 mg/ 10 ml		2.25 mg/ 0.15 ml	Physically compatible	55	**C**
Thiopental sodium	AB	75 mg/ 3 ml		2.25 mg/ 0.15 ml	Physically compatible for at least 30 min	21	**C**
	AB	75 mg/ 3 ml		2.25 mg/ 0.15 ml	Physically compatible	55	**C**

Additional Compatibility Information

Alkaline Solutions— Because of the high pH of barbiturates, a precipitate may form if a barbiturate is combined with tubocurarine chloride (1-11/90; 1-11/24/92; 4).

A haze forms in 15 minutes when tubocurarine chloride is mixed with methohexital sodium (4).

Tubocurarine chloride 9 mg/L has been reported to be conditionally compatible with thiopental sodium (Abbott) 25 g/L. The mixture is physically incompatible in most Abbott infusion solutions except as noted below (3):

Dextran 6% in dextrose 5%	Physically compatible
Dextran 6% in sodium chloride 0.9%	Physically compatible
Dextrose 2½% in sodium chloride 0.45%	Physically compatible
Dextrose 2½% in sodium chloride 0.9%	Physically compatible

Dextrose 5% in sodium chloride 0.225%	Physically compatible
Dextrose 5% in sodium chloride 0.45%	Physically compatible
Dextrose 2½% in water	Physically compatible
Dextrose 5% in water	Physically compatible
Ionosol PSL (Darrow's)	Physically compatible
Sodium chloride 0.45%	Physically compatible
Sodium chloride 0.9%	Physically compatible
Sodium lactate ⅙ M	Physically compatible

Tubocurarine chloride 15 mg/ml has been reported to be conditionally compatible with thiopental sodium 2.5% in a 1:19 ratio. This mixture is usually satisfactory, but occasional precipitation occurs if the pH of the tubocurarine chloride is at its lower pH limit. The overall pH of the mixture is then reduced below 9.7, resulting in thiopental precipitation. As long as the final pH is above 9.7, no precipitate forms over 48 hours (40).

UROKINASE
AHFS 20:40

Abbokinase   **Abbott**
Abbokinase Open-Cath   **Abbott**

Products—— Urokinase manufacturing and distribution have been temporarily discontinued in the United States because of manufacturing difficulties. The following product information reflects approved products that were previously marketed and which may reappear on the market when manufacturing and distribution resume.

Urokinase for injection (Abbokinase, Abbott) is available as a lyophilized product containing 250,000 I.U. of urokinase activity, mannitol 25 mg, human albumin 250 mg, and sodium chloride 50 mg in each vial. The pH of the product is adjusted with sodium hydroxide and/or hydrochloric acid. Reconstitute with 5 ml of sterile water for injection without preservatives, rolling and tilting the vial to effect dissolution. To minimize filament formation, do not shake the vial. The reconstituted solution contains, in each milliliter, 50,000 I.U. of urokinase activity with mannitol 0.5%, human albumin 5%, and sodium chloride 1% (2; 4).

For use in catheter clearance, 1 ml of the injection is diluted with 9 ml of sterile water for injection without preservatives to yield a concentration of 5000 I.U./ml (4).

Alternatively, urokinase for catheter clearance (Abbokinase Open-Cath, Abbott) is available in lyophilized form in 1- and 1.8-ml dual chamber vials with diluent. After reconstitution, each milliliter of solution contains 5000 I.U. of urokinase activity with gelatin 5 mg, mannitol 15 mg, sodium chloride 1.7 mg, and monobasic sodium phosphate anhydrous 4.6 mg. The pH is adjusted with sodium hydroxide and/or hydrochloric acid. Reconstitute with the diluent provided in the upper chamber of the dual-chamber vial. Roll and tilt the vial to effect dissolution but do not shake it vigorously (2; 4).

pH—— From 6 to 7.5 (4).

Osmolality—— Urokinase 5000 I.U./ml in sterile water for injection has an osmolality of 391 mOsm/kg (1689).

Administration—— Urokinase may be infused intravenously by means of an infusion pump, or it may be administered into an occluded coronary artery. For intravenous infusion, reconstituted drug in vials is usually diluted to about 200 ml with dextrose 5% in water or sodium chloride 0.9%. For intracoronary administration, 750,000 I.U. may be added to 500 ml of dextrose 5% in water to provide a solution containing 1500 I.U./ml (2; 4).

To restore the patency of an occluded intravenous catheter, a volume of urokinase equal to the volume of the catheter (up to 1 ml) may be injected slowly and gently in a concentration of 5000 I.U./ml; wait 5 minutes, then attempt to aspirate. If unsuccessful, repeat at five-minute intervals for 30 minutes. If the catheter is not open within that time, the solution may be left in the catheter for 30 to 60 minutes. A second injection may be necessary (2; 4).

Stability—— Intact vials of urokinase should be refrigerated at 2 to 8 °C. The product for catheter clearance may be stored at below 25 °C, but freezing should be avoided (2; 4).

The manufacturer recommends using the reconstituted solution immediately after preparation and discarding any unused solution because the products contain no antibacterial preservatives. Only sterile water for injection (containing no preservatives) should be used for reconstitution. Diluents that contain preservatives should not be used because of possible incompatibilities (2; 4).

Abbokinase, diluted for catheter clearance, is stated to be stable for 24 hours at room temperature after reconstitution (1181).

The reconstituted solution should be practically colorless. Solutions with a significant color should not be administered. The solution may contain thin translucent filaments. The manufacturer states that the formation of such filaments does not indicate a decrease in potency and does not seem to be associated with adverse effects. The formation of filaments can be minimized by not shaking the vial during reconstitution (2; 4).

pH Effects—— The pH range of maximum stability is about 6 to 7 (1602).

Syringes—— Urokinase (Abbott) 5000 I.U./ml in dextrose 5% in water and sodium chloride 0.9% was stored in glass and polypropylene syringes (Becton-Dickinson and Sherwood). No loss of urokinase activity occurred in 24 hours at room temperature (1536).

Sorption— No apparent loss of urokinase activity was observed when urokinase (Abbott) 2500 I.U./ml in sodium chloride 0.9% was flushed through administration sets (McGaw) containing parenteral nutrition solutions. Furthermore, adding Silastic catheters to the administration sets did not result in urokinase sorption (1046).

However, Patel reported instantaneous urokinase loss from a 1500-I.U./ml solution due to adsorption to PVC bags. The extent of this loss, from 3% at 100,000 I.U./mg of protein to 15% at 155,000 I.U./mg of protein, depended on the specific activity of the urokinase (1602).

Urokinase 100 I.U./ml in 0.1 M phosphate buffer, pH 7.4, lost approximately 50% of its activity by bioactivity assay when placed in a glass test tube. Each subsequent transfer of the same solution also resulted in an approximate 50% loss. The authors indicated that urokinase was being adsorbed on the glass. Siliconizing the glass tubes reduced the extent of sorption but did not eliminate it. However, this effect was not observed when human serum albumin was present (1588). A comparison of urokinase maintenance doses administered from glass and plastic containers found that a significantly higher maintenance dose was necessary from glass containers (1070 I.U./kg/hr) compared to plastic containers (760 I.U./kg/hr) (1589).

Filtration— Urokinase solutions may be filtered through 0.45 μm or smaller cellulose ester membrane filters before administration (2; 4).

Compatibility Information

Solution Compatibility

Urokinase

Solution	Mfr	Mfr	Conc/L	Remarks	Ref	C/I
Dextrose 5% in water	AB[a]	AB	1.5 and 5 million I.U.	No urokinase loss in 30 min at room temperature	1536	C
	AB, BA[b]	AB	1.5 million I.U.	Approximately 20% urokinase loss in 2 min due to sorption	1536	I
	AB, BA[b]	AB	5 million I.U.	6% or less urokinase loss in 30 min at room temperature due to sorption	1536	C
Sodium chloride 0.9%	AB, BA[c]	AB	1.5 and 5 million I.U.	Little or no urokinase loss in 30 min at room temperature	1536	C

[a]Tested in glass containers.
[b]Tested in PVC containers.
[c]Tested in both glass and PVC containers.

Y-Site Injection Compatibility (1:1 Mixture)

Urokinase

Drug	Mfr	Conc	Mfr	Conc	Remarks	Ref	C/I
TPN #55 and #56[a]			AB	2500 I.U./ml[b]	No loss of urokinase activity when assayed immediately after mixing	1046	C

[a]Refer to Appendix I for the composition of parenteral nutrition solutions. TPN indicates a 2-in-1 admixture.
[b]Tested in sodium chloride 0.9%.

Additional Compatibility Information

The manufacturer recommends that urokinase be infused only in dextrose 5% in water or sodium chloride 0.9%. No other medication should be added to the infusion solution (2).

Heparin— To simulate an admixture used to maintain patency in implantable vascular-access devices, heparin (Burgess) 100 units/ml was used to reconstitute urokinase (Leo) to a concentration of 6250 units/ml. The mixture was stored for 21 days at 37 °C. No visible precipitation and no loss of anticoagulant activity occurred. An apparent decline in urokinase thrombolytic activity was noted, however. Nevertheless, marked fibrinolytic activity still remained after 21 days of incubation. The authors concluded that the mixture could be used in implantable vascular-access devices for up to three weeks (1174).

VANCOMYCIN HCL
AHFS 8:12.28

Vancocin Hydrochloride   **Lilly**

Products— Vancomycin HCl (Lilly) is available in vials containing drug equivalent to 500 mg or 1 g of vancomycin base. Reconstitute the vials with 10 or 20 ml, respectively, of sterile water for injection to yield a solution containing 50 mg of base (as the hydrochloride) per milliliter. Vancomycin HCl (Lilly) is also available in 5- and 10-g pharmacy bulk packages (2; 4; 29).

Vancomycin HCl is also available as a frozen premixed infusion solution containing 500 mg in 100 ml of dextrose 5% in water; the pH is adjusted with hydrochloric acid and/or sodium hydroxide. The frozen solution should not be thawed by warming in a water bath or exposure to microwave radiation. A precipitate may form during freezing, but it should redissolve upon warming to room temperature. After thawing, the bag should be checked for leaks by squeezing. The bag should be discarded if any leaks are found or if a precipitate or discoloration occurs (4).

pH— Vancomycin HCl (Lilly) in distilled water or sodium chloride 0.9% has a pH of about 3.9 (143). A 5% solution in water has a pH of 2.5 to 4.5. The commercial frozen vancomycin HCl premixed solution has a pH of 3 to 5 (4).

Osmolality— Vancomycin HCl (Lilly) 50 mg/ml in sterile water for injection has an osmolality of 57 mOsm/kg (50).

The osmolality of vancomycin HCl (Lederle) 5 mg/ml was determined to be 249 mOsm/kg in dextrose 5% in water and 291 mOsm/kg in sodium chloride 0.9% (1375).

Administration— Vancomycin HCl is administered by intermittent (2; 4) or continuous (4) intravenous infusion. The drug is extremely irritating to tissue and may cause necrosis. Therefore, it should not be given by intramuscular injection, and extravasation should be avoided during intravenous administration. For intermittent intravenous infusion, 500 mg to 1 g should be added to 100 to 200 ml, respectively, of dextrose 5% in water or sodium chloride 0.9% and administered over at least one hour (2; 4). For continuous infusion, 1 to 2 g may be added to a fluid volume sufficient to permit administration of the daily dose over 24 hours (4). Thrombophlebitis can be minimized by using dilute solutions of 2.5 to 5 mg/ml and rotating injection sites (2; 4).

Stability— Intact vials should be stored at controlled room temperature. The manufacturer indicates that reconstituted solutions of vancomycin HCl are stable for 14 days under refrigeration (2); other information indicates that the drug is also stable in solution for 14 days at room temperature (4; 141).

The frozen premixed infusion solution should be stored at –20 °C and is stable for 90 days from the date of shipping. The frozen solutions should be thawed at room temperature or under refrigeration. After thawing, they should not be refrozen. The thawed solutions are stable for 72 hours at room temperature and 30 days under refrigeration (4).

pH Effects— In the pH range of 2 to 10, vancomycin HCl degradation is principally deamidation (1927). Vancomycin HCl has been reported to be most stable at pH 3 to 5 (141) and at pH 5.5 (1927), with relatively pH-independent decomposition in the range of 3 to 8 (1927). The stability of a 1-mg/ml concentration was evaluated in buffer solutions having pH values of 1.4, 5.6, and 7.1 at 24 °C. Little or no loss occurred in 24 hours in any solution. However, the pH 1.4 buffer had a 19% loss in five days, the pH 5.6 buffer had a 10% loss in 17 days, and the pH 7.1 buffer had an 11% loss in five days (1134).

Vancomycin HCl has a low pH and may cause a physical incompatibility with other drugs, especially drugs with an alkaline pH (2; 4; 873).

In an accelerated study at 66 °C, the half-life of vancomycin B (the largest component of the commercial product) was 400 minutes in a phosphate buffer with a pH of 2.2 and 650 minutes in a phosphate buffer with a pH of 7 (1354).

Freezing Solutions— Vancomycin HCl (Lilly) at a concentration of 5 mg/ml in dextrose 5% in water or sodium chloride 0.9% exhibited no loss after 63 days of storage when frozen at −10 °C. However, neither did a loss occur in the same time period when the solution was stored at 5 °C (1134).

Vancomycin HCl (Elkins-Sinn) 5 mg/ml in dextrose 5% in water and sodium chloride 0.9% frozen at −20 °C for 12 weeks exhibited 4% or less loss of potency by HPLC analysis in latex elastomeric reservoirs (Secure Medical) and in glass containers (1970).

Syringes— Nahata et al. studied the stability of vancomycin HCl (Lilly) 5 mg/ml in dextrose concentrations ranging from 5 to 30% and packaged in plastic syringes. The syringes were stored at 4 °C for 24 hours followed by two hours at room temperature. Little or no change in the vancomycin concentration occurred during the study period (1301).

Wood et al. reported the stability of vancomycin HCl (Lilly) reconstituted to a concentration of 10 mg/ml with sterile water for injection, dextrose 5% in water, and 0.9% sodium chloride repackaged into plastic syringes. Five milliliters of the solutions were filled into three-piece Plastipak (Becton-Dickinson) and two-piece Injekt (Braun) syringes that were then sealed with Luer-Lok hubs (Vigon) and stored at 4 and 25 °C for 84 days. Under refrigeration, vancomycin HCl prepared with all three solutions and packaged in both kinds of syringes was physically and chemically stable for the 84-day period; losses determined by HPLC analysis were 4% or less for all samples.

However, stored at 25 °C in the Plastipak syringes, 10% loss occurred in about 47 days in water, 55 days in dextrose 5% in water, and 62 days in sodium chloride 0.9%. In the Injekt syringes, stability was less; 10% loss occurred in 29 days in water, 33 days in dextrose 5% in water, and 34 days in sodium chloride 0.9%. In addition, a degradation product appeared as a white flocculent precipitate in all room temperature samples after about eight weeks of storage (1893).

Implantable Pump— Vancomycin HCl (Lilly) 1 mg/ml in water in an implantable pump (Infusaid model 100) was incubated in a water bath at 37 °C for 28 days. Vancomycin losses were substantial—about 25% in seven days and 40% in 28 days. At the end of the test period, a colloidal precipitate also was found in the pumps (1302).

Portable Pumps— Stiles et al. evaluated the stability of vancomycin HCl (Elkins-Sinn) 10 mg/ml in sterile water for injection and sodium chloride 0.9% in 100-ml portable pump reservoirs (Pharmacia Deltec) during simulated administration for 24 hours. The drug solutions were tested by HPLC analysis when administered immediately after preparation and after storage for 24 hours at 5 °C before 24-hour administration. During simulated administration, some reservoirs were kept at 30 °C; others were placed in insulated pouches with frozen (−20 °C) gel packs to keep them chilled below the ambient temperature. The vancomycin HCl solutions exhibited little or no loss by HPLC under all study conditions throughout the observation periods. To complete the infusions, chilling of the drug reservoirs was not necessary nor did it enhance stability during the study period (1779).

Vancomycin HCl (Abbott) 20 and 40 mg/ml in dextrose 5% in water stored in SIMS Deltec Medication Cassette reservoirs exhibited little or no loss by HPLC analysis after 96 hours of storage at 25 °C and 30 days stored at 5 °C (2097).

Elastomeric Reservoir Pumps— Vancomycin HCl (Elkins-Sinn) 5 mg/ml in dextrose 5% in water and sodium chloride 0.9% 100 ml was packaged in latex elastomeric reservoirs (Secure Medical). Little or no loss by HPLC analysis occurred in 24 hours at 25 °C and in 14 days at 5 °C (1970).

Vancomycin HCl (Lilly) 10 mg/ml in both dextrose 5% in water

and sodium chloride 0.9% was evaluated for binding potential to natural rubber elastomeric reservoirs (Baxter). No loss was found after storage for two weeks at 35 °C with gentle agitation (2014).

Sorption— Vancomycin HCl (Lilly) 15 mg/ml in dextrose 5% in water is reported to undergo substantial sorption to Teflon tubing used in an automatic dilutor (Syva). The vancomycin HCl was apparently released from the tubing into subsequent solutions resulting in vancomycin toxicity (2153).

Filtration— Vancomycin HCl (Lilly) 2 mg/ml in dextrose 5% in water or sodium chloride 0.9% was filtered through a 0.22-μm cellulose ester filter (Ivex-HP, Millipore) over six hours. No significant drug loss due to binding to the filter was noted (1034).

Compatibility Information

Solution Compatibility

Vancomycin HCl

Solution	Mfr	Mfr	Conc/L	Remarks	Ref	C/I
Dextran 6% in sodium chloride 0.9%		LI	5 g	Physically compatible	143	C
Dextrose 5% in sodium chloride 0.9%		LI	1 g	Physically compatible	74	C
Dextrose 5% in water		LI	1 g	Physically compatible	74	C
		LI	5 g	Potency retained for at least 7 days at 5 and 25 °C	141	C
	TR[a]	LI	5 g	Physically compatible and potency retained for 24 hr at room temperature	518	C
	TR[b]	LI	5 g	Physically compatible with no vancomycin loss in 7 days and 5% loss in 17 days at 24 °C. In glass containers, no loss in 63 days at 5 °C	1134	C
	TR	LI	4 and 5 g	Physically compatible with 8% loss in 17 days at 23 °C and 11% loss in 30 days at 4 °C	1354	C
	AB[c]	ES	5 g	Little or no loss of drug by HPLC in 24 hr at 25 °C and in 14 days at 5 °C	1970	C
	AB[f]	AB	20 and 40 g	Little or no loss by HPLC in 96 hr at 25 °C and in 30 days at 5 °C	2097	C
	[a]	QLM	8 g	Visually compatible and no loss by HPLC during a 24 hr simulated infusion at 22 °C	2148	C
	[a]	QLM	5 g	Visually compatible and no loss by HPLC during a 1 hr simulated infusion at 22 °C	2148	C
	[a]	QLM	5 g	Visually compatible and no loss by HPLC during storage for 48 hr at 22 °C exposed to light and 7 days at 4 °C protected from light	2148	C
Dextrose 10% in water		LI	5 g	Physically compatible	143	C
Ringer's injection, lactated		LI	5 g	Physically compatible	143	C
		LI	1 g	Physically compatible	74	C
Sodium bicarbonate 3.75%		LI	5 g	Physically compatible	143	C
Sodium chloride 0.9%		LI	5 g	Potency retained for at least 7 days at 5 and 25 °C	141	C
		LI	1 g	Physically compatible	74	C
	TR[a]	LI	5 g	Physically compatible and potency retained for 24 hr at room temperature	518	C
	TR[b]	LI	5 g	Physically compatible with no vancomycin loss in 7 days and 5% loss in 17 days at 24 °C. In glass containers, no loss in 63 days at 5 °C	1134	C
	TR	LI	4 and 5 g	Physically compatible with 9% loss in 24 days at 23 °C and 5 to 6% loss in 30 days at 4 °C	1354	C

Solution Compatibility (Cont.)

Vancomycin HCl

Solution	Mfr	Mfr	Conc/L	Remarks	Ref	C/I
	AB[d]	ES	10 g	Little or no drug loss by HPLC with 24-hr storage at 5 °C followed by 24-hr simulated administration at 30 °C via portable pump	1779	C
	AB[c]	ES	5 g	Little or no loss of drug by HPLC in 24 hr at 25 °C and in 14 days at 5 °C	1970	C
	[a]	QLM	8 g	Visually compatible and no loss by HPLC during a 24 hr simulated infusion at 22 °C	2148	C
	[a]	QLM	5 g	Visually compatible and no loss by HPLC during a 1 hr simulated infusion at 22 °C	2148	C
	[a]	QLM	5 g	Visually compatible and no loss by HPLC during storage for 48 hr at 22 °C exposed to light and 7 days at 4 °C protected from light	2148	C
Sodium lactate ⅙ M		LI	5 g	Physically compatible	143	C
TPN #95 and #96[e]		LE	400 mg	Physically compatible and vancomycin content retained for 8 days at room temperature and under refrigeration, with and without heparin, by TDx	1321	C
TPN #105 and #106[e]		LI	1 and 6 g	Physically compatible with little or no vancomycin loss in 4 hr at 22 °C by HPLC	1325	C
TPN #107[e]			200 mg	Physically compatible and vancomycin content retained for 24 hr at 21 °C by microbiological assay	1326	C
TPN #202[a,e]		LI	500 mg and 1 g	Visually compatible and vancomycin activity by bioassay and immunoassay retained for 35 days at 4 °C and an additional 24 hr at 22 °C	1933	C

[a]*Tested in PVC containers.*
[b]*Tested in both glass and PVC containers.*
[c]*Tested in glass containers and latex elastomeric reservoirs (Secure Medical).*
[d]*Tested in portable pump reservoirs (Pharmacia Deltec).*
[e]*Refer to Appendix I for the composition of parenteral nutrition solutions. TPN indicates a 2-in-1 admixture.*
[f]*Tested in SIMS Deltec Medication Cassette reservoirs.*

Additive Compatibility

Vancomycin HCl

Drug	Mfr	Conc/L	Mfr	Conc/L	Test Soln	Remarks	Ref	C/I
Amikacin sulfate	BR	5 g	LI	2 g	D5LR, D5R, D5S, D5W, D10W, IS10, LR, NS, R, SL	Physically compatible and amikacin potency retained for 24 hr at 25 °C. Vancomycin not tested	293	C
Aminophylline		250 mg	LI	1 g	D5W	Physically compatible	74	C
	SE	1 g	LI	5 g	D5W	Physically incompatible	15	I
Amobarbital sodium			LI			Physically incompatible	9	I
	LI	1 g	LI	5 g	D5W	Physically incompatible	15	I
Atracurium besylate	BW	500 mg		5 g	D5W	Physically compatible and atracurium chemically stable for 24 hr at 5 and 30 °C	1694	C

Additive Compatibility (Cont.)

Vancomycin HCl

Drug	Mfr	Conc/L	Mfr	Conc/L	Test Soln	Remarks	Ref	C/I
Aztreonam	SQ	40 g	AB	10 g	D5W, NS	Microcrystalline precipitate forms immediately. Gross turbidity and precipitate form over 24 hr	1848	I
	SQ	4 g	AB	1 g	D5W	Physically compatible with little or no loss of either drug in 31 days at 4 °C. 8 to 10% aztreonam loss in 14 days at 23 °C and 7 days at 32 °C	1848	C
	SQ	4 g	AB	1 g	NS	Physically compatible with little or no loss of either drug in 31 days at 4 °C. About 5 to 8% aztreonam loss in 31 days at 23 °C and 7 days at 32 °C	1848	C
Calcium gluconate		1 g	LI	1 g	D5W	Physically compatible	74	C
Cefepime HCl	BR	4 g	LI	5 g	D5W, NS	4% cefepime loss by HPLC in 24 hr at room temperature exposed to light and 2% loss in 7 days at 5 °C. No vancomycin loss by HPLC, but cloudiness develops in 5 days at 5 °C	1682	C
	BR	40 g	LI	1 g	D5W, NS	4% cefepime loss by HPLC in 24 hr at room temperature exposed to light and 2% loss in 7 days at 5 °C. No vancomycin loss by HPLC and no cloudiness	1682	C
Chloramphenicol sodium succinate	PD	10 g	LI	5 g	D5W	Physically incompatible	15	I
Chlorothiazide sodium	MSD		LI			Physically incompatible	9	I
Cimetidine HCl	SKF	3 g	LI	5 g	D5W	Physically compatible and cimetidine chemically stable for 24 hr at room temperature. Vancomycin not tested	551	C
Corticotropin		500 units	LI	1 g	D5W	Physically compatible	74	C
Dexamethasone sodium phosphate			LI			Physically incompatible	9	I
Dimenhydrinate	SE	50 mg	LI	1 g	D5W	Physically compatible	74	C
Famotidine	YAM	200 mg	AB	5 g	D5W[d]	Visually compatible with 9% vancomycin loss and 6% famotidine loss by HPLC in 14 days at 25 °C. At 4 °C, 3 to 4% loss of both drugs occurred in 14 days	2111	C
Heparin sodium		12,000 units	LI	1 g	D5W	Immediate precipitate	74	I
	IX	1000 units	LE	400 mg	TPN #95[a]	Physically compatible and vancomycin content retained for 8 days at room temperature and under refrigeration by TDx	1321	C
	OR	500 to 14,300 units	LI	15 mg to 5.3 g	[b]	Physically compatible for 24 hr at 25 °C	1322	C
	OR	500 to 14,300 units	LI	6.9 to 14.3 g	[b]	Immediate white precipitation	1322	I
Hydrocortisone sodium succinate	UP	100 mg	LI	1 g	D5W	Physically compatible	74	C
Meropenem	ZEN	1 and 20 g	LI	1 g	NS	Visually compatible for 4 hr at room temperature	1994	C

Additive Compatibility (Cont.)

Vancomycin HCl

Drug	Mfr	Conc/L	Mfr	Conc/L	Test Soln	Remarks	Ref	C/I
Ofloxacin	HO	1.67 g	LI	4.2 g	W	Visually compatible with little or no loss of either drug by HPLC in 48 hr	1613	**C**
Pentobarbital sodium		LI				Physically incompatible	9	**I**
Phenobarbital sodium	WI	LI				Physically incompatible	9	**I**
Potassium chloride		3 g	LI	1 g	D5W	Physically compatible	74	**C**
Ranitidine HCl	GL	100 mg	DI	1 g	D5W	Physically compatible for 24 hr at ambient temperature under fluorescent light	1151	**C**
	GL	50 mg and 2 g		5 g	D5W	Physically compatible and ranitidine chemically stable by HPLC for 24 hr at 25 °C. Vancomycin not tested	1515	**C**
Sodium bicarbonate		LI				Physically incompatible	9	**I**
	AB	2.4 mEq[c]	LI	500 mg	D5W	Physically compatible for 24 hr	772	**C**
Verapamil HCl	KN	80 mg	LI	1 g	D5W, NS	Physically compatible for 24 hr	764	**C**
Vitamin B complex with C		1 vial	LI	1 g	D5W	Physically compatible	74	**C**

[a]Refer to Appendix I for the composition of parenteral nutrition solutions. TPN indicates a 2-in-1 admixture.
[b]Tested in Dianeal with dextrose 2.5 and 4.25%.
[c]One vial of Neut added to a liter of admixture.
[d]Tested in methyl-methacrylate-butadiene-styrene plastic containers.

Drugs in Syringe Compatibility

Vancomycin HCl

Drug (in syringe)	Mfr	Amt	Mfr	Amt	Remarks	Ref	C/I
Heparin sodium		2500 units/ 1 ml	LI	500 mg	Turbidity or precipitate forms within 5 min	1053	**I**

Y-Site Injection Compatibility (1:1 Mixture)

Vancomycin HCl

Drug	Mfr	Conc	Mfr	Conc	Remarks	Ref	C/I
Acyclovir sodium	BW	5 mg/ml[a]	LI	5 mg/ml[a]	Physically compatible for 4 hr at 25 °C	1157	**C**
Albumin		0.1 and 1%[b]		20 mg/ml[a]	Heavy turbidity forms immediately and precipitate develops subsequently	1701	**I**
Allopurinol sodium	BW	3 mg/ml[b]	LY	10 mg/ml[b]	Physically compatible with no change in measured turbidity or increase in particle content in 4 hr at 22 °C	1686	**C**
Amifostine	USB	10 mg/ml[a]	AB	10 mg/ml[a]	Physically compatible with no change in measured turbidity or increase in particle content in 4 hr at 23 °C	1845	**C**
Amiodarone HCl	LZ	4 mg/ml[c]	LI	5 mg/ml[c]	Physically compatible for 4 hr at room temperature	1444	**C**
Ampicillin sodium	SKB	250 mg/ml[d]	AB	20 mg/ml[a]	Transient precipitate forms followed by clear solution	2189	**?**
	SKB	1, 10, 50 mg/ml[b]	AB	20 mg/ml[a]	Physically compatible with no change in measured turbidity or increase in particle content in 4 hr at 23 °C	2189	**C**

Y-Site Injection Compatibility (1:1 Mixture) (Cont.)

Vancomycin HCl

Drug	Mfr	Conc	Mfr	Conc	Remarks	Ref	C/I
	SKB	1[b], 10[b], 50[b], 250[d] mg/ml	AB	2 mg/ml[a]	Physically compatible with no change in measured turbidity or increase in particle content in 4 hr at 23 °C	2189	**C**
Ampicillin sodium–sulbactam sodium	PF	250 + 125 mg/ml[d]	AB	20 mg/ml[a]	Transient precipitate forms followed by clear solution	2189	**?**
	PF	1 + 0.5, 10 + 5, and 50 + 25 mg/ml[b]	AB	20 mg/ml[a]	Physically compatible with no change in measured turbidity or increase in particle content in 4 hr at 23 °C	2189	**C**
	PF	1 + 0.5[b], 10 + 5[b], and 50 + 25[b], and 250 + 125[d] mg/ml	AB	2 mg/ml[a]	Physically compatible with no change in measured turbidity or increase in particle content in 4 hr at 23 °C	2189	**C**
Amphotericin B cholesteryl sulfate complex	SEQ	0.83 mg/ml[a]	AB	10 mg/ml[a]	Gross precipitate forms	2117	**I**
Amsacrine	NCI	1 mg/ml[a]	LI	10 mg/ml[a]	Physically compatible for 4 hr at room temperature under fluorescent light	1381	**C**
Atracurium besylate	BW	0.5 mg/ml[a]	ES	5 mg/ml[a]	Physically compatible for 24 hr at 28 °C	1337	**C**
Aztreonam	SQ	200 mg/ml[b]	LI	67 mg/ml[b]	White granular precipitate forms immediately in tubing when given sequentially	1364	**I**
	SQ	40 mg/ml[a]	AB	10 mg/ml[a]	Physically compatible with no subvisual haze or particle formation in 4 hr at 23 °C	1758	**C**
Cefazolin sodium	SKB	200 mg/ml[d]	AB	20 mg/ml[a]	Transient precipitate forms followed by clear solution	2189	**?**
	SKB	10 and 50 mg/ml[a]	AB	20 mg/ml[a]	Gross white precipitate forms immediately	2189	**I**
	SKB	1 mg/ml[a]	AB	20 mg/ml[a]	Physically compatible with no change in measured turbidity or increase in particle content in 4 hr at 23 °C	2189	**C**
	SKB	200 mg/ml[d]	AB	2 mg/ml[a]	Physically compatible with no change in measured turbidity or increase in particle content in 4 hr at 23 °C	2189	**C**
	SKB	50 mg/ml[a]	AB	2 mg/ml[a]	Subvisual measured haze forms immediately	2189	**I**
	SKB	1 and 10 mg/ml[a]	AB	2 mg/ml[a]	Physically compatible with no change in measured turbidity or increase in particle content in 4 hr at 23 °C	2189	**C**
Cefepime HCl	BR	20 mg/ml[a]	AB	10 mg/ml[a]	Haze forms immediately and flocculent precipitate forms in 4 hr	1689	**I**
Cefotaxime sodium		100 mg/ml[d]		12.5, 25, 30, 50 mg/ml[d]	White precipitate forms immediately	1721	**I**
		100 mg/ml[d]		5 mg/ml[d]	No precipitate visually observed over 7 days at room temperature, but nonvisual incompatibility cannot be ruled out	1721	**?**
	HO	200 mg/ml[d]	AB	20 mg/ml[a]	Transient precipitate forms followed by clear solution	2189	**?**
	HO	50 mg/ml[a]	AB	20 mg/ml[a]	White cloudiness forms immediately	2189	**I**
	HO	1 and 10 mg/ml[a]	AB	20 mg/ml[a]	Physically compatible with no change in measured turbidity or increase in particle content in 4 hr at 23 °C	2189	**C**

Y-Site Injection Compatibility (1:1 Mixture) (Cont.)

Vancomycin HCl

Drug	Mfr	Conc	Mfr	Conc	Remarks	Ref	C/I
	HO	1[a], 10[a], 50[a], 200[d] mg/ml	AB	2 mg/ml[a]	Physically compatible with no change in measured turbidity or increase in particle content in 4 hr at 23 °C	2189	C
Cefotetan sodium	ZEN	200 mg/ml[d]	AB	20 mg/ml[a]	Transient precipitate forms followed by clear solution. White precipitate forms in 4 hr	2189	I
	ZEN	10 and 50 mg/ml[a]	AB	20 mg/ml[a]	Gross white precipitate forms immediately	2189	I
	ZEN	1 mg/ml[a]	AB	20 mg/ml[a]	Subvisual measured haze forms immediately followed by white precipitate in 4 hr	2189	I
	ZEN	1[a], 10[a], 50[a], 200[d] mg/ml	AB	2 mg/ml[a]	Physically compatible with no change in measured turbidity or increase in particle content in 4 hr at 23 °C	2189	C
Cefoxitin sodium	ME	180 mg/ml[d]	AB	20 mg/ml[a]	Transient precipitate forms followed by clear solution	2189	?
	ME	50 mg/ml[a]	AB	20 mg/ml[a]	Gross white precipitate forms immediately	2189	I
	ME	10 mg/ml[a]	AB	20 mg/ml[a]	Visible haze forms in 4 hr at 23 °C	2189	I
	ME	1 mg/ml[a]	AB	20 mg/ml[a]	Physically compatible with no change in measured turbidity or increase in particle content in 4 hr at 23 °C	2189	C
	ME	1[a], 10[a], 50[a], 180[d] mg/ml	AB	2 mg/ml[a]	Physically compatible with no change in measured turbidity or increase in particle content in 4 hr at 23 °C	2189	C
Cefpirome sulfate	HO	50 mg/ml[e]	AB	5 mg/ml[e]	Visually and microscopically compatible with little or no cefpirome and vancomycin loss by HPLC in 8 hr at 23 °C	2044	C
Ceftazidime	GL[p]	25 and 60 mg/ml[a]	AB	3 mg/ml[a]	Physically compatible with no subvisual haze or particle formation in 4 hr at 23 °C	1563	C
	GL[p]	25 mg/ml[a]	AB	10 mg/ml[a]	Subvisual haze forms immediately	1563	I
	GL[p]	60 mg/ml[a]	AB	10 mg/ml[a]	Dense turbidity and white particles form immediately and become gross precipitate in 1 hr	1563	I
	SKB[p]	10[a], 50[a], 200[d] mg/ml	AB	20 mg/ml[a]	Gross white precipitate forms immediately	2189	I
	SKB[p]	1 mg/ml[a]	AB	20 mg/ml[a]	Physically compatible with no change in measured turbidity or increase in particle content in 4 hr at 23 °C	2189	C
	SKB[p]	1[a], 10[a], 50[a], 200[d] mg/ml	AB	2 mg/ml[a]	Physically compatible with no change in measured turbidity or increase in particle content in 4 hr at 23 °C	2189	C
Ceftizoxime sodium	FUJ	280 mg/ml[d]	AB	20 mg/ml[a]	Transient precipitate forms followed by clear solution	2189	?
	FUJ	1, 10, 50 mg/ml[a]	AB	20 mg/ml[a]	Physically compatible with no change in measured turbidity or increase in particle content in 4 hr at 23 °C	2189	C
	FUJ	1[a], 10[a], 50[a], 280[d] mg/ml	AB	2 mg/ml[a]	Physically compatible with no change in measured turbidity or increase in particle content in 4 hr at 23 °C	2189	C
Ceftriaxone sodium	RC	250 mg/ml[d]	AB	20 mg/ml[a]	Transient precipitate forms followed by clear solution	2189	?

Y-Site Injection Compatibility (1:1 Mixture) (Cont.)

Vancomycin HCl

Drug	Mfr	Conc	Mfr	Conc	Remarks	Ref	C/I
	RC	10 and 50 mg/ml[a]	AB	20 mg/ml[a]	Gross white precipitate forms immediately	2189	**I**
	RC	1 mg/ml[a]	AB	20 mg/ml[a]	Subvisual measured haze forms immediately	2189	**I**
	RC	1[a], 10[a], 50[a], 250[d] mg/ml	AB	2 mg/ml[a]	Physically compatible with no change in measured turbidity or increase in particle content in 4 hr at 23 °C	2189	**C**
Cefuroxime sodium	GW	150 mg/ml[d]	AB	20 mg/ml[a]	Transient precipitate forms followed by a subvisual measured haze	2189	**I**
	GW	50 mg/ml[a]	AB	20 mg/ml[a]	Gross white precipitate forms immediately	2189	**I**
	GW	10 mg/ml[a]	AB	20 mg/ml[a]	Subvisual measured haze forms immediately	2189	**I**
	GW	1 mg/ml[a]	AB	20 mg/ml[a]	Physically compatible with no change in measured turbidity or increase in particle content in 4 hr at 23 °C	2189	**C**
	GW	1[a], 10[a], 50[a], 150[d] mg/ml	AB	2 mg/ml[a]	Physically compatible with no change in measured turbidity or increase in particle content in 4 hr at 23 °C	2189	**C**
Cisatracurium besylate	GW	0.1, 2, 5 mg/ml[a]	AB	10 mg/ml[a]	Physically compatible with no change in measured turbidity or increase in particle content in 4 hr at 23 °C	2074	**C**
Clarithromycin	AB	4 mg/ml[a]	DB	10 mg/ml[a]	Visually compatible for 72 hr at both 30 and 17 °C	2174	**C**
Cyclophosphamide	MJ	20 mg/ml[a]	LI	5 mg/ml[a]	Physically compatible for 4 hr at 25 °C	1194	**C**
Diltiazem HCl	MMD	5 mg/ml	LI	5 and 50 mg/ml[b]	Visually compatible	1807	**C**
Docetaxel	RPR	0.9 mg/ml[a]	LI	10 mg/ml[a]	Physically compatible with no change in measured turbidity or increase in particle content in 4 hr at 23 °C	2224	**C**
Doxorubicin HCl liposome injection	SEQ	0.4 mg/ml[a]	AB	10 mg/ml[a]	Physically compatible with little or no change in measured turbidity and no increase in particle content in 4 hr at 23 °C	2087	**C**
Enalaprilat	MSD	0.05 mg/ml[b]	LE	5 mg/ml[a]	Physically compatible for 24 hr at room temperature under fluorescent light	1355	**C**
Esmolol HCl	DCC	10 mg/ml[a]	LE	5 mg/ml[a]	Physically compatible for 24 hr at 22 °C	1169	**C**
Etoposide phosphate	BR	5 mg/ml[a]	LI	10 mg/ml[a]	Physically compatible with no change in measured turbidity or increase in particle content in 4 hr at 23 °C	2218	**C**
Filgrastim	AMG	30 μg/ml[a]	AB	10 mg/ml[a]	Physically compatible with no change in measured turbidity or increase in particle content in 4 hr at 22 °C	1687	**C**
Fluconazole	RR	2 mg/ml	LY	20 mg/ml	Physically compatible for 24 hr at 25 °C	1407	**C**
Fludarabine phosphate	BX	1 mg/ml[a]	LI	10 mg/ml[a]	Physically compatible for 4 hr at room temperature under fluorescent light	1439	**C**
Foscarnet sodium	AST	24 mg/ml	LE	20 mg/ml	Immediate precipitation	1335	**I**
	AST	24 mg/ml	LE	15 mg/ml[c]	Physically compatible for 24 hr at 25 °C under fluorescent light by visual and microscopic examination	1393	**C**

Y-Site Injection Compatibility (1:1 Mixture) (Cont.)

Vancomycin HCl

Drug	Mfr	Conc	Mfr	Conc	Remarks	Ref	C/I
	AST	24 mg/ml	LE	10 mg/ml[b]	Visually compatible for 24 hr at room temperature in test tubes. No precipitate found on filter	2063	**C**
Gemcitabine HCl	LI	10 mg/ml[b]	LI	10 mg/ml[b]	Physically compatible with no change in measured turbidity or increase in particle content in 4 hr at 23 °C	2226	**C**
Granisetron HCl	SKB	0.05 mg/ml[a]	AB	10 mg/ml[a]	Physically compatible with no change in measured turbidity or increase in particle content in 4 hr at 23 °C	2000	**C**
Heparin sodium	TR	50 units/ml	LI	6.6 mg/ml[a]	Visually incompatible within 6 hr at 25 °C	1793	**I**
	ES	100 units/ml[c]	LE	10 mg/ml[b]	Precipitate forms	2063	**I**
Hydromorphone HCl	WY	0.2 mg/ml[a]	LI	5 mg/ml[a]	Physically compatible for at least 4 hr at 25 °C under fluorescent light	987	**C**
Idarubicin HCl	AD	1 mg/ml[b]	AD	4 mg/ml[a]	Color changes immediately	1525	**I**
Insulin, regular	LI	0.2 unit/ml[b]	LI	4 mg/ml[a]	Physically compatible for 2 hr at 25 °C	1395	**C**
Labetalol HCl	SC	1 mg/ml[a]	LE	5 mg/ml[a]	Physically compatible for 24 hr at 18 °C	1171	**C**
Lorazepam	WY	0.33 mg/ml[b]	LI	5 mg/ml	Visually compatible for 24 hr at 22 °C	1855	**C**
Magnesium sulfate	IX	16.7, 33.3, 66.7, 100 mg/ml[a]	LI	5 mg/ml[a]	Physically compatible for at least 4 hr at 32 °C	813	**C**
Melphalan HCl	BW	0.1 mg/ml[b]	LY	10 mg/ml[b]	Physically compatible with no change in measured turbidity or increase in particle content in 3 hr at 22 °C	1557	**C**
Meperidine HCl	WY	10 mg/ml[a]	LI	5 mg/ml[a]	Physically compatible for at least 4 hr at 25 °C under fluorescent light	987	**C**
Meropenem	ZEN	1 and 50 mg/ml[b]	LI	5 mg/ml[d]	Visually compatible for 4 hr at room temperature	1994	**C**
Methotrexate sodium	LE	[a,f]	AB	510 mg[g]	Physically compatible during 1-hr simultaneous infusion	1405	**C**
		30 mg/ml		5 mg/ml[a]	Visually compatible for 2 hr at room temperature. Dark yellow precipitate forms in 4 hr	1788	**I**
Midazolam HCl	RC	1 mg/ml[a]	LI	5 mg/ml[a]	Visually compatible for 24 hr at 23 °C	1847	**C**
	RC	5 mg/ml	LI	5 mg/ml	Visually compatible for 24 hr at 22 °C	1855	**C**
Morphine sulfate	WI	1 mg/ml[a]	LI	5 mg/ml[a]	Physically compatible for at least 4 hr at 25 °C under fluorescent light	987	**C**
Nafcillin sodium	BE	250 mg/ml[d]	AB	20 mg/ml[a]	Transient precipitate forms followed by a visibly hazy solution	2189	**I**
	BE	10 and 50 mg/ml[b]	AB	20 mg/ml[a]	Gross white precipitate forms immediately	2189	**I**
	BE	1 mg/ml[b]	AB	20 mg/ml[a]	Physically compatible with no change in measured turbidity or increase in particle content in 4 hr at 23 °C	2189	**C**
	BE	10[b], 50[b], 250[d] mg/ml	AB	2 mg/ml[a]	Subvisual measured haze forms immediately	2189	**I**
	BE	1 mg/ml[b]	AB	2 mg/ml[a]	Physically compatible with no change in measured turbidity or increase in particle content in 4 hr at 23 °C	2189	**C**

Y-Site Injection Compatibility (1:1 Mixture) (Cont.)

Vancomycin HCl

Drug	Mfr	Conc	Mfr	Conc	Remarks	Ref	C/I
Omeprazole		4 mg/ml		10 mg/ml[a]	White precipitate forms within 5 min	2173	**I**
Ondansetron HCl	GL	1 mg/ml[b]	LI	10 mg/ml[a]	Physically compatible for 4 hr at 22 °C	1365	**C**
Paclitaxel	NCI	1.2 mg/ml[a]		10 mg/ml[a]	Physically compatible with no change in measured turbidity in 4 hr at 22 °C	1528	**C**
Pancuronium bromide	ES	0.05 mg/ml[a]	ES	5 mg/ml[a]	Physically compatible for 24 hr at 28 °C	1337	**C**
Perphenazine	SC	0.02 mg/ml[a]	LI	5 mg/ml[a]	Physically compatible for 4 hr at 25 °C	1155	**C**
Piperacillin sodium	LE	200 mg/ml[d]	AB	20 mg/ml[a]	Transient precipitate forms followed by clear solution	2189	**?**
	LE	10 and 50 mg/ml[a]	AB	20 mg/ml[a]	Gross white precipitate forms immediately	2189	**I**
	LE	1 mg/ml[a]	AB	20 mg/ml[a]	Physically compatible with no change in measured turbidity or increase in particle content in 4 hr at 23 °C	2189	**C**
	LE	1[a], 10[a], 50[a], 200[d] mg/ml	AB	2 mg/ml[a]	Physically compatible with no change in measured turbidity or increase in particle content in 4 hr at 23 °C	2189	**C**
Piperacillin sodium–tazobactam sodium	LE	40 + 5 mg/ml[a]	AB	10 mg/ml[a]	White turbidity forms immediately and white precipitate forms in 4 hr	1688	**I**
	LE	200 + 25 mg/ml[d]	AB	20 mg/ml[a]	Transient precipitate forms followed by clear solution	2189	**?**
	LE	10 + 1.25 and 50 + 6.25 mg/ml[a]	AB	20 mg/ml[a]	Gross white precipitate forms immediately	2189	**I**
	LE	1 + 0.125 mg/ml[a]	AB	20 mg/ml[a]	Physically compatible with no change in measured turbidity or increase in particle content in 4 hr at 23 °C	2189	**C**
	LE	1 + 0.125[a], 10 + 1.25[a], 50 + 6.25[a], and 200 + 25[d] mg/ml	AB	2 mg/ml[a]	Pysically compatible with no change in measured turbidity or increase in particle content in 4 hr at 23 °C	2189	**C**
Propofol	ZEN	10 mg/ml	AB	10 mg/ml[a]	Physically compatible for 1 hr at 23 °C with no increase in particle content	2066	**C**
Remifentanil HCl	GW	0.025 and 0.25 mg/ml[b]	AB	10 mg/ml[a]	Physically compatible with no change in measured turbidity or increase in particle content in 4 hr at 23 °C	2075	**C**
Sargramostim	IMM	10 μg/ml[b]	LI	10 mg/ml[b]	Physically compatible for 4 hr at 22 °C	1436	**C**
	IMM	15 μg/ml[b]	LI	20 mg/ml[c]	Visually compatible for 2 hr	1618	**C**
	IMM	6 μg/ml[b,h]	LI	20 mg/ml[c]	Haze forms within 15 min and increases due to vancomycin incompatibility with albumin	1618; 1701	**I**
Sodium bicarbonate		1.4%		5 mg/ml[a]	Visually compatible for 4 hr at room temperature	1788	**C**
Tacrolimus	FUJ	1 mg/ml[b]	LI	5 mg/ml[a]	Visually compatible for 24 hr at 25 °C	1630	**C**
Teniposide	BR	0.1 mg/ml[a]	AB	10 mg/ml[a]	Physically compatible with no subvisual haze or particle formation in 4 hr at 23 °C	1725	**C**

Y-Site Injection Compatibility (1:1 Mixture) (Cont.)

Vancomycin HCl

Drug	Mfr	Conc	Mfr	Conc	Remarks	Ref	C/I
Theophylline	TR	4 mg/ml	LI	6.6 mg/ml[a]	Visually compatible for 6 hr at 25 °C	1793	**C**
Thiotepa	IMM[i]	1 mg/ml[a]	AB	10 mg/ml[a]	Physically compatible with no change in measured turbidity or increase in particle content in 4 hr at 23 °C	1861	**C**
Ticarcillin disodium	SKB	50[a] and 200[d] mg/ml	AB	20 mg/ml[a]	Transient precipitate forms followed by clear solution	2189	**?**
	SKB	1 and 10 mg/ml[a]	AB	20 mg/ml[a]	Gross white precipitate forms immediately	2189	**I**
	SKB	1[a], 10[a], 50[a] 200[d] mg/ml	AB	2 mg/ml[a]	Physically compatible with no change in measured turbidity or increase in particle content in 4 hr at 23 °C	2189	**C**
Ticarcillin disodium–clavulanate potassium	SKB	206.7 mg/ml[d]	AB	20 mg/ml[a]	Transient precipitate forms followed by clear solution	2189	**?**
	SKB	1.034, 10.335, and 51.675 mg/ml[a]	AB	20 mg/ml[a]	Gross white precipitate forms	2189	**I**
	SKB	31 mg/ml[b]		5 mg/ml[b]	White precipitate formed sporadically	2167	**I**
	SKB	1.034[a], 10.335[a], 51.675[a], and 206.7[d] mg/ml	AB	2 mg/ml[a]	Physically compatible with no change in measured turbidity or increase in particle content in 4 hr at 23 °C	2189	**C**
Tolazoline HCl		0.1 mg/ml[a]	LE	5 mg/ml[a]	Physically compatible for 24 hr at 22 °C	1363	**C**
TNA #218 to #226[j]			AB	10 mg/ml[a]	Visually compatible with no precipitate or emulsion damage apparent in 4 hr at 23 °C	2215	**C**
TPN #61[j]		[k]	LI	50 mg/1 ml[l]	Physically compatible	1012	**C**
		[m]	LI	300 mg/6 ml[l]	Physically compatible	1012	**C**
TPN #91[j]		[n]	LI	30 mg[o]	Physically compatible	1170	**C**
TPN #189[j]			DB	10 mg/ml[b]	Visually compatible for 24 hr at 22 °C	1767	**C**
TPN #212 to #215[j]			AB	10 mg/ml[a]	Physically compatible with no change in measured turbidity or increase in particle content in 4 hr at 23 °C	2109	**C**
Vecuronium bromide	OR	0.1 mg/ml[a]	ES	5 mg/ml[a]	Physically compatible for 24 hr at 28 °C	1337	**C**
Vinorelbine tartrate	BW	1 mg/ml[b]	LY	10 mg/ml[b]	Physically compatible with no change in measured turbidity or increase in particle content in 4 hr at 22 °C	1558	**C**
Warfarin sodium	DU	2 mg/ml[d]	LI	4 mg/ml[a]	Haze forms immediately	2010	**I**
	DU	0.1 mg/ml[c]	AB	10 mg/ml[c]	Physically compatible with no change in measured turbidity or increase in particle content in 24 hr at 23 °C	2011	**C**
	DU	2 mg/ml[d]	AB	10 mg/ml[c]	Heavy white turbidity forms immediately	2011	**I**
	DME	2 mg/ml[d]	LI	4 mg/ml[a]	Haze forms immediately	2078	**I**

Y-Site Injection Compatibility (1:1 Mixture) (Cont.)

Vancomycin HCl

Drug	Mfr	Conc	Mfr	Conc	Remarks	Ref	C/I
Zidovudine	BW	4 mg/ml[a]	LI	15 mg/ml[a]	Physically compatible for 4 hr at 25 °C under fluorescent light by visual and microscopic examination	1193	C

[a]*Tested in dextrose 5% in water.*
[b]*Tested in sodium chloride 0.9%.*
[c]*Tested in both dextrose 5% in water and sodium chloride 0.9%.*
[d]*Tested in sterile water for injection.*
[e]*Tested in dextrose 5% in water, Ringer's injection, lactated, sodium chloride 0.45%, and sodium chloride 0.9%.*
[f]*Concentration unspecified.*
[g]*Infused over one hour simultaneously with methotrexate.*
[h]*Tested with 0.1% albumin (human) added.*
[i]*Lyophilized formulation tested.*
[j]*Refer to Appendix I for the composition of parenteral nutrition solutions. TNA indicates a 3-in-1 admixture, and TPN indicates a 2-in-1 admixture.*
[k]*Run at 21 ml/hr.*
[l]*Given over 30 minutes by syringe pump.*
[m]*Run at 94 ml/hr.*
[n]*Run at 10 ml/hr.*
[o]*Given over one hour by syringe pump.*
[p]*Sodium carbonate–containing formulation tested.*

Additional Compatibility Information

pH and Concentration Dependency— The concentration dependency of compatibility or incompatibility of vancomycin HCl mixed with or administered simultaneously with a number of penicillins and cephalosporins has been demonstrated (2189). See Y-Site Injection Compatibility table above. Vancomycin HCl has a low pH and is variably compatible with drugs having neutral to mildly alkaline pH, including cephalosporins and penicillins. The compatibility may depend on a number of factors including concentration of each drug, dilution vehicle, actual pH of solutions, and completeness of mixing during administration. Combinations that are compatible when well mixed may result in precipitation if only partially mixed, presumably due to regionally different concentrations and pH values. If attempting to administer vancomycin HCl with another drug product, care should be taken to ensure that the specific combination and concentrations are compatible under the exact administration conditions to be used. An inline filter should be used as a final safety measure (2189).

Solutions— Dextrose 5% in water and sodium chloride 0.9% are recommended as diluents for the intravenous infusion of vancomycin HCl. The manufacturer indicates that vancomycin HCl, at a concentration of no more than 5 mg/ml, is stable for 14 days under refrigeration in either of these solutions (2).

Vancomycin HCl 5 mg/ml is stated to be stable for 96 hours under refrigeration in the following solutions (2):

Acetated Ringer's injection
Dextrose 5% in Ringer's injection, lactated
Dextrose 5% in sodium chloride 0.9%
Isolyte E
Normosol M in dextrose 5%
Ringer's injection, lactated

Peritoneal Dialysis Solutions— The activity of vancomycin 15 mg/L was evaluated in peritoneal dialysis fluids containing dextrose 1.5 or 4.25% (Dianeal 137, Travenol). Storage at 25 °C resulted in virtually no loss of antimicrobial activity in 24 hours (738).

Vancomycin HCl with aztreonam admixed in Dianeal 137 with dextrose 4.25% is stated to be stable for 24 hours at room temperature (2p738).

Vancomycin HCl (Lilly) 10 and 50 mg/L in peritoneal dialysis concentrate with dextrose 50% (McGaw) retained 93 to 100% of its initial activity (by microbiological assay) after 24 hours of storage at room temperature (1044).

The stability of vancomycin HCl (Lilly) 20 mg/L in peritoneal dialysis solutions (Dianeal 137 and PD2) with heparin sodium 500 units/L was evaluated by microbiological assay. Approximately 95 ± 12% activity remained after 24 hours at 25 °C (1228).

Drake et al. evaluated the retention of antimicrobial activity, using a disc diffusion bioassay, of vancomycin HCl (Lilly) 1 g/L alone and with each of the aminoglycosides gentamicin sulfate (SoloPak) 120 mg/L and tobramycin sulfate (Lilly) 120 mg/L in Dianeal PD-2 (Travenol) with dextrose 1.5%. Little or no loss of any antibiotic occurred in eight hours at 37 °C. Vancomycin HCl alone retained activity for at least 48 hours at 4 and 25 °C. In combination with gentamicin sulfate and tobramycin sulfate, antimicrobial activity of both vancomycin and the aminoglycosides was retained for up to 48 hours. However, the authors recommended refrigeration at 4 °C for storage periods greater than 24 hours (1414).

The stability of vancomycin HCl (Lilly) 25 mg/L in Dianeal 137 (Baxter) with dextrose 1.36 and 3.86%, while protected from direct sunlight, was evaluated by HPLC and enzyme immunoassay. At both dextrose concentrations, less than 4% vancomycin HCl was lost in 42 days at 4 °C. At 20 °C, a 5% or less loss occurred in 28 days. At 37 °C, a 10% loss occurred in six to seven days (1654).

Vancomycin HCl (Lilly) 1 mg/ml admixed with ceftazidime (sodium carbonate–containing formulation) (Lilly) 0.5 mg/ml in Dianeal PD-2 (Baxter) with 1.5% and also 4.25% dextrose were evaluated for compatibility and stability. Samples were stored under fluorescent light at 4 and 24 °C for 24 hours and at 37 °C for 12 hours. No precipitation or other change was observed by visual inspection in any sample. HPLC analysis found no loss of either drug in the samples stored at 4 °C and no loss of vancomycin HCl and about 4 to 5% ceftazidime loss in the samples stored at 24 °C in 24 hours. Vancomycin HCl losses of 3% or less and ceftazidime loss of about 6% were found in the samples stored at 37 °C for 12 hours. No difference in stability was found between samples at either dextrose concentration (2217).

Chloramphenicol and Penicillin G— Chloramphenicol sodium succinate and high concentrations of penicillin G in combination with vancomycin HCl may result in the formation of a precipitate. Five to 10 million units of penicillin G added to vancomycin HCl, especially in dextrose solutions, cause precipitation (143).

Ceftazidime— A precipitate formed instantaneously when ceftazidime 2 g/50 ml in sterile water for injection was added to a burette previously used to administer vancomycin HCl 1 g/100 ml in dextrose 5% in water. The authors suggested that vancomycin may have precipitated because of the alkaline pH due to the sodium carbonate in the ceftazidime formulation (873). However, the manufacturer of Ceptaz also notes precipitation with vancomycin HCl, even though no sodium carbonate is present in the Ceptaz formulation (2).

The concentration dependency of precipitation for these drugs has been demonstrated (2189). For more information, see pH and Concentration Dependency and also the Y-Site Injection Compatibility table above.

Heparin— Heparin sodium approximately 5000 units/L has been reported to be conditionally compatible with vancomycin HCl 2 g/L. A satisfactory solution is obtained if the infusion solution used is sodium chloride 0.9%. However, if dextrose 5% in water is used, a precipitate may form (143).

Vancomycin HCl (Lilly) 15 mg/L to 5.3 g/L in Dianeal with dextrose 2.5 or 4.25% was physically compatible with heparin sodium (Organon) 500 to 14,300 units/L for 24 hours at 25 °C under fluorescent light. However, a white precipitate formed immediately in combinations of heparin sodium with vancomycin HCl 6.9 to 14.3 g/L (1322).

Vancomycin HCl (Lilly) 25 µg/ml and heparin sodium (Elkins-Sinn) 100 units/ml in 0.9% sodium chloride injection as a catheter flush solution was evaluated for stability when stored at 4 °C for 14 days. The flush solution was visually clear, and the vancomycin activity (by bioassay and immunoassay) and heparin activity (by colorimetric assay) were retained throughout the storage period. However, an additional 24 hours at 37 °C to simulate use conditions resulted in losses of both agents ranging from 20 to 37% (1933).

Ticarcillin— Sequential administration of ticarcillin disodium 4.25 g/50 ml and then vancomycin HCl 500 mg/50 ml in dextrose 5% in sodium chloride 0.3% through a calibrated chamber set (Buretrol) has resulted in a white precipitate. The precipitate did not appear during the initial infusion but formed after repeated administration through the same set. The sequence of administration (ticarcillin first, followed by vancomycin), drug concentrations, and repetitive administration all appear to affect the appearance of the precipitate (972).

The concentration dependency of precipitation for these drugs has been demonstrated (2189). For more information, see pH and Concentration Dependency and also the Y-Site Injection Compatibility table above.

Ticarcillin Disodium–Clavulanate Potassium— Vancomycin HCl when admixed with ticarcillin disodium–clavulanate potassium has been reported to exhibit occasional precipitate formation. This observation from practice was made with a combination of vancomycin HCl 5 mg/ml and ticarcillin disodium–clavulanate potassium 30 + 1 mg/ml and also with combinations at variable but unrecorded concentrations. The occurrence of precipitate formation was characterized as sporadic and unpredictable (2167).

The concentration dependency of precipitation for these drugs has been demonstrated (2189). For more information, see pH and Concentration Dependency and also the Y-Site Injection Compatibility table above.

Concentrated Solutions— The following incompatibility determinations were performed with concentrated solutions. The drugs in dry form were reconstituted according to manufacturers' recommendations. One milliliter of vancomycin HCl (Lilly) was added to 5 ml of sterile distilled water along with 1 ml of each of the following drugs. Particulate matter was noted within two hours (28):

Aminophylline
Chloramphenicol sodium succinate (Parke-Davis)
Dexamethasone sodium phosphate (MSD)
Heparin sodium
Hydrocortisone sodium succinate (Upjohn)
Penicillin G potassium
Phenytoin sodium (Parke-Davis)
Vitamin B complex with C (Lederle)

Other Information

Plasticizer Leaching— Vancomycin HCl (Qualimed Laboratories) 8 mg/ml in dextrose 5% in water and sodium chloride 0.9% in PVC containers (Macropharma) did not leach detectable amounts of DEHP plasticizer during simulated administration over 24 hours. If any DEHP was present, the concentration was less than 1 µg/ml, the limit of detection in this study (2148).

VASOPRESSIN
AHFS 68:28

American Regent

Products— Vasopressin (American Regent) is available in 0.5-, 1-, and 10-ml vials. Each milliliter of solution contains vasopressin 20 pressor units, sodium chloride 0.9%, chlorobutanol 0.5%, in water for injection. Acetic acid may have been used to adjust pH during manufacture (1-2/96).

pH— From 2.5 to 4.5 (4).

Osmolality— Vasopressin 20 units/ml has an osmolality of 30 mOsm/kg (1689).

Administration— Vasopressin may be given subcutaneously or intramuscularly (1-2/96; 4) or by continuous intravenous or intra-arterial infusion using a controlled infusion device. For infusion, the drug is usually diluted to a concentration of 0.1 to 1 unit/ml with sodium chloride 0.9% or dextrose 5% in water (4).

Stability— Vasopressin injection is a clear, colorless or practically colorless solution. It should be stored at room temperature, 15 to 30 °C, but not frozen (1-2/96; 4).

Compatibility Information

Additive Compatibility

Vasopressin

Drug	Mfr	Conc/L	Mfr	Conc/L	Test Soln	Remarks	Ref	C/I
Verapamil HCl	KN	80 mg	PD	40 units	D5W, NS	Physically compatible for 24 hr	764	**C**

VECURONIUM BROMIDE
AHFS 12:20

Norcuron   **Organon**

Products— Vecuronium bromide (Organon) is available in 10-ml vials as a lyophilized cake, both with and without accompanying bacteriostatic water for injection with benzyl alcohol 0.9% for use as a diluent. It also is available in 20-ml vials without a diluent. The vials contain (2):

Component	10 ml	20 ml
Vecuronium bromide	10 mg	20 mg
Citric acid anhydrous	20.75 mg	41.5 mg
Mannitol	97 mg	194 mg
Sodium phosphate dibasic anhydrous	16.25 mg	32.5 mg

Sodium hydroxide and/or phosphoric acid also may be present to adjust the pH (2).

The 10- and 20-mg vials should be reconstituted with 10 and 20 ml, respectively, of the accompanying bacteriostatic water for injection or sterile water for injection to yield a 1-mg/ml solution (2; 4). The bacteriostatic water for injection, which contains benzyl alcohol 0.9%, is not for use in newborns (2).

pH— Approximately 4 (2; 4).

Osmolality— The osmolality of vecuronium bromide 4 mg/ml was determined to be 292 mOsm/kg (1233).

Administration— Vecuronium bromide may be administered by rapid intravenous injection or by intravenous infusion using an infusion control device after dilution to a concentration of 0.1 to 0.2 mg/ml in a compatible infusion solution (4).

Stability— Vecuronium bromide should be stored at room temperature and protected from light. The reconstituted solution is clear and colorless. When reconstituted with bacteriostatic water for injection, the solution may be used for up to five days when stored at room temperature or under refrigeration. When reconstituted with sterile water for injection, the vial is a single-use container and should be stored under refrigeration and used within 24 hours (2).

pH Effects— Vecuronium bromide is unstable in the presence of bases and should not be combined with alkaline drugs or simultaneously administered through the same line as an alkaline solution (4).

Syringes— Vecuronium solutions reconstituted with sterile water for injection are stable for 48 hours at room temperature or under refrigeration, but the manufacturer recommends that they be used within 24 hours (4).

Compatibility Information

Y-Site Injection Compatibility (1:1 Mixture)

Vecuronium bromide

Drug	Mfr	Conc	Mfr	Conc	Remarks	Ref	C/I
Aminophylline	AB	1 mg/ml[a]	OR	0.1 mg/ml[a]	Physically compatible for 24 hr at 28 °C	1337	**C**
Amphotericin B cholesteryl sulfate complex	SEQ	0.83 mg/ml[a]	MAR	1 mg/ml[a]	Gross precipitate forms	2117	**I**
Cefazolin sodium	LY	10 mg/ml[a]	OR	0.1 mg/ml[a]	Physically compatible for 24 hr at 28 °C	1337	**C**
Cefuroxime sodium	GL	7.5 mg/ml[a]	OR	0.1 mg/ml[a]	Physically compatible for 24 hr at 28 °C	1337	**C**

Y-Site Injection Compatibility (1:1 Mixture) (Cont.)

Vecuronium bromide

Drug	Mfr	Conc	Mfr	Conc	Remarks	Ref	C/I
Cimetidine HCl	SKF	6 mg/ml[a]	OR	0.1 mg/ml[a]	Physically compatible for 24 hr at 28 °C	1337	C
Clarithromycin	AB	4 mg/ml[a]	ORG	2 mg/ml[a]	Visually compatible for 72 hr at both 30 and 17 °C	2174	C
Diazepam	ES	5 mg/ml[a]	OR	0.1 mg/ml[a]	Cloudy solution forms immediately	1337	I
Diltiazem HCl	MMD	1 mg/ml[a]	OR	1 mg/ml	Visually compatible for 4 hr at 27 °C	2062	C
Dobutamine HCl	LI	1 mg/ml[a]	OR	0.1 mg/ml[a]	Physically compatible for 24 hr at 28 °C	1337	C
	LI	4 mg/ml[a]	OR	1 mg/ml	Visually compatible for 4 hr at 27 °C	2062	C
Dopamine HCl	SO	1.6 mg/ml[a]	OR	0.1 mg/ml[a]	Physically compatible for 24 hr at 28 °C	1337	C
	AB	3.2 mg/ml[a]	OR	1 mg/ml	Visually compatible for 4 hr at 27 °C	2062	C
Epinephrine HCl	AB	4 μg/ml[a]	OR	0.1 mg/ml[a]	Physically compatible for 24 hr at 28 °C	1337	C
	AB	0.02 mg/ml[a]	OR	1 mg/ml	Visually compatible for 4 hr at 27 °C	2062	C
Esmolol HCl	DCC	10 mg/ml[a]	OR	0.1 mg/ml[a]	Physically compatible for 24 hr at 28 °C	1337	C
Etomidate	AB	2 mg/ml	OR	1 mg/ml	Slight turbidity and white particles form	1801	I
Fentanyl citrate	ES	10 μg/ml[a]	OR	0.1 mg/ml[a]	Physically compatible for 24 hr at 28 °C	1337	C
	ES	0.05 mg/ml	OR	1 mg/ml	Visually compatible for 4 hr at 27 °C	2062	C
Fluconazole	RR	2 mg/ml	OR	1 mg/ml[a]	Visually compatible for 24 hr at 28 °C under fluorescent light	1760	C
Furosemide	AMR	10 mg/ml	OR	1 mg/ml	Precipitate forms immediately	2062	I
Gentamicin sulfate	ES	2 mg/ml[a]	OR	0.1 mg/ml[a]	Physically compatible for 24 hr at 28 °C	1337	C
Heparin sodium	SO	40 units/ml[a]	OR	0.1 mg/ml[a]	Physically compatible for 24 hr at 28 °C	1337	C
	ES	100 units/ml[a]	OR	1 mg/ml	Visually compatible for 4 hr at 27 °C	2062	C
Hydrocortisone sodium succinate	AB	1 mg/ml[a]	OR	0.1 mg/ml[a]	Physically compatible for 24 hr at 28 °C	1337	C
Hydromorphone HCl	KN	1 mg/ml	OR	1 mg/ml	Visually compatible for 4 hr at 27 °C	2062	C
Isoproterenol HCl	ES	4 μg/ml[a]	OR	0.1 mg/ml[a]	Physically compatible for 24 hr at 28 °C	1337	C
Labetalol HCl	AH	2 mg/ml[a]	OR	1 mg/ml	Visually compatible for 4 hr at 27 °C	2062	C
Lorazepam	WY	0.5 mg/ml[a]	OR	0.1 mg/ml[a]	Physically compatible for 24 hr at 28 °C	1337	C
	WY	0.33 mg/ml[a]	OR	4 mg/ml	Visually compatible for 24 hr at 22 °C	1855	C
	WY	0.5 mg/ml[a]	OR	1 mg/ml	Visually compatible for 4 hr at 27 °C	2062	C
Midazolam HCl	RC	0.05 mg/ml[a]	OR	0.1 mg/ml[a]	Physically compatible for 24 hr at 28 °C	1337	C
	RC	5 mg/ml	OR	4 mg/ml	Visually compatible for 24 hr at 22 °C	1855	C
	RC	2 mg/ml[a]	OR	1 mg/ml	Visually compatible for 4 hr at 27 °C	2062	C
Milrinone lactate	SW	0.2 mg/ml[a]	OR	1 mg/ml	Visually compatible for 4 hr at 27 °C	2062	C
	SW	0.4 mg/ml[a]	OR	1 mg/ml[a]	Visually compatible with little or no loss of either drug by HPLC in 4 hr at 23 °C	2214	C
Morphine sulfate	WY	1 mg/ml[a]	OR	0.1 mg/ml[a]	Physically compatible for 24 hr at 28 °C	1337	C
	SCN	2 mg/ml[a]	OR	1 mg/ml	Visually compatible for 4 hr at 27 °C	2062	C
Nicardipine HCl	WY	1 mg/ml[a]	OR	1 mg/ml	Visually compatible for 4 hr at 27 °C	2062	C
Nitroglycerin	SO	0.4 mg/ml[a]	OR	0.1 mg/ml[a]	Physically compatible for 24 hr at 28 °C	1337	C
	AB	0.4 mg/ml[a]	OR	1 mg/ml	Visually compatible for 4 hr at 27 °C	2062	C
Norepinephrine bitartrate	AB	0.128 mg/ml[a]	OR	1 mg/ml	Visually compatible for 4 hr at 27 °C	2062	C
Propofol	ZEN	10 mg/ml	OR	1 mg/ml	Physically compatible for 1 hr at 23 °C with no increase in particle content	2066	C

Y-Site Injection Compatibility (1:1 Mixture) (Cont.)

Vecuronium bromide

Drug	Mfr	Conc	Mfr	Conc	Remarks	Ref	C/I
Ranitidine HCl	GL	0.5 mg/ml[a]	OR	0.1 mg/ml[a]	Physically compatible for 24 hr at 28 °C	1337	**C**
	GL	1 mg/ml[a]	OR	1 mg/ml	Visually compatible for 4 hr at 27 °C	2062	**C**
Sodium nitroprusside	ES	0.2 mg/ml[a]	OR	0.1 mg/ml[a]	Physically compatible for 24 hr at 28 °C	1337	**C**
Thiopental sodium	AB	25 mg/ml	OR	1 mg/ml	White particles form immediately	1801	**I**
	AB	25 mg/ml[d]	OR	1 mg/ml	Precipitate forms immediately	2062	**I**
TPN #189[c]			OR	2 mg/ml[b]	Visually compatible for 24 hr at 22 °C	1767	**C**
Trimethoprim–sulfamethoxazole	ES	0.64 + 3.2 mg/ml[a]	OR	0.1 mg/ml[a]	Physically compatible for 24 hr at 28 °C	1337	**C**
Vancomycin HCl	ES	5 mg/ml[a]	OR	0.1 mg/ml[a]	Physically compatible for 24 hr at 28 °C	1337	**C**

[a]*Tested in dextrose 5% in water.*
[b]*Tested in sodium chloride 0.9%.*
[c]*Refer to Appendix I for the composition of parenteral nutrition solutions. TPN indicates a 2-in-1 admixture.*
[d]*Tested in sterile water for injection.*

Additional Compatibility Information

Solutions— Vecuronium bromide is physically compatible and chemically stable for at least 24 hours in the following solutions (2; 4):

Dextrose 5% in sodium chloride 0.9%
Dextrose 5% in water
Ringer's injection, lactated
Sodium chloride 0.9%

VERAPAMIL HCL
AHFS 24:04
Abbott

Products— Verapamil HCl (Abbott) is available in single-dose containers including 2-ml ampuls, vials, and syringes and in 4-ml vials and syringes. Each milliliter contains verapamil HCl 2.5 mg with sodium chloride 8.5 mg in water for injection. Hydrochloric acid may have been used to adjust pH during manufacture (1-5/97).

pH— From 4 to 6.5. Target pH is 4.9 (1-5/97).

Osmolality— The osmolality of verapamil HCl 2.5 mg/ml was determined to be 290 mOsm/kg (1233).

Administration— Verapamil HCl is administered slowly intravenously. Direct intravenous injection should be performed over at least two minutes and at least three minutes in older patients (1-5/97; 4). Intravenous infusion has also been performed (4).

Stability— Verapamil HCl should be stored at controlled room temperature and protected from light (1-5/97). Freezing should be avoided (4). Infusion solution stability studies indicate that verapamil HCl does not adsorb to glass, PVC, or polyolefin containers (548). It is physically compatible in solution over a pH range of 3 to 6 but may precipitate in solutions having a pH greater than 6 (1-5/97; 4) or 7 (1384).

Compatibility Information

Solution Compatibility

Verapamil HCl

Solution	Mfr	Mfr	Conc/L	Remarks	Ref	C/I
Dextran 40 10% in sodium chloride 0.9%	TR	KN	80 mg	Physically compatible for 24 hr	764	**C**
Dextran 75 6% in sodium chloride 0.9%	TR	KN	80 mg	Physically compatible for 24 hr	764	**C**
Dextrose 5% in Ringer's injection	MG	KN	40 mg	Physically compatible and chemically stable for 48 hr at 25 °C protected from light	548	**C**

Solution Compatibility (Cont.)

Verapamil HCl

Solution	Mfr	Mfr	Conc/L	Remarks	Ref	C/I
Dextrose 5% in Ringer's injection, lactated	MG	KN	40 mg	Physically compatible and chemically stable for 24 hr at 25 °C protected from light	548	C
Dextrose 5% in sodium chloride 0.45%	MG	KN	40 mg	Physically compatible and chemically stable for 24 hr at 25 °C protected from light	548	C
Dextrose 5% in sodium chloride 0.9%	MG	KN	40 mg	Physically compatible and chemically stable for 24 hr at 25 °C protected from light	548	C
Dextrose 5% in water	CU	KN	40 mg	Physically compatible and chemically stable for 48 hr at 25 °C protected from light	548	C
	MG[a]	KN	40 mg	Physically compatible and chemically stable for 24 hr at 25 °C protected from light	548	C
	TR[b]	KN	40 mg	Physically compatible and chemically stable for 24 hr at 25 °C protected from light	548	C
	TR[b]	KN	160 mg	Physically compatible with no drug loss in 7 days at 24 °C	811	C
	AB	KN	100 and 400 mg	Physically compatible with no drug loss in 24 hr at 24 °C under fluorescent light	1198	C
Ringer's injection	MG	KN	40 mg	Physically compatible and chemically stable for 24 hr at 25 °C protected from light	548	C
Ringer's injection, lactated	MG	KN	40 mg	Physically compatible and chemically stable for 24 hr at 25 °C protected from light	548	C
Sodium chloride 0.45%	MG	KN	40 mg	Physically compatible and chemically stable for 24 hr at 25 °C protected from light	548	C
		LY	1.25 and 2 g	Physically compatible with no drug loss in 4 hr at 22 °C	1419	C
Sodium chloride 0.9%	CU	KN	40 mg	Physically compatible and chemically stable for 48 hr at 25 °C protected from light	548	C
	MG[a]	KN	40 mg	Physically compatible and chemically stable for 24 hr at 25 °C protected from light	548	C
	TR[b]	KN	40 mg	Physically compatible and chemically stable for 24 hr at 25 °C protected from light	548	C
	TR[b]	KN	160 mg	Physically compatible with little or no drug loss in 7 days at 24 °C	811	C
Sodium lactate ⅙ M	MG	KN	40 mg	Physically compatible and chemically stable for 48 hr at 25 °C protected from light	548	C

[a]Tested in polyolefin containers.
[b]Tested in PVC containers.

Additive Compatibility

Verapamil HCl

Drug	Mfr	Conc/L	Mfr	Conc/L	Test Soln	Remarks	Ref	C/I
Albumin	ARC	25 g	KN	80 mg	D5W, NS	Cloudiness develops within 8 hr	764	I
Amikacin sulfate	BR	2 g	KN	80 mg	D5W, NS	Physically compatible for 24 hr	764	C
Aminophylline	SE	1 g	KN	80 mg	D5W, NS	Transient precipitate clears rapidly. Solution physically compatible for 48 hr	739	C
	SE	1 g	KN	400 mg	D5W	Visible turbidity forms immediately. Filtration removes all verapamil	1198	I

Additive Compatibility (Cont.)

Verapamil HCl

Drug	Mfr	Conc/L	Mfr	Conc/L	Test Soln	Remarks	Ref	C/I
	SE	1 g	KN	100 mg	D5W	Visually clear, but precipitate found by microscopic examination. Filtration removes all verapamil	1198	I
Amiodarone HCl	LZ	1.8 g	KN	50 mg	D5W, NS[a]	Physically compatible with 8% or less amiodarone loss in 24 hr at 24 °C under fluorescent light	1031	C
Amphotericin B	SQ	100 mg	KN	80 mg	D5W	Physically incompatible after 8 hr	764	I
	SQ	100 mg	KN	80 mg	NS	Physically incompatible immediately	764	I
Ampicillin sodium	BR	4 g	KN	80 mg	D5W, NS	Physically compatible for 24 hr	764	C
	WY	40 g	SE	[b]	D5W, NS	Cloudy solution clears with agitation	1166	?
Ascorbic acid	LI	1 g	KN	80 mg	D5W, NS	Physically compatible for 24 hr	764	C
Atropine sulfate	IX	0.8 mg	KN	80 mg	D5W, NS	Physically compatible for 24 hr	764	C
Bretylium tosylate	ACC	2 g	KN	80 mg	D5W, NS	Physically compatible for 48 hr	739	C
Calcium chloride	ES	2 g	KN	80 mg	D5W, NS	Physically compatible for 24 hr	764	C
Calcium gluconate	IX	2 g	KN	80 mg	D5W, NS	Physically compatible for 48 hr	739	C
Cefamandole nafate	LI	4 g	KN	80 mg	D5W, NS	Physically compatible for 24 hr	764	C
Cefazolin sodium	SKF	2 g	KN	80 mg	D5W, NS	Physically compatible for 24 hr	764	C
Cefotaxime sodium	HO	4 g	KN	80 mg	D5W, NS	Physically compatible for 24 hr	764	C
Cefoxitin sodium	MSD	4 g	KN	80 mg	D5W, NS	Physically compatible for 24 hr	764	C
Chloramphenicol sodium succinate	PD	2 g	KN	80 mg	D5W, NS	Physically compatible for 24 hr	764	C
Cimetidine HCl	SKF	2.4 g	KN	80 mg	D5W, NS	Physically compatible for 24 hr	764	C
Clindamycin phosphate	UP	1.2 g	KN	80 mg	D5W, NS	Physically compatible for 24 hr	764	C
Dexamethasone sodium phosphate	MSD	40 mg	KN	80 mg	D5W, NS	Physically compatible for 24 hr	764	C
Diazepam	RC	20 mg	KN	80 mg	D5W, NS	Physically compatible for 24 hr	764	C
Digoxin	BW	2 mg	KN	80 mg	D5W, NS	Physically compatible for 48 hr	739	C
Dobutamine HCl	LI	500 mg	KN	80 mg	D5W, NS	Slight pink color develops after 24 hr because of dobutamine oxidation	764	I
	LI	250 mg	KN	160 mg	D5W	No decomposition of either drug in 48 hr at 24 °C or 7 days at 5 °C. Transient light pink color noted	811	C
	LI	250 mg	KN	160 mg	NS	No verapamil decomposition and 3% dobutamine loss in 48 hr at 24 °C. Initially colorless solution becomes pink with time. At 5 °C, no loss of either drug in 7 days	811	C
	LI	1 g	KN	1.25 g	D5W, NS	Physically compatible for 24 hr at 21 °C	812	C
Dopamine HCl	ES	400 mg	KN	80 mg	D5W, NS	Physically compatible for 24 hr	764	C
Epinephrine HCl	PD	2 mg	KN	80 mg	D5W, NS	Physically compatible for 24 hr	764	C
Erythromycin lactobionate	AB	2 g	KN	80 mg	D5W, NS	Physically compatible for 24 hr	764	C
Floxacillin sodium	BE	20 g	AB	500 mg	NS	Haze and precipitate form in 24 hr at 30 °C. No change at 15 °C	1479	I
Furosemide	HO	200 mg	KN	80 mg	D5W, NS	Physically compatible for 24 hr	764	C
	HO	1 g	AB	500 mg	NS	Slight precipitate forms but dissipates	1479	?

Additive Compatibility (Cont.)

Verapamil HCl

Drug	Mfr	Conc/L	Mfr	Conc/L	Test Soln	Remarks	Ref	C/I
Gentamicin sulfate	SC	160 mg	KN	80 mg	D5W, NS	Physically compatible for 24 hr	764	**C**
Heparin sodium	ES	20,000 units	KN	80 mg	D5W, NS	Physically compatible for 24 hr	764	**C**
Hydralazine HCl	CI	40 mg	KN	80 mg	D5W, NS	Yellow discoloration	764	**I**
Hydrocortisone sodium phosphate	MSD	200 mg	KN	80 mg	D5W, NS	Physically compatible for 24 hr	764	**C**
Hydrocortisone sodium succinate	UP	200 mg	KN	80 mg	D5W, NS	Physically compatible for 24 hr	764	**C**
Hydromorphone HCl	KN	16 mg	KN	80 mg	D5W, NS	Physically compatible for 24 hr	764	**C**
Insulin, regular	SQ	200 units	KN	80 mg	D5W, NS	Physically compatible for 48 hr	739	**C**
Isoproterenol HCl	BN	10 mg	KN	80 mg	D5W, NS	Physically compatible for 24 hr	764	**C**
Lidocaine HCl	IMS	2 g	KN	80 mg	D5W, NS	Physically compatible for 48 hr	739	**C**
Magnesium sulfate	IX	10 g	KN	80 mg	D5W, NS	Physically compatible for 24 hr	764	**C**
Mannitol	IX	25 g	KN	80 mg	D5W, NS	Physically compatible for 24 hr	764	**C**
Meperidine HCl	WI	150 mg	KN	80 mg	D5W, NS	Physically compatible for 24 hr	764	**C**
Metaraminol bitartrate	MSD	20 mg	KN	80 mg	D5W, NS	Physically compatible for 24 hr	764	**C**
Methyldopate HCl	MSD	500 mg	KN	80 mg	D5W, NS	Physically compatible for 24 hr	764	**C**
Methylprednisolone sodium succinate	UP	250 mg	KN	80 mg	D5W, NS	Physically compatible for 24 hr	764	**C**
Metoclopramide HCl	RB	20 mg	KN	80 mg	D5W, NS	Physically compatible for 24 hr	764	**C**
Morphine sulfate	KN	30 mg	KN	80 mg	D5W, NS	Physically compatible for 24 hr	764	**C**
Multivitamins	USV	10 ml	KN	80 mg	D5W, NS	Physically compatible for 24 hr	764	**C**
Nafcillin sodium	WY	4 g	KN	80 mg	D5W, NS	Physically compatible for 24 hr	764	**C**
	WY	40 g	SE	[b]	D5W, NS	Cloudy solution clears with agitation	1166	**?**
Naloxone HCl	EN	0.8 mg	KN	80 mg	D5W, NS	Physically compatible for 24 hr	764	**C**
Nitroglycerin	ACC	100 mg	KN	80 mg	D5W, NS	Physically compatible for 24 hr	764	**C**
Norepinephrine bitartrate	BN	8 mg	KN	80 mg	D5W, NS	Physically compatible for 24 hr	764	**C**
Oxacillin sodium	BR	4 g	KN	80 mg	D5W, NS	Physically compatible for 24 hr	764	**C**
	BR	40 g	SE	[b]	D5W, NS	Cloudy solution clears with agitation	1166	**?**
Oxytocin	SZ	40 units	KN	80 mg	D5W, NS	Physically compatible for 24 hr	764	**C**
Pancuronium bromide	OR	8 mg	KN	80 mg	D5W, NS	Physically compatible for 24 hr	764	**C**
Penicillin G potassium	SQ	10 million units	KN	80 mg	D5W, NS	Physically compatible for 24 hr	764	**C**
	PD	62.5 g	SE	[b]	D5W, NS	Physically compatible for 24 hr at 21 °C under fluorescent light	1166	**C**
Penicillin G sodium	SQ	10 million units	KN	80 mg	D5W, NS	Physically compatible for 24 hr	764	**C**
Pentobarbital sodium	AB	200 mg	KN	80 mg	D5W, NS	Physically compatible for 24 hr	764	**C**
Phenobarbital sodium	ES	260 mg	KN	80 mg	D5W, NS	Physically compatible for 24 hr	764	**C**
Phentolamine mesylate	RC	10 mg	KN	80 mg	D5W, NS	Physically compatible for 24 hr	764	**C**
Phenytoin sodium	PD	500 mg	KN	80 mg	D5W, NS	Physically compatible for 48 hr	739	**C**

Additive Compatibility (Cont.)

Verapamil HCl

Drug	Mfr	Conc/L	Mfr	Conc/L	Test Soln	Remarks	Ref	C/I
Piperacillin sodium	LE	40 g	SE	b	D5W, NS	Physically compatible for 24 hr at 21 °C	1166	C
Potassium chloride	TR	80 mEq	KN	80 mg	D5W, NS	Physically compatible for 24 hr	764	C
Potassium phosphates	AB	88 mEq	KN	80 mg	D5W, NS	Physically compatible for 24 hr	764	C
Procainamide HCl	SQ	2 g	KN	80 mg	D4W, NS	Physically compatible for 48 hr	739	C
Propranolol HCl	AY	4 mg	KN	80 mg	D5W, NS	Physically compatible for 24 hr	764	C
Protamine sulfate	LI	100 mg	KN	80 mg	D5W, NS	Physically compatible for 24 hr	764	C
Quinidine gluconate	LI	800 mg	KN	80 mg	D5W, NS	Physically compatible for 48 hr	739	C
Sodium bicarbonate	BR	89.2 mEq	KN	80 mg	D5W, NS	Physically compatible for 24 hr	764	C
Sodium nitroprusside	RC	100 mg	KN	80 mg	D5W, NS	Physically compatible for 24 hr	764	C
Theophylline	AB	400 mg and 4 g[c]	KN	100 and 400 mg	D5W	Physically compatible both visually and microscopically with little or no loss of either drug in 24 hr at 24 °C under fluorescent light	1172	C
Ticarcillin disodium	BE	6 g	KN	80 mg	D5W, NS	Physically compatible for 24 hr	764	C
	BE	40 g	SE	b	D5W, NS	Physically compatible for 24 hr at 21 °C	1166	C
Tobramycin sulfate	LI	160 mg	KN	80 mg	D5W, NS	Physically compatible for 24 hr	764	C
Tolazoline HCl	CI	160 mg	KN	80 mg	D5W, NS	Physically compatible for 24 hr	764	C
Trimethoprim–sulfamethoxazole	BW	160 + 800 mg	KN	80 mg	D5W, NS	Transient precipitate	764	I
Vancomycin HCl	LI	1 g	KN	80 mg	D5W, NS	Physically compatible for 24 hr	764	C
Vasopressin	PD	40 units	KN	80 mg	D5W, NS	Physically compatible for 24 hr	764	C
Vitamin B complex with C	RC	4 ml	KN	80 mg	D5W, NS	Physically compatible for 24 hr	764	C

[a]Tested in both polyolefin and PVC containers.
[b]Final concentration unspecified.
[c]Premixed theophylline infusion.

Drugs in Syringe Compatibility

Verapamil HCl

Drug (in syringe)	Mfr	Amt	Mfr	Amt	Remarks	Ref	C/I
Amrinone lactate	WI	5 mg/1 ml	LY	10 mg/4 ml	Physically compatible with little or no loss of either drug in 4 hr at 22 °C	1419	C
Heparin sodium		2500 units/1 ml	KN	5 mg/2 ml	Physically compatible for at least 5 min	1053	C
Milrinone lactate	WI	3.5 mg/3.5 ml	KN	10 mg/4 ml	Brought to 10 ml total volume with D5W. Physically compatible with no loss of either drug in 4 hr at 23 °C	1191	C

Y-Site Injection Compatibility (1:1 Mixture)

Verapamil HCl

Drug	Mfr	Conc	Mfr	Conc	Remarks	Ref	C/I
Albumin	HY	250 mg/ml[a]	LY	0.2 mg/ml[a]	Slight haze in 1 hr	1316	I
	HY	250 mg/ml[b]	LY	0.2 mg/ml[b]	Slight haze in 3 hr	1316	I

Y-Site Injection Compatibility (1:1 Mixture) (Cont.)

Verapamil HCl

Drug	Mfr	Conc	Mfr	Conc	Remarks	Ref	C/I
Amphotericin B cholesteryl sulfate complex	SEQ	0.83 mg/ml[a]	AMR	2.5 mg/ml	Gross precipitate forms	2117	I
Ampicillin sodium	WY	40 mg/ml[c]	SE	2.5 mg/ml	White milky precipitate forms immediately and persists. 91% of verapamil precipitated	1166	I
Amrinone lactate	WB	3 mg/ml[b]	SE	0.1 mg/ml[a]	Physically compatible for at least 4 hr at 25 °C under fluorescent light	992	C
	WI	2.5 mg/ml[d]	LY	2.5 mg/ml	Physically compatible with little or no loss of either drug in 4 hr at 22 °C	1419	C
Ciprofloxacin	MI	2 mg/ml[c]	KN	2.5 mg/ml	Visually compatible for 24 hr at 24 °C	1655	C
Clarithromycin	AB	4 mg/ml[a]	BKN	2.5 mg/ml	Visually compatible for 72 hr at both 30 and 17 °C	2174	C
Dobutamine HCl	LI	4 mg/ml[c]	LY	0.2 mg/ml[c]	Physically compatible for 3 hr	1316	C
Dopamine HCl				[e]	Physically compatible	840	C
Famotidine	MSD	0.2 mg/ml[a]	KN	0.1 mg/ml[a]	Physically compatible for 4 hr at 25 °C	1188	C
Hydralazine HCl	SO	1 mg/ml[c]	LY	0.2 mg/ml[c]	Physically compatible for 3 hr	1316	C
Meperidine HCl	AB	10 mg/ml	DU	2.5 mg/ml	Physically compatible for 4 hr at 25 °C	1397	C
Milrinone	WI	200 μg/ml[a]	KN	2.5 mg/ml[a]	Physically compatible with no loss of either drug in 4 hr at 23 °C	1191	C
Nafcillin sodium				[f]	White milky precipitate forms immediately	840; 1303	I
	WY	40 mg/ml[c]	SE	2.5 mg/ml	White milky precipitate forms immediately and persists. 20% of verapamil precipitated	1166	I
Oxacillin sodium	BR	40 mg/ml[c]	SE	2.5 mg/ml	White milky precipitate forms immediately and persists. 39% of verapamil precipitated	1166	I
Penicillin G potassium	PD	62.5 mg/ml[c]	SE	2.5 mg/ml	Physically compatible for 15 min at 21 °C under fluorescent light	1166	C
Piperacillin sodium	LE	40 mg/ml[c]	SE	2.5 mg/ml	Physically compatible for 15 min at 21 °C under fluorescent light	1166	C
Propofol	AMR	2.5 mg/ml	ZEN	10 mg/ml	Emulsion broke and oiled out	1916	I
Sodium bicarbonate		88 mEq/L[d]	SE	5 mg/2 ml	Crystalline precipitate forms when verapamil injected into infusion line	839	I
Ticarcillin disodium	BE	40 mg/ml[c]	SE	2.5 mg/ml	Physically compatible for 15 min at 21 °C under fluorescent light	1166	C

[a]*Tested in dextrose 5% in water.*
[b]*Tested in sodium chloride 0.9%.*
[c]*Tested in both dextrose 5% in water and sodium chloride 0.9%.*
[d]*Tested in sodium chloride 0.45%.*
[e]*Injected into a line being used to infuse dopamine HCl in dextrose 5% in sodium chloride 0.3% with potassium chloride 20 mEq.*
[f]*Injected into a line being used to infuse nafcillin sodium.*

VINBLASTINE SULFATE
AHFS 10:00

Velban   **Lilly**

Products— Vinblastine sulfate (Lilly) is available in 10-ml vials containing 10 mg of lyophilized drug without excipients. It should be reconstituted with 10 ml of sodium chloride 0.9% or bacteriostatic sodium chloride 0.9% (preserved with benzyl alcohol) to yield a 1-mg/ml solution (2).

pH— The pH of the reconstituted solution is 3.5 to 5 (2).

Osmolality— Vinblastine sulfate 1 mg/ml in sodium chloride 0.9% has an osmolality of 278 mOsm/kg (1689).

Administration— Vinblastine sulfate is administered intravenously only. It should not be given by any other route. The container holding an individual dose prepared for a patient must be enclosed in an overwrap bearing these statements:

> *"Do not remove covering until moment of injection.*
> *Fatal if given intrathecally. For intravenous use only."*

The drug may be administered over one minute directly into a vein or into the tubing of a running infusion solution. Generally, dilution of vinblastine sulfate in larger amounts of intravenous fluid and administration over longer time periods are not recommended. Extravasation should be avoided (2; 4).

Stability— The vials should be refrigerated to ensure extended stability (2). Room temperature stability of intact vials has been variously reported for the Lilly product to be at least one month (853) and only 14 days (1433). The Lyphomed product has been reported to be stable for up to three months (1181) and for less than two months (1433). The solution reconstituted with bacteriostatic sodium chloride injection is stable under refrigeration for 28 days. If reconstituted with unpreserved sodium chloride injection, any remaining unused drug should be discarded immediately (2).

Vinblastine sulfate, reconstituted according to the manufacturer's instructions, was cultured with human lymphoblasts to determine whether its cytotoxic activity was retained. The solution retained cytotoxicity for 24 hours at 4 °C and room temperature (1575).

pH Effects— The range of maximum stability for vinblastine sulfate in aqueous solutions was determined to be pH 2 to 4. Vinblastine sulfate in solution at pH 3 retained 90% potency after 39 days at 20 °C (1307).

Vinblastine sulfate in solutions having a pH above 6 may form a precipitate of vinblastine base (1369).

Effects of Light— It is recommended that vinblastine sulfate, both in the dry state and in solution, be protected from light (4).

Black et al. studied the effects of light exposure on a 1.197-mg/ml vinblastine sulfate solution in sterile water for injection. Samples at 25 °C were exposed to indirect incandescent (not fluorescent) light intermittently for at least 12 hours each day; another group was exposed to direct incandescent light intermittently for 12 hours daily with at least two additional hours of exposure to sunlight. A third group of samples at 30 °C were exposed to continuous direct incandescent light. Both groups of samples exposed directly to light showed substantial losses of vinblastine sulfate. Samples exposed to continuous direct light sustained a 10% loss in about one day and a 71% loss in 14 days. Samples intermittently exposed to direct light and sunlight sustained a 10% loss in eight days and a 23% loss in

15 days. However, samples exposed to intermittent indirect light showed no drug loss in 70 days (1306).

McElnay et al. found less than a 6% vinblastine loss in 48 hours from a 3-μg/ml solution in sodium chloride 0.9% contained as a static solution in polybutadiene tubing when exposed to normal mixed daylight and fluorescent light. The authors concluded that photodegradation is not a problem with vinblastine sulfate (1378).

Freezing Solutions— Vinblastine sulfate (Lilly) 20 μg/ml in dextrose 5% in water, Ringer's injection, lactated, and sodium chloride 0.9% underwent no degradation after four weeks when frozen at −20 °C (1195).

Syringes— Vinblastine sulfate (David Bull Laboratories) 10 mg/ml in polypropylene syringes was stable by HPLC for 31 days at 8 °C and for at least 23 days at 21 °C in the dark; little or no loss occurred (1566).

Vinblastine sulfate (Lilly) 1 mg/ml in sodium chloride 0.9% was packaged in polypropylene syringes (Plastipak, Becton-Dickinson) and stored at 25 °C protected from light. HPLC analysis found no vinblastine sulfate loss after storage for 30 days (2155).

Elastomeric Reservoir Pumps— Vinblastine sulfate 0.2 mg/ml in both dextrose 5% in water and sodium chloride 0.9% was evaluated for binding potential to natural rubber elastomeric reservoirs (Baxter). Less than 1% loss was found after storage for two weeks at 35 °C with gentle agitation (2014).

Implantable Infusion Pump— Vinblastine sulfate (Lilly) 1 mg/ml in bacteriostatic sodium chloride 0.9% was evaluated for stability in an implantable pump (Infusaid model 400). In this in vitro assessment, a 24% vinblastine loss occurred in 24 hours at 37 °C with mild agitation. In 12 days, the loss totaled 48%. In comparison, control solutions in glass vials had no drug loss in 24 hours and a 20% loss in 12 days at 37 °C. The authors believed that this result indicated an acute interaction of vinblastine with some component of the Infusaid model 400, rendering it unsuitable for administration with this infusion device (767).

Sorption— McElnay et al. evaluated the stability of vinblastine sulfate (Lilly) 3 μg/ml in methacrylate butadiene styrene (Avon A2001 Sureset) and cellulose propionate (Avon A200 standard and A2000 Amberset) when exposed to normal mixed daylight and fluorescent light for up to 48 hours. A maximum vinblastine loss of about 5% resulted in the Sureset, with as little as a 2.25% loss occurring with foil wrapping. However, significant losses occurred in both cellulose propionate burettes in 24 hours, and losses of 15 to 20% occurred in 48 hours. The vinblastine sulfate solution in the polybutadiene tubing of the Sureset showed no more than a 6% drug loss with or without light protection. However, in the PVC tubing of the standard or Amberset, losses were significant within four hours; at 48 hours, losses were 42 to 44% (1378).

Vinblastine sulfate (Lilly) 10 mg/250 ml in dextrose 5% in water or sodium chloride 0.9%, in PVC bags at 22 °C with protection from light, was infused over two hours at 2.08 ml/min through PVC sets. HPLC analysis of the effluent solution found no loss due to sorption (1631).

Vinblastine sulfate (Lederle) 250 μg/ml in sodium chloride 0.9% exhibited no loss by UV spectroscopy due to sorption to PVC and polyethylene administration lines during simulated infusions at 0.875 ml/hr for 2.5 hours via a syringe pump (1795).

Filtration— Vinblastine sulfate (Lilly) 10 mg/50 ml in dextrose 5% in water and sodium chloride 0.9%, filtered at a rate of about 3

ml/min through a 0.22-μm cellulose ester membrane filter (Ivex-2), showed no significant reduction in potency due to binding to the filter (533).

Vinblastine sulfate 10 to 300 μg/ml exhibited no loss due to sorption to either cellulose nitrate/cellulose acetate ester (Millex OR) or Teflon (Millex FG) filters (1415; 1416).

Vinblastine sulfate (Lederle) 250 μg/ml in sodium chloride 0.9% exhibited no loss by UV spectroscopy due to sorption to cellulose acetate (Minisart 45, Sartorius) and polysulfone (Acrodisc 45, Gelman) filters. However, a 10 to 20% loss due to sorption occurred during the first 30 to 60 minutes of infusion through nylon filters (Nylaflo, Gelman, and Utipore, Pall). About a 30% loss was found during the first hour using a positively-charged nylon filter (Posidyne ELD96, Pall). The delivered concentrations gradually returned to the full concentrations within 2 to 2.5 hours (1795).

Compatibility Information

Solution Compatibility

Vinblastine sulfate

Solution	Mfr	Mfr	Conc/L	Remarks	Ref	C/I
Dextrose 5% in water	TR[a]	LI	170 mg	Less than 10% decrease in 24 hr at room temperature	519	**C**
		LI	20 mg	Physically compatible with little or no drug loss in 21 days at 4 and 25 °C in the dark	1195	**C**
	[b]	LI	100 mg	6 to 8% loss by HPLC in 7 days at 4 °C protected from light	1631	**C**
	MG[c]		170 mg	Less than 10% loss by HPLC in 24 hr at room temperature exposed to light	1658	**C**
Ringer's injection, lactated		LI	20 mg	Physically compatible with 2 to 3% drug loss in 21 days at 4 and 25 °C in the dark	1195	**C**
Sodium chloride 0.9%		LI	20 mg	Physically compatible with little or no drug loss in 21 days at 4 and 25 °C in the dark	1195	**C**
	[b]	LI	100 mg	No loss by HPLC in 7 days at 4 °C protected from light	1631	**C**

[a]Tested in both glass and PVC containers.
[b]Tested in PVC containers.
[c]Tested in both glass and polyolefin containers.

Additive Compatibility

Vinblastine sulfate

Drug	Mfr	Conc/L	Mfr	Conc/L	Test Soln	Remarks	Ref	C/I
Bleomycin sulfate	BR	20 and 30 mg	LI	10 and 100 mg	NS	Physically compatible and bleomycin activity retained for 1 week at 4 °C. Vinblastine not tested	763	**C**
Doxorubicin HCl	AD	500 mg	LI	75 mg	NS[a]	Physically compatible for at least 10 days at 8, 25, and 32 °C. HPLC assays highly erratic	838	**?**
	AD	1.5 g	LI	150 mg	NS[a]	Physically compatible for at least 10 days at 8, 25, and 32 °C. HPLC assays highly erratic	838	**?**

[a]Tested in PVC containers.

Drugs in Syringe Compatibility

Vinblastine sulfate

Drug (in syringe)	Mfr	Amt	Mfr	Amt	Remarks	Ref	C/I
Bleomycin sulfate		1.5 units/ 0.5 ml		0.5 mg/ 0.5 ml	Physically compatible for 5 min at room temperature followed by 8 min of centrifugation	980	**C**

Drugs in Syringe Compatibility (Cont.)

Vinblastine sulfate

Drug (in syringe)	Mfr	Amt	Mfr	Amt	Remarks	Ref	C/I
Cisplatin		0.5 mg/ 0.5 ml		0.5 mg/ 0.5 ml	Physically compatible for 5 min at room temperature followed by 8 min of centrifugation	980	C
Cyclophosphamide		10 mg/ 0.5 ml		0.5 mg/ 0.5 ml	Physically compatible for 5 min at room temperature followed by 8 min of centrifugation	980	C
Doxorubicin HCl	AD	45 mg/ 22.5 ml	LI	4.5 mg/ 4.5 ml	(Brought to 30-ml total volume with NS) Physically compatible for at least 10 days at 8, 25, and 32 °C. HPLC assays highly erratic	838	?
	AD	15 mg/ 7.5 ml	LI	2.25 mg/ 2.25 ml	(Brought to 30-ml total volume with NS) Physically compatible for at least 10 days at 8, 25, and 32 °C. HPLC assays highly erratic	838	?
		1 mg/ 0.5 ml		0.5 mg/ 0.5 ml	Physically compatible for 5 min at room temperature followed by 8 min of centrifugation	980	C
Droperidol		1.25 mg/ 0.5 ml		0.5 mg/ 0.5 ml	Physically compatible for 5 min at room temperature followed by 8 min of centrifugation	980	C
Fluorouracil		25 mg/ 0.5 ml		0.5 mg/ 0.5 ml	Physically compatible for 5 min at room temperature followed by 8 min of centrifugation	980	C
Furosemide		5 mg/ 0.5 ml		0.5 mg/ 0.5 ml	Immediate precipitation	980	I
Heparin sodium		200 units/ 1 ml[a]		1 mg/ 1 ml	Turbidity appears in 2 to 3 min	767	I
		500 units/ 0.5 ml		0.5 mg/ 0.5 ml	Physically compatible for 5 min at room temperature followed by 8 min of centrifugation	980	C
Leucovorin calcium		5 mg/ 0.5 ml		0.5 mg/ 0.5 ml	Physically compatible for 5 min at room temperature followed by 8 min of centrifugation	980	C
Methotrexate sodium		12.5 mg/ 0.5 ml		0.5 mg/ 0.5 ml	Physically compatible for 5 min at room temperature followed by 8 min of centrifugation	980	C
Metoclopramide HCl		2.5 mg/ 0.5 ml		0.5 mg/ 0.5 ml	Physically compatible for 5 min at room temperature followed by 8 min of centrifugation	980	C
Mitomycin		0.25 mg/ 0.5 ml		0.5 mg/ 0.5 ml	Physically compatible for 5 min at room temperature followed by 8 min of centrifugation	980	C
Vincristine sulfate		0.5 mg/ 0.5 ml		0.5 mg/ 0.5 ml	Physically compatible for 5 min at room temperature followed by 8 min of centrifugation	980	C

[a]*Tested in bacteriostatic sodium chloride 0.9%.*

Y-Site Injection Compatibility (1:1 Mixture)

		Vinblastine sulfate					
Drug	Mfr	Conc	Mfr	Conc	Remarks	Ref	C/I
Allopurinol sodium	BW	3 mg/ml[b]	LI	0.12 mg/ml[b]	Physically compatible with no change in measured turbidity or increase in particle content in 4 hr at 22 °C	1686	**C**
Amifostine	USB	10 mg/ml[a]	LI	0.12 mg/ml[a]	Physically compatible with no change in measured turbidity or increase in particle content in 4 hr at 23 °C	1845	**C**
Amphotericin B cholesteryl sulfate complex	SEQ	0.83 mg/ml[a]	FAU	0.12 mg/ml[a]	Physically compatible with little or no change in measured turbidity or increase in particle content in 4 hr at 23 °C under fluorescent light	2117	**C**
Aztreonam	SQ	40 mg/ml[a]	LI	0.12 mg/ml[a]	Physically compatible with no subvisual haze or particle formation in 4 hr at 23 °C	1758	**C**
Bleomycin sulfate		3 units/ml		1 mg/ml	Drugs injected sequentially into Y-site with no flush between. No visually apparent precipitate	980	**C**
Cefepime HCl	BR	20 mg/ml[a]	LI	0.12 mg/ml[a]	Haze with numerous particles forms immediately	1689	**I**
Cisplatin		1 mg/ml		1 mg/ml	Drugs injected sequentially into Y-site with no flush between. No visually apparent precipitate	980	**C**
Cyclophosphamide		20 mg/ml		1 mg/ml	Drugs injected sequentially into Y-site with no flush between. No visually apparent precipitate	980	**C**
Doxorubicin HCl		2 mg/ml		1 mg/ml	Drugs injected sequentially into Y-site with no flush between. No visually apparent precipitate	980	**C**
Doxorubicin HCl liposome injection	SEQ	0.4 mg/ml[a]	FAU	0.12 mg/ml[a]	Physically compatible with little or no change in measured turbidity and no increase in particle content in 4 hr at 23 °C	2087	**C**
Droperidol		2.5 mg/ml		1 mg/ml	Drugs injected sequentially into Y-site with no flush between. No visually apparent precipitate	980	**C**
Etoposide phosphate	BR	5 mg/ml[a]	FAU	0.12 mg/ml[b]	Physically compatible with no change in measured turbidity or increase in particle content in 4 hr at 23 °C	2218	**C**
Filgrastim	AMG	30 μg/ml[a]	LI	0.12 mg/ml[a]	Physically compatible with no change in measured turbidity or increase in particle content in 4 hr at 22 °C	1687	**C**
Fludarabine phosphate	BX	1 mg/ml[a]	LY	0.12 mg/ml[a]	Physically compatible for 4 hr at room temperature under fluorescent light	1439	**C**
Fluorouracil		50 mg/ml		1 mg/ml	Drugs injected sequentially into Y-site with no flush between. No visually apparent precipitate	980	**C**
Furosemide		10 mg/ml		1 mg/ml	Drugs injected sequentially into Y-site with no flush between. Immediate precipitation	980	**I**

Y-Site Injection Compatibility (1:1 Mixture) (Cont.)

		Vinblastine sulfate					
Drug	*Mfr*	*Conc*	*Mfr*	*Conc*	*Remarks*	*Ref*	*C/I*
Gemcitabine HCl	LI	10 mg/ml[b]	FAU	0.12 mg/ml[b]	Physically compatible with no change in measured turbidity or increase in particle content in 4 hr at 23 °C	2226	C
Granisetron HCl	SKB	0.05 mg/ml[a]	LI	0.12 mg/ml[a]	Physically compatible with no change in measured turbidity or increase in particle content in 4 hr at 23 °C	2000	C
Heparin sodium		1000 units/ml		1 mg/ml	Drugs injected sequentially into Y-site with no flush between. No visually apparent precipitate	980	C
Leucovorin calcium		10 mg/ml		1 mg/ml	Drugs injected sequentially into Y-site with no flush between. No visually apparent precipitate	980	C
Melphalan HCl	BW	0.1 mg/ml[b]	LI	0.12 mg/ml[b]	Physically compatible with no change in measured turbidity or increase in particle content in 3 hr at 22 °C	1557	C
Methotrexate sodium		25 mg/ml		1 mg/ml	Drugs injected sequentially into Y-site with no flush between. No visually apparent precipitate	980	C
Metoclopramide HCl		5 mg/ml		1 mg/ml	Drugs injected sequentially into Y-site with no flush between. No visually apparent precipitate	980	C
Mitomycin HCl		0.5 mg/ml		1 mg/ml	Drugs injected sequentially into Y-site with no flush between. No visually apparent precipitate	980	C
Ondansetron HCl	GL	1 mg/ml[b]	LY	0.12 mg/ml[a]	Physically compatible for 4 hr at 22 °C	1365	C
Paclitaxel	NCI	1.2 mg/ml[a]	LI	0.12 mg/ml[b]	Physically compatible with no change in measured turbidity in 4 hr at 22 °C	1556	C
Piperacillin sodium–tazobactam sodium	LE	40 + 5 mg/ml[a]	LI	0.12 mg/ml[a]	Physically compatible with no change in measured turbidity or increase in particle content in 4 hr at 22 °C	1688	C
Sargramostim	IMM	10 μg/ml[b]	LY	0.12 mg/ml[b]	Physically compatible for 4 hr at 22 °C	1436	C
Teniposide	BR	0.1 mg/ml[a]	LI	0.12 mg/ml[a]	Physically compatible with no subvisual haze or particle formation in 4 hr at 23 °C	1725	C
Thiotepa	IMM[c]	1 mg/ml[a]	LI	0.12 mg/ml[b]	Physically compatible with no change in measured turbidity or increase in particle content in 4 hr at 23 °C	1861	C
Vincristine sulfate		1 mg/ml		1 mg/ml	Drugs injected sequentially into Y-site with no flush between. No visually apparent precipitate	980	C
Vinorelbine tartrate	BW	1 mg/ml[b]	LI	0.12 mg/ml[b]	Physically compatible with no change in measured turbidity or increase in particle content in 4 hr at 22 °C	1558	C

[a]*Tested in dextrose 5% in water.*
[b]*Tested in sodium chloride 0.9%.*
[c]*Lyophilized formulation tested.*

Additional Compatibility Information

Aluminum— Ogawa et al. reported that immersion of a needle with an aluminum component in vinblastine sulfate (Lilly) 1 mg/ml resulted in no visually apparent reaction after seven days at 24 °C (988).

Dacarbazine— No alteration in the ultraviolet/visible spectra was observed when dacarbazine was combined in solution with vinblastine sulfate (492).

Other Information

Bacterial Inhibition— Vinblastine sulfate (Lilly) 0.015 and 0.5 mg/ml in sodium chloride 0.9% did not inhibit the growth of deliberately inoculated *Staphylococcus epidermidis* (10^6 to 10^7 CFU/ml) during 21 days at 35 °C (representing near body temperature) (1659).

Inactivation— In the event of spills or leaks, Lilly recommends the use of sodium hypochlorite 5% (household bleach) to inactivate vinblastine sulfate (1200).

VINCRISTINE SULFATE
AHFS 10:00

Oncovin   **Lilly**

Products— Vincristine sulfate (Lilly) is available as a ready-to-use solution in a 1-mg/ml concentration. Each milliliter also contains mannitol 100 mg, methylparaben 1.3 mg, propylparaben 0.2 mg, and acetic acid and sodium acetate to adjust the pH in water for injection. The solution is provided in 1-, 2-, and 5-ml multiple-dose vials and 1- and 2-ml disposable syringes (2).

pH— From 3.5 to 5.5 (2).

Osmolality— Vincristine sulfate 1 mg/ml has an osmolality of 610 mOsm/kg (1689).

Administration— Vincristine sulfate is administered intravenously only. It should not be given by any other route. The container holding an individual dose prepared for a patient must be enclosed in an overwrap bearing these statements:

*"Do not remove covering until moment of injection.
Fatal if given intrathecally. For intravenous use only."*

The drug may be administered over one minute directly into a vein or into the tubing of a running infusion solution (2; 4). It can also be diluted in dextrose 5% in water or sodium chloride 0.9% and given by intermittent or continuous intravenous infusion (4). Extravasation should be avoided (2; 4).

Stability— The ready-to-use solution should be stored under refrigeration and protected from light (2; 4). Vincristine sulfate and its solutions are light sensitive; light protection has been recommended (4). The pH range of maximum stability is 4 to 6 (1195). Precipitation may occur at alkaline pH values (1369).

Room temperature stability has been variously reported for the Lilly product to be at least one month (853) and only three days (1433). The Adria product has been stated to be stable at room temperature for seven days, while the Lyphomed product is stable for 30 days (1433). These differences are likely due more to varying study periods and regulatory changes than real stability variations of such magnitudes.

Vincristine sulfate was cultured with human lymphoblasts to determine whether its cytotoxic activity was retained. The solution retained cytotoxicity for 24 hours at 4 °C and room temperature (1575).

Freezing Solutions— Vincristine sulfate (Lilly) 20 µg/ml in dextrose 5% in water, Ringer's injection, lactated, and sodium chloride 0.9% underwent no degradation after four weeks when frozen at −20 °C (1195).

Sorption— Vincristine sulfate (Lilly) 2 mg/250 ml in dextrose 5% in water or sodium chloride 0.9%, in PVC bags at 22 °C with protection from light, was infused over two hours at 2.08 ml/min through PVC sets. HPLC analysis of the effluent solution found no loss due to sorption (1631).

Vincristine sulfate (David Bull Laboratories) 25 µg/ml in sodium chloride 0.9% exhibited no loss by UV spectroscopy due to sorption to a polyethylene administration line (Vygon) during simulated infusions at 0.875 ml/hr for 2.5 hours via a syringe pump. However, about a 9% loss of delivered concentration due to sorption occurred during the first hour using a PVC administration line (Baxter). The delivered concentration returned to the full concentration within 1.5 hours (1795).

Filtration— Vincristine sulfate (Lilly) 1 mg/50 ml in dextrose 5% in water and sodium chloride 0.9% was filtered at about 3 ml/min through a 0.22-µm cellulose ester membrane filter (Ivex-2). Losses of vincristine sulfate due to binding to the filters were noted in both solutions. In dextrose 5% in water, about 6.5% of the vincristine sulfate was bound; about 12% of the drug was lost from the sodium chloride 0.9% solution (533).

In static equilibrium experiments, 100 mg of 0.22-µm cellulose ester membrane filter (Ivex-2) was soaked in 25 ml of vincristine sulfate (Lilly) 10 and 20 µg/ml in both dextrose 5% in water and sodium chloride 0.9%. The higher concentration exhibited about 20 to 30% binding to the filter in 24 to 48 hours. The lower concentration had about 30 to 45% binding in the same period (533).

In a followup study, a filter material specially treated with a proprietary agent was evaluated for a reduction in vincristine sulfate binding. Vincristine sulfate (Lilly) 1 mg/50 ml in dextrose 5% in water and sodium chloride 0.9% was run through an administration set with a treated 0.22-µm cellulose ester inline filter at a rate of 3 ml/min. Cumulative vincristine sulfate losses of about 1% occurred from both solutions compared to the much higher losses previously reported for untreated cellulose ester filter material. Furthermore, equilibrium binding studies showed five- and sevenfold reductions in binding from dextrose 5% in water and sodium chloride 0.9%, respectively (904). All Abbott Ivex integral filter and extension sets currently use this treated filter material (1074).

Vincristine sulfate 1.5 mg/3 ml was injected as a bolus through a 0.2-µm nylon, air-eliminating, filter (Ultipor, Pall) to evaluate the effect of filtration on simulated intravenous push delivery. Spectrophotometric evaluation showed that about 90% of the drug was delivered through the filter after flushing with 10 ml of sodium chloride 0.9% (809).

Vincristine sulfate 10 to 200 µg/ml exhibited a 10 to 15% loss due to sorption to both cellulose nitrate/cellulose acetate ester (Millex OR) and Teflon (Millex FG) filters (1415; 1416).

Vincristine sulfate (David Bull Laboratories) 250 µg/ml in sodium chloride 0.9% exhibited little or no loss by UV spectroscopy due to sorption to cellulose acetate (Minisart 45, Sartorius) and polysulfone (Acrodisc 45, Gelman) filters. However, a 5 to 20% loss due to sorption occurred during the first 30 to 60 minutes of infusion through nylon filters (Nylaflo, Gelman, and Utipore, Pall). About a 20 to 25% loss was found during the first hour using a nylon filter (Posidyne ELD96, Pall). The delivered concentrations gradually returned to the full concentrations within 2 to 2.5 hours (1795).

Compatibility Information

Solution Compatibility

Vincristine sulfate

Solution	Mfr	Mfr	Conc/L	Remarks	Ref	C/I
Dextrose 5% in water	TR[a]	LI	16.7 mg	No loss of vincristine in 24 hr at room temperature	806	C
		LI	20 mg	Physically compatible with 3 to 5% drug loss in 21 days at 4 and 25 °C in the dark	1195	C
	[b]	LI	20 mg	Little or no loss by HPLC in 7 days at 4 °C protected from light	1631	C
	MG, TR[c]		20 mg	Less than 10% loss by HPLC in 24 hr at room temperature exposed to light	1658	C
Ringer's injection, lactated		LI	20 mg	Physically compatible with little or no drug loss in 21 days at 4 and 25 °C in the dark	1195	C
Sodium chloride 0.9%		LI	20 mg	Physically compatible with little or no drug loss in 21 days at 4 and 25 °C in the dark	1195	C
	[b]	LI	20 mg	8% or less loss by HPLC in 7 days at 4 °C protected from light	1631	C

[a]Tested in both glass and PVC containers.
[b]Tested in PVC containers.
[c]Tested in glass, polyolefin, and PVC containers.

Additive Compatibility

Vincristine sulfate

Drug	Mfr	Conc/L	Mfr	Conc/L	Test Soln	Remarks	Ref	C/I
Bleomycin sulfate	BR	20 and 30 units	LI	50 and 100 mg	NS	Physically compatible and bleomycin activity retained for 1 week at 4 °C	763	C
Cytarabine	UP	16 mg	LI	4 mg	D5W	Physically compatible. No alteration in UV spectra in 8 hr at room temperature	207	C
Doxorubicin HCl with ondansetron HCl	AD GL	400 mg 480 mg	LI	14 mg	D5W[b]	Visually compatible with >90% potency of all drugs by HPLC after 5 days at 4 °C followed by 24 hr at 30 °C	2092	C
Doxorubicin HCl with ondansetron HCl	AD GL	800 mg 960 mg	LI	28 mg	D5W[a]	Visually compatible with >90% potency of all drugs by HPLC after 120 hr at 30 °C	2092	C
Fluorouracil	RC	10 mg	LI	4 mg	D5W	Physically compatible. No alteration in UV spectra in 8 hr at room temperature	207	C

Additive Compatibility (Cont.)

Vincristine sulfate

Drug	Mfr	Conc/L	Mfr	Conc/L	Test Soln	Remarks	Ref	C/I
Methotrexate sodium	LE	100 mg	LI	10 mg	D5W	Physically compatible	15	C
	LE	8 mg	LI	4 mg	D5W	Physically compatible. No alteration in UV spectra in 8 hr at room temperature	207	C

[a]Tested in PVC containers.
[b]Tested in polyisoprene infusion pump reservoirs.

Drugs in Syringe Compatibility

Vincristine sulfate

Drug (in syringe)	Mfr	Amt	Mfr	Amt	Remarks	Ref	C/I
Bleomycin sulfate		1.5 units/ 0.5 ml		0.5 mg/ 0.5 ml	Physically compatible for 5 min at room temperature followed by 8 min of centrifugation	980	C
Cisplatin		0.5 mg/ 0.5 ml		0.5 mg/ 0.5 ml	Physically compatible for 5 min at room temperature followed by 8 min of centrifugation	980	C
Cyclophosphamide		10 mg/ 0.5 ml		0.5 mg/ 0.5 ml	Physically compatible for 5 min at room temperature followed by 8 min of centrifugation	980	C
Doxapram HCl	RB	400 mg/ 20 ml		1 mg/ 10 ml	Physically compatible with 7% doxapram loss in 24 hr	1177	C
Doxorubicin HCl		1 mg/ 0.5 ml		0.5 mg/ 0.5 ml	Physically compatible for 5 min at room temperature followed by 8 min of centrifugation	980	C
Droperidol		1.25 mg/ 0.5 ml		0.5 mg/ 0.5 ml	Physically compatible for 5 min at room temperature followed by 8 min of centrifugation	980	C
Fluorouracil		25 mg/ 0.5 ml		0.5 mg/ 0.5 ml	Physically compatible for 5 min at room temperature followed by 8 min of centrifugation	980	C
Furosemide		5 mg/ 0.5 ml		0.5 mg/ 0.5 ml	Immediate precipitation	980	I
Heparin sodium		500 units/ 0.5 ml		0.5 mg/ 0.5 ml	Physically compatible for 5 min at room temperature followed by 8 min of centrifugation	980	C
Leucovorin calcium		5 mg/ 0.5 ml		0.5 mg/ 0.5 ml	Physically compatible for 5 min at room temperature followed by 8 min of centrifugation	980	C
Methotrexate sodium		12.5 mg/ 0.5 ml		0.5 mg/ 0.5 ml	Physically compatible for 5 min at room temperature followed by 8 min of centrifugation	980	C
Metoclopramide HCl		2.5 mg/ 0.5 ml		0.5 mg/ 0.5 ml	Physically compatible for 5 min at room temperature followed by 8 min of centrifugation	980	C
Mitomycin		0.25 mg/ 0.5 ml		0.5 mg/ 0.5 ml	Physically compatible for 5 min at room temperature followed by 8 min of centrifugation	980	C

Drugs in Syringe Compatibility (Cont.)

Vincristine sulfate

Drug (in syringe)	Mfr	Amt	Mfr	Amt	Remarks	Ref	C/I
Vinblastine sulfate		0.5 mg/ 0.5 ml		0.5 mg/ 0.5 ml	Physically compatible for 5 min at room temperature followed by 8 min of centrifugation	980	C

Y-Site Injection Compatibility (1:1 Mixture)

Vincristine sulfate

Drug	Mfr	Conc	Mfr	Conc	Remarks	Ref	C/I
Allopurinol sodium	BW	3 mg/ml[b]	LI	0.05 mg/ml[b]	Physically compatible with no change in measured turbidity or increase in particle content in 4 hr at 22 °C	1686	C
Amifostine	USB	10 mg/ml[a]	LI	0.05 mg/ml[a]	Physically compatible with no change in measured turbidity or increase in particle content in 4 hr at 23 °C	1845	C
Amphotericin B cholesteryl sulfate complex	SEQ	0.83 mg/ml[a]	FAU	0.05 mg/ml[a]	Physically compatible with little or no change in measured turbidity or increase in particle content in 4 hr at 23 °C under fluorescent light	2117	C
Aztreonam	SQ	40 mg/ml[a]	LI	0.05 mg/ml[a]	Physically compatible with no subvisual haze or particle formation in 4 hr at 23 °C	1758	C
Bleomycin sulfate		3 units/ml		1 mg/ml	Drugs injected sequentially into Y-site with no flush between. No visually apparent precipitate	980	C
Cefepime HCl	BR	20 mg/ml[b]	LI	0.05 mg/ml[b]	Small particles form immediately	1689	I
Cisplatin		1 mg/ml		1 mg/ml	Drugs injected sequentially into Y-site with no flush between. No visually apparent precipitate	980	C
Cladribine	ORT	0.015[b] and 0.5[c] mg/ml	LI	0.05 mg/ml[b]	Physically compatible with no change in measured turbidity or increase in particle content in 4 hr at 23 °C	1969	C
Cyclophosphamide		20 mg/ml		1 mg/ml	Drugs injected sequentially into Y-site with no flush between. No visually apparent precipitate	980	C
Doxorubicin HCl		2 mg/ml		1 mg/ml	Drugs injected sequentially into Y-site with no flush between. No visually apparent precipitate	980	C
Doxorubicin HCl liposome injection	SEQ	0.4 mg/ml[a]	FAU	0.05 mg/ml[a]	Physically compatible with little or no change in measured turbidity and no increase in particle content in 4 hr at 23 °C	2087	C
Droperidol		2.5 mg/ml		1 mg/ml	Drugs injected sequentially into Y-site with no flush between. No visually apparent precipitate	980	C
Etoposide phosphate	BR	5 mg/ml[a]	FAU	0.05 mg/ml[a]	Physically compatible with no change in measured turbidity or increase in particle content in 4 hr at 23 °C	2218	C

Y-Site Injection Compatibility (1:1 Mixture) (Cont.)

Vincristine sulfate

Drug	Mfr	Conc	Mfr	Conc	Remarks	Ref	C/I
Filgrastim	AMG	30 μg/ml[a]	LI	0.05 mg/ml[a]	Physically compatible with no change in measured turbidity or increase in particle content in 4 hr at 22 °C	1687	**C**
Fludarabine phosphate	BX	1 mg/ml[a]	LY	1 mg/ml[a]	Physically compatible for 4 hr at room temperature under fluorescent light	1439	**C**
Fluorouracil		50 mg/ml		1 mg/ml	Drugs injected sequentially into Y-site with no flush between. No visually apparent precipitate	980	**C**
Furosemide		10 mg/ml		1 mg/ml	Drugs injected sequentially into Y-site with no flush between. Immediate precipitation	980	**I**
Gemcitabine HCl	LI	10 mg/ml[b]	FAU	0.05 mg/ml[b]	Physically compatible with no change in measured turbidity or increase in particle content in 4 hr at 23 °C	2226	**C**
Granisetron HCl	SKB	1 mg/ml	LI	0.34 mg/ml[b]	Physically compatible with little or no loss of either drug by HPLC in 4 hr at 22 °C	1883	**C**
	SKB	1 mg/ml	LI	0.01 mg/ml[b]	Physically compatible with little or no loss of granisetron by HPLC in 4 hr at 22 °C	1883	**C**
Heparin sodium		1000 units/ml		1 mg/ml	Drugs injected sequentially into Y-site with no flush between. No visually apparent precipitate	980	**C**
Idarubicin HCl	AD	1 mg/ml[b]	AD	1 mg/ml	Color changes immediately	1525	**I**
Leucovorin calcium		10 mg/ml		1 mg/ml	Drugs injected sequentially into Y-site with no flush between. No visually apparent precipitate	980	**C**
Melphalan HCl	BW	0.1 mg/ml[b]	LI	0.05 mg/ml[b]	Physically compatible with no change in measured turbidity or increase in particle content in 3 hr at 22 °C	1557	**C**
Methotrexate sodium		25 mg/ml		1 mg/ml	Drugs injected sequentially into Y-site with no flush between. No visually apparent precipitate	980	**C**
		30 mg/ml	LI	0.1 mg/ml	Visually compatible for 4 hr at room temperature	1788	**C**
Metoclopramide HCl		5 mg/ml		1 mg/ml	Drugs injected sequentially into Y-site with no flush between. No visually apparent precipitate	980	**C**
Mitomycin		0.5 mg/ml		1 mg/ml	Drugs injected sequentially into Y-site with no flush between. No visually apparent precipitate	980	**C**
Ondansetron HCl	GL	1 mg/ml[b]	LY	0.05 mg/ml[a]	Physically compatible for 4 hr at 22 °C	1365	**C**
Paclitaxel	NCI	1.2 mg/ml[a]	LI	0.05 mg/ml[a]	Physically compatible with no change in measured turbidity in 4 hr at 22 °C	1556	**C**
Piperacillin sodium–tazobactam sodium	LE	40 + 5 mg/ml[a]	LI	0.05 mg/ml[a]	Physically compatible with no change in measured turbidity or increase in particle content in 4 hr at 22 °C	1688	**C**
Sargramostim	IMM	10 μg/ml[b]	LY	0.05 mg/ml[b]	Physically compatible for 4 hr at 22 °C	1439	**C**

Y-Site Injection Compatibility (1:1 Mixture) (Cont.)

Vincristine sulfate

Drug	Mfr	Conc	Mfr	Conc	Remarks	Ref	C/I
Sodium bicarbonate		1.4%	LI	0.1 mg/ml	White precipitate forms in 30 min at room temperature	1788	I
Teniposide	BR	0.1 mg/ml[a]	LI	0.05 mg/ml[a]	Physically compatible with no subvisual haze or particle formation in 4 hr at 23 °C	1725	C
Thiotepa	IMM[d]	1 mg/ml[a]	LI	0.05 mg/ml[a]	Physically compatible with no change in measured turbidity or increase in particle content in 4 hr at 23 °C	1861	C
Vinblastine sulfate		1 mg/ml		1 mg/ml	Drugs injected sequentially into Y-site with no flush between. No visually apparent precipitate	980	C
Vinorelbine tartrate	BW	1 mg/ml[b]	LI	0.05 mg/ml[b]	Physically compatible with no change in measured turbidity or increase in particle content in 4 hr at 22 °C	1558	C

[a]*Tested in dextrose 5% in water.*
[b]*Tested in sodium chloride 0.9%.*
[c]*Tested in bacteriostatic sodium chloride 0.9% preserved with benzyl alcohol 0.9%.*
[d]*Lyophilized formulation tested.*

Additional Compatibility Information

The manufacturer recommends that vincristine sulfate not be added to solutions that would raise or lower the pH outside the 3.5 to 5.5 range. Only dextrose 5% in water and sodium chloride 0.9% are recommended (2).

Doxorubicin— The compatibility of doxorubicin HCl (Farmitalia) 1.4 mg/ml with vincristine sulfate (Lilly) 0.033 mg/ml in three infusion solutions, under conditions simulating prolonged infusion via an implanted device (37 °C) or via a pump kept under clothing (30 °C) as well as at 25 °C, has been reported. In sodium chloride 0.9% and dextrose 2.5% in sodium chloride 0.45%, there was no precipitate or color change; the concentration of both drugs showed 10% or less loss after 14 days of storage at any of the temperatures. The greatest losses of doxorubicin HCl and vincristine sulfate were about 10 and 6 to 8%, respectively, in the 37 °C samples (1030).

However, when sodium chloride 0.45% and Ringer's acetate was used as the infusion solution, the stability of both drugs was much worse, probably because of the substantially higher solution pH. At 37 °C, a red-pink precipitate formed after two to three days, with about 40% doxorubicin HCl and 14% vincristine sulfate losses occurring in four days. The lower temperatures showed 17 to 27% doxorubicin HCl losses in four days, followed eventually by opalescence in the solutions. Also, the degradation products of doxorubicin adsorbed extensively to the walls of the low density polyethylene–polysiloxane bags (1030).

Increasing the concentration of doxorubicin HCl from 1.4 to 1.88 and 2.37 mg/ml increased the extent of decomposition at 37 °C from 10% at the lowest concentration to 12 and 16%, respectively, after 14 days. Increasing the vincristine sulfate concentration to 0.05 mg/ml did not alter the stability of either drug (1030).

Doxorubicin HCl (Nycomed) was combined with vincristine sulfate (Lilly) in both PVC (Pharmacia Deltec) and polyisoprene (Infusor, Baxter) infusion reservoirs. The drug solution concentrates were diluted slightly with sodium chloride 0.9% to yield a doxorubicin HCl concentration of 1.67 mg/ml and a vincristine sulfate concentration of 0.036 mg/ml. The reservoirs were stored at 4 °C for seven days. This was followed by incubation for four days at 35 °C to simulate near-body temperature during use. No visible changes occurred and neither drug sustained any loss by HPLC analysis throughout the course of the study in either reservoir (1874).

Aluminum— Ogawa et al. reported that immersion of a needle with an aluminum component in vincristine sulfate (Lilly) 1 mg/ml resulted in no visually apparent reaction after seven days at 24 °C (988).

Other Information

Inactivation— In the event of spills or leaks, Lilly recommends the use of sodium hypochlorite 5% (household bleach) to inactivate vincristine sulfate (1200).

VINORELBINE TARTRATE
AHFS 10:00

Navelbine   **Glaxo Wellcome**

Products—— Vinorelbine tartrate (Glaxo Wellcome) is available in a 10-mg/ml concentration in water for injection in 1- and 5-ml single-use vials. No preservatives or other additives are present (2).

Vinorelbine tartrate should be diluted with a compatible diluent for administration. Because skin reactions may occur, gloves should be worn during preparation (2).

pH— The injection has a pH of approximately 3.5 (2).

Administration—— Vinorelbine tartrate is administered intravenously, after dilution, from a syringe (at a concentration of 1.5 to 3 mg/ml) or infusion solution minibag (at a concentration of 0.5 to 2 mg/ml) over six to 10 minutes into the side port of a free-flowing infusion solution closest to the infusion container. After administration, 75 to 125 ml of solution should be used as a flush. Extravasation should be avoided due to tissue irritation, necrosis, and thrombophlebitis (2).

Intrathecal injection of other vinca alkaloids has resulted in death. When vinorelbine tartrate is dispensed in a syringe containing an individual dose, the syringe must be labeled with this statement (2; 4):

"Warning: Navelbine for intravenous use only.
Fatal if given intrathecally"

Stability—— Vinorelbine tartrate injection is a colorless to pale yellow clear solution. Intact vials should be refrigerated at 2 to 8 °C and protected from light (by storage in the carton) and freezing. Intact vials are stable at room temperature (up to 25 °C) for up to 72 hours (2).

When diluted to 1.5 to 3 mg/ml in polypropylene syringes or to 0.5 to 2 mg/ml in PVC infusion containers, vinorelbine tartrate is stable for 24 hours at 5 to 30 °C with exposure to normal room light (2).

Sorption—— Vinorelbine tartrate (Pierre Fabre) 50 mg/250 ml in dextrose 5% in water or sodium chloride 0.9% in PVC bags was infused through PVC sets over two hours at 2.08 ml/min at 22 °C with protection from light. HPLC analysis of the effluent solution found no loss due to sorption to plastic (1631).

Compatibility Information

Solution Compatibility

Vinorelbine tartrate

Solution	Mfr	Mfr	Conc/L	Remarks	Ref	C/I
Dextrose 5% in water	a		500 mg	Little or no loss by HPLC in 7 days at 4 °C protected from light	1631	C
	a	GW	0.5 and 2 g	Visually compatible with 6% or less loss by HPLC in 120 hr at 24 °C under fluorescent light	2213	C
Sodium chloride 0.9%	a		500 mg	4% loss in 3 days and 14% loss in 7 days by HPLC at 4 °C protected from light	1631	C
	a	GW	0.5 and 2 g	Visually compatible with 3% or less loss by HPLC in 120 hr at 24 °C under fluorescent light	2213	C

[a]Tested in PVC containers.

Y-Site Injection Compatibility (1:1 Mixture)

Vinorelbine tartrate

Drug	Mfr	Conc	Mfr	Conc	Remarks	Ref	C/I
Acyclovir sodium	BW	7 mg/ml[b]	BW	1 mg/ml[b]	Heavy white precipitate forms immediately	1558	I
Allopurinol sodium	BW	3 mg/ml[b]	BW	1 mg/ml[b]	Heavy gelatinous white precipitate forms immediately	1686	I
Amikacin sulfate	BR	5 mg/ml[b]	BW	1 mg/ml[b]	Physically compatible with no change in measured turbidity or increase in particle content in 4 hr at 22 °C	1558	C
Aminophylline	AB	2.5 mg/ml[b]	BW	1 mg/ml[b]	Initial light haze becomes visible in room light along with large particles in 1 hr	1558	I
Amphotericin B	SQ	0.6 mg/ml[a,b]	BW	1 mg/ml[b]	Heavy yellow precipitate forms immediately	1558	I
Amphotericin B cholesteryl sulfate complex	SEQ	0.83 mg/ml[a]	BW	1 mg/ml[a]	Gross precipitate forms	2117	I

Y-Site Injection Compatibility (1:1 Mixture) (Cont.)

Vinorelbine tartrate

Drug	Mfr	Conc	Mfr	Conc	Remarks	Ref	C/I
Ampicillin sodium	WY	20 mg/ml[b]	BW	1 mg/ml[b]	Tiny particles form immediately, becoming large white particles in cloudy solution in 1 hr	1558	**I**
Aztreonam	SQ	40 mg/ml[b]	BW	1 mg/ml[b]	Physically compatible with no change in measured turbidity or increase in particle content in 4 hr at 22 °C	1558	**C**
Bleomycin sulfate	BR	1 unit/ml[b]	BW	1 mg/ml[b]	Physically compatible with no change in measured turbidity or increase in particle content in 4 hr at 22 °C	1558	**C**
Bumetanide	RC	0.04 mg/ml[b]	BW	1 mg/ml[b]	Physically compatible with no change in measured turbidity or increase in particle content in 4 hr at 22 °C	1558	**C**
Buprenorphine HCl	RKC	0.04 mg/ml[b]	BW	1 mg/ml[b]	Physically compatible with no change in measured turbidity or increase in particle content in 4 hr at 22 °C	1558	**C**
Butorphanol tartrate	BR	0.04 mg/ml[b]	BW	1 mg/ml[b]	Physically compatible with no change in measured turbidity or increase in particle content in 4 hr at 22 °C	1558	**C**
Calcium gluconate	AMR	40 mg/ml[b]	BW	1 mg/ml[b]	Physically compatible with no change in measured turbidity or increase in particle content in 4 hr at 22 °C	1558	**C**
Carboplatin	BR	5 mg/ml[b]	BW	1 mg/ml[b]	Physically compatible with no change in measured turbidity or increase in particle content in 4 hr at 22 °C	1558	**C**
Carmustine	BR	1.5 mg/ml[b]	BW	1 mg/ml[b]	Physically compatible with no change in measured turbidity or increase in particle content in 4 hr at 22 °C	1558	**C**
Cefazolin sodium	GEM	20 mg/ml[b]	BW	1 mg/ml[b]	Large increase in measured turbidity occurs immediately and grows over 4 hr at 22 °C	1558	**I**
Cefoperazone sodium	RR	40 mg/ml[b]	BW	1 mg/ml[b]	Heavy white flocculent precipitate forms immediately	1558	**I**
Cefotaxime sodium	HO	20 mg/ml[b]	BW	1 mg/ml[b]	Physically compatible with no change in measured turbidity or increase in particle content in 4 hr at 22 °C	1558	**C**
Cefotetan disodium	STU	20 mg/ml[b]	BW	1 mg/ml[b]	Tiny particles form immediately, becoming numerous in cloudy solution in 4 hr at 22 °C	1558	**I**
Ceftazidime	LI[c]	40 mg/ml[b]	BW	1 mg/ml[b]	Physically compatible with no change in measured turbidity or increase in particle content in 4 hr at 22 °C	1558	**C**
Ceftizoxime sodium	FUJ	20 mg/ml[b]	BW	1 mg/ml[b]	Physically compatible with no change in measured turbidity or increase in particle content in 4 hr at 22 °C	1558	**C**
Ceftriaxone sodium	RC	20 mg/ml[b]	BW	1 mg/ml[b]	Tiny particles form immediately, becoming more numerous in 4 hr at 22 °C	1558	**I**
Cefuroxime sodium	GL	20 mg/ml[b]	BW	1 mg/ml[b]	Large increase in measured turbidity occurs immediately and grows over 4 hr at 22 °C	1558	**I**

Y-Site Injection Compatibility (1:1 Mixture) (Cont.)

		Vinorelbine tartrate					
Drug	*Mfr*	*Conc*	*Mfr*	*Conc*	*Remarks*	*Ref*	*C/I*
Chlorpromazine HCl	RU	2 mg/ml[b]	BW	1 mg/ml[b]	Physically compatible with no change in measured turbidity or increase in particle content in 4 hr at 22 °C	1558	**C**
Cimetidine HCl	SKB	12 mg/ml[b]	BW	1 mg/ml[b]	Physically compatible with no change in measured turbidity or increase in particle content in 4 hr at 22 °C	1558	**C**
Cisplatin	BR	1 mg/ml	BW	1 mg/ml[b]	Physically compatible with no change in measured turbidity or increase in particle content in 4 hr at 22 °C	1558	**C**
Clindamycin phosphate	AB	10 mg/ml[b]	BW	1 mg/ml[b]	Physically compatible with no change in measured turbidity or increase in particle content in 4 hr at 22 °C	1558	**C**
Cyclophosphamide	MJ	10 mg/ml[b]	BW	1 mg/ml[b]	Physically compatible with no change in measured turbidity or increase in particle content in 4 hr at 22 °C	1558	**C**
Cytarabine	CET	50 mg/ml	BW	1 mg/ml[b]	Physically compatible with no change in measured turbidity or increase in particle content in 4 hr at 22 °C	1558	**C**
Dacarbazine	MI	4 mg/ml[b]	BW	1 mg/ml[b]	Physically compatible with no change in measured turbidity or increase in particle content in 4 hr at 22 °C	1558	**C**
Dactinomycin	MSD	0.01 mg/ml[b]	BW	1 mg/ml[b]	Physically compatible with no change in measured turbidity or increase in particle content in 4 hr at 22 °C	1558	**C**
Daunorubicin HCl	WY	1 mg/ml[b]	BW	1 mg/ml[b]	Physically compatible with little change in measured turbidity or increase in particle content in 4 hr at 22 °C	1558	**C**
Dexamethasone sodium phosphate	LY	1 mg/ml[b]	BW	1 mg/ml[b]	Physically compatible with no change in measured turbidity or increase in particle content in 4 hr at 22 °C	1558	**C**
Diphenhydramine HCl	ES	2 mg/ml[b]	BW	1 mg/ml[b]	Physically compatible with no change in measured turbidity or increase in particle content in 4 hr at 22 °C	1558	**C**
Doxorubicin HCl	CET	2 mg/ml	BW	1 mg/ml[b]	Physically compatible with no change in measured turbidity or increase in particle content in 4 hr at 22 °C	1558	**C**
Doxorubicin HCl liposome injection	SEQ	0.4 mg/ml[a]	BW	1 mg/ml[a]	Physically compatible with little or no change in measured turbidity and no increase in particle content in 4 hr at 23 °C	2087	**C**
Doxycycline hyclate	ES	1 mg/ml[b]	BW	1 mg/ml[b]	Physically compatible with no change in measured turbidity or increase in particle content in 4 hr at 22 °C	1558	**C**
Droperidol	JN	0.4 mg/ml[b]	BW	1 mg/ml[b]	Physically compatible with no change in measured turbidity or increase in particle content in 4 hr at 22 °C	1558	**C**
Enalaprilat	MSD	0.1 mg/ml[b]	BW	1 mg/ml[b]	Physically compatible with no change in measured turbidity or increase in particle content in 4 hr at 22 °C	1558	**C**

Y-Site Injection Compatibility (1:1 Mixture) (Cont.)

Vinorelbine tartrate

Drug	Mfr	Conc	Mfr	Conc	Remarks	Ref	C/I
Etoposide	BR	0.4 mg/ml[b]	BW	1 mg/ml[b]	Physically compatible with no change in measured turbidity or increase in particle content in 4 hr at 22 °C	1558	C
Famotidine	MSD	2 mg/ml[b]	BW	1 mg/ml[b]	Physically compatible with no change in measured turbidity or increase in particle content in 4 hr at 22 °C	1558	C
Filgrastim	AMG	30 μg/ml[a]	BW	1 mg/ml[b]	Physically compatible with no change in measured turbidity or increase in particle content in 4 hr at 22 °C	1687	C
Floxuridine	RC	3 mg/ml[b]	BW	1 mg/ml[b]	Physically compatible with no change in measured turbidity or increase in particle content in 4 hr at 22 °C	1558	C
Fluconazole	RR	2 mg/ml	BW	1 mg/ml[b]	Physically compatible with no change in measured turbidity or increase in particle content in 4 hr at 22 °C	1558	C
Fludarabine phosphate	BX	1 mg/ml[b]	BW	1 mg/ml[b]	Physically compatible with no change in measured turbidity or increase in particle content in 4 hr at 22 °C	1558	C
Fluorouracil	RC	16 mg/ml[b]	BW	1 mg/ml[b]	Heavy white precipitate forms immediately	1558	I
Furosemide	ES	3 mg/ml[b]	BW	1 mg/ml[b]	Heavy white precipitate forms immediately	1558	I
Ganciclovir sodium	SY	20 mg/ml[b]	BW	1 mg/ml[b]	White turbid solution with precipitate forms immediately	1558	I
Gemcitabine HCl	LI	10 mg/ml[b]	GW	1 mg/ml[b]	Physically compatible with no change in measured turbidity or increase in particle content in 4 hr at 23 °C	2226	C
Gentamicin sulfate	ES	5 mg/ml[b]	BW	1 mg/ml[b]	Physically compatible with no change in measured turbidity or increase in particle content in 4 hr at 22 °C	1558	C
Granisetron HCl	SKB	0.05 mg/ml[a]	BW	1 mg/ml[a]	Physically compatible with no change in measured turbidity or increase in particle content in 4 hr at 23 °C	2000	C
Haloperidol lactate	MN	0.2 mg/ml[b]	BW	1 mg/ml[b]	Physically compatible with no change in measured turbidity or increase in particle content in 4 hr at 22 °C	1558	C
Heparin sodium	ES	100 units/ml[b]	BW	1 mg/ml[b]	Physically compatible with no change in measured turbidity or increase in particle content in 4 hr at 22 °C	1558	C
Hydrocortisone sodium phosphate	MSD	1 mg/ml[b]	BW	1 mg/ml[b]	Physically compatible with no change in measured turbidity or increase in particle content in 4 hr at 22 °C	1558	C
Hydrocortisone sodium succinate	UP	1 mg/ml[b]	BW	1 mg/ml[b]	Physically compatible with no change in measured turbidity or increase in particle content in 4 hr at 22 °C	1558	C
Hydromorphone HCl	KN	0.5 mg/ml[b]	BW	1 mg/ml[b]	Physically compatible with no change in measured turbidity or increase in particle content in 4 hr at 22 °C	1558	C

Y-Site Injection Compatibility (1:1 Mixture) (Cont.)

Vinorelbine tartrate

Drug	Mfr	Conc	Mfr	Conc	Remarks	Ref	C/I
Hydroxyzine HCl	ES	4 mg/ml[b]	BW	1 mg/ml[b]	Physically compatible with no change in measured turbidity or increase in particle content in 4 hr at 22 °C	1558	**C**
Idarubicin HCl	AD	0.5 mg/ml[b]	BW	1 mg/ml[b]	Increase in measured turbidity no greater than dilution of idarubicin with sodium chloride 0.9%. No increase in particle content in 4 hr at 22 °C	1558; 1675	**C**
Ifosfamide	MJ	25 mg/ml[b]	BW	1 mg/ml[b]	Physically compatible with no change in measured turbidity or increase in particle content in 4 hr at 22 °C	1558	**C**
Imipenem–cilastatin sodium	MSD	10 mg/ml[b]	BW	1 mg/ml[b]	Physically compatible with no change in measured turbidity or increase in particle content in 4 hr at 22 °C	1558	**C**
Lorazepam	WY	0.1 mg/ml[b]	BW	1 mg/ml[b]	Physically compatible with no change in measured turbidity or increase in particle content in 4 hr at 22 °C	1558	**C**
Mannitol	BA	15%	BW	1 mg/ml[b]	Physically compatible with no change in measured turbidity or increase in particle content in 4 hr at 22 °C	1558	**C**
Mechlorethamine HCl	MSD	1 mg/ml	BW	1 mg/ml[b]	Physically compatible with no change in measured turbidity or increase in particle content in 4 hr at 22 °C	1558	**C**
Melphalan HCl	BW	0.1 mg/ml[b]	BW	1 mg/ml[b]	Physically compatible with no change in measured turbidity or increase in particle content in 4 hr at 22 °C	1558	**C**
Meperidine HCl	WY	4 mg/ml[b]	BW	1 mg/ml[b]	Physically compatible with no change in measured turbidity or increase in particle content in 4 hr at 22 °C	1558	**C**
Mesna	MJ	10 mg/ml[b]	BW	1 mg/ml[b]	Physically compatible with no change in measured turbidity or increase in particle content in 4 hr at 22 °C	1558	**C**
Methotrexate sodium	LE	15 mg/ml[b]	BW	1 mg/ml[b]	Physically compatible with no change in measured turbidity or increase in particle content in 4 hr at 22 °C	1558	**C**
Methylprednisolone sodium succinate	AB	5 mg/ml[b]	BW	1 mg/ml[b]	Heavy white precipitate forms immediately	1558	**I**
Metoclopramide HCl	RB	5 mg/ml	BW	1 mg/ml[b]	Physically compatible with no change in measured turbidity or increase in particle content in 4 hr at 22 °C	1558	**C**
Metronidazole	BA	5 mg/ml	BW	1 mg/ml[b]	Physically compatible with no change in measured turbidity or increase in particle content in 4 hr at 22 °C	1558	**C**
Minocycline HCl	LE	0.2 mg/ml[b]	BW	1 mg/ml[b]	Physically compatible with no change in measured turbidity or increase in particle content in 4 hr at 22 °C	1558	**C**
Mitomycin	BR	0.5 mg/ml	BW	1 mg/ml[b]	Color changes from pale blue to reddish purple in 1 hr	1558	**I**

Y-Site Injection Compatibility (1:1 Mixture) (Cont.)

					Vinorelbine tartrate		
Drug	*Mfr*	*Conc*	*Mfr*	*Conc*	*Remarks*	*Ref*	*C/I*
Mitoxantrone HCl	LE	0.5 mg/ml[b]	BW	1 mg/ml[b]	Physically compatible with little change in measured turbidity or increase in particle content in 4 hr at 22 °C	1558	C
Morphine sulfate	WI	1 mg/ml[b]	BW	1 mg/ml[b]	Physically compatible with no change in measured turbidity or increase in particle content in 4 hr at 22 °C	1558	C
Nalbuphine HCl	AST	10 mg/ml	BW	1 mg/ml[b]	Physically compatible with no change in measured turbidity or increase in particle content in 4 hr at 22 °C	1558	C
Netilmicin sulfate	SC	5 mg/ml[b]	BW	1 mg/ml[b]	Physically compatible with no change in measured turbidity or increase in particle content in 4 hr at 22 °C	1558	C
Ondansetron HCl	GL	1 mg/ml[b]	BW	1 mg/ml[b]	Physically compatible with no change in measured turbidity or increase in particle content in 4 hr at 22 °C	1558	C
Piperacillin sodium	LE	40 mg/ml[b]	BW	1 mg/ml[b]	Heavy white turbidity forms immediately, becoming white flocculent precipitate in 4 hr at 22 °C	1558	I
Plicamycin	MI	0.01 mg/ml[b]	BW	1 mg/ml[b]	Physically compatible with no change in measured turbidity or increase in particle content in 4 hr at 22 °C	1558	C
Sodium bicarbonate	AB	1 mEq/ml	BW	1 mg/ml[b]	Tiny particles and light blue haze form immediately, developing into large particles in 4 hr at 22 °C	1558	I
Streptozocin	UP	40 mg/ml[b]	BW	1 mg/ml[b]	Physically compatible with no change in measured turbidity or increase in particle content in 4 hr at 22 °C	1558	C
Teniposide	BR	0.1 mg/ml[a]	BW	1 mg/ml[a]	Physically compatible with no change in measured turbidity or increase in particle content in 4 hr at 23 °C	1725	C
Thiotepa	LE	10 mg/ml[b]	BW	1 mg/ml[b]	Cloudy solution with particles forms immediately	1558	I
Ticarcillin disodium	BE	30 mg/ml[b]	BW	1 mg/ml[b]	Physically compatible with no change in measured turbidity or increase in particle content in 4 hr at 22 °C	1558	C
Ticarcillin disodium–clavulanate potassium	SKB	31 mg/ml[b]	BW	1 mg/ml[b]	Physically compatible with no change in measured turbidity or increase in particle content in 4 hr at 22 °C	1558	C
Tobramycin sulfate	LI	5 mg/ml[b]	BW	1 mg/ml[b]	Physically compatible with no change in measured turbidity or increase in particle content in 4 hr at 22 °C	1558	C
Trimethoprim–sulfamethoxazole	ES	0.8 + 4 mg/ml[b]	BW	1 mg/ml[b]	Heavy white turbidity forms immediately, developing particles in 1 hr	1558	I
Vancomycin HCl	LY	10 mg/ml[b]	BW	1 mg/ml[b]	Physically compatible with no change in measured turbidity or increase in particle content in 4 hr at 22 °C	1558	C
Vinblastine sulfate	LI	0.12 mg/ml[b]	BW	1 mg/ml[b]	Physically compatible with no change in measured turbidity or increase in particle content in 4 hr at 22 °C	1558	C

Y-Site Injection Compatibility (1:1 Mixture) (Cont.)

Vinorelbine tartrate

Drug	Mfr	Conc	Mfr	Conc	Remarks	Ref	C/I
Vincristine sulfate	LI	0.05 mg/ml[b]	BW	1 mg/ml[b]	Physically compatible with no change in measured turbidity or increase in particle content in 4 hr at 22 °C	1558	C
Zidovudine	BW	4 mg/ml[b]	BW	1 mg/ml[b]	Physically compatible with no change in measured turbidity or increase in particle content in 4 hr at 22 °C	1558	C

[a]*Tested in dextrose 5% in water.*
[b]*Tested in sodium chloride 0.9%.*
[c]*Sodium carbonate–containing formulation tested.*

Additional Compatibility Information

Solutions— Vinorelbine tartrate, diluted to between 1.5 and 3 mg/ml in dextrose 5% in water or sodium chloride 0.9% for intravenous injection from a syringe, is reported to be stable for 24 hours at 5 to 30 °C when exposed to normal room light (2).

Vinorelbine tartrate injection, diluted to between 0.5 and 2 mg/ml for intravenous infusion, is reported to be stable for up to 24 hours at 5 to 30 °C when exposed to normal room light in the following infusion solutions (2):

Dextrose 5% in sodium chloride 0.45%
Dextrose 5% in water
Ringer's injection
Ringer's injection, lactated
Sodium chloride 0.45%
Sodium chloride 0.9%

Other Information

Bacterial Challenge— Vinorelbine tartrate (Pierre Fabre) 0.1 mg/ml diluted in sodium chloride 0.9% and stored at 22 °C did not exhibit an antimicrobial effect on the growth of four organisms (*Enterococcus faecium*, *Staphylococcus aureus*, *Pseudomonas aeruginosa*, and *Candida albicans*) inoculated into the solution. The author recommended that diluted solutions of vinorelbine tartrate be stored under refrigeration whenever possible and that the potential for microbiological growth be considered when assigning expiration periods (2160).

VITAMIN A
AHFS 88:04

Aquasol A Parenteral   **Astra**

Products— Vitamin A (Astra) is available in 2-ml single-dose vials. Each milliliter contains (2):

Vitamin A (retinol present as the palmitate)	50,000 I.U.
Polysorbate 80	12%
Chlorobutanol	0.5%
Citric acid	0.1%
Butylated hydroxyanisole	0.03%
Butylated hydroxytoluene	0.03%
Sodium hydroxide	to adjust pH

pH— From 6.5 to 7.1 (4).

Equivalency— Vitamin A activity is usually expressed in USP or International Units or retinol equivalents. The USP and International Units are equivalent and are equal to the biological activity of 300 ng of all-*trans*-retinol, 334 ng of all-*trans*-retinol acetate, or 600 ng of β-carotene. One retinol equivalent equals 1 μg of all-*trans*-retinol, 6 μg of β-carotene, or 12 μg of other provitamin A carotenoids (4).

Administration— Vitamin A is administered intramuscularly (2; 4). Intravenous administration is not recommended (2).

Stability— Vitamin A is a light yellow to amber or red oil. It is sensitive to, and should be protected from, light and air (4). Intact vials should be stored under refrigeration and protected from light and freezing (2; 4).

Photodecomposition— Kishi et al. reported on a parenteral nutrition solution in glass bottles exposed to sunlight. Vitamin A decomposed rapidly, losing more than 50% in three hours. The decomposition could be slowed to approximately a 25% loss in three hours by covering the bottle with a light-resistant vinyl bag (1040).

Allwood found that vitamin A was rapidly and significantly decomposed when exposed to daylight. The extent and rate of loss were dependent on the degree of exposure to daylight which, in turn, depended on various factors such as the direction of the radiation, time of day, and climatic conditions. Delivery of less than 10% of the expected amount was reported (1047). In controlled light experiments, the decomposition initially progressed exponentially. Subsequently, the rate of decomposition slowed. This result was attributed to a protective effect of the degradation products on the remaining vitamin A. The presence of amino acids provided greater protection. Compared to degradation rates in dextrose 5% in water, decomposition was reduced by up to 50% in some amino acid mixtures (1048).

In a parenteral nutrition solution composed of amino acids, dextrose, electrolytes, trace elements, and multivitamins in PVC bags stored at 4 and 25 °C, vitamin A rapidly deteriorated to 10% of the initial concentration in eight hours at 25 °C while exposed to light. The decomposition was slowed by light protection and refrigeration, with a loss of about 25% in four days (1063).

Billion-Rey et al. reported substantial loss by HPLC analysis of retinol all-*trans* palmitate and phytonadione from both TPN and TNA admixtures due to exposure to sunlight. In three hours' exposure to sunlight, essentially total loss of retinol and 50% loss of phytonadione had occurred. The presence or absence of lipids did not affect stability. In contrast, tocopherol concentrations remained essentially unchanged by exposure to sunlight through 12 hours. The container material used to store the nutrition admixtures affected the concentration of the vitamins as well. Losses were greatest (10 to 25%) in PVC containers and were slightly better in EVA and glass containers (2049).

Sorption— Vitamin A (as the acetate) (Sigma) 7.5 mg/L displayed 66.7% sorption to a PVC plastic test strip in 24 hours. The presence of dextrose 5% and sodium chloride 0.9% increased the extent of sorption (12).

In another study, vitamin A acetate displayed 78% sorption to 200-ml PVC containers after 24 hours at 25 °C with gentle shaking. The initial concentration was 3 mg/L. The sorption was increased by approximately 10% in sodium chloride 0.9% and by 20% in dextrose 5% in water (133).

However, Nedich noted that vitamin A delivery is also reduced in glass intravenous containers. At a concentration of 10,000 units/L in glass and PVC plastic containers protected from light with aluminum foil, 77 and 71%, respectively, of the vitamin A were delivered in 10 hours. Without light protection, 61% was delivered from glass and 49% from PVC plastic containers over a 10-hour period (290).

In another test using multivitamin infusion (USV), one ampul/L of sodium chloride 0.9% in glass and PVC containers not protected from light, 69.4 and 67.9% of the vitamin A were delivered from the glass and PVC containers, respectively, in 10 hours. The amount of vitamin A was constant over this test period, not decreasing with time (282).

Similar results were observed in a parenteral nutrition solution composed of protein hydrolysate 2%, dextrose 20%, electrolytes, and multivitamin infusion (USV) 10 ml in 1-L glass containers. Approximately 50 to 65% of the vitamin A content in the solution was lost in 24 hours, and then it remained stable for three to seven days. When added to the cellulose propionate burette chambers of infusion sets, about 60% of the vitamin A was lost in six hours. Further, the effluent from the PVC tubing of the set was even worse. The concentration dropped from an initial 3 µg/ml to 1 µg/ml in two hours. Wrapping foil around the chambers to exclude light did not alter the vitamin A disappearance. About 50% of the lost vitamin A was recovered by hexane extraction of the administration sets (438).

Gillis et al. evaluated the delivery of vitamins A, D, and E from a parenteral nutrition solution composed of 3% amino acid solution (Pharmacia) in dextrose 10% with electrolytes, trace elements, vitamin K, folate, and vitamin B_{12}. To this solution was added 6 ml of multivitamin infusion (USV). The solution was prepared in PVC bags (Travenol), and administration was simulated through a fluid chamber (Buretrol) and infusion tubing with a 0.5-µm filter at 10 ml/hr. During the first 60 to 90 minutes, minimal delivery of the vitamins occurred. Then a rise and a plateau in the delivered vitamins followed and were attributed to an increasing saturation of adsorptive binding sites in the tubing. Total amounts delivered over 24 hours were: vitamin A, 31%; vitamin D, 68%; and vitamin E, 64%. Sorption of the vitamins was found in the PVC bag, fluid chamber, and tubing. Decomposition was not a factor (836).

Howard et al. reported on a patient receiving 3000 I.U. of retinol daily in a parenteral nutrition solution; nevertheless, this patient experienced two episodes of night blindness. The pharmacy prepared the parenteral nutrition solution in 1-L PVC bags in weekly batches and stored them at 4 °C in the dark until use. A subsequent in vitro study showed losses of vitamin A of 23 and 77% in three- and 14-day periods, respectively, under these conditions. About 30% of the lost vitamin A could be extracted from the PVC bag (1038).

Shenai et al. reported on losses of vitamin A from neonatal parenteral nutrition solutions containing multivitamins (USV). The solution was prepared in colorless glass bottles and run through an administration set with a burette (Travenol). The total loss of vitamin A was 75% in 24 hours, with about 16% as decomposition in the glass bottle. The decomposition was not noticeable during the first 12 hours, but then vitamin A levels fell rather precipitously to about one-third of the initial amount. The balance of the loss, averaging about 59%, occurred during transit through the administration set. Removal of the inline filter and treatment of the set with albumin had no effect on vitamin A delivery. The authors recommended a three- to fourfold increase in the amount of vitamin A to compensate for the losses (1039).

Riggle et al. noted a 50% loss of vitamin A from a bottle of parenteral nutrition solution prepared with multivitamin infusion (USV) after 5.5 hours of infusion. The amount delivered through an Ivex-2 filter set was only 6.3% of the added amount. Similar quantities were found after 20 hours of infusion. A reduced light exposure and use of ^{3}H-labeled vitamin A confirmed binding to the infusion bottles and tubing (704).

Subsequently, Riggle and Brandt incubated solutions containing multivitamins (USV) spiked with ^{3}H-labeled retinol in intravenous tubing protected from light and agitated to simulate flow for five hours. About half of the vitamin A was lost in 30 minutes, and 88 to 96% was lost in five hours. Spectrophotometric assays correlated closely with the radioisotope assays. Hexane rinses and radioactivity determinations on the tubing accounted for the decrease in radioactivity (1049).

In another experiment, neonatal parenteral nutrition solutions containing multivitamins prepared in bags were delivered at 10 ml/hr through Buretrol sets (Travenol). The bags and sets were protected from light. Spectrophotometric and radioisotope assays showed that about 26% of the vitamin A was lost before the flow was started. At 10 ml/hr, about 67% was lost from the effluent. More rapid flow reduced the extent of loss. Analysis of clinical samples of parenteral nutrition solutions showed losses of 21 to 57% after 20 hours. Because losses after five hours were of the same magnitude, the authors concluded that the loss occurs fairly rapidly and is not due to gradual decomposition (1049).

Dahl et al. reported the stability of numerous vitamins in parenteral nutrition solutions composed of amino acids (Kabi-Vitrum), dextrose 30%, and fat emulsion 20% (Kabi-Vitrum) in a 2:1:1 ratio with electrolytes, trace elements, and both fat- and water-soluble vitamins. The admixtures were stored in darkness at 2 to 8 °C for 96 hours with no significant loss of retinyl palmitate, alpha-tocopherol, thiamine mononitrate, sodium riboflavin-5′-phosphate, pyridoxine HCl, nicotinamide, folic acid, biotin, sodium pantothenate, and cyanocobalamin. Sodium ascorbate and its biologically active degradation product, dehydroascorbic acid, totaled 59 and 42% of the nominal starting concentration at 24 and 96 hours, respectively. However, the actual initial concentration was only 66% of the nominal concentration (1225).

When the admixture was subjected to simulated infusion over 24 hours at 20 °C, either exposed to room light or light protected, or stored for six days in the dark under refrigeration and then subjected to the same simulated infusion, once again the retinyl palmitate, alpha-tocopherol, and sodium riboflavin-5′-phosphate did not undergo significant loss. However, sodium ascorbate and its degradation product, dehydroascorbic acid, had initial combined concentrations of 51 to 65% of the nominal initial concentration, with further declines during infusion. Light protection did not significantly alter the loss of total ascorbic acid (1225).

McKenna and Bieri reported that 40% retinol losses occurred in two hours and 60% in five hours from parenteral nutrition solutions pumped at 10 ml/hr through standard infusion sets at room temperature. The retinol concentration in the bottle remained constant while the retinol in the effluent decreased. Antioxidants had no effect. Much of the vitamin A was recoverable from hexane washings of the tubing (1050).

Smith et al. reported the stability of several vitamins from M.V.I.-12 (Armour) admixed in parenteral nutrition solutions composed of different amino acid products, with or without Intralipid 10%, when stored in glass bottles and PVC bags at 25 and 5 °C for 48 hours. No vitamin A was lost from any formula in glass bottles, but samples in PVC containers lost as much as 35 and 60% at 5 and 25 °C, respectively, in 48 hours (1431).

Bluhm et al. studied the stability of vitamin A in two parenteral nutrition solutions. In TPN #172 (see Appendix I), a 10% loss of vitamin A palmitate by HPLC occurred in about 20 days in PVC bags while no loss occurred in Buretrol chambers in 21 days at 30 °C with exposure to normal ward light. In TPN #173 (see Appendix I), a 10% loss of vitamin A palmitate occurred in about 12 days in both glass and PVC containers at 2 to 8 °C with protection from light (1606).

Bluhm et al. also evaluated the effects of the fat emulsion concentration on vitamin A stability in several parenteral nutrition solutions. Vitamin A palmitate was not absorbed into PVC containers from Intralipid 10%. Among TPN solutions with lower Intralipid contents, no correlation existed between the fat emulsion content and the extent of vitamin A loss during refrigerated storage. The fat emulsion content afforded vitamin A some protection from decomposition due to light exposure at 30 °C (1607).

The quantity of retinol delivered from an M.V.I.-containing 2-in-1 parenteral nutrition solution and when M.V.I. was added to Intralipid 10% was evaluated during simulated administration through a PVC administration set. The parenteral nutrition solution was composed of amino acids 2.8%, dextrose 10%, and standard electrolytes; M.V.I. was added to yield a nominal retinol concentration of 455 μg/150 ml. Retinol losses were about 80% of the admixed amount after being delivered through the PVC set. When M.V.I. was added to Intralipid 10% in a retinol concentration of 455 μg/20 ml, retinol losses were reduced to about 10% of the admixed amount. As in the study by Bluhm et al. (1607), the fat emulsion provided retinol protection from sorption to the PVC administration set (2027).

Substantially higher amounts of retinol were found to be delivered using polyolefin administration set tubing than with PVC tubing during simulated neonatal intensive care administration. Retinol was added to a 2-in-1 parenteral nutrition solution (TPN #206) in concentrations of 25 and 50 I.U./ml and run at 4 and 10 ml/hr through three meter lengths of polyolefin (MiniMed) and PVC (Baxter) intravenous extension set tubing protected from light and passed through a 37 °C water bath. Using HPLC analysis, delivered quantities of retinol varied from 19 to 74% through the PVC tubing and 47 to 87% through the polyolefin tubing. The authors noted that the loss of retinol to the PVC tubing appeared to be saturable. Even so, the use of polyolefin tubing increases the amount of retinol delivered during simulated neonatal administration (2028).

Interestingly, no loss of vitamin A to PVC delivery systems of *enteral* feeding solutions, after six hours of storage without protection from light and with exposure to ambient temperature, was reported by Bryant and Neufeld. The authors attributed this result to the presence of other (undefined) substances in the enteral feeding mixtures (1051).

To minimize the importance of this sorption, Allwood suggested using vitamin A palmitate, which he and others have noted does not sorb as extensively to PVC (1033; 1606; 2026), instead of the acetate. However, this change does not alter the problem of degradation from exposure to light. Alternatively, an excess of vitamin A could be used (1033).

Plasticizer Leaching— Vitamin A leached significant amounts of diethylhexyl phthalate (DEHP) plasticizer from PVC bags and administration set tubing (1621).

Compatibility Information

Solution Compatibility

Vitamin A

Solution	Mfr	Mfr	Conc/L	Remarks	Ref	C/I
Fat emulsion 10%, intravenous	KA	KA[a]	101 mg	Physically compatible for 24 hr at 26 °C with little loss of retinol and of most other vitamins by HPLC; up to 52% ascorbate loss	2050	C

[a]*From multivitamins.*

WARFARIN SODIUM
AHFS 20:12.04

Coumadin   **Du Pont Pharma**

Products— Warfarin sodium (Du Pont Pharma) is available as a lyophilized powder in vials containing a total of 5.4 mg of drug. When reconstituted with 2.7 ml of sterile water for injection, each milliliter of solution contains (2):

Warfarin sodium	2 mg
Sodium phosphate, dibasic, heptahydrate	4.98 mg
Sodium phosphate, monobasic, monohydrate	0.194 mg
Sodium chloride	0.1 mg
Mannitol	38 mg
Sodium hydroxide	to adjust pH

The maximum amount of withdrawable solution is about 2.5 ml (2).

pH— From 8.1 to 8.3 (2).

Administration— Warfarin sodium is administered by slow intravenous injection over one to two minutes into a peripheral vein. It should not be given intramuscularly (2).

Stability— Intact vials should be stored at controlled room temperature and protected from exposure to light. After reconstitution, warfarin sodium is physically and chemically stable for only four hours at room temperature. The reconstituted solution should not be refrigerated. If either particulates or discoloration is noted, the drug should be discarded. Unused solution also should be discarded (2).

pH Effects— A precipitate may form in solution due to formation of the poorly soluble enol form of warfarin at pH values below 8. At pH 8 or higher, clear stable solutions result because the warfarin is in the soluble enolate form (964).

Sorption— Warfarin sodium (Abbott) 25 mg/L displayed 11.7% sorption to a PVC plastic test strip in 24 hours. The presence of dextrose 5% increased the extent of the sorption (12).

Warfarin sodium 22 mg/L in sodium chloride 0.9% (Travenol) in PVC bags exhibited approximately a 15% loss in one week at room temperature (15 to 20 °C) due to sorption. However, when the solution was buffered from its initial pH of 6.7 to 7.4, no significant loss of drug due to sorption was observed over the one-week study period (536).

In another study, warfarin sodium 22 mg/L in sodium chloride 0.9% did not exhibit any loss due to sorption during a seven-hour simulated infusion through an infusion set (Travenol) consisting of a cellulose propionate burette chamber and 170 cm of PVC tubing (606).

The drug was also tested as a simulated infusion over at least one hour by a syringe pump system. A glass syringe on a syringe pump was fitted with 20 cm of polyethylene tubing or 50 cm of Silastic tubing. No loss of drug due to sorption was observed with either tubing (606).

Table 1. Extent of Equilibrium Sorption of Warfarin Sodium in Sodium Chloride 0.9% in PVC Bags (770)

Initial Concentration (mg/ml)	pH	Extent of Sorption (%)
1.31	6.95	4
0.433	6.55	6
0.190	6.27	18
0.093	6.04	24
0.048	5.90	30
0.024	5.78	45
0.009	5.65	66

In addition, a 25-ml aliquot of warfarin sodium 22 mg/L in sodium chloride 0.9% was stored in all-plastic syringes composed of polypropylene barrels and polyethylene plungers for 24 hours at room temperature in the dark. No loss due to sorption occurred (606).

The sorption of warfarin sodium 20 mg/L in sodium chloride 0.9% was evaluated in 100-ml PVC infusion bags (Travenol). After eight hours at 20 to 24 °C, 29% of the warfarin was lost. Adjusting the pH of the solution to 2 or 4 increased the sorption in eight hours to 49% because of the increased amount of unionized warfarin present in the solution at these low pH values. The unionized form is most favorably sorbed by the plastic. The concentration of warfarin sodium in solution also affects the pH and, thereby, the extent of sorption. Table 1 shows that as the warfarin sodium concentration is reduced, small changes in the pH of the solution occur. Even these small pH changes result in a greatly increased extent of sorption at equilibrium (about 100 hours of exposure) (770).

Like the old formulation, the new phosphate-buffered formulation of warfarin sodium (DuPont) undergoes sorption to PVC containers and administration sets. At a concentration of 0.02 mg/ml in dextrose 5% in water in PVC containers, about 2.4% loss occurred in six hours. In sodium chloride 0.9% in PVC containers, the loss was only 1% in six hours. At 0.6 mg/ml, no potency loss was found in either solution. Similarly, a 0.02-mg/ml concentration exhibited a 6% loss in dextrose 5% in water and a 2% loss in sodium chloride 0.9% to PVC administration sets in two hours of contact; potency continued to decrease at four and six hours of contact. Once again, the 0.6-mg/ml concentration did not exhibit potency loss due to sorption in six hours in either solution. It would appear that low concentrations and dextrose 5% in water used as the infusion vehicle may increase loss due to sorption to PVC (2010).

Warfarin sodium showed a negligible (less than 3%) loss if the aqueous solutions at pH 2 to 7 were stored in polypropylene infusion bags (770).

Warfarin sodium (Orion) 25 μg/ml in sodium chloride 0.9% exhibited no loss by UV spectroscopy and HPLC analysis due to sorption in 120 hours at 21 °C in glass bottles and polypropylene trilayer bags (Softbag, Orion). However, about a 70% loss due to sorption occurred under these conditions in PVC bags (1796).

Compatibility Information

Solution Compatibility

Warfarin sodium

Solution	Mfr	Mfr	Conc/L	Remarks	Ref	C/I
Dextrose 5% in Ringer's injection, lactated	BA	DU	100 mg	Physically compatible with no change in measured turbidity or increase in particle content in 24 hr at 23 °C	2011	C
Dextrose 5% in sodium chloride 0.45%	BA	DU	100 mg	Physically compatible with no change in measured turbidity or increase in particle content in 24 hr at 23 °C	2011	C
Dextrose 5% in sodium chloride 0.9%	BA	DU	100 mg	Physically compatible with no change in measured turbidity or increase in particle content in 24 hr at 23 °C	2011	C
Dextrose 5% in water	[a]	DU	20 mg	Visually compatible with about 2.4% loss due to sorption in 6 hr	2010	C
	[b]	DU	20 mg	Visually compatible with no loss in 6 hr	2010	C
	[a]	DU	600 mg	Visually compatible with no loss in 6 hr	2010	C
	MG	DU	100 mg	Physically compatible with no change in measured turbidity or increase in particle content in 24 hr at 23 °C	2011	C
Dextrose 10% in water	BA	DU	100 mg	Physically compatible with no change in measured turbidity or increase in particle content in 24 hr at 23 °C	2011	C
Ringer's injection		DU	1 g	Haze forms immediately	2010	I
	BA	DME	1 g	Haze forms immediately	2078	I
Ringer's injection, lactated	BA	DU	100 mg	Physically compatible with no change in measured turbidity or increase in particle content in 24 hr at 23 °C	2011	C
	BA	DME	1 g	Slight haze may form in 1 hr	2078	I
Sodium chloride 0.9%	[c]	ON	100 mg	Visually compatible with no drug loss by UV and HPLC in 24 hr at 21 °C	1796	C
	[a]	ON	100 mg	Visually compatible but 50% drug loss in 24 hr and 70% loss in 120 hr by UV and HPLC at 21 °C due to sorption	1796	I
	[a]	DU	20 mg	Visually compatible with about 1% loss due to sorption in 6 hr	2010	C
	[b]	DU	20 mg	Visually compatible with no loss in 6 hr	2010	C
	[a]	DU	600 mg	Visually compatible with no loss in 6 hr	2010	C
	MG	DU	100 mg	Physically compatible with no change in measured turbidity or increase in particle content in 24 hr at 23 °C	2011	C
	AB	DME	1 g	Haze may form in 24 hr	2078	I

[a]Tested in PVC containers.
[b]Tested in glass containers.
[c]Tested in glass containers and polypropylene trilayer containers.

Drugs in Syringe Compatibility

Warfarin sodium

Drug (in syringe)	Mfr	Amt	Mfr	Amt	Remarks	Ref	C/I
Heparin sodium	ES	5000 units/ 1 ml	DU	2 mg/ 1 ml[a]	Low-level haze forms immediately and becomes visible in ambient light in 1 hr	2010	I

[a]Tested in sterile water for injection.

Y-Site Injection Compatibility (1:1 Mixture)

Warfarin sodium

Drug	Mfr	Conc	Mfr	Conc	Remarks	Ref	C/I
Amikacin sulfate	AB	5 mg/ml[a,b]	DU	0.1[a,b] and 2[d] mg/ml	Physically compatible with no change in measured turbidity or increase in particle content in 24 hr at 23 °C	2011	**C**
Aminophylline	ES	4 mg/ml[a]	DME	2 mg/ml[d]	Haze forms in 4 hr	2078	**I**
Ammonium chloride	AB	5 mEq/ml	DU	0.1 mg/ml[a]	Subvisual haze forms immediately	2011	**I**
	AB	5 mEq/ml	DU	0.1 mg/ml[b]	Physically compatible with no change in measured turbidity or increase in particle content in 24 hr at 23 °C	2011	**C**
	AB	5 mEq/ml	DU	2 mg/ml[d]	Heavy white turbidity forms immediately and becomes flocculent precipitate in 24 hr at 23 °C	2011	**I**
Ascorbic acid injection	SCN	0.5 mg/ml[a,b]	DU	0.1[a,b] and 2[d] mg/ml	Physically compatible with no change in measured turbidity or increase in particle content in 24 hr at 23 °C	2011	**C**
Bretylium tosylate	FAU	10 mg/ml[a]	DU	2 mg/ml[d]	Haze forms immediately	2010	**I**
	DU	10 mg/ml[a]	DME	2 mg/ml[d]	Haze forms immediately	2078	**I**
Cefazolin sodium	SKB	20 mg/ml[a]	DU	2 mg/ml[d]	Visually compatible with no warfarin loss by HPLC in 30 min	2010	**C**
	SKB	20 mg/ml[a]	DME	2 mg/ml[d]	Visually compatible for 24 hr at 24 °C	2078	**C**
Ceftazidime	SKB[c]	20 mg/ml[a]	DME	2 mg/ml[d]	Haze forms in 24 hr at 24 °C	2078	**I**
Ceftriaxone sodium	RC	20 mg/ml[a]	DME	2 mg/ml[d]	Visually compatible for 24 hr at 24 °C	2078	**C**
Cimetidine HCl	SKB	3.6 mg/ml[a]	DU	2 mg/ml[d]	Haze forms in 1 hr	2010	**I**
	EN	3.6 mg/ml[a]	DU	2 mg/ml[d]	Haze forms immediately	2010	**I**
	SKB	3.6 mg/ml[a]	DME	2 mg/ml[d]	Haze forms in 1 hr	2078	**I**
Ciprofloxacin	MI	2 mg/ml[a]	DU	2 mg/ml[d]	Haze forms immediately; crystals form in 1 hr	2010	**I**
	MI	2 mg/ml[a]	DME	2 mg/ml[d]	Haze forms immediately; crystals form in 1 hr	2078	**I**
Dobutamine HCl	LI	1 mg/ml[a]	DU	2 mg/ml[d]	Haze and precipitate form immediately	2010	**I**
	LI	1 mg/ml[a]	DME	2 mg/ml[d]	Haze and precipitate form immediately	2078	**I**
Dopamine HCl	FAU	1.6 mg/ml[a]	DU	2 mg/ml[d]	Visually compatible with no warfarin loss by HPLC in 30 min	2010	**C**
	DU	1.6 mg/ml[a]	DME	2 mg/ml[d]	Visually compatible for 24 hr at 24 °C	2078	**C**
Epinephrine HCl	AMR	0.1 mg/ml[a,b]	DU	0.1[a,b] and 2[d] mg/ml	Physically compatible with no change in measured turbidity or increase in particle content in 24 hr at 23 °C	2011	**C**
Esmolol HCl	OHM	10 mg/ml[a]	DU	2 mg/ml[d]	Haze forms immediately	2010	**I**
	OHM	10 mg/ml[a]	DME	2 mg/ml[d]	Haze forms immediately	2078	**I**
Gentamicin sulfate	SCH	1.6 mg/ml[a]	DU	2 mg/ml[d]	Haze forms immediately	2010	**I**
	SC	1.6 mg/ml[a]	DME	2 mg/ml[b]	Haze forms immediately	2078	**I**
Heparin sodium	AB	100 units/ml[a]	DU	2 mg/ml[d]	Visually compatible with no warfarin loss by HPLC in 30 min	2010	**C**
	AB	100 units/ml[a]	DME	2 mg/ml[d]	Visually compatible for 24 hr at 24 °C	2078	**C**
Labetalol HCl	SCH	0.8 mg/ml[a]	DU	2 mg/ml[d]	Haze forms immediately	2010	**I**
	SC	0.8 mg/ml[a]	DME	2 mg/ml[d]	Haze forms immediately	2078	**I**
Lidocaine HCl	AST	2 mg/ml[a]	DU	2 mg/ml[d]	Visually compatible with no warfarin loss by HPLC in 30 min	2010	**C**
	AST	2 mg/ml[a]	DME	2 mg/ml[d]	Visually compatible for 24 hr at 24 °C	2078	**C**

Y-Site Injection Compatibility (1:1 Mixture) (Cont.)

Warfarin sodium

Drug	Mfr	Conc	Mfr	Conc	Remarks	Ref	C/I
Metaraminol tartrate	MSD	0.2 mg/ml[a,b]	DU	0.1[a,b] and 2[d] mg/ml	Physically compatible with no change in measured turbidity or increase in particle content in 24 hr at 23 °C	2011	C
Metronidazole HCl	SCS	5 mg/ml[b]	DME	2 mg/ml[d]	Slight haze forms in 24 hr at 24 °C	2078	I
Morphine sulfate	ES	2 mg/ml[a]	DU	2 mg/ml[d]	Visually compatible with no warfarin loss by HPLC in 30 min	2010	C
	ES	2 mg/ml[a]	DME	2 mg/ml[d]	Visually compatible for 24 hr at 24 °C	2078	C
Nitroglycerin	FAU	0.4 mg/ml[a]	DU	2 mg/ml[d]	Visually compatible with no warfarin loss by HPLC in 30 min	2010	C
	DU	0.4 mg/ml[a]	DME	2 mg/ml[d]	Visually compatible for 24 hr at 24 °C	2078	C
Oxytocin	FUJ	1 unit/ml[a,b]	DU	0.1[a,b] and 2[d] mg/ml	Physically compatible with no change in measured turbidity or increase in particle content in 24 hr at 23 °C	2011	C
Potassium chloride	BA	0.04 mEq/ml[e]	DME	2 mg/ml[d]	Visually compatible for 24 hr at 24 °C	2078	C
Promazine HCl	WY	5 mg/ml[a,b]	DU	0.1[a,b] and 2[d] mg/ml	Heavy white turbidity forms immediately	2011	I
Ranitidine HCl	GL	1 mg/ml[a]	DU	2 mg/ml[d]	Visually compatible with no warfarin loss by HPLC in 30 min	2010	C
	GL	1 mg/ml[a]	DME	2 mg/ml[d]	Visually compatible for 24 hr at 24 °C	2078	C
Ringer's injection	BA		DU	2 mg/ml[d]	Haze forms immediately	2010	I
Vancomycin HCl	LI	4 mg/ml[a]	DU	2 mg/ml[d]	Haze forms immediately	2010	I
	AB	10 mg/ml[a,b]	DU	0.1 mg/ml[a,b]	Physically compatible with no change in measured turbidity or increase in particle content in 24 hr at 23 °C	2011	C
	AB	10 mg/ml[a,b]	DU	2 mg/ml[d]	Heavy white turbidity forms immediately	2011	I
	LI	4 mg/ml[a]	DME	2 mg/ml[d]	Haze forms immediately	2078	I

[a]Tested in dextrose 5% in water.
[b]Tested in sodium chloride 0.9%.
[c]Sodium carbonate–containing formulation tested.
[d]Tested in sterile water for injection.
[e]Tested in dextrose 5% in sodium chloride 0.45%.

ZIDOVUDINE
AHFS 8:18.08

Retrovir   **Glaxo Wellcome**

Products— Zidovudine (Glaxo Wellcome) is available in 20-ml single-use vials. Each milliliter of solution contains zidovudine 10 mg in water for injection. Hydrochloric acid and/or sodium hydroxide may be present to adjust the pH (2).

pH— Approximately 5.5 (2).

Osmolality— Zidovudine 10 mg/ml has an osmolality of 34 mOsm/kg (1689).

Administration— Zidovudine must be diluted in dextrose 5% in water to a concentration no greater than 4 mg/ml prior to administration. The drug is administered by intravenous infusion at a constant rate over one hour (2; 4). Zidovudine has also been administered by continuous intravenous infusion (4). Intramuscular injection, intravenous bolus, and rapid intravenous infusion should be avoided (2; 4).

Stability— Intact vials of zidovudine should be stored at 15 to 25 °C and protected from light (2).

Compatibility Information

Solution Compatibility

Zidovudine

Solution	Mfr	Mfr	Conc/L	Remarks	Ref	C/I
Dextrose 5% in water	a	BW	4 g	Physically compatible with no drug loss in 8 days at 4 and 25 °C	1411	**C**
Sodium chloride 0.9%	a	BW	4 g	Physically compatible with no drug loss in 8 days at 4 and 25 °C	1411	**C**

[a]Tested in PVC containers.

Additive Compatibility

Zidovudine

Drug	Mfr	Conc/L	Mfr	Conc/L	Test Soln	Remarks	Ref	C/I
Meropenem	ZEN	1 g	BW	4 g	NS	Visually compatible for 4 hr at room temperature	1994	**C**
	ZEN	20 g	BW	4 g	NS	Dark yellow discoloration forms in 4 hr at room temperature	1994	**I**

Y-Site Injection Compatibility (1:1 Mixture)

Zidovudine

Drug	Mfr	Conc	Mfr	Conc	Remarks	Ref	C/I
Acyclovir sodium	BW	7 mg/ml[a]	BW	4 mg/ml[a]	Physically compatible for 4 hr at 25 °C under fluorescent light by visual and microscopic examination	1193	**C**
Allopurinol sodium	BW	3 mg/ml[b]	BW	4 mg/ml[b]	Physically compatible with no change in measured turbidity or increase in particle content in 4 hr at 22 °C	1686	**C**
Amifostine	USB	10 mg/ml[a]	BW	4 mg/ml[a]	Physically compatible with no change in measured turbidity or increase in particle content in 4 hr at 23 °C	1845	**C**
Amikacin sulfate	BR	4 mg/ml[a]	BW	4 mg/ml[a]	Physically compatible for 4 hr at 25 °C under fluorescent light by visual and microscopic examination	1193	**C**
Amphotericin B	SQ	600 μg/ml[a]	BW	4 mg/ml[a]	Physically compatible for 4 hr at 25 °C under fluorescent light by visual and microscopic examination	1193	**C**
Amphotericin B cholesteryl sulfate complex	SEQ	0.83 mg/ml[a]	BW	4 mg/ml[a]	Physically compatible with little or no change in measured turbidity or increase in particle content in 4 hr at 23 °C under fluorescent light	2117	**C**
Aztreonam	SQ	40 mg/ml[a]	BW	4 mg/ml[a]	Physically compatible for 4 hr at 25 °C under fluorescent light by visual and microscopic examination	1193	**C**
	SQ	40 mg/ml[a]	BW	4 mg/ml[a]	Physically compatible with no subvisual haze or particle formation in 4 hr at 23 °C	1758	**C**
Cefepime HCl	BR	20 mg/ml[a]	BW	4 mg/ml[a]	Physically compatible with no change in measured turbidity or increase in particle content in 4 hr at 22 °C	1689	**C**

Y-Site Injection Compatibility (1:1 Mixture) (Cont.)

Zidovudine

Drug	Mfr	Conc	Mfr	Conc	Remarks	Ref	C/I
Ceftazidime	GL[g]	20 mg/ml[a]	BW	4 mg/ml[a]	Physically compatible for 4 hr at 25 °C under fluorescent light by visual and microscopic examination	1193	C
Ceftriaxone sodium	RC	20 mg/ml[a]	BW	4 mg/ml[a]	Physically compatible for 4 hr at 25 °C under fluorescent light by visual and microscopic examination	1193	C
Cimetidine HCl	SKF	6 mg/ml[a]	BW	4 mg/ml[a]	Physically compatible for 4 hr at 25 °C under fluorescent light by visual and microscopic examination	1193	C
Cisatracurium besylate	GW	0.1, 2, 5 mg/ml[a]	BW	4 mg/ml[a]	Physically compatible with no change in measured turbidity or increase in particle content in 4 hr at 23 °C	2074	C
Clindamycin phosphate	UP	12 mg/ml[a]	BW	4 mg/ml[a]	Physically compatible for 4 hr at 25 °C under fluorescent light by visual and microscopic examination	1193	C
Dexamethasone sodium phosphate	ES	0.16 mg/ml[a]	BW	4 mg/ml[a]	Physically compatible for 4 hr at 25 °C under fluorescent light by visual and microscopic examination	1193	C
Dobutamine HCl	LI	5 mg/ml[a]	BW	4 mg/ml[a]	Physically compatible for 4 hr at 25 °C under fluorescent light by visual and microscopic examination	1193	C
Docetaxel	RPR	0.9 mg/ml[a]	GW	4 mg/ml[a]	Physically compatible with no change in measured turbidity or increase in particle content in 4 hr at 23 °C	2224	C
Dopamine HCl	AB	1.6 mg/ml[a]	BW	4 mg/ml[a]	Physically compatible for 4 hr at 25 °C under fluorescent light by visual and microscopic examination	1193	C
Doxorubicin HCl liposome injection	SEQ	0.4 mg/ml[a]	BW	4 mg/ml[a]	Physically compatible with little or no change in measured turbidity and no increase in particle content in 4 hr at 23 °C	2087	C
Erythromycin lactobionate	AB	20 mg/ml[a,c]	BW	4 mg/ml[a]	Physically compatible for 4 hr at 25 °C under fluorescent light by visual and microscopic examination	1193	C
Etoposide phosphate	BR	5 mg/ml[a]	BW	4 mg/ml[a]	Physically compatible with no change in measured turbidity or increase in particle content in 4 hr at 23 °C	2218	C
Filgrastim	AMG	30 μg/ml[a]	BW	4 mg/ml[a]	Physically compatible with no change in measured turbidity or increase in particle content in 4 hr at 22 °C	1687	C
Fluconazole	RR	2 mg/ml	BW	10 mg/ml	Physically compatible for 24 hr at 25 °C	1407	C
Fludarabine phosphate	BX	1 mg/ml[a]	BW	4 mg/ml[a]	Physically compatible for 4 hr at room temperature under fluorescent light	1439	C
Gemcitabine HCl	LI	10 mg/ml[b]	GW	4 mg/ml[b]	Physically compatible with no change in measured turbidity or increase in particle content in 4 hr at 23 °C	2226	C
Gentamicin sulfate	IMS	2 mg/ml[a]	BW	4 mg/ml[a]	Physically compatible for 4 hr at 25 °C under fluorescent light by visual and microscopic examination	1193	C

Y-Site Injection Compatibility (1:1 Mixture) (Cont.)

Drug	Mfr	Conc	Mfr	Conc	Remarks	Ref	C/I
				Zidovudine			
Granisetron HCl	SKB	0.05 mg/ml[a]	BW	4 mg/ml[a]	Physically compatible with no change in measured turbidity or increase in particle content in 4 hr at 23 °C	2000	**C**
Heparin sodium	LY	100 units/ml[a]	BW	4 mg/ml[a]	Physically compatible for 4 hr at 25 °C under fluorescent light by visual and microscopic examination	1193	**C**
Imipenem–cilastatin sodium	MSD	5 mg/ml[a]	BW	4 mg/ml[a]	Physically compatible for 4 hr at 25 °C under fluorescent light by visual and microscopic examination	1193	**C**
Lorazepam	WY	80 μg/ml[a]	BW	4 mg/ml[a]	Physically compatible for 4 hr at 25 °C under fluorescent light by visual and microscopic examination	1193	**C**
Melphalan HCl	BW	0.1 mg/ml[b]	BW	4 mg/ml[b]	Physically compatible with no change in measured turbidity or increase in particle content in 3 hr at 22 °C	1557	**C**
Meropenem	ZEN	1 mg/ml[b]	BW	4 mg/ml[d]	Visually compatible for 4 hr at room temperature	1994	**C**
	ZEN	50 mg/ml[b]	BW	4 mg/ml[d]	Yellow discoloration forms in 4 hr at room temperature	1994	**I**
Metoclopramide HCl	RB	2 mg/ml[a]	BW	4 mg/ml[a]	Physically compatible for 4 hr at 25 °C under fluorescent light by visual and microscopic examination	1193	**C**
Morphine sulfate	ES	1 mg/ml[a]	BW	4 mg/ml[a]	Physically compatible for 4 hr at 25 °C under fluorescent light by visual and microscopic examination	1193	**C**
Nafcillin sodium	BR	20 mg/ml[a]	BW	4 mg/ml[a]	Physically compatible for 4 hr at 25 °C under fluorescent light by visual and microscopic examination	1193	**C**
Ondansetron HCl	GL	1 mg/ml[b]	BW	4 mg/ml[a]	Physically compatible for 4 hr at 22 °C	1365	**C**
Oxacillin sodium	BR	20 mg/ml[a]	BW	4 mg/ml[a]	Physically compatible for 4 hr at 25 °C under fluorescent light by visual and microscopic examination	1193	**C**
Paclitaxel	NCI	1.2 mg/ml[a]	BW	4 mg/ml[a]	Physically compatible with no change in measured turbidity in 4 hr at 22 °C under fluorescent light	1556	**C**
Pentamidine isethionate	LY	6 mg/ml[a]	BW	4 mg/ml[a]	Physically compatible for 4 hr at 25 °C under fluorescent light by visual and microscopic examination	1193	**C**
Phenylephrine HCl	WI	1 mg/ml[a]	BW	4 mg/ml[a]	Physically compatible for 4 hr at 25 °C under fluorescent light by visual and microscopic examination	1193	**C**
Piperacillin sodium	LE	4 mg/ml[a]	BW	4 mg/ml[a]	Physically compatible for 4 hr at 25 °C under fluorescent light by visual and microscopic examination	1193	**C**
Piperacillin sodium–tazobactam sodium	LE	40 + 5 mg/ml[a]	BW	4 mg/ml[a]	Physically compatible with no change in measured turbidity or increase in particle content in 4 hr at 22 °C	1688	**C**

Y-Site Injection Compatibility (1:1 Mixture) (Cont.)

			Zidovudine				
Drug	*Mfr*	*Conc*	*Mfr*	*Conc*	*Remarks*	*Ref*	*C/I*
Potassium chloride	IMS	0.67 mEq/ml[a]	BW	4 mg/ml[a]	Physically compatible for 4 hr at 25 °C under fluorescent light by visual and microscopic examination	1193	**C**
Ranitidine HCl	GL	1 mg/ml[a]	BW	4 mg/ml[a]	Physically compatible for 4 hr at 25 °C under fluorescent light by visual and microscopic examination	1193	**C**
Remifentanil HCl	GW	0.025 and 0.25 mg/ml[b]	BW	4 mg/ml[a]	Physically compatible with no change in measured turbidity or increase in particle content in 4 hr at 23 °C	2075	**C**
Sargramostim	IMM	10 μg/ml[b]	BW	4 mg/ml[b]	Physically compatible for 4 hr at 22 °C	1436	**C**
Teniposide	BR	0.1 mg/ml[a]	BW	4 mg/ml[a]	Physically compatible with no subvisual haze or particle formation in 4 hr at 23 °C	1725	**C**
Thiotepa	IMM[e]	1 mg/ml[a]	BW	4 mg/ml[a]	Physically compatible with no change in measured turbidity or increase in particle content in 4 hr at 23 °C	1861	**C**
TNA #218 to #226[f]			GW	4 mg/ml[a]	Visually compatible with no precipitate or emulsion damage apparent in 4 hr at 23 °C	2215	**C**
Tobramycin sulfate	LI	2 mg/ml[a]	BW	4 mg/ml[a]	Physically compatible for 4 hr at 25 °C under fluorescent light by visual and microscopic examination	1193	**C**
TPN #212 to #215[f]			BW	4 mg/ml[a]	Physically compatible with no change in measured turbidity or increase in particle content in 4 hr at 23 °C	2109	**C**
Trimethoprim–sulfamethoxazole	BW	0.53 + 2.6 mg/ml[a]	BW	4 mg/ml[a]	Physically compatible for 4 hr at 25 °C under fluorescent light by visual and microscopic examination	1193	**C**
Trimetrexate	WL	1 mg/ml[a]	BW	4 mg/ml[a]	Physically compatible for 4 hr at 25 °C under fluorescent light by visual and microscopic examination	1193	**C**
Vancomycin HCl	LI	15 mg/ml[a]	BW	4 mg/ml[a]	Physically compatible for 4 hr at 25 °C under fluorescent light by visual and microscopic examination	1193	**C**
Vinorelbine tartrate	BW	1 mg/ml[b]	BW	4 mg/ml[b]	Physically compatible with no change in measured turbidity or increase in particle content in 4 hr at 22 °C	1558	**C**

[a]*Tested in dextrose 5% in water.*
[b]*Tested in sodium chloride 0.9%.*
[c]*Sodium bicarbonate 2.5 mEq added to adjust pH.*
[d]*Tested in sterile water for injection.*
[e]*Lyophilized formulation tested.*
[f]*Refer to Appendix I for the composition of parenteral nutrition solutions. TNA indicates a 3-in-1 admixture, and TPN indicates a 2-in-1 admixture.*
[g]*Sodium carbonate–containing formulation tested.*

Additional Compatibility Information

Solutions—— The manufacturer indicates that zidovudine is physically and chemically stable in dextrose 5% in water for 24 hours at room temperature and 48 hours under refrigeration at 2 to 8 °C. However, the manufacturer also recommends that zidovudine diluted for infusion be administered within eight hours if stored at 25 °C or 24 hours if refrigerated because no antibacterial preservative is present in the formulation (2; 4). Other information indicates that the drug is chemically stable diluted for infusion for longer time periods (1411). See Solution Compatibility table above.

DRUGS AVAILABLE
OUTSIDE UNITED STATES

The monographs in this section describe drugs available in much of the world, but not the United States, for which substantial stability and/or compatibility information has been published. The drug names cited in this section are primarily those in use in the United Kingdom. The drug names in use in the United States have been cross-referenced elsewhere in the book.

L-ALANYL-L-GLUTAMINE

Dipeptiven   **Fresenius-Kabi**

Products— Dipeptiven (Fresenius-Kabi) contains the dipeptide *N*(2)-L-alanyl-L-glutamine. The product is available in 50- and 100-ml glass bottles. Each milliliter of solution contains 200 mg of the dipeptide and provides the equivalent of 82 mg of L-alanine and 134.6 mg of L-glutamine. L-Alanyl-L-glutamine solution is a concentrate that must be diluted for administration. For infusion, the product is diluted with at least five times its volume of a suitable amino acid solution or parenteral nutrition solution. The concentration of L-alanyl-L-glutamine should not exceed 3.5% (1-4/96).

pH— From 5.4 to 6.0 (1-4/96).

Osmolarity— The osmolarity of L-alanyl-L-glutamine solution is 921 mOsm/L (1-4/96).

Administration— L-Alanyl-L-glutamine may be administered intravenously after dilution to a concentration not exceeding 3.5%. Each 100 ml of L-alanyl-L-glutamine should be mixed with at least 500 ml of amino acid solution or parenteral nutrition admixture (1-4/96).

Stability— Intact containers of L-alanyl-L-glutamine solution should be stored at room temperature (20 °C) (1-4/96).

Compatibility Information

Solution Compatibility

L-Alanyl-L-glutamine solution

Solution	Mfr	Mfr	Conc/L	Remarks	Ref	C/I
AKE 4 GX		FRE	50 ml	Compatible for 24 hr at room temperature	2047	C
AKE 1100 with glucose		FRE	50 ml	Compatible for 24 hr at room temperature	2047	C
Aminomel 10%		FRE	100 ml	Compatible for 24 hr at room temperature	2047	C
Aminosteril KE 10%		FRE	100 ml	Compatible for 24 hr at room temperature	2047	C
Aminosteril 10%		FRE	100 ml	Compatible for 24 hr at room temperature	2047	C
Combiplasmal 4,5 GXE		FRE	50 ml	Compatible for 24 hr at room temperature	2047	C
Intrafusin 10%		FRE	100 ml	Compatible for 24 hr at room temperature	2047	C
Nutriflex 32/125 G-E		FRE	100 ml	Compatible for 24 hr at room temperature	2047	C
Nutriflex 48/150 G-E		FRE	100 ml	Compatible for 24 hr at room temperature	2047	C
Nutri Twin Forte		FRE	100 ml	Compatible for 24 hr at room temperature	2047	C
Nutri Twin G		FRE	100 ml	Compatible for 24 hr at room temperature	2047	C
Nutri Twin GX		FRE	100 ml	Compatible for 24 hr at room temperature	2047	C
Salviamin 3,5 G-E		FRE	50 ml	Compatible for 24 hr at room temperature	2047	C
Salviamin 3,5 GX-E		FRE	50 ml	Compatible for 24 hr at room temperature	2047	C
Salviamin 3,5 X-E		FRE	50 ml	Compatible for 24 hr at room temperature	2047	C

Additional Compatibility Information

Parenteral Nutrition Admixtures— L-Alanyl-L-glutamine solution in amounts up to 200 ml/L per liter has been reported to be compatible with a wide and varied array of parenteral nutrition admixtures for nine days under refrigeration followed by one day at room temperature. The parenteral nutrition admixtures contained 500 to 1000 ml of the amino acid sources Aminosteril KE 10%, Vamin 14, Vamin 14 EF, Vamin 18 EF, Vamin glucose, and Vamin N. Dextrose sources ranged from 10 to 70%. Lipovenoes 10% PLR or Lipovenoes 20% was incorporated in some combinations. The following electrolytes were also included (2047):

Sodium chloride	20 to 120 mmol/L
Potassium chloride	20 to 90 mmol/L
Sodium glycerophosphate	6.3 to 25 mmol/L
Calcium chloride	1.5 to 7.5 mmol/L
Magnesium sulfate	1.23 to 6.0 mmol/L

AMOXYCILLIN SODIUM

Amoxil   **Bencard**

Products— Amoxycillin sodium (Bencard) is available in vials containing the equivalent of amoxycillin 250 mg, 500 mg, and 1 g (1442).

For intramuscular injection, reconstitute the vials with the following volumes of sterile water for injection (1442):

Vial Size	Volume of Diluent	Final Volume
250 mg	1.5 ml	1.7 ml
500 mg	2.5 ml	2.9 ml
1 g	2.5 ml	3.3 ml

Alternatively, the 1-g vial may be reconstituted with lignocaine HCl 1% or procaine HCl 0.5% (1442).

For intravenous injection, reconstitute the vials with the following volumes of sterile water for injection (1442):

Vial Size	Volume of Diluent	Final Volume
250 mg	5 ml	5.2 ml
500 mg	10 ml	10.4 ml
1 g	20 ml	20.8 ml

For intravenous infusion, the reconstituted drug may be added to an intravenous solution in a minibag or burette chamber of an administration set (1442).

Sodium Content— Amoxycillin sodium contains 3.2 mEq of sodium per gram of drug (1442).

Administration— Amoxycillin sodium may be administered by intramuscular injection, direct intravenous injection over three to four minutes, or intermittent intravenous infusion over 30 to 60 minutes (1442).

Stability— After reconstitution with sterile water for injection, a transient pink color or slight opalescence may appear. Reconstituted solutions are normally a pale straw color (1-9/86). The manufacturers state that the reconstituted solution should be administered or diluted immediately in a suitable infusion solution (1442).

Concentration Effects— Amoxycillin sodium 50 mg/ml is substantially less stable in all infusion solutions than at lower concentrations of 10 or 20 mg/ml (1469).

Freezing Solutions— Amoxycillin sodium 10 mg/ml in sterile water for injection was unstable when stored frozen at between 0 and −20 °C but was stable for 13 days when stored below −30 °C. Amoxycillin sodium 10 mg/ml in sterile water for injection was stable for only two days at 0 °C in the unfrozen state (1470).

McDonald et al. showed that amoxycillin sodium 10 mg/ml in sodium chloride 0.9% was stable for 10.5 days at 0 °C (unfrozen) and for 14 hours when frozen at −19 °C; in dextrose 5% in water, the comparative times were 12.5 and 8.4 hours, respectively (1471).

The processes of freezing and thawing increase the degradation rate of amoxycillin sodium 10 mg/ml in sodium chloride 0.9% in PVC bags (Travenol). Freezing and thawing (natural or microwave) could account for a 5 to 10% loss of amoxycillin; the losses will be affected by the time to reach the equilibrium frozen temperature (1472).

Sorption— Amoxycillin trihydrate (Beecham) 400 mg/L in sodium chloride 0.9% (Travenol) in PVC bags did not exhibit significant sorption to the plastic during one week at room temperature (15 to 20 °C) (536).

Amoxycillin sodium (Beecham) 400 mg/L in sodium chloride 0.9% did not exhibit any loss due to sorption during a seven-hour simulated infusion through an infusion set (Travenol) consisting of a cellulose propionate burette chamber and 170 cm of PVC tubing (606).

The drug also was tested as a simulated infusion over at least one hour by a syringe pump system. A glass syringe on a syringe pump was fitted with 20 cm of polyethylene tubing or 50 cm of Silastic tubing. No drug loss due to sorption was observed with either tubing (606).

A 25-ml aliquot of amoxycillin sodium (Beecham) 400 mg/L in sodium chloride 0.9% was stored in all-plastic syringes composed of polypropylene barrels and polyethylene plungers for 24 hours at room temperature in the dark. The solution did not exhibit any loss due to sorption (606).

Picard et al. reported little or no loss due to sorption of amoxycillin sodium (Beecham) 1 g/100 ml in sodium chloride 0.9% in trilayer solution bags (Bieffe Medital) composed of polyethylene, polyamide, and polypropylene. The admixtures were evaluated by HPLC analysis up to two hours after preparation. Similarly, no loss was found after one hour of simulated infusion (1918).

Filtration— Amoxycillin sodium 1.98 mg/ml in sodium chloride 0.9% was filtered through a 0.22-μm cellulose ester membrane filter (Ivex-HP, Millipore) over five hours. No significant drug loss due to sorption to the filter was noted (1034).

Compatibility Information

Solution Compatibility

Amoxycillin sodium

Solution	Mfr	Mfr	Conc/L	Remarks	Ref	C/I
Compound sodium lactate			10, 20, 50 g	5, 9, and 22% losses at 10, 20, and 50 g/L, respectively, in 6 hr at 25 °C	1469	I
Dextran 40 10% in dextrose 5% in water			10, 20, 50 g	9 to 12% loss in 1 hr at 25 °C	1469	I
Dextran 40 10% in sodium chloride 0.9%			10, 20, 50 g	12, 14, and 20% losses at 10, 20, and 50 g/L, respectively, in 3 hr at 25 °C	1469	I

Solution Compatibility (Cont.)

Amoxycillin sodium

Solution	Mfr	Mfr	Conc/L	Remarks	Ref	C/I
Dextrose 5% in water			1 g	9% loss in 4 hr and 34% loss in 24 hr at room temperature	768	I
			10, 20, 50 g	14 and 18% losses in 3 hr at 10 and 20 g/L, respectively, and 14% loss in 1.5 hr at 50 g/L at 25 °C	1469	I
	a	BE	20 g	No drug loss by HPLC during 2-hr storage and 1-hr simulated infusion	1774	C
Sodium bicarbonate 2.74%			10, 20, 50 g	9% loss in 6 and 4 hr at 10 and 20 g/L, respectively, and 15% loss in 4 hr at 50 g/L at 25 °C	1469	I
Sodium bicarbonate 8.4%			10, 20, 50 g	10 and 13% losses in 4 hr at 10 and 20 g/L, respectively, and 17% loss in 3 hr at 50 g/L at 25 °C	1469	I
Sodium chloride 0.9%			1 g	10% loss in 24 hr at room temperature	768	C
			10, 20, 50 g	3 and 7% losses in 6 hr at 10 and 20 g/L, respectively, and 12% loss in 4 hr at 50 g/L at 25 °C	1469	I
	TR	PR	10 g	Less than 3% loss in 24 hr at 0 °C	1472	C
Sodium chloride 0.9% with potassium chloride 0.3%			10, 20, 50 g	4 and 9% losses in 8 hr at 10 and 20 g/L, respectively, and 9% loss in 3 hr at 50 g/L at 25 °C	1469	I
Sodium lactate ⅙ M			10, 20, 50 g	10% loss in 6 hr at 10 and 20 g/L and 14% loss in 4 hr at 50 g/L at 25 °C	1469	I
Sorbitol 30%			10 and 20 g	11 and 16% losses in 1 hr at 10 and 20 g/L, respectively, at 25 °C	1469	I

[a]*Tested in PVC containers.*

Additive Compatibility

Amoxycillin sodium

Drug	Mfr	Conc/L	Mfr	Conc/L	Test Soln	Remarks	Ref	C/I
Ciprofloxacin		2 g		10 g	a	Immediate precipitation	1473	I
Ofloxacin	HO	1.67 g	BE	8.3 g	W	Visually compatible with little or no loss of either drug by HPLC in 48 hr	1613	C
Pefloxacin		4 g		10 g	D5W, NS	Precipitate forms within 1 hr	1473	I

[a]*Amoxycillin sodium added to ciprofloxacin solution.*

Y-Site Injection Compatibility (1:1 Mixture)

Amoxycillin sodium

Drug	Mfr	Conc	Mfr	Conc	Remarks	Ref	C/I
Lorazepam	WY	0.33 mg/ml[a]	SKB	50 mg/ml	Visually compatible for 24 hr at 22 °C	1855	C
Midazolam HCl	RC	5 mg/ml	SKB	50 mg/ml	White precipitate forms immediately	1855	I
TPN #189[b]				50 mg/ml[a]	Visually compatible for 24 hr at 22 °C	1767	C

[a]*Tested in sodium chloride 0.9%.*
[b]*Refer to Appendix I for the composition of parenteral nutrition solutions. TPN indicates a 2-in-1 admixture.*

Additional Compatibility Information

Solutions— The manufacturer states that amoxycillin sodium is stable in infusion solutions at 25 °C, exhibiting less than 10% degradation in variable time periods depending on concentration (1-9/86):

Intravenous Solution	Amoxycillin Concentration		
	1%	2%	3%
Dextran 40 10% in dextrose 5% in water	1 hr	1 hr	1 hr
Dextran 40 10% in sodium chloride 0.9%	2 hr	1.5 hr	1.5 hr
Dextrose 5% in water	2 hr	1.5 hr	1 hr
Ringer's injection, lactated	6 hr	6 hr	3 hr
Sodium chloride 0.18% in dextrose 4%	2 hr	1.5 hr	1 hr
Sodium chloride 0.9%	8 hr	8 hr	3 hr
Sodium chloride 0.9% with potassium chloride 0.3%	8 hr	8 hr	3 hr
Sodium lactate ⅙ M	6 hr	6 hr	3 hr

Aminoglycosides— The manufacturers state that amoxycillin sodium should not be mixed with aminoglycoside antibiotics in the same syringe, intravenous infusion container, or set because aminoglycoside activity may be lost (1442).

AMOXYCILLIN SODIUM–CLAVULANIC ACID (CO-AMOXICLAV)

Augmentin Intravenous   **SmithKline Beecham**

Products— Amoxycillin sodium–clavulanic acid (SmithKline Beecham) is available in 600-mg vials containing amoxycillin sodium 500 mg and clavulanic acid 100 mg as the potassium salt and in 1.2-g vials containing amoxycillin sodium 1 g and clavulanic acid 200 mg as the potassium salt. Reconstitute the 600-mg vials with 10 ml and the 1.2-g vials with 20 ml of sterile water for injection (1442).

Sodium and Potassium Content— Amoxycillin sodium–clavulanic acid contains 3.1 mEq of sodium and 1 mEq of potassium in 1.2 g of drug product (1442).

Administration— Amoxycillin sodium–clavulanic acid may be administered by intravenous injection or intermittent infusion. It is not suitable for intramuscular administration. When given by intravenous injection directly into a vein or via a drip tube, it should be injected slowly over three to four minutes. For intravenous infusion, add the contents of the 600-mg or 1.2-g vial to 50 or 100 ml, respectively, of sterile water for injection or sodium chloride 0.9% and then infuse over 30 to 40 minutes, completing the administration within four hours of reconstitution (1442).

Stability— The manufacturer states that the injection should be used within 20 minutes after reconstitution with sterile water for injection (1442).

Ashwin et al. reported that the stability of amoxycillin sodium–clavulanic acid is governed by the more rapid degradation of clavulanic acid compared with amoxycillin. Amoxycillin sodium–clavulanic acid 1.2 g reconstituted with 20 ml of sterile water for injection and added to 100 ml of sodium chloride 0.9% in PVC bags showed 10% degradation of amoxycillin in 390 minutes and of clavulanic acid in 261 minutes at 25 °C. However, the drug was more stable when stored at 5 °C. Amoxycillin sodium–clavulanic acid 1.2 g reconstituted with 20 ml of sterile water for injection and added to 100 ml of sterile water for injection, sodium chloride 0.9%, or dextrose 5% in water lost 10% activity in 15, 12.5, and 1.2 hours, respectively, when stored at 5 °C (1474).

Stability is also concentration dependent; amoxycillin sodium–clavulanic acid is less stable in high concentrations. Therefore, it is suggested that reconstituted solutions be used immediately or diluted without delay (1474).

Freezing Solutions— Amoxycillin sodium–clavulanic acid 1.2 g reconstituted with 20 ml and diluted in 100 ml of sterile water for injection was frozen at −20 °C for four hours, followed by microwave thawing. Solutions retained only 65% of the initial clavulanic acid content (1474).

Sorption— Amoxycillin sodium–clavulanic acid 1.2 g in 100 ml of sodium chloride 0.9% stored at 25 °C in PVC bags (Baxter) did not show evidence of sorption compared to solutions stored in glass containers. Furthermore, identical solutions infused at 1 ml/min through a standard administration set (Continuflo, Baxter) did not show drug loss due to sorption (1474).

Compatibility Information

Solution Compatibility

Amoxycillin sodium–clavulanic acid

Solution	Mfr	Mfr	Conc/L	Remarks	Ref	C/I
Dextrose 5% in water	BT[a]	BE	8.33 + 1.67 g	Physically compatible with 10% loss within 30 min at 25 °C and 1.2 hr at 5 °C	1474	I

Solution Compatibility (Cont.)

Amoxycillin sodium–clavulanic acid

Solution	Mfr	Mfr	Conc/L	Remarks	Ref	C/I
Ringer's injection	BT[a]	BE	8.33 + 1.67 g	Physically compatible with 10% loss in 4.1 hr at 25 °C	1474	I[b]
Ringer's injection, lactated	BT[a]	BE	8.33 + 1.67 g	Physically compatible with 10% loss in 4.1 hr	1474	I[b]
Sodium chloride 0.9%	BT[a]	BE	8.33 + 1.67 g	Physically compatible with 10% loss in 4.4 hr at 25 °C and 12.5 hr at 5 °C	1474	I[b]
Sodium chloride 0.9% with potassium chloride 0.3%	BT[a]	BE	8.33 + 1.67 g	Physically compatible with 10% loss in 3.9 hr at 25 °C	1474	I[b]
Sodium lactate ⅙ M	BT[a]	BE	8.33 + 1.67 g	Physically compatible with 10% loss in 4.3 hr at 25 °C	1474	I[b]

[a]*Tested in polyethylene containers.*
[b]*Incompatible by conventional standards; may be used in shorter time periods.*

Additive Compatibility

Amoxycillin sodium–clavulanic acid

Drug	Mfr	Conc/L	Mfr	Conc/L	Test Soln	Remarks	Ref	C/I
Ciprofloxacin		2 g		10 + 2 g	[a]	Immediate precipitation	1473	I
Metronidazole	BAY	5 g	BE	20 + 2 g		Physically compatible with 8% clavulanate loss in 2 hr and 25% loss in 6 hr at 21 °C by HPLC. 7 to 8% amoxycillin and no metronidazole loss in 6 hr at 21 °C.	1920	I
Ofloxacin	HO	1.67 g	BE	8.33 + 1.67 g	W	Visually compatible with little or no loss of either drug by HPLC in 48 hr	1613	C
Pefloxacin		4 g		10 + 2 g	D5W, NS	Precipitate forms within 1 hr	1473	I

[a]*Amoxycillin sodium–clavulanic acid added to ciprofloxacin solution.*

Y-Site Injection Compatibility (1:1 Mixture)

Amoxycillin sodium–clavulanic acid

Drug	Mfr	Conc	Mfr	Conc	Remarks	Ref	C/I
Clarithromycin	AB	4 mg/ml[a]	BE	20 + 4 mg/ml[a]	Visually compatible for 72 hr at both 30 and 17 °C	2174	C
Lorazepam	WY	0.33 mg/ml[b]	SKB	20 + 2 mg/ml	Visually compatible for 24 hr at 22 °C	1855	C
Midazolam HCl	RC	5 mg/ml	SKB	20 + 2 mg/ml	White precipitate formed immediately	1855	I

[a]*Tested in dextrose 5% in water.*
[b]*Tested in sodium chloride 0.9%.*

Additional Compatibility Information

Solutions—— Amoxycillin sodium–clavulanic acid should not be added to infusion solutions containing dextrose, dextran, sodium bicarbonate, blood products, proteinaceous fluids, or intravenous fat emulsions (1442).

Ashwin et al. reported that administration should be completed within the following periods after further dilution in infusion solutions and storage at room temperature (25 °C) (1474):

Ringer's injection	3 hr
Ringer's injection, lactated	3 hr
Sodium chloride 0.9%	4 hr

Sodium chloride 0.9% with potassium chloride 0.3%	3 hr
Sodium lactate ⅙ M	4 hr

The manufacturer indicates that infusions of amoxycillin sodium–clavulanic acid in sterile water for injection or sodium chloride 0.9% are stable at 5 °C for up to eight hours. Amoxycillin sodium–clavulanic acid is less stable in dextrose, dextran, or bicarbonate-containing infusion solutions and should not be added to them. However, it may be injected into the tubing of running infusions of these solutions (1442).

Aminoglycosides—— The manufacturer states that amoxycillin sodium–clavulanic acid should not be mixed in a syringe, intravenous fluid container, or administration set with aminoglycosides because of possible aminoglycoside activity loss (1).

AMSACRINE
(ACRIDINYL ANISIDIDE; m-AMSA)

Amsidine Concentrate for Infusion   **Gold Shield**

Products—— Amsacrine (Gold Shield) is available in ampuls containing 1.5 ml of a 50-mg/ml solution (75 mg total) in anhydrous N,N-dimethylacetamide. It is packaged with a vial containing 13.5 ml of 0.0353 M L-lactic acid diluent (1442).

To prepare the drug for use, aseptically add 1.5 ml of the amsacrine solution to the vial of L-lactic acid diluent. The resulting orange-red solution contains amsacrine 5 mg/ml in 10% (v/v) N,N-dimethylacetamide and 0.0318 M L-lactic acid. This concentrated solution must be diluted in dextrose 5% in water for infusion; do not use chloride-containing solutions (234; 1442).

Direct contact of amsacrine solutions with skin or mucous membranes may result in skin sensitization and should be avoided (234).

Administration—— Amsacrine is administered intravenously over 60 to 90 minutes after the dose is diluted in 500 ml of dextrose 5% in water (1442).

Stability—— In intact ampuls, amsacrine is stable for three years at room temperature when protected from light (1442). When mixed with the L-lactic acid diluent, the amsacrine solution is physically and chemically stable for at least 48 hours at room temperature under ambient light (234).

Effects of Light— The effect of diffuse daylight and fluorescent light on amsacrine 150 μg/ml in dextrose 5% in water was studied for 48 hours at 19 to 21 °C; no loss due to light exposure occurred. The authors concluded that light protection has no relevance to the normal clinical use of amsacrine (1308). Nevertheless, protection from direct sunlight is recommended (1442).

Sorption— Amsacrine 150 μg/ml in dextrose 5% in water was evaluated for sorption to cellulose propionate and methacrylate butadiene styrene burette chambers and PVC and polybutadiene tubing. No amsacrine loss due to sorption was found during 48 hours at 19 to 21 °C (1308).

Compatibility Information

Solution Compatibility

Amsacrine

Solution	Mfr	Mfr	Conc/L	Remarks	Ref	C/I
Dextrose 5% in water		PD	150 mg[a]	Physically compatible with little or no loss in 48 hr at 20 °C exposed to light	1308	C
		NCI	150 mg	Physically compatible and chemically stable for at least 48 hours at room temperature under ambient light	234	C

[a]*Tested in burette chambers composed of cellulose propionate, PVC, or methacrylate butadiene styrene.*

Additive Compatibility

Amsacrine

Drug	Mfr	Conc/L	Mfr	Conc/L	Test Soln	Remarks	Ref	C/I
Sodium bicarbonate		2 mEq	NCI	a	D5W	Amsacrine chemically stable for 96 hr at room temperature	234	**C**

aConcentration unspecified.

Y-Site Injection Compatibility (1:1 Mixture)

Amsacrine

Drug	Mfr	Conc	Mfr	Conc	Remarks	Ref	C/I
Acyclovir sodium	BW	7 mg/ml[a]	NCI	1 mg/ml[a]	Immediate dark orange turbidity, becoming brownish orange in 1 hr	1381	**I**
Amikacin sulfate	BR	5 mg/ml[a]	NCI	1 mg/ml[a]	Physically compatible for 4 hr at room temperature under fluorescent light	1381	**C**
Amphotericin B	SQ	0.6 mg/ml[a]	NCI	1 mg/ml[a]	Immediate light yellow turbidity, becoming yellow flocculent precipitate in 15 min	1381	**I**
Aztreonam	SQ	40 mg/ml[a]	NCI	1 mg/ml[a]	Immediate light yellow-orange turbidity, developing into flocculent precipitate in 4 hr	1381	**I**
Ceftazidime	GL[c]	40 mg/ml[a]	NCI	1 mg/ml[a]	Light flocculent orange precipitate forms immediately, becoming heavier with time	1381	**I**
Ceftriaxone sodium	RC	40 mg/ml[a]	NCI	1 mg/ml[a]	Immediate orange turbidity, developing into flocculent precipitate in 4 hr	1381	**I**
Chlorpromazine HCl	ES	2 mg/ml[a]	NCI	1 mg/ml[a]	Physically compatible for 4 hr at room temperature under fluorescent light	1381	**C**
Cimetidine HCl	SKF	12 mg/ml[a]	NCI	1 mg/ml[a]	Initially clear, but yellow-orange turbidity develops in 1 hr, becoming flocculent precipitate in 4 hr	1381	**I**
Clindamycin phosphate	UP	10 mg/ml[a]	NCI	1 mg/ml[a]	Physically compatible for 4 hr at room temperature under fluorescent light	1381	**C**
Cytarabine	QU	50 mg/ml	NCI	1 mg/ml[a]	Physically compatible for 4 hr at room temperature under fluorescent light	1381	**C**
Dexamethasone sodium phosphate	QU	1 mg/ml[a]	NCI	1 mg/ml[a]	Physically compatible for 4 hr at room temperature under fluorescent light	1381	**C**
Diphenhydramine HCl	PD	2 mg/ml[a]	NCI	1 mg/ml[a]	Physically compatible for 4 hr at room temperature under fluorescent light	1381	**C**
Famotidine	MSD	2 mg/ml[a]	NCI	1 mg/ml[a]	Physically compatible for 4 hr at room temperature under fluorescent light	1381	**C**
Fludarabine phosphate	BX	1 mg/ml[a]	NCI	1 mg/ml[a]	Physically compatible for 4 hr at room temperature under fluorescent light	1439	**C**
Furosemide	ES	3 mg/ml[a]	NCI	1 mg/ml[a]	Heavy yellow-orange turbidity forms initially, becoming colorless liquid with yellow precipitate	1381	**I**
Ganciclovir sodium	SY	20 mg/ml[a]	NCI	1 mg/ml[a]	Immediate dark orange turbidity	1381	**I**
Gentamicin sulfate	SO	5 mg/ml[a]	NCI	1 mg/ml[a]	Physically compatible for 4 hr at room temperature under fluorescent light	1381	**C**

Y-Site Injection Compatibility (1:1 Mixture) (Cont.)

Amsacrine

Drug	Mfr	Conc	Mfr	Conc	Remarks	Ref	C/I
Granisetron HCl	SKB	0.05 mg/ml[a]	NCI	1 mg/ml[a]	Physically compatible with no change in measured turbidity or increase in particle content in 4 hr at 23 °C. Precipitate forms in 24 hr	2000	C
Haloperidol lactate	MN	0.2 mg/ml[a]	NCI	1 mg/ml[a]	Physically compatible for 4 hr at room temperature under fluorescent light	1381	C
Heparin sodium	SO	40 units/ml[a]	NCI	1 mg/ml[a]	Light flocculent orange precipitate forms immediately	1381	I
Hydrocortisone sodium succinate	UP	1 mg/ml[a]	NCI	1 mg/ml[a]	Physically compatible for 4 hr at room temperature under fluorescent light	1381	C
Hydromorphone HCl	AST	0.5 mg/ml[a]	NCI	1 mg/ml[a]	Physically compatible for 4 hr at room temperature under fluorescent light	1381	C
Lorazepam	WY	0.1 mg/ml[a]	NCI	1 mg/ml[a]	Physically compatible for 4 hr at room temperature under fluorescent light	1381	C
Methylprednisolone sodium succinate	UP	5 mg/ml[a]	NCI	1 mg/ml[a]	Immediate orange turbidity and precipitate in 4 hr	1381	I
Metoclopramide HCl	RB	2.5 mg/ml[a]	NCI	1 mg/ml[a]	Yellow-orange turbidity develops in 15 min, becoming heavy flocculent orange precipitate in 1 hr	1381	I
Morphine sulfate	ES	1 mg/ml[a]	NCI	1 mg/ml[a]	Physically compatible for 4 hr at room temperature under fluorescent light	1381	C
Ondansetron HCl	GL	1 mg/ml[a]	NCI	1 mg/ml[a]	Orange precipitate forms within 30 min	1365	I
Prochlorperazine edisylate	SKF	0.5 mg/ml[a]	NCI	1 mg/ml[a]	Physically compatible for 4 hr at room temperature under fluorescent light	1381	C
Promethazine HCl	ES	2 mg/ml[a]	NCI	1 mg/ml[a]	Physically compatible for 4 hr at room temperature under fluorescent light	1381	C
Ranitidine HCl	GL	2 mg/ml[a]	NCI	1 mg/ml[a]	Physically compatible for 4 hr at room temperature under fluorescent light	1381	C
Sargramostim	IMM	10 μg/ml[a]	NCI	1 mg/ml[a]	Physically compatible for 4 hr at 22 °C under fluorescent light	1436	C
	IMM	10 μg/ml[b]	NCI	1 mg/ml[a]	Immediate haze with heavy yellow flocculent precipitate in 30 min	1436	I
Tobramycin sulfate	LI	5 mg/ml[a]	NCI	1 mg/ml[a]	Physically compatible for 4 hr at room temperature under fluorescent light	1381	C
Vancomycin HCl	LI	10 mg/ml[a]	NCI	1 mg/ml[a]	Physically compatible for 4 hr at room temperature under fluorescent light	1381	C

[a]*Tested in dextrose 5% in water.*
[b]*Tested in sodium chloride 0.9%.*
[c]*Sodium carbonate–containing formulation tested.*

Additional Compatibility Information

Chloride-Containing Solutions— Amsacrine is physically incompatible with sodium chloride 0.9% and other chloride-containing solutions. The hydrochloride salt is poorly soluble, and precipitation may result (234; 1442).

Evacuated flasks may contain a small amount of chloride-containing solution from the manufacturing process. This residual chloride ion caused precipitation when amsacrine solutions were prepared in evacuated flasks (234).

Other Information

Glass Syringes— Glass syringes are recommended for the transfer of amsacrine concentrate to the L-lactic acid diluent (1442). The *N,N*-dimethylacetamide solvent may extract UV-absorbing species from plastics and rubber used in plastic syringes (967).

AZLOCILLIN SODIUM

Securopen   **Bayer**

Products— Azlocillin sodium (Bayer) is available in vials and infusion bottles containing 1, 2, or 5 g. Reconstitute each gram of drug with at least 10 ml of sterile water for injection, dextrose 5% in water, or sodium chloride 0.9%. For infusion, the reconstituted drug is diluted further to the desired volume with a compatible diluent (1442).

pH— From 6 to 8 (1442).

Osmolality— The osmolality of azlocillin sodium 3 and 4 g was calculated for the following dilutions (1054):

Diluent	Osmolality (mOsm/kg)	
	50 ml	100 ml
3 g		
Dextrose 5% in water	490	372
Sodium chloride 0.9%	554	426
4 g		
Dextrose 5% in water	568	411
Sodium chloride 0.9%	622	465

Robinson et al. recommended the following maximum azlocillin sodium concentrations to achieve osmolalities suitable for peripheral infusion in fluid-restricted patients (1180):

Diluent	Maximum Concentration (mg/ml)	Osmolality (mOsm/kg)
Dextrose 5% in water	82	519
Sodium chloride 0.9%	74	508
Sterile water for injection	148	408

Sodium Content— Each gram of azlocillin contains 2.17 mEq (49.8 mg) of sodium (1442).

Administration— Azlocillin sodium is administered intermittently by slow intravenous injection over five minutes or longer or by intravenous infusion over 20 to 30 minutes in about 50 to 100 ml of compatible infusion solution (1442).

Stability— Azlocillin sodium is a white to pale yellow powder, which yields a colorless to pale yellow solution on reconstitution. Reconstituted solutions are stable for six hours at room temperature (1442).

Freezing Solutions— Tidy el al. reported the stability of azlocillin sodium (Bayer) 50 mg/ml in sodium chloride 0.9% frozen at −20 °C for up to six months and thawed by exposure to microwaves while rotating in the horizontal and vertical axes simultaneously. HPLC analysis showed little or no loss after six months, with no extraction of plasticizer or increase in subvisual particulates (1440).

Compatibility Information

Solution Compatibility

Azlocillin sodium

Solution	Mfr	Mfr	Conc/L	Remarks	Ref	C/I
Dextrose 5% in water	TR[a], GRI[b]	BAY	10 g	More than 10% loss in 24 hr at 25 °C by UV spectroscopy	1900	**I**
Fructose 5% in water	TR[a], GRI[b]	BAY	10 g	10% loss in about 4 days at 25 °C by UV spectroscopy	1900	**C**
Ringer's injection, lactated	TR[a], GRI[b]	BAY	10 g	More than 10% loss in 24 hr at 25 °C by UV spectroscopy	1900	**I**

Solution Compatibility (Cont.)

Azlocillin sodium

Solution	Mfr	Mfr	Conc/L	Remarks	Ref	C/I
Sodium chloride 0.9%	TR[a], GRI[b]	BAY	10 g	10% loss in about 6 days at 25 °C by UV spectroscopy	1900	**C**
TPN #107[c]			2 g	26% azlocillin loss in 24 hr at 21 °C by microbiological assay	1326	**I**

[a]Tested in PVC containers.
[b]Tested in glass containers.
[c]Refer to Appendix I for the composition of parenteral nutrition solutions. TPN indicates a 2-in-1 admixture.

Additive Compatibility

Azlocillin sodium

Drug	Mfr	Conc/L	Mfr	Conc/L	Test Soln	Remarks	Ref	C/I
Verapamil HCl	SE	[a]	MI	40 g	D5W, NS	Physically compatible for 24 hr at 21 °C under fluorescent light	1166	**C**

[a]Final concentration unspecified.

Drugs in Syringe Compatibility

Azlocillin sodium

Drug (in syringe)	Mfr	Amt	Mfr	Amt	Remarks	Ref	C/I
Heparin sodium		2500 units/ 1 ml		2 g	Physically compatible for at least 5 min	1053	**C**

Y-Site Injection Compatibility (1:1 Mixture)

Azlocillin sodium

Drug	Mfr	Conc	Mfr	Conc	Remarks	Ref	C/I
Cyclophosphamide	MJ	20 mg/ml[a]	MI	20 mg/ml[a]	Physically compatible for 4 hr at 25 °C	1194	**C**
Perphenazine	SC	0.02 mg/ml[a]	MI	20 mg/ml[a]	Physically compatible for 4 hr at 25 °C	1155	**C**
TPN #54[b]				133 and 200 mg/ml	Physically compatible and azlocillin activity retained over 6 hr at 22 °C by microbiological assay	1045	**C**
TPN #61[b]		[c]	MI	250 mg/ 2.5 ml[d]	Physically compatible	1012	**C**
		[e]	MI	1.5 mg/ 15 ml[d]	Physically compatible	1012	**C**
Verapamil HCl	SE	2.5 mg/ml	MI	40 mg/ml[a]	Physically compatible for 15 min at 21 °C under fluorescent light	1166	**C**

[a]Tested in dextrose 5% in water.
[b]Refer to Appendix I for the composition of parenteral nutrition solutions. TPN indicates a 2-in-1 admixture.
[c]Run at 21 ml/hr.
[d]Given over five minutes by syringe pump.
[e]Run at 94 ml/hr.

Additional Compatibility Information

Vehicles— Azlocillin sodium is stated to be stable and compatible with the following infusion solutions (1442):

Dextrose 5 and 10% in water
Fructose 5%
Ringer's injection
Sodium chloride 0.9%

Peritoneal Dialysis Solutions— The stability of azlocillin sodium (Miles) 200 mg/L in peritoneal dialysis solutions (Dianeal 137 and PD2) with heparin sodium 500 units/L was evaluated at 25 °C by microbiological assay. Approximately 95 ± 7% activity remained after 24 hours (1228).

Aminoglycosides— Mixing azlocillin sodium with aminoglycoside antibiotics is not recommended by the manufacturer (2).

Pickering and Rutherford evaluated several aminoglycosides combined with a number of penicillins. Gentamicin sulfate, netilmicin sulfate, and tobramycin sulfate 5 and 10 μg/ml and amikacin 10 and 20 μg/ml were combined in human serum with 125, 250, and 500 μg/ml of azlocillin, carbenicillin disodium, amdinocillin, mezlocillin, and piperacillin individually. Tobramycin and gentamicin sustained greater losses than netilmicin and amikacin at each of the penicillin concentrations. Significant decomposition of all aminoglycosides occurred in 24 hours at 37 °C at a penicillin concentration of 500 μg/ml. Tobramycin and gentamicin had losses of 40 to 60%, while 15 to 30% losses occurred for netilmicin. Amikacin sustained the least inactivation with losses of about 10 to 20%. At penicillin concentrations of 125 to 250 μg/ml, smaller losses of aminoglycosides were observed (68).

Several aminoglycosides were evaluated in combination with several penicillins. Gentamicin sulfate, netilmicin sulfate, and tobramycin sulfate, 5 μg/ml, were combined with carbenicillin disodium, azlocillin sodium, and mezlocillin sodium, 50, 250, and 500 μg/ml, in human plasma. Samples were evaluated over nine days at 27 and 37 °C. All of the aminoglycosides underwent significant inactivation during the study. Aminoglycoside decomposition of 17 to 61% in 24 hours occurred at the higher two concentrations of penicillins—the highest inactivation was sustained by tobramycin and the lowest by netilmicin. Little if any aminoglycoside inactivation occurred at 50 μg/ml of penicillin. Carbenicillin caused a greater degree of aminoglycoside decomposition than did azlocillin or mezlocillin (616).

Roberts et al. studied the stability of azlocillin sodium 500 mg/L combined with the aminoglycosides amikacin sulfate 20 mg/L, gentamicin sulfate 8 mg/L, and netilmicin sulfate 7.5 mg/L in peritoneal dialysis solution (Dianeal 1.36%) stored at 37 °C. No azlocillin sodium loss occurred by HPLC during the eight-hour study period. However, the aminoglycosides tested by the enzyme-multiplied immunoassay technique (EMIT) showed 10% losses in about six hours for gentamicin sulfate and netilmicin sulfate and in about 30 minutes for amikacin sulfate (1179).

The inactivation of gentamicin, tobramycin, and amikacin, each 5 μg/ml, by seven β-lactam antibiotics, 250 and 500 μg/ml, in serum at 25 °C over 24 hours was studied using bioassay, enzyme-mediated immunoassay (EMIT), fluorescence polarization immunoassay (TDx), and radioimmunoassay (RIA) techniques. Results with the penicillins varied, depending on the assay technique used. The bioassay was the most sensitive to loss, TDx and RIA were intermediate, and EMIT was the least sensitive. Azlocillin, carbenicillin, mezlocillin, and piperacillin all cause variable but extensive inactivation (up to 70%) of gentamicin and tobramycin in 24 hours. Amikacin, however, had only minor losses compared to the other aminoglycosides (654).

The clinical significance of these interactions in patients appears to be primarily confined to those with renal failure (218; 334; 361; 364; 616; 814; 847). Literature reports of greatly reduced aminoglycoside levels in such patients have appeared frequently (303; 365–367; 614; 615; 962). In addition, the interaction may be clinically important if assays for aminoglycoside levels in serum are sufficiently delayed (576; 618; 824; 847; 1052).

Most authors believe that in vitro mixing of penicillins such as azlocillin sodium with aminoglycoside antibiotics should be avoided but that clinical use of the drugs in combination can be of great value. It is generally recommended that the drugs be given separately in such combined therapy (157; 218; 222; 224; 361; 364; 368–370).

CEFPIROME SULFATE

Cefrom **Aventis**

Products— Cefpirome sulfate (Aventis) is available in 1- and 2-g vials for intravenous injection. Each vial also contains anhydrous sodium carbonate 242 mg per gram of cefpirome (1442).

For intravenous use, reconstitute the vials with the following volumes of sterile water for injection. The reconstituted drug may be diluted further in a compatible infusion solution (1442):

Vial Size	Volume of Diluent	Final Volume
1 g	10 ml	10.7 ml
2 g	20 ml	21.4 ml

The 1- and 2-g intravenous infusion bottles should be reconstituted with 100 ml of sterile water for injection or other compatible infusion solution (1442).

Although the vials have a slight negative pressure, reconstitution releases carbon dioxide, increasing the pressure in the vial. Effervescence occurs during dissolution, and the container should be tipped gently from side to side for approximately one minute to assure complete dissolution of the drug. The reconstituted solution may still retain some bubbles of carbon dioxide, but these have no adverse effects on efficacy (1442).

Sodium Content— Cefpirome sulfate contains 4.7 mEq (107 mg) of sodium per gram of drug (1442).

Administration— Cefpirome sulfate may be administered by intravenous injection over three to five minutes or by intermittent intravenous infusion over 20 to 30 minutes (1442).

Stability— Intact containers of cefpirome sulfate should be stored at 25 °C or below and protected from light. The drug is a white to pale yellow powder that becomes a faint yellow to yellow solution upon reconstitution. Some color intensification of both the powder and its solutions may occur during storage. However, this does not indicate a change in potency or safety (1442).

The manufacturer recommends storage of the reconstituted solution under refrigeration at 2 to 8 °C and use within 24 hours.

Compatibility Information

Y-Site Injection Compatibility (1:1 Mixture)

		Cefpirome sulfate					
Drug	Mfr	Conc	Mfr	Conc	Remarks	Ref	C/I
Amikacin sulfate	APC	0.5 mg/ml[a]	HO	50 mg/ml[a]	Visually and microscopically compatible with less than 6% cefpirome loss and less than 10% amikacin loss by HPLC in 8 hr at 23 °C	2044	C
Amphotericin B	SQ	0.1 mg/ml[a]	HO	50 mg/ml[a]	Little or no cefpirome loss but up to 45% amphotericin B loss by HPLC in 4 hr at 23 °C	2044	I
Cefazolin sodium	LI	10 mg/ml[a]	HO	50 mg/ml[a]	Visually and microscopically compatible with 7% or less cefpirome loss and little or no cefazolin loss by HPLC in 8 hr at 23 °C	2044	C
Clindamycin phosphate	AB	12 mg/ml[a]	HO	50 mg/ml[a]	Visually and microscopically compatible with 5% or less cefpirome loss and 4% or less clindamycin loss by HPLC in 8 hr at 23 °C	2044	C
Dexamethasone sodium phosphate	LY	4 mg/ml[a]	HO	50 mg/ml[a]	Visually and microscopically compatible with 5% or less cefpirome loss and little or no dexamethasone loss by HPLC in 8 hr at 23 °C	2044	C
Dopamine HCl	AB	0.8 mg/ml[a]	HO	50 mg/ml[a]	Visually and microscopically compatible with 7% or less cefpirome loss and 6% or less dopamine loss by HPLC in 8 hr at 23 °C	2044	C
Fluconazole	RR	2 mg/ml[a]	HO	50 mg/ml[a]	Visually and microscopically compatible with little or no cefpirome loss and 8% or less fluconazole loss by HPLC in 8 hr at 23 °C	2044	C
Gentamicin sulfate	LY	1 mg/ml[a]	HO	50 mg/ml[a]	Visually and microscopically compatible with little or no cefpirome and cefazolin loss by HPLC in 8 hr at 23 °C	2044	C
Vancomycin HCl	AB	5 mg/ml[a]	HO	50 mg/ml[a]	Visually and microscopically compatible with little or no cefpirome and vancomycin loss by HPLC in 8 hr at 23 °C	2044	C

[a]Tested in dextrose 5% in water, Ringer's injection, lactated, sodium chloride 0.45%, and sodium chloride 0.9%.

Additional Compatibility Information

Infusion Solutions— The manufacturer states that cefpirome sulfate is chemically stable and physically compatible for 24 hours stored under refrigeration at 2 to 8 °C in the following solutions (1442):
Dextrose 5% in water
Dextrose 10% in water
Fructose 5% in water
Ringer's injection
Sodium chloride 0.9%
Sterile water for injection

Cefpirome sulfate should not be administered in sodium bicarbonate injection (1442).

CHLORMETHIAZOLE EDISYLATE

Heminevrin 0.8% Infusion **AstraZeneca**

Products— Chlormethiazole edisylate (AstraZeneca) is available in 500-ml glass infusion bottles. Each milliliter contains (1442):

Chlormethiazole edisylate	8 mg
Dextrose	40 mg
Sodium hydroxide	to adjust pH

Sodium Content— Chlormethiazole edisylate contains 0.032 mEq of sodium per milliliter (1442).

Administration— Chlormethiazole edisylate 0.8% is administered by infusion using an infusion pump or other apparatus to control the flow rate. In general, the infusion is given as a loading dose followed by a maintenance dose (1442).

Stability— Chlormethiazole edisylate 0.8% infusion is stored under refrigeration (1442).

Sorption— The manufacturer states that chlormethiazole edisylate is sorbed to PVC administration sets, resulting in some concentration loss before the drug reaches the patient (1442).

Chlormethiazole edisylate (Astra) 8 g/L in the infusion solution supplied by the manufacturer and placed into PVC bags (Travenol) exhibited approximately a 33% loss in 24 hours and a 43% loss in one week at room temperature (15 to 20 °C) due to sorption (536).

Chlormethiazole edisylate (Astra) 8 g/L in the infusion solution supplied by the manufacturer was delivered through a polyethylene administration set (Tridilset) over eight hours at 15 to 20 °C. The flow rate was 1 ml/min. No appreciable loss due to sorption occurred (769).

This result is in contrast to that of a study using conventional PVC sets. Chlormethiazole edisylate (Astra) 8 g/L in the infusion solution supplied by the manufacturer exhibited a cumulative 34% loss due to sorption during a seven-hour simulated infusion through an infusion set (Travenol) consisting of a cellulose propionate burette chamber and 170 cm of PVC tubing. Both the burette chamber and the tubing contributed to the loss. The extent of sorption increased with increasing concentration (606).

Chlormethiazole edisylate (Astra) 8 g/L in the infusion solution supplied by the manufacturer was delivered at a flow rate of 0.8 ml/min through a polybutadiene set, with and without a methacrylate butadiene styrene burette chamber (Avon Medical). For tests in the burette sets, 150 ml was run into the burette before simulated administration was begun. Losses of chlormethiazole to polybutadiene sets were 7 to 13%. Drug delivery was not affected by the burette. In contrast, losses up to 50% to PVC sets were observed (1027).

In a similar study, losses due to sorption of chlormethiazole edisylate infusion to a volume infusion set (Ivac), blood administration set (Travenol), and Metriset (McGaw) were investigated. Flow rates were 1.25 to 2.5 ml/min. Following 500 ml of infusion, the average recoveries of chlormethiazole were 78.5, 82.2, and 71.2%, respectively (1446).

The drug was also tested as a simulated infusion over at least one hour by a syringe pump system. A glass syringe on a syringe pump was fitted with 20 cm of polyethylene tubing or 50 cm of Silastic tubing. A negligible amount of drug was lost with the polyethylene tubing, but a cumulative 32% loss occurred during the one-hour infusion through the Silastic tubing (606).

A 25-ml aliquot of chlormethiazole edisylate (Astra) 8 g/L in the supplied infusion solution, stored in all-plastic syringes composed of polypropylene barrels and polyethylene plungers (Pharma-Plast, AHS Australia) for 24 hours at room temperature in the dark, did not exhibit any loss due to sorption (606). These same syringes were compared with glass containers in an investigation of the possible sorption of the drug. After 24 hours of storage of aqueous solutions of chlormethiazole edisylate (concentration unspecified), no drug loss was found in either the plastic syringes or glass containers. The authors indicated that these plastic syringes could be substituted for glass syringes for use with syringe pumps (782).

Other Information

It was reported that PVC bags containing chlormethiazole edisylate solutions become softer and more pliable during storage. The distinctive odor of the solution was also detectable in the immediate vicinity of the bags (536). Penetration of chlormethiazole edisylate through the walls of silicone catheters might be responsible for the high incidence of thrombophlebitis (1447). The manufacturer recommends that a glass syringe connected to a Teflon intravenous cannula using a polyethylene extension set be used for administration to small children (1442).

CHLORPHENIRAMINE MALEATE (CHLORPHENAMINE MALEATE)

Piriton **Link Pharmaceuticals**

Products— Chlorpheniramine maleate (Link Pharmaceuticals) is available in 1-ml ampuls containing 10 mg/ml of drug along with sodium chloride in water for injection (1442).

pH— From 4 to 5.2 (4).

Osmolality— Chlorpheniramine maleate 10 mg/ml has an osmolality of 44 mOsm/kg (1689).

Administration— Chlorpheniramine maleate 10 mg/ml may be administered by subcutaneous, intramuscular, or intravenous injection slowly over a period of one minute (1442). Intradermal injection is not recommended (4). The 100-mg/ml injection should not be given intravenously (154).

Stability— Intact containers of chlorpheniramine maleate should be stored below 25 °C and protected from light (1442). The injection may be stored at room temperature or under refrigeration; freezing should be avoided (4).

Compatibility Information

Additive Compatibility

Chlorpheniramine maleate

Drug	Mfr	Conc/L	Mfr	Conc/L	Test Soln	Remarks	Ref	C/I
Amikacin sulfate	BR	5 g	SC	40 mg	D5LR, D5R, D5S, D5W, D10W, IS10, LR, NS, R, SL	Physically compatible and potency of both retained for 24 hr at 25 °C	294	C
Calcium chloride						Physically incompatible	9	I
	UP	1 g	SC	100 mg	D5W	Physically incompatible	15	I
Kanamycin sulfate	BR	4 g	SC	100 mg	D5W	Physically incompatible	15	I
Norepinephrine bitartrate	WI					Physically incompatible	9	I
	WI	2 mg	SC	100 mg	D5W	Physically incompatible	15	I
Pentobarbital sodium						Physically incompatible	9	I
	AB	1 g	SC	100 mg	D5W	Physically incompatible	15	I

Drugs in Syringe Compatibility

Chlorpheniramine maleate

Drug (in syringe)	Mfr	Amt	Mfr	Amt	Remarks	Ref	C/I
Diatrizoate meglumine 52%, diatrizoate sodium 8% (Renografin-60)	SQ	40 to 1 ml	SC	1 ml[a]	Physically compatible for 48 hr	530	C
Diatrizoate meglumine 34.3%, diatrizoate sodium 35% (Renovist)	SQ	40 to 1 ml	SC	1 ml[a]	Physically compatible for 48 hr	530	C
Diatrizoate sodium 75% (Hypaque)	WI	40 to 1 ml	SC	1 ml[a]	Physically compatible for 48 hr	530	C
Iodipamide meglumine 52% (Cholografin)	SQ	40 to 5 ml	SC	1 ml[a]	Forms a precipitate initially but clears within 1 hr and remains clear for 48 hr	530	I
	SQ	2 and 1 ml	SC	1 ml[a]	Forms a precipitate initially but clears within 1 hr. Precipitate reforms within 48 hr	530	I
Iothalamate meglumine 60% (Conray)	MA	40 to 1 ml	SC	1 ml[a]	Physically compatible for 48 hr	530	C
Iothalamate sodium 80% (Angio-Conray)	MA	40 to 1 ml	SC	1 ml[a]	Physically compatible for 48 hr	530	C

[a]Chlorpheniramine maleate concentration unspecified.

Additional Compatibility Information

Miscellaneous— Chlorpheniramine maleate is reportedly compatible with most intravenous infusion solutions (4).

Chlorpheniramine maleate (Schering) was found to be compatible with diatrizoate meglumine products (Squibb) but incompatible with iodipamide meglumine (Squibb) (40).

CLARITHROMYCIN

Klaricid   **Abbott Laboratories**

Products— Clarithromycin (Abbott) is available in 500-mg vials with lactobionic acid as a solubilizing agent. Reconstitute with 10 ml of sterile water for injection, and shake to dissolve the powder. Do not use diluents containing preservatives or inorganic salts. Each milliliter of the resultant solution contains 50 mg of clarithromycin. This solution must be diluted before use. See Administration below (1442).

Administration— Clarithromycin is administered by intravenous infusion after dilution in an appropriate infusion solution. See Additional Compatibility Information below. It should not be given by intravenous bolus or intramuscular injection. The reconstituted drug solution (500 mg) is added to 250 ml of compatible infusion solution yielding a 2-mg/ml final solution. The final diluted solution is administered by intravenous infusion over 60 minutes into one of the larger proximal veins (1442).

Stability— Intact containers of the white to off-white lyophilized powder should be stored at 30 °C or below and protected from light. When reconstituted as directed, the 50-mg/ml solution may be stored at temperatures from 5 to 25 °C and should be used within 24 hours. After final dilution to a 2-mg/ml concentration for administration, the solution should be used within six hours stored at room temperature (25 °C) or 24 hours if stored under refrigeration at 5 °C (1442).

Compatibility Information

Y-Site Injection Compatibility (1:1 Mixture)

	Clarithromycin						
Drug	Mfr	Conc	Mfr	Conc	Remarks	Ref	C/I
Aminophylline	EV	2 mg/ml[a]	AB	4 mg/ml[a]	Needle-like crystals form in 2 hr at 30 °C and 4 hr at 17 °C	2174	I
Amiodarone HCl	SW	3 mg/ml[a]	AB	4 mg/ml[a]	Visually compatible for 72 hr at both 30 and 17 °C	2174	C
Amoxicillin sodium–clavulanate potassium	BE	20 + 4 mg/ml[a]	AB	4 mg/ml[a]	Visually compatible for 72 hr at both 30 and 17 °C	2174	C
Ampicillin sodium	BE	40 mg/ml[a]	AB	4 mg/ml[a]	Visually compatible for 72 hr at both 30 and 17 °C	2174	C
Atracurium besylate	GW	1 mg/ml[a]	AB	4 mg/ml[a]	Visually compatible for 72 hr at both 30 and 17 °C	2174	C
Bumetanide	LEO	0.5 mg/ml	AB	4 mg/ml[a]	Visually compatible for 72 hr at both 30 and 17 °C	2174	C
Cefuroxime sodium	GW	60 mg/ml[a]	AB	4 mg/ml[a]	White precipitate forms in 3 hr at 30 °C and 24 hr at 17 °C	2174	I
Cimetidine HCl	SKB	8 mg/ml[a]	AB	4 mg/ml[a]	Visually compatible for 72 hr at both 30 and 17 °C	2174	C
Ciprofloxacin	BAY	2 mg/ml[a]	AB	4 mg/ml[a]	Visually compatible for 72 hr at both 30 and 17 °C	2174	C
Dobutamine HCl	BI	2 mg/ml[a]	AB	4 mg/ml[a]	Visually compatible for 72 hr at both 30 and 17 °C	2174	C
Dopamine HCl	DB	3.2 mg/ml[a]	AB	4 mg/ml[a]	Visually compatible for 72 hr at both 30 and 17 °C	2174	C
Flucloxacillin sodium	BE	40 mg/ml[a]	AB	4 mg/ml[a]	Translucent precipitate forms in 1 to 2 hr becoming a gel in 3 hr at both 30 and 17 °C	2174	I
Frusemide	ANT	10 mg/ml	AB	4 mg/ml[a]	White cloudiness forms immediately becoming an obvious precipitate in 15 min	2174	I
Gentamicin sulfate	RS	40 mg/ml	AB	4 mg/ml[a]	Visually compatible for 72 hr at both 30 and 17 °C	2174	C
Heparin sodium	CPP	1000 units/ml[a]	AB	4 mg/ml[a]	White cloudiness forms immediately	2174	I

Y-Site Injection Compatibility (1:1 Mixture) (Cont.)

Clarithromycin

Drug	Mfr	Conc	Mfr	Conc	Remarks	Ref	C/I
Hydrocortisone sodium phosphate	GL	100 mg/ml	AB	4 mg/ml[a]	Visually compatible for 72 hr at both 30 and 17 °C	2174	C
Insulin, human	NOV	4 units/ml[a]	AB	4 mg/ml[a]	Visually compatible for 72 hr at both 30 and 17 °C	2174	C
Lignocaine HCl	ANT	4 mg/ml[a]	AB	4 mg/ml[a]	Visually compatible for 72 hr at both 30 and 17 °C	2174	C
Metoclopramide HCl	ANT	5 mg/ml	AB	4 mg/ml[a]	Visually compatible for 72 hr at both 30 and 17 °C	2174	C
Metronidazole	PRK	5 mg/ml	AB	4 mg/ml[a]	Visually compatible for 72 hr at both 30 and 17 °C	2174	C
Penicillin G sodium	BRT	24 mg/ml[a]	AB	4 mg/ml[a]	Visually compatible for 72 hr at both 30 and 17 °C	2174	C
Phenytoin sodium	ANT	20 mg/ml[a]	AB	4 mg/ml[a]	White cloudiness forms immediately becoming a white precipitate in 1 hr at both 30 and 17 °C	2174	I
Prochlorperazine (salt unspecified)	ANT	12.5 mg/ml	AB	4 mg/ml[a]	Visually compatible for 72 hr at both 30 and 17 °C	2174	C
Potassium chloride	ANT	0.08 mmol/ml[a]	AB	4 mg/ml[a]	Visually compatible for 72 hr at both 30 and 17 °C	2174	C
Ranitidine HCl	GW	5 mg/ml[a]	AB	4 mg/ml[a]	Visually compatible for 72 hr at both 30 and 17 °C	2174	C
Ticarcillin disodium–clavulanate potassium	BE	32 mg/ml[a]	AB	4 mg/ml[a]	Visually compatible for 72 hr at both 30 and 17 °C	2174	C
Vancomycin HCl	DB	10 mg/ml[a]	AB	4 mg/ml[a]	Visually compatible for 72 hr at both 30 and 17 °C	2174	C
Vecuronium bromide	ORG	2 mg/ml[a]	AB	4 mg/ml[a]	Visually compatible for 72 hr at both 30 and 17 °C	2174	C
Verapamil HCl	BKN	2.5 mg/ml	AB	4 mg/ml[a]	Visually compatible for 72 hr at both 30 and 17 °C	2174	C

[a]*Tested in dextrose 5% in water.*

Additional Compatibility Information

Solutions— The following diluents are recommended by the manufacturer for the preparation of the final dilution of clarithromycin to 2 mg/ml (1442):

Dextrose 5% in Ringer's injection, lactated
Dextrose 5% in sodium chloride 0.3%
Dextrose 5% in sodium chloride 0.45%
Dextrose 5% in water
Normosol M in dextrose 5%
Normosol R in dextrose 5%
Ringer's injection, lactated
Sodium chloride 0.9%

CLOMIPRAMINE HCL

Anafranil   **Novartis Pharmaceuticals**

Products— Clomipramine HCl (Novartis) is available as a 12.5-

mg/ml solution in 2-ml ampuls containing 25 mg of drug with glycerine in water. The ampuls are pressurized with carbon dioxide (1442).

For intravenous administration, the drug should be diluted in dextrose 5% in water or sodium chloride 0.9%. After addition of the drug, the admixture should be agitated to ensure even distribution (1442).

Administration—— Clomipramine HCl is administered by intramuscular injection or intravenous infusion. By intravenous infusion, the dose should initially be diluted in 250 to 500 ml of infusion solution and infused over 1.5 to 3 hours. If tolerated satisfactorily, the volume of fluid for subsequent doses may be reduced to 125 ml and the infusion time decreased to 45 minutes (1442).

Stability—— Intact ampuls of clomipramine HCl should be stored protected from light (1442).

Sorption—— Clomipramine HCl (Ciba-Geigy) (concentration unspeci-fied) in dextrose 5% in water in PVC containers was delivered over four hours through PVC administration sets. Loss due to sorption ranged from about 1 to 8% determined by UV spectroscopy (2045).

The manufacturer states that any standard administration set can be used to deliver clomipramine HCl (1442).

Compatibility Information

Infusion Solutions—— The manufacturer recommends dextrose 5% in water or sodium chloride 0.9% for preparing intravenous infusion admixtures (1442).

CLONAZEPAM

Rivotril   **Roche**

Products—— Clonazepam (Roche) is available in 1-ml ampuls containing 1 mg of drug in a solvent composed of absolute alcohol, glacial acetic acid, benzyl alcohol, and propylene glycol. An ampul containing 1 ml of sterile water for injection is included as a diluent (1442).

pH—— Clonazepam (Roche) 0.125, 0.222, and 0.5 mg/ml in sodium chloride 0.9% for continuous subcutaneous infusion had pH values of 3.6, 3.5, and 3.6, respectively (2161).

Administration—— Clonazepam is administered by slow intravenous injection. For bolus administration, the content of the diluent ampul is added to the drug immediately before administration. The injection is administered over not less than 30 seconds into a large vein of the antecubital fossa. Clonazepam is also administered as a slow intravenous infusion; up to 3 mg of clonazepam is added to 250 ml of dextrose 5 or 10% in water, sodium chloride 0.9%, or dextrose 2.5% in sodium chloride 0.45% (1442).

Stability—— The colorless solution in intact ampuls should be stored below 30 °C and protected from light. The manufacturer recommends that the drug be used immediately after mixing with the supplied diluent. After dilution in any recommended infusion solution, the infusion should be completed within 12 hours (1442).

Syringes—— Clonazepam (Roche) 5 and 10 mg, diluted to 48 ml with sodium chloride 0.9% and stored in polyethylene syringes, was physically compatible and exhibited no clonazepam loss in 10 hours at room temperature (1708).

In another study, the stability of reconstituted clonazepam (Roche) 0.5 mg/ml packaged in polypropylene syringes was evaluated. HPLC analysis found less than 2% clonazepam loss in 48 hours stored at room temperature exposed to normal room light (2172).

Sorption—— Clonazepam shows evidence of sorption losses when in contact with PVC bags or tubing. It is recommended that glass containers be used for infusions. If PVC bags are used, the admixture should be infused without delay after preparation and over a period no longer than two hours (1442).

Nation et al. reported that clonazepam (Roche) 3 mg in 500 ml of dextrose 5% in water or sodium chloride 0.9%, stored at room temperature and protected from light in PVC bags, showed losses of 17 to 20% after 24 hours and 31 to 33% after six days (1707).

It was further reported that clonazepam 3 mg in 500 ml of dextrose 5% in water or sodium chloride 0.9% in glass bottles, delivered through PVC infusion sets at 40 ml/hr, had losses of approximately 20 to 25% in delivered potency over 20 to 30 minutes. Thereafter, the effluent concentrations increased over time to stabilize at 92 to 94% of the original concentration. An even greater loss of delivered potency, but in a similar pattern, was reported when admixtures were prepared in PVC bags. Losses of 25 to 30% occurred over the first 20 to 30 minutes but decreased to about a 16 to 20% loss of delivered potency over 6.5 hours (1707).

Hooymans et al. compared losses of clonazepam to PVC and polyethylene-lined infusion tubing. Clonazepam (Roche) 5 and 10 mg, diluted in sodium chloride 0.9% to a final volume of 48 ml in polyethylene syringes, was delivered at room temperature through tubing at flow rates of 2 or 4 ml/hr (5 mg in 48 ml) and 2 ml/hr (10 mg in 48 ml). No losses were observed in the plastic syringes or to the polyethylene-lined tubing over 10 hours. Losses to the PVC tubing depended on the flow rate and concentration, being greater at 2 ml/hr and at 5 mg/48 ml, respectively. Potency decreased to approximately 40 and 55% of the original strength after 0.6 hour for the 5-mg/48 ml concentration at 2 and 4 ml/hr, respectively. After 0.6 hour, the 10-mg/48 ml concentration was at 55% of original potency when delivered at 2 ml/hr. Effluent concentrations gradually increased after the first hour, reaching approximately 80 to 90% of original concentrations after 10 hours (1708).

Clonazepam (Roche) (concentration unspecified) in dextrose 5% in water in PVC containers was delivered over four hours through PVC administration sets. Losses due to sorption ranged from about 13 to 18% determined by UV spectroscopy (2045).

Compatibility Information

Solution Compatibility

	Clonazepam					

Solution	Mfr	Mfr	Conc/L	Remarks	Ref	C/I
Dextrose 5% in water	AB[a]	RC	6 mg	Physically compatible with no loss in 10 hr	1707	C
	TR[b]	RC	6 mg	7% loss in 7 hr, 17 to 20% loss in 24 hr, and 31 to 33% loss in 6 days at room temperature protected from light	1707	I
Sodium chloride 0.9%	AB[a]	RC	6 mg	Physically compatible with no loss in 10 hr	1707	C
	TR[b]	RC	6 mg	14% loss in 7 hr, 17 to 20% loss in 24 hr, and 31 to 33% loss in 6 days at room temperature protected from light	1707	I

[a]Tested in glass containers.
[b]Tested in PVC containers.

Y-Site Injection Compatibility (1:1 Mixture)

			Clonazepam				

Drug	Mfr	Conc	Mfr	Conc	Remarks	Ref	C/I
TPN #189[a]			RC	10 mg/ml[b]	Visually compatible for 24 hr at 22 °C	1767	C

[a]Refer to Appendix I for the composition of parenteral nutrition solutions. TPN indicates a 2-in-1 admixture.
[b]Tested in sterile water for injection.

Additional Compatibility Information

Solutions— Dextrose 2.5% in sodium chloride 0.45%, dextrose 5 or 10% in water, and sodium chloride 0.9% have been recommended as diluents for the intravenous infusion of clonazepam. Infusions should be completed within 12 hours of preparation (1442).

CYCLIZINE LACTATE

Valoid   **Glaxo Wellcome**

Products— Cyclizine lactate (Glaxo Wellcome) is available in 1-ml ampuls containing 50 mg of drug (1442).

pH— From 3.3 to 3.7 (176).

Administration— Cyclizine lactate is administered by intramuscular or intravenous injection. When administered intravenously, it should be injected slowly, with minimal withdrawal of blood in the syringe (1442).

Stability— Cyclizine lactate injection, a colorless solution, should be stored below 25 °C and protected from light (1442). Although a slight yellow tint may develop during storage, this color change is stated not to indicate a potency loss (19).

pH Effects— Cyclizine lactate is incompatible with any solution having a pH of 6.8 or greater (19).

Solubility— Cyclizine lactate has an aqueous solubility of 8 mg/ml. When the drug was diluted to concentrations of 7.5 and 3.75 mg/ml in water or dextrose 5% in water, it remained in solution for at least 24 hours at 23 °C. However, when these dilutions were made with sodium chloride 0.9%, crystals formed within 24 hours at 23 °C (1761).

Compatibility Information

Drugs in Syringe Compatibility

Cyclizine lactate

Drug (in syringe)	Mfr	Amt	Mfr	Amt	Remarks	Ref	C/I
Diamorphine HCl	MB	10, 25, 50 mg/ 1 ml	CA	5 mg/ 1 ml[a]	Physically compatible and diamorphine potency retained for 24 hr at room temperature	1454	**C**
	EV	15 mg/ 1 ml	CA	15 mg/ 1 ml	Physically compatible for 24 hr at room temperature	1455	**C**
	EV	37.5 to 150 mg/ 1 ml	CA	12.5 to 50 mg/ 1 ml	Precipitate forms within 24 hr	1455	**I**
	HC	25 to 100 mg/ ml	CA	10 mg/ ml	Visually incompatible	1672	**I**
	HC	20 mg/ ml	CA	10 mg/ ml	Visually compatible for 48 hr at 5 and 20 °C	1672	**C**
	HC	100 mg/ml	CA	6.7 mg/ ml	Visually compatible for 48 hr at 5 and 20 °C	1672	**C**
	HC	2 mg/ml	CA	6.7 mg/ ml	5% diamorphine loss by HPLC in 9.9 days at 20 °C. Cyclizine potency by HPLC retained for at least 45 days	1672	**C**
	HC	20 mg/ ml	CA	6.7 mg/ ml	5% diamorphine loss by HPLC in 13.6 days at 20 °C. Cyclizine potency by HPLC retained for at least 45 days	1672	**C**
	BP	6 mg/ml	WEL	51 mg/ ml	Physically compatible with 10% diamorphine loss in 1.7 days and little or no cyclizine loss by HPLC at 23 °C	2071	**C**
	BP	9 mg/ml	WEL	32 mg/ ml	Physically compatible with less than 10% diamorphine loss and little or no cyclizine loss by HPLC in 4 days at 23 °C	2071	**C**
	BP	10 mg/ ml	WEL	39 mg/ ml	Physically compatible with less than 10% diamorphine loss and little or no cyclizine loss by HPLC in 4 days at 23 °C	2071	**C**
	BP	10 mg/ ml	WEL	28 mg/ ml	Physically compatible with 10% diamorphine loss in 3.1 days and little or no cyclizine loss by HPLC at 23 °C	2071	**C**
	BP	12 mg/ ml	WEL	51 mg/ ml	Physically compatible with 10% diamorphine loss in 2.2 days and little or no cyclizine loss by HPLC at 23 °C	2071	**C**
	BP	14 mg/ ml	WEL	40 mg/ ml	Crystals form	2071	**I**
	BP	17 mg/ ml	WEL	26 mg/ ml	Physically compatible with 10% diamorphine loss in 1.1 days and 10% cyclizine loss in 2.5 days by HPLC at 23 °C	2071	**C**
	BP	18 mg/ ml	WEL	52 mg/ ml	Crystals form	2071	**I**
	BP	20 mg/ ml	WEL	10 mg/ ml	Physically compatible with less than 10% diamorphine loss and little or no cyclizine loss by HPLC in 7 days at 23 °C	2071	**C**
	BP	20 mg/ ml	WEL	15 mg/ ml	Physically compatible with little or no diamorphine loss and 10% cyclizine loss in 0.5 days by HPLC at 23 °C	2071	**I**
	BP	21 mg/ ml	WEL	26 mg/ ml	Physically compatible with 10% diamorphine loss in 4.9 days and 10% cyclizine loss in 3.2 days by HPLC at 23 °C	2071	**C**

Drugs in Syringe Compatibility (Cont.)

Cyclizine lactate

Drug (in syringe)	Mfr	Amt	Mfr	Amt	Remarks	Ref	C/I
	BP	18 mg/ml	WEL	23 mg/ml	Physically compatible with little or no diamorphine loss and 10% cyclizine loss by HPLC in 3.2 days at 23 °C	2071	**C**
	BP	26 mg/ml	WEL	23 mg/ml	Physically compatible with 10% diamorphine loss in 1.9 days and 10% cyclizine loss in 0.4 days by HPLC at 23 °C	2071	**I**
	BP	30 mg/ml	WEL	30 mg/ml	Physically compatible with 10% diamorphine loss in 0.9 days and 10% cyclizine loss in 0.4 days by HPLC at 23 °C	2071	**I**
	BP	49 mg/ml	WEL	10 mg/ml	Physically compatible with little or no diamorphine loss and 10% cyclizine loss in 5.5 days by HPLC at 23 °C	2071	**C**
	BP	51 mg/ml	WEL	4 mg/ml	Physically compatible with little or no diamorphine or cyclizine loss in 7 days by HPLC at 23 °C	2071	**C**
	BP	61 mg/ml	WEL	8 mg/ml	Physically compatible with 10% diamorphine loss in 1.4 days and 10% cyclizine loss in 1.1 days by HPLC at 23 °C	2071	**C**
	BP	65 mg/ml	WEL	13 mg/ml	Physically compatible with 10% diamorphine loss in 1.6 days and 10% cyclizine loss in 0.5 days by HPLC at 23 °C	2071	**I**
	BP	92 mg/ml	WEL	10 mg/ml	Physically compatible with little or no diamorphine loss and 10% cyclizine loss in 2.4 days by HPLC at 23 °C	2071	**C**
	BP	99 mg/ml	WEL	4 mg/ml	Physically compatible with little or no diamorphine or cyclizine loss in 7 days by HPLC at 23 °C	2071	**C**
Diamorphine HCl with haloperidol lactate	BP JC	11 mg/ml 2.2 mg/ml	WEL	16 mg/ml	Physically compatible with less than 10% loss of any drug by HPLC in 7 days at 23 °C	2071	**C**
Diamorphine HCl with haloperidol lactate	BP JC	25 mg/ml 2.2 mg/ml	WEL	16 mg/ml	Physically compatible with less than 10% loss of any drug by HPLC in 7 days at 23 °C	2071	**C**
Diamorphine HCl with haloperidol lactate	BP JC	40 mg/ml 2.2 mg/ml	WEL	11 mg/ml	Physically compatible with less than 10% loss of any drug by HPLC in 7 days at 23 °C	2071	**C**
Diamorphine HCl with haloperidol lactate	BP JC	42 mg/ml 2.1 mg/ml	WEL	13 mg/ml	Physically compatible with less than 10% loss of any drug by HPLC in 6 days at 23 °C	2071	**C**
Diamorphine HCl with haloperidol lactate	BP JC	55 mg/ml 2.1 mg/ml	WEL	9 mg/ml	Physically compatible with less than 10% loss of any drug by HPLC in 7 days at 23 °C	2071	**C**
Diamorphine HCl with haloperidol lactate	BP JC	56 mg/ml 2.1 mg/ml	WEL	13 mg/ml	Physically compatible with less than 10% loss of any drug by HPLC in 7 days at 23 °C	2071	**C**
Haloperidol lactate	SE	1.5 mg/0.3 ml	WEL	150 mg/3 ml	Diluted with 17 ml of NS. Crystals of cyclizine form within 24 hr at 25 °C	1761	**I**
	SE	1.5 mg/0.3 ml	WEL	150 mg/3 ml	Diluted with 17 ml of D5W or W. Visually compatible for 24 hr at 25 °C	1761	**C**

Drugs in Syringe Compatibility (Cont.)

Cyclizine lactate

Drug (in syringe)	Mfr	Amt	Mfr	Amt	Remarks	Ref	C/I
Ranitidine HCl	GL	50 mg/ 2 ml	CA	50 mg/ 1 ml	Physically compatible for 1 hr at 25 °C both macroscopically and microscopically	978	C

aDiluted with sterile water for injection.

Additional Compatibility Information

Diamorphine— Grassby and Hutchings reported that cyclizine lactate is conditionally compatible with diamorphine HCl, depending on the concentrations of the two drugs. Diamorphine HCl to cyclizine lactate concentration ratios of 1:1 are stable in concentrations up to 20 mg/ml. However, an increase in the diamorphine HCl concentration necessitates a reduction in the cyclizine lactate concentration to 10 mg/ml. Similarly, an increase in the cyclizine lactate concentration necessitates a reduction in the diamorphine HCl concentration to 15 mg/ml for the combinations to remain stable for at least 24 hours at room temperature (2071). See Compatibility Information above.

DIAMORPHINE HCL

Evans Medical

Products— Diamorphine HCl (Evans Medical) is available as a lyophilized product in 5-, 10-, 30-, 100-, and 500-mg ampuls (1442).

Diamorphine HCl is very soluble in water. Up to 100 mg can be reconstituted in 1 ml of diluent; a minimum of 2 ml of diluent is recommended for the 500-mg size. The preferred diluent is dextrose 5% in water, but sodium chloride 0.9% also may be used (1442).

Administration— Diamorphine HCl is given by intramuscular, intravenous, or subcutaneous injection. Administration can also be by slow continuous subcutaneous or intravenous injection with an infusion control device (1442).

Stability— Ampuls of lyophilized diamorphine HCl should be stored below 25 °C (1442).

Diamorphine HCl 1 mg/ml as a simple aqueous solution in flint glass ampuls stored at 25 °C exhibited a 10% loss in about 50 days (1958).

The stability of diamorphine HCl was determined in PVC bags and glass syringes. Solutions containing 1 or 20 mg/ml in sodium chloride 0.9% were stable for at least 15 days at 4 °C. At ambient temperature, diamorphine HCl in glass syringes was stable for only seven days at 1 mg/ml and for 12 days at 20 mg/ml. Stability was also assessed in two disposable infusion devices, Infusor (Travenol) and Intermate 200 (I.S.C.). The drug was stable for 15 days in most cases. However, solutions containing diamorphine HCl 1 mg/ml in the Intermate reservoir stored at 31 °C were only stable for two days (1449).

Solutions containing diamorphine HCl 250 mg/ml in an Act-a-Pump (Pharmacia) reservoir were stable for at least 14 days during simulated patient use (1450). Jones et al. also reported that degradation was both temperature and concentration dependent. Solutions of diamorphine HCl 1 mg/ml in water stored at 21 °C for 42 days in the Act-a-Pump reservoir showed 10.6% degradation. At 37 °C, 32.6% degradation occurred (1451).

Diamorphine HCl (Evans Medical) 5 mg/ml in sterile water for injection was stable in Parker Micropump PVC reservoirs for 14 days at 4 °C, exhibiting no loss by HPLC analysis. At 37 °C, about a 2% loss occurred in seven days and a 7% loss occurred in 14 days (1696).

However, at a concentration of 250 mg/ml, diamorphine HCl losses of 11 and 85.8% at 21 and 37 °C, respectively (1451), were partially attributed to precipitation (1452).

Solutions of diamorphine HCl in sterile water for injection at concentrations greater than 15 mg/ml exhibited precipitation when stored at 21 and 37 °C for longer than two weeks. At concentrations of 1 to 250 mg/ml in sterile water for injection in glass containers, diamorphine HCl was stable for eight weeks at −20 °C, exhibiting less than 10% degradation. At 4 °C, degradation was inversely related to concentration. Diamorphine HCl 31 and 250 mg/ml was stable, but solutions containing 1 and 7.81 mg/ml showed 15 and 12% losses, respectively, after eight weeks of storage (1452).

Diamorphine HCl stability also was investigated in plastic syringes. Gove et al. reported the stability of diamorphine HCl solutions to be 14 days at room temperature and greater than 40 days at 4 °C, although no details of concentrations were cited (982).

Diamorphine HCl (Hillcross) 2 and 20 mg/ml in water for injection also was stored in plastic syringes (Becton-Dickinson) sealed with blind hubs. HPLC showed a 5% potency loss in about 18 days at 20 °C (1672).

In another study, diamorphine HCl up to 50 mg/ml in sterile water for injection was stable for longer than two days at ambient temperature when protected from light (1454).

pH Effects— The stability of the reconstituted injection depends on its pH; it is most stable at acidic pH, around pH 3.8 to 4.4 (1442) to pH 4.5 (1958). Degradation increases greatly at neutral or basic pH (1448).

Diamorphine HCl exhibits a pH-dependent incompatibility in sodium chloride injection. To remain in solution, the pH must be below 6 (1458). Solutions containing up to 250 mg/ml of diamorphine HCl have been shown to be compatible in sodium chloride 0.9% (1457–1459).

Compatibility Information

Solution Compatibility

Diamorphine HCl

Solution	Mfr	Mfr	Conc/L	Remarks	Ref	C/I
Sodium chloride 0.9%	TR	EV	1 and 20 g	Little or no loss in 15 days at 4 and 24 °C	1449	C

Additive Compatibility

Diamorphine HCl

Drug	Mfr	Conc/L	Mfr	Conc/L	Test Soln	Remarks	Ref	C/I
Bupivacaine HCl	GL	1.25 g		0.125 g	NS	Visually compatible with 8% diamorphine loss and no bupivacaine loss by HPLC in 28 days at room temperature	1791	C
	AST	150 mg	NAP	20 mg	NS[a]	5% diamorphine and no bupivacaine loss by HPLC in 14 days at 7 °C. Both drugs were stable for 6 months at −20 °C	2070	C
Flucloxacillin sodium	BE	20 g	EV	500 mg	W	Physically compatible for 24 hr at 15 and 30 °C. Haze forms in 48 hr at 30 °C. No change at 15 °C	1479	C
Frusemide	HO	1 g	EV	500 mg	W	Physically compatible for 72 hr at 15 and 30 °C	1479	C

[a]Tested in PVC containers.

Drugs in Syringe Compatibility

Diamorphine HCl

Drug (in syringe)	Mfr	Amt	Mfr	Amt	Remarks	Ref	C/I
Bupivacaine HCl	AST	0.5%	EV	1 and 10 mg/ml	10 to 11% diamorphine loss by HPLC in 5 weeks at 20 °C and 3 to 7% loss in 8 weeks at 6 °C. Little or no bupivacaine loss at 6 or 20 °C in 8 weeks	1952	C
Cyclizine lactate	CA	5 mg/1 ml[a]	MB	10, 25, 50 mg/1 ml	Physically compatible and diamorphine potency retained for 24 hr at room temperature	1454	C
	CA	15 mg/1 ml	EV	15 mg/1 ml	Physically compatible for 24 hr at room temperature	1455	C
	CA	12.5 to 50 mg/1 ml	EV	37.5 to 150 mg/1 ml	Precipitate forms within 24 hr	1455	I
	CA	10 mg/ml	HC	25 to 100 mg/ml	Visually incompatible	1672	I
	CA	10 mg/ml	HC	20 mg/ml	Visually compatible for 48 hr at 5 and 20 °C	1672	C
	CA	6.7 mg/ml	HC	≤100 mg/ml	Visually compatible for 48 hr at 5 and 20 °C	1672	C
	CA	6.7 mg/ml	HC	2 mg/ml	5% diamorphine loss by HPLC in 9.9 days at 20 °C. Cyclizine potency by HPLC retained for at least 45 days	1672	C

Drugs in Syringe Compatibility (Cont.)

Diamorphine HCl

Drug (in syringe)	Mfr	Amt	Mfr	Amt	Remarks	Ref	C/I
	CA	6.7 mg/ml	HC	20 mg/ml	5% diamorphine loss by HPLC in 13.6 days at 20 °C. Cyclizine potency by HPLC retained for at least 45 days	1672	**C**
	WEL	51 mg/ml	BP	6 mg/ml	Physically compatible with 10% diamorphine loss in 1.7 days and little or no cyclizine loss by HPLC at 23 °C	2071	**C**
	WEL	32 mg/ml	BP	9 mg/ml	Physically compatible with less than 10% diamorphine loss and little or no cyclizine loss by HPLC in 4 days at 23 °C	2071	**C**
	WEL	39 mg/ml	BP	10 mg/ml	Physically compatible with less than 10% diamorphine loss and little or no cyclizine loss by HPLC in 4 days at 23 °C	2071	**C**
	WEL	28 mg/ml	BP	10 mg/ml	Physically compatible with 10% diamorphine loss in 3.1 days and little or no cyclizine loss by HPLC at 23 °C	2071	**C**
	WEL	51 mg/ml	BP	12 mg/ml	Physically compatible with 10% diamorphine loss in 2.2 days and little or no cyclizine loss by HPLC at 23 °C	2071	**C**
	WEL	40 mg/ml	BP	14 mg/ml	Crystals form	2071	**I**
	WEL	26 mg/ml	BP	17 mg/ml	Physically compatible with 10% diamorphine loss in 1.1 days and 10% cyclizine loss in 2.5 days by HPLC at 23 °C	2071	**C**
	WEL	52 mg/ml	BP	18 mg/ml	Crystals form	2071	**I**
	WEL	10 mg/ml	BP	20 mg/ml	Physically compatible with less than 10% diamorphine loss and little or no cyclizine loss by HPLC in 7 days at 23 °C	2071	**C**
	WEL	15 mg/ml	BP	20 mg/ml	Physically compatible with little or no diamorphine loss and 10% cyclizine loss in 0.5 days by HPLC at 23 °C	2071	**I**
	WEL	26 mg/ml	BP	21 mg/ml	Physically compatible with 10% diamorphine loss in 4.9 days and 10% cyclizine loss in 3.2 days by HPLC at 23 °C	2071	**C**
	WEL	23 mg/ml	BP	18 mg/ml	Physically compatible with little or no diamorphine loss and 10% cyclizine loss by HPLC in 3.2 days at 23 °C	2071	**C**
	WEL	23 mg/ml	BP	26 mg/ml	Physically compatible with 10% diamorphine loss in 1.9 days and 10% cyclizine loss in 0.4 days by HPLC at 23 °C	2071	**I**
	WEL	30 mg/ml	BP	30 mg/ml	Physically compatible with 10% diamorphine loss in 0.9 days and 10% cyclizine loss in 0.4 days by HPLC at 23 °C	2071	**I**
	WEL	10 mg/ml	BP	49 mg/ml	Physically compatible with little or no diamorphine loss and 10% cyclizine loss in 5.5 days by HPLC at 23 °C	2071	**C**
	WEL	4 mg/ml	BP	51 mg/ml	Physically compatible with little or no loss of either drug by HPLC in 7 days at 23 °C	2071	**C**
	WEL	8 mg/ml	BP	61 mg/ml	Physically compatible with 10% diamorphine loss in 1.4 days and 10% cyclizine loss in 1.1 days by HPLC at 23 °C	2071	**C**
	WEL	13 mg/ml	BP	65 mg/ml	Physically compatible with 10% diamorphine loss in 1.6 days and 10% cyclizine loss in 0.5 days by HPLC at 23 °C	2071	**I**

Drugs in Syringe Compatibility (Cont.)

Diamorphine HCl

Drug (in syringe)	Mfr	Amt	Mfr	Amt	Remarks	Ref	C/I
	WEL	10 mg/ml	BP	92 mg/ml	Physically compatible with little or no diamorphine loss and 10% cyclizine loss in 2.4 days by HPLC at 23 °C	2071	C
	WEL	4 mg/ml	BP	99 mg/ml	Physically compatible with little or no loss of either drug by HPLC in 7 days at 23 °C	2071	C
Cyclizine lactate with haloperidol lactate	WEL JC	16 mg/ml 2.2 mg/ml	BP	11 mg/ml	Physically compatible with less than 10% loss of any drug by HPLC in 7 days at 23 °C	2071	C
Cyclizine lactate with haloperidol lactate	WEL JC	16 mg/ml 2.2 mg/ml	BP	25 mg/ml	Physically compatible with less than 10% loss of any drug by HPLC in 7 days at 23 °C	2071	C
Cyclizine lactate with haloperidol lactate	WEL JC	11 mg/ml 2.2 mg/ml	BP	40 mg/ml	Physically compatible with less than 10% loss of any drug by HPLC in 7 days at 23 °C	2071	C
Cyclizine lactate with haloperidol lactate	WEL JC	13 mg/ml 2.1 mg/ml	BP	42 mg/ml	Physically compatible with less than 10% loss of any drug by HPLC in 6 days at 23 °C	2071	C
Cyclizine lactate with haloperidol lactate	WEL JC	9 mg/ml 2.1 mg/ml	BP	55 mg/ml	Physically compatible with less than 10% loss of any drug by HPLC in 7 days at 23 °C	2071	C
Cyclizine lactate with haloperidol lactate	WEL JC	13 mg/ml 2.1 mg/ml	BP	56 mg/ml	Physically compatible with less than 10% loss of any drug by HPLC in 7 days at 23 °C	2071	C
Haloperidol lactate	SE	1.5 mg/1 ml[a]	MB	10, 25, 50 mg/1 ml	Physically compatible and diamorphine content retained for 24 hr at room temperature	1454	C
	SE	2 mg/1 ml	EV	20 mg/1 ml	Crystallization with 58% haloperidol loss in 7 days at room temperature	1455	I
	SE	5 mg/1 ml	EV	50 and 150 mg/1 ml	Immediate precipitation	1455	I
	SE	2.5 mg/8 ml	EV	100 mg/8 ml	Physically compatible for 24 hr at room temperature and 7 days at 6 °C	1456	C
	SE	0.75 mg/ml	HC	20 to 100 mg/ml	Visually compatible for 48 hr at 5 and 20 °C	1672	C
	SE	0.75 mg/ml	HC	2 mg/ml	5% diamorphine loss by HPLC in 14.8 days at 20 °C. Haloperidol potency by HPLC retained for at least 45 days	1672	C
	SE	0.75 mg/ml	HC	20 mg/ml	5% diamorphine loss by HPLC in 20.7 days at 20 °C. Haloperidol potency by HPLC retained for at least 45 days	1672	C
	JC	2 mg/ml	BP	20, 50, 100 mg/ml	Physically compatible with no loss of either drug by HPLC in 7 days at 23 °C	2071	C
	JC	3 mg/ml	BP	20, 50, 100 mg/ml	Physically compatible with no loss of either drug by HPLC in 7 days at 23 °C	2071	C

Drugs in Syringe Compatibility (Cont.)

Drug (in syringe)	Mfr	Amt	Diamorphine HCl Mfr	Diamorphine HCl Amt	Remarks	Ref	C/I
	JC	4 mg/ml	BP	20 and 50 mg/ml	Physically compatible with no loss of either drug by HPLC in 7 days at 23 °C	2071	**C**
Hyoscine butylbromide	BI	20 mg/1 ml	EV	50 and 150 mg/1 ml	Physically compatible with no hyoscine loss and 4% diamorphine loss in 7 days at room temperature	1455	**C**
Hyoscine HBr	EV	60 μg/1 ml[a]	MB	10, 25, 50 mg/1 ml	Physically compatible and diamorphine content retained for 24 hr at room temperature	1454	**C**
	EV	0.4 mg/1 ml	EV	50 and 150 mg/1 ml	Physically compatible with 7% diamorphine loss in 7 days at room temperature	1455	**C**
Methotrimeprazine	MB	2.5 and 1.25 mg/1 ml[a]	MB	50 mg/1 ml	Physically compatible and diamorphine content retained for 24 hr at room temperature	1454	**C**
Metoclopramide HCl	BK	5 mg/1 ml	MB	10, 25, 50 mg/1 ml	Physically compatible and diamorphine content retained for 24 hr at room temperature	1454	**C**
	LA	5 mg/1 ml	EV	50 and 150 mg/1 ml	Slight discoloration with 8% metoclopramide loss and 9% diamorphine loss in 7 days at room temperature	1455	**C**
Midazolam HCl	RC	10[b] and 75[c] mg	EV	10 mg	Visually compatible with 10% diamorphine loss and no midazolam loss by HPLC in 15.9 days at 22 °C	1792	**C**
	RC	10[b] and 75[c] mg	EV	500 mg	Visually compatible with 10% diamorphine loss and no midazolam loss by HPLC in 22.2 days at 22 °C	1792	**C**
Prochlorperazine edisylate	MB	1.25 mg/1 ml[a]	MB	10, 25, 50 mg/1 ml	Physically compatible and diamorphine content retained for 24 hr at room temperature	1454	**C**

[a]*Diluted with sterile water for injection.*
[b]*Diluted with sterile water to 15 ml.*
[c]*Diamorphine HCl constituted with midazolam injection.*

Additional Compatibility Information

The manufacturer indicates that hyoscine HBr, methotrimeprazine, and metoclopramide HCl are stable and compatible with diamorphine HCl. Chlorpromazine HCl and prochlorperazine edisylate also are stated to be compatible (1442).

FLUCLOXACILLIN SODIUM (FLOXACILLIN SODIUM)

Floxapen Injection   **SmithKline Beecham**
Ladropen   **Berck**

Products— Fluucloxacillin sodium (SmithKline Beecham) is available in vials containing 250 mg, 500 mg, and 1 g of flucloxacillin as the sodium salt. To reconstitute for intramuscular use, add 1.5 ml of sterile water for injection to the 250-mg vial or 2 ml to the 500-mg vial (1442).

For intravenous use, reconstitute the 250- or 500-mg vial with 5 to 10 ml of sterile water for injection; reconstitute the 1-g vial with 15 to 20 ml of sterile water for injection. For intravenous infusion, the solution may be diluted further in a compatible infusion fluid (1442). (See Compatibility Information.)

For intrapleural use, reconstitute the 250-mg vial with 5 to 10 ml of sterile water for injection. For intra-articular use, reconstitute the 250- or 500-mg vial with up to 5 ml of sterile water for injection or lignocaine HCl 0.5% injection (1442).

Sodium Content— Each gram of flucloxacillin sodium contains 2.17 mEq of sodium (89).

Administration— Flucloxacillin sodium may be administered by intramuscular injection, direct intravenous injection slowly over three to four minutes, continuous intravenous infusion, and intrapleural and intra-articular injection (1442).

Stability— The reconstituted flucloxacillin sodium injection should be stored under refrigeration and used within 24 hours (1442).

Lynn reported losses of 8% in three days for reconstituted solutions containing flucloxacillin sodium (Beecham) 100 mg/ml stored at 20 to 25 °C (89).

Syringes— Flucloxacillin sodium (Berck) 125 mg/ml in sterile water for injection, packaged as 0.16 ml in 1-ml Injekt syringes (Braun) sealed with blind hubs and stored at about 6 °C, retained antibiotic activity against *Staphylococcus aureus* for nine days but lost 13% by day 14 (1697).

Freezing Solutions— Flucloxacillin sodium (Beecham) 10 mg/ml in sodium chloride 0.9% or dextrose 5% in water in PVC bags (Travenol) retained greater than 90% potency after being frozen and stored at −27 °C for up to 270 days. Thawing by microwave radiation and subsequent storage for 24 hours at 4 °C did not cause drug potency to fall below 90% of the stated concentration. However, a distinct yellow discoloration was produced after 90 days of storage, rendering the solutions unacceptable (1176).

Flucloxacillin sodium (Beecham) 1 g in 50 ml of sodium chloride 0.9% or dextrose 5% in water in PVC bags (Travenol) was stored at −20 °C for 30 days, followed by natural thawing and storage at 5 °C for 21 hours. The drug was stable under these conditions for the duration of the study (299).

Ambulatory Pumps— Flucloxacillin sodium at a concentration of 120 mg/ml in sodium chloride 0.9% and packaged in polyvinyl chloride bags (Baxter) for use in ambulatory and in-home treatment was evaluated for stability. After preparation, the containers were stored under refrigeration at about 4 °C for six days followed by 24 hours at 37 °C to simulate use conditions. HPLC analysis found that the flucloxacillin sodium solutions remained stable during refrigerated storage, but about 28% loss occurred during the 24-hour simulated in-use condition. The authors recommended not administering flucloxacillin sodium infusions as single 24-hour infusions. The use of divided dose reservoirs, which expose the drug solution to elevated temperatures for shorter time periods, was recommended (2206).

Sorption— Flucloxacillin sodium (Beecham) 200 mg/L in sodium chloride 0.9% (Travenol) in PVC bags did not exhibit significant sorption to the plastic during one week at room temperature (15 to 20 °C) (536).

Flucloxacillin sodium (Beecham) 200 mg/L in sodium chloride 0.9% did not exhibit any loss due to sorption during a seven-hour simulated infusion through an infusion set (Travenol) consisting of a cellulose propionate burette chamber and 170 cm of PVC tubing (606).

The drug also was tested as a simulated infusion over at least one hour by a syringe pump system. A glass syringe on a syringe pump was fitted with 20 cm of polyethylene tubing or 50 cm of Silastic tubing. No drug loss due to sorption was observed with either tubing (606).

Furthermore, a 25-ml aliquot of flucloxacillin sodium (Beecham) 200 mg/L in sodium chloride 0.9% was stored in all-plastic syringes composed of polypropylene barrels and polyethylene plungers for 24 hours at room temperature in the dark. The solution did not exhibit any loss due to sorption (606).

Compatibility Information

Solution Compatibility

Flucloxacillin sodium

Solution	Mfr	Mfr	Conc/L	Remarks	Ref	C/I
Dextrose 2.5% in sodium chloride 0.45%		BE	1 g	6% loss in 24 hr at 20 to 25 °C	89	C
Dextrose 5% in water		BE	1 g	1% loss in 24 hr at 20 to 25 °C	89	C
Sodium chloride 0.9%		BE	1 g	3% loss in 24 hr at 20 to 25 °C	89	C
	BA	BE	20 g	Visually compatible with 3% drug loss in 14 days and 9% loss in 28 days by HPLC at 5 °C	1844	C
	BA	BE	10 g	Visually compatible with 3% drug loss in 14 days and 8% loss in 28 days by HPLC at 5 °C	1844	C
	BA	BE	5 g	Visually compatible with 2% drug loss in 14 days and 7% loss in 28 days by HPLC at 5 °C	1844	C
	BA[a]		120 g	Stable for at least 6 days at 4 °C by HPLC analysis. 28% loss in 24 hours at 37 °C	2206	C
Sodium lactate ⅙ M		BE	1 g	4% loss in 24 hr at 20 to 25 °C	89	C

[a] *Tested in PVC containers.*

Additive Compatibility

Flucloxacillin sodium

Drug	Mfr	Conc/L	Mfr	Conc/L	Test Soln	Remarks	Ref	C/I
Aminophylline	ANT	1 g	BE	20 g	NS	Physically compatible for 72 hr at 15 and 30 °C	1479	C
Amiodarone HCl	LZ	4 g	BE	20 g	D5W	Immediate precipitation	1479	I
Ampicillin sodium	BE	20 g	BE	20 g	NS	Physically compatible for 72 hr at 15 and 30 °C	1479	C
Atropine sulphate	ANT	60 mg	BE	20 g	W	Haze forms in 24 hr and precipitate forms in 48 hr at 30 °C. No change at 15 °C	1479	I
Bumetanide	LEO	6 mg	BE	20 g	NS	Physically compatible for 72 hr at 15 and 30 °C	1479	C
Buprenorphine HCl		75 mg	BE	20 g	W	Thick haze forms in 24 hr and precipitate forms in 47 hr at 30 °C. No change at 15 °C	1479	I
Calcium gluconate	ANT	2 g	BE	20 g	NS	Thick white precipitate forms immediately	1479	I
Cefamandole nafate	DI	20 g	BE	20 g	W	Physically compatible for 24 hr at 15 and 30 °C. Haze forms in 48 hr and precipitate forms in 72 hr at 30 °C. No change at 15 °C	1479	C
Cefuroxime sodium	GL	37.5 g	BE	20 g	W	Physically compatible for 72 hr at 15 and 30 °C	1479	C
	GL	7.5 g	BE	10 g	D5W, NS	Physically compatible for 48 hr. Potency of both drugs retained when assayed after 1 hr at room temperature	1036	C
Chlorpromazine HCl	ANT	5 g	BE	20 g	W	Sticky yellow precipitate forms immediately	1479	I
Cimetidine HCl	SKF	4 g	BE	20 g	NS	Physically compatible for 72 hr at 15 and 30 °C	1479	C
Ciprofloxacin		2 g	BE	10 g	a	Immediate precipitation	1473	I
Dexamethasone sodium phosphate	MSD	4 g	BE	20 g	NS	Physically compatible for 72 hr at 15 and 30 °C	1479	C
Diamorphine HCl	EV	500 mg	BE	20 g	W	Physically compatible for 24 hr at 15 and 30 °C. Haze forms in 48 hr at 30 °C. No change at 15 °C	1479	C
Diazepam	PHX	1 g	BE	20 g	D5W	Haze forms in 7 hr at 30 °C and 48 hr at 15 °C	1479	I
Digoxin	BW	25 mg	BE	20 g	NS	Physically compatible for 72 hr at 15 and 30 °C	1479	C
Dobutamine HCl	LI	500 mg	BE	20 g	NS	Haze forms immediately and precipitate forms in 24 to 48 hr at 15 and 30 °C	1479	I
Epinephrine HCl	ANT	8 mg	BE	20 g	W	Physically compatible for 72 hr at 15 and 30 °C	1479	C
Erythromycin lactobionate	AB	5 g	BE	20 g	NS	Immediate precipitation. Crystals form in 5 hr at 15 °C	1479	I
Gentamicin sulphate	RS	8 g	BE	20 g	NS	Haze forms immediately and precipitate forms in 2 hr	1479	I
	EX	8 g	BE	10 g	NS	Physically compatible for 48 hr. Potency of both drugs retained when assayed after 1 hr at room temperature	1036	C

Additive Compatibility (Cont.)

Flucloxacillin sodium

Drug	Mfr	Conc/L	Mfr	Conc/L	Test Soln	Remarks	Ref	C/I
	EX	8 g	BE	10 g	D5W	Immediate precipitation	1036	I
Heparin sodium	WED	20,000 units	BE	20 g	NS	Physically compatible for 24 hr at 15 and 30 °C. Haze forms in 48 hr at 30 °C. No change at 15 °C	1479	C
Hydrocortisone sodium succinate	UP	50 g	BE	20 g	NS	Physically compatible for 72 hr at 15 and 30 °C	1479	C
Hyoscine butylbromide	BI	2 g	BE	20 g	W	Physically compatible for 24 hr at 15 and 30 °C. Precipitate forms in 48 hr. No change at 15 °C	1479	C
Isoprenaline HCl	PX	4 mg	BE	20 g	D5W	Physically compatible for 24 hr at 15 and 30 °C. Haze forms in 48 hr and precipitate forms in 72 hr	1479	C
Isosorbide dinitrate		1 g	BE	20 g		Physically compatible for 24 hr at 15 and 30 °C. Haze forms in 48 hr and precipitate forms in 72 hr at 30 °C. No change at 15 °C	1479	C
Lignocaine HCl	ANT	2 g	BE	20 g	NS	Physically compatible for 72 hr at 15 and 30 °C	1479	C
Metoclopramide HCl	ANT	1 g	BE	20 g	NS	White precipitate forms immediately	1479	I
Metronidazole		5 g	BE	10 g		Physically compatible for 48 hr. Potency of both drugs retained when assayed after 1 hr at room temperature	1036	C
Morphine sulphate	EV	1 g	BE	20 g	W	Haze forms in 24 hr and precipitate forms in 48 hr at 30 °C. No change at 15 °C	1479	I
Netilmicin sulphate	EX	1 g	BE	10 g	NS	Physically compatible for 48 hr. Potency of both drugs retained when assayed after 1 hr at room temperature	1036	C
	EX	1 g	BE	10 g	D5W	Immediate precipitation	1036	I
Ofloxacin	HO	1.67 g	BE	8.3 g	W	Visually compatible for 7 hr. Precipitate forms by 24 hr with about 75% ofloxacin loss and 20% flucloxacillin loss by HPLC	1613	I
Papaveretum	RC	2 g	BE	20 g	W	White precipitate forms immediately	1479	I
Pefloxacin		4 g	BE	10 g	D5W, NS	Immediate precipitation	1473	I
Penicillin G	GL	12 g	BE	20 g	NS	Haze forms in 24 hr and precipitate forms in 48 hr at 30 °C. No change at 15 °C	1479	I
Pethidine HCl	RC	5 g	BE	20 g	W	Haze forms immediately and precipitate forms in 5 to 24 hr	1479	I
Piperacillin sodium	LE	120 g	BE	50 g	W	10% piperacillin loss and 6% flucloxacillin loss by HPLC in 12 days at 5 °C. 3% piperacillin loss and 6% flucloxacillin loss by HPLC in 1 day at 30 °C	1748	C
Potassium chloride	ANT	40 mM	BE	20 g	W	Physically compatible for 72 hr at 15 and 30 °C	1479	C
Prochlorperazine edisylate	MB	1.25 g	BE	20 g	W	Immediate precipitation	1479	I
Promethazine HCl	MB	5 g	BE	20 g	W	White precipitate forms immediately	1479	I

Additive Compatibility (Cont.)

Flucloxacillin sodium

Drug	Mfr	Conc/L	Mfr	Conc/L	Test Soln	Remarks	Ref	C/I
Ranitidine HCl	GL	500 mg	BE	20 g	NS	Physically compatible for 72 hr at 15 and 30 °C	1479	**C**
Sodium bicarbonate	IMS	84 g	BE	20 g		Physically compatible for 72 hr at 15 and 30 °C	1479	**C**
Sulphadimidine	ICI	100 g	BE	20 g	W	Crystals form in 48 hr and globular precipitate forms in 72 hr at 30 °C. No change at 15 °C	1479	**I**
Tobramycin sulphate	LI	8 g	BE	20 g	NS	White precipitate forms in 7 hr	1479	**I**
Verapamil HCl	AB	500 mg	BE	20 g	NS	Haze and precipitate form in 24 hr at 30 °C. No change at 15 °C	1479	**I**

[a]*Flucloxacillin sodium added to ciprofloxacin solvent.*

Y-Site Injection Compatibility (1:1 Mixture)

Flucloxacillin sodium

Drug	Mfr	Conc	Mfr	Conc	Remarks	Ref	C/I
Clarithromycin	AB	4 mg/ml[a]	BE	40 mg/ml[a]	Translucent precipitate forms in 1 to 2 hr becoming a gel in 3 hr at both 30 and 17 °C	2174	**I**
Lorazepam	WY	0.33 mg/ml[b]	SKB	50 mg/ml	White opalescence forms in 4 hr	1855	**I**
Midazolam HCl	RC	5 mg/ml	SKB	50 mg/ml	White precipitate forms immediately	1855	**I**
TPN #189[c]			BE	50 mg/ml[b]	Visually compatible for 24 hr at 22 °C	1767	**C**

[a]*Tested in dextrose 5% in water.*
[b]*Tested in sodium chloride 0.9%.*
[c]*Refer to Appendix 1 for the composition of parenteral nutrition solutions. TPN indicates a 2-in-1 admixture.*

Additional Compatibility Information

Solutions— Flucloxacillin sodium is stated to be stable over 24 hours at room temperature, exhibiting less than a 10% potency loss when administered with the following intravenous infusion fluids (1475):

> Dextran 40 10% in dextrose 5%
> Dextran 40 10% in sodium chloride 0.9%

> Dextrose 5% in water
> Ringer's injection, lactated
> Sodium chloride 0.18% in dextrose 4%
> Sodium chloride 0.9%
> Sodium lactate ⅙ M

Aminoglycosides— Flucloxacillin sodium and aminoglycosides should not be mixed in the same syringe, intravenous fluid container, or administration set because precipitation may occur (1442).

ISOSORBIDE DINITRATE

Isoket **Schwartz Pharma**

Products— Isosorbide dinitrate (Schwartz Pharma) is available as a 0.1% solution in 10-ml ampuls and 50-ml and 100-ml bottles. Each milliliter contains isosorbide dinitrate 1 mg. It also is available as a 0.05% solution in 50-ml bottles. Each milliliter contains isosorbide dinitrate 0.5 mg in sodium chloride 0.9% (1442).

Administration— Isosorbide dinitrate is administered only by intravenous infusion when diluted to a maximum concentration of 0.05% in sodium chloride 0.9% or dextrose 5% in water. The delivery rate should be controlled using an infusion or syringe pump (1442).

Stability— Isosorbide dinitrate injections are colorless and stable in the intact ampuls or bottles when stored at room temperature.

Syringes— Isosorbide dinitrate (Rhone-Poulenc) 10 mg/ml was repackaged in polypropylene syringes (Plastipak, Becton-Dickinson) and stored for eight hours at room temperature and 4 °C. HPLC analysis found no loss of drug (1799).

Sorption— Isosorbide dinitrate is readily sorbed to PVC; sorption to polyethylene, polypropylene, and glass appears to be negligible. Consequently, it is recommended that nonabsorbing polyethylene or polybutadiene administration sets and polyethylene bags or glass containers be used for infusion. Alternatively, glass or polypropylene syringes can be used with a syringe pump to control the delivery rate. Sorption losses are affected by many factors, especially concentration, flow rate, time of infusion, and length of the administration set. The greatest amount of sorption occurs early in the infusion. Losses are greater if the flow rate is slow and the tubing is long. Simple calculations or corrections cannot be applied to this complex phenomenon to determine or control the actual delivery rate of isosorbide dinitrate if PVC bags or sets are used. However, losses of 15 to 30% can occur (1442).

Several articles have described or evaluated isosorbide dinitrate sorption characteristics. Lee and Fenton-May reported on losses of isosorbide dinitrate from an 80-mg/L solution in sodium chloride 0.9% to PVC (Viaflex, Steriflex), glass containers, and polyethylene (Polyfusor) bags. Losses of 20 to 30% in PVC bags were recorded after six hours at room temperature. Losses to glass or polyethylene bags were negligible. Isosorbide dinitrate injection was not sorbed to polypropylene syringes over six hours at room temperature. In addition, sorption to conventional PVC administration sets during simulated infusion at 1.5 ml/min accounted for 70 to 80% losses during the first 15 to 30 minutes of the infusion. Delivery then increased slowly as the set became partially saturated (1464).

Kowaluk et al. reported on isosorbide dinitrate 50 mg/ml in sodium chloride 0.9% in glass bottles delivered through a polyethylene administration set (Tridilset) over eight hours at 15 to 20 °C. The flow rate was 1 ml/min. No appreciable loss due to sorption occurred (769). This result is in contrast to the 30% loss that occurred using a conventional PVC administration set. The same authors reported losses up to 50% in a PVC bag with conventional PVC administration set combination, depending on the flow rate. The delivered dose of isosorbide dinitrate fell rapidly over the first hour and then became almost constant as the infusion continued (795).

Lee reported on isosorbide dinitrate 100 mg/L in sodium chloride 0.9% in glass bottles delivered at 0.8 ml/min through conventional PVC and polybutadiene administration sets (Avon Medical). While losses of isosorbide dinitrate of 15 to 25% to PVC sets over a four-hour period were observed, there was no appreciable loss to polybutadiene sets. Tests were also conducted in burette administration sets with polybutadiene tubing and acrylate butadiene styrene burette chambers (Avon Medical). Each chamber was primed with 100 ml of isosorbide dinitrate 100-mg/L solution, and the flow rate was 0.7 ml/min. Losses of isosorbide dinitrate were negligible over 90 minutes (1027).

Martens et al. stored isosorbide dinitrate 100 mg/L in PVC bags, Clear-Flex bags (laminated polyethylene, nylon, and polypropylene), and glass bottles at 21 °C in the dark for 24 hours. Losses due to sorption amounted to 9% in two hours and 23% in 24 hours in the PVC containers but were negligible in the Clear-Flex and glass containers (1392).

De Muynck et al. also studied the sorption of isosorbide dinitrate 100 mg/L in sodium chloride 0.9% and dextrose 10% in water at room temperature to various containers and administration sets. Losses due to sorption of less than 1 and 10% were observed for glass and high density polyethylene, respectively, while losses to PVC and polyamide bags amounted to 20 to 26%. Isosorbide dini-

trate solutions containing 250 mg/L exhibited variable losses to burette chambers after seven hours of storage, depending on the burette composition. The loss to methacrylate butadiene styrene burettes was less than 2%, while burettes composed of cellulose propionate yielded 13 to 16% losses. Butadiene styrene burettes yielded 22 to 26% losses. During simulated infusion of isosorbide dinitrate solutions containing 250 mg/L in sodium chloride 0.9% at a flow rate of 20 ml/hr, sorption to administration set tubing composed of polybutadiene was 2 to 4%. However, sorption to the Venisystem (Abbott) and Dosifix (B. Braun) was 50 to 60% (1465).

Struhar et al. reported that the infusion of isosorbide dinitrate 50 mg/L from glass containers through PVC administration sets resulted in an accumulated drug loss of about 16% over three hours. The maximum loss occurred in the first hour (1466).

Lee and Fenton-May investigated the sorption of isosorbide dinitrate to syringes and extension sets used when administering the drug via syringe pump. Sabre (Gillette), Plastipak (Becton-Dickinson), and Brunswick (Sherwood) plastic syringes containing isosorbide dinitrate 1 mg/ml were stored for six hours. No drug loss due to sorption was observed (1464).

Pharma-Plast (AHS Australia) plastic syringes having polypropylene barrels and polyethylene plungers were compared to glass containers for the possible sorption of isosorbide dinitrate. After 24 hours of storage of aqueous solutions of the drug (concentration unspecified), no drug loss was found in either plastic syringes or glass containers. The authors indicated that these plastic syringes could be substituted for glass syringes for use with syringe pumps (782).

Allwood also investigated the sorption of isosorbide dinitrate during simulated syringe pump injection. Solutions containing drug concentrations of 100 mg/L to 1 g/L in Plastipak (Becton-Dickinson) plastic syringes were administered at 0.75 ml/hr through PVC (Kimel), nylon (Portex), and polyethylene (Lectrocath) extension sets. Losses of up to 90% were observed when the solution was delivered through the PVC sets, but sorption to nylon and polyethylene sets was negligible over 24 hours. There was no detectable sorption to plastic syringes during the study (1467).

DeMuynck et al. studied isosorbide dinitrate 250 µg/ml in sodium chloride 0.9% and dextrose 10% in water delivered at 20 ml/hr through PVC tubing. The tubing was plasticized with diethylhexyl phthalate (DEHP). Losses due to sorption varied from 5.5 to 35% and were directly related to the hardness (and DEHP content) of the PVC. The harder the PVC, the lower was the loss. Similar results were noted with triethyl trimellitate plasticized PVC. The sorption to polybutadiene tubing was small (1 to 2%) but increased to 9% in some polybutadiene–PVC laminates. Polyethylene tubing also sorbed little isosorbide dinitrate, with losses of 1.6 to 1.9% (1619).

Isosorbide dinitrate 1 mg/ml was delivered by syringe pump at 5 ml/hr through Terumo administration sets 100 cm in length with an internal diameter of 2.1 mm. HPLC analysis of the effluent found about 70% loss during the first hour, gradually changing to about 40% loss over eight hours. Administration tubing of greater length resulted in more isosorbide dinitrate loss, whereas shorter tubing caused less loss (2143).

Filtration— Losses due to sorption of isosorbide dinitrate 250 mg/L in sodium chloride 0.9% delivered at 20 ml/hr through cellulose acetate filters (Sterifix, Ivex HP) were 15 to 26%. Losses to polyamide filters (Pall) were 9 to 13% under the same conditions (1465).

The loss of isosorbide dinitrate due to sorption to filters extends to filters used in hemodialysis. HPLC analysis of isosorbide dinitrate 0.1 mg/ml in sodium chloride 0.9% during simulated hemodialysis using five different filter media found substantial drug losses from the solution and binding to some of the filters. Losses of approximately 86% with polysulfone (Fresenius), 72% with cellulose acetate (Baxter), 43% with polyacrylonitrile (Hospal), and 12% cuprophan (Gambro) were found. However, with hemophan filters (Gambro), no loss of drug due to sorption occurred (2138).

Compatibility Information

Solution Compatibility

Isosorbide dinitrate

Solution	Mfr	Mfr	Conc/L	Remarks	Ref	C/I
Sodium chloride 0.9%	TR[a], BT[a]	TL	80 mg	44% loss in 24 hr at room temperature	1464	**I**
	TR[b], BT[c]	TL	80 mg	Physically compatible with little or no loss in 6 hr at room temperature	1464	**C**
	TR[a]	TL	100 mg	9% loss in 2 hr and 23% loss in 24 hr at 21 °C in the dark	1392	**I**
	[b,d]	TL	100 mg	Physically compatible with little or no loss in 24 hr at 21 °C in the dark	1392	**C**

[a]*Tested in PVC containers.*
[b]*Tested in glass containers.*
[c]*Tested in polyethylene containers.*
[d]*Tested in Clear-Flex polyethylene-lined laminated containers.*

Additive Compatibility

Isosorbide dinitrate

Drug	Mfr	Conc/L	Mfr	Conc/L	Test Soln	Remarks	Ref	C/I
Flucloxacillin sodium	BE	20 g		1 g		Physically compatible for 24 hr at 15 and 30 °C. Haze forms in 48 hr and precipitate forms in 72 hr at 30 °C. No change at 15 °C	1479	**C**
Frusemide	HO	1 g		1 g		Physically compatible for 72 hr at 15 and 30 °C	1479	**C**

Y-Site Injection Compatibility (1:1 Mixture)

Isosorbide dinitrate

Drug	Mfr	Conc	Mfr	Conc	Remarks	Ref	C/I
Heparin sodium	LEO	300 units/ml[a]	RP	10 mg/ml[a]	Erratic availability of both drugs delivered through PVC tubing	1799	**I**

[a]*Tested in dextrose 5% in water.*

LENOGRASTIM

Granocyte   **Chugai Pharma**

Products— Lenograstim (rHuG-CSF) (Chugai Pharma) is available as a lyophilized powder in single-use vials containing 13.4 million I.U. (Granocyte-13) or 33.6 million I.U. (Granocyte-34). In addition to lenograstim, each vial of the product contains human albumin 1 mg, mannitol 50 mg, polysorbate 20 0.1 mg, and disodium phosphate and sodium dihydrogen phosphate to adjust pH (1442).

Lenograstim vials of either strength should be reconstituted with 1.05 ml of the accompanying water for injection diluent. Gently mix to effect dissolution, usually about 5 seconds. Do not shake the vials vigorously. Both the lenograstim vials and the diluent are overfilled by 5% to permit withdrawal of a full 1 ml of the reconstituted product containing 13.4 or 33.6 million I.U. (1442).

Units— Each 13.4-million I.U. vial contains 105 μg of lenograstim. Each 33.6-million I.U. vial contains 263 μg of lenograstim (1442).

pH— The reconstituted solution has a pH buffered to 6.5 (1442).

Administration— Lenograstim is administered by intravenous infusion after dilution in sodium chloride 0.9%. Granocyte-13 should not be diluted to a concentration lower than 0.26 million I.U. per milliliter (2 μg/ml); Granocyte-34 should not be diluted to a concentration lower than 0.32 million I.U. per milliliter (2.5 μg/ml). The dilution volume should not exceed 50 ml for each vial of Granocyte-13 and 100 ml for each vial of Granocyte-34 (1442).

Stability— Intact vials of lenograstim should be stored under refrigeration at 2 to 8 °C. However, a brief single exposure to temperatures up to 30 °C for a period of not more than two weeks does not affect product stability. When reconstituted as directed and diluted for administration to concentrations not less than 0.26 million I.U. (Granocyte-13) or 0.32 million I.U. (Granocyte-34) per milliliter, lenograstim is stable for up to 24 hours at 5 or 25 °C (1442).

Portable Pumps— The stability of lenograstim (Rhône-Poulenc Rorer)

33.6 million I.U. (263 μg) and 67.2 million I.U. (526 μg) each in 100 ml of sodium chloride 0.9% filled into Intermate elastomeric infusion devices (Baxter) was evaluated stored at 4 °C for 14 days. Bioassay of the solutions found no loss of lenograstim (2048).

Sorption— The manufacturer states that lenograstim prepared in sodium chloride 0.9% as directed for administration is compatible with common administration sets, including PVC sets (1442).

Compatibility Information

Infusion Solutions— At concentrations not less than 0.26 million I.U. (Granocyte-13) or 0.32 million I.U. (Granocyte-34) per milliliter, lenograstim (Chugai Pharma) is stable for up to 24 hours at 5 or 25 °C (1442).

METHOTRIMEPRAZINE
(LEVOMEPROMAZINE HCL)

Nozinan   **Link Pharmaceuticals**

Products— Methotrimeprazine (Link Pharmaceuticals) is available in 1-ml ampuls as a 2.5% (w/v) solution. The injection also contains ascorbic acid, sodium sulphite, and sodium chloride (1442).

pH— From 3 to 5 (17).

Osmolality— Methotrimeprazine is an isotonic solution (1442).

Administration— Methotrimeprazine is administered by intramuscular injection or intravenously after dilution with an equal volume of sodium chloride 0.9% immediately before use. It may also be given by continuous subcutaneous infusion diluted with the appropriate volume of sodium chloride 0.9% (1442).

Stability— Methotrimeprazine injection is a clear, transparent solution. It should be stored at controlled room temperature and protected from light. On exposure to light, methotrimeprazine HCl rapidly develops a pink or yellow discoloration; discolored solutions should be discarded. The drug is incompatible with alkaline solutions (1442).

Compatibility Information

Drugs in Syringe Compatibility

				Methotrimeprazine			
Drug (in syringe)	*Mfr*	*Amt*	*Mfr*	*Amt*	*Remarks*	*Ref*	*C/I*
Butorphanol tartrate	BR	4 mg/ 2 ml		25 mg/ 1 ml	Physically compatible for 30 min at room temperature both microscopically and macroscopically	566	C
Diamorphine HCl	MB	50 mg/ 1 ml	MB	1.25 and 2.5 mg/ 1 ml[a]	Physically compatible and diamorphine potency retained for 24 hr at room temperature	1454	C
Heparin sodium		2500 units/ 1 ml		25 mg/ 1 ml	Turbidity or precipitate forms within 5 min	1053	I
Hydroxyzine HCl	PF	50 mg/ 1 ml	LE	20 mg/ 1 ml	Physically compatible	771	C
	PF	100 mg/ 2 ml	LE	10 mg/ 0.5 ml	Physically compatible	771	C
Metoclopramide HCl	NO	10 mg/ 2 ml	RP	10 mg/ 2 ml	Physically compatible for 15 min at room temperature both microscopically and macroscopically	565	C

Drugs in Syringe Compatibility (Cont.)

Methotrimeprazine

Drug (in syringe)	Mfr	Amt	Mfr	Amt	Remarks	Ref	C/I
Perphenazine	SC	5 mg/ 1 ml		25 mg/ 1 ml	Physically compatible for 30 min at room temperature both microscopically and macroscopically	566	**C**
Ranitidine HCl	GL	50 mg/ 2 ml	RP	25 mg/ 1 ml	Immediate white turbidity	978	**I**
Sufentanil citrate	JN	50 μg/ml	LE	20 mg/ ml	Physically compatible with no subvisual haze or particle formation in 24 hr at 23 °C	1711	**C**

[a]*Diluted with sterile water for injection.*

Y-Site Injection Compatibility (1:1 Mixture)

Methotrimeprazine

Drug	Mfr	Conc	Mfr	Conc	Remarks	Ref	C/I
Heparin sodium		50 units/ml/ min		25 mg/1 ml[a]	White precipitate forms	1053	**I**
Sufentanil citrate	JN	12.5 μg/ml[b]	LE	0.2 mg/ml[b]	Physically compatible with no subvisual haze or particle formation in 24 hr at 23 °C	1711	**C**

[a]*Given over three minutes via Y-site into a running infusion solution of heparin sodium in sodium chloride 0.9%.*
[b]*Tested in dextrose 5% in water.*

Additional Compatibility Information

Atropine sulfate or scopolamine hydrobromide may be mixed in the same syringe with methotrimeprazine for intramuscular administration (19).

Methotrimeprazine is stated to be stable and compatible with diamorphine HCl for 24 hours (1442).

NIZATIDINE

Axid   **Lilly**

Products— Nizatidine (Lilly) is available as a 25-mg/ml solution in 4-ml ampuls (1442).

pH— From 6.5 to 7.5 (1442).

Administration— Nizatidine is administered by continuous intravenous infusion; the manufacturer recommends diluting 300 mg of drug in 150 ml of compatible diluent and infusing at a rate of 10 mg/hr. The drug is also given by intermittent intravenous infusion; the manufacturer recommends diluting 100 mg of drug in 50 ml of compatible diluent and infusing over 15 minutes (1442).

Stability— Intact containers of nizatidine should be stored below 25 °C and protected from light. Nizatidine injection is a clear and colorless to yellow solution. It may tend to darken slightly, but this does not adversely affect potency (1442).

Freezing Solutions— Nizatidine (Lilly) 0.75 and 3 mg/ml in dextrose 5% in water, sodium chloride 0.9%, and sterile water for injection in PVC containers was stored frozen at −20 °C for 30 days. Little or no nizatidine loss was found using HPLC analysis after frozen storage. An additional seven days of storage under refrigeration at 4 °C resulted in no additional loss of drug (1533).

Sorption— Nizatidine (Lilly) 0.75, 1.5, and 3 mg/ml in dextrose 5% in water, sodium chloride 0.9%, and sterile water for injection exhibited no loss due to sorption during seven days of storage at 4 and 25 °C in both glass and PVC containers (1533).

Compatibility Information

Solution Compatibility

Nizatidine

Solution	Mfr	Mfr	Conc/L	Remarks	Ref	C/I
Amino acids 8.5%	TR[a]	LI	0.75 and 1.5 g	Visually compatible and nizatidine potency by HPLC retained for 7 days at 4 and 25 °C. Amino acids not tested	1533	C
	TR[a]	LI	3 g	Visually compatible with 8% nizatidine loss in 3 days and 13% loss in 7 days at 25 °C by HPLC. 5% nizatidine loss in 7 days at 4 °C. Amino acids not tested	1533	C
Dextrose 5% in Ringer's injection, lactated	TR[a]	LI	0.75, 1.5, 3 g	Visually compatible with 5% or less loss by HPLC in 7 days at 4 and 25 °C	1533	C
Dextrose 5% in sodium chloride 0.2%	TR[a]	LI	0.75, 1.5, 3 g	Visually compatible with little or no loss by HPLC in 7 days at 4 and 25 °C	1533	C
Dextrose 5% in sodium chloride 0.45%	TR[a]	LI	0.75, 1.5, 3 g	Visually compatible with 6% or less loss by HPLC in 7 days at 25 °C and little or no loss in 7 days at 4 °C	1533	C
Dextrose 5% in sodium chloride 0.45% with potassium chloride 0.15%	TR[a]	LI	0.75, 1.5, 3 g	Visually compatible with 7% or less loss by HPLC in 7 days at 4 and 25 °C	1533	C
Dextrose 5% in sodium chloride 0.9%	TR[a]	LI	0.75, 1.5, 3 g	Visually compatible with little or no loss by HPLC in 7 days at 4 and 25 °C	1533	C
Dextrose 5% in water	TR[a,b]	LI	0.75, 1.5, 3 g	Visually compatible with little or no loss by HPLC in 7 days at 4 and 25 °C	1533	C
Dextrose 10% in water	TR[a]	LI	0.75, 1.5, 3 g	Visually compatible with little or no loss by HPLC in 7 days at 4 and 25 °C	1533	C
Mannitol 20%	MG[a]	LI	0.75, 1.5, 3 g	Visually compatible with little or no loss by HPLC in 7 days at 4 and 25 °C	1533	C
Plasma-Lyte 56 with dextrose 5%	TR[a]	LI	0.75, 1.5, 3 g	Visually compatible with 7% or less loss by HPLC at 25 °C in 7 days and little or no loss at 4 °C in 7 days	1533	C
Ringer's injection, lactated	TR[a]	LI	0.75, 1.5, 3 g	Visually compatible with little or no loss by HPLC in 7 days at 4 and 25 °C	1533	C
Sodium bicarbonate 5%	TR[a]	LI	0.75, 1.5, 3 g	Visually compatible with little or no loss by HPLC in 7 days at 4 and 25 °C	1533	C
Sodium chloride 0.9%	TR[a,b]	LI	0.75, 1.5, 3 g	Visually compatible with little or no loss by HPLC in 7 days at 4 and 25 °C	1533	C
Sodium lactate ⅙ M	TR[a]	LI	0.75, 1.5, 3 g	Visually compatible with little or no loss by HPLC in 7 days at 4 and 25 °C	1533	C

Solution Compatibility (Cont.)

Nizatidine

Solution	Mfr	Mfr	Conc/L	Remarks	Ref	C/I
TNA #135 to #138 and TPN #134[c]		LI	150 mg	Physically compatible with no increase in fat particle size and 2 to 7% nizatidine loss by HPLC in 48 hr at 22 °C under fluorescent light	1534; 1921	C

[a]Tested in glass containers.
[b]Tested in PVC containers.
[c]Refer to Appendix I for the composition of parenteral nutrition solutions. TNA indicates a 3-in-1 admixture, and TPN indicates a 2-in-1 admixture.

Additional Compatibility Information

Infusion Solutions— The manufacturer states that nizatidine admixtures in the following solutions are stable for 24 hours stored under refrigeration at 2 to 8 °C. However, other information indicates the drug may be stable for longer periods. See the following solutions in the Solution Compatibility table above (1442):

Dextrose 5% in water
Ringer's injection, lactated (Compound sodium lactate injection)
Sodium bicarbonate 5%
Sodium chloride 0.9%

OMEPRAZOLE

Losec Infusion   **AstraZeneca**

Products— Omeprazole infusion (AstraZeneca) is available in vials containing 40 mg of drug as the sodium salt. Also present in the formulation are sodium hydroxide and disodium edetate. Reconstitute the vials with 5 ml of sodium chloride 0.9% or dextrose 5% in water. The reconstituted drug should be diluted to 100 ml with the same diluent for administration (1442).

Administration— After dilution to 100 ml with sodium chloride 0.9% or dextrose 5% in water, omeprazole is administered only as a 20- to 30-minute intravenous infusion. Omeprazole must not be given by any other route (1442).

Stability— Intact vials of omeprazole infusion should be stored at room temperature not exceeding 25 °C. Dilution with sodium chloride 0.9% or dextrose 5% in water results in a solution that is stable for 12 hours or 3 hours, respectively. Other solutions must not be used for dilution of omeprazole. Do not use the reconstituted solution if particles are present (1442).

Compatibility Information

Y-Site Injection Compatibility (1:1 Mixture)

Omeprazole

Drug	Mfr	Conc	Mfr	Conc	Remarks	Ref	C/I
Lorazepam	WY	0.33 mg/ml[b]	AST	4 mg/ml	Yellow discoloration forms	1855	I
Midazolam HCl	RC	5 mg/ml	AST	4 mg/ml	Brown discoloration forms, followed by brown precipitate	1855	I
Vancomycin HCl		10 mg/ml[a]		4 mg/ml	White precipitate forms within 5 min	2173	I

[a]Tested in dextrose 5% in water.
[b]Tested in sodium chloride 0.9%.

PROMAZINE HCL

Genus

Products— Promazine HCl is available in a concentration of 50 mg/ml in 1-ml ampuls (30).

pH— From 4 to 5.5 (17).

Administration— Promazine HCl is administered by deep intramuscular injection (4; 30) or slowly by direct intravenous injection at a concentration not exceeding 25 mg/ml. Extravasation should be avoided. It should not be given intra-arterially (4).

Stability— The product should be stored at controlled room temperature and protected from freezing and light (4). Promazine HCl is maximally stable at pH 6.5 (67). It oxidizes after prolonged exposure to air (4). A slight yellowish discoloration does not affect potency or efficacy, but markedly discolored solutions or solutions containing a precipitate should not be used (4).

Sorption— Promazine HCl (Wyeth) 6.4 mg/L in sodium chloride 0.9% (Travenol) in PVC bags did not exhibit significant sorption to the plastic during one week of storage at room temperature (15 to 20 °C). However, when the solution was buffered from its initial pH of 5 to 7.4, approximately 48% of the drug was lost in one week due to sorption (536).

Promazine HCl (Wyeth) 6.4 mg/L in sodium chloride 0.9% exhibited a cumulative 11% loss during a seven-hour simulated infusion through an infusion set (Travenol) consisting of a cellulose propionate burette chamber and 170 cm of PVC tubing due to sorption. Both the burette and the tubing contributed to the loss. The extent of sorption was found to be independent of concentration (606).

The drug was also tested as a simulated infusion over at least one hour by a syringe pump system. A glass syringe on a syringe pump was fitted with 20 cm of polyethylene tubing or 50 cm of Silastic tubing. A negligible amount of drug was lost with the polyethylene tubing, but a cumulative loss of 59% occurred during the one-hour infusion through the Silastic tubing (606).

A 25-ml aliquot of promazine HCl (Wyeth) 6.4 mg/L in sodium chloride 0.9%, stored in all-plastic syringes composed of polypropylene barrels and polyethylene plungers for 24 hours at room temperature in the dark, did not exhibit any loss due to sorption (606).

Compatibility Information

Solution Compatibility

Promazine HCl

Solution	Mfr	Mfr	Conc/L		Remarks	Ref	C/I
Dextran 6% in dextrose 5%	AB	WY	300	mg	Physically compatible	3	C
Dextran 6% in sodium chloride 0.9%	AB	WY	300	mg	Physically compatible	3	C
Dextrose–Ringer's injection combinations	AB	WY	300	mg	Physically compatible	3	C
Dextrose–Ringer's injection, lactated, combinations	AB	WY	300	mg	Physically compatible	3	C
Dextrose–saline combinations	AB	WY	300	mg	Physically compatible	3	C
Dextrose 2½% in water	AB	WY	300	mg	Physically compatible	3	C
Dextrose 5% in water	AB	WY	300	mg	Physically compatible	3	C
	TR	WY	1	g	10% loss in 3 days at room temperature exposed to daylight. No loss in 6 days at room temperature or 4 °C in the dark	1149	C
Dextrose 10% in water	AB	WY	300	mg	Physically compatible	3	C
Fructose 10% in sodium chloride 0.9%	AB	WY	300	mg	Physically compatible	3	C
Fructose 10% in water	AB	WY	300	mg	Physically compatible	3	C
Invert sugar 5 and 10% in sodium chloride 0.9%	AB	WY	300	mg	Physically compatible	3	C
Invert sugar 5 and 10% in water	AB	WY	300	mg	Physically compatible	3	C
Ionosol products (except as noted below)	AB	WY	300	mg	Physically compatible	3	C
Ionosol B with dextrose 5%	AB	WY	300	mg	Haze or precipitate forms within 6 hr	3	I
Ringer's injection	AB	WY	300	mg	Physically compatible	3	C
Ringer's injection, lactated	AB	WY	300	mg	Physically compatible	3	C
Sodium chloride 0.45%	AB	WY	300	mg	Physically compatible	3	C
Sodium chloride 0.9%	AB	WY	300	mg	Physically compatible	3	C
	TR	WY	1	g	8% loss in 8 hr and 15% in 24 hr at room temperature exposed to daylight	1149	I

Solution Compatibility (Cont.)

Promazine HCl

Solution	Mfr	Mfr	Conc/L	Remarks	Ref	C/I
	TR	WY	1 g	10% loss in 6 days at room temperature or 4 °C in the dark	1149	C
Sodium lactate ⅙ M	AB	WY	300 mg	Physically compatible	3	C

Additive Compatibility

Promazine HCl

Drug	Mfr	Conc/L	Mfr	Conc/L	Test Soln	Remarks	Ref	C/I
Aminophylline	SE	1 g	WY	1 g	D5W	Physically incompatible	15	I
	BP	1 g	BP	200 mg	D5W, NS	Immediate precipitation	26	I
Chloramphenicol sodium succinate	PD	1 g	WY	100 mg		Physically compatible	6	C
Chlorothiazide sodium	BP	2 g	BP	200 mg	D5W, NS	Immediate precipitation	26	I
Erythromycin lactobionate	AB	1 g	WY	100 mg		Physically compatible	20	C
Ethacrynate sodium	MSD	50 mg	WY	50 mg	NS	Little alteration of UV spectra in 8 hr at room temperature	16	C
Fibrinogen	CU	2 g	WY	1 g	D5W	Physically incompatible	11	I
Fibrinolysin, human	MSD	2 g	WY	1 g	D5W	Physically incompatible	11	I
Heparin sodium	AB	20,000 units	WY	100 mg		Physically compatible	21	C
Lidocaine HCl	AST	2 g	WY	100 mg		Physically compatible	24	C
Metaraminol bitartrate	MSD	100 mg	WY	100 mg		Physically compatible	7	C
Methohexital sodium	BP	2 g	BP	200 mg	D5W, NS	Immediate precipitation	26	I
Methyldopate HCl	MSD	1 g	WY	100 mg	D, D–S, S	Physically compatible	23	C
Nafcillin sodium	WY	500 mg	WY	100 mg		Physically compatible for only 6 hr	27	I
Penicillin G potassium	PF	20 million units	WY	1 g	D5W	Physically incompatible	11	I
Pentobarbital sodium	AB	200 mg	WY	1 g	D5W	Physically incompatible	11	I
Phenobarbital sodium	BP	800 mg	BP	200 mg	NS	Immediate precipitation	26	I
Sodium bicarbonate	AB	3.75 g	WY	1 g	D5W	Physically incompatible	11	I
	AB	2.4 mEq[a]	WY	100 mg	D5W	Physically compatible for 24 hr	772	C
Thiopental sodium	AB	2.5 g	WY	1 g	D5W	Physically incompatible	11	I
	AB	2.5 g	WY	100 mg	D5W	Precipitate forms within 1 hr	21	I

[a]One vial of Neut added to a liter of admixture.

Drugs in Syringe Compatibility

Promazine HCl

Drug (in syringe)	Mfr	Amt	Mfr	Amt	Remarks	Ref	C/I
Atropine sulfate	ST	0.4 mg/ 1 ml	WY	50 mg/ 1 ml	Physically compatible for at least 15 min	326	C
Chlorpromazine HCl	PO	50 mg/ 2 ml	WY	50 mg/ 1 ml	Physically compatible for at least 15 min	326	C

Drugs in Syringe Compatibility (Cont.)

Promazine HCl

Drug (in syringe)	Mfr	Amt	Mfr	Amt	Remarks	Ref	C/I
Cimetidine HCl	SKF	300 mg/ 2 ml	WY	25 mg/ 1 ml	Physically compatible for 4 hr at 25 °C	25	C
Dimenhydrinate	HR	50 mg/ 1 ml	WY	50 mg/ 1 ml	Physically incompatible within 15 min	326	I
Diphenhydramine HCl	PD	50 mg/ 1 ml	WY	50 mg/ 1 ml	Physically compatible for at least 15 min	326	C
Droperidol	MN	2.5 mg/ 1 ml	WY	50 mg/ 1 ml	Physically compatible for at least 15 min	326	C
Fentanyl citrate	MN	0.05 mg/ 1 ml	WY	50 mg/ 1 ml	Physically compatible for at least 15 min	326	C
Glycopyrrolate	RB	0.2 mg/ 1 ml	WY	50 mg/ 1 ml	Physically compatible and pH in stability range for glycopyrrolate for 48 hr at 25 °C	331	C
	RB	0.2 mg/ 1 ml	WY	100 mg/ 2 ml	Physically compatible and pH in stability range for glycopyrrolate for 48 hr at 25 °C	331	C
	RB	0.4 mg/ 2 ml	WY	50 mg/ 1 ml	Physically compatible and pH in stability range for glycopyrrolate for 48 hr at 25 °C	331	C
Hydroxyzine HCl	PF	50 mg/ 1 ml	WY	50 mg/ 1 ml	Physically compatible for at least 15 min	326	C
Meperidine HCl	WI	50 mg/ 1 ml	WY	50 mg/ 1 ml	Physically compatible for at least 15 min	326	C
Metoclopramide HCl	NO	10 mg/ 2 ml	MY	50 mg/ 1 ml	Physically compatible both macroscopically and microscopically for 15 min at room temperature	565	C
Midazolam HCl	RC	5 mg/ 1 ml	WY	50 mg/ 1 ml	Physically compatible for 4 hr at 25 °C under fluorescent light	1145	C
Morphine sulfate	ST	15 mg/ 1 ml	WY	50 mg/ 1 ml	Physically compatible for at least 15 min	326	C
Pentazocine lactate	WI	30 mg/ 1 ml	WY	25 mg/ 1 ml	Potency retained for 3 months at room temperature in Tubex	13	C
	WI	30 mg/ 1 ml	WY	50 mg/ 1 ml	Potency retained for 3 months at room temperature in Tubex	13	C
	WI	30 mg/ 1 ml	WY	50 mg/ 1 ml	Physically compatible for at least 15 min	326	C
Pentobarbital sodium	AB	50 mg/ 1 ml	WY	50 mg/ 1 ml	Physically incompatible within 15 min	326	I
Prochlorperazine edisylate	PO	5 mg/ 1 ml	WY	50 mg/ 1 ml	Physically compatible for at least 15 min	326	C
Promethazine HCl	PO	50 mg/ 2 ml	WY	50 mg/ 1 ml	Physically compatible for at least 15 min	326	C
Scopolamine HBr	ST	0.4 mg/ 1 ml	WY	50 mg/ 1 ml	Physically compatible for at least 15 min	326	C

Y-Site Injection Compatibility (1:1 Mixture)

Promazine HCl

Drug	Mfr	Conc	Mfr	Conc	Remarks	Ref	C/I
Warfarin sodium	DU	0.1[a,b] and 2[c] mg/ml	WY	5 mg/ml[a,b]	Heavy white turbidity forms immediately	2011	I

[a]Tested in dextrose 5% in water.
[b]Tested in sodium chloride 0.9%.
[c]Tested in sterile water for injection.

Additional Compatibility Information

Concentrated Solutions— The following incompatibility determinations were performed with concentrated solutions. The drugs in dry form were reconstituted according to manufacturers' recommendations. One milliliter of promazine HCl was added to 5 ml of sterile distilled water along with 1 ml of each of the following drugs. Particulate matter was noted within two hours (28):

Aminophylline
Chloramphenicol sodium succinate (Parke-Davis)
Dimenhydrinate (Searle)
Heparin sodium
Hydrocortisone sodium succinate (Upjohn)
Penicillin G potassium
Phenobarbital sodium (Winthrop)
Phenytoin sodium (Parke-Davis)
Vitamin B complex with C (Lederle)

PROPAFENONE HCL

Rhythmol **Knoll AG**
Rytmonorm **Knoll AG**

Products— Propafenone HCl (Knoll) is available as a 3.5-mg/ml solution in 20-ml (70-mg) ampuls. Each milliliter of solution also contains dextrose monohydrate 53.8 mg in water for injection (411; 412; 441).

pH— Propafenone HCl (Knoll) 70 mg/20 ml injection has a pH of 4.7 to 6 (411; 412).

Administration— Propafenone HCl is administered by intravenous injection as a bolus given slowly over three to five minutes. Intervals between doses should be about 90 to 120 minutes. Blood pressure and electrocardiogram parameters should be monitored (441).

Propafenone HCl may also be given as a short-term infusion over one to three hours or as a long-term infusion continuously over periods up to several days. The drug is diluted in dextrose 5% in water or fructose 5% in water for intravenous infusion (441).

Stability— The manufacturer indicates that propafenone HCl is incompatible with chloride-containing infusion solutions because of the potential for precipitation (441).

Syringes— Propafenone HCl (Knoll) at concentrations of 0.5, 1, and 2 mg/ml in dextrose 5% in water and in dextrose 5% in 0.2% sodium chloride was packaged as 7 ml of solution in 10-ml polypropylene syringes (Becton-Dickinson). The solutions were visually compatible and HPLC analysis found 4% or less loss in 48 hours stored at 21 °C exposed to fluorescent light (411).

Freezing Solutions— Propafenone HCl (Knoll) 2 mg/ml in dextrose 5% in 0.2% sodium chloride in PVC bags was found to have precipitated on thawing of frozen solutions. Precipitation was not observed when lower drug concentrations (0.5 and 1 mg/ml) in polypropylene syringes (Becton-Dickinson) were frozen and when dextrose 5% in water was used as the diluent for concentrations of 0.5, 1, and 2 mg/ml. Nevertheless, avoiding the freezing of propafenone HCl solutions should be considered (411).

Solution Compatibility

Propafenone HCl

Solution	Mfr	Mfr	Conc/L	Remarks	Ref	C/I
Dextrose 5% in water	BA[a]	KN	0.5, 1, and 2 g	Visually compatible with 4% or less loss by HPLC in 48 hr at 21 °C under fluorescent light	411	C
Dextrose 5% in 0.2% sodium chloride	BA[a]	KN	0.5 and 1 g	Visually compatible with no loss by HPLC in 48 hr at 21 °C under fluorescent light	411	C

[a]Tested in PVC containers.

Additive Compatibility

Propafenone HCl

Drug	Mfr	Conc/L	Mfr	Conc/L	Test Soln	Remarks	Ref	C/I
Amiodarone HCl	LZ	1.25 g[a]	KN	0.625 g	D5W	Visually compatible with no propafenone loss by HPLC in 24 hr at 22 °C exposed to fluorescent light. Amiodarone not tested	412	C
Amrinone lactate	SW	1 and 2.5 g[a]	KN	0.5 g	NS	Visually compatible with little or no propafenone loss by HPLC in 24 hr at 22 °C exposed to fluorescent light. Amrinone not tested	412	C
Dopamine HCl	DU	0.9 and 2.3 g[a]	KN	0.54 g	D5W	Visually compatible with little or no propafenone loss by HPLC in 24 hr at 22 °C exposed to fluorescent light. Dopamine not tested	412	C
Lidocaine HCl	AST	4.5 g[a]	KN	0.54 g	D5W	Visually compatible with little or no propafenone loss by HPLC in 24 hr at 22 °C exposed to fluorescent light. Lidocaine not tested	412	C
Potassium chloride	AST	18 mmol[a]	KN	0.54 g	D5W	Visually compatible for 24 hr at 22 °C exposed to fluorescent light	412	C

[a]*Approximate concentration.*

SALBUTAMOL SULPHATE

Ventolin   **Allen and Hanburys**

Products— Salbutamol (Allen and Hanburys) is available as a 50-μg/ml solution in 5-ml ampuls and as a 500-μg/ml solution in 1-ml ampuls as the sulphate. In addition, the products contain sodium chloride, sodium hydroxide, and sulfuric acid (1442).

Tonicity— Salbutamol injection is isotonic (1442).

Administration— Salbutamol is administered by subcutaneous, intramuscular, or intravenous injection. For intravenous administration, it may be diluted in a compatible infusion solution (1442).

Stability— Salbutamol is a clear, colorless, or pale straw-colored solution. The intact containers should be stored below 30 °C and protected from light (1442).

Compatibility Information

Drugs in Syringe Compatibility

Salbutamol

Drug (in syringe)	Mfr	Amt	Mfr	Amt	Remarks	Ref	C/I
Hydromorphone HCl	KN	1 mg/ 0.5 ml	GL	2.5 mg/ 2.5 ml[a]	Visually compatible for 1 hr both macroscopically and microscopically	1904	C
Morphine sulfate	AB	5 mg/ 0.5 ml	GL	2.5 mg/ 2.5 ml[a]	Visually compatible for 1 hr both macroscopically and microscopically	1904	C

[a]*Both preserved (benzyl alcohol 0.9%; benzalkonium chloride 0.01%) and unpreserved sodium chloride 0.9% were used as a diluent.*

Additional Compatibility Information

Dextrose 5% in water
Sodium chloride 0.18% and dextrose 4%
Sodium chloride 0.9%
Sterile water for injection

Infusion Solutions— The manufacturer states that salbutamol is stable for use within 24 hours diluted in the following infusion solutions (1442):

SODIUM FUSIDATE

Fucidin for Intravenous Infusion   Leo Pharmaceuticals

Products— Sodium fusidate (Leo Pharmaceuticals) is available as a dry powder in vials containing 500 mg (equivalent to 480 mg of fusidic acid). It is packaged with a diluent vial containing 10 ml of phosphate–citrate buffer (pH 7.4 to 7.6). The drug should be reconstituted with the diluent to provide a 4.8-mg/ml concentration (1442).

Sodium and Phosphate Content— Each vial of reconstituted sodium fusidate contains 3.1 mmol of sodium and 1.1 mmol of phosphate (1442).

Administration— Sodium fusidate is administered by slow intravenous infusion over not less than six hours if a superficial vein is employed. If a central venous line is used, the infusion should be given over two hours. The reconstituted sodium fusidate in 10 ml of buffer solution is diluted in 500 ml of compatible infusion solution for administration (1442).

Stability— Sodium fusidate should be stored below 25 °C (1442).

Freezing Solutions— Sodium fusidate (Leo) 1 mg/ml in sodium chloride 0.9%, dextrose 5% in water, and sodium chloride 0.18% and dextrose 4% is stated to be stable frozen at −20 °C for 24 hours followed by thawing in a microwave oven (1800).

Fusidic acid (Leo) 500 mg, reconstituted in buffer and diluted to 550 ml in sodium chloride 0.9% in PVC bags, was stored frozen at −20 °C. No loss was found by HPLC after 12 months of storage followed by microwave thawing. Furthermore, the solution was physically compatible, with no increase in subvisual particles. In addition, there was no loss of sodium fusidate after six months of storage at −20 °C followed by three freeze–thaw cycles (1612).

Compatibility Information

Solution Compatibility

Sodium fusidate

Solution	Mfr	Mfr	Conc/L	Remarks	Ref	C/I
Compound sodium lactate intravenous infusion (Ringer's lactate)	BP	LEO	1 g	Physically compatible and chemically stable for 48 hr at room temperature	1800	C
Darrow-glucose intravenous infusion		LEO	2 g	Physically compatible and chemically stable for 48 hr at room temperature	1800	C
Dextrose 5% in water	BA[a]	LEO	1.16 and 2.32 g	Physically compatible with less than 10% loss in 162 days at 4 °C and 10% loss in 10.4 days at 25 °C or 2.1 days at 37 °C	1709	C
	BP	LEO	1 or 2 g	Physically compatible and chemically stable for 48 hr at room temperature	1800	C
Electrolyte Solution B with dextrose 20%	TR	LEO	1 g	Physically incompatible	1800	I
Fat emulsion, intravenous 10% (Intralipid)		LEO	1 g	Physically incompatible	1800	I
Potassium chloride 0.3% and dextrose 5%	BP	LEO	1 g	Physically compatible and chemically stable for 48 hr at room temperature	1800	C
Potassium chloride 0.3% and sodium chloride 0.9%	BP	LEO	1 and 2 g	Physically compatible and chemically stable for 48 hr at room temperature	1800	C
Sodium chloride 0.9%	BP	LEO	1 and 2 g	Physically compatible and chemically stable for 48 hr at room temperature	1800	C
Sodium chloride 0.18% and dextrose 4%	BP	LEO	1 g	Physically compatible and chemically stable for 48 hr at room temperature	1800	C

Solution Compatibility (Cont.)

Sodium fusidate

Solution	Mfr	Mfr	Conc/L	Remarks	Ref	C/I
Sodium lactate intravenous infusion	BP	LEO	1 g	Physically compatible and chemically stable for 48 hr at room temperature	1800	C

^aTested in PVC containers.

Additive Compatibility

Sodium fusidate

Drug	Mfr	Conc/L	Mfr	Conc/L	Test Soln	Remarks	Ref	C/I
Amdinocillin		50 g	LEO	500 mg	D-S	Physically incompatible	1800	I
Cefotaxime sodium		2.5 g	LEO	500 mg	D-S	Physically compatible and chemically stable for 48 hr at room temperature	1800	C
Erythromycin lactobionate		5 g	LEO	1 g	D-S	Physically compatible and chemically stable for 48 hr at room temperature	1800	C
Flucloxacillin sodium		2.5 g	LEO	500 mg	D-S	Physically compatible and chemically stable for 48 hr at room temperature	1800	C
Gentamicin sulphate		160 mg	LEO	1 g	D-S	Physically compatible and chemically stable for 48 hr at room temperature	1800	C
		1.5 g	LEO	1 g	D-S	Physically incompatible	1800	I
Vancomycin HCl		25 g	LEO	500 mg	D-S	Physically incompatible	1800	I

Additional Compatibility Information

Peritoneal Dialysis Solutions— Sodium fusidate (Leo) at a concentration of 0.125 mg/ml is stated to be physically incompatible with the following peritoneal dialysis solutions (1800):

Dianeal PD2 with dextrose 1.36%
Dianeal PD3 with dextrose 1.36%
Dianeal with dextrose 3.86%
Peritoneal Dialysis Solution 6.36%
Peritoneal Dialysis Solution 6.36% + acetate
Peritoneal Dialysis Solution with dextrose 2.27%

TEICOPLANIN

Targocid   **Aventis**

Products— Teicoplanin (Aventis) is available as a lyophilized powder in vials containing teicoplanin 200 and 400 mg. The vials are accompanied by an ampul of water for injection for use as a diluent. Reconstitute by adding the diluent slowly to the vial of teicoplanin and then rolling the vial gently until the powder is completely dissolved. Care should be taken to avoid the formation of foam; if foam does form, the solution should stand for about 15 minutes for the foam to subside. The teicoplanin vials contain a calculated excess so that when reconstituted as directed the full amount of drug can be withdrawn from the vial using a syringe and needle. The concentration of teicoplanin is 100 mg in 1.5 ml (from the 200-mg vials) and 400 mg in 3 ml (from the 400-mg vial) (1442).

Administration— Teicoplanin may be administered after reconstitution either intramuscularly or by direct intravenous injection as a bolus. It may also be administered as an intravenous infusion over 30 minutes after dilution of the reconstituted solution in a compatible infusion solution (1442).

Stability— Intact vials of teicoplanin should be stored below 25 °C. The manufacturer recommends that reconstituted teicoplanin be used immediately after preparation and any unused portion be discarded. However, the manufacturer also states that the reconstituted solution may be stored under refrigeration at 4 °C for up to 24 hours if the situation makes discarding the reconstituted drug impractical (1442).

Compatibility Information

Solution Compatibility

Teicoplanin

Solution	Mfr	Mfr	Conc/L	Remarks	Ref	C/I
Dextrose 5% in water	BA[a]	HO	2 g	Visually compatible with no loss of teicoplanin by HPLC and microbiological assays in 24 hr at 25 °C	2165	C
Sodium chloride 0.9%	BA[a]	HO	2 g	Visually compatible with no loss of teicoplanin by HPLC and microbiological assays in 24 hr at 25 °C	2165	C

[a]Tested in glass containers.

Additive Compatibility

Teicoplanin

Drug	Mfr	Conc/L	Mfr	Conc/L	Test Soln	Remarks	Ref	C/I
Heparin sodium	CPP	20,000 and 40,000 units	HO	2 g	DSW, NS	Visually compatible with no loss of teicoplanin by HPLC and microbiological assay and no loss of heparin activity in 24 hr at 25 °C	2165	C

Y-Site Injection Compatibility (1:1 Mixture)

Teicoplanin

Drug	Mfr	Conc	Mfr	Conc	Remarks	Ref	C/I
Ciprofloxacin	BAY	2 mg/ml[a]	GRP	60 mg/ml	White precipitate forms immediately but disappears with shaking	1934	?

[a]Tested in sodium chloride 0.9%.

Additional Compatibility Information

Infusion Solutions— The manufacturer recommends the following infusion solutions for diluting teicoplanin for intravenous infusion (1442):

Dextrose 5% in water

Ringer's injection, lactated (Compound sodium lactate injection)

Sodium chloride 0.18% and dextrose 4%

Sodium chloride 0.9%

Dextrose-Containing Solutions— Teicoplanin forms dextrose aldehyde adducts when diluted in dextrose-containing solutions. Equilibrium is reached faster at room temperature (seven days) than with refrigerated storage (30 days). The equilibrium concentration of the adduct is directly related to the dextrose concentration. The reaction is reversible with dilution (2046).

Peritoneal Dialysis Solutions— The manufacturer recommends use of peritoneal dialysis solutions containing 1.36 or 3.86% dextrose (1442).

Teicoplanin (Marion Merrell Dow) 0.025 mg/ml in Dianeal PD-2 with dextrose 1.5% in PVC containers was physically and chemically stable by HPLC analysis for 24 hours at 25 °C exposed to light, exhibiting no loss; additional storage for eight hours at 37 °C resulted in losses of 6% or less. Under refrigeration at 4 °C protected from light, no loss occurred in seven days. Additional storage for 16 hours at 25 °C followed by eight hours at 37 °C resulted in about 7% loss (1989).

Ceftazidime (sodium carbonate formulation) (Glaxo) 0.1 mg/ml admixed with teicoplanin (Marion Merrell Dow) 0.025 mg/ml in Dianeal PD-2 with dextrose 1.5% in PVC containers did not result in a stable mixture. Using HPLC analysis, large (but variable) teicoplanin losses generally in the 20% range were noted in as little as two hours at 25 °C exposed to light. Ceftazidime losses of about 9% occurred in 16 hours. Refrigeration and protection from light of the peritoneal dialysis admixture reduced losses of both drugs to negligible levels. Even so, the authors did not recommend admixing these two drugs because of the high levels of teicoplanin loss at room temperature (1989).

Teicoplanin (Merrell Dow) 25 mg/L in Dianeal 137 with dextrose 1.36% (Baxter) was evaluated for stability over 42 days using a stability-indicating bioassay. Stored at 4 °C, teicoplanin retained stability with a loss of less than 5% in 42 days. At 20 °C, 10% loss occurred in about 25 days with 17% loss in 42 days. At an elevated temperature of 37 °C, a much greater rate of decomposition occurs with over 40% loss occurring in 42 days (2145).

Heparin Sodium— The stability of catheter flush solutions composed of teicoplanin 133 mg/ml in water for injection, or heparin sodium 10 units/ml or 100 units/ml, was evaluated in Hickman catheters at

25 °C over 24 hours. No decomposition products formed by HPLC analysis, and no loss was found by HPLC or microbiological assays. Indeed, a small (11%) increase in teicoplanin concentration was observed which the authors attributed to loss of water (2165).

Aminoglycosides— Solutions of teicoplanin and aminoglycosides are incompatible and should not be directly mixed prior to injection (1442).

TRAMADOL HCL

Zamadol	**Asta Medica**
Zydol	**Searle**

Products— Tramadol HCl is available as a 50-mg/ml aqueous solution in 2-ml (100 mg) ampuls. Sodium acetate is also present in the formulation (1442).

Osmolarity— Tramadol HCl (Asta Medica) has an osmolarity of 320 to 380 mOsm/L (1442).

Administration— Tramadol HCl is administered intramuscularly, by direct intravenous injection slowly over two to three minutes, or by intravenous infusion after dilution (1442).

Stability— Tramadol HCl is a clear, colorless solution. The intact ampuls should be stored below 30 °C (1442).

Exposure to or protection from light did not affect the stability of tramadol HCl 0.5- and 4-mg/ml infusion solutions in dextrose 5% in water or sodium chloride 0.9% (434).

Portable Infusion Pump— Tramadol HCl (Mundipharma) 0.5 and 4 mg/ml in dextrose 5% in water or sodium chloride 0.9% was evaluated by HPLC analysis for stability in PVC portable infusion pump reservoirs (Ultraflow, Fresenius). No visible changes were observed, and HPLC analysis found little or no loss of tramadol HCl in 14 days at 4 °C followed by six hours at room temperature and in seven days stored at room temperature. At 40 °C, 3 to 5% loss was found in sodium chloride 0.9% but little or no loss occurred in dextrose 5% in water (434).

Compatibility Information

Solution Compatibility

Tramadol HCl

Solution	Mfr	Mfr	Conc/L	Remarks	Ref	C/I
Dextrose 5% in water	a	MUN	0.5 and 4 g	Visually compatible with no loss by HPLC in 14 days at 4 °C and 7 days at room temperature or 40 °C	434	**C**
Sodium chloride 0.9%	a	MUN	0.5 and 4 g	Visually compatible with little or no loss by HPLC in 14 days at 4 °C and 7 days at room temperature. 3 to 5% loss in 7 days at 40 °C	434	**C**

a Tested in PVC containers.

Additional Compatibility Information

Solutions— Tramadol HCl (Searle) is stated to be physically compatible and chemically stable for up to five days in the following infusion solutions (1442):

    Compound sodium lactate (Ringer's lactate)
    Dextrose 5% in water
    Haemaccel

    Sodium chloride 0.9%
    Sodium chloride 0.18% and dextrose 4%

Tramadol HCl is stated to be physically compatible and chemically stable for up to 24 hours in Ringer's solution and sodium bicarbonate 4.2% (1442).

Other Drugs— Tramadol HCl should not be mixed in the same syringe with diazepam, diclofenac sodium, indomethacin sodium, midazolam, and piroxicam (1442).

TROPISETRON HCL

Navoban	**Novartis Pharmaceuticals**

Products— Tropisetron HCl (Novartis) is available as an aqueous solution in 2- and 5-ml ampuls. Each milliliter of solution provides

1 mg of tropisetron (present as 1.13 mg of the hydrochloride). Also present in the formulation are acetic acid, sodium acetate, sodium chloride, and water for injection (1442).

Administration— Tropisetron HCl is administered either as a slow injection over greater than 30 seconds or as an infusion of 5 mg in 100 ml of infusion solution over 15 minutes (1442).

Stability— Tropisetron HCl injection is a colorless or faintly brown-yellow solution. Intact ampules should be stored at room temperature (1442).

Tropisetron HCl is stated to be physically compatible and chemically stable for 24 hours under refrigeration diluted in several common infusion solutions. (See Additional Compatibility Information below.) However, the manufacturer recommends use within eight hours of preparing the infusion because of microbiological contamination concerns (1442).

Sorption— The manufacturer indicates that tropisetron HCl solutions are compatible with both glass and PVC containers and infusion sets (1442).

Compatibility Information

Solution Compatibility

Tropisetron HCl

Solution	Mfr	Mfr	Conc/L	Remarks	Ref	C/I
Dextrose 5% in water	AGT[a], BFM[b]	SZ	50 mg	Visually compatible with no loss by HPLC in 90 days at 4 and −20 °C	470	C
Sodium chloride 0.9%	AGT[a], BFM[b]	SZ	50 mg	Visually compatible with no loss by HPLC in 90 days at 4 and −20 °C	470	C

[a]*Tested in PVC containers.*
[b]*Tested in three-layer (Clear-Flex) laminate containers having a polyethylene inner surface.*

Additional Compatibility Information

Solutions— Tropisetron HCl is physically compatible and chemically stable for 24 hours under refrigeration with the following infusion solutions (1442):

Dextrose 5% in water
Fructose 5% in water
Ringer's injection
Sodium chloride 0.9%

VINDESINE SULFATE

Eldisine   **Lilly**

Products— Vindesine sulfate (Lilly) is available in lyophilized form in vials containing 5 mg with mannitol 25 mg and sodium hydroxide and/or sulfuric acid to adjust the pH. A 5-ml vial of sterile diluent containing, in each milliliter, sodium chloride 9 mg, benzyl alcohol 2%, and hydrochloric acid and/or sodium hydroxide to adjust the pH in water for injection is also provided. The drug should be reconstituted with 5 ml of the sterile diluent to yield a 1-mg/ml solution (1442).

pH— From 4.2 to 4.5 (234).

Administration— Vindesine sulfate is administered intravenously. It must not be given intramuscularly, subcutaneously, or intrathecally. Administration of the reconstituted injection directly into a vein or into the tubing of a running intravenous solution is recommended. Extravasation must be avoided because of possible severe tissue irritation (1442).

Stability— Intact vials should be refrigerated at 2 to 8 °C. The reconstituted solution is stable under refrigeration for 30 days (1442).

Vindesine sulfate, reconstituted according to the manufacturer's instructions, was cultured with human lymphoblasts to determine whether its cytotoxic activity was retained. The solution retained cytotoxicity for 24 hours at 4 °C and room temperature (1575).

pH Effects— Vindesine sulfate is most stable at pH 1.9 (1369). It may precipitate in a solution with a pH greater than 6. Therefore, multielectrolyte solutions such as Ringer's injection, lactated, are not recommended (234).

Freezing Solutions— Vindesine sulfate (Lilly) 20 μg/ml in dextrose 5% in water, Ringer's injection, lactated, or sodium chloride 0.9% underwent no degradation after four weeks when frozen at −20 °C (1195).

Sorption— Vindesine sulfate (Lilly) 4 mg/250 ml in dextrose 5% in water or sodium chloride 0.9% in PVC bags was infused over two hours at 2.08 ml/min through PVC sets at 22 °C while protected from light. HPLC of the effluent solution found no loss due to sorption to the plastic (1631).

Compatibility Information

Solution Compatibility

Vindesine sulfate

Solution	Mfr	Mfr	Conc/L	Remarks	Ref	C/I
Dextrose 5% in water		LI	20 mg	Physically compatible with little or no loss in 21 days at 4 and 25 °C in the dark	1195	C
	[a]	LI	20 mg	Little or no loss by HPLC in 7 days at 4 °C protected from light	1631	C
	MG, TR[b]	LI	47.6 mg	Less than 10% loss by HPLC in 24 hr at room temperature exposed to light	1658	C
Ringer's injection, lactated		LI	20 mg	Physically compatible with little or no loss in 21 days at 4 and 25 °C in the dark	1195	C
Sodium chloride 0.9%		LI	20 mg	Physically compatible with little or no loss in 21 days at 4 and 25 °C in the dark	1195	C
	[a]	LI	20 mg	No loss by HPLC in 7 days at 4 °C protected from light	1631	C

[a]*Tested in PVC containers.*
[b]*Tested in both glass and PVC containers.*

APPENDIX I

APPENDIX I: Parenteral Nutrition Formulas

The following tables summarize the composition of the total parenteral nutrition mixtures that are referenced throughout the *Handbook on Injectable Drugs*. Each unique formula that has been tested for stability and/or compatibility characteristics, alone or in combination with other drugs, is described and assigned a code number. These code numbers are used in the drug monographs to denote the TNA (3-in-1) or TPN (2-in-1) formulation being discussed (i.e., TPN #183, TPN #184, etc.). The TNA and TPN formulations are described as completely as possible from the original published sources.

The consolidation of the formulations into a single appendix is designed to avoid unnecessary repetition and to facilitate comparisons among different mixtures.

| Component | Mfr | Concentration per Liter |||||||||| |
		#1	#2	#3	#4	#5	#6	#7	#8	#9	#10
Amino acids	CU	4%	4%	4%	4%	4%	4%	4%	4%	4%	4%
Dextrose	CU	25%	25%	25%	25%	25%	25%	25%	25%	25%	25%
Calcium gluconate	PR	10 mEq	20 mEq	15 mEq	10 mEq	20 mEq	15 mEq	10 mEq	20 mEq	15 mEq	
Potassium phosphate	MG	20 mEq	25 mEq	40 mEq	20 mEq	25 mEq	40 mEq	20 mEq	25 mEq	40 mEq	
Folic acid	LE				5 mg	5 mg	5 mg	5 mg	5 mg	5 mg	
Cyanocobalamin	SQ				1 mg	1 mg	1 mg	1 mg	1 mg	1 mg	
Multivitamin concentrate	USV								5 ml	5 ml	5 ml
Vitamin B complex with C	UP				10 ml	10 ml	10 ml				

| Component | Mfr | Concentration per Liter |||||||||| |
		#11	#12	#13	#14	#15	#16	#17	#18	#19	#20
Amino acids	CU	4%	4%	4%	4%	4%	4%	4%	4%	4%	4%
Dextrose	CU	25%	25%	25%	25%	25%	25%	25%	25%	25%	25%
Calcium gluconate	PR	10 mEq	20 mEq	25 mEq	15 mEq	40 mEq	10 mEq	20 mEq	25 mEq	15 mEq	40 mEq
Potassium phosphate	MG	10 mEq	25 mEq	20 mEq	40 mEq	15 mEq	10 mEq	25 mEq	20 mEq	40 mEq	15 mEq
Folic acid	LE	5 mg	5 mg	5 mg	5 mg	5 mg					
Cyanocobalamin	SQ	1 mg	1 mg	1 mg	1 mg	1 mg					
Phytonadione	MSD	10 mg	10 mg	10 mg	10 mg	10 mg					
Multivitamin concentrate	USV										
or			10 ml	10 ml	10 ml	10 ml	10 ml				
Vitamin B complex with C	UP										

| Component | Mfr | Concentration per Liter |||| |
		#21	#22	#23	#24
Amino acids	MG	200 ml			
Amino acids 8.5%	TR		500 ml		
Amino acids 8.5% with electrolytes	TR			500 ml	500 ml
Dextrose 50% in water		400 ml		500 ml	500 ml
Dextrose 33.3% in water			500 ml		
Phosphate		15 mEq[a]	30 mEq		30 mEq[a]
Acetate		15 mEq[a]	67.5 mEq		
Calcium gluconate		2 g	9 mEq	1 g	
Calcium chloride			7.2 mEq		
Potassium chloride			70 mEq		20 mEq
Sodium chloride		40 mEq	55 mEq		60 mEq
Magnesium sulfate		8.1 mEq			
Multivitamins		10 ml			
Multivitamin concentrate				5 ml	
Water for injection		qs 1000 ml			
Trace elements			present		

[a]*Potassium salt.*

Component	Mfr	Concentration per Liter					
		#25	#26	#27	#28	#29	#30
Amino acids (Aminosyn)	AB	3.5%			1%		
Amino acids (FreAmine III)	MG		4.25%			1%	
Amino acids (Travasol)	TR			4.25%			1%
Dextrose		25%	25%	25%	25%	25%	25%
Sodium phosphate	AB	10 mmol	10 mmol	10 mmol	10 mmol	10 mmol	10 mmol
Multivitamins (M.V.I.-12)	USV	10 ml	10 ml	10 ml	10 ml	10 ml	10 ml
Multielectrolyte concentrate[a]	SE	25 ml	25 ml	25 ml	25 ml	25 ml	25 ml
Trace mineral injection[b]		3.5 ml	3.5 ml	3.5 ml	3.5 ml	3.5 ml	3.5 ml

[a]*Each 25 ml provides: sodium, 25 mEq; potassium, 40.5 mEq; calcium, 5 mEq; magnesium, 8 mEq; chloride, 33.5 mEq; acetate, 40.6 mEq; and gluconate, 5 mEq.*
[b]*Each 3.5 ml provides: zinc, 2 mg; copper, 1 mg; manganese, 0.5 mg; and chromium, 10 μg.*

Component	Mfr	Concentration per Liter						
		#31	#32	#33	#34	#35	#36	#37
Amino acids	TR	4.2%	4.2%	4.2%	4.2%	4.2%	4.2%	4.2%
Dextrose		25%	25%	25%	25%	25%	25%	25%
Sodium		29 mEq	29 mEq	29 mEq	29 mEq	69 mEq	69 mEq	69 mEq
Potassium		25 mEq	25 mEq	25 mEq	25 mEq	46 mEq	46 mEq	46 mEq
Calcium		9 mEq	9 mEq	9 mEq	4.5 mEq	9.5 mEq	9.5 mEq	9.5 mEq
Magnesium		4 mEq	4 mEq	4 mEq	4 mEq	12 mEq	12 mEq	12 mEq
Phosphorus		388 mg	388 mg	388 mg	388 mg	388 mg	388 mg	388 mg
Chloride		29 mEq	29 mEq	29 mEq	29 mEq	103 mEq	103 mEq	103 mEq
Acetate		63 mEq	63 mEq	63 mEq	63 mEq	63 mEq	63 mEq	63 mEq
Trace elements			a,b	a		a,b	a,b	a,b
Multivitamins	USV			10 ml			5 ml	5 ml
Vitamin B complex with C plus folic acid (Soluzyme)	UP			5 ml				5 ml

[a]*Trace elements: selenium, 120 μg; chromium, 2 μg; zinc, 3 mg; and manganese, 0.7 mg.*
[b]*Trace elements: iodine, 120 μg; and copper, 1 mg.*

Component	Mfr	Concentration per Liter									
		#38	#39	#40	#41	#42	#43	#44	#45	#46	#47
Amino acids	CU	4%	4%	4%	4%	4%	4%	4%	4%	4%	4%
Dextrose	CU	25%	25%	25%	25%	25%	25%	25%	25%	25%	25%
Calcium gluconate	PR	10 mEq	20 mEq	25 mEq	15 mEq	40 mEq	10 mEq	20 mEq	25 mEq	15 mEq	40 mEq
Potassium phosphate	MG	10 mEq	25 mEq	20 mEq	40 mEq	15 mEq	10 mEq	25 mEq	20 mEq	40 mEq	15 mEq
Folic acid	LE						5 mg	5 mg	5 mg	5 mg	5 mg
Cyanocobalamin	SQ						1 mg	1 mg	1 mg	1 mg	1 mg
Phytonadione	MSD						10 mg	10 mg	10 mg	10 mg	10 mg
Multivitamin concentrate	USV										
or		5 and	5 and	5 and	5 and	5 and	10 ml	10 ml	10 ml	10 ml	10 ml
Vitamin B complex with C	UP	10 ml	10 ml	10 ml	10 ml	10 ml					

Component	Concentration per Liter			
	#48	#49	#50	#51
Amino acids	5%	5%	5%	5%
Dextrose	5%	5%	25%	25%
Vitamins	present		present	
Trace elements		present		present

Component	Mfr	Concentration per Liter				
		#52	#53	#54	#55	#56
Amino acids	VT	7%	2.3%			
Amino acids	AB			1.5%		
Amino acids (FreAmine III)	MG				3%	3%
Dextrose			6.5%	15%	25%	25%
Fructose		10%	3.2%			
Sodium		50 mmol	16.2 mmol	[a]	35 mEq	35 mEq
Potassium		20 mmol	18.4 mmol	[a]		
Calcium		2.5 mmol	4.9 mmol	300 mg	5 mEq[b]	5 mEq[b]
Magnesium		1.5 mmol	2.1 mmol		8 mEq	8 mEq
Phosphorus				155 mg		
Phosphate			12.1 mmol[c]		40 mEq[d]	40 mEq[d]
Chloride		55 mmol	17.8 mmol	[e]	35 mEq	35 mEq
Laevulate calcium			9.8 mmol			
Folic acid				0.5 mg		
Cyanocobalamin				[f]		
Phytonadione				0.2 mg		
Multivitamins			present	4 ml		10 ml
Vitamin B complex with C (Berocca-C)				0.2 ml		

[a]*Adjusted to provide 2.5 mEq/kg/day.*
[b]*Present as the gluconate.*
[c]*Anion not specified.*
[d]*Present as the potassium salt.*
[e]*Adjusted to provide 5 mEq/kg/day.*
[f]*Present but concentration not specified.*

Component	Mfr	Concentration per Liter				
		#57	#58[a]	#59	#60	#61
Amino acids	MG	2.125%	4.25%			
Amino acids	TR				2.125%	
Amino acids	AB					3%
Amino acids with electrolytes	TR			4.25%		
Dextrose		10%	25%	25%	25%	20%
Sodium		40 mEq	100 mmol	50 mEq	50 mEq	30 mEq
Potassium		30 mEq	60 to 80 mmol			25 mEq
Calcium		15 mEq	5 mmol	5 mEq	5 mEq	15 mEq
Magnesium		12.5 mEq	5 mmol	5 mEq	5 mEq	10 mEq
Phosphorus		6 mmol	10 mmol	465 mg	465 mg	15 mmol
Chloride		40 mEq	100 mmol	50 mEq	50 mEq	
Heparin sodium			1000 units	500 units	500 units	
Phytonadione				1 mg	1 mg	
Multivitamins			10 ml	10 ml	10 ml	2 ml
Multivitamin concentrate		2 ml				
Iron			1 mg			
Trace elements		present	present	present	present	present

[a]*Concentration per 1200 ml.*

Component	Mfr	Concentration per Liter						
		#62	#63	#64	#65	#66	#67	#68
Amino acids 8.5% (FreAmine III)	MG	500 ml	500 ml			500 ml		
Amino acids 5.4% (Nephramine)	MG			500 ml			500 ml	
Amino acids 5.2% (Aminosyn RF)	AB				500 ml			500 ml
Dextrose 50%	MG	500 ml	500 ml	500 ml	500 ml	500 ml	500 ml	500 ml
Hyperlyte (electrolyte) concentrate	MG		25 ml					
Fat emulsion 10%, intravenous	CU					500 ml	500 ml	500 ml
Multivitamins (M.V.I.-12)	USV	[a]	[a]	[a]	[a]	[a]	[a]	[a]

[a]*Tested both with and without multivitamins.*

Component	Mfr	Concentration per Liter		
		#69	#70	#71
Amino acids 8.5% (FreAmine II)	MG	1000 ml		
Amino acids 8.5% with electrolytes	TR			1500 ml[a]
Amino acids 7%	AB		500 ml	
Dextrose 50% in water		500 ml	500 ml	1500 ml
Dextrose 20% with electrolyte pattern A	TR	500 ml[b]		
Dextrose 20% in water		500 ml		
Sodium chloride 0.9%		500 ml		
Potassium chloride		20 mmol		
Calcium gluconate 10%				30 ml
Multivitamins		1 ampul		10 ml
Multivitamin concentrate			5 ml	
Folic acid		1 mg	0.25, 0.5, 0.75, 1 mg	
Trace elements				present

[a]Each 1500 ml provides: sodium, 105 mEq; potassium, 90 mEq; magnesium, 15 mEq; chloride, 105 mEq; acetate, 203 mEq; and phosphate, 45 mmol.
[b]Each 500 ml provides: magnesium, 14 mmol; calcium, 13 mmol; chloride, 54 mmol; acetate, 0.08 mmol; zinc, 0.04 mmol; and manganese, 0.02 mmol.

Component	Mfr	Concentration per Liter			
		#72	#73	#74	#75
Amino acids 10%	TR	750 ml	750 ml		
Amino acids 8.5%	TR			500 ml	
Amino acids 8.5%	MG				500 ml
Dextrose 70%		429 ml	429 ml		300 ml
Dextrose 50%				500 ml	
Fat emulsion 20%, intravenous	TR	225 ml	225 ml		
Sterile water for injection		24.2 ml	15 ml		300 ml
Calcium gluconate 10%		20 ml	20 ml		
Calcium gluceptate					8 mEq
Sodium phosphate			15 mmol		
Potassium phosphate		20 mmol		30 mEq	18 mEq
Potassium chloride		30 mEq	40 mEq	20 mEq	20 mEq
Magnesium sulfate 50%		2 ml	2 ml		8 mEq
Sodium chloride		60 mEq	60 mEq	40 mEq	60 mEq
Sodium acetate					5 mEq
Heparin sodium			6000 units		
Multivitamins		10 ml	10 ml		
Trace elements		present	present		

Component	Mfr	Concentration per Liter				
		#76	#77	#78	#79	#80
Amino acids	CU	4%	4%	4%	4%	4%
Dextrose	CU	25%	25%	25%	25%	25%
Calcium gluconate	PR	10 mEq	20 mEq	25 mEq	15 mEq	40 mEq
Potassium phosphate	MG	10 mEq	25 mEq	20 mEq	40 mEq	15 mEq
Cyanocobalamin	SQ	0.5 and 1 mg	0.5 and 1 mg	0.5 and 1 mg	0.5 and 1 mg	0.5 and 1 mg

Component	Mfr	Concentration per Liter				
		#81	#82	#83	#84	#85
Amino acids	CU	4%	4%	4%	4%	4%
Dextrose	CU	25%	25%	25%	25%	25%
Calcium gluconate	PR	10 mEq	20 mEq	25 mEq	40 mEq	15 mEq
Potassium phosphate	MG	10 mEq	25 mEq	20 mEq	15 mEq	40 mEq
Other components		[a]	[a]	[a]	[a]	[a]

[a]Tested with each of the following individually: folic acid (Lederle), 2.5 and 5 mg; cyanocobalamin (Squibb), 0.5 and 1 mg; phytonadione (MSD), 5 and 10 mg; multivitamin concentrate (USV), 5 and 10 ml; and vitamin B complex with C (Upjohn), 5 and 10 ml.

		Concentration per Liter		
Component	Mfr	#86	#87	#88
Amino acids (Aminosyn)	AB	2.5%	4.25%	5%
Dextrose		10%	25%	35%
Calcium		4.5 mEq	4.5 mEq	4.5 mEq
Magnesium		5 mEq	5 mEq	5 mEq
Potassium		23 mEq	40 mEq	40 mEq
Sodium		47 mEq	35 mEq	35 mEq
Acetate		82 mEq	74.5 mEq	74.5 mEq
Chloride		35 mEq	52.5 mEq	52.5 mEq
Phosphorus		9 mmol	12 mmol	12 mmol
Heparin sodium		1000 units	1000 units	1000 units
Insulin		[a]	[a]	[a]

[a]Insulin 10 to 40 units/L.

	Concentration per Liter	
Component	#89	#90
Amino acids (Travasol)	4.25%	
Amino acids with electrolytes (Travasol with electrolytes)		4.25%
Dextrose	25%	25%

		Concentration per 100 ml	Concentration per 2L
Component	Mfr	#91	#92
Amino acids 10%		1.6 ml	
Nitrogen (from amino acids)	PFM		14 g
Dextrose 5% in water		15 ml	
Dextrose 50% in water			500 ml
Fat emulsion 20%, intravenous	KA		500 ml
Sodium		3 mEq	150 mEq
Potassium		2.2 mEq	120 mEq
Calcium		1 mEq	15 mEq
Magnesium		0.3 mEq	30 mEq
Phosphate		0.5 mmol	30 mmol
Chloride		2.5 mEq	150 mEq
Sulfate			30 mEq
Acetate			90 mEq
Pediatric multivitamins		5 ml	
Multivitamins			present
Trace elements		[a]	present
Heparin sodium		100 units	
Water for injection			qs 2000 ml

[a]Trace elements: zinc, 600 μg; copper, 40 μg; manganese, 10 μg; and chromium, 0.4 μg.

Component	Mfr	Concentration per Liter			
		#93	#94	#95	#96
Amino acids	TR	4.25%	4.25%		
Amino acids	AB			3%	3%
Dextrose		25%	25%	20%	20%
Potassium chloride		15 mEq	15 mEq	25 mEq	25 mEq
Sodium chloride		15 mEq	15 mEq	30 mEq	30 mEq
Calcium gluconate		4.7 mEq	4.7 mEq	15 mEq	15 mEq
Magnesium sulfate		4.05 mEq	4.05 mEq	10 mEq	10 mEq
Potassium phosphate		5 mEq	5 mEq	15 mmol	15 mmol
Sodium phosphate		10 mEq	10 mEq		
Zinc		1.5 mg	1.5 mg	3 mg	3 mg
Manganese		150 µg	150 µg	50 µg	50 µg
Chromium		6 µg	6 µg	2 µg	2 µg
Selenium		30 µg	30 µg		
Copper			600 µg	200 µg	200 µg
Multivitamins	LY			2 ml	2 ml
Heparin sodium	IX			1000 units	

Component	Mfr	Milliliters per Container							
		#97	#98	#99	#100	#101	#102	#103	#104
Amino acids 8.5% (FreAmine III)	MG	10	10	10	10	75	75	75	75
Dextrose 70%		89	36	89	36	89	36	89	36
Fat emulsion 20%, intravenous (Intralipid)	KV	5	5	75	75	5	5	50	50
Sterile water qs ad		250	250	250	250	250	250	250	250
Other components		a	a	a	a	a	a	a	a

[a]Each TNA admixture also contained: sodium, 25 mEq; potassium, 25 mEq; calcium, 5 mEq; magnesium, 25 mEq; chloride, 30 mEq; acetate, 7.5 mEq; lactate, 10.5 mEq; phosphate 1.5 mmol; multivitamins (M.V.I. Pediatric), 2.5 ml; trace elements; and heparin sodium, 250 units.

Component	Mfr	Concentration per Liter			
		#105	#106	#107	#108
Amino acids	TR	1.65%	4.25%	1.5%	1.5%
Dextrose		10%	10%	15%	15%
Sodium		21 mEq	35 mEq		
Potassium		18 mEq	30 mEq		
Magnesium		3 mEq	5 mEq		
Calcium		15 mEq	10 mEq		
Phosphate		10 mmol	15 mmol		
Chloride		21 mEq	35 mEq		
Acetate		30 mEq	68 mEq		
Pediatric multivitamins		1 ml	1 ml		
Trace elements		0.1 ml	0.1 ml		
Unspecified electrolytes and vitamins				present	present

Component	Mfr	Concentration per Liter				
		#109	#110	#111	#112	#113
Amino acids (FreAmine III)	MG	4.25%	2%	4.25%	2.125%	
Amino acids (Travasol)	TR					4.25%
Fat emulsion 20%, intravenous (Intralipid)	KV			200 ml	125 ml	
Dextrose		25%	25%	20%	25%	25%
Sodium		50 mEq	50 mEq	50 mEq	50 mEq	35 mEq
Potassium		40 mEq	40 mEq	40 mEq	40 mEq	30 mEq
Chloride		40 mEq	40 mEq	a	a	35 mEq
Phosphorus		13 mmol	13 mmol	6 mmol	6 mmol	15 mmol
Acetate		31 mEq	31 mEq	a	a	70.5 mEq
Calcium		16.7 mEq	16.7 mEq	10 mEq	10 mEq	4.7 mEq
Magnesium		10 mEq	10 mEq	5 mEq	5 mEq	5 mEq
Multivitamins		4 ml	4 ml	3.33 ml	3.33 ml	
Trace elements		present	present	present	present	present
Heparin sodium		1000 units	1000 units	1000 units	1000 units	
Sterile water		qs	qs	qs	qs	

[a] Not cited.

Component	Concentration per Liter				
	#114	#115	#116	#117	#118
Nitrogen (from amino acids)	7 g				
Amino acids (Travasol)		3.5%	3.5%	4.5%	3.7%
Dextrose	12.5%	17.5%	35%	22.7%	18.5%
Fat emulsion, intravenous	50 g[a]				3.7%
Sodium	75 mEq	66.7 mmol	66.7 mmol	45 mEq	45 mEq
Potassium	60 mEq	50 mmol	50 mmol	40 mEq	40 mEq
Magnesium	15 mEq	4.16 mmol	4.16 mmol	8 mEq	8 mEq
Calcium	7.5 mEq	4.16 mmol	4.16 mmol	5 mEq	5 mEq
Chloride	75 mEq	66.7 mmol	66.7 mmol	53 mEq	53 mEq
Phosphorus	15 mmol	8.3 mmol	8.3 mmol	15 mmol	15 mmol
Sulfate	15 mEq				
Acetate	45 mEq	90.8 mmol	90.8 mmol	84 mEq	84 mEq
Trace elements	present	present	present		
Multivitamins	present	8.3 ml	8.3 ml		
Sterile water for injection	qs				
Iron		833 µg	833 µg		
Heparin sodium		1000 units	1000 units		

[a] Both Intralipid (long-chain triglycerides) and MCT/LCT (medium- and long-chain triglycerides) tested.

Component	Mfr	Concentration per Liter						
		#119	#120	#121	#122	#123	#124	#125
Amino acids	TR	4.25%	4.25%	5%	5%	1%	2%	
Amino acids (TrophAmine)	MG							2%
Dextrose		35%	35%	20%	14.3%	10%	10%	10%
Fat emulsion					5.7%			
Sodium chloride		50 mEq	50 mEq	20 mEq	4 mEq	16 mEq	16 mEq	16 mEq
Potassium chloride				20 mEq	30 mEq	5 mEq	5 mEq	5 mEq
Potassium phosphate		30 mEq	30 mEq		3 mmol	10 to 40 mmol	10 to 40 mmol	10 to 40 mmol
Magnesium sulfate		10 mEq	10 mEq	8 mEq	12 mEq	4 mEq	4 mEq	4 mEq
Calcium gluconate		4.7 mEq	4.7 mEq	4.8 mEq	4 mEq	10 to 40 mEq	10 to 40 mEq	10 to 40 mEq
Sodium phosphates				20 mEq				
Sodium acetate					20 mEq	10 mEq	10 mEq	10 mEq
Cysteine HCl								1 g
Mixed electrolytes	LY				27 ml			
Trace Elements		1 ml	1 ml	present	3 ml			
Heparin sodium			1000 units					
Multivitamins				10 ml	10 ml			
Phytonadione					1 mg			
Cimetidine HCl					1 g			

Component	Mfr	Concentration per Liter							
		#126	#127	#128	#129	#130	#131	#132	#133
Amino acids (Aminosyn II)	AB	2%	3.3%	3.6%	3.6%	5%	3.5%	3.5%	
Amino acids (Travasol)	TR								4.25%
Dextrose		14.8%	3.3%	23.3%	20.8%	10%	25%	25%	25%
Fat emulsion, intravenous (Liposyn II)	AB	1.2%	3.3%	3.3%	2%	7.1%			
Sodium		39.5 mEq	51.7 mEq	48.4 mEq	96.3 mEq	49.4 mEq	33.6 mEq	33.6 mEq	75 mEq
Potassium		27 mEq	13.3 mEq	21.4 mEq	60 mEq	78.6 mEq	35.6 mEq	35.6 mEq	20 mEq
Calcium		6.6 mEq	3 mEq	6.7 mEq	10 mEq	13.4 mEq	4.5 mEq	4.5 mEq	9.6 mEq
Magnesium		3.2 mEq	3.3 mEq	10 mEq	12 mEq	14.5 mEq	5 mEq	5 mEq	10 mEq
Phosphate		5.5 mmol	10 mmol	10 mmol	15 mmol	21.4 mmol	12 mmol	12 mmol	10 mEq
Chloride		57.9 mEq	23.3 mEq	40 mEq	80 mEq	73.9 mEq	35 mEq	35 mEq	85 mEq
Acetate		21.9 mEq	43.6 mEq	23.9 mEq	65.8 mEq	35.9 mEq	35.7 mEq	35.7 mEq	
Trace elements		present	present	present	present	present		present	3 ml
Multivitamins (M.V.I.-12)								present	10 ml

Component	Mfr	Concentration per Liter						
		#134	#135	#136	#137	#138	#139	#140
Amino acids (Travasol)	BA	5.8%	5.8%	5.8%	5.8%	5.8%	5.7%	6%
Dextrose	BA	23.7%	23.7%	23.7%	23.7%	23.7%	23.4%	25%
Fat emulsion, intravenous (Intralipid)	KV		3%	5%			3%	
Fat emulsion, intravenous (Liposyn II)	AB					3%	5%	
Potassium chloride		54.2 mEq	54.2 mEq	54.2 mEq	54.2 mEq	54.2 mEq	32.2 mEq	30 mEq
Sodium chloride		108 mEq	108 mEq	108 mEq	108 mEq	108 mEq	64.4 mEq	110 mEq
Calcium gluconate 10%		13.6 ml	13.6 ml	13.6 ml	13.6 ml	13.6 ml	8 ml	10 ml
Magnesium sulfate 50%		1.4 ml	1.4 ml	1.4 ml	1.4 ml	1.4 ml	0.8 ml	4 ml
Potassium phosphate		20.3 mmol	20.3 mmol	20.3 mmol	20.3 mmol	20.3 mmol	36 mmol	
Multivitamins		6.8 ml	6.8 ml	6.8 ml	6.8 ml	6.8 ml	4 ml	1 vial
Trace elements		present	present	present	present	present	present	present
Phytonadione								1 mg

Component	Mfr	Concentration per Liter			
		#141	#142	#143	#144
Amino acids	AB		2.5%	5%	
Amino acids (Travasol)	TR				4.25%
Dextrose		25%	25%	25%	25%
Sodium		50 mEq	50 mEq	50 mEq	22.5 mEq
Potassium		40 mEq	40 mEq	40 mEq	20 mEq
Magnesium		5 mEq	5 mEq	5 mEq	2.85 mEq
Calcium		5 mEq	5 mEq	5 mEq	4.25 mEq
Phosphorus		15 mmol	15 mmol	15 mmol	15.75 mmol
Chloride		58 mEq	58 mEq	58 mEq	17 mEq
Acetate					58 mEq
Multivitamins		10 ml	10 ml	10 ml	
Trace elements		1 ml	1 ml	1 ml	present
Heparin sodium	UP	500 units	500 units	500 units	
Sterile water for injection					qs

Component	Mfr	Concentration per Liter			
		#145	#146	#147	#148
Amino acids (Travasol)	BA	5%			
Amino acids	AB		5%	2.5%	1%
Dextrose		15%	25%	25%	25%
Sodium		45 mEq	35 mEq	35 mEq	35 mEq
Potassium		15 mEq	40 mEq	40 mEq	40 mEq
Chloride		20 mEq	35 mEq	35 mEq	35 mEq
Phosphorus		16 mmol	12 mmol	12 mmol	12 mmol
Acetate		81 mEq	82 mEq	82 mEq	82 mEq
Calcium		20 mEq	9 mEq	9 mEq	9 mEq
Magnesium			5 mEq	5 mEq	5 mEq

Component	Concentration per Liter									
	#149	#150	#151	#152	#153	#154	#155	#156	#157	#158
Amino acids 10% (TrophAmine)	50 ml	50 ml	50 ml	50 ml	350 ml	350 ml	350 ml	350 ml	50 ml	350 ml
Dextrose	10%	10%	10%	10%	25%	25%	25%	25%	25%	25%
Fat emulsion 20%, intravenous[a]	25 ml	25 ml	70 ml	70 ml	25 ml	25 ml	70 ml	70 ml	100 ml	100 ml
Sodium	25 mEq	100 mEq	25 mEq	100 mEq	25 mEq	100 mEq	25 mEq	100 mEq	100 mEq	100 mEq
Potassium	15 mEq	80 mEq	15 mEq	80 mEq	15 mEq	80 mEq	15 mEq	80 mEq	80 mEq	80 mEq
Chloride	25 mEq	100 mEq	25 mEq	100 mEq	25 mEq	100 mEq	25 mEq	100 mEq	100 mEq	100 mEq
Calcium	7 mEq	18 mEq	7 mEq	18 mEq	7 mEq	18 mEq	7 mEq	18 mEq	18 mEq	18 mEq
Magnesium	2.5 mEq	13 mEq	2.5 mEq	13 mEq	2.5 mEq	13 mEq	2.5 mEq	13 mEq	13 mEq	13 mEq
Phosphate	3.4 mmol	9 mmol	3.4 mmol	9 mmol	3.4 mmol	9 mmol	3.4 mmol	9 mmol	9 mmol	9 mmol
Trace elements	present	present	present	present	present	present	present	present	present	present
Multivitamins (M.V.I. Pediatric)	5 ml	5 ml	5 ml	5 ml	5 ml	5 ml	5 ml	5 ml	5 ml	5 ml
Heparin	1000 units	1000 units	1000 units	1000 units	1000 units	1000 units	1000 units	1000 units	1000 units	1000 units

[a]*Intralipid 20%, Liposyn II 20%, and Nutrilipid 20% were each tested.*

Component	Mfr	Concentration per Liter							
		#159	#160	#161	#162	#163	#164	#165	#166
Amino acids 5.5% with electrolytes (Travasol)	BA	100 ml	100 ml	400 ml	400 ml	400 ml	400 ml	100 ml	100 ml
Fat emulsion 20%, intravenous (Intralipid)	KV	100 ml		200 ml		100 ml		200 ml	
Fat emulsion 20%, intravenous (Liposyn II)	AB		100 ml		200 ml		100 ml		200 ml
Heparin sodium 1000 units/ml	ES	5 ml	5 ml	5 ml	5 ml	5 ml	5 ml	5 ml	5 ml
Dextrose 10%		795 ml	795 ml					695 ml	695 ml
Dextrose 20%				395 ml	395 ml	495 ml	495 ml		

Component	Concentration per Liter						
	#167	#168	#169	#170	#171	#172	#173
Aminoplex 12			500 ml		1000 ml		
Aminoplex 24	500 ml	500 ml	500 ml	500 ml			
Vamin glucose							1000 ml
Lipofundin S 20%	500 ml	500 ml	500 ml	500 ml	500 ml		
Fat emulsion 10%, intravenous (Intralipid)						300 ml	
Glucoplex 1000	1000 ml						
Glucoplex 1600		1000 ml	1000 ml		500 ml		
Dextrose 5%					1000 ml		
Dextrose 50%				500 ml			1000 ml
Potassium chloride 15%		37.5 ml		10 ml			
Potassium phosphate 17%	20 ml	20 ml	20 ml	20 ml	10 ml		
Sodium chloride 30%		27 ml		15 ml			
Addamel	10 ml	10 ml	10 ml	10 ml	10 ml		10 ml
Soluvit						7.5 ml	
Vitalipid infant						15 ml	
Pancebrin							10 ml

Component	Mfr	Concentration per Liter					
		#174	#175	#176	#177	#178	#179
Amino acids	AB	25 g	50 g	15 g			
Amino acids	TR				3%		
Nitrogen						7.9 g	7 g
Dextrose		125 g	250 g	100 g	5%	100 g	125 g
Fat emulsion, intravenous (Intralipid)	KV					50 g	5 g
TPN II electrolytes	AB	20 ml	20 ml				
Sodium		26.3 mEq	37.5 mEq	40 mEq	46 mEq	24 mmol	75 mEq
Potassium		35.5 mEq	40 mEq	50 mEq	40 mEq	12.5 mmol	60 mEq
Magnesium		5 mEq	5 mEq	10 mEq	8 mEq	2.5 mmol	15 mEq
Calcium		9 mEq	4.5 mEq	10 mEq	5 mEq		7.5 mEq
Phosphorus		12 mmol	45 mmol	5 mmol	12 mmol	4.5 mmol	15 mmol
Chloride		35 mEq	35 mEq	47.6 mEq	57 mEq	7 mmol	75 mEq
Acetate		25 mEq	43 mEq	31.8 mEq	61 mEq	40.5 mmol	45 mEq
Gluconate					10 mEq		
Sulfate					10 mEq		15 mEq
Trace elements			present	present	present	present	present
Multivitamins (M.V.I. Pediatric)		3 ml		present	3 ml		
Multivitamins (M.V.I. 9+3)			10 ml				
Multivitamins						10 ml	present	present
Vitamin K			5 mg				
Heparin sodium		1000 units	1000 units	1000 units	1000 units		
Sterile water qs ad		1000 ml	1000 ml	1000 ml		1000 ml	1000 ml

Component	Concentration per Liter	
	#180	#181
Amino acids 10%	1000 ml	400 ml
Dextrose 50% in water	500 ml	500 ml
Fat emulsion 20%, intravenous (Intralipid)	500 ml	
Sodium	40 mmol	41 mEq
Potassium	70 mmol	22.7 mEq
Calcium	4.6 mmol	5 mEq
Magnesium	5 mmol	5 mEq
Phosphorus	17.5 mmol	12 mmol
Chloride	120 mmol	30 mEq
Acetate	45 mmol	89 mEq
Trace elements		present
Multivitamins		10 ml

Component	Mfr	Concentration per Liter
		#182
Amino acids	KV	5%
Dextrose		25%
Fat emulsion, intravenous (Intralipid)	KV	2.25%
Potassium phosphate		10 mmol
Potassium chloride		45 mEq
Sodium chloride		75 mEq
Magnesium sulfate		8 mEq
Calcium gluconate		47 mg
Trace elements		present
Multivitamins		5 ml
Sterile water qs ad		1000 ml

Component	Mfr	Concentration per Liter						
		#183	#184	#185	#186[a]	#187[b]	#188[c]	#189
Amino acids (Aminosyn II)	AB	1%	2.5%	5%				
Amino acids (Aminosyn)	AB				15 g	25 g	50 g	
Amino acids 10% with electrolytes (Synthamin 17 with electrolytes)								500 ml
Dextrose	AB	10%	10%	25%	125 g	125 g	250 g	
Dextrose 50%								500 ml
TPN II electrolytes							1 ml	1 ml
Calcium		9 mEq	4.4 mEq	5 mEq	1 mEq	9 mEq	4.5 mEq	2.2 mmol
Magnesium		5 mEq	5 mEq	5 mEq	1 mEq	5 mEq	5 mEq	2.5 mmol
Potassium		27 mEq	18 mEq	40 mEq	5 mEq	30 mEq	40 mEq	42.5 mmol
Sodium		24 mEq	38 mEq	42 mEq	4 mEq	35 mEq	37.65 mEq	45 mmol
Phosphorus		6 mmol	9 mmol	15 mmol	2 mmol	6 mmol	12 mmol	15 mmol
Chloride		35 mEq	35 mEq	43 mEq	5.7 mEq	46.9 mEq	39.4 mEq	55.65 mmol
Acetate		22 mEq	25 mEq	38 mEq	11.1 mEq	25.6 mEq	43.5 mEq	81.25 mmol
Gluconate					1.1 mEq	2.5 mEq	0.05 mEq	
Sulfate					1.1 mEq			
Trace elements		1 ml	1 ml	1 ml	0.6 ml	1 ml	1 ml	present
Multivitamins (M.V.I. Pediatric)	AST				3 ml	3 ml		
Multivitamins (M.V.I. 9+3)	AST						10 ml	
Heparin sodium	ES				1000 units	1000 units	1000 units	
Sterile water					qs	qs	qs	

[a]Neonatal formula.
[b]Pediatric formula.
[c]Adult formula.

Component	Mfr	Concentration per Liter		
		#190	#191	#192
Amino acids (Aminosyn II 15%)	AB	333 ml		
Amino acids (Azonutril 25)			500 ml	
Amino acids				17 g
Dextrose 70%		500 ml		
Dextrose 50%			250 ml	
Dextrose 30%			750 ml	
Dextrose				42.4 g
Fat emulsion 20%, intravenous (Intralipid)			500 ml	24.2 g
Fat emulsion 20%, intravenous (Liposyn II)	AB	400 ml		
Sterile water		133 ml		
Sodium				55.7 mmol
Potassium				19.4 mmol
Magnesium				2.3 mmol
Calcium				1.5 to 150 mmol
Phosphate				21 to 300 mmol
Unspecified electrolytes		present		
Vitamins		present		present
Trace elements			present	present

Component	Mfr	Concentration per Liter #193
Amino acids 10%	CL	1000 ml
Dextrose 50%	CL	750 ml
Sodium chloride	AB	140 mEq
Potassium phosphates	AB	20 mmol
Calcium gluconate		4.8 mEq
Magnesium sulfate		40 mEq
Multivitamins	AST	10 ml
Trace elements	LY	3 ml
Famotidine		40 mg

Component	Concentration per Liter	
	#194	#195
Amino acids	2.2%	2.2%
Dextrose	12.5%	20%
Sodium chloride	26 mEq	26 mEq
Potassium phosphates	15 mmol	15 mmol
Calcium gluconate	25 mEq	25 mEq
Magnesium sulfate	8 mEq	8 mEq
Potassium chloride	2 mEq	2 mEq
Heparin sodium	1000 units	1000 units
Cysteine	660 mg	660 mg
Trace elements	present	present
Multivitamins	20 ml	20 ml

Component	Mfr	Concentration per Liter				
		#196	#197	#198	#199	#200
Amino acids	BA	6%	6%	6%	6%	6%
Dextrose	BA	24%	24%	24%	24%	24%
Intralipid	KV		3%	5%		
Liposyn II	AB				3%	5%
Sodium chloride	LY	108 mEq	108 mEq	108 mEq	108 mEq	108 mEq
Potassium phosphates	AB	20 mmol	20 mmol	20 mmol	20 mmol	20 mmol
Calcium gluconate	LY	6.3 mEq	6.3 mEq	6.3 mEq	6.3 mEq	6.3 mEq
Magnesium sulfate	AST	5.6 mEq	5.6 mEq	5.6 mEq	5.6 mEq	5.6 mEq
Potassium chloride	AB	54 mEq	54 mEq	54 mEq	54 mEq	54 mEq
Trace elements	SO	present	present	present	present	present
Multivitamins	AR	6.8 ml	6.8 ml	6.8 ml	6.8 ml	6.8 ml

Component	Mfr	Concentration per Liter			
		#201	#202	#203[a]	#204[b]
Amino acids	BA	4.25%			
Amino acids	AB		4.25%		
Amino acids (TrophAmine)	MG			2%	3%
Dextrose		25%	25%	10%	20%
Sodium		35 mEq	35 mEq	38 mEq	77 mEq
Potassium		30 mEq	30 mEq	20 mEq	40 mEq
Calcium		5 mEq	9.4 mEq	600 mg	600 mg
Magnesium		3 mEq	10 mEq	2.5 mEq	2.5 mEq
Chloride		47 mEq	[c]	38 mEq	77 mEq
Phosphate		14.3 mEq	15 mmol	400 mg	400 mg
Acetate		67 mEq	50 mEq	29 mEq	58 mEq
L-cysteine				200 mg	300 mg
Trace elements			present	present	present
Multivitamins			present	present	present
Heparin					500 units

[a]Calculated quantities from a pediatric peripheral line formula.
[b]Calculated quantities from a pediatric central line formula.
[c]Unspecified.

Component	Mfr	Concentration per Liter	
		#205	#206
Amino acids	BA	5%	
Aminosyn	AB		2.125%
Dextrose		25%	20%
Intralipid	KA		
Liposyn II	AB		
Sodium chloride		75 mEq	30 mEq
Potassium chloride		60 mEq	30 mEq
Potassium phosphates		20 mmol	
Sodium phosphates			15 mmol
Calcium gluconate		10 mEq	14 mEq
Magnesium sulfate		10 mEq	50 mg
Trace elements		present	present
Multivitamins			
Heparin sodium		3000 to 20,000 units	

Component	Mfr	Concentration per Liter				
		#207	#208	#209	#210	#211
Amino acids (TrophAmine)	MG	0.5%	1%	1.5%	2%	2.5%
Dextrose		10%	10%	10%	10%	10%
Sodium chloride		20 mEq	20 mEq	20 mEq	20 mEq	20 mEq
Sodium acetate		10 mEq	10 mEq	10 mEq	10 mEq	10 mEq
Potassium acetate		5 mEq	5 mEq	5 mEq	5 mEq	5 mEq
Potassium phosphates		10 mmol	10 mmol	10 mmol	10 mmol	10 mmol
Calcium gluconate		20 mEq	20 mEq	20 mEq	20 mEq	20 mEq
Magnesium sulfate		4 mEq	4 mEq	4 mEq	4 mEq	4 mEq
Trace elements	FUJ	[a]	[a]	[a]	[a]	[a]
Multivitamins	AST	[b]	[b]	[b]	[b]	[b]
Heparin sodium		1000 units	1000 units	1000 units	1000 units	1000 units
L-Cysteine[c]		200 mg	400 mg	600 mg	800 mg	1 g

[a]*Tested with and without trace elements (Neotrace, Fujisawa).*

[b]*Tested with and without multivitamins (M.V.I. Pediatric, Astra) 3.5 ml/L.*

[c]*40 mg/g of protein.*

Component	Mfr	Concentration per Liter				
		#212	#213	#214	#215	#216[a]
Amino acids (Aminosyn II)	AB	3.5%		4.25%		
Amino acids (FreAmine III)	MG		3.5%		4.25%	
Amino acids (Travasol)	BA					0.5 to 5%
Dextrose		5%	5%	25%	25%	10 to 20%
Sterile water for injection		516.8 ml	516.75 ml	161 ml	158.6 ml	q.s.
Potassium phosphates		3.5 mmol	[b]	15 mmol	5.75 mmol[c]	0 to 20 mEq K[d]
Sodium chloride		25 mEq	37.5 mEq	25 mEq	40 mEq	0 to 44 mEq
Sodium acetate						0 to 40 mEq
Potassium chloride		35 mEq	40 mEq	18 mEq	25 mEq	0 to 20 mEq
Magnesium sulfate		8 mEq	8 mEq	8 mEq	8 mEq	4 mEq
Calcium gluconate		9.3 mEq	5 mEq	9.15 mEq	7.5 mEq	19.2 to 28.8 mEq
Multivitamins	AST	10 ml	10 ml	10 ml	10 ml	14 ml
Trace elements		present	present	present	present	present
Heparin sodium	ES					500 units
Ranitidine (as HCl)	GL					0 to 84 mg

[a]*Forty parenteral nutrition formulations within the ranges cited were tested. Specific formulations were not reported.*

[b]*No phosphates added. Phosphates from FreAmine III formulation yielded 3.5 mmol/L.*

[c]*Added phosphates indicated. All phosphates from addition plus FreAmine III formulation totaled 10 mmol/L.*

[d]*Reported as potassium concentration.*

Component	Mfr	Concentration per Liter			
		#217	#218	#219	#220
Amino acids		5%			
Amino acids	MG		3%	3%	
Amino acids	AB				3%
Dextrose		25%	5%	5%	5%
Intralipid	KA		2%		
Liposyn II	AB			2%	
Liposyn III	AB				2%
Sodium		50 mEq	43 mEq	43 mEq	41.6 mEq
Potassium		40 mEq	40 mEq	40 mEq	40 mEq
Chloride		58 mEq	45 mEq	45 mEq	35 mEq
Phosphorus		15 mmol	7.5 mmol	7.5 mmol	15 mmol
Calcium		5 mEq	5 mEq	5 mEq	9.15 mEq
Magnesium		8 mEq	8 mEq	8 mEq	8 mEq
Acetate			51.7 mEq	51.7 mEq	42 mEq
Heparin sodium		1000 units			
Multivitamins		10 ml	10 ml	10 ml	10 ml
Phytonadione		1 mg			
Trace elements		2 ml	1 ml	1 ml	1 ml
Sterile water for injection			qs	qs	qs

Component	Mfr	Concentration per Liter					
		#221	#222	#223	#224	#225	#226
Amino acids	MG	4.9%	4.9%			6%	6%
Amino acids	AB			4.9%	6%		
Dextrose		20%	20%	20%	11%	10.7%	10.7%
Intralipid	KA		3.5%	3.5%			4%
Liposyn II	AB	3.5%				4%	
Liposyn III	AB			3.5%	4%		
Sodium		39.8 mEq	39.8 mEq	39.7 mEq	45 mEq	45 mEq	45 mEq
Potassium		40 mEq	40 mEq	40 mEq	40 mEq	40.2 mEq	40.2 mEq
Calcium		7.5 mEq	7.5 mEq	9.15 mEq	9.15 mEq	7.5 mEq	7.5 mEq
Magnesium		8 mEq	8 mEq	8 mEq	8 mEq	8 mEq	8 mEq
Chloride		45 mEq	45 mEq	35 mEq	35 mEq	51 mEq	51 mEq
Acetate		67.7 mEq	67.7 mEq	45 mEq	53.2 mEq	78.4 mEq	78.4 mEq
Phosphate		10 mmol	10 mmol	15 mmol	15 mmol	10 mmol	10 mmol
Multivitamins		10 ml	10 ml	10 ml	10 ml	10 ml	10 ml
Trace elements		1 ml	1 ml	1 ml	1 ml	1 ml	1 ml

REFERENCES

REFERENCES

1. Package insert (for brands listed after the nonproprietary name heading a monograph; date of package insert given as part of citation).
2. Physicians' Desk Reference, 53rd edition, Medical Economics Company, Montvale, New Jersey, 1999.
3. Kirkland WD, Jones RW, Ellis JR, et al.: Compatibility studies of parenteral admixtures, *Am J Hosp Pharm 18*:694–699 (Dec) 1961.
4. McEvoy GK (ed): American hospital formulary service drug information 99, American Society of Health-System Pharmacists, Bethesda, Maryland, 1999.
5. Reynolds JEF (ed): Martindale: the extra pharmacopoeia, 30th ed, The Pharmaceutical Press, London, England, 1993.
6. Parker EA: Compatibility digest, *Am J Hosp Pharm 27*:67–69 (Jan) 1970.
7. Parker EA: Compatibility digest, *Am J Hosp Pharm 27*:672–673 (Aug) 1970.
8. Rapp RP, Butts JD, and Piecoro JJ: Guidelines for the administration of commonly used intravenous drugs—1988 update, *J Pharm Tech 4*:15–32 (Jan–Feb) 1988.
9. Patel JA and Phillips GL: Guide to physical compatibility of intravenous drug admixtures, *Am J Hosp Pharm 23*:409–411 (Aug) 1966.
10. Bogash RC: Compatibilities and incompatibilities of some parenteral medication, *Bull Am Soc Hosp Pharm 12*:445–448 (July–Aug) 1955.
11. Dunworth RD and Kenna FR: Preliminary report: incompatibility of combinations of medications in intravenous solutions, *Am J Hosp Pharm 22*:190–191 (Apr) 1965.
12. Moorhatch P and Chiou WL: Interactions between drugs and plastic intravenous fluid bags, part i: sorption studies on 17 drugs, *Am J Hosp Pharm 31*:72–78 (Jan) 1974.
13. Levin HJ, Fieber RA, and Levi RS: Stability data for Tubex filled by hospital pharmacists, *Hosp Pharm 8*:310–311, 314 (Oct) 1973.
14. Powers S: Incompatibilities of pre-op medications, *Hosp Formul Manage 5*:22 (May) 1970.
15. Anon: Intravenous additive incompatibilities, Pharmacy Department, National Institutes of Health (Jan) 1970.
16. Cantina PN and King JC: Physico-chemical incompatibilities of selected cardiovascular and psychotherapeutic agents with sodium ethacrynate, *Am J Hosp Pharm 29*:141–146 (Feb) 1972.
17. The United States Pharmacopeia, 24th rev, United States Pharmacopeial Convention, Rockville, Maryland, 2000.
18. Kramer W, Inglott A, and Cluxton R: Some physical and chemical incompatibilities of drugs for i.v. administration, *Drug Intell Clin Pharm 5*:211–228 (July) 1971.
19. McEvoy GK (ed): American hospital formulary service drug information 97, American Society of Health-System Pharmacists, Bethesda, Maryland, 1997.
20. Parker EA: Compatibility digest, *Am J Hosp Pharm 26*:412–413 (July) 1969.
21. Parker EA: Compatibility digest, *Am J Hosp Pharm 26*:653–655 (Nov) 1969.
22. Parker EA: Compatibility digest, *Am J Hosp Pharm 27*:327–329 (Apr) 1970.
23. Parker EA: Compatibility digest, *Am J Hosp Pharm 31*:1076 (Nov) 1974.
24. Parker EA: Compatibility digest, *Am J Hosp Pharm 28*:805 (Oct) 1971.
25. Souney PF, Solomon MA, and Stancher D: Visual compatibility of cimetidine hydrochloride with common preoperative injectable medications, *Am J Hosp Pharm 41*:1840–1841 (Sep) 1984.
26. Riley BB: Incompatibilities in intravenous solutions, *J Hosp Pharm 28*:228–240 (Aug) 1970.
27. Parker EA and Levin HJ: Compatibility digest, *Am J Hosp Pharm 32*:943–944 (Sep) 1975.
28. Misgen R: Compatibilities and incompatibilities of some intravenous solution admixtures, *Am J Hosp Pharm 22*:92–94 (Feb) 1965.
29. Drug Topics Red Book, Medical Economics Company, Montvale, New Jersey, 1999.
30. Mehta DK (ed.): British National Formulary 38, British Medical Association and Royal Pharmaceutical Society of Great Britain, London, England, September, 1999.
31. Ohio State University Hospitals Pharmacy and Therapeutics Committee: Restrictive list of i.v. push medications which qualified registered nurses may administer, *Am J IV Ther 3*:45–49 (Apr–May) 1976.
32. Frank JT: Intralipid compatibility study, *Drug Intell Clin Pharm 7*:351–352 (Aug) 1973.
33. Yeo MT, Gazzaniga AB, Bartlett RH, et al.: Total intravenous nutrition experience with fat emulsions and hypertonic glucose, *Arch Surg 106*:792–796 (June) 1973.
34. Melly MA, Meng HC, and Schaffner W: Microbial growth in lipid emulsions used in parenteral nutrition, *Arch Surg 110*:1479–1481 (Dec) 1975.
35. Deitel M and Kaminsky V: Total nutrition by peripheral vein—the lipid system, *Can Med Assoc J 111*:152–154 (July 20) 1974.
36. Cashore WJ, Sedaghatian MR, and Usher RA: Nutritional supplements with intravenously administered lipid, protein hydrolysate, and glucose in small premature infants, *Pediatrics 56*:8–16 (July) 1975.
37. Lynn B: Intralipid compatibility study, *Drug Intell Clin Pharm 8*:75, 78 (Feb) 1974.
38. Griffin JP and D'Arcy PF: Manual of adverse drug reactions, John Wright & Sons Ltd., Bristol, England, 1975.
39. Fortner CL, Grove WR, Bowie D, et al.: Fat emulsion vehicle for intravenous administration of an aqueous insoluble drug, *Am J Hosp Pharm 32*:582–584 (June) 1975.
40. Riffkin C: Incompatibilities of manufactured parenteral products, *Am J Hosp Pharm 20*:19–22 (Jan) 1963.
41. Edward M: *p*H—an important factor in the compatibility of additives in intravenous therapy, *Am J Hosp Pharm 24*:440–449 (Aug) 1967.
42. Turner FE and King JC: Spectrophotometric analysis of intravenous admixtures containing metaraminol and corticosteroids, *Am J Hosp Pharm 27*:540–547 (July) 1970.
43. Anderson RW and Latiolais CJ: Physico-chemical incompatibilities of parenteral admixtures—Aramine and Solu-Cortef, *Am J Hosp Pharm 30*:128–133 (Feb) 1973.
44. Smith MC: The dextrans, *Am J Hosp Pharm 22*:273–275 (May) 1965.
45. Stokes TF, Sumner ED, and Needham TE: Particulate contamination and stability of three additives in 0.9% sodium chloride injection in plastic and glass large-volume containers, *Am J Hosp Pharm 32*:821–826 (Aug) 1975.
46. Parker EA: Solution additive chemical incompatibility study, *Am J Hosp Pharm 24*:434–439 (Aug) 1967.
47. Parker EA: Compatibility digest, *Am J Hosp Pharm 26*:543–544 (Sep) 1969.
48. Parker EA: Parenteral incompatibilities, *Hosp Pharm 4*:14–22 (Aug) 1969.
49. Beatrice MG, Stanaszek WF, Allen LV, et al.: Physicochemical stability of a preanesthetic mixture of hydroxyzine hydrochloride and atropine sulfate, *Am J Hosp Pharm 32*:1133–1137 (Nov) 1975.
50. Leff RD and Roberts RJ: Effect of intravenous fluid and drug solution coadministration on final-infusate osmolality, specific gravity, and pH, *Am J Hosp Pharm 39*:468–471 (Mar) 1982.
51. Crevar GE and Slotnick IJ: A note on the stability of actinomycin D, *J Pharm Pharmacol 16*:429, 1964.
52. Coles CLJ and Lees KA: Additives to intravenous fluids, *Pharm J 206*:153–154 (Mar 27) 1971.
53. Prasad VK, Granatek AP, and Mihotic MM: Physical compatibility and chemical stability of cephapirin sodium in combination with non-antibiotic drugs in large-volume parenteral solutions, part ii, *Curr Ther Res Clin Exp 16*:540–572 (May) 1974.
54. Webb JW: A *p*H pattern for i.v. additives, *Am J Hosp Pharm 26*:31–35 (Jan) 1969.
55. Jones RW, Stanko GL, and Gross HM: Pharmaceutical compatibilities of Pentothal and Nembutal, *Am J Hosp Pharm 18*:700–704 (Dec) 1961.
56. Turco SJ, Sherman NE, Zagar L, et al.: Stability of aminophylline in 5% dextrose in water, *Hosp Pharm 10*:374–375 (Sep) 1975.
57. Hodby ED, Hirsch J, and Adeniyi-Jones C: Influence of drugs upon the anticoagulant activity of heparin, *Can Med Assoc J 106*:562–564 (Mar 4) 1972.
58. Piafsky KM and Ogilvie RI: Dosage of theophylline in bronchial asthma, *N Engl J Med 292*:1218–1222 (June 5) 1975.
59. Parker EA: Compatibility digest, *Am J Hosp Pharm 31*:775 (Aug) 1974.
60. Wolfert RR and Cox RM: Room temperature stability of drug products labeled for refrigerated storage, *Am J Hosp Pharm 32*:585–587 (June) 1975.
61. Anon: Intravenous fat, *Lancet 1*:1059–1060 (May 15) 1976.
62. Sachtler G: Dilantin for i.v. use, *Drug Intell Clin Pharm 7*:418 (Sep) 1973.
63. Burke WA: I.V. drug incompatibilities—Dilantin, *Am J IV Ther 2*:16–18 (Oct/Nov) 1975.
64. Baldwin J and Amerson AB: Intramuscular use of diphenylhydantoin, *Am J Hosp Pharm 30*:837–838 (Sep) 1973.
65. Tobias DC and Kellick KA: Dilantin for i.v. use, *Drug Intell Clin Pharm 7*:418 (Sep) 1973.
66. Chan NL: Dilantin for i.v. use, *Drug Intell Clin Pharm 7*:419 (Sep) 1973.
67. Ammar HO, Salama HA, and El-Nimr AE: Studies on the stability of injectable solutions of some phenothiazines, part i: effect of *p*H and buffer

systems, *Pharmazie 30*:368–369 (June) 1975.

68. Pickering LK and Rutherford I: Effect of concentration and time upon inactivation of tobramycin, gentamicin, netilmicin, and amikacin by azlocillin, carbenicillin, mecillinam, mezlocillin, and piperacillin, *J Pharmacol Exp Ther 217*:345–349 (May) 1981.

69. Ho NFH and Goeman JA: Prediction of pharmaceutical stability of parenteral solutions, *Drug Intell Clin Pharm 4*:69–71 (Mar) 1970.

70. Wilson CO and Jones TE: American drug index, J.B. Lippincott Company, Philadelphia, Pennsylvania, 1975.

71. Product Information Office (Astra Pharmaceutical Products, Westborough, Massachusetts): Personal communication, October 16, 1991.

72. Trissel LA, Davignon JP, Kleinman LM, et al.: NCI investigational drugs pharmaceutical data, National Cancer Institute, Bethesda, Maryland, 1988.

73. Muhlhauser I, Broermann C, Tsotsalas M, et al.: Miscibility of human and bovine ultralente insulin with soluble insulin, *Br Med J 289*:1656–1657 (Dec 15) 1984.

74. Grant HR: Compatibilities of intravenous admixtures, *Hosp Pharmacist 15*:67–70, 94 (Mar–Apr) 1962.

75. Hanson DB and Hendeles L: Guide to total dose intravenous iron dextran therapy, *Am J Hosp Pharm 31*:592–595 (June) 1974.

76. Duke AB, Kelleher J, Bauminger BB, et al.: Serum iron and iron binding capacity after total dose infusion of iron–dextran for iron deficiency anaemia in pregnancy, *J Obstet Gynaecol Br Commonwealth 81*:895–900 (Nov) 1974.

77. Parker EA: Compatibility digest, *Am J Hosp Pharm 32*:214 (Feb) 1975.

78. Gardella LA, Kesler H, Carter JE, et al.: Intropin (dopamine hydrochloride) intravenous admixture compatibility, part ii: stability with some commonly used antibiotics in 5% dextrose injection, *Am J Hosp Pharm 33*:537–540 (June) 1976.

79. Gardella LA, Zaroslinski JF, and Possley LH: Intropin (dopamine hydrochloride) intravenous admixture compatibility, part i: stability with common intravenous fluids, *Am J Hosp Pharm 32*:575–578 (June) 1975.

80. Garnett W: Diluents for antineoplastic drugs, *Drug Intell Clin Pharm 5*:261 (Aug) 1971.

81. Landersjo L, Stjernstrom G, and Lundgren P: Studies on the stability and compatibility of drugs in infusion fluids V. Effect of lactate and metal ions on the stability of benzylpenicillin, *Acta Pharm Suec 15*:161–168 (3) 1978.

82. Notari RE, Chin ML, and Wittebort R: Arabinosylcytosine stability in aqueous solutions: *p*H profile and shelf life predictions, *J Pharm Sci 61*:1189–1196 (Aug) 1972.

83. Murty BSR and Kapoor JN: Properties of mannitol injection (25%) after repeated autoclavings, *Am J Hosp Pharm 32*:826–827 (Aug) 1975.

84. Rosch JM, Pazin GJ, and Fireman P: Reduction of amphotericin B nephrotoxicity with mannitol, *J Am Med Assoc 235*:1995–1996 (May 3) 1976.

85. Bergman N and Vellar ID: Potential life-threatening variations of drug concentrations in intravenous infusion systems—potassium chloride, insulin, and heparin, *Med J Aust 2*:270–272 (Sep 18) 1982.

86. Parker EA: Compatibility digest, *Am J Hosp Pharm 27*:492–493 (June) 1970.

87. Feigen RD, Moss KS, and Shackelford PG: Antibiotic stability in solutions used for intravenous nutrition and fluid therapy, *Pediatrics 51*:1016–1026 (June) 1973.

88. Zost ED and Yanchick VA: Compatibility and stability of disodium carbenicillin in combination with other drugs and large volume parenteral solutions, *Am J Hosp Pharm 29*:135–140 (Feb) 1972.

89. Lynn B: Recent work on parenteral penicillins, *J Hosp Pharm 29*:183–194 (July) 1971.

90. Tourville J: Sodium nitroprusside, *Drug Intell Clin Pharm 9*:361–364 (July) 1975.

91. Anon: Sodium nitroprusside in anaesthesia, *Br Med J 2*:524–525 (June 7) 1975.

92. Hargrave RE: Degradation of solutions of sodium nitroprusside, *J Hosp Pharm 32*:188–189, 191 (Oct) 1974.

93. Anon: Sodium nitroprusside for hypertensive crisis, *Med Letter Drug Ther 17*:82–83 (Sep 26) 1975.

94. Anderson RA and Rae W: Stability of sodium nitroprusside solutions, *Aust J Pharm Sci NS1*:45–46 (July) 1972.

95. Schumacher GE: Sodium nitroprusside injection, *Am J Hosp Pharm 23*:532 (Sep) 1966.

96. Johnson DE: Nitroprusside in hypertensive emergencies, *Hosp Formul 10*:272–273 (June) 1975.

97. Thomas R: Meperidine HCl and heparin sodium precipitation, *Hosp Pharm 9*:356 (Sep) 1974.

98. Fleischer NM: Promethazine hydrochloride–morphine sulfate incompatibility, *Am J Hosp Pharm 30*:665 (Aug) 1973.

99. Lynn B: Pharmaceutical aspects of semi-synthetic penicillins, *J Hosp Pharm 28*:71–86 (Mar) 1970.

100. Meisler JM and Skolaut MW: Extemporaneous sterile compounding in intravenous additives, *Am J Hosp Pharm 23*:557–563 (Oct) 1966.

101. Guthaus MR (Medical Services, The Upjohn Company, Kalamazoo, Michigan): Personal communication, August 9, 1973.

102. Hamlin WE, Riebe KW, Scothorn WW, et al.: Pharmacy profile of Cleocin Phosphate, Presented at 10th Annual ASHP Midyear Clinical Meeting, December 11, 1975, Washington, D.C.

103. Riebe KW and Oesterling TO: Parenteral development of clindamycin-2-phosphate, *Bull Parenter Drug Assoc 26*:139–145 (May–June) 1972.

104. Anon: Therapeutic profile: Cleocin Phosphate, The Upjohn Company, Kalamazoo, Michigan, 1973.

105. Wyatt RG, Okamato GA, and Feigen RD: Stability of antibiotics in parenteral solutions, *Pediatrics 49*:22–29 (Jan) 1972.

106. Murty BSR, Kapoor JN, and DeLuca PP: Compliance with USP osmolarity labeling requirements, *Am J Hosp Pharm 33*:546–551 (June) 1976.

107. Whiting DA: Treatment of chromoblastomycosis with local concentrations of amphotericin B, *Br J Dermatol 79*:345–351, 1967.

108. Kirschenbaum BE and Latiolais CJ: Injectable medications—a guide to stability and reconstitution, McMahon Group, New York, New York, 1993.

109. Bair JN and Carew DP: Therapeutic availability of antibiotics in parenteral solutions, *Bull Parenter Drug Assoc 19*:153–163 (Nov–Dec) 1965.

110. Dancey JW and Carew DP: Availability of antibiotics in combination with other additives in intravenous solutions, *Am J Hosp Pharm 23*:543–551 (Oct) 1966.

111. Prasad VK, Granatek AP, and Mihotic MM: Physical compatibility and chemical stability of cephapirin sodium in combination with antibiotics and large-volume parenteral solutions, part i, *Curr Ther Res Clin Exp 16*:505–539 (May) 1974.

112. Lynn B: Carbenicillin plus gentamicin, *Lancet 1*:654 (Mar 27) 1971.

113. Jacobs J, Kletter D, Superstine E, et al.: Intravenous infusions of heparin and penicillins, *J Clin Pathol 26*:742–746, 1973.

114. Lynn B: Penicillin instability in infusions, *Br Med J 1*:174 (Jan 16) 1971.

115. Product information, Aminosyn II 5% in 25% Dextrose Injection, Abbott Laboratories, North Chicago, Illinois, January 1987.

116. Product information, Aminosyn II, Abbott Laboratories, North Chicago, Illinois, March 1993.

117. McEvoy GK (ed): American hospital formulary service drug information 95, American Society of Health-System Pharmacists, Bethesda, Maryland, 1995.

118. Harrison DC: Practical guidelines for the use of lidocaine, *J Am Med Assoc 233*:1202–1204 (Sep 15) 1975.

119. Collinsworth K: Clinical pharmacology of lidocaine as an antiarrhythmic drug, *West J Med 124*:36–43 (Jan) 1976.

120. Anon: Prophylactic use of lidocaine in myocardial infarction, *Med Letter Drug Ther 18*:1–2 (Jan 2) 1976.

121. Dundee JW, Gamble JAS, and Assaf RAE: Plasma diazepam levels following intramuscular injection by nurses and doctors, *Lancet 2*:1461 (Dec 14) 1974.

122. Product information, Trophamine, McGaw, Irvine, California, March 1992.

123. Tortorici MP: Stability data on frozen i.m. and i.v. solutions, *Pharm Times 41*:68–72 (Aug) 1975.

124. Barbara AC, Clemente C, and Wagman E: Physical incompatibility of sulfonamide compounds and polyionic solutions, *N Engl J Med 274*:1316–1317 (June 9) 1966.

125. Brooke D, Bequette RJ, and Davis RE: Chemical stability of cyclophosphamide in parenteral solutions, *Am J Hosp Pharm 30*:134–137 (Feb) 1973.

126. Brooke D, Scott JA, and Bequette RJ: Effect of briefly heating cyclophosphamide solutions, *Am J Hosp Pharm 32*:44–45 (Jan) 1975.

127. Gallelli JF: Stability studies of drugs used in intravenous solutions, part i, *Am J Hosp Pharm 24*:425–433 (Aug) 1967.

128. Anon: Nubain, physical compatibility, Dupont Pharmaceuticals, Wilmington, Delaware.

129. Kramer W, Tanja JJ, and Harrison WL: Precipitates found in admixtures of potassium chloride and dextrose 5% in water, *Am J Hosp Pharm 27*:548–553 (July) 1970.

130. Lawson DH: Clinical use of potassium supplements, *Am J Hosp Pharm 32*:708–711 (July) 1975.

131. Lundgren P and Landersjo L: Studies on the stability and compatibility of drugs in infusion fluids, ii: factors affecting the stability of benzylpenicillin, *Acta Pharm Suec 7*:509–526 (Nov) 1970.

132. Weber CR and Gupta VD: Stability of phenylephrine hydrochloride in intravenous solutions, *J Hosp Pharm 28*:200–208 (July) 1970.

133. Chiou WL and Moorhatch P: Interaction between vitamin A and plastic

intravenous fluid bags, *J Am Med Assoc 223*:328 (Jan 15) 1973.

134. Komesaroff D and Field JE: Pancuronium bromide: a new non-depolarizing muscle relaxant, *Med J Aust 1*:908–911 (May 3) 1969.

135. Simberkoff MS, Thomas L, McGregor D, et al.: Inactivation of penicillins by carbohydrate solutions at alkaline *p*H, *N Engl J Med 283*:116–119 (July 16) 1970.

136. Hicks CI, Gallardo JPB, and Guillory JK: Stability of sodium bicarbonate injection stored in polypropylene syringes, *Am J Hosp Pharm 29*:210–216 (Mar) 1972.

137. DeLuca PP and Kowalski RJ: Problems arising from the transfer of sodium bicarbonate injection from ampuls to plastic disposable syringes, *Am J Hosp Pharm 29*:217–222 (Mar) 1972.

138. D'Arcy PF and Thompson KM: Stability of chlorpromazine hydrochloride added to intravenous infusion fluids, *Pharm J 210*:28 (Jan 13) 1973.

139. Bergstrom RF and Fites AL: Stability of erythromycin glucepate in sodium chloride injection and dextrose injection, *Am J Hosp Pharm 32*:241 (Mar) 1975.

140. Murabito AS (Medical Correspondence, Smith Kline & French Laboratories, Philadelphia, Pennsylvania): Personal communication, December 15, 1986.

141. Mann JM, Coleman DL, and Boylan JC: Stability of parenteral solutions of sodium cephalothin, cephaloridine, potassium penicillin G (buffered), and vancomycin HCl, *Am J Hosp Pharm 28*:760–763 (Oct) 1971.

142. Appleby DH and John JF: Effect of peritoneal dialysis solution on the antimicrobial activity of cephalosporins, *Nephron 30*:341–344, 1982.

143. Upshaw MD (Medical Information Services, Eli Lilly and Company, Indianapolis, Indiana): Personal communication, January 10, 1972.

144. Gallelli JF, MacLowry JD, and Skolaut MW: Stability of antibiotics in parenteral solutions, *Am J Hosp Pharm 26*:630–635 (Nov) 1969.

145. Dienstag JL and Neu HC: Tobramycin: new aminoglycoside antibiotic, *Clin Med 82*:13–19 (Dec) 1975.

146. McCracken GH and Nelson JD: Commentary: an appraisal of tobramycin usage in pediatrics, *J Pediatr 88*:315–317 (Feb) 1976.

147. Bergstrom RF, Fites AL, and Lamb JW: Stability of parenteral solutions of tobramycin sulfate, *Am J Hosp Pharm 32*:887–888 (Sep) 1975.

148. Huber RC and Riffkin C: Inline final filters for removing particles from amphotericin B infusions, *Am J Hosp Pharm 32*:173–176 (Feb) 1975.

149. Rebagay T, Rapp R, Bivins B, et al.: Residues in antibiotic preparations, i: scanning electron microscopic studies of surface topography, *Am J Hosp Pharm 33*:433–443 (May) 1976.

150. Gallelli JF: Assay and stability of amphotericin B in aqueous solutions, *Drug Intell 1*:102–105 (Mar) 1967.

151. Piecoro JJ, Goodman NL, Wheeler WE, et al.: Particulate matter in reconstituted amphotericin B and assay of filtered solutions of amphotericin B, *Am J Hosp Pharm 32*:381–384 (Apr) 1975.

152. Gotz V and Simon W: Inline filtration of amphotericin B infusions, *Am J Hosp Pharm 32*:458 (May) 1975.

153. Chatterji D, Hiranaka PK, and Gallelli JF: Stability of sodium oxacillin in intravenous solutions, *Am J Hosp Pharm 32*:1130–1132 (Nov) 1975.

154. Drug Facts and Comparisons, St. Louis, MO, Facts and Comparisons, 1999.

155. Parodi JF: Stability of frozen antibiotic solutions in Viaflex infusion containers, *Hosp Pharm 11*:178–179 (May) 1976.

156. Larsen SS: Studies on stability of drugs in frozen systems, iv: the stability of benzylpenicillin sodium in frozen aqueous solutions, *Dansk Tidsskr Farm 45*:307–316 (9) 1971.

157. Noone P and Pattison JR: Therapeutic implications of interaction of gentamicin and penicillins, *Lancet 2*:575–578 (Sep 11) 1971.

158. Boulet M, Marier JR, and Rose D: Effect of magnesium on formation of calcium phosphate precipitates, *Arch Biochem Biophys 96*:629–636, 1962.

159. van den Berg L and Soliman FS: Composition and pH changes during freezing of solutions containing calcium and magnesium phosphate, *Cryobiology 6*:10–14 (1) 1969.

160. Ong JTH and Kostenbauder HB: Effect of self-association on rate of penicillin G degradation in concentrated aqueous solutions, *J Pharm Sci 64*:1378–1380 (Aug) 1975.

161. Shoup LK and Thur MP: Stability of frozen buffered penicillin G potassium injection, *Hosp Formul Manage 3*:38–39 (May) 1968.

162. Boylan JC, Simmons JL, and Winely CL: Stability of frozen solutions of sodium cephalothin and cephaloridine, *Am J Hosp Pharm 29*:687–689 (Aug) 1972.

163. Grant NH, Clark DE, and Alburn HE: Imidazole- and base-catalyzed hydrolysis of penicillin in frozen systems, *J Am Chem Soc 83*:4476–4477 (Nov) 1961.

164. Lindsay RE and Hem SL: Dosage form for potassium penicillin G intravenous infusion solutions, *Drug Devel Commun 1*:211–222 (3) 1974–1975.

165. Im S and Latiolais CJ: Physico-chemical incompatibilities of parenteral admixtures—penicillin and tetracyclines, *Am J Hosp Pharm 23*:333–343 (July) 1966.

166. Pfeifer HJ and Webb JW: Compatibility of penicillin and ascorbic acid injection, *Am J Hosp Pharm 33*:448–450 (May) 1976.

167. Rusmin S and DeLuca PP: Effect of inline filtration on the potency of potassium penicillin G, *Bull Parenter Drug Assoc 30*:64–71 (Mar–Apr) 1976.

168. Stolar MH, Carlin HS, and Blake MI: Effect of freezing on the stability of sodium methicillin injection, *Am J Hosp Pharm 25*:32–35 (Jan) 1968.

169. Lynn B: Stability of methicillin in dextrose solutions at alkaline *p*H, *J Hosp Pharm 30*:81–83 (Mar) 1972.

170. Lynn B: Pharmaceutics of the semi-synthetic penicillins, *Chem Drug 187*:134–136 (Feb 11) 1967.

171. Lynn B: Inactivation of methicillin in dextrose solutions at alkaline *p*H, *N Engl J Med 285*:690 (Sep 16) 1971.

172. Mattson CJ, Clark ST, and Colangelo A: Stability of clindamycin phosphate in plastic syringes, Presented at 20th Annual ASHP Midyear Clinical Meeting, December 1985, New Orleans, Louisiana.

173. Clark ST and Colangelo A: Stability of clindamycin phosphate in plastic syringes, Presented at 20th Annual ASHP Midyear Clinical Meeting, December 1985, New Orleans, Louisiana.

174. Cohon MS (Drug Information Services, Upjohn Company, Kalamazoo, Michigan): Personal communications, December 12, 1986, January 27, 1988, February 3, 1988.

175. Trissel LA: Unpublished data.

176. Owen RT (UK Medical Information Section, The Wellcome Foundation Ltd., Cheshire, England): Personal communication, August 19, 1993.

177. Lesson LJ and Weidenheimer JF: Stability of tetracycline and riboflavin, *J Pharm Sci 58*:355–357 (Mar) 1969.

178. Turco SJ and Burke WA: Methods of ordering and use of intravenous phosphate (mEq vs mM), *Hosp Pharm 10*:320, 322, 326 (Aug) 1975.

179. Pinkus TF and Jeffrey LP: Incompatibility of calcium and phosphate in parenteral alimentation solutions, *Am J IV Ther 3*:22–24 (Feb–Mar) 1976.

180. Kaminski MV, Harris DF, Collin CF, et al.: Electrolyte compatibility in synthetic amino acid hyperalimentation solution, *Am J Hosp Pharm 31*:244–246 (Mar) 1974.

181. Package insert, Calcium Gluconate Injection, USP, American Regent, Shirley, New York, January 1990.

182. Package insert, Calcium Gluconate Injection, USP, The Upjohn Company, Kalamazoo, Michigan, August 1985.

183. Lee FA and Gwinn JL: Roentgen patterns of extravasation of calcium gluconate in the tissues of the neonate, *J Pediatr 86*:598–601 (Apr) 1975.

184. Weiss Y, Ackerman C, and Shmilovitz L: Localized necrosis of scalp in neonates due to calcium gluconate infusions: a cautionary note, *Pediatrics 56*:1084–1086 (Dec) 1975.

185. Ramamurthy RS, Harris V, and Pildes RS: Subcutaneous calcium deposition in the neonate associated with intravenous administration of calcium gluconate, *Pediatrics 55*:802–806 (June) 1975.

186. Laegeler WL, Tio JM, and Blake MI: Stability of certain amino acids in a parenteral nutrition solution, *Am J Hosp Pharm 31*:776–779 (Aug) 1974.

187. Kleinman LM, Tangrea JA, Gallelli JF, et al.: Stability of solutions of essential amino acids, *Am J Hosp Pharm 30*:1054–1057 (Nov) 1973.

188. Rowlands DA: Compatibility of calcium and phosphate in amino acids solution, *Am J Hosp Pharm 32*:360 (Apr) 1975.

189. FreAmine brochure, McGaw Laboratories, Santa Ana, California, April 1971.

190. Rowlands DA, Wilkinson WR, and Yoshimura N: Storage stability of mixed hyperalimentation solutions, *Am J Hosp Pharm 30*:436–438 (May) 1973.

191. Ravin RL: Parenteral hyperalimentation, *Drug Intell Clin Pharm 6*:186–189 (May) 1972.

192. Hull RL: Physicochemical considerations in intravenous hyperalimentation, *Am J Hosp Pharm 31*:236–243 (Mar) 1974.

193. Dryps JS and Hoffman RP: Hyperalimentation review, *Drug Intell Clin Pharm 7*:413–417 (Sep) 1973.

194. Hull RL: Use of trace elements in intravenous hyperalimentation solutions, *Am J Hosp Pharm 31*:759–761 (Aug) 1974.

195. Johnson C, Cloyd J, and Rapp RP: Parenteral hyperalimentation, *Drug Intell Clin Pharm 9*:493–499 (Sep) 1975.

196. Hankins DA, Riella MC, Scribner BH, et al.: Whole blood trace element concentrations during total parenteral nutrition, *Surgery 79*:674–677 (June) 1976.

197. Hamann MA: Trace element requirements in hyperalimentation, *Am J Hosp Pharm 31*:1035, 1038 (Nov) 1974.

198. Hull RL: Trace element requirements in hyperalimentation, *Am J Hosp*

Pharm 31:1038 (Nov) 1974.

199. Heird WC and Winters RW: Total intravenous alimentation in pediatric patients, *South Med J 68*:1173–1176 (Sep) 1975.

200. Baker JA, Kirkman H, Woodley C, et al.: Computer-assisted pediatric hyperalimentation, *Am J Hosp Pharm 31*:752–758 (Aug) 1974.

201. Parish R: Hyperalimentation procedures, *Am J Hosp Pharm 31*:1160, 1166 (Dec) 1974.

202. Pomerance HH and Rader RE: Crystal formation: a new complication of total parenteral nutrition, *Pediatrics 52*:864–866 (Dec) 1973.

203. Bohart RD and Ogawa G: An observation on the stability of cis-dichlorodiammineplatinum (II): a caution regarding its administration, *Cancer Treat Rep 63*:2117–2118 (Nov–Dec) 1979.

204. Prestayko AW, Cadiz M, and Crooke ST: Incompatibility of aluminum-containing iv administration equipment with cis-dichlorodiammineplatinum (II) administration, *Cancer Treat Rep 63*:2118–2119 (Nov–Dec) 1979.

205. Shils ME: Minerals in total parenteral nutrition, *Drug Intell Clin Pharm 6*:385–393 (Nov) 1972.

206. Flack HL, Gans VA, Serlick SE, et al.: Current status of parenteral hyperalimentation, *Am Hosp Pharm 28*:326–335 (May) 1971.

207. McRae MP and King JC: Compatibility of antineoplastic, antibiotic, and corticosteroid drugs in intravenous admixtures, *Am J Hosp Pharm 33*:1010–1013 (Oct) 1976.

208. Warren E, Synder RJ, Thompson CO, et al.: Stability of ampicillin in intravenous solutions, *Mayo Clin Proc 47*:34–35 (Jan) 1972.

209. Raffanti EF and King JC: Effect of *pH* on the stability of sodium ampicillin solutions, *Am J Hosp Pharm 31*:745–751 (Aug) 1974.

210. Savello DR and Shangraw RF: Stability of sodium ampicillin solutions in the frozen and liquid states, *Am J Hosp Pharm 28*:754–759 (Oct) 1971.

211. Jacobs J, Nathan I, Superstine E, et al.: Ampicillin and carbenicillin stability in commonly used infusion solutions, *Drug Intell Clin Pharm 4*:204–208 (Aug) 1970.

212. Hiranaka P, Frazier AG, and Gallelli JF: Stability of ampicillin in aqueous solutions, *Am J Hosp Pharm 29*:321–322 (Apr) 1972.

213. Stratton M and Sandmann BJ: Stability studies of ampicillin sodium in intravenous fluids using optical activity, *Bull Parenter Drug Assoc 29*:286–295 (Nov–Dec) 1975.

214. Pincock RE and Kiovsky TE: Kinetics of reactions in frozen solutions, *J Chem Educ 43*:358–360 (July) 1966.

215. Hou JP and Poole JW: Kinetics and mechanism of degradation of ampicillin in solution, *J Pharm Sci 58*:447–454 (Apr) 1969.

216. Shils ME, Wright WL, Turnbull A, et al.: Long-term parenteral nutrition through an external arteriovenous shunt, *N Engl J Med 283*:341–344 (Aug 13) 1970.

217. Zia H, Tehrani M, and Zargarbashi R: Kinetics of carbenicillin degradation in aqueous solutions, *Can J Pharm Sci 9*:112–117 (4) 1974.

218. Riff LJ and Jackson GG: Laboratory and clinical conditions for gentamicin inactivation by carbenicillin, *Arch Intern Med 130*:887–891 (Dec) 1972.

219. McLaughlin JE and Reeves DS: Clinical and laboratory evidence for inactivation of gentamicin by carbenicillin, *Lancet 1*:261–264 (Feb 6) 1971.

220. Klastersky J: Carbenicillin plus gentamicin, *Lancet 1*:653–654 (Mar 27) 1971.

221. Levison ME and Kaye D: Carbenicillin plus gentamicin, *Lancet 2*:45–46 (July 3) 1971.

222. Eykyn S, Phillips I, and Ridley M: Gentamicin plus carbenicillin, *Lancet 1*:545–546 (Mar 13) 1971.

223. Riff L and Jackson GG: Gentamicin plus carbenicillin, *Lancet 1*:592 (Mar 20) 1971.

224. Zost ED and Yanchick VA: Stability of gentamicin in combination with carbenicillin, *Am J Hosp Pharm 29*:388–390 (May) 1972.

225. Jacoby GA: Carbenicillin and gentamicin, *N Engl J Med 284*:1096–1098 (May 13) 1971.

226. Saudek EC (Pharmaceutical Production, The Upjohn Company, Kalamazoo, Michigan): Personal communication, January 3, 1973.

227. Baldini JT (Professional Services, Schering Laboratories, Kenilworth, New Jersey): Personal communication, February 11, 1972.

228. Koup JR and Gerbracht L: Combined use of heparin and gentamicin in peritoneal dialysis solutions, *Drug Intell Clin Pharm 9*:388 (July) 1975.

229. Reeves DS, Bywater MJ, Wise R, et al.: Availability of three antibiotics after intramuscular injection into thigh and buttock, *Lancet 2*:1421–1422 (Dec 14) 1974.

230. Jackson GG: Gentamicin, *Practitioner 198*:855–866 (June) 1967.

231. Preskey D and Kayes JB: Stability of sulfadiazine sodium as used in admixture with intravenous infusion fluids, *J Clin Pharm 1*:39–48 (Mar) 1976.

232. Physicians' desk reference, 49th ed, Medical Economics Company, Oradell, New Jersey, 1995.

233. Larsen SS and Jensen VG: Studies on the stability of drugs in frozen systems, ii: the stabilities of hexobarbital sodium and phenobarbital sodium in frozen aqueous solutions, *Dansk Tidsskr Farm 44*:21–31 (2) 1970.

234. NCI investigational drugs pharmaceutical data, National Cancer Institute, Bethesda, Maryland, 1988, 1990, 1994.

235. Shapiro WR, Young DF, and Mehta BM: Methotrexate: distribution in cerebrospinal fluid after intravenous, ventricular and lumbar injections, *N Engl J Med 293*:161–165 (July 24) 1975.

236. Anon: Kidney toxicity—main source of methotrexate complications, *J Am Med Assoc 223*:1036–1037, 1040 (Sep 8) 1975.

237. Frei E, Jaffe N, Tattersall MHN, et al.: New approaches to cancer chemotherapy with methotrexate, *N Engl J Med 292*:846–851 (Apr 17) 1975.

238. Rosen G, Ghavimi F, Vanucci R, et al.: Pontine glioma—high-dose methotrexate and leucovorin rescue, *J Am Med Assoc 230*:1149–1152 (Nov 25) 1974.

239. Jaffe N, Frei E, Traggis D, et al.: Adjuvant methotrexate and citrovorum-factor treatment of osteogenic sarcoma, *N Engl J Med 291*:994–997 (Nov 7) 1974.

240. Rosen G, Suwansirikul S, Kwon C, et al.: High-dose methotrexate with citrovorum factor rescue and adriamycin in childhood osteogenic sarcoma, *Cancer (Philadelphia) 33*:1151–1163 (Apr) 1974.

241. Lapidas B: Cautions regarding the preparation of high-dose methotrexate infusions, *Am J Hosp Pharm 33*:760 (Aug) 1976.

242. Pelsor FR: Cautions regarding the preparation of high-dose methotrexate infusions, *Am J Hosp Pharm 33*:760 (Aug) 1976.

243. Pritchard J: Stability of heparin solutions, *J Pharm Pharmacol 16*:487–489 (July) 1964.

244. Turco SJ: I.V. drug incompatibilities—heparin sodium USP, *Am J IV Ther 3*:16–19 (Dec–Jan) 1976.

245. Kakkar VV, Corrigan TP, and Fossard DP: Prevention of fatal postoperative pulmonary embolism by low doses of heparin: an international multicentre trial, *Lancet 2*:45–51 (July 12) 1975.

246. Sherry S: Low-dose heparin prophylaxis for postoperative venous thromboembolism, *N Engl J Med 293*:300–302 (Aug 7) 1975.

247. Gallus AS, Hirsch J, O'Brien SE, et al.: Prevention of venous thrombosis with small, subcutaneous doses of heparin, *J Am Med Assoc 235*:1980–1982 (May 3) 1976.

248. Hopefl AW: Low-dose heparin for the prevention of venous thromboembolism, *Hosp Pharm 11*:223, 226 (June) 1976.

249. Wessler S: Heparin as an antithrombotic agent, *J Am Med Assoc 236*:389–391 (July 26) 1976.

250. Erdi A, Kakkar VV, Thomas DP, et al.: Effect of low-dose subcutaneous heparin on whole-blood viscosity, *Lancet 2*:342–344 (Aug 14) 1976.

251. Hadgraft JW: Adding drugs to intravenous infusions, *Lancet 2*:1254 (Dec 12) 1970.

252. Stock SL and Warner N: Heparin in acid solutions, *Br Med J 3*:307 (July 31) 1971.

253. Chessells JM, Braithwaite TA, and Chamberlain DA: Dextrose and sorbitol as diluents for continuous intravenous heparin infusion, *Br Med J 2*:81–82 (Apr 8) 1972.

254. Mitchell JF, Barger RC, and Cantwell L: Heparin stability in 5% dextrose and 0.9% sodium chloride, *Am J Hosp Pharm 33*:540–542 (June) 1976.

255. Thomas RB and Salter FJ: Heparin locks: their advantages and disadvantages, *Hosp Formul 10*:536–538 (Nov) 1975.

256. Deeb EN and DiMattia PE: The key question: how much heparin in the lock?, *Am J IV Ther 3*:22–26 (Dec–Jan) 1976.

257. DeFina E: How we use heparin locks, *Am J IV Ther 3*:27, 33 (Dec–Jan) 1976.

258. Hanson RL, Grant AM, and Majors KR: Heparin-lock maintenance with ten units of sodium heparin in one milliliter of normal saline solution, *Surg Gynecol Obstet 142*:373–376 (Mar) 1976.

259. Rebagay T and DeLuca PP: Residues in antibiotic preparations, ii: effect of *pH* on the nature and level of particulate matter in sodium cephalothin intravenous solutions, *Am J Hosp Pharm 33*:443–448 (May) 1976.

260. Gaines K (Parenteral Products Development, Eli Lilly and Company, Indianapolis, Indiana): Personal communication, August 13, 1976.

261. Hopefl AW: Room temperature stability of drug products, *Am J Hosp Pharm 32*:1084, 1089 (Nov) 1975.

262. Barger RC: Room temperature stability of drug products, *Am J Hosp Pharm 32*:1089 (Nov) 1975.

263. Rosenbloom AL: Advances in commercial insulin preparations, *Am J Dis Child 128*:631–633 (Nov) 1974.

264. Rosenberg JM, Simon WA, Sangkachand P, et al.: Mixing insulin preparations, *Hosp Pharm 11*:186, 191 (May) 1976.

265. Shainfeld FJ: Errors in insulin doses due to the design of insulin syringes,

Pediatrics 56:302–303 (Aug) 1975.

266. Weisenfeld S, Podolsky S, Goldsmith L, et al.: Adsorption of insulin to infusion bottles and tubing, *Diabetes 17*:766–771 (Dec) 1968.

267. Petty C and Cunningham NL: Insulin adsorption by glass infusion bottles, polyvinylchloride infusion containers, and intravenous tubing, *Anesthesiology 40*:400–404 (Apr) 1974.

268. Kraegen EW, Lazarus L, Meler H, et al.: Carrier solutions for low-level intravenous insulin infusion, *Br Med J 3*:464–466 (Aug 23) 1975.

269. Semple P, Ratcliffe JG, and Manderson WG: Carrier solutions for low-level intravenous insulin infusion, *Br Med J 4*:228–229 (Oct 25) 1975.

270. Hays DP and Mehl B: I.V. drug incompatibilities—insulin, *Am J IV Ther 3*:30–32 (Apr–May) 1976.

271. Owen JA: The insulin revolution, *Hosp Formul 11*:343 (July) 1976.

272. Galloway JA (Medical Research Division, Eli Lilly and Company, Indianapolis, Indiana): Personal communication, August 29, 1967.

273. Kaplan MA and Granatek AP: Stability of frozen solutions of cephapirin sodium, *Curr Ther Res Clin Exp 16*:573–579 (May) 1974.

274. Prasad VK, Johns WH, Wingate MW, et al.: Pharmaceutics of cephapirin sodium (Cefadyl) a new semisynthetic cephalosporin part iii, *Curr Ther Res Clin Exp 16*:1214–1237 (Nov) 1974.

275. Kochevar M and Fry LK: Insulin and dead space volume, *Drug Intell Clin Pharm 8*:33–34 (Jan) 1974.

276. Bornstein M, Thomas PN, Coleman DL, et al.: Stability of parenteral solutions of cefazolin sodium, *Am J Hosp Pharm 31*:296–298 (Mar) 1974.

277. Carone SM, Bornstein M, Coleman DL, et al.: Stability of frozen solutions of cefazolin sodium, *Am J Hosp Pharm 33*:639–641 (July) 1976.

278. Royston DA (Consumer Technical Services, Eli Lilly and Company, Indianapolis, Indiana): Personal communication, February 19, 1976.

279. Brudney N, Eustace BT, and Gilmour WN: Some formulations and compatibility problems with dimenhydrinate (Gravol), *Can Pharm J 96*:470–471, 1963.

280. Acred P, Brown DM, Knudsen ET, et al.: New semi-synthetic penicillin active against pseudomonas pyocyanea, *Nature (London) 215*:25–30 (July) 1967.

281. Schwartz MA and Buckwalter FH: Pharmaceutics of penicillin, *J Pharm Sci 51*:1119–1128 (Dec) 1962.

282. Thur MP (Parenteral Products, Travenol Laboratories, Deerfield, Illinois): Personal communication, September 20, 1976.

283. Ziemba LJ (Medical Information, ICI Pharmaceuticals Group, Wilmington, Delaware): Personal communication, March 15, 1990.

284. Yamana T and Tsuji A: Comparative stability of cephalosporins in aqueous solution: kinetics and mechanisms of degradation, *J Pharm Sci 65*:1563–1574 (Nov) 1976.

285. Kleinman LM, Davignon JP, Cradock JC, et al.: Investigational drug information, *Drug Intell Clin Pharm 10*:48–49 (Jan) 1976.

286. Chang SY, Evans TL, and Alberts DS: The stability of melphalan in the presence of chloride ion, *J Pharm Pharmacol 31*:853–854, 1979.

287. Mitenko PA and Ogilvie RI: Rational intravenous doses of theophylline, *N Engl J Med 289*:600–603 (Sep 20) 1973.

288. Simons FER, Pierson WE, and Bierman CW: Current status of the use of intravenously administered aminophylline, *South Med J 68*:802–804 (July) 1975.

289. Weinberger MW, Matthay RA, Ginchansky EJ, et al.: Intravenous aminophylline dosage use of serum theophylline measurement for guidance, *J Am Med Assoc 235*:2110–2113 (May 10) 1976.

290. Nedich RL: Vitamin A absorption from plastic i.v. bags, *J Am Med Assoc 224*:1531–1532 (June 11) 1973.

291. Kaplan MA, Coppola WP, Nunning BC, et al.: Pharmaceutical properties and stability of amikacin, part i, *Curr Ther Res Clin Exp 20*:352–358 (Oct) 1976.

292. Nunning BC and Granatek AP: Physical compatibility and chemical stability of amikacin sulfate in large-volume parenteral solutions, part ii, *Curr Ther Res Clin Exp 20*:359–368 (Oct) 1976.

293. Nunning BC, Granatek AP, and Ricci RA: Physical compatibility and chemical stability of amikacin sulfate in combination with antibiotics in large-volume parenteral solutions, part iii, *Curr Ther Res Clin Exp 20*:369–416 (Oct) 1976.

294. Nunning BC and Granatek AP: Physical compatibility and chemical stability of amikacin sulfate in combination with non-antibiotic drugs in large-volume parenteral solutions, part iv, *Curr Ther Res Clin Exp 20*:417–491 (Oct) 1976.

295. Koup JR and Gerbracht L: Reduction in heparin activity by gentamicin, *Drug Intell Clin Pharm 9*:568 (Oct) 1975.

296. McKinley JD (M.D. Anderson Hospital and Tumor Institute, Houston, Texas): Personal communication, August 23, 1976.

297. Weiner B, McNeely DJ, Kluge RM, et al.: Stability of gentamicin sulfate following unit dose repackaging, *Am J Hosp Pharm 33*:1254–1259 (Dec) 1976.

298. Dinel BA, Ayotte DL, Behme RJ, et al.: Comparative stability of antibiotic admixtures in minibags and minibottles, *Drug Intell Clin Pharm 11*:226–239 (Apr) 1977.

299. Dinel BA, Ayotte DL, Behme RJ, et al.: Stability of antibiotic admixtures frozen in minibags, *Drug Intell Clin Pharm 11*:542–548 (Sep) 1977.

300. Lynn B: Pharmaceutics of the semi-synthetic penicillins, *Chem Drug 187*:157–160 (Feb 18) 1967.

301. Stanaszek WF and Pan IH: Analysis of hydroxyzine hydrochloride, meperidine hydrochloride and atropine sulfate in glass and plastic syringes, *Am J Hosp Pharm 35*:1084–1087 (Sep) 1978.

302. Fraser GL: Incompatibility of magnesium sulfate and hydrocortisone sodium succinate, *Am J Hosp Pharm 35*:783 (July) 1978.

303. Kresel JJ, McDermott JS, Huffer LM, et al.: Stability of carbenicillin and oxacillin frozen in syringes, *Am J Hosp Pharm 35*:310–312 (Mar) 1978.

304. Manning RE: Predicted expiration times for penicillin G in combination with multivitamin injections, *Am J Hosp Pharm 33*:870, 874 (Sep) 1976.

305. Cloyd JC, Bosch DE, and Sawchuk RJ: Concentration–time profile of phenytoin after admixture with small volumes of intravenous fluids, *Am J Hosp Pharm 35*:45–48 (Jan) 1978.

306. Bauman JL, Siepler JK, and Fitzloff J: Phenytoin crystallization in intravenous fluids, *Drug Intell Clin Pharm 11*:646–649 (Nov) 1977.

307. Ashwin J and Lynn B: Ampicillin stability in saline or dextrose infusions, *Pharm J 214*:487–489 (May 31) 1975.

308. O'Brien MJ, Portnoff JB, and Cohen EM: Cefoxitin sodium compatibility with intravenous infusions and additives, *Am J Hosp Pharm 36*:33–38 (Jan) 1979.

309. Stevens JS: Incompatibility of diphenhydramine hydrochloride (Benadryl) with meglumine iodipamide (Cholografin), *Radiology 117*:224–225 (Oct) 1975.

310. Petrick RJ, Wolleben JE, and Vargas TA: Stability of frozen solutions of doxycycline hyclate for injection, *Am J Hosp Pharm 35*:1386–1387 (Nov) 1978.

311. Chrai SS, Phelan KR, Speicher ER, et al.: Stability of gentamicin sulfate admixture, *Am J Hosp Pharm 34*:348 (Apr) 1977.

312. Gardella LA, Kesler H, Amann A, et al.: Intropin (dopamine hydrochloride) intravenous admixture compatibility, part 3: stability with miscellaneous additives, *Am J Hosp Pharm 35*:581–584 (May) 1978.

313. Schuetz DH and King JC: Compatibility and stability of electrolytes, vitamins and antibiotics in combination with 8% amino acids solution, *Am J Hosp Pharm 35*:33–44 (Jan) 1978.

314. El-Nakeeb MA, Souccar N, and Yousef RT: Inactivation of various antibiotics by some vitamins, *Can J Pharm Sci 11*:85–89 (July) 1976.

315. Dixon FW and Weshalek J: Physical compatibility of nine drugs in various intavenous solutions, *Am J Hosp Pharm 29*:822–823 (Oct) 1972.

316. Earhart RH: Instability of cis-dichlorodiammineplatinum in dextrose solution, *Cancer Treat Rep 62*:1105–1106 (July) 1978.

317. Greene RF, Chatterji DC, Hiranaka PK, et al.: Stability of cisplatin in aqueous solution, *Am J Hosp Pharm 36*:38–43 (Jan) 1979.

318. Morrison RA, Oseekey KB, and Fung HL: 5-Fluorouracil and methotrexate sodium: an admixture incompatibility?, *Am J Hosp Pharm 35*:15, 18 (Jan) 1978.

319. King JC: 5-Fluorouracil and methotrexate sodium: an admixture incompatibility?, *Am J Hosp Pharm 35*:18 (Jan) 1978.

320. Rusmin S, Welton S, DeLuca P, et al.: Effect of inline filtration on the potency of drugs administered intravenously, *Am J Hosp Pharm 34*:1071–1074 (Oct) 1977.

321. Morris ME: Compatibility and stability of diazepam injection following dilution with intravenous fluids, *Am J Hosp Pharm 35*:669–672 (June) 1978.

322. Allen LV, Levinson RS, and Phisutsinthop D: Compatibility of various admixtures with secondary additives at Y-injection sites of intravenous administration sets, *Am J Hosp Pharm 34*:939–943 (Sep) 1977.

323. Arnold TR, Eder J, and Lower B: Compatibility of primary-piggyback solution combinations, *Am J Hosp Pharm 35*:249–250 (Mar) 1978.

324. Jansen JR: Volume control sets and incompatibilities, *Am J Hosp Pharm 32*:1225 (Dec) 1975.

325. Aisenstein A and Kahn S: Study of the stability of some frozen antibiotics, *Hosp Pharm 4*:17–21 (Feb) 1969.

326. Parker WA: Physical compatibilities of preanesthetic medications, *Can J Hosp Pharm 29*:91–92 (May–June) 1976.

327. Cradock JC, Kleinman LM, and Rahman A: Evaluation of some pharmaceutical aspects of intrathecal methotrexate sodium, cytarabine and hydro-

cortisone sodium succinate, *Am J Hosp Pharm 35*:402–406 (Apr) 1978.

328. Sarubbi FA, Wilson MB, Lee M, et al.: Noscomial meningitis and bacteremia due to contaminated amphotericin B, *J Am Med Assoc 239*:416–418 (Jan 30) 1978.

329. The Upjohn Company, Solu-Medrol IV admixture, dilution, and compatibility information, August 1978.

330. Parker WA, Morris ME, and Shearer CA: Incompatibility of diazepam injection in plastic intravenous bags, *Am J Hosp Pharm 36*:505–507 (Apr) 1979.

331. Ingallinera T, Kapadia AJ, Hagman D, et al.: Compatibility of glycopyrrolate injection with commonly used infusion solutions and additives, *Am J Hosp Pharm 36*:508–510 (Apr) 1979.

332. Bateman NE and Graham MD: Solubility of an ephedrine–phenobarbitone complex in water, *Australas J Pharm 48*:S68–S69 (June 30) 1967.

333. Chang CH, Ashford WR, Ives DAJ, et al.: Stability of oxytocin in various infusion solutions, *Can J Hosp Pharm 25*:152 (July–Aug) 1972.

334. Lynn B: Administration of carbenicillin and ticarcillin—pharmaceutical aspects, *Europ J Cancer 9*:425–433 (June) 1973.

335. Block ER and Bennett JE: Stability of amphotericin B in infusion bottles, *Antimicrob Agents Chemother 4*:648–649 (Dec) 1973.

336. Prue B and Elliott RK: Bethesda Hospital IV reference, *Am J IV Ther 4*:22–34 (Dec–Jan) 1977.

337. Anon: Label changes on albumin—a reminder, *FDA Drug Bull 8*:32 (Oct–Nov) 1978.

338. Van Der Linde LP, Campbell RK, and Jackson E: Guidelines for the intravenous administration of drugs, *Drug Intell Clin Pharm 11*:30–55 (Jan) 1977.

339. Koup JR, Schentag JJ, Vance JW, et al.: System for clinical pharmacokinetic monitoring of theophylline therapy, *Am J Hosp Pharm 33*:949–956 (Sep) 1976.

340. Jusko WJ, Koup JR, Vance JW, et al.: Intravenous theophylline therapy: nomogram guidelines, *Ann Intern Med 86*:400–404 (Apr) 1977.

341. Product information, Travasol, Travenol Laboratories, Deerfield, Illinois, January 1994.

342. Product information, FreAmine III, McGaw Laboratories, Irvine, California, September 1991.

343. Odne MAL, Lee SC, and Jeffrey LP: Rationale for adding trace elements to total parenteral nutrient solutions—a brief review, *Am J Hosp Pharm 35*:1057–1059 (Sep) 1978.

344. Jeejeebhoy KN, Langer B, Tsallas G, et al.: Total parenteral nutrition at home: studies in patients surviving 4 months to 5 years; *Gastroenterology 71*:943–953 (Dec) 1976.

345. Hull RL and Cassidy D: Trace element deficiencies during total parenteral nutrition, *Drug Intell Clin Pharm 11*:536–541 (Sep) 1977.

346. Shils ME: More on trace elements in total parenteral nutrition solutions, *Am J Hosp Pharm 32*:141–142 (Feb) 1975.

347. Okada A, Takagi Y, Itakura T, et al.: Skin lesions during intravenous hyperalimentation: zinc deficiency, *Surgery 80*:629–635 (Nov) 1976.

348. Matoi JR and Jeffreys LP: Formulation of a trace element solution for long-term parenteral nutrition, *Am J Hosp Pharm 35*:165–168 (Feb) 1978.

349. Athanikar N, Boyer B, Deamer R, et al: Visual compatibility of 30 additives with a parenteral nutrient solution, *Am J Hosp Pharm 36*:511–513 (Apr) 1979.

350. Finlayson JS: The birth and demise of "salt-poor" albumin, *Am J Hosp Pharm 35*:898–900 (Aug) 1978.

351. Winsnes M, Jeppsson R, and Sjoberg B: Diazepam adsorption to infusion sets and plastic syringes, *Acta Anaesthesiol Scand 25*:93–96 (Apr) 1981.

352. Bonner DP, Mechlinski W, and Schaffner CP: Stability studies with amphotericin B and amphotericin B methyl ester, *J Antibiotics 28*:132–135 (Feb) 1975.

353. Shadomy S, Brummer DL, and Ingroff AV: Light sensitivity of prepared solutions of amphotericin B, *Am Rev Resp Dis 107*:303–304, 1973.

354. Fields BT, Bates JH, and Abernathy RS: Effect of rapid intravenous infusion on serum concentrations of amphotericin B, *App Microbiol 22*:615–617 (Oct) 1971.

355. Barreuther AD, Dodge RR, and Blondeaux AM: Administration of amphotericin B, *Drug Intell Clin Pharm 11*:368–369 (June) 1977.

356. Arbuthnot R, Dullea A, and Rippel S: Controlling thrombophlebitis from amphotericin B, *Am J Hosp Pharm 35*:129 (Feb) 1978.

357. Rosch JM, Pazin G, and Fireman P: Mannitol and amphotericin B, *J Am Med Assoc 237*:27 (Jan 3) 1977.

358. Package insert, Cenolate, Abbott Laboratories, North Chicago, Illinois, December 1991.

359. Roberts JR: Cutaneous and subcutaneous complications of calcium infusions, *J Am Col Emerg Phys 6*:16–20 (Jan) 1977.

360. Product information, Tagamet, Smith Kline & French Laboratories, Philadelphia, Pennsylvania, October 1978.

361. Winters RE, Chow AW, Hecht RH, et al.: Combined use of gentamicin and carbenicillin, *Ann Intern Med 75*:925–927 (Dec) 1971.

362. Waitz JA, Drube CG, Moss EL, et al.: Biological aspects of the interaction between gentamicin and carbenicillin, *J Antibiot 25*:219–225 (Apr) 1972.

363. Ervin FR, Bullock WE, and Nuttall CE: Inactivation of gentamicin by penicillins in patients with renal failure, *Antimicrob Agents Chemother 9*:1004–1011 (June) 1976.

364. Peterson CD, Kaatz BL, and Angaran DM: Ticarcillin and carbenicillin, *Drug Intell Clin Pharm 11*:482–486 (Aug) 1977.

365. Davies M, Morgan JR, and Anand C: Interactions of carbenicillin and ticarcillin with gentamicin, *Antimicrob Agents Chemother 7*:431–434 (Apr) 1975.

366. Weibert R, Keane W, and Shapiro F: Carbenicillin inactivation of aminoglycosides in patients with severe renal failure, *Trans Am Soc Artif Int Organs 22*:439–443 1976.

367. Weibert RT and Keane WF: Carbenicillin–gentamicin interaction in acute renal failure, *Am J Hosp Pharm 34*:1137–1139 (Oct) 1977.

368. Bodey GP, Feld R, and Burgess MA: β-Lactam antibiotics alone or in combination with gentamicin for therapy of gram-negative bacillary infections in neutropenic patients, *Am J Med Sci 271*:179–186 (Mar–Apr) 1976.

369. Schimpff S, Satterlee W, Young UM, et al.: Empiric therapy with carbenicillin and gentamicin for febrile patients with cancer and granulocytopenia, *N Eng J Med 284*:1061–1065 (May 13) 1971.

370. Hendeles L: Are carbenicillin and gentamicin synergists or antagonists? *Hosp Pharm 7*:297–298 (Sep) 1972.

371. Kole-James A: Electrolyte content of common intravenous solutions and antibiotics, *Hosp Pharm 12*:394 (Aug) 1977.

372. Anon: Correction: Sodium in ticarcillin and carbenicillin, *Med Letter Drug Ther 19*:28 (Mar 25) 1977.

373. Turco SJ and Hasan I: Comparison of features of Kefzol and Ancef, *Hosp Pharm 11*:482, 484 (Nov) 1976.

374. Vukovich RA, Sugerman AA, and Fields LA: Effect of 2% procaine hydrochloride solution on the bioavailability of cephradine after intramuscular injection, *Curr Ther Res Clin Exp 18*:711–719 (Nov) 1975.

375. Stennett DJ, Simonson W, and Ayres JW: Effect of membrane filtration on 10-mg/ml cefazolin admixtures, *Am J Hosp Pharm 36*:657–660 (May) 1979.

376. Klink PR, Frable RA, and Bornstein M: Stability of Mandol in parenteral fluids, frozen solutions and admixtures containing other drugs, Presented at 13th Annual ASHP Midyear Clinical Meeting, December 1978, San Antonio, Texas.

377. Henney JE, Von Hoff DD, Rozencweig M, et al.: Thrombophlebitic potential of intravenous cytotoxic agents, *Drug Intell Clin Pharm 11*:266–267 (May) 1977.

378. Sillers BR: Irritant properties of diazepam, *Br Dent J 124*:295 (Apr 2) 1968.

379. Roche Products Ltd: Irritant properties of diazepam—reply, *Br Dent J 124*:295 (Apr 2) 1968.

380. Friedenberg W and Barker JD: Intravenous diazepam administration, *J Am Med Assoc 224*:901 (May 7) 1973.

381. Jusko WJ, Gretch M, and Gassett R: Precipitation of diazepam from intravenous preparations, *J Am Med Assoc 225*:176 (July 9) 1973.

382. Kortilla K, Sothman A, and Andersson P: Polyethylene glycol as a solvent for diazepam: bioavailability and clinical effects after intramuscular administration, comparison of oral, intramuscular and rectal administration, and precipitation from intravenous solutions, *Acta Pharmacol Toxicol 39*:104–117 (Aug) 1976.

383. Hillestad L, Hansen T, Melsome H, et al.: Diazepam metabolism in normal man I. Serum concentrations and clinical effects after intravenous, intramuscular and oral administration, *Clin Pharmacol Ther 16*:479–484 (Sep) 1974.

384. Assaf RAE, Dundee JW, and Gamble JAS: Influence of route of administration on the clinical action of diazepam, *Anesthesia 30*:152–158 (Mar) 1975.

385. Baxter MT, McKenzie DD, and Mikish RA: Dilution of diazepam in intravenous fluids, *Am J Hosp Pharm 34*:124 (Feb) 1977.

386. Thong YH and Abramson DC: Continuous infusion of diazepam in infants with severe recurrent convulsions, *Med Ann DC 43*:63–65 (Feb) 1974.

387. Khalid MS and Schultz H: Treatment and management of emergency status epilepticus, *Epilepsia 17*:73–76 (Mar) 1976.

388. Gibberd FB: Diseases of the central nervous system—epilepsy, *Br Med J 4*:270–272 (Nov 1) 1975.

389. Kawathekar P, Anusuya SR, Sriniwas P, et al.: Diazepam (Calmpose) in eclampsia: a preliminary report of 16 cases, *Curr Ther Res Clin Exp 15*:845–855 (Nov) 1973.

390. Baskett TF and Bradford CR: Active management of severe pre-eclampsia, *Can Med Assoc J 109*:1209–1211 (Dec 15) 1973.

391. Prensky AL, Raff MC, Moore MJ, et al.: Intravenous diazepam in the treatment of prolonged seizure activity, *N Eng J Med 276*:779–784 (Apr 6) 1967.

392. Tehrani JB and Cavanaugh A: Diazepam infusion in the treatment of tetanus, *Drug Intell Clin Pharm 11*:491 (Aug) 1977.

393. McLean WN: Safety of diazepam infusion questioned, *Drug Intell Clin Pharm 11*:690 (Nov) 1977.

394. Trissel LA, Kleinman LM, Davignon JP, et al.: Investigational drug information—daunorubicin hydrochloride and streptozotocin, *Drug Intell Clin Pharm 12*:404–406 (July) 1978.

395. Elsberry VA, Grangeia JM, Giorgianni SJ, et al.: The lipid phase in TPN, *Am J IV Ther 4*:22–28 (Apr–May) 1977.

396. Belin RP, Bivins BA, Jona JZ, et al.: Fat overload with a 10% soybean oil emulsion, *Arch Surg 111*:1391–1393 (Dec) 1976.

397. McNiff BL: Clinical use of 10% soybean oil emulsion, *Am J Hosp Pharm 34*:1080–1086 (Oct) 1977.

398. Roche Laboratories, Personal communication.

399. Anon: McGaw compatibility studies. A preliminary report, McGaw Laboratories, Irvine, California, 1978.

400. Cooperman LB and Rubin I: Toxicity of ethacrynic acid and furosemide, *Am Heart J 85*:831–834 (June) 1973.

401. Kresel JJ, Smith AL, and Siber GR: Stability of gentamicin in plastic syringes, *Am J Hosp Pharm 34*:570 (June) 1977.

402. McNeely DJ, Weiner B, Stewart RB, et al.: Stability of gentamicin in plastic syringes, *Am J Hosp Pharm 34*:570, 575 (June) 1977.

403. Chrai SS and Ambrosio TJ: Gentamicin sulfate injection repackaging in syringes, *Am J Hosp Pharm 34*:920 (Sep) 1977.

404. Product information, Heparin Lock Flush Solution, Wyeth Laboratories, Philadelphia, Pennsylvania, 1978.

405. Sohn C and Cupit GC: Concentration of heparin in heparin-locks, *Drug Intell Clin Pharm 12*:112 (Feb) 1978.

406. Okuno T and Nelson CA: Anticoagulant activity of heparin in intravenous fluids, *J Clin Pathol 28*:494–497 (June) 1975.

407. Joy RT, Hyneck ML, Berardi RR, et al.: Effect of pH on the stability of heparin in 5% dextrose solutions, *Am J Hosp Pharm 36*:618–621 (May) 1979.

408. Brown J and Stead K: Anti-human lymphocyte globulin-heparin precipitate, *Drug Intell Clin Pharm 10*:654 (Nov) 1976.

409. Raab WP and Windisch J: Antagonism of neomycin by heparin, *Drug Res 23*:1326–1328 (9) 1973.

410. Stella VJ: A case for prodrugs: Fosphenytoin, *Adv Drug Del Rev 19*:311–330, 1996.

411. Dupuis LL, Wong B, and Trope A: Stability of propafenone hydrochloride in i.v. solutions, *Am J Health-Syst Pharm 54*:1293–1295 (June 1) 1997.

412. Dupuis LL, Trope A, Giesbrecht E, and Wong B: Compatibility and stability of propafenone hydrochloride with five critical-care medications, *Can J Hosp Pharm 51*:55–57 (Apr) 1998.

413. Storvick WO and Henry HJ: Effect of storage temperature on stability of commercial insulin preparations, *Diabetes 17*:499–502 (Aug) 1968.

414. Jackson RL, Storvick WO, Hollinden CS, et al.: Neutral regular insulin, *Diabetes 21*:235–245 (Apr) 1972.

415. Page MM, Alberti KGMM, Greenwood R, et al.: Treatment of diabetic coma with continuous low-dose infusion of insulin, *Br Med J 2*:687–690 (June 29) 1974.

416. Kidson W, Casey J, Kraegen E, et al.: Treatment of severe diabetes mellitus by insulin infusion, *Br Med J 2*:691–694 (June 29) 1974.

417. Semple PF, White C, and Manderson WG: Continuous intravenous infusion of small doses of insulin in treatment of diabetic ketoacidosis, *Br Med J 2*:694–698 (June 29) 1974.

418. Campbell LV, Lazarus L, Casey JH, et al.: Routine use of low-dose intravenous insulin infusion in severe hyperglycaemia, *Med J Aust 2*:519–522 (Oct 2) 1976.

419. Martin MM and Martin ALA: Continuous low-dose infusion of insulin in the treatment of diabetic ketoacidosis in children, *J Pediatr 89*:560–564 (Oct) 1976.

420. Drop SLS, Duval-Arnould BJM, Gober AE, et al.: Low-dose intravenous insulin infusion versus subcutaneous insulin injection: A controlled comparative study of diabetic ketoacidosis, *Pediatrics 59*:733–738 (May) 1977.

421. Fisher JN, Shahshahani MN, and Kitabchi AE: Diabetic ketoacidosis: low-dose insulin therapy by various routes, *N Engl J Med 297*:238–241 (Aug 4) 1977.

422. Goldberg NJ and Levin SR: Insulin adsorption to an inline membrane filter, *N Engl J Med 298*:1480 (June 29) 1978.

423. Kristofferson J, Skobba TJ, and Johansen T: Adsorption of insulin to infusion equipment, *Nor Farm Tidsskr 85*:220–224 (7) 1977.

424. Hirsch JI, Fratkin MJ, Wood JH, et al.: Clinical significance of insulin adsorption by polyvinyl chloride infusion systems, *Am J Hosp Pharm 34*:583–588 (June) 1977.

425. Weber SS, Wood WA, and Jackson EA: Availability of insulin from parenteral nutrient solutions, *Am J Hosp Pharm 34*:353–357 (Apr) 1977.

426. Whalen FJ, LeCain WK, and Latiolais CJ: Availability of insulin from continuous low-dose insulin infusions, *Am J Hosp Pharm 36*:330–337 (Mar) 1979.

427. Clarke BF, Campbell IW, Fraser DM, et al.: Direct addition of small doses of insulin to intravenous infusion in severe uncontrolled diabetes, *Br Med J 2*:1395–1396 (Nov 26) 1977.

428. Peterson L, Caldwell J, and Hoffman J: Insulin adsorbance to polyvinyl chloride surfaces with implications for constant-infusion therapy, *Diabetes 25*:72–74 (Jan) 1976.

429. Sadeghi A, Mehrbanpour J, Behmard S, et al.: A trial of total dose infusion iron therapy as an outpatient procedure in rural Iranian villages (a three month follow-up), *Curr Ther Res Clin Exp 19*:595–602 (June) 1976.

430. Leach JK, Strickland RD, Millis DL, et al.: Biological activity of dilute isoproterenol solution stored for long periods in plastic bags, *Am J Hosp Pharm 34*:709–712 (July) 1977.

431. Browning ML: IM MgSO₄ ampuls for IV use, *Hosp Pharm 11*:325 (Aug) 1976.

432. Epperson E and Nedich RL: Mannitol crystallization in plastic containers, *Am J Hosp Pharm 35*:1337 (Nov) 1978.

433. Chatterji DC and Gallelli JF: Thermal and photolytic decomposition of methotrexate in aqueous solutions, *J Pharm Sci 67*:526–531 (Apr) 1978.

434. Muller HJ and Berg J: Stabilitatsstudie zu tramadolhydrochlorid im PVC-infusionbeutel, *Krankenhauspharmazie 18*:75–79, 1997.

435. Duttera MJ, Gallelli JF, Kleinman LM, et al.: Intrathecal methotrexate, *Lancet 2*:540 (Mar 4) 1972.

436. Hartshorn EA: Oxidation of methyldopa hydrochloride in alkaline media, *Am J Hosp Pharm 32*:244 (Mar) 1975.

437. Parker EA: Oxidation of methyldopa hydrochloride in alkaline media, *Am J Hosp Pharm 32*:244 (Mar) 1975.

438. Hartline JV and Zachman RD: Vitamin A delivery in total parenteral nutrition solution, *Pediatrics 58*:448–451 (Sep) 1976.

439. Sina A, Youssef MK, Kassem AA, et al.: Stability of oxytetracycline in solutions and injections, *Can J Pharm Sci 9*:44–49 (2) 1974.

440. Colding H and Anderson GE: Stability of antibiotics and amino acids in two synthetic L-amino acid solutions commonly used for total parenteral nutrition in children, *Antimicrob Agents Chemother 13*:555–558 (Apr) 1978.

441. Schneider E (Knoll AG, Milan, Italy): Personal communication, February 25, 2000.

442. Perrier D, Rapp R, Young B, et al.: Maintenance of therapeutic phenytoin plasma levels via intramuscular administration, *Ann Intern Med 85*:318–321 (Sep) 1976.

443. Sellers EM and Kalant H: Alcohol intoxication and withdrawal, *N Eng J Med 294*:757–762, 1976.

444. Greenblatt DJ and Shader RI: Treatment of the alcohol withdrawal syndrome, *in* Manual of psychiatric therapeutics, Little, Brown and Company, Boston, Massachusetts, 1975, pp 211–235.

445. Cooper PE: Intravenous phenytoin, *N Eng J Med 295*:1078 (Nov 4) 1976.

446. Greenblatt DJ and Shader RI: Intravenous phenytoin, *N Eng J Med 295*:1078 (Nov 4) 1976.

447. Frank JT: Author's response, *Drug Intell Clin Pharm 7*:419 (Sep) 1973.

448. Woo E and Greenblatt DJ: Choosing the right phenytoin dosage, *Drug Ther 7*:131–139 (Oct) 1977.

449. Bighley LD, Wille J, and Lach JL: Mixing of additives in glass and plastic intravenous fluid containers, *Am J Hosp Pharm 31*:736–739 (Aug) 1974.

450. Schondelmeyer S, Gatlin L, and Gwilt P: Intravenous phenytoin (concluded), *N Eng J Med 296*:111 (Jan 13) 1977.

451. Bauman JL and Siepler JK: Intravenous phenytoin (concluded), *N Eng J Med 296*:111 (Jan 13) 1977.

452. Sistare F and Greene R: Phenytoin crystallization in intravenous fluids, *Drug Intell Clin Pharm 12*:120 (Feb) 1978.

453. Biberdorf RI and Spurbeck GH: Phenytoin in IV fluids: results endorsed, *Drug Intell Clin Pharm 12*:300–301 (May) 1978.

454. Williams RHP: Potassium overdosage: a potential hazard of non-rigid parenteral fluid containers, *Br Med J 1*:714–715 (Mar 24) 1973.

455. Woodside W, King JA, and Barr A: Addition of potassium to non-rigid plastic intravenous infusion containers: a potential hazard, *J Hosp Pharm 31*:192–194 (Sep) 1973.

456. Lankton JW, Siler JN, and Neigh JL: Hyperkalemia after administration of potassium from nonrigid parenteral-fluid containers, *Anesthesiology*

39:660–661, 1973.

457. Vrabel RB and Amerson AB: Reconstitution of sodium nitroprusside, *Am J Hosp Pharm 32*:140–141 (Feb) 1975.

458. Challen RG: Stability of sodium nitroprusside solutions, *Australas J Pharm 48*:S110 (Oct 30) 1967.

459. Martin T and Patel JA: Determination of sodium nitroprusside in aqueous solution, *Am J Hosp Pharm 26*:51–53 (Jan) 1969.

460. Frank MJ, Johnson JB, and Rubin SH: Spectrophotometric determination of sodium nitroprusside and its photodegradation products, *J Pharm Sci 65*:44–48 (Jan) 1976.

461. Ammar HO: Stability of injection solutions of vitamin B₁, *Pharmazie 31*:373–374 (June) 1976.

462. Anon: Correction: sodium in ticarcillin and carbenicillin, *Med Letter Drug Ther 19*:28 (Mar 25) 1977.

463. Yamaji A, Yasuko F, Okuda H, et al.: Photodegradation of vitamin K^1 and vitamin K^2 injections in preservation and in intravenous admixtures, *J Nippon Hosp Pharm Assoc Sci Ed 4*:7–11 (5) 1978.

464. Kobayashi NH and King JC: Compatibility of common additives in protein hydrolysate/dextrose solutions, *Am J Hosp Pharm 34*:589–594 (June) 1977.

465. Humphreys A, Marty JJ, Gooey SL, et al.: Stability of methotrexate in an intravenous fluid, *Aust J Hosp Pharm 8*:66–67 (2) 1978.

466. Clayton SK: Stability of intravenous additive preparations; studies on hydralazine as an additive, *J Clin Pharm 2*:247–256 (4) 1978.

467. Anon: Mixing chlorpromazine and morphine, *Br Med J 3*:681 (Sep 14) 1974.

468. Crapper JB: Mixing chlorpromazine and morphine, *Br Med J 1*:33 (Jan 4) 1975.

469. Baird GM and Willoughby MLN: Photodegradation of dacarbazine, *Lancet 2*:681 (Sep 23) 1978.

470. Georget S, Vigneron J, Blaise N, et al.: Stability of refrigerated and frozen solutions of tropisetron in either polyvinylchloride or polyolefin infusion bags, *J Clin Pharm Ther 22*:257–260, 1997.

471. Bergman HD: Cefamandole, *Drug Intell Clin Pharm 13*:144–149 (Mar) 1979.

472. Indelicato JM, Wilham WL, and Cerimele BJ: Conversion of cefamandole nafate to cefamandole sodium, *J Pharm Sci 65*:1175–1178 (Aug) 1976.

473. Palmer MA and Fraterrigo CC: Production of carbon dioxide gas after reconstitution of cefamandole nafate, *Am J Hosp Pharm 36*:596–597 (May) 1979.

474. Klink PR and McKeechan CW: Production of carbon dioxide gas after reconstitution of cefamandole nafate, *J Pharm 36*:597 (May) 1979.

475. Bornstein M, Klink PR, Farrell BT, et al.: Stability of frozen solutions of cefamandole nafate, *Am J Hosp Pharm, 37*:98–101 (Jan) 1980.

476. Buckles J and Walters V: Stability of amitriptyline hydrochloride in aqueous solution, *J Clin Pharm 1*:107–112 (June) 1976.

477. Enever RP, Po ALW, Millard BJ, et al.: Decomposition of amitriptyline hydrochloride in aqueous solution: identification of decomposition products, *J Pharm Sci 64*:1497–1499 (Sep) 1975.

478. Enever RP, Po ALW, and Shotton E: Factors influencing decomposition rate of amitriptyline hydrochloride in aqueous solution, *J Pharm Sci 66*:1087–1089 (Aug) 1977.

479. Holman BL and Dewanjee MK: Potential pH incompatibility of pharmacological and isotopic adjuncts to arteriography, *Radiology 110*:722–723 (Mar) 1974.

480. Kawilarang CRT, Georghiou K, and Groves MJ: The effect of additives on the physical properties of a phospholipid-stabilized soybean oil emulsion, *J Clin Hosp Pharm 5*:151–160, 1980.

481. Anon: Stadol Q&A, Bristol Laboratories, Syracuse, New York, November 1978, p 7.

482. Jacobs RS: Calcitonin-Salmon, *Drug Intell Clin Pharm 9*:557–559 (Oct) 1975.

483. Honda DH, Jansen JR, Minor DR, et al.: Preprinted physician's order form for intravenous cisplatin therapy, *Am J Hosp Pharm 36*:742–743 (June) 1979.

484. Davignon JP, Yang KW, Wood HB, et al.: Formulation of three nitrosoureas for intravenous use, *Cancer Chemother Rep*, Part 3, *4*:7–11 (May) 1973.

485. Buckles J and Walters V: Stability of imipramine hydrochloride solutions, *J Clin Pharm 1*:113–118 (June) 1976.

486. Shand DG: Propranolol, *N Eng J Med 293*:280–285 (Aug 7) 1975.

487. Vidarabine monohydrate for infusion, *Fed Register 44*:1374 (Jan 5) 1979.

488. Lauper RD: Leucovorin calcium administration and preparation, *Am J Hosp Pharm 35*:377 (Apr) 1978.

489. Tavoloni N, Guarino AM, and Berk PD: Photolytic degradation of adriamycin, *J Pharm Pharmacol 32*:860–862, 1980.

490. Black CD and Popovich NG: Stability of intravenous fat emulsions, *Arch Surg 115*:891 (July) 1980.

491. Bacon L: A review of two safety factors in the use of paraldehyde, *J Royal Col Gen Pract 30*:622–624 (Oct) 1980.

492. Horton JK and Stevens MFG: Search for drug interactions between the antitumor agent DTIC and other cytotoxic agents, *J Pharm Pharmacol 31(Suppl)*:64P, 1979.

493. Anon: Monistat I.V. product monograph, Ortho Pharmaceutical Company, Raritan, New Jersey, October 1978.

494. Kuehnle C and Moore TD: Sodium chloride residue provides potential for drug incompatibilities, *Am J Hosp Pharm 36*:881 (July) 1979.

495. Trissel LA, Kleinman LM, Cradock JC, et al.: Investigational drug information—ifosfamide and semustine, *Drug Intell Clin Pharm 13*:340–343 (June) 1979.

496. Kohno M, Haneda I, Koyama Y, et al.: Basic studies on the stability of the high molecular weight antineoplastic agent neocarzinostatin. I. The stability of aqueous solutions of neocarzinostatin, *Japan J Antibiotics 27*:707–714 (6) 1974.

497. Dean TW and Baun DC: Preparation and standardization of nitroglycerin injection, *Am J Hosp Pharm 32*:1036–1038 (Oct) 1975.

498. Fung HL and Rhodes CT: Preparation of intravenous nitroglycerin solutions, *Am J Hosp Pharm 32*:139–140 (Feb) 1975.

499. Christensson B, Nordenfelt I, Westling H, et al.: Intravenous infusion of nitroglycerin in normal subjects, *Scand J Clin Lab Invest 23*:49–53, 1969.

500. Flaherty JT, Reid PR, Kelly DT, et al.: Intravenous nitroglycerin in acute myocardial infarction, *Circulation 51*:132–139 (Jan) 1975.

501. Kaplan JA and Treasure RL: Intravenous nitroglycerin during coronary artery surgery, *Mil Med 142*:152–153 (Feb) 1977.

502. Kaplan JA, Dunbar RW, and Jones EL: Nitroglycerin infusion during coronary-artery surgery, *Anesthesiology 45*:14–21 (July) 1976.

503. McNiff BL, McNiff EF, and Fung HL: Potency and stability of extemporaneous nitroglycerin infusions, *Am J Hosp Pharm 36*:173–177 (Feb) 1979.

504. Stach PE: Stability of nitroglycerin in aqueous solution, *Am J Hosp Pharm 30*:579 (July) 1973.

505. Cottrell JE and Turndorff H: Intravenous nitroglycerin, *Am Heart J 96*:550–553 (Oct) 1978.

506. Sturek JK, Sokolski TD, Winsley WT, et al.: Stability of nitroglycerin injection determined by gas chromatography, *Am J Hosp Pharm 35*:537–541 (May) 1978.

507. Fung HL: Potency and stability of extemporaneously prepared nitroglycerin intravenous solutions (editorial), *Am J Hosp Pharm 35*:528–529 (May) 1978.

508. Crouthamel WG, Dorsch B, and Shangraw R: Loss of nitroglycerin from plastic intravenous bags, *N Eng J Med 299*:262 (Aug 3) 1978.

509. Cossum PA, Galbraith AJ, Roberts MS, et al.: Loss of nitroglycerin from intravenous infusion sets, *Lancet 2*:349–350 (Aug 12) 1978.

510. Boylan JC, Robison RL, and Terrill PM: Stability of nitroglycerin solutions in Viaflex plastic containers, *Am J Hosp Pharm 35*:1031 (Sep) 1978.

511. Ludwig DJ and Ueda CT: Apparent stability of nitroglycerin in dextrose 5% in water, *Am J Hosp Pharm 35*:541–544 (May) 1978.

512. Brillaud AR: Interaction of Platinol (cisplatin) and the metal aluminum, Bristol Laboratories, Syracuse, New York, July 1979.

513. Product information, Intralipid 10% and 20%, Clintec Nutrition Company, Deerfield, Illinois, August 1991.

514. Product information, Liposyn II 10% and 20%, Abbott Laboratories, North Chicago, Illinois, August 1989.

515. Sewell DL and Golper TA: Stability of antimicrobial agents in peritoneal dialysate, *Antimicrob Agents Chemother 21*:528–529 (Mar) 1982.

516. El-Mallakh R: Incompatibilities with cimetidine hydrochloride injection, *Am J Hosp Pharm 36*:1024 (Aug) 1979.

517. Cutie MR: Letters, *Hosp Formul 15*:502–503 (June) 1980.

518. Tung EC, Gurwich EL, Sula JA, et al.: Stability of five antibiotics in plastic intravenous solution containers of dextrose and sodium chloride, *Drug Intell Clin Pharm 14*:848–850 (Dec) 1980.

519. Benvenuto JA, Anderson RW, Kerkof K, et al.: Stability and compatibility of antitumor agents in glass and plastic containers, *Am J Hosp Pharm 38*:1914–1918 (Dec) 1981.

520. Jhunjhunwala VP and Bhalla HL: Compatibility of mephentermine sulfate with hydrocortisone sodium succinate or aminophylline in 5% dextrose injection, *Am J Hosp Pharm 38*:1922–1924 (Dec) 1981.

521. Jhunjhunwala VP and Bhalla HL: Compatibility of aminophylline with hydrocortisone sodium succinate or dexamethasone sodium phosphate in 5% dextrose injection, *Am J Hosp Pharm 38*:900–901 (June) 1981.

522. Lee YC, Malick AW, Amann AH, et al.: Bretylium tosylate intravenous admixture compatibility. II. Dopamine, lidocaine, procainamide and nitroglycerin, *Am J Hosp Pharm 38*:183–187 (Feb) 1981.

523. Colvin M, Hartner J, and Summerfield M: Stability of carmustine in the presence of sodium bicarbonate, *Am J Hosp Pharm 37*:677–678 (May) 1980.

524. Dorr RT: Incompatibilities with parenteral anticancer drugs, *Am J IV Ther 6*:42, 45, 46, 52 (Feb–Mar) 1979.

525. Das Gupta V and Stewart KR: Stability of cefamandole nafate and cefoxitin sodium solutions, *Am J Hosp Pharm 38*:875–879 (June) 1981.

526. Poochikian GK, Cradock JC, and Flora KP: Stability of anthracycline antitumor agents in four infusion fluids, *Am J Hosp Pharm 38*:483–486 (Apr) 1981.

527. Newton DW, Fung EYY, and Williams DA: Stability of five catecholamines and terbutaline sulfate in 5% dextrose injection in the absence and presence of aminophylline, *Am J Hosp Pharm 38*:1314–1319 (Sep) 1981.

528. Neil JM: A rational approach to intravenous additives, *Proc Guild 7*:3–33 (Winter) 1979.

529. Otterman GE and Samuelson DW: Incompatibility between carbenicillin injection and promethazine injection, *Am J Hosp Pharm 36*:1156 (Sep) 1979.

530. Marshall TR, Ling IT, Follis G, et al.: Pharmacological incompatibility of contrast media with various drugs and agents, *Radiology 84*:536–539 (Mar) 1965.

531. Monder C: Stability of corticosteroids in aqueous solutions, *Endocrinology 82*:318–326 (Feb) 1968.

532. Kleinberg ML, Stauffer GL, Prior RB, et al.: Stability of antibiotics frozen and stored in disposable hypodermic syringes, *Am J Hosp Pharm 37*:1087–1088 (Aug) 1980.

533. Butler LD, Munson JM, and DeLuca PP: Effect of inline filtration on the potency of low-dose drugs, *Am J Hosp Pharm 37*:935–941 (July) 1980.

534. Allen LV and Stiles ML: Compatibility of various admixtures with secondary additives at Y-injection sites of intravenous administration sets. Part 2, *Am J Hosp Pharm 38*:380–381 (Mar) 1981.

535. Kleinberg, ML, Stauffer GL, and Latiolais CJ: Stability of five liquid drug products after unit dose repackaging, *Am J Hosp Pharm 37*:680–682 (May) 1980.

536. Kowaluk EA, Roberts MS, Blackburn HD, et al.: Interactions between drugs and polyvinyl chloride infusion bags, *Am J Hosp Pharm 38*:1308–1314 (Sep) 1981.

537. Zatz L, Sethia P, and Sherman NE: Stability of refrigerated aminophylline in 5% dextrose in water: a 96-hour study, *Hosp Pharm 16*:548 (Oct) 1981.

538. Scott KR, Bell AF, and Telang VG: Drug interactions I: Folic acid and calcium gluconate, *J Pharm Sci 69*:234 (Feb) 1980.

539. Jurgens RW, DeLuca PP, and Papadimitriou D: Compatibility of amphotericin B with certain large-volume parenterals, *Am J Hosp Pharm 38*:377–378 (Mar) 1981.

540. Gotz VP, Mar DD, and Roche JJ: Compatibility of amphotericin B with drugs used to reduce adverse reactions, *Am J Hosp Pharm 38*:378–379 (Mar) 1981.

541. Lee YC, Baaske DM, Amann AH, et al.: Bretylium tosylate intravenous admixture compatibility. I. Stability in common large-volume parenteral solutions, *Am J Hosp Pharm 37*:803–808 (June) 1980.

542. Yuhas EM, Lofton FT, Baldinus JG, et al.: Cimetidine hydrochloride compatibility with preoperative medications, *Am J Hosp Pharm 38*:1173–1174 (Aug) 1981.

543. Smith FM and Nuessle NO: Stability of lidocaine hydrochloride in 5% dextrose injection in plastic bags, *Am J Hosp Pharm 38*:1745–1747 (Nov) 1981.

544. Finch ME: Sodium thiopental in 5% dextrose in lactated Ringer's precipitate, *Hosp Pharm 14*:559–560 (Sep) 1979.

545. Kirschenbaum HL, Lesko LJ, Mendes RW, et al.: Stability of procainamide in 0.9% sodium chloride or dextrose 5% in water, *Am J Hosp Pharm 36*:1464–1465 (Nov) 1979.

546. Baaske DM, Malick AW, and Carter JE: Stability of procainamide hydrochloride in dextrose solutions, *Am J Hosp Pharm 37*:1050–1052 (Aug) 1980.

547. Jeglum EL, Winter E, and Kotos M: Nafcillin sodium incompatibility with acidic solutions, *Am J Hosp Pharm 38*:462, 464 (Apr) 1981.

548. Cutie MR and Lordi NG: Compatibility of verapamil hydrochloride injection in commonly used large-volume parenterals, *Am J Hosp Pharm 37*:675–676 (May) 1980.

549. Rosenberg HA, Dougherty JT, Mayron D, et al.: Cimetidine hydrochloride compatibility I: Chemical aspects and room temperature stability in intravenous infusion fluids, *Am J Hosp Pharm 37*:390–393 (Mar) 1980.

550. Yuhas EM, Lofton FT, Mayron D, et al.: Cimetidine hydrochloride compatibility II: Room temperature stability in intravenous infusion fluids, *Am J Hosp Pharm 38*:879–881 (June) 1981.

551. Yuhas EM, Lofton FT, Rosenberg HA, et al.: Cimetidine hydrochloride compatibility III: Room temperature stability in drug admixtures, *Am J Hosp Pharm 38*:1919–1922 (Dec) 1981.

552. Dahlin PA and Paredes SM: Visual compatibility of dobutamine with seven parenteral drug products, *Am J Hosp Pharm 37*:460, 464 (Apr) 1980.

553. Lesko LJ, Marion A, Ericson J, et al.: Stability of trimethoprim-sulfamethoxazole injection in two infusion fluids, *Am J Hosp Pharm 38*:1004–1006 (July) 1981.

554. Holmes CJ, Ausman RK, Walter CW, et al.: Activity of antibiotic admixtures subjected to different freeze-thaw treatments, *Drug Intell Clin Pharm 14*:353–357 (May) 1980.

555. Holmes CJ, Ausman RK, Kundsin RB, et al.: Effect of freezing and microwave thawing on the stability of six antibiotic admixtures in plastic bags, *Am J Hosp Pharm 39*:104–108 (Jan) 1982.

556. Boddapati S, Yang K, and Murty R: Physiochemical properties of aminophylline–dextrose injection admixtures, *Am J Hosp Pharm 39*:108–112 (Jan) 1982.

557. Canton EM and Baluch WM: Effect of freezing on particle formation in three antibiotic injections, *Am J Hosp Pharm 39*:124–125 (Jan) 1982.

558. Chaudry IA, Bruey KP, Hurlburt LE, et al.: Compatibility of netilmicin sulfate injection with commonly used intravenous injections and additives, *Am J Hosp Pharm 38*:1737–1742 (Nov) 1981.

559. Cutie MR: Effects of cold and freezing temperatures on pharmaceutical dosage forms, *US Pharmacist 4*:38–40, 48 (Oct) 1979.

560. Gove L, Walls ADF, and Scott W: Mixing parenteral nutrition products, *Pharm J 223*:587 (Dec 8) 1979.

561. Lauder AD: Mixing parenteral nutrition products, *Pharm J 223*:587 (Dec 8) 1979.

562. Hardin TC and Clibon U: Stability of 5-fluorouracil in a crystalline amino acid solution, *Am J IV Ther Clin Nutr 9*:39–40, 43 (Jan) 1982.

563. Yamaji A, Fujii Y, Kurata Y, et al.: Stability of pyridoxine hydrochloride in infusion solution under practical circumstances in wards, *Yakuzaigaku 40*:143–150 (Oct 20) 1980.

564. Dony J and Devleeschouwer MJ: Etude de la degradation photochimique de macrolides en presence de riboflavine, *J Pharm Belg 31*:479–484 (Sep–Oct) 1976.

565. Parker WA and Shearer CA: Metoclopramide compatibility, *Can J Hosp Pharm 32*:38 (Mar–Apr) 1979.

566. Parker WA: Compatibility of perphenazine and butorphanol admixtures, *Can J Hosp Pharm 33*:152 (Sep–Oct) 1980.

567. Stiles ML and Allen LV: Retention of drugs during inline filtration of parenteral solutions, *Infusion 3*:67–69 (May–June) 1979.

568. Somani P, Leathem WD, and Barlow AL: Safflower oil emulsion: single and multiple infusions with or without added heparin in normal human volunteers, *J Parenter Enter Nutr 4*:307–311 (May–June) 1980.

569. Giorgianni SJ (Scientific Information, Roerig Division, Pfizer Pharmaceuticals, New York, New York): Personal communication, March 27, 1980.

570. Moore RA, Feldman S, Treuting J, et al.: Cimetidine and parenteral nutrition, *J Parenter Enter Nutr 5*:61–63 (Jan–Feb) 1981.

571. Das Gupta V and Stewart KR: Stability of haloperidol in 5% dextrose injection, *Am J Hosp Pharm 39*:292–294 (Feb) 1982.

572. Cutie MR and Waranis R: Compatibility of hydromorphone hydrochloride in large-volume parenterals, *Am J Hosp Pharm 39*:307–308 (Feb) 1982.

573. Mirtallo JM, Caryer K, Schneider PJ, et al.: Growth of bacteria and fungi in parenteral nutrition solutions containing albumin, *Am J Hosp Pharm 38*:1907–1910 (Dec) 1981.

574. Holt HA, Broughall JM, McCarthy MM, et al.: Interactions between aminoglycoside antibiotics and carbenicillin or ticarcillin, *Infection 4*:107–109 (2) 1976.

575. Pickering LK and Gearhart P: Effect of time and concentration upon interaction between gentamicin, tobramycin, netilmicin, or amikacin and carbenicillin or ticarcillin, *Antimicrob Agents Chemother 15*:592–596 (Apr) 1979.

576. Pieper JA, Vidal RA, and Schentag JJ: Animal model distinguishing in vitro from in vivo carbenicillin–aminoglycoside interactions, *Antimicrob Agents Chemother 18*:604–609 (Oct) 1980.

577. Sturgeon RJ, Athanikar NK, Henry RS, et al.: Titratable acidities of crystalline amino acid admixtures, *Am J Hosp Pharm 37*:388–390 (Mar) 1980.

578. Ausman RK, Kerkhof K, Holmes CJ, et al.: Frozen storage and microwave thawing of parenteral nutrition solutions in plastic containers, *Drug Intell Clin Pharm 15*:440–443 (June) 1981.

579. Tortorici MP, Fearing D, Inman M, et al.: Photoreaction involving essential amino acid injection, *Am J Hosp Pharm 35*:1030 (Sep) 1978.

580. West KR, Sansom LN, Cosh DG, et al.: Some aspects of the stability of parenteral nutrition solutions, *Pharm Acta Helv 5*:19–22 (1–2) 1976.

581. Jurgens RW, Henry RS, and Welco A: Amino acid stability in a mixed

parenteral nutrition solution, *Am J Hosp Pharm* 38:1358–1359 (Sep) 1981.

582. Mirtallo JM, Rogers KR, Johnson JA, et al.: Stability of amino acids and the availability of acid in total parenteral nutrition solutions containing hydrochloric acid, *Am J Hosp Pharm* 38:1729–1731 (Nov) 1981.

583. Rusho WJ, Standish R, and Bair JN: A comparison of crystalline amino acid solutions for total parenteral nutrition, *Hosp Formul* 16:29–33 (Jan) 1981.

584. Shils ME, Burke AW, Greene HL, et al.: Guidelines for essential trace element preparations for parenteral use: A statement by an expert panel, *J Am Med Assoc* 241:2051–2054 (May 11) 1979.

585. Freund H, Atamian S, and Fischer JE: Chromium deficiency during total parenteral nutrition, *J Am Med Assoc* 241:496–498 (Feb 2) 1979.

586. Heller RM, Kirchner SG, O'Neill JA, et al.: Skeletal changes of copper deficiency in infants receiving prolonged total parenteral nutrition, *J Pediatr* 92:947–949 (June) 1978.

587. Moran DM, Russo J, and Bell LV: Zinc deficiency dermatitis accompanying parenteral nutrition supplemented with trace elements, *Clin Pharm* 1:169–176 (Mar–Apr) 1982.

588. Askari A, Long CL, and Blakemore WS: Zinc, copper and parenteral nutrition in cancer: a review, *J Parenter Enter Nutr* 4:561–571 (Nov–Dec) 1980.

589. Wolman SL, Anderson GH, Marliss EB, et al.: Zinc in total parenteral nutrition: requirements and metabolic effects, *Gastroenterology* 76:458–467 (Mar) 1979.

590. Fliss DM and Lamy PP: Trace elements and total parenteral nutrition, *Hosp Formul* 14:698–717 (July) 1979.

591. Schneider PJ: Total parenteral nutrition: Part II: What goes into parenteral nutrition solutions?, *J Postgrad Pharm (Hosp Ed)* 1:18–27 (Mar) 1979.

592. Isaacs JW, Millikan WJ, Stackhouse J, et al.: Parenteral nutrition of adults with a 900 milliosmolar solution via peripheral veins, *Am J Clin Nutr* 30:552–559 1977.

593. Romankiewicz JA, McManus J, Gotz VP, et al.: Medications not to be refrigerated, *Am J Hosp Pharm* 36:1541–1545 (Nov) 1979.

594. Swerling R: Dilution of oral and intravenous aminophylline preparations, *Am J Hosp Pharm* 38:1359–1360 (Sep) 1981.

595. Alcorn BT, Barnes SG, and du Plessis DJ: Pharmacy-initiated intravenous infusion guidelines, *Hosp Pharm* 17:60–76 (Feb) 1982.

596. Bowtle WJ, Heasman MJ, Prince AP, et al.: Compatibility of the cephalosporin, cefamandole nafate, with injections, *Int J Pharm* 4:263–265 (Jan) 1980.

597. Anon: I.V. dosage guidelines for theophylline products, *FDA Drug Bulletin* 10:4–5 (Feb) 1980.

598. Tipple M, Shadomy S, and Espinel-Ingroff A: Availability of active amphotericin B after filtration through membrane filters, *Am Rev Resp Dis* 115:879–881, 1977.

599. Maddux MS and Barriere SL: A review of complications of amphotericin B therapy: recommendations for prevention and management, *Drug Intell Clin Pharm* 14:177–181 (Mar) 1980.

600. Lufter CH and Ball WD: Activity of amphotericin B after filtration, *Drug Intell Clin Pharm* 14:719 (Oct) 1980.

601. Kuchinskas EJ and Levy GN: Comparative stabilities of ampicillin and hetacillin in aqueous solutions, *J Pharm Sci* 61:727–729 (May) 1972.

602. Schwartz MA and Hayton WL: Relative stability of hetacillin and ampicillin in solution, *J Pharm Sci* 61:906–909 (June) 1972.

603. Bundgaard H: Polymerization of penicillins: kinetics and mechanism of di- and polymerization of ampicillin in aqueous solution, *Acta Pharm Suec* 13:9–26, 1976.

604. Stjernstrom G, Olson OT, Nyqvist H, et al.: Studies on the stability and compatibility of drugs in infusion fluids 6. Factors affecting the stability of ampicillin, *Acta Pharm Suec* 15:33–50, 1978.

605. Johnson CA and Porter WA: Compatibility of azathioprine sodium with intravenous fluids, *Am J Hosp Pharm* 38:871–875 (June) 1981.

606. Kowaluk EA, Roberts MS, and Polack AE: Interactions between drugs and intravenous delivery systems, *Am J Hosp Pharm* 39:460–467 (Mar) 1982.

607. Bryan CK and Darby MH: Bretylium tosylate: a review, *Am J Hosp Pharm* 36:1189–1192 (Sep) 1979.

608. Henry RS, Jurgens RW, Sturgeon R, et al.: Compatibility of calcium chloride and calcium gluconate with sodium phosphate in a mixed TPN solution, *Am J Hosp Pharm* 37:673–674 (May) 1980.

609. Eggert LD, Rusho WJ, MacKay MW, et al.: Calcium and phosphorus compatibility in parenteral nutrition solutions for neonates, *Am J Hosp Pharm* 39:49–53 (Jan) 1982.

610. Robinson LA and Wright BT: Central venous catheter occlusion caused by body-heat-mediated calcium phosphate precipitation, *Am J Hosp Pharm* 39:120–121 (Jan) 1982.

611. Tuttle CB: Guidelines for phenytoin infusions, *Can J Hosp Pharm* 37:137–

139 (4) 1984.

612. Stewart P, Lourwood D, and Skolly S: Guidelines for the administration of a phenytoin loading dose via IVPB, *Hosp Pharm* 21:1003–1004 (Oct) 1986.

613. Goldschmied S: An evaluation of the stability and safety of phenytoin infusion, *NY State J Pharm* 7:45–47 (2) 1987.

614. Kradjan WA and Burger R: In vivo inactivation of gentamicin by carbenicillin and ticarcillin, *Arch Intern Med* 140:1668–1670 (Dec) 1980.

615. Young LS, Decker G, and Hewitt WL: Inactivation of gentamicin by carbenicillin in the urinary tract, *Chemotherapy* 20:212–220, 1974.

616. Henderson JL, Polk RE, and Kline BJ: In vitro inactivation of gentamicin, tobramycin, and netilmicin by carbenicillin, azlocillin, or mezlocillin, *Am J Hosp Pharm* 38:1167–1170 (Aug) 1981.

617. Flournoy DJ: Inactivation of netilmicin by carbenicillin, *Infection* 6:241 (5) 1978.

618. Russo ME: Penicillin–aminoglycoside inactivation: another possible mechanism of interaction, *Am J Hosp Pharm* 37:702–704 (May) 1980.

619. Laskar PA and Ayres JW: Degradation of carmustine in aqueous media, *J Pharm Sci* 66:1073–1076 (Aug) 1977.

620. Cardi V and Willcox GS: Reconstituting cefamandole and protecting from light, *Am J Hosp Pharm* 37:334 (Mar) 1980.

621. Kaiser GV, Gorman M, and Webber JA: Cefamandole—a review of chemistry and microbiology, *J Infect Dis* 137:S10–S16 (May) 1978.

622. Wold JS, Joost RR, Black HR, et al.: Hydrolysis of cefamandole nafate to cefamandole in vivo, *J Infect Dis* 137:S17–S24 (May) 1978.

623. Palmer MA and Fraterrigo CC: Clarification of "explosive-like" reaction occurring when reconstituted cefamandole nafate was stored in syringes, *Am J Hosp Pharm* 36:1025 (Aug) 1979.

624. Fites AL: Reconstituting cefamandole and protecting from light, *Am J Hosp Pharm* 37:334 (Mar) 1980.

625. Foster TS, Shrewsbury RP, and Coonrod JD: Bioavailability and pain study of cefamandole nafate, *J Clin Pharm* 20:526–533 (Aug–Sep) 1980.

626. Indelicato JM, Stewart BA, and Engel GL: Formylation of glucose by cefamandole nafate at alkaline pH, *J Pharm Sci* 69:1183–1188 (Oct) 1980.

627. Tomecko GW, Kleinberg ML, Latiolais CL, et al.: Stability of cefazolin sodium admixtures in plastic bags after thawing by microwave radiation, *Am J Hosp Pharm* 37:211–215 (Feb) 1980.

628. Janousek JP and Minisci MP: An evaluation of cefazolin sodium injection in an IV piggyback bottle, *Infusion* 2:67–73 (Mar–Apr) 1978.

629. Stiles ML: Effect of microwave radiation on the stability of frozen cefoxitin sodium solution in plastic bags, *Am J Hosp Pharm* 38:1743–1745 (Nov) 1981.

630. Oberholtzer ER and Brenner GS: Cefoxitin sodium: solution and solid state chemical stability studies, *J Pharm Sci* 68:863–866 (July) 1979.

631. Dreiman RK: Filtering cephalothin sodium i.v. piggyback doses, *Am J Hosp Pharm* 38:305–310 (Mar) 1981.

632. Walker SE, Paton TW, Fabian TM, et al.: Stability and sterility of cimetidine admixtures frozen in minibags, *Am J Hosp Pharm* 38:881–883 (June) 1981.

633. Cohen MR: Error 148—More on cisplatin storage, *Hosp Pharm* 15:158–159 (Mar) 1980.

634. LeRoy AF: Some quantitative data on cis-dichlorodiammineplatinum (II) species in solution, *Cancer Treat Rep* 63:231–233 (Feb) 1979.

635. Hincal AA, Long DF, and Repta AJ: Cis-platin stability in aqueous parenteral vehicles, *J Parenter Drug Assoc* 33:107–116 (May–June) 1979.

636. Mariani EP, Southard BJ, Woolever JT, et al.: Physical compatibility and chemical stability of cisplatin in various diluents and in large-volume parenteral solutions, *in* Cisplatin current status and new developments, Prestayko AW, Crooke ST, and Carter SK (eds), Academic Press, New York, New York, 1980, pp 305–316.

637. Repta AJ, Long DF, and Hincal AA: cis-Dichlorodiammineplatinum (II) stability in aqueous vehicles, *Cancer Treat Rep* 63:229–230 (Feb) 1979.

638. Gamble JAS, Dundee JW, and Assaf RAE: Plasma diazepam levels after single dose oral and intramuscular administration, *Anesthesia* 30:164–169, 1975.

639. Langdon DE, Harlan JR, and Bailey RL: Thrombophlebitis with diazepam used intravenously, *J Am Med Assoc* 223:184–185 (Jan 8) 1973.

640. Dam M and Christiansen J: Diazepam: intravenous infusion in the treatment of status epilepticus, *Acta Neurol Scandinav* 54:278–280, 1976.

641. Huber JW and Raymond GG: Additional conclusions on diazepam injectable precipitate: GC–MS confirmation, *Clin Toxicol* 14:439–444 (4) 1979.

642. Raymond G and Huber JW: Identification of injectable Valium precipitate, *Drug Intell Clin Pharm* 13:612 (Oct) 1979.

643. Newton DW, Driscoll DF, Goudreau JL, et al.: Solubility characteristics of diazepam in aqueous admixture solutions: theory and practice, *Am J Hosp Pharm* 38:179–182 (Feb) 1981.

644. Mason NA, Cline S, Hyneck ML, et al.: Factors affecting diazepam infu-

sion: solubility, administration-set composition, and flow rate, *Am J Hosp Pharm* 38:1449–1454 (Oct) 1981.

645. MacKichan J, Duffner PK, and Cohen ME: Adsorption of diazepam to plastic tubing, *N Eng J Med* 301:332–333 (Aug 9) 1979.

646. Parker WA and MacCara ME: Compatibility of diazepam with intravenous fluid containers and administration sets, *Am J Hosp Pharm* 37:496–500 (Apr) 1980.

647. Cloyd JC, Vezeau C, and Miller KW: Availability of diazepam from plastic containers, *Am J Hosp Pharm* 37:492–496 (Apr) 1980.

648. Cloyd JC: Diluting diazepam injection, *Am J Hosp Pharm* 38:32 (Jan) 1981.

649. Dasta JF, Brier K, and Schonfield S: Loss of diazepam to drug delivery systems, *Am J Hosp Pharm* 37:1176, 1178 (Sep) 1980.

650. Boatman JA and Johnson JB: A four-stage approach to new-drug development, *Pharm Tech* 5:46–56 (Jan) 1981.

651. Martin CM: Chemical incompatibility of Renografin 76 and protamine sulfate, *Am Heart J* 91:675–677 (May) 1976.

652. Hoffman DM, Grossano DD, Damin L, et al.: Stability of refrigerated and frozen solutions of doxorubicin hydrochloride, *Am J Hosp Pharm* 36:1536–1538 (Nov) 1979.

653. Gardiner WA: Possible incompatibility of doxorubicin hydrochloride with aluminum, *Am J Hosp Pharm* 38:1276 (Sep) 1981.

654. Pfaller MA, Granich GG, Valdes R, et al.: Comparative study of the ability of four aminoglycoside assay techniques to detect the inactivation of aminoglycosides by β-lactam antibiotics, *Diag Microbiol Infect Dis* 2:93–100, 1984.

655. Product information, Liposyn III 10% and 20%, Abbott Laboratories, North Chicago, Illinois, June 1989.

656. Black CD and Popovich NG: Study of intravenous emulsion compatibility: effects of dextrose, amino acids and selected electrolytes, *Drug Intell Clin Pharm* 15:184–193 (Mar) 1981.

657. Black CD and Popovich NG: Comment on intravenous emulsion compatibility, *Drug Intell Clin Pharm* 15:908–909 (Nov) 1981.

658. Pelham LD: Rational use of intravenous fat emulsions, *Am J Hosp Pharm* 38:198–208 (Feb) 1981.

659. Solussol C, et al: Long-term parenteral nutrition: an artificial gut, *Int Surg* 61:266–270, 1976.

660. Wretlind A: Current status of Intralipid and other fat emulsions, *in* Fat emulsion in parenteral nutrition, Meng HC and Wilmore DW (eds), American Medical Association, Chicago, Illinois, 1975, pp 109–119.

661. Higbee KC and Lamy PP: Use of Intralipid in neonates and infants, *Hosp Formul* 15:117–119, 122, 127 (Feb) 1980.

662. Kleinberg ML, Stauffer GL, and Latiolais CJ: Effect of microwave radiation on redissolving precipitated matter in fluorouracil injection, *Am J Hosp Pharm* 37:678–679 (May) 1980.

663. Driessen O, deVos D, and Timmermans PJA: Adsorption of fluorouracil on glass surfaces, *J Pharm Sci* 67:1494–1495 (Oct) 1978.

664. Ghanekar AG, Das Gupta V, and Gibbs CW: Stability of furosemide in aqueous systems, *J Pharm Sci* 67:808–811 (June) 1978.

665. McLaughlin JE and Reeves DS: Gentamicin plus carbenicillin, *Lancet* 1:864–865 (Apr 24) 1971.

666. Young LS, Decker G, and Hewitt WL: Inactivation of gentamicin by carbenicillin in the urinary tract, *Chemotherapy* 20:212–220, 1974.

667. Murillo J, Standiford HC, Schimpff SC, et al.: Gentamicin and ticarcillin serum levels, *J Amer Med Assoc* 241:2401–2403 (June 1) 1979.

668. Gomez-Perez F: Anticoagulant activity of two commercially available heparin preparations: a controlled study, *J Clin Pharm* 12:413–416 (Oct) 1972.

669. Bangham DR and Woodward PM: Collaborative study of heparins from different sources, *Bull WHO* 42:129–149, 1972.

670. Baltes BJ, Diamond S, and D'Agostino RJ: Comparison of anticoagulant activity of two preparations of purified heparin, *Clin Pharmacol Ther* 14:287–290 (2) 1973.

671. McMahon FG, Jain AK, Ryan JR, et al.: Anticoagulant potency of mucosal and lung heparin, *Clin Pharmacol Ther* 17:79–80 (1) 1975.

672. Jain AK, McMahon FG, and Ryan JR: Comparison of anticoagulant activity of three preparations of heparin, *Curr Ther Res* 22:427–432 (Sep) 1977.

673. Hoover RC and Binus MH: Types of heparin used in renal dialysis units, *Am J Hosp Pharm* 38:1516–1517 (Oct) 1981.

674. Anderson W, Harthill JE, Couper IA, et al.: Heparin stability in dextrose solutions, *J Pharm Pharmacol* 29:31P (Dec) 1977.

675. Bowie HM and Haylor V: Stability of heparin in sodium chloride solution, *J Clin Pharm* 3:211–214 (3) 1978.

676. Tunbridge LJ, Lloyd JV, Penhall RK, et al.: Stability of diluted heparin sodium stored in plastic syringes, *Am J Hosp Pharm* 38:1001–1004 (July) 1981.

677. Deeb EN and DiMattia PE: Standardization of heparin-lock maintenance

678. Holford NHG, Vozeh S, Coates P, et al.: More on heparin lock, *N Eng J Med* 296:1300–1301 (June 2) 1977.

679. Lynch CL, Linder GE, and Scheller JC: Frequently asked questions about insulin, *Hosp Pharm* 15:213–214 (Apr) 1980.

680. Graham DT and Pomeroy AR: Effects of freezing on commercial insulin suspensions, *Int J Pharm* 1:315–322, 1978.

681. Hill JB: Adsorption of insulin to glass, *Proc Soc Exp Biol Med* 102:75–77 (Oct) 1959.

682. Hill JB: The adsorption of I^{131}-insulin to glass, *Endocrinology* 65:515–517 (Sep) 1959.

683. Wiseman R and Baltz BE: Prevention of insulin-I^{131} adsorption to glass, *Endocrinology* 68:354–356 (Feb) 1961.

684. Sonksen PH, Ellis JP, Lowy C, et al.: Quantitative evaluation of the relative efficiency of gelatine and albumin in preventing insulin adsorption to glass, *Diabetologia* 1:208–210, 1965.

685. Suess V and Froesch ER: Zur therapie des coma diabeticum: quantitative bedeutung des insulinuerlusts am infusionsbesteck, *Schweizer Med Wochanschr* 105:1315–1318, 1975.

686. Okamoto H, Kikuchi T, and Tanizawa H: Adsorption of insulin to infusion bottles and plastic intravenous tubing, *Yakuzaigaku* 39:107–111 (July 30) 1979.

687. Wingert TD and Levin SR: Insulin adsorption to an air-eliminating inline filter, *Am J Hosp Pharm* 38:382–383 (Mar) 1981.

688. Hirsch JI, Wood JH, and Thomas RB: Insulin adsorption to polyolefin infusion bottles and polyvinyl chloride administration sets, *Am J Hosp Pharm* 38:995–997 (July) 1981.

689. Kerchner J, Cocaluca DM, and Juhl RP: Effect of whole blood on insulin adsorption onto intravenous infusion systems, *Am J Hosp Pharm* 37:1323–1325 (Oct) 1980.

690. Galloway JA and Bressler R: Insulin treatment in diabetes, *Med Clinics N Amer* 62:663–680 (July) 1978.

691. Sonksen P: Carrier solutions for low-level intravenous insulin infusion, *Br Med J* 1:151–152 (Jan 17) 1976.

692. Wan KK and Tsallas G: Dilute iron dextran formulation for addition to parenteral nutrient solutions, *Am J Hosp Pharm* 37:206–210 (Feb) 1980.

693. Bornstein M, Lo AY, Thomas PN, et al.: Moxalactam disodium compatibility with intramuscular and intravenous diluents, *Am J Hosp Pharm* 39:1495–1498 (Sep) 1982.

694. Kleinberg ML, Latiolais CJ, and Stauffer GL: Use of a microwave oven to redissolve crystallized mannitol injection (25%) in ampuls, *Hosp Pharm* 14:391–392 (July) 1979.

695. Hanson GG: Microwave oven explosion, *Hosp Pharm* 14:612 (Oct) 1979.

696. Kleinberg ML, Latiolais CJ, and Stauffer GL: Microwave oven explosion, *Hosp Pharm* 14:612 (Oct) 1979.

697. Kana MJ: Microwave oven explosion, *Hosp Pharm* 15:104 (Feb) 1980.

698. Post RE, Stephen SP, and McKinley JD: A warming cabinet for storing mannitol ampuls, *Hosp Pharm* 10:102–103 (Mar) 1975.

699. Scott KR, Bell AF, and Thomas AJ: Warming kettle for storing mannitol injection, *Am J Hosp Pharm* 37:16, 19, 22 (Jan) 1980.

700. Herring P: Keeping mannitol in solution, *Hosp Pharm* 15:530–531 (Oct) 1980.

701. Church JJ: Continuous narcotic infusions for relief of postoperative pain, *Br Med J* 1:977–979 (Apr 14) 1979.

702. Townsend RJ, Puchala AH, and Nail SL: Stability of methylprednisolone sodium succinate in small volumes of 5% dextrose and 0.9% sodium chloride injections, *Am J Hosp Pharm* 38:1319–1322 (Sep) 1981.

703. Knutsen CV, Epps DR, McCormick DC, et al.: Total nutrient admixture guidelines, *Drug Intell Clin Pharm* 18:253–254 (Mar) 1984.

704. Riggle MA, Brandt RB, and Mueller DG: Decomposition of TPN solutions, *J Pediatr* 100:670 (Apr) 1982.

705. Gralla RJ, Itri LM, Pisko SH, et al.: Antiemetic efficacy of high-dose metoclopramide: randomized trials with placebo and prochlorperazine in patients with chemotherapy-induced nausea and vomiting, *N Eng J Med* 305:905–909 (Oct 15) 1981.

706. Cohen MR: Hazard warning—Flagyl IV (metronidazole hydrochloride) product reconstitution, *Hosp Pharm* 16:398, 400 (July) 1981.

707. Little GB and Boylan JC: I.V. Flagyl reacts with aluminum, *Hosp Pharm* 16:627 (Nov) 1981.

708. Carmichael RR, Mahoney CD, and Jeffrey LP: Solubility and stability of phenytoin sodium when mixed with intravenous solutions, *Am J Hosp Pharm* 37:95–98 (Jan) 1980.

709. Salem RB, Yost RL, Torosian G, et al.: Investigation of the crystallization of phenytoin in normal saline, *Drug Intell Clin Pharm* 14:605–608 (Sep) 1980.

710. Pfeifle CE, Adler DS, and Gannaway WL: Phenytoin sodium solubility in three intravenous solutions, *Am J Hosp Pharm* 38:358–362 (Mar) 1981.

711. Wilensky AJ and Lowden JA: Inadequate serum levels after intramuscular administration of diphenylhydantoin, *Neurology* 23:318–324 (Mar) 1973.

712. Serrano EE, Roye DB, Hammer RH, et al.: Plasma diphenylhydantoin values after oral and intramuscular administration of diphenylhydantoin, *Neurology* 23:311–317 (Mar) 1973.

713. Newton DW and Kluza RB: Prediction of phenytoin solubility in intravenous admixtures: physicochemical theory, *Am J Hosp Pharm* 37:1647–1651 (Dec) 1980.

714. Cohen MR: Make sure your nurses mix drug additions to infusing I.V. solutions, *Hosp Pharm* 16:164 (Mar) 1981.

715. Schuna A, Nappi J, and Kolstad J: Potassium pooling in non-rigid parenteral fluid containers, *J Parenter Drug Assn* 33:184–186 (July–Aug) 1979.

716. McCloskey WW and Jeffrey LP: Rational ordering of phosphate supplements, *Hosp Pharm* 14:486–487 (Aug) 1979.

717. Herman JJ: Phosphate: its valence and methods of quantification in parenteral solutions, *Drug Intell Clin Pharm* 13:579–585 (Oct) 1979.

718. Benderev K: Hypophosphatemia and phosphorus supplementation, *Hosp Pharm* 15:611–613 (Dec) 1980.

719. Swerling R: Use and preparation of cardioplegic solutions in cardiac surgery, *Hosp Pharm* 15:497–503 (Oct) 1980.

720. Loucas SP, Mehl B, Maager P, et al.: Stability of procaine HCl in a buffered cardioplegia formulation, *Am J Hosp Pharm* 38:1924–1928 (Dec) 1981.

721. Amann AH, Baaske DM, and Wagenknecht DM: Plastic i.v. container for nitroglycerin, *Am J Hosp Pharm* 37:618 (May) 1980.

722. Cacace LG, Harralson A, and Clougherty T: Stability of NTG, *Am Heart J* 97:816–818 (June) 1979.

723. Yuen PH, Denman SL, Sokoloski TD, et al.: Loss of nitroglycerin from aqueous solution into plastic intravenous delivery systems, *J Pharm Sci* 68:1163–1166 (Sep) 1979.

724. Baaske DM, Amann AH, Wagenknecht DM, et al.: Nitroglycerin compatibility with intravenous fluid filters, containers, and administration sets, *Am J Hosp Pharm* 37:201–205 (Feb) 1980.

725. Roberts MS, Cossum PA, Galbraith AJ, et al.: Availability of nitroglycerin from parenteral solutions, *J Pharm Pharmacol* 32:237–244, 1980.

726. Christiansen H, Skobba TJ, Andersen R, et al.: Nitroglycerin infusion—factors influencing the concentration of nitroglycerin available to the patient, *J Clin Hosp Pharm* 5:209–215 (Sep) 1980.

727. Sokoloski TD, Wu CC, and Burkman AM: Rapid adsorptive loss of nitroglycerin from aqueous solution to plastic, *Int J Pharm* 6:63–76 (July) 1980.

728. Baaske DM, Amann AH, Karnatz NN, et al.: Administration set for use with intravenous nitroglycerin, *Am J Hosp Pharm* 39:121–122 (Jan) 1982.

729. Little LA and Hatheway GJ: Problems with administration devices for commercially available nitroglycerin injection, *Am J Hosp Pharm* 39:400 (Mar) 1982.

730. Schad RF and Jennings R: Problems with administration devices for commercially available nitroglycerin injection, *Am J Hosp Pharm* 39:400 (Mar) 1982.

731. Turco SJ: Problems with administration devices for commercially available nitroglycerin injection, *Am J Hosp Pharm* 39:977 (June) 1982.

732. Vesey CJ and Batistoni GA: Determination and stability of sodium nitroprusside in aqueous solutions (determination and stability of SNP), *J Clin Pharm* 2:105–117 (2) 1977.

733. Milewski B and Jones D: Photodecomposition, *Hosp Pharm* 16:178 (Mar) 1981.

734. Nolly RJ, Stach PE, Latiolais CJ, et al.: Stability of thiamine hydrochloride repackaged in disposable syringes, *Am J Hosp Pharm* 39:471–474 (Mar) 1982.

735. Polk RE and Kline BJ: Mail order tobramycin serum levels: low values caused by ticarcillin, *Am J Hosp Pharm* 37:920, 922 (July) 1980.

736. Seitz DJ, Archambault JR, Kresel JJ, et al.: Stability of tobramycin sulfate in plastic syringes, *Am J Hosp Pharm* 37:1614–1615 (Dec) 1980.

737. Levison ME, Knight R, and Kaye D: In vitro evaluation of tobramycin, a new aminoglycoside antibiotic, *Antimicrob Agents Chemother* 1:381–384 (May) 1972.

738. Svensson LA: Stressed oxidative degradation of terbutaline in aqueous solution, *Acta Pharm Suec* 9:141–146 (Apr) 1972.

739. Cutie MR: Compatibility of verapamil with other additives, *Am J Hosp Pharm* 38:231 (Feb) 1981.

740. Anon: Hospital formulary monograph—Pipracil, Lederle Laboratories, Wayne, New Jersey, November 1981.

741. Chan KK, Giannini DD, Staroscik JA, et al.: 5-Azacytidine hydrolysis kinetics measured by high-pressure liquid chromatography and ^{13}C-NMR spectroscopy, *J Pharm Sci* 68:807–812 (July) 1979.

742. Poochikian GK and Cradock JC: 2,5-Diaziridinyl-3,6-bis(carboethoxy amino)-1,4-benzoquinone I: Kinetics in aqueous solutions by high-performance liquid chromatography, *J Pharm Sci* 70:159–162 (Feb) 1981.

743. Flora KP, Smith SL, and Cradock JC: Application of a simple high-performance liquid chromatographic method for the determination of melphalan in the presence of its hydrolysis products, *J Chromatogr* 177:91–97, 1979.

744. Kohno M, Ishii F, Haneda I, et al.: Studies on the stability of the high molecular weight antineoplastic antibiotic neocarzinostatin. II. The stability of neocarzinostatin injection, *Jap J Antibiot* 27:715–724 (6) 1974.

745. Morris ME and Parker WA: Compatibility of chlordiazepoxide HCl injection following dilution, *Can J Pharm Sci* 16:43–45 (1) 1981.

746. Cummings DS, Park MK, and Howard AB: Compatibility of propranolol hydrochloride injection with intravenous infusion fluids in plastic containers, *Am J Hosp Pharm* 39:1685–1687 (Oct) 1982.

747. Deans KW, Lang JR, and Smith DE: Stability of trimethoprim-sulfamethoxazole injection in five infusion fluids, *Am J Hosp Pharm* 39:1681–1684 (Oct) 1982.

748. Munson JW, Kubiak EJ, and Cohon MS: Cytosine arabinoside stability in intravenous admixtures with sodium bicarbonate and in plastic syringes, *Drug Intell Clin Pharm* 16:765–767 (Oct) 1982.

749. Kirschenbaum HL, Aronoff W, Perentesis GP, et al.: Stability of dobutamine hydrochloride in selected large-volume parenterals, *Am J Hosp Pharm* 39:1923–1925 (Nov) 1982.

750. Ray JB, Newton DW, Nye MT, et al.: Droperidol stability in intravenous admixtures, *Am J Hosp Pharm* 40:94–97 (Jan) 1983.

751. Das Gupta V, Stewart KR, and Gunter JM: Stability of cefotaxime sodium and moxalactam disodium in 5% dextrose and 0.9% sodium chloride injections, *Am J IV Ther Clin Nutr* 10:20, 27–29 (Jan) 1983.

752. Jett S, Eng SS, and Milewski B: Prochlorperazine edisylate incompatibility, *Am J Hosp Pharm* 40:210 (Feb) 1983.

753. Porter WR, Johnson CA, Cohon MS, et al.: Compatibility and stability of clindamycin phosphate with intravenous fluids, *Am J Hosp Pharm* 40:91–94 (Jan) 1983.

754. Hittel WP, Iafrate RP, Karnes HT, et al.: Stability of pentobarbital sodium in 5% dextrose injection and 0.9% sodium chloride injection, *Am J Hosp Pharm* 40:294–296 (Feb) 1983.

755. Niemiec PW, Vanderveen TW, Hohenwarter MW, et al.: Stability of aminophylline injection in three parenteral nutrition solutions, *Am J Hosp Pharm* 40:428–432 (Mar) 1983.

756. Perentesis GP, Piltz GW, Kirschenbaum HL, et al.: Stability and visual compatibility of bretylium tosylate with selected large-volume parenterals and additives, *Am J Hosp Pharm* 40:1010–1012 (June) 1983.

757. Yuen PC, Taddei CR, Wyka BE, et al.: Compatibility and stability of labetalol hydrochloride in commonly used intravenous solutions, *Am J Hosp Pharm* 40:1007–1009 (June) 1983.

758. Pyter RA, Hsu LCC, and Buddenhagen JD: Stability of methylprednisolone sodium succinate in 5% dextrose and 0.9% sodium chloride injection, *Am J Hosp Pharm* 40:1329–1333 (Aug) 1983.

759. Gannon PM and Sesin GP: Stability of cytarabine following repackaging in plastic syringes and glass containers, *Am J IV Ther Clin Nutr* 10:11–16 (June) 1983.

760. Sesin GP, Millette LA, and Weiner B: Stability study of 5-fluorouracil following repackaging in plastic disposable syringes and multidose vials, *Am J IV Ther Clin Nutr* 9:23–25, 29–30 (Sep) 1982.

761. Parker WA: Compatibility of perphenazine and butorphanol admixtures, *Can J Hosp Pharm* 34:38 (Mar–Apr) 1981.

762. Jump WG, Plaza VM, and Poremba A: Compatibility of nalbuphine hydrochloride with other preoperative medications, *Am J Hosp Pharm* 39:841–843 (May) 1982.

763. Dorr RT, Peng YM, and Alberts DS: Bleomycin compatibility with selected intravenous medications, *J Med* 13:121–130 (1–2) 1982.

764. Cutie MR: Compatibility of verapamil hydrochloride injection with commonly used additives, *Am J Hosp Pharm* 40:1205–1207 (July) 1983.

765. Shively CD, Redford A, and Mancini A: Flagyl I.V., drug–drug physical compatibility, *Am J IV Ther Clin Nutr* 8:9–16 (Aug) 1981.

766. Souney PF, Steele L, and Polk BF: Effect of vitamin B complex and ascorbic acid on the antimicrobial activity of cefazolin sodium, *Am J Hosp Pharm* 39:840–841 (May) 1982.

767. Keller JH and Ensminger WD: Stability of cancer chemotherapeutic agents in a totally implanted drug delivery system, *Am J Hosp Pharm* 39:1321–1323 (Aug) 1982.

768. Rodanelli R, Comelli M, Pascale W, et al.: Clinical pharmacology of some antibiotics: problems relating to their intravenous use in hospitals, *Farmaco Ed Prat* 37:185–188 (June) 1982.

769. Kowaluk EA, Roberts MS, and Polack AE: Drug loss in polyolefin infusion systems, *Am J Hosp Pharm* 40:118–119 (Jan) 1983.

770. Illum L and Bundgaard H: Sorption of drugs by plastic infusion bags, *Int J Pharm* 10:339–351, 1982.

771. Anon: Vistaril IM, table of physical compatibilities, Pfizer Laboratories, New York, New York, July 1979.

772. Package insert, Neut, Abbott Laboratories, North Chicago, Illinois, October 1988.

773. Jhunjhuowala VP and Bhalla HL: Sodium ampicillin: its stability in some large volume parenteral solutions, *Indian J Hosp Pharm* 8:55–57 (Mar–Apr) 1981.

774. Scheiner JM, Araujo MM, and DeRitter E: Thiamine destruction by sodium bisulfite in infusion solutions, *Am J Hosp Pharm* 38:1911–1913 (Dec) 1981.

775. Kirschenbaum HL, Aronoff W, Perentesis GP, et al.: Stability and compatibility of lidocaine hydrochloride with selected large-volume parenterals and drug additives, *Am J Hosp Pharm* 39:1013–1015 (June) 1982.

776. Lackner TE, Baldus D, Butler CD, et al.: Lidocaine stability in cardioplegic solution stored in glass bottles and polyvinyl chloride bags, *Am J Hosp Pharm* 40:97–101 (Jan) 1983.

777. Armes DA, Townsend IR, and Pickering LK: Effect of temperature and time on the stability of mezlocillin in 5% dextrose injection and human serum, *Am J Hosp Pharm* 39:1536–1537 (Sep) 1982.

778. Shank WA and Coupal JJ: Stability of digoxin in common large-volume injections, *Am J Hosp Pharm* 39:844–846 (May) 1982.

779. Solomon DA and Nasinnyk KK: Compatibility of haloperidol lactate and heparin sodium, *Am J Hosp Pharm* 39:843–844 (May) 1982.

780. Elliott GT, McKenzie MW, Curry SH, et al.: Stability of cimetidine hydrochloride in admixtures after microwave thawing, *Am J Hosp Pharm* 40:1002–1006 (June) 1983.

781. Tsallas G and Allen LC: Stability of cimetidine hydrochloride in parenteral nutrition solutions, *Am J Hosp Pharm* 39:484–485 (Mar) 1982.

782. Roberts MS, Cossum PA, Kowaluk EA, et al.: Plastic syringes and intravenous infusions, *Med J Aust* 2:580–581 (Nov 28) 1981.

783. Das Gupta V and Stewart KR: Effect of tobramycin on the stability of carbenicillin disodium, *Am J Hosp Pharm* 40:1013–1016 (June) 1983.

784. Simmons A and Allwood MC: Sorption to plastic syringes of drugs administered by syringe pump, *J Clin Hosp Pharm* 6:71–73 (Mar) 1981.

785. Nicholas E, Hess G, and Colten HR: Degradation of penicillin, ticarcillin and carbenicillin resulting from storage of unit doses, *N Eng J Med* 306:547–548 (Mar 4) 1982.

786. Carpenter JP, Gomez EA, and Levin HJ: Administration of lorazepam injection through intravenous tubing, *Am J Hosp Pharm* 38:1514–1516 (Oct) 1981.

787. Newton DW, Narducci WA, Leet WA, et al.: Lorazepam solubility in and sorption from intravenous admixture solutions, *Am J Hosp Pharm* 40:424–427 (Mar) 1983.

788. Frable RA, Klink PR, Engel GL, et al.: Stability of cefamandole nafate injection with parenteral solutions and additives, *Am J Hosp Pharm* 39:622–627 (Apr) 1982.

789. Kirschenbaum HL, Aronoff W, Piltz GW, et al.: Compatibility and stability of dobutamine hydrochloride with large-volume parenterals and selected additives, *Am J Hosp Pharm* 40:1690–1691 (Oct) 1983.

790. Product information, Ivadantin, Norwich-Eaton Pharmaceuticals, Norwich, New York, June 1980.

791. Intralipid admixture manual, Cutter Medical, Berkeley, California, September 1982.

792. Roney JV (Scientific Services, Hoechst-Roussel Pharmaceuticals, Somerville, New Jersey): Personal communication, December 4, 1983.

793. Berge SM, Henderson NL, and Frank MJ: Kinetics and mechanism of degradation of cefotaxime sodium in aqueous solution, *J Pharm Sci* 72:59–63 (Jan) 1983.

794. Smith FM and Nuessle NO: Stability of diazepam injection repackaged in glass unit-dose syringes, *Am J Hosp Pharm* 39:1687–1690 (Oct) 1982.

795. Cossum PA and Roberts MS: Availability of isosorbide dinitrate, diazepam and chlormethiazole from I.V. delivery systems, *Eur J Clin Pharmacol* 19:181–185 (3) 1981.

796. Smith A and Bird G: Compatibility of diazepam with infusion fluids and their containers, *J Clin Hosp Pharm* 7:181–186 (Sep) 1982.

797. Yliruusi JK, Sothmann AG, Laine RH, et al.: Sorptive loss of diazepam and nitroglycerin from solutions to three types of containers, *Am J Hosp Pharm* 39:1018–1021 (June) 1982.

798. Kuhlman J, Abshagen U, and Rietbrock N: Cleavage of glycosidic bonds of digoxin and derivatives as function of pH and time, *Naunyn Schmiedebergs Arch Pharmacol* 276:149–156, 1973.

799. Gault MH, Charles JD, Sugden DL, et al.: Hydrolysis of digoxin by acid, *J Pharm Pharmacol* 29:27–32 (Jan) 1977.

800. Sternson LA and Shaffer RD: Kinetics of digoxin stability in aqueous solution, *J Pharm Sci* 67:327–330 (Mar) 1978.

801. Khalil SA and El-Masry S: Instability of digoxin in acid medium using a nonisotopic method, *J Pharm Sci* 67:1358–1360 (Oct) 1978.

802. Fagerman KE and Dean RE: Daily digoxin administration in parenteral nutrition solution, *Am J Hosp Pharm* 38:1955 (Dec) 1981.

803. Patterson MJ, Tjokrosetio R, and Hett KF: Stability of adrenaline injection BP following resterilization, *Aust J Hosp Pharm* 11:21–22 (Mar) 1981.

804. Nazeravich DR and Otlen NHH: Effect of inline filtration on delivery of gentamicin at a slow infusion rate, *Am J Hosp Pharm* 40:1961–1964 (Nov) 1983.

805. Zell M and Paone RP: Stability of insulin in plastic syringes, *Am J Hosp Pharm* 40:637–638 (Apr) 1983.

806. Benvenuto JA: Errors in oncolytic agent stability study, *Am J Hosp Pharm* 40:1628 (Oct) 1983.

807. Bisaillon S and Sarrazin R: Compatibility of several antibiotics or hydrocortisone when added to metronidazole solution for intravenous infusion, *J Parenter Sci Technol* 37:129–132 (July–Aug) 1983.

808. Gove L: Antibiotic interactions, *Pharm J* 231:233 (Sep 3) 1983.

809. Ennis CE, Merritt RJ, and Neff ON: In vitro study of inline filtration of medications commonly administered to pediatric cancer patients, *J Parenter Enter Nutr* 7:156–158 (Mar–Apr) 1983.

810. Buxton PC, Conduit SM, and Hathaway J: Stability of parentrovite in infusion fluids, *Br J IV Ther* 4:5, 12 (Jan) 1983.

811. Das Gupta V and Stewart KR: Stability of dobutamine hydrochloride and verapamil hydrochloride in 0.9% sodium chloride and 5% dextrose injections, *Am J Hosp Pharm* 41:686–689 (Apr) 1984.

812. Hasegawa GR and Eder JF: Visual compatibility of dobutamine hydrochloride with other injectable drugs, *Am J Hosp Pharm* 41:949–951 (May) 1984.

813. Souney PF, Colucci RD, Mariani G, et al.: Compatibility of magnesium sulfate solutions with various antibiotics during simulated Y-site injection, *Am J Hosp Pharm* 41:323–324 (Feb) 1984.

814. Lundergan FS, Lombardi TP, Neilan GE, et al.: Stability of tobramycin sulfate mixed with oxacillin sodium and nafcillin sodium in human serum, *Am J Hosp Pharm* 41:144–145 (Jan) 1981.

815. Parker WA: Physical compatibility update of preoperative medications, *Hosp Pharm* 19:475–478 (July) 1984.

816. Hale DC, Jenkins R, and Matsen JM: In-vitro inactivation of aminoglycoside antibiotics by piperacillin and carbenicillin, *Am J Clin Pathol* 74:316–319 (Sep) 1980.

817. Rank DM, Packer AM, and Tierney MG: In vitro inactivation of tobramycin by penicillins, *Am J Hosp Pharm* 41:1187–1188 (June) 1984.

818. Karlsen J, Thonnesen HH, Olsen IR, et al.: Stability of cytotoxic intravenous solutions subjected to freeze–thaw treatment, *Nor Pharm Acta* 45:61–67 (2) 1983.

819. Cheung YW, Vishnuvajjala BR, and Flora KP: Stability of cytarabine, methotrexate sodium, and hydrocortisone sodium succinate admixtures, *Am J Hosp Pharm* 41:1802–1806 (Sep) 1984.

820. Bundgaard H and Larsen C: Influence of carbohydrates and polyhydric alcohols on the stability of cephalosporins in aqueous solution, *Int J Pharm* 16:319–325 (Oct) 1983.

821. Hamilton G: Adverse reactions to intravenous pyelography contrast agents, *Can Med Assoc J* 129:405–406 (Sep 1) 1983.

822. Miller B and Pesko L: Effect of freezing on particulate matter concentrations in five antibiotic solutions, *Am J IV Ther Clin Nutr* 11:19–22 (Mar) 1984.

823. Wagman GH, Bailey JV, and Weinstein MJ: Binding of aminoglycoside antibiotics to filtration materials, *Antimicrob Agents Chemother* 7:316–319 (Mar) 1975.

824. Tindula RJ, Ambrose PJ, and Harralson AF: Aminoglycoside inactivation by penicillins and cephalosporins and its impact on drug-level monitoring, *Drug Intell Clin Pharm* 17:906–908 (Dec) 1983.

825. Gillies IR: Physical stability of Intralipid following drug addition, *Aust J Hosp Pharm* 10:118–120 (Sep) 1980.

826. Hardin TC, Clibon U, Page CP, et al.: Compatibility of 5-fluorouracil and total parenteral nutrition solutions, *J Parenter Enter Nutr* 6:163–165 (Mar–Apr) 1982.

827. Gaj E, Sesin GP, and Griffin RE: Evaluation of growth of five microorganisms in doxorubicin and floxuridine media, *Pharm Manufacturing* 1:50, 52–53 (Mar) 1984.

828. Gaj E and Griffin RE: Evaluation of growth of six microorganisms in fluorouracil, bacteriostatic sodium chloride 0.9% and sodium chloride 0.9% media, *Hosp Pharm* 18:348–349 (July) 1983.

829. Turco SJ: Drug adsorption to membrane filters, *Am J IV Ther Clin Nutr* 9:6,

9 (May) 1982.

830. Robinson WA and Krebs LU: The "real stuff" for intrathecal injection during leukaemia therapy, *Lancet 1*:283 (Jan 30) 1982.

831. Frear RS: Cefoperazone–aminoglycoside incompatibility, *Am J Hosp Pharm 40*:564 (Apr) 1983.

832. O'Bey KA, Jim LK, Gee JP, et al.: Temperature dependence of the stability of tobramycin mixed with penicillins in human serum, *Am J Hosp Pharm 39*:1005–1008 (June) 1982.

833. Bhatia J, Mims LC, and Roesel RA: Effect of phototherapy on amino acid solutions containing multivitamins, *J Pediatr 96*:284–286 (Feb) 1980.

834. Koshiro A and Fujita T: Interaction of penicillins with the components of plasma expanders, *Drug Intell Clin Pharm 17*:351–356 (May) 1983.

835. Szucsova S, Slana M, and Lehky M: Stability of infusion mixtures of 5% glucose solution with injection solutions, *Farm Obzor 52*:209–213 (May) 1983.

836. Gillis J, Jones G, and Pencharz P: Delivery of vitamin A, D, and E in total parenteral nutrition solutions, *J Parenter Enter Nutr 7*:11–14 (Jan–Feb) 1983.

837. Farago S: Compatibility of antibiotics and other drugs in total parenteral nutrition solutions, *Can J Hosp Pharm 36*:43–51 (2) 1983.

838. Gaj E and Sesin GP: Compatibility of doxorubicin hydrochloride and vinblastine sulfate—stability of a solution stored in Cormed reservoir bags or Monoject plastic syringes, *Am J IV Ther Clin Nutr 11*:8–9, 13–14, 19–20 (May) 1984.

839. Bar-Or D, Kulig K, Marx JA, et al.: Precipitation of verapamil, *Ann Intern Med 97*:619 (Oct) 1982.

840. Tucker R and Gentile JF: Precipitation of verapamil with nafcillin, *Am J Hosp Pharm 41*:2588 (Dec) 1984.

841. Hasegawa GR and Eder JF: Dobutamine–heparin mixture inadvisable, *Am J Hosp Pharm 41*:2588, 2590 (Dec) 1984.

842. Chen MF, Boyce HW, and Triplett L: Stability of B vitamins in mixed parenteral nutrition solution, *J Parenter Enter Nutr 7*:462–464 (Sep–Oct) 1983.

843. Bowman BB and Nguyen P: Stability of thiamine in parenteral nutrition solutions, *J Parenter Enter Nutr 7*:567–568 (Nov–Dec) 1983.

844. Newton DW: Physicochemical determinants of incompatibility and instability in injectable drug solutions and admixtures, *Am J Hosp Pharm 35*:1213–1222 (Oct) 1978.

845. Newton DW: Physicochemical determinants of incompatibility and instability of drugs for injection and infusion, *in* Trissel LA: Handbook on injectable drugs, 3rd ed, American Society of Hospital Pharmacists, Bethesda, Maryland, 1983, pp XI–XXI.

846. Raymond G, Day P, and Rabb M: Sodium content of commonly administered intravenous drugs, *Hosp Pharm 17*:560–561 (Oct) 1982.

847. Rich DS: Recent information about inactivation of aminoglycosides by carbenicillin and ticarcillin: clinical implications, *Hosp Pharm 18*:41–43 (Jan) 1983.

848. Lawrence RI, Flukes WK, Rust VJ, et al.: Total parenteral nutrition using a combined nutrient solution, *Aust J Hosp Pharm 11*:540–542 (4) 1981.

849. Davis SS and Galloway M: Total parenteral nutrition, *Pharm J 230*:6 (Jan 1 & 8) 1983.

850. Anon: 3-in-1 admixture guide from Travenol, Travenol Laboratories, November 1983.

851. Chan JCM, Malekzadeh M, and Hurley J: pH and titratable acidity of amino acid mixtures used in hyperalimentation, *J Am Med Assoc 220*:1119–1120 (May 22) 1972.

852. Kirk B and Sprake JM: Stability of aminophylline, *Br J IV Ther 3*:4, 6, 8 (Nov) 1982.

853. Vogenberg FR and Souney PF: Stability guidelines for routinely refrigerated drug products, *Am J Hosp Pharm 40*:101–102 (Jan) 1983.

854. Niemiec PW and Vanderveen TW: Compatibility considerations in parenteral nutrient solutions, *Am J Hosp Pharm 41*:893–911 (May) 1984.

855. Irving JD and Reynolds PV: Disposable syringe danger, *Lancet 1*:362 (Feb 12) 1966.

856. Salter F (Bristol Myers Squibb, Princeton, New Jersey): Personal communication, February 27, 1991.

857. Hopefl AW: Clinical use of intravenous acyclovir, *Drug Intell Clin Pharm 17*:623–628 (Sep) 1983.

858. Larsen C and Bundgaard H: Polymerization of penicillins VI. Time-course of formation of antigenic di- and polymerization products in aqueous ampicillin sodium solutions, *Arch Pharm Chemi Sci Ed 5*:201–209, 1977.

859. Carthy BJ and Hill GT: Some aspects of the analysis and stability of atracurium besylate, *Anal Proc 20*:177–179 (Apr) 1983.

860. D'Arcy PF: Comment on handling of anticancer drugs, *Drug Intell Clin Pharm 18*:417 (May) 1984.

861. Adams J, Wilson JP, and Solimando DA: Instability of bleomycin in plastic containers, *Am J Hosp Pharm 39*:1636 (Oct) 1982.

862. Levin VA, Zackheim HS, and Liu J: Stability of carmustine for topical application, *Arch Dermatol 118*:450–451 (July) 1982.

863. Chan KK and Zackheim HS: Stability of nitrosourea solutions, *Arch Dermatol 107*:298, 1973.

864. Teil SM, Arwood LL, and Visconti JA: Stability of gentamicin and cefamandole in serum, *Am J Hosp Pharm 39*:485–486 (Mar) 1982.

865. Portnoff JB, Henley MW, and Restaino FA: Development of sodium cefoxitin as a dosage form, *J Parenter Sci Technol 37*:180–185 (Sep–Oct) 1983.

866. Hilleman DE, McEvoy GK, Bailey RT, et al.: Stability of cephapirin sodium admixtures after freezing and conventional or microwave thaw techniques, *Hosp Pharm 19*:202, 207, 211–213 (Mar) 1984.

867. Wang YJ and Monkhouse DC: Solution stability of cephradine neutralized with arginine or sodium bicarbonate, *Am J Hosp Pharm 40*:432–434 (Mar) 1983.

868. Sorkin EM and Darvey DC: Review of cimetidine drug interactions, *Drug Intell Clin Pharm 17*:110–120 (Feb) 1983.

869. Raymond G and Day P: Multiple sources of sodium in injectable drugs, *Drug Intell Clin Pharm 16*:703 (Sep) 1982.

870. Eshaque M, McKay MJ, and Theophanides T: D-Mannitol platinum complexes, *Wadley Med Bull 7*:338–348 (1) 1977.

871. Ferguson DE: Degradation of clindamycin in frozen admixtures, *Am J Hosp Pharm 38*:1156 (July) 1982.

872. Ausman RK, Holmes CJ, Kundsin RB, et al.: Degradation of clindamycin in frozen admixtures, *Am J Hosp Pharm 39*:1156 (July) 1982.

873. Cairns CJ and Robertson J: Incompatibility of ceftazidime and vancomycin, *Pharm J 238*:577 (May 9) 1987.

874. Anon: Sandimmune—pharmacy fact sheet, Sandoz, East Hanover, New Jersey, November 1983.

875. Senholzi CS and Kerus MP: Crystal formation after reconstituting cefazolin sodium with 0.9% sodium chloride injection, *Am J Hosp Pharm 42*:129–130 (Jan) 1985.

876. Thompson DF, Allen LV, Desai SR, et al.: Compatibility of furosemide with aminoglycoside admixtures, *Am J Hosp Pharm 42*:116–119 (Jan) 1985.

877. Geary TG, Akood MA, and Jensen JB: Characteristics of chloroquine binding to glass and plastic, *Am J Trop Med Hyg 32*:19–23 (Jan) 1984.

878. Yayon A and Ginsburg A: A method for the measurement of chloroquin uptake in erythrocytes, *Anal Biochem 107*:332–336, 1980.

879. D'Arcy PF: Drug interactions with medical plastics, *Drug Intell Clin Pharm 17*:726–731 (Oct) 1983.

880. Kowaluk EA, Roberts MS, and Polack AE: Factors affecting the availability of diazepam stored in plastic bags and administered through intravenous sets, *Am J Hosp Pharm 40*:417–423 (Mar) 1983.

881. Kasahara K and Ruiz-Torres A: Einwirkung der verdauungssäfe auf die beständigkeit des digoxin-und digitoxin-moleküls, *Klin Wochenschr 47*:1109–1111, 1969.

882. Berman W, Whitman V, Marks KH, et al.: Inadvertent overadministration of digoxin to low-birth-weight infants, *J Pediatr 92*:1024–1025 (June) 1978.

883. Berman W, Dubynsky O, Whitman V, et al.: Digoxin therapy in low-birth-weight infants with patent ductus arteriosus, *J Pediatr 93*:652–655 (Oct) 1978.

884. Hajratwala BR: Stability of prostaglandins, *Aust J Pharm Sci NS5*:39–41 (June) 1975.

885. Roseman TJ, Sims B, and Stehle RG: Stability of prostaglandins, *Am J Hosp Pharm 30*:236–239 (Mar) 1973.

886. Gupta VD and Stewart KR: Stability of cefsulodin in aqueous buffered solutions and some intravenous admixtures, *J Clin Hosp Pharm 9*:21–27 (Jan) 1984.

887. Williamson MJ, Luce JK, and Hausmann WK: Doxorubicin hydrochloride–aluminum interaction, *Am J Hosp Pharm 40*:214 (Feb) 1983.

888. Chin TH (Professional Services, Miles Inc., West Haven, Connecticut): Personal communication, December 3, 1993.

889. Hausrani PK, Davis SS, and Groves J: Preparation and properties of sterile intravenous emulsions, *J Parenter Sci Technol 37*:145–150 (July–Aug) 1983.

890. Gray MS and Singleton WS: Creaming of phosphatide stabilized fat emulsions by electrolyte solutions, *J Pharm Sci 56*:1428–1431 (Nov) 1967.

891. Knutsen C, Miller P, and Kaminski MV: Compatibility, stability, and effect of mixing 10% fat emulsion in TPN solutions, *J Parenter Enter Nutr 5*:579 (Nov–Dec) 1981.

892. Burnham WR, Hansrani PK, Knott CE, et al.: Stability of a fat emulsion based intravenous feeding mixture, *Int J Pharm 13*:9–22 (Dec) 1983.

893. Hardin TC: Complex parenteral nutrition solutions: II. Addition of fat emul-

sions, *Nutr Supp Serv* 3:50–51 (May) 1983.

894. Quebbeman EJ, Hamid AAR, Hoffman NE, et al.: Stability of fluorouracil in plastic containers used for continuous infusion at home, *Am J Hosp Pharm* 41:1153–1156 (June) 1984.

895. Barker A, Hebron BS, Beck PR, et al.: Folic acid and total parenteral nutrition, *J Parenter Enter Nutr* 8:3–7 (Jan–Feb) 1984.

896. Louie N and Stennett DJ: Stability of folic acid in 25% dextrose, 3.5% amino acids, and multivitamin solutions, *J Parenter Enter Nutr* 8:421–426 (July–Aug) 1984.

897. Koshiro A, Oie S, Harima Y, et al.: Compatibility of gentamicin sulfate injection in parenteral solutions, *Jap J Hosp Pharm* 7:377–380 (6) 1982.

898. Godefroid RJ: Intravenous gentamicin dilution requirements, *Am J Hosp Pharm* 39:1457, 1459 (Sep) 1982.

899. Godefroid RJ: Comment on IV guidelines, *Drug Intell Clin Pharm* 18:925 (Nov) 1984.

900. Matthews H: Heparin anticoagulant activity in intravenous fluids utilising a chromagenic substrate assay method, *Aust J Hosp Pharm* 12:S17–S22 (June) 1982.

901. Turco SJ: Heparin locks, *Am J IV Ther Clin Nutr* 10:9, 12 (Jan) 1983.

902. Swerling R: Normal saline or dilute heparin for heparin lock flush? *Infusion* 6:123–124 (July–Aug) 1982.

903. Epperson EL: Efficacy of 0.9% sodium chloride injection with and without heparin for maintaining indwelling intermittent injection sites, *Clin Pharm* 3:626–629 (Nov–Dec) 1984.

904. Kanke M, Eubanks JL, and DeLuca PP: Binding of selected drugs to a "treated" inline filter, *Am J Hosp Pharm* 40:1323–1328 (Aug) 1983.

905. Anderson W and Harthill JE: Anticoagulant activity of heparins in dextrose solutions, *J Pharm Pharmacol* 34:90–96 (Feb) 1982.

906. Enderlin G: Discoloration of hydralazine injection, *Am J Hosp Pharm* 41:634 (Apr) 1984.

907. Pingel M and Volund A: Stability of insulin preparations, *Diabetes* 21:805–813 (July) 1972.

908. Weber SS and Wood WA: Insulin adsorption controversy, *Drug Intell Clin Pharm* 10:232–233 (Apr) 1976.

909. Schildt B, Ahlgren T, Berghem L, et al.: Adsorption of insulin by infusion materials, *Acta Anaesthesiol Scand* 22:556–562, 1978.

910. Mitrano FP and Newton DW: Factors affecting insulin adherence to type I glass bottles, *Am J Hosp Pharm* 39:1491–1495 (Sep) 1982.

911. Twardowski ZJ, Nolph KD, McGary TJ, et al.: Insulin binding to plastic bags: a methodologic study, *Am J Hosp Pharm* 40:575–579 (Apr) 1983.

912. Twardowski ZJ, Nolph KD, McGary TJ, et al.: Nature of insulin binding to plastic bags, *Am J Hosp Pharm* 40:579–582 (Apr) 1983.

913. Twardowski ZJ, Nolph KD, McGary TJ, et al.: Influence of temperature and time on insulin adsorption to plastic bags, *Am J Hosp Pharm* 40:583–586 (Apr) 1983.

914. Sato S, Ebert CD, and Kim SW: Prevention of insulin self-association and surface adsorption, *J Pharm Sci* 72:228–232 (Mar) 1983.

915. Phillips NC and Lauper RD: Review of etoposide, *Clin Pharm* 2:112–119 (Mar–Apr) 1983.

916. McCollam PL and Garrison TJ: Etoposide: A new chemotherapeutic agent, *Am J IV Ther Clin Nutr* 11:24, 27–28 (Mar) 1984.

917. Stroup JW and Mighton-Eryou LM: Expiry date guidelines for a centralized IV admixture service, *Can J Hosp Pharm* 39:57–59 (June) 1986.

918. Bishop BG: Adsorption of iron-dextran on membrane filters, *NZ Pharm* 1:49 (Mar) 1981.

919. Reed MD, Bertino JS, and Halpin TC: Use of intravenous iron dextran injection in children receiving total parenteral nutrition, *Am J Dis Child* 135:829–831 (Sep) 1981.

920. Halpin TC: Use of intravenous iron dextran in sick patients receiving TPN, *Nutr Supp Serv* 2:19–20 (Jan) 1982.

921. Shimada A: Adverse reactions to total-dose infusion of iron dextran, *Clin Pharm* 1:248–249 (May–June) 1982.

922. Thompson DF and Shimanek M: Stability of sterility study with magnesium sulfate admixtures, *Infusion* 7:83, 86 (May–June) 1983.

923. Ausman RK, Crevar GE, Hagedorn H, et al.: Studies in the pharmacodynamics of mechlorethamine and AB100, *J Am Med Assoc* 178:143–146 (Nov 18) 1961.

924. Anon: Compatibility chart for Reglan injectable 5 mg/ml, A.H. Robins Pharmaceutical Division, Richmond, Virginia, October 1983.

925. Das Gupta V: Stability of mezlocillin sodium as determined by high-performance liquid chromatography, *J Pharm Sci* 72:1479–1481 (Dec) 1983.

926. Feroz RM, Puppala S, Chaudhry MA, et al.: Compatibility of M.V.C. 9+3 (multivitamin concentrate for infusion) in different large volume parenteral solutions, LyphoMed, Inc., 1984.

927. Alam AS: Identification of labetalol precipitate, *Am J Hosp Pharm* 41:74 (Jan) 1984.

928. Wagenknecht DM, Baaske DM, Alam AS, et al.: Stability of nitroglycerin solutions in polyolefin and glass containers, *Am J Hosp Pharm* 41:1807–1811 (Sep) 1984.

929. Klamerus KJ, Ueda CT, and Newton DW: Stability of nitroglycerin in intravenous admixtures, *Am J Hosp Pharm* 41:303–305 (Feb) 1984.

930. Scheife AH, Grisafe JA, and Shargel L: Stability of intravenous nitroglycerin solutions, *J Pharm Sci* 71:55–59 (Jan) 1982.

931. Ingram JK and Miller JD: Plastic absorption adsorption of nitroglycerin solution, *Anesthesiology* 51:S132 (Sep) 1979.

932. Mathot F, Bonnard J, Hans P, et al.: Les perfusions de nitroglycerine: Etude de l'absorption par differents materiaux plastiques, *J Pharm Belg* 35:389–393 (Sep–Oct) 1980.

933. Sokoloski TD and Wu CC: Nitroglycerin stability: effects on bioavailability, assay and biological dissolution, *J Clin Hosp Pharm* 6:227–232 (Dec) 1981.

934. Cawello VW and Bonn R: Bioverfugbarkeitseinflusse durch die wahl des infusionsmaterials bei der therapie mit nitroglycerin, *Arzneim-Forsch* 33:595–597 (4) 1983.

935. Rock CM and Gull J: Reducing IV-nitroglycerin loss to an intravenous administration set by preliminary preparation, *Am J IV Ther Clin Nutr* 9:36, 40–42 (Oct) 1982.

936. Nix DE, Tharpe WN, and Francisco GE: Effects of presaturation on nitroglycerin delivery by polyvinyl chloride infusion sets, *Am J Hosp Pharm* 41:1835–1837 (Sep) 1984.

937. Jacobi J, Dasta JF, Reilley TE, et al.: Loss of nitroglycerin to pulmonary artery delivery systems, *Am J Hosp Pharm* 40:1980–1982 (Nov) 1983.

938. Jacobi J, Dasta JF, Wu LS, et al.: Loss of nitroglycerin to central venous pressure catheter, *Drug Intell Clin Pharm* 16:331–332 (Apr) 1982.

939. Dasta JF, Jacobi J, Sokolowski TD, et al.: Loss of nitroglycerin to cardiopulmonary bypass apparatus, *Crit Care Med* 11:50–52, 1983.

940. Dasta JF, Jacobi J, Sokoloski TD, et al.: Extraction of nitroglycerin by a membrane oxygenator, *J Extra-Corp Tech* 15:101–103 (4) 1983.

941. St. Peter JV and Cochran TG: Nitroglycerin loss from intravenous solutions administered with a volumetric infusion pump, *Am J Hosp Pharm* 39:1328–1330 (Aug) 1982.

942. Hola ET: Loss of nitroglycerin during microinfusion, *Am J Hosp Pharm* 41:142–144 (Jan) 1984.

943. Yacobi J, Amann AH, and Baaske DM: Pharmaceutical considerations of nitroglycerin, *Drug Intell Clin Pharm* 17:255–263 (Apr) 1983.

944. Malick AW, Amann AH, Baaske DM, et al.: Loss of nitroglycerin from solutions to intravenous plastic containers: a theoretical treatment, *J Pharm Sci* 70:798–800 (July) 1981.

945. Amann AH and Baaske DM: Loss of nitroglycerin from intravenous administration sets during infusion: a theoretical treatment, *J Pharm Sci* 71:473–474 (Apr) 1982.

946. Neftel KA, Walti M, Spengler H, et al.: Effect of storage of penicillin G solutions on sensitization to penicillin G after intravenous administration, *Lancet* 1:986–988 (May 1) 1982.

947. Salem RB, Wilder BJ, Yost RL, et al.: Rapid infusion of phenytoin sodium loading doses, *Am J Hosp Pharm* 38:354–357 (Mar) 1981.

948. Gannaway WL, Wilding DC, Siepler JK, et al.: Clinical use of intravenous phenytoin sodium infusions, *Clin Pharm* 2:135–138 (Mar–Apr) 1983.

949. Boike SC, Rybak MJ, Tintinalli JE, et al.: Evaluation of a method for intravenous phenytoin infusion, *Clin Pharm* 2:444–446 (Sep–Oct) 1983.

950. Earnest MP, Marx JA, and Drury LR: Complications of intravenous phenytoin for acute treatment of seizures, *J Am Med Assoc* 249:762–765 (Feb 11) 1983.

951. Giacona N, Bauman JL, and Siepler JK: Crystallization of three phenytoin preparations in intravenous solutions, *Am J Hosp Pharm* 39:630–634 (Apr) 1982.

952. Lau A, Lee M, Flascha S, et al.: Effect of piperacillin on tobramycin pharmacokinetics in patients with normal renal function, *Antimicrob Agents Chemother* 24:533–537 (Oct) 1983.

953. Autian J and Dhorda CN: Evaluation of disposable plastic syringes as to physical incompatibilities with parenteral products, *Am J Hosp Pharm* 16:176–179, 1959.

954. Addy DP, Alesbury P, and Winter L: Paraldehyde and plastic syringes, *Br Med J* 2:1434 (Nov 18) 1978.

955. Fenton-May VT and Lee F: Paraldehyde and plastic syringes, *Br Med J* 2:1166 (Oct 21) 1978.

956. Evans RJ: Effect of paraldehyde on disposable syringes and needles, *Lancet* 2:1451 (Dec 30) 1961.

957. Johnson CE and Vigoreaux JA: Compatibility of paraldehyde with plastic syringes and needle hubs, *Am J Hosp Pharm* 41:306–308 (Feb) 1984.

958. Mahony C, Brown JE, Starget WW, et al.: In vitro stability of sodium nitroprusside solutions for intravenous administration, *J Pharm Sci* 73:838–839 (June) 1984.

959. Fricker MP and Swerling R: Sodium nitroprusside reconstitution and administration, *Infusion* 5:56 (2–3) 1981.

960. Boehm JJ, Dutton DM, and Poust RI: Shelf life of unrefrigerated succinylcholine chloride injection, *Am J Hosp Pharm* 41:300–302 (Feb) 1984.

961. Roach M: IV tetracycline, *Pharm J* 220:143 (Feb 18) 1978.

962. Chow MSS, Qwintiliani R, and Nightingale CH: In vivo inactivation of tobramycin by ticarcillin, *J Am Med Assoc* 247:658–659 (Feb 5) 1982.

963. Baumgartner TG and Russell WL: Intravenous trimethoprim–sulfamethoxazole administration alert, *Am J IV Ther Clin Nutr* 10:14–15 (Feb) 1983.

964. Hiskey CF, Bullock E, and Whitman G: Spectrophotometric study of aqueous solutions of warfarin sodium, *J Pharm Sci* 51:43–46 (Jan) 1962.

965. Nahata MC: Stability of ceftriaxone sodium in intravenous solutions, *Am J Hosp Pharm* 40:2193–2194 (Dec) 1983.

966. Smith BR: Effect of storage temperature and time on stability of cefmenoxime, ceftriaxone, and cefotetan in 5% dextrose injection, *Am J Hosp Pharm* 40:1024–1025 (June) 1983.

967. Vishnuvajjala BR and Cradock JC: Compatibility of plastic infusion devices with diluted *N*-methylformamide and *N,N*-dimethylacetamide, *Am J Hosp Pharm* 41:1160–1163 (June) 1984.

968. Godefroid RJ: Vindesine: A new antineoplastic drug, *Cancer Chemother Update* 2:4–7 (Jan–Feb) 1984.

969. Cheung YW, Vishnuvajjala BR, Morris NL, et al.: Stability of azacitidine in infusion fluids, *Am J Hosp Pharm* 41:1156–1159 (June) 1984.

970. Bosanquet AG: Stability of melphalan solutions during preparation and storage, *J Pharm Sci* 74:348–351 (Mar) 1985.

971. Tabibi SE and Cradock JC: Stability of melphalan in infusion fluids, *Am J Hosp Pharm* 41:1380–1382 (July) 1984.

972. Teresi M and Allison J: Interaction between vancomycin and ticarcillin, *Am J Hosp Pharm* 42:2420, 2422 (Nov) 1985.

973. Jorgensen JH and Crawford SA: Selective inactivation of aminoglycosides by newer beta-lactam antibiotics, *Curr Ther Res Clin Exp* 32:25–35 (July) 1982.

974. Bhatia J, Stegink LD, and Zeigler EE: Riboflavin enhances photo-oxidation of amino acids under simulated clinical conditions, *J Parenter Enter Nutr* 7:277–279 (May–June) 1983.

975. Smith G, Hasson K, and Clements JA: Effects of ascorbic acid and disodium edetate on the stability of isoprenaline hydrochloride injection, *J Clin Hosp Pharm* 9:209–215 (Sep) 1984.

976. Hutchinson SMW: Heparin and aminoglycosides instability, *Drug Intell Clin Pharm* 20:886 (Nov) 1986.

977. Johnston-Early A, McKenzie MA, Krasnow SH, et al.: Drug trapping in intravenous infusion side arms, *J Am Med Assoc* 252:2392 (Nov 2) 1984.

978. Parker WA: Physical compatibility of ranitidine HCl with preoperative injectable medications, *Can J Hosp Pharm* 38:160–161 (Dec) 1985.

979. Das Gupta V, Stewart KR, and Torre MD: Chemical stabilities of cefamandole nafate and metronidazole when mixed together for intravenous infusion, *J Clin Hosp Pharm* 10:379–383 (Dec) 1985.

980. Cohen MH, Johnston-Early A, Hood MA, et al.: Drug precipitation within iv tubing: a potential hazard of chemotherapy administration, *Cancer Treat Rep* 69:1325–1326 (Nov) 1985.

981. Marble DA, Bosso JA, and Townsend RJ: Compatibility of clindamycin phosphate with amikacin sulfate at room temperature and with gentamicin sulfate and tobramycin sulfate under frozen conditions, *Drug Intell Clin Pharm* 20:960–963 (Dec) 1986.

982. Gove LF, Gordon NH, Miller J, et al.: Pre-filled syringes for self-administration of epidural opiates, *Pharm J* 234:378–379 (Mar 23) 1985.

983. Bosso JA and Townsend RJ: Stability of clindamycin phosphate and ceftizoxime sodium, cefoxitin sodium, cefamandole nafate, or cefazolin sodium in two intravenous solutions, *Am J Hosp Pharm* 42:2211–2214 (Oct) 1985.

984. Nahata MC and Durrell DE: Stability of tobramycin sulfate in admixtures with calcium gluconate, *Am J Hosp Pharm* 42:1987–1988 (Sep) 1985.

985. Baker DE, Yost GS, Craig VL, et al.: Compatibility of heparin sodium and morphine sulfate, *Am J Hosp Pharm* 42:1352–1355 (June) 1985.

986. Carlson GH and Matzke GR: Particle formation of third-generation cephalosporin injections, *Am J Hosp Pharm* 42:1578–1579 (July) 1985.

987. Nieves-Cordero AL, Luciw HM, and Souney PF: Compatibility of narcotic analgesic solutions with various antibiotics during simulated Y-site injection, *Am J Hosp Pharm* 42:1108–1109 (May) 1985.

988. Ogawa GS, Young R, and Munar M: Dispensing-pin problems, *Am J Hosp Pharm* 42:1042, 1045 (May) 1985.

989. Conklin CA, Kerege JF, and Christensen JM: Stability of an analgesic-sedative combination in glass and plastic single-dose syringes, *Am J Hosp Pharm* 42:339–342 (Feb) 1985.

990. Thompson M, Smith M, Gragg R, et al.: Stability of nitroglycerin and dobutamine in 5% dextrose and 0.9% sodium chloride injection, *Am J Hosp Pharm* 42:361–362 (Feb) 1985.

991. Rhodes RS, Rhodes PJ, and McCurdy HH: Stability of meperidine hydrochloride, promethazine hydrochloride, and atropine sulfate in plastic syringes, *Am J Hosp Pharm* 42:112–115 (Jan) 1985.

992. Kiel D, Connolly BJ, and Souney PF: Visual compatibility of amrinone lactate with various i.v. secondary additives, *Parenterals* 3:1, 5–6 (May–June) 1985.

993. Das Gupta V and Stewart KR: Chemical stabilities of hydrocortisone sodium succinate and several antibiotics when mixed with metronidazole injection for intravenous infusion, *J Parenter Sci Technol* 39:145–148 (May–June) 1985.

994. Foley PT, Bosso JA, Bair JN, et al.: Compatibility of clindamycin phosphate with cefotaxime sodium or netilmicin sulfate in small-volume admixtures, *Am J Hosp Pharm* 42:839–843 (Apr) 1985.

995. Mansur JM, Abramowitz PW, Lerner SA, et al.: Stability and cost analysis of clindamycin–gentamicin admixtures given every eight hours, *Am J Hosp Pharm* 42:332–335 (Feb) 1985.

996. Quock JR and Sakai RI: Stability of cytarabine in a parenteral nutrient solution, *Am J Hosp Pharm* 42:592–594 (Mar) 1985.

997. Walker SE and Bayliff CD: Stability of ranitidine hydrochloride in total parenteral nutrient solution, *Am J Hosp Pharm* 42:590–592 (Mar) 1985.

998. Baptista RJ, Palumbo JD, Tahan SR, et al.: Stability of cimetidine hydrochloride in a total nutrient admixture, *Am J Hosp Pharm* 42:2208–2210 (Oct) 1985.

999. Das Gupta V and Stewart KR: pH-Dependent effect of magnesium sulfate on the stability of penicillin G potassium solution, *Am J Hosp Pharm* 42:598–602 (Mar) 1985.

1000. Macias JM, Martin WJ, and Lloyd CW: Stability of morphine sulfate and meperidine hydrochloride in a parenteral nutrient formulation, *Am J Hosp Pharm* 42:1087–1094 (May) 1985.

1001. James MJ and Riley CM: Stability of intravenous admixtures of aztreonam and ampicillin, *Am J Hosp Pharm* 42:1095–1110 (May) 1985.

1002. James MJ and Riley CM: Stability of intravenous admixtures of aztreonam and clindamycin phosphate, *Am J Hosp Pharm* 42:1984–1986 (Sep) 1985.

1003. Thompson DF, Thompson GD, and Hedrick PJ: Effect of inline filtration on pediatric doses of gentamicin and tobramycin, *Infusion* 8:31–32 (Jan–Feb) 1984.

1004. Alexander SR and Arena R: Predicting calcium phosphate precipitation in premature infant parenteral nutrition solutions, *Hosp Pharm* 20:656–658 (Sep) 1985.

1005. Spruill WJ, McCall CY, and Francisco GE: In vitro inactivation of tobramycin by cephalosporins, *Am J Hosp Pharm* 42:2506–2509 (Nov) 1985.

1006. Stevenson JG and Patriarca C: Incompatibility of morphine sulfate and prochlorperazine edisylate in syringes, *Am J Hosp Pharm* 42:2651 (Dec) 1985.

1007. Beijnen JH, Rosing H, deVries PA, et al.: Stability of anthracycline antitumor agents in infusion fluids, *J Parenter Sci Technol* 39:220–222 (Nov–Dec) 1985.

1008. Baptista RJ and Lawrence RW: Compatibility of total nutrient admixtures and secondary antibiotic infusions, *Am J Hosp Pharm* 42:362–363 (Feb) 1985.

1009. Baptista RJ, Dumas GJ, Bistrian BR, et al.: Compatibility of total nutrient admixtures and secondary cardiovascular medications, *Am J Hosp Pharm* 42:777–778 (Apr) 1985.

1010. Bullock L, Parks RB, Lampasona V, et al.: Stability of ranitidine hydrochloride and amino acids in parenteral nutrient solutions, *Am J Hosp Pharm* 42:2683–2687 (Dec) 1985.

1011. Henann NE and Jacks TT: Compatibility and availability of sodium bicarbonate in total parenteral nutrient solutions, *Am J Hosp Pharm* 42:2718–2720 (Dec) 1985.

1012. Watson D: Piggyback compatibility of antibiotics with pediatric parenteral nutrition solutions, *J Parenter Enter Nutr* 9:220–224 (Mar–Apr) 1985.

1013. Turner SA: Stability and clinical use of intravenous admixtures containing lipid emulsion, *Pharm J* 234:799–800 (June 22) 1985.

1014. El Eini D and Knott CE: Stability of iv lipid emulsions, *Pharm J* 235:170 (Aug 10) 1985.

1015. Hobbiss JH: Stability of iv lipid emulsions, *Pharm J* 235:170 (Aug 10) 1985.

1016. Allwood MC: Drop size of infusions containing fat emulsion, *Br J Parenter Ther* 5:113–114, 116 (May) 1984.

1017. Iliano L, Delanghe M, van Den Baviere H, et al.: Effect of electrolytes in the presence of some trace elements on the stability of all-in-one emulsion mixtures for total parenteral nutrition, *J Clin Hosp Pharm* 9:87–93 (June) 1984.

1018. Whateley TL, Steele G, Urwin J, et al.: Particle size stability of Intralipid and mixed total parenteral nutrition mixtures, *J Clin Hosp Pharm* 9:113–126 (June) 1984.

1019. Harrie KR, Jacob M, McCormick D, et al.: Comparison of total nutrient admixture stability using two intravenous fat emulsions, Soyacal and Intralipid 20%, *J Parenter Enter Nutr* 10:381–387 (July–Aug) 1986.

1020. Riley CM and James MJ: Stability of intravenous admixtures containing aztreonam and cefazolin, *Am J Hosp Pharm* 43:925–927 (Apr) 1986.

1021. Kuhn RJ and Nahata MC: Stability of netilmicin sulfate in admixtures with calcium gluconate and aminophylline, *Am J Hosp Pharm* 43:1241–1242 (May) 1986.

1022. Johnson CE, Cohen IA, Craft DA, et al.: Compatibility of aminophylline and methylprednisolone sodium succinate intravenous admixtures, *Am J Hosp Pharm* 43:1482–1485 (June) 1986.

1023. Bell RG, Lipford LC, Massanari MJ, et al.: Stability of intravenous admixtures of aztreonam and cefoxitin, gentamicin, metronidazole, or tobramycin, *Am J Hosp Pharm* 43:1444–1453 (June) 1986.

1024. Fitzgerald KA and MacKay MW: Calcium and phosphate solubility in neonatal parenteral nutrient solutions containing TrophAmine, *Am J Hosp Pharm* 43:88–93 (Jan) 1986.

1025. Sayeed FA, Johnson HW, Sukumaran KB, et al.: Stability of Liposyn II fat emulsion in total nutrient admixtures, *Am J Hosp Pharm* 43:1230–1235 (May) 1986.

1026. Marble DA, Bosso JA, and Townsend RJ: Stability of clindamycin phosphate with aztreonam, ceftazidime sodium, ceftriaxone sodium, or piperacillin sodium in two intravenous solutions, *Am J Hosp Pharm* 43:1732–1736 (July) 1986.

1027. Lee MG: Sorption of four drugs to polyvinyl chloride and polybutadiene intravenous administration sets, *Am J Hosp Pharm* 43:1945–1950 (Aug) 1986.

1028. Riley CM and Lipford LC: Interaction of aztreonam with nafcillin in intravenous admixtures, *Am J Hosp Pharm* 43:2221–2224 (Sep) 1986.

1029. Walker PC, Kaufmann RE, and Massoud N: Compatibility of cefazolin and gentamicin in peritoneal dialysis solutions, *Drug Intell Clin Pharm* 20:697–700 (Sep) 1986.

1030. Beijnen JH, Neef C, Menwissen OJAT, et al.: Stability of intravenous admixtures of doxorubicin and vincristine, *Am J Hosp Pharm* 43:3022–3027 (Dec) 1986.

1031. Campbell S, Nolan PE, Bliss M, et al.: Stability of amiodarone hydrochloride in admixtures with other injectable drugs, *Am J Hosp Pharm* 43:917–921 (Apr) 1986.

1032. Hasegawa GR and Eder JF: Visual compatibility of amiodarone hydrochloride injection with other injectable drugs, *Am J Hosp Pharm* 41:1379–1380 (July) 1984.

1033. Allwood MC: Sorption of drugs to intravenous delivery systems, *Pharm Int* 4:83–85 (Apr) 1983.

1034. Khue NV and Jung L: Study of the retention of child-dose drugs on cellulose ester membranes during inline intravenous filtration, *S-T-P-Pharma* 1:201–207 (Mar) 1985.

1035. Das Gupta V, Shah KA, and de la Torre M: Stability of ampicillin sodium and penicillin G potassium solutions using high-pressure liquid chromatography, *Can J Pharm Sci* 16:61–65 (1) 1981.

1036. Janknegt R and Neil MJLE: De verenigbaarheid van antimicrobiele middelen in infusievloeistoffen, *Pharm Weekbl* 120:638–640 (Aug) 1985.

1037. Bouma J, Beijnen JH, Bult A, et al.: Anthracycline antitumor agents, a review of physicochemical, analytical and stability properties, *Pharm Weekbl Sci Ed* 8:109–133, 1986.

1038. Howard L, Chu R, Feman S, et al.: Vitamin A deficiency from long-term parenteral nutrition, *Ann Intern Med* 93:576–577 (Oct) 1980.

1039. Shenai JP, Stahlman MT, and Chytil F: Vitamin A delivery from parenteral alimentation solution, *J Pediatr* 99:661–663 (Oct) 1981.

1040. Kishi H, Yamaji A, Kataoka K, et al.: Vitamin A and E requirements during total parenteral nutrition, *J Parenter Enter Nutr* 5:420–423 (Sep–Oct) 1981.

1041. Knight P, Heer D, and Abdenour G: CaXP and Ca/P in the parenteral feeding of preterm infants, *J Parenter Enter Nutr* 7:110–114 (Mar–Apr) 1983.

1042. Poole RK, Rupp CA, and Kerner JA: Calcium and phosphorus in neonatal parenteral nutrition solutions, *J Parenter Enter Nutr* 7:358–360 (July–Aug) 1983.

1043. Ritschel WA, Alcorn GJ, Streng WH, et al.: Cimetidine–theophylline complex formation, *Methods Find Exp Clin Pharmacol* 5:55–58 (1) 1983.

1044. Glew RH and Pavuk RA: Stability of vancomycin and aminoglycoside antibiotics in peritoneal dialysis concentrate, *Nephron* 28:241–243, 1981.

1045. Kamen BA, Gunther N, Sowinsky N, et al.: Analysis of antibiotic stability in a parenteral nutrition solution, *Pediatr Infect Dis* 4:387–389 (July) 1985.

1046. Baumgartner TG, Sitren HS, Hall J, et al.: Stability of urokinase in parenteral nutrition solutions, *Nutr Supp Serv* 5:41–43 (Jan) 1985.

1047. Allwood MC: Influence of light on vitamin A degradation during administration, *Clin Nutr* 1:63–70, 1982.

1048. Allwood MC and Plane JH: Degradation of vitamin A exposed to ultraviolet radiation, *Int J Pharm* 19:207–213 (Apr) 1984.

1049. Riggle MA and Brandt RB: Decrease of available vitamin A in parenteral nutrition solutions, *J Parenter Enter Nutr* 10:388–392 (July–Aug) 1986.

1050. McKenna MC and Bieri JC: Loss of vitamin A from total parenteral nutrition (TPN) solutions, *Fed Proc* 39:561, 1980.

1051. Bryant CA and Neufeld NJ: Differences in vitamin A content of enteral feeding solutions following exposure to a polyvinyl chloride enteral feeding system, *J Parenter Enter Nutr* 6:403–405 (Sep–Oct) 1982.

1052. Riff LJ and Thomason JL: Comparative aminoglycoside inactivation by beta-lactam antibiotics—effect of cephalosporin and six penicillins on five aminoglycosides, *J Antibiot (Tokyo)* 35:850–857 (July) 1982.

1053. Schutz VH and Schroder F: Heparin–natrium kompatibilitat bei gleichzeitiger applikation anderer pharmaka, *Krankenhauspharmazie* 6:7–11 (Jan) 1985.

1054. Wermeling DP, Rapp RP, DeLuca PP, et al.: Osmolality of small-volume intravenous admixtures, *Am J Hosp Pharm* 42:1739–1744 (Aug) 1985.

1055. Johnston SJ: Stability of tryptophan in total parenteral nutrient solutions, *Am J Hosp Pharm* 43:1424 (June) 1986.

1056. Allwood MC: Factors influencing the stability of ascorbic acid in total parenteral nutrition solutions, *J Clin Hosp Pharm* 9:75–85 (June) 1984.

1057. Parr MD, Bertch KE, and Rapp RP: Amino acid stability and microbial growth in total parenteral nutrient solutions, *Am J Hosp Pharm* 42:2688–2691 (Dec) 1985.

1058. Nordfjeld K, Rasmussen M, and Jensen VG: Storage of mixtures for total parenteral nutrition: long-term stability of a total parenteral nutrition mixture, *J Clin Hosp Pharm* 8:265–274 (Sep) 1983.

1059. Nordfjeld K, Pedersen JL, Rasmussen M, et al.: Storage of mixtures for total parenteral nutrition III. Stability of vitamins in TPN mixtures, *J Clin Hosp Pharm* 9:293–301 (Dec) 1984.

1060. Das Gupta V: Stability of vitamins in total parenteral nutrient solutions, *Am J Hosp Pharm* 43:2132 (Sep) 1986.

1061. Allwood MC: Stability of vitamins in total parenteral nutrient solutions, *Am J Hosp Pharm* 43:2138 (Sep) 1986.

1062. Louie N: Stability of vitamins in total parenteral nutrient solutions, *Am J Hosp Pharm* 43:2138, 2143 (Sep) 1986.

1063. Shine B and Farwell JA: Stability and compatibility in parenteral nutrition solutions, *Br J Parenter Ther* 5:4, 44–46, 50 (Mar) 1984.

1064. Pamperl H and Kleinberger G: Stability of intravenous fat emulsions, *Arch Surg* 117:859–860 (June) 1982.

1065. Hardy G, Cotter R, and Dawe R: The stability and comparative clearance of TPN mixtures with lipid, in: *Advances in Clinical Nutrition—Selected Proceedings of the 2nd International Symposium*, Johnson ID (ed), MTP Press, Lancaster, England, 1983, pp 241–260.

1066. Hardy G and Klim RA: Stability studies of parenteral nutrition mixtures with lipids, *J Parenter Enter Nutr* 5:569 (Nov–Dec) 1981.

1067. Jeppsson RI and Sjoberg B: Compatibility of parenteral nutrition solutions when mixed in a plastic bag, *Clin Nutr* 2:149–158, 1984.

1068. Parry VA, Harrie KR, and McIntosh-Lowe NL: Effect of various nutrient ratios on the emulsion stability of total nutrient admixtures, *Am J Hosp Pharm* 43:3017–3022 (Dec) 1986.

1069. Bettner FS and Stennett DJ: Effects of pH, temperature, concentration, and time on particle counts in lipid-containing total parenteral nutrition admixtures, *J Parenter Enter Nutr* 10:375–380 (July–Aug) 1986.

1070. Schneider PJ: Three-in-one TPN formulations, *Infusion* 8:94–95, 101 (May–June) 1984.

1071. Ernst JA, Williams JM, Glick MR, et al.: Osmolality of substances used in the intensive care nursery, *Pediatrics* 72:347–352 (Sep) 1983.

1072. Connors KA, Amidon GL, and Stella VJ: *Chemical Stability of Pharmaceuticals, A Handbook for Pharmacists*, John Wiley & Sons, New York, 1986.

1073. Bosanquet AG: Stability of solutions of antineoplastic agents during preparation and storage for in vitro assays II. Assay methods, adriamycin and the other antitumor antibiotics, *Cancer Chemother Pharmacol* 17:1–10, 1986.

1074. Grant AM (Manager, Medical Affairs, Abbott Laboratories, Abbott Park, Illinois): Personal communication, March 23, 1987.

1075. Bornstein M and Templeton RJ: Crystal formation after reconstituting cefazolin sodium with 0.9% sodium chloride injection, *Am J Hosp Pharm* 42:2436 (Nov) 1985.

1076. Wong WW, Maderich AB, Polli GP, et al.: Stability of cefonicid sodium in infusion fluids, *Am J Hosp Pharm* 42:1980–1983 (Sep) 1985.

1077. Das Gupta V: Stability of cefotaxime sodium as determined by high-performance liquid chromatography, *J Pharm Sci* 73:565–567 (Apr) 1984.

1078. Carlson GH and Matzke GR: Particle formation of ceftizoxime sodium injections, *Am J Hosp Pharm* 42:2651–2652 (Dec) 1985.

1079. Swenson E, Gooch WM, and Higbee MD: Visual compatibility of ceftizoxime sodium in four electrolyte injections, *Am J Hosp Pharm* 43:2242–2244 (Sep) 1986.

1080. Barbero JR, Marino EL, and Dominguez-Gil A: Accelerated stability studies on Rocephin by high-efficiency liquid chromatography, *Int J Pharm* 19:199–206 (Apr) 1984.

1081. Smith RC: Overfill in cefuroxime sodium vials, *Am J Hosp Pharm* 42:1045–1046 (May) 1985.

1082. Smith RC: No more overfill in cefuroxime sodium vials, *Am J Hosp Pharm* 43:2154 (Sep) 1986.

1083. DeVane CL and Wailand LA: Stability of chlorpromazine in five milliliter vials, *Can J Hosp Pharm* 37:9 (1) 1984.

1084. Mu-Chow KJ and Baptista RJ: Cost-effectiveness of parenteral nutrient solutions containing cimetidine hydrochloride, *Am J Hosp Pharm* 41:1321, 1324 (July) 1984.

1085. Parasrampuria J, Das Gupta V, and Stewart KR: Stability of acetazolamide sodium in 5% dextrose or 0.9% sodium chloride injection, *Am J Hosp Pharm* 44:358–360 (Feb) 1987.

1086. Zuber DEL: Compatibility of morphine sulfate injection and prochlorperazine edisylate injection, *Am J Hosp Pharm* 44:67 (Jan) 1987.

1087. Cheung YW, Cradock JC, Vishnuvajjala BR, et al.: Stability of cisplatin, iproplatin, carboplatin, and tetraplatin in commonly used intravenous infusion solutions, *Am J Hosp Pharm* 44:124–130 (Jan) 1987.

1088. LaFollette JM, Arbus MH, and Lauper RD: Stability of cisplatin admixtures in polyvinyl chloride bags, *Am J Hosp Pharm* 42:2652 (Dec) 1985.

1089. Hussain AA, Haddadin M, and Iga K: Reaction of cis-platinum with sodium bisulfite, *J Pharm Sci* 69:364 (Mar) 1980.

1090. Kirk B, Melia CD, Wilson JV, et al.: Chemical stability of cyclophosphamide injection, *Br J Parenter Ther* 5:90–97 (May) 1984.

1091. Ptachcinski RJ, Logue LW, Burckart GJ, et al.: Stability and availability of cyclosporine in 5% dextrose injection or 0.9% sodium chloride injection, *Am J Hosp Pharm* 43:94–97 (Jan) 1986.

1092. Venkataramanan R, Burckart GJ, Ptachcinski RJ, et al.: Leaching of diethylhexyl phthalate from polyvinyl chloride bags into intravenous cyclosporine solution, *Am J Hosp Pharm* 43:2800–2802 (Nov) 1986.

1093. Stevens MFG and Peatey L: Photodegradation of solutions of the antitumor drug DTIC, *J Pharm Pharmacol* 30(Suppl):47P, 1978.

1094. Williams BA and Tritton TR: Photoinactivation of anthracyclines, *Photochem Photobiol* 34:131–134, 1981.

1095. Maloney TJ: Dilution of diazepam injection prior to intravenous administration, *Aust J Hosp Pharm* 13:79 (June) 1983.

1096. Hancock BG and Black CD: Effect of polyethylene-lined administration set on the availability of diazepam injection, *Am J Hosp Pharm* 42:335–339 (Feb) 1985.

1097. Yliruusi JK, Uotila JA, and Kristoffersson ER: Effect of tubing length on adsorption of diazepam to polyvinyl chloride administration sets, *Am J Hosp Pharm* 43:2789–2794 (Nov) 1986.

1098. Yliruusi JK, Uotila JA, and Kristoffersson ER: Effect of flow rate and type of i.v. container on adsorption of diazepam to i.v. administration systems, *Am J Hosp Pharm* 43:2795–2799 (Nov) 1986.

1099. Bell HE and Bertino JS: Constant diazepam infusion in the treatment of continuous seizure activity, *Drug Intell Clin Pharm* 18:965–970 (Dec) 1984.

1100. Dandurand KR and Stennett DJ: Stability of dopamine hydrochloride exposed to blue-light phototherapy, *Am J Hosp Pharm* 42:595–597 (Mar) 1985.

1101. Pluta PL and Morgan PK: Stability of erythromycin in intravenous admixtures, *Am J Hosp Pharm* 43:2732, 2738 (Nov) 1986.

1102. Deitel M, Faksa M, Kaminsky VM, et al.: Growth of microorganisms in soybean oil emulsion and clinical implications, *Int Surg* 64:27–32, 1979.

1103. Keammerer D, Mayhall CG, Hall GO, et al.: Microbial growth patterns in intravenous fat emulsions, *Am J Hosp Pharm* 40:1650–1653 (Oct) 1983.

1104. Kim CH, Lewis DE, and Kumar A: Bacterial and fungal growth in intravenous fat emulsions, *Am J Hosp Pharm* 40:2159–2161 (Dec) 1983.

1105. Allwood MC: Release of DEHP plasticizer into fat emulsion from iv administration sets, *Pharm J* 235:600 (Nov 2) 1985.

1106. Driscoll DF, Baptista RJ, Bistrian BR, et al.: Practical considerations regarding the use of total nutrient admixtures, *Am J Hosp Pharm* 43:416–419 (Feb) 1986.

1107. Morgan DE, Bergdale S, and Zeigler EE: Effect of syringe-pump position on infusion of fat emulsion with a primary solution, *Am J Hosp Pharm* 42:1110–1111 (May) 1985.

1108. Neil JM, Fell AF, and Smith G: Evaluation of the stability of frusemide in intravenous infusions by reversed-phase high-performance liquid chromatography, *Int J Pharm* 22:105–126 (Nov) 1984.

1109. Dean T and Ridley P: Use of 0.9% sodium chloride injection without heparin for maintaining indwelling intermittent injection sites, *Clin Pharm* 4:488 (Sep–Oct) 1985.

1110. Chantelau EA and Berger M: Pollution of insulin with silicone oil, a hazard of disposable plastic syringes, *Lancet* 1:1459 (June 22) 1985.

1111. Furberg H, Jensen AK, and Salbu B: Effect of pretreatment with 0.9% sodium chloride or insulin solutions on the delivery of insulin from an infusion system, *Am J Hosp Pharm* 43:2209–2213 (Sep) 1986.

1112. Kane M, Jay M, and DeLuca PP: Binding of insulin to a continuous ambulatory peritoneal dialysis system, *Am J Hosp Pharm* 43:81–88 (Jan) 1986.

1113. Hutchinson KG: Assessment of gelling in insulin solutions for infusion pumps, *J Pharm Pharmacol* 37:528–531, 1985.

1114. Kamerman B: Dissolving mannitol crystals, *Hosp Pharm* 20:360 (May) 1985.

1115. Cano SB and Glogiewicz FL: Storage requirements for metronidazole injection, *Am J Hosp Pharm* 43:2983, 2985 (Dec) 1986.

1116. Schell KH and Copland JR: Metronidazole hydrochloride–aluminum interaction, *Am J Hosp Pharm* 42:1040, 1042 (May) 1985.

1117. Struthers BJ and Parr RJ: Clarifying the metronidazole hydrochloride–aluminum interaction, *Am J Hosp Pharm* 42:2660 (Dec) 1985.

1118. Quebbeman EJ, Hoffman NE, Ausman RK, et al.: Stability of mitomycin admixtures, *Am J Hosp Pharm* 42:1750–1754 (Aug) 1985.

1119. Edwards D, Selkirk AB, and Taylor RB: Determination of the stability of mitomycin C by high-performance liquid chromatography, *Int J Pharm* 4:21–26, 1979.

1120. Young JB, Pratt CM, Farmer JA, et al.: Specialized delivery systems for intravenous nitroglycerin—are they necessary?, *Am J Med* 75:27–37 (June 22) 1984.

1121. Nix DE, Tharpe WN, and Francisco GE: Intravenous nitroglycerin delivery: dynamics and cost considerations, *Hosp Pharm* 20:230–232 (Apr) 1985.

1122. Schaber DE, Uden DL, and McCoy HG: Nitroglycerin adsorption to a combination polyvinyl chloride, polyethylene intravenous administration set, *Drug Intell Clin Pharm* 19:572–575 (July–Aug) 1985.

1123. Mendel S and Green JA: Comment: Nitroglycerin iv tubing adsorption, *Drug Intell Clin Pharm* 19:946–947 (Dec) 1985.

1124. Clarke AJ and Watkins RE: Nitroglycerin injection manufactured by a hospital pharmacy, *Am J Hosp Pharm* 42:1542–1546 (July) 1985.

1125. Rayani S and Fakhreddin J: Stability of penicillin G sodium in 5% dextrose in water minibags after freezing, *Can J Hosp Pharm* 38:162–163 (Dec) 1985.

1126. Das Gupta V, Davis DD, and Stewart KR: Stability of piperacillin sodium in dextrose 5% and sodium chloride 0.9% injections, *Am J IV Ther Clin Nutr* 11:14–15, 18–19 (Feb) 1984.

1127. Deardorff DL and Schmidt CN: Mixing additives by squeezing plastic bags, *Am J Hosp Pharm* 42:533–534 (Mar) 1985.

1128. Synave R, Vergote A, and Remon JP: Stability of procaine hydrochloride in a cardioplegic solution containing bicarbonate, *J Clin Hosp Pharm* 10:385–388 (Dec) 1985.

1129. Raymond G and DeGennaro M: Effect of Neut on the pH of some commercially available intravenous solutions, *Infusion* 9:144–146 (Sep–Oct) 1985.

1130. Sewell GJ, Forbes DR, and Munton TJ: Stability of sodium nitroprusside infusion during the administration by motorized syringe-pump, *J Clin Hosp Pharm* 10:351–360 (Dec) 1985.

1131. Baaske DM, Smith MD, Karnatz N, et al.: High-performance liquid chromatographic determination of sodium nitroprusside, *J Chromatogr* 212:339–346, 1981.

1132. Elenbaas JK, Lander RD, and Elenbaas RM: Effect of inline filtration on tobramycin delivery, *Drug Intell Clin Pharm* 19:122–125 (Feb) 1985.

1133. Mehta J, Searcy CJ, and Jung DT: Stability of terbutaline sulfate admixtures stored in polyvinyl chloride bags, *Am J Hosp Pharm* 43:1760–1762 (July) 1986.

1134. Das Gupta V, Stewart KR, and Nohria S: Stability of vancomycin hydrochloride in 5% dextrose and 0.9% sodium chloride injections, *Am J Hosp Pharm* 43:1729–1731 (July) 1986.

1135. Hopefl AW: Comment: Acyclovir iv, *Drug Intell Clin Pharm* 21:548–549 (June) 1987.

1136. Richardson BL, Woodford JD, and Andrews GD: Pharmacy of ceftazidime, *J Antimicrob Chemother* 8:233–236 (Suppl B) 1981.

1137. Cox ME, Roesner M, and McAllister JC: Production of carbon dioxide gas after reconstitution of ceftazidime, *Am J Hosp Pharm 43*:1422 (June) 1986.

1138. Fites AL: Production of carbon dioxide gas after reconstitution of ceftazidime, *Am J Hosp Pharm 43*:1422–1423 (June) 1986.

1139. Marwaha RK, Johnson BF, and Wright GE: Simple stability-indicating assay for histamine solutions, *Am J Hosp Pharm 42*:1568–1571 (July) 1985.

1140. Marwaha RK and Johnson BF: Long-term stability study of histamine in sterile bronchoprovocation solutions, *Am J Hosp Pharm 43*:380–383 (Feb) 1986.

1141. Bigley FP, Forsyth RJ, and Henley MW: Compatibility of imipenem–cilastatin sodium with commonly used intravenous solutions, *Am J Hosp Pharm 43*:2803–2809 (Nov) 1986.

1142. De NC, Alam AS, and Kapoor JN: Stability of pentamidine isethionate in 5% dextrose and 0.9% sodium chloride injections, *Am J Hosp Pharm 43*:1486–1488 (June) 1986.

1143. Lampasona V, Mullins RE, and Parks RB: Stability of ranitidine admixtures frozen and refrigerated in minibags, *Am J Hosp Pharm 43*:921–925 (Apr) 1986.

1144. Gralla RJ, Tyson LB, Kris MG, et al.: Management of chemotherapy-induced nausea and vomiting, *Med Clinics N Am 71*:289–301 (Mar) 1987.

1145. Forman JK and Souney PF: Visual compatibility of midazolam hydrochloride with common preoperative injectable medications, *Am J Hosp Pharm 44*:2298–2299 (Oct) 1987.

1146. Thompson DF and Thompson GD: Visual compatibility of esmolol hydrochloride and furosemide in 5% dextrose or 0.9% sodium chloride injections, *Am J Hosp Pharm 44*:2740 (Dec) 1987.

1147. Ahmed I and Day P: Stability of cefazolin sodium in various artificial tear solutions and aqueous vehicles, *Am J Hosp Pharm 44*:2287–2290 (Oct) 1987.

1148. McSherry TJ: Incompatibility between chlorpromazine and metacresol, *Am J Hosp Pharm 44*:1574 (July) 1987.

1149. Tebbett IR, Melrose E, and Reeves DE: Stability of promazine as an intravenous infusion, *Pharm J 237*:172, 174 (Aug 9) 1986.

1150. Johnson CE, Cohen IA, Michelini TJ, et al.: Compatibility of premixed theophylline and methylprednisolone sodium succinate intravenous admixtures, *Am J Hosp Pharm 44*:1620–1624 (July) 1987.

1151. Marti E and Cervera P: Compatibility of ranitidine hydrochloride with other injectable pharmaceuticals in common use, *Rev Assoc Esp Farm Hosp 9*:169–172 (Oct–Dec) 1985.

1152. Navarro JN, Aznar MT, Ruiz MD, et al.: Stability of 5-fluorouracil in large volume intravenous solutions, *Rev Assoc Esp Farm Hosp 9*:69–72 (Apr–June) 1985.

1153. Biondi L and Nairn JG: Stability of 5-fluorouracil and flucytosine in parenteral solutions, *Can J Hosp Pharm 39*:60–63, 66 (June) 1986.

1154. Parr MD, Barton SD, Haver VM, et al.: Cyclosporine binding to components in medication administration sets, *Drug Intell Clin Pharm 22*:173–174 (Feb) 1988.

1155. Gasca M, Fanikos J, and Souney PF: Visual compatibility of perphenazine with various antimicrobials during simulated Y-site injection, *Am J Hosp Pharm 44*:574–575 (Mar) 1987.

1156. Nolte MS, Poon V, Grodsky GM, et al.: Reduced solubility of short-acting soluble insulins when mixed with longer-acting insulins, *Diabetes 32*:1177–1181 (Dec) 1983.

1157. Forman JK, Lachs JR, and Souney PF: Visual compatibility of acyclovir sodium with commonly used intravenous drugs during simulated Y-site injection, *Am J Hosp Pharm 44*:1408–1409 (June) 1987.

1158. Nelson RW, Young R, and Lamnin M: Visual incompatibility of dacarbazine and heparin, *Am J Hosp Pharm 44*:2028 (Sep) 1987.

1159. Zbrozek AS, Marble DA, Bosso JA, et al.: Compatibility and stability of clindamycin phosphate–aminoglycoside combinations within polypropylene syringes, *Drug Intell Clin Pharm 21*:806–810 (Oct) 1987.

1160. Perry M, Khalidi N, and Sanders CA: Stability of penicillins in total parenteral nutrient solution, *Am J Hosp Pharm 44*:1625–1628 (July) 1987.

1161. Tu YH, Allen LV, and Wang DP: Stability of papaverine hydrochloride and phentolamine mesylate in injectable mixtures, *Am J Hosp Pharm 44*:2524–2527 (Nov) 1987.

1162. Seargeant LE, Kobrinsky NL, Sus CJ, et al.: In vitro stability and compatibility of daunorubicin, cytarabine, and etoposide, *Cancer Treat Rep 71*:1189–1192 (Dec) 1987.

1163. Baumgartner TG, Knudsen AK, Dunn AJ, et al.: Norepinephrine stability in saline solutions, *Hosp Pharm 23*:44, 49, 59 (Jan) 1988.

1164. Marble DA, Bosso JA, and Townsend RJ: Compatibility of clindamycin phosphate with aztreonam in polypropylene syringes and with cefoperazone sodium, cefonicid sodium, and cefuroxime sodium in partial-fill glass bottles, *Drug Intell Clin Pharm 22*:54–57 (Jan) 1988.

1165. Welty TE, Cloyd JC, and Abdel-Monem MM: Delivery of paraldehyde in

1166. 5% dextrose and 0.9% sodium chloride injections through polyvinyl chloride i.v. sets and burettes, *Am J Hosp Pharm 45*:131–135 (Jan) 1988.

1166. Thompson DF, Stiles ML, Allen LV, et al.: Compatibility of verapamil hydrochloride with penicillin admixtures during simulated Y-site injection, *Am J Hosp Pharm 45*:142–145 (Jan) 1988.

1167. Pesko LJ, Arend KA, Hagman DE, et al.: Physical compatibility and stability of metoclopramide injection, *Parenterals 5*:1–3, 6–8 (Dec–Jan) 1988.

1168. Karnatz NN, Wong J, Kesler H, et al.: Compatibility of esmolol hydrochloride with morphine sulfate and fentanyl citrate during simulated Y-site administration, *Am J Hosp Pharm 45*:368–371 (Feb) 1988.

1169. Colucci RD, Cobuzzi LE, and Halpern NA: Visual compatibility of esmolol hydrochloride and various injectable drugs during simulated Y-site injection, *Am J Hosp Pharm 45*:630–632 (Mar) 1988.

1170. Schilling CG: Compatibility of drugs with a heparin-containing neonatal total parenteral nutrient solution, *Am J Hosp Pharm 45*:313–314 (Feb) 1988.

1171. Colucci RD, Cobuzzi LE, and Halpern NA: Visual compatibility of labetalol hydrochloride injection with various injectable drugs during simulated Y-site injection, *Am J Hosp Pharm 45*:1357–1358 (June) 1988.

1172. Johnson CE, Lloyd CW, Aviles AI, et al.: Compatibility of premixed theophylline and verapamil intravenous admixtures, *Am J Hosp Pharm 45*:609–612 (Mar) 1988.

1173. Askerud L, Finholt P, and Karlsen J: Intravenous infusion of theophylline in 5% dextrose solution—formulation and stability, *Medd Nor Farm Selsk 43*:17–24, 1981.

1174. Morgan GJ, McClellan JD, and Hutton RD: Stability of a heparin urokinase mixture, *Br J Parenter Ther 8*:89 (May–June) 1987.

1175. Garren KW and Repta AJ: Incompatibility of cisplatin and Reglan injectable, *Int J Pharm 24*:91–99, 1985.

1176. Sanburg AL, Lyndon RC, and Sunderland B: Effects of freezing, long-term storage and microwave thawing on the stability of three antibiotics reconstituted in minibags, *Aust J Hosp Pharm 17*:31–34 (Mar) 1987.

1177. Murase S, Ochiai K, Aoki M, et al.: Study on compatibility of dopram with other drugs, *Jap J Hosp Pharm 13*:244–260 (Aug) 1987.

1178. Borst DL, Sesin GP, and Cersosimo RJ: Stability of selected beta-lactam antibiotics stored in plastic syringes, *NITA 10*:368–372 (Sep–Oct) 1987.

1179. Roberts DE, Cross MD, Thomas PH, et al.: Azlocillin–aminoglycoside combinations in CAPD fluid, *Br J Pharm Pract 9*:98–99 (Apr) 1987.

1180. Robinson DC, Cookson TL, and Grisafe JA: Concentration guidelines for parenteral antibiotics in fluid-restricted patients, *Drug Intell Clin Pharm 21*:985–989 (Dec) 1987.

1181. Sterchele JA: Update on stability guidelines for routinely refrigerated drug products, *Am J Hosp Pharm 44*:2698, 2701 (Dec) 1987.

1182. Dahl JM, Roche VF, and Hilleman DE: Visual compatibility of cibenzoline succinate with commonly used acute care medications, *Am J Hosp Pharm 44*:1123–1125 (May) 1987.

1183. Cano SM, Montoro JB, Pastor C, et al.: Stability of ranitidine hydrochloride in total nutrient admixtures, *Am J Hosp Pharm 45*:1100–1102 (May) 1988.

1184. Jimenez MD: Visual compatibility of nalbuphine hydrochloride and promethazine hydrochloride, *Am J Hosp Pharm 45*:1278 (June) 1988.

1185. Pereira-Rosario R, Utamura T, and Perrin JH: Interaction of heparin sodium and dopamine hydrochloride in admixtures studied by microcalorimetry, *Am J Hosp Pharm 45*:1350–1352 (June) 1988.

1186. Baptista RJ and Mitrano FP: Stability and compatibility of cimetidine hydrochloride and aminophylline in dextrose 5% in water injection, *Drug Intell Clin Pharm 22*:592–593 (July–Aug) 1988.

1187. Holmes CJ, Kubey WY, and Love DI: Viability of microorganisms in fluorouracil and cisplatin small-volume injections, *Am J Hosp Pharm 45*:1089–1091 (May) 1988.

1188. Jay GT, Fanikos J, and Souney PF: Visual compatibility of famotidine with commonly used critical-care medications during simulated Y-site injection, *Am J Hosp Pharm 45*:1556–1557 (July) 1988.

1189. Tucker DR and Sieradzan R: Visual compatibility of ciprofloxacin lactate with five broad-spectrum antimicrobial agents during simulated Y-site injection, *Am J Hosp Pharm 45*:1910–1911 (Sep) 1988.

1190. Marquardt ED: Visual compatibility of hydroxyzine hydrochloride with various antineoplastic agents, *Am J Hosp Pharm 45*:2127 (Oct) 1988.

1191. Riley CM: Stability of milrinone and digoxin, furosemide, procainamide hydrochloride, propranolol hydrochloride, quinidine gluconate, or verapamil hydrochloride in 5% dextrose injection, *Am J Hosp Pharm 45*:2079–2091 (Oct) 1988.

1192. Awang DVC and Graham KC: Microwave thawing of frozen drug solutions, *Am J Hosp Pharm 44*:2256 (Oct) 1987.

1193. Bashaw ED, Amantea MA, Minor JR, et al.: Visual compatibility of zidovudine with other injectable drugs during simulated Y-site administration, *Am J Hosp Pharm 45*:2532–2533 (Dec) 1988.

1194. Souney PF, Fanikos J, and Gasca M: Compatibility of cyclophosphamide solution with antibiotics during simulated Y-site injection, *Parenterals* 6:1, 2, 8 (Aug–Sep) 1988.

1195. Beijnen JH, Vendrig DEMM, and Underberg WJM: Stability of Vinca alkaloid anticancer drugs in three commonly used infusion fluids, *J Parenter Sci Technol* 43:84–87 (Mar–Apr) 1989.

1196. Fong PA and Ward J: Visual compatibility of intravenous famotidine with selected drugs, *Am J Hosp Pharm* 46:125–126 (Jan) 1989.

1197. Karnatz NN, Wong J, Baaske DM, et al.: Stability of esmolol hydrochloride and sodium nitroprusside in intravenous admixtures, *Am J Hosp Pharm* 46:101–104 (Jan) 1989.

1198. Johnson CE, Lloyd CW, Mesaros JL, et al.: Compatibility of aminophylline and verapamil in intravenous admixtures, *Am J Hosp Pharm* 46:97–100 (Jan) 1989.

1199. Parti R and Wolf W: Caveats with respect to storage of cisplatin and flurouracil admixtures, *Am J Hosp Pharm* 46:259 (Feb) 1989.

1200. Johnson EG and Janosik JE: Manufacturer's recommendations for handling spilled antineoplastic agents, *Am J Hosp Pharm* 46:318–319 (Feb) 1989.

1201. Jarosinski PF, Kennedy PF, and Gallelli JF: Stability of concentrated trimethoprim–sulfamethoxazole admixtures, *Am J Hosp Pharm* 46:732–737 (Apr) 1989.

1202. Bosanquet AG: Stability of solutions of antineoplastic agents during preparation and storage for in vitro assays III. Antimetabolites, tubulin-binding agents, platinum drugs, amsacrine, L-asparaginase, interferons, steroids and other miscellaneous antitumor agents, *Cancer Chemother Pharmacol* 23:197–207, 1989.

1203. Beijnen JH and Underberg WJM: Degradation of mitomycin C in acidic solution, *Int J Pharm* 24:219–229, 1985.

1204. Beijnen JH, den Hartigh J, and Underberg WJM: Quantitative aspects of the degradation of mitomycin C in alkaline solution, *J Pharm Biomed Anal* 3:59–69, 1985.

1205. Beijnen JH, Rosing H, and Underberg WJM: Stability of mitomycins in infusion fluids, *Arch Pharm Chemi Sci Ed* 13:58–66, 1985.

1206. Janssen MJH, Crommelin DJA, Storm G, et al.: Doxorubicin decomposition on storage. Effect of pH, type of buffer and liposome encapsulation, *Int J Pharm* 23:1–11, 1985.

1207. Beijnen JH, van der Houwen OAGJ, Voskuilen MCH, et al.: Aspects of the degradation kinetics of daunorubicin in aqueous solution, in: Chemical stability of mitomycin and anthracycline antineoplastic drugs, Beijnen JH (ed), Drukkerij Elkinkwijk BV, Utrecht, The Netherlands, 1986, pp 245–260.

1208. Beijnen JH, van der Houwen OAGJ, and Underberg WJM: Aspects of the degradation kinetics of doxorubicin in aqueous solution, *Int J Pharm* 32:123–131, 1986.

1209. Fritz BL, Lockhart HE, and Giacin JR: Chemical stability of selected pharmaceuticals repackaged in glass and plastic, *Pharm Tech* 12:44, 46, 48, 50–52 (Nov) 1988.

1210. Venkataraman PS, Brissie EO, and Tsang RC: Stability of calcium and phosphorus in neonatal parenteral nutrition solutions, *J Pediatr Gastroenterol Nutr* 2:640–643 (4) 1983.

1211. Fitzgerald KA and MacKay MW: Calcium and phosphate solubility in neonatal parenteral nutrient solutions containing Aminosyn PF, *Am J Hosp Pharm* 44:1396–1400 (June) 1987.

1212. Mikrut BA: Calcium and phosphate solubility in neonatal parenteral nutrient solutions containing Aminosyn PF or TrophAmine, *Am J Hosp Pharm* 44:2702–2704 (Dec) 1987.

1213. Lenz GT and Mikrut BA: Calcium and phosphate solubility in neonatal parenteral nutrient solutions containing Aminosyn-PF or TrophAmine, *Am J Hosp Pharm* 45:2367–2371 (Nov) 1988.

1214. Raupp P, von Kries R, Schmidt E, et al.: Incompatibility between fat emulsion and calcium plus heparin in parenteral nutrition of premature babies, *Lancet* 1:700 (Mar 26) 1988.

1215. Waller DJ and Smith SR: Use of infusion devices with total nutrient admixtures, *Am J Hosp Pharm* 44:1570, 1574 (July) 1987.

1216. Gilbert M, Gallagher SC, Eads M, et al.: Microbial growth patterns in a total parenteral nutrition formulation containing lipid emulsion, *J Parenter Enter Nutr* 10:494–497 (Sep–Oct) 1986.

1217. Barat AC, Harrie K, Jacob M, et al.: Effect of amino acid solutions on total nutrient admixture stability, *J Parenter Enter Nutr* 11:384–388 (July–Aug) 1987.

1218. Cripps AL: Stability studies on total parenteral nutrition mixtures containing fat emulsions, *Br J Pharm Pract* 6:187–195 (June) 1984.

1219. Davis SS and Galloway M: Studies on fat emulsions in combined nutrition solutions, *J Clin Hosp Pharm* 11:33–45 (Feb) 1986.

1220. Ang SD, Canham JE, and Daly JM: Parenteral infusion with an admixture of amino acids, dextrose, fat emulsion solution: compatibility and clinical safety, *J Parenter Enter Nutr* 11:23–27 (Jan–Feb) 1987.

1221. du Plessis J, Van Wyk CJ, and Ackermann C: The stability of parenteral fat emulsions in nutrition admixtures, *J Clin Pharm Ther* 12:307–318 (Oct) 1987.

1222. Sayeed FA, Tripp MG, Sukumaran KB, et al.: Stability of total nutrient admixtures using various intravenous fat emulsions, *Am J Hosp Pharm* 44:2271–2280 (Oct) 1987.

1223. Sayeed FA, Tripp MG, Sukumaran KB, et al.: Stability of various total nutrient admixture formulations using Liposyn II and Aminosyn II, *Am J Hosp Pharm* 44:2280–2286 (Oct) 1987.

1224. McGee CD, Mascarenhas MG, Ostro MJ, et al.: Selenium and vitamin E stability in parenteral solutions, *J Parenter Enter Nutr* 9:568–570 (Sep–Oct) 1985.

1225. Dahl GB, Jeppsson RI, and Tengborn HJ: Vitamin stability in a TPN mixture stored in an EVA plastic bag, *J Clin Hosp Pharm* 11:271–279 (Aug) 1986.

1226. Shenkin A, Fraser WD, McLelland AJD, et al.: Maintenance of vitamin and trace element status in intravenous nutrition using a complete nutritive mixture, *J Parenter Enter Nutr* 11:238–242 (May–June) 1987.

1227. Yamaoka K, Nakajima Y, Okinaga S, et al.: Variation by combination of hyperalimentation with fat emulsion, *Jap J Hosp Pharm* 13:211–215 (Aug) 1987.

1228. Sewell DL, Golper TA, Brown SD, et al.: Stability of single and combination antimicrobial agents in various peritoneal dialysates in the presence of insulin and heparin, *Am J Kidney Dis* 111:209–212 (Nov) 1983.

1229. Nance KS and Matzke GR: Stability of gentamicin and tobramycin in concentrate solutions for automated peritoneal dialysis, *Am J Nephrol* 4:240–243, 1984.

1230. Das Gupta V and Parasrampuria J: Quantitation of acetazolamide in pharmaceutical dosage forms using high-performance liquid chromatography, *Drug Dev Ind Pharm* 13:147–157 (1) 1987.

1231. Boak LR: Aminophylline stability, *Can J Hosp Pharm* 40:155 (5) 1987.

1232. Moore BR and Tindula R: Incompatibility between amphotericin B and evacuated i.v. containers, *Am J Hosp Pharm* 44:1312 (June) 1987.

1233. Bretschneider H: Osmolalities of commercially supplied drugs often used in anesthesia, *Anaesth Analg* 66:361–362, 1987.

1234. Odgers C: Drug/nutrient interactions and incompatibilities complicating TPN, *N.Z. Pharm* 6:64–68 (Jan) 1986.

1235. Kedzierewicz F, Finance C, Nicolas A, et al.: Etude comparative de la stabilite de solutions de carbenicilline en fonction de la temperature. Interet du cycle congelation-decongelation au four a micro-ondes, *Pharm Acta Helv* 62:109–115 (4) 1987.

1236. Arbus MH: Room temperature stability guidelines for carmustine, *Am J Hosp Pharm* 45:531 (Mar) 1988.

1237. Frederiksson K, Lundgren P, and Landersjo L: Stability of carmustine—kinetics and compatibility during administration, *Acta Pharm Suec* 23:115–124 (2) 1986.

1238. Sewell GJ, Riley CM, and Rowland CG: The stability of carboplatin in ambulatory continuous infusion regimes, *J Clin Pharm Ther* 12:427–432, 1987.

1239. Ross MB: Additional stability guidelines for routinely refrigerated drug products, *Am J Hosp Pharm* 45:1498–1499 (July) 1988.

1240. Goodell JA, Harry DJ, and Low JR: More on production of a carbon dioxide gas after reconstitution of ceftazidime, *Am J Hosp Pharm* 44:510, 512 (Mar) 1987.

1241. Savello DR: More on production of carbon dioxide gas after reconstitution of ceftazidime, *Am J Hosp Pharm* 44:512 (Mar) 1987.

1242. Rovers JP, Menielly G, Souney PF, et al.: The use of stability-indicating assays to determine the in vitro compatibility and stability of metronidazole/gentamicin admixtures, *Can J Hosp Pharm* 42:143–146 (Aug) 1989.

1243. Walker SE and Dranitsaris G: Stability of reconstituted ceftriaxone in dextrose and saline solutions, *Can J Hosp Pharm* 40:161–166 (Oct) 1987.

1244. Martinez-Pancheco R, Vila-Jato JL, and Gomez-Amoza JL: Effect of different factors on stability of ceftriaxone in solution, *Farmaco Ed Prat* 42:131–137 (May) 1987.

1245. Kedzierewicz F, Finance C, Nicolas A, et al.: Stability of parenteral ceftriaxone disodium solutions in frozen and liquid states: effect of freezing and microwave thawing, *J Pharm Sci* 78:73–77 (Jan) 1988.

1246. Kristjansson F, Sternson LA, and Lindenbaum S: An investigation on possible oligomer formation in pharmaceutical formulations of cisplatin, *Int J Pharm* 41:67–74 (Jan) 1988.

1247. Anon: High-dose Maxolon mixes with cisplatin, *Pharm J* 234:593 (May 11) 1985.

1248. Kirk B: The evaluation of a light-protective giving set. The photosensitivity of intravenous dacarbazine solutions, *Br J Parenter Ther* 8:78, 81–82,

85–86 (May–June) 1987.

1249. Bosanquet AG: Stability of solutions of antineoplastic agents during preparation and storage for in vitro assays. General considerations, the nitrosoureas and alkylating agents, *Cancer Chemother Pharmacol 14*:83–95, 1985.

1250. Beijnen JH, Potman RP, van Ooijen RD, et al.: Structure elucidation and characterization of daunorubicin degradation products, *Int J Pharm 34*:247–257, 1987.

1251. Haronikova K, Pikulikova Z, Kral L, et al.: Sorption of diazepam on the surface of the plastic infusion unit, part 2, *Farm Obz 55*:485–494 (11) 1986.

1252. Mathot F, Bonnard J, Paris P, et al.: Influence des materiaux de perfusion sur les solutions de diazepam, *J Pharm Belg 37*:153–156 (Mar–Apr) 1982.

1253. Murphy A, Maltby S, and Launchbury AP: Dissolution time, on reconstitution, of a new parenteral formulation of doxorubicin (Doxorubicin Rapid Dissolution), *Int J Pharm 38*:257–259, 1987.

1254. Baumann TJ, Smythe MA, Kaufmann K, et al.: Dissolution times of Adriamycin and Adriamycin RDF, *Am J Hosp Pharm 45*:1667 (Aug) 1988.

1255. Vogelzang NJ, Ruane M, and DeMeester TR: Phase I trial of an implanted battery-powered, programmable drug delivery system for continuous doxorubicin administration, *J Clin Oncol 3*:407–414 (Mar) 1985.

1256. Keusters L, Stolk LML, Umans R, et al.: Stability of solutions of doxorubicin and epirubicin in plastic minibags for intravesical use after storage at −20 °C and thawing by microwave radiation, *Pharm Weekbl Sci Ed 8*:194–197 (June 20) 1986.

1257. Williamson M and Luce JK: Microwave thawing of doxorubicin hydrochloride admixtures not recommended, *Am J Hosp Pharm 44*:505, 510 (Mar) 1987.

1258. Adams S and Fernandez F: Intravenous use of haloperidol, *Hosp Pharm 22*:306–307 (Mar) 1987.

1259. Thoma K and Struve M: Untersuchungen zur photo- und thermostabilitat von adrenalin-losungen, *Pharm Acta Helv 61*:2–9 (1) 1986.

1260. David LM: Phlebitis with intravenous erythromycin, *Am J Hosp Pharm 44*:732, 738 (Apr) 1987.

1261. Schwinghammer TL, Reilly M, and Rosenfeld CS: Cracking of ABS plastic devices used to infuse undiluted etoposide injection, *Am J Hosp Pharm 45*:1277 (June) 1988.

1262. Beijnen JH, Holthuis JJM, Kerkdijk HG, et al.: Degradation kinetics of etoposide in aqueous solution, *Int J Pharm 41*:169–178, 1988.

1263. Brown DH and Simkover RA: Maximum hang times for i.v. fat emulsions, *Am J Hosp Pharm 44*:282, 284 (Feb) 1987.

1264. Allwood MC: The release of phthalate ester plasticizer from intravenous administration sets into fat emulsion, *Int J Pharm 29*:233–236, 1986.

1265. Nahata MC, Hipple TF, and Strausbaugh SD: Stability of gentamicin diluted in 0.9% sodium chloride injection in glass syringes, *Hosp Pharm 22*:1131–1132 (Nov) 1987.

1266. Dunn DL and Lenihan SF: The case for the saline flush, *Am J Nurs 87*:798–799 (June) 1987.

1267. Shearer J: Normal saline flush versus dilute heparin flush. A study of peripheral intermittent I.V. devices, *NITA 10*:425–427 (Nov–Dec) 1987.

1268. Hamilton RA, Plis JM, Clay C, et al.: Heparin sodium versus 0.9% sodium chloride injection for maintaining patency of indwelling intermittent infusion devices, *Clin Pharm 7*:439–443, 1988.

1269. Lombardi TP, Gundersen B, Zammett LO, et al.: Efficacy of 0.9% sodium chloride injection with or without heparin sodium for maintaining patency of intravenous catheters in children, *Clin Pharm 7*:832–836, 1988.

1270. Cyganski JM, Donahue JM, and Heaton JS: The case for the heparin flush, *Am J Nurs 87*:796–797 (June) 1987.

1271. Bullock LS, Fitzgerald JF, and Glick MR: Stability of famotidine in minibags refrigerated and/or frozen, *DICP, Ann Pharmacother 23*:132–135 (Feb) 1989.

1272. Swanson DJ, DeAngelis C, Smith IL, et al.: Degradation kinetics of imipenem in normal saline and human serum, *Antimicrob Agents Chemother 29*:936–937 (May) 1986.

1273. Smith GB and Schoenewaldt EF: Stability of N-formimidoylthienamycin in aqueous solution, *J Pharm Sci 70*:272–276 (Mar) 1981.

1274. McElnay JC, Elliott DS, and D'Arcy PF: Binding of human insulin to burette administration sets, *Int J Pharm 36*:199–203 (May) 1987.

1275. Adams PS, Haines-Nutt RF, and Town R: Stability of insulin mixtures in disposable plastic insulin syringes, *J Pharm Pharmacol 39*:158–163 (Mar) 1987.

1276. Mozzi G, Conegliani B, Lomi R, et al.: Stabilita del calcio folinato in soluzioni acquose in funzione del pH e delta temperatura, *Boll Chim Farm 125*:424–428 (Dec) 1986.

1277. Powell MF: Stability of lidocaine in aqueous solution: effect of temperature,

pH, buffer, and metal ions on amide hydrolysis, *Pharm Res 4*:42–45 (Feb) 1987.

1278. Das Gupta V and Stewart KR: Chemical stabilities of lignocaine hydrochloride and phenylephrine hydrochloride in aqueous solution, *J Clin Hosp Pharm 11*:449–452 (Dec) 1986.

1279. Kirk B: Stability of reconstituted mustine injection BP during storage, *Br J Parenter Ther 7*:86–87, 90–92 (July–Aug) 1986.

1280. Wright MP and Newton JM: Stability of methotrexate injection in prefilled, plastic disposable syringes, *Int J Pharm 45*:237–244 (3) 1988.

1281. Dyvik O, Grislingaas AL, Tonnesen HH, et al.: Methotrexate in infusion solutions—a stability test for the hospital pharmacy, *J Clin Hosp Pharm 11*:343–348 (5) 1986.

1282. McGookin AG, Millership JS, and Scott EM: Miconazole sorption to intravenous infusion sets, *J Clin Pharm Ther 12*:433–437, 1987.

1283. Beijnen JH, Fokkens RH, Rosing H, et al.: Degradation of mitomycin C in acid phosphate and acetate buffer solutions, *Int J Pharm 32*:111–121, 1986.

1284. Beijnen JH, Lingeman H, Van Munster HA, et al.: Mitomycin antitumor agents: a review of their physico-chemical and analytical properties and stability, *J Pharm Biomed Anal 4*:275–295, 1986.

1285. Stolk LML, Fruijtier A, and Umans R: Stability after freezing and thawing of solutions of mitomycin C in plastic minibags for intravesical use, *Pharm Weekbl Sci Ed 8*:286–288, 1986.

1286. Depiero D, Rekhi GS, Souney PF, et al.: Stability of morphine sulfate solutions frozen in polyvinyl chloride intravenous bags, *Pharm Pract News 14*:1, 39–40 (Oct) 1987.

1287. Hung CT, Young M, and Gupta PK: Stability of morphine solutions in plastic syringes determined by reversed-phase ion-pair liquid chromatography, *J Pharm Sci 77*:719–723 (Aug) 1988.

1288. Visor GC, Lin LH, Jackson SE, et al.: Stability of ganciclovir sodium (DHPG sodium) in 5% dextrose or 0.9% sodium chloride injections, *Am J Hosp Pharm 43*:2810–2812 (Nov) 1986.

1289. Behme RJ, Brooke D, Kensler TT, et al.: Incompatibility of ifosfamide with benzyl-alcohol-preserved bacteriostatic water for injection, *Am J Hosp Pharm 45*:627–628 (Mar) 1988.

1290. Rowland CG, Bradford E, Adams P, et al.: Infusion of ifosfamide plus mesna, *Lancet 2*:468 (Aug 25) 1984.

1291. Anon: Mesnex (Mesna), Bristol-Myers Oncology Division, Evansville, Indiana, June 1989.

1292. Dorr RT: Mesnex dosing and administration guide, Bristol Myers Company, Evansville, Indiana, 1989.

1293. Anon: Novantrone, Lederle Laboratories, American Cyanamid Company, Pearl River, New York, 1988.

1294. Nahata MC, Hipple TF, and Strausbaugh SD: Stability of phenobarbital sodium diluted in 0.9% sodium chloride injection, *Am J Hosp Pharm 43*:384–385 (Feb) 1986.

1295. Dela Cruz FG, Kanter MZ, Fischer JH, et al.: Efficacy of individualized phenytoin sodium loading doses administered by intravenous infusion, *Clin Pharm 7*:219–224 (Mar) 1988.

1296. Davidson SW and Lyall D: Sodium nitroprusside stability in light-protective administration sets, *Pharm J 239*:599–601 (Nov 14) 1987.

1297. Saunders A: Stability and light sensitivity of sodium nitroprusside infusions, *Aust J Hosp Pharm 16*:55–56 (Mar) 1986.

1298. Glascock JC, DiPiro JT, Cadwallader DE, et al.: Stability of terbutaline sulfate repackaged in disposable plastic syringes, *Am J Hosp Pharm 44*:2291–2293 (Oct) 1987.

1299. Raymond GG: Stability of terbutaline sulfate injection stored in plastic tuberculin syringes, *Drug Intell Clin Pharm 22*:303–305 (Apr) 1988.

1300. Das Gupta V, Gardner SN, Jalowsky CM, et al.: Chemical stability of thiopental sodium injection in disposable plastic syringes, *J Clin Pharm Ther 12*:339–342 (Oct) 1987.

1301. Nahata MC, Miller MA, and Durrell DE: Stability of vancomycin hydrochloride in various concentrations of dextrose injection, *Am J Hosp Pharm 44*:802–804 (Apr) 1987.

1302. Greenberg RN, Saeed AMK, Kennedy DJ, et al.: Instability of vancomycin in Infusaid drug pump model 100, *Antimicrob Agents Chemother 31*:610–611 (Apr) 1987.

1303. Tucker R and Gentile JF: Precipitation of verapamil in an intravenous line, *Ann Intern Med 101*:880 (Dec) 1984.

1304. Patel SD and Yalkowsky SH: Development of an intravenous formulation for the antiviral drug 9-(beta-D-arabinofuranosyl)-adenine, *J Parenter Sci Technol 41*:15–20 (Jan–Feb) 1987.

1305. Stolk LML, Huisman W, Nordemann HD, et al.: Formulation of a stable vidarabine infusion fluid, *Pharm Weekbl Sci Ed 5*:57–60 (Apr 29) 1983.

1306. Black J, Buechter DD, and Thurston DE: Stability of vinblastine sulfate when exposed to light, *Drug Intell Clin Pharm* 22:634–636 (July–Aug) 1988.

1307. Vindrig DEMM, Smeets BPGH, Beijnen JH, et al.: Degradation kinetics of vinblastine sulphate in aqueous solutions, *Int J Pharm* 43:131–138, 1988.

1308. Cartwight-Shamoon JM, McElnay JC, and D'Arcy PF: Examination of sorption and photodegradation of amsacrine during storage in intravenous burette administration sets, *Int J Pharm* 42:41–46, 1988.

1309. Bosanquet AG: Instability of solutions of diaziquone stored at negative temperatures, *Int J Pharm* 47:215–221, 1988.

1310. Kleinberg ML, Oberdier J, Muller RJ, et al.: Stability of gallium nitrate and mitoguazone dihydrochloride in commonly used intravenous fluids, *Hosp Pharm* 24:929–934 (Nov) 1989.

1311. Leigh PH and Buddle GC: Pentamidine infusion stability, *Br J Pharm Pract* 10:22–23 (Jan) 1988.

1312. Toledo MM, Cadwallader DE, Trissel LA, et al.: Stability of pibenzimol hydrochloride in commonly used infusion solutions and after filtration, *Am J Hosp Pharm* 46:2043–2046 (Oct) 1989.

1313. Wohlford JG and Fowler MD: Visual compatibility of hetastarch with injectable critical-care drugs, *Am J Hosp Pharm* 46:995–996 (May) 1989.

1314. Wohlford JG: Clarification of visual compatibility of hetastarch and ranitidine hydrochloride, *Am J Hosp Pharm* 46:1772 (Sep) 1989.

1315. Wohlford JG, Wright JC, and Wilson MR: More information on the visual compatibility of hetastarch with injectable critical-care drugs, *Am J Hosp Pharm* 47:297–298 (Feb) 1990.

1316. Dasta JF, Hale KN, Stauffer GL, et al.: Comparison of visual and turbidimetric methods for determining short-term compatibility of intravenous critical-care drugs, *Am J Hosp Pharm* 45:2361–2366 (Nov) 1988.

1317. Smith JA, Morris A, Duafala ME, et al.: Stability of floxuridine and leucovorin calcium admixtures for intraperitoneal administration, *Am J Hosp Pharm* 46:985–989 (May) 1989.

1318. Perrin JH, Pereira-Rosario R, and Utamura T: The interaction of dobutamine hydrochloride and heparin sodium in parenteral fluids, *Drug Dev Indust Pharm* 14:1617–1622 (11) 1988.

1319. Lesko AB, Sesin GP, and Cersosimo RJ: Ceftizoxime stability in iv solutions, *DICP, Ann Pharmacother* 23:615, 617–618 (July–Aug) 1989.

1320. Mitrano FP and Baptista RJ: Stability of cimetidine HCl and copper sulfate in a TPN solution, *DICP, Ann Pharmacother* 23:429–430 (May) 1989.

1321. Schilling CG, Watson DM, McCoy HG, et al.: Stability and delivery of vancomycin hydrochloride when admixed in a total parenteral nutrition solution, *J Parenter Enter Nutr* 13:63–64 (1) 1989.

1322. Strong DK, Ho W, and Nairn JG: Visual compatibility of vancomycin and heparin in peritoneal dialysis solutions, *Am J Hosp Pharm* 46:1832–1833 (Sep) 1989.

1323. Chilvers MR and Lysne JM: Visual compatibility of ranitidine hydrochloride with commonly used critical-care medications, *Am J Hosp Pharm* 46:2057–2058 (Oct) 1989.

1324. Bullock L, Clark JH, Fitzgerald JF, et al.: The stability of amikacin, gentamicin, and tobramycin in total nutrient admixture, *J Parenter Enter Nutr* 13:505–509 (Sep–Oct) 1989.

1325. Nahata MC: Stability of vancomycin hydrochloride in total parenteral nutrient solutions, *Am J Hosp Pharm* 46:2055–2057 (Oct) 1989.

1326. Fox AS, Boyer KM, and Sweeney HM: Antibiotic stability in a pediatric parenteral alimentation solution, *J Pediatr* 112:813–817 (May) 1988.

1327. Raymond GG, Reed MT, Teagarden JR, et al.: Stability of procainamide hydrochloride in neutralized 5% dextrose injection, *Am J Hosp Pharm* 45:2513–2517 (Dec) 1988.

1328. Zbrozek AS, Marble DA, and Bosso JA: Compatibility and stability of cefazolin sodium, clindamycin phosphate, and gentamicin sulfate in two intravenous solutions, *Drug Intell Clin Pharm* 22:873–875 (Nov) 1988.

1329. Stewart CF and Hampton EM: Stability of cisplatin and etoposide in intravenous admixtures, *Am J Hosp Pharm* 46:1400–1404 (July) 1989.

1330. Shea BF, Ptachcinski RJ, O'Neill S, et al.: Stability of cyclosporine in 5% dextrose injection, *Am J Hosp Pharm* 46:2053–2055 (Oct) 1989.

1331. Bullock L, Fitzgerald JF, Glick MR, et al.: Stability of famotidine 20 and 40 mg/L and amino acids in total parenteral nutrient solutions, *Am J Hosp Pharm* 46:2321–2325 (Nov) 1989.

1332. Bullock L, Fitzgerald JF, and Glick MR: Stability of famotidine 20 and 50 mg/L in total nutrient admixtures, *Am J Hosp Pharm* 46:2326–2329 (Nov) 1989.

1333. Montoro JB, Pou L, Salvador P, et al.: Stability of famotidine 20 and 40 mg/L in total nutrient admixtures, *Am J Hosp Pharm* 46:2329–2332 (Nov) 1989.

1334. DiStefano JE, Mitrano FP, Baptista RJ, et al.: Long-term stability of famotidine 20 mg/L in a total parenteral nutrient solution, *Am J Hosp Pharm* 46:2333–2335 (Nov) 1989.

1335. Lor E and Takagi J: Visual compatibility of foscarnet with other injectable drugs, *Am J Hosp Pharm* 47:157–159 (Jan) 1990.

1336. Scott SM: Incompatibility of cefoperazone and promethazine, *Am J Hosp Pharm* 47:519 (Mar) 1990.

1337. Savitsky ME: Visual compatibility of neuromuscular blocking agents with various injectable drugs during simulated Y-site injection, *Am J Hosp Pharm* 47:820–821 (Apr) 1990.

1338. Smythe MA, Patel MA, and Gasloli RA: Visual compatibility of narcotic analgesics with selected intravenous admixtures, *Am J Hosp Pharm* 47:819–820 (Apr) 1990.

1339. Stewart CF and Fleming RA: Compatibility of cisplatin and fluorouracil in 0.9% sodium chloride injection, *Am J Hosp Pharm* 47:1373–1377 (June) 1990.

1340. Lee CY, Mauro VF, and Alexander KS: Visual and spectrophotometric determination of compatibility of alteplase and streptokinase with other injectable drugs, *Am J Hosp Pharm* 47:606–608 (Mar) 1990.

1341. Gupta VD, Bethea C, and dela Torre M: Chemical stabilities of cefoperazone sodium and ceftazidime in 5% dextrose and 0.9% sodium chloride injections, *J Clin Pharm Ther* 13:199–205 (June) 1988.

1342. Gupta VD, Parasrampuria J, and Bethea C: Chemical stabilities of famotidine and ranitidine hydrochloride in intravenous admixtures, *J Clin Pharm Ther* 13:329–334 (Oct) 1988.

1343. Gupta VD, Pramar Y, and Bethea C: Stability of acyclovir sodium in dextrose and sodium chloride injections, *J Clin Pharm Ther* 14:451–456 (6) 1989.

1344. Underberg WJM, Koomen JM, and Beijnen JH: Stability of famotidine in commonly used nutritional infusion fluids, *J Parenter Sci Technol* 42:94–97 (May–June) 1988.

1345. Messerschmidt W: Pharmazeutische kompatibilitat von ceftazidim und metronidazol, *Pharm Ztg* 135:36–38 (Mar 8) 1990.

1346. Messerschmidt W: Kompatibilitat von ciprofloxacin und metronidazol in mischinfusionen, *Pharm Ztg* 133:26, 28 (May 26) 1988.

1347. Murdoch JM and Garner ST: Calcium gluconate compatibility, *Pharm J* 242:634 (June 3) 1989.

1348. Stoberski P, Zakrzewski Z, and Szulc A: Bandanie stabilnosci furosemidu i soli sodowej hemibursztynianu hydrokortyzonu metoda RP-HPLC w wybranych plynach infuzyjnych, *Farm Pol* 44:398–401 (7) 1988.

1349. Veechio M, Walker SE, Iazzetta J, et al.: The stability of morphine intravenous infusion solutions, *Can J Hosp Pharm* 41:5–9, 43 (Feb) 1988.

1350. Walker SE and Kirby K: Stability of ranitidine hydrochloride admixtures refrigerated in polyvinyl chloride minibags, *Can J Hosp Pharm* 41:105–108 (June) 1988.

1351. Gupta VD, Parasrampuria J, Bethea C, et al.: Stability of clindamycin phosphate in dextrose and saline solutions, *Can J Hosp Pharm* 42:109–112 (June) 1989.

1352. Walker SE, Iazzetta J, Lau DWC, et al.: Famotidine stability in total parenteral nutrient solutions, *Can J Hosp Pharm* 42:97–103 (June) 1989.

1353. Walker SE and Dranitsaris G: Ceftazidime stability in normal saline and dextrose 5% in water, *Can J Hosp Pharm* 41:65–71 (Apr) 1988.

1354. Walker SE and Birkhans B: Stability of intravenous vancomycin, *Can J Hosp Pharm* 41:233–238, 242 (Oct) 1988.

1355. Halpern NA, Colucci RD, Alicea M, et al.: Visual compatibility of enalaprilat with commonly used critical care medications during simulated Y-site injection, *Int J Clin Pharmacol Ther Toxicol* 27:294–297 (June) 1989.

1356. Allen LV Jr, Stiles ML, and Tu YH: Stability of fentanyl citrate in 0.9% sodium chloride solution in portable infusion pumps, *Am J Hosp Pharm* 47:1572–1574 (July) 1990.

1357. Kowalski SR and Gourlay GK: Stability of fentanyl citrate in glass and plastic containers and in a patient-controlled delivery system, *Am J Hosp Pharm* 47:1584–1587 (July) 1990.

1358. Schaaf LJ, Robinson DH, Vogel GJ, et al.: Stability of esmolol hydrochloride in the presence of aminophylline, bretylium tosylate, heparin sodium, and procainamide hydrochloride, *Am J Hosp Pharm* 47:1567–1571 (July) 1990.

1359. Rosenberg LS, Hostetler CK, Wagenknecht DM, et al.: An accurate prediction of the pH change due to degradation: correction for a "produced" secondary buffering system, *Pharm Res* 5:514–517 (Aug) 1988.

1360. Williams MF, Hak LJ, and Dukes G: In vitro evaluation of the stability of ranitidine hydrochloride in total parenteral nutrient mixtures, *Am J Hosp Pharm* 47:1574–1579 (July) 1990.

1361. Galante LJ, Stewart JT, Warren FW, et al.: Stability of ranitidine hydrochloride with eight medications in intravenous admixtures, *Am J Hosp Pharm* 47:1606–1610 (July) 1990.

1362. Galante LJ, Stewart JT, Warren FW, et al.: Stability of ranitidine hydrochloride at dilute concentration in intravenous infusion fluids at room temperature, *Am J Hosp Pharm* 47:1580–1584 (July) 1990.

1363. Marquardt ED: Visual compatibility of tolazoline hydrochloride with various medications during simulated Y-site injection, *Am J Hosp Pharm* 47:1802–1803 (Aug) 1990.

1364. Chandler SW, Folstad J, and Trissel LA: Aztreonam–vancomycin incompatibility, *Am J Hosp Pharm* 47:1970 (Sep) 1990.

1365. Trissel LA, Tramonte SM, and Grilley BJ: Visual compatibility of ondansetron hydrochloride with other selected drugs during simulated Y-site injection, *Am J Hosp Pharm* 48:988–992 (May) 1991.

1366. Leak RE and Woodford JD: Pharmaceutical development of ondansetron injection, *Eur J Cancer Clin Oncol 25 (Suppl 1)*:S67–S69, 1989.

1367. MacKinnon JWM and Collin DT: The chemistry of ondansetron, *Eur J Cancer Clin Oncol 25 (Suppl 1)*:S61, 1989.

1368. Anon: Idamycin—hospital formulary product information form, Adria Laboratories, Columbus, Ohio, October 19, 1990.

1369. Allwood M, Stanley A, and Wright P: The cytotoxics handbook, 3rd ed, Radcliffe Medical Press, Oxford, England, 1997.

1370. Garinot O, Vitzling C, Mottu R, et al.: Sandostatine: compatibility of Sandostatine 100 μg/ml and 500 μg/ml infusions with various plastic syringes and infusion apparatus, Sandoz Pharmaceutical Research Center, Basle, Switzerland, September 1988.

1371. Anon: Sandostatin—compatibility between octreotide in the infusion and the giving set/container, Sandoz Laboratories, Basle, Switzerland, April 3, 1986.

1372. Anon: Sandostatin—stability in physiological salt solutions, Sandoz Laboratories, Basle, Switzerland, March 26, 1986.

1373. Marchiarullo M: Stability of octreotide in various infusion supplies, Sandoz Pharmaceuticals Corporation, East Hanover, New Jersey, March 20, 1990.

1374. Beijnen JH, Beijnen-Bandhoe AU, Dubbelman AC, et al.: Chemical and physical stability of etoposide and teniposide in commonly used infusion fluids, *J Parenter Sci Technol* 45:108–112 (Mar–Apr) 1991.

1375. Santiero ML, Sagraves R, and Allen LV Jr: Osmolality of small-volume i.v. admixtures for pediatric patients, *Am J Hosp Pharm* 47:1359–1364 (June) 1990.

1376. Messerschmidt W: Kompatibilitat von cefuroxim mit metronidazole, *Krankenhauspharmazie* 8:45–47 (2) 1987.

1377. Rosen GH: Potential incompatibility of insulin and octreotide in total parenteral nutrient solutions, *Am J Hosp Pharm* 46:1128 (June) 1989.

1378. McElnay JC, Elliott DS, Cartwright-Shamoon J, et al.: Stability of methotrexate and vinblastine in burette administration sets, *Int J Pharm* 47:239–247 (Nov) 1988.

1379. Williams DA: Stability and compatibility of admixtures of antineoplastic drugs, *in* Lokich JJ (ed), Cancer chemotherapy by infusion, 2nd ed, Precept Press, Chicago, Illinois, 1990, pp 52–73.

1380. Adams PS, Haines-Nutt RF, Bradford E., et al.: Pharmaceutical aspects of home infusion therapy for cancer patients, *Pharm J* 11:476–478, 1987.

1381. Trissel LA, Chandler SW, and Folstad JT: Visual compatibility of amsacrine with selected drugs during simulated Y-site injection, *Am J Hosp Pharm* 47:2525–2528 (Nov) 1990.

1382. Townsend RS: In vitro inactivation of gentamicin by ampicillin, *Am J Hosp Pharm* 46:2250–2251 (Nov) 1989.

1383. Vaughn LM, Small C, and Plunkett V: Incompatibility of iron dextran and a total nutrient admixture, *Am J Hosp Pharm* 47:1745–1746 (Aug) 1990.

1384. Cutie MR: Verapamil precipitation, *Ann Intern Med* 98:672 (May) 1983.

1385. Garner SS and Wiest DB: Compatibility of drugs separated by a fluid barrier in a retrograde intravenous infusion system, *Am J Hosp Pharm* 47:604–606 (Mar) 1990.

1386. Lokich J, Anderson N, Bern M, et al.: Combined floxuridine and cisplatin in a 14-day infusion, *Cancer* 62:2309–2312 (Dec 1) 1988.

1387. Anderson N, Lokich J, Bern M, et al.: A phase I clinical trial of combined fluoropyrimidines with leucovorin in a 14-day infusion, *Cancer* 63:233–237 (Jan 15) 1989.

1388. Lokich J, Anderson N, Bern M, et al.: Etoposide admixed with cisplatin, *Cancer* 63:818–821 (Mar 1) 1989.

1389. Lokich J, Bern M, Anderson N, et al.: Cyclophosphamide, methotrexate, and 5-fluorouracil in a three-drug admixture, *Cancer* 63:822–824 (Mar 1) 1989.

1390. Anderson N, Lokich J, Bern M, et al.: Combined 5-fluorouracil and floxuridine administered as a 14-day infusion, *Cancer* 63:825–827 (Mar 1) 1989.

1391. Stiles ML, Tu YH, and Allen LV Jr: Stability of cefazolin sodium, cefoxitin sodium, ceftazidime, and penicillin G sodium in portable pump reservoirs, *Am J Hosp Pharm* 46:1408–1412 (July) 1989.

1392. Martens HJ, De Goede PN, and van Loenen AC: Sorption of various drugs in polyvinyl chloride, glass, and polyethylene-lined infusion containers, *Am*

1393. Baltz JK, Kennedy P, Minor JR, et al.: Visual compatibility of foscarnet with other injectable drugs during simulated Y-site administration, *Am J Hosp Pharm* 47:2075–2077 (Sep) 1990.

1394. Walker SE, Coons C, Matte D, et al.: Hydromorphone and morphine stability in portable infusion pump casettes and minibags, *Can J Hosp Pharm* 41:177–182 (Aug) 1988.

1395. Smythe M and Malouf E: Visual compatibility of insulin with secondary intravenous drugs in admixtures, *Am J Hosp Pharm* 48:125–126 (Jan) 1991.

1396. Tu YH, Stiles ML, and Allen LV Jr: Stability of fentanyl citrate and bupivacaine hydrochloride in portable pump reservoirs, *Am J Hosp Pharm* 47:2037–2040 (Sep) 1990.

1397. Pugh CB, Pabis DJ, and Rodriguez C: Visual compatibility of morphine sulfate and meperidine hydrochloride with other injectable drugs during simulated Y-site injection, *Am J Hosp Pharm* 48:123–125 (Jan) 1991.

1398. Pritts D and Hancock D: Incompatibility of ceftriaxone with vancomycin, *Am J Hosp Pharm* 48:77 (Jan) 1991.

1399. DeMuynck C, De Vroe C, Remon JP, et al.: Binding of drugs to end-line filters: a study of four commonly administered drugs in intensive care units, *J Clin Pharm Ther* 13:335–340 (Oct) 1988.

1400. Aki H, Sawai N, Yamamoto K, et al.: Structural confirmation of ampicillin polymers formed in aqueous solution, *Pharm Res* 8:119–122 (Jan) 1991.

1401. Bonhomme L, Postaire E, Touratier S, et al.: Chemical stability of lignocaine (lidocaine) and adrenaline (epinephrine) in pH-adjusted parenteral solutions, *J Clin Pharm Ther* 13:257–261, 1988.

1402. Lee DKT, Lee A, and Wang DP: Compatibility of cefoperazone sodium and furosemide in 5% dextrose injection, *Am J Hosp Pharm* 48:108–110 (Jan) 1991.

1403. Lee DKT, Wang DP, and Lee A: Compatibility of cefoperazone sodium and cimetidine hydrochloride in 5% dextrose injection, *Am J Hosp Pharm* 48:111–113 (Jan) 1991.

1404. Kirkpatrick AE, Holcome BJ, and Sawyer WT: Effect of retrograde aminophylline administration on calcium and phosphate solubility in neonatal total parenteral nutrient solutions, *Am J Hosp Pharm* 46:2496–2500 (Dec) 1989.

1405. Seay R and Bostrom B: Apparent compatibility of methotrexate and vancomycin, *Am J Hosp Pharm* 47:2656, 2658 (Dec) 1990.

1406. Johnson OL, Washington C, Davis SS, et al.: The destabilization of parenteral feeding emulsions by heparin, *Int J Pharm* 53:237–240 (Aug 1) 1989.

1407. Lor E, Sheybani T, and Takagi J: Visual compatibility of fluconazole with commonly used injectable drugs during simulated Y-site administration, *Am J Hosp Pharm* 48:744–746 (Apr) 1991.

1408. Tol A, Quik RFP, and Thyssen JHH: Adsorption of human and porcine insulins to intravenous administration sets, *Pharm Weekbl Sci Ed* 10:213–216 (Oct 14) 1988.

1409. Thompson DF, Allen LV Jr, and Stiles ML: Visual compatibility of enalaprilat with selected intravenous medications during simulated Y-site injection, *Am J Hosp Pharm* 47:2530–2531 (Nov) 1990.

1410. Wilson TD and Forde MD: Stability of milrinone and epinephrine, atropine sulfate, lidocaine hydrochloride, or morphine sulfate injection, *Am J Hosp Pharm* 47:2504–2507 (Nov) 1990.

1411. Lam NP, Kennedy PE, Jarosinski PF, et al.: Stability of zidovudine in 5% dextrose injection and 0.9% sodium chloride injection, *Am J Hosp Pharm* 48:280–282 (Feb) 1991.

1412. Horrow JC, Digregorio GJ, Barbieri EJ, et al.: Intravenous infusions of nitroprusside, dobutamine, and nitroglycerin are compatible, *Crit Care Med* 18:858–861 (Aug) 1990.

1413. Halstead DC, Guzzo J, Giardina JA, et al.: In vitro bactericidal activities of gentamicin, cefazolin, and imipenem in peritoneal dialysis fluids, *Antimicrob Agents Chemother* 33:1553–1556 (Sep) 1989.

1414. Drake JM, Myre SA, Staneck JL, et al.: Antimicrobial activity of vancomycin, gentamicin, and tobramycin in peritoneal dialysis solution, *Am J Hosp Pharm* 47:1604–1606 (July) 1990.

1415. Pavlik EJ, van Nagell JR, Hanson MB, et al.: Sensitivity to anticancer agents in vitro: standardizing the cytotoxic response and characterizing the sensitivities of a reference cell line, *Gynecol Oncol* 14:243–261 (Oct) 1982.

1416. Pavlik EJ, Kenady DE, van Nagell JR, et al.: Properties of anticancer agents relevant to in vitro determinations of human tumor cell sensitivity, *Cancer Chemother Pharmacol* 11:8–15 (1) 1983.

1417. Gora ML, Seth S, Visconti JA, et al.: Stability of dobutamine hydrochloride in peritoneal dialysis solutions, *Am J Hosp Pharm* 48:1234–1237 (June) 1991.

1418. Strom JG Jr and Miller SW: Stability and compatibility of methylprednisolone sodium succinate and cimetidine hydrochloride in 5% dextrose injection, *Am J Hosp Pharm* 48:1237–1241 (June) 1991.

J Hosp Pharm 47:369–373 (Feb) 1990.

1419. Riley CM and Junkin P: Stability of amrinone and digoxin, procainamide hydrochloride, propranolol hydrochloride, sodium bicarbonate, potassium chloride, or verapamil hydrochloride in intravenous admixtures, *Am J Hosp Pharm* 48:1245–1252 (June) 1991.

1420. Pennell AT, Allington DR, and Chandler MHH: Effect of ceftazidime, cefotaxime, and cefoperazone on serum tobramycin concentrations, *Am J Hosp Pharm* 48:520–522 (Mar) 1991.

1421. Collins JL and Lutz RJ: In vitro study of simultaneous infusion of incompatible drugs in multilumen catheters, *Heart Lung* 20:271–277 (May) 1991.

1422. Gupta VD: Complexation of procainamide with dextrose, *J Pharm Sci* 71:994–996 (Sep) 1982.

1423. Gupta VD: Complexation of procainamide with hydroxide-containing compounds, *J Pharm Sci* 72:205–207 (Feb) 1983.

1424. Parasrampuria J and Gupta VD: Preformulation studies of acetazolamide: effect of pH, two buffer species, ionic strength, and temperature on its stability, *J Pharm Sci* 78:855–857 (Oct) 1989.

1425. Franzin BS: Maximal dilution of Activase, *Am J Hosp Pharm* 47:1016 (May) 1990.

1426. Tripp MG: Automated 3-in-1 admixture compounding: a comparative study of simultaneous versus sequential pumping of core substrates on admixture stability, *Hosp Pharm* 25:1090–1093, 1096 (Dec) 1990.

1427. Knowles JB, Cusson G, Smith M, et al.: Pulmonary deposition of calcium phosphate crystals as a complication of home total parenteral nutrition, *J Parenter Enter Nutr* 13:209–213 (Mar–Apr) 1989.

1428. Knight PJ, Buchanan S, and Clatworthy HW: Calcium and phosphate requirements of preterm infants who require prolonged hyperalimentation, *J Am Med Assoc* 243:1244–1246, 1980.

1429. Stennett DJ, Gerwick WH, Egging PK, et al.: Precipitate analysis from an indwelling total parenteral nutrition catheter, *J Parenter Enter Nutr* 12:88–92, 1988.

1430. Mazur HI, Stennett DJ, and Egging PK: Extraction of diethylhexylphthalate from total nutrient solution-containing polyvinyl chloride bags, *J Parenter Enter Nutr* 13:59–62 (Jan–Feb) 1989.

1431. Smith JL, Canham JE, Kirkland WD, et al.: Effect of Intralipid, amino acids, container, temperature, and duration of storage on vitamin stability in total parenteral nutrition admixtures, *J Parenter Enter Nutr* 12:478–483 (Sep–Oct) 1988.

1432. Tripp MG, Menon SK, and Mikrut BA: Stability of total nutrient admixtures in a dual-chamber flexible container, *Am J Hosp Pharm* 47:2496–2503 (Nov) 1990.

1433. Dalton-Bunnow MF and Halvacks FJ: Update on room-temperature stability of drug products labeled for refrigerated storage, *Am J Hosp Pharm* 47:2522–2524 (Nov) 1990.

1434. Kintzel PE and Kennedy PE: Stability of amphotericin B in 5% dextrose injection at concentrations used for administration through a central venous line, *Am J Hosp Pharm* 48:283–285 (Feb) 1991.

1435. Rice JK: Visual compatibility of amphotericin B and flush solutions, *Am J Hosp Pharm* 46:2461 (Dec) 1989.

1436. Trissel LA, Bready BB, Kwan JW, et al.: The visual compatibility of sargramostim with selected chemotherapeutic drugs, anti-infectives, and other drugs during simulated Y-site injection, *Am J Hosp Pharm* 49:402–406 (Feb) 1992.

1437. Pilla TJ, Beshany SE, and Shields JB: Incompatibility of Hexabrix and papaverine, *Am J Roentgenol* 146:1300–1301 (June) 1986.

1438. Irving HD and Burbridge BE: Incompatibility of contrast agents with intravascular medications, *Radiology* 173:91–92, 1989.

1439. Trissel LA, Parks NPT, and Santiago NM: Visual compatibility of fludarabine phosphate with antineoplastic drugs, anti-infectives, and other selected drugs during simulated Y-site injection, *Am J Hosp Pharm* 48:2186–2189 (Oct) 1991.

1440. Tidy PJ, Sewell GJ, and Jeffries TM: Microwave freeze–thaw studies on azlocillin infusion, *Pharm J* 241:R22–R23 (Nov 12 Suppl) 1988.

1441. Koberda M, Zieske PA, Raghavan NV, et al.: Stability of bleomycin sulfate reconstituted in 5% dextrose injection or 0.9% sodium chloride injection stored in glass vials or polyvinyl chloride containers, *Am J Hosp Pharm* 47:2528–2529 (Nov) 1990.

1442. Anon: ABPI compendium of data sheets and summaries of product characteristics 1999/2000, Datapharm Publications Ltd., London, England, 1999.

1443. Weir SJ, Szucs Myers VA, Bengston KD, et al.: Sorption of amiodarone to polyvinyl chloride infusion bags and administration sets, *Am J Hosp Pharm* 42:2679–2683 (Dec) 1985.

1444. Benedict MK, Roche VF, Banakar UV, et al.: Visual compatibility of amiodarone hydrochloride with various antimicrobial agents during simulated Y-site injection, *Am J Hosp Pharm* 45:1117–1118 (May) 1988.

1445. Capps PA and Robertson AL: Influence of amiodarone injection on delivery rate of intravenous fluids, *Pharm J* 234:14–15 (Jan 5) 1985.

1446. Tsuei SE, Nation RL, and Thomas J: Sorption of chlormethiazole by intravenous infusion giving sets, *Eur J Clin Pharmacol* 18:333–338 (Aug) 1980.

1447. Lingam S, Bertwistle H, Elliston HM, et al.: Problems with intravenous chlormethiazole (Heminevrin) in status epilepticus, *Br Med J* 1:155–156 (Jan) 1980.

1448. Beaumont IM: Stability study of aqueous solutions of diamorphine and morphine using HPLC, *Pharm J* 229:39–41 (July 10) 1982.

1449. Kleinberg ML, Duafala ME, Nacov C, et al.: Stability of heroin hydrochloride in infusion devices and containers for intravenous administration, *Am J Hosp Pharm* 47:377–381 (Feb) 1990.

1450. Jones VA and Hanks GW: New portable infusion pump for prolonged subcutaneous administration of opiod analgesics in patients with advanced cancer, *Br Med J* 292:1496 (June 7) 1986.

1451. Jones VA, Hoskin PJ, Omar OA, et al.: Diamorphine stability in aqueous solution for subcutaneous infusion, *Abs Br Soc Pharmacol Meet* 66 (Dec) 1986.

1452. Omar OA, Hoskin PJ, Johnston A, et al.: Diamorphine stability in aqueous solution for subcutaneous infusion, *J Pharm Pharmacol* 41:275–277 (Apr) 1989.

1453. Al-Razzak LA, Benedetti AE, Waugh WN, et al.: Chemical stability of pentostatin (NSC-218321), a cytotoxic and immunosuppressive agent, *Pharm Res* 7:452–460 (May) 1990.

1454. Allwood MC: Diamorphine mixed with antiemetic drugs in plastic syringes, *Br J Pharm Prac* 6:88–90 (Mar) 1984.

1455. Regnard C, Pashley S, and Westrope F: Anti-emetic/diamorphine mixture compatibility in infusion pumps, *Br J Pharm Pract* 8:218–220 (Aug) 1986.

1456. Collins AJ, Abathell JA, Holmes SG, et al.: Stability of diamorphine hydrochloride with haloperidol in prefilled syringes for continuous subcutaneous administration, *J Pharm Pharmacol* 38(S):51P (Nov) 1986.

1457. Page J and Hudson SA: Diamorphine hydrochloride compatibility with saline, *Pharm J* 228:238–239 (Feb 27) 1982.

1458. Kirk B and Hain WR: Diamorphine injection BP incompatibility, *Pharm J* 235:171 (Aug 10) 1985.

1459. Jones V, Murphy A, and Hanks GW: Solubility of diamorphine, *Pharm J* 235:426 (Oct 5) 1985.

1460. Wood MJ, Irwin WJ, and Scott DK: Stability of doxorubicin, daunorubicin and epirubicin in plastic syringes and minibags, *J Clin Pharm Ther* 15:279–289, 1990.

1461. Targett PL, Keefe PA, and Merridew CG: Stability of two concentrations of morphine tartrate in 10 ml polypropylene syringes, *Aust J Hosp Pharm* 27:452–454 (6) 1997.

1462. Keusters L, Stolk LML, Umans R, et al.: Stability of solutions of doxorubicin and epirubicin in plastic minibags for intravesical use after storage at −20 °C and thawing by microwave radiation, *Pharm Weekbl Sci Ed* 8:194–197 (June) 1986.

1463. Wood MJ, Irwin WJ, and Scott DK: Photodegradation of doxorubicin, daunorubicin, and epirubicin measured by high-performance liquid chromatography, *J Clin Pharm Ther* 35:291–300, 1990.

1464. Lee MG and Fenton-May V: Absorption of isosorbide dinitrate by PVC infusion bags and administration sets, *J Clin Hosp Pharm* 6:209–211 (Sep) 1981.

1465. DeMuynck C, Remon JP, and Colardyn F: The sorption of isosorbide dinitrate to intravenous delivery systems, *J Pharm Pharmacol* 40:601–604 (Sep) 1988.

1466. Struhar M, Mandak M, Heinrich J, et al.: Sorption of isosorbide dinitrate on infusion sets, *Farm Obz* 58:443–446 (Oct) 1989.

1467. Allwood MC: Sorption of parenteral nitrates during administration with a syringe pump and extension set, *Int J Pharm* 39:183–186 (Feb) 1987.

1468. Wilson TD, Forde MD, Crain AVR, et al.: Stability of milrinone in 0.45% sodium chloride, 0.9% sodium chloride, or 5% dextrose injections, *Am J Hosp Pharm* 43:2218–2220 (Sep) 1986.

1469. Cook B, Hill SA, and Lynn B: The stability of amoxycillin sodium in intravenous infusion fluids, *J Clin Hosp Pharm* 7:245–250 (Dec) 1982.

1470. Concannon J, Lovitt H, Ramage M, et al.: Stability of aqueous solutions of amoxicillin sodium in the frozen and liquid states, *Am J Hosp Pharm* 43:3027–3030 (Dec) 1986.

1471. McDonald C, Sunderland VB, Lau H, et al.: The stability of amoxicillin sodium in normal saline and glucose (5%) solutions in the liquid and frozen states, *J Clin Pharm Ther* 14:45–52 (Feb) 1989.

1472. McDonald C, Sunderland VB, Marshall CA, et al.: Freezing rates of 50-ml infusion bags and some implications for drug stability as shown with amoxycillin, *Aust J Hosp Pharm* 19:194–197 (Apr) 1989.

1473. Janknegt R, Schrouff GGM, Hooymans PM, et al.: Quinolones and penicillins incompatibility, *DICP, Ann Pharmacother 23*:91–92 (Jan) 1989.

1474. Ashwin J, Lynn B, and Taskis CB: Stability and administration of intravenous Augmentin, *Pharm J 238*:116–118 (Jan 24) 1987.

1475. Lynn B: The stability and administration of intravenous penicillins, *Br J IV Ther 2*:22–39 (Mar) 1981.

1476. Landersjo L, Kallstrand G, and Lundgren P: Studies on the stability and compatibility of drugs in infusion fluids III. Factors affecting the stability of cloxacillin, *Acta Pharm Suec 11*:563–580 (Dec) 1974.

1477. Bundgaard H and Ilver K: Kinetics of degradation of cloxacillin sodium in aqueous solution, *Dansk Tidsskr Farm 44*:365–380, 1970.

1478. Brown AF, Harvey DA, Hoddinott DJ, et al.: Freeze–thaw stability of antibiotics used in an IV additive service, *Br J Parenter Ther 7*:42–44 (Mar–Apr) 1986.

1479. Beatson C and Taylor A: A physical compatibility study of frusemide and flucloxacillin injections, *Br J Pharm Pract 9*:223–226, 236 (July) 1987.

1480. Nahata MC and Ahalt PA: Stability of cefazolin sodium in peritoneal dialysis solutions, *Am J Hosp Pharm 48*:291–292 (Feb) 1991.

1481. Paap CM and Nahata MC: Stability of cefotaxime in two peritoneal dialysis solutions, *Am J Hosp Pharm 47*:147–150 (Jan) 1990.

1482. Mehta AC, McCarty M, and Calvert RT: The chemical stability of cephradine injection solutions, *Intensive Ther Clin Monit 9*:195–196 (Oct) 1988.

1483. Lyall D and Blythe J: Ciprofloxacin lactate infusion, *Pharm J 238*:290 (Mar 7) 1987.

1484. Veljkovic VB, Lazic ML, and Cakic MD: Stability of bottled dextran solutions with respect to insoluble particle formations: a review, *Pharmazie 44*:305–310 (May) 1989.

1485. Veljkovic VB, Lazic ML, and Cakic MD: Mechanism of insoluble particle formation in bottled dextran solutions, *Pharmazie 43*:840–842 (Dec) 1988.

1486. Shea BF and Souney PF: Stability of famotidine frozen in polypropylene syringes, *Am J Hosp Pharm 47*:2073–2074 (Sep) 1990.

1487. Bullock LS, Fitzgerald JF, and Mazur HI: Stability of intravenous famotidine stored in polyvinyl-chloride syringes, *DICP, Ann Pharmacother 23*:588–590 (July–Aug) 1989.

1488. Thomas SMB: Stability of Intralipid in a parenteral nutrition solution, *Aust J Hosp Pharm 17*:115–117 (July) 1987.

1489. Stiles ML, Allen LV Jr, and Tu YH: Stability of fluorouracil administered through four portable infusion pumps, *Am J Hosp Pharm 46*:2036–2040 (Oct) 1989.

1490. Tu YH, Stiles ML, Allen LV Jr, et al.: Stability study of gentamicin sulfate administered via Pharmacia Deltec CADD-VT pump, *Hosp Pharm 25*:843–845 (Sep) 1990.

1491. Parkinson R, Wilson JV, Ross M, et al.: Stability of low-dosage heparin in pre-filled syringes, *Br J Pharm Pract 11*:34, 36 (Jan) 1989.

1492. Menzies AR, Benoliel DM, and Edwards HE: The effects of autoclaving on the physical properties and biological activity of parenteral heparin preparations, *J Pharm Pharmacol 41*:512–516, 1989.

1493. Anon: Stability of 4-demethoxydaunorubicin hydrochloride reconstituted solutions with water for injections, sodium chloride, dextrose, and sodium chloride with dextrose injections, Farmitalia Carlo Erba, June 1985.

1494. Radford JA, Margison JM, Swindell R, et al.: The stability of ifosfamide in aqueous solution and its suitability for continuous 7-day infusion by ambulatory pump, *Cancer Chemother Pharmacol 26*:144–146 (May) 1990.

1495. Shaw IC and Rose JWP: Infusion of ifosfamide plus mesna, *Lancet 1*:1353–1354 (June 16) 1984.

1496. Anon: IFEX (Ifosfamide), Bristol Myers Oncology, Evansville, Indiana, February 1990.

1497. Doglietto GB, Bellantone R, Bossola M, et al.: Insulin adsorption to three-liter ethylene vinyl acetate bags during 24-hour infusion, *J Parenter Enter Nutr 13*:539–543 (Sep–Oct) 1989.

1498. Donnelly RF: Immune globulin solubility in 5% dextrose injection, *Am J Hosp Pharm 47*:1976 (Sep) 1990.

1499. Prouix SM: Reconstitution of intravenous immunoglobulins, *Hosp Pharm 22*:1133–1134 (Nov) 1987.

1500. Denson DD, Crews JC, Grummich KW, et al.: Stability of methadone hydrochloride in 0.9% sodium chloride injection in single-dose plastic containers, *Am J Hosp Pharm 48*:515–517 (Mar) 1991.

1501. Anderson BD and Taphouse V: Initial rate studies of hydrolysis and acyl migration in methylprednisolone 21-hemisuccinate and 17-hemisuccinate, *J Pharm Sci 70*:181–186 (Feb) 1981.

1502. Bogardus JB, Kaplan MA, and Carpenter JP: Precipitation of teniposide during infusion, *Am J Hosp Pharm 48*:518 (Mar) 1990.

1503. Beijnen JH, van Gijn R, and Underberg WJM: Chemical stability of the antitumor drug mitomycin C in solutions for intravesical installation, *J Parenter Sci Technol 44*:332–335 (Nov–Dec) 1990.

1504. Duafala ME, Kleinberg ML, Nacov C, et al.: Stability of morphine sulfate in infusion devices and containers for intravenous administration, *Am J Hosp Pharm 47*:143–146 (Jan) 1990.

1505. Walker SE, Iazetta J, and Lau DWC: Stability of sulfite free high potency morphine sulfate solutions in portable infusion pump casettes, *Can J Hosp Pharm 42*:195–200, 218–219 (Oct) 1989.

1506. Altman L, Hopkins RJ, Ahmed S, et al.: Stability of morphine sulfate in Cormed III (Kalex) intravenous bags, *Am J Hosp Pharm 47*:2040–2042 (Sep) 1990.

1507. Stiles ML, Tu YH, and Allen LV Jr: Stability of morphine sulfate in portable pump reservoirs during storage and simulated administration, *Am J Hosp Pharm 46*:1404–1407 (July) 1989.

1508. Cante B, Monsarrat B, Lazorthes Y, et al.: The stability of morphine in isobaric and hyperbaric solutions in a drug delivery system, *J Pharm Pharmacol 40*:644–645, 1988.

1509. Martens HJ: Stabilitat wasserloslicher vitamine in verschiedenen infusionsbenteln, *Krankenhauspharmazie 10*:359–361 (Sep) 1989.

1510. Tracy TS, Bowman L, and Black CD: Nitroglycerin delivery through a polyethylene-lined intravenous administration set, *Am J Hosp Pharm 46*:2031–2035 (Oct) 1989.

1511. Loucas SP, Maager P, Mehl B, et al.: Effect of vehicle ionic strength on sorption on nitroglycerin to a polyvinyl chloride administration set, *Am J Hosp Pharm 47*:1559–1562 (July) 1990.

1512. DeRudder D, Remon JP, and Neyt EN: The sorption of nitroglycerin by infusion sets, *J Pharm Pharmacol 39*:556–558 (July) 1987.

1513. Jarosinski PF and Hirschfield S: Precipitation of ondansetron in alkaline solutions, *N Engl J Med 325*:1315–1316 (Oct 31) 1991.

1514. Markowsky SJ, Kohls PR, Ehresman D, et al.: Compatibility and pH variability of four injectable phenytoin sodium products, *Am J Hosp Pharm 48*:510–514 (Mar) 1991.

1515. Stolshek BS (Professional Services, Glaxo Inc.): Personal communication, August 27, 1990.

1516. Stewart JT, Warren FW, Johnson SM, et al.: Stability of ranitidine in intravenous admixtures stored frozen, refrigerated, and at room temperature, *Am J Hosp Pharm 47*:2043–2046 (Sep) 1990.

1517. Thibault L: Streptokinase flocculation in evacuated glass bottles, *Am J Hosp Pharm 42*:278, 280 (Feb) 1985.

1518. Camacho-Sanchez MA, Torres-Suarez AI, and Sanz MP: Stability of amonafide solutions in front of light and temperature, *Cienc Ind Farm 8*:104–109 (Mar–Apr) 1989.

1519. Den Hartigh J, Brandenburg HCR, and Vermeij P: Stability of azacitidine in lactated Ringer's injection frozen in polypropylene syringes, *Am J Hosp Pharm 46*:2500–2505 (Dec) 1989.

1520. Waugh WN, Trissel LA, and Stella VJ: Stability, compatibility, and plasticizer extraction of taxol (NSC-125973) injection diluted in infusion solutions and stored in various containers, *Am J Hosp Pharm 48*:1520–1524 (July) 1991.

1521. Strong DK and Morris LA: Precipitation of teniposide during infusion, *Am J Hosp Pharm 47*:512 (Mar) 1990.

1522. Outman WR, Mitrano FP, and Baptista RJ: Visual compatibility of ganciclovir sodium and total parenteral nutrient solution during simulated Y-site injection, *Am J Hosp Pharm 48*:1538–1539 (July) 1991.

1523. Outman WR and Monolakis J: Visual compatibility of haloperidol lactate with 0.9% sodium chloride injection or injectable critical-care drugs during simulated Y-site injection, *Am J Hosp Pharm 48*:1539–1541 (July) 1991.

1524. Neels JT: Compatibility of hydromorphone hydrochloride and tetracaine hydrochloride, *Am J Hosp Pharm 48*:1682–1683 (Aug) 1991.

1525. Turowski RC and Durthaler JM: Visual compatibility of idarubicin hydrochloride with selected drugs during simulated Y-site injection, *Am J Hosp Pharm 48*:2181–2184 (Oct) 1991.

1526. Woloschuk DMM, Wermeling JR, and Pruemer JM: Stability and compatibility of fluorouracil and mannitol during simulated Y-site administration, *Am J Hosp Pharm 48*:2158–2160 (Oct) 1991.

1527. Ishisaka DY, van Fleet J, and Marquardt E: Visual compatibility of indomethacin sodium trihydrate with drugs given to neonates by continuous infusion, *Am J Hosp Pharm 48*:2442–2443 (Nov) 1991.

1528. Trissel LA and Bready BB: Turbidimetric assessment of the compatibility of taxol with selected other drugs during simulated Y-site injection, *Am J Hosp Pharm 49*:1716–1719 (July) 1992.

1529. DiStefano JE and Outman WR: Additional data on visual compatibility of foscarnet sodium with morphine sulfate, *Am J Hosp Pharm 49*:1672 (July) 1992.

1530. Farquhar Zanetti LA: Visual compatibility of diltiazem with commonly used injectable drugs during simulated Y-site administration, *Am J Hosp Pharm 49*:1911 (Aug) 1992.

1531. Martin KM (Product Information Services, Lederle Laboratories, Pearl

River, New York): Personal communication, January 14, 1992.

1532. Walker SE, DeAngelis C, and Iazzetta J: Stability and compatibility of combinations of hydromorphone and a second drug, *Can J Hosp Pharm* 44:289–295 (Dec) 1991.

1533. Raineri DL, Cwik MJ, Rodvold KA, et al.: Stability of nizatidine in commonly used intravenous fluids and containers, *Am J Hosp Pharm* 45:1523–1529 (July) 1988.

1534. Hatton J, Holstad SG, Rosenbloom AD, et al.: Stability of nizatidine in total nutrient admixtures, *Am J Hosp Pharm* 48:1507–1510 (July) 1991.

1535. Wade CS, Lampasona V, Mullins RE, et al.: Stability of ceftazidime and amino acids in parenteral nutrient solutions, *Am J Hosp Pharm* 48:1515–1519 (July) 1991.

1536. Patel JP, Tran LT, Sinai WJ, et al.: Activity of urokinase diluted in 0.9% sodium chloride injection or 5% dextrose injection and stored in glass or plastic syringes, *Am J Hosp Pharm* 48:1511–1514 (July) 1991.

1537. Kintzel PE and Kennedy PE: Stability of amphotericin B in 5% dextrose injection at 25 °C, *Am J Hosp Pharm* 48:1681 (Aug) 1991.

1538. Stiles ML and Allen LV: Stability of doxorubicin hydrochloride in portable pump reservoirs, *Am J Hosp Pharm* 48:1976–1977 (Sep) 1991.

1539. Sarkar MA, Rogers E, Reinhard M, et al.: Stability of clindamycin phosphate, ranitidine hydrochloride, and piperacillin sodium in polyolefin containers, *Am J Hosp Pharm* 48:2184–2186 (Oct) 1991.

1540. Ritchie DJ, Holstad SG, Westrich TJ, et al.: Activity of octreotide acetate in a total nutrient admixture, *Am J Hosp Pharm* 48:2172–2175 (Oct) 1991.

1541. Goodwin SD, Nix DE, Heyd A, et al.: Compatibility of ciprofloxacin injection with selected drugs and solutions, *Am J Hosp Pharm* 48:2166–2171 (Oct) 1991.

1542. Walker SE, DeAngelis C, Iazzetta J, et al.: Compatibility of dexamethasone sodium phosphate with hydromorphone hydrochloride or diphenhydramine hydrochloride, *Am J Hosp Pharm* 48:2161–2166 (Oct) 1991.

1543. Harkness BJ, Williams D, Stewart MC, et al.: Change needed for i.v. rifampin preparation instructions, *Am J Hosp Pharm* 48:2127–2128 (Oct) 1991.

1544. Wiest DB, Maish WA, Garner SS, et al.: Stability of amphotericin B in four concentrations of dextrose injection, *Am J Hosp Pharm* 48:2430–2433 (Nov) 1991.

1545. Silvestri AP, Mitrano FP, Baptista RJ, et al.: Stability and compatibility of ganciclovir sodium in 5% dextrose injection over 35 days, *Am J Hosp Pharm* 48:2641–2643 (Dec) 1991.

1546. Mitrano FP, Outman WR, Baptista RJ, et al.: Chemical and visual stability of amphotericin B in 5% dextrose injection stored at 4 °C for 35 days, *Am J Hosp Pharm* 48:2635–2637 (Dec) 1991.

1547. Rivers TE, McBride HA, and Trang JM: Stability of cefotaxime sodium and metronidazole in an i.v. admixture at 8 °C, *Am J Hosp Pharm* 48:2638–2640 (Dec) 1991.

1548. Rochard EB, Barthes DMC, and Courtois PY: Stability of fluorouracil, cytarabine, or doxorubicin hydrochloride in ethylene vinyl acetate portable infusion-pump reservoirs, *Am J Hosp Pharm* 49:619–623 (Mar) 1992.

1549. Letourneau M, Milot L, and Souney PF: Visual compatibility of magnesium sulfate with narcotic analgesics, *Am J Hosp Pharm* 49:838–839 (Apr) 1992.

1550. Thompson DF and Heflin NR: Incompatibility of injectable indomethacin with gentamicin sulfate or tobramycin sulfate, *Am J Hosp Pharm* 49:836, 838 (Apr) 1992.

1551. Munoz M, Girona V, Pujol M, et al.: Stability of ifosfamide in 0.9% sodium chloride solution or water for injection in a portable i.v. pump cassette, *Am J Hosp Pharm* 49:1137–1139 (May) 1992.

1552. Anderson PM, Rogosheske JR, Ramsay NKC, et al.: Biological activity of recombinant interleukin-2 in intravenous admixtures containing antibiotic, morphine sulfate, or total parenteral nutrient solution, *Am J Hosp Pharm* 49:608–612 (Mar) 1992.

1553. Stiles ML, Allen LV, and Fox JL: Stability of ondansetron hydrochloride in portable infusion-pump reservoirs, *Am J Hosp Pharm* 49:1471–1473 (June) 1992.

1554. Couch P, Jacobson P, and Johnson CE: Stability of fluconazole and amino acids in parenteral nutrient solutions, *Am J Hosp Pharm* 49:1459–1462 (June) 1992.

1555. McDonald C and Faridah: Solubilities of trimethoprim and sulfamethoxazole at various pH values and crystallization of trimethoprim from infusion fluids, *J Parenter Sci Tech* 45:147–151 (May–June) 1991.

1556. Trissel LA and Martinez JF: Turbidimetric assessment of the compatibility of taxol with 42 drugs during simulated Y-site injection, *Am J Hosp Pharm* 50:300–304 (Feb) 1993.

1557. Trissel LA and Martinez JF: Melphalan physical compatibility with selected drugs during simulated Y-site administration, *Am J Hosp Pharm* 50:2359–2363 (Nov) 1993.

1558. Trissel LA and Martinez JF: Visual, turbidimetric, and particle-content assessment of compatibility of vinorelbine tartrate with selected drugs during simulated Y-site injection, *Am J Hosp Pharm* 51:495–499 (Feb 15) 1994.

1559. Pearson SD and Trissel LA: Stability and compatibility of minocycline hydrochloride and rifampin in intravenous solutions at various temperatures, *Am J Hosp Pharm* 50:698–702 (Apr) 1993.

1560. Graham CL, Dukes GE, Kao CF, et al.: Stability of ondansetron in large-volume parenteral solutions, *Ann Pharmacother* 26:768–771 (June) 1992.

1561. Halasi S and Nairn JG: Stability of hydralazine hydrochloride in parenteral solutions, *Can J Hosp Pharm* 43:237–241 (Oct) 1990.

1562. Speaker TJ, Turco SJ, Nardone DA, et al.: A study of the interaction of selected drugs and plastic syringes, *J Parenter Sci Tech* 45:212–217 (Sep–Oct) 1991.

1563. Trissel LA, Martinez JF, and Gilbert D: Data on file, Pharmaceutical Analysis Laboratory, University of Texas, M. D. Anderson Cancer Center, Houston, Texas, August 1995.

1564. Adams PS, Haines-Nutt RF, Bradford E, et al.: Pharmaceutical aspects of home infusion therapy for cancer patients, *Pharm J* 238:476–478, 1987.

1565. Barnes AR: Chemical stabilities of cefuroxime sodium and metronidazole in an admixture for intravenous infusion, *J Clin Pharm Ther* 15:187–196, 1990.

1566. Weir PJ and Ireland DS: Chemical stability of cytarabine and vinblastine injections, *Br J Pharm Pract* 12:53, 54, 60 (Feb) 1990.

1567. Vincke BJ, Verstraeten AE, El Eini DID, et al.: Extended stability of 5-fluorouracil and methotrexate solutions in PVC containers, *Int J Pharm* 54:181–189, 1989.

1568. Stevens RF and Wilkins KM: Use of cytotoxic drugs with an end-line filter—a study of four drugs commonly administered to paediatric patients, *J Clin Pharm Ther* 14:475–479, 1989.

1569. Garner ST and Murdoch JM: Dopamine dilutions, *Pharm J* 244:218 (Feb 24) 1990.

1570. Schroder F and Schutz H: Kompatibilitat von heparin und gentamicin sulfat, *Pharm Ztg* 134:24–26 (July 27) 1989.

1571. Adams PS, Haines-Nutt RF, and Ross ID: The stability of aminophylline intravenous infusion solutions, *Proc Guild* 25:41–44 (Autumn) 1988.

1572. Schaaf LJ, Tremel LC, Wulf BG, et al.: Compatibility of enalaprilat with dopamine, dopamine, heparin, nitroglycerin, potassium chloride, and nitroprusside, *J Clin Pharm Ther* 15:371–376 (5) 1990.

1573. Kern JW, Lee KJ, Martinoff JT, et al.: The in vivo availability of gentamicin when admixed with total nutrient solutions: a comparative study, *J Parenter Enter Nutr* 14:523–526 (Sep–Oct) 1990.

1574. Montoro JB, Galard R, Catalan R, et al.: Stability of somatostatin in total parenteral nutrition, *Pharm Weekbl Sci Ed* 12:240–242 (Dec 14) 1990.

1575. Sauer H: Aufbewahrung von zytostatika-losungen, *Krankenhauspharmazie* 11:373–375 (Sep) 1990.

1576. Shea BF and Souney PF: Stability of famotidine in a 3-in-1 total nutrient admixture, *DICP Ann Pharmacother* 24:232–235 (Mar) 1990.

1577. De Vroe C, De Muynck C, Remon JP, et al.: A study on the stability of three antineoplastic drugs and on their sorption by i.v. delivery systems and end-line filters, *Int J Pharm* 65:49–56 (Nov 28) 1990.

1578. Raymond GG and Davis RL: Physical compatibility and chemical stability of amphotericin B in combination with magnesium sulfate in 5% dextrose injection, *DICP Ann Pharmacother* 25:123–126 (Feb) 1991.

1579. Prammar Y, Gupta VD, Gardner SN, et al.: Stabilities of dobutamine, dopamine, nitroglycerin, and sodium nitroprusside in disposable plastic syringes, *J Clin Pharm Ther* 16:203–207 (3) 1991.

1580. Stewart JT, Warren FW, Johnson SM, et al.: Stability of ceftazidime in plastic syringes and glass vials under various storage conditions, *Am J Hosp Pharm* 49:2765–2768 (Nov) 1992.

1581. Stiles ML, Allen LV Jr, and Fox JL: Stability of ceftazidime (with arginine) and cefuroxime sodium in infusion-pump reservoirs, *Am J Hosp Pharm* 49:2761–2764 (Nov) 1992.

1582. Kaufman MB, Scavone JM, and Foley JJ: Stability of undiluted trimethoprim–sulfamethoxazole for injection in plastic syringes, *Am J Hosp Pharm* 49:2782–2783 (Nov) 1992.

1583. Nahata MC, Morosco RS, and Hipple TF: Stability of morphine sulfate in bacteriostatic 0.9% sodium chloride injection stored in glass vials at two temperatures, *Am J Hosp Pharm* 49:2785–2786 (Nov) 1992.

1584. Nahata MC, Morosco RS, and Fox JF: Stability of ceftazidime (with arginine) stored in plastic syringes at three temperatures, *Am J Hosp Pharm* 49:2954–2956 (Dec) 1992.

1585. Mawhinney WM, Adair CG, Gorman SP, et al.: Stability of ciprofloxacin in peritoneal dialysis solutions, *Am J Hosp Pharm* 49:2956–2959 (Dec) 1992.

1586. Nahata MC, Morosco RS, and Hipple TF: Stability of aminophylline in bacteriostatic water for injection stored in plastic syringes at two temperatures, *Am J Hosp Pharm* 49:2962–2963 (Dec) 1992.

1587. Allwood MC: The influence of buffering on the stability of erythromycin injection in small-volume infusions, *Int J Pharm* 80:R7–R9 (Feb 10) 1992.

1588. Toki N: Glass adsorption of highly purified urokinase, *Thromb Haemost* 43:67, 1980.

1589. Zimmerman R, Schoffel G, and Harenberg J: Urokinase therapy: dose reduction by administration in plastic material, *Thromb Haemost* 45:296 (3) 1981.

1590. Walker SE and Iazzetta J: Compatibility and stability of pentobarbital infusions, *Anesthesiology* 55:487–489 (Oct) 1981.

1591. Walker SE and Iazzetta J: Cefotetan stability in normal saline and five percent dextrose in water, *Can J Hosp Pharm* 45:9–13, 37 (1) 1992.

1592. Nahata MC: Stability of ceftriaxone sodium in peritoneal dialysis solutions, *DICP Ann Pharmacother* 25:741–742 (July–Aug) 1991.

1593. Walker SE, Lau DWC, DeAngelis C, et al.: Mitoxantrone stability in syringes and glass vials and evaluation of chemical contamination, *Can J Hosp Pharm* 44:143–151 (June) 1991.

1594. Walker S, Lau D, DeAngelis C, et al.: Doxorubicin stability in syringes and glass vials and evaluation of chemical contamination, *Can J Hosp Pharm* 44:71–78, 88 (Apr) 1991.

1595. Peterson GM, Khoo BHC, Galloway JG, et al.: A preliminary study of the stability of midazolam in polypropylene syringes, *Aust J Hosp Pharm* 21:115–118 (Apr) 1991.

1596. Lecompte D, Bousselet M, Gayrard D, et al.: Stability study of reconstituted and diluted solutions of calcium folinate, *Pharm Ind* 53:90–94 (1) 1991.

1597. Allwood MC: The stability of erythromycin injection in small-volume infusions, *Int J Pharm* 62:R1–R3 (July 15) 1990.

1598. Gupta VD, Pramar Y, Odom C, et al.: Chemical stability of cefotetan disodium in 5% dextrose and 0.9% sodium chloride injections, *J Clin Pharm Ther* 15:109–114, 1990.

1599. Poggi GL: Compatibility of morphine tartrate admixtures in polypropylene syringes, *Aust J Hosp Pharm* 21:316 (Oct) 1991.

1600. McLaughlin JP and Simpson C: The stability of reconstituted aztreonam, *Br J Pharm Pract* 12:328, 330, 334 (Oct) 1990.

1601. Biejnen JH, van Gijn R, Horenblas S, et al.: Chemical stability of suramin in commonly used infusion fluids, *DICP Ann Pharmacother* 24:1056–1058 (Nov) 1990.

1602. Patel JP: Urokinase: stability studies in solution and lyophilized formulations, *Drug Dev Ind Pharm* 16:2613–2626, 1990.

1603. Driver AG and Worden JP Jr: Intravenous streptomycin, *DICP Ann Pharmacother* 24:826–828 (Sep) 1990.

1604. Bosso JA: Clindamycin stability, *DICP Ann Pharmacother* 24:1008–1009 (Oct) 1990.

1605. Theuer H, Scherbel G, Distler F, et al.: Cisplatin-injektionslosung, *Krankenhauspharmazie* 11:288–291 (July) 1990.

1606. Bluhm DP, Summers RS, Lowes MMJ, et al.: Influence of container on vitamin A stability in TPN admixtures, *Int J Pharm* 68:281–283 (Feb 1) 1991.

1607. Bluhm DP, Summers RS, Lowes MMJ, et al.: Lipid emulsion content and vitamin A stability in TPN admixtures, *Int J Pharm* 68:277–280 (Feb 1) 1991.

1608. Beijnen J and Koks CHW: Visual compatibility of ondansetron and dexamethasone, *DICP Ann Pharmacother* 25:869 (July–Aug) 1991.

1609. Lawson WA, Longmore RB, McDonald C, et al.: Stability of hyoscine in mixtures with morphine for continuous subcutaneous administration, *Aust J Hosp Pharm* 21:395–396 (Dec) 1991.

1610. Allwood MC: The stability of four catecholamines in 5% glucose infusions, *J Clin Pharm Ther* 16:337–340 (5) 1991.

1611. Van Asten P, Glerum JH, Spaanderman ER, et al.: Compatibility of bupivacaine and iohexol in two mixtures for paediatric regional anaesthesia, *Pharm Weekbl Sci Ed* 13:254–256 (6) 1991.

1612. Sewell GJ and Palmer AJ: The chemical and physical stability of three intravenous infusions subjected to frozen storage and microwave thawing, *Int J Pharm* 72:57–63 (May 13) 1991.

1613. Janknegt R, Stratermans T, Cilissen J, et al.: Ofloxacin intravenous—compatibility with other antibacterial agents, *Pharm Weekbl Sci Ed* 13:207–209 (Oct 18) 1991.

1614. Dunham B, Marcuard S, Khazanie PG, et al.: The solubility of calcium and phosphorus in neonatal total parenteral nutrition solutions, *J Parenter Enter Nutr* 15:608–611 (Nov–Dec) 1991.

1615. Delaney RA, Mikkelsen SL, and Jackson MB: Effects of heat treatment on selected plasma therapeutic drug concentrations, *Ann Pharmacother* 26:338–340 (Mar) 1992.

1616. McLeod HL, McGuire TR, and Yee GC: Stability of cyclosporine in dextrose 5%, NaCl 0.9%, dextrose/amino acid solution, and lipid emulsion, *Ann Pharmacother* 26:172–175 (Feb) 1992.

1617. Andreu A, Cardona D, Pastor C, et al.: Intravenous aminophylline: in vitro stability in fat-containing TPN, *Ann Pharmacother* 26:127–128 (Jan) 1992.

1618. Matsuura G: Visual compatibility of sargramostim (GM-CSF) during simulated Y-site administration with selected agents, *Hosp Pharm* 27:200, 202, 209 (Mar) 1992.

1619. De Muynck C, Colardyn F, and Remon JP: Influence of intravenous administration set composition on the sorption of isosorbide dinitrate, *J Pharm Pharmacol* 43:601–604 (Sep) 1991.

1620. Bullock L, Fitzgerald JF, and Walter WV: Emulsion stability in total nutrient admixtures containing a pediatric amino acid formulation, *J Parenter Enter Nutr* 16:64–68 (Jan–Feb) 1992.

1621. Olbrich A: Weichmacher als problematische bestandteile von mischinfusionen, *Krankenhauspharmazie* 12:192–194 (May) 1991.

1622. Cano SM, Montoro JB, Pastor C, et al.: Stability of cimetidine in total parenteral nutrition, *J Clin Nutr Gastroenter* 2:40–43 (1) 1987.

1623. Loeppky C, Tarka E, and Everett ED: Compatibility of cephalosporins and aminoglycosides in peritoneal dialysis fluid, *Perit Dial Bull* 3:128–129, 1983.

1624. Bhatt-Mehta V, Rosen DA, King RS, et al.: Stability of midazolam hydrochloride in parenteral nutrient solutions, *Am J Hosp Pharm* 50:285–288 (Feb) 1993.

1625. Jacobson PA, Maksym CJ, Landvay A, et al.: Compatibility of cyclosporine with fat emulsion, *Am J Hosp Pharm* 50:687–690 (Apr) 1993.

1626. Johnson CE, Jacobson PA, Pillen HA, et al.: Stability and compatibility of fluconazole and aminophylline in intravenous admixtures, *Am J Hosp Pharm* 50:703–706 (Apr) 1993.

1627. Allen LV Jr, Stiles ML, Wang DP, et al.: Stability of bupivacaine hydrochloride, epinephrine hydrochloride, and fentanyl citrate in portable infusion-pump reservoirs, *Am J Hosp Pharm* 50:714–715 (Apr) 1993.

1628. Percy LA and Rho JP: Visual compatibility of ciprofloxacin with selected components of total parenteral nutrient solutions during simulated Y-site injection, *Am J Hosp Pharm* 50:715–716 (Apr) 1993.

1629. Nieforth KA, Shea BF, Souney PF, et al.: Stability of cyclosporine with magnesium sulfate in 5% dextrose injection, *Am J Hosp Pharm* 50:470–472 (Mar) 1993.

1630. Min DI, Brown T, and Hwang GC: Visual compatibility of tacrolimus with commonly used drugs during simulated Y-site injection, *Am J Hosp Pharm* 49:2964–2966 (Dec) 1992.

1631. Dine T, Luyckx M, Cazin JC, et al.: Stability and compatibility studies of vinblastine, vincristine, vindesine and vinorelbine with PVC infusion bags, *Int J Pharm* 77:279–285 (Nov 15) 1991.

1632. Inagaki K, Gill MA, Okamoto MP, et al.: Stability of ranitidine hydrochloride with aztreonam, ceftazidime, or piperacillin sodium during simulated Y-site administration, *Am J Hosp Pharm* 49:2769–2772 (Nov) 1992.

1633. Mitra AK and Narurkar MM: Kinetics of azathioprine degradation in aqueous solution, *Int J Pharm* 35:165–171, 1986.

1634. Snyder RL: Filter clogging caused by albumin in i.v. nutrient solution, *Am J Hosp Pharm* 50:63–64 (Jan) 1993.

1635. Feldman F and Bergman G: Filter clogging caused by albumin in i.v. nutrient solution, *Am J Hosp Pharm* 50:64 (Jan) 1993.

1636. Bornstein M, Kao SH, Mercorelli M, et al.: Stability of an ofloxacin injection in various infusion fluids, *Am J Hosp Pharm* 49:2756–2760 (Nov) 1992.

1637. Heni J: Rekonstituierte ganciclovirlosung, *Krankenhauspharmazie* 12:342–344 (Aug) 1991.

1638. Theuer H, Scherbel G, and Windsheimer U: Stabilitatsuntersuchungen von fentanylcitrat i.v., *Krankenhauspharmazie* 12:233–245 (June) 1991.

1639. Burger DM, Brandjes DPM, Koks CHW, et al.: Heparine in het heparineslot? *Pharm Weekbl* 126:624–627 (July 5) 1991.

1640. Witmer DR: Heparin lock flush solution versus 0.9% sodium chloride injection for maintaining patency, *Am J Hosp Pharm* 50:241 (Feb) 1993.

1641. Weber DR: Is heparin really necessary in the lock and, if so, how much? *DICP Ann Pharmacother* 25:399–407 (Apr) 1991.

1642. Bosso JA, Prince RA, and Fox JL: Stability of ondansetron hydrochloride in injectable solutions at −20, 5, and 25 °C, *Am J Hosp Pharm* 49:2223–2225 (Sep) 1992.

1643. Parasrampuria J, Li LC, Stelmach AH, et al.: Stability of ganciclovir sodium in 5% dextrose injection and in 0.9% sodium chloride injection over 35 days, *Am J Hosp Pharm* 49:116–118 (Jan) 1992.

1644. Guo-jie JL: Compatibility of bumetanide injection and dextrose injection, *Yaoxue Tongbao* 24:86–87 (Feb) 1989.

1645. Buck GW and Wolfe KR: Interaction of sodium ascorbate with stainless steel particulate-filter needles, *Am J Hosp Pharm* 48:1191 (June) 1991.

1646. Floy BJ, Royko CG, and Fleitman JS: Compatibility of ketorolac tromethamine injection with common infusion fluids and administration sets, *Am J Hosp Pharm* 47:1097–1100 (May) 1990.

1647. Zieske PA, Koberda M, Hines JL, et al.: Characterization of cisplatin degradation as affected by pH and light, *Am J Hosp Pharm* 48:1500–1506 (July) 1991.

1648. Tu YH, Knox NL, Biringer JM, et al.: Compatibility of iron dextran with total nutrient admixtures, *Am J Hosp Pharm* 49:2233–2235 (Sep) 1992.

1649. Rivers TE, McBride HA, and Trang JM: Stability of cefazolin sodium and metronidazole at 8 °C for use as an IV admixture, *J Parenter Sci Tech* 47:135–137 (May–June) 1993.

1650. Inagaki K, Gill MA, Okamoto MP, et al.: Chemical compatibility of cefmetazole sodium with ranitidine hydrochloride during simulated Y-site administration, *J Parenter Sci Tech* 47:35–39 (Jan–Feb) 1993.

1651. Washington C and Sizer T: Stability of TPN mixtures compounded from Lipofundin S and Aminoplex amino-acid solutions: comparison of laser diffraction and Coulter counter droplet size analysis, *Int J Pharm* 83:227–231 (June 30) 1992.

1652. Mason NA, Johnson CE, and O'Brien MA: Stability of ceftazidime and tobramycin sulfate in peritoneal dialysis solution, *Am J Hosp Pharm* 49:1139–1142 (May) 1992.

1653. Corbo DC, Suddith RL, Sharma B, et al.: Stability, potency, and preservative effectiveness of epoetin alfa after addition of a bacteriostatic diluent, *Am J Hosp Pharm* 49:1455–1458 (June) 1992.

1654. Mawhinney WM, Adair CG, Gorman SP, et al.: Stability of vancomycin hydrochloride in peritoneal dialysis solution, *Am J Hosp Pharm* 49:137–139 (Jan) 1992.

1655. Cervenka P, DeJong DJ, Butler BL, et al.: Visual compatibility of injectable ciprofloxacin lactate with selected injectable drugs during simulated Y-site administration, *Hosp Pharm* 27:957–958, 961–962 (Nov) 1992.

1656. Garrelts JC, LaRocca J, Ast D, et al.: Comparison of heparin and 0.9% sodium chloride injection in the maintenance of indwelling intermittent i.v. devices, *Clin Pharm* 8:34–39 (Jan) 1989.

1657. Lewis JS: Justification for use of 1.2 micron end-line filters on total nutrient admixtures, *Hosp Pharm* 28:656–658, 697 (July) 1993.

1658. Benvenuto JA, Adams SC, Vyas HM, et al.: Pharmaceutical issues in infusion chemotherapy stability and compatibility, *in* Lokich JJ (ed), Cancer chemotherapy by infusion, Precept Press, Chicago, Illinois, 1987, pp 100–113.

1659. Briceland LL, Fudin J, and Johnson KR: Evaluation of microbial growth in select inoculated antineoplastic solutions, *Hosp Pharm* 25:338–340, 359 (Apr) 1990.

1660. Neels JT: Compatibility of bupivacaine hydrochloride with hydromorphone hydrochloride or morphine sulfate, *Am J Hosp Pharm* 49:2149 (Sep) 1992.

1661. Hauser AR, Trissel LA, and Martinez JF: Ondansetron compatible with sodium acetate, *J Clin Oncol* 11:197 (Jan) 1993.

1662. Pecosky DA, Parasrampuria J, Li LC, et al.: Stability and sorption of calcitriol in plastic tuberculin syringes, *Am J Hosp Pharm* 49:1463–1466 (June) 1992.

1663. Gregory R, Edwards S, and Yateman NA: Demonstration of insulin transformation products in insulin vials by high-performance liquid chromatography, *Diabetes Care* 14:42–48 (Jan) 1991.

1664. Seres DS: Insulin adsorption to parenteral infusion systems: case report and review of the literature, *Nutr Clin Pract* 5:111–117 (June) 1990.

1665. Lazorova L, Haronikova K, and Mandak M: Studium sorpcie inzulinu v priebehu infuznej terapie, *Farm Obz* 59:157–164 (Apr) 1990.

1666. Stolk LML and Chandi LS: Stabiliteit van fluorouracil (0,55 mg) in polypropyleen spuiten bij −20 °C, *Ziekenhuisfarmacie* 7:12–13 (1) 1991.

1667. de Vogel EM, Hendrikx MMP, van Dellen RT, et al.: Adsorptie van sufentanil aan bacteriefilters, *Ziekenhuisfarmacie* 7:65–70 (3) 1991.

1668. Hehenberger H: Fettemulsionen kompatibilitat wahrend der bypass-infusion, *Krankenhauspharmazie* 10:513–518 (Dec) 1989.

1669. Carstens G: Calcium-folinat uberlegungen zur stabilitat und zum einsatz verschiedener zubereitungen, *Krankenhauspharmazie* 10:478–482 (Nov) 1989.

1670. Washington C: The stability of intravenous fat emulsions in total parenteral nutrition mixtures, *Int J Pharm* 66:1–21 (Dec 1) 1990.

1671. Allwood MC and Brown PW: The effect of buffering on the stability of reconstituted benzylpenicillin injection, *Int J Pharm Pract* 1:242–244 (Aug) 1992.

1672. Allwood MC: The stability of diamorphine alone and in combination with anti-emetics in plastic syringes, *Palliative Med* 5:330–333, 1991.

1673. Lober CA and Dollard PA: Visual compatibility of gallium nitrate with selected drugs during simulated Y-site injection, *Am J Hosp Pharm* 50:1208–1210 (June) 1993.

1674. Jahns BE and Bakst CM: Extension of expiration time for lorazepam in-

jection at room temperature, *Am J Hosp Pharm* 50:1134 (June) 1993.

1675. Trissel LA and Martinez JF: Idarubicin hydrochloride turbidity versus incompatibility, *Am J Hosp Pharm* 50:1134, 1137 (June) 1993.

1676. Hunt-Fugate AK, Hennessey CK, and Kazarian CM: Stability of fluconazole injectable solutions, *Am J Hosp Pharm* 50:1186–1187 (June) 1993.

1677. Inagaki K, Takagi J, Lor E, et al.: Stability of fluconazole in commonly used intravenous antibiotic solutions, *Am J Hosp Pharm* 50:1206–1208 (June) 1993.

1678. Liao E, Fox JL, and Dukes GE: Inline filtration of ondansetron hydrochloride during simulated i.v. administration, *Am J Hosp Pharm* 50:906, 909 (May) 1993.

1679. Belliveau PP, Shea BF, and Scavone JM: Stability of metoprolol tartrate in 5% dextrose injection or 0.9% sodium chloride injection, *Am J Hosp Pharm* 50:950–952 (May) 1993.

1680. Ringwood MA: Stability of cefepime for injection for IM or IV use following constitution/dilution, Bristol-Myers Company, Syracuse, New York, August 16, 1990.

1681. Ringwood MA and Vance VH: Cefepime IM, IV, and compatibility studies for U.S. registrational filing, Bristol-Myers Squibb Company, Syracuse, New York, May 13, 1992.

1682. Vance VH: Stability of cefepime admixed with vancomycin, metronidazole, ampicillin, clindamycin, tobramycin, netilmicin, TPN solution, and PD solution, Bristol-Myers Squibb Company, Syracuse, New York, October 14, 1992.

1683. Pearson SD and Trissel LA: Leaching of diethylhexyl phthalate from polyvinyl chloride containers by selected drugs and formulation components, *Am J Hosp Pharm* 50:1405–1409 (July) 1993.

1684. Trissel LA and Pearson SD: Storage of lorazepam in three injectable solutions in polyvinyl chloride and polyolefin bags, *Am J Hosp Pharm* 51:368–372 (Feb 1) 1994.

1685. Reilly MD and Trissel LA: Visual compatibility of cisplatin, cyclophosphamide, doxorubicin HCl, and methotrexate sodium with selected drugs during simulated Y-site injection, Data on file, Pharmaceutical Analysis Laboratory, University of Texas, M. D. Anderson Cancer Center, Houston, Texas, January 15, 1990.

1686. Trissel LA and Martinez JF: Compatibility of allopurinol sodium with selected drugs during simulated Y-site administration, *Am J Hosp Pharm* 51:792–799 (July 15) 1994.

1687. Trissel LA and Martinez JF: Compatibility of filgrastim with selected drugs during simulated Y-site administration, *Am J Hosp Pharm* 51:1907–1913 (Aug 1) 1994.

1688. Trissel LA and Martinez JF: Compatibility of piperacillin sodium plus tazobactam sodium with selected drugs during simulated Y-site injection, *Am J Hosp Pharm* 51:672–678 (Mar 1) 1994.

1689. Trissel LA, Martinez JF, and Xu Q: Data on file, Pharmaceutical Analysis Laboratory, University of Texas, M. D. Anderson Cancer Center, Houston, Texas, January 24, 1994.

1690. Trissel LA, Xu Q, Martinez JF, et al.: Compatibility and stability of ondansetron hydrochloride with morphine sulfate and hydromorphone hydrochloride in 0.9% sodium chloride injection at various temperatures, *Am J Hosp Pharm* 51:2138–2142 (Sep 1) 1994.

1691. Belliveau PP, Nightingale CH, and Quintiliani R: Stability of aztreonam and ampicillin/sulbactam in 0.9% saline for injection, *Am J Hosp Pharm* 51:901–904 (Apr 1) 1994.

1692. Fisher DM, Canfell C, and Miller RD: Stability of atracurium administered by infusion, *Anesthesiology* 61:347–348 (Sep) 1984.

1693. Harper NJN, Pollard BJ, Edwards D, et al.: Stability of atracurium in dilute solutions, *Br J Anaeth* 60:344P–345P (Feb) 1988.

1694. Talton MA (Drug Information, Burroughs Wellcome Company, Research Triangle Park, North Carolina): Personal communication, June 11, 1993.

1695. Perrone RK, Kaplan MA, and Bogardus JB: Extent of cisplatin formation in carboplatin admixtures, *Am J Hosp Pharm* 46:258–259 (Feb) 1989.

1696. Northcott M, Allsopp MA, Powell H, et al.: The stability of carboplatin, diamorphine, 5-fluorouracil and mitozantrone infusions in an ambulatory pump under storage and prolonged "in-use" conditions, *J Clin Pharm Ther* 16:123–129, 1991.

1697. Ahmed ST and Parkinson R: The stability of drugs in pre-filled syringes: flucloxacillin, ampicillin, cefuroxime, cefotaxime, and ceftazidime, *Hosp Pharm Pract* 2:285–289 (Apr) 1992.

1698. Faouzi MA, Dine T, Luyckx M, et al.: Stability and compatibility studies of pefloxacin, ofloxacin and ciprofloxacin with PVC infusion bags, *Int J Pharm* 89:125–131, 1993.

1699. Stiles ML, Allen LV Jr, and Fox JL: Gas production of three brands of ceftazidime, *Am J Hosp Pharm* 48:1727–1729 (Aug) 1991.

1700. Dine T, Cazin JC, Gressier B, et al.: Stability and compatibility of four anthracyclines: doxorubicin, epirubicin, daunorubicin, and pirarubicin with PVC infusion bags, *Pharm Weekbl Sci Ed 14*:365–369 (6) 1992.

1701. Trissel LA and Martinez JF: Sargramostim incompatibility, *Hosp Pharm 27*:929 (Oct) 1992.

1702. Trissel LA: Alternative interpretation for data, *Am J Hosp Pharm 49*:570 (Mar) 1992.

1703. Knapp AJ, Mauro VF, and Alexander KS: Incompatibility of ketorolac tromethamine with selected postoperative drugs, *Am J Hosp Pharm 49*:2960–2962 (Dec) 1992.

1704. Trissel LA: Data on file, Pharmaceutical Analysis Laboratory, University of Texas, M. D. Anderson Cancer Center, Houston, Texas, October 29, 1993.

1705. Cohon MS (Clinical Development and Medical Affairs, The Upjohn Company, Kalamazoo, Michigan): Personal communication, December 6, 1993.

1706. DeArmond B (Medical Affairs Divison, Syntex Laboratories, Inc., Palo Alto, California): Personal communication, December 28, 1993.

1707. Nation RL, Hackett LP, and Dusci LJ: Uptake of clonazepam by plastic intravenous infusion bags and administration sets, *Am J Hosp Pharm 40*:1692–1693 (Oct) 1983.

1708. Hooymans PM, Janknegt R, and Lohman JJHM: Comparison of clonazepam sorption to polyvinyl chloride-coated and polyethylene-coated tubings, *Pharm Weekbl Sci Ed 12*:188–189 (July) 1990.

1709. McLaughlin JP and Simpson C: The stability of reconstituted diethanolamine fusidate in a 5% dextrose infusion, *Hosp Pharm Pract 2*:59–62 (Jan) 1992.

1710. Olsen KM, Gurley BJ, Davis GA, et al.: Stability of flumazenil with selected drugs in 5% dextrose injection, *Am J Hosp Pharm 50*:1907–1912 (Sep) 1993.

1711. Trissel LA and Martinez JF: Sufentanil data on file, Pharmaceutical Analysis Laboratory, University of Texas, M. D. Anderson Cancer Center, Houston, Texas, February 1995.

1712. Larson PO, Ragi G, Swandby M, et al.: Stability of buffered lidocaine and epinephrine used for local anesthesia, *J Dermatol Surg Oncol 17*:411–414, 1991.

1713. Stewart JH, Cole GW, and Klein JA: Neutralized lidocaine with epinephrine for local anesthesia, *J Dermatol Surg Oncol 15*:1081–1083 (Oct) 1989.

1714. Nahata MC, Morosco RS, and Hipple TF: Stability of cimetidine hydrochloride and of clindamycin phosphate in water for injection stored in glass vials at two temperatures, *Am J Hosp Pharm 50*:2559–2561 (Dec) 1993.

1715. Zeisler J and Alagna C: Incompatibility of labetalol hydrochloride and furosemide, *Am J Hosp Pharm 50*:2521–2522 (Dec) 1993.

1716. Pfeifer RW and Hale KN: Precipitation of paclitaxel during infusion by pump, *Am J Hosp Pharm 50*:2518, 2521 (Dec) 1993.

1717. Hagan RL, Jacobs LF, Pimsler M, et al.: Stability of midazolam hydrochloride in 5% dextrose injection or 0.9% sodium chloride injection over 30 days, *Am J Hosp Pharm 50*:2379–2381 (Nov) 1993.

1718. Jones JW and Davis AT: Stability of bupivacaine hydrochloride in polypropylene syringes, *Am J Hosp Pharm 50*:2364–2365 (Nov) 1993.

1719. Vogt C, Skipper PM, and Ruggaber S: Compatibility of magnesium sulfate and morphine sulfate in 0.9% sodium chloride injection, *Am J Hosp Pharm 50*:2311 (Nov) 1993.

1720. Bailey LC, Tang KT, and Medwick T: Stability of ceftriaxone sodium in infusion-pump syringes, *Am J Hosp Pharm 50*:2092–2094 (Oct) 1993.

1721. Szof C and Walker PC: Incompatibility of cefotaxime sodium and vancomycin sulfate during Y-site administration, *Am J Hosp Pharm 50*:2054, 2057 (Oct) 1993.

1722. Jhee SS, Jeong EW, Chin A, et al.: Stability of ondansetron hydrochloride stored in a disposable, elastomeric infusion device at 4 °C, *Am J Hosp Pharm 50*:1918–1920 (Sep) 1993.

1723. Bartfield JM, Homer PJ, Ford DT, et al.: Buffered lidocaine as a local anesthetic: an investigation of shelf life, *Ann Emerg Med 21*:16–19 (Jan) 1992.

1724. Peterfreund RA, Datta S, and Ostheimer GW: pH adjustment of local anesthetic solutions with sodium bicarbonate: laboratory evaluation of alkalinization and precipitation, *Reg Anesth 14*:265–270 (Nov–Dec) 1989.

1725. Trissel LA and Martinez JF: Screening teniposide for Y-site physical incompatibilities, *Hosp Pharm 29*:1012–1014, 1017 (Nov) 1994.

1726. Woods K, Steinman W, Bruns L, et al.: Stability of foscarnet sodium in 0.9% sodium chloride injection, *Am J Hosp Pharm 51*:88–90 (Jan 1) 1994.

1727. Parrish MA, Bailey LC, and Medwick T: Stability of ceftriaxone sodium and aminophylline or theophylline in intravenous admixtures, *Am J Hosp Pharm 51*:92–94 (Jan 1) 1994.

1728. Lee MD, Hess MM, Boucher BA, et al.: Stability of amphotericin B in 5% dextrose injection stored at 4 or 25 °C for 120 hours, *Am J Hosp Pharm 51*:394–396 (Feb 1) 1994.

1729. Trissel LA and Martinez JF: Data on file, Pharmaceutical Analysis Laboratory, University of Texas, M. D. Anderson Cancer Center, Houston, Texas, November 1994.

1730. Pompilio FM, Fox JL, Inagaki K, et al.: Stability of ranitidine hydrochloride with ondansetron hydrochloride or fluconazole during simulated Y-site administration, *Am J Hosp Pharm 51*:391–394 (Feb 1) 1994.

1731. Wolff DJ, Kline SS, and Mauro LS: Stability of amikacin, gentamicin, or tobramycin in 10% dextrose injection, *Am J Hosp Pharm 51*:518–519 (Feb 15) 1994.

1732. Bosso JA, Prince RA, and Fox JL: Compatibility of ondansetron hydrochloride with fluconazole, ceftazidime, aztreonam, and cefazolin sodium under simulated Y-site conditions, *Am J Hosp Pharm 51*:389–391 (Feb 1) 1994.

1733. Stiles ML, Allen LV Jr, Prince SJ, et al.: Stability of dexamethasone sodium phosphate, diphenhydramine hydrochloride, lorazepam, and metoclopramide hydrochloride in portable infusion-pump reservoirs, *Am J Hosp Pharm 51*:514–517 (Feb 15) 1994.

1734. Messerschmidt W: Kompatibilitat von ofloxacin mit ampicillin, *Krankenhauspharmazie 15*:337–340 (6) 1994.

1735. Messerschmidt W: Kompatibilitat von cefotaxim mit ofloxacin, *Pharmazie 136*:42–44 (Sep) 1991.

1736. Trissel LA, Gilbert D, and Martinez JF: Data on file, Pharmaceutical Analysis Laboratory, University of Texas, M. D. Anderson Cancer Center, Houston, Texas, August 1995.

1737. Messerschmidt W: Kompatibilitat von cefotiam mit metronidazol, *Krankenhauspharmazie 7*:263–265 (6) 1986.

1738. Messerschmidt W: Pharmazeutische kompatibilitat der kombination cefotiam und ampicillin, *Krankenhauspharmazie 13*:98–100 (3) 1992.

1739. Cronquist SE and Daniels M: Precipitation of paclitaxel during infusion by pump, *Am J Hosp Pharm 50*:2521 (Dec) 1993.

1740. Fraser GL and Riker RR: Visual compatibility of haloperidol lactate with injectable solutions, *Am J Hosp Pharm 51*:905–906 (Apr 1) 1994.

1741. Burm JP, Jhee SS, Chin A, et al.: Stability of paclitaxel with ondansetron hydrochloride or ranitidine hydrochloride during simulated Y-site administration, *Am J Hosp Pharm 51*:1201–1204 (May 1) 1994.

1742. Mulye NV, Turco SJ, and Speaker TJ: Stability of ganciclovir sodium in an infusion-pump syringe, *Am J Hosp Pharm 51*:1348–1349 (May 15) 1994.

1743. Bonhomme L, Benhamou D, Comoy E, et al.: Stability of adrenaline pH-adjusted solutions of local anaesthetics, *J Pharm Biomed Anal 9*:497–499 (6) 1991.

1744. Johnson CE, Jacobson PA, and Chan E: Stability of ganciclovir sodium and amino acids in parenteral nutrient solutions, *Am J Hosp Pharm 51*:503–508 (Feb 15) 1994.

1745. Abubakar AA, Mustapha A, and Wambebe OC: An in vitro chemical interaction between promethazine hydrochloride and chloroquine phosphate, *Int J Pharm 7*:14–19 (1) 1993.

1746. Xu Q, Trissel LA, and Martinez JF: Stability of paclitaxel in 5% dextrose injection or 0.9% sodium chloride injection at 4, 22, or 32 °C, *Am J Hosp Pharm 51*:3058–3060 (Dec 15) 1994.

1747. Kearney AS, Patel K, and Palepu NR: Preformulation studies to aid in the development of a ready-to-use injectable solution of the antitumor agent, topotecan, *Int J Pharm 127*:229–237 (Feb 17) 1996.

1748. Cilissen J, Hooymans PM, and Lohman JJHM: Indicatie van de stabiliteit van een mengsel van piperacilline en flucloxacilline in een reservoir voor een draagbare infusiepomp, *Ziekenhuisfarmacie 10*:10–11, 1994.

1749. Banerjee PS, Ghosh LK, and Gupta BK: Studies on the effects of some additives on the stability of injectable formulations of diazepam, *Indian Drugs 29*:361–364 (8) 1992.

1750. Lorillon P, Corbel JC, Mordelet MF, et al.: Photosensibilite du 5-fluorouracile et du methotrexate dans des perfuseurs translucides ou opaques, *J Pharm Clin 11*:285–295, 1992.

1751. Brouwers JRBJ, van Doorne H, Meevis RF, et al.: Stability of sufentanil citrate and sufentanil citrate/bupivacaine mixture in portable infusion pump reservoirs, *Eur Hosp Pharm 1*:12–14 (Jan) 1995.

1752. Chung KC, Moon YSK, Chin A, et al.: Compatibility of ondansetron hydrochloride and piperacillin sodium–tazobactam sodium during simulated Y-site administration, *Am J Health-Syst Pharm 52*:1554–1556 (July 15) 1995.

1753. Erickson SH and Ulici D: Incompatibility of cefotetan disodium and promethazine hydrochloride, *Am J Health-Syst Pharm 52*:1347 (June 15) 1995.

1754. Belliveau PP, Nightingale CH, and Quintiliani R: Stability of cefotaxime sodium and metronidazole in 0.9% sodium chloride injection or in ready-to-use metronidazole bags, *Am J Health-Syst Pharm 52*:1561–1563 (July 15) 1995.

1755. Roos PJ, Glerum JH, and Meilink JW: Stability of sufentanil citrate in a portable pump reservoir, a glass container and a polyethylene container, *Pharm Weekbl Sci Ed 14*:196–200 (4) 1992.

1756. Roos PJ, Glerum JH, and Schroeders MJH: Effect of glucose 5% solution and bupivacaine hydrochloride on adsorption of sufentanil citrate in a portable pump reservoir during storage and simulated infusion by an epidural catheter, *Pharm World Sci 15*:269–275 (6) 1993.

1757. Benaji B, Dine T, Luyckx M, et al.: Stability and compatibility of cisplatin and carboplatin with PVC infusion bags, *J Clin Pharm Ther 19*:95–100, 1994.

1758. Trissel LA and Martinez JF: Compatibility of aztreonam with selected drugs during simulated Y-site administration, *Am J Health-Syst Pharm 52*:1086–1090 (May 15) 1995.

1759. Choi JS, Burm JP, Jhee SS, et al.: Stability of piperacillin sodium–tazobactam sodium and ranitidine hydrochloride in 0.9% sodium chloride injection during simulated Y-site administration, *Am J Hosp Pharm 51*:2273–2276 (Sep 15) 1994.

1760. Ishisaka DY: Visual compatibility of fluconazole with drugs given by continuous infusion, *Am J Hosp Pharm 51*:2290, 2292 (Sep 15) 1994.

1761. Fawcett JP, Woods DJ, Munasiri B, et al.: Compatibility of cyclizine lactate and haloperidol lactate, *Am J Hosp Pharm 51*:2292 (Sep 15) 1994.

1762. Hassan E, Leslie J, and Martir-Herrero ML: Stability of labetalol hydrochloride with selected critical care drugs during simulated Y-site injection, *Am J Hosp Pharm 51*:2143–2145 (Sep 1) 1994.

1763. Wang DP, Chang LC, Wong CY, et al.: Stability of cefazolin sodium–famotidine admixture, *Am J Hosp Pharm 51*:2205, 2209 (Sep 1) 1994.

1764. Singh RF, Corelli RL, and Guglielmo BJ: Sterility of unit dose syringes of filgrastim and sargramostim, *Am J Hosp Pharm 51*:2811–2812 (Nov 15) 1994.

1765. Kleinberg ML: Sterility of repackaged filgrastim and sargramostim, *Am J Health-Syst Pharm 52*:1101 (May 15) 1995.

1766. Kirkham JC, Rutherford ET, Cunningham GN, et al.: Stability of ondansetron hydrochloride in a total parenteral nutrient admixture, *Am J Health-Syst Pharm 52*:1557–1558 (July 15) 1995.

1767. Gilbar PJ and Groves CF: Visual compatibility of total parenteral nutrition solution (Synthamin 17 premix) with selected drugs during simulated Y-site injection, *Aust J Hosp Pharm 24*:167–170 (2) 1994.

1768. Moon YSK, Chung KC, Chin A, et al.: Stability of piperacillin sodium–tazobactam sodium in polypropylene syringes and polyvinyl chloride minibags, *Am J Health-Syst Pharm 52*:999–1001 (May 1) 1995.

1769. Lumpkin MM and Burlington DB: Safety alert: hazards of precipitation associated with parenteral nutrition, *Am J Hosp Pharm 51*:1427–1428 (June 1) 1994.

1770. Hasegawa GR: Caring about stability and compatibility, *Am J Hosp Pharm 51*:1533–1534 (June 15) 1994.

1771. Trissel LA: Compounding our problems, *Am J Hosp Pharm 51*:1534 (June 15) 1994.

1772. Mirtallo JM: The complexity of mixing calcium and phosphate, *Am J Hosp Pharm 51*:1535–1536 (June 15) 1994.

1773. Koorenhof MJC and Timmer JG: Stability of total parenteral nutrition supplied as "all-in-one" for children with chemotherapy-linked hyperhydration, *Pharm Weekbl Sci Ed 14*:50–54 (2) 1992.

1774. Picard C, Brazier M, Hary L, et al.: Stabilite de quatre solutions de penicillines dans des poches et tubulures de perfusion en PVC plastifie, *J Pharm Clin 11*:302–305, 1992.

1775. Szucsova S and Sykora J: Stablita injekcneho pripravku celaskon v infuznych zmesiach, *Farm Obzor 61*:109–112, 1992.

1776. Walker SE, Iazzetta J, De Angelis C, et al.: Stability and compatibility of combinations of hydromorphone and dimenhydrinate, lorazepam or prochlorperazine, *Can J Hosp Pharm. 46*:61–65 (Apr) 1993.

1777. Maswoswe JJ, Okpara AU, and Hilliard MA: An old nemesis: calcium and phosphate interaction in TPN admixtures, *Hosp Pharm 30*:579–580, 582–586 (July) 1995.

1778. Deardorff DL, Schmidt CN, and Wiley RA: Effect of preparation techniques on mixing of additives in intravenous fluids in nonrigid containers, *Hosp Pharm 28*:306, 309–310, 312–313 (Apr) 1993.

1779. Stiles ML, Allen LV Jr, and Prince SJ: Stability of various antibiotics kept in an insulated pouch during administration via portable infusion pump, *Am J Health-Syst Pharm 52*:70–74 (Jan 1) 1995.

1780. Wang DP, Chang LC, Lee DKT, et al.: Stability of fluorouracil–metoclopramide hydrochloride admixture, *Am J Health-Syst Pharm 52*:98–99 (Jan 1) 1995.

1781. Jackson CW and Cunningham K: Compatibility of haloperidol lactate with benztropine mesylate, *Am J Hosp Pharm 51*:2962–2963 (Dec 1) 1994.

1782. Mirtallo JM: Should the use of total nutrient admixtures be limited? *Am J Hosp Pharm 51*:2831–2834 (Nov 15) 1994.

1783. Driscoll DF, Newton DW, and Bistrian BR: Precipitation of calcium phosphate from parenteral nutrient fluids, *Am J Hosp Pharm 51*:2834–2836 (Nov 15) 1994.

1784. Gibler B, Kim MS, and Raleigh F: Visual compatibility of neuroleptics with anticholinergics or antihistamines in polyethylene syringes, *Am J Hosp Pharm 51*:2709–2710 (Nov 1) 1994.

1785. Huang E and Anderson RP: Compatibility of hydromorphone hydrochloride with haloperidol lactate and ketorolac tromethamine, *Am J Hosp Pharm 51*:2963 (Dec 1) 1994.

1786. Mendenhall A and Hoyt DB: Incompatibility of ketorolac tromethamine with haloperidol lactate and thiethylperazine maleate, *Am J Hosp Pharm 51*:2964 (Dec 1) 1994.

1787. Harraki B, Guiraud P, Rochat MH, et al.: Influence of copper, iron, and zinc on the physicochemical properties of parenteral admixture, *J Parenter Sci Technol 47*:199–204 (Sep–Oct) 1993.

1788. Aujoulat P, Coze C, Braguer D, et al.: Compatibilite physico-chimique du methotrexate avec les medicaments co-administres dans les protocols de chimiotherapie, *J Pharm Clin 12*:31–35, 1993.

1789. Johnson CE, Bhatt-Mehta V, Mancari SC, et al.: Stability of midazolam hydrochloride and morphine sulfate during simulated intravenous coadministration, *Am J Hosp Pharm 51*:2812–2813 (Nov 15) 1994.

1790. Burm JP, Choi JS, Jhee SS, et al.: Stability of paclitaxel and fluconazole during simulated Y-site administration, *Am J Hosp Pharm 51*:2704–2706 (Nov 1) 1994.

1791. Grassby PF and Roberts DE: Stability of epidural opiate solutions in 0.9 per cent sodium chloride infusion bags, *Int J Pharm Pract 3*:174–177 (July) 1995.

1792. Allwood MC, Brown PW, and Lee M: Stability of injections containing diamorphine and midazolam in plastic syringes, *Int J Pharm Pract 3*:57–59 (Oct) 1994.

1793. Kershaw BP, Monnier HL, and Mason JH: Visual compatibility of premixed theophylline or heparin with selected drugs for i.v. administration, *Am J Hosp Pharm 50*:1360, 1362–1363 (July) 1993.

1794. Trissel LA: Were the bubbles evolved or entrained? *Am J Health-Syst Pharm 52*:757 (Apr 1) 1995.

1795. Francomb MM, Ford JL, and Lee MG: Adsorption of vincristine, doxorubicin and mitoxantrone to in-line intravenous filters, *Int J Pharm 103*:87–92 (Feb 25) 1994.

1796. Salomies HEM, Heinonen RM, and Toppila MAI: Sorptive loss of diazepam, nitroglycerin and warfarin sodium to polypropylene-lined infusion bags (Softbags), *Int J Pharm 110*:197–201 (Sep 19) 1994.

1797. Haginaka J, Nakagawa T, and Uno T: Stability of clavulanic acid in aqueous solutions, *Chem Pharm Bull 29*:3334–3341 (11) 1981.

1798. Bianchi C, Airaudo CB, and Gayte-Sorbier A: Sorption studies of dipotassium clorazepate salt (Tranxene) and midazolam hydrochloride (Hypnovel) in polyvinyl chloride and glass infusion containers, *J Clin Pharm Ther 17*:223–227, 1992.

1799. Sautou V, Chopineau J, Gremeau I, et al.: Compatibility with medical plastics and stability of continuously and simultaneously infused isosorbide dinitrate and heparin, *Int J Pharm 107*:111–119 (July 4) 1994.

1800. Mitchell CL (Medical Information Officer, Leo Pharmaceuticals, Buckinghamshire, United Kingdom): Personal Communication, September 11, 1998.

1801. Hadzija BW and Lubarsky DA: Compatibility of etomidate, thiopental sodium, and propofol injections with drugs commonly administered during induction of anesthesia, *Am J Health-Syst Pharm 52*:997–999 (May 1) 1995.

1802. Stewart JT, Warren FW, and King AD: Stability of ranitidine hydrochloride and seven medications, *Am J Hosp Pharm 51*:1802–1807 (July 15) 1994.

1803. Palmquist KL, Quattrocchi FP, and Looney LA: Compatibility of furosemide with 20% mannitol, *Am J Health-Syst Pharm 52*:648, 650 (Mar 15) 1995.

1804. Trissel LA and Martinez JF: Compatibility of granisetron hydrochloride with selected alkaline drugs, *Am J Health-Syst Pharm 52*:208 (Jan 15) 1995.

1805. Bhatt-Mehta V, Paglia RE, and Rosen DA: Stability of propofol with parenteral nutrient solutions during simulated Y-site injection, *Am J Health-Syst Pharm 52*:192–196 (Jan 15) 1995.

1806. Hagan RL, Carr-Lopez SM, and Strickland JS: Stability of nafcillin sodium in the presence of lidocaine hydrochloride, *Am J Health-Syst Pharm 52*:521–523 (Mar 1) 1995.

1807. Gayed AA, Keshary PR, and Hinkle RL: Visual compatibility of diltiazem injection with various diluents and medications during simulated Y-site injection, *Am J Health-Syst Pharm 52*:516–520 (Mar 1) 1995.

1808. Trissel LA: Amphotericin B does not mix with fat emulsion, *Am J Health-Syst Pharm 52*:1463–1464 (July 1) 1995.

1809. Kirsch R, Goldstein R, Tarloff J, et al.: An emulsion formulation of amphotericin B improves the therapeutic index when treating systemic murine candidiasis, *J Infect Dis 158*:1065–1070, 1988.

1810. Chavenet PY, Garry I, Charlier N, et al.: Trial of glucose versus fat emulsion in preparation of amphotericin for use in HIV infected patients with candidiasis, *Br Med J 305*:921–925, 1992.

1811. Caillot D, Casanova O, Solary E, et al.: Efficacy and tolerance of an amphotericin B lipid (Intralipid) emulsion in the treatment of candidaemia in neutropenic patients, *J Antimicrob Chemother 31*:161–169, 1993.

1812. Fleming RA, Olsen DJ, Savage PD, et al.: Stability of ondansetron hydrochloride and cyclophosphamide in injectable solutions, *Am J Health-Syst Pharm 52*:514–516 (Mar 1) 1995.

1813. Bhatt-Mehta V, Johnson CE, Leininger N, et al.: Stability of fentanyl citrate and midazolam hydrochloride during simulated intravenous coadministration, *Am J Health-Syst Pharm 52*:511–513 (Mar 1) 1995.

1814. Driscoll DF, Bhargava HN, Li L, et al.: Physicochemical stability of total nutrient admixtures, *Am J Health-Syst Pharm 52*:623–634 (Mar 15) 1995.

1815. Pettei MJ, Israel D, and Levine J: Serum vitamin K concentration in pediatric patients receiving total parenteral nutrition, *J Parenter Enter Nutr 17*:465–467 (5) 1993.

1816. Trissel LA, Martinez JF, and Xu QA: Incompatibility of fluorouracil with leucovorin calcium or levoleucovorin calcium, *Am J Health-Syst Pharm 52*:710–715 (Apr 1) 1995.

1817. Montoya Garcia-Reol C, Sevilla Azzati E, Negro Vega E, et al.: Estudio de la estabilidad de la mezcla fluorouracilo/folinato calcico en fluidos intravenosos, *Farm Hosp 17*:99–103 (2) 1993.

1818. Ward GH and Yalkowsky SH: Studies in phlebitis VI: dilution-induced precipitation of amiodarone HCl, *J Parenter Sci Technol 47*:161–165 (July–Aug) 1993.

1819. Ward GH and Yalkowsky SH: Studies in phlebitis IV: injection rate and amiodarone-induced phlebitis, *J Parenter Sci Technol 47*:40–43 (Jan–Feb) 1993.

1820. Allwood MC and Brown PW: Stability of ampicillin infusions in unbuffered and buffered saline, *Int J Pharm 97*:219–222, 1993.

1821. Lauper RD (Director, Professional Services, Cetus Oncology Corporation, Emeryville, California): Personal communication, December 20, 1993.

1822. Allen LV: Plasminogen activator, *US Pharmacist 17*:64–65, 70–71, 1992.

1823. Rochard E, Barthes D, and Courtois P: Stability and compatibility of carboplatin with three portable infusion pump reservoirs, *Int J Pharm 101*:257–262 (Jan 25) 1994.

1824. Bailey LC, Cappel KM, and Orosz ST Jr: Stability of ceftriaxone sodium in injectable solutions stored frozen in syringes, *Am J Hosp Pharm 51*:2159–2161 (Sep 1) 1994.

1825. Mazzo DJ, Nguyen-Huu JJ, Pagniez S, et al.: Compatibility of docetaxel and paclitaxel in intravenous solutions with polyvinyl chloride infusion materials, *Am J Health-Syst Pharm 54*:566–569 (Mar 1) 1997.

1826. Kane MP, Bailie GR, Moon DG, et al.: Stability of ciprofloxacin injection in peritoneal dialysis solutions, *Am J Hosp Pharm 51*:373–377 (Feb 1) 1994.

1827. Rochard E, Barthes D, and Courtois P: Stability of cisplatin in ethylene vinylacetate portable infusion-pump reservoirs, *J Clin Pharm Ther 17*:315–318, 1992.

1828. Cubells MP, Aixela JP, Brumos VG, et al.: Stability of cisplatin in sodium chloride 0.9% intravenous solution related to the container's material, *Pharm World Sci 15*:34–36 (1) 1993.

1829. Islam MS and Asker AF: Photostabilization of dacarbazine with reduced glutathione, *J Pharm Sci Technol 48*:38–40 (Jan–Feb) 1994.

1830. Wiest DB, Garner SS, and Childress LM: Stability of esmolol hydrochloride in 5% dextrose injection, *Am J Health-Syst Pharm 52*:716–718 (Apr 1) 1995.

1831. Baaske DM, Dykstra SD, Wagenknecht DM, et al.: Stability of esmolol hydrochloride in intravenous solutions, *Am J Hosp Pharm 51*:2693–2696 (Nov 1) 1994.

1832. Woloschuk DMM and Nazeravich DR: Etoposide precipitation, *Can J Hosp Pharm 45*:136 (Aug) 1992.

1833. Barthes DMC, Rochard EB, Pouliquen IJ, et al.: Stability and compatibility of etoposide in 0.9% sodium chloride injection in three containers, *Am J Hosp Pharm 51*:2706–2709 (Nov 1) 1994.

1834. Mathew M, Gupta VD, and Bethea C: Stability of foscarnet sodium in 5% dextrose and 0.9% sodium chloride injections, *J Clin Pharm Ther 19*:35–36, 1994.

1835. Stolk LM, Hendrikse H, and Chandi LS: Autoclave and long-term sterility of foscarnet sodium admixtures, *Am J Health-Syst Pharm 52*:103 (Jan 1) 1995.

1836. Phaypradith S, Vigneron J, Perrin A, et al.: Stabilite des solutions diluees de ganciclovir sodique (Cymevan) en seringues polypropylene et en poches PVC pour perfusions, *J Pharm Belg 47*:494–498 (6) 1992.

1837. Chung KC, Chin A, and Gill MA: Stability of granisetron hydrochloride in a disposable elastomeric infusion device, *Am J Health-Syst Pharm 52*:1541–1543 (July 15) 1995.

1838. Flahive E (Medical Information, Ortho-McNeil, Raritan, New Jersey): Personal communication, April 6, 1995.

1839. Anon: ASHP therapeutic position statement on the institutional use of 0.9% sodium chloride injection to maintain patency of peripheral indwelling intermittent infusion devices, *Am J Hosp Pharm 51*:1572–1574 (June 15) 1994.

1840. Nahata MC, Morosco RS, and Hipple TF: Stability of lorazepam diluted in bacteriostatic water for injection at two temperatures, *J Clin Pharm Ther 18*:69–71, 1993.

1841. Pinguet F, Martel P, Rouanet P, et al.: Effect of sodium chloride concentration and temperature on melphalan stability during storage and use, *Am J Hosp Pharm 51*:2701–2704 (Nov 1) 1994.

1842. Chin A, Ramakrishnan RR, Yoshimura NN, et al.: Paclitaxel stability and compatibility in polyolefin containers, *Ann Pharmacother 28*:35–36 (Jan) 1994.

1843. Trissel LA, Xu Q, Kwan J, et al.: Compatibility of paclitaxel injection vehicle with intravenous administration and extension sets, *Am J Hosp Pharm 51*:2804–2810 (Nov 15) 1994.

1844. McLaughlin JP, Simpson C, and Taylor RA: When is flucloxacillin stable? *Hosp Pharm Pract 553*–556 (Nov) 1993.

1845. Trissel LA and Martinez JF: Compatibility of amifostine with selected drugs during simulated Y-site administration, *Am J Health-Syst Pharm 52*:2208–2212 (Oct 15) 1995.

1846. Henry DW, Marshall JL, Nazzaro D, et al.: Stability of cisplatin and ondansetron hydrochloride in admixtures for continuous infusion, *Am J Health-Syst Pharm 52*:2570–2573 (Nov 15) 1995.

1847. Mantong ML and Marquardt ED: Visual compatibility of midazolam hydrochloride with selected drugs during simulated Y-site injection, *Am J Health-Syst Pharm 52*:2567–2568 (Nov 15) 1995.

1848. Trissel LA, Xu QA, and Martinez JF: Compatibility and stability of aztreonam and vancomycin hydrochloride, *Am J Health-Syst Pharm 52*:2560–2564 (Nov 15) 1995.

1849. Rivers TE and Webster AA: Stability of ceftizoxime sodium, ceftriaxone sodium, and ceftazidime with metronidazole in ready-to-use metronidazole bags, *Am J Health-Syst Pharm 52*:2568–2570 (Nov 15) 1995.

1850. Wulf H, Gleim M, and Mignat C: The stability of mixtures of morphine hydrochloride, bupivacaine hydrochloride, and clonidine hydrochloride in portable pump reservoirs for the management of chronic pain syndromes, *J Pain Symptom Manage 9*:308–311 (July) 1994.

1851. Korth-Bradley JM, Ludwig S, and Callaghan C: Incompatibility of amiodarone hydrochloride and sodium bicarbonate injections, *Am J Health-Syst Pharm 52*:2340 (Oct 15) 1995.

1852. Bhatt-Mehta V, Johnson CE, Leininger N, et al.: Stability of fentanyl citrate and midazolam hydrochloride during simulated intravenous coadministration, *Am J Health-Syst Pharm 52*:511–513 (Mar 1) 1995.

1853. Matuschka PR, Smith WR, and Vissing RS: Compatibility of mannitol and sodium bicarbonate in injectable fluids, *Am J Health-Syst Pharm 52*:320–321 (Feb 1) 1995.

1854. Ku YM, Min DI, Kumar V, et al.: Compatibility of tacrolimus injection with cimetidine hydrochloride injection in 0.9% sodium chloride injection, *Am J Health-Syst Pharm 52*:2024–2025 (Sep 15) 1995.

1855. Swart EL, Mooren RAG, and van Loenen AC: Compatibility of midazolam hydrochloride and lorazepam with selected drugs during simulated Y-site administration, *Am J Health-Syst Pharm 52*:2020–2022 (Sep 15) 1995.

1856. Lam XM, Ward CA, and de C de Mee CPR: Stability and activity of alteplase with injectable drugs commonly used in cardiac therapy, *Am J Health-Syst Pharm 52*:1904–1909 (Sep 1) 1995.

1857. Alex S, Gupta SL, Minor JR, et al.: Compatibility and activity of aldesleukin (recombinant interleukin-2) in presence of selected drugs during simulated Y-site administration: evaluation of three methods, *Am J Health-Syst Pharm 52*:2423–2426 (Nov 1) 1995.

1858. Mancano MA, Boullata JI, Gelone SP, et al.: Availability of lorazepam after simulated administration from glass and polyvinyl chloride containers, *Am J Health-Syst Pharm 52*:2213–2216 (Oct 15) 1995.

1859. McMullin ST, Burns Schaif RA, and Dietzen DJ: Stability of midazolam hydrochloride in polyvinyl chloride bags under fluorescent light, *Am J Health-Syst Pharm 52*:2018–2020 (Sep 15) 1995.

1860. Bednar DA, Klutman NE, Henry DW, et al.: Stability of ceftazidime (with arginine) in an elastomeric infusion device, *Am J Health-Syst Pharm 52*:1912–1914 (Sep 1) 1995.

1861. Trissel LA and Martinez JF: Compatibility of thiotepa (lyophilized) with selected drugs during simulated Y-site administration, *Am J Health-Syst*

Pharm 53:1041–1045 (May 1) 1996.

1862. Xu QA, Trissel LA, and Fox JL: Compatibility of ondansetron hydrochloride with meperidine hydrochloride for combined administration, *Ann Pharmacother 29*:1106–1109 (Nov) 1995.

1863. Bleasel MD, Peterson GM, and Jestrimski KW: Stability of midazolam in sodium chloride infusion packs, *Aust J Hosp Pharm 23*:260–262 (4) 1993.

1864. Taormina D, Abdallah HY, Venkataramanan R, et al.: Stability and sorption of FK 506 in 5% dextrose injection and 0.9% sodium chloride injection in glass, polyvinyl chloride, and polyolefin containers, *Am J Hosp Pharm 49*:119–122 (Jan) 1992.

1865. Stiles ML, Allen LV Jr, and Prince SJ: Stability of ranitidine hydrochloride during simulated home-care use, *Am J Hosp Pharm 51*:1706–1707 (July 1) 1994.

1866. Dorr RT and Likkil JD: Stability of mitomycin C in different infusion fluids: compatibility with heparin and glucocorticoids, *J Oncol Pharm Pract 1*:19–24 (3) 1995.

1867. Benaji B, Dine T, Goudaliez F, et al.: Compatibility study of methotrexate with PVC bags after repackaging into two types of infusion admixtures, *Int J Pharm 105*:83–87 (Apr 25) 1994.

1868. Sanchez Alcaraz A, Quintana Vergara B, and Sangrador Garcia G: Estabilidad del midazolam en soluciones intravenosas gran volumen, *Farm Hosp 16*:393–398 (6) 1992.

1869. Trissel LA: Concentration-dependent precipitation of sodium bicarbonate with ciprofloxacin lactate, *Am J Health-Syst Pharm 53*:84–85 (Jan 1) 1996.

1870. Christen C, Johnson CE, and Walters JR: Stability of bupivacaine hydrochloride and hydromorphone hydrochloride during simulated epidural coadministration, *Am J Health-Syst Pharm 53*:170–173 (Jan 15) 1996.

1871. Mewborn AL, Kessler JM, and Joyner KA: Compatibility and activity of enoxaparin sodium in 0.9% sodium chloride injection for 48 hours, *Am J Health-Syst Pharm 53*:167–169 (Jan 15) 1996.

1872. Ericsson O, Hallmen AC, and Wikstrom I: Amphotericin B incompatible with lipid emulsion, *Ann Pharmacother 30:*298 (Mar) 1996.

1873. Hoey LL, Vance-Bryan K, Clarens DM, et al.: Lorazepam stability in parenteral solutions for continuous intravenous administration, *Ann Pharmacother 30*:343–346 (Apr) 1996.

1874. Nyhammar EK, Johansson SG, and Seiving BE: Stability of doxorubicin hydrochloride and vincristine sulfate in two portable infusion-pump reservoirs, *Am J Health-Syst Pharm 53*:1171–1173 (May 15) 1996.

1875. Chin A, Moon YSK, Chung KC, et al.: Stability of granisetron hydrochloride with dexamethasone sodium phosphate for 14 days, *Am J Health-Syst Pharm 53*:1174–1176 (May 15) 1996.

1876. Stewart JT, Warren FW, King DT, et al.: Stability of ondansetron hydrochloride and five antineoplastic medications, *Am J Health-Syst Pharm 53*:1297–1300 (June 1) 1996.

1877. Yamashita SK, Walker SE, Choudhury T, et al.: Compatibility of selected critical care drugs during simulated Y-site administration, *Am J Health-Syst Pharm 53*:1048–1051 (May 1) 1996.

1878. Ohls RK and Christensen RD: Stability of human recombinant epoetin alfa in commonly used neonatal intravenous solutions, *Ann Pharmacother 30*:466–468 (May) 1996.

1879. Nahata MC, Edmonds JJ, and Morosco RS: Stability of metronidazole and ceftizoxime sodium in ready-to-use metronidazole bags stored at 4 and 25°C, *Am J Health-Syst Pharm 53*:1046–1048 (May 1) 1996.

1880. Lewis JD and El-Gendy A: Cephalosporin-pentamidine isethionate incompatibilities, *Am J Health-Syst Pharm 53*:1461–1462 (June 15) 1996.

1881. Tanque N, Ueda H, Moriyama Y, et al.: Compatibility of irinotecan hydrochloride injection with other injections, *Jpn J Hosp Pharm 22*:457–465 (5) 1996.

1882. Hagan RL, Mallett MS, and Fox JL: Stability of ondansetron hydrochloride and dexamethasone sodium phosphate in infusion bags and syringes for 32 days, *Am J Health-Syst Pharm 53*:1431–1435 (June 15) 1996.

1883. Mayron D and Gennaro AR: Stability and compatibility of granisetron hydrochloride in i.v. solutions and oral liquids and during simulated Y-site injection with selected drugs, *Am J Health-Syst Pharm 53*:294–304 (Feb 1) 1996.

1884. Pinguet F, Rouanet P, Martel P, et al.: Compatibility and stability of granisetron, dexamethasone, and methylprednisolone in injectable solutions, *J Pharm Sci 84*:267–268 (Feb) 1995.

1885. Lindsay CA, Dang K, Adams JM, et al.: Stability and activity of intravenous immunoglobulin with neonatal dextrose and total parenteral nutrient solutions, *Ann Pharmacother 28*:1014–1017 (Sep) 1994.

1886. Ukhun IA: Compatibility of haloperidol and diphenhydramine in a hypodermic syringe, *Ann Pharmacother 29*:1168–1169 (Nov) 1995.

1887. Melonakos TK: Ciprofloxacin-ampicillin sulbactam incompatibility, *Ann Pharmacother 30*:87 (Jan) 1996.

1888. Digel S: Cefamandolnafat und metronidazol, *Krankenhauspharmazie 16*:9–12 (Jan) 1995.

1889. Heni J and Strehl E: Kompatibilitat von cefotiam, *Krankenhauspharmazie 15*:187–192 (Apr) 1994.

1890. Tham A (Drug Information Associate, Medical Affairs, Chiron Therapeutics, Emeryville, CA): Personal Communication, November 1, 1999.

1891. Mathew M, Gupta VD, and Zerai T: Stability of ciprofloxacin in 5% dextrose and normal saline injections, *J Clin Pharm Ther 19*:397–399 (6) 1994.

1892. Pramar YV, Moniz D, and Hobbs D: Chemical stability and adsorption of succinylcholine chloride injections in disposable plastic syringes, *J Clin Pharm Ther 19*:195–198, 1994.

1893. Wood MJ, Lund R, and Beavan M: Stability of vancomycin in plastic syringes measured by high-performance liquid chromatography, *J Clin Pharm Ther 20*:319–325 (6) 1995.

1894. Strong ML, Schaaf LJ, Pankaskie MC, et al.: Shelf-lives and factors affecting the stability of morphine sulphate and meperidine (pethidine) hydrochloride in plastic syringes for use in patient-controlled analgesic devices, *J Clin Pharm Ther 19*:361–369 (6) 1994.

1895. Giordano F, Bettinetti G, Cursano R, et al.: A physicochemical approach to the investigation of the stability of trimethoprim-sulfamethoxazole (Co-Trimoxazole) mixtures for injectables, *J Pharm Sci 84*:1254–1258 (Oct) 1995.

1896. Sianipar A, Parkin JE, and Sunderland VB: Chemical incompatibility between procainamide hydrochloride and glucose following intravenous admixture, *J Pharm Pharmacol 46*:951–955 (Dec) 1994.

1897. Lau DWC, Law S, Walker SE, et al.: Dexamethasone phosphate stability and contamination of solutions stored in syringes, *PDA J Pharm Sci Technol 50*:261–267 (July–Aug) 1996.

1898. Ambados F: Incompatibility between aminophylline and elemental zinc injections, *Aust J Hosp Pharm 26*:370–371 (3) 1996.

1899. Ambados F: Compatibility of morphine and ketamine for subcutaneous infusion, *Aust J Hosp Pharm 25*:352 (4) 1995.

1900. Boldu SP, Cubells MP, Brumos VG, et al.: Stability study of azlocillin sodium in glass bottles and PVC bags containing intravenous admixtures, *Boll Chim Farm 134*:467–471 (Sep) 1995.

1901. LeBelle MJ, Savard C, and Gagnon A: Compatibility of morphine and midazolam or haloperidol in parenteral admixtures, *Can J Hosp Pharm 48*:155–160 (June) 1995.

1902. Donnelly RF and Yen M: Epinephrine stability in plastic syringes and glass vials, *Can J Hosp Pharm 49*:62–65 (2) 1996.

1903. Sadjak A and Wintersteiger R: Compatibility of morphine, baclofen, floxuridine and fluorouracil in an implantable medication pump, *Arzneim Forsch 45*:93–98 (1) 1995.

1904. Donnelly RF and Farncombe M: Compatibility of morphine or hydromorphone with salbutamol in a syringe, *Can J Hosp Pharm 47*:252 (Dec) 1994.

1905. Corbo DC, Suddith RL, Sharma B, et al.: Stability, potency, and preservative effectiveness of epoetin alfa after addition of a bacteriostatic diluent, *Am J Hosp Pharm 49*:1455–1458 (June) 1992.

1906. Lane G and Waite N: Erythropoietin stability, *Can J Hosp Pharm 47*:182 (Aug) 1994.

1907. Walker SE and Lau DWC: Compatibility and stability of hyaluronidase and hydromorphone, *Can J Hosp Pharm 45*:187–192 (Oct) 1992.

1908. Sastre Gervas I and Ferrandiz Gosalbez JR: Estabilidad fisica y quimica del sulfate magnesico combinado con heparina sodica en solucion salina al 0,9 por 100, *Farm Hosp 19*:38–40 (1) 1995.

1909. Halkiewicz A, Barteczko I, and Janicki S: Interakcje fizykochemiczne izotonicznego roztworu teofiliny do wlewu dozylnego z niektorymi lekami do wstrzykiwan, *Farm Polska 49*:11–15, 1993.

1910. Gila Azanedo JA, Mengual Sendra A, Fernandez Barral C, et al.: Estudio de la estabilidad de una solucion de clorhidrato de morfina mas anestesicos locales en solucion salina 0,9 por 100 sin conservantes para uso epidural, *Farm Hosp 18*:261–264 (Sep–Oct) 1994.

1911. Sitaram BR, Tsui M, Rawicki HB, et al.: Stability and compatibility of baclofen and morphine admixtures for use in an implantable infusion pump, *Int J Pharm 118*:181–189 (May 16) 1995.

1912. Allwood MC and Martin H: The extraction of diethylhexylphthalate (DEHP) from polyvinyl chloride components of intravenous infusion containers and administration sets by paclitaxel injection, *Int J Pharm 127*:65–71 (Jan 15) 1996.

1913. Jacolot A, Arnaud P, Lecompte D, et al.: Stability and compatibility of 2.5 mg/ml methotrexate solution in plastic syringes over 7 days, *Int J Pharm 128*:283–286 (Feb 29) 1996.

1914. Wright A and Hecker J: Long term stability of heparin in dextrose-saline intravenous fluids, *Int J Pharm Pract 3*:253–255 (Nov) 1995.

1915. Kawano K, Matsunaga A, Terada K, et al.: Loss of diltiazem hydrochloride in solutions in polyvinyl chloride containers or intravenous administration set—hydrolysis and sorption, *Jpn J Hosp Pharm* 20:537–541 (6) 1994.

1916. Trissel LA and Gilbert DL: Data on file. Pharmaceutical Analysis Laboratory, University of Texas, M. D. Anderson Cancer Center, Houston, Texas, January 14, 2000.

1917. Kawano K, Takamatsu S, Yamashita J, et al.: Effect of pH on the sorption of in-solution diazepam into the ethylene-vinylacetate copolymer membrane, *Jpn J Hosp Pharm* 20:404–409 (5) 1994.

1918. Picard C, Brazier M, Bou P, et al.: Stabilite de quatre solutions de penicillines dans les poches de perfusion multicouches, *J Pharm Clin* 13:45–49 (1) 1994.

1919. Theuer H, Scherbel G, Balzulat S, et al.: Herstellung und stabilitatuntersuchungen von carboplatin i.v., *Krankenhauspharmazie* 15:120–130 (Mar) 1994.

1920. Strehl E and Heni J: Amoxicillin, clavulansaure und metronidazol in kombination, *Krankenhauspharmazie* 15:592–595 (Oct) 1994.

1921. Hatton J, Luer M, Hirsch J, et al.: Histamine receptor antagonists and lipid stability in total nutrient admixtures, *J Parenter Enter Nutr* 18:308–312 (July–Aug) 1994.

1922. Ku YM, Min DI, Kumar V, et al.: Stability of tacrolimus injection in total parenteral nutrition solution, *J Pharm Technol* 12:58–61 (Mar–Apr) 1996.

1923. Martinelli E and Muhlebach S: Kunststoffumbeutel als lichtschutz fur infusionen, *Krankenhauspharmazie* 16:286–289 (July) 1995.

1924. Teraoka K, Minakuchi K, Tsuchiya K, et al.: Compatibility of ciprofloxacin infusion with other injections, *Jpn J Hosp Pharm* 21:541–550 (6) 1995.

1925. Asahara K, Goda Y, Shimomura Y, et al.: Stability of thiamine in intravenous hyperalimentation containing multivitamin, *Jpn J Hosp Pharm* 21:15–21 (1) 1995.

1926. Namika Y, Fujiwara A, Kihara N, et al.: Factors affecting tautomeric phenomenon of a novel potent immunosuppressant (FK506) on the design for injectable formulation, *Drug Dev Ind Pharm* 21:809–822 (7) 1995.

1927. Antipas AS, Vander Velde D, Stella VJ: Factors affecting the deamidation of vancomycin in aqueous solutions, *Int J Pharm* 109:261–269, 1994.

1928. King AD, Stewart JT, and Warren FW: Stability of cefmetazole-doxycycline mixtures in sodium chloride and dextrose injections, *J Clin Pharm Ther* 19:317–325 (5) 1994.

1929. Hughes IE and Smith JA: The stability of noradrenaline in physiologic saline solutions, *J Pharm Pharmacol* 30:124–126, 1978.

1930. Anon: Infections linked to lax handling of propofol, *Am J Health-Syst Pharm* 52:2061, 2066 (Oct 1) 1995.

1931. Ordovas Baines JP, Ronchera Oms CL, Jimenez Torres NV, et al.: Mezclas iv binarias de metronidazol y aminoglycosidos, *Revista AEFH* 12:119–123 (2) 1988.

1932. Nitescu P, Hultman E, Appelgren L, et al.: Bacteriology, drug stability and exchange of percutaneous delivery systems and antibacterial filters in long-term intrathecal infusion of opioid drugs and bupivacaine in "refractory" pain, *Clin J Pain* 8:324–337 (4) 1992.

1933. Yao JDC, Arkin CF, and Karchmer AW: Vancomycin stability in heparin and total parenteral nutrition solutions: novel approach to therapy of central venous catheter-related infections, *J Parenter Enter Nutr* 16:268–274 (May–June) 1992.

1934. Jim LK: Physical and chemical compatibility of intravenous ciprofloxacin with other drugs, *Ann Pharmacother* 27:704–707 (June) 1993.

1935. Paesen J, Khan K, Roets E, et al.: Study of the stability of erythromycin in neutral and alkaline solutions by liquid chromatography on poly(styrene-divinylbenzene), *Int J Pharm* 113:215–222, 1994.

1936. Keyi X, Gagnon N, Bisson C, et al.: Stability of famotidine in polyvinyl chloride minibags and polypropylene syringes and compatibility of famotidine with selected drugs, *Ann Pharmacother* 27:422–426 (Apr) 1993.

1937. Pleasants RA, Vaughan LM, Williams DM, et al.: Compatibility of ceftazidime and aminophylline admixtures for different methods of intravenous infusion, *Ann Pharmacother* 26:1221–1226 (Oct) 1992.

1938. Nahata MC, Morosco RS, and Hipple TF: Stability of diluted methylprednisolone sodium succinate injection at two temperatures, *Am J Hosp Pharm* 51:2157–2159 (Sep 1) 1994.

1939. Nixon AR, O'Hare MCB, and Chisakuta AM: The stability of morphine sulphate and metoclopramide hydrochloride in various delivery presentations, *Pharm J* 254:153–155, 1995.

1940. Lugo RA and Nahata MC: Stability of diluted dexamethasone sodium phosphate injection at two temperatures, *Ann Pharmacother* 28:1018–1019 (Sep) 1994.

1941. Hanff PAJM and Van den Biggelaar JPFA: Stabiliteitsonderzoek van nitroglycerine-oplossingen voor parenteraal gebruik, *Ziekenhuisfarmacie* 10:134–138 (4) 1994.

1942. Forte FJ, Caravone D, Coyne MJ, et al.: Albumin dilution as a cause of hemolysis during plasmapheresis, *Am J Health-Syst Pharm* 52:207 (Jan 15) 1995.

1943. Little G (Drug Information, Wyeth-Ayerst Laboratories, Philadelphia, Pennsylvania): Personal communication, March 25, 1996.

1944. Andersin R and Tammilehto S: Photochemical decomposition of midazolam, part iv: study of pH-dependent stability by high-performance liquid chromatography, *Int J Pharm* 123:229–235 (Sep 12) 1995.

1945. Boullata JI, Gelone SP, Mancano MA, et al.: Precipitation of lorazepam infusion, *Ann Pharmacother* 30:1037–1038 (Sep) 1996.

1946. Taylor RB, Richards RME, Low AS, et al.: Chemical stability of polymyxin B in aqueous solution, *Int J Pharm* 102:201–206 (Feb 7) 1994.

1947. Allwood MC and Brown PW: The effect of buffering on the stability of reconstituted benzylpenicillin injection, *Int J Pharm Pract* 1:242–244 (Aug) 1992.

1948. Katakam M and Banga AK: Aggregation of insulin and its prevention by carbohydrate excipients, *PDA J Pharm Sci Technol* 49:160–165 (July–Aug) 1995.

1949. Woloschuk DMM: Drug precipitation and peristaltic pumps, *Am J Hosp Pharm* 51:1473 (June 1) 1994.

1950. Hehenberger H: Prednisolon-21-hemisuccinat-natrium, *Krankenhauspharmazie* 7:128–132 (Apr) 1986.

1951. Driscoll DF, Bacon M, Provost PS, et al.: Automated compounders for parenteral nutrition admixtures, *J Parenter Enter Nutr* 18:385–386 (July–Aug) 1994.

1952. Mehta AC and Kay EA: Admixtures' storage is extended, *Pharm Pract* 6:113–114 (Apr) 1996.

1953. Faouzi MA, Dine T, Luyckx M, et al.: Stability and compatibility studies of cephaloridine, cefuroxime and ceftazidime with PVC infusion bags, *Pharmazie* 49:425–429 (June) 1994.

1954. Williams DA and Lokich J: A review of the stability and compatibility of antineoplastic drugs for multiple-drug infusions, *Cancer Chemother Pharmacol* 31:171–181, 1992.

1955. Chevrier R, Sautou V, Pinon V, et al.: Stability and compatibility of a mixture of the anti-cancer drugs etoposide, cytarabine and daunorubicine for infusion, *Pharm Acta Helv* 70:141–148, 1995.

1956. Christie JM, Jones CW, and Markowsky SJ: Chemical compatibility of regional anesthetic drug combinations, *Ann Pharmacother* 26:1078–1080 (Sep) 1992.

1957. Abdel-Moety EM, Al-Rashood KA, Rauf A, et al.: Photostability-indicating HPLC method for determination of trifluoperazine in bulk form and pharmaceutical formulations, *J Pharm Biomed Anal* 14:1639–1644 (Aug) 1996.

1958. Poochikian GK, Cradock JC, and Davignon JP: Heroin: stability and formulation approaches, *Int J Pharm* 13:219–226, 1983.

1959. Kamitomo V and Olson K: Using normal saline to lock peripheral intravenous catheters in ambulatory cancer patients, *J Intraven Nurs* 19:75–78 (Mar–Apr) 1996.

1960. Burnakis TG: Insulin syringes: more than a one-shot deal, *Hosp Pharm* 31:410, 414 (Apr) 1996.

1961. Sautou-Miranda V, Gremeau I, Chamard I, et al.: Stability of dopamine hydrochloride and of dobutamine hydrochloride in plastic syringes and administration sets, *Am J Health-Syst Pharm* 53:186, 193 (Jan 15) 1996.

1962. Murthey SS and Brittain HG: Stability of revex, nalmefene hydrochloride injection, in injectable solutions, *J Pharm Biomed Anal* 15:221–226 (Nov) 1996.

1963. Yuan LC, Samuels GJ, and Visor GC: Stability of cidofovir in 0.9% sodium chloride injection and in 5% dextrose injection, *Am J Health-Syst Pharm* 53:1939–1943 (Aug 15) 1996.

1964. Leader WG: Incompatibility between ceftriaxone sodium and labetalol hydrochloride, *Am J Health-Syst Pharm* 53:2639 (Nov 1) 1996.

1965. Nahata MC, Morosco RS, and Fox J: Stability of ranitidine hydrochloride in water for injection in glass vials and plastic syringes, *Am J Health-Syst Pharm* 53:1588–1590 (July 1) 1996.

1966. Lee DKT, Wong CY, and Wang DP: Stability of cefazolin sodium and meperidine hydrochloride, *Am J Health-Syst Pharm* 53 :1608, 1610 (July 1) 1996.

1967. Stiles ML, Allen LV Jr, and Prince SJ: Stability of deferoxamine mesylate, floxuridine, fluorouracil, hydromorphone hydrochloride, lorazepam, and midazolam hydrochloride in polypropylene infusion-pump syringes, *Am J Health-Syst Pharm* 53:1583–1588 (July 1) 1996.

1968. Quercia RA, Zhang J, Fan C, et al.: Stability of granisetron hydrochloride in polypropylene syringes, *Am J Health-Syst Pharm* 53:2744–2746 (Nov 15) 1996.

1969. Trissel LA, Martinez JF, and Gilbert DL: Screening cladribine for Y-site physical compatibility with selected drugs, *Hosp Pharm* 31:1425–1428 (Nov) 1996.

1970. Allen LV Jr, Stiles ML, Prince SJ, et al.: Stability of 14 drugs in the latex reservoir of an elastomeric infusion device, *Am J Health-Syst Pharm* 53:2740–2743 (Nov 15) 1996.

1971. Benjamin BE: Ciprofloxacin and sodium phosphates not compatible during actual Y-site injection, *Am J Health-Syst Pharm* 53:1850–1851 (Aug 1) 1996.

1972. Trissel LA: Everything in a compatibility study is important, *Am J Health-Syst Pharm* 53:2990 (Dec 1) 1996.

1973. Matuschka PR, Hill LJ, and Canada CA: More on the compatibility of mannitol and sodium bicarbonate in injectable fluids, *Am J Health-Syst Pharm* 53:2639 (Nov 1) 1996.

1974. Veltri M and Lee CKK: Compatibility of neonatal parenteral nutrient solutions with selected intravenous drugs, *Am J Health-Syst Pharm* 53:2611–2613 (Nov 1) 1996.

1975. Ritter H, Trissel LA, Anderson RW, et al.: Electronic balance as quality assurance for cytotoxic drug admixtures, *Am J Health-Syst Pharm* 53:2318–2320 (Oct 1) 1996.

1976. Zhang Y, Xu QA, Trissel LA, et al.: Physical and chemical stability of methotrexate sodium, cytarabine, and hydrocortisone sodium succinate in Elliott's B solution, *Hosp Pharm* 31:965–970 (Aug) 1996.

1977. Xu QA, Trissel LA, and Martinez JF: Stability and compatibility of fluorouracil with morphine sulfate and hydromorphone hydrochloride, *Ann Pharmacother* 30:756–761 (July–Aug) 1996.

1978. Kohut J III, Trissel LA, and Leissing NC: Don't ignore the details of drug-compatibility reports, *Am J Health-Syst Pharm* 53:2339 (Oct 1) 1996.

1979. Grillo JA and Barie PS: Precipitation of lorazepam during infusion by volumetric pump, *Am J Health-Syst Pharm* 53:1850 (Aug 1) 1996.

1980. Volles DF: More on usability of lorazepam admixtures for continuous infusion, *Am J Health-Syst Pharm* 53:2753–2754 (Nov 15) 1996.

1981. Boullata JI and Gelone SP: More on usability of lorazepam admixtures for continuous infusion, *Am J Health-Syst Pharm* 53:2754 (Nov 15) 1996.

1982. Strozyk WR, Williamson R, and Thompson D: Incompatibility of amiodarone hydrochloride and evacuated glass bottles, *Am J Health-Syst Pharm* 53:184 (Jan 15) 1996.

1983. Baud-Camus F, Crauste-Manciet S, Klein E, et al.: Stability of fluorouracil in polypropylene syringes and ethylene vinyl acetate infusion-pump reservoirs, *Am J Health-Syst Pharm* 53:1457, 1461 (June 15) 1996.

1984. Chernin EL, Stewart JT, and Smiler B: Stability of thiopental sodium and propofol in polypropylene syringes at 23 and 4 °C, *Am J Health-Syst Pharm* 53:1576–1579 (July 1) 1996.

1985. Prankerd RJ and Jones RD: Physicochemical compatibility of propofol with thiopental sodium, *Am J Health-Syst Pharm* 53:2606–2610 (Nov 1) 1996.

1986. Williams NA, Bornstein M, and Johnson K: Stability of levofloxacin in intravenous solutions in polyvinyl chloride bags, *Am J Health-Syst Pharm* 53:2309–2313 (Oct 1) 1996.

1987. Cleary JD: Amphotericin B formulated in a lipid emulsion, *Ann Pharmacother* 30:409–412 (Apr) 1996.

1988. Lopez RM, Ayestaran A, Pou L, et al.: Stability of amphotericin B in an extemporaneously prepared i.v. fat emulsion, *Am J Health-Syst Pharm* 53:2724–2727 (Nov 15) 1996.

1989. Manduru M, Fariello A, White RL, et al.: Stability of ceftazidime sodium and teicoplanin sodium in a peritoneal dialysis solution, *Am J Health-Syst Pharm* 53:2731–2734 (Nov 15) 1996.

1990. Plumridge RJ, Rieck AM, Annus TP, et al.: Stability of ceftriaxone sodium in polypropylene syringes at −20, 4, and 20 °C, *Am J Health-Syst Pharm* 53:2320–2323 (Nov 15) 1996.

1991. Plumridge RJ, Rieck AM, Annus TP, et al.: Stability of ceftriaxone sodium reconstituted with lidocaine hydrochloride and stored in polypropylene syringes, *Am J Health-Syst Pharm* 53:2323–2325 (Oct 1) 1996.

1992. Henderson F: 21-Day compatibility of hydromorphone hydrochloride and promethazine hydrochloride in a casette, *Am J Health-Syst Pharm* 53:2338–2339 (Nov 1) 1996.

1993. Lima HA, Lennon J, Sesterhenn K, et al.: Stability of dextrose and sodium chloride in injectable solutions stored in an elastomeric infusion device, *Am J Health-Syst Pharm* 53:794–795 (Apr 1) 1996.

1994. Patel PR: Compatibility of meropenem with commonly used injectable drugs, *Am J Health-Syst Pharm* 53:2853–2855 (Dec 1) 1996.

1995. Lougheed WD, Albisser AM, Martindale HM, et al.: Physical stability of insulin formulations, *Diabetes* 32:424–432 (May) 1983.

1996. Gupta VD: Quantitation of papaverine hydrochloride in a discoloured injection, *Drug Stability* 1:132–134 (2) 1996.

1997. Akimoto K, Kawai A, Ohya K, et al.: Photodegradation reactions of CPT-11, a derivative of camptothecin, part i: chemical structure of main degradation products in aqueous solution, *Drug Stability* 1:118–122 (2) 1996.

1998. Akimoto K, Kawai A, and Ohya K: Photodegradation reactions of CPT-11, a derivative of camptothecin, part ii: photodegradation behaviour of CPT-11 in aqueous solution, *Drug Stability* 1:141–146 (3) 1996.

1999. O'Connell C, Sabra K, and Scott K: Stability of reconstituted ceftriaxone solution in polypropylene syringes, *Eur Hosp Pharm* 2:47–48 (May) 1996.

2000. Trissel LA, Gilbert DL, and Martinez JF: Compatibility of granisetron hydrochloride with selected drugs during simulated Y-site administration, *Am J Health-Syst Pharm* 54:56–60 (Jan 1) 1997.

2001. Zhang Y, Trissel LA, Martinez JF, et al.: Stability of metoclopramide hydrochloride in plastic syringes, *Am J Health-Syst Pharm* 53:1300–1302 (June 1) 1996.

2002. Kaijser GP, Aalbers T, Beijnen JH, et al.: Chemical stability of cyclophosphamide, trofosfamide, and 2- and 3-dechloroethylifosfamide in aqueous solutions, *J Oncol Pharm Pract* 2:15–21 (1) 1996.

2003. Nelson TJ and Graves SM: 0.9% Sodium chloride injection with and without heparin for maintaining peripheral indwelling intermittent-infusion devices in infants, *Am J Health-Syst Pharm* 55:570–573 (Mar 15) 1998.

2004. Martel P, Petit I, Pinguet F, et al.: Long-term stability of 5-fluorouracil stored in PVC bags and in ambulatory pump reservoirs, *J Pharm Biomed Anal* 14:395–399 (Feb) 1996.

2005. Darbar D, Dell'Orto S, Wilkinson GR, et al.: Loss of quinidine gluconate injection in a polyvinyl chloride infusion system, *Am J Health-Syst Pharm* 53:655–658 (Mar 15) 1996.

2006. Erkkila DM (Professional Services, Immunex Corporation): Personal communication, March 6, 1996.

2007. Xu QA, Trissel LA, Zhang Y, et al.: Stability of thiotepa (lyophilized) in 5% dextrose injection at 4 and 23 °C, *Am J Health-Syst Pharm* 53:2728–2730 (Nov 15) 1996.

2008. van Doorne H, Bernaards J, and de Jonge P: Ceftazidime degradation rates for predicting stability in a portable infusion-pump reservoir, *Am J Health-Syst Pharm* 53:1302–1305 (June 1) 1996.

2009. Celesk RA (Medical Services, Bayer Pharmaceutical Division): Personal communication, May 7, 1996.

2010. Grandison D (Worldwide Medical Affairs, Du Pont Pharma): Personal communication, December 4, 1995.

2011. Martinez JF, Trissel LA, and Gilbert DL: Compatibility of warfarin sodium with selected drugs and large-volume parenteral solutions, *Int J Pharm Compound* 1:356–358 (Sep–Oct) 1997.

2012. Williams DA: Zwitterions and pH-dependent solubility, *Am J Health-Syst Pharm* 53:1732 (July 15) 1996.

2013. Ariano RE, Kassum DA, Meatherhill RC, et al.: Lack of in vitro inactivation of tobramycin by imipenem/cilastatin, *Ann Pharmacother* 26:1075–1077 (Sep) 1992.

2014. Jenke DR: Drug binding by reservoirs in elastomeric devices, *Pharm Res* 11:984–989 (7) 1994.

2015. McCollom RA, Lange B, Bryson SM, et al.: Polyvinylchloride containers do not influence the hemodynamic response to intravenous nitroglycerin, *Can J Hosp Pharm* 46:165–170 (Aug) 1993.

2016. Altavela JL, Haas CE, Nowak DR, et al.: Clinical response to intravenous nitroglycerin infused through polyethylene or polyvinyl chloride tubing, *Am J Hosp Pharm* 51:490–494 (Feb 15) 1994.

2017. McCullough JM, Sprentall-Nankervis E, Potcova CA, et al.: Recovery and biological activity of filgrastim after injection through silicone rubber catheters, *Am J Health-Syst Pharm* 52:186–188 (Jan 15) 1995.

2018. Park TW, Le-Bui LPK, Chung KC, et al.: Stability of piperacillin sodium–tazobactam sodium in peritoneal dialysis solutions, *Am J Health-Syst Pharm* 52:2022–2024 (Sep 15) 1995.

2019. Young D, Fadiran EO, Chang KT, et al.: Stability of ticarcillin disodium in polypropylene syringes, *Am J Health-Syst Pharm* 52:890, 892 (Apr 15) 1996.

2020. Stiles ML, Allen LV Jr, Resztak KE, et al.: Stability of octreotide acetate in polypropylene syringes, *Am J Hosp Pharm* 50:2356–2358 (Nov) 1993.

2021. Ripley RG, Ritchie DJ, and Holstad SG: Stability of octreotide acetate in polypropylene syringes at 5 and −20 °C, *Am J Health-Syst Pharm* 52:1910–1911 (Sep 1) 1995.

2022. Schepart BS, Burns BA, Evans S, et al.: Long-term stability of interferon alfa-2b diluted to 2 million units/mL, *Am J Health-Syst Pharm* 52:2128–2130 (Oct 1) 1995.

2023. Ikeda S, Frank PA, Schweiss JF, et al.: In vitro cyanide release from sodium nitroprusside in various intravenous solutions, *Anesth Analg* 67:360–362, 1988.

2024. Webster LK, Crinis NA, Davis JR, et al.: Conversion of etoposide phosphate to etoposide under ambulatory infusion conditions, *J Oncol Pharm Pract* 1:33–36 (3) 1995.

2025. Hensrud DD, Burritt MF, and Hall LG: Stability of heparin anticoagulant activity over time in parenteral nutrition solutions, *J Parenter Enter Nutr*

20:219–221 (May–June) 1996.

2026. Gutcher GR, Lax AA, and Farrell PM: Vitamin A losses to plastic intravenous infusion devices and an improved method of delivery, *Am J Clin Nutr* 40:8–13 (July) 1984.

2027. Greene HL, Phillips BL, Franck L, et al.: Persistently low blood retinol levels during and after parenteral feeding of very low birth weight infants: examination of losses into intravenous administration sets and a method of prevention by addition to a lipid emulsion, *Pediatrics* 79:894–900 (June) 1987.

2028. Henton DH and Merrott RJ: Vitamin A sorption to polyvinyl and polyolefin intravenous tubing, *J Parenter Enter Nutr* 14:79–81 (Jan–Feb) 1990.

2029. Washington C, Ferguson JA, and Irwin SE: Computational prediction of the stability of lipid emulsions in total nutrient admixtures, *J Pharm Sci* 82:808–812 (Aug) 1993.

2030. Li LC and Sampogna TP: A factorial design study on the physical stability of 3-in-1 admixtures, *J Pharm Pharmacol* 45:985–987, 1993.

2031. Foresta K: Use of total nutrient admixtures should not be limited, *Am J Health-Syst Pharm* 52:893 (Apr 15) 1995.

2032. Driscoll DF: Use of total nutrient admixtures should not be limited, *Am J Health-Syst Pharm* 52:893–894 (Apr 15) 1995.

2033. Mirtallo JM: Use of total nutrient admixtures should not be limited, *Am J Health-Syst Pharm* 52:894–895 (Apr 15) 1995.

2034. Trissel LA: Use of total nutrient admixtures should not be limited, *Am J Health-Syst Pharm* 52:895 (Apr 15) 1995.

2035. Driscoll DF: Debate on total nutrient admixtures continues, *Am J Health-Syst Pharm* 52:1921–1922 (Sep 1) 1995.

2036. Trissel LA: Debate on total nutrient admixtures continues, *Am J Health-Syst Pharm* 52:1921–1922 (Sep 1) 1995.

2037. Hill SE, Heldman LS, Goo EDH, et al.: Fatal microvascular pulmonary emboli from precipitation of a total nutrient admixture solution, *J Parenter Enter Nutr* 20:81–87 (Jan–Feb) 1996.

2038. MacKay MW, Fitzgerald KA, and Jackson D: The solubility of calcium and phosphate in two specialty amino acid solutions, *J Parenter Enter Nutr* 20:63–66 (Jan–Feb) 1996.

2039. Shatsky F, McFeely EJ, and Takahashi D: A table for estimating calcium and phosphorus compatibility in parenteral nutrition formulas that contain Trophamine plus cysteine, *Hosp Pharm* 30:690–692, 723 (Aug) 1995.

2040. Grassby PF and Hutchings L: Factors affecting the physical and chemical stability of morphine sulphate solutions stored in syringes, *Int J Pharm Pract* 2:39–43 (Mar) 1993.

2041. Xu QA, Zhang YP, Trissel LA, et al.: Stability of busulfan injection admixtures in 5% dextrose injection and 0.9% sodium chloride injection, *J Oncol Pharm Pract* 2:101–105 (2) 1996.

2042. Roos PJ, Glerum JH, Meilink JW, et al.: Effect of pH on absorption of sufentanil citrate in a portable pump reservoir during storage and administration under simulated epidural conditions, *Pharm World News* 15:139–144 (3) 1993.

2043. Trissel LA and Xu QA: Data on file, Pharmaceutical Analysis Laboratory, University of Texas, M. D. Anderson Cancer Center, Houston, Texas, July 30, 1997.

2044. Allen LV Jr, Stiles ML, Prince SJ, et al.: Stability of cefpirome sulfate in the presence of commonly used intensive care drugs during simulated Y-site injection, *Am J Health-Syst Pharm* 52:2427–2433 (Nov 1) 1995.

2045. Bureau A, Lahet JJ, D'Athis P, et al.: Compatibilite PVC-psychotropes au cours d'une perfusion, *J Pharm Clin* 14:26–30 (Mar) 1995.

2046. Streng WH and Brake NW: Dextrose adduct formation in aqueous teicoplanin solutions, *Pharm Res* 6:1032–1038 (Dec) 1989.

2047. Hixt U: L-Alanyl-L-glutamine dipeptide for parenteral nutrition, *Eur Hosp Pharm* 2:72–76 (May) 1996.

2048. Tivnann H, Gaines-Gas R, Thorpe R, et al.: An evaluation of the stability of granulocyte colony stimulating factor on the short-term storage and delivery from an elastomeric infusion system, *J Oncol Pharm Pract* 2:107–112 (2) 1996.

2049. Billion-Rey F, Guillaumont M, Frederich A, et al.: Stability of fat-soluble vitamins A (retinol palmitate), E (tocopherol acetate), and K1 (phylloquinone) in total parenteral nutrition at home, *J Parenter Enter Nutr* 17:56–60 (Jan–Feb) 1993.

2050. Dahl GB, Svensson L, Kinnander NJG, et al.: Stability of vitamins in soybean oil fat emulsion under conditions simulating intravenous feeding of neonates and children, *J Parenter Enter Nutr* 18:234–239 (May–June) 1994.

2051. Henry DW, Lacerte JA, Klutman NE, et al.: Irreversibility of procainamide-dextrose complex in plasma in vitro, *Am J Hosp Pharm* 48:2426–2429 (Nov) 1991.

2052. Martin M and Bepko R: Paclitaxel diluent and the case of the slippery spike, *Am J Hosp Pharm* 51:3078, 3080 (Dec 15) 1994.

2053. Faouzi MA, Dine T, Luyckx M, et al.: Leaching of diethylhexyl phthalate from PVC bags into intravenous teniposide solution, *Int J Pharm* 105:89–93 (Apr 25) 1994.

2054. Haas CE, Nowak DR, and Mabb WA: Effect of using a standard polyvinyl chloride intravenous infusion set on patient response to nitroglycerin, *Am J Hosp Pharm* 49:1135–1137 (May) 1992.

2055. Driver PS, Jarvi EJ, and Gratzer PL: Stability of nitroglycerin as nitroglycerin concentrate for injection stored in plastic syringes, *Am J Hosp Pharm* 50:2561–2563 (Nov) 1993.

2056. Casto DT: Stability of ondansetron stored in polypropylene syringes, *Ann Pharmacother* 28:712–714 (June) 1994.

2057. Bailey LC, Tang KT, and Rogozinski BA: Effect of syringe filter and i.v. administration set on delivery of propofol emulsion, *Am J Hosp Pharm* 48:2627–2630 (Dec) 1991.

2058. Johnson CE, Christen C, Perez MM, et al.: Compatibility of bupivacaine hydrochloride and morphine sulfate, *Am J Health-Syst Pharm* 54:61–64 (Jan 1) 1997.

2059. Ambados F: Compatibility of ketamine hydrochloride and meperidine hydrochloride, *Am J Health-Syst Pharm* 54:205 (Jan 15) 1997.

2060. Hall PD, Yui D, Lyons S, et al.: Compatibility of filgrastim with selected antimicrobial drugs during simulated Y-site administration, *Am J Health-Syst Pharm* 54:185–189 (Jan 15) 1997.

2061. Fausel CA, Newton DW, Driscoll DF, et al.: Effect of fat emulsion and supersaturation on calcium phosphate solubility in parenteral nutrient admixtures, *Int J Pharm Compound* 1:54–59 (Jan–Feb) 1997.

2062. Chiu MF and Schwartz ML: Visual compatibility of injectable drugs used in the intensive care unit, *Am J Health-Syst Pharm* 54:64–65 (Jan 1) 1997.

2063. Najari Z and Rusho WJ: Compatibility of commonly used bone marrow transplant drugs during Y-site delivery, *Am J Health-Syst Pharm* 54:181–184 (Jan 15) 1997.

2064. Xu QA, Trissel LA, and Martinez JF: Rapid loss of fentanyl citrate admixed with fluorouracil in polyvinyl chloride containers, *Ann Pharmacother* 31:297–302 (Mar) 1997.

2065. Gilbert DL Jr, Trissel LA, and Martinez JF: Compatibility of ciprofloxacin lactate with sodium bicarbonate during simulated Y-site administration, *Am J Health-Syst Pharm* 54:1193–1195 (May 15) 1997.

2066. Trissel LA, Gilbert DL, and Martinez JF: Compatibility of propofol injectable emulsion with selected drugs during simulated Y-site administration, *Am J Health-Syst Pharm* 54:1287–1292 (June 1) 1997.

2067. Asker AF and Ferdous AJ: Photodegradation of furosemide solutions, *PDA J Pharm Sci Technol* 50:158–162 (May–June) 1996.

2068. Correction notice. Compatibility of meropenem with commonly used injectable drugs, *Am J Health-Syst Pharm*, 1998; 55: in press.

2069. Schobelock MJ (Medical Affairs Department, Roxane Laboratories, Inc.): Personal communication, November 4, 1997.

2070. Barnes AR and Nash S: Stability of bupivacaine hydrochloride and diamorphine hydrochloride in an epidural infusion, *Pharm World Sci* 17:87–92 (Mar) 1995.

2071. Grassby PF and Hutchings L: Drug combinations in syringe drivers: the compatibility and stability of diamorphine with cyclizine and haloperidol, *Palliat Med* 11:217–224, 1997.

2072. Cohen MR: Volume limitations for IV drug infusions when sterile water for injection is used as a diluent, *Hosp Pharm* 33:274–277 (March) 1998.

2073. Pierce LR, Gaines A. Hemolysis and renal failure associated with use of sterile water for injection to dilute 25% human albumin, *Am J Health-Syst Pharm* 55:1057, 1062, 1070 (May 15) 1998.

2074. Trissel LA, Martinez JF, and Gilbert DL: Compatibility of cisatracurium besylate with selected drugs during simulated Y-site administration, *Am J Health-Syst Pharm* 54:1735–1741 (Aug 1) 1997.

2075. Trissel LA, Gilbert DL, Martinez JF, et al.: Compatibility of remifentanil hydrochloride with selected drugs during simulated Y-site administration, *Am J Health-Syst Pharm* 54:2192–2196 (Oct 1) 1997.

2076. Ennis RD and Dahl TC: Stability of cidofovir in 0.9% sodium chloride injection for five days. *Am J Health-Syst Pharm* 54:2204–2206 (Oct 1) 1997.

2077. Murray KM, Erkkila D, Gombotz WR, et al.: Stability of thiotepa (lyophilized) in 0.9% sodium chloride injection, *Am J Health-Syst Pharm* 54:2588–2591 (Nov 15) 1997.

2078. Bahal SM, Lee TJ, McGinnes M, et al.: Visual compatibility of warfarin sodium injection with selected medications and solutions, *Am J Health-Syst Pharm* 54:2599–2600 (Nov 15) 1997.

2079. Nolan PE, Hoyer GL, LeDoux JH, et al.: Stability of ranitidine hydrochloride and human insulin in 0.9% sodium chloride injection, *Am J Health-Syst Pharm* 54:1304–1306 (June) 1997.

2080. Stiles ML and Allen LV: Stability of nafcillin sodium, oxacillin sodium, penicillin G potassium, penicillin G sodium, and tobramycin sulfate in polyvinyl chloride drug reservoirs, *Am J Health-Syst Pharm 54:*1068–1070 (May 1) 1997.

2081. Pujol M, Munoz M, Prat J, et al.: Stability study of epirubicin in NaCl 0.9% injection, *Ann Pharmacother 31:*992–995 (Sep) 1997.

2082. Walker SE, DeAngelis C, and Iazetta J: Stability and compatibility of combinations of hydromorphone and a second drug, *Can J Hosp Pharm 44:*289–295 (Dec) 1991.

2083. Fischer JH, Cwik MJ, Luer MS, et al.: Stability of fosphenytoin sodium with intravenous solutions in glass bottles, polyvinyl chloride bags, and polypropylene syringes, *Ann Pharmacother 31:*553–559 (May) 1997.

2084. Evrard B, Ceccato A, Gaspard O, et al.: Stability of ondansetron hydrochloride and dexamethasone sodium phosphate in 0.9% sodium chloride injection and in 5% dextrose injection, *Am J Health-Syst Pharm 54:*1065–1068 (May 1) 1997.

2085. Peddicord TE, Olsen KM, ZumBrunnen TL, et al.: Stability of high-concentration dopamine hydrochloride, norepinephrine bitartrate, epinephrine hydrochloride, and nitroglycerin in 5% dextrose injection, *Am J Health-Syst Pharm 54:*1417–1419 (June 15) 1997.

2086. Walker SE, Meinders A, and Tailor H: Stability and compatibility of reconstituted sterile hydromorphone with midazolam, *Can J Hosp Pharm 49:*290–298 (Dec) 1996.

2087. Trissel LA, Gilbert DL, and Martinez JF: Compatibility of doxorubicin hydrochloride liposome injection with selected other drugs during simulated Y-site administration, *Am J Health-Syst Pharm 54:*2708–2713 (Dec 1) 1997.

2088. Pramar YV, Loucas VA, and El-Rachidi A: Stability of midazolam hydrochloride in syringes and i.v. fluids, *Am J Health-Syst Pharm 54:*913–915 (Apr 15) 1997.

2089. Patel PR and Cook SE: Stability of meropenem in intravenous solutions, *Am J Health-Syst Pharm 54:*412–421 (Feb 15) 1997.

2090. Cornish LA, Montgomery PA, and Johnson CE: Stability of bumetanide in 5% dextrose injection, *Am J Health-Syst Pharm 54:*422–423 (Feb 15) 1997.

2091. Bailey LC and Orosz ST: Stability of ceftriaxone sodium and metronidazole hydrochloride, *Am J Health-Syst Pharm 54:*424–427 (Feb 15) 1997.

2092. Stewart JT, Warren FW, King DT, et al.: Stability of ondansetron hydrochloride, doxorubicin hydrochloride, and dacarbazine or vincristine sulfate in elastomeric portable infusion devices and polyvinyl chloride bags, *Am J Health-Syst Pharm 54:*915–920 (Apr 15) 1997.

2093. Owens D, Fleming RA, Restino MS, et al.: Stability of amphotericin B 0.05 and 0.5 mg/ml in 20% fat emulsion, *Am J Health-Syst Pharm 54:*683–686 (Mar 15) 1997.

2094. Zhang YP, Xu QA, Trissel LA, et al.: Compatibility and stability of paclitaxel combined with cisplatin and with carboplatin in infusion solutions, *Ann Pharmcother 31:*1465–1470 (Dec) 1997.

2095. Gupta VD, Maswoswe J, and Bailey RE: Stability of ketorolac tromethamine in 5% dextrose injection and 0.9% sodium chloride injections, *Int J Pharm Compound 1:*206–207 (May–June) 1997.

2096. Zhang YP and Trissel LA: Stability of aminocaproic acid injection admixtures in 5% dextrose injection and 0.9% sodium chloride injection, *Int J Pharm Compound 1:*132–134 (Mar–Apr) 1997.

2097. Allen LV and Stiles ML: Stability of vancomycin hydrochloride in medication cassette reservoirs, *Int J Pharm Compound 1:*123–124 (Mar–Apr) 1997.

2098. Zhang YP, Trissel LA, Martinez JF, et al.: Stability of acyclovir sodium 1, 7, and 10 mg/ml in 5% dextrose injection and 0.9% sodium chloride injection, *Am J Health-Syst Pharm 55:*574–577 (Mar 15) 1998.

2099. Amador FD, Azzati ES, Lopez-Coterilla AHT: Stability of carboplatin in polyvinyl chloride bags, *Am J Health-Syst Pharm 55:*602, 604 (Mar 15) 1998.

2100. Gupta VD, Maswoswe J, and Bailey RE: Stability of cefmetazole sodium in 5% dextrose injection and 0.9% sodium chloride injection, *Int J Pharm Compound 1:*208–209 (May–June) 1997.

2101. Gupta VD, Maswoswe J, and Bailey RE: Stability of ceftriaxone sodium when mixed with metronidazole injection, *Int J Pharm Compound 1:*280–281 (July–Aug) 1997.

2102. Gupta VD, Maswoswe J, and Bailey RE: Stability of cefepime hydrochloride in 5% dextrose injection and 0.9% sodium chloride injection, *Int J Pharm Compound 1:*435–436 (Nov–Dec) 1997.

2103. Mayhew SL and Quick MW: Compatibility of iron dextran with neonatal parenteral nutrient solutions, *Am J Health-Syst Pharm 54:*570–571 (Mar 1) 1997.

2104. Moshfeghi M and Ciuffo JD: Visual compatibility of fentanyl citrate with parenteral nutrient solutions, *Am J Health-Syst Pharm 55:*1194, 1197 (June 1) 1998.

2105. Gupta VD and Maswoswe J: Stability of indomethacin in 0.9% sodium chloride injection, *Int J Pharm Compound 2:*170–171 (Mar–Apr) 1998.

2106. Wong F and Gill MA: Stability of milrinone lactate 200 µg/mL in 5% dextrose injection and 0.9% sodium chloride injection, *Int J Pharm Compound 2:*168–169 (Mar–Apr) 1998.

2107. Nguyen D, Gill MA, and Wong F: Stability of milrinone lactate in 5% dextrose injection and 0.9% sodium chloride injection at concentrations of 400, 600, and 800 µg/mL, *Int J Pharm Compound 2:*246–248 (May–June) 1998.

2108. Montgomery PA, Cornish LA, Johnson CE, et al.: Stability of torsemide in 5% dextrose injection, *Am J Health-Syst Pharm 55:*1042–1043 (May 15) 1998.

2109. Trissel LA, Gilbert DL, Martinez JF, et al.: Compatibility of parenteral nutrient solutions with selected drugs during simulated Y-site administration, *Am J Health-Syst Pharm 54:*1295–1300 (June 1) 1997.

2110. Pramar YV: Chemical stability of amiodarone hydrochloride in intravenous fluids, *Int J Pharm Compound 1:*347–348 (Sep–Oct) 1997.

2111. Wang DP, Wang MT, Wong CY, et al.: Compatibility of vancomycin hydrochloride and famotidine in 5% dextrose injection, *Int J Pharm Compound 1:*354–355 (Sep–Oct) 1997.

2112. Bhatt-Mehta V and Hirata S: Physical compatibility and chemical stability of atracurium besylate and midazolam hydrochloride during intravenous coinfusion, *Int J Pharm Compound 2:*79–82 (Jan–Feb) 1998.

2113. Stendal TL, Klem W, Tonnesen HH, et al.: Drug stability and pyridine generation in ceftazidime injection stored in an elastomeric infusion device, *Am J Health-Syst Pharm 55:*683–685 (Apr 1) 1998.

2114. Ketkar VA, Kolling WM, Nardviriyakul N, et al.: Stability of undiluted and diluted adenosine at three temperatures in syringes and bags, *Am J Health-Syst Pharm 55:*466–470 (Mar 1) 1998.

2115. Naud C, Marti B, Fernandez C, et al.: Stability of adenosine 6 µg/ml in 0.9% sodium chloride solution, *Am J Health-Syst Pharm 55:*1161–1164 (June 1) 1998.

2116. Xu QA, Zhang YP, Trissel LA, et al.: Stability of cisatracurium besylate in vials, syringes, and infusion admixtures, *Am J Health-Syst Pharm 55:*1037–1041 (May 15) 1998.

2117. Trissel LA, Gilbert DL, and Martinez JF: Incompatibility and compatibility of amphotericin B cholsteryl sulfate complex with selected other drugs during simulated Y-site administration, *Hosp Pharm 33:*284–292 (Mar) 1998.

2118. Allwood MC and Martin J: How does storage affect propofol? The stability of propofol in plastic syringes, *Pharm Pract 7:*15–16 (Jan) 1997.

2119. Harris MC and Como JA: Heparin flush solutions: how much is enough? *South J Health-Syst Pharm 2:*10–14 (Fall) 1997.

2120. Meyer BA, Little CJ, Thorp JA, et al.: Heparin versus normal saline as a peripheral line flush in maintenance of intermittent intravenous lines in obstetric patients, *Obstet Gynecol 5:*433–436 (Mar) 1995.

2121. Danek GD and Noris EM: Pediatric IV catheters: efficacy of saline flush, *Ped Nurs 8:*111–113 (Mar–Apr) 1992.

2122. Hok ML, Reuling J, Luettgen ML, et al.: Comparison of the patency of arterial lines maintained with heparinized and nonheparinized infusions, *Heart & Lung 16:*693–699 (Nov) 1987.

2123. Kulkarni M, Elsner C, Ouellet D, et al.: Heparinized saline versus normal saline in maintaining patency of the radial artery catheter, *Can J Surg 37:*37–42 (Feb) 1994.

2124. Clifton GD, Branson P, Kelly HJ, et al.: Comparison of normal saline and heparin solutions for maintenance of arterial catheter patency, *Heart & Lung 20:*115–118 (Mar) 1991.

2125. Butt W, Shann F, McDonnell G, et al.: Effect of heparin concentration and infusion rate on the patency of arterial catheters, *Crit Care Med 15:*230–232 (Mar) 1987.

2126. Smith S, Dawson S, Hennessey R, et al.: Maintenance of the patency of indwelling central venous catheters: is heparin necessary? *Am J Ped Hem/Onc 13:*141–143 (2) 1991.

2127. O'Neill TJ, Tierney LM, and Proulx RJ: Heparin lock-induced alterations in the activated partial thromboplastin time, *J Am Med Assoc 227:*1297–1298 (Mar 18) 1974.

2128. Passannante A and Macik BG: Case report: the heparin flush syndrome: a cause of iatrogenic hemorrhage, *Am J Med Sci 296:*71–73 (July) 1988.

2129. Heeger PS and Backstrom JT: Heparin flushes and thrombocytopenia, *Ann Intern Med 105:*143 (July) 1986.

2130. Laster J, Cikrit D, Walker N, et al.: The heparin-induced thrombocytopenia syndrome: an update, *Surgery 102:*763–770 (Oct) 1987.

2131. Rizzoni WE, Miller K, Rick M, et al.: Heparin-induced thrombocytopenia and thromboembolism in the postoperative period, *Surgery 103:*470–476 (Apr) 1988.

2132. Doty JR, Alving BM, McDonnell DE, et al.: Heparin-associated thrombocytopenia in the neurosurgical patient, *Neurosurgery 19:*69–72, 1986.

2133. Mehta AC and Kay EA: Storage time can be extended, *Pharm Pract* 7:305, 306, 308 (June) 1997.

2134. Brittain HG, Lafferty L, Bousserski P, et al.: Stability of Revex, nalmefene hydrochloride injection, *PDA J Pharm Sci Technol* 50:35–39 (Jan–Feb) 1996.

2135. McKinnon BT: FDA Safety Alert: hazards of precipitation associated with parenteral nutrition, *Nutr Clin Pract* 11:59–65 (Apr) 1996.

2136. Seidner DL, Speerhas R, and Trexler K: Can octreotide be added to parenteral nutrition? Point-counterpoint, *Nutr Clin Pract* 13:84–88 (Apr) 1998.

2137. Dodds HM, Craik DJ, and Rivory LP: Photodegradation of irinotecan (CPT-11) in aqueous solutions: identification of fluorescent products and influence of solution composition, *J Pharm Sci* 86:1410–1416 (Dec) 1997.

2138. Gremeau I, Sautou-miranda V, Picq F, et al.: Influence de la nature de la membrane sur le passage du nitrate d'isosorbide et de son metabolite actif au cours d'une dialyse, *J Pharm Clin* 16:19–23 (1) 1997.

2139. Graham AE, Speicher E, and Williamson B: Analysis of gentamicin sulfate and a study of its degradation in dextrose solution, *J Pharm Biomed Anal* 15:537–543, 1997.

2140. Craig SB, Bhatt UH, and Patel K: Stability and compatibility of topotecan hydrochloride for injection with common infusion solutions and containers, *J Pharm Biomed Anal* 16:199–205, 1997.

2141. Pramar YV, Loucas VA, and Word D: Chemical stability and adsorption of atracurium besylate injections in disposable plastic syringes, *J Clin Pharm Ther* 21:173–175, 1996.

2142. Galanti LM, Hecq JD, Vanbeckbergen D, et al.: Long-term stability of cefuroxime and cefazolin sodium in intravenous infusions, *J Clin Pharm Ther* 21:185–189, 1996.

2143. Kawano K, Takamatsu S, Mochizuku C, et al.: Loss of isosorbide dinitrate or nitroglycerin solution content in practice injection or precision continuous drip infusion, *Jpn J Hosp Pharm* 22:167–172 (2) 1996.

2144. Yoshida H, Takaba D, Uchida Y, et al.: Research for the crystal material produced in the continuous infusion line of midazloam (Dormicium) and butorphanol (Stadol), *Jpn J Hosp Pharm* 23:531–538 (6) 1997.

2145. Mawhinney WM, Adair CG, Gorman SP, et al.: Long-term stability of teicoplanin in dialysis fluid: implications for the home-treatment of CAPD peritonitis, *Int J Pharm Pract* 1:90–93 (Oct) 1991.

2146. Allwood MC and Martin H: The extraction of diethylhexylphthalate (DEHP) from polyvinyl chloride components of intravenous infusion containers and administration sets by paclitaxel injection, *Int J Pharm* 127:65–71, 1996.

2147. Valiere C, Arnaud P, Caroff E, et al.: Stability and compatibility study of a carboplatin solution in syringes for continuous ambulatory infusion, *Int J Pharm* 138:125–128, 1996.

2148. Khalfi F, Dine T, Gressier B, et al.: Compatibility and stability of vancomycin hydrochloride with PVC infusion material in various conditions using stability-indicating high-performance liquid chromatographic assay, *Int J Pharm* 139:243–247, 1996.

2149. Hourcade F, Sautou-Miranda V, Normand B, et al.: Compatibility of granisetron towards glass and plastics and its stability under various storage conditions, *Int J Pharm* 154:95–102, 1997.

2150. Rabouan-Guyon SM, Guet AF, Courtois PY, et al.: Stability study of cefepime in different infusion solutions, *Int J Pharm* 154:185–190, 1997.

2151. Anon: How I survived a direct injection of potassium chloride, *Hosp Pharm* 32:298–300 (Mar) 1997.

2152. Kramer I: Stability of meropenem in elastomeric portable infusion devices, *Eur Hosp Pharm* 3:168–171 (Dec) 1997.

2153. Uges DRA and Ruige M: Vancomycin adsorption to teflon tubing, *Eur Hosp Pharm* 2:38 (Feb) 1996.

2154. Daouphars M, Vigneron J, Perrin A, et al.: Stability of cladribine in either polyethylene containers or polyvinyl chloride bags, *Europ Hosp Pharm* 3:154–156 (Sep) 1997.

2155. Girona V, Prat J, Pujol M, et al.: Stability of vinblastine sulphate in 0.9% sodium chloride in polypropylene syringes, *Boll Chim Farm* 135:413–414 (7) 1996.

2156. Smith BA, Hilmi SC, McDonald C, et al.: The stability of foscarnet in the presence of potassium, *Aust J Hosp Pharm* 26:560–561 (5) 1996.

2157. Jaffe GJ, Green GDJ, and Abrams GW: Stability of recombinant tissue plasminogen activator, *Am J Ophthal* 108:90–91 (July) 1989.

2158. Ward C and Weck S: Dilution and storage of recombinant tissue plasminogen activator (Activase) in balanced salt solutions, *Am J Ophthal* 109:98–99 (Jan) 1990.

2159. Grewing R, Mester U, and Low M: Clinical experience with tissue plasminogen activator stored at –20 °C, *Ophthal Surg* 23:780–781 (Nov) 1992.

2160. Kramer I: Viability of microorganisms in novel antineoplastic and antiviral drug solutions, *J Oncol Pharm Pract* 4:32–37 (Mar) 1998.

2161. Schneider JJ, Wilson KM, and Ravenscroft PJ: A study of the osmolality and pH of subcutaneous drug infusion solutions, *Aust J Hosp Pharm* 27:29–31 (1) 1997.

2162. Vermeire A and Remon JP: The solubility of morphine and the stability of concentrated morphine solutions in glass, polypropylene syringes and PVC containers, *Int J Pharm* 146:213–223, 1997.

2163. Kearney MCJ, Allwood MC, Martin H, et al.: The influence of amino acid source on the stability of ascorbic acid in TPN mixtures, *Nutrition* 14:173–178 (2) 1998.

2164. Casasin Edo T, Roca Massa M, and Soy Munne D: Sistema de distribucion de medicamentos utilizados en anestesia mediante jeringas precargadas. Estudio de estabilidad, *Farm Hosp* 20:55–59 (1) 1996.

2165. Malcomson C, Zilka S, Saum J, et al.: Investigations into the compatibility of teicoplanin with heparin, *Eur J Parenter Sci* 2:51–55 (2) 1997.

2166. Walker SE, Walshaw PR, and Grad H: Imipenem stability and staining of teeth, *Can J Hosp Pharm* 50:61–67 (Apr) 1997.

2167. Gilbar P and McAllan Z: Ticarcillin-potassium clavulanate and vancomycin incompatibility, *Aust J Hosp Pharm* 27:470 (6) 1997.

2168. Burm JP: Stability of ondansetron and fluconazole in 5% dextrose injection and normal saline during Y-site administration, *Arch Pharm Res* 20:171–175 (2) 1997.

2169. Truelle-Hugon B, Tourrette G, Couineaux B, et al.: Etude de stabilite du chlorhydrate de morphine Lavoisier dans differents systemes actifs pour perfusion apres reconstitution dans divers solvents, *Ann Pharm Fr* 55:216–223 (5) 1997.

2170. Sitaram BR, Tsui M, Rawicki HB, et al.: Stability and compatibility of intrathecal admixtures containing baclofen and high concentrations of morphine, *Int J Pharm* 153:13–24, 1997.

2171. Trinkle R: Compatibility of hydromorphone and prochlorperazine, and irritation due to subcutaneous prochlorperazine infusion, *Ann Pharmacother* 31:789–790 (Jun) 1997.

2172. Guchelar HJ and Hartog ME: De stabiliteit van clonazepaminjectievloeistof, *Ziekenhuisfarmacie* 13:21–23 (1) 1997.

2173. Leboucher G and Charpiat B: Incompatibilite physico-chimique entre l'omeprazole et la vancomycine, *Pharm Hosp Fr* 121:124, 1997.

2174. Taylor A: Review of clarithromycin mixtures, *Pharm Pract* 7:473, 474, 476 (Oct) 1997.

2175. Farhang-Asnafi S, Callaert S, Barre J, et al.: Influence du solvant de dilution sur la stabilite de la nouvelle forme de 5-fluorouracile en perfusion, *J Pharm Clin* 16:45–48 (1) 1997.

2176. Oustric-Mendes AC, Huart B, Le Hoang MD, et al.: Study protocol: stability of morphine injected without preservative, delivered with a disposable infusion device, *J Clin Pharm Ther* 22:283–290, 1997.

2177. Schoffski P, Freund M, Wunder R, et al.: Safety and toxicity of amphotericin B in glucose 5% or Intralipid 20% in neutropenic patients with pneumonia or fever of unknown origin: randomised study, *Br Med J* 317:379–384 (Aug 8) 1998.

2178. Heinemann V, Kahny B, Jehn U, et al.: Serum pharmacology of amphotericin B applied in lipid emulsions, *Antimicrob Agents Chemother* 41:728–732 (Apr) 1997.

2179. Gupta VD and Maswoswe J: Stability of mitomycin aqueous solution when stored in tuberculin syringes, *Int J Pharm Compound* 1:282–283 (July–Aug) 1997.

2180. Targett PL, Keefe PA, and Merridew CG: Compatibility and stability of drug adjuvants and morphine tartrate in 10 ml polypropylene syringes, *Aust J Hosp Pharm* 27:207–212 (3) 1997.

2181. Goren MP, Lyman BA, and Li JT: The stability of mesna in beverages and syrup for oral administration, *Cancer Chemother Pharmacol* 28:298–301, 1991.

2182. Xu QA, Trissel LA, and Davis MR: Compatibility of paclitaxel in 5% glucose and 0.9% sodium chloride injections with EVA minibags, *Aust J Hosp Pharm* 28:156–159 (3) 1998.

2183. Xu QA, Zhang YP, Trissel LA, et al.: Stability of busulfan injection admixtures in 5% dextrose injection and 0.9% sodium chloride injection, *J Oncol Pharm Pract* 2:101–105 (2) 1996.

2184. Sarver JG, Pryka R, Alexander KS, et al.: Stability of magnesium sulfate in 0.9% sodium chloride and lactated Ringer's solutions, *Int J Pharm Compound* 2:385–388 (Sep–Oct) 1998.

2185. Jobet-Hermelin I, Mallvais ML, Jacquot C, et al.: Proposition d'une concentration limite acceptable du plastifiant librere par le poly(chlorure de vinyle) dans les solutions injectables aqueuses, *J Pharm Clin* 15:132–136 (2) 1996.

2186. Jacobsen PA, West NJ, Spadoni V, et al.: Sterility of filgrastim (G-CSF) in syringes, *Ann Pharmacother* 30:1238–1242 (Nov) 1996.

2187. Trissel LA and Spadoni VT: Comment: filgrastim sterility in syringes, *Ann*

*Pharmacother 31:*500–501 (Apr) 1997.

2188. Appenheimer MM, Schepart BS, Poleon GP, et al.: Stability of albumin-free interferon alfa-2b for 42 days, *Am J Health-Syst Pharm 55:*1602–1605 (Aug 1) 1998.

2189. Trissel LA, Gilbert DL, and Martinez JF: Concentration dependency of vancomycin hydrochloride compatibility with beta-lactam antibiotics during simulated Y-site administration, *Hosp Pharm 33:*1515–1522 (Dec) 1998.

2190. McLaughlin JP, Simpson C, and Taylor RA: How stable is acyclovir in PVC bags? The stability of reconstituted acyclovir sodium in a 0.9% w/v sodium chloride infusion when stored at room temperature, *Pharm Pract 5:*53–58 (Feb) 1995.

2191. Mehta AC and Kay EA: How stable is alfentanil? Stability of alfentanil hydrochloride in 5% dextrose stored in syringes, *Pharm Pract 5:*303–304 (July–Aug) 1995.

2192. McLaughlin JP, Simpson C, and Taylor RA: How stable are Zinacef & Metrovex? The stability of cefuroxime sodium and metronidazole infusion when stored in a refrigerator, *Pharm Pract 5:*100–106 (Mar) 1995.

2193. Bonferoni MC, Mellerio G, Giunchedi P, et al.: Photostability evaluation of nicardipine HCl solutions, *Int J Pharm 80:*109–117, 1992.

2194. Erdman SH, McElwee CL, Kramer JM, et al.: Central line occlusion with three-in-one nutrition admixtures administered at home, *J Parenter Enter Nutr 18:*177–181 (2) 1994.

2195. Allwood MC and Martin H: Factors influencing the stability of ranitidine in TPN mixtures, *Clin Nutr 14:*171–176, 1995.

2196. Hoie EB and Narducci WA: Laser particle analysis of calcium phosphate precipitate in neonatal TPN admixtures, *J Ped Pharm Pract 1:*163–167 (Nov–Dec) 1996.

2197. Ambados F and Brealey J: Incompatibilities with trace elements during TPN solution admixture, *Aust J Hosp Pharm 28:*112–114 (2) 1998.

2198. Xu QA and Trissel LA: Compatibility of paclitaxel injection diluent with two reduced-phthalate administration sets for the Acclaim pump, *Int J Pharm Compound 2:*382–384 (Sep–Oct) 1998.

2199. Stewart JT, Warren FW, King DT, et al.: Stability of ondansetron hydrochloride and 12 medications in plastic syringes, *Am J Health-Syst Pharm 55:*2630–2634 (Dec 15) 1998.

2200. Donnelly RF and Bushfield TL: Chemical stability of meperidine hydrochloride in polypropylene syringes, *Int J Pharm Compound 2:*463–465 (Nov–Dec) 1998.

2201. Jappinen AL, Kokki H, Rasi AS, et al.: Stability of sufentanil in a syringe pump under simulated epidural infusion, *Int J Pharm Compound 2:*466–468 (Nov–Dec) 1998.

2202. Wilson KM, Schneider JJ, and Ravenscroft PJ: Stability of midazolam and fentanyl in infusion solutions, *J Pain Symptom Manage 16:*52–58 (July) 1998.

2203. Gupta VD and Pramar Y: Stability of lorazepam in 5% dextrose injection, *Int J Pharm Compound 2:*322–324 (July–Aug) 1998.

2204. Heide PE: Precipitation of amphotericin B from i.v. fat emulsion, *Am J Health-Syst Pharm 54:*1449 (June 15) 1997.

2205. Heide PE and Hehenberger H: Tensiometrische und konduktometrische stabilitatuntersuchungen von amphotericin B in fettmulsionen, *Oesterreichische Krankenhaus Pharmazie 10:*36–43 (3) 1996.

2206. To TP and Garrett MK: Stability of flucloxacillin in a hospital in the home program, *Aust J Hosp Pharm 28:*289–290 (4) 1998.

2207. Levanda M: Noticeable difference in admixtures prepared from lorazepam 2 and 4 mg/ml, *Am J Health-Syst Pharm 55:*2305 (Nov 1) 1998.

2208. Share MJ, Harrison RD, Folstad J, et al.: Stability of lorazepam 1 and 2 mg/ml in glass bottles and polypropylene syringes, *Am J Health-Syst Pharm 55:*2013–2015 (Oct 1) 1998.

2209. Inagaki K, Kambara M, Mizuno M, et al.: Compatibility and stability of ranitidine hydrochloride with six cephalosporins during simulated Y-site administration, *Int J Pharm Compound 2:*318–321 (July–Aug) 1998.

2210. Ray LR and Chen DA: Stability of somatropin stored in plastic syringes for 28 days, *Am J Health-Syst Pharm 55:*1508–1511 (Jul 15) 1998.

2211. Patel K, Craig SB, McBride MG, et al.: Microbial inhibitory properties and stability of topotecan hydrochloride injection, *Am J Health-Syst Pharm 55:*1584–1587 (Aug 1) 1998.

2212. English BA, Riggs RM, Webster AA, et al.: Y-site stability of fosphenytoin and sodium phenobarbital, *Int J Pharm Compound 3:*64–66 (Jan–Feb) 1999.

2213. Lieu CL, Chin A, and Gill MA: Five-day stability of vinorelbine in 5% dextrose injection and in 0.9% sodium chloride injection at room temperature, *Int J Pharm Compound 3:*67–68 (Jan–Feb) 1999.

2214. Akkerman SR, Zhang H, Mullins RE, et al.: Stability of milrinone lactate in the presence of 29 critical care drugs and 4 i.v. solutions, *Am J Health-Syst Pharm 56:*63–68 (Jan 1) 1999.

2215. Trissel LA, Gilbert DL, Martinez JF, et al.: Compatibility of medications with 3-in-1 parenteral nutrition admixtures, *J Parenter Enter Nutr 23:*67–74 (2) 1999.

2216. Johnson CE, vandenBussche HL, Chio CC, et al.: Stability of tacrolimus with morphine sulfate, hydromorphone hydrochloride, and ceftazidime during simulated intravenous coadministration, *Am J Health-Syst Pharm 56:*164–169 (Jan 15) 1999.

2217. Stamatakis MK, Leader WG, and Tracy TS: Stability of high-dose vancomycin and ceftazidime in peritoneal dialysis solutions, *Am J Health-Syst Pharm 56:*246–248 (Feb 1) 1999.

2218. Trissel LA, Martinez JF, and Simmons M: Compatibility of etoposide phosphate with selected drugs during simulated Y-site injection, *J Am Pharm Assoc 39:*141–145 (Mar–Apr) 1999.

2219. Zhang Y and Trissel LA: Physical and chemical stability of etoposide phosphate solutions, *J Am Pharm Assoc 39:*146–150 (Mar–Apr) 1999.

2220. Stewart JT, Warren FW, and Maddox FC: Stability of cefepime hydrochloride injection in polypropylene syringes at –20 °C, 4 °C, and 22–24 °C, *Am J Health Syst Pharm 56:*457–459 (Mar 1) 1999.

2221. Stewart JT, Maddox FC, and Warren FW: Stability of cefepime hydrochloride in polypropylene syringes, *Am J Health-Syst Pharm 56:*1134 (June 1) 1999.

2222. Burkiewicz JS: Incompatibility of ceftriaxone sodium with lactated Ringer's injection, *Am J Health-Syst Pharm 56:*384 (Feb 15) 1999.

2223. Riggs RM, English BA, Webster AA, et al.: Fosphenytoin Y-site stability studies with lorazepam and midazolam hydrochloride, *Int J Pharm Compound 3:*235–238 (May–June) 1999.

2224. Trissel LA, Gilbert DL, and Wolkin AC: Compatibility of docetaxel with selected drugs during simulated Y-site administration, *Int J Pharm Compound 3:*241–244 (May–Jun) 1999.

2225. Johnson CE and Truong NM: Stability and compatibility of tacrolimus and fluconazole in 0.9% sodium chloride, *J Am Pharm Assoc 39:*505–508 (July–Aug) 1999.

2226. Trissel LA, Martinez JF, and Gilbert DL: Compatibility of gemcitabine hydrochloride with 107 selected drugs during simulated Y-site injection, *J Am Pharm Assoc 39:*514–518 (July–Aug) 1999.

2227. Xu Q, Zhang Y, and Trissel LA: Physical and chemical stability of gemcitabine hydrochloride solutions, *J Am Pharm Assoc 39:*509–513 (July–Aug) 1999.

2228. Walker SE, Gray S, and Schmidt B: Stability of reconstituted indomethacin sodium trihydrate in original vials and polypropylene syringes, *Am J Health-Syst Pharm 55:*154–158 (Jan 15) 1998.

2229. Schlatter J and Saulnier JL: Inline filtration of ranitidine hydrochloride solutions, *Am J Health-Syst Pharm 55:*840, 843 (Apr 15) 1998.

2230. Zhang Y, Trissel LA, and Xu QA: Paclitaxel compatibility with a triple-lumen polyurethane central catheter, *Hosp Pharm 33:*547–551 (May) 1998.

2231. Xu QA, Trissel LA, and Zhang Y: Paclitaxel compatibility with the IV Express filter unit, *Int J Pharm Compound 2:*243–245 (May–Jun) 1998.

2232. Xu QA, Trissel LA, and Gilbert DL: Paclitaxel compatibility with a TOTM-plasticized PVC administration set, *Hosp Pharm 32:*1635–1638 (Dec) 1997.

INDEX

INDEX

Nonproprietary drug names appear in **bold** type and trade names in regular type.